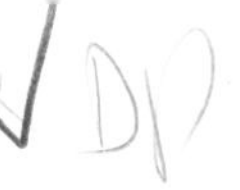

Second Edition

Oncologic Imaging

A Multidisciplinary Approach

Paul M. Silverman, MD
Editor-in-Chief
Professor of Radiology (Ret.)
Gerald D. Dodd, Jr., Distinguished Chair and Director of Academic Development for Diagnostic Imaging
Department of Diagnostic Radiology
The University of Texas MD Anderson Cancer Center
Houston, Texas

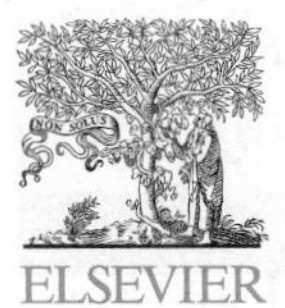
ELSEVIER

Elsevier
1600 John F. Kennedy Blvd.
Ste 1800
Philadelphia, PA 19103-2899

ONCOLOGIC IMAGING: A MULTIDISCIPLINARY APPROACH,
SECOND EDITION ISBN: 978-0-323-69538-1

Notice

Practitioners and researchers must always rely on their own experience and knowledge in evaluating and using any information, methods, compounds, or experiments described herein. Because of rapid advances in the medical sciences, in particular, independent verification of diagnoses and drug dosages should be made. To the fullest extent of the law, no responsibility is assumed by Elsevier, authors, editors, or contributors for any injury and/or damage to persons or property as a matter of products liability, negligence or otherwise, or from any use or operation of any methods, products, instructions, or ideas contained in the material herein.

Executive Content Strategist: Robin R. Carter
Senior Content Development Specialist: Mary Hegeler
Content Development Specialist: Rebecca Corradetti
Senior Project Manager: Manchu Mohan
Publishing Services Manager: Deepthi Unni
Design: Patrick C. Ferguson
Marketing Manager: Kate Bresnahan

Printed in India

Last digit is the print number: 9 8 7 6 5 4 3 2 1

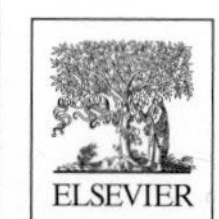

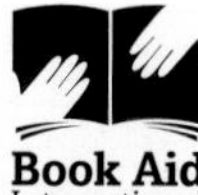

To my wife, Amy

Ani L'Dodi, v'Dodi Li

"I am My Beloved's, and My Beloved is Mine"

Contributors

Eddie K. Abdalla, MD
Medical Director
Liver and Pancreas Program
Northside Hospital Cancer Institute
Atlanta, Georgia

Jitesh Ahuja, MBBS, MD
Assistant Professor
Cardiothoracic Radiology
Department of Chest Radiology
The University of Texas
MD Anderson Cancer Center
Houston, Texas

Felipe Aluja-Jaramillo, MD
Professor Ad Honorem
Department of Radiology
Hospital Universitario San Ignacio - Pontificia Universidad Javeriana, Bogotá
Radiologist
Bogotá, Colombia

Rodabe N. Amaria, MD
Associate Professor
Melanoma Medical Oncology
The University of Texas
MD Anderson Cancer Center
Houston, Texas

Behrang Amini, MD, PhD
Associate Professor
Department of Musculoskeletal Radiology, Division of Imaging
The University of Texas
MD Anderson Cancer Center
Houston, Texas

Anca Avram, MD
Professor of Radiology
Radiology/Nuclear Medicine
University of Michigan
Ann Arbor, Michigan

Rony Avritscher, MD
Associate Professor
Interventional Radiology
The University of Texas
MD Anderson Cancer Center
Houston, Texas

Isabelle Bedrosian, MD
Professor
Breast Surgical Oncology
Division of Surgery
The University of Texas
MD Anderson Cancer Center
Houston, Texas

Sonia L. Betancourt-Cuellar, MD
Professor of Radiology
Thoracic Imaging Department
The University of Texas
MD Anderson Cancer Center
Houston, Texas

Priya R. Bhosale, MD
Professor
Department of Abdominal Radiology
The University of Texas
MD Anderson Cancer Center
Houston, Texas

Andrew J. Bishop, MD
Assistant Professor
Radiation Oncology
The University of Texas
MD Anderson Cancer Center
Houston, Texas

Yulia Bronstein, MD
Associate Radiologist
Virtual Radiologic
Eden Prairie, Minnesota

Constantine M. Burgan, MD
Assistant Professor
Department of Radiology, Abdominal Imaging Section
University of Alabama-Birmingham
Birmingham, Alabama

Hop S. Tran Cao, MD
Assistant Professor
Department of Surgical Oncology
The University of Texas
MD Anderson Cancer Center
Houston, Texas

Sudpreeda Chainitikun, MD
Postdoctoral Fellow
Department of Medical Oncology
MedPark Hospital
Bangkok, Thailand

Joe Y. Chang, MD
Professor
Department of Radiation Oncology
The University of Texas
MD Anderson Cancer Center
Houston, Texas

Lisly J. Chery, MD
Assistant Professor
Department of Urology
The University of Texas
MD Anderson Cancer Center
Houston, Texas

Hubert H. Chuang, MD, PhD
Associate Professor
Department of Nuclear Medicine
The University of Texas
MD Anderson Cancer Center
Houston, Texas

Aaron Coleman, MD
Resident Physician
Department of Radiology
University of Alabama at Birmingham
Birmingham, Alabama

Colleen M. Costelloe, MD
Professor of Radiology
Department of Musculoskeletal Radiology
The University of Texas
MD Anderson Cancer Center
Houston, Texas

Prajnan Das, MD, MS, MPH
Professor
Radiation Oncology
The University of Texas
MD Anderson Cancer Center
Houston, Texas

Reordan DeJesus, MD
Associate Professor and Division Chief, Neuroradiology
University of Florida
Gainesville, Florida

Catherine Devine, MD
Professor
Department of Abdominal Imaging
The University of Texas
MD Anderson Cancer Center
Houston, Texas

Patricia J. Eifel, MD
Professor of Radiation Oncology
Radiation Oncology
The University of Texas
MD Anderson Cancer Center
Houston, Texas

Jeremy J. Erasmus, MD
Professor
Diagnostic Radiology
The University of Texas
MD Anderson Cancer Center
Houston, Texas

Silvana C. Faria, MD, PhD
Professor
Abdominal Imaging
The University of Texas
MD Anderson Cancer Center
Houston, Texas

Jason B. Fleming, MD
Professor
Department of Surgical Oncology
Moffitt Cancer Center
Tampa, Florida

Samuel J. Galgano, MD
Assistant Professor
Department of Radiology
Abdominal Imaging Section
University of Alabama at Birmingham
Birmingham, Alabama

Dhakshinamoorthy Ganeshan, MD
Associate Professor
Department of Diagnostic Radiology
The University of Texas
MD Anderson Cancer Center
Houston, Texas

Naveen Garg, MD
Associate Professor
Abdominal Imaging
The University of Texas
MD Anderson Cancer Center
Houston, Texas

Patrick B. Garvey, MD
Associate Professor
Department of Plastic and Reconstructive Surgery
The University of Texas
MD Anderson Cancer Center
Houston, Texas

Gregory Gladish, MD
Professor
Thoracic Imaging
The University of Texas
MD Anderson Cancer Center
Houston, Texas

Chunxiao Guo, MD, PhD
Resident
Department of Radiology
The University of Minnesota
Minneapolis, Minnesota

Fernando R. Gutiérrez, MD
Professor of Radiology
Cardiothoracic Imaging Section
Mallinckrodt Institute of Radiology - Washington University in St. Louis
St. Louis, Missouri

Daniel M. Halperin, MD
Assistant Professor
Department of GI Medical Oncology
The University of Texas
MD Anderson Cancer Center
Houston, Texas

Abdelrahman K. Hanafy, MD
Resident
Diagnostic Radiology
The University of Texas
Health Science Center at San Antonio
San Antonio, Texas

Karen Hoffman, MD
Associate Professor
Radiation Oncology
The University of Texas
MD Anderson Cancer Center
Houston, Texas

Wayne L. Hofstetter, MD
Professor of Surgery and Deputy Chair
Thoracic and Cardiovascular Surgery
The University of Texas
MD Anderson Cancer Center
Houston, Texas

Wen-Jen Hwu, MD, PhD
Professor
Department of Melanoma Medical Oncology
The University of Texas
MD Anderson Cancer Center
Houston, Texas

Juan J. Ibarra Rovira, MD
Assistant Professor of Radiology
Diagnostic Radiology
The University of Texas
MD Anderson Cancer Center
Houston, Texas

Mohannad Ibrahim, MD
University of Michigan
Ann Arbor, Michigan

Naruhiko Ikoma, MD
Assistant Professor
Surgical Oncology
The University of Texas
MD Anderson Cancer Center
Houston, Texas

Revathy B. Iyer, MD
Professor
Diagnostic Radiology
The University of Texas
MD Anderson Cancer Center
Houston, Texas

Sanaz Javadi, MD
Assistant Professor
Department of Abdominal Imaging
The University of Texas
MD Anderson Cancer Center
Houston, Texas

Milind Javle, MD
Professor
Department of Gastrointestinal Medical Oncology
The University of Texas
MD Anderson Cancer Center
Houston, Texas

Corey T. Jensen, MD
Associate Professor
Abdominal Radiology
The University of Texas
MD Anderson Cancer Center
Houston, Texas

Eric Jonasch, MD
Professor
Department of Genitourinary Medical Oncology
Division of Cancer Medicine
The University of Texas
MD Anderson Cancer Center
Houston, Texas

Aparna Kamat, MD
Associate Professor
Gynecologic Oncology
Methodist, Weill Cornell Medical College
Houston, Texas

Ashish Kamat, MD, MBBS, FACS
Professor
Urology
The University of Texas
MD Anderson Cancer Center
Houston, Texas

Avinash R. Kambadakone, MD, DNB, FRCR
Clinical Fellow
Division of Abdominal Imaging and Intervention
Massachusetts General Hospital
Boston, Massachusetts

Gregory P. Kaufman, MD
Assistant Professor
Department of Lymphoma/Myeloma
Division of Cancer Medicine
The University of Texas
MD Anderson Cancer Center
Houston, Texas

Amritjot Kaur, MBBS
Medical Officer
Emergency
Columbia Asia Hospital, Patiala
Punjab, India
Observer
Body Imaging
The University of Texas
MD Anderson Cancer Center
Houston, Texas

Harmeet Kaur, MBBS, MD
Professor
Diagnostic Radiology
The University of Texas
MD Anderson Cancer Center
Houston, Texas

Brinda Rao Korivi, MD, MPH
Associate Professor
Abdominal Imaging
The University of Texas
MD Anderson Cancer Center
Houston, Texas

Rajendra Kumar, MD, FACR
Professor of Radiology
Department of Musculoskeletal Radiology
The University of Texas
MD Anderson Cancer Center
Houston, Texas

Vikas Kundra, MD, PhD
Professor
Diagnostic Radiology
The University of Texas
MD Anderson Cancer Center
Houston, Texas

Marcelo F. Kuperman Benveniste, MD
Associate Professor
Thoracic Imaging Department
The University of Texas
MD Anderson Cancer Center
Houston, Texas

Ott Le, MD
Abdominal Imaging
The University of Texas
MD Anderson Cancer Center
Houston, Texas

Jeffrey H. Lee, MD
Professor
Department of Gastroenterology, Hepatology, and Nutrition
The University of Texas
MD Anderson Cancer Center
Houston, Texas

Huang LePetross, MD, FRCPC, FSBI
Professor
Department of Breast Imaging, Division of Radiology
The University of Texas
MD Anderson Cancer Center
Houston, Texas

Patrick P. Lin, MD
Professor of Orthopaedic Oncology
Department of Orthopaedic Oncology
The University of Texas
MD Anderson Cancer Center
Houston, Texas

Joseph A. Ludwig, MD
Associate Professor
Department of Sarcoma Medical Oncology
The University of Texas
MD Anderson Cancer Center
Houston, Texas
United States
Adjunct Professor
Department of Bioengineering
Rice University
Houston, Texas

Homer A. Macapinlac, MD
Chair
Department of Nuclear Medicine
The University of Texas
MD Anderson Cancer Center
Houston, Texas

John E. Madewell, MD
Professor, Chair-ad-Interim
Department of Musculoskeletal Imaging
The University of Texas
MD Anderson Cancer Center
Houston, Texas

Paul Mansfield, MD
Professor
Department of Surgical Oncology
The University of Texas
MD Anderson Cancer Center
Houston, Texas

Leonardo P. Marcal, MD
Associate Professor
Department of Abdominal Imaging
The University of Texas
MD Anderson Cancer Center
Houston, Texas

Edith M. Marom, MD
Professor of Radiology
Department of Diagnostic Imaging
The Chaim Sheba Medical Center
Affiliated with the Tel Aviv University
Ramat Gan, Israel

Tara Massini, MD
Clinical Assistant Professor and Program Director
Neuroradiology
University of Florida
Gainesville, Florida

Aurelio Matamoros Jr., MD
Professor
Department of Abdominal Imaging, Division of Diagnostic Imaging
The University of Texas
MD Anderson Cancer Center
Houston, Texas

Mary Frances McAleer, MD, PhD
Professor
Radiation Oncology Department
MD Anderson Cancer Center
Houston, Texas

Reza J. Mehran, MD
Professor
Thoracic and Cardiovascular Surgery
The University of Texas
MD Anderson Cancer Center
Houston, Texas

Christine Menias, MD
Professor of Radiology
Department of Radiology
Mayo Clinic
Scottsdale, Arizona
United States
Adjunct Professor of Radiology
Department of Radiology
Washington University in St. Louis
St. Louis, Missouri

Ajaykumar C. Morani, MD
Associate Professor
Abdominal Radiology
The University of Texas
MD Anderson Cancer Center
Houston, Texas

Van K. Morris, MD
Associate Professor
GI Medical Oncology
The University of Texas
MD Anderson Cancer Center
Houston, Texas

Stacy L. Moulder-Thompson, MD
Breast Medical Oncology
The University of Texas
MD Anderson Cancer Center
Houston, Texas

Bilal Mujtaba, MD
Assistant Professor
Department of Musculoskeletal Imaging
Division of Diagnostic Imaging
The University of Texas
MD Anderson Cancer Center
Houston, Texas

Suresh K. Mukherji, MD, MBA, FACR
University of Michigan
Ann Arbor, Michigan

Sameh Nassar, MD
Research Assistant
Diagnostic Radiology
The University of Texas
MD Anderson Cancer Center
Houston, Texas

Quynh-Nhu Nguyen, MD
Professor
Radiation Oncology
The University of Texas
MD Anderson Cancer Center
Houston, Texas

Yoshifumi Noda, MD
Department of Radiology
Massachusetts General Hospital
Boston, Massachusetts

Amir Onn, MD
Head, Institute of Pulmonary Oncology
The Chaim Sheba Medical Center
Affiliated with the Tel Aviv University
Ramat Gan, Israel

Michael J. Overman, MD
Professor
Gastrointestinal Medical Oncology
The University of Texas
MD Anderson Cancer Center
Houston, Texas

Lance C. Pagliaro, MD
Professor of Oncology
Mayo Clinic
Rochester, Minnesota

Diana P. Palacio, MD
Professor of Radiology
Department of Medical Imaging
University of Texas Medical Branch
Galveston, Texas

Anushri Parakh, MBBS, MD
Postdoctoral Research Fellow
Department of Radiology
Massachusetts General Hospital
Boston, Massachusetts

Hemant A. Parmar, MD
Professor of Radiology
Radiology
University of Michigan
Ann Arbor, Michigan

Shreyaskumar Patel, MD
RR Herring Distinguished Professor
Sarcoma Medical Oncology
The University of Texas
MD Anderson Cancer Center
Houston, Texas

Madhavi Patnana, MD
Professor
Department of Abdominal Imaging
The University of Texas
MD Anderson Cancer Center
Houston, Texas

Alexandria Phan, MD
Professor
University of Texas Health Center at Tyler
Tyler, Texas

Halyna Pokhylevych, MD
Imaging Research Specialist
Quantitative Imaging Analysis Core, Division of Diagnostic Imaging
The University of Texas
MD Anderson Cancer Center
Houston, Texas

Kristin K. Porter, MD, PhD
Associate Professor, MR Modality Chief
Department of Radiology, Abdominal Imaging Section
University of Alabama at Birmingham
Birmingham, Alabama

Gaiane M. Rauch, MD, PhD
Associate Professor
Department of Abdominal Imaging, Division of Diagnostic Imaging
The University of Texas
MD Anderson Cancer Center
Houston, Texas

Bharat Raval, MB,ChB, FRCP(C), FACR
Professor (Retired)
Diagnostic Radiology
The University of Texas
MD Anderson Cancer Center
Houston, Texas

Miguel Rodriguez-Bigas, MD
Professor of Surgery
Department of Colorectal Surgery
The University of Texas
MD Anderson Cancer Center
Houston, Texas

Eric M. Rohren, MD, PhD
Professor and Chair
Department of Radiology
Baylor College of Medicine
Houston, Texas

Christina L. Roland, MD, MS
Associate Professor; Chief, Sarcoma Surgery
Surgical Oncology
The University of Texas
MD Anderson Cancer Center
Houston, Texas

Jeremy Ross, MD
Physician
Radiology
University of Michigan
Ann Arbor, Michigan

Bradley S. Sabloff, MD
Professor
Thoracic Imaging Department
The University of Texas
MD Anderson Cancer Center
Houston, Texas

Tara Sagebiel, MD
Associate Professor
Abdominal Imaging
The University of Texas
MD Anderson Cancer Center
Houston, Texas

Dushant V. Sahani, MD
Chairman
Radiology
University of Washington
Seattle, Washington

Kathleen M. Schmeler, MD
Associate Professor
Department of Gynecologic Oncology
The University of Texas
MD Anderson Cancer Center
Houston, Texas

Girish Shroff, MD
Associate Professor
Thoracic Imaging Department
The University of Texas
MD Anderson Cancer Center
Houston, Texas

Arlene O. Siefker-Radtke, MD
Professor
Genitourinary Medical Oncology
The University of Texas
MD Anderson Cancer Center
Houston, Texas

Elainea N. Smith, MD
Resident Physician
Department of Radiology
University of Alabama at Birmingham
Birmingham, Alabama

R. Jason Stafford, PhD, DABR, FAAPM
Professor
Imaging Physics
The University of Texas
MD Anderson Cancer Center
Houston, Texas

David J. Stewart, MD, FRCPC
Professor
Division of Medical Oncology
University of Ottawa and The Ottawa Hospital
Ottawa, Ontario
Canada

Chad D. Strange, MD
Assistant Professor
Department of Chest Radiology
The University of Texas
MD Anderson Cancer Center
Houston, Texas

Stephen G. Swisher, MD
Professor
Thoracic Surgery
The University of Texas
MD Anderson Cancer Center
Houston, Texas

Ahmed Taher, MD
Postdoctoral Research Fellow
Department of Musculoskeletal Imaging
Division of Diagnostic Imaging
The University of Texas
MD Anderson Cancer Center
Houston, Texas

Cher Heng Tan, MBBS, FRCR
Department of Diagnostic Radiology
Tan Tock Seng Hospital
Lee Kong Chian School of Medicine
Nanyang Technological University
Singapore

Mylene T. Truong, MD
Professor
Department of Chest Radiology,
Diagnostic Imaging
The University of Texas
MD Anderson Cancer Center
Houston, Texas

Naoto T. Ueno, MD, PhD, FACP
Professor
Department of Breast Medical Oncology
The University of Texas
MD Anderson Cancer Center
Houston, Texas

Gauri R. Varadhachary, MD
Professor
Gastrointestinal Medical Oncology
The University of Texas
MD Anderson Cancer Center
Houston, Texas

Aradhana M. Venkatesan, MD
Associate Professor of Radiology and Director of Translational Research
Department of Abdominal Imaging, Division of Diagnostic Imaging
The University of Texas
MD Anderson Cancer Center
Houston, Texas

Claire F. Verschraegen, MD
Medical Oncologist
Ohio State University Wexner Medical Center
Columbus, Ohio

Raghunandan Vikram, MD, MBA
Professor
Department of Abdominal Imaging
The University of Texas
MD Anderson Cancer Center
Houston, Texas

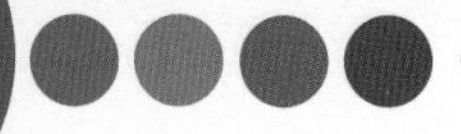

Sarah J. Vinnicombe, BSc, MBBS, MRCP, FRCR
Consultant Radiologist
Department of Radiology
Gloucestershire NHS Foundation Trust, Cheltenham
Gloucestershire
United Kingdom

Mayur K. Virarkar, MD
Fellow
Department of Diagnostic Imaging
The University of Texas
MD Anderson Cancer Center
Houston, Texas

Chitra Viswanathan, MD
Professor
Diagnostic Radiology
The University of Texas
MD Anderson Cancer Center
Houston, Texas

Jason R. Westin, MD, MS, FACP
Director, Lymphoma Clinical Research; Section Chief, Aggressive Lymphoma
Department of Lymphoma and Myeloma
The University of Texas
MD Anderson Cancer Center
Houston, Texas

Wendy A. Woodward, MD, PhD
Professor
Radiation Oncology
The University of Texas
MD Anderson Cancer Center
Houston, Texas

T. Kuan Yu, PhD
(Formerly of MD Anderson Cancer Center and currently practicing at the Houston Precision Cancer Center)
Houston, Texas

Foreword

This textbook explains how imaging technology and knowledge contribute to the management of patients with cancer. It is comprehensive in that it considers the discovery of cancer's presence, staging of the extent of disease, and evaluation of response to treatment; and it also describes, separately, the use of imaging for evaluation of cancer at each site in the body.

The great majority of chapters in this book were written by faculty at The University of Texas MD Anderson Cancer Center. Care at our institution is delivered by multidisciplinary teams of specialists for each type of cancer, which include surgeons, radiation oncologists, medical oncologists, pathologists, and imaging specialists. Therefore, each author was able to provide his or her expertise both as a specialist in imaging the type of cancer under consideration and in the context of collaboration with a team of treating physicians.

As a result, the chapters are informative not only for radiologists in general or specialized practices, but also for oncologists who are directly caring for patients with cancers. Today, at each stage in the course of managing a cancer patient, input from diagnostic imaging is becoming critical for making most clinical decisions.

Successes in developing new drugs and antibodies that target aberrant genetic functioning in each individual patient's tumor make it imperative to characterize the genetic abnormalities in individual cancers. This is especially important in situations in which a malignancy continues to metastasize and spread in spite of standard treatment.

The importance of radiologists in oncology will continue to expand as new imaging techniques become effective at detecting genetic abnormalities and the aberrant functioning of cancer cells in patients. Imaging studies will join genetic and molecular pathology studies in identifying targets for treatment of an individual patient.

Cancer care is a collaborative enterprise, and this excellent textbook is making a major contribution to enhancing the ability of the cancer care team to provide the very best care for patients. I highly recommend it to all physicians who must deal with the challenge of providing the right treatment to the right patient at the right time.

John Mendelsohn, MD
Past President
Codirector
Khalifa Institute for Personalized Cancer Therapy
The University of Texas
MD Anderson Cancer Center
Houston, Texas

Acknowledgments

I wish to take this opportunity to extend a note of appreciation to those individuals who have been instrumental in my career in radiology and those who have been fundamental to this project.

It was during medical school when I had my first exposure to radiology. I had an opportunity to spend some time at a local hospital, where I met Dr. Murray Janower. His commanding personality captivated my interest. I distinctly remember our meeting more than a quarter of a century later. He walked in, nodded hello, and went to read his alternator of studies. He stepped on the pedal and started dictating. I was not quite sure if his foot ever came off that pedal. When he finished he shifted gears and patiently reviewed cases on my alternator, asking me what I thought about them and adding pertinent teaching points. This was the beginning of a mentorship and friendship that has lasted to the present time.

At Stanford University Medical Center, during my residency, I was fortunate to meet Dr. Ronald Castellino. Residents rotated on the chest and oncologic radiology service, "CTO," or as the residents fondly referred to it "Castellino and three others." It was at this time that I had the opportunity to observe a radiologist interact with clinicians, including medical and radiation oncologists, as an equal partner in the evaluation and management of cancer patients. At lymphoma conferences, Dr. Castellino would fill out detailed sheets that described the contribution of imaging studies to the extent of disease, which he meticulously edited with multicolor pens (and which formed the basis for much of his clinical research on imaging of the lymphomas). This was my first exposure to an important opportunity and responsibility and part of what I later understood as a multidisciplinary approach to patient care.

Following residency, as a fellow at Duke University Medical Center, I had the opportunity to work with Dr. Melvyn Korobkin. In the early 1980s, body computed tomography had become a major imaging modality. Dr. Korobkin was the first person who took me "under his wing" to teach me about academic medicine and academic radiology in particular. His clinical knowledge was substantial, but more importantly his academic knowledge and great patience were instrumental in teaching me how to compose an abstract and write successful scientific publications.

I have been at MD Anderson Cancer Center now for more than a decade. It has, without a doubt, been the most rewarding time in my career. When I arrived, I realized that, no matter how experienced one was, the many and highly complex cases were a challenge to all of us. I was fortunate to be surrounded by talented and dedicated clinical radiologists who shared their knowledge and experience. I also was fortunate to be immersed in a dedicated multidisciplinary care environment. Radiologists work closely with the clinicians, and, unlike in many traditional medical centers, the discussions about imaging findings occur directly between attending radiologists and the referring clinicians, providing for an immediate and rewarding relationship. One important link between all the physicians and patients is the work of the highly skilled physician assistants and nurse practitioners who are involved in all layers of patient care and contribute so importantly to the personalized therapies at MD Anderson.

It is this multidisciplinary approach that encouraged me to develop a series of postgraduate courses in oncologic imaging featuring radiologists, surgeons, and medical oncologists. This was a departure from traditional radiology courses, which limit presentations to radiologists. It was a result of positive feedback about this approach from course registrants that I established a Core Lecture Series for radiologists and trainees at MD Anderson. This series features medical oncologists, surgeons, and radiation oncologists speaking with a focus on "what the clinician needs to know from the radiologist." These talks have evolved to have a permanent status, with their content archived as Video Podcasts. It was these experiences that prompted me to take a similar approach for a textbook in oncologic imaging. Although the traditional target audience for such a textbook is practicing radiologists, the material is equally relevant to all clinicians who actually order the imaging studies. I am truly indebted to all of my colleagues participating in the project, and especially my colleagues at MD Anderson for their incredible level of commitment to patients living with cancer.

I also have some special acknowledgments to the individuals who brought this textbook from concept to a physical reality. There are a liberal number of hand-drawn, full-color original illustrations within the textbook. These were all created by a skilled graphic artist, David Bier, who devoted significant time and effort to this project. Great appreciation is also due to Kelly Duggan, who spent significant hours working with the images; his expertise was invaluable. I also want to acknowledge my senior administrative assistant, Charita Scott, who was tirelessly committed to keeping all of this material organized and working with me from its inception to the final product. Her great instincts, complemented by her tremendous work ethic, made it the rewarding experience that it was.

Paul M. Silverman, MD

Table of Contents

PART I GENERAL PRINCIPLES

CHAPTER 1 A Multidisciplinary Approach to Cancer: A Radiologist's View

Eric M. Rohren, M.D., Ph.D.

INTRODUCTION

Multidisciplinary care teams are those that are composed of members from multiple different medical specialties working together to achieve the highest quality of care for the patient. Such teams are particularly needed in complex environments such as cancer hospitals. Frequently patients and their physicians are faced with different options for workup and therapy that cross the boundaries of specialties. These multidisciplinary teams may be comprised of medical oncologists, radiation oncologists, surgeons, radiologists, pathologists, and representatives from a variety of supportive services including nutrition, rehabilitation, and chaplaincy. In order for such a diverse group to work effectively together, communication and mutual understanding are critical.

Imaging plays a central role in the care of patients with cancer. Subsequent chapters deal with some of the specifics regarding the use of imaging in the multidisciplinary environment, such as tumor staging, lesion respectability, and treatment-related complications. Many clinical decisions are influenced by the results of imaging studies, and the radiologist must, therefore, be a central member of the multidisciplinary care team. The significant role of imaging can be seen in the continued growth in the numbers of scans performed each year, particularly in the advanced imaging studies such as x-ray computed tomography (CT), magnetic resonance imaging (MRI), and positron emission tomography with x-ray CT (PET/CT).[1]

One of the major challenges for radiologists in the multidisciplinary environment is that imaging intersects with nearly all aspects of patient care. Scans ordered by a radiation oncologist for the purpose of treatment planning may be interpreted with a different emphasis and perspective than scans ordered by a surgeon before planned curative resection or by a medical oncologist in anticipation of systemic chemotherapy. The radiologist needs to be aware of the clinical scenario in which the scan is being ordered and should have an understanding of the implications of the scan results for the patient. To provide the most relevant information, the radiologist must have direct and frequent interaction with the other members of the care team through participation in tumor boards or other multidisciplinary activities.

Central to the role radiologists play in the management of patients with cancer is communication. Results need to be conveyed in an understandable and clinically relevant fashion, and preferably in a timely manner. The following sections describe the radiologist's perspective on multidisciplinary cancer care and discuss ways to effectively communicate in such an environment.

MULTIDISCIPLINARY CANCER IMAGING: THE ROLE OF THE RADIOLOGIST

The field of radiology has grown in complexity as the technology of imaging has advanced. Plain x-ray, fluoroscopy, and radionuclide scintigraphy have been a part of medical practice for many decades, whereas CT, MRI, ultrasound, and PET/CT are more recent additions to the field. Even within imaging modalities, techniques continue to evolve. CT studies are now often performed in a multiphasic fashion, using multispectral scanners. Clinical MRI is now performed on both 1.5- and 3.0-T systems, with an ever-increasing array of sequences and coils. In addition, 7.0-T MRI systems are now clinically approved in many environments, and oncologic applications of this technology are being explored.

Advances are not confined solely to the diagnostic arena, but are also seen in the fields of intervention and therapy. In the field of nuclear radiology, there has been rapid expansion in the clinical availability of positron-emitting radiopharmaceutical agents beyond F-18 fluorodeoxyglucose, including agents used for the imaging of neuroendocrine tumors and prostate carcinoma. For many of these compounds, a therapeutic radioisotope can be employed in lieu of the imaging radioisotope, repurposing the compound from a diagnostic imaging study to a therapeutic procedure.[2] Furthermore, the imaging study can often serve as a predictor of response to the therapeutic agent. This framework has been termed "theranostics."

The field of interventional radiology has also seen significant advances in cancer care. Anticancer agents may be administered via catheter, including chemotherapy and radiolabeled microspheres. Percutaneous ablations using radiofrequency ablation or microwave technology can be used to treat some tumors. Also, as the field of oncology moves toward molecular diagnosis and prediction of response, the acquisition of tumor tissue at multiple phases of therapy becomes a critical need. The increasing engagement of interventional radiology in the field of cancer care has led some to use the term "Interventional Oncology" to describe these efforts.[3]

This increase in the breadth and complexity of radiology and nuclear medicine has necessitated a shift in practice patterns at many sites. To effectively function in the multidisciplinary environment of an academic cancer hospital, radiologists have needed to specialize. Radiology specialization has traditionally been either by modality (e.g., ultrasound, CT) or by system (e.g., body imaging, neuroradiology, thoracic radiology). The clinical specialties, conversely, have trended toward specialization according to disease. At MD Anderson Cancer Center, there are multidisciplinary care teams devoted to the care of patients with various malignancies. Each care team is composed of multiple members from various disciplines, including surgery, medical oncology, and radiation therapy. To adapt to the multidisciplinary paradigm, imaging has had to adapt from the traditional modality-based and system-based approaches to a disease-oriented framework (Fig. 1.1).

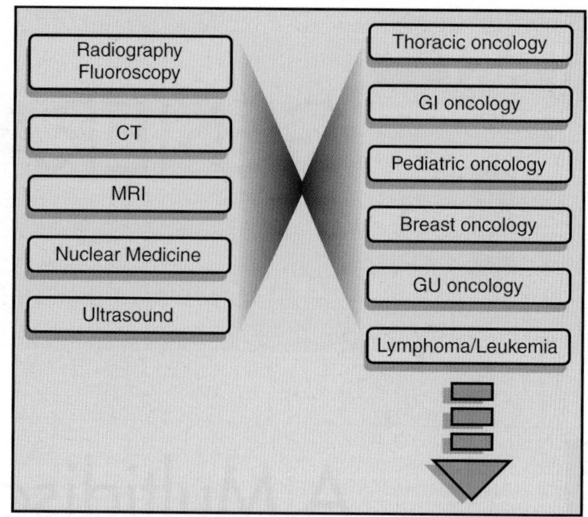

FIGURE 1.1. In the multidisciplinary cancer care environment, the emphasis in imaging shifts from modality-based practice to disease-based practice. *CT*, Computed tomography; *GI*, gastrointestinal; *GU*, genitourinary; *MRI*, magnetic resonance imaging.

The challenge for the radiologist is that diagnostic imaging within each of the multidisciplinary centers crosses the boundaries between traditional imaging specialties. To take an example, a woman with newly diagnosed, locally advanced breast cancer presents for workup (Fig. 1.2). Breast imaging plays a central role in her evaluation, starting with mammography and moving to breast ultrasound and/or MRI as needed. Her pathologic diagnosis and tumor genetic markers will likely be established by a guided biopsy procedure. Further imaging workup of such a patient may include a contrast-enhanced CT of the chest and abdomen or a radionuclide bone scan for detection of osseous metastatic disease. The workup may stop there, but depending on many clinical factors such as signs and symptoms and serum tumor markers, additional imaging may be requested including PET/CT with 2-[^{18}F] fluoro-2-deoxy-D-glucose (FDG), or brain MRI.

All of these imaging studies will be taken into account to decide whether the patient should proceed to surgery, undergo neoadjuvant chemotherapy or chemoradiation, or undergo chemotherapy or radiotherapy either alone or in combination. Imaging may guide specific intervention that is not part of the overall treatment strategy, such as radiotherapy or surgical fixation of a bone metastasis with impending pathologic fracture. In this fairly straightforward example, there is potentially a need for imaging specialists in the fields of breast imaging, body imaging, nuclear medicine, and neuroradiology.

In response to this shift in clinical practice toward multidisciplinary care, radiology at many cancer hospitals has moved toward a disease-based approach. This has required a shift in traditional boundaries, as well as close cooperation between radiologists of different subspecialties. In many cases, one of the radiology subspecialties fits in well with one or more of the clinical care centers. For the patient undergoing workup and care by the breast cancer team described previously, the breast imaging section plays a major role, interacting directly with the clinicians and offering guidance with regards to additional imaging. The thoracic imaging group provides direct interface with the lung cancer, esophageal cancer, and mesothelioma teams. Within each of these sections, radiologists may develop areas of interest and become, for example, specialists in the imaging of pancreatic cancer or gynecologic malignancies.

The radiologists associated with various disease-based care centers should be familiar with the role of imaging in the workup and management of their patients, including the role of imaging studies outside their traditional boundaries. One could use The University of Texas MD Anderson Cancer Center as an example of this approach in imaging, specifically with regards to the interpretation of oncologic FDG PET scans. These studies were traditionally interpreted by a small group of physicians with training in nuclear medicine. With the advent of PET/CT and the additional anatomic information provided by the CT component of the study, radiologists began to show greater and greater interest in the modality. Currently, many sites are performing PET/CT with intravenous and oral contrast, making the CT portion of the examination nearly identical to a traditional diagnostic-quality CT scan. As a result, PET/CT has developed into one of the central

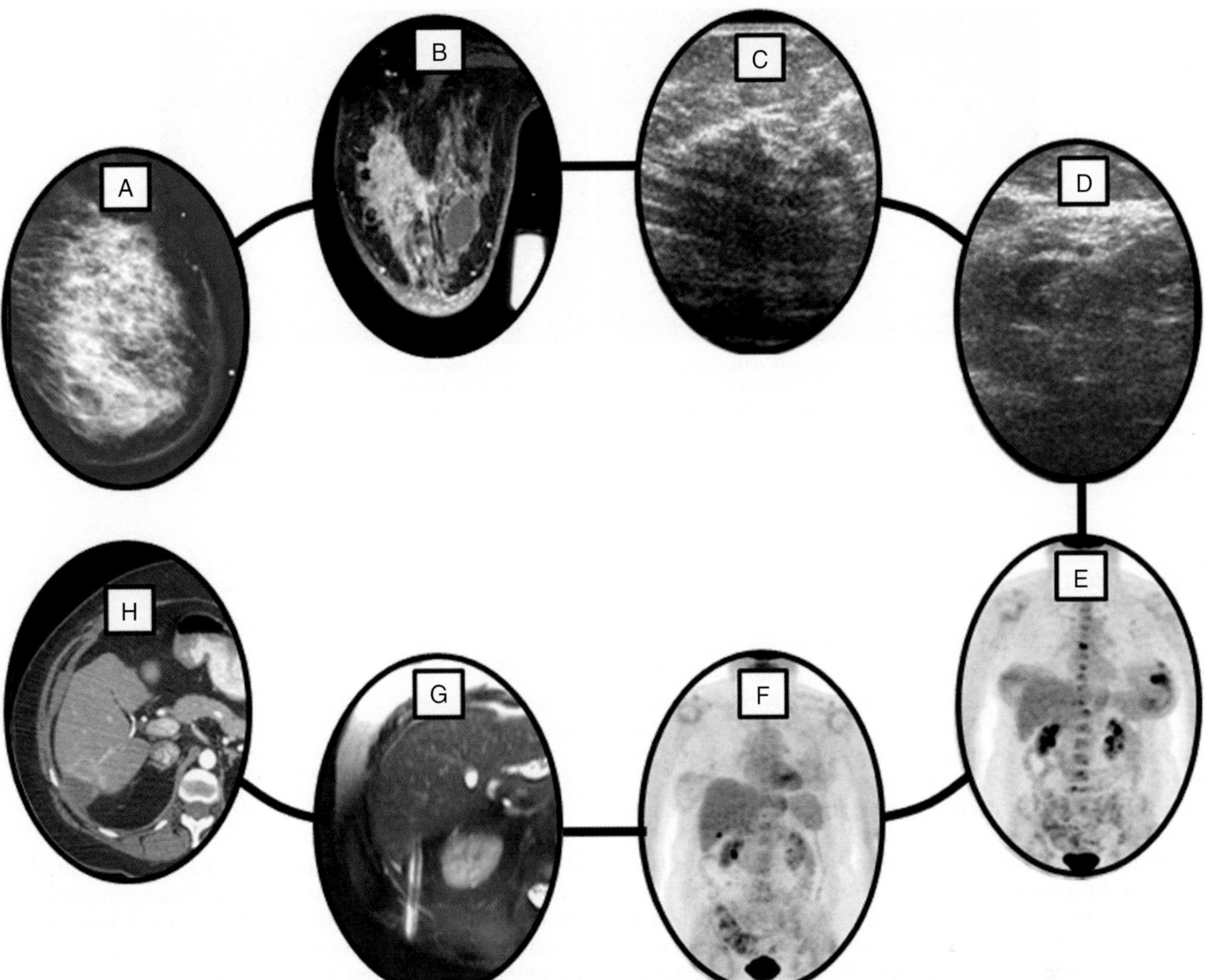

FIGURE 1.2. Imaging can play a role at all stage of the patient care cycle. In this patient with a new breast lump, the diagnosis of breast cancer was first suspected on mammography (**A**) and magnetic resonance imaging (**B**), and was subsequently confirmed on ultrasound (**C**) with ultrasound-guided biopsy (**D**). **E**, A fluoro-2-deoxy-D-glucose (FDG)–positron emission tomography/computed tomography (PET/CT) showed the primary tumor and axillary metastases, but also numerous osseous metastases. **F**, The patient subsequently received chemoradiation for stage IV disease. A follow-up FDG PET/CT showed complete metabolic response of the primary tumor, nodal metastases, and osseous metastases, but a new hypermetabolic lesion in the liver. **G**, This lesion was confirmed and biopsied under ultrasound guidance, after which a limited hepatectomy was performed. **H**, Follow-up CT scan shows evolving postoperative changes and no evidence of recurrence.

imaging strategies in the evaluation of patients with a variety of malignancies.

In response to these changes, the FDG PET/CT readership at MD Anderson was expanded to include specialist radiologists (abdominal, thoracic, neuro, etc.) with advanced training and credentials in FDG PET/CT. The section of PET/CT has, therefore, become a "virtual section," with members from nuclear medicine, body imaging, thoracic imaging, musculoskeletal imaging, and neuroradiology. The section benefits from the diversity of its membership, with each physician bringing knowledge and insight to the community.

The need for a broad fund of knowledge in a well-integrated multidisciplinary environment is balanced by the need for specialization. No one radiologist in an academic cancer center can be familiar enough with each and every imaging test to provide the level of expertise and consultation required. Radiology, therefore, also needs teams. The primary radiology section interfacing with a multidisciplinary care center serves as the anchor and a point of contact. The other sections provide backup and consultation as needed for particular patients. A bone scan performed in nuclear medicine using single-photon emission computed tomography/CT, for example, may show an unsuspected finding in the pancreas, and the advice of a member of the body imaging section may be requested to provide a differential diagnosis.

Cancer imaging in a multidisciplinary environment provides the opportunity to become directly involved in the decision-making processes of patient care and to learn about the role and relevance of imaging within the broad clinical picture. There are challenges in adapting from the traditional modality-based or region-based practice of imaging to a disease-based approach, but these challenges can be met with adaptation and communication.

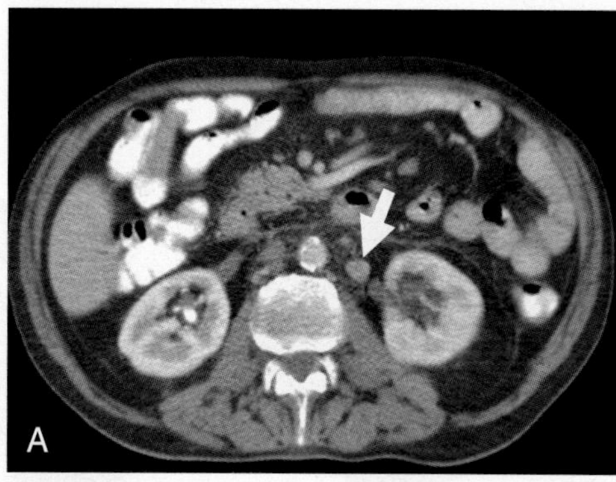

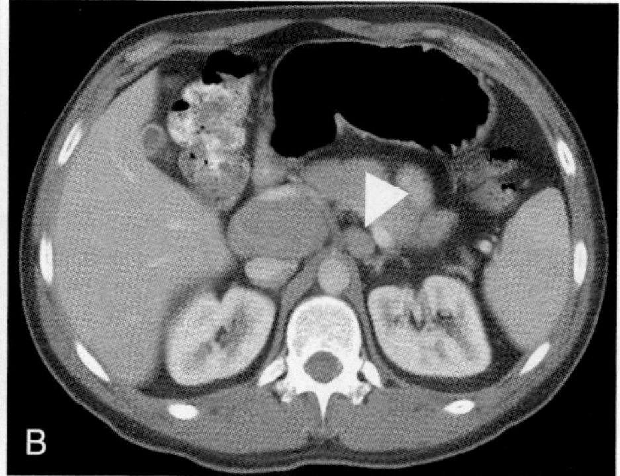

FIGURE 1.3. Similar imaging findings may have very different significance depending on the clinical scenario. **A**, In a patient with newly diagnosed esophageal cancer, computed tomography (CT) showed a suspicious lymph node in the left retroperitoneum (arrow), subsequently biopsied and shown to be owing to metastatic disease. This node significantly altered patient management from neoadjuvant chemoradiation followed by surgery to palliative chemotherapy. **B**, In a patient with newly diagnosed non-Hodgkin lymphoma, a similar node was seen in the left retroperitoneum (arrowhead) on CT. In this case, the presence of this node had no impact on management, because many larger nodes were seen throughout the abdomen and pelvis.

THE VALUE OF COMMUNICATION

Central to the role of the radiologist in the multidisciplinary environment is the ability to communicate effectively. This must occur in direct interactions with colleagues and through the written radiology report. Although verbal communication has many advantages, it is simply not feasible to personally discuss each and every case with the clinical team, and the written report is, therefore, the avenue through which the information obtained from the scan is conveyed in the majority of cases. For this to be done effectively, careful attention should be given to reporting skills.

First and foremost, any radiologic report should answer the clinical question. Scans are ordered with a particular question in mind, from the general ("What is the patient's disease status following treatment?") to the specific ("What is the cause of the abdominal fullness felt on abdominal examination?"). Effective reports directly answer these questions, in either the positive or the negative. For this to happen, the radiologist must understand the clinical question being asked. Sometimes this information is contained in the scan order, but at other times it may be necessary to probe the patient's history to find the rationale for the scan in question.

In the setting of multidisciplinary cancer care, the challenge for the radiologist is to fully understand the clinical questions for different disease types. The information relevant to the care of patients with different types of malignancies can be quite diverse. As an example (Fig. 1.3), patient A has newly diagnosed esophageal cancer, verified by endoscopic biopsy. Patient B has newly diagnosed large B-cell lymphoma, diagnosed by retroperitoneal lymph node biopsy of a known retroperitoneal mass. Both patients undergo FDG PET/CT, and each is found to have a hypermetabolic nodal mass in the left paraaortic space of the retroperitoneum below the celiac trunk. In patient B, in which this additional node is almost certainly a manifestation of retroperitoneal lymphoma, it has little additional significance because it does not change the stage of the patient's disease. In patient A, however, this node is a critical finding, changing management from chemoradiation and potentially curative surgery to palliative chemotherapy or chemoradiation. An identical finding in these two patients has markedly different significance in terms of the fundamental clinical question of tumor stage and appropriate therapy, and the reporting should reflect this.

Box 1.1 The Eight Cs of Effective Radiology Reporting

Correctness	**C**larity
Completeness	**C**onfidence
Consistency	**C**oncision
Communication	**C**onsultation

From Reiner BI, Knight N, Siegel EL. Radiology reporting, past, present, and future: the radiologist's perspective. *J Am Coll Radiol.* 2007;4:313-319.

Answering the clinical question, therefore, becomes a matter of first understanding the disease process enough to appreciate the relative importance of various radiologic findings and then, of reporting those findings in an effective manner. A helpful framework for high-quality radiology reporting is the eight Cs of effective reporting (Box 1.1). This framework was initially put forward by Armas[4] as six Cs, and was expanded to eight Cs by Reiner and colleagues.[5] The eight Cs are Correctness, Completeness, Consistency, Communication, Clarity, Confidence, Concision, and Consultation. These are useful measures of effective reporting, particularly in the setting of a multidisciplinary cancer care system.

Correctness is perhaps the most basic of these concepts, but at the same time it is not as absolute as it seems. Everyone strives for the correct diagnosis in radiology reporting, yet given the complexities of imaging it is not always possible to arrive at the correct diagnosis. In fact, there are situations in which the best scan interpretation may not contain the correct diagnosis. For example, a patient with prior non–small cell lung cancer presents with a new, slowly enlarging speculated pulmonary nodule. The report of the chest CT appropriately suggests metastatic disease, and a percutaneous biopsy is performed. The biopsy shows inflammatory reaction and fungal elements, and a diagnosis of *Nocardia* infection is made. In this case, the CT report was not "correct" in the sense of making the appropriate diagnosis; however, the workup generated by the CT report was appropriate, and the diagnosis of fungal infection was made, allowing for treatment with antibiotics. The emphasis might, therefore, be better placed on interpreting studies in the correct fashion (i.e., up to the standards of good medical practice) rather than focusing on the correct diagnosis.[6]

Completeness and consistency are related parameters. Completeness is defined as containing all the parts and elements necessary for a high-quality report, and consistency implies structure to the report, applied over time. Both of these elements can be achieved through the use of reporting templates or standardized reporting. A representative guideline for reporting of PET/CT scans is provided by the Society of Nuclear Medicine's PET Center of Excellence, outlining the components of an effective PET/CT report in oncology.[7] Other guidelines and templates exist for other imaging modalities.

Communication is the core of quality in the field of imaging. The best images obtained on the newest scanner and interpreted by the best-trained radiologist can be clinically useless if the results are not effectively communicated to the referring clinician. Often, the written report is the only interface between the radiologist and the clinician. Special care must, therefore, be given to the structuring of the report to ensure the message is delivered in an appropriate fashion. The final four Cs can be seen as tools to achieve that effective communication.

Clarity means that the opinion of the radiologist is clearly stated in the report. In the arena of oncologic imaging, this may mean definitively categorizing into one of the four criteria outlined in the World Health Organization and Response Evaluation Criteria In Solid Tumors criteria[8–10]: complete response, partial response, stable disease, or progressive disease. Clarity does not necessarily imply a single diagnosis, because many radiologic findings require an organized and logically ordered differential diagnosis. Further clarity can be achieved with the addition of next steps, if appropriate.

Confidence is a measure of how much faith the radiologist has in his or her conclusions. Again, it is entirely appropriate to give a differential diagnosis when imaging findings are not conclusive for a single process (as is often the case). A warning sign of low confidence is the overuse of qualifiers such as "likely," "possible," and "cannot exclude." When such words are used frequently in reports, it waters down the message and leaves the clinician lacking in guidance as to how to manage the patient.

Concision means brevity; it is desirable in radiology reports for several reasons. First, from a pragmatic and economical standpoint, many practices pay for dictation by the word or by the line, so there can be significant cost savings associated with shortening the length of reports. Second, concision tends to lead to clarity in that, to achieve it, care must be given to the choice of wording and how the message is to be spelled out. Finally, most clinicians are busy and may skim over lengthy reports to pull out the "bottom line," leaving room for misinterpretation. When possible, it is best to distill the findings from imaging studies into a series of short, declarative sentences. This may not always be possible, particularly with complex modalities such as PET/CT and complex clinical scenarios, but should be striven for.

Consultation is where all of the Cs are pulled together. Radiologists are members of the multidisciplinary team and should view themselves as imaging consultants, rendering advice and opinion as to the significance of imaging findings in the care of each patient. The role of consultant should be maintained whether presenting cases at a tumor board or when reading cases at the workstation. It is here that knowledge of the clinical scenarios and questions becomes paramount. Effective consultation sometimes requires anticipating what questions may arise in a patient's care and proactively answering those questions in the report, including both pertinent positive findings and pertinent negative findings. One of the phrases that is often used in radiology reporting can undermine the role of consultant: "clinical correlation is recommended." When used in the context of a differential diagnosis in which there are certain signs and/or symptoms that may confirm the diagnosis, the use of the phrase may be appropriate. For example, in a patient whose CT shows inflammatory changes surrounding the sigmoid colon, a report reading "these changes may represent acute diverticulitis, correlate clinically" gives guidance and direction. In other settings, however, its use can be vague and may lead to confusion. In a patient with a subcentimeter pulmonary nodule, a report reading "this nodule could be inflammatory or malignant, correlate clinically" provides no guidance or advice, because no sign, symptom, or laboratory test will significantly change estimation of the likelihood of malignancy. If follow-up scanning is indicated to determine the stability of the nodule, this should be stated. If the findings are more concerning, and the nodule is amenable to biopsy, this information should be conveyed.

PARTICIPATION

The eight Cs described previously are helpful tools in the construction of effective and useful radiology reports. Many of the studies that are interpreted are acted upon based on that report without further interaction by the radiologist. However, in the true multidisciplinary care environment, keeping in mind the role of the radiologist as imaging consultant, person-to-person interaction is a requirement. This can range from phone consultation to participation in tumor boards or other multidisciplinary conferences. Despite best efforts to appreciate and answer clinical questions, it is not always possible to fully understand or anticipate the information required by the clinician in a particular patient's care. Even at centers in which the radiologist has access to the patient's medical record and clinic notes, the most recent notes indicating the precise reason the examination was performed may not be available at the time of dictation.

Personal consultation with clinicians is highly beneficial to the practice of radiology, and the benefits flow in both directions. Through discussions with the surgeons, medical oncologists, and radiation oncologists, the radiologist expands her or his knowledge of the medical field, improving their quality of interpretation and reporting for future patients. The clinician, by understanding more about the strengths and weaknesses of imaging studies, will improve his or her appropriate utilization of the modalities. Finally, personal interactions ensure that the radiologist is viewed as a colleague, a member of the multidisciplinary team.

SUMMARY

The practice of oncologic imaging in the multidisciplinary setting presents challenges for the radiologist. Because of the nature of the disease, therapies, and imaging technologies, there is a high degree of complexity in patient imaging. Adherence to the eight Cs of effective reporting can help ensure effective communication, and an understanding of the diseases and therapeutic options aids in crafting a clinically relevant report. Finally, the radiologist must be an active and participating member of the multidisciplinary team, providing insight into and perspective on the value and limitations of imaging in the care of patients with malignancy.

REFERENCES

1. IMV 2006 CT Market Summary Report. Des Plaines, IL: IMV Medical Information Division; 2006.
2. Farolfi A, Fendler W, Iravani A, et al. Theranostics for advanced prostate cancer: current indications and future developments. *Eur Urol Oncol*. 2019;2(2):152-162.
3. Schoenberg SO, Attenberger UI, Solomon SB, Weissleder R. Developing a roadmap for interventional oncology. *Oncologist*. 2018;23(10):1162-1170.
4. Armas RR. Qualities of a good radiology report. *AJR Am J Roentgenol*. 1998;170:1110.
5. Reiner BI, Knight N, Siegel EL. Radiology reporting, past, present, and future: the radiologist's perspective. *J Am Coll Radiol*. 2007;4:313-319.
6. Gunderman RB, Nyce JM. The tyranny of accuracy in radiologic education. *Radiology*. 2002;222:297-300.
7. Available at http://interactive.snm.org/docs/PET_PROS/ElementsofPETCTReporting.pdf
8. Miller AB, Hoogstraten B, Staquet M, Winkler A. Reporting results of cancer treatment. *Cancer*. 1981;47:208-214.
9. Therasse P, Arbuck SG, Eisenhauer EA, et al. New guidelines to evaluate the response to treatment in solid tumors. European Organization for Research and Treatment of Cancer, National Cancer Institute of the United States, National Cancer Institute of Canada. *J Natl Cancer Inst*. 2000;92:205-216.
10. Eisenhauer EA, Therasse P, Bogaerts J, et al. New response evaluation criteria in solid tumours: revised RECIST guideline (version 1.1). *Eur J Cancer*. 2009;45:228-247.

CHAPTER 2

A Multidisciplinary Approach to Cancer: A Surgeon's View

Eddie K. Abdalla, M.D.

INTRODUCTION

Surgery remains a pillar of multimodality therapy for long-term survival in virtually all patients with solid tumors. For surgery to be effective, however, patients must be selected properly so that nontherapeutic surgery is avoided. In the current era of cancer surgery and imaging, "exploratory surgery" should, with the rarest of exceptions, not exist as a diagnostic modality. Both survival and resectability rates are rising based on many factors, including improved preoperative staging, but no test (biologic or radiologic) can tell the surgeon whether the patient should be operated. As an example, high-quality computed tomography (CT) imaging can predict degree of abutment versus encasement of the superior mesenteric artery with virtually 100% accuracy in pancreatic adenocarcinoma,[1] yet other tumor–vessel relationships cannot be defined with 100% radioogical–clinical correlative accuracy (e.g., hilar cholangiocarcinoma abutment or involvement of a sectoral hepatic artery),[2] and small volume peritoneal disease may not be detected on even the best preoperative imaging, regardless of modality. These anatomic factors do not define whether a patient should be resected but rather what anatomical considerations define the resection planes. Clinically relevant underlying liver disease is inadequately assessed by imaging (steatosis, cirrhosis, hemochromatosis can be assessed and graded, for example), yet, despite radiological grading, the clinical relevance of underlying liver disease to a given planned procedure does not correlate well to imaging findings.[3] Furthermore, the interaction between different treatments, including chemotherapy with and without biologically active agents, radiotherapy, intraarterial therapies, and surgery, require that treatment sequencing, timing, and duration be considered carefully. Together, these factors contribute to the constant movement in the line defining resectability for many tumors. Tumors (and liver parenchyma) may change character on imaging over time as some treatments are delivered, changing the sensitivity and specificity of radiologic findings as treatment progresses. Before patients embark on complex treatment plans, treatment sequence/timing issues must be considered by a team of physicians. Importantly, such multidisciplinary discussion and appropriate imaging must be completed before "palliative" treatments render potentially curable patients incurable (e.g., patients with resectable disease can be rendered unresectable if overtreatment with chemotherapy leads to liver toxicity). Open communication between surgeons and radiologists changes the way surgeons operate and changes the way radiologists report their findings to optimize patient care. Patient care is just that, patient care. If the focus of the radiologist, surgeon, radiotherapist, oncologist, and others in the care team is constantly on the patient, the best outcomes can be achieved. If the surgeon operates, the oncologist gives chemotherapy, and the radiation oncologist delivers radiotherapy based on a piece of paper (e.g., a radiology report), the best care may not be delivered. If the radiologist is integrated into the treatment team, modern, rapidly improving patient outcomes can be achieved more widely. Finally, goals of care differ in different patients. In some the goal is prevention, in others diagnosis and treatment. Imaging has a major role in screening and risk assessment in cohorts with a genetic tendency to develop hepatobiliary and other gastrointestinal cancers (e.g., BRCA1 and 2 for pancreatic cancer) or in assessing risk related to existing imaging findings (e.g., mucinous pancreatic cysts). In yet others, the goal may be palliation. Achieving these goals requires the members of the treatment team to work together in a patient-focused way.

Candidacy for "potentially curative" therapy is rapidly changing. As an example, multiple bilateral liver metastases from colorectal or neuroendocrine primary cancers can be treated with curative intent by surgery or by integration of interventional, percutaneous, and surgical approaches, leading to survival rates exceeding 50% at 5 years postresection.[4–6] In such cases, radiology reports of "multiple bilateral liver metastases" may be accurate, but may also be misleading to the patient or oncologist/gastroenterologist reading the report (discussed later). Not every clinician is willing or able to review and understand imaging studies for every patient seen in the clinic. Surgeons should review every image on every patient, but primary care physicians, gastroenterologists, and medical oncologists are the gateways to surgeons, often encountering patients first and initiating treatment plans. Thus, clear assessment of imaging and clearly written reports are frequently the starting point for medical providers caring for patients with many tumor types. Multidisciplinary conferences help to overcome some of these problems because images are reviewed directly, but the vast majority of treated patients nationwide and worldwide will not be presented in multidisciplinary conferences. These factors contribute to the need for communication between members of the care team to optimize the value of imaging, as well as optimize patient care. This chapter will outline the following areas:

- Diagnosis
- Staging

- Surgical Planning
- Surgical Treatment
- Screening and follow-up in high-risk patients

DIAGNOSIS

Accurate diagnosis may be based on patient history, clinical findings, imaging, biopsy or a combination of these elements. In rare cases, diagnosis may be made accurately with clinical history, tumor markers, and imaging, whereas pathology may be confusing (e.g., hepatic hemangioendothelioma, some cystic lesions in the liver and pancreas). Functional treatment modalities such as 2-[^{18}F] fluoro-2-deoxy-D-glucose positron emission tomography (FDG PET) and magnetic resonance imaging (MRI) can help clinicians in the correct clinical scenario but may also confuse the picture (by missing lesions in patients undergoing effective chemotherapy, and by highlighting nonmalignant areas of inflammation or postoperative change in other cases) unless the multidisciplinary team members work together to interpret studies in the proper context. Correct cancer diagnosis can often be made by review of imaging, depending on the disease site and type, as described in detail elsewhere in this book.

In many cases, however, pathologic diagnosis is needed, whether to confirm the clinical/radiological suspicion, as a requirement for treatment by radiotherapy or chemotherapy, or as a requirement for protocol-based therapy. In these cases, the initial imaging will often define whether a percutaneous or endoscopic approach to biopsy is needed. When percutaneous biopsy is planned, the presumed tumor type and location impact biopsy planning. For liver tumors, biopsy technique significantly impacts needle tract seeding, which should be an extremely rare event (<1%), even with primary liver tumors such as hepatocellular carcinoma.[7,8] Ultrasound-guided lymph node biopsy with core biopsy can provide diagnosis of lymphoma, although excisional biopsy may be needed and is guided by both clinical examination and cross-sectional imaging; more recently, FDG PET may demonstrate the most active nodes and guide biopsy planning as well. Seeding is exceptionally rare with endoscopic ultrasound–guided biopsy and remains the standard of care for many tumors such as pancreatic and lower biliary lesions. Thus even at the level of obtaining diagnosis, consideration as to the probable diagnosis and possible treatments must often be given, reemphasizing the need for a multidisciplinary approach when treating cancer patients, including accurate prebiopsy imaging. Finally, interventions (percutaneous, endoscopic, or surgical) create artifacts that can impair quality of imaging; thus proper imaging before biopsy is critical for many reasons.

STAGING

Once the diagnosis is made, the disease must be staged. Staging differs based not only on disease site but disease type, as treatments differ depending on findings (e.g., pancreatic adenocarcinoma with liver metastases is not treated surgically, whereas well-differentiated pancreatic neuroendocrine tumors with multiple bilateral liver metastases may be treated surgically with the expectation of very long-term survival); and the sensitivity of tests (and agents used such as FDG vs. gallium-68 for PET) differs based on disease subtype, such as mucinous versus nonmucinous gastric tumors, or tumor grade, such as well-differentiated versus poorly differentiated neuroendocrine tumors. Indications for chemo- and radiotherapy differ depending on the presence, absence, and often extent of distant disease (and sometimes imaging findings, as discussed later). Solid tumors are typically staged using the TNM system, although many elements of TNM staging are not typically assessed by cross-sectional imaging. T classification describes the primary tumor, and may relate to size (well-defined on cross-sectional imaging), but also may relate to depth of penetration through the layers of the organ (as with the gastrointestinal tract for esophagogastric, small bowel, and colorectal tumors), which is not evaluated on CT or MRI. Other factors such as invasion of adjacent organs and perforation may be seen well on imaging. Endoluminal MRI may classify invasion in rectal tumors, but otherwise CT and MRI are not used to assess whether layers of the gastrointestinal tract are invaded. N classification consistently relates to nodal involvement, although the N classifications differ from disease to disease based on the number and location of suspected or known nodal metastases. Imaging is central to further assessment of suspicious nodes based on nodal size, location, enhancement, diffusion restriction, and metabolic activity, and all contribute to surgical planning. M classification relates to metastases in all cases. Suspicious findings on any imaging study may be pursued, again given different impacts of metastases based on disease type. Treatments for different diseases with the same T, N, or M classification differ widely. Thus coordination between the imaging radiologist, interventional radiologist/gastroenterologist, and treating physician helps to ensure that the needed staging information is conveyed (and that the proper staging studies are obtained) to facilitate optimal patient care. In addition to classical staging information, surgical planning requires assessment of tumor–vessel relationships and anatomical variations, as discussed later.

SURGICAL PLANNING

Surgical planning depends on more than staging *per se*. Tumors in different locations are approached differently, and information about tumor–vessel and tumor–organ associations may not simply define resectability, but enable proper surgical planning:

- Tumor location/extent
- Tumor–vessel relationships
- Tumor–organ relationships
- Anatomical variations

Two different examples are described here. First, in the case of pancreatic adenocarcinoma, whether in the head, body, or tail of the pancreas, critical anatomical relationships define surgical resectability, including vascular abutment, vascular encasement, and occlusion by the tumor. Vascular involvement provokes significantly different treatment approaches (these are discussed in subsequent chapters and summarized here).[9] Further, the vessel involved is important—arterial (superior mesenteric artery, celiac trunk, hepatic artery, splenic artery, left gastric artery, accessory, or replaced hepatic arteries) and mesenteric/portal venous involvement have significantly different surgical and oncologic implications. In the case of no vascular abutment or encasement based on multiphasic thin-cut CT or MRI, straightforward pancreatectomy is generally planned, with pre- or postoperative chemoradiotherapy. In the case of venous involvement, an entirely different operative plan is made to include vascular resection and reconstruction; this picture can change with neoadjuvant therapy. Venous abutment and encasement may not exclude resectability, whereas venous occlusion is considered "borderline" and may be resectable in selected cases. In the case of arterial involvement, preoperative therapy is generally advised, and in the case of extensive involvement (>180 degree encasement of the artery) surgery may not be indicated (again, this is a moving bar: the superior mesenteric artery and celiac artery are resected and replaced with venous and synthetic conduits with increasing frequency and improving results, so reports providing degree of involvement/encasement are most helpful to surgeons).[9] The finding of liver metastasis virtually excludes the therapeutic value of surgery, even for the smallest resectable primary pancreatic adenocarcinoma. Regional adenopathy does not exclude resectability. Clear peritoneal carcinomatosis is a contraindication to surgery and to locoregional therapy; suggestion of peritoneal disease, which may not definitive (e.g., indistinct nodularity of peritoneum, mesenteric stranding, trace ascites) may prompt staging laparoscopy. Thus accurate staging and reporting of findings relevant to surgery for the specific disease are critical to surgical planning and result from communication between imaging and treating physicians. Primary tumor type impacts the requirements of the report—primary pancreatic adenocarcinoma with a single liver metastasis is not a surgical disease; primary colorectal cancer with 17 bilateral liver metastases may be treated with curative intent, as described later.

As a different example, issues in liver surgery can be even more complex. Resectable liver tumor(s) are often defined based on liver that will remain after resection, including preservation of adequate inflow and outflow to the preserved segments, with adequate liver remnant volumes.[10,11] Tumor–vessel relationships within the liver impact resectability differently than for pancreatic or other gastrointestinal, thoracic, head and neck, or extremity tumors. Vascular resection (portal, hepatic venous, caval, and arterial) is increasingly performed in many centers, depending on disease type and often therapy response. Tumors may involve two of three outflow vessels (hepatic veins) in the liver and abut the inferior vena cava but be resectable with standard techniques and excellent results.[12] Rarely, involvement of all three hepatic veins, traditionally considered a sign of unresectablity, is not an impediment to complete resection either, because vascular resection/reconstruction can be considered,[13] or because venous anomalies may permit otherwise impossible resections such as subtotal hepatectomy based on the presence of a dominant inferior right hepatic vein.[14] Major hepatectomy includes resection of tumors involving major hepatic and portal branches routinely, as long as vessels supplying and draining the liver remnant are free of tumor. In other cases, major resection is possible because of other anatomic variations in the liver, such as a staged portal bifurcation allowing resection of tumors involving the central liver. Arterial and biliary anomalies contribute to assessment of resectability in a significant proportion of patients.

Thus surgeons and radiologists must understand the anatomy of the liver (the hepatic veins, portal veins, and hepatic arteries) and must remark variations including replaced or accessory hepatic arteries (present in up to 55% of patients)[15] or even the existence of important venous variants (e.g. inferior hepatic veins). Segmental liver volume is highly variable, which impacts surgical planning[16]; and tumor involvement of intrahepatic vessels or portal structures, as well as therapy changes, can alter volume distribution among hepatic segments. Systematic liver volumetry based on cross-sectional imaging and/or functional imaging is a critical tool to surgical planning for major liver resection, reiterating the intersection of radiologists and surgeons in surgical planning, although liver volumetry is typically requested by the surgeon to facilitate surgical planning that leaves specific adjacent anatomical liver segments intact.[10,11,17] Radiologists and surgeons who work together are aware of the importance of anatomic variations and tumor–vessel relationships, and that these factors can lead to different radiological reports that guide patients and clinicians with the help of high-quality imaging and interpretation. An example synthesizing these issues in a patient with multiple bilateral colorectal liver metastases is illustrated in Fig. 2.1.

Finally, advances in imaging have advanced the correlation between imaging findings and patient outcomes. Two examples warrant comment, both of which relate to treatment of solid tumors with "biologic" agents and assessment of response on CT (and/or PET). The first is gastrointestinal stromal tumor (GIST), which treated with imatinib mesylate, an inhibitor of KIT and PDGFRa tyrosine kinases. Traditional methods of assessing response such as Response Evaluation Criteria in Solid Tumors (RECIST)[18] are not always sufficient to capture the effects of this class of new agents, which cause less size change and more cystic change and loss of vascularity in GIST tumors than traditional treatments, leading to a shift in assessment of response in these tumors that is based on different radiologic criteria.[19] Even in colorectal liver metastases, RECIST is a poor indicator of response to newer agents such as bevacizumab, a vascular endothelial growth factor antagonist. One study has shown that morphologic criteria that focus not on tumor size changes but on changes in vascularity and the margin between the tumor and the liver predict survival in patients with resectable and unresectable colorectal liver metastases treated with bevacizumab, and that the morphologic radiologic response (but not RECIST) correlates with pathologic response to chemotherapy, a true survival predictor.[20] MRI with diffusion-weighted imaging may also provide information as to the degree of activity of liver metastases after chemotherapy (or intraarterial therapy). MRI may have an advantage in lesion detection after chemotherapy as well, owing to changes in the character of the tumor and the liver impacting the "contrast" between lesion and normal underlying liver.[21] These examples of advances in imaging, as well

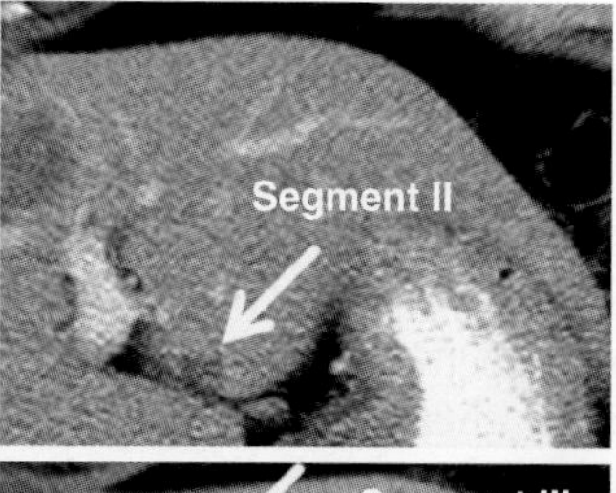

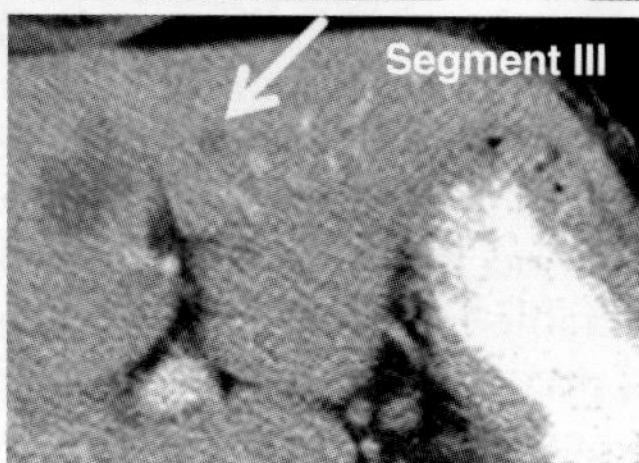

FIGURE 2.1. This patient with a synchronous presentation of obstructing colon cancer and multiple bilateral colorectal liver metastases presented with a total of 16 tumors involving every anatomic segment of the liver, including the caudate (segment I). Resection was possible because the lateral liver was relatively spared; after chemotherapy with response, he underwent first-stage wedge resections of the segment II and III lesions, followed by right portal vein embolization extended to segment IV, followed by second-stage extended right hepatectomy with caudate lobectomy. He never experienced recurrence in the liver.

as the correlation between newer imaging findings and outcomes, are important to physicians and surgeons who determine treatment plans. At the same time, shortcomings of even the most modern imaging techniques must be considered. The absence of PET activity or arterial enhancement of a GIST or colorectal liver metastasis almost never (<10%) indicates cure,[22] so again, oncologists, surgeons, and radiologists must avoid overinterpretation of findings on imaging before treatment decisions are made.

SURGICAL TREATMENT

Treatment objectives differ depending on tumor types, stages, and locations.

- Definitive resection of primary tumors
- Definitive resection of metastatic tumors
- Debulking surgery
- Palliative and emergency surgery
- Reconstruction

Definitive Resection of Primary Tumors

Treatment with curative or definitive intent is often the goal of surgical therapy, whether surgery is a standalone treatment or part of a multipronged approach to cancer in combination with chemotherapy and/or radiotherapy. Treatments of many primary tumors (e.g., craniofacial tumors, extremity tumors, gastrointestinal/genitourinary tumors) impact quality of life because they cause permanent deformity or other alterations to the patient such as ostomy. Oncologic surgery typically implies surgery along anatomic planes (perhaps excluding some soft tissue tumors); most solid tumors are resected with regional lymph nodes. Some lymph node basins are of significant interest because metastases in distant basins may indicate advanced disease and contraindicate surgery (e.g., interaortocaval nodal metastasis from gallbladder cancer). Many solid tumors can be resected along with adjacent structures/organs with curative intent (T4 colon tumors, some pancreatic neoplasms). Some primary tumors are appropriately resected despite the presence or even unresectability of metastatic tumors (e.g., small bowel neuroendocrine tumors without peritoneal metastases but with unresectable but controllable liver metastases, and increasingly colorectal tumors with liver-only metastases), especially with the advent of other approaches to control liver metastases such as intraarterial therapies and systemic radionuclide treatments. The appropriate margin of resection may be a specific distance (millimeters of normal liver for a liver tumor, millimeters of esophagus or pharynx for an upper gastrointestinal tumor) or simply an anatomic plane (a fat plane along the superior mesenteric artery for a pancreatic adenocarcinoma), and millimeters may be the difference between leaving a patient with a permanent ostomy or with a continuous gastrointestinal tract (as for low rectal cancer). Relevant disease- and tumor-specific concepts are brought to the forefront when surgeons and radiologists work together.

Definitive Resection of Metastatic Tumors

As mentioned, many metastatic tumors require surgery. Colorectal, neuroendocrine, other endocrine, and noncolorectal, nonendocrine primary cancers that metastasize to the liver and lung can be resected with expectation of long-term survival[23,24] or even cure.[25] Barriers to resectability have been shattered in the best studied subgroup, those with liver metastases from colorectal cancer, with survival following resection exceeding 50% at 5 years.[10] In addition, the criteria for resectability of this and other tumors that metastasize to the liver no longer consider the number or size of tumors. Rather, resectability is defined by:[10]

- Fitness for surgery
- Potential for definitive treatment of the primary tumor
- Potential to remove all tumor deposits with adequate margin
- Potential to leave adequate liver remnant postresection (based on three-dimensional liver volumetry and/or volumetry with functional imaging)
- Potential to preserve adequate inflow, outflow, and biliary drainage of the future liver remnant (FLR)

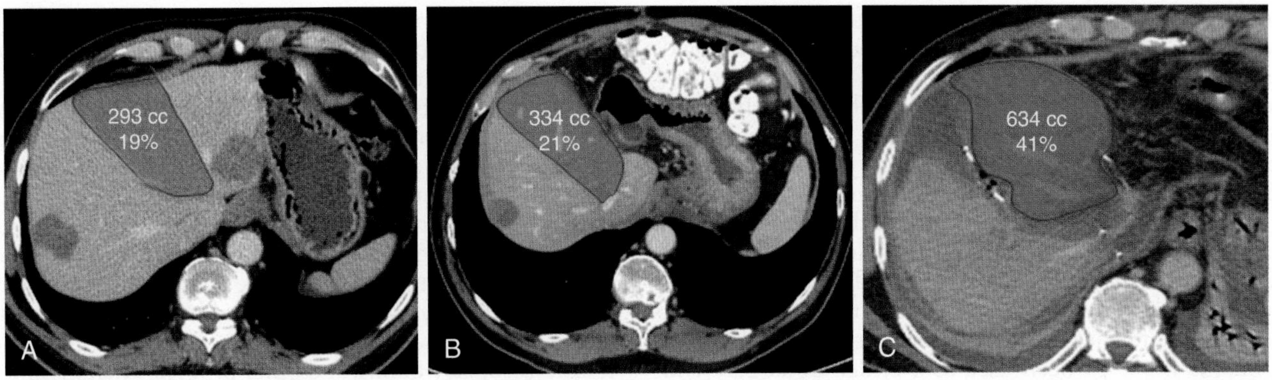

Figure 2.2. This patient underwent lateral bisegment resection and right portal vein embolization in preparation for right hepatectomy and total caudate lobectomy. The planned future liver remnant (FLR) was segment IV only. Preoperative measurement of the FLR volume indicated that it was 19% of the standardized total liver volume **(A)**. Unfortunately, postembolization there was inadequate growth of the FLR (reaching only 21% of the total liver volume) **(B)**. Salvage Associating Liver Partition and Portal vein ligation for Staged hepatectomy was performed: the transection plane between segment IV and V/VIII was divided, with division of the right portal vein but preservation of the right hepatic artery, right bile duct, and right hepatic vein. The resulting plane is seen, with doubling of the size of the FLR (to 41%) as a result **(C)**. Subsequent right hepatectomy rendered the patient free of disease.

Resectability is no longer defined by counting tumors or measuring the size of tumors *per se* (though these factors may be relevant to determine whether resection is oncologically appropriate); rather, the search is made for an anatomical region of the liver that has been relatively spared by disease that can be preserved as the FLR.[26] If resection is oncologically appropriate, and if the anticipated FLR will be too small to support postresection liver function, modern interventional radiologic techniques permit percutaneous embolization of the portal branches supplying the part of the liver to be resected. This diverts portal flow to the FLR and leads to a shift in liver function, from that part of the liver containing tumors that is to be resected to the disease-free part of the liver that will remain, before resection is performed.[26,27] Extended hepatic resection is safe following portal flow diversion.[12] Patients with bilateral liver tumors can also be treated with curative intent. Some patients with bilateral liver tumors can be treated with curative intent by a totally resective approach (two separate, sequential operations, one to address disease on the left, one to address disease on the right). Classical two-stage liver resection involves two operations separated by weeks with interval portal vein embolization performed by the interventional radiologist. During the first laparotomy (or laparoscopy), the liver is surgically staged and all tumors in the planned future liver remnant (FLR) are resected using parenchymal-preserving techniques to render the FLR free of disease. After recovery, the patient undergoes an intervening percutaneous portal vein embolization (if needed to divert portal flow to the now disease-free FLR, inducing hypertrophy), and about 4-6 weeks later, a second laparotomy (or laparoscopy) is performed to complete major hepatectomy (hemihepatectomy or extended hepatectomy) assuring complete tumor resection, leaving patients with preserved liver function and normal performance status. Some patients are candidates for a more compressed two-stage approach called Associating Liver Partition and Portal vein ligation for Staged hepatectomy (ALPPS)[4,28] (Fig. 2.2). During the first stage of ALPPS, 3 objectives are completed including 1) complete, parenchymal-sparing resection of the disease in the planned FLR, 2) intraoperative portal ligation/embolization to immediately divert portal flow to the newly disease-free FLR, and 3) initiate the parenchymal transection normally associated with the second stage resection. This combined portal flow diversion plus partial parenchymal transection can induce more rapid and complete FLR hypertrophy and, upon only brief recovery, allow second-stage laparotomy/laparoscopy within 2 weeks of the first-stage resection, rather than 1 to 2 months required by classical two-stage surgery. ALPSS also eliminates the inter-stage need for a separate procedure in interventional radiology. Long-term outcomes are excellent with both techniques; the preferred approach in a given case is guided by FLR volume assessment, anatomical and patient factors, and availability of intraoperative imaging for selective PVE. Complex liver operations and procedures such as portal embolization or ALPPS for liver remodeling impact anatomy, liver lesions, and the parenchyma, requiring continuous communication between the radiologist and the surgeon to understand what was done and what is needed in radiologic reporting. Findings after the first stage (whether conventional or ALPPS) cannot be interpreted by radiologists if they are not aware of what was done at initial surgery. The safety of extended liver resection, whether for primary liver tumors, biliary tumors, or secondary (metastatic) tumors, relies uniformly on liver remnant function, which is interpreted on the basis of liver volume, along with presence and degree of underlying liver disease. Imaging evidence of liver disease such as cirrhosis, portal hypertension, varices, fatty liver, and treatment-related changes in the liver over time are evaluated by surgeons considering major liver surgery.

Other methods of tumor destruction can be considered for primary and metastatic liver tumors. Percutaneous ablation or transarterial embolization alone or in combination with ablation can be considered in selected patients, especially those with hepatocellular carcinoma with cirrhosis. Some patients undergo simultaneous intraoperative resection of some tumors and ablation of others to preserve adequate liver parenchyma. Selection of patients for resection versus ablation requires evaluation and assessment by qualified hepatobiliary surgeons and skilled interventional radiologists. Referral directly by oncologists to radiologists may lead to overutilization of ablation when resection would be a better choice, further reinforcing the need for comprehensive multidisciplinary evaluation in these patients.[23] In some cases, ablative techniques are the best choice (e.g., hepatocellular carcinoma in severe cirrhosis) because other options (transplantation or resection) are contraindicated; in others, ablation may help to control disease or systemic manifestation of disease (such as carcinoid, which produces a systemic hormonal syndrome). The advent of "radiation segmentectomy" with high-dose yttrium-90 intraarterial radiotherapy further expands options for patients, and this technique has even been used as a bridge to surgery and transplantation.[29,30] Conventional transarterial chemoembolization or bland embolization combined with percutaneous ablation may increase efficacy and expand the population of individuals with various liver tumors that can be treated.[31] This expansion of surgical, arterial, and ablative treatment options, combinations, and sequences reinforces the need for comprehensive multidisciplinary discussion before treatment plans are made to optimize patient care.

Debulking Surgery

Debulking is rarely indicated for solid tumors. In virtually all tumor types amenable to debulking, chemotherapy is also used. The best-studied cancers in which debulking significantly benefits patients are peritoneal surface malignancies, such as mucinous appendiceal cancers and ovarian cancers.[32] Selected patients undergo peritonectomy and debulking, often with resection of bowel, stomach, spleen, colorectum—followed in some cases by hyperthermic peritoneal chemotherapy.[32] Rarely, metastatic liver tumors such as small bowel carcinoid or functional pancreatic neuroendocrine tumors may require debulking by partial hepatectomy with or without *in situ* ablation when they create intolerable hormonal syndrome,[33] although not all centers agree with this approach, and many prefer to resect/ablate when all disease can be completely resected, even if only with a close margin.[6]

Palliative and Emergency Surgery

Palliative surgery is an art and is less and less commonly performed, even at major cancer centers. Bypass of gastric outlet obstruction, the biliary tract, or the rectum has largely been supplanted by percutaneous and endoscopic measures to intubate and dilate symptomatic strictures or place draining tubes such as percutaneous gastrectomy or percutaneous transhepatic catheters, avoiding the need for surgery in patients with unresectable disease. Many strictures can be palliated with metallic totally internal stents inserted by endoscopic or percutaneous routes. Further, more effective chemotherapy and radiotherapy may resolve or control some malignant problems to be avoided or ameliorated, such as malignant obstruction and bleeding. The decision to perform bypass surgery or ostomy is made after careful clinical consideration and complementary radiographic assessment to assure that surgery to bypass a stricture will achieve the goal of improving the patient's condition (e.g., a gastroenterostomy performed for "gastric outlet obstruction," which is not a physical obstruction but is related to a tumor invading the celiac plexus, creating a functional obstruction, will not significantly improve the patient's ability to eat).

Emergency surgery in is even more rarely needed in patients with cancer. Ruptured/bleeding hepatic tumors should almost always be embolized, and surgery considered only when the patient is stable.[34] Surgery for malignant obstruction in a patient with carcinomatosis may or may not be appropriate, as it may potentiate the patient's decline rather than palliate the obstructive symptoms (carcinomatosis in some cases makes it impossible to safely enter the abdomen or create an internal bypass; rather, surgery leads to fistulas, open wounds, and other problems that in no way achieve the goal of treatment). Perforation of the gastrointestinal tract may indicate urgent surgery in patients who have treatment options (e.g., obstructing rectal tumors), but even in these cases the operation conducted (tumor resection with ostomy vs. diverting ostomy only) must be considered based on the clinical scenario and imaging.

In short, palliative and emergent surgery requires the convergence of judgment, experience, and data (clinical and imaging) so that the best interests of the specific patient can be met. Comprehensive description of radiologic findings is tantamount to proper surgical planning to avoid surgery in a patient with little reserve to tolerate a nontherapeutic procedure.

Reconstructive Surgery

Reconstructive surgery is a critical element of cancer surgery. Craniofacial, abdominal, pelvic, skin/soft tissue, and extremity surgeons often create defects that require reconstruction. Tissue transfer, including rotational and free flaps, may be indicated to ensure healing and cosmetic or anatomic recovery from cancer surgery. Craniofacial, breast, abdominal wall, vaginal, pelvic floor, and extremity reconstructions are common in major cancer centers. In these settings, surgical planning may be complex in terms of assessing candidate flaps for the plastic and reconstructive members of the surgical team, and the postoperative rehabilitation often requires a further team of physical therapists, occupational therapists, and psychologists.

CONCLUSIONS

Cancer care is advancing rapidly and requires interaction between members of the care team to optimize treatment. Treatment timing, duration, and sequencing significantly impact outcomes. For solid tumors, long-term survival and "cure" virtually always rely on surgical excision or other forms of destruction of the tumor(s), although these approaches are very frequently combined with neoadjuvant and/or postoperative adjuvant therapy. Selection of patients for surgery remains a challenge, particularly as those with more advanced cancers or larger tumors and those requiring complex reconstructions are routinely operated on, with excellent outcomes. Advances in selection have come largely with improved preoperative treatments such as effective chemotherapy, but will always rely heavily on accurate imaging, not only to select patients for surgery, but also to plan critical aspects of resection and reconstruction. Staging, response assessment, and communication between imaging radiologists and surgeons will impact patients, surgeons, and radiologists and propel treatment and outcomes forward in the future.

SUMMARY

- Surgery remains the pillar of treatment for "cure" of solid tumors, but does not stand alone in this endeavor, which requires a skilled multidisciplinary team that communicates effectively to optimize patient care.
- Patient selection is critical to ensure optimal surgical outcomes, which depend in turn on high-quality preoperative imaging and accurate reading and reporting of findings.
- Diagnosis, staging, and careful reporting of relevant anatomic findings are the critical elements surgeons seek in preoperative imaging studies and reports.
- "Exploratory" surgery should be a thing of the past—surgery should be conducted with specific objectives, for definitive resection of primary or metastatic tumors, debulking for certain tumor types, palliation when nonsurgical alternatives do not exist, rarely in emergency situations, and for reconstruction at the time of resection or at a separate stage to restore function or cosmesis after cancer surgery.

REFERENCES

1. Fuhrman GM, Charnsangavej C, Abbruzzese JL, et al. Thin-section contrast-enhanced computed tomography accurately predicts the resectability of malignant pancreatic neoplasms. *Am J Surg*. 1994;167(1):104-111. discussion 111-113.
2. Aloia TA, Charnsangavej C, Faria S, et al. High-resolution computed tomography accurately predicts resectability in hilar cholangiocarcinoma. *Am J Surg*. 2007;193(6):702-706.
3. Cho CS, Curran S, Schwartz LH, et al. Preoperative radiographic assessment of hepatic steatosis with histologic correlation. *J Am Coll Surg*. 2008;206:480-488.
4. Chun YS, Vauthey JN, Ribero D, et al. Systemic chemotherapy and two-stage hepatectomy for extensive bilateral colorectal liver metastases: perioperative safety and survival. *J Gastrointest Surg*. 2007;11(11):1498-1504.
5. Frilling A, Sotiropoulos GC, Li J, Kornasiewicz O, Plockinger U. Multimodal management of neuroendocrine liver metastases. *HPB (Oxford)*. 2010;12(6):361-379.
6. Glazer ES, Tseng JF, Al-Refaie W, et al. Long-term survival after surgical management of neuroendocrine hepatic metastases. *HPB (Oxford)*. 2010;12(6):427-433.
7. Abdalla EK, Vauthey JN. Technique and patient selection, not the needle, determine outcome of percutaneous intervention for hepatocellular carcinoma. *Ann Surg Oncol*. 2004;11(3):240-241.
8. Azoulay D, Johann M, Raccuia JS, Castaing D, Bismuth H. "Protected" double needle biopsy technique for hepatic tumors. *J Am Coll Surg*. 1996;183(2):160-163.
9. Katz MH, Pisters PW, Evans DB, et al. Borderline resectable pancreatic cancer: the importance of this emerging stage of disease. *J Am Coll Surg*. 2008;206(5):833-846. discussion 846-848.
10. Abdalla EK, Adam R, Bilchik AJ, Jaeck D, Vauthey JN, Mahvi D. Improving resectability of hepatic colorectal metastases: expert consensus statement. *Ann Surg Oncol*. 2006;13(10):1271-1280.
11. Vauthey JN, Dixon E, Abdalla EK, et al. Pretreatment assessment of hepatocellular carcinoma: expert consensus statement. *HPB (Oxford)*. 2010;12(5):289-299.
12. Kishi Y, Abdalla EK, Chun YS, et al. Three hundred and one consecutive extended right hepatectomies: evaluation of outcome based on systematic liver volumetry. *Ann Surg*. 2009;250(4):540-548.
13. Hemming AW, Reed AI, Langham MR, Fujita S, van der Werf WJ, Howard RJ. Hepatic vein reconstruction for resection of hepatic tumors. *Ann Surg*. 2002;235(6):850-858.
14. Zorzi D, Abdalla EK, Pawlik TM, Brown TD, Vauthey JN. Subtotal hepatectomy following neoadjuvant chemotherapy for a previously unresectable hepatocellular carcinoma. *J Hepatobiliary Pancreat Surg*. 2006;13(4):347-350.
15. Michels NA. Newer anatomy of the liver and its variant blood supply and collateral circulation. *Am J Surg*. 1966;112(3):337-347.
16. Abdalla EK, Denys A, Chevalier P, Nemr RA, Vauthey JN. Total and segmental liver volume variations: implications for liver surgery. *Surgery*. 2004;135(4):404-410.
17. Rassam F, Olthof P, Bennick RJ, van Gulik TM. Current modalities for assessment of future remnant liver function. *Visc Med*. 2017;33:442-448.
18. Therasse P, Arbuck SG, Eisenhauer EA, et al. New guidelines to evaluate the response to treatment in solid tumors. European Organization for Research and Treatment of Cancer, National Cancer Institute of the United States, National Cancer Institute of Canada. *J Natl Cancer Inst*. 2000;92(3):205-216.
19. Choi H, Charnsangavej C, de Castro Faria S, et al. CT evaluation of the response of gastrointestinal stromal tumors after imatinib mesylate treatment: a quantitative analysis correlated with FDG PET findings. *AJR Am J Roentgenol*. 2004;183(6):1619-1628.
20. Chun YS, Vauthey JN, Boonsirikamchai P, et al. Association of computed tomography morphologic criteria with pathologic response and survival in patients treated with bevacizumab for colorectal liver metastases. *JAMA*. 2009;302(21):2338-2344.
21. Granata V, Fusco R, de Lutio di Castelguidone E, et al. Diagnostic performance of gadoxetic acid-enhanced liver MRI versus multidetector CT in the assessment of colorectal liver metastases compared to hepatic resection. *BMC Gastroenterol*. 2019;19(1):129.
22. Blazer 3rd DG, Kishi Y, Maru DM, et al. Pathologic response to preoperative chemotherapy: a new outcome end point after resection of hepatic colorectal metastases. *J Clin Oncol*. 2008;26(33):5344-5351.
23. Abdalla EK, Vauthey JN, Ellis LM, et al. Recurrence and outcomes following hepatic resection, radiofrequency ablation, and combined resection/ablation for colorectal liver metastases. *Ann Surg*. 2004;239(6):818-825.
24. Adam R, Chiche L, Aloia T, et al. Hepatic resection for noncolorectal nonendocrine liver metastases: analysis of 1,452 patients and development of a prognostic model. *Ann Surg*. 2006;244(4):524-535.
25. Tomlinson JS, Jarnagin WR, DeMatteo RP, et al. Actual 10-year survival after resection of colorectal liver metastases defines cure. *J Clin Oncol*. 2007;25(29):4575-4580.
26. Abdalla EK, Hicks ME, Vauthey JN. Portal vein embolization: rationale, technique and future prospects. *Br J Surg*. 2001;88(2):165-175.
27. Madoff DC, Abdalla EK, Vauthey JN. Portal vein embolization in preparation for major hepatic resection: evolution of a new standard of care. *J Vasc Interv Radiol*. 2005;16(6):779-790.
28. Rosok BI, Bjornsson B, Sparrelid E, Hasselgren K, et al. Scandinavian multicenter study on the safety and feasibility of the associating liver partition and portal vein ligation for staged hepatectomy procedure. *Surgery*. 2016;159:1279-1286.
29. Gulec SA, Pennington K, Hall M, Fong Y. Preoperative Y-90 microsphere selective internal radiation treatment for tumor downsizing and future liver remnant recruitment: a novel approach to improving the safety of major hepatic resections. *World J Surg Oncol*. 2009;7:6.
30. Titano J, Voutsinas N, Kim E. The role of radioembolization in bridging and downstaging hepatocellular carcinoma to curative therapy. *Semin Nucl Med*. 2019;49(3):189-196.
31. Peng ZW, Zhang YJ, Chen MS, et al. Radiofrequency ablation with or without transcatheter arterial chemoembolization in the treatment of hepatocellular carcinoma: A prospective randomized trial. *J Clin Oncol*. 2013;31:426-432.
32. Glockzin G, Schlitt HJ, Piso P. Peritoneal carcinomatosis: patients selection, perioperative complications and quality of life related to cytoreductive surgery and hyperthermic intraperitoneal chemotherapy. *World J Surg Oncol*. 2009;7:5.
33. Sarmiento JM, Heywood G, Rubin J, Ilstrup DM, Nagorney DM, Que FG. Surgical treatment of neuroendocrine metastases to the liver: a plea for resection to increase survival. *J Am Coll Surg*. 2003;197(1):29-37.
34. Liu CL, Fan ST, Lo CM, et al. Management of spontaneous rupture of hepatocellular carcinoma: single-center experience. *J Clin Oncol*. 2001;19(17):3725-3732.

CHAPTER 3 A Multidisciplinary Approach to Cancer: A Medical Oncologist's View

Jason R. Westin, M.D.

INTRODUCTION

As our understanding of cancer has grown, medical oncology has evolved as a subspecialty of internal medicine since the 1960s. Initially, few treatments beyond surgery and a handful of toxic chemotherapy agents were available to cancer patients. Medical oncologists now have hundreds of chemotherapeutic agents and hundreds of targeted agents ranging from small molecules to monoclonal antibodies to genetically engineered cellular therapy to choose from for hundreds of separate diseases, with countless new agents in development.

The primary tool of the medical oncologist is chemotherapy; however, cancer treatment is best accomplished when a multidisciplinary approach is used. The medical oncologist must work closely with the surgical oncologist, radiation oncologist, radiologist, pathologist, and primary care physician.

The medical oncologist is typically involved in the final decisions concerning management, and frequently coordinates implementation of these decisions. The decision whether to take a curatively aggressive or a palliative measured approach, or to transition from one approach to another, decisions about the timing of localized therapies, such as surgery and radiotherapy, and the decision regarding therapy is required or whether supportive care is most appropriate are often made by the medical oncologist. The oncologist must also strike the balance between expected treatment sequelae and potential to cure. If there is a reasonable expectation for cure, treatment-related toxicity becomes more acceptable. If there is a reasonable expectation for prolonging survival or improving quality of life, some toxicity is acceptable. If the chance of significantly altering the course of the disease is low, most oncologists and their patients will feel that only minimal toxicity is acceptable, but these decisions are based on individualized conversations weighing the unique situation of each patient and his or her family.

EPIDEMIOLOGY

As medicine, nutrition, and improved sanitation continue to further extend the average life expectancy, more people are surviving long enough to develop a malignancy. Thankfully, this is being tempered with an overall decrease in the incidence of and mortality from the most common cancers.[1]

Cancer screening has become a routine part of the health maintenance performed on healthy individuals. Mammograms, fecal occult blood tests, colonoscopy, Papanicolaou smear, and digital rectal examinations have the potential to detect a malignancy at an early, asymptomatic stage and perhaps change the disease outcome. With increased screening, more early-stage, potentially curable cancers are being detected. Many of these cancers are amenable to local therapy (surgery and/or radiation), but a large portion continue to require systemic therapy.

THE RATIONALE FOR CHEMOTHERAPY

In most cancers, only 20% to 40% of cells are active at any one time, which explains why the doubling time for a tumor is significantly longer than the duration of a single cell cycle. Tumor growth would be exponential if all cells were dividing, or constant if the fraction of actively cycling cells remained fixed; however, this does not correspond to clinically observed tumor doubling times. In 1825, Benjamin Gompertz described the nonexponential growth pattern of disease that he observed in cancer patients. He noted that the doubling time increased steadily as the tumor grew larger, a phenomenon now described as Gompertzian growth. This has been postulated to occur owing to decreased cell production, possibly related to relative lack of oxygen and of growth factors in the central portion of the large mass.[2] A smaller tumor, conversely, would have a larger portion of actively cycling cells and, thus, be potentially more sensitive to cytotoxic chemotherapy.

A clinically or radiographically detectible tumor that measures at least 1 cm in diameter already contains 10^8 to 10^9 cells and weighs approximately 1 g. If derived from a single progenitor cell, it would have undergone at least 30 doublings before detection. Further growth to a potentially lethal mass would only take 10 further doublings. Thus, the clinically apparent portion of the growth of the tumor represents only a fraction of the total life history of the tumor. Given the long period of time during which growth of the tumor can go undetected, occult micrometastases have often developed by the time of diagnosis.

Cytotoxic chemotherapy has the ability to kill more cancer cells than normal tissue, likely because of impaired DNA damage repair mechanisms in the former. This is relevant because most cytotoxic agents damage actively cycling cells. Typically, the more aggressive the cancer, the higher the proportion of its tumor cells that are in active phases of the cell cycle.

As a result of the enhanced efficacy of chemotherapy against rapidly dividing malignant cells, rapidly proliferating cancers that, in the past, were associated with shorter survival may have a better chance for cure from systemic chemotherapy than more indolent disease, as long as the tumor cells are sensitive to the chemotherapeutic agents. An example of this paradox is Burkitt lymphoma, which is sensitive to chemotherapeutic agents and is curable in the majority of patients, despite having an extremely rapid proliferation rate. Conversely, a slow-growing follicular lymphoma, even when sensitive to chemotherapy as defined by the complete disappearance of the tumor, will relapse and ultimately cause death.

Early studies of the ability of chemotherapy to kill cancer cells were conducted in leukemia cell lines in the 1960s.[3] These studies noted log-kill kinetics, meaning if 99% of cells were killed, tumor cell number would decrease from 10^{10} to 10^8 or from 10^5 to 10^3, for example. The fraction of cells killed was proportional, regardless of tumor size; thus, even though a given treatment would appear to have eradicated the tumor, both clinically and radiographically, there would be a high probability of residual cells that would eventually proliferate and show up as a clinically evident tumor (relapse). One explanation for the achievement of sustainable complete remission following this argument would be that other factors such as host immune response may be important at low levels of residual tumoral cells.[4]

Clinical prognostic models are, in part, based on risk of disease relapse and thus take into account features that might suggest micrometastatic undetectable disease at the time of diagnosis. As an example, a large tumor may suggest a longer clinically silent tumor lifetime or a higher doubling rate. Clinically apparent nodal involvement demonstrates that the tumor has gained the capability to spread, at least regionally.

INDICATIONS FOR CHEMOTHERAPY

If the decision is made that the patient will benefit from chemotherapy, the treatment strategy devised by the medical oncologist will be largely determined by the stage of the cancer. The initial medical treatment of cancer can be thought of as requiring (1) preoperative (neoadjuvant) chemotherapy, (2) postoperative (adjuvant) chemotherapy, or (3) chemotherapy without localized therapy, either for metastatic, inoperable disease (attributed to locally advanced stage and/or comorbid medical conditions) or a hematologic malignancy. Chemotherapy without surgical therapy was historically thought of as a palliative measure; however, improved efficacy of chemotherapy and radiotherapy is changing this notion. Many hematologic and epithelial malignancies are now approached in curative fashion with chemotherapy alone or combined with radiotherapy.

Adjuvant Chemotherapy

When the first chemotherapies were developed, they were used only in patients with advanced disease who were failing other therapies. This was largely because of poor efficacy of therapy, and chemotherapy in this setting was usually associated with significant treatment-related morbidity. The therapeutic index (benefit opposed to morbidity) and associated supportive care measures of chemotherapy today tip this balance in favor of treating patients earlier, even with no objective evidence of postsurgical disease.

Miraculous progress has been made in surgical and radiotherapeutic treatments for localized disease; however, many cancers have metastatic spread at diagnosis. Surgically or radiotherapeutically treated tumors may fail locally, but they often recur at distant sites. When considering the previously discussed undetectable period of tumor growth, it becomes apparent how a completely resected tumor may have significant occult residual disease, either locally or at distant sites. In this situation, chemotherapy is given as an adjuvant to augment the effect of surgery; hence the name adjuvant chemotherapy. Many patients who receive adjuvant therapy are without evidence of disease after local therapy. The pathologic margins of surgical specimens may be negative, and imaging may reveal no abnormality; however, significant relapse potential from residual local disease or micrometastases may exist. Adjuvant therapy aims to eradicate this subclinical disease before it reaches a critical threshold at which cure becomes difficult. Breast, lung, and colon cancer are a few examples of the many cancers that benefit from adjuvant therapy.[5–7]

Neoadjuvant Chemotherapy

Treating with chemotherapy before surgery is a newer concept. With more effective chemotherapy, neoadjuvant treatment approaches are occasionally used in appropriate-stage breast, lung, and resectable metastatic colorectal cancers.[8–10]

Neoadjuvant chemotherapy has three main advantages. Micrometastases are exposed to chemotherapy earlier in the treatment course, which may more effectively lead to their eradication before becoming clinically apparent (based on log-kill theory). Second, a primary lesion that fails to respond indicates micrometastatic disease that is also likely resistant, allowing a change in therapy.[11] Without neoadjuvant therapy, this knowledge would become apparent only after micrometastatic disease becomes clinically apparent and, thus, the potential for cure at that time would be very unlikely. Third, a primary tumor may regress sufficiently to facilitate a less morbid surgical procedure or occasionally obviate the need for surgical resection.[12,13]

Chemotherapy for Metastatic Cancer

The large portion of chemotherapy is given for clinically evident metastatic cancer, often as part of a palliation strategy to prolong survival and improve quality of life. However, some malignancies, including lymphoma and testicular cancers, may be cured even when they present with advanced metastatic disease. Other cancers, including ovarian and breast cancer, may demonstrate great sensitivity to chemotherapy in the metastatic setting, with long-term disease control or disappearance of all detectable disease. An additional number of cancers, such as lung or pancreatic, may have brief stabilization or minor response to chemotherapy, but long-term control is uncommon.

CHEMOTHERAPY SCHEDULES

Dose Intensity

In tumors that follow the Gompertzian growth model, the fraction of cycling cells will increase as a tumor mass shrinks from chemotherapy. Each exposure to chemotherapy creates selection pressure; thus, the remaining cells are more likely to develop resistance. As a result, adequate dose intensity is required for tumor eradication. If chemotherapy doses are too small or too infrequent, the proportion of cell kill will gradually decrease as resistant clones emerge. If doses are too large or frequent, treatment-related morbidity will limit how much therapy a patient will tolerate, possibly leading to treatment delays and resistant clone development. Dose density strives to increase doses of chemotherapy and frequency so as to find the limits of toxicity with as much antitumor activity as possible. Still, many effective chemotherapeutic agents with myelotoxicity could be made more effective by further increasing their doses, at the risk of ablating the marrow. The use of high-dose chemotherapy with autologous stem cell rescue has been successfully attempted in selected malignancies such as lymphomas and multiple myeloma to benefit from this fact. In solid tumors, however, success has been minimal, suggesting there is a threshold at which tumor response becomes nonlinear.

Combination Chemotherapy

Tumors are more genetically unstable than benign cells, leading to a high rate of random mutation and possible chemotherapy resistance. Mutations occur at a high rate; thus, at the time of a tumor becoming clinically apparent, several drug-resistant clones may already exist. This would explain why a tumor with a dominant clone sensitive to chemotherapy may initially respond but subsequently relapse after therapy. Other tumors are largely chemotherapy-resistant at presentation—for example, melanoma and pancreatic cancer—even with low-volume disease. A possible explanation for *de novo* resistance is that a slower-growing tumor will take longer to become clinically apparent and thus may have undergone a longer undetectable growth phase. This longer period of time could allow more mutation opportunities, and thus, once diagnosed, the dominant portion of the tumor may already be resistant to standard therapies. It is also possible that a slower-growing tumor could be better able to repair DNA damage or less prone to developing damage in the first place. In other malignancies such as gastrointestinal neoplasms, tumors might shed cells into the lumen and thus require additional doubling times and genetic mutations before it achieves a given size.

The rationale for combination chemotherapy was adapted from observations of tuberculosis therapy in the 1950s. If a single agent was used, resistance would eventually develop. If multiple agents with different mechanisms of action were used concurrently, resistance was less common. Frei and coworkers[14] published a study of combinatorial chemotherapy for leukemia in 1958, one of the first randomized clinical trials. They demonstrated transient responses in adult and pediatric leukemia patients achieved by combining methotrexate and 6-mercaptopurine, thus ushering in the modern era of combinatorial chemotherapy. Today, most patients treated with curative intent are given combination chemotherapy.

Intermittent Chemotherapy

Because tumors have impaired DNA repair mechanisms and are thus more sensitive than normal tissue, they take longer to recover from the insult of chemotherapy. As a result, cytotoxic chemotherapy given at the appropriate interval will allow normal tissue, including hematopoietic stem cells, to recover, whereas tumor tissue will not have sufficient time to recuperate (Fig. 3.1). Most cytotoxic therapies are dosed every 2 or 3 weeks based on this observation.

Continuous Therapy

Cytostatic agents, such as many of the newer targeted agents, require continuous exposure to maintain disease control. Drugs that have a potent, although short-lived, effect on a tumor will not work well with intermittent dosing, because when the drug is removed the tumor will move from a static to an active phase. Imatinib, an oral agent taken daily, inhibits the BCR-ABL tyrosine kinase, resulting in blood count normalization and excellent long-term control in the vast majority of patients with chronic-phase chronic myelogenous leukemia (CML). If the medicine is withdrawn, the majority of patients will again develop the hematologic abnormalities of chronic-phase CML. These agents hold the promise of turning cancer that is currently incurable into a chronic disease, such as diabetes or hypertension.

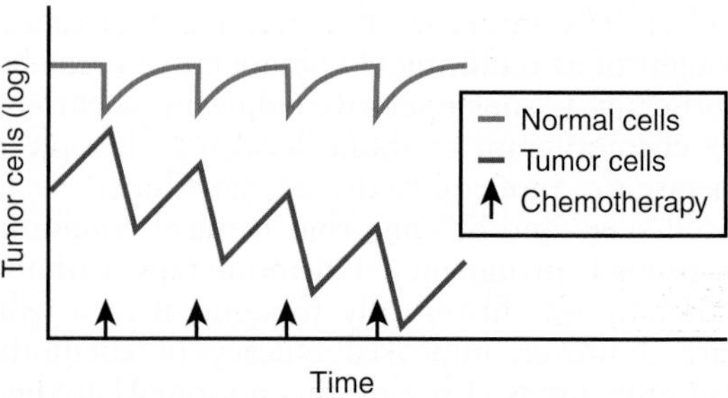

FIGURE 3.1. The effect of intermittent chemotherapy on tumor and normal cell populations.

Targeted Therapy

The field of medical oncology is rapidly changing owing to a convergence of factors. With an improved understanding of disease biology, many new drugs have been created that specifically target a tumor-specific aberrancy. There has also been a revival of the idea that the immune system can impact and even eradicate cancers. These targeted therapies can target specific tyrosine kinases involved in cell survival–relevant signaling or target benign immune cells to activate an antitumor response. The dosing schedule and side effect profile of targeted therapies are variable and based on the specific target, but usually targeted therapy is less toxic and can be administered for a longer period of time than cytotoxic chemotherapy because of its increased specificity. The evolution of targeted therapy has revolutionized outcomes for patients with many cancers that historically were difficult to treat, including metastatic melanoma and lung cancer, leading to significantly longer survival. The future prospects for targeted therapy are incredible, with more and more advances that would have sounded like science fiction to the earliest generations of medical oncologists becoming reality. As an example, there are now several U.S. Food and Drug Administration (FDA)–approved products based on genetically modified autologous immune cells—the patient's own immune cells are weaponized to eradicated chemotherapy-refractory cancers like lymphomas or leukemias.

Route of Administration

The majority of chemotherapy is administered intravenously, in an attempt to eliminate erratic gastrointestinal absorption as well as compliance issues. Chemotherapeutic agents can be given as a bolus (over a very short interval), short infusion (over a period of hours), or continuous infusion (usually administered as an inpatient or with a preprogrammed pump for home administration). The advantages of intravenous administration include more standardized absorption, documented compliance, and use of concurrent intravenous hydration or supportive medications.

Many of the newer chemotherapeutic agents target a specific cellular metabolic pathway, and some of these have eliminated the problems of erratic absorption that occur when they are administered orally, which has advantages for the patient, including not requiring an intravenous catheter. Other routes of administration include intrathecal (e.g., methotrexate to treat central nervous system leukemia relapse), subcutaneous (e.g., rituximab to treat B-cell non-Hodgkin lymphoma), intraarterial (e.g., cisplatin to treat sarcoma), intravesical (e.g., bacillus Calmette–Guérin to treat bladder dysplasia), intraocular (e.g., bevacizumab to treat macular degeneration), and intraperitoneal (e.g., to treat ovarian cancer).

DRUG DEVELOPMENT

Historically, many drugs were developed in the same serendipitous fashion as Alexander Fleming's penicillin discovery. Currently, the vast majority of new agents are engineered to attack a specific tumor-related target, which requires understanding of disease mechanisms. New agents are created as novel chemical entities based on knowledge of the molecular basis of their action or by modifying an existing agent. Drug companies perform *in vitro* screening of multiple similar compounds to evaluate for potential efficacy. Once a lead molecule is identified, nonhuman animal studies are conducted to evaluate for potential toxicity. Once an agent has fulfilled these requirements, clinical trials in humans may begin.

CLINICAL DEVELOPMENT

Phase I studies are the first in-human studies of a new agent and have the goal of determining the maximum tolerated dose by using dose escalation and evaluating dose-limiting toxicities. Response rates are typically low, because adequate dosing is unknown and patients typically have refractory disease, but a significant portion of patients do receive benefit.[15] Pharmacokinetic and pharmacodynamic studies are performed during early clinical development to better understand the *in vivo* properties of the drug. Phase II studies use doses and schedules from the phase I data to assess efficacy with response as the primary endpoint. Patients are typically less heavily pretreated and must have measurable disease for response monitoring. Phase II trials typically enroll 20 to 50 patients, are designed for early termination if a significant number of responses are not seen, and may evaluate a new agent alone or in combination with standard chemotherapy.

Phase III trials are larger, typically randomized, and evaluate the experiment treatment against a standard of care regimen. Endpoints are usually progression-free survival (PFS) and/or overall survival (OS). Evaluation of OS may be confounded by patients receiving subsequent effective therapies, and hence PFS is usually thought to be the more reliable endpoint. Quality-of-life and comparative toxicity data are usually collected. These trials usually require hundreds of patients or more to participate to achieve their statistical goals, and may lead to FDA approval of the new agent.

SUMMARY

Historically, chemotherapy was used only after other methods had failed to control cancer. Chemotherapy and targeted therapies are now used as a primary weapon against many cancers, but can also improve surgical outcomes, eradicate micrometastases, control metastatic disease, and occasionally obviate the need for local therapy. Rapidly increasing understanding of tumorigenesis and discovery of new molecular targets has increased our comprehension of how to better treat patients with cancer. These rationally designed targeted agents hold promise to either eradicate cancers or convert cancer into another chronic disease, such as diabetes or hypertension.

REFERENCES

1. Edwards BK, Ward E, Kohler BA, et al. Annual report to the nation on the status of cancer, 1975-2006, featuring colorectal cancer trends and impact of interventions (risk factors, screening, and treatment) to reduce future rates. *Cancer*. 2010;116:544-573.
2. Watson JV. The cell proliferation kinetics of the EMT6/M/AC mouse tumour at four volumes during unperturbed growth in vivo. *Cell Tissue Kinet*. 1976;9:147-156.
3. Skipper HE, Schabel Jr. FM, Wilcox WS. Experimental evaluation of potential anticancer agents. XIII. On the criteria and kinetics associated with "curability" of experimental leukemia. *Cancer Chemother Rep*. 1964;35:1-111.
4. Rockall T, Lowndes S, Johnson P, et al. Multidisciplinary treatment of cancer: surgery, chemotherapy and radiotherapy. In: Husband JE, Reznek RH, eds. *Imaging in Oncology*. London: Taylor & Francis; 2004:43-63.
5. Early Breast Cancer Trialists' Collaborative Group (EBCTCG). Effects of chemotherapy and hormonal therapy for early breast cancer on recurrence and 15-year survival: an overview of the randomised trials. *Lancet*. 2005;365:1687-1717.
6. Pignon J-P, Tribodet H, Scagliotti GV, et al. Lung adjuvant cisplatin evaluation: a pooled analysis by the LACE Collaborative Group. *J Clin Oncol*. 2008;26:3552-3559.
7. Sun W, Haller DG. Adjuvant therapy of colon cancer. *Semin Oncol*. 2005;32:95-102.
8. Carlson RW, Allred DC, Anderson BO, et al. Breast cancer. Clinical practice guidelines in oncology. *J Natl Compr Canc Netw*. 2009;7:122-192.
9. Gray J, Sommers E, Alvelo-Rivera M, et al. Neoadjuvant chemotherapy for resectable non-small-cell lung cancer. *Oncology (Huntingt)*. 2009;23:879-886.
10. Chau I, Chan S, Cunningham D. Overview of preoperative and postoperative therapy for colorectal cancer: the European and United States perspectives. *Clin Colorectal Cancer*. 2003;3:19-33.
11. Rosen G, Caparros B, Huvos AG, et al. Preoperative chemotherapy for osteogenic sarcoma: selection of postoperative adjuvant chemotherapy based on the response of the primary tumor to preoperative chemotherapy. *Cancer*. 1982;49:1221-1230.
12. Jacquillat C, Weil M, Baillet F, et al. Results of neoadjuvant chemotherapy and radiation therapy in the breast-conserving treatment of 250 patients with all stages of infiltrative breast cancer. *Cancer*. 1990;66:119-129.
13. The Department of Veterans Affairs Laryngeal Cancer Study Group Induction chemotherapy plus radiation compared with surgery plus radiation in patients with advanced laryngeal cancer. *N Engl J Med*. 1991;324:1685-1690.
14. Frei III E, Holland JF, Schneiderman MA, et al. A comparative study of two regimens of combination chemotherapy in acute leukemia. *Blood*. 1958;13:1126-1148.
15. Wheler J, Tsimberidou AM, Hong D, et al. Survival of patients in a phase 1 clinic. *Cancer*. 2009;115:1091-1099.

CHAPTER 4

A Multidisciplinary Approach to Cancer: A Radiation Oncologist's View

Patricia J. Eifel, M.D.

Radiation therapy forms an integral part of the care of 50% to 60% of cancer patients in the United States. It plays a key role in the multidisciplinary curative treatment of many patients with head and neck, thoracic, genitourinary, gynecologic, and gastrointestinal cancers, lymphoma, sarcoma, brain tumors, and other malignancies. Radiation therapy also provides highly effective palliation of cancer symptoms, including pain, bleeding, and other symptoms of progressive or metastatic cancer.

Although early cancers of the prostate, head and neck, cervix, and other sites are commonly cured with radiation alone, more advanced cancers are usually treated with radiation in combination with surgery, chemotherapy, or other systemic treatments.

In many clinical situations, postoperative radiation therapy after surgical resection improves local control. Frequently the use of radiation before or after surgical resection also permits use of less-radical, organ-preserving operations, without any associated reduction in—and sometimes even with improvement in—local tumor control and survival rates.

For many disease sites, the combination of radiation and chemotherapy has also been demonstrated to improve local disease control, enhance the effectiveness of organ-sparing approaches, and improve the curative potential of local treatments, presumably by sterilizing micrometastatic disease that would otherwise lead to the appearance of distant metastases. Randomized trials have proven that addition of concurrent chemotherapy to radiation improves local control and survival in patients with cervical, head and neck, lung, gastrointestinal, and other types of cancer.[1–4]

The goal of the radiation oncologist and his or her multidisciplinary team is to sterilize tumor while also minimizing treatment-related side effects and optimizing the patient's quality of life. The best results depend on a well-integrated team that includes radiation oncologists, medical oncologists, and surgeons, as well as experienced pathologists, diagnostic imagers, nutritionists, radiation physicists, nursing specialists, therapists, and others. Frequent face-to-face communication in tumor boards, multidisciplinary clinics, and sidebars over individual cases is vital to the development of a common language and an understanding of the needs and concerns of each member of the multidisciplinary team.

The relationship and the quality of communication between radiation oncologist and diagnostic imager are particularly crucial. The desire to reduce treatment-related side effects while maintaining or improving local disease control rates has led to increasingly precise, tightly conforming radiation dose delivery methods such as intensity-modulated radiation therapy and proton therapy. The theoretical advantages of these approaches can be realized only through precise understanding of the distribution of disease and regional anatomy as revealed in the patient's imaging evaluation.

RADIATION BIOLOGY

Most radiation-induced cell death is caused by damage to nuclear DNA and is referred to as mitotic cell death. The interaction of photons or charged particles with water produces highly reactive free radicals that interact with DNA, causing breaks that can interfere with cell division. Although cells are equipped with very effective mechanisms for repair of the damage caused by free radicals, accumulated injury can lead to irrecoverable DNA breaks that prevent successful mitosis. Oxygen in the environment enhances the lethal effects of radiation by fixing free radical damage. Damaged cells that have lost their ability to reproduce indefinitely may continue to be metabolically active or even undergo several divisions before losing their integrity. For this reason, radiation-induced damage to tumors may not be expressed morphologically for days or even weeks after the radiation exposure.

Another type of radiation-induced cell death is referred to as apoptosis or programmed cell death. Apoptosis can occur before or after mitosis and appears to play an important role in the radiation response of some tumors and in certain normal tissues such as salivary glands and lymphocytes.[5]

In vitro studies of the relationship between radiation dose and cell survival demonstrate that mammalian cells differ widely in their inherent radiosensitivity. These differences contribute to the wide range of doses required to cure tumors of different cell types. Even bulky lymphomas can typically be controlled with doses of 25 to 35 Gy, whereas 2- to 3-cm carcinomas usually require doses of more than 60 Gy. Melanomas and most sarcomas require even higher doses and usually cannot be controlled with tolerable radiation doses if there is more than microscopic residual disease after surgery.

A number of factors influence cellular radiosensitivity and tumor responsiveness. These include the cells' capacity to repair radiation injury, the effects of cellular repopulation, and the influence of sensitizing agents, including oxygen.

Normal tissues typically have a greater capacity to accumulate and repair radiation damage than cancers; this difference is responsible for the "therapeutic window" that makes it possible to cure cancers without causing unacceptable damage to irradiated normal tissues. However, some normal cells—particularly those that are rapidly proliferating—have relatively little repair capacity, and some tumors, such as prostate cancer, are able to accumulate and repair damage as effectively as most normal tissues. These variations influence the approaches used to treat various tumor types and sites.

Experimental and clinical evidence suggests that most repair is accomplished within 4 to 6 hours. For this reason, schedules that involve more than one daily fraction of radiation are usually designed with a minimum interfraction interval of approximately 6 hours.

The effect of cellular proliferation during a course of radiation therapy depends on the doubling time of the neoplastic cells and the duration of treatment. Although the tolerable weekly dose of radiation is limited by normal tissue effects, many studies demonstrate that unnecessary protraction compromises tumor control rates.[6–8] Also, evidence suggests that radiation therapy, as well as other cytotoxic treatments and even surgery, can accelerate the rate of repopulation. This enhances the detrimental effects of delayed postoperative radiation and may explain why neoadjuvant chemotherapy has often proven less effective than expected.[9]

Because oxygen is needed to fix the free radicals that mediate radiation-induced DNA damage, the dose of sparsely ionizing radiation required to effect a given level of cell killing is about three times greater under anoxic conditions than under fully oxygenated conditions. Although regions of hypoxia are present in many solid tumors, the clinical importance of hypoxia is diminished by reoxygenation that occurs as initially hypoxic cells become better oxygenated during a course of fractionated radiation therapy.[10]

NORMAL TISSUE EFFECTS OF RADIATION

The extent, nature, and likelihood of radiation-related normal tissue effects depend on the structure of the irradiated tissue, the dose and the volume of tissue irradiated, and other clinical factors.

Normal tissues can be categorized as "serial" or "parallel" according to the organization of their functional subunits. Serial structures, such as the spinal cord, small bowel, and ureter, may fail when even a small portion of the organ is irradiated to a high dose. In contrast, parallel structures, such as liver, kidney, and lung, can sustain very high doses to partial volumes but are less tolerant of moderate whole-organ doses.

Tissues and cells that have a rapid turnover rate (e.g., bone marrow stem cells, skin, oral mucosa, hair follicles, and gastrointestinal epithelium) tend to exhibit side effects during or soon after a course of fractionated radiation therapy; these are referred to as acutely responding tissues. The renewal rate of acutely responding tissues typically limits the rate at which radiation therapy can be safely delivered to 900 to 1000 cGy/week. However, most acute side effects resolve within weeks of the completion of a course of radiation therapy.

Tissues that are more slowly proliferating are referred to as late-responding tissues and tend to manifest side effects weeks or months after radiation therapy. These effects may reflect direct damage to parenchymal cells or damage to vascular stroma, and the dose–response relationship varies according to the tissue irradiated and other factors. Table 4.1 presents some of the conclusions of a 1991 task force[11] charged with summarizing relevant data concerning the effect of ionizing radiation on normal tissues. A more detailed update was subsequently published in 2010.[12] Although these summaries provide some guidance as to the risks of radiation-related side effects, analyses of treatments using modern conformal image-based planning methods will continue to refine our understanding of the relationships between the dose and volume of radiated tissues and the risk of adverse effects.

Patient characteristics can also strongly influence the risks of treatment-related side effects. Tissues that have been compromised by injury or illness may be more susceptible to radiation injury than healthy tissues. A history of smoking or other substance abuse, infection, poor nutrition, and other factors can increase the likelihood of serious treatment-related side effects.[13] Surgery, chemotherapy, and other treatments may also enhance the acute and late effects of radiation. An understanding of the complex relationships between these factors and normal tissue effects is critical in radiation therapy treatment planning.

The duration of a course of radiation therapy has little impact on the incidence of late complications, but the dose per fraction has a major impact. In general, radiation schedules that involve fractional doses of 2 Gy or less permit maximal recovery of sublethal damage to normal tissues. For this reason, and because acute side effects usually limit the weekly dose of radiation to no more than approximately 10 Gy, radiation therapy is most commonly delivered with a schedule of 1.8 to 2 Gy per fraction, five times per week. Because most tumors repair cellular damage less effectively than late-responding normal tissues, the differential effect on tumor versus normal tissues is increased when a dose of radiation is fractionated. This is referred to as the fractionation effect.

Under certain circumstances, alternate fractionation schedules may be used to reduce the overall duration of treatment. Hypofractionation, the use of daily fractional doses of more than 2 Gy per fraction, is routinely used for palliative radiation therapy to optimize convenience, cost, and the rapidity of symptom relief. Common schedules used for palliation include 30 Gy in 10 fractions, 20 Gy in five fractions, and in some cases 8 to 10 Gy in a single dose of radiation. The development of highly conforming radiation technique has also led investigators to explore the value of hypofractionated radiation therapy for curative radiation therapy in certain situations. This approach is most effective if adjacent critical structures receive a significantly lower dose and dose per fraction than the target. Stereotactic body radiation therapy is a form of ultrahypofractionated radiation therapy in which very large daily doses of radiation are delivered with great precision

TABLE 4.1 Approximate Dose/Volume/Outcome Data for Several Organs After Conventionally Fractionated Radiation Therapy

ORGAN	DOSE (Gy) OR DOSE/ VOLUME PARAMETERS	RATE (%)	ENDPOINT
Brain	$D_{max} < 60$	<3	Symptomatic necrosis Data at 72 and 90 Gy extrapolated from BED model
	$D_{max} = 72$	5	
	$D_{max} = 90$	10	
Brainstem	$D_{1\text{-}10\,cc} \leq 59$ Gy	<5	Permanent cranial neuropathy or necrosis
Optic nerve/chiasm	$D_{max} < 55$	<3	Optic neuropathy
	$D_{max} = 55–60$	3–7	
Spinal cord[a]	$D_{max} = 50$	0.2	Myelopathy
	$D_{max} = 60$	6	
	$D_{max} = 69$	50	
Parotid[b]	Mean dose < 25	<20	Long-term salivary function < 25% of preradiation level
Lung[b]	V20 ≤ 30%	<20	Symptomatic pneumonitis
	Mean dose = 7	5	
	Mean dose = 13	10	
	Mean dose = 24	30	
Esophagus	Mean dose < 34	5–20	Grade ≥ 3 acute esophagitis
Heart	V25 < 10%	<1[c]	Long-term cardiac mortality
Liver[d]	Mean dose < 30–32	<5	Classic RILD; does not apply to patients with preexisting liver disease or hepatocellular cancer
	Mean dose < 42	<50	
Kidney[b]	Mean dose < 15–18	<5	Clinically relevant renal dysfunction
	Mean dose < 28	<50	
Stomach	$D_{max} < 45$	<7	Ulceration
Small bowel	V45 < 195 cc[e]		Grade ≥ 3 acute toxicity
Rectum	V50 < 50%	<10	Grade ≥ 3 late toxicity; based on current RTOG recommendations for prostate cancer treatment
	V65 < 25%	<15	
	V75 < 15%	<15	
Bladder	$D_{max} < 65$	<6	Grade ≥ 3, RTOG scoring

BED, Biologic effective dose; *RILD*, radiation-induced liver disease; *RTOG*, radiation therapy oncology group.
[a]Partial length; including full cord cross-section.
[b]Bilateral whole organ(s).
[c]Believed to be an overly safe risk estimate based on model predictions.
[d]Excludes patients with preexisting liver disease or hepatocellular carcinoma because tolerance doses are lower in these patients.
[e]Based on segmentation of the entire potential bowel space within the peritoneal cavity.

under image guidance. In contrast, hyperfractionation is the delivery of small doses of radiation two or more times daily (usually with a minimum interfraction interval of 5–6 hours). This approach is most useful when repopulation is considered to be an important factor in tumor curability, but proximate late-reacting normal tissues prohibit the use of hypofractionation.

THERAPEUTIC GAIN

The goal of radiation therapy is to sterilize tumor with the fewest possible side effects. The difference between the rate of tumor control and the rate of normal tissue complications is referred to as the therapeutic gain or therapeutic ratio (Fig. 4.1). The probabilities of tumor control and late normal tissue effects can generally be described by two sigmoid dose–response relationships. Below a threshold dose, the probability of tumor control is very low; it then rises steeply to a dose above which little additional benefit can be achieved by further increases in dose. The shape and slope of the curve are related to the type and size of the tumor and other factors, including the use of concurrent systemic treatments. The likelihood of complication-free tumor control is determined by the separation between the tumor control and the late effects dose–response curves. The most successful treatment strategies are those that maximize the separation between these curves. Strategies that combine surgery or chemotherapy with radiation in a way that shifts the tumor control dose–response curve to the left without a commensurate shift in the complication curve probability increase the likelihood of a good result.

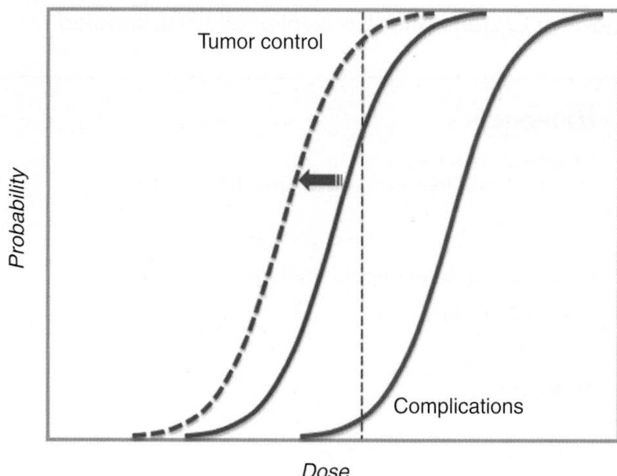

Figure 4.1. The difference between the rate of tumor control and the rate of normal tissue complications is referred to as the therapeutic gain or therapeutic ratio.

Conversely, multidisciplinary treatments that increase the risk of complications without significant improvement in the probability of tumor control should be avoided.

The position of the tumor control probability curve is also related to the volume of disease. For carcinomas, microscopic nodal disease can usually be controlled with a dose of 40 to 45 Gy. However, for most carcinomas, the likelihood of controlling a 1- to 2-cm tumor is negligible with doses less than 55 Gy, but may be as high as 90% to 95% after doses greater than 60 Gy. The steepness of this dose–response relationship highlights the importance of diagnostic accuracy. An entire course of treatment can be rendered ineffective if a single grossly involved node fails to receive the necessary added dose.

SURGERY AND RADIATION THERAPY

In some cases, the close proximity of critical structures prohibits delivery of a dose of radiation sufficient to eradicate gross disease. In other cases, surgical resection leaves microscopic disease that could lead to future recurrence. In cases such as these, judicious combinations of surgical resection and radiation therapy may significantly improve local control and survival and preserve organ function. Postoperative radiation therapy is often used to prevent local recurrence after gross total resection.[14–16] In some cases preoperative radiation therapy is used to "downstage" tumor, improve local control, or enable the surgeon to use organ-sparing operations. This approach has been particularly effective in the treatment of rectal cancers.[15] However, unnecessary multimodality treatment can increase complications, and poorly chosen surgical procedures can, in some cases, compromise the ability to deliver curative radiation therapy.

The information gained from surgery can also help guide planning of radiation therapy. Operative findings frequently provide critical information about local and regional disease extent that can guide the radiation oncologist in target volume definition. However, optimal combined-modality treatment requires careful communication between surgeon and radiation oncologist, preferably before any treatment has been initiated.

CHEMOTHERAPY AND RADIATION THERAPY

During the past several decades, randomized trials have demonstrated the benefit of combining radiation therapy and chemotherapy in the curative treatment of many cancers. A number of cytotoxic agents have been demonstrated to potentiate the effects of radiation when given concurrently with a course of radiation therapy. Drugs that have proved to be particularly effective radiation sensitizers include cisplatin, 5-fluorouracil, and mitomycin-C. Concurrent chemoradiation schedules are most effective if the dose-limiting toxic effects of the drugs differ from those of radiation and if the sensitizing effect on the tumor is greater than that on normal tissues.

Concurrent or sequential combinations of drugs and radiation may also improve the cure through spatial cooperation. For example, chemotherapy may be used to sterilize minimal microscopic disease in distant sites, whereas radiation is used to treat areas of gross or high-risk microscopic local and regional disease. The use of neoadjuvant chemotherapy before radiation therapy has been explored in a number of settings. Unfortunately, when neoadjuvant chemotherapy followed by radiation therapy has been tested in clinical trials, impressive chemotherapy responses have rarely translated into significant improvements in survival. Large metaanalyses of outcome in patients with head and neck or cervical cancers suggest much smaller benefits with this approach than with concurrent chemoradiation.[2,17,18] However, neoadjuvant chemotherapy has been used effectively in patients with breast cancer and continues to be explored in other settings.[19]

Adjuvant chemotherapy is also used after local treatment to control metastatic disease in a number of disease sites.

RADIATION TECHNIQUES

External Beam Radiation Therapy

Photons

Most modern external beam radiation treatments are delivered using linear accelerators that generate high-energy (6–20 MV) photon beams by bombarding a target (usually tungsten) with accelerated electrons. Photons in this energy range interact with tissues primarily through the mechanism referred to as Compton scatter; absorption is independent of atomic number but is related to the density of the absorbing material. The number of scattered electrons and ionizations increases as the photons penetrate the surface, resulting in a relative sparing of superficial tissues referred to as skin sparing.

The photon source is located in the head of a gantry that rotates around the treatment table (Fig. 4.2). Collimators in the treatment head govern the radiation field size and rotation; a secondary, electronically controlled, multileaved collimator can be used to shape the field to

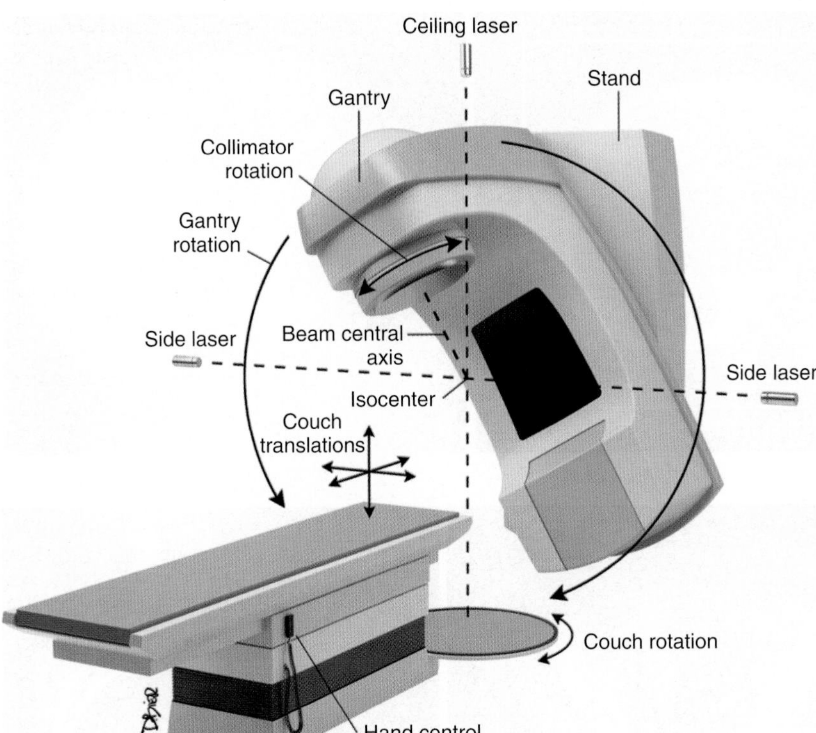

Figure 4.2. The photon source is located in the head of a gantry that rotates around the treatment table.

the irregular contours of a treatment target volume. The energy of the beam, the distance from the source to the patient, the depth of the target, and the density of intervening tissue also determine the doses delivered to the targets and normal tissues. The depth of penetration and the amount of skin sparing are correlated with the energy of the photons.

Electrons and Protons

Several types of particle beams have also been used in radiation therapy. Most modern linear accelerators are equipped to produce electron beams of several energies in addition to photon beams. The absorbed dose from an electron beam is relatively homogeneous to a certain depth and then falls rapidly to nearly zero; the depth of penetration is related to the energy of the electrons and typically ranges from approximately 2 to 6 cm for electron energies between 6 and 18 MV, respectively. Electrons are used primarily to treat targets on or just below the skin surface.

Protons are positively charged particles that deposit most of their energy at a tissue depth determined by the energy of the protons. The rapid deposition of energy is referred to as a Bragg peak. For most clinical applications, the proton energy is modulated to spread out the peak, creating a dose distribution characterized by a relatively low entrance dose, a homogeneous dose within the target, and very little exit dose. Although proton beams have been studied in a small number of facilities for several decades, there has been a dramatic increase in interest in proton therapy and in the number of facilities providing this therapy as the cost of proton accelerators has declined somewhat during the past 10 to 15 years. The tumors that have so far been of greatest interest are prostate, skull base, ocular, and pediatric tumors, although proton beam use is being explored in many other settings.[20] There are few randomized trials comparing proton therapy with more conventional treatments, although early results are encouraging.[21,22] The reduced volume of tissue receiving intermediate doses of radiation is undoubtedly beneficial for the treatment of a variety of pediatric cancers.[23] However, proton therapy continues to be a very expensive, complex technology that requires highly skilled physics and technical support. The best applications for proton beam therapy are still being determined.[20,24]

Several other types of particle beams, including neutrons, carbon ions, and pi-mesons, have been explored for their clinical potential but currently are not in common use.[20,24]

Treatment Planning

For the first step in external beam treatment planning, patients are usually imaged on a computed tomography (CT) simulator in the same position that would be used for treatment. The center of the treatment field is marked on the patient and identified on the CT using radiopaque markers. These images are then transferred to a computer equipped with specialized treatment planning software that is used by the physician to designate treatment fields or treatment planning goals; the images and the physician's directives are then used by a medical dosimetrist to design a treatment plan. Once the plan is approved, it undergoes rigorous quality assurance checks before the treatment parameters are transferred to the treatment machine.

Two major approaches are used to plan treatments—forward planning and inverse planning. With forward planning, the physician designates the treatment fields directly, drawing them on radiographs (more recently on digitally reconstructed radiographs) that simulate the "beam's eye

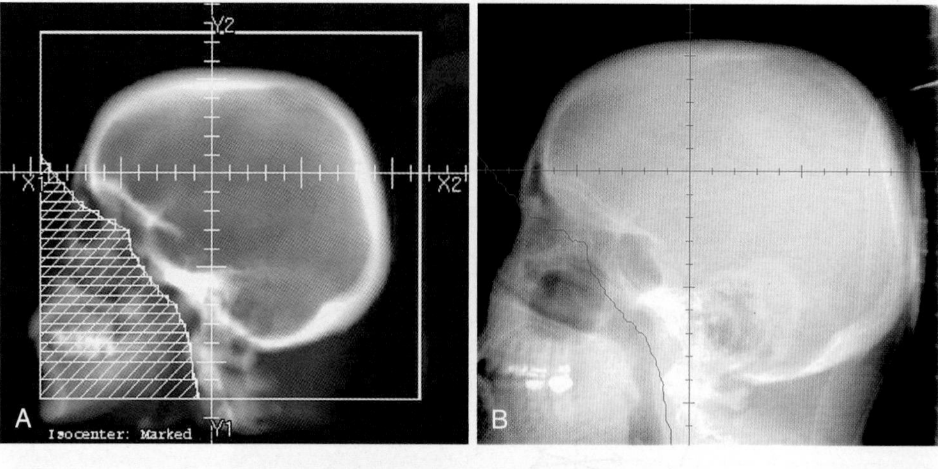

FIGURE 4.3. Radiation treatment fields may be drawn on digitally reconstructed radiographs (DRRs) generated from a planning computed tomography scan **(A)**. In the past, these were compared periodically with "port films" taken using the MV treatment beam. Today, most linear accelerators are equipped with KV imaging units that produce high-quality images for daily comparison with DRRs **(B)**.

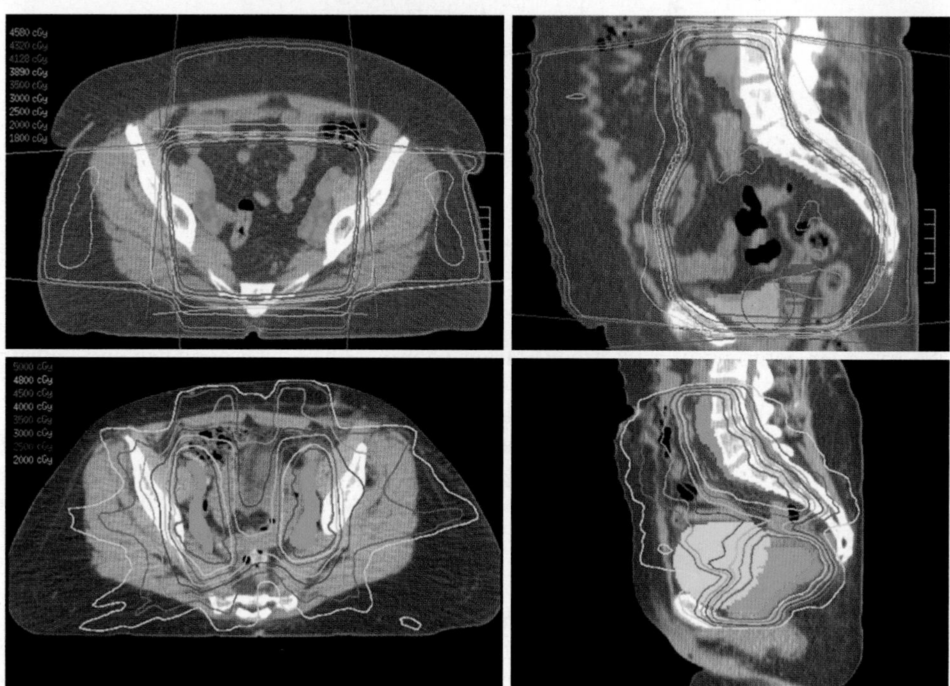

FIGURE 4.4. Top panels: Multiple-field techniques can be used to minimize the volume of uninvolved tissue treated to a high dose. Bottom panels: Intensity-modulated radiation therapy can generate plans that conform even more closely to the target volume, sparing adjacent critical structures.

view" of each treatment field. The field design is informed by the patient's history and physical examination, diagnostic imaging studies, and an understanding of anatomy and typical patterns of disease progression; however, treatments derived through forward planning necessarily involve fairly simple, standardized beam arrangements, usually with four radiation fields or fewer (Fig. 4.3). Until the mid 2000s, nearly all treatments were forward-planned, although the radiation dose distributions were increasingly calculated in three dimensions with corrections for the tissue heterogeneities revealed in planning CTs. (Fig. 4.4).

More recently, modern inverse planning technology has made it possible to take treatment planning one step further. With this approach, the radiation oncologist does not define treatment fields *per se* but rather designates target volumes and structures that are carefully contoured on a planning CT scan. Advanced computer algorithms are then used to design treatment plans that deliver the desired dose to the target volumes while minimizing the collateral dose to critical structures. The resulting plans are usually far more complex than could be conceived with a forward-planned approach, typically consisting of six to nine modulated treatment fields (e.g., intensity-modulated radiation therapy) or modulated rotational treatments (e.g., volumetric modulated arc therapy). Field shapes are modulated through the dynamic use of multileaf collimators.

These modern approaches can produce highly conforming treatment plans that usually permit the delivery of a greater dose to targets or greater protection of normal structures than is possible with simpler techniques. However, the opportunity for error is also greater. The demands upon the radiation oncologist to understand normal anatomy and to correctly transmit the findings of diagnostic studies to contoured target volumes are much greater than with forward-planned techniques. Incorrectly defined target volumes lead to underdosage of the

TABLE 4.2 Sources Commonly Used in Sealed-Source Brachytherapy

ELEMENT	ISOTOPES	HALF-LIFE (DAYS)	Eγ (MeV)	Eβ (MeV)
Iodine	^{125}I	60.2	0.028 (average)	None
Cesium	^{137}Cs	30	0.662	0.514, 1.17
Iridium	^{192}Ir	74	0.32–0.61	0.24, 0.67
Palladium	^{103}Pd	17	0.021 (average)	None
Radium	^{226}Ra	1620	0.19–0.6	3.26 (max)
Cobalt	^{60}Co	5.26	1.17–1.33	0.313 (max)

target, risking unnecessary tumor recurrences. For these reasons, accurate communication between the diagnostic imager and radiation oncologist is more important than ever. Patient positioning and understanding internal organ motion also become more important when these very highly conforming treatments are used. Because treatments are entirely dependent on accurate computer control of the treatment machine, meticulous quality assurance methods are required to ensure that treatments are being delivered as prescribed.

Brachytherapy

Brachytherapy refers to treatments that involve placement of radiation sources directly in or adjacent to the area to be treated. Brachytherapy that involves placement of sources directly into the tissues, usually via needles, is termed interstitial therapy. Treatment that involves placement of sources in a body cavity (e.g., uterus, bronchus, or esophagus) is termed intracavitary therapy. The use of sources placed in a surface applicator to treat superficial targets is termed mold therapy.

Because the dose of radiation in tissue declines in proportion to the square of the distance from the source of radiation, brachytherapy doses tend to fall off very rapidly as the distance from the sources increases; this provides excellent opportunities for sparing of adjacent tissues. Also, because brachytherapy sources usually move with the target in which they are inserted, the uncertainties caused by internal organ motion and patient motion are less of a problem than with external beam irradiation. Brachytherapy doses may be delivered at a continuous rate over several days (low dose rate irradiation), in short, fractionated doses (high dose rate), or in periodic pulses over hours or days (pulsed dose rate).

Typical applications for intracavitary brachytherapy are treatment of intact cervical cancer and endobronchial therapy for lung cancer. One of the most frequent applications for interstitial brachytherapy is treatment of prostate cancer. Interstitial brachytherapy is also used to treat head and neck cancers, gynecologic cancers, sarcomas, and other tumors.

A number of different isotopes have been used in brachytherapy (Table 4.2). Radium and cesium were once the primary isotope used for brachytherapy but have, for the most part, been abandoned in favor of safer isotopes with shorter half-lives. Iridium-192 has a half-life of 74 days and is used for most high dose rate and pulsed dose rate brachytherapy. Iodine-125 and palladium-103 are frequently used for brachytherapy for prostate cancer.

ROLE OF IMAGING IN RADIATION THERAPY

The effectiveness of radiation therapy is heavily dependent on the quality, accuracy, and interpretation of the images that form the basis of most treatment plans and that document the accuracy of radiation delivery. Most radiation treatments are planned directly using CT scans that are obtained in the treatment position. The specialized scanners designed for this purpose are termed "CT simulators." Some facilities are also equipped with magnetic resonance imaging (MRI) simulators that can facilitate target definition in selected cases. To improve the accuracy of transferred information, planning CT scans may also be digitally fused with MRI, positron emission tomography/CT, or other tomographic imaging studies obtained in the course of the patient's diagnostic evaluation. Once a plan has been finalized, the actual treatment delivery is also guided by periodic imaging. At a minimum, the accuracy of treatment is documented with weekly portal images taken with the treatment beam. However, daily image guidance with kilovoltage imaging (see Fig. 4.3), ultrasonography, or CT has become increasingly routine as a means of optimizing the accuracy of daily setup for intensity-modulated radiation therapy, proton therapy, and other tightly conforming treatments. Most recently, clinical researchers have been exploring the use of MRI guidance for linear accelerator treatments; with these specialized "MRI-linac" units, treatment plans can be modified daily to adjust to changes in the target position or configuration.

With these increasingly conformal, image-based treatments, close, effective communication between radiation oncologist and diagnostic imager has never been more critical (Fig. 4.5). Even small misunderstandings about the location or significance of radiographic abnormalities can result in serious errors in treatment design. Diagnostic imagers greatly assist their radiation oncology colleagues by providing specific information about the location, size, and relevance of abnormal or potentially suspicious findings. Diagnostic uncertainties should be discussed openly to allow clinicians to weigh the risks and benefits of expanding radiation target volumes to encompass such regions.

Diagnostic radiologists can improve communication of their findings by specifying the series and slice number corresponding to the best views of each finding. Additional

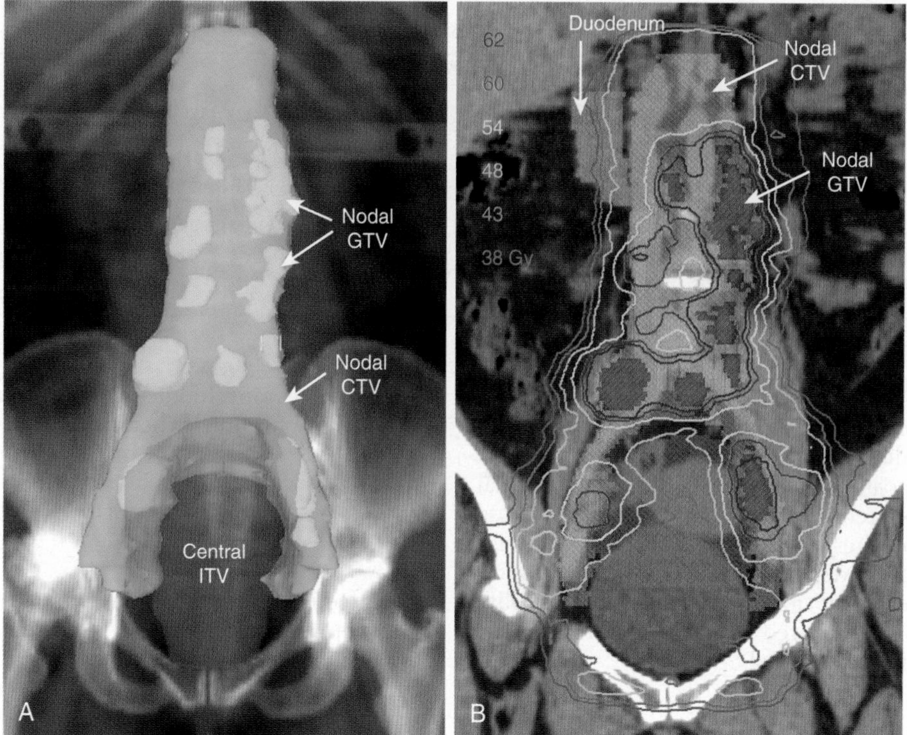

FIGURE 4.5. Even patients with extensive lymphadenopathy can be successfully treated if an adequate dose can be delivered to gross disease without exceeding normal tissue tolerance doses. However, this requires the clinician to have a precise understanding of the location and extent of every pathologic node. This patient was diagnosed with a squamous carcinoma of the cervix metastatic to multiple pelvic and paraaortic nodes **(A)**. Using intensity-modulated radiation therapy **(B)**, the clinical target volume, including the primary site and all nodes at risk for microscopic disease, was treated to a dose of 45 Gy; the nodal gross target volume was treated to 62 Gy. This highly conformal treatment plan allowed a tumoricidal dose to be delivered without exceeding the tolerated dose to critical structures such as the duodenum. The cervix received additional dose with brachytherapy. At 8 years after treatment, the patient had no evidence of disease and no treatment-related side effects. *CTV, GTV, ITV*

anatomic information about the laterality, vertebral level, and proximity to easily identifiable structures often helps the radiation oncologist to accurately transfer diagnostic imaging information to treatment planning studies. Radiation oncologists also often depend on their imaging colleagues' suggestions for ways of obtaining the most accurate depiction of disease. However, in very difficult cases, no amount of written communication can replace direct discussion between the imager and the radiation oncologist through tumor boards, face-to-face reviews, or telephone discussions while both the radiation oncologist and the diagnostic imager review the patient's images. In this context, radiation oncologists have a responsibility to ask for help and to confirm that their understanding of images and reports is accurate.

Radiation oncologists can also provide their imaging colleagues with important information to assist in accurate posttreatment diagnoses. In particular, the differential diagnosis of posttreatment abnormalities in bowel, lung, bone, and other structures can often be narrowed if the imager understands whether these structures were included in previous radiation fields. Close communication can also help the imager, radiation oncologist, and other members of the multidisciplinary team determine whether recurrences are inside, outside, or marginal to radiation therapy treatment fields. This has important implications as radiation oncologists attempt to determine whether a patient can be treated with additional radiation therapy; such information also provides radiation oncologists with important information about the reasons for treatment failure, helping to improve treatment for future patients.

REFERENCES

1. Eifel PJ, Winter K, Morris M, et al. Pelvic irradiation with concurrent chemotherapy versus pelvic and para-aortic irradiation for high-risk cervical cancer: an update of radiation therapy oncology group trial (RTOG) 90-01. *J Clinical Oncol.* 2004;22:872-880.
2. Pignon JP, le Maitre A, Maillard E, et al. Meta-analysis of chemotherapy in head and neck cancer (MACH-NC): an update on 93 randomised trials and 17,346 patients. *Radiother Oncol.* 2009;92:4-14.
3. O'Connell MJ, Martenson JA, Wieand HS, et al. Improving adjuvant therapy for rectal cancer by combining protracted-infusion fluorouracil with radiation therapy after curative surgery. *N Engl J Med.* 1994;331:502-507.
4. Cummings BJ, Keane TJ, O'Sullivan B, et al. Epidermoid anal cancer: treatment by radiation alone or by radiation and 5-fluorouracil with and without mitomycin C. *Int J Radiat Oncol Biol Phys.* 1991;21:1115-1125.
5. Dewey WC, Ling CC, Meyn RE. Radiation-induced apoptosis: relevance to radiotherapy. *Int J Radiat Oncol Biol Phys.* 1995;33:781-796.
6. Fyles A, Keane TJ, Barton M, et al. The effect of treatment duration in the local control of cervix cancer. *Radiotherapy and Oncology.* 1992;25:273-279.
7. Suwinski R, Sowa A, Rutkowski T, et al. Time factor in postoperative radiotherapy: a multivariate locoregional control analysis in 868 patients. *Int J Radiat Oncol Biol Phys.* 2003;56:399-412.

8. Koukourakis M, Hlouverakis G, Kosma L, et al. The impact of overall treatment time on the results of radiotherapy for nonsmall cell lung carcinoma. *Int J Radiat Oncol Biol Phys*. 1996;34:315-322.
9. Eifel PJ. Chemordiotherapy: neoadjuvant, concomitant, sequential or monomodality treatment?. In: Ayhan A, Reed N, Gultekin M, eds. *Textbook of Gynaecological Oncology*. Ankara: Gunes Publishing; 2016:1405-1412.
10. Kallman RF. The phenomenon of reoxygenation and its implications for fractionated radiotherapy. *Radiology*. 1972;105:135-142.
11. Emami B, Lyman J, Brown A, et al. Tolerance of normal tissue to therapeutic irradiation. *Int J Radiat Oncol Biol Phys*. 1991;21:109-122.
12. Marks LB, Ten Haken RK, Martel MK. Guest editor's introduction to QUANTEC: a users guide. *Int J Radiat Oncol Biol Phys*. 2010;76:S1-2.
13. Eifel PJ, Jhingran A, Bodurka DC, et al. Correlation of smoking history and other patient characteristics with major complications of pelvic radiation therapy for cervical cancer. *J Clin Oncol*. 2002;20:3651-3657.
14. Rotman M, Sedlis A, Piedmonte MR, et al. A phase III randomized trial of postoperative pelvic irradiation in Stage IB cervical carcinoma with poor prognostic features: follow-up of a gynecologic oncology group study. *Int J Radiat Oncol Biol Phys*. 2006;65:169-176.
15. Ceelen WP, Van Nieuwenhove Y, Fierens K. Preoperative chemoradiation versus radiation alone for stage II and III resectable rectal cancer. *Cochrane Database Syst Rev*. 2009:CD006041.
16. Garden AS, Reddy JP. Postoperative radiation therapy for metastatic cervical adenopathy. *Semin Radiat Oncol*. 2019;29:144-149.
17. Chemoradiotherapy for Cervical Cancer Meta-Analysis Collaboration. Reducing uncertainties about the effects of chemoradiotherapy for cervical cancer: a systematic review and meta-analysis of individual patient data from 18 randomized trials. *J Clin Oncol*. 2008;26:5802-5812.
18. Neoadjuvant Chemotherapy for Cervical Cancer Meta-Analysis Collaboration. Neoadjuvant chemotherapy for locally advanced cervix cancer. *Cochrane Database Syst Rev*. 2004:CD001774.
19. Mauri D, Pavlidis N, Ioannidis JP. Neoadjuvant versus adjuvant systemic treatment in breast cancer: a meta-analysis. *J Natl Cancer Inst*. 2005;97:188-194.
20. Rackwitz T, Debus J. Clinical applications of proton and carbon ion therapy. *Semin Oncol*. 2019;46:226-232.
21. Liao Z, Lee JJ, Komaki R, et al. Bayesian adaptive randomization trial of passive scattering proton therapy and intensity-modulated photon radiotherapy for locally advanced non-small-cell lung cancer. *J Clin Oncol*. 2018;36:1813-1822.
22. Zietman AL, Bae K, Slater JD, et al. Randomized trial comparing conventional-dose with high-dose conformal radiation therapy in early-stage adenocarcinoma of the prostate: long-term results from proton radiation oncology group/American College of Radiology 95-09. *J Clin Oncol*. 2010;28:1106-1111.
23. Weber DC, Habrand JL, Hoppe BS, et al. Proton therapy for pediatric malignancies: Fact, figures and costs. A joint consensus statement from the pediatric subcommittee of PTCOG, PROS and EPTN. *Radiother Oncol*. 2018;128:44-55.
24. Durante M, Flanz J. Charged particle beams to cure cancer: Strengths and challenges. *Semin Oncol*. 2019;46:219-225.

CHAPTER 5

Assessing Response to Therapy

Mayur K. Virarkar, M.D.; Homer A. Macapinlac, M.D.; Halyna Pokhylevych, M.D.; and Priya R. Bhosale, M.D.

INTRODUCTION

Cancer continues to be a major health problem, as one in four deaths in the United States is attributed to cancer. However, we continue to see incremental improvements over time, with the relative 5-year survival rate for cancer in the United States at 68%, up from 50% in the mid-1970s. Cancer death rates fell 21.0% among men and 12.3% among women from 1991 to 2006 in the United States. The American Cancer Society estimates that the cancer incidence decreased 1.3% per year among men from 2000 to 2006 and 0.5% per year from 1998 to 2006 among women. This decline is attributed mainly to falling smoking rates, improved cancer treatments, and earlier detection of cancer.[1]

Oncologic imaging is recognized as an integral part of the management of cancer patients. Continued improvement in survival and the introduction of novel and multimodality therapies demand greater contributions from imaging to assess the presence of tumor, its extent, and response to therapy.

Improved understanding of the basic mechanisms of tumor biology, immunology, carcinogenesis, and genetics provides a rich foundation for translating these findings into enhancing efforts to reduce the impact of cancer. Some of these areas include understanding inherited or acquired genetic mutations or malfunctions; elucidating the molecular pathways of cell proliferation; acknowledging the effects of immune response and vascular proliferation; and taking advantage of more effective clinical cancer detection modalities, including magnetic resonance imaging (MRI), computed tomography (CT), and molecular imaging techniques paired with gene screening arrays to identify molecular abnormalities in individual patients' cancer cells.

The challenges to imaging are continuously evolving as novel personalized therapies and multimodality regimens are developed. However, scientific limitations and economic realities mean there is a need to provide proof of principle of the ways in which imaging can be an integral part of daily care and the design of various clinical trials to treat cancer patients.

The ability of imaging to provide indices to response such as tumor size and perfusion, as well as the more recent advent of functional imaging, makes imagining a standard component of clinical practice and the assessment of novel therapies. This central role is best exemplified by the multidisciplinary approach to the management of cancer patients. The integration of surgery, pathology, imaging, medical oncology, radiation oncology, and medical physics to cancer patient care attests to the complex nature of the disease and the need to bring together the expertise of a group in lieu of the traditional models on which individual patient–physician relationships are developed, followed by subspecialist referrals.

The traditional subspecialty designations in diagnostic imaging have and continue to be anatomic regions—for example, neuroradiology (head and/or neck), thoracic (chest), body (abdomen/pelvis), and others. However, cancer imaging demands expertise not only of specific anatomic areas but also in other modalities such as ultrasound, MRI, CT, x-ray plain films, and nuclear medicine, including positron emission tomography (PET)/CT. This multimodality ability is now supported by the ready availability of images via picture archiving and communication systems and electronic medical records and, when necessary, ready access to other imaging specialists, because it may be difficult to manage expertise in so many modalities. Easier access to referring physicians for consultation is also aided by fast communications via smartphones, the web, or the traditional page and phone system. Finally, the availability and use of voice-recognition systems and web access allows rapid turnaround of report results to both referring physicians and patients. The transparency of these imaging reports should remind us all to avoid causing unnecessary anxiety by ensuring the proper use of language that is accurate and concise and hopefully answers the clinical question being posed.

For both the individual patient and clinical trial patients, close communication between the interpreting doctor and the referring physician is necessary for deciding the most appropriate imaging technique to use and when to perform a follow-up study to assess response. Appropriate care in planning the imaging component of clinical trials is essential, and may include proper imaging techniques, analysis, reporting, image transfer, and the design of forms that may need to be filled out for these studies. Ideally, these imaging modalities and measurements are identical in both individual and trial patients, which may make it easier to perform clinical imaging research or even to incorporate an individual patient into a clinical trial. Such planning will avoid added costs of repeat imaging or the need to go back and reanalyze images. Many of these imaging strategies could be made easier by accreditation of the imaging facility by the American College of Radiology, which ensures that the imaging equipment and the staff and physicians' qualifications are registered, which then makes it easier to participate in collaborative groups that carry out clinical imaging trials such as the American College of Radiology Imaging Network. Ensuring the high quality of imaging primarily benefits our patients but also allows easy participation in clinical research, which is the foundation of continuing improvement in our various specialties.

GENERAL IMAGING STRATEGIES

KEY POINTS

- A multidisciplinary approach to cancer care will require multimodality, subspecialty imaging.
- Novel therapies will require improved imaging indices to assess extent of disease and response.
- Multimodality imaging expertise and rapid communication between physicians and reporting are a must.
- Integration of imaging into clinical trial planning and accreditation is encouraged.

WHY DO WE NEED TO MONITOR TUMOR RESPONSE?

The need for monitoring response became apparent in the early days of chemotherapy, particularly for conducting clinical comparative trials for various experimental chemotherapeutic agents in multiple cancer types. The typical development pathway for cancer therapeutic drugs is evolution from phase I to phase II and to phase III clinical trials. In phase I trials, the toxicity of the agent is assessed to determine what dose is appropriate for subsequent trials. In phase II trials, evidence of antitumor activity is obtained. Phase II trials can be done in several ways. One way is to examine tumor response rate versus a historical control population treated with an established drug. New drugs with a low response rate are typically not moved forward to advanced clinical testing under such a design. In such trials, tumor response has traditionally been determined with anatomic imaging techniques. An alternative approach is to use a larger sample size and have a randomized phase II trial, in which the new treatment is given in one treatment arm and compared with a standard treatment. Once drug activity is shown in phase II, phase III trials are then performed. Phase III trials are larger and usually have a control arm treated with a standard therapy. Therefore, imaging is expected to have a major role not only in the individual patient care but also in designing clinical trials to select which therapies should be advanced to progressively larger trials and become standard of care.

History of an Evolving Imaging-Based Response Assessment

Moertel and Hanley performed an early study to assess response,[2] in which 16 experienced oncologists were asked to measure 12 simulated tumors, placed underneath foam, using their clinical methods, which entailed physical examination with a ruler or caliper. Although seemingly crude, this was an appropriate simulation of the clinical setting in which a physician will palpate a tumor and then estimate its size before and after administering the treatment. This paper suggested that a 50% reduction in the perpendicular diameters of the tumors at approximately 2 months is an acceptable objective response rate. This 50% reduction in bidimensional measurement of a single lesion was adopted in the World Health Organization (WHO) guidelines in 1979. Miller[3] and coworkers recommended that a partial response (PR) be defined as a 50% reduction in the bidimensional measure of tumor area or, if multiple tumors are present, the sum of the product of the diameters. This study also described unidimensional measurements for "measurable" disease, assessment of the presence of bone metastases, and criteria for "nonmeasurable" disease. Tumor volume estimates were based on conventional radiography techniques by measuring the two longest perpendicular diameters and calculating their product. Although widely used, obvious shortcomings of the WHO guidelines were the clinical foundation of the criteria without accounting for the improvements in imaging to determine tumor volumes. Tumors are rarely round or symmetrical, thus making these measurements difficult to implement, particularly by using a ruler or calipers. The lack of distinction between a complete response (CR) versus a PR in 50% to 90% decrease in tumor volume was an obvious flaw.

The European Organization of Research and Treatment of Cancer and the National Cancer Institute (NCI) of the United States and Canada set up a study group (RECIST)[4] to standardize assessment criteria in cancer treatment trials. The objective was to simplify and standardize the methods used to assess tumor response by more precisely defining tumor targets, with proposed guidelines for imaging methods. The criteria for CR, PR, stable disease (SD), and progressive disease (PD) were revised. Unidimensional measurements were established for lesions of 2 cm or larger for CT, MRI, plain film, and physical examination and 1 cm or larger for spiral CT scan. The sum of the unidimensional tumor measurements was used for evaluation of response, which may decrease sources of error.

RECIST criteria were adopted by multiple investigators, cooperative groups, and industry and government entities for assessing the treatment outcomes. However, a number of questions and issues have arisen that have led to the development of the revised RECIST 1.1 guidelines.

RECIST 1.1: The Current Standard

The major change in RECIST 1.1 is that the number of lesions required to assess tumor burden for response determination has been reduced to a maximum of five total (and two per organ, maximum). Pathologic lymph nodes with a short axis of 15 mm are considered measurable and assessable as target lesions. The short-axis measurement should be included in the sum of lesions in calculation of tumor response. Nodes that shrink to less than 10 mm on the short axis are considered normal. Confirmation of response is required for trials with response as the primary endpoint but is no longer required in randomized studies because the control arm serves as an appropriate means of interpreting the data. Disease progression is clarified in several aspects: in addition to the previous definition of progression in target disease as a 20% increase in sum, a 5-mm absolute increase is now required as well to guard against overcalling PD when the total sum is very small. Furthermore, guidance is offered on what constitutes "unequivocal progression" of nonmeasurable/nontarget disease, a source of confusion in the original RECIST guidelines. Finally, a section on detection of new lesions, including the interpretation of 2-[^{18}F] fluoro-2-deoxy-D-glucose (FDG)–PET scan assessment is included. Finally, the revised RECIST 1.1 guidelines include a new imaging appendix with updated recommendations on the optimal anatomical assessment of lesions.[5]

TABLE 5.1 Response Evaluation Criteria in Solid Tumors 1.1 Target Lesions Response Criteria

Objective response	Response Evaluation Criteria in Solid Tumors (RECIST) 1.1 target lesions[a] change in sum of LDs, maximum of two per organ up to five total.
Complete response	Disappearance of all target lesions, confirmed at ≥4 weeks. Reduction in short axis of target lymph nodes to <10 mm.
Partial response	Decrease in target LD sum ≥30%, confirmed at 4 weeks.
Progressive disease	Increase in target LD sum ≥20%. Overall ≥5-mm increase in target LD sum. New, malignant FDG uptake in the absence of other indications of progressive disease or an anatomically preexisting lesion and confirmed on contemporaneous or follow-up CT.
Stable disease	Does not meet other criteria.

[a]Measurable lesion, unidimensional (LD only: size measured by conventional techniques ≥20 mm, measured with spiral CT ≥10 mm; nodes: target short axis ±15 mm, nontarget 10- to 15-mm nodes, normal <10 mm). Nonmeasurable: all other lesions, including small lesions; evaluation is not recommended.
CT, Computed tomography; *FDG*, 2-[^{18}F] fluoro-2-deoxy-D-glucose; *LD*, long-axis diameter.
From Eisenhauer EA, Therasse P, Bogaerts J, et al. New response evaluation criteria in solid tumours: revised RECIST guideline (version 1.1). *Eur J Cancer*. 2009;45:228-247.

In developing RECIST 1.1, the RECIST Working Group concluded that, at present, there is not sufficient standardization or evidence to abandon unidimensional anatomic (vs. volumetric) assessment of tumor burden. The only exception to this is in the use of FDG-PET imaging as an adjunct to determination of progression.

Although use of these anatomic criteria has been evolving to develop better response criteria, the RECIST criteria, and now, quite likely, the RECIST 1.1 criteria, are or will be used in virtually every clinical trial of new solid tumor therapeutics, because response is essentially always measured. Regulatory agencies have accepted RECIST as the standard in response assessment for clinical trials in most countries. Familiarity with the implications of trials in which response is measured using the WHO, RECIST, and RECIST 1.1 criteria is essential, because they are not identical and do not produce identical results. Table 5.1 presents RECIST 1.1 overall response criteria for both measurable and nonmeasurable lesions.

HIGHLIGHTING SOURCES OF ERRORS IN RESPONSE EVALUATION

Possible Problems Related to Image Acquisition

Multiple imaging modalities are used and are continuously updated over time, presenting differences in equipment capabilities from within a manufacturer and across competing imaging equipment makers. CT has undergone significant evolution in a short period of time, and it is the most commonly used modality for therapeutic clinical trials. Image acquisition protocols vary as to body region or organ being evaluated. The proper phase of contrast has to be consistently used, as does proper windowing, and it is important to ensure that the entire tumor or organ is imaged (Fig. 5.1).

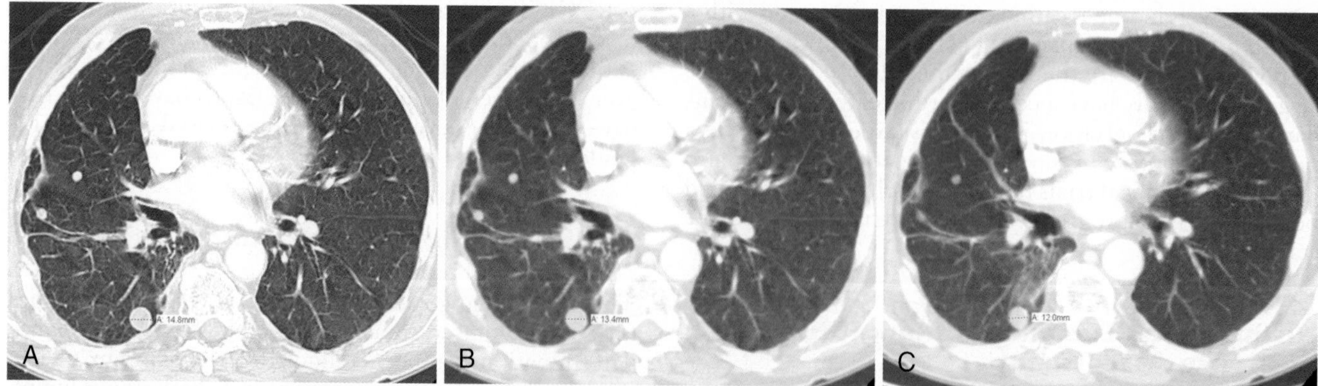

FIGURE 5.1. A, Importance of imaging consistency and windowing. Computed tomography (CT) of the chest shows a 1.48-cm nodule, correct window lung 2.5-mm slice thickness. **B,** CT of chest shows incorrect soft tissue window selection. Note how the nodule measurement is now 1.34 cm, which is smaller than the actual measurement and therefore wrong. **C,** CT of chest shows wrong soft tissue window and wrong slice thickness selection at 5 mm. Note how the nodule measures 1.20 cm, smaller than the correct measurement shown in panel **A**.

Breathing and cardiac motion can induce variations in tumor measurement. MRI is commonly used in certain tumor types not amenable to CT evaluation. There is a wide range of MRI acquisition techniques, which can make comparisons between studies difficult. Rigorous attention to protocol has to be enforced to prevent these problems, particularly if repeated examinations are performed using the same or, worse, different machines. It is imperative that patients who are recruited for clinical trials or individual patients who are referred for response evaluation are identified, and that the appropriate imaging acquisition parameters are applied. Most important for clinical trials incorporating imaging for response is the proper consultation and selection of imaging experts up front to ensure that the proper endpoints for both baseline and follow-up for response are identified, that the imaging protocol is consistent, and that the time and effort needed to make these measurements, fill out forms, and transfer images be properly anticipated and funded.

Errors Resulting From Target Selection

There are very few well-demarcated, uniform, round tumors. Most tumors are difficult to measure precisely and reproducibly. Tumors can be difficult to delineate from normal structures, including blood vessels. Intravenous contrast administration, timing of acquisition, proper phase selection, and windowing are crucial in minimizing this problem. A potential problem would be using a chest CT to measure liver lesions or, conversely, using abdominal scans to measure lung base lesions. Some tumors are difficult to measure because they are heterogenous and cystic (Fig. 5.2). Complex tumor spread, such as that seen in peritoneal carcinomatosis, is difficult to incorporate into measurements, but this may be used to assess for progression and/or response. Tumor involvement of organs such as the ovary present complex problems because it may be difficult to distinguish tumor from normal tissue after therapy; thus, CR is difficult or impossible to assess. Bone metastases should not be included as measurable lesions because they calcify and enlarge. Certain tumors such as gastrointestinal stromal tumor may respond to therapy with cystic changes, and sometimes enlargement of these cystic lesions. Pleural and peritoneal lesions may have a predominantly liquid component and can be loculated, making them difficult to measure and assess for response.

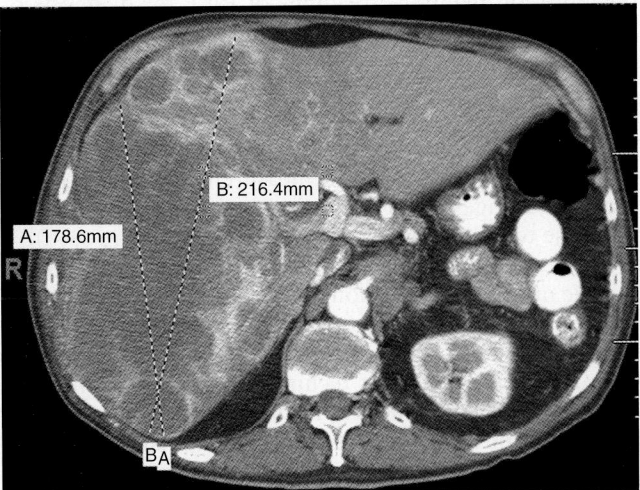

FIGURE 5.2. Selecting target lesions. The abdominal computed tomography scan shows multiple metastases. The 17.8-cm target is correct, and the 21.6-cm measurement is incorrect because it incorporates two adjacent lesions as one.

Errors in Tumor Measurement

Minimum size requirements (usually 10 mm) and the need to measure the largest cross-section of the tumor should be kept in mind. Liver lesions should be measured using the proper enhancement or even nonenhancement technique consistently. Cystic and necrotic components of tumors will evolve and may have a different response from that of the solid component of the tumor. Thus, it may be difficult to assess response in these heterogeneous tumors (Fig. 5.3).

Errors Related to Nontumor Conditions

Patients may develop postobstructive pneumonia or intercurrent pulmonary infarction, or lung cancer patients may present with a significant atelectatic component, making it difficult to distinguish tumor from collapsed lung.

FDG-PET imaging has become the standard functional molecular imaging technique; it is based on the measurement of the increased glycolytic activity of tumors. Integration of FDG-PET and CT has further improved the accuracy of this modality in the malignancy diagnosis of, staging, and response evaluation.

How Is Response Determined on Positron Emission Tomography?

Qualitative Technique. FDG-PET scans for diagnosis and staging of cancer in clinical practice are typically interpreted using qualitative methods, in which the distribution and intensity of FDG uptake in potential tumor foci are compared with tracer uptake in normal structures such as the blood pool, muscle, brain, and liver. This "visual" interpretation requires a great deal of clinical experience, knowledge of disease spread patterns for various tumors, and knowledge of normal variants and artifacts. An FDG-positive PET scan turning completely negative is easy to interpret, as is the appearance of new lesions. Difficulties arise if there is residual activity after therapy or is the new lesions are areas of active infection.

The best implementation of the qualitative technique is found in the Revised Response Criteria for Malignant Lymphoma, developed through the International Harmonization Project. Juweid and colleagues[6] classified FDG-PET results into visual findings as positive or negative relative to the intensity of tumor tracer uptake as compared with the blood pool or nearby normal structures. These dichotomized findings are used for interpretation of scans at the end of standard therapy and specify minimum times after treatment to avoid inflammatory changes. Interpretation guidance is provided for specific areas such

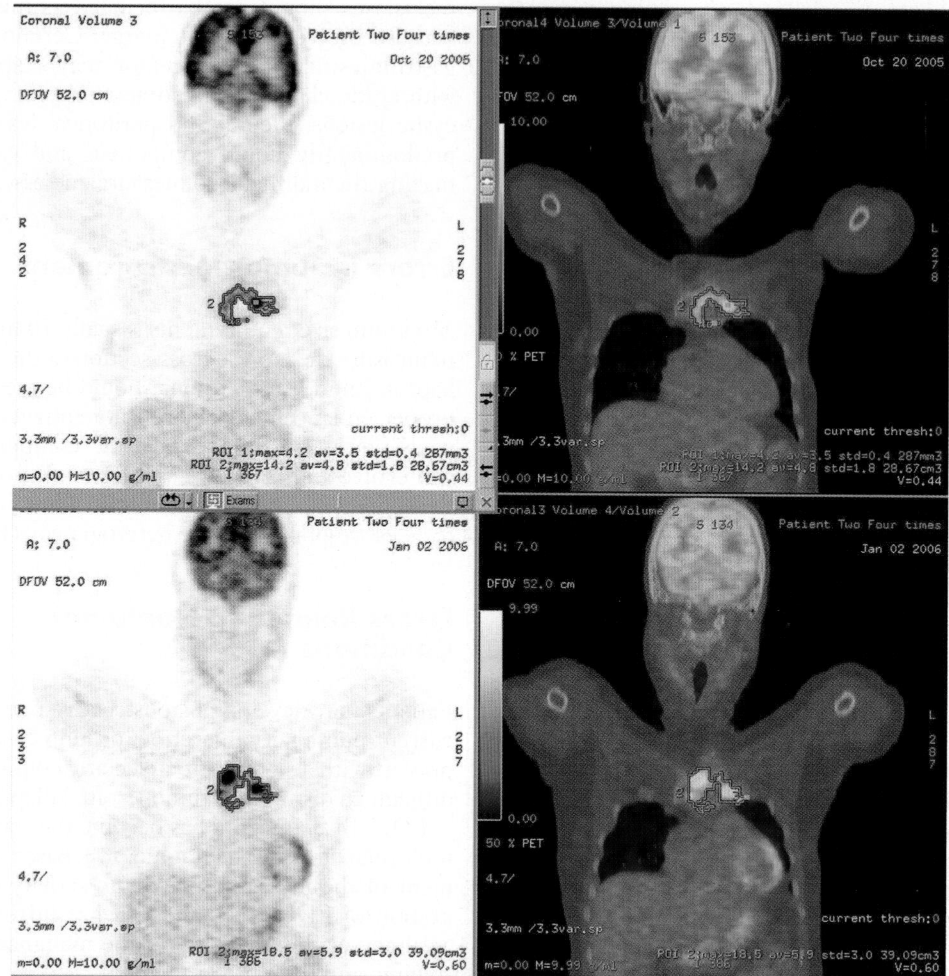

FIGURE 5.3. Volumetric positron emission tomography (PET)/computed tomography (CT) measurement. **Top left,** Baseline 2-[^{18}F] fluoro-2-deoxy-D-glucose (FDG)–PET scan. **Top right,** PET/CT scan shows residual mediastinal mass with FDG uptake average standardized uptake value (SUV) of 4.8 and maximum SUV of 14.2. **Bottom left,** FDG-PET 3 months later shows increasing FDG uptake. **Bottom right,** FDG-PET/CT of increasing mass on CT and FDG uptake average SUV has increased to 5.9, and maximum SUV is measured at 5.9.

as the lungs, liver, and bone marrow, and can provide consistency in response evaluation, but recognize the limitations of FDG-PET in identifying low-grade tumors, such as those in the marrow.

However, the difficulty still lies in the intermediate pattern or minimal residual uptake described by Mikhaeel and associates.[7] In this study of 102 patients evaluated with FDG-PET at midtreatment for aggressive lymphoma, 19 patients had scans with minimal residual uptake and had an estimated 5-year progression-free survival of 59.3%, closer to the 88.8% observed in the PET-negative group ($n = 50$) than the 16.2% observed for the PET-positive group ($n = 52$).

Hicks and MacManus and coworkers[8,9] have used the visual qualitative analysis criteria to predict outcomes at the end of therapy for non–small cell lung cancer, with excellent risk stratification capability between FDG-positive and FDG-negative scans. Hicks[10] has argued for qualitative assessments and has emphasized that a reduction in tissue FDG retention, however it is measured and at whatever time after treatment it is recorded, is more likely to be associated with both a pathologic response and improved survival than is a lack of change.

There are, however, surprisingly little data on the reproducibility of qualitative readings of PET for diagnosis or for treatment response. This points out the weakness of this technique that is hindering its wider application in clinical trials.

Quantitative Technique. PET is inherently a quantitative imaging technique, and the measurement of treatment-induced changes is an attractive tool for assessing early response to therapy (before anatomic changes are seen).[11]

Numerous quantitative techniques have been developed, but the model involving nonlinear regression (NLR) of the full compartment is theoretically the most accurate quantitative measure of glucose metabolic rate. It may be the best, but is also the most technically demanding, because it requires dynamic imaging for 60 minutes (imaging over the area of interest) during tracer injection, taking multiple blood samples to measure whole blood, assessing plasma FDG concentration (in a well counter), and determining arterial input function from either images or arterial blood samples. The Amsterdam Group performed an illustrative study in 20 women with advanced breast cancer and compared NLR with 10 simplified quantitative techniques. They noted that the Patlak method, the Simplified Kinetic Method, and the standardized uptake value (SUV) normalized for lean body mass and blood glucose were the most promising alternatives to the NLR technique.[12]

The SUV is a widely used metric for assessing tissue accumulation of tracers, defined as the ratio of radioactivity in tissue per milliliter (in mCi/mL) divided by the decay corrected activity injected to the patient (in mCi/body weight in g). Body weight is the most commonly used parameter, but body surface area (BSA), standardized uptake value corrected for lean body mass (SUL), and others may also be employed.[13] BSA and SUL are less dependent on body habitus across populations than SUV, which is based on total body mass. The determination of SUV is dependent on identical patient preparation and adequate scan quality, which must be similar between baseline and follow-up studies. Absolute and rigorous standardization of the protocol for PET is required to achieve reproducible SUVs. Differences between image reconstruction parameters, as well as imaging pediatric patients, can also result in significant SUV changes. Ramos and colleagues[14] demonstrated that the use of different reconstruction methods, such as iterative reconstruction and segmented attenuation correction, seem to generate more accurate SUVs than are obtained from conventional filtered backprojection images. Yeung and associates[15] demonstrated that SUVs calculated based on BSA are a more uniform parameter than SUVs calculated based on body weight in pediatric patients, and that this approach is probably most appropriate for use in the follow-up of these patients. Remember that significant differences occur in SUV measurements between dedicated PET scans and PET/CT scans. More recently, FDG-PET/CT studies are being acquired in conjunction with intravenous contrast, which can alter SUVs. It is worth noting that studies have shown no significant difference in the diagnostic accuracy of scan interpretation when readers are blinded to the reconstruction method, using CT with or without intravenous contrast.[16] Recent software reconstruction enhancements mean that FDG-PET/CT scans are less susceptible to the effects of orally administered contrast or the presence of prosthetic devices.[17] Motion correction techniques such as average CT have been proposed to allow correction for both pulmonary and cardiac motion.[18] These SUV changes appear magnified at the lung bases, where obviously the motion is largest. These motion correction techniques not only allow more accurate SUV measurement but also improve PET and CT tumor matching, which may facilitate interpretation. These are applicable not only to lung lesions, but also to esophageal cancers and lesions involving the upper abdominal organs such as the liver, adrenals, and spleen.[19] These motion correction techniques have had applications in radiotherapy planning, particularly for tumor volume delineation in thoracic tumors.[20]

Standardization has been well summarized in guidelines set by the Society of Nuclear Medicine and the European Association of Nuclear Medicine for FDG-PET/CT imaging in oncology. This is a concerted effort to standardize imaging performance, including developing quality assurance/quality control procedures in an effort to improve the consistency of imaging and interpretation and, more importantly, improve quantification of response using SUVs.[21,22]

PERCIST 1.0 was drafted by Wahl and coworkers[23] as a framework that may be useful for consideration in clinical trials or individual patients. An important premise offered by PERCIST is that cancer response assessed by PET is a continuous and time-dependent variable. An important concept is that reduced uptake of FDG by tumors is expected to decline after effective therapy; hence, the change from baseline, as well as the timepoint at which the PET image was obtained, is important. RECIST confines us to four bins (CR, PR, SD, and PD) in a dynamic, continuous process of response assessment.

PERCIST mandates standardized imaging as outlined by Shankar and colleagues[24] on the recommendations of the NCI for the performance of FDG-PET scans for clinical trials. This would require standard FDG doses (±20%), uptake time (50–70 minutes), patient preparation (fasting 4–6 hours), fasting blood sugar less than 200 mg/dL, and uniform image acquisition and reconstruction parameters.

Wahl and coworkers[23] suggest that early after treatment (i.e., after one cycle, just before the next cycle) may be a reasonable time for monitoring response to determine whether the tumor shows no primary resistance to the treatment. This was supported by multiple studies, one on ovarian cancer, showing that 60% to 70% of the total SUV decline occurs after just one cycle of effective treatment.[25] Performing the PET scan at the end of treatment can provide evidence that resistance to therapy was present during treatment. End-of-therapy PET scans are most commonly performed as restaging examinations to determine whether additional treatment is needed.[26]

PERCIST requires that SUV measurements be corrected for lean body mass (SUL) and that normal background activity be determined based on a 3-cm-diameter spherical region of interest in the right lobe of the liver. If the tumor involves the liver, then blood pool activity in the descending aorta is an alternate background site.

No more than five lesions are assessed, similar to RECIST 1.1. For PERCIST 1.0, it is suggested that only the percentage difference in SUL between the tumor with the most intense SUL on the first study and the tumor with the most intense SUL on the second study should be used as a classifier for response. Given the uncertainty about the best metric, it is suggested that SUL peak data be determined and summed before and after treatment for up to the five hottest lesions, and that the ratio of the sums before and after treatment be compared as a secondary analysis. Obvious progression of any tumor (e.g., >30% increase) or new lesions would negate a PR.

For PERCIST 1.0, complete metabolic response should be assessed visually, and would be defined as complete resolution of FDG uptake in the target lesion, less than the mean liver activity and indistinguishable from surrounding blood pool activity.

Partial metabolic response (PMR) would be a reduction by a minimum of 30% in target measurable tumor FDG SUL peak. This measurement is commonly taken from the same lesion as the baseline measurement, but can be taken from another lesion if that lesion was previously present and is the most active lesion after treatment. Reduction in the extent of tumor FDG uptake is not a requirement for

TABLE 5.2 Positron Emission Tomography Response Evaluation Criteria In Solid Tumors 1.0 Response Criteria

CATEGORY OF RESPONSE	POSITRON EMISSION TOMOGRAPHY RESPONSE EVALUATION CRITERIA IN SOLID TUMORS (PERCIST) 1.0
Complete metabolic response	Normalization of all lesions (target and nontarget) to SUL less than mean liver SUL and equal to normal surrounding tissue SUL. Verification with follow-up study in 1 month if anatomic criteria indicate disease progression.
Partial metabolic response	>30% decrease in SUL peak; minimum 0.8-unit decrease. Verification with follow-up study if anatomic criteria indicate disease progression.
Progressive metabolic disease	>30% increase in SUL peak; minimum 0.8-unit increase in SUL peak. >75% increase in TLG of the five most active lesions. Visible increase in extent of FDG uptake. New lesions. Verification with follow-up study if anatomic criteria indicate complete or partial response.
Stable metabolic disease	Does not meet other criteria.

FDG, 2-[^{18}F] fluoro-2-deoxy-D-glucose; *SUL*, standardized uptake value corrected for lean body mass; *TLG*, total lesion glycolysis.

PMR. The percentage decline in SUL should be recorded, as well as the time in weeks after treatment was begun and after the last new lesions appeared.

Progressive metabolic disease (PMD) requires a 30% increase in FDG SUL peak, with a greater than 0.8 SUL unit increase in tumor SUV peak from baseline scan. This may be documented with a visible increase in the extent of FDG tumor uptake or the appearance of new FDG-avid lesions that are typical of cancer and not related to treatment effect or infection. PMD other than new visceral lesions should be confirmed on follow-up study within 1 month unless PMD also is clearly associated with PD as defined by RECIST 1.1. Additional clarification on the nuances of assessing progression can be found in the article, and a summary of the response categories is presented in Table 5.2.

Bone metastases are a common manifestation of advanced disease and can be detected by plain films, bone scanning, CT, MRI, and FDG-PET. RECIST 1.1 currently considers bone metastases with soft tissue masses greater than 10 mm to be measurable disease. The University of Texas MD Anderson Cancer Center criteria (MDA criteria) were developed specifically for bone metastases and can be used to assess response (Table 5.3). The MDA criteria divide response into four standard categories (CR, PR, PD, and SD) and include quantitative and qualitative assessments of the behavior of bone metastases (Table 5.4). A recent review by Costelloe and associates[27] showed that, in some studies, the MDA criteria better differentiate responders from nonresponders after chemotherapy. The MDA criteria can also show correlation with

TABLE 5.3 Response Evaluation Criteria in Solid Tumors 1.1 Nontarget Lesion Response Criteria

Objective response	Response Evaluation Criteria In Solid Tumors (RECIST) 1.1 nontarget lesions
Complete response	Disappearance of all nontarget lesions and normalization of tumor markers, confirmed at ≥4 weeks.
Nonprogressive disease	Persistence of one or more nontarget lesions or tumor markers above normal limits.
Progressive disease	Unequivocal progression of nontarget lesions or appearance of new lesion New "positive PET" scan with confirmed anatomic progression.[a]

[a]Stably positive PET is not progressive disease if it corresponds to anatomic nonprogressive disease.

PET, Positron emission tomography.

From Costelloe CM, Chuang HH, Madewell JE, Ueno NT. Cancer response criteria and bone metastases: RECIST 1.1, MDA and PERCIST. *J Cancer.* 2010;1:80-92.

TABLE 5.4 MD Anderson Response Criteria for Bone Metastases

CATEGORY OF RESPONSE	MD ANDERSON CRITERIA FOR BONE METASTASES
Complete response	Complete sclerotic fill-in of lytic lesions on x-ray or CT. Normalization of bone density on x-ray or CT. Normalization of signal intensity on MRI. Normalization of tracer uptake on SS.
Partial response	Development of a sclerotic rim or partial sclerotic fill-in of lytic lesions on x-ray or CT. Osteoblastic flare: interval visualization of lesions with sclerotic rims or new sclerotic lesions in the setting of other signs of PR and absence of progressive bony disease. ≥50% decrease in measurable lesions on x-ray, CT, or MRI. ≥50% subjective decrease in the size of ill-defined lesions on x-ray, CT, or MRI. ≥50% subjective decrease in tracer uptake on SS.
Progressive disease	≥25% increase in size of measurable lesions on x-ray, CT, or MRI. ≥25% subjective increase in the size of ill-defined lesions on x-ray, CT, or MRI ≥25% subjective increase in tracer uptake on SS. New bone metastases.
Stable disease	No change. <25% increase or <50% decrease in size of measurable lesions. <25% subjective increase or <50% subjective decrease in size of ill-defined lesions. No new bone metastases.

CT, Computed tomography; *MRI*, magnetic resonance imaging; *PR*, partial response; *SS*, skeletal scintigraphy.

From Costelloe CM, Chuang HH, Madewell JE, Ueno NT. Cancer response criteria and bone metastases: RECIST 1.1, MDA and PERCIST. *J Cancer.* 2010;1:80-92.

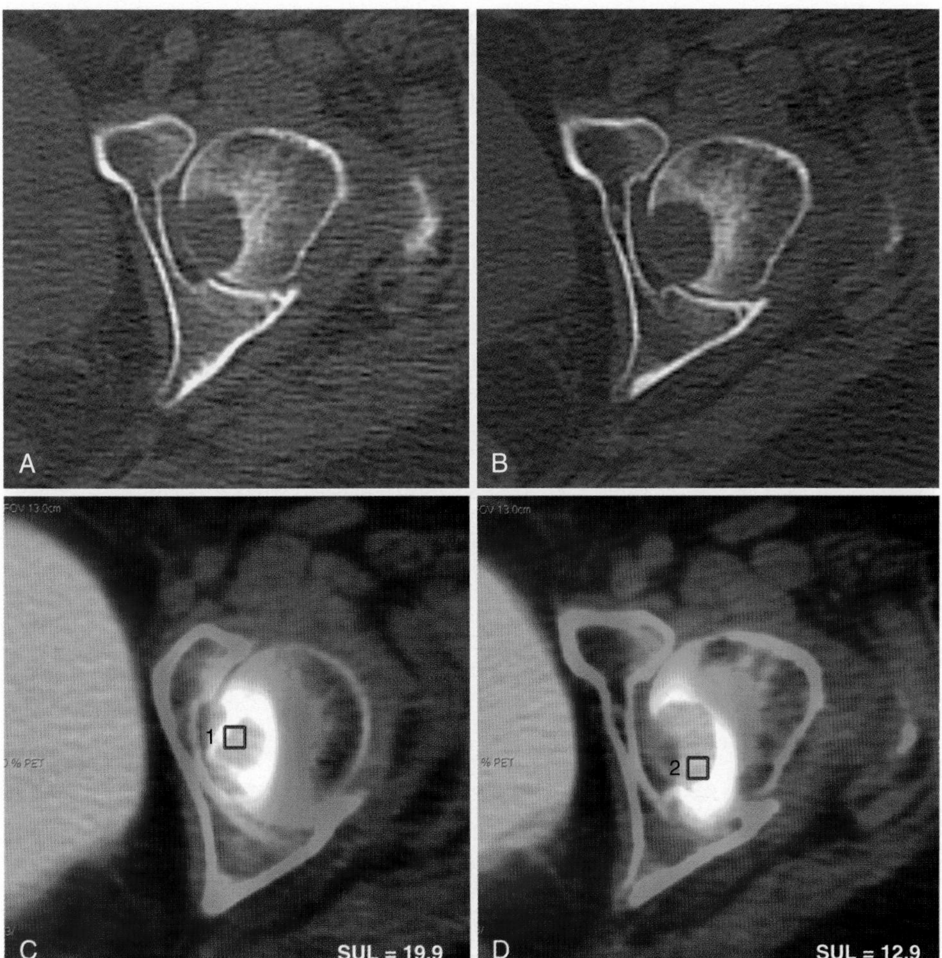

FIGURE 5.4. Metabolic response according to the Positron Emission Tomography Response Evaluation Criteria in Solid Tumors (PERCIST) criteria in the absence of anatomic response. **A,** The computed tomography (CT) portion of an 2-[^{18}F] fluoro-2-deoxy-D-glucose–positron emission tomography (PET)/CT scan in a patient with lung cancer demonstrates a lytic metastasis in the left femoral head. **B,** The CT from a PET/CT scan 2 months later demonstrates no anatomic change. The standardized uptake value corrected for lean body mass (SUL) peak (average SUL in a 1-cm^3 region of interest centered at the most active part of each tumor) changes from 19.8 **(C)** to 12.9 **(D),** representing a 35% decrease, which satisfies the minimal requirements for partial response (>30%) according to PERCIST. Assessment of tumor metabolism allowed therapeutic response to be measured in the absence of any other indication of change. (From Costelloe CM, Chuang HH, Madewell JE, Ueno NT. Cancer response criteria and bone metastases: RECIST 1.1, MDA and PERCIST. *J Cancer.* 2010;1:80-92.)

progression-free survival in breast cancer patients. MDA bone response criteria more closely reflect the behavior of bone metastases on radiography and CT, and can be used as guidelines for the interpretation of these studies, whether or not a patient is enrolled in a therapeutic trial (Fig. 5.4).

Beyond the indices discussed, which are essentially CT and FDG-PET parameters, multiple new techniques, including a range of functional MRI techniques, CT perfusion, novel PET/single-photon emission CT tracers, and microbubble ultrasonography are being developed. These new techniques may be selectively incorporated in the future as standards in evaluating response to therapy.[28]

IMMUNE-RELATED RESPONSE CRITERIA

There has been a tremendous progress in the field of oncological immunotherapy. Currently, multiple cancer immunotherapy trials are being conducted in the United States, and a few of the drugs have been approved by U.S. Food and Drug Administration for clinical application.[29] These include an anti–PD-1 antibody (Pembrolizumab), anti–PD-L1 and anti–PD-L2 antibodies (Nivolumab, Atezolizumab, Durvalumab), and an anti–CTLA-4 antibody (Ipilimumab). The adoption of immunotherapy has resulted in new findings regarding response to treatment.[30–32] Conventional response assessment criteria such as RECIST may not be sufficient in evaluating response to these therapies. Hence, newer imaging response criteria such as immune-related response evaluation criteria (irRC) and immune-related Response Evaluation Criteria In Solid Tumors (irRECIST) are being developed and implemented in many clinical trials to evaluate accurate treatment response to immune therapies.[33,34]

In 2004 to 2005, an integrative group of experts developed the irRC.[35] The irRC were adapted from the WHO criteria and designed to evaluate treatment response and recommendations on follow-up imaging of patients receiving immunotherapy (Fig. 5.5). Subsequently, the irRECIST criteria were implemented based on irRC for evaluating tumor burden in patients treated with immunotherapies.[36] Similar to RECIST, irRECIST uses unidimensional measurement of the lesion.[37] Most recently, consensus immune RECIST (iRECIST) guidelines were formulated for use in oncological immunotherapy trials, so as to facilitate data collection and evaluate treatment effect.[38] The concept of the iRECIST guidelines is very similar to that of RECIST 1.1 and irRECIST. Table 5.5 summarizes the key concepts of immune-related response criteria.

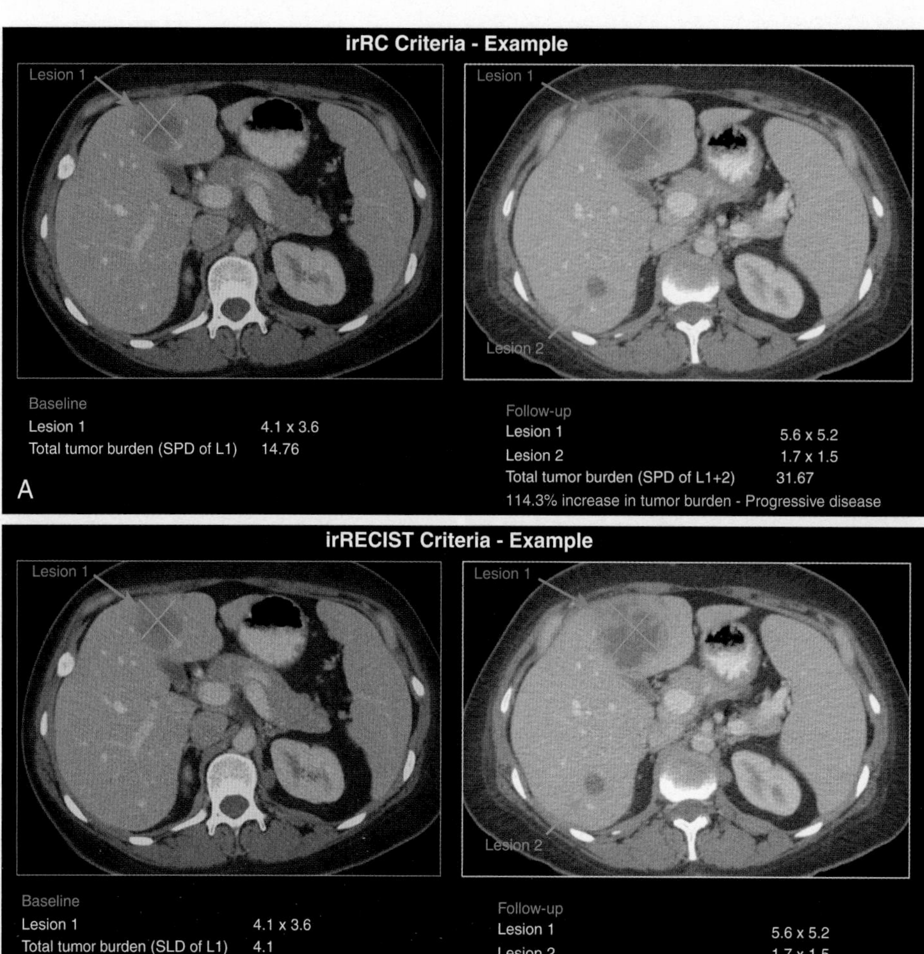

FIGURE 5.5. Progression of disease according to the immune-related response criteria (irRC) and immune-related Response Evaluation Criteria in Solid Tumors (irRECIST) criteria. A 25-year-old female with malignant metastatic melanoma in a phase 2 trial of lymphodepletion plus adoptive cell transfer with or without dendritic cell immunization. Panels **A** and **B** show case examples of baseline and follow-up study (14 weeks later) assessed by irRC and irRECIST criteria, respectively. The patient developed several new lesions (liver metastasis) on follow-up. Based on irRC criteria **(A)** a total of 10 new lesions (five per organ) can be assessed as "new target lesions." Hence, new liver lesions were assessed as a "new lesions," and total tumor burden was calculated from the sum of the product of diameters of the old and new target lesions. Based on irRECIST criteria **(B)** a total of five new lesions (two per organ) can be assessed as "new target lesions." Hence, a new liver lesion was assessed as a "new lesion," and the total tumor burden was calculated from the sum of the long-axis diameters of the old and new target lesions.

TABLE 5.5 Summary of Immune-Related Response Criteria

CATEGORY	IMMUNE-RELATED RESPONSE CRITERIA (irRC)	IMMUNE-RELATED RESPONSE EVALUATION CRITERIA IN SOLID TUMORS (irRECIST)	IMMUNE RESPONSE EVALUATION CRITERIA IN SOLID TUMORS (iRECIST)
Complete response	Complete disappearance of lesions. Confirmed by repeat, consecutive assessment at ≥4 weeks from initial assessment.	Complete disappearance of nonnodal lesions and <10-mm short axis for lymph nodes. Confirmation is not necessary.	Complete resolution of lesions. Confirmed ≥4 weeks.
Partial response	≥50% decrease in tumor burden relative to baseline. Confirmed by repeat, consecutive assessment at ≥4 weeks from initial assessment.	≥30% decrease in tumor burden relative to baseline.	≥30% decrease in tumor burden relative to baseline without new lesions or progression of nontarget lesions.
Stable disease	Does not meet other group criteria.	Does not meet other group criteria.	Does not meet other group criteria.
Progressive disease	≥25% increase in tumor burden relative to minimum recorded disease burden. Confirmed by repeat, consecutive assessment at ≥4 weeks from initial assessment.	Minimum 20% increase and a minimum absolute increase of 5 mm in tumor burden relative to nadir. Confirmed after 4 weeks from first progression.	Unconfirmed: New lesions, or ≥20% increase in tumor burden relative to first progression. Confirmed: New lesions, further increase in previous lesion size, or lesion from prior unconfirmed progressive disease on follow up scan after 4–8 weeks.

(*Continued*)

Table 5.5 Summary of Immune-Related Response Criteria *(Continued)*

CATEGORY	IMMUNE-RELATED RESPONSE CRITERIA (irRC)	IMMUNE-RELATED RESPONSE EVALUATION CRITERIA IN SOLID TUMORS (irRECIST)	IMMUNE RESPONSE EVALUATION CRITERIA IN SOLID TUMORS (iRECIST)
New lesions	Added into the tumor burden.	Greatest dimension of nonnodal lesion, short axis dimension of a node to be added to the tumor burden.	Assessed according to Response Evaluation Criteria in Solid Tumors 1.1 guidelines. New lesions constitute unconfirmed progressive disease. Confirmed progressive disease is only achieved if additional new lesions appear or there is an increase in size of prior new lesions or the presence of new lesions when none have previously been recorded
New nonmeasurable lesions	Not added into the tumor burden. Do not define progression, but exclude complete response.	New nonmeasurable lesions and to be followed quantitatively. Clear progression of nonmeasurable lesions leads to progressive disease. Persisting nonmeasurable lesions excludes complete response.	-

Key Points

- RECIST 1.1 criteria will be adopted by multiple investigators, cooperative groups, and industry and government entities in assessing treatment outcomes.
- PERCIST 1.0 is a proposed plan to use FDG-PET in assessing treatment response, and may be adopted and incorporated into clinical trials.
- Familiarity with and use of RECIST and PERCIST criteria will allow participation in clinical trials, and application of similar guidelines may improve individual patient care.
- Newer criteria such as irRC and iRECIST have been developed for assessment of response to immunotherapy.

REFERENCES

1. Jemal A, Siegel R, Xu J, Ward E. Cancer statistics, 2010. *CA Cancer J Clin*. 2010;60:277-300.
2. Moertel CG, Hanley JA. The effect of measuring error on the results of therapeutic trials in advanced cancer. *Cancer*. 1976;38:388-394.
3. Miller AB, Hoogstraten B, Staquet M, Winkler A. Reporting results of cancer treatment. *Cancer*. 1981;47:207-214.
4. Therasse P, Arbuck SG, Eisenhauer EA, et al. New guidelines to evaluate the response to treatment in solid tumors. European Organization for Research and Treatment of Cancer, National Cancer Institute of the United States, National Cancer Institute of Canada. *J Natl Cancer Inst*. 2000;92:205-216.
5. Eisenhauer EA, Therasse P, Bogaerts J, et al. New response evaluation criteria in solid tumours: revised RECIST guideline (version 1.1). *Eur J Cancer*. 2009;45:228-247.
6. Juweid ME, Wiseman GA, Vose JM, et al. Response assessment of aggressive non-Hodgkin's lymphoma by integrated International Workshop Criteria and fluorine-18-fluorodeoxyglucose positron emission tomography. *J Clin Oncol*. 2005;23:4652-4661.
7. Mikhaeel NG, Hutchings M, Fields PA, et al. FDG-PET after two to three cycles of chemotherapy predicts progression-free and overall survival in high-grade non-Hodgkin lymphoma. *Ann Oncol*. 2005;16:1514-1523.
8. Hicks RJ, MacManus MP, Matthews JP, et al. Early FDG-PET imaging after radical radiotherapy for non-small-cell lung cancer: inflammatory changes in normal tissues correlate with tumor response and do not confound therapeutic response evaluation. *Int J Radiat Oncol Biol Phys*. 2004;60:412-418.
9. MacManus MP, Hicks RJ, Matthews JP, et al. Positron emission tomography is superior to computed tomography scanning for response-assessment after radical radiotherapy or chemoradiotherapy in patients with non-small-cell lung cancer. *J Clin Oncol*. 2003;21:1285-1292.
10. Hicks RJ. Role of 18F-FDG PET in assessment of response in non-small cell lung cancer. *J Nucl Med*. 2009;50(suppl 1):S31-S42.
11. Weber WA, Wieder H. Monitoring chemotherapy and radiotherapy of solid tumors. *Eur J Nucl Med Mol Imaging*. 2006;33(suppl 1):27-37.
12. Krak NC, van der Hoeven JJ, Hoekstra OS, et al. Measuring [^{18}F] FDG uptake in breast cancer during chemotherapy: comparison of analytical methods. *Eur J Nucl Med Mol Imaging*. 2003;30:674-681.
13. Graham MM, Peterson LM, Hayward RM. Comparison of simplified quantitative analyses of FDG uptake. *Nucl Med Biol*. 2000;27:647-655.
14. Ramos CD, Erdi YE, Gonen M, et al. FDG-PET standardized uptake values in normal anatomical structures using iterative reconstruction segmented attenuation correction and filtered back-projection. *Eur J Nucl Med*. 2001;28:155-164.
15. Yeung HW, Sanches A, Squire OD, et al. Standardized uptake value in pediatric patients: an investigation to determine the optimum measurement parameter. *Eur J Nucl Med Mol Imaging*. 2002;29:61-66.
16. Mawlawi O, Erasmus JJ, Munden RF, et al. Quantifying the effect of IV contrast media on integrated PET/CT: clinical evaluation. *AJR Am J Roentgenol*. 1862006308-319.
17. Mawlawi O, Pan T, Macapinlac HA. PET/CT imaging techniques, considerations, and artifacts. *J Thorac Imaging*. 2006;21:99-110.
18. Pan T, Mawlawi O, Luo D, et al. Attenuation correction of PET cardiac data with low-dose average CT in PET/CT. *Med Phys*. 2006;33:3931-3938.
19. Tonkopi E, Chi PC, Mawlawi O, et al. Average CT in PET studies of colorectal cancer patients with metastasis in the liver and esophageal cancer patients. *J Appl Clin Med Phys*. 2010;11:3073.
20. Chi PC, Mawlawi O, Luo D, et al. Effects of respiration-averaged computed tomography on positron emission tomography/computed tomography quantification and its potential impact on gross tumor volume delineation. *Int J Radiat Oncol Biol Phys*. 2008;71:890-899.
21. Delbeke D, Coleman RE, Guiberteau MJ, et al. Procedure guideline for tumor imaging with 18F-FDG PET/CT 1.0. *J Nucl Med*. 2006;47:885-895.
22. Boellaard R, O'Doherty MJ, Weber WA, et al. FDG PET and PET/CT: EANM procedure guidelines for tumour PET imaging: version 1.0. *Eur J Nucl Med Mol Imaging*. 2010;37:181-200.
23. Wahl RL, Jacene H, Kasamon Y, Lodge MA. From RECIST to PERCIST: evolving considerations for PET response criteria in solid tumors. *J Nucl Med*. 2009;50(suppl 1):S122-S150.
24. Shankar LK, Hoffman JM, Bacharach S, et al. Consensus recommendations for the use of 18F-FDG PET as an indicator of therapeutic

response in patients in National Cancer Institute Trials. *J Nucl Med.* 2006;47:1059-1066.
25. Avril N, Sassen S, Schmalfeldt B, et al. Prediction of response to neoadjuvant chemotherapy by sequential F-18-fluorodeoxyglucose positron emission tomography in patients with advanced-stage ovarian cancer. *J Clin Oncol.* 2005;23:7445-7453.
26. Cheson BD, Pfistner B, Juweid ME, et al. Revised response criteria for malignant lymphoma. *J Clin Oncol.* 2007;25:579-586.
27. Costelloe CM, Chuang HH, Madewell JE, Ueno NT. Cancer response criteria and bone metastases: RECIST 1.1, MDA and PERCIST. *J Cancer.* 2010;1:80-92.
28. Padhani AR, Miles KA. Multiparametric imaging of tumor response to therapy. *Radiology.* 2010;256:348-364.
29. Hoos A. Development of immuno-oncology drugs - from CTLA4 to PD1 to the next generations. *Nat Rev Drug Discov.* 2016;15(4):235-247.
30. Hodi FS, Butler M, Oble DA, et al. Immunologic and clinical effects of antibody blockade of cytotoxic T lymphocyte-associated antigen 4 in previously vaccinated cancer patients. *Proc Natl Acad Sci U S A.* 2008;105(8):3005-3010.
31. Hodi FS, Oble DA, Drappatz J, et al. CTLA-4 blockade with ipilimumab induces significant clinical benefit in a female with melanoma metastases to the CNS. *Nat Clin Pract Oncol.* 2008;5(9):557-561.
32. Hoos A, Parmiani G, Hege K, et al. A clinical development paradigm for cancer vaccines and related biologics. *J Immunother.* 2007;30(1):1-15.
33. Carter BW, Bhosale PR, Yang WT. Immunotherapy and the role of imaging. *Cancer.* 2018;124(14):2906-2922.
34. Somarouthu B, Lee SI, Urban T, Sadow CA, Harris GJ, Kambadakone A. Immune-related tumour response assessment criteria: a comprehensive review. *Br J Radiol.* 2018;91(1084):20170457.
35. Wolchok JD, Hoos A, O'Day S, et al. Guidelines for the evaluation of immune therapy activity in solid tumors: immune-related response criteria. *Clin Cancer Res.* 2009;15(23):7412-7420.
36. Nishino M, Jagannathan JP, Krajewski KM, et al. Personalized tumor response assessment in the era of molecular medicine: cancer-specific and therapy-specific response criteria to complement pitfalls of RECIST. *AJR Am J Roentgenol.* 2012;198(4):737-745.
37. Nishino M, Giobbie-Hurder A, Gargano M, Suda M, Ramaiya NH, Hodi FS. Developing a common language for tumor response to immunotherapy: immune-related response criteria using unidimensional measurements. *Clin Cancer Res.* 2013;19(14):3936-3943.
38. Seymour L, Bogaerts J, Perrone A, et al. iRECIST: guidelines for response criteria for use in trials testing immunotherapeutics. *Lancet Oncol.* 2017;18(3):e143-e152.

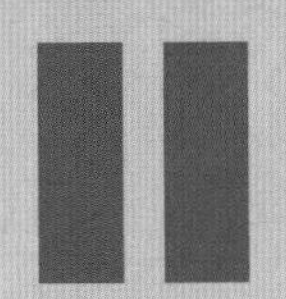

PART II HEAD AND NECK

CHAPTER 6 Head and Neck Cancer

Tara Massini, M.D.; and Reordan DeJesus, M.D.

INTRODUCTION

Head and neck cancer is a topic that at first glance can be somewhat formidable, but has considerable shared risk factors as other tumors, and is often found synchronously or incidentally on workup for other lesions. Recognizing that many radiologists prefer to keep their focus at or below the level of the clavicles, we aim to make head and neck cancer less of an enigma. In this chapter, we will present a brief overview of the types of tumors encountered and their patterns of spread. We will focus on tumors arising in the oral cavity, pharynx, and larynx, as these are the most commonly encountered. We will also briefly address lesions arising in the nasal cavity, paranasal sinuses, and salivary gland tumors, as well as spread patterns of skin cancer as it relates to this region in the workup of an unknown primary, and finally some unique examples of lymphoma isolated to the head and neck. Primary intracranial, intraorbital, and temporal bone tumors are beyond the scope of this chapter. Thyroid neoplasms will be discussed separately in another chapter.

EPIDEMIOLOGY AND CLINICAL PRESENTATION

Approximately 63,000 new cases of oral, pharyngeal, or laryngeal head and neck cancer are diagnosed each year, and head and neck cancer is responsible for over 14,000 cancer deaths per year.[1] Men have a slightly higher incidence of developing head and neck cancer.

A high percentage of head and neck cancers are found when patients present with palpable lymphadenopathy, and localizing a potential primary site with imaging can help direct inspection by the otolaryngologist (ENT). The primary mass may also be palpable when arising in the salivary glands.

Patients with head and neck cancers frequently present with localized and referred pain, otalgia being a well-recognized presenting symptom in patients with hypopharyngeal and oropharyngeal pathology. Tumors also cause dysfunction of the affected and adjacent structures. Nasopharyngeal masses may obstruct the Eustachian tube and present with a unilateral middle ear and mastoid effusion, with or without ear pain and fullness or generalized headache (Fig. 6.1). Dysphagia and dysphonia are also frequent complaints that may lead to workup for malignancy.

PATHOLOGY AND RISK FACTORS

Mucosal Squamous Cell Carcinoma

Squamous cell carcinoma (SCC) forms the vast majority of primary head and neck tumors, as the mucosal surface throughout the head and neck region is lined by squamous epithelium. SCCs comprise about 90% of all visceral compartment lesions and follow a characteristic progression, from worsening grades of dysplasia to carcinoma *in situ* to invasive disease. Invasive disease diagnosis requires adequate sampling of the lesion.

Historically, the greatest risk factor for SCC has been tobacco use. Hence, a large number of patients with head and neck cancers overlap with the lung cancer screening population, and their head and neck tumors may be found incidentally during workup for lung nodules, with one example shown in Fig. 6.2. Thankfully, as tobacco use has slightly declined, this has also affected the rates of tobacco-associated cancers.

FIGURE 6.1. Nasopharyngeal carcinoma. Noncontrast head computed tomography for headache shows unilateral mastoid opacification (**A**, blue arrow) with ipsilateral soft tissue fullness in the nasopharynx (**A** and **B**, orange arrows) and probable infiltration of the parapharyngeal space.

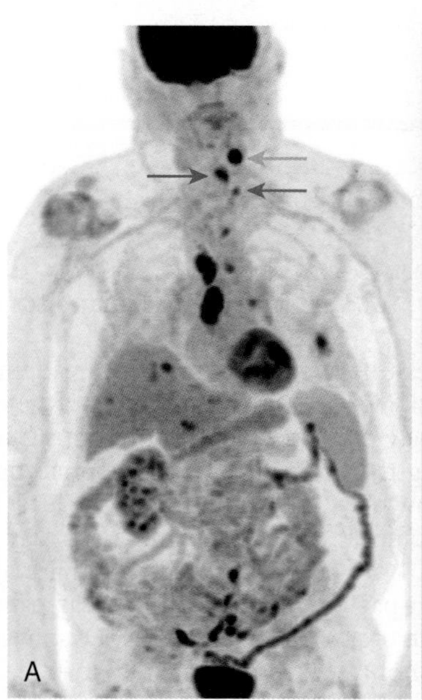

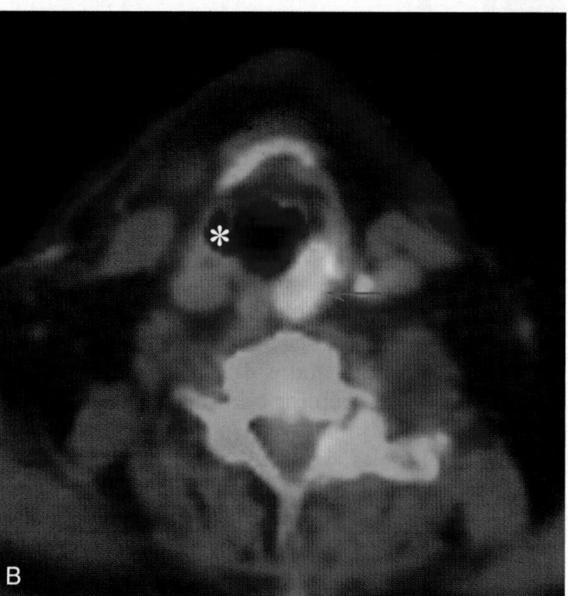

FIGURE 6.2. Squamous cell carcinoma of the hypopharynx. **A**, Maximum intensity projection image from 2-[18F] fluoro-2-deoxy-D-glucose–positron emission tomography for staging of lung cancer shows multiple foci of activity in the left side of the neck (arrows) in addition to the primary lung mass, mediastinal adenopathy, and liver and bone metastases. **B**, The axial fused images through the neck localize one of these foci to the entrance of the left pyriform sinus (dark blue arrow), with ipsilateral level III and level IV lymph nodes (**A**, orange and red arrows). The normal right pyriform sinus (star) has a thin mucosal lining and is air-filled.

However, in the last couple of decades there has been an increasingly recognized association between multiple subtypes of the human papillomavirus (HPV) and SCCs, particularly of the oral cavity and oropharynx,[2,3] with ongoing research looking into the role of HPV in SCC at other subsites.[4,5] Oropharyngeal SCCs have become the most common HPV-associated tumors, surpassing cervical and anal cancers.[6] HPV-associated tumors are identified by positive immunohistochemistry staining for overexpression of p16. The importance of this distinction will be discussed in more detail later in the chapter.

Skin Cancers

Skin cancers, although not unique to the head and neck, are frequently encountered in this region. Sun exposure is associated with 90% of nonmelanoma skin cancers, of which basal cell carcinomas and SCCs are the most frequent types, and it is estimated that 85% of these occur in the head and neck.[7] They present as a superficial lesion or, in patients who do not provide or recognize a history of skin cancer, in a region where "something" was previously cut/lasered/frozen off or with regional metastatic disease (Fig. 6.3). Skin cancers have a high risk of developing at multiple sites in patients with a history of long-term sun exposure or in immunosuppressed patients (i.e., posttransplant or autoimmune disease treatment or human immunodeficiency virus infection).

Neglected basal cell carcinomas can have exhibit full-thickness invasion through the skin, scalp, skull, and dura and into the brain, as shown in Fig. 6.4, but are unlikely to have nodal metastases.[8,9] Melanoma is unfortunately common at all sites, but will be discussed in more detail in a later chapter.

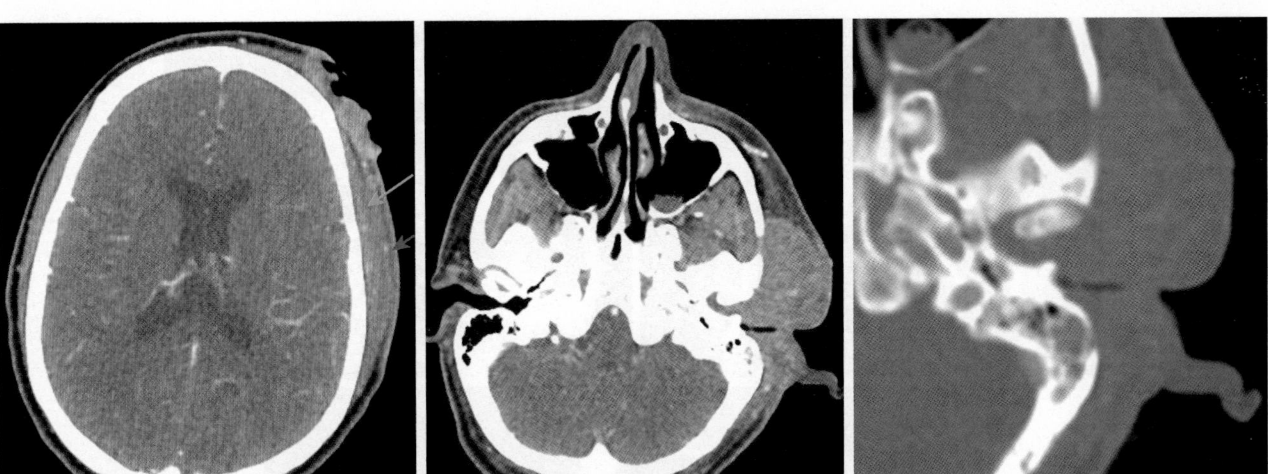

FIGURE 6.3. Cutaneous squamous cell carcinoma. **A**, There is a large ulcerated cutaneous and subcutaneous mass in the left frontal scalp, abutting bone on its deep margin. There is marked thickening of the temporalis muscle (orange arrow) and infiltration of the subcutaneous fat (blue arrow) posterior to the dominant lesion. **B**, There is also marked infiltration of the ipsilateral periauricular soft tissues and parotid gland reflecting a large nodal conglomerate with extranodal extension. **C**, Coned-in images on bone window at the same level as in **(B)** show early invasion of the mastoid, as well as widening of the left temporomandibular joint owing to tumor invasion.

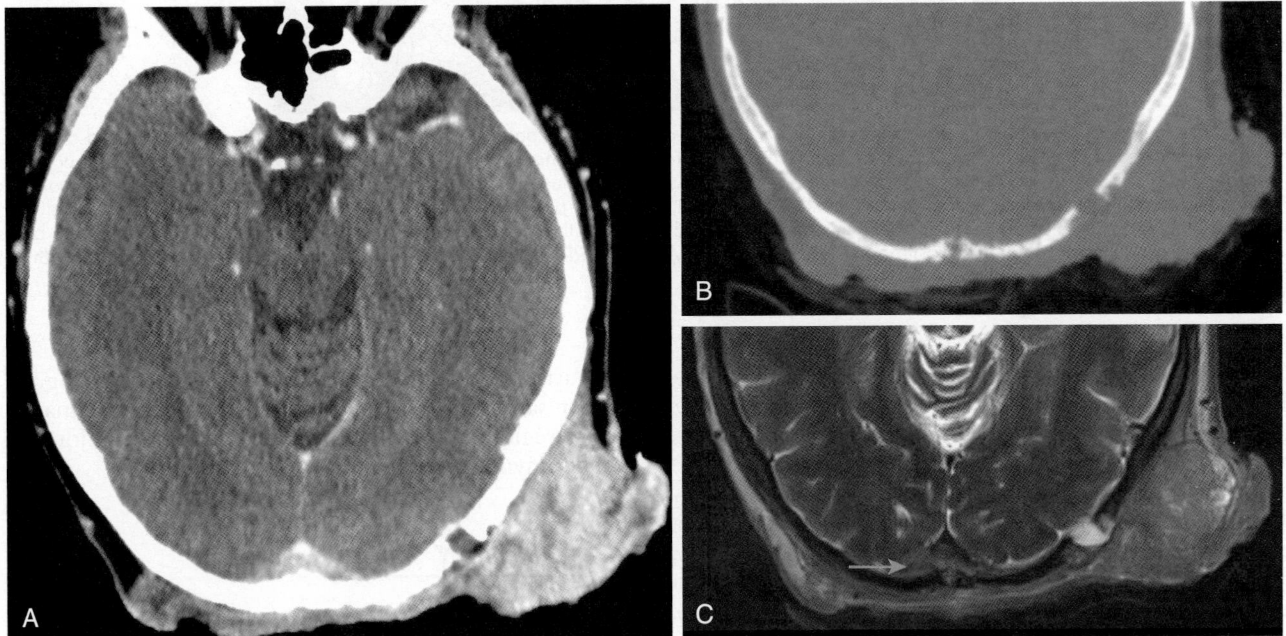

FIGURE 6.4. Basal cell carcinoma, direct intracranial invasion. Axial computed tomography with contrast **(A)** shows a large cutaneous mass with cortical irregularity and motheaten appearance through the diploic space of the adjacent calvarium on bone window **(B)**. Subsequent magnetic resonance imaging **(C)** confirmed tumor invasion of the superior sagittal sinus.

Lymphoma

Lymphoma is common in the cervical region because of the relatively high concentration of lymph nodes in the neck in relation to the rest of the body, as well as the presence of lymphoid tissue throughout the pharynx, concentrating in Waldeyer's ring from the level of the adenoids in the nasopharynx to the palatine tonsils and the lingual tonsillar tissue in the oropharynx. Lymphoma can also present as an extranodal infiltrative mass almost anywhere in the head and neck region, much like in the rest of the body. An example is shown in Fig. 6.5.

Salivary Gland Tumors

Adenocarcinoma, adenoid cystic carcinoma, and mucoepidermoid carcinoma are the most common tumors to arise from the glandular tissue in the major salivary glands—the parotid, submandibular, and sublingual glands—and in submucosal minor salivary glands just deep to the mucosal surface in the visceral compartment. Other malignant lesions such as acinic cell carcinoma, malignant mixed tumor, or oncocytic carcinomas are extremely rare.

In the parotid glands, the majority (80%) of incidental or palpable nodules are benign.[10] These can frequently be

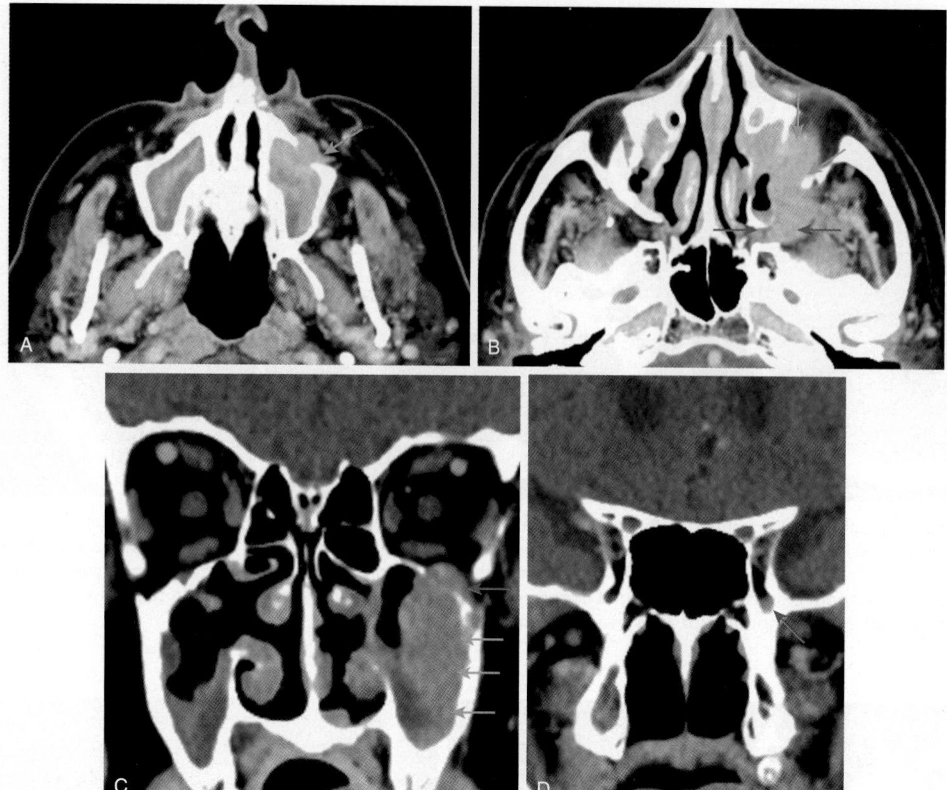

FIGURE 6.5. Extranodal lymphoma, left maxillary sinus. This patient presented with palpable fullness over the left face initially noticed after a fall with facial trauma and progressing for several months. Axial **(A** and **B)** and coronal **(C** and **D)** images from contrasted maxillofacial computed tomography (CT) showed an enhancing infiltrative mass deep to the superficial musculoaponeurotic system on the left near the infraorbital canal and invading through the anterior wall of the left maxillary sinus **(A)**, extending posteriorly along the canal for V2 **(B** and **C)** to the level of the pterygopalatine fossa **(B**, blue arrows**)** and subtle involvement as far posterior as the foramen rotundum **(D**, blue arrow**)**. Percutaneous core biopsy yielded a high-grade B-cell lymphoma. Positron emission tomography/CT showed no other sites of disease, and the patient was treated with both chemotherapy and localized radiation.

found incidentally on staging 2-[^{18}F] fluoro-2-deoxy-D-glucose (FDG)–positron emission tomography (PET)/computed tomography (CT) for unrelated pathologies as metabolically active lesions, and include oncocytic (Warthin) tumors (as in Fig. 6.6) and benign mixed tumors (pleomorphic adenomas). Benign mixed tumors, however, do have a low malignant potential of approximately 5%. Additionally, it is important to consider metastatic adenopathy from a cutaneous malignancy in the differential for parotid nodules.

Miscellaneous

Less common cancers include esthesioneuroblastoma and sinonasal undifferentiated carcinoma. Nasopharyngeal carcinomas, as well as some forms of aggressive lymphomas, have been associated with Epstein–Barr virus (EBV). Nasal SCCs are associated with woodworking and other inhaled substances (e.g., formaldehyde) that contribute to chronic irritation.

Primary and metastatic osseous or cartilaginous tumors can also occur in the calvarium and cervical spine, as well as the skull base, and osseous metastases will be covered in detail in a later chapter. Interestingly, primary osteosarcomas or chondrosarcomas also occasionally occur in the paranasal sinuses or nasal cavity, and chondrosarcomas can arise in the laryngeal skeleton, as seen in Fig. 6.7. Other sarcomas can also occur in the neck and maxillofacial region, primarily in the pediatric population (e.g., rhabdomyosarcomas).

ANATOMY

Mucosal Surfaces

The visceral compartment in the head and neck can be simplistically thought of as the entryway for the aerodigestive tract. This can be separated into subsites that ultimately separate below the plane of the hyoid bone into the aero- (larynx→trachea) and the -digestive (hypopharynx→esophagus) pathways.

The most anterior and superior subsite is the nasal cavity. The paranasal sinuses surround and drain into the nasal cavity from anteriorly, laterally, posteriorly, and superiorly. The nasopharynx is located posterior to the nasal cavity from the level of the posterior choanae and anterior and inferior to the skull base. It is separated from the more inferior oropharynx by the soft palate and uvula.

The oropharynx is located posterior to the oral cavity from the level of the anterior tonsillar pillar and anterior to the upper cervical spine. It is separated from the more

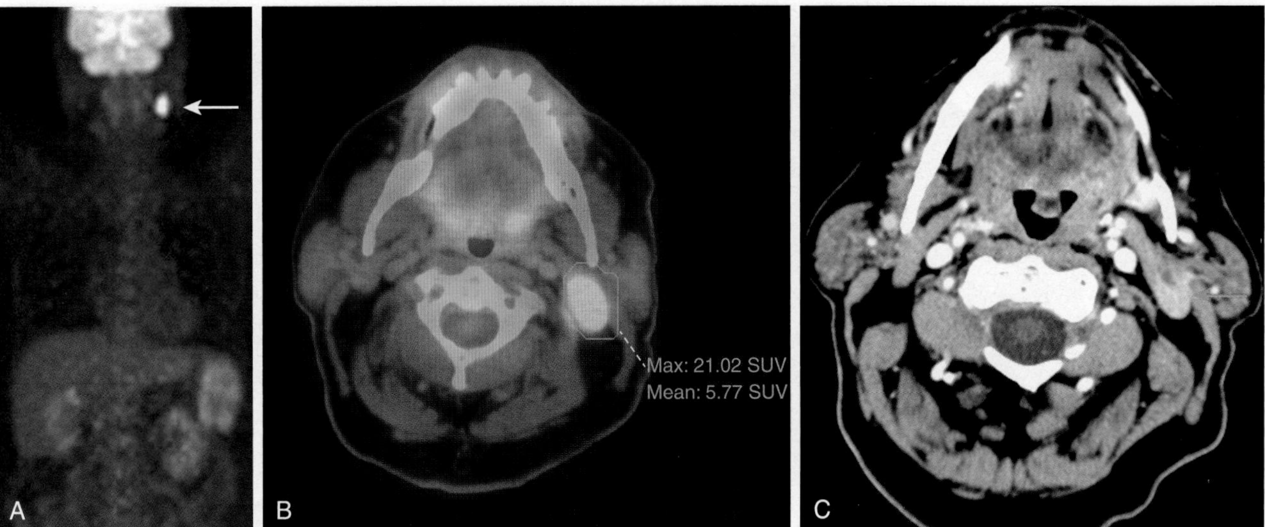

FIGURE 6.6. Warthin tumor on positron emission tomography (PET). **A**, Maximum intensity projection image from 2-[^{18}F] fluoro-2-deoxy-D-glucose–PET shows an incidental hypermetabolic focus in the neck. **B**, Fused axial PET/computed tomography (CT) image localizes this activity to a nodule deep to the sternocleidomastoid muscle, mimicking a level II lymph node, with a maximum standardized uptake value of 21. **C**, Comparison with a CT from 6 years earlier shows that this nodule had not significantly changed in size, slightly hyperenhancing relative to the adjacent posterior belly of the digastric muscle. Fine needle aspiration confirmed a benign Warthin tumor, exophytic from the deep lobe of the parotid gland.

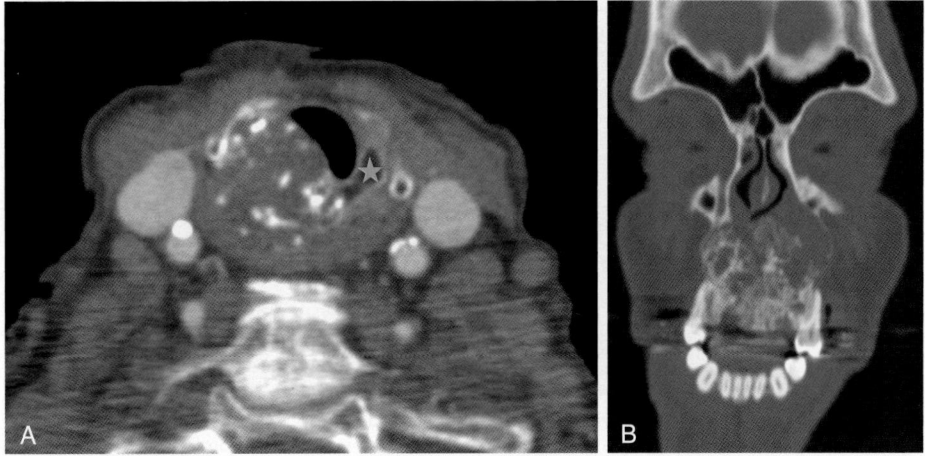

FIGURE 6.7. Chondrosarcoma. **A**, This patient with hoarseness had a chondroid lesion expanding the right side of the cricoid cartilage. The relatively normal left side is marked with a star. **B**, Different patient with chondrosarcoma of the nose and involving the full thickness of the hard palate and maxillary alveolar ridge.

inferior hypopharynx and larynx by the plane of the hyoid bone. The oropharynx includes the tonsillar pillars, the palatine tonsils, the base of tongue, the glossotonsillar sulcus, and the vallecula.

The oral cavity is inferior to the nasal cavity, and they are separated from each other by the hard palate. The oral cavity includes the buccal and gingival mucosa, the alveolar ridge and teeth, the retromolar trigone, the hard palate, the oral (moveable) tongue, and the floor of the mouth. An example of an oral cavity mass is shown in Fig. 6.8. The floor of the mouth is separated from the submandibular space by the sling-like mylohyoid muscle and its attachments.

The larynx and the posteriorly located hypopharynx are separated by the laryngeal inlet, formed by the free border of the epiglottis and the aryepiglottic folds. The larynx can be separated into the supraglottic, glottic, and subglottic larynx. The supraglottic larynx includes the epiglottis, the false vocal cords, and the laryngeal ventricle. The epiglottis is a supraglottic laryngeal structure with a mobile suprahyoid portion that moves to cover the entry to the larynx and diverting food from entering the respiratory tract during swallowing, and a fixed infrahyoid portion, forming the anterior aspect of the supraglottic cavity, that terminates in a petiole, with the thyroepiglottic ligament attaching it to the thyroid cartilage just above the false vocal folds. The pharyngoepiglottic and aryepiglottic folds run from the lateral margin of the epiglottis to the lateral walls of the pharynx and the arytenoid cartilages, respectively. The false vocal cords (also known as the vestibular folds) are a mucosal fold covering the vestibular ligament, which is surrounded by fat (paraglottic fat). The laryngeal ventricle is a small air-filled structure that separates the false vocal folds from the true vocal folds (glottis). A supraglottic mass is shown in Fig. 6.9.

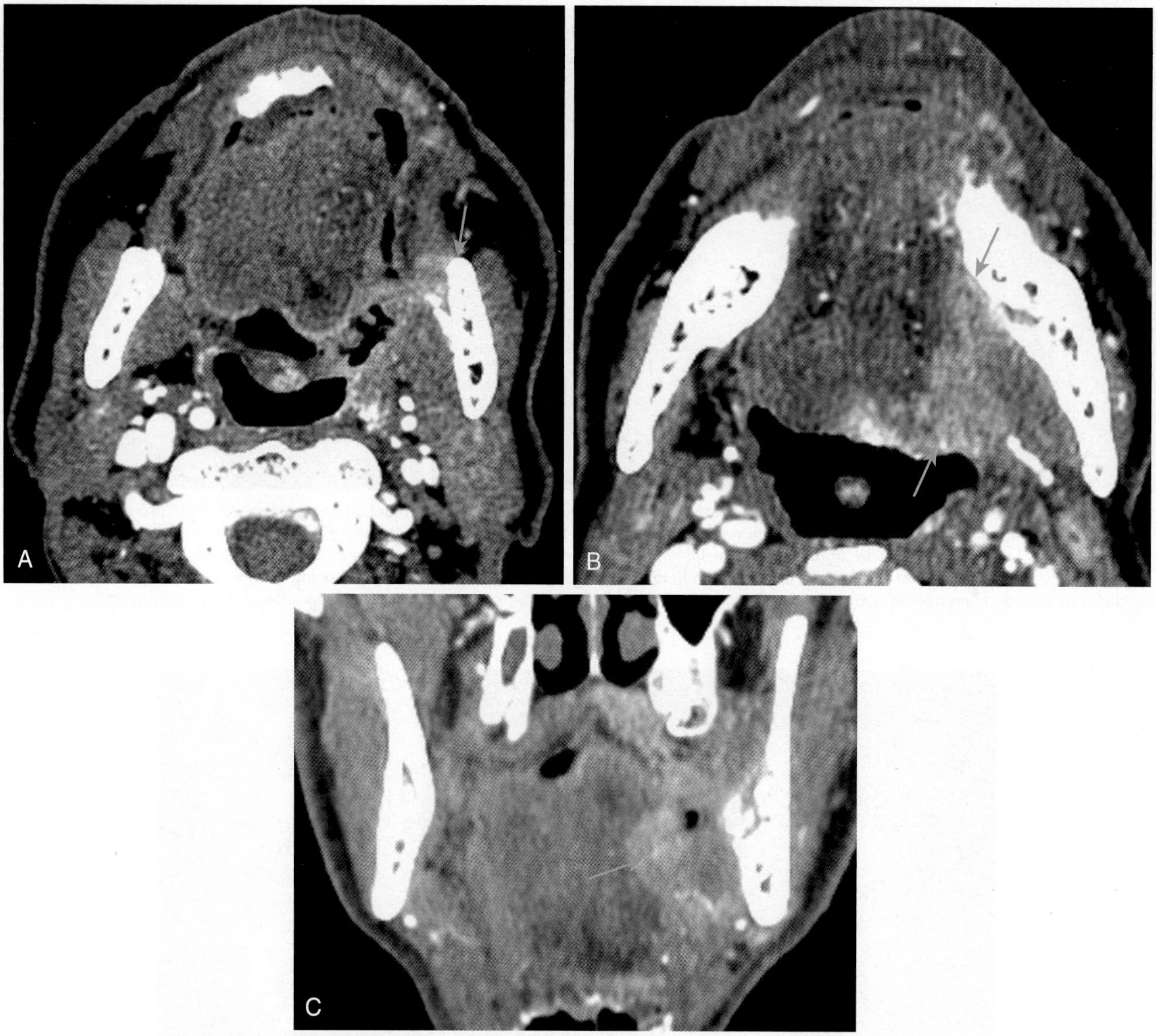

Figure 6.8. Squamous cell carcinoma of the oral cavity. Contrast computed tomography images show an enhancing tumor **(A)** at the left retromolar trigone with invasion of the mandible. There is involvement of the posterior and lateral oral tongue seen on axial **(B)** and coronal **(C)** images. Bone invasion defines T4 disease.

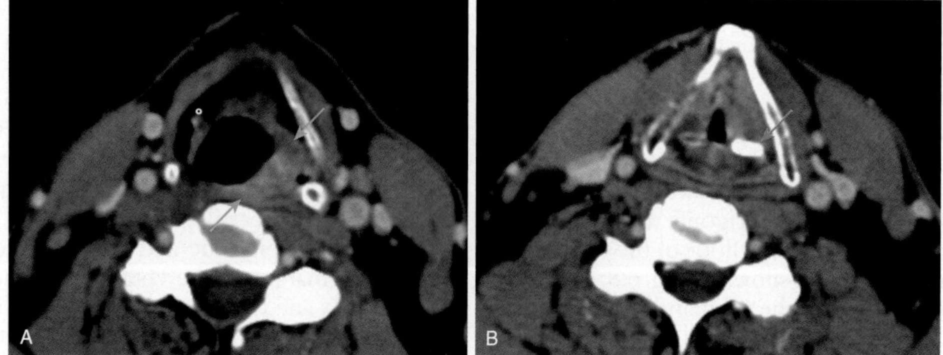

Figure 6.9. Squamous cell carcinoma of the supraglottic larynx. **A**, There is marked thickening of the left aryepiglottic fold extending to the posterior pharyngeal wall. This narrows the entrance site of the left pyriform sinus but does not circumferentially involve the mucosa of the pyriform sinus. **B**, Note the marked asymmetric sclerosis of the ipsilateral arytenoid cartilage, which may be reactive but remains nonspecific.

The glottis is formed by the true vocal folds, which are a mucosal fold covering the vocal ligaments, which is surrounded by muscle (vocalis and thyroarytenoid muscles). The subglottic portion of the larynx is a short segment of the larynx below the glottis that becomes contiguous with the cervical trachea.

The hypopharynx can be separated into the paired pyriform sinuses, the posterior pharyngeal wall, and the postcricoid region, which leads to the esophageal verge and becomes contiguous with the cervical esophagus.

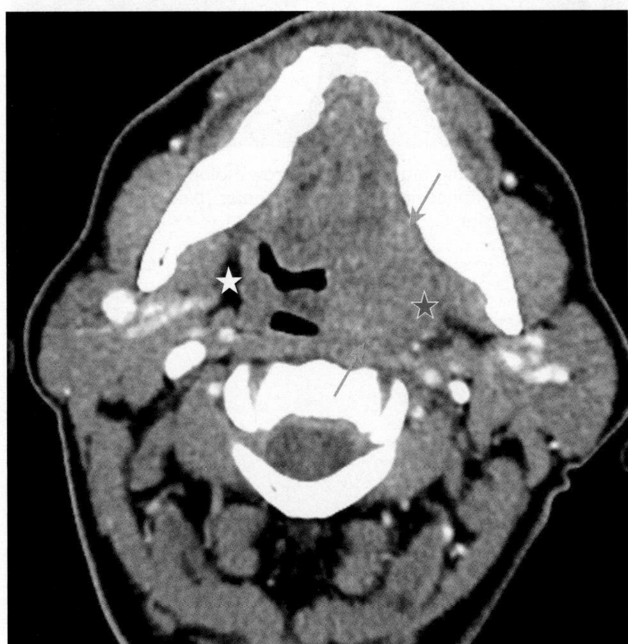

Figure 6.10. Parapharyngeal space. Computed tomography at time of diagnosis shows a large, locally infiltrative left tonsillar mass (orange arrows) invading the base of tongue, and early invasion of the floor of the mouth. There was infiltration of the left parapharyngeal space (PPS) (blue star). Normal right PPS (white star).

Parapharyngeal and Retropharyngeal Spaces

The parapharyngeal space is lateral to the pharynx and at risk of direct invasion by tumor in the pharynx (Fig. 6.10). This can be separated into prestyloid and retrostyloid regions in relation to the styloid process. The carotid sheath runs in the retrostyloid parapharyngeal space.

The retropharyngeal space is a thin fat plane posterior to the pharynx and forms a potential space that is contiguous inferiorly with the posterior mediastinum. It contains retropharyngeal lymph nodes which receive lymphatic drainage from the pharynx and the thyroid.

Salivary glands

The parotid glands are the largest of the major salivary glands and track from the preauricular region to approximately the level of the angle of the mandible. The main parotid duct runs roughly parallel to the zygomatic arch, slightly deeper and more inferiorly, posterior to the facial vein (Fig. 6.11), and crosses through a gap in the buccinator muscle across from the second maxillary molar tooth.

The submandibular glands are paired glands in the submandibular space, inferolateral to the mylohyoid muscle. The ducts drain anteromedially through the floor of the mouth to drain anteriorly at the puncta just behind the mandibular symphysis.

The sublingual glands lie lateral to the submandibular duct in the anterior one-third to one-half of the floor of the mouth. The ducts mostly open in the mouth (plica sublingualis), but some may partially join the submandibular ducts.

Minor salivary gland tissue can be found deep to the epithelial surface, in greatest concentration along the hard and soft palate (Fig. 6.12), the oral cavity, and the pharynx.

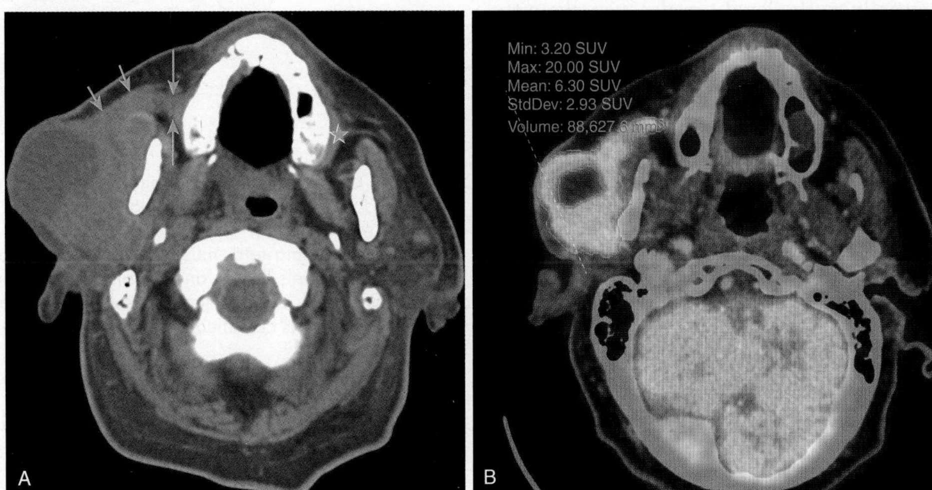

Figure 6.11. Tumor growth along the parotid duct. Computed tomography (**A**) and positron emission tomography (**B**) demonstrate extension of tumor along the markedly thickened and hypermetabolic right parotid duct, contiguous with bulky metastatic adenopathy in the parotid in this patient with a history of regional skin cancer.

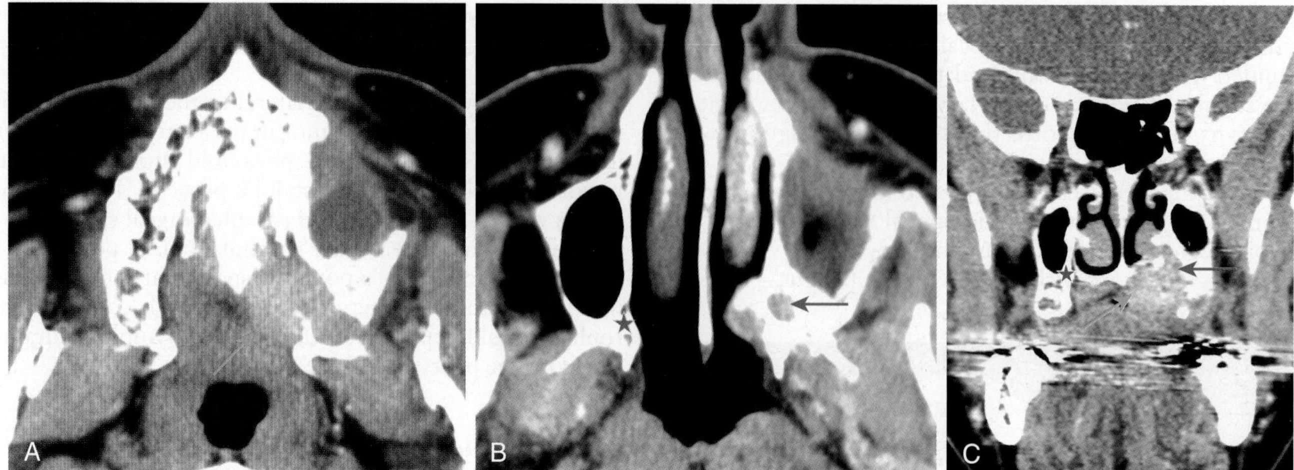

FIGURE 6.12. Mucoepidermoid carcinoma of the hard palate. There is a submucosal enhancing mass (orange arrows) along the posterior aspect of the hard palate, with bone erosion. There is marked enlargement of the foramina and enhancement along the greater (*blue arrows*) and lesser palatine nerves. The contralateral normal palatine neural foramina are adjacent to the blue star.

Lymphatics

Lymphoid tissue is present in abundance within the pharynx, lining Waldeyer's ring circumferentially from the posterior nasopharynx (adenoids) to the palatine tonsils and the lingual tonsillar tissue along the base of tongue and tapering out toward the vallecula.

Cervical lymph nodes are also numerous, and the location of nodes is important both in the evaluation of suspected primary sites for a patient presenting with adenopathy and in accurate staging of at-risk nodes from a known primary.[11,12] The standard cervical nodal stations are denoted by levels I through VI, as detailed later and as per the diagram shown in Fig. 6.13.

Level I lymph nodes are the most anteriorly located, situated below the mylohyoid muscle and above the hyoid bone, anterior to the posterior border of the submandibular glands. Level I is subdivided into level IA (submental) and level IB (submandibular) by the medial margins of the anterior belly of the digastric muscles. The lips and oral cavity drain preferentially to the level I nodes, usually with subsequent sequential drainage to levels II through IV.

Level II lymph nodes make up the superior internal jugular chain. These extend from the skull base to the lower margin of the body of hyoid bone, posterior to the posterior edge of the submandibular glands and anterior to the posterior edge of the sternocleidomastoid (SCM) muscle. Level II is conventionally subdivided into level IIA and level IIB by the jugular vein; level IIA nodes lie adjacent to the vein (Fig. 6.14), and level IIB nodes lie posterior to and separated by an identifiable fat plane from the vein, but still deep to the SCM.

Level III lymph nodes are also deep to the SCM and run along the course of the internal jugular vein, below the inferior border of the body of the hyoid bone and above the inferior margin of the cricoid cartilage.

Level IV nodes make up the lowest internal jugular chain lymph nodes, located inferior to the inferior margin of the cricoid cartilage and anterior to the posterior edge of the SCM.

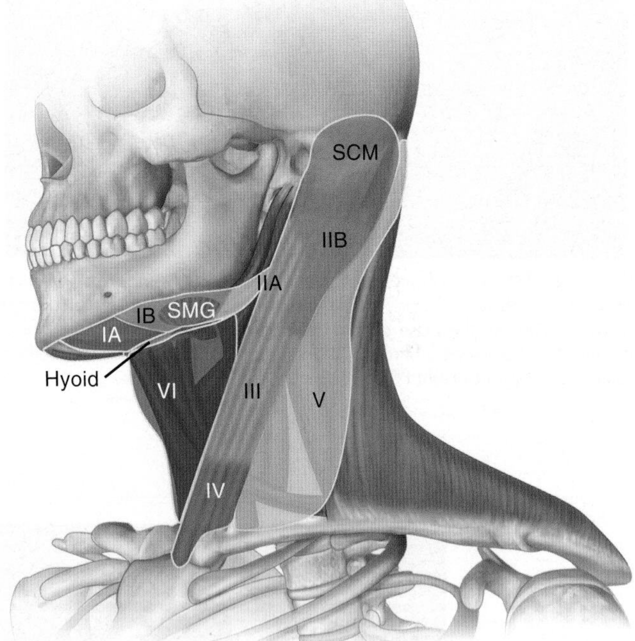

FIGURE 6.13. Cervical lymph node stations. Volume-rendered computed tomography with nodal stations as marked. Note that level II begins posterior to the submandibular gland (*SMG*), and the sternocleidomastoid muscle ([*SCM*]; denoted in lavender) lies superficial to levels IIB, III, and IV (and most of level IIA). Intraparotid, retropharyngeal, external jugular, suboccipital, and facial nodes are not included in this classification system.

Level V denotes the posterior cervical chain (posterior triangle), posterior to the posterior border of the SCM. This chain has rich drainage from the skin. This level can be further subdivided into levels VA and VB by the inferior margin of the cricoid cartilage, but this is not generally necessary unless pathology is isolated to one or the other,

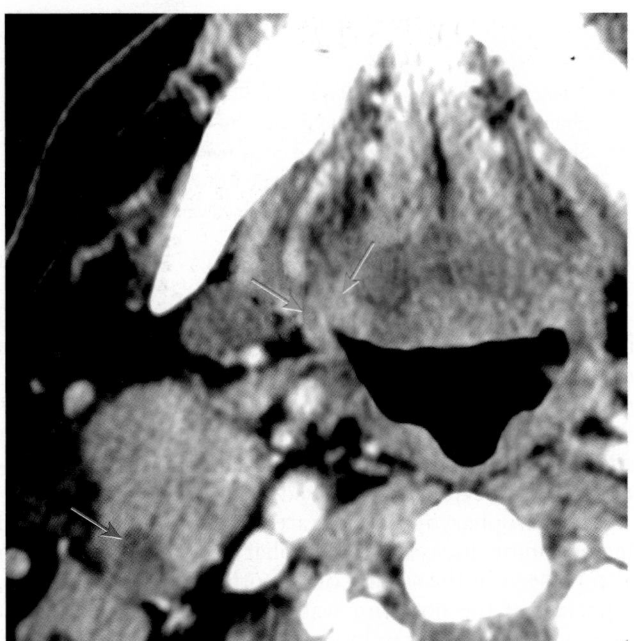

Figure 6.14. Human papillomavirus–associated squamous cell carcinoma of the oropharynx. An axial image through the oropharynx shows subtle a small-volume tumor as asymmetric enhancement and fullness projecting laterally at the right glossotonsillar sulcus (orange arrows) and bulky ipsilateral adenopathy at level IIA with an internal filling defect reflecting necrosis in a metastatic deposit (blue arrow). The study was performed for palpable adenopathy.

implying a more likely upper or lower primary source. It should be noted that some authors advocate including the level IIB nodes (deep to the SCM and separate from the internal jugular vein [IJV]) into the level V station, as they more closely follow the typical spinal accessory drainage pathway and are frequently abnormal, without involving the level IIA nodes in the setting of metastatic cutaneous malignancies. However, for the purposes of this book, we will keep these divided into level IIB and V as we do in our practice.

Level VI nodes are in the anterior compartment in the neck, inferior to the inferior border of the hyoid body, medial to the medial borders of the common carotid arteries and cervical internal carotid arteries, above the top of the sternal manubrium, and deep to the platysma. The eponym for a level VI prelaryngeal/precricoid node is Delphian node, which receives lymphatic drainage from the thyroid gland and the larynx.

Some authors include an additional designation of level VII to denote lymph nodes that arise between the superior border of the manubrium and the upper border of the innominate vein, as well as the medial border of the common carotid arteries. However, this nodal station is not standard nomenclature used by ENT surgeons and does not match the intrathoracic numbering system. We prefer to use descriptive terms for localization of superior mediastinal nodes when seen in the setting of head and neck disease (e.g., pretracheal, paratracheal, tracheoesophageal groove).

Similarly, other lymph nodes in the neck do not fall within the numbered nodal stations, and other authors have proposed numbering systems to include as many as 10 stations,[12] several with smaller subsets. Although this numbering system is not standard, these other stations are still important to evaluate. Retropharyngeal nodes receive drainage from the pharynx and also can be abnormal in the setting of thyroid carcinoma because of its embryologic descent through the neck. Intraparotid lymph nodes receive drainage from the scalp and face in addition to the periauricular soft tissues and are frequently abnormal. Lymphatic drainage from the posterior scalp may also involve the retroauricular and suboccipital lymph nodes. Buccal and facial nodes are only rarely identified and, when seen, should be presumed to be pathologic; drainage is from the regional skin or oral cavity.

IMAGING

The main role of imaging is determining extent of disease. This can include evaluation of local invasion or metastatic disease in patients with visible mucosal abnormalities, as well as identification of a primary lesion in the case of a patient presenting with adenopathy, either not yet evaluated by a clinician or with an occult primary site.

Computed Tomography

Contrast CT is the test of choice for in the initial evaluation of primary head and neck malignancies, as well as nodal metastasis. CT is also fairly readily available and lower cost than magnetic resonance imaging (MRI) or PET. Images are acquired helically in the axial plane and reformatted into coronal and sagittal planes. The entire neck can be evaluated quickly with a single acquisition. Some centers use dual-energy CT to increase specificity, but this may vary with CT vendor and is not standard practice at our institution.

CT does have some limitations. Patients with dental amalgam often have significant metallic streak artifact related to beam hardening. This may obscure evaluation of the oral cavity and even the oropharynx if dense enough. Metal suppression techniques or separately acquired angled images may be helpful for evaluation of small lesions, especially in the buccal space, oral tongue, or anterior floor of the mouth.

In the larynx, acquiring or reformatting images along the plane of the true vocal folds is similarly helpful for identifying subtle areas of asymmetric thickening or ulceration. Motion related to patient swallowing can degrade evaluation, as can a closed glottis at the time of the scan. Technologists should be alert to identify these possibilities and rescan immediately if needed.

Positron Emission Tomography

At our institutions, PET/CT with FDG is used primarily for identification of distant metastatic disease and as a baseline examination for comparison to posttreatment surveillance studies. In cases of an unknown primary, PET can sometimes identify a suspicious site not seen on CT and help guide targeted biopsies at the time of direct laryngoscopy. It may also help confirm status of regional lymph node involvement. PET does have relatively lower spatial resolution than CT, which may limit evaluation of small lesions and perineural tumor spread.

Magnetic Resonance Imaging

MRI is primarily used as a problem-solving tool in head and neck cancers. Its higher contrast resolution compared with CT results in greater sensitivity for evaluating the full extent of involvement of the primary site and the adjacent structures, such as extension to the esophagus, as well as evaluation of perineural spread and bone marrow/cartilaginous involvement.

MRI is also a critical part in the complete initial staging of lesions with a high propensity for intracranial extension with meningeal/brain invasion, including nasopharyngeal and olfactory masses.

Ultrasound

We do not routinely use ultrasound for diagnostic characterization or staging of lesions, but we do perform ultrasound-guided percutaneous sampling as a part of the workup of the patient, both in newly diagnosed disease and suspected recurrence of tumor.

PATTERNS OF NODAL METASTASES AND WORKUP OF THE "UNKNOWN PRIMARY"

There is rich lymphatic drainage from most of the mucosa of the head and neck. When a primary lesion is identified, the at-risk nodal stations need to be identified and specifically addressed. The converse is also true when a patient presents with palpable adenopathy, which is a frequent indication for imaging. The "unknown primary" evaluation begins with a CT and requires accurate determination of the location of the adenopathy.[13]

As mentioned, lesions of the lips or oral cavity tend to drain first to level I nodes, as do lesions of the submandibular or sublingual glands. From there, adenopathy can extend sequentially to levels II, III, and occasionally IV in high-volume, aggressive tumors.

The presence of adenopathy beginning at or isolated to level IIA is highly suggestive of an oropharyngeal primary in the palatine tonsils or tongue base. Even if a lesion is not found on imaging or in-office inspection, this should prompt a panendoscopy for full visualization of the oropharynx, targeted biopsies of any mucosal abnormalities, blind biopsies of the base of tongue, and consideration for tonsillectomies if appropriate. If all workup is negative, the treatment would still include radiation to the ipsilateral oropharynx in this situation. When advanced disease is present starting at level IIA, it also tends to spread sequentially through levels III and IV, but it is rare for an oropharyngeal lesion to spread to the level I nodes.

KEY POINTS

- Adenopathy beginning at level IIA raises suspicion for an oropharyngeal abnormality, even if one is not seen on imaging.
- Skin cancer from the scalp and face tends to drain to lymph nodes in the superficial parotid or tail, followed by posterior cervical nodes (levels IIB and V), without involvement of the anterior cervical nodes.

Isolated level III adenopathy, although occasionally related to upper pharyngeal disease, is more suggestive of a lesion in the hypopharynx or the supraglottic larynx. Because of the relative lack of lymphatic drainage from the glottis, tumors limited to the true vocal cords are less likely to present with adenopathy until they extend to the supraglottic or subglottic larynx or deeply invade the adjacent paraglottic fat.

The retropharyngeal nodes are most commonly involved by metastatic disease from nasopharyngeal tumors, but can also be seen in the setting of any other pharyngeal lesion, especially if the posterior wall is involved. As mentioned previously, thyroid carcinoma is also a consideration for pathologic retropharyngeal adenopathy.

Intraparotid adenopathy and/or posterior cervical (level V± level IIB) adenopathy with sparing of the more anterior deep cervical chains (levels IIA, III, or IV) is most typically associated with cancers of cutaneous origin, particularly SCC and melanoma. The primary site in those cases may or may not be apparent on imaging or even present at the time of development of adenopathy because it may have been removed or ablated without pathologic evaluation to confirm malignancy. Close questioning of the patient with this pattern of adenopathy may obviate the need for other invasive evaluations for an "unknown primary."

PATTERNS OF TUMOR SPREAD AND STAGING OF DISEASE

Similar to the remainder of the body, and regardless of tumor type, the main pathways for tumor spread are direct local invasion and metastatic disease by lymphatic vs. hematogenous routes. Staging for both prognostic and treatment determination is routinely classified by the tumor-node-metastasis (TNM) staging system of the American Joint Committee on Cancer (AJCC). For head and neck cancer, the most recent update (8th edition) of the TNM staging included major changes because of new and increasing understanding of viral-mediated cancer as it relates to HPV and EBV, and the differences between viral-mediated cancers and the typical tobacco-associated SCCs in terms of prognosis. This also has implications for treatment planning.

KEY POINTS

- TNM staging varies for each subsite in the head and neck, and in the oropharynx is now dependent on the HPV/p16 status of the tumor.
- Increasing size of the tumor increases the T stage. At most sites, T1 is a tumor with a maximum diameter <2 cm, and T3 is 4 to 6 cm.
- Bone or cartilage invasion defines T4 disease in the oral cavity and larynx.

Direct Invasion by Primary Tumor (T Stage)

The vast majority of head and neck cancers arising along the mucosa of the visceral compartment have a propensity to be locally invasive (Fig. 6.15). Rarely, a lesion may be exophytic from the mucosa, which portends a better prognosis because of better likelihood for a complete and curative surgical resection with good margins. Unfortunately, it is much more common that the tumors grow endophytically, invading the neighboring structures. This is one reason that imaging in head and neck cancer is so important; although the superficial lesions are easily visualized and biopsied on endoscopy, this may only be the tip of the iceberg, and determining the full extent of the tumor is critical for staging and determining appropriate therapy. Additionally, some lesions primarily arise submucosally, only causing regional fullness that is invisible on direct inspection.

In each subsite, tumoral invasion into specific structures changes the local tumor (T) stage in the TNM staging system.[14] As representation of concept, the local disease T stage for tumors arising in the oral cavity is automatically a T4a (moderately advanced) if there is invasion of the mandible, maxillary sinus, or facial skin, and is upstaged to T4b if there is masticator space invasion or invasion of the pterygoid plates or skull base, or if the tumor encases the internal carotid artery. Staging of glottis cancers does not specifically include tumor volume or diameter, but is entirely based on the extent of involvement of nearby structures. Immobilization/fixation of the vocal cords (a clinical finding) may increase staging of what is apparent on imaging to at least T3 disease. Invasion of the outer thyroid cartilage or the cricoid cartilage or extralaryngeal spread increases the stage to T4.

Note that bone and cartilaginous involvement immediately increases the stage to T4 disease, even for otherwise relatively small-volume tumors in these sites (with the exception of the inner cortex of the thyroid cartilage, which is still defined as T3). It is also important to recognize that invasion of these structures may not result in aggressive erosion. In the larynx in particular increased density of the cartilage may reflect tumor invasion or reactive changes, but should be reported, particularly when other confirmatory findings are present (Figs. 6.16 and 6.17). The loss of mobility of the tongue or the vocal cords also impacts staging, reflecting a functional denervation that may or may not be apparent radiographically.

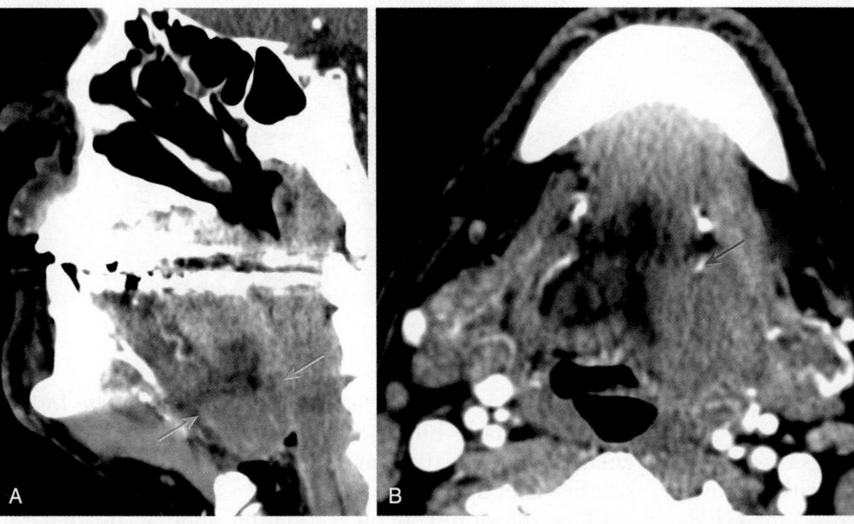

Figure 6.15. Squamous cell carcinoma of the oropharynx, local invasion. **A**, Sagittal computed tomography image shows a soft tissue mass arising at the left base of tongue (*orange arrows*). **B**, There is invasion of the floor of the mouth around the posterior aspect of the lingual neurovascular bundle (*blue arrow*).

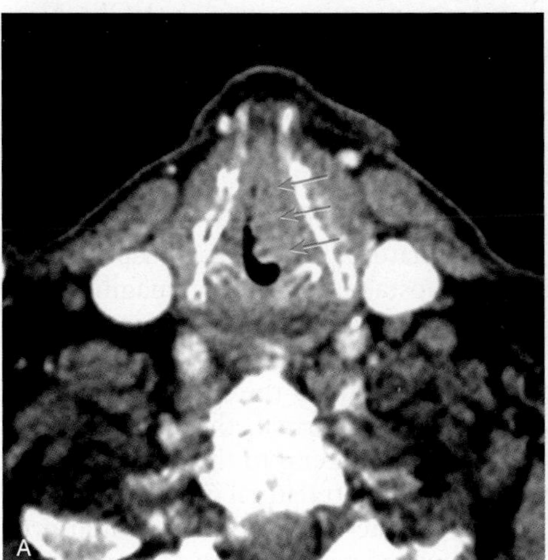

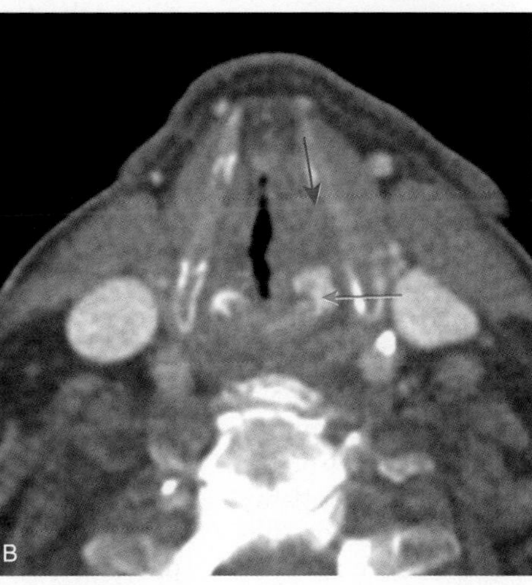

Figure 6.16. Squamous cell carcinoma of the larynx. **A**, Nodular glottic thickening along the entire length of the left true vocal cord (orange arrows). **B**, Sclerosis of the left arytenoid cartilage (*orange arrow*) is suspicious for tumor infiltration, nonspecific on its own but also with expansion and irregular margins. There is early infiltration of the paraglottic fat on the left (*blue arrow*), making this at least T3 disease, but cartilage invasion would increase to T4.

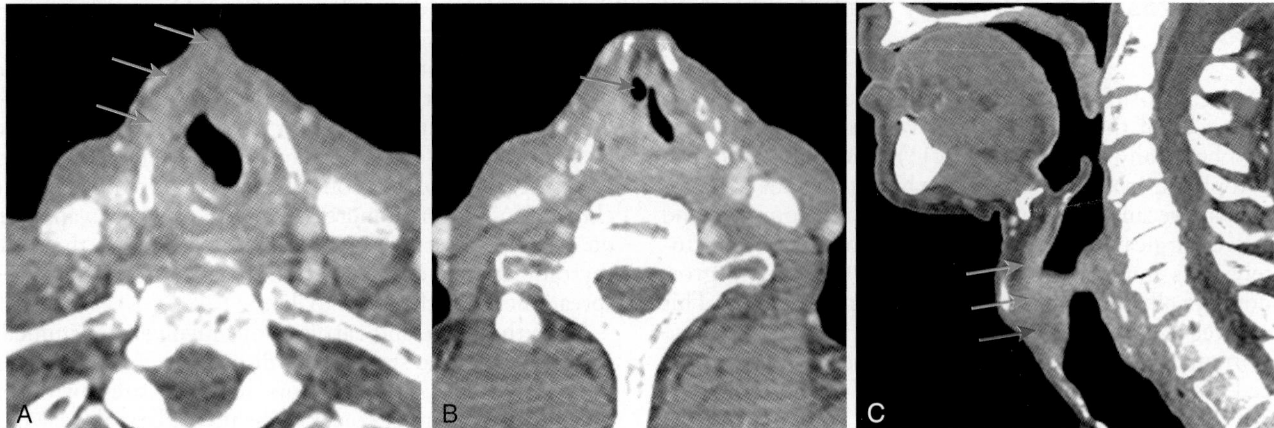

FIGURE 6.17. Squamous cell carcinoma of the larynx, transglottic (T4). There is a large and locally invasive transglottic tumor. **A**, There is invasion through the thyroid cartilage bilaterally and infiltration of the strap muscles. Tumor extends nearly to the skin surface. **B**, There is a small air-filled laryngocele on the right. **C**, Sagittal reformation shows the involvement of the infrahyoid epiglottis and true and false vocal cords (orange arrows) and the subglottic extent anteriorly (blue arrow).

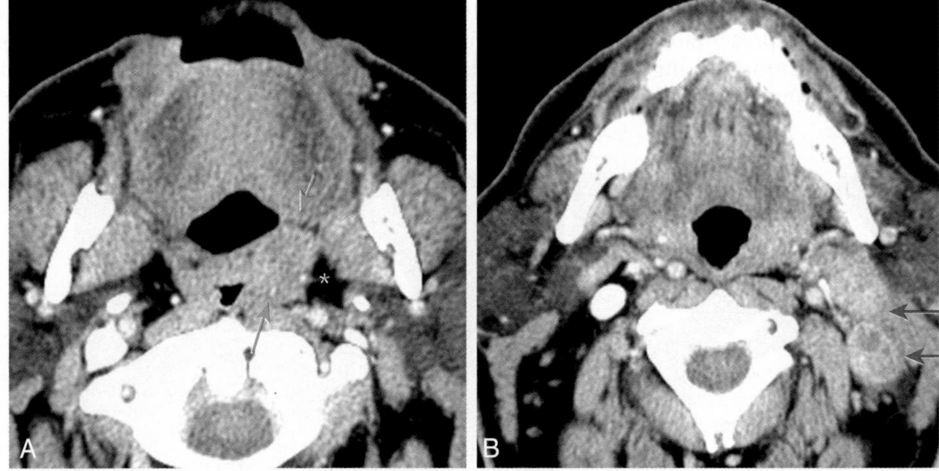

FIGURE 6.18. Human papillomavirus–associated squamous cell carcinoma of the oropharynx. **A**, This patient had a small-volume T2 (>2 cm) tumor of the left palatine tonsil (*orange arrows*) without infiltration of the parapharyngeal space (star). **B**, There was ipsilateral metastatic adenopathy at level IIA and IIB (*blue arrows*) with internal necrosis.

For the oropharynx, there is evidence that the HPV-associated tumors in general have a better prognosis,[4] and the latest consensus TNM staging incorporates this difference into both the T stage and the N stage, with removal of the T4b designation (advanced local disease) for HPV-associated tumors.

Cervical Lymphadenopathy (N Stage)

Nodal evaluation is, in general, best evaluated with a contrast CT owing to the greater spatial resolution of this imaging methodology. Many authors have posited different threshold sizes for distinguishing normal from abnormal lymph nodes in the neck.[12] In most of the nodal stations, we would consider a maximum "short axis" dimension of over 1 cm on CT as abnormal, or 1.5 cm for level IB and IIA. However, the morphology and enhancement of a lymph node are also important clues for determining tumor involvement in the earlier stages, sometimes before the node reaches size criteria for pathologic adenopathy. The presence of even minute intranodal necrosis or "filling defects" is abnormal (Fig. 6.18), as is a more rounded configuration, which is usually associated with the loss of the normal fatty hilum or bean shape.[14,15] Conversely, an enlarged node with maintained fatty hilum may reflect reactive adenopathy.

Once the tumor involves a lymph node, it also has the potential to spread extranodally into the surrounding soft tissues through direct extracapsular extension (ECE). Normal lymph nodes should have well-circumscribed margins with maintenance of the surrounding fat.[13,16] If the margins become irregular or there is infiltration of the fat around a pathologic lymph node, this is suspicious for ECE, which should be reported as such (Fig. 6.19), as well as suspicion for invasion into nearby structures such as the carotid sheath, vessels, or musculature.[16] However, suspicion for ECE is not adequate to upstage a patient by imaging alone in the latest TNM staging unless there is clear invasion of adjacent structures,[14,17] most commonly the SCM or IJV.

For staging purposes, the larger the lymph nodes and the more of them that are abnormal, the higher the N stage. Isolated adenopathy ipsilateral to the primary site is generally a lower stage than contralateral involvement. For all head and neck cancer other than HPV-mediated oropharyngeal or EBV-associated nasopharyngeal carcinomas,

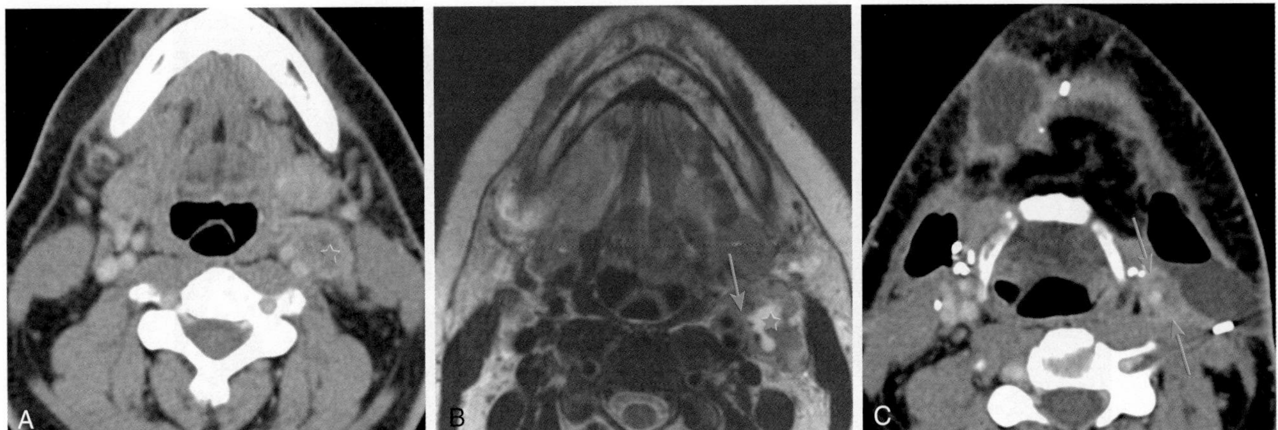

FIGURE 6.19. Extracapsular extension. Metastatic adenopathy in the setting of T4 squamous cell carcinoma of the oral tongue. **A**, On computed tomography this representative level IIA node (*star*) has suspicious ill-defined margins and lack of a fat plane between the node and the adjacent carotid sheath more medially. **B**, On magnetic resonance imaging invasion of the carotid sheath is confirmed (arrow), with soft tissue encasing the proximal internal and external carotid arteries. **C**, Adherence or encasement of vessels limits resectability. Immediate postoperative imaging shows residual disease around the distal common carotid artery.

the (clinical) N stage is subdivided based on size thresholds of 3 and 6 cm, single vs. multiple nodes, and ipsilateral or contralateral, and takes some account of overt extranodal extension. For example, an N2c designation indicates metastatic adenopathy in bilateral nodes (or unilateral but contralateral to the primary tumor), none over 6 cm, and without extranodal extension. For HPV-associated oropharynx tumors, the N stage is much more straightforward: cN1 includes any ipsilateral nodes up to 6 cm, cN2 for the presence of contralateral or bilateral nodes up to 6 cm, and cN3 for adenopathy over 6 cm.

In our institution, abnormal retropharyngeal lymph nodes are denoted with R1, in addition to potentially changing the N stage in the TNM designation. This station is not included in traditional lymph node dissection and requires specific targeting at the time of radiation therapy and follow-up imaging.

Hematogenous Dissemination, Distant Metastases (M stage)

The most common site for extracervical metastatic disease is the lungs, followed by the mediastinal lymph nodes. In patients with aggressive tumors, disseminated disease can occur in the liver and bones, with other sites possible but much less likely. Any of these extranodal metastases would be staged as M1 (and therefore stage IV) disease in the TNM staging, regardless of tumor type.

Of note, hematogenous intracranial metastases are much less common from SCC of the head and neck than from other tumor sites elsewhere in the body. Intracranial involvement, however, can occur from other causes such as direct extension through the skull base, for example from nasopharyngeal tumors or esthesioneuroblastoma, or perineural tumor spread to the level of the cavernous sinuses and/or brainstem, which is why MRI is so important in staging in those cases, as mentioned previously; but this would increase the T stage of these specific tumors rather than define M1 disease.

Perineural Tumor Spread

Perineural tumor spread along regional nerves is a somewhat more unique spread pattern that is also frequently encountered in the head and neck,[18] and although this is considered an adjuvant prognostic factor and may impact treatment[19] it is not directly incorporated into TNM staging.

Macroscopic spread of tumor along a nerve is seen as thickening and enhancement along the course of a nerve (Fig. 6.20). When large or extensive enough, it is easily visible on CT, but MRI does have higher sensitivity.[20] PET/CT is variable for detection of perineural involvement, primarily because of the relatively poor spatial resolution in comparison with other cross-sectional imaging currently available, but high-grade tumors may be metabolically active enough to be appreciated even when small.

In the head and neck, perineural spread is most commonly seen along branches of the facial and trigeminal nerves. The greater and lesser palatine nerves or the Vidian nerve may be involved by lesions arising along the hard or soft palate, as seen previously (see Fig. 6.12). Less commonly encountered, perineural tumor spread may also occur along the superior laryngeal neurovascular bundle from laryngeal tumors.

Although adenoid cystic carcinomas are overwhelmingly less common than SCCs, a much higher percentage of these tumors will be associated with perineural tumor spread.[21] In contrast, it is much less common to identify clinical or pathologic perineural invasion in basal cell carcinomas.[22]

The detection of perineural spread depends on close inspection of fat planes along the course of the nerves and particularly at the known fixed entry sites of various branches. For example, the stylomastoid foramen contains the main trunk of the facial nerve as it exits the temporal bone and tracks toward the parotid gland. In the absence of pathology, there should be visible fat surrounding the nerve in this foramen. Similarly, there should be fat in the foramen rotundum and the infraorbital foramen along the maxillary (V2) division of the trigeminal nerve (see Fig. 6.5), and the

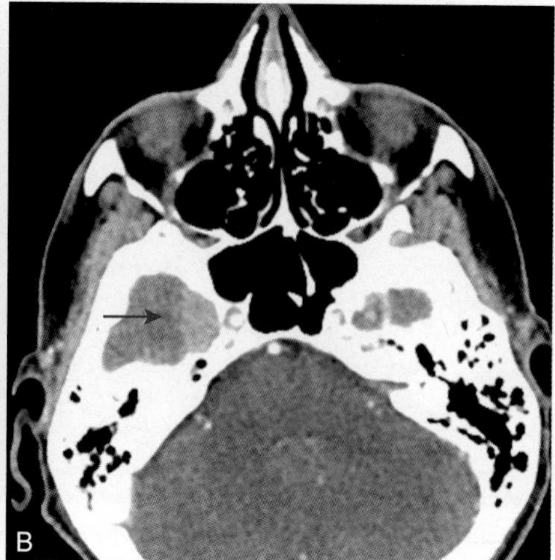

Figure 6.20. A, Coronal image from follow-up neck contrast computed tomography for the patient with nasopharyngeal carcinoma shown in Fig. 6.1 shows invasion along V3 with widening of foramen ovale (orange arrow). There was also significant parapharyngeal space invasion and infiltration of the medial and lateral pterygoid muscles (light blue arrows). The intracranial extent of disease is seen on both coronal and axial **(B)** images, denoted with dark blue arrows.

mental and mandibular foramina and foramen ovale should have symmetric fat around the mandibular (V3) branches. Fat can even be seen along the greater and lesser palatine nerves to the hard palate in normal subjects. Infiltration of fat or widening of foramina would be considered positive. Similarly, the presence of secondary signs of nerve dysfunction can be helpful, such as denervation atrophy of the muscles of mastication when there is V3 involvement, or atrophy of the extraocular muscles if disease extends to the cavernous sinus and affects cranial nerves III, IV, or VI.[22,23]

Importantly, neoplastic cells may track retrograde along one nerve and then at a ganglion or branch point may subsequently have antegrade extension along another branch remote from the primary site.

Also important to remember, the absence of macroscopic perineural tumor spread on imaging does not ensure lack of microscopic invasion. Lastly, the presence of perineural invasion on surgical resection may be a factor in whether a patient receives adjuvant radiation and/or chemotherapy.

TREATMENT

Treatment options for head and neck cancer are determined by tumor stage and site(s) of involvement. There can also be some regional variability in preference between surgery and chemoradiation depending on the experience and preference of the referring ENT.

In low-risk, low-volume lesions for certain subsites, external beam radiation therapy (XRT) can be used in isolation, with high control rates. This is particularly true in the larynx, where preservation of laryngeal function is a usual concern.

The likelihood of cure with radiation alone decreases with size and extent of invasion (T stage) of the primary tumor, and concomitant chemotherapy may increase rate of control in higher-stage disease. Ultimately, for T3 and T4 disease in the larynx surgery has the highest rate of control but is usually followed by adjuvant radiation without chemotherapy, depending on other high-risk features on histologic evaluation (perineural or lymphovascular invasion, positive or close margins, etc.). Additionally, laryngectomy would be offered in the salvage setting for patients with local tumor recurrence after other therapies.

Conversely, for oral cavity lesions the treatment of choice with highest likelihood of cure remains surgical resection. Radiation can be offered as a second-line therapy but may significantly decrease quality of life because of mucositis.

For small-volume tumors of the palatine tonsils, tonsillectomy is generally associated with low morbidity and is frequently performed as both a diagnostic and potentially therapeutic procedure for patients presenting with cervical adenopathy from an unknown primary. Transoral resection has also been advocated by some surgeons for improved clearance of the deep margin in this location and the ability to safely decrease adjuvant therapy doses.[24] However, there is also a high control rate of oropharyngeal tumors with chemoradiation alone. This is particularly true in the setting of HPV-associated tumors, which have a better overall survival and prognosis when other risk factors such as tobacco use are not present, as is now reflected in the latest AJCC TNM staging. Related to this difference in prognosis, "dose deintensification" with lower radiation dose has become the standard of care for HPV-associated tumors at our institution[25,26] to minimize side effects while maintaining the effectiveness of therapy.

Some of the newer immunotherapy agents do have some effectiveness in head and neck cancers, but this is evaluated on a case-by-case basis, including testing of the tumoral tissue for specific ligands such as PDL-1.

Chemotherapy alone is usually less effective and is reserved for palliative/noncurative intent when other options are unavailable. Intraarterial chemotherapy may be offered rarely for localized recurrences when it is not possible to provide more radiation.

SURVEILLANCE

Monitoring Tumor Response and Detecting Recurrence

This a controversial topic, and there are no consensus guidelines for follow-up of asymptomatic patients. However, a common recommendation in all patients is a baseline PET/CT with a diagnostic contrast CT, which should be obtained at 12 weeks following completion of treatment. If there are findings highly suspicious for residual disease at that time, the standard is to undergo surgical resection, especially in patients treated with radiation with or without chemotherapy with a curative intent.

PET/CT obtained earlier than 12 weeks is limited by the potential for residual metabolic activity in treated tumor that is undergoing necrosis but has not completely resolved. A standard 1 month posttreament diagnostic CT is also often equivocal, improving but not yet meeting criteria for tumor control, and we no longer routinely acquire these unless there is a change in patient's clinical status.

Initial posttreatment evaluation at greater than 3 months is not standard, as the degree of fibrosis becomes significantly greater over time, which can increase the difficulty of the procedure for the ENT surgeon and increase the risk to the patient.

However, in patients with HPV-associated oropharyngeal tumors taken to surgery, there is a pathologically proven low positive predictive value of a positive or equivocal 12-week PET/CT.[27] If the initial 12-week PET is abnormal but equivocal, or if the patient is a poor surgical candidate, a repeat PET/CT with diagnostic neck may be considered at 4 to 6 months from completion of therapy to ensure continued decrease in activity.[28]

If the initial posttreatment imaging shows apparent control of disease, most patients can be followed using protocols established by the clinical service in their respective institution, most using a combination of clinical examination and imaging every 3 to 6 months for at least 2 years. Some only reserve subsequent imaging for patients who develop new clinical symptoms or new mucosal abnormalities, or in patients with trismus or other factors that limit a full clinical evaluation. Others use imaging as an adjunct to the clinical examination.

Patients with new symptoms should have clinical evaluation for direct inspection as well as repeat imaging, given high concern for recurrence and risks of new primary tumor (Fig. 6.21).

Suspected recurrence on imaging usually requires histologic confirmation for discussion of additional treatment options and subsequent prognosis. This may be with surgical resection as a "salvage" procedure, but if surgery is not an option tissue sampling can also be frequently done percutaneously with imaging guidance, either with CT/ultrasound in the radiology department or with in-office ultrasound by the ENT surgeons.

Unfortunately, regardless of underlying etiology, a "field effect" exists, such that a patient who has had head and neck cancer is at risk for not just local tumor recurrence (particularly if the disease was tobacco-related and the patient continues smoking) but also development of a new primary at different sites exposed to the carcinogen. Similarly, a patient with an HPV-associated tumor is potentially at risk for development of other sites of disease, as the patient's entire body has been exposed to the virus.[29]

Complications of Therapy

Radiation therapy is highly effective and provides excellent cure rates for many tumors. However, it also incites a brisk inflammatory response in the adjacent normal tissues. This can lead to patient discomfort secondary to mucositis and ulceration in the visceral compartment. Irradiated oral cavity cancers can cause trismus and fibrosis, impairing the opening of the jaw and a full clinical evaluation of the primary site.

At the same time that the radiation is inciting inflammation, it is also working to intentionally decrease vascularity to the area of tumor and the rest of the radiation field. This

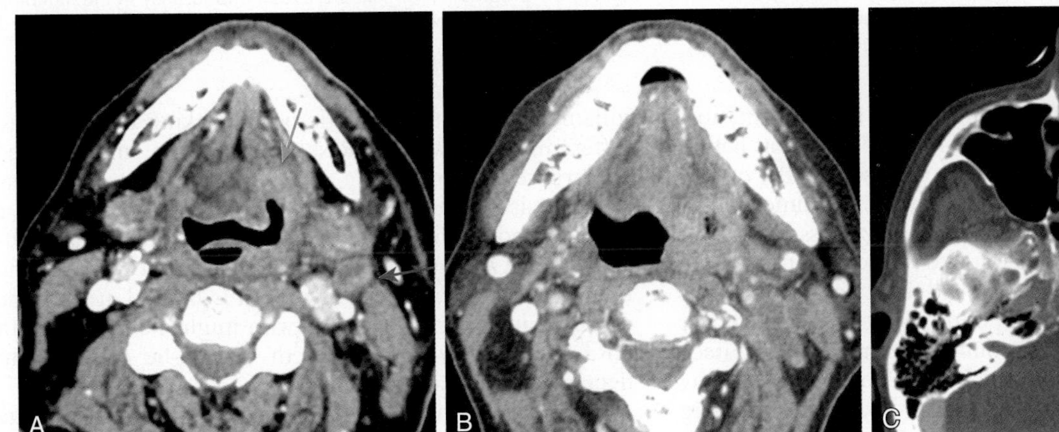

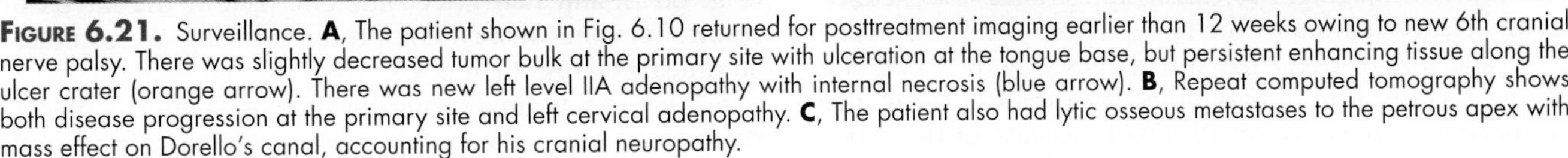

FIGURE 6.21. Surveillance. **A**, The patient shown in Fig. 6.10 returned for posttreatment imaging earlier than 12 weeks owing to new 6th cranial nerve palsy. There was slightly decreased tumor bulk at the primary site with ulceration at the tongue base, but persistent enhancing tissue along the ulcer crater (orange arrow). There was new left level IIA adenopathy with internal necrosis (blue arrow). **B**, Repeat computed tomography shows both disease progression at the primary site and left cervical adenopathy. **C**, The patient also had lytic osseous metastases to the petrous apex with mass effect on Dorello's canal, accounting for his cranial neuropathy.

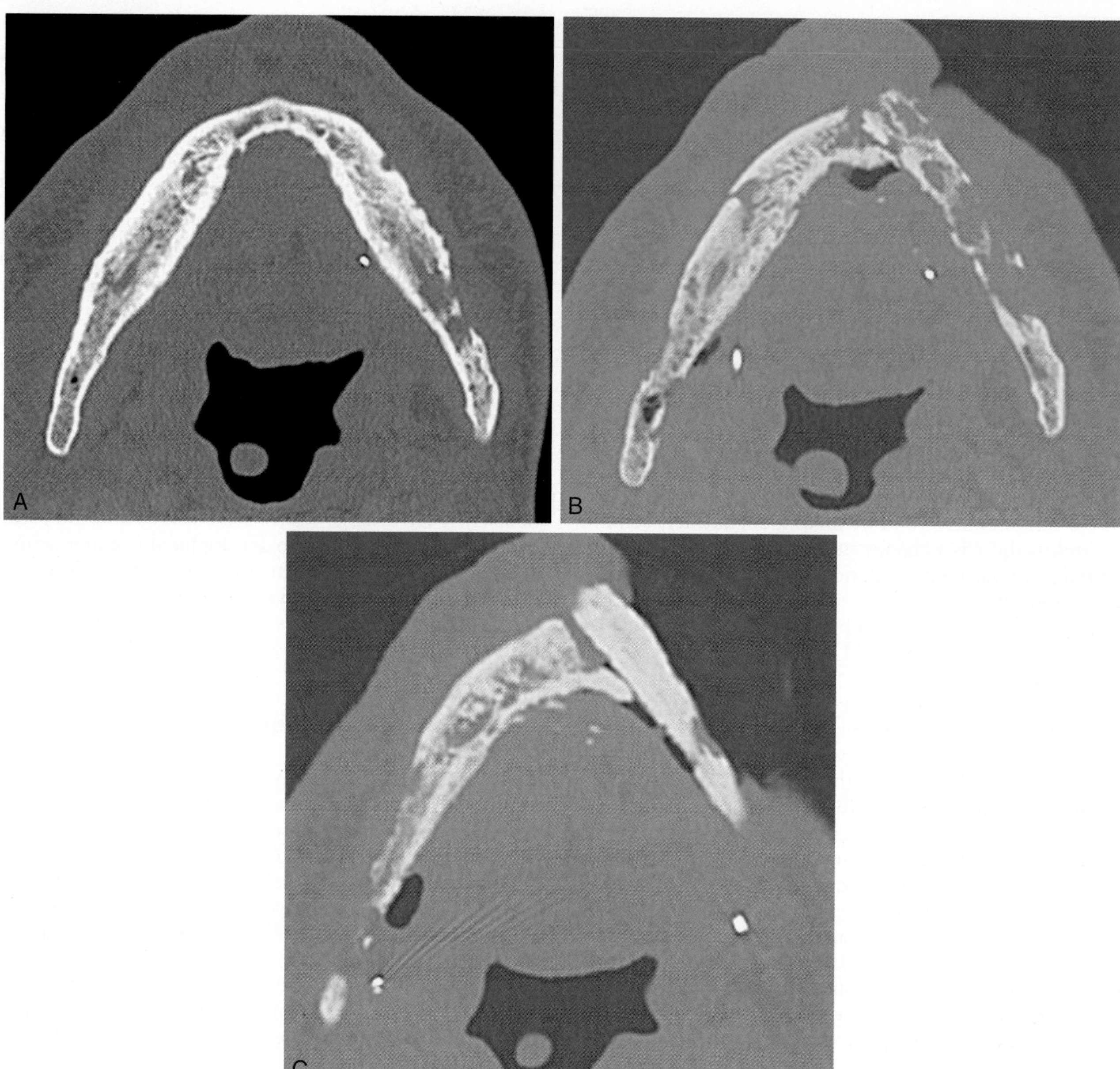

FIGURE 6.22. Severe osteoradionecrosis of the mandible. Three axial images show progression of mixed sclerosis and lucency in the mandible (**A** - early), progressive fragmentation with eventual pathologic fracture (**B** - moderate), and development of marked tissue necrosis (**C** - advanced) with large area of exposed bone on clinical examination.

can result in poor wound healing or in fistula formation. This is a higher risk if patients undergo radiation before surgery or if they have an underlying vasculopathy or diabetes. This risk also increases if a patient has tumor recurrence and receives additional radiation to a tissue that was previously irradiated in the initial treatment field.

Osteoradionecrosis (ORN) and chondroradionecrosis are additional potential complications of radiation therapy that are more commonly encountered in the head and neck than in some other sites in the body. Clinically, ORN may manifest as exposed bone with loss of devitalized overlying mucosa. On imaging, the classic appearance is of sclerosis and fragmentation of the bone, with possible air in the bone and loss of overlying soft tissues (Fig. 6.22). When severe, this can lead to pathologic fracture. ORN can also be metabolically active on PET/CT because of the active inflammation in the necrotic bone, making it difficult to differentiate between ORN, osteomyelitis, and infected tumoral recurrence.

There is potential for ORN to occur in any bone in a radiation portal, but the mandible and maxilla are at highest risk of ORN particularly in the setting of preexisting dental decay. Attention to the teeth is helpful at the time of initial imaging for patients who might be treated with XRT, as severely decayed teeth should be extracted to decrease this risk.

Chondroradionecrosis is fragmentation of cartilage (Fig. 6.23), and may affect just one part of the larynx or result in acute airway compromise owing to complete laryngeal collapse.[30,31]

For patients treated surgically, there is a high risk of local recurrence at the margins of previous resection. In patients

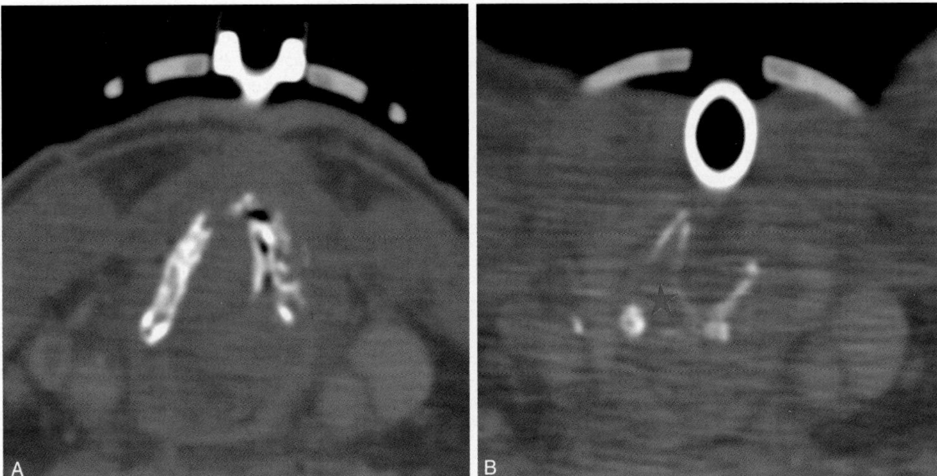

Figure 6.23. Severe chondroradionecrosis of the larynx. **A**, There is sclerosis, fragmentation, and air in the distorted thyroid cartilage, with complete collapse of the airway. **B**, There is also partial absence of the cricoid cartilage on the left, with the right side grossly preserved (*star*).

who have undergone flap reconstruction, the greatest risk is to the anastomotic sites, but tumor can potentially recur anywhere along the flap. If a neck dissection is undertaken to remove lymph nodes with extranodal tumor extension, the risk of local recurrence is higher. Similarly, vascular encasement or adherence to other critical structures, or disease high near the skull base where there is limited exposure of tissues, may result in small amounts of residual tumor that may blossom on surveillance imaging.

Lymphoma is typically treated with systemic chemotherapy, and patients are followed with whole-body surveillance imaging. Radiation is occasionally useful for isolated sites of high-grade lymphoma. It is otherwise rare for our patient population to receive curative-intent chemotherapy in the absence of other therapies, but CT surveillance would be evaluated the same as any other treatment modality, with attention to the primary site and potential metastatic sites.

It is becoming increasingly common to see patients treated with immunotherapies when they have exhausted other options. Imaging findings are not as predictable on those surveillance scans, because of the immune response, with some small degree of apparent "increase" in tumor volume ("pseudoprogression") at initiation of therapy that does not preclude them from continuing. We have seen patients develop diffuse nodal prominence and FDG uptake outside of the expected lymphatic sites at risk. For these complex patients, surveillance studies are often undertaken at shorter intervals, and changes are discussed at length in multidisciplinary conferences before altering therapy.

SUMMARY

Head and neck cancer is a common disease that is often treatable when identified early and staged appropriately. An important take-home point is that the understanding of tumor biology is in flux, and that HPV-related tumors are now staged differently from conventional tobacco-related tumors in the oropharynx, with many centers also treating these differently. CT remains a mainstay in staging, with PET bring important in restaging of disease, and MRI having a more complementary role for addressing specific questions. Some unique features of head and neck cancer are the predictable patterns of nodal spread from the mucosa of the visceral compartment, the high propensity for perineural tumor spread, and the possibility for high T stage even for small-volume tumors that are locally infiltrative into bone, cartilage, or surrounding structures.

REFERENCES

1. Siegel RL, Miller KD, Jemal A. Cancer Statistics, 2019. *CA Cancer J Clin*. 2019;69:7-34.
2. McDermott JD, Bowles DW. Epidemiology of Head and Neck Squamous Cell Carcinomas: Impact on Staging and Prevention Strategies. *Curr Treat Options in Oncol*. 2019;20:43.
3. Aldalwg MAH, Brestovac B. Human papillomavirus associated cancers of the head and neck: an australian perspective. *Head and Neck Pathol*. 2017;11:377-384.
4. Li H, Torabi SJ, Yarbrough WG, et al. Association of human papillomavirus status at head and neck carcinoma subsites with overall survival. *JAMA Otolaryngol Head Neck Surg*. 2018;144(6):519-525.
5. Apalla Z, Lallas A, Sotiriou E, et al. Epidemiological Trends in Skin Cancer. *Dermatology Practical & Conceptual*. 2017;7(2):1.
6. Senkomago V, Henley SJ, Thomas CC, et al. Human papillomavirus-attributable cancers – United States, 2012-2016. *MMWR Morb Mortal Wkly Rep*. 2019;68(33):724-728.
7. Leiter U, Garbe C. Epidemiology of melanoma and nonmelanoma skin cancer—the role of sunlight. *Adv Exp Med Biol*. 2008;624:89-103.
8. Berlin JM, Warner MR, Bailin PL. Metastatic basal cell carcinoma presenting as unilateral axillary lymphadenopathy: report of a case and review of the literature. *Dermatol Surg*. 2002;28:1082-1084.
9. Mehta KS, Mahajan VK, Chauhan PS, et al. Metastatic basal cell carcinoma: a biological continuum of basal cell carcinoma? *Case Rep Dermatol Med*. 2012;2012:157187.
10. Thielker J, Grosheva M, Ihrler S, et al. Contemporary Management of Benign and Malignant Parotid Tumors. *Front Surg*. 2018;5:39.
11. Mukherji SK, Gujar MD, Londy FJ. A simplified approach to the lymph nodes of the neck. *Neurographics*. 2003;2(2).
12. Gregoire V, Ang K, Budach W, et al. Delineation of the neck node levels for head and neck tumors: a 2013 update. DAHANCA, EORTC, HKNPCSG, NCIC CTG, NCRI, RTOG, TROG Consensus Guidelines. *Radiother Oncol*. 2014;110:172-181.

13. Mancuso AA, Hanafee WN. *Head and Neck Radiology*. Lippincott Williams & Wilkins; 2010.
14. American Joint Committee on Cancer, American College of Surgeons. *AJCC Cancer Staging Manual, Eighth Edition Staging Form Supplement*. 2016.
15. Van den Brekel MWM, Castelijns JA, Snow GB. The size of lymph nodes in the neck on sonograms as a radiologic criterion for metastasis: how reliable is it? *AJNR Am J Neuroradiol*. 1998;19:695-700.
16. Hermans R, ed. *Head and Neck Cancer Imaging*. Springer; 2016.
17. Lydiatt W, O'Sullivan B, Patel S. Major changes in head and neck staging for 2018. *Am Soc Clin Oncol Educ Book*. 2018;38:505-514.
18. Badger D, Aygun N. Imaging of perineural spread in head and neck cancer. *Radiol Clin N Am*. 2017;55:139-149.
19. Mendenhall WM, Amdur RJ, Williams LS, et al. Carcinoma of the skin of the head and neck with perineural invasion. *Head Neck*. 2002;24(1):78-83.
20. Williams LS, Mancuso AA, Mendenhall WM. Perineural spread of cutaneous squamous and basal cell carcinoma: CT and MR detection and its impact on patient management and prognosis. *Int J Radiat Oncol Biol Phys*. 2001;49(4):1061-1069.
21. Balamucki CJ, Amdur RJ, Werning JW, et al. Adenoid cystic carcinoma of the head and neck. *Am J Otolaryngol*. 2012;33(5):510-518.
22. Ashraf DC, Kalin-Hajdu E, Levin MH, et al. Mixed cranial neuropathies due to occult perineural invasion of basal cell carcinoma. *Am J Ophthalmol Case Rep*. 2019;13:136-139.
23. Mullen SJ, Coret-Simon J, Rodriguez AR. Perineural spread of skin cancer presenting as diplopia. *CMAJ*. 2018;190:E13-16.
24. Baskin RM, Boyce BJ, Amdur RJ, et al. Transoral robotic surgery for oropharyngeal cancer: patient selection and special considerations. *Cancer Manage Res*. 2018;10:839-846.
25. Cheraghlou S, Yu PK, Otremba MD, et al. Treatment deintensification in human papillomavirus-positive oropharynx cancer: outcomes from the National Cancer Data Base. *Cancer*. 2018;124:717-826.
26. Chera BS, Amdur RJ, Tepper JE, et al. Mature results of a prospective study of deintensified chemoradiotherapy for low-risk human papillomavirus-associated oropharyngeal squamous cell carcinoma. *Cancer*. 2018;124:2347-2354.
27. Wang K, Wong TZ, Amdur RJ, et al. Pitfalls of post-treatment PET after de-intensified chemoradiotherapy for HPV-associated oropharynx cancer: secondary analysis of a phase 2 trial. *Oral Oncol*. 2018;78:108-113.
28. Liu HY, Milne R, Lock G, et al. Utility of a repeat PET/CT scan in HPV-associated oropharyngeal cancer following incomplete nodal response from (chemo)radiotherapy. *Oral Oncol*. 2019;88:153-159.
29. Suk R, Mahale P, Sonawane K, et al. Trends in risks for second primary cancers associated with index human papillomavirus-associated cancers. *JAMA Netw Open*. 2018;1(5):e181999.
30. Hermans R, Pameijer FA, Mancuso AA, et al. CT Findings in chondroradionecrosis of the larynx. *AJNR Am J Neuroradiol*. 1988;19:711-718.
31. Halkud R, Shenoy AM, Naik SM, et al. Chondroradionecrosis of larynx a delayed complication of radiotherapy: management and review of literature. *Indian J Surg Oncol*. 2014;5(2):128-133.

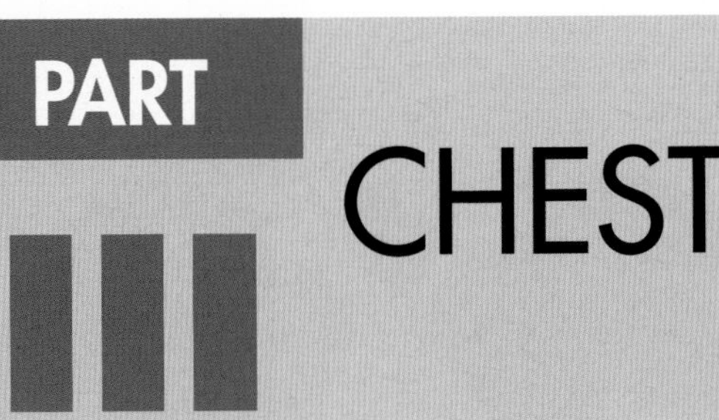

PART III CHEST

CHAPTER 7 Lung Cancer

Jeremy J. Erasmus, M.D.; Quynh-Nhu Nguyen, M.D.; David J. Stewart, M.D., F.R.C.P.C.; and Stephen G. Swisher, M.D.

INTRODUCTION

Lung cancer is a common malignancy, and imaging is an integral part of the detection, diagnosis, and staging of the disease, as well as assessing response to therapy and monitoring for tumor recurrence after treatment. This chapter will review the appropriate use of computed tomography (CT), magnetic resonance imaging (MRI), and positron emission tomography (PET) imaging and management in patients with nonsmall cell lung carcinoma (NSCLC) and small cell lung carcinoma (SCLC).

Epidemiology and Risk Factors

It is estimated that 235,760 new cases of lung cancer will be diagnosed in the United States in 2021[1,1a]. Although higher incidence rates have recently been reported in young women, the incidence is overall declining in both men and women. However, lung cancer remains the leading cause of cancer-related deaths in both men and women in the United States, accounting for an estimated 22% of all cancer deaths in men and 22% in woman in 2021.

The strongest risk factor for the development of lung cancer is cigarette smoking, and it is estimated that 85% to 90% of lung cancers in men and 80% in women are attributable to smoking.[1] Involuntary smoke exposure is also associated with an increased risk of lung cancer, and a metaanalysis analyzing 22 studies showed a 24% increase in lung cancer risk among workers exposed to environmental tobacco smoke.[2] Environmental and occupational exposure to particulate and chemical substances are additional risk factors, as well as exposure to the naturally occurring radioactive gas radon, which is the most important lung cancer risk factor after cigarette smoking.[1,3–5] Additional risk factors for the development of lung cancer include exposure to ionizing radiation, arsenic, chloromethyl ethers, chromium, isopropyl oil, mustard gas, nickel, beryllium, lead, copper, chloroprene, and vinyl chloride.[6,7] Finally, genetic susceptibility to lung cancer may be an important risk factor. A number of different gene mutations are common in lung cancer, and there is a strong association between *KRAS* mutations and smoking in lung adenocarcinoma.[8] In addition, mutations of the epidermal growth factor receptor gene have a strong association with adenocarcinoma.[9,10]

Pathology

Lung cancer is divided by the World Health Organization classification into two major histologic categories: NSCLC and SCLC. NSCLC is subdivided into histologic types (squamous cell carcinoma, adenocarcinoma, and large cell carcinoma) according to the most differentiated portion of the tumor. Adenocarcinoma is the most common histologic type. To appropriately describe these tumors, a new adenocarcinoma classification was introduced in 2011 by a joint working group of the International Association for the Study of Lung Cancer (IASLC), the American Thoracic Society, and the European Respiratory Society (Box 7.1).[11,12] This new classification strategy is based on a multidisciplinary approach to the diagnosis of lung adenocarcinoma that incorporates clinical, molecular, radiologic, and surgical issues, but it is primarily based on histology. This new classification provides uniform terminology and diagnostic criteria, especially for tumors formerly known as bronchioloalveolar carcinoma (a term that has now been eliminated). For resection specimens, the new histologic classification

Box 7.1 International Association for the Study of Lung Cancer/ American Thoracic Society/European Respiratory Society Pathologic Classification of Lung Adenocarcinoma

Preinvasive lesions
Atypical adenomatous hyperplasia
Adenocarcinoma *in situ* (≤3 cm, pure lepidic growth without invasion, formerly bronchioloalveolar cell carcinoma [BAC])
Nonmucinous
Mucinous
Mixed mucinous/nonmucinous
Minimally invasive adenocarcinoma (≤3 cm lepidic predominant tumor with >5 mm invasion)
Nonmucinous
Mucinous
Mixed mucinous/nonmucinous
Invasive adenocarcinoma
Lepidic predominant (formerly nonmucinous BAC pattern, with >5 mm invasion)
Acinar predominant
Papillary predominant
Micropapillary predominant
Solid predominant with mucin production
Variants of invasive adenocarcinoma
Invasive mucinous adenocarcinoma (formerly mucinous BAC)
Colloid
Fetal (low- and high-grade)
Enteric

(Modified from Van Schil PE, Sihoe AD, Travis WD. Pathologic classification of adenocarcinoma of lung. *J Surg Oncol.* 2013;108(5):320-326.)

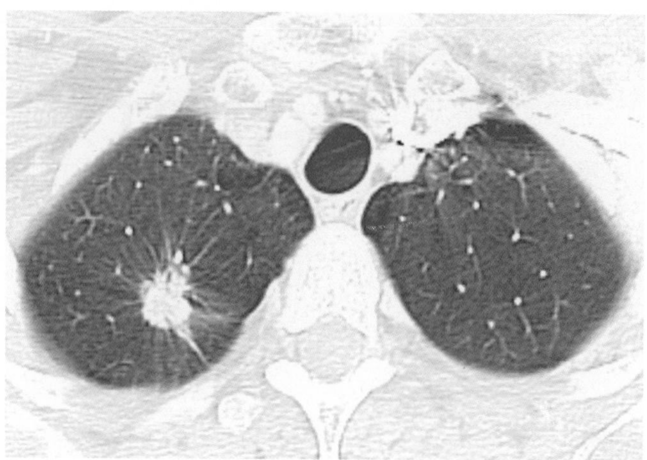

FIGURE 7.1. A 59-year-old woman with adenocarcinoma manifesting as small peripheral pulmonary nodule. Computed tomography shows a spiculated nodule (*arrow*) in the right upper lobe. The spiculated margin is typical of lung cancer.

comprises preinvasive lesions (adenocarcinoma *in situ* (≤3 cm, solitary, pure lepidic growth, formerly bronchioloalveolar cell carcinoma), minimally invasive adenocarcinoma (≤3 cm with predominant lepidic growth and ≤5 mm invasion), and invasive adenocarcinomas (classified by predominant pattern: lepidic, acinar, papillary, micropapillary, solid).

A histologic classification has also been proposed by Noguchi et al., whereby small (≤2 cm) peripheral adenocarcinomas are classified into six types, A through F, based on tumor growth patterns.[13] The soft-tissue attenuation component tends to be absent or less than a third of the opacity with type A and greater in extent (more than two-thirds) in types D to F.[14] The likelihood of invasive adenocarcinoma and more advanced stage of lung cancer has been reported to be higher with mixed and solid opacities.[15]

Adenocarcinoma

These tumors commonly manifest as a peripheral, solitary pulmonary nodule with irregular or spiculated margins as a result of parenchymal invasion and associated fibrotic response (Fig. 7.1). The nodules are usually of soft-tissue attenuation, and cavitation is rare. However, adenocarcinomas manifesting as purely ground-glass or part-solid (ground-glass and solid) are being detected with increasing frequency (Figs. 7.2 and 7.3).

Squamous Cell Carcinoma

These tumors typically occur as a central endobronchial mass and frequently manifest as postobstructive pneumonia or atelectasis (Fig. 7.4) Approximately one-third of squamous cell carcinomas occur beyond the segmental bronchi, and usually range in size from 1 to 10 cm. Squamous cell carcinomas are more likely to cavitate than the other histologic cell types of lung cancer (Fig. 7.5).

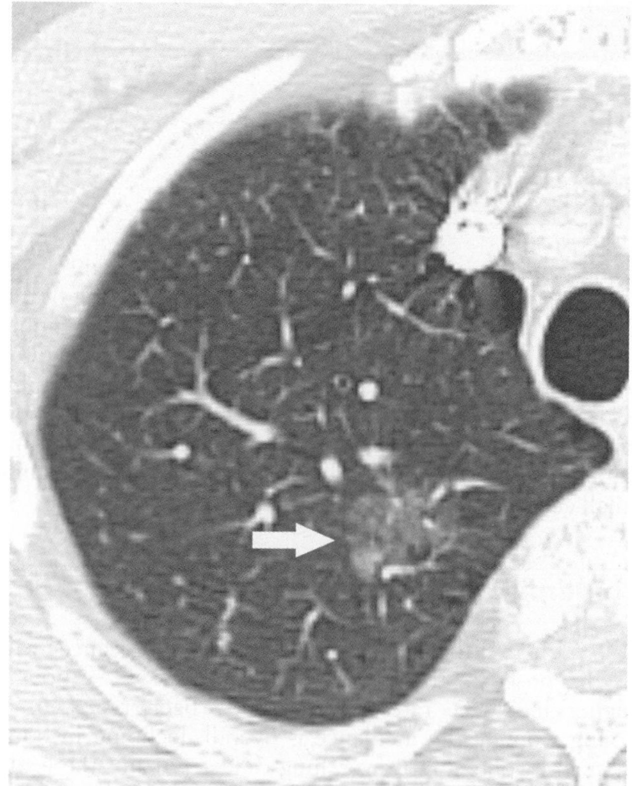

FIGURE 7.2. A 78-year-old man with adenocarcinoma manifesting as a pulmonary nodule with ground-glass attenuation (arrow). Computed tomography shows a poorly marginated ground-glass opacity in the left upper lobe. Note that these malignancies are typically indolent.

Large Cell Carcinoma

These tumors are usually peripheral, poorly marginated masses greater than 7 cm in diameter.

Small Cell Lung Cancer

These constitute 15% to 20% of all lung cancers. SCLC is a neuroendocrine tumor with 10 mitoses/2 mm^2 that manifests histologically as sheets of small, oval to slightly spindled-shaped cells with scant cytoplasm and hyperchromatic nuclei with small to absent nucleoli. The primary tumor is typically small and often central in location, and extensive hilar and mediastinal adenopathy is common (Fig. 7.6). Rarely, SCLC manifests as a small, peripheral solitary pulmonary nodule.

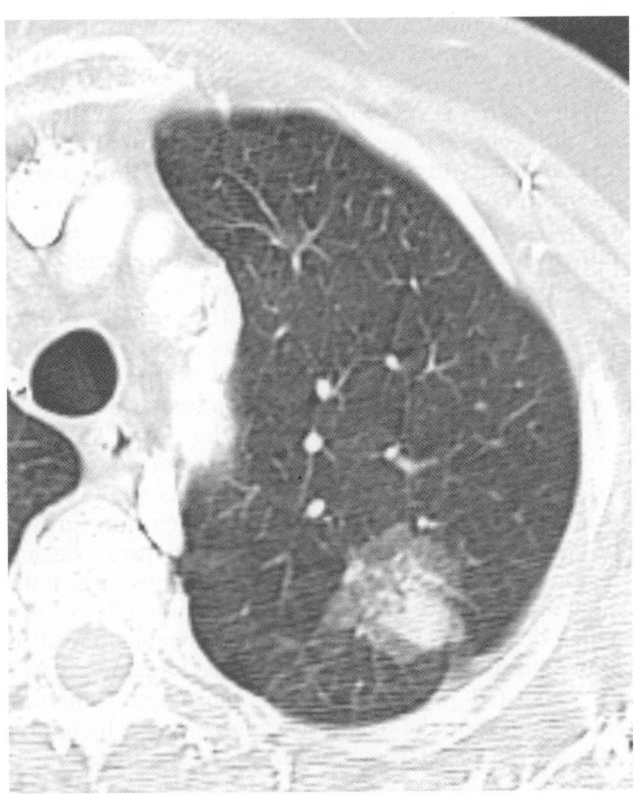

FIGURE 7.3. A 76-year-old woman with adenocarcinoma manifesting as a pulmonary nodule with mixed ground-glass and solid attenuation. Computed tomography shows a poorly marginated ground-glass opacity containing a focal solid component in the left upper lobe. The likelihood of invasive adenocarcinoma is high in part-solid nodules.

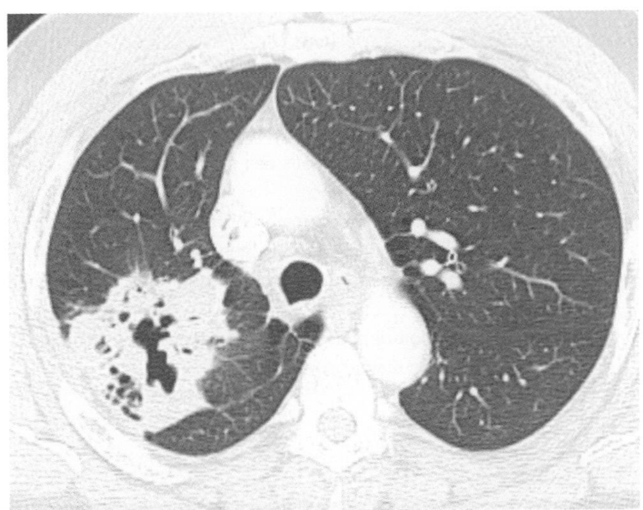

FIGURE 7.5. A 52-year-old man with squamous cell carcinoma manifesting as a large cavitary mass. Computed tomography shows a large irregular cavitary mass in the right upper lobe. Note that cavitation is more common with squamous cell carcinomas than the other histologic subtypes of lung cancer.

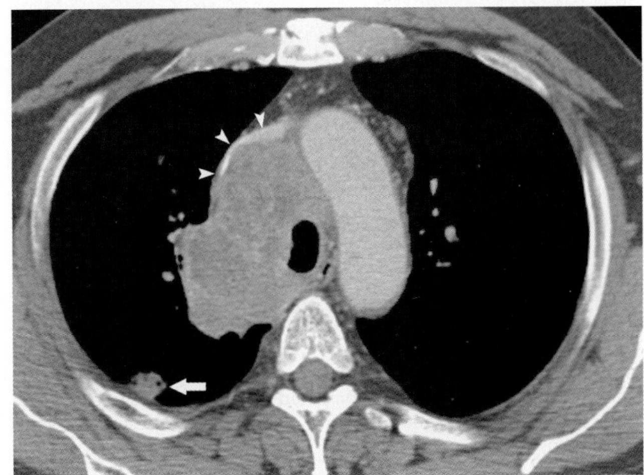

FIGURE 7.6. A 52-year-old man with small cell lung cancer manifesting as a small lung nodule and extensive mediastinal adenopathy. Computed tomography shows a small lung nodule (*arrow*) and mediastinal adenopathy that compresses and narrows the left brachiocephalic vein and superior vena cava (*arrowheads*).

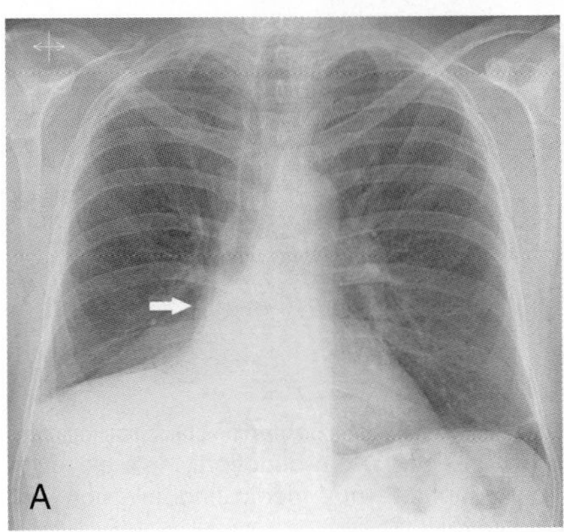

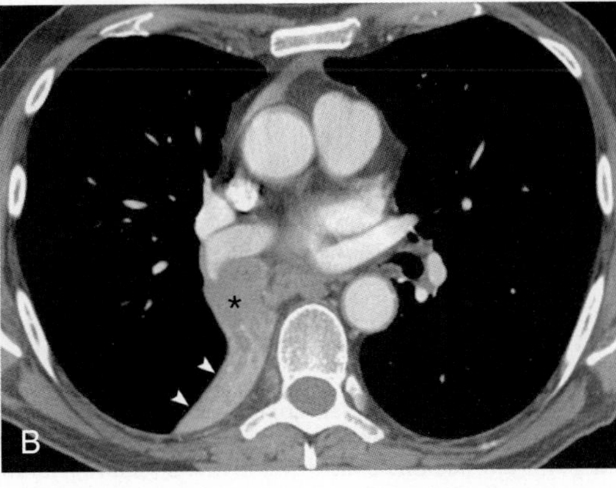

FIGURE 7.4. A 62-year-old man with squamous cell lung cancer manifesting as a central endobronchial mass. **A**, Posteroanterior chest radiograph shows complete atelectasis of the middle and right lower lobes. Convexity in the atelectatic lung (*arrow*) is the result of a central mass. **B**, Computed tomography confirms an endobronchial mass (*) that occludes the bronchus intermedius and causes complete atelectasis of the middle and lower lobes distal to the mass (*arrowheads*).

KEY POINTS

Pathology

- Two major histologic categories: nonsmall cell lung carcinoma (NSCLC) and small cell lung carcinoma (SCLC).
- NSCLC subdivided into squamous cell carcinoma, adenocarcinoma, and large cell carcinoma.
- Adenocarcinoma is the most common histologic subtype and is classified into adenocarcinoma *in situ*, minimally invasive adenocarcinoma, invasive adenocarcinoma, and variants of invasive adenocarcinoma.
- Noguchi classification applies to small peripheral adenocarcinomas and is based on tumor growth patterns.

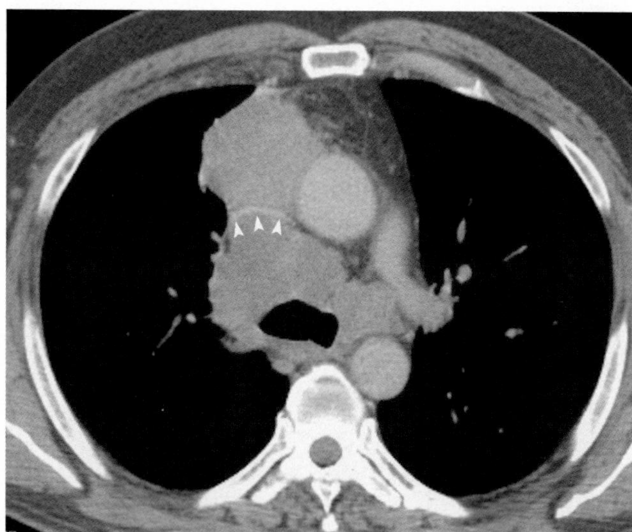

FIGURE 7.7. A 57-year-old man with nonsmall cell lung cancer presenting with superior vena cava syndrome (dyspnea, upper extremity and facial swelling). Computed tomography shows extensive, multicompartmental adenopathy and obstruction of the superior vena cava (*arrowheads*).

Clinical Manifestations

At presentation most patients are in their fifth and sixth decades and are symptomatic. Symptoms are variable and depend on the local effects of the primary mass, the presence of regional or distant metastases, and the coexistence of paraneoplastic syndromes. Central endobronchial carcinomas can manifest as cough, hemoptysis, and dyspnea. Symptoms that can occur as a result of local growth and invasion of adjacent nerves, vessels, and mediastinal structures include superior vena cava syndrome (Fig. 7.7), chest pain attributed to peribronchial nerve or chest wall involvement, vocal cord paralysis and hoarseness, dyspnea attributed to diaphragmatic paralysis (Fig. 7.8), and Horner syndrome (ptosis, miosis, anhidrosis attributed to sympathetic chain and stellate ganglion involvement by superior sulcus tumors).

Many patients present with symptoms related to extrathoracic metastases, most commonly bone pain or central nervous system abnormalities. Clinical signs and symptoms can also be caused by tumor excretion of a bioactive substance or hormone, or as a result of immune-mediated neural tissue destruction caused by antibody- or cell-mediated immune responses. These paraneoplastic syndromes occur in 10% to 20% of lung cancer patients and are usually associated with SCLC. Antidiuretic and adrenocorticotropin hormones are the more frequently excreted hormones and can result in hyponatremia and serum hypoosmolarity and in Cushing syndrome (central obesity, hypertension, glucose intolerance, plethora, hirsutism), respectively. Other hormones that can be elevated are calcitonin, growth hormone, human chorionic gonadotropin, prolactin, and serotonin. Neurologic paraneoplastic syndromes (Lambert–Eaton myasthenic syndrome, paraneoplastic cerebellar degeneration, paraneoplastic encephalomyelitis, paraneoplastic sensory neuropathy) are rare and are usually associated with SCLC. The neurologic symptoms typically precede the diagnosis of lung cancer by up to 2 years, are incapacitating, and progress rapidly, although

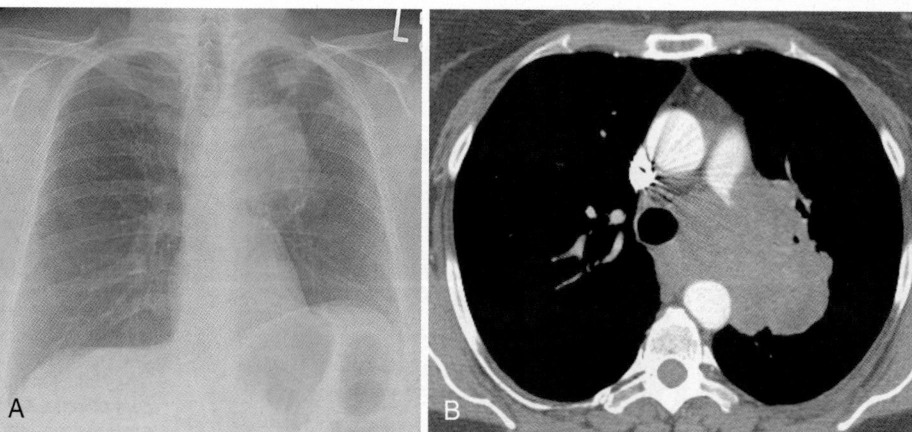

FIGURE 7.8. A 61-year-old woman with nonsmall cell lung cancer presenting with hoarseness and dyspnea. **A**, Posteroanterior chest radiograph shows a left perihilar mass and opacities more peripherally in the left upper lobe because of obstructive atelectasis/consolidation. Note elevation of the left hemidiaphragm because of paralysis as a result of phrenic nerve invasion. **B**, Computed tomography reveals mediastinal invasion with extension of the mass into the aortopulmonary window (the anatomic location of the recurrent laryngeal nerve).

improvement can occur after treatment. Miscellaneous paraneoplastic syndromes associated with lung cancer include acanthosis nigricans, dermatomyositis, disseminated intravascular coagulation, and hypertrophic pulmonary osteoarthropathy.

Patterns of Tumor Spread

Lung cancers usually invade the pulmonary arterial and venous systems, and hematogenously disseminated metastases to the lung, pleura, adrenals, liver, brain, and bones are common (Fig. 7.9). There is evidence that dissemination of cells or fragments of tumor from the primary malignancy occurs at an early stage of the malignancy, and tumor emboli or micrometastasis in bone marrow and circulating cancer cells in blood have been detected in localized NSCLC. However, the clinical relevance of this minimal hematogenous tumor cell dissemination is controversial. Nonetheless, these shed cells may represent true micrometastasis, as they are an independent prognostic factor for overall survival.[16] The pathogenesis of metastatic disease once tumor emboli have disseminated is complex and multifactorial. Although there is considerable variation among tumors, there is a relationship between the incidence of hematogenously disseminated metastases and the cell type of the lung cancer. In this regard, squamous cell carcinoma tends to grow slowly and remain localized to the lung, and hematogenous dissemination of extrathoracic metastases usually occurs late. Because adenocarcinomas are histologically a very diverse group of malignancies, there is variability in their propensity for hematogenous dissemination. Generally, the likelihood of early hematogenous dissemination of metastases is high with poorly differentiated, invasive adenocarcinomas (Noguchi types D, E, and F) and low with localized and indolent adenocarcinomas (Noguchi types A, B, and C).[15,17] Large cell carcinoma and SCLC have a high propensity for early vascular invasion, and hematogenous dissemination of distant metastases to liver, bone marrow, adrenals, and brain is common.

Similar to hematogenous dissemination, lymphatic dissemination to lymph nodes is broadly related to tumor location and tumor cell type. There is a greater frequency of nodal metastasis in patients with central tumors compared with those with peripheral tumors, and lymphatic dissemination of metastasis tends to occurs late in patients with squamous cell carcinomas and early and frequently in patients with invasive adenocarcinomas, large cell carcinomas, and SCLCs. Additionally, besides a higher prevalence of mediastinal nodal metastases in these malignancies compared with squamous cell carcinoma, there is also a much higher frequency of mediastinal metastases without lobar or hilar involvement reported in adenocarcinomas.

Lymphatic dissemination of tumor emboli in the lungs, more frequently seen with adenocarcinomas, is termed lymphangitic carcinomatosis (Fig. 7.10). Lymphangitic carcinomatosis is preceded by hematogenous dissemination of metastases. After hematogenous dissemination of metastasis in the lung parenchyma, tumor growth remains localized to the perivascular interstitium, with subsequent growth toward the hilum or periphery of the lung along pulmonary lymphatics in the perivenous and bronchoarterial interstitium and interlobular septa.

Lastly, to account for the multifocality of primary adenocarcinoma, dissemination by aerosolization has been proposed. In this regard, the origin of adenocarcinoma may either be monoclonal (with multifocality because of dissemination by aerosolization, intrapulmonary lymphatics, and intraalveolar growth) or polyclonal (with multifocality owing to *de novo* tumor growth at multiple sites) (Fig. 7.11).

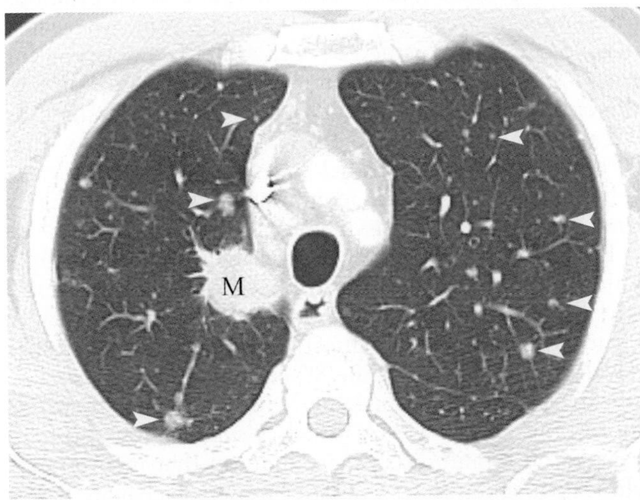

FIGURE 7.9. A 55-year-old man with nonsmall cell lung cancer and hematogenously disseminated lung metastases. Chest computed tomography scan shows the primary malignancy in the right upper lobe (*M*) and numerous small discrete nodules both lungs (*arrowheads*). Note sharp margination and variability is size is typical of hematogenous dissemination.

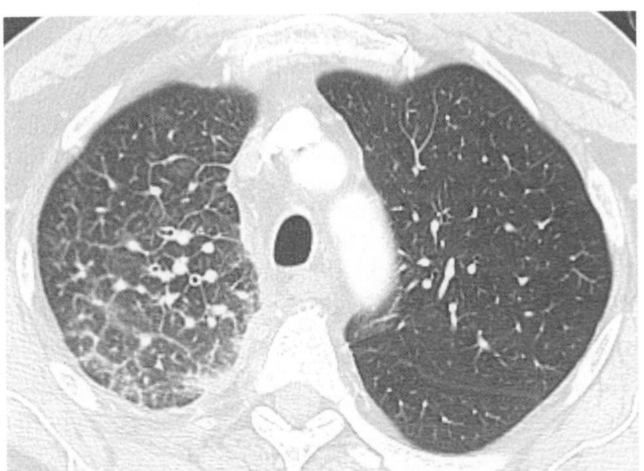

FIGURE 7.10. A 66-year-old man with a right upper nonsmall cell lung cancer (not shown) and lymphangitic carcinomatosis. Chest computed tomography shows thickening of the interlobular septa and peribronchovascular interstitium and visualization of the polygonal shape of the secondary pulmonary lobules.

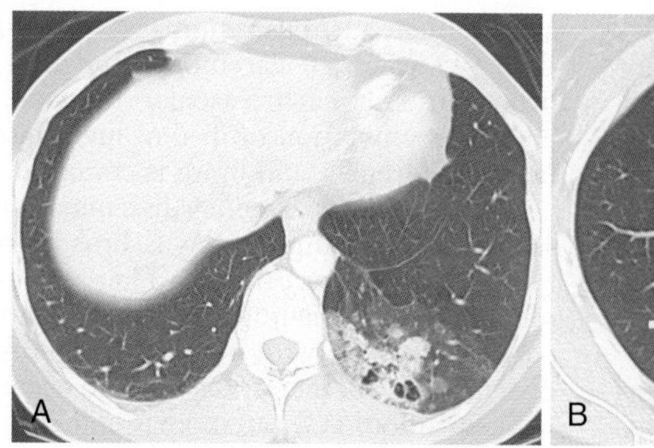

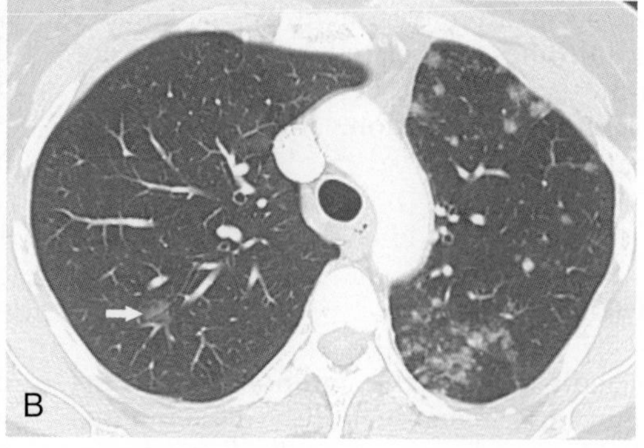

FIGURE 7.11. A 39-year-old woman with adenocarcinoma of the lung. **A**, Chest computed tomography shows a poorly marginated, cavitary mass with mixed solid and ground-glass attenuation. Note adjacent diffuse and nodular ground glass opacities consistent with multifocal malignancy. The patient underwent lower lobe resection confirming multifocal primary adenocarcinoma of the lung. **B**, Chest computed tomography 6 years after **A** shows interval development of multifocal discrete and ground glass nodular opacities in the left upper lobe and a focal ground-glass nodular opacity in the right upper lobe (*arrow*) consistent with malignancy. Note dissemination of malignancy may be by aerosolization, intrapulmonary lymphatics, and intraalveolar growth or because of *de novo* tumor growth at multiple sites.

KEY POINTS

Tumor Spread

- Dissemination of cancer cells from the primary malignancy occurs early. Tumor emboli are common and are a prognostic factor for overall survival.
- Incidence of hematogenously disseminated metastases is related to cell type.
- Hematogenous dissemination occurs late with squamous cell carcinoma.
- Hematoneous dissemination is high with invasive adenocarcinoma, large cell carcinoma, and small cell carcinoma and low with localized/indolent adenocarcinoma.
- Lymphatic dissemination of metastasis occurs late with squamous cell carcinoma and early and frequently in patients with invasive adenocarcinoma, large cell carcinoma, and small cell carcinoma.

IMAGING EVALUATION

Nonsmall Cell Lung Cancer Tumor-Node-Metastasis Staging

The treatment and prognosis of patients with NSCLC depends on the anatomic extent of disease or stage of disease at presentation. The tumor-node-metastasis (TNM) descriptors and stage-grouping of the American Joint Committee on Cancer (AJCC) TNM-8 staging system, based on analysis of the IASLC databases, are used to stage patients with lung cancer.[18–20]

Primary Tumor (T Descriptor)

The T descriptor defines the size (typically measured along the greatest long-axis diameter), location, and extent of the primary tumor (Table 7.1, Fig. 7.12).[18,21]

T1 tumors are subdivided into three groups, at 1-cm thresholds: T1a nodules (≤1 cm), T1b tumors (>1 and ≤2 cm), and T1c tumors (>2 and ≤3 cm). T2 tumors are subdivided into two groups: T2a tumors (>3 and ≤4 cm) and T2b lesions (>4 and ≤5 cm or any of the following: invade the visceral pleura or involve a main bronchus without direct invasion of the carina or partial or complete lung atelectasis/obstructive pneumonitis). T3 tumors are >5 and ≤7 cm or directly invade any of the following structures: parietal pleura, chest wall (including superior sulcus tumors), phrenic nerve, parietal pericardium, or separate tumor nodule(s) in the same lobe. T4 tumors are >7 cm or invade any of the following structures: mediastinum, diaphragm, heart, great vessels, trachea, recurrent laryngeal nerve, esophagus, vertebral body, or carina; or are separate tumor nodule(s) in a different lobe of the same lung.

In lung cancer, the T descriptor has been traditionally based on total tumor size. However, in nonmucinous adenocarcinomas manifesting as subsolid lesions, the solid component (which typically corresponds to the invasive component of the tumor) is used to determine the T descriptor.[22] If the adenocarcinoma manifests as a pure ground-glass lesion on CT it is classified as carcinoma *in situ* Tis if it is >0.5 and ≤3 cm, whereas if it is >3 cm it is classified as T1a. The T descriptor for part-solid nodules is determined by the largest size of the solid component: nodules ≤0.5 cm are classified as T1 minimally invasive (T1mi), >0.5 and ≤1 cm as T1a, >1 and ≤2 cm as T1b, and >2 and ≤3 cm as T1c. If a part-solid nodule has a solid component ≤0.5 cm but has a total size >3 cm, it is classified as cT1a.[22]

Patients with lung cancer that manifests as multiple pulmonary sites of disease have been challenging to classify. The International Association for the Study of Lung Cancer Staging and Prognostic Factors Committee has developed proposals for the 8th edition of the TNM classification to address this issue.[23] In this regard, if two or more lung lesions are classified as synchronous primary cancers on a multidisciplinary opinion that incorporates clinical, imaging, and pathologic findings, each malignancy should be staged separately within the TNM staging system, with each being assigned distinct T descriptors and overall stage group.[24,25] Furthermore, lung cancers manifesting as multiple pulmonary lesions with ground-glass

Table 7.1 International Association for the Study of Lung Cancer Lung Cancer Staging Project T, N, and M Descriptors for the TNM-8 Classification of Lung Cancer

T – PRIMARY TUMOR		
CATEGORY	**SUBCATEGORY**	**DESCRIPTORS**
TX		Primary tumor cannot be assessed, or tumor proven by the presence of malignant cells in sputum or bronchial washings but not visualized by imaging or bronchoscopy
T0		No evidence of primary tumor
Tis		Carcinoma *in situ*: Tis (adenocarcinoma *in situ*): adenocarcinoma Tis(SCIS): squamous cell carcinoma
T1		Tumor ≤3 in greatest dimension, surrounded by lung or visceral pleura, without bronchoscopic evidence of invasion more proximal than the lobar bronchus (i.e., not in the main bronchus). The uncommon superficial spreading tumor of any size with its invasive component limited to the bronchial wall, which may extend proximal to the main bronchus, is also classified as T1a.
	T1mi	Minimally invasive adenocarcinoma
	T1a	Tumor ≤1 cm in greatest dimension
	T1b	Tumor >1 cm but <2 cm in greatest dimension
	T1c	Tumor >2 cm but <3 cm in greatest dimension
T2		Tumor >3 cm but <5 cm; or tumor with any of the following features. T2 tumors with these features are classified T2a if ≤4 cm, or if size cannot be determined; and T2b if >4 cm but not >5 cm. Involves main bronchus regardless of distance to the carina, but without involving the carina Invades visceral pleura Associated with atelectasis or obstructive pneumonitis that extends to the hilar region, involving either part of the lung or the entire lung
	T2a	Tumor >3 cm but <4 cm in greatest dimension
	T2b	Tumor >4 cm but <5 cm in greatest dimension
T3		Tumor >5 cm but <7 cm in greatest dimension or one that directly invades any of the following: parietal pleura (PL3), chest wall (including superior sulcus tumors), phrenic nerve, parietal pericardium; or associated separate tumor nodule(s) in the same lobe as the primary
T4		Tumors >7 cm or one that invades any of the following: diaphragm, mediastinum, heart, great vessels, trachea, recurrent laryngeal nerve, esophagus, vertebral body, carina; separate tumor nodule(s) in a different ipsilateral lobe to that of the primary

Modified from Goldstraw P, Crowley J, Chansky K, et al. The IASLC Lung Cancer Staging Project: proposals for the revision of the TNM stage groupings in the forthcoming (seventh) edition of the TNM Classification of malignant tumors. *J Thorac Oncol.* 2007;2(8):706-714.

or lepidic features are generally multifocal adenocarcinomas and are classified by the lesion with the highest-level T descriptor and the number of lesions (#) or simply (m) for multiple indicated in parentheses.[26] The lesion size is determined by the largest diameter of the solid component. The T (#/m) multifocal classification should be used regardless of whether these lesions are suspected on imaging or are pathologically proven, and regardless of whether lesions are in the same lobe or in different ipsilateral or contralateral lobes. The N and M categories that apply to all of the tumor foci collectively should be used. Lung cancer manifesting as diffuse consolidation is assigned a T category as follows: the T descriptor of consolidation confined to a single lobe is determined by the size of the lesion, and, if difficult to measure, the T3 descriptor is assigned; if multiple sites of lung involvement are present, the T category is determined by location: T3 if confined to one lobe, T4 if affecting different lobes in the same lung, and M1a if involving both lungs. When tumor is present within both lungs, the T category is based on the appropriate T category for the lung with the greatest extent of tumor involvement. For instance, if one or multiple lobes of the same lung are affected, the designation is T3 or T4, respectively. The N and M categories that apply to all of the tumor foci collectively should be used.

Regional Lymph Nodes (N Status)

The presence and location of nodal metastasis are of major importance in determining management and prognosis in patients with NSCLC. In contrast to the primary lung cancer, the short-axis diameter is typically used for lymph node measurement. N0 is defined as the absence of lymph node involvement; N1 includes ipsilateral peripheral or hilar lymph node metastases; N2 includes ipsilateral mediastinal (upper, aorticopulmonary, lower) or subcarinal lymph node metastases; and N3 includes ipsilateral or contralateral supraclavicular lymph node or contralateral mediastinal, hilar/interlobar, or peripheral lymph node metastases (see Table 7.2).[19]

To enable a consistent and standardized description of N status, lymph node "maps" are used to describe the location of nodal metastases. The International Association for the Study of Lung Cancer has proposed a lymph node map that reconciles differences among currently used maps and provides precise anatomic definitions for all lymph node stations. The IASLC map assigns lymph nodes to seven specific zones: the upper,

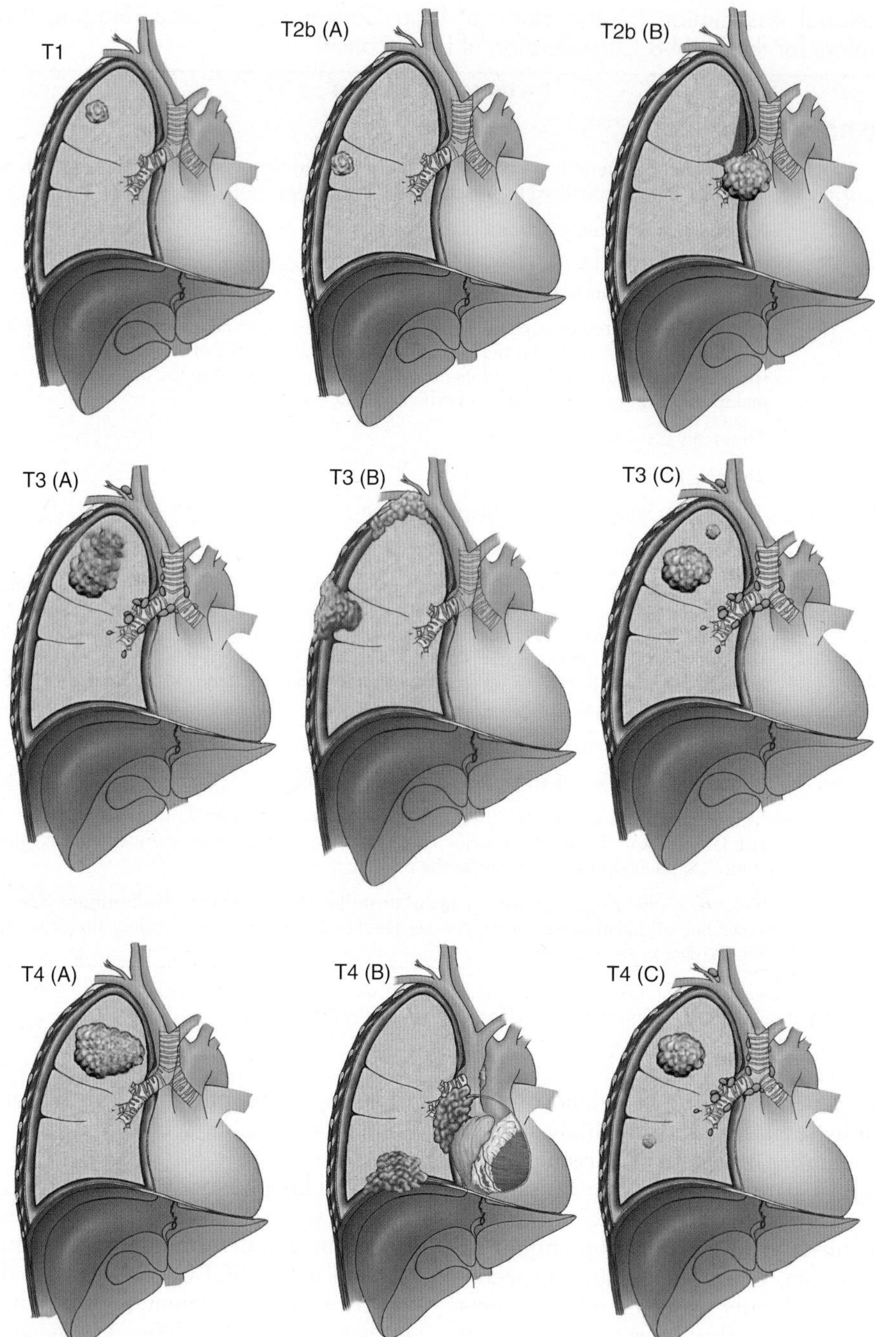

FIGURE 7.12. T1: tumor <3-cm surrounded by lung or visceral pleura without evidence of invasion proximal to a lobar bronchus. T1 tumors are subdivided into three groups at 1-cm thresholds: **T1a** nodules ≤1-cm, **T1b** tumors >1 and ≤2-cm, and **T1c** lesions >2 and ≤3-cm (not shown). **T2** tumors are subdivided into two groups: **T2a** tumors >3 and ≤4-cm and **T2b** tumors >4 and ≤5-cm (not shown) or tumor of any size with any of the following: invades visceral pleura (A), involves a main bronchus without direct invasion of the carina (B), or partial or complete lung atelectasis/obstructive pneumonia (not shown). **T3**, Tumor >5 and ≤7-cm (A), or tumor of any size with any of the following: invades parietal pleura or chest wall including superior sulcus tumors (B), phrenic nerve, parietal pericardium or separate tumor nodule(s) in same lobe as the primary (C). **T4**, Tumors >7-cm (A), or invades any of the following structures: mediastinum diaphragm, heart, great vessels, trachea, recurrent laryngeal nerve, esophagus, vertebral body, carina (B); or separate tumor nodule(s) in a different lobe of the same lung (C).

Table 7.2 Regional Lymph Node Stations for Lung Cancer Staging

N – REGIONAL LYMPH NODES	
NX	Regional lymph nodes cannot be assessed
N0	No regional lymph node metastasis
N1	Metastasis in ipsilateral peribronchial and/or ipsilateral hilar lymph nodes and intrapulmonary nodes, including involvement by direct extension
N2	Metastasis in ipsilateral mediastinal and/or subcarinal lymph node(s)
N3	Metastasis in contralateral mediastinal, contralateral hilar, ipsilateral or contralateral scalene, or supraclavicular lymph node(s)
M- DISTANT METASTASIS	
M0	No distant metastasis
M1	Distant metastasis
M1a	Separate tumor nodule(s) in a contralateral lobe; tumor with pleural nodules or malignant pleural or pericardial effusion. Most pleural (pericardial) effusions with lung cancer are attributed to tumor. In a few patients, however, multiple microscopic examinations of pleural (pericardial) fluid are negative for tumor, and the fluid is nonbloody and is not an exudate. Where these elements and clinical judgment dictate that the effusion is not related to the tumor, the effusion should be excluded as a staging descriptor.
M1b	Single extrathoracic metastasis in a single organ and involvement of a single distant (nonregional) node
M1c	Multiple extrathoracic metastases in one or several organs

Besides the descriptor "tumor size,", it should be indicated that, for part-solid tumors, the size of the solid component on computed tomography and the size of the invasive component at pathologic examination are the ones to be used to define the T category based on tumor size.

aorticopulmonary, subcarinal, lower, hilar/interlobar, and peripheral zones (Table 7.2).[27]

Metastatic Disease (M Status)

Patients with NSCLC commonly have metastases to the lung, adrenals, liver, brain, bones, and extrathoracic lymph nodes at presentation. The M1 descriptor is subclassified into M1a (additional nodules in the contralateral lung, malignant pleural/pericardial effusions/nodules), M1b (single extrathoracic metastasis in a single distant organ), and M1c (multiple extrathoracic metastases in one or more distant organs).[20]

The International Staging System for Lung Cancer combines the T descriptors with the N and M descriptors into subsets or stages that have similar treatment options and prognosis.[21]

Key Points

Staging

- Size of the tumor is important in determining the T descriptor.
- The solid component is used to determine the T descriptor in nonmucinous adenocarcinomas manifesting as subsolid lesions.
- Additional nodules in the lung (primary lobe) are classified as T3; additional nodules in the ipsilateral lung (different lobe) are classified as T4.
- Lung cancers manifesting as multiple pulmonary lesions with ground-glass attenuation are classified by the lesion with the highest level T descriptor and the number of lesions (#), or simply (m) for multiple, indicated in parentheses.
- The N descriptor describes the location of nodal metastases.
- The M1 descriptor is subclassified into M1a (additional nodules in the contralateral lung, malignant pleural/pericardial effusions/nodules), M1b (single extrathoracic metastasis in a single distant organ), and M1c (multiple extrathoracic metastases in one or more distant organs).

Small Cell Lung Cancer Staging

SCLC is generally staged according to the Veteran's Administration Lung Cancer Study Group recommendations as limited disease (LD) or extensive disease (ED).[28] LD defines tumor confined to a hemithorax and the regional lymph nodes. Unlike the TNM classification for NSCLC, metastases to the ipsilateral supraclavicular, contralateral supraclavicular, and mediastinal lymph nodes are considered local disease. ED includes tumor with noncontiguous metastases to the contralateral lung and distant metastases.[28]

The AJCC TNM staging system is also applicable to SCLC, but is used less frequently in clinical practice, because only a small percentage of patients with SCLC present at a stage for which surgery is appropriate. Nevertheless, small published series of resected SCLCs have suggested that the TNM pathologic staging correlates with the survival of resected patients. An analysis of the 8088 cases of SCLC in the IASLC database demonstrated the usefulness of clinical TNM staging in this malignancy.[29] The TNM-8 classification has prognostic value in SCLC, and it is proposed that TNM staging should be the standard for all SCLC cases.[30]

Key Points

Staging

- Small cell lung cancer (SCLC) is traditionally staged as limited disease (confined to one hemithorax) or extensive disease (noncontiguous metastases).
- The International Association for the Study of Lung Cancer Lung Cancer Staging Project proposes that tumor-node-metastasis staging becomes the standard for SCLC.

IMAGING

Nonsmall Cell Lung Cancer

Imaging is a major component of clinical TNM staging. However, there is currently little consensus on the imaging that should be performed for appropriate staging evaluation in patients presenting with NSCLC. The American Society of Clinical Oncology (ASCO) has published evidence-based guidelines for the diagnostic evaluation of patients with NSCLC.[31] In the staging of locoregional disease these guidelines recommend that a chest radiograph and contrast-enhanced chest CT that includes the liver and adrenals should be performed. In addition, whole-body imaging with 2-[^{18}F] fluoro-2-deoxy-D-glucose (FDG)-PET should be performed when there is no evidence of distant metastatic disease on CT.[31] This recommendation is based on the fact that FDG-PET imaging improves the detection of nodal and distant metastases and frequently alters patient management.[32,33] Although not addressed in the guidelines, whole-body MRI has been advocated as an alternative to standard imaging for staging cancer, as accuracy is similar and staging efficiency is better.[34]

CT and MRI are often performed to more optimally assess the primary tumor, because the extent of the primary tumor can determine therapeutic management (surgical resection, radiotherapy, or chemotherapy). Evaluation of the primary tumor (size, location, proximity to critical structures) is important and provides information to surgeons and radiation oncologists that can affect therapeutic management. For instance, centrally located tumors close to the spinal cord impose radiation dose-volume constraints, and determination of tumor margins is important and can affect the delivery of radiotherapy. This is especially important with the increasing use of precision radiation therapy (RT) including stereotactic body RT (SBRT) and proton therapy, techniques that generate dose distributions that conform tightly to target volumes. The determination of the degree of pleural, chest wall, and mediastinal invasion, as well as involvement of the central airways and pulmonary arteries, is also important not only to radiation oncologists, but also to surgeons evaluating patients for resectability. For instance, involvement of the main pulmonary artery may require a pneumonectomy rather than a lobectomy to obtain clear surgical margins. Additionally, involvement of the origin of the lobar bronchus or main bronchus may require a sleeve resection or pneumonectomy. Because patients treated by medical oncologists generally have metastatic disease, and treatment is directed both at local and systemic disease, accurate determination of tumor location and extent is only important if there is a potential risk for a significant complication such as invasion of a vascular structure that could result in significant bleeding.

CT is useful in defining the T descriptors of the primary tumor, but in many patients this assessment has limitations. For instance, CT is useful in confirming gross chest wall invasion but is inaccurate in differentiating between anatomic contiguity and subtle invasion. Determining the presence and extent of chest wall invasion is important from a surgical perspective, as the surgical approach may be altered to include an *en bloc* resection of the primary malignancy and chest wall. Although MRI offers superior soft-tissue contrast resolution compared with CT, the sensitivity and specificity in identifying chest wall invasion are not optimal. CT or MRI is also useful in confirming gross invasion of the mediastinum, but these modalities, similar to chest wall assessment, are inaccurate in determining subtle invasion. However, MRI is particularly useful in the evaluation of cardiac invasion and superior sulcus tumors. In superior sulcus tumors MRI helps determine the degree of involvement of the brachial plexus, subclavian vessels, and vertebral bodies (Fig. 7.13).[35,36] Importantly, absolute contraindications to surgery (invasion of the brachial plexus roots or trunks above the level of T1, invasion of greater than 50% of a vertebral body, and invasion of the esophagus or trachea) are often accurately assessed by MRI.[37,38]

Because surgical resection and potential use of adjuvant therapy are dependent on the patient's N descriptor, attempts have been made to improve the accuracy of detection of nodal metastases. Importantly, ipsilateral peribronchial or hilum (N1) nodes are usually resectable, and it is the presence of mediastinal adenopathy that has a major impact on resectability. Specifically, ipsilateral nonbulky,

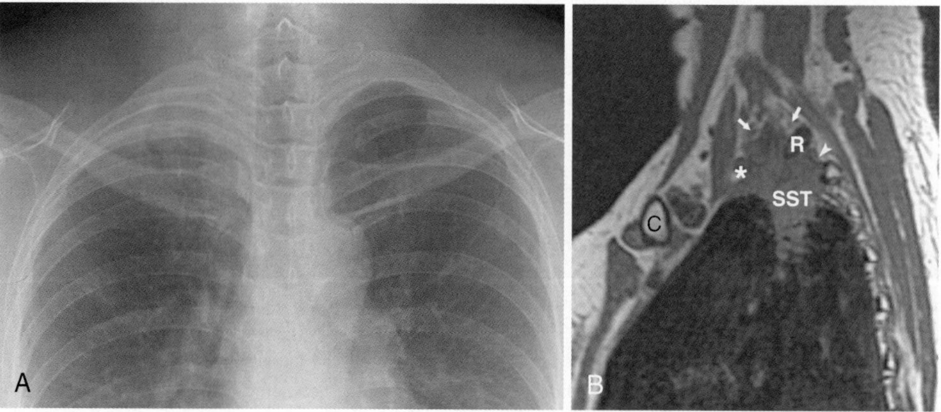

FIGURE 7.13. A 49-year-old woman with a superior sulcus nonsmall cell lung cancer presenting with shoulder pain and Horner syndrome (ptosis, miosis, anhidrosis). **A**, Posteroanterior chest radiograph shows a soft tissue mass in the right lung apex. There are no findings of rib or vertebral body invasion. **B**, Sagittal T1-weighted magnetic resonance imaging scan shows the superior sulcus tumor (*SST*) extending posteriorly into the T1/T2 neurovertebral foramen (*arrowhead*) and causing obliteration of the exiting T1 nerve root. The C7 and C8 nerve root are preserved (*arrows*). Note that limited involvement of the brachial plexus does not preclude surgical resection. *C*, Clavicle; *R*, first rib; *, subclavian artery.

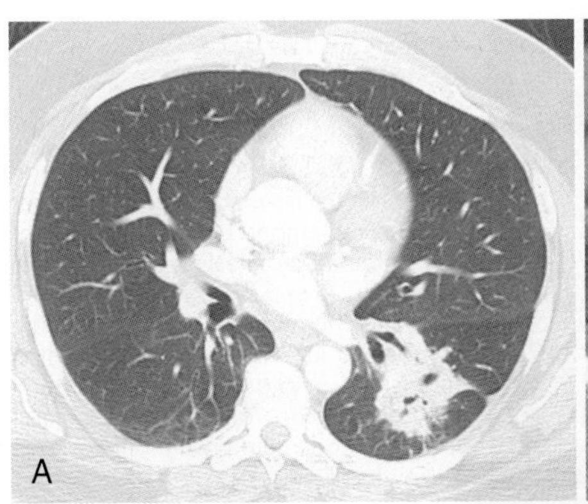

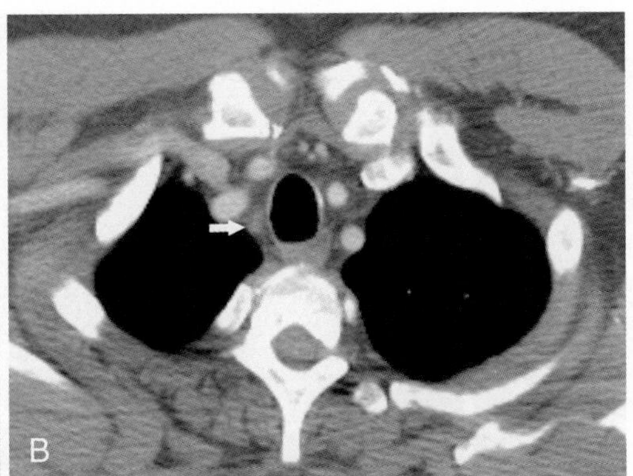

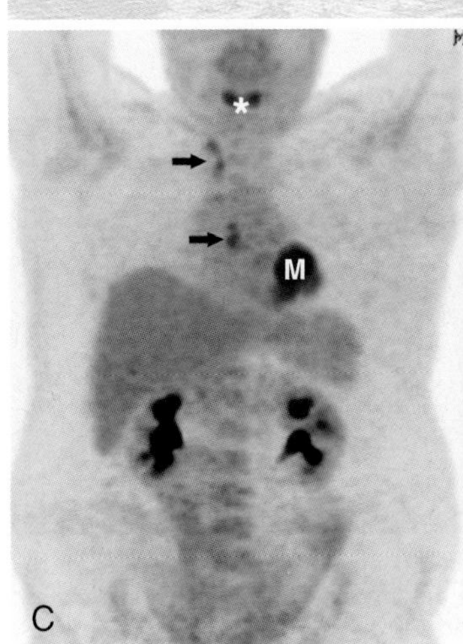

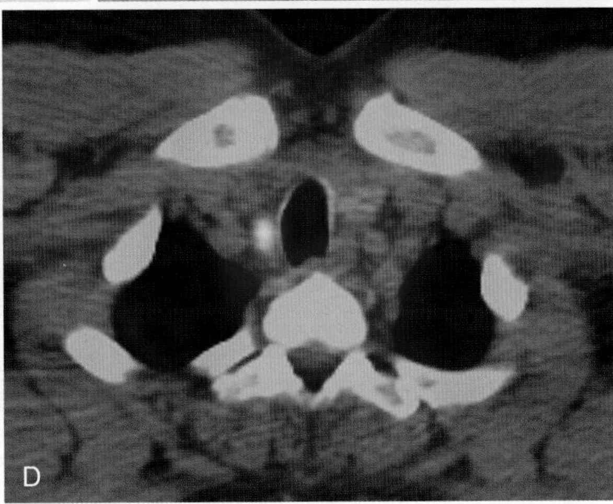

FIGURE 7.14. A 51-year-old man with a left lower lobe nonsmall cell lung cancer being evaluated for surgical resection. **A** and **B**, Computed tomography (CT) shows a left lower lobe mass and small node in the contralateral superior mediastinum (*arrow*). **C**, Whole-body coronal positron emission tomography (PET) shows focal increased 2-[^{18}F] fluoro-2-deoxy-D-glucose (FDG) uptake in the left lower lobe mass (*M*) and in subcarinal and contralateral mediastinal nodes (*arrow*); *, normal uptake of FDG in vocal cords. **D**, Positron emission tomography shows increased uptake of FDG in a right superior mediastinal node. Biopsy confirmed metastatic disease (N3), and the patient was treated palliatively.

single-station mediastinal or subcarinal adenopathy (N2) may be resectable (usually after induction chemotherapy or chemoradiation), whereas contralateral mediastinal adenopathy and scalene or supraclavicular adenopathy (N3) are felt to be unresectable. The detection of nodal metastases is also important to the radiation oncologist, as incorporation of these nodes into the radiation treatment plan is important in appropriate treatment. In the imaging evaluation of nodal metastasis, size is the only criterion used to diagnose metastases, with nodes greater than 1 cm on the short-axis diameter considered abnormal. However, lymph node size is not a reliable parameter for the evaluation of nodal metastatic disease in patients with NSCLC. In a metaanalysis of 3438 patients evaluating CT accuracy for staging the mediastinum, there was a pooled sensitivity of 57%, specificity of 82%, positive predictive value of 56%, and negative predictive value of 83%.[39] Furthermore, Prenzel et al. reported that, in 2891 resected hilar and mediastinal nodes obtained from 256 patients with NSCLC, 77% of the 139 patients with no nodal metastases had at least one node greater than 1 cm in diameter, and 12% of the 127 patients with nodal metastases had no nodes greater than 1 cm.[40]

FDG-PET improves the accuracy of nodal staging (Fig. 7.14).[41,42] In a meta-analysis (17 studies, 833 patients) comparing PET and CT in nodal staging in patients with NSCLC, the sensitivity and specificity of FDG-PET for detecting mediastinal lymph node metastases ranged from 66% to 100% (overall 83%) and 81% to 100% (overall 92%), respectively, compared with sensitivity and specificity of CT of 20% to 81% (overall 59%) and 44% to 100% (overall 78%), respectively.[41] Because of the improvements of nodal staging when PET/CT is incorporated into the imaging algorithm, all patients with potentially resectable NSCLC, regardless of the size of mediastinal nodes, should undergo PET/CT to direct nodal sampling, as well as to detect distant occult metastasis. Importantly, although FDG-PET is cost effective for nodal staging and can reduce the likelihood that a patient with mediastinal nodal metastases (N3) will undergo unneeded surgery, the number of false-positive results because of infectious or inflammatory etiologies is too high to preclude the necessity of invasive mediastinal sampling.

The detection of metastases is important in determining whether the patient will be a candidate for surgical resection or receive palliative radiation and chemotherapy. For instance, the diagnosis of a malignant pleural effusion or pleural metastases is important in patient management, because these metastases preclude surgical resection (Fig. 7.15). However, the role of imaging in detecting M1 disease is not clearly defined. For instance, patients with early-stage (T1, N0) NSCLC have a very low incidence of occult metastasis, and extensive evaluation for metastasis in these patients is not warranted.[43] However, in patients with more advanced disease, whole-body FDG-PET/CT can improve the accuracy of staging. FDG-PET/CT has a higher sensitivity and specificity than CT in detecting metastases to the adrenals, bones, and extrathoracic lymph nodes (Figs. 7.16 and 7.17). In this regard, the American College of Surgeons Oncology Trial reports a sensitivity, specificity, positive predictive value, and negative predictive value of 83%, 90%, 36%, and 99%, respectively, for M1 disease.[33]

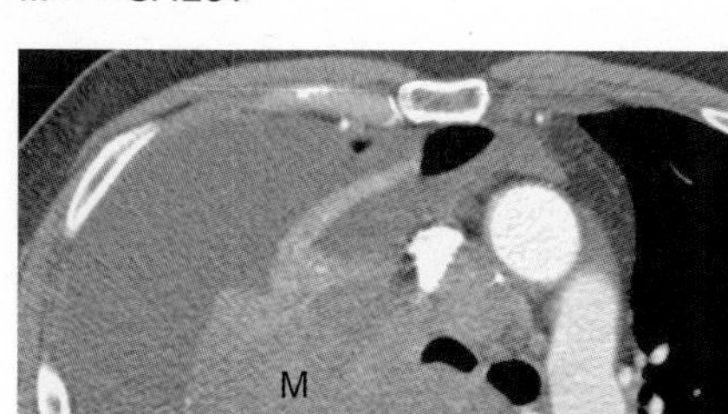

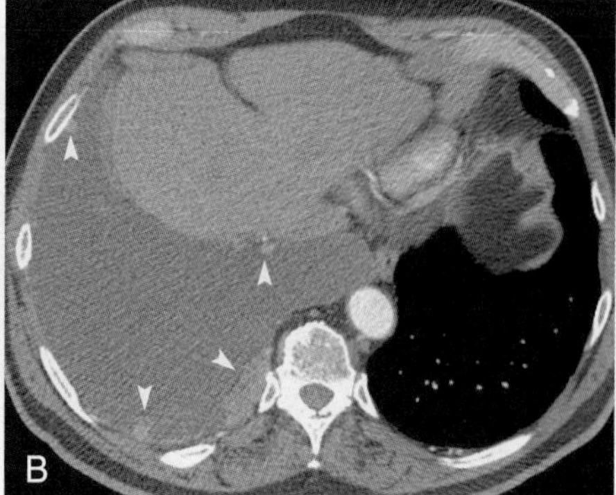

FIGURE 7.15. A 64-year-old man with primary nonsmall cell lung cancer and a malignant pleural effusion at presentation manifesting as shortness of breath. **A** and **B**, Contrast-enhanced computed tomography shows a large right upper lobe mass (*M*) with invasion into the mediastinum, large right pleural effusion, and nodular pleural lesions consistent with metastases (*arrowheads*).

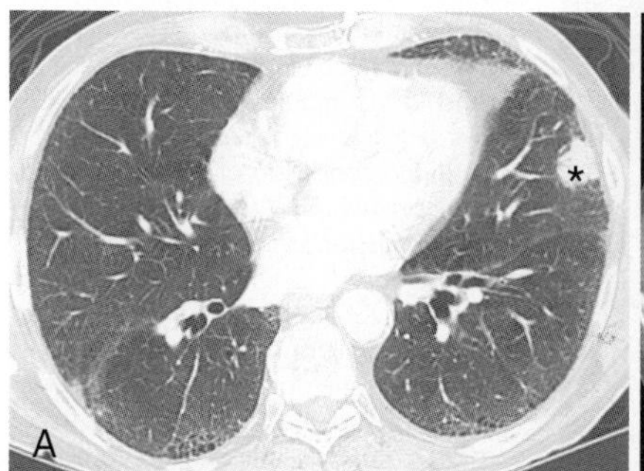

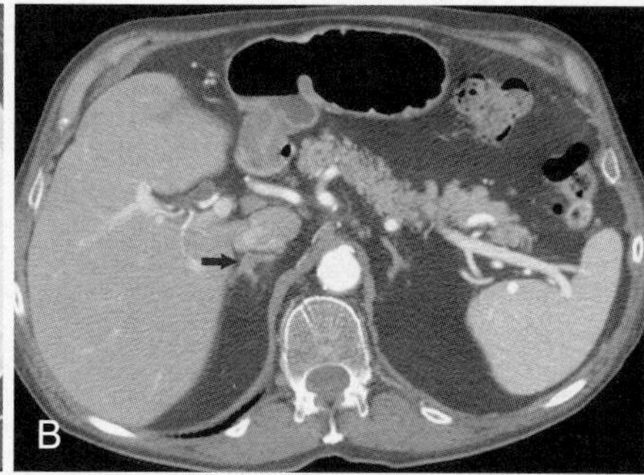

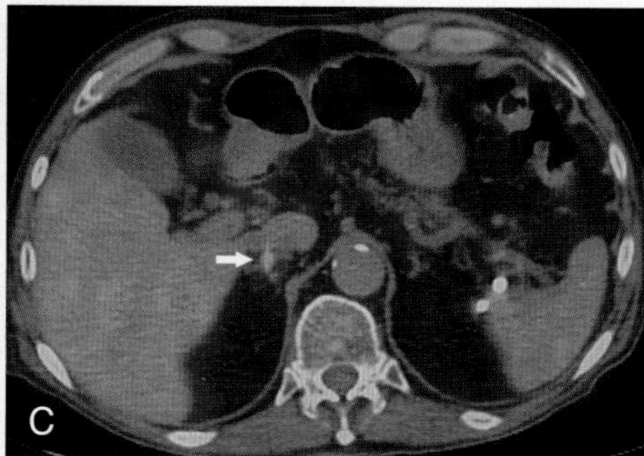

FIGURE 7.16. An 83-year-old man with nonsmall cell cancer of the left upper lobe. **A** and **B**, Contrast-enhanced computed tomography (CT) shows a left upper lobe nodule (*) and a small region of focal nodularity of the right adrenal gland (*arrow*). Note emphysema and fibrosis. **C**, Positron emission tomography-CT shows increased uptake of 2-[^{18}F] fluoro-2-deoxy-D-glucose in the right adrenal gland (*arrow*) suspicious for a metastasis. Repeat CT (*not shown*) revealed increase in size consistent with progression of metastatic disease.

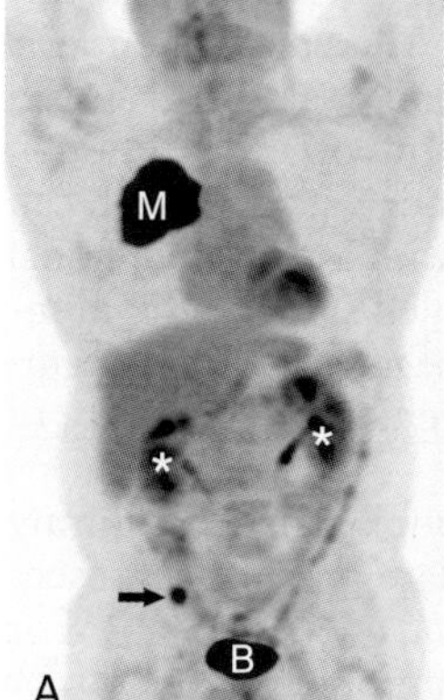

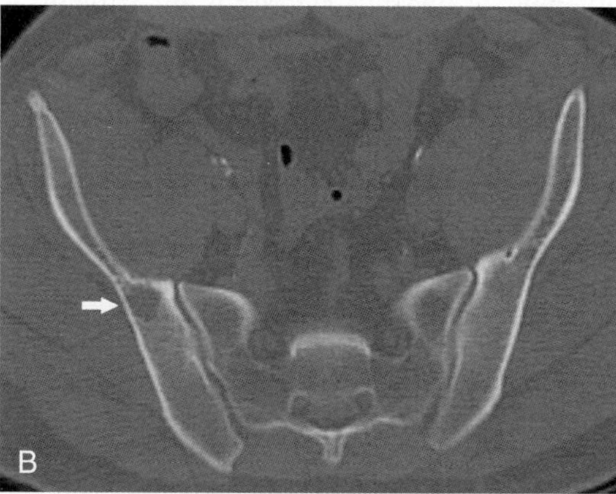

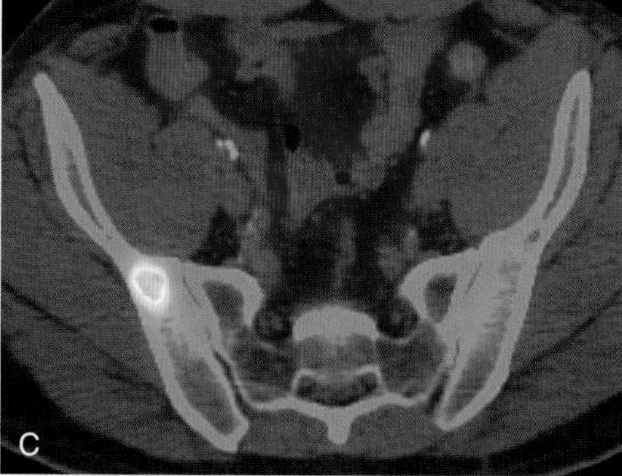

FIGURE 7.17. A 52-year-old man with nonsmall cell lung cancer presenting with a solitary bone metastasis. **A**, Coronal whole-body positron emission tomography (PET) shows increased 2-[^{18}F] fluoro-2-deoxy-D-glucose (FDG) uptake within the primary malignancy (*M*). There is focal abnormal FDG uptake (*arrow*) in the region of the pelvis suspicious for a metastasis. **B**, Accumulation of FDG in the bladder; *, renal excretion of FDG. Computed tomography (CT) (**B**) and PET-CT (**C**) show lytic lesion in the right iliac bone (*arrow*) with focal increased uptake of FDG. Biopsy confirmed metastatic disease, and the patient was treated palliatively.

Whole-body PET imaging stages intra- and extrathoracic disease in a single study and detects occult extrathoracic metastases in up to 24% of patients selected for curative resection.[32,33,44] The incidence of detection of occult metastases has been reported to increase as the staging T and N descriptors increase, (i.e., 7.5% in early stage disease to 24% in advanced disease).[44] In two studies with a relatively high proportion of more advanced lung cancers considered resectable by standard clinical staging, PET imaging prevented nontherapeutic surgery in one in five patients.[32,33] It is important to emphasize that, although whole-body FDG-PET imaging improves the accuracy of staging, false-positive uptake of FDG can mimic distant metastases, and therefore all focal lesions with increased FDG uptake should biopsied if they potentially would alter patient management.

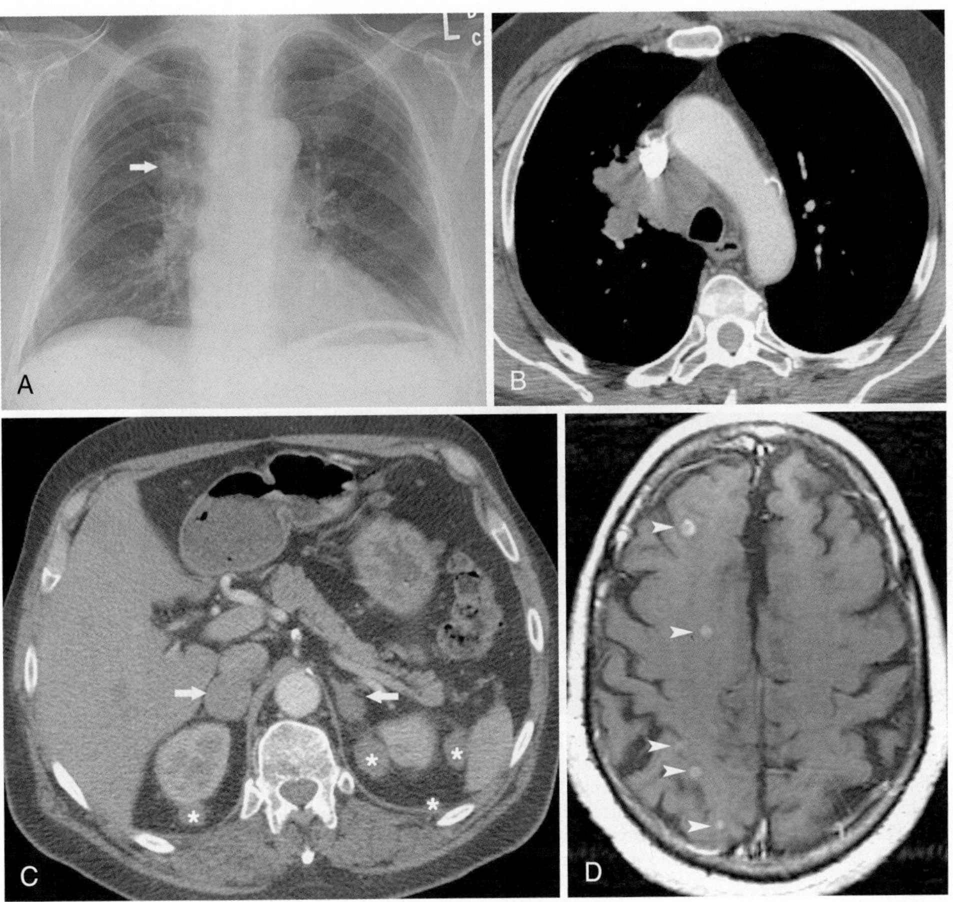

FIGURE 7.18. A 61-year-old man with extensive small cell lung cancer presenting with seizures. **A**, Posteroanterior chest radiograph shows a poorly marginated right lung mass (*arrow*). **B**, Chest computed tomography (CT) confirms a poorly marginated right upper lobe mass and reveals confluent mediastinal adenopathy. **C**, Contrast-enhanced abdominal CT shows bilateral adrenal metastases (*arrows*) and perirenal soft tissue metastases (*). **D**, T1-weighted contrast-enhanced axial magnetic resonance image of the brain reveals numerous small metastases (*arrowheads*).

KEY POINTS

What the Surgeon Needs to Know

- The size, location, and presence of locoregional invasion (T descriptor) is necessary to determine the appropriate surgical resection plan.
- Degree of pleural, chest wall, and mediastinal invasion, as well as involvement of the central airways and pulmonary arteries, is important in determining not only potential resectability but also surgical approach.
- Involvement of the main pulmonary artery may require pneumonectomy or sleeve resection with pulmonary arterioplasty rather than a lobectomy.
- Involvement of the lobar or main bronchi without main pulmonary artery involvement may require a sleeve resection or pneumonectomy.
- Ipsilateral peribronchial/hilar (N1) nodes are usually resectable.
- Ipsilateral nonbulky single-station (N2) nodes may be resectable after induction chemotherapy or chemoradiation.
- Contralateral or supraclavicular nodes (N3) typically preclude resection.
- Distant metastasis usually precludes local treatment such as surgical resection or radiation therapy, unless oligometastatic (one to three lesions).

What the Medical Oncologist Needs to Know

- Treatment is usually directed at both local and systemic disease.
- Accurate determination of tumor location and extent usually is not important.
- Imaging is important in the determination of the effectiveness of treatment.

What the Radiation Oncologist Needs to Know

- Size and location of the primary tumor, as well as the proximity of tumor to critical structures in cases where radiation tolerance imposes dose-volume constraints.
- Determination of tumor margins is important because of increasing use of radiation techniques where dose distributions conform tightly to target volumes.
- Detection and incorporation of nodal metastasis into the radiation treatment is required for appropriate treatment.

Small Cell Lung Cancer

Most patients with SCLC have widely disseminated disease at presentation. Common sites of metastatic disease include the liver, bone, bone marrow, brain, and retroperitoneal lymph nodes (Fig. 7.18). Although there is no consensus regarding the imaging and invasive procedures that should be performed in the staging evaluation of patients with SCLC, appropriate staging workup for patients with SCLC has traditionally included contrast-enhanced CT of the chest and abdomen, technitium-99m methyl diphosphonate bone scintigraphy, and MRI or CT scan of the brain. MRI has been advocated to assess the liver, adrenals, brain, and axial skeleton in a single study.[45] Whole-body PET imaging has been also been reported to improve the accuracy of staging of patients with SCLC (Fig. 7.19).[46]

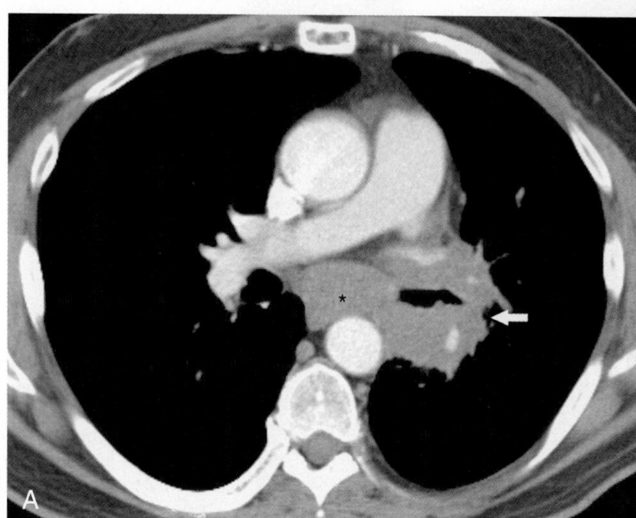

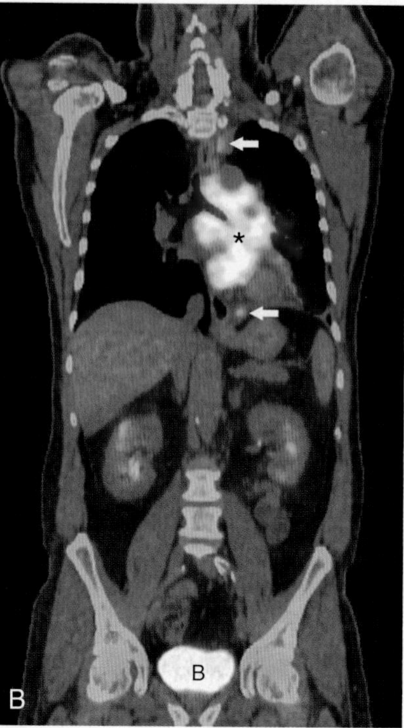

Figure 7.19. A 63-year-old man with small cell lung cancer who presented with a history of hemoptysis. **A**, Contrast-enhanced computed tomography (CT) shows a large left lower lobe mass (*arrow*) surrounding the left lower lobe bronchus, as well as subcarinal adenopathy (*). Extensive multicompartmental mediastinal adenopathy was also present (*not shown*). **B**, Whole-body coronal positron emission tomography-CT shows increased uptake of 2-[^{18}F] fluoro-2-deoxy-D-glucose (FDG) within confluent multicompartmental mediastinal nodes (*) and superior paratracheal and peri-esophageal nodes (*arrows*). There are no FDG-avid extrathoracic metastases. Because the patient had limited disease (disease confined to the thorax), treatment was concurrent chemoradiation. *B*, Accumulation of FDG in the bladder.

TREATMENT

Nonsmall Cell Lung Cancer

Surgical resection is typically the treatment of choice in patients with localized NSCLC in which the tumor size is larger than 2 cm. In those patients who are potential candidates for surgical resection, clinical and physiologic assessment should be performed to determine the patient's ability to tolerate resection. Spirometry is a good initial test to quantify a patient's pulmonary reserve and assess the ability to tolerate surgical resection. A postoperative forced expiratory volume in the first second of less than 0.8 liters or less than 35% of predicted is associated with an increased risk of perioperative complications, respiratory insufficiency, and death. Additional risk factors for lung resection include a predicted postoperative diffusing capacity or maximum ventilatory ventilation of less than 40%, hypercarbia (greater than 45 mm CO_2), or hypoxemia (less than 60 mm O_2) on preoperative arterial blood gases.

Surgical resection can be curative in patients with early-stage (stage I or II) NSCLC, and in those who are physiologically fit surgery alone is usually the treatment of choice (Figs. 7.20 and 7.21). Unfortunately, most patients present with locally advanced or metastatic disease for which surgery alone is not a therapeutic option. The population of patients with locally advanced NSCLC is heterogenous. Overall survival for this group of patients is poor because of the high risk of both locoregional and metastatic recurrence. However, patients whose disease is resectable with a multidisciplinary approach (surgery, chemotherapy, and RT), such as patients with T4 tumors with N0 or N1 nodes or nonbulky single-station N2, may benefit from resection in combination with chemotherapy or chemoradiation. Postoperative adjuvant chemotherapy is the standard treatment for most patients with advanced NSCLC

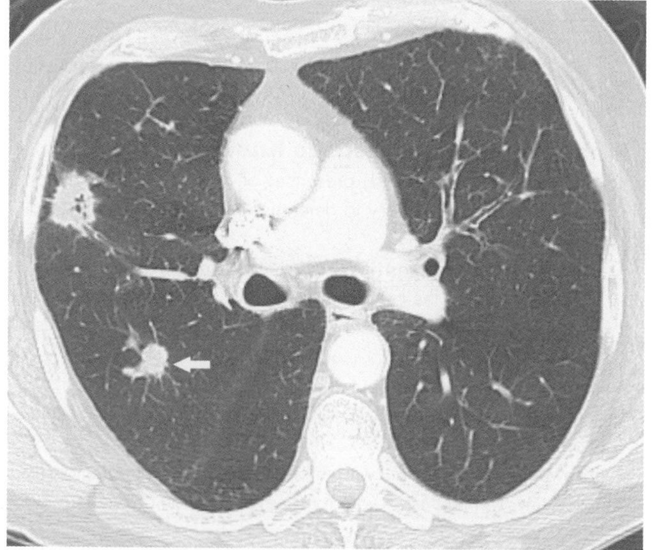

Figure 7.20. A 79-year-old man with nonsmall cell lung cancer. Contrast-enhanced computed tomography shows a cavitary nodule in the right upper lobe and a smaller satellite nodule (*arrow*). Note that when there is an additional nodule in the same lobe as the primary tumor the tumor-node-metastasis staging system designates a T3 descriptor (potentially resectable). The patient was T3N0 on staging and underwent curative surgical resection.

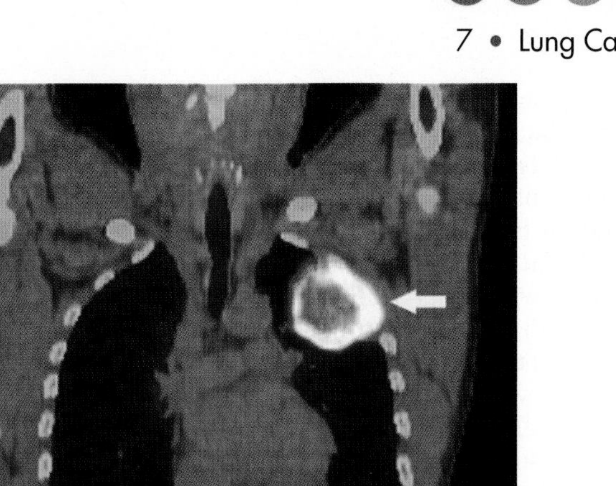
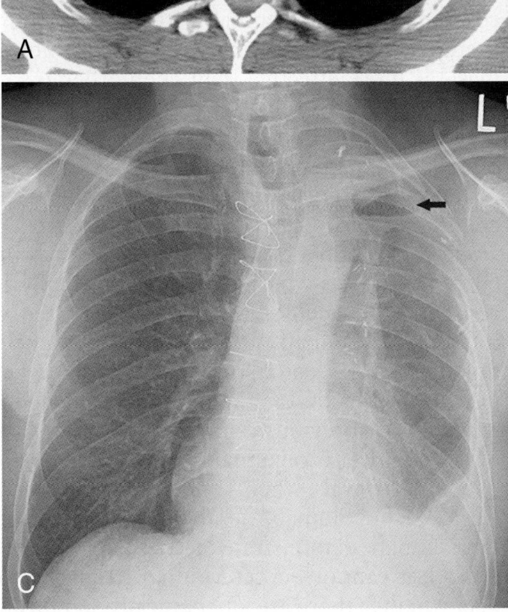
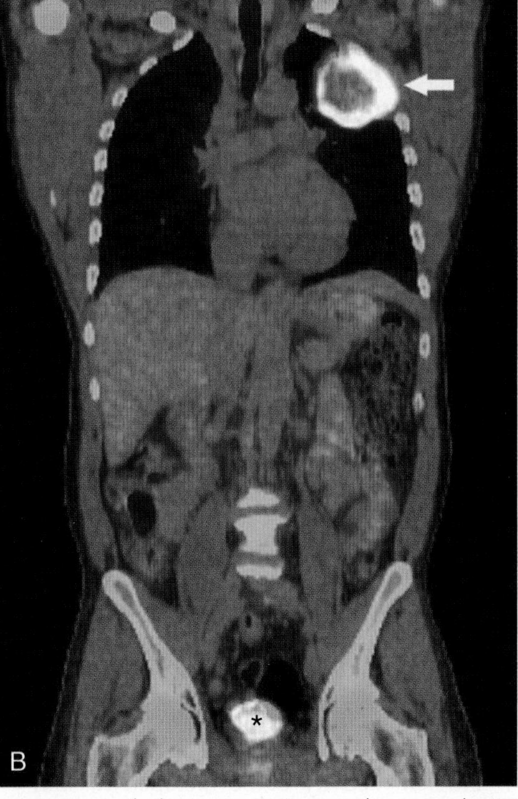

FIGURE 7.21. A 49-year-old man with primary nonsmall cell lung cancer presenting with chest pain. **A**, Computed tomography (CT) shows a large left upper lobe lung mass containing amorphous calcification. There is locoregional chest wall invasion and focal destruction of the adjacent rib (T3). **B**, Whole-body coronal positron emission tomography-CT shows increased 2-[^{18}F] fluoro-2-deoxy-D-glucose (FDG) uptake within the primary malignancy (*arrow*). FDG uptake in the mediastinum is normal, and there is no focal abnormal extrathoracic FDG uptake. The findings are indicative of T3N0M0 disease. Mediastinoscopy confirmed absence of nodal metastasis, and the patient underwent surgical resection. *, Accumulation of FDG in the bladder. **C**, Posteroanterior chest radiograph shows postsurgical changes after left upper lobe lobectomy and *en bloc* chest wall resection of the 2nd, 3rd, and 4th ribs. Note small air and fluid collection in the pleural space (arrow).

who undergo surgical resection. In these patients administration of adjuvant chemotherapy improves long-term survival rates.[47,48] The efficacy of this adjuvant chemotherapy appears to be comparable whether it is administered before surgery (neoadjuvant chemotherapy) or postoperatively.[48,49]

Patients with tumors involving the contralateral mediastinal nodes (N3) and T4 tumors that invade the mediastinum, heart, great vessels, trachea, esophagus, or vertebral body and who have ipsilateral mediastinal (N2) nodes are better treated with chemoradiation rather than with surgery. Patients with metastatic disease typically are treated with systemic therapy such as chemotherapy and/or immunotherapy, but can be treated surgically, such as in the scenario of isolated brain metastases with a node-negative lung primary.

In the majority of patients with metastatic NSCLC, chemotherapy and/or immunotherapy can improve symptoms, as well as quality of life.[50,51] In addition, chemotherapy and/or immunotherapy induces an objective response in approximately 35% of patients and modestly prolongs median survival.[50] In front-line therapy for advanced NSCLC, immunotherapy or chemoimmunotherapy have become the new standard of treatment in patients who do not have driver mutations in key genes (*EGFR, ALK, RET, ROS1, NTRK*) or contraindications to immunotherapy (i.e., autoimmune disease). In this regard, the treatment strategy in advanced NSCLC is rapidly evolving from the use of chemotherapy to a more personalized approach based on histology and molecular markers. This rapid evolution precludes a comprehensive review of current and evolving novel therapies being used to treat advanced NSCLC, and the discussion is limited to broad principles of treatment. Targeted therapies are directed at the products of gene mutations and come in the form of receptor monoclonal antibodies (mAbs) or tyrosine kinase inhibitors (TKIs). Common targets include mutated forms of epidermal growth factor receptor (EGFR) and anaplastic lymphoma kinase (ALK). Mutated forms of EGFR are well-known biomarkers for response to targeted therapy, and EGFR TKIs are most effective in patients with an activating *EGFR* mutation.[52,53] Patients who have never smoked and East Asian patients are more likely to have an activating mutation than are other patients, and patients with an activating mutation can have very rapid, dramatic responses that in some cases can be prolonged.[54] In addition, single-agent EGFR inhibitors are more effective than combination chemotherapy as front-line therapy for metastatic NSCLC if an *EGFR* activating mutation is present.[55] Unfortunately, despite the high response rate to the first-generation EGFR TKIs, disease progression is common because of the development of resistance to therapy. Osimertinib, a third-generation EGFR TKI, has much longer progression-free survival and better efficacy, as well as decreased toxicity, compared with other EGFR TKIS and is currently being used as both first- and second-line therapy.

Targeted therapy is also being directed at mutations of the ALK gene, which occur in 3% to 5% of NSCLCs. Crizotinib, a small-molecule TKI of the ALK, MET, and ROS1 kinases, is superior to standard first-line pemetrexed-plus-platinum chemotherapy in patients with previously untreated advanced ALK-positive NSCLC, and is the current standard first-line treatment for advanced NSCLC harboring ALK rearrangement. The third-generation ALK TKIs alectinib[56] and brigatininib[57] have been demonstrated to be superior to crizotinib, with better efficacy and comparable or decreased toxicity. These agents and others such as ceritinib[58] and lorlatinib[59] may also be effective in patients whose tumors have progressed on prior crizotinib therapy. Targeted agents may also be effective in NSCLC patients whose tumors harbor other mutations such as the *ROS1*,[60] *RET*,[61] *NTRK* fusion genes,[62] or with *MET*[63] or *BRAF* mutations.[64]

Immunotherapy is being used more frequently to treat patients with advanced NSCLC, although challenges including immune-related toxicities and primary/adaptive resistance to immunotherapy are ongoing issues.[65,66] mAbs directed at proteins overexpressed on the surface of tumor cells have also been explored but have not yet demonstrated sufficient activity to be included in standard therapy for lung cancer. Immunomodulatory mAbs can be directed against targets, including programmed death protein 1/programmed death receptor ligand 1 (PD-1/PD-L1) and cytotoxic T-lymphocyte antigen-4 (CTLA-4). mAbs targeting these molecules are referred to as immune checkpoint inhibitors and act by interfering with the interaction between a ligand on tumor cells (e.g., PD-L1) and its receptor (e.g., PD-1) on T-cells. The interaction between the ligand and the receptor turns off T-cell function so that the T-cell cannot kill the tumor cell, and mAbs targeting the ligand or the receptor can prevent this interaction, thereby increasing the possibility that a T-cell may be able to kill a tumor cell. Overall, across a broad range of solid tumors, PD-1/PD-L1 inhibitors have had a broader impact than any class of agents since the introduction of cisplatin in the late 1970s, and their optimal used has still to be determined. Particularly relevant to lung cancer, the agents nivolumab and pembrolizumab target PD-1, whereas atezolizumab and durvalumab target PD-L1. Although these agents generally appear to be more effective if tumor cells have high PD-L1 expression, they may be effective in some patients even with very low PD-L1 expression.[67,68] Similarly, tumors with a high mutation burden appear to be more sensitive to PD-1/PD-L1 inhibitors than are tumors with a low mutation burden, presumably because a high tumor mutation burden might be associated with a higher expression of neoantigens that can be targeted by the immune system.[69]

For reasons that are unclear, tumors that harbor a known activating mutation such as an *EGFR* or *ALK* mutation appear to be less sensitive to PD-1/PD-L1 inhibitors than wild-type tumors, even if tumor cell PD-L1 expression is high.[70] In randomized trials, nivolumab was shown to be more effective than standard chemotherapy as second-line treatment for both adenocarcinomas[67] and squamous cell carcinomas[68] of the lung. Atezolizumab was also more effective than chemotherapy in previously-treated patients with advanced NSCLC.[71]

In patients who express PD-L1 in 50% or more of tumor cells, pembrolizumab is more effective than chemotherapy as first-line treatment for advanced NSCLC,[72] and combining pembrolizumab with chemotherapy as first-line therapy for lung nonsquamous[73] or squamous cell carcinomas[74] is more effective than chemotherapy alone, even in patients with low PD-L1 expression. Similarly, combining the CTLA-4 inhibitor ipilimumab with nivolumab is more effective in patients with previously-untreated advanced NSCLC than is chemotherapy.[75] Adding atezolizumab to chemotherapy is also more effective than chemotherapy alone for treating NSCLC.[76] Durvalumab improves outcome in patients with locally-advanced NSCLC who have responded to chemoradiation administered with curative intent.[77] Nivolumab and nivolumab combined with ipilimumab have also demonstrated activity in previously-treated patients with SCLC,[78] as has single-agent pembrolizumab.[79] In previously-untreated patients with advanced SCLC, both atezolizumab[80] and durvalumab[81] improved overall survival when combined with chemotherapy. Although nivolumab, pembrolizumab, atezolizumab, and durvalumab demonstrate activity in both NSCLC and SCLC, it cannot be determined from currently available data whether there are any clinically significant differences between these agents.

RT is an important modality in the management of patients with NSCLC, and it has been estimated that approximately 45% of patients with lung cancer receive radiotherapy as initial treatment.[82] SBRT alone is being used for curative intent in medically inoperable patients with early-stage NSCLC. It has also been suggested that SBRT may have a role in the treatment of medically operable patients with early-stage disease. A pooled analysis of two randomized trials comparing SBRT with surgery in operable patients with early-stage NSCLC showed that 5-year local recurrence rates and overall survival were comparable in both groups, but surgery resulted in an increased rate of procedure-related mortality and morbidity compared with SBRT (30- to 90-day postoperative mortality for video-assisted thoracoscopic surgery lobectomy 2%; open thoracotomy lobectomy, 5.4%; SBRT, 0.7%).[83] Patients with early-stage NSCLC and N1 are typically treated with surgery, followed by adjuvant chemotherapy. However, after resection, if the patients have positive mediastinal nodes (N2) or multiple or large hilar nodes (N1) with extracapsular involvement, postoperative radiotherapy is a therapeutic option, and adjuvant cisplatin-based chemotherapy is given before or after RT. Patients with early-stage NSCLC and N1 who are medically inoperable receive intensity-modulated radiation therapy or proton RT with or without chemotherapy. Patients with microscopic N2 or nodes less than 1.5 cm in size are usually treated by induction chemotherapy, followed by surgery and postoperative RT. In patients with multiple-level positive mediastinal nodes or nodes larger than 1.5 cm, patients with T3 to T4 lesions requiring pneumonectomy, or patients with surgically unresectable advanced disease, the treatment is concurrent chemoradiotherapy. Importantly, in inoperable patients undergoing radiotherapy with curative intent, chemotherapy given concurrently with the radiotherapy increases cure rates by a few percentage points by reducing metastatic disease and increasing the efficiency of tumor cell killing by radiotherapy.[84]

Key Points

Therapy

- Surgical resection is the treatment of choice in patients with localized nonsmall cell lung cancer (NSCLC) >2 cm.
- Resection may be an option in patients with locally advanced (T4) disease without N2/3 involvement.
- Postoperative adjuvant chemotherapy is the standard treatment for most patients with advanced NSCLC who undergo surgical resection.
- Surgery alone is not a therapeutic option for advanced or metastatic disease.
- Chemotherapy and/or immunotherapy is the new standard to treat patients with distant metastasis who do not have driver mutations or contraindications to immunotherapy.
- Oligometastatic lung cancer patients (less than or equal to three sites) may benefit from the addition of local consolidation therapy (surgery and/or radiation therapy).
- Cisplatin-based (cisplatin or carboplatin) regimens are standard therapy for metastatic patients who do not have driver mutations or contraindications to immunotherapy.
- Overall, combination chemotherapy is superior to single-agent chemotherapy.
- Patients with driver mutations in key genes (*EGFR, ALK, ROS1, RET, NTRK*) are treated initially with targeted agents rather than chemotherapy or immunotherapy.
- Stereotactic body radiation therapy alone is being used for curative intent in medically inoperable patients with early-stage NSCLC.
- Patients with early-stage NSCLC who are medically inoperable receive intensity-modulated radiation therapy or proton radiation therapy with or without chemotherapy.
- Concurrent chemoradiotherapy can be used to treat patients with locoregionally advanced (stage IIIB/IIIC) NSCLC.

Small Cell Lung Cancer

SCLC tends to be disseminated at the time of presentation and is therefore not typically amenable to cure with surgical resection. However, there is a small role for surgical resection of SCLC. Solitary peripheral pulmonary nodules without distant metastatic disease can be treated with surgical resection. In these select patients, 5-year survivals of 50% have been achieved for T1N0, T2N0, and completely resected N1 disease (Fig. 7.22). Generally, limited-stage SCLC is treated with concurrent chemoradiotherapy, whereas patients with ED are treated with systemic chemotherapy. Chemotherapy is very effective at inducing tumor regression in SCLC and can cure approximately 10% of patients with LD (confined to one hemithorax); and radiotherapy increases the probability of cure by about 5% when added to chemotherapy.[85] In extensive SCLC (distant metastases), median survival is only approximately 6 weeks without chemotherapy, and increases to 7 to 11 months with chemotherapy; but long-term survival is uncommon.[86,87] A large majority of SCLC patients will respond to chemotherapy, with symptomatic and radiologic improvement often seen within a few days of therapy initiation.[88] The standard chemotherapy choice for SCLC is a combination of cisplatin or carboplatin with the topoisomerase II inhibitor etoposide.[87] Addition of the topoisomerase I inhibitor irinotecan to platinum yields outcomes comparable to those seen with the combination of etoposide and platinum. Enhancing tumor-specific T-cell immunity by inhibiting PD-L1–PD-1 signaling has shown promise in the treatment of extensive-stage SCLC. In this regard, atezolizumab was approved in 2019 by the U.S. Food and Drug Administration, in combination with the chemotherapy drugs carboplatin and etoposide, for the initial treatment of patients with extensive-stage SCLC.[80]

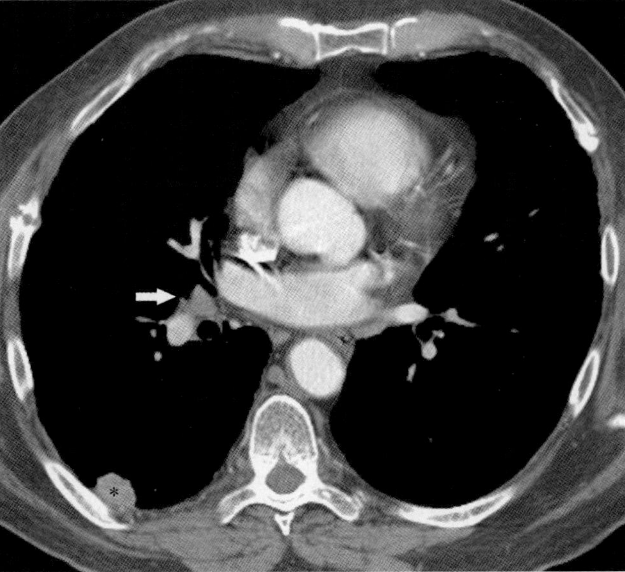

Figure 7.22. A 72-year-old man with small cell lung cancer. Contrast-enhanced computed tomography shows a left lower nodule (*) and 1- to 1.5-cm left infrahilar node (*arrow*). Using tumor-node-metastasis descriptors the patient was considered to have early-stage disease and underwent surgical resection. The resected primary tumor showed visceral pleural invasion, and the infrahilar nodes were negative for metastatic disease. Note bilateral posttraumatic rib fractures.

Key Points

Therapy

- Limited-stage small cell lung cancer (SCLC) is usually treated with concurrent chemoradiotherapy.
- Extensive-stage SCLC is usually treated with systemic chemotherapy.
- Standard chemotherapy is the combination of cisplatin or carboplatin with etoposide.
- Checkpoint inhibition (using atezolizumab) combined with cytotoxic therapy is being used in the initial treatment of patients with extensive-stage SCLC.

SURVEILLANCE

In an attempt to prolong survival of patients with recurrent malignancy after attempted curative treatment of NSCLC, patients can be treated with repeat surgery, salvage chemotherapy, or radiotherapy. Unfortunately, two-thirds of patients with lung cancer who relapse present with incurable metastases. However, recent prospective data from patients who present with limited metastases suggests that improved survival benefit is possible following local ablative therapy and provides the impetus for aggressive treatment of early recurrence.[89,90] Relying on patient symptomatology to determine persistent or early local recurrence of NSCLC can delay diagnosis and compromise retreatment. However, CT or MRI is unreliable in distinguishing persistent or recurrent tumor from necrosis, posttreatment scarring, or fibrosis. FDG-PET can be useful in detecting local recurrence of tumor after definitive treatment with surgery, chemotherapy, or radiotherapy before conventional imaging (Fig. 7.23). However, diagnostic difficulties over the presence or absence of persistent or recurrent cancer are frequent after radiotherapy. In this regard, three-dimensional conformal radiotherapy is particularly likely to manifest as opacities on CT that can be difficult to differentiate from tumor recurrence, and the associated radiation-induced inflammatory changes can result in false-positive uptake of FDG.

Presently there is no standardized clinical algorithm established to monitor patients with NSCLC for recurrence of disease using imaging. Although imaging is an integral component of this evaluation, there is considerable variability in the imaging performed to evaluate for disease because of a lack of evidence in the published literature regarding optimal follow-up after treatment. Nevertheless, specific follow-up strategies have been advocated, and several guidelines, including those from the American Society of Clinical Oncology, the American College of Radiology, and the National Comprehensive Cancer Network, have been published that include recommendations for a posttreatment surveillance program. The guidelines and institutional practices are similar. Each recommends more frequent visits during the first 2 years following curative-intent therapy and a decrease to a minimal level after year 5. Recently published ASCO guidelines regarding lung cancer surveillance after definitive curative-intent therapy address numerous common questions regarding surveillance, including:

1. What should be the frequency of surveillance imaging? Patients should undergo surveillance imaging for recurrence every 6 months for 2 years and annually thereafter for the detection of new primary lung cancers.[91]
2. What is the optimal imaging modality? Diagnostic chest CT that includes the adrenals, with contrast (preferred) or without contrast, when conducting surveillance for recurrence during the first 2 years posttreatment, and low-dose screening chest CT thereafter. FDG-PET imaging should not be used for surveillance.[91]

However, little is known about the effectiveness of follow-up regimens. Walsh et al., in a retrospective study following curative-intent surgical resection for NSCLC, concluded that intensive surveillance was not cost effective and suggested a reduced surveillance approach consisting of a chest radiograph every 6 months for the first year following curative-intent surgery, and annually thereafter.[92] However, there are concerns regarding the validity of the conclusions of the studies advocating limited surveillance that include the limitations of retrospective analyses, the small size and heterogenous nature of the study groups, and the different treatments and imaging evaluations that the patients received. In this regard, Westeel et al., performed a prospective study to determine the feasibility of an intensive surveillance program and the influence on patient survival and concluded that intensive follow-up is feasible and may improve survival by detecting asymptomatic recurrences after surgery.[93]

Key Points

Detection of Recurrence

- Recurrent malignancy can occasionally be treated with repeat surgery, salvage chemotherapy, or radiotherapy.
- Computed tomography (CT) and magnetic resonance imaging can be unreliable in distinguishing persistent or recurrent tumor from necrosis and posttreatment fibrosis.

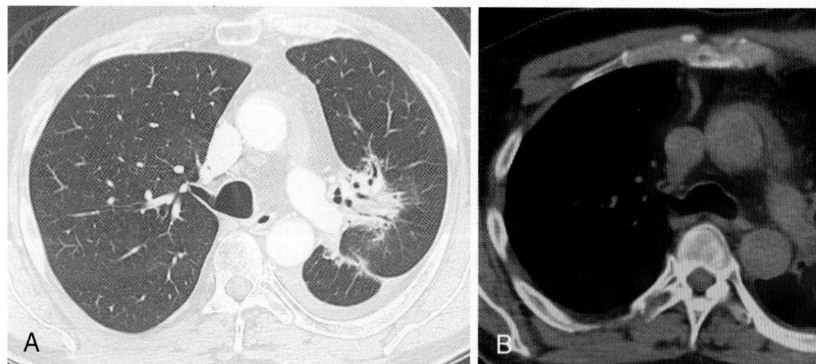

Figure 7.23. A 74-year-old woman with history of left upper lobe nonsmall cell lung cancer 1 year after resection and chemoradiation therapy. **A**, Axial contrast-enhanced computed tomography (CT) shows atelectatic and consolidative opacities in the left perihilar region because of radiation-induced lung injury. Note air bronchograms and no CT findings of recurrence of malignancy. **B**, Axial positron emission tomography-CT shows focal increased 2-[^{18}F] fluoro-2-deoxy-D-glucose uptake in radiation fibrosis. Recurrence of malignancy was confirmed by transthoracic needle aspiration biopsy.

- 2-[^{18}F] fluoro-2-deoxy-D-glucose positron emission tomography can detect local recurrence of tumor before conventional imaging.
- There is no standardized clinical algorithm to monitor patients with nonsmall cell lung cancer for recurrence of disease after treatment.
- Reasonable imaging surveillance approach would use chest CT every 6 months for 2 years and then annually.

CONCLUSION

TNM staging of lung cancer is important in determining therapeutic management and prognosis. CT, PET, and MRI are an integral component of this evaluation. However, there is considerable variability in the imaging performed to evaluate for nodal and extrathoracic disease. Chest CT is almost universally used to stage patients with lung cancer and is typically performed to assess the primary tumor, perform direct mediastinoscopy, and detect intra- and extrathoracic metastases. MRI is particularly useful in the evaluation of superior sulcus tumors. Whereas whole-body MRI can be used to stage patients, MRI is generally used as an adjunct to CT in evaluating patients whose CT findings are equivocal. PET complements conventional radiologic assessment of lung cancer and is routinely used to improve the detection of nodal and extrathoracic metastases.

REFERENCES

1. Alberg AJ, Ford JG, Samet JM, et al. Epidemiology of lung cancer: ACCP evidence-based clinical practice guidelines (2nd edition). *Chest*. 2007;132(3 Suppl):29S–55S.

1a. Rebecca L, Siegel MPH, Kimberly D, et al. Cancer Statistics, 2021. *CA Cance J Clin*. 2021;71:7–33.

2. Samet JM, Avila-Tang E, Boffetta P, et al. Lung cancer in never smokers: clinical epidemiology and environmental risk factors. *Clin Cancer Res*. 2009;15(18):5626–5645.
3. Al-Zoughool M, Krewski D. Health effects of radon: a review of the literature. *Int J Radiat Biol*. 2009;85(1):57–69.
4. Erren TC, Jacobsen M, Piekarski C. Synergy between asbestos and smoking on lung cancer risks. *Epidemiology*. 1999;10(4):405–411.
5. Goodman M, Morgan RW, Ray R, et al. Cancer in asbestos-exposed occupational cohorts: a meta-analysis. *Cancer Causes Control*. 1999;10(5):453–465.
6. Wild P, Bourgkard E, Paris C. Lung cancer and exposure to metals: the epidemiological evidence. *Methods Mol Biol*. 2009;472:139–167.
7. Clapp RW, Jacobs MM, Loechler EL. Environmental and occupational causes of cancer: new evidence 2005-2007. *Rev Environ Health*. 2008;23(1):1–37.
8. Le Calvez F, Mukeria A, Hunt JD, et al. TP53 and KRAS mutation load and types in lung cancers in relation to tobacco smoke: distinct patterns in never, former, and current smokers. *Cancer Res*. 2005;65(12):5076–5083.
9. Jackman DM, Miller VA, Cioffredi LA, et al. Impact of epidermal growth factor receptor and KRAS mutations on clinical outcomes in previously untreated non-small cell lung cancer patients: results of an online tumor registry of clinical trials. *Clin Cancer Res*. 2009;15(16):5267–5273.
10. van Zandwijk N, Mathy A, Boerrigter L, et al. EGFR and KRAS mutations as criteria for treatment with tyrosine kinase inhibitors: retro- and prospective observations in non-small-cell lung cancer. *Ann Oncol*. 2007;18(1):99–103.
11. Travis WD, Brambilla E, Noguchi M, et al. International Association for the Study of Lung Cancer/American Thoracic Society/European Respiratory Society International multidisciplinary classification of lung adenocarcinoma. *J Thorac Oncol*. 2011;6(2):244–285.
12. Van Schil PE, Sihoe AD, Travis WD. Pathologic classification of adenocarcinoma of lung. *J Surg Oncol*. 2013;108(5):320–326.
13. Noguchi M, Morikawa A, Kawasaki M, et al. Small adenocarcinoma of the lung. Histologic characteristics and prognosis. *Cancer*. 1995;75(12):2844–2852.
14. Kishi K, Homma S, Kurosaki A, et al. Small lung tumors with the size of 1cm or less in diameter: clinical, radiological, and histopathological characteristics. *Lung Cancer*. 2004;44(1):43–51.
15. Suzuki K, Kusumoto M, Watanabe S, et al. Radiologic classification of small adenocarcinoma of the lung: radiologic-pathologic correlation and its prognostic impact. *Ann Thorac Surg*. 2006;81(2):413–419.
16. Passlick B. Micrometastases in non-small cell lung cancer (NSCLC). *Lung Cancer*. 2001;34(Suppl 3):S25–S29.
17. Kondo T, Yamada K, Noda K, et al. Radiologic-prognostic correlation in patients with small pulmonary adenocarcinomas. *Lung Cancer*. 2002;36(1):49–57.
18. Rami-Porta R, Bolejack V, Crowley J, et al. The IASLC Lung Cancer Staging Project: proposals for the revisions of the t descriptors in the eighth edition of the TNM Classification for lung cancer. *J Thorac Oncol*. 2015;10(7):990–1003.
19. Asamura H, Chansky K, Crowley J, et al. The International Association for the Study of Lung Cancer Lung Cancer Staging Project: proposals for the revision of the N descriptors in the eighth edition of the TNM Classification for lung cancer. *J Thorac Oncol*. 2015;10(12):1675–1684.
20. Eberhardt WE, Mitchell A, Crowley J, et al. The IASLC Lung Cancer Staging Project: proposals for the revision of the m descriptors in the eighth edition of the TNM Classification of lung cancer. *J Thorac Oncol*. 2015;10(11):1515–1522.
21. Goldstraw P, Crowley J, Chansky K, et al. The IASLC Lung Cancer Staging Project: proposals for the revision of the TNM stage groupings in the (seventh) edition of the TNM Classification of malignant tumors. *J Thorac Oncol*. 2007;2(8):706–714.
22. Travis WD, Asamura H, Bankier AA, et al. The IASLC Lung Cancer Staging Project: proposals for coding t categories for subsolid nodules and assessment of tumor size in part-solid tumors in the eighth edition of the TNM Classification of lung cancer. *J Thorac Oncol*. 2016;11(8):1204–1223.
23. Detterbeck FC, Nicholson AG, Franklin WA, et al. The IASLC Lung Cancer Staging Project: summary of proposals for revisions of the classification of lung cancers with multiple pulmonary sites of involvement in the eighth edition of the TNM Classification. *J Thorac Oncol*. 2016;11(5):639–650.
24. Detterbeck FC, Bolejack V, Arenberg DA, et al. The IASLC Lung Cancer Staging Project: background data and proposals for the classification of lung cancer with separate tumor nodules in the eighth edition of the TNM Classification for lung cancer. *J Thorac Oncol*. 2016;11(5):681–692.
25. Detterbeck FC, Franklin WA, Nicholson AG, et al. The IASLC Lung Cancer Staging Project: background data and proposed criteria to distinguish separate primary lung cancers from metastatic foci in patients with two lung tumors in the eighth edition of the TNM Classification for lung cancer. *J Thorac Oncol*. 2016;11(5):651–665.
26. Detterbeck FC, Marom EM, Arenberg DA, et al. The IASLC Lung Cancer Staging Project: background data and proposals for the application of TNM staging rules to lung cancer presenting as multiple nodules with ground glass or lepidic features or a pneumonic type of involvement in the eighth deition of the TNM Classification. *J Thorac Oncol*. 2016;11(5):666–680.
27. Rusch VW, Crowley J, Giroux DJ, et al. The IASLC Lung Cancer Staging Project: proposals for the revision of the N descriptors in the seventh edition of the TNM classification for lung cancer. *J Thorac Oncol*. 2007;2(7):603–612.
28. Darling GE. Staging of the patient with small cell lung cancer. *Chest Surg Clin N Am*. 1997;7(1):81–94.
29. Vallieres E, Shepherd FA, Crowley J, et al. The IASLC Lung Cancer Staging Project: proposals regarding the relevance of TNM in the pathologic staging of small cell lung cancer in the (seventh) edition of the TNM Classification for lung cancer. *J Thorac Oncol*. 2009;4(9):1049–1059.
30. Shirasawa M, Fukui T, Kusuhara S, et al. Prognostic significance of the 8th edition of the TNM classification for patients with extensive disease small cell lung cancer. *Cancer Manag Res*. 2018;10:6039–6047.

31. Pfister DG, Johnson DH, Azzoli CG, et al. American Society of Clinical Oncology treatment of unresectable non-small-cell lung cancer guideline: update 2003. *J Clin Oncol*. 2004;22(2):330–353.
32. van Tinteren H, Hoekstra OS, Smit EF, et al. Effectiveness of positron emission tomography in the preoperative assessment of patients with suspected non-small-cell lung cancer: the PLUS multicentre randomised trial. *Lancet*. 2002;359(9315):1388–1393.
33. Reed CE, Harpole DH, Posther KE, et al. Results of the American College of Surgeons Oncology Group Z0050 trial: the utility of positron emission tomography in staging potentially operable non-small cell lung cancer. *J Thorac Cardiovasc Surg*. 2003;126(6):1943–1951.
34. Taylor SA, Mallett S, Miles A, et al. Whole-body MRI compared with standard pathways for staging metastatic disease in lung and colorectal cancer: the Streamline diagnostic accuracy studies. *Health Technol Assess*. 2019;23(66):1–270.
35. Bruzzi JF, Komaki R, Walsh GL, et al. Imaging of non-small cell lung cancer of the superior sulcus: part 2: initial staging and assessment of resectability and therapeutic response. *Radiographics*. 2008;28(2):561–572.
36. Bruzzi JF, Komaki R, Walsh GL, et al. Imaging of non-small cell lung cancer of the superior sulcus: part 1: anatomy, clinical manifestations, and management. *Radiographics*. 2008;28(2):551–560. quiz 620.
37. Bilsky MH, Vitaz TW, Boland PJ, et al. Surgical treatment of superior sulcus tumors with spinal and brachial plexus involvement. *J Neurosurg*. 2002;97(3 Suppl):301–309.
38. Dartevelle P, Macchiarini P. Surgical management of superior sulcus tumors. *Oncologist*. 1999;4(5):398–407.
39. Toloza EM, Harpole L, Detterbeck F, et al. Invasive staging of non-small cell lung cancer: a review of the current evidence. *Chest*. 2003;123(1 Suppl):157S–166S.
40. Prenzel KL, Monig SP, Sinning JM, et al. Lymph node size and metastatic infiltration in non-small cell lung cancer. *Chest*. 2003;123(2):463–467.
41. Birim O, Kappetein AP, Stijnen T, et al. Meta-analysis of positron emission tomographic and computed tomographic imaging in detecting mediastinal lymph node metastases in nonsmall cell lung cancer. *Ann Thorac Surg*. 2005;79(1):375–382.
42. Gould MK, Kuschner WG, Rydzak CE, et al. Test performance of positron emission tomography and computed tomography for mediastinal staging in patients with non-small-cell lung cancer: a meta-analysis. *Ann Intern Med*. 2003;139(11):879–892.
43. Tanaka K, Kubota K, Kodama T, et al. Extrathoracic staging is not necessary for non-small-cell lung cancer with clinical stage T1-2 N0. *Ann Thorac Surg*. 1999;68(3):1039–1042.
44. MacManus MP, Hicks RJ, Matthews JP, et al. High rate of detection of unsuspected distant metastases by pet in apparent stage III non-small-cell lung cancer: implications for radical radiation therapy. *Int J Radiat Oncol Biol Phys*. 2001;50(2):287–293.
45. Meyer M, Budjan J. Whole-body MRI for lung cancer staging: a step in the right direction. *Lancet Respir Med*. 2019;7(6):471–472.
46. Kalemkerian GP. Advances in the treatment of small-cell lung cancer. *Semin Respir Crit Care Med*. 2011;32(1):94–101.
47. Higgins MJ, Ettinger DS. Chemotherapy for lung cancer: the state of the art in 2009. *Expert Rev Anticancer Ther*. 2009;9(10):1365–1378.
48. Lim E, Harris G, Patel A, et al. Preoperative versus postoperative chemotherapy in patients with resectable non-small cell lung cancer: systematic review and indirect comparison meta-analysis of randomized trials. *J Thorac Oncol*. 2009;4(11) 1380-138.
49. Song WA, Zhou NK, Wang W, et al. Survival benefit of neoadjuvant chemotherapy in non-small cell lung cancer: an updated meta-analysis of 13 randomized control trials. *J Thorac Oncol*. 2010;5(4):510–516.
50. Vansteenkiste J. Improving patient management in metastatic non-small cell lung cancer. *Lung Cancer*. 2007;57(Suppl 2):S12–S17.
51. Dooms C, Verbeken E, Stroobants S, et al. Prognostic stratification of stage IIIA-N2 non-small-cell lung cancer after induction chemotherapy: a model based on the combination of morphometric-pathologic response in mediastinal nodes and primary tumor response on serial 18-fluoro-2-deoxy-glucose positron emission tomography. *J Clin Oncol*. 2008;26(7):1128–1134.
52. Costa DB, Kobayashi S, Tenen DG, et al. Pooled analysis of the prospective trials of gefitinib monotherapy for EGFR-mutant non-small cell lung cancers. *Lung Cancer*. 2007;58(1):95–103.
53. Gazdar AF. Activating and resistance mutations of EGFR in non-small-cell lung cancer: role in clinical response to EGFR tyrosine kinase inhibitors. *Oncogene*. 2009;28(Suppl 1):S24–S31.
54. Riely GJ, Pao W, Pham D, et al. Clinical course of patients with non-small cell lung cancer and epidermal growth factor receptor exon 19 and exon 21 mutations treated with gefitinib or erlotinib. *Clin Cancer Res*. 2006;12(3 Pt 1):839–844.
55. Mok TS, Wu YL, Thongprasert S, et al. Gefitinib or carboplatin-paclitaxel in pulmonary adenocarcinoma. *N Engl J Med*. 2009;361(10):947–957.
56. Peters S, Camidge DR, Shaw AT, et al. Alectinib versus Crizotinib in Untreated ALK-Positive Non-Small-Cell Lung Cancer. *N Engl J Med*. 2017;377(9):829–838.
57. Camidge DR, Kim HR, Ahn MJ, et al. Brigatinib versus Crizotinib in ALK-Positive Non-Small-Cell Lung Cancer. *N Engl J Med*. 2018;379(21):2027–2039.
58. Shaw AT, Kim TM, Crino L, et al. Ceritinib versus chemotherapy in patients with ALK-rearranged non-small-cell lung cancer previously given chemotherapy and crizotinib (ASCEND-5): a randomised, controlled, open-label, phase 3 trial. *Lancet Oncol*. 2017;18(7):874–886.
59. Solomon BJ, Besse B, Bauer TM, et al. Lorlatinib in patients with ALK-positive non-small-cell lung cancer: results from a global phase 2 study. *Lancet Oncol*. 2018;19(12):1654–1667.
60. Shaw AT, Ou SH, Bang YJ, et al. Crizotinib in ROS1-rearranged non-small-cell lung cancer. *N Engl J Med*. 2014;371(21):1963–1971.
61. Drilon A, Rekhtman N, Arcila M, et al. Cabozantinib in patients with advanced RET-rearranged non-small-cell lung cancer: an open-label, single-centre, phase 2, single-arm trial. *Lancet Oncol*. 2016;17(12):1653–1660.
62. Doebele RC, Drilon A, Paz-Ares L, et al. Entrectinib in patients with advanced or metastatic NTRK fusion-positive solid tumours: integrated analysis of three phase 1-2 trials. *Lancet Oncol*. 2020 Feb;21(2):271–282. doi: 10.1016/S1470-2045(19)30691-6. Epub 2019 Dec 11.
63. Paik PK, Drilon A, Fan PD, et al. Response to MET inhibitors in patients with stage IV lung adenocarcinomas harboring MET mutations causing exon 14 skipping. *Cancer Discov*. 2015;5(8):842–849.
64. Planchard D, Besse B, Groen HJM, et al. Dabrafenib plus trametinib in patients with previously treated BRAF(V600E)-mutant metastatic non-small cell lung cancer: an open-label, multicentre phase 2 trial. *Lancet Oncol*. 2016;17(7):984–993.
65. Zhang C, Leighl NB, Wu YL, et al. Emerging therapies for non-small cell lung cancer. *J Hematol Oncol*. 2019;12(1):45.
66. Shroff GS, de Groot PM, Papadimitrakopoulou VA, et al. Targeted therapy and immunotherapy in the treatment of non-small cell lung cancer. *Radiol Clin North Am*. 2018;56(3):485–495.
67. Borghaei H, Paz-Ares L, Horn L, et al. Nivolumab versus docetaxel in advanced nonsquamous non-small-cell lung cancer. *N Engl J Med*. 2015;373(17):1627–1639.
68. Brahmer J, Reckamp KL, Baas P, et al. Nivolumab versus docetaxel in advanced squamous-cell non-small-cell lung cancer. *N Engl J Med*. 2015;373(2):123–135.
69. Samstein RM, Lee CH, Shoushtari AN, et al. Tumor mutational load predicts survival after immunotherapy across multiple cancer types. *Nat Genet*. 2019;51(2):202–206.
70. Berghoff AS, Bellosillo B, Caux C, et al. Immune checkpoint inhibitor treatment in patients with oncogene- addicted non-small cell lung cancer (NSCLC): summary of a multidisciplinary round-table discussion. *ESMO Open*. 2019;4(3):e000498.
71. Rittmeyer A, Barlesi F, Waterkamp D, et al. Atezolizumab versus docetaxel in patients with previously treated non-small-cell lung cancer (OAK): a phase 3, open-label, multicentre randomised controlled trial. *Lancet*. 2017;389(10066):255–265.
72. Reck M, Rodriguez-Abreu D, Robinson AG, et al. Pembrolizumab versus chemotherapy for pd-l1-positive non-small-cell lung cancer. *N Engl J Med*. 2016;375(19):1823–1833.
73. Gandhi L, Rodriguez-Abreu D, Gadgeel S, et al. Pembrolizumab plus chemotherapy in metastatic non-small-cell lung cancer. *N Engl J Med*. 2018;378(22):2078–2092.
74. Paz-Ares L, Luft A, Vicente D, et al. Pembrolizumab plus chemotherapy for squamous non-small-cell lung cancer. *N Engl J Med*. 2018;379(21):2040–2051.
75. Hellmann MD, Paz-Ares L, Bernabe Caro R, et al. Nivolumab plus ipilimumab in advanced non-small-cell lung cancer. *N Engl J Med*. 2019;381(21):2020–2031.
76. Socinski MA, Jotte RM, Cappuzzo F, et al. Atezolizumab for first-line treatment of metastatic nonsquamous NSCLC. *N Engl J Med*. 2018;378(24):2288–2301.

77. Antonia SJ, Villegas A, Daniel D, et al. Overall survival with durvalumab after chemoradiotherapy in stage III NSCLC. *N Engl J Med*. 2018;379(24):2342–2350.
78. Antonia SJ, Lopez-Martin JA, Bendell J, et al. Nivolumab alone and nivolumab plus ipilimumab in recurrent small-cell lung cancer (CheckMate 032): a multicentre, open-label, phase 1/2 trial. *Lancet Oncol*. 2016;17(7):883–895.
79. Ott PA, Elez E, Hiret S, et al. Pembrolizumab in patients with extensive-stage small-cell lung cancer: results from the phase ib KEYNOTE-028 Study. *J Clin Oncol*. 2017;35(34):3823–3829.
80. Horn L, Mansfield AS, Szczesna A, et al. First-line atezolizumab plus chemotherapy in extensive-stage small-cell lung cancer. *N Engl J Med*. 2018;379(23):2220–2229.
81. Paz-Ares L, Dvorkin M, Chen Y, et al. Durvalumab plus platinum-etoposide versus platinum-etoposide in first-line treatment of extensive-stage small-cell lung cancer (CASPIAN): a randomised, controlled, open-label, phase 3 trial. *Lancet*. 2019;394(10212):1929–1939.
82. Tyldesley S, Boyd C, Schulze K, et al. Estimating the need for radiotherapy for lung cancer: an evidence-based, epidemiologic approach. *Int J Radiat Oncol Biol Phys*. 2001;49(4):973–985.
83. Chang JY, Senan S, Paul MA, et al. Stereotactic ablative radiotherapy versus lobectomy for operable stage I non-small-cell lung cancer: a pooled analysis of two randomised trials. *Lancet Oncol*. 2015;16(6):630–637.
84. Kepka L, Sprawka A, Casas F, et al. Combination of radiotherapy and chemotherapy in locally advanced NSCLC. *Expert Rev Anticancer Ther*. 2009;9(10):1389–1403.
85. Sandler AB. Chemotherapy for small cell lung cancer. *Semin Oncol*. 2003;30(1):9–25.
86. Rosti G, Carminati O, Monti M, et al. Chemotherapy advances in small cell lung cancer. *Ann Oncol*. 2006;17(Suppl 5) v99-102.
87. Murray N, Turrisi 3rd AT. A review of first-line treatment for small-cell lung cancer. *J Thorac Oncol*. 2006;1(3):270–278.
88. Rosti G, Bevilacqua G, Bidoli P, et al. Small cell lung cancer. *Ann Oncol*. 2006;17(Suppl 2) ii5-10.
89. Gomez DR, Tang C, Zhang J, et al. Local consolidative therapy vs. maintenance therapy or observation for patients with oligometastatic non-small-cell lung cancer: long-term results of a multi-institutional, phase ii, randomized study. *J Clin Oncol*. 2019;37(18):1558–1565.
90. Palma DA, Olson R, Harrow S, et al. Stereotactic ablative radiotherapy versus standard of care palliative treatment in patients with oligometastatic cancers (SABR-COMET): a randomised, phase 2, open-label trial. *Lancet*. 2019;393(10185):2051–2058.
91. Schneider BJ, Ismaila N, Aerts J, et al. Lung cancer surveillance after definitive curative-intent therapy: ASCO guideline. *J Clin Oncol*. 2019 JCO1902748.
92. Walsh GL, O'Connor M, Willis KM, et al. Is follow-up of lung cancer patients after resection medically indicated and cost-effective? *Ann Thorac Surg*. 1995;60(6):1563–1570. discussion 70-72.
93. Westeel V, Choma D, Clement F, et al. Relevance of an intensive postoperative follow-up after surgery for non-small cell lung cancer. *Ann Thorac Surg*. 2000;70(4):1185–1190.

ABBREVIATED REFERENCES

1. Travis WD, Brambilla E, Noguchi M, et al. International Association for the Study of Lung Cancer/American Thoracic Society/European Respiratory Society international multidisciplinary classification of lung adenocarcinoma. *J Thorac Oncol*. 2011;6(2):244–285.
2. Van Schil PE, Sihoe AD, Travis WD. Pathologic classification of adenocarcinoma of lung. *J Surg Oncol*. 2013;108(5):320–326.
3. Noguchi M, Morikawa A, Kawasaki M, et al. Small adenocarcinoma of the lung. Histologic characteristics and prognosis. *Cancer*. 1995;75(12):2844–2852.
4. Suzuki K, Kusumoto M, Watanabe S, et al. Radiologic classification of small adenocarcinoma of the lung: radiologic-pathologic correlation and its prognostic impact. *Ann Thorac Surg*. 2006;81(2):413–419.
5. Rami-Porta R, Bolejack V, Crowley J, et al. The IASLC Lung Cancer Staging Project: proposals for the revisions of the T descriptors in the eighth edition of the TNM Classification for lung cancer. *J Thorac Oncol*. 2015;10(7):990–1003.
6. Asamura H, Chansky K, Crowley J, et al. The International Association for the Study of Lung Cancer lung cancer staging project: proposals for the revision of the N descriptors in the 8th edition of the TNM classification for lung cancer. *J Thorac Oncol*. 2015;10(12):1675–1684.
7. Eberhardt WE, Mitchell A, Crowley J, et al. The IASLC Lung Cancer Staging Project: Proposals for the revision of the M descriptors in the eighth edition of the TNM Classification of lung cancer. *J Thorac Oncol*. 2015;10(11):1515–1522.
8. Goldstraw P, Crowley J, Chansky K, et al. The IASLC Lung Cancer Staging Project: proposals for the revision of the TNM stage groupings in the (seventh) edition of the TNM classification of malignant tumours. *J Thorac Oncol*. 2007;2(8):706–714.
9. Travis WD, Asamura H, Bankier AA, et al. The IASLC Lung Cancer Staging Project: Proposals for coding T categories for subsolid nodules and assessment of tumor size in part-solid tumors in the eighth edition of the TNM Classification of lung cancer. *J Thorac Oncol*. 2016;11(8):1204–1223.
10. Detterbeck FC, Nicholson AG, Franklin WA, Marom EM, et al. The IASLC Lung Cancer Staging Project: summary of proposals for revisions of the classification of lung cancers with multiple pulmonary sites of involvement in the eighth edition of the TNM Classification. *J Thorac Oncol*. 2016;11(5):639–650.
11. Detterbeck FC, Bolejack V, Arenberg DA, et al. The IASLC Lung Cancer Staging Project: background data and proposals for the classification of lung cancer with separate tumor nodules in the eighth edition of the TNM Classification for lung cancer. *J Thorac Oncol*. 2016;11(5):681–692.
12. Detterbeck FC, Franklin WA, Nicholson AG, et al. The IASLC Lung Cancer Staging Project: background data and proposed criteria to distinguish separate primary lung cancers from metastatic foci in patients with two lung tumors in the eighth edition of the TNM Classification for lung cancer. *J Thorac Oncol*. 2016;11(5):651–665.
13. Detterbeck FC, Marom EM, Arenberg DA, et al. The IASLC Lung Cancer Staging Project: background data and proposals for the application of TNM staging rules to lung cancer presenting as multiple nodules with ground glass or lepidic features or a pneumonic type of involvement in the eighth edition of the TNM Classification. *J Thorac Oncol*. 2016;11(5):666–680.
14. Rusch VW, Crowley J, Giroux DJ, et al. The IASLC Lung Cancer Staging Project: proposals for the revision of the N descriptors in the seventh edition of the TNM classification for lung cancer. *J Thorac Oncol*. 2007;2(7):603–612.
15. Vallieres E, Shepherd FA, Crowley J, et al. The IASLC Lung Cancer Staging Project: proposals regarding the relevance of TNM in the pathologic staging of small cell lung cancer in the (seventh) edition of the TNM Classification for lung cancer. *J Thorac Oncol*. 2009;4(9):1049–1059.
16. Shirasawa M, Fukui T, Kusuhara S, et al. Prognostic significance of the 8th edition of the TNM classification for patients with extensive disease small cell lung cancer. *Cancer Manag Res*. 2018; 10:6039–6047.
17. van Tinteren H, Hoekstra OS, Smit EF, et al. Effectiveness of positron emission tomography in the preoperative assessment of patients with suspected non-small-cell lung cancer: the PLUS multicentre randomised trial. *Lancet*. 2002;359(9315):1388–1393.
18. Reed CE, Harpole DH, Posther KE, et al. Results of the American College of Surgeons Oncology Group Z0050 trial: the utility of positron emission tomography in staging potentially operable non-small cell lung cancer. *J Thorac Cardiovasc Surg*. 2003;126(6):1943–1951.
19. Taylor SA, Mallett S, Miles A, et al. Whole-body MRI compared with standard pathways for staging metastatic disease in lung and colorectal cancer: the Streamline diagnostic accuracy studies. *Health Technol Assess*. 2019;23(66):1–270.
20. Bruzzi JF, Komaki R, Walsh GL, et al. Imaging of non-small cell lung cancer of the superior sulcus: part 2: initial staging and assessment of resectability and therapeutic response. *Radiographics*. 2008;28(2):561–572.
21. Bruzzi JF, Komaki R, Walsh GL, et al. Imaging of non-small cell lung cancer of the superior sulcus: part 1: anatomy, clinical manifestations, and management. *Radiographics*. 2008;28(2):551–560. quiz 620.
22. Prenzel KL, Monig SP, Sinning JM, et al. Lymph node size and metastatic infiltration in non-small cell lung cancer. *Chest*. 2003;123(2):463–467.

23. Birim O, Kappetein AP, Stijnen T, et al. Meta-analysis of positron emission tomographic and computed tomographic imaging in detecting mediastinal lymph node metastases in nonsmall cell lung cancer. *Ann Thorac Surg*. 2005;79(1):375–382.
24. Gould MK, Kuschner WG, Rydzak CE, et al. Test performance of positron emission tomography and computed tomography for mediastinal staging in patients with non-small-cell lung cancer: a meta-analysis. *Ann Intern Med*. 2003;139(11):879–892.
25. MacManus MP, Hicks RJ, Matthews JP, et al. High rate of detection of unsuspected distant metastases by pet in apparent stage III non-small-cell lung cancer: implications for radical radiation therapy. *Int J Radiat Oncol Biol Phys*. 2001;50(2):287–293.
26. Meyer M, Budjan J. Whole-body MRI for lung cancer staging: a step in the right direction. *Lancet Respir Med*. 2019;7(6):471–472.
27. Kalemkerian GP. Advances in the treatment of small-cell lung cancer. *Semin Respir Crit Care Med*. 2011;32(1):94–101.
28. Lim E, Harris G, Patel A, et al. Preoperative versus postoperative chemotherapy in patients with resectable non-small cell lung cancer: systematic review and indirect comparison meta-analysis of randomized trials. *J Thorac Oncol*. 2009;4(11):1380–1388.
29. Song WA, Zhou NK, Wang W, et al. Survival benefit of neoadjuvant chemotherapy in non-small cell lung cancer: an updated meta-analysis of 13 randomized control trials. *J Thorac Oncol*. 2010;5(4):510–516.
30. Baldwin CM, Perry CM. Pemetrexed: a review of its use in the management of advanced non-squamous non-small cell lung cancer. *Drugs*. 2009;69(16):2279–2302.
31. Soon YY, Stockler MR, Askie LM, et al. Duration of chemotherapy for advanced non-small-cell lung cancer: a systematic review and meta-analysis of randomized trials. *J Clin Oncol*. 2009;27(20):3277–3283.
32. Gazdar AF. Activating and resistance mutations of EGFR in non-small-cell lung cancer: role in clinical response to EGFR tyrosine kinase inhibitors. *Oncogene*. 2009;28(Suppl 1):S24–S31.
33. Shroff GS, de Groot PM, Papadimitrakopoulou VA, et al. Targeted therapy and immunotherapy in the treatment of non-small cell lung cancer. *Radiol Clin North Am*. 2018;56(3):485–495.
34. Berghoff AS, Bellosillo B, Caux C, et al. Immune checkpoint inhibitor treatment in patients with oncogene- addicted non-small cell lung cancer (NSCLC): summary of a multidisciplinary round-table discussion. *ESMO Open*. 2019;4(3):e000498.
35. Socinski MA, Jotte RM, Cappuzzo F, et al. Atezolizumab for first-line treatment of metastatic nonsquamous NSCLC. *N Engl J Med*. 2018;378(24):2288–2301.
36. Horn L, Mansfield AS, Szczesna A, et al. First-line atezolizumab plus chemotherapy in extensive-stage small-cell lung cancer. *N Engl J Med*. 2018;379(23):2220–2229.
37. Chang JY, Senan S, Paul MA, et al. Stereotactic ablative radiotherapy versus lobectomy for operable stage I non-small-cell lung cancer: a pooled analysis of two randomised trials. *Lancet Oncol*. 2015;16(6):630–637.
38. Palma DA, Olson R, Harrow S, et al. Stereotactic ablative radiotherapy versus standard of care palliative treatment in patients with oligometastatic cancers (SABR-COMET): a randomised, phase 2, open-label trial. *Lancet*. 2019;393(10185):2051–2058.
39. Schneider BJ, Ismaila N, Aerts J, et al. Lung cancer surveillance after definitive curative-intent therapy: ASCO guideline. *J Clin Oncol*. 2019 JCO1902748.
40. Westeel V, Choma D, Clement F, et al. Relevance of an intensive postoperative follow-up after surgery for non-small cell lung cancer. *Ann Thorac Surg*. 2000;70(4):1185–1190.

CHAPTER

8 Primary Mediastinal Neoplasms

Fernando R. Gutiérrez, M.D.; Felipe Aluja-Jaramillo, M.D.; and Jeremy J. Erasmus, M.D.

INTRODUCTION

The mediastinum can be the site of a variety of neoplastic conditions that can include both benign and malignant entities. Most neoplasms of the mediastinum are metastases, typically from lung cancer, although extrathoracic neoplasms such as breast cancer and melanoma have a predilection for spread to the mediastinum. Primary neoplasms of the mediastinum are uncommon, and whereas the majority in adults are benign, those in children tend to be malignant.[1] In terms of primary neoplasms, the most common prevascular or anterior compartment neoplasms include thymomas, teratomas, and lymphomas. Neoplasms of the visceral or middle compartment are typically congenital cysts, including foregut and pericardial cysts, whereas those that arise in the posterior or paravertebral compartment are often tumors of neurogenic origin.

This chapter discusses mediastinal neoplasms, with particular emphasis on those primary neoplasms that are frequently encountered in an oncologic medical practice. Computed tomography (CT), magnetic resonance imaging (MRI), and positron emission tomography (PET)/CT will be emphasized as the tools of choice in the characterization of these neoplastic entities to help referring physicians, oncologists, and surgeons deliver proper care and follow-up of afflicted patients.

EPIDEMIOLOGY AND RISK FACTORS

Thymic neoplasms account for 17%, lymphomas 16%, and neurogenic neoplasms 14% of all cases of primary mediastinal neoplasms.[2] Germ cell tumors (teratomas, seminomas, embryonal carcinomas, endodermal sinus tumors, and choriocarcinomas) account for approximately 15% of all mediastinal tumors in adults and 24% in children.[3] The remainder of the neoplasms in the mediastinum represent a substantial group of miscellaneous entities, including mediastinal cysts (bronchogenic, esophageal, pericardial, thymic, and neurenteric), which account for 15% to 20% of all mediastinal masses.

Thymomas are the most common thymic epithelial neoplasms, and characteristically are located in the prevascular or anterior compartment. Thymomas typically occur in patients older than 40 years, are rare in children, and affect men and women with equal frequency.[4–6] Thymic neuroendocrine tumors (carcinoid, small cell carcinoma, and large cell carcinoma) are uncommon. Thymic carcinoid tumors represents the most common of this group of tumors. Affected patients are typically in the fourth and fifth decades of life, with a male predominance.

Germ cell tumors usually occur in young adults (mean age 27 years).[7] Most malignant germ cell neoplasms (>90%) occur in men.[7] Teratomas are the most common germ cell neoplasm, representing 70% of all germ cell tumors in children and 60% in adults.[7] Men and women are affected with equal frequency. Malignant germ cell neoplasms are divided into seminomas and nonseminomatous neoplasms. Seminomas are the most common pure histologic type, accounting for 40% of such neoplasms, usually occurring in men in the third and fourth decades of life.[7] The nonseminomatous germ cell tumors of the mediastinum include embryonal cell carcinoma, endodermal sinus tumor, choriocarcinoma, and mixed germ cell tumors. Teratoma with embryonal cell carcinoma (teratocarcinoma) is the most common subtype, whereas pure endodermal sinus tumors, choriocarcinomas, and embryonal carcinomas are less common.

Neurogenic neoplasms represent 75% of primary paravertebral or posterior compartment masses.[8] These neoplasms are classified as tumors of peripheral nerves (neurofibromas, schwannomas, and malignant tumors of nerve sheath origin), sympathetic ganglia (ganglioneuromas, ganglioneuroblastomas, and neuroblastomas), or parasympathetic ganglia (paraganglioma and pheochromocytoma). Peripheral nerves are more commonly involved in adults, and schwannomas constitute 75% of this group, whereas sympathetic ganglia neoplasms are more common in children. Schwannomas and neurofibromas typically occur with equal frequency in men and women, most commonly in the third and fourth decades of life. Some 30% to 45% of neurofibromas[9] occur in patients with neurofibromatosis (NF), and multiple neurogenic tumors or a single plexiform neurofibroma are considered pathognomonic for the disease.[10] Malignant tumors of nerve sheath origin (also termed malignant neurofibromas, malignant schwannomas, or neurofibrosarcomas) are rare and typically develop from solitary or plexiform neurofibromas in the third to fifth decades of life. Up to 50% occur in patients with type 1 NF (NF-1), and in these patients tumors occur at an earlier age (typically adolescents) and with a higher incidence than in the general population.[4,11] Neuroblastomas are the most common extracranial solid neoplasms in children, accounting for 10% of all childhood neoplasms. Neuroblastomas are typically diagnosed at a median age of younger than 2 years, ganglioneuroblastomas at 5.5 years of age, and ganglioneuromas at 10 years.[12]

ANATOMY AND PATHOLOGY

The mediastinum is located in the central portion of the thorax, sandwiched between the two pleural cavities and extending from the diaphragm to the thoracic inlet in the longitudinal axis. The mediastinum is generally divided into three anatomic regions or compartments: prevascular (anterior), visceral (middle), and paravertebral (posterior).[13] Although there are no fascial planes that separate these compartments from each other, this division facilitates tumor localization and is useful in limiting the differential diagnosis.

The prevascular compartment is bounded anteriorly by the sternum, posteriorly by the anterior portion of the pericardium, superiorly by the thoracic inlet, and inferiorly by the diaphragm. Its contents include the thymus, lymph nodes, and fat. The visceral compartment is bounded anteriorly by the pericardium and posteriorly by a vertical line through the vertebral bodies 1 cm posterior to their anterior margin, and its contents include the heart, aorta, vena cava, brachiocephalic vessels, pulmonary vessels, trachea and main bronchi, esophagus, lymph nodes, and phrenic, vagus, and left recurrent laryngeal nerves. The paravertebral compartment is bounded anteriorly by the visceral compartment, inferiorly by the diaphragm, posteriorly by the vertebral transverse processes, and superiorly by the thoracic inlet. The contents of the paravertebral compartment include the paravertebral soft tissues and the thoracic spine.[13]

A significant proportion of the neoplasms that occur in the prevascular compartment arise from the thymus. An understanding of the normal size, appearance, and location of the thymus at different ages is important. Anatomically, the thymus consists of two lobes in close contact with each other along the midline extending from the fourth costal cartilage superiorly, as high as the lower border of the thyroid gland. However, ectopic thymic tissue can occur at any level in the pathway of normal thymic descent, which extends from the angle of the mandible to the upper prevascular compartment more inferiorly. The two lobes generally differ in size; the left lobe is usually larger than the right and extends more inferiorly. Thymic hyperplasia, an increase in weight and size, has two distinct histologic forms: true and lymphoid hyperplasia. True hyperplasia occurs in children and young adults recovering from severe illness or trauma or after chemotherapy (Fig. 8.1). Lymphoid hyperplasia occurs most commonly in patients with myasthenia gravis, but also in association with other diseases such as hyperthyroidism, Graves disease, rheumatoid arthritis, and scleroderma.[14]

Thymic epithelial neoplasms include thymomas and carcinomas. Most thymomas are solid neoplasms that are encapsulated and anatomically limited to the thymus. However, one-third have necrosis, hemorrhage, or cystic components; invasion of the capsule and involvement of the surrounding structures occurs in approximately one-third of cases.[15] Thymomas have a wide variety of histologic features, and there is a strong association between the histologic findings and prognosis.[16] Thymic carcinomas usually manifest histologically as large, solid, and infiltrating masses with cystic and necrotic areas. They are histologically classified as low or high grade, with squamous cell–like or lymphoepithelioma-like variants being the most common cell types.[4] Thymic neuroendocrine neoplasms are uncommon. These tumors typically present as a large, lobulated, and usually invasive prevascular mediastinal mass that can exhibit areas of hemorrhage and necrosis.[4,17] Malignant potential ranges from relatively benign (thymic carcinoid) to highly malignant (small cell/large cell carcinoma of the thymus). The typical carcinoid has low mitotic activity (<2 mitoses/2 mm^2) without necrosis, whereas atypical carcinoids have a higher rate of mitosis (2–10 mitoses/2 mm^2) and/or necrosis. Small cell and large cell neuroendocrine carcinomas have a higher rate of mitotic activity (>10 mitoses/2 mm^2) and associated necrosis.

Germ cell tumors arise from mediastinal remnants of embryonal cell migration. The mediastinum is the most common extragonadal primary site of these neoplasms and can account for 60% of all germ cell tumors in adults. Teratomas, the most common mediastinal germ cell tumors, are composed of elements that arise from one or more of the three primitive germ cell layers (ectoderm, mesoderm, and endoderm). Mediastinal teratomas are classified as mature, immature, or malignant; most teratomas are composed of well-differentiated or mature tissue and are usually benign. Mature or benign teratomas are composed of ectoderm, endoderm, or mesoderm, with ectodermal derivatives predominating. Teratomas are spherical, lobulated, and encapsulated neoplasms that are frequently cystic and multiloculated. These neoplasms can contain sebaceous material, as well as

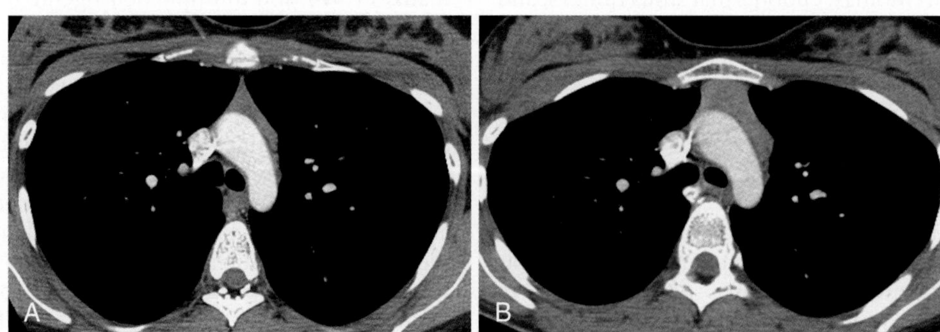

FIGURE 8.1. Thymic hyperplasia in a 15-year-old girl with a right femoral osteosarcoma. **A,** Axial computed tomography (CT) image shows decrease in thymic volume during chemotherapy. **B,** Axial CT image shows increase in thymic size 6 months after completion of chemotherapy. Note diffuse, symmetrical enlargement with preservation of the normal shape of the thymus.

hair and teeth. Respiratory and intestinal epithelium may also be present. Nonteratomatous tumors include seminomas and nonseminomatous types. Seminomas, also known as germinomas or dysgerminomas, are the second most common mediastinal germ cell tumor. These tumors typically present as solid masses with lobulated contours. Nonseminomatous neoplasms are divided into embryonal carcinoma, endodermal sinus tumor, choriocarcinoma, and mixed types, which include any combination of these histologic types.

In the paravertebral or posterior compartment, most of the neoplasms are of neurogenic origin. Nerve sheath tumors are schwannomas, neurofibromas, or malignant tumors of nerve sheath origin (malignant neurofibroma, malignant schwannoma, and neurogenic fibrosarcoma). From a histologic perspective, schwannomas are encapsulated tumors that arise from Schwann cells located in the nerve sheath and extend along the nerve, causing extrinsic compression.[11] They are heterogeneous in composition and can have low cellularity, areas of cystic degeneration, and hemorrhage, as well as small calcifications. Neurofibromas differ from schwannomas in that they are unencapsulated and result from proliferation of all nerve elements, including Schwann cells, nerve fibers, and fibroblasts. Neurofibromas grow by diffusely expanding the nerve, whereas plexiform neurofibromas, variants of neurofibromas, infiltrate along nerve trunks or plexuses.[18] Ganglion cell tumors arise from the autonomic nervous system rather than nerve sheaths and range from benign encapsulated neoplasms (ganglioneuromas) to moderately aggressive neoplasms (ganglioneuroblastomas) to malignant unencapsulated masses (neuroblastomas). These tumors derive from cells of embryologic origin or from sympathetic ganglia. After the abdomen, the thorax is the second most common location of neuroblastomas,[19] whereas ganglioneuromas and ganglioneuroblastomas are more common in the sympathetic chain of the paravertebral compartment. Ganglioneuromas are benign tumors composed of one or more mature ganglionic cells. Ganglioneuroblastomas, the least common type of neurogenic tumors, have histologic features of both ganglioneuromas and neuroblastomas. Neuroblastomas are the most aggressive type and are composed of small round cells arranged in sheets or pseudorosettes.[20,21]

KEY POINTS Anatomy: Prevascular Mediastinal Masses

- Thymic origin: thymic hyperplasia, thymic epithelial tumors and cyst.
- Germ cell tumors: teratoma (mature, immature, malignant), seminoma, nonseminomatous.
- Lymphoma: Hodgkin and non-Hodgkin.
- Thyroid mass: goiter, thyroid cancer.
- Miscellaneous: adenopathy, parathyroid adenoma, mesenchymal tumors (lymphangioma, hemangioma).

KEY POINTS Pathology

- Thymic neoplasms: epithelial (thymomas and carcinoma); neuroendocrine tumors (carcinoid-typical and atypical, small and large cell neuroendocrine carcinoma).
- Germ cell tumors: teratoma (mature, immature, and malignant); nonteratomatous tumors (seminomas and nonseminomas); seminomas (germinomas); nonseminomatous germ cell tumors (embryonal carcinoma, endodermal sinus tumor, choriocarcinoma, and mixed type).
- Neurogenic sheath tumors: schwannomas or neurofibromas.
- Ganglion cell tumors: ganglioneuromas, ganglioneuroblastomas, and neuroblastomas arise from the autonomic nervous system rather than the nerve sheath.

CLINICAL PRESENTATION

Most patients are asymptomatic at the time of diagnosis. Symptoms are usually related to local effects, which can include compression, displacement, and invasion, and can manifest clinically as respiratory distress, dysphagia, diaphragm paralysis, or superior vena cava (SVC) syndrome. Systemic symptoms and paraneoplastic syndromes occur occasionally and are caused by secretion of hormones, antibodies, or cytokines by the tumor.

Thymomas usually are an incidental finding, but patients can present with chest pain, cough, or dyspnea in up to one-third of cases.[22] Myasthenia gravis, which is characteristically associated with thymomas, occurs most frequently in women. Some 30% to 50% of patients with thymomas have myasthenia gravis, whereas 10% to 15% of patients with myasthenia gravis have a hymoma.[23] Some 10% of patients with a thymoma have hypogammaglobulinemia, and 5% of patients have pure red cell aplasia. Thymomas are also associated with various autoimmune disorders such as systemic lupus erythematosus, polymyositis, or myocarditis.[2] Thymic carcinomas are frequently symptomatic at presentation owing to marked local invasion of mediastinal structures. Symptoms include SVC syndrome, usually are attributed to compression or invasion of the SVC; paraneoplastic syndromes are rare. Thymic neuroendocrine tumors are also associated with ectopic secretion of hormones. Up to 50% of affected patients with thymic carcinoid tumors have hormonal abnormalities, and up to 35% have Cushing syndrome as a result of tumoral production of adrenocorticotropic hormone. Nonfunctioning thymic carcinoids may be seen in association with multiple endocrine neoplasia syndrome type 1.

Patients with germ cell tumors are often asymptomatic. Large tumors, however, can lead to the development of clinical symptoms depending on the location and the adjacent structures. Seminomas can manifest as SVC syndrome in 10% of cases. β-human chorionic gonadotropin (β-hCG) and α-fetoprotein (AFP) levels are usually normal. However, 7% to 8% of patients with pure seminomas are reported to have elevated serum levels of β-hCG, and elevation of serum lactate dehydrogenase (LDH) levels can occur in up to 80% of patients with advanced seminomas. Importantly, elevation of AFP indicates a nonseminomatous component of the tumor. Most (90%) patients with nonseminomatous germ cell tumors of the mediastinum exhibit symptoms at the time of diagnosis including weight loss and fever, 71% of affected patients have elevated AFP levels, and 54% have elevated β-hCG levels.[24] There is an association between malignant nonseminomatous germ cell tumors of the mediastinum and hematologic malignancies, and approximately 20% of cases are associated with Klinefelter syndrome.

Nerve sheath tumors are usually asymptomatic. The development of pain often indicates malignant transformation (malignant neurofibromas, schwannomas, or neurofibrosarcomas). Mediastinal neuroblastomas can cause symptoms caused by local mass effect or spinal cord compression. Neuroblastomas and, less frequently, ganglioneuroblastoma and ganglioneuroma can produce metabolically active catecholamines that can be responsible for hypertension, flushing, and watery diarrhea syndrome.[25,26] Catecholamine derivatives, such as vanilmandelic acid and homovanilic acid, can be secreted.

KEY Points Visceral and Paravertebral Mediastinal Masses

- Vascular: aorta (aneurysm, dissection, and congenital abnormalities), pulmonary artery (aneurysm and pulmonary hypertension), and venous abnormalities (left superior vena cava and azygos/hemiazygos system abnormalities).
- Adenopathy: infectious (tuberculosis, histoplasmosis, and coccidioidomycosis), sarcoidosis, lymphoma, metastatic disease (head and neck, melanoma, breast, and genitourinary), Castleman disease.
- Cysts: pericardial, esophageal, bronchogenic, meningocele, pancreatic pseudocyst, neurenteric, cystic tumors.
- Esophageal: megaesophagus, esophageal varices, neoplasms.
- Neurogenic tumors: nerve sheath (neurofibroma, schwannoma, and malignant tumors of nerve sheath origin), ganglion cell (neuroblastoma, ganglioneuroma, and ganglioneuroblastoma), paraganglia cell (paraganglioma).
- Miscellaneous: hematoma, abscess, hiatal hernia, congenital hernia.

STAGING

Several classification schemes and staging systems for thymic epithelial tumors have been proposed; however, because thymomas are composed of a mixture of neoplastic epithelial cells and nonneoplastic lymphocytes, there is a marked variability in the histology of these tumors, both within the same tumor and between different thymomas.

In 1999, the World Health Organization (WHO) Consensus Committee published a histologic classification of tumors of the thymus. In this scheme, thymomas are classified the morphology of the neoplastic epithelial cells and the lymphocyte to epithelial cell ratio. Updates to the WHO classification were published in 2004 and 2015.[27,28] This classification outlines six separate histologic subtypes of thymomas (types A, AB, B1, B2, and B3) (Table 8.1). The type C term is no longer used. The neuroendocrine thymic carcinomas are included in the thymic carcinomas, except for thymic paraganglioma. A new addition in the 2015 classification is the “atypical type A thymoma variant,” which can show increased cellularity and mitotic activity. Immunohistochemical features are included as criteria for diagnosis of thymomas with ambiguous histology. Most type A and type AB thymomas

TABLE 8.1 World Health Organization Classification Scheme for Thymic Epithelial Tumors

TUMOR TYPE	DESCRIPTION
A	Medullary
Atypical type A	Comedo-type tumor necrosis
AB	Mixed
B1	Lymphocyte-rich, predominantly cortical
B2	Cortical
B3	Epithelial (well-differentiated thymic carcinoma)
Thymic carcinoma	

tend to have no local invasion, are completely resectable, and have no recurrence or tumor-related deaths. There is an increasing tendency to local invasion, incomplete resection, and recurrence after resection from types B1 and B2 to type B3. In this regard, most thymic carcinomas are locally invasive, many are incompletely resected, and there is a high early relapse rate and poor prognosis. The WHO histologic subtype classification and the Masaoka staging system provide the clinician and surgeon the information needed to provide a prognosis. The Masaoka staging system is a pathologic staging system that is based on the presence of capsular invasion and is currently the system that is most widely used to determine therapy.[29] In this staging system, the stages are defined as follows: stage I, macroscopically encapsulated and microscopically no capsular invasion; stage II, macroscopic invasion into surrounding fatty tissue of mediastinal pleura or microscopic invasion into capsule; stage III, macroscopic invasion into a neighboring organ; stage IVa, pleural or pericardial dissemination; and stage IVb, lymphogenous or hematogenous metastasis.

Neuroblastomas are currently staged according to the International Neuroblastoma Risk Group (INRG) (pretreatment)[30] and International Neuroblastoma Staging System (INSS) (postsurgical).[31] INRG classification is based on clinical and imaging features, whereas INSS classification is based on surgical findings, as well as lymph node and metastatic involvement. Both of these staging systems have an important role in the determination of appropriate treatment and prediction of outcome in patients with neuroblastoma (Table 8.2).

KEY POINTS Staging Thymic Neoplasms

- The World Health Organization classification is based on histologic findings.
- The Masaoka classification is based on surgical and pathologic findings.
- The Masaoka staging system is currently the system that is most widely used to determine therapy.
- Neuroblastoma is staged according to the International Neuroblastoma Risk Group (INRG) and International Neuroblastoma Staging System (INSS) systems.
- The INRG is based on imaging and clinical features, and the INSS is based on surgical findings and tumor spread.

TABLE 8.2 Comparison Between International Neuroblastoma Staging System and International Neuroblastoma Risk Group Staging System

INTERNATIONAL NEUROBLASTOMA STAGING SYSTEM	INTERNATIONAL NEUROBLASTOMA RISK GROUP STAGING SYSTEM
Stage 1: Localized tumor with complete gross excision; ± microscopic residual disease; representative ipsilateral lymph node negative for tumor microscopically.	Stage L1: Localized tumor not involving vital structures as defined by imaging-defined risk factors (IDRFs) and confined to one body compartment.
Stage 2A: Localized tumor with incomplete gross excision; representative ipsilateral lymph node negative for tumor microscopically.	Stage L2: Locoregional tumor with presence of one or more IDRFs.
Stage 2B: Localized tumor with or without complete gross excision; ipsilateral lymph node positive for tumor microscopically; enlarged contralateral lymph nodes should be negative microscopically.	Equals stage L2.
Stage 3: Unresectable unilateral tumor infiltrating across the midline; ± regional lymph node involvement; or localized unilateral tumor with contralateral regional lymph node involvement or midline tumor with bilateral extension by infiltration (unresectable) or by lymph node involvement.	Equals stage L2.
Stage 4: Any primary tumor with dissemination to distant lymph nodes, bone, bone marrow, liver, skin, or other organs.	Stage M: Distant metastatic disease (except stage MS). Distant lymph node involvement is metastatic disease. Ascites and pleural effusion, even if malignant cells are present, do not constitute metastatic disease unless they are remote from the primary tumor.
Stage 4S: Localized primary tumor in infants <1 years old (localized as in stage 1, 2A, or 2B) with dissemination limited to skin, liver, or bone marrow (<10% malignant cells).	Stage MS: Metastatic disease in children <547 days (18 months) of age with metastases confined to skin, liver, and/or bone marrow (<10% malignant cells); metaiodobenzylguanidine scan must be negative in bone and bone marrow. Primary tumor can be L1 or L2 with no limitations in terms of crossing or infiltration of the midline.

(Modified from Monclair T, Brodeur GM, Ambros PF, et al. The International Neuroblastoma Risk Group (INRG) staging system: an INRG Task Force report. *J Clin Oncol.* 2009;27:298-303.)

PATTERNS OF SPREAD

Thymomas can remain localized or can spread through the mediastinum in a contiguous fashion. Dissemination into the pleural space can result in solitary, multiple, or diffuse metastases distant to the primary mass, an occurrence referred to as drop metastases (Fig. 8.2). Pleural effusions are not common. Transdiaphragmatic spread has been reported in up to one-third of patients.[32] Pericardial involvement is common and can manifest as nodular or diffuse thickening, as well as pericardial effusion. Systemic dissemination is rare, although lung metastases can occur. Thymic carcinomas are aggressive malignancies that often exhibit marked local invasion and early dissemination. In 40% of cases, there is invasion of adjacent organs, 40% present with nodal metastatic disease, and 10% have pleural or pericardial involvement. Distant metastases to lung, liver, adrenal glands, brain, and bone occur in 40% of patients.

Mature teratomas are benign, although rare cases of tumor rupture into adjacent structures have been reported. Seminomas usually have lymphatic or systemic dissemination, and local invasion of adjacent structures is rare. Metastases to regional nodes, as well as metastatic involvement of cervical (25%) and abdominal lymph nodes (8%), has been reported.[33] In cases of nonseminomatous tumors, invasion of the adjacent structures such as lung and mediastinal pleura is frequent.[34] Pleural and pericardial effusions are common as a result of local and direct invasion. Chest wall invasion is more frequently associated with larger masses. Hematogenous disseminated metastases to lungs, liver, brain, and bones are common and can occur in up to 50% of patients. Metastatic spread to the lymph nodes is less frequent.

Intraspinal extension in neurogenic tumors is common. Some 10% of paravertebral neurofibromas and schwannomas extend into the neural foramina and spinal canal.[11] Compression and destruction of adjacent structures can occur as a result of aggressive local tumor invasion. Ganglioneuromas are encapsulated benign tumors without evidence of local or distant dissemination. Ganglioneuroblastomas and neuroblastomas are more aggressive, with evidence of local and intraspinal invasion. Neuroblastomas have a tendency to grow across the midline, and lymph node involvement can occur. Lymphatic and hematogenous dissemination are common, and sites of metastatic involvement include bone (60%), regional lymph nodes (45%), orbit (20%), liver (15%), brain (14%), and lung (10%).

KEY POINTS Patterns of Spread

- Thymoma. Most have slow growth and remain localized. In one-third of cases contiguous invasion of adjacent structures occurs. Drop metastasis can occur.
- Thymic carcinoma. Local invasion and hematogenous dissemination to brain, lung, liver, adrenal glands, and bones are common.
- Germ cell tumor. Teratomas are typically benign, although rarely malignant transformation and local invasion occurs. With seminomas, local invasion does not occur, and hematogenous dissemination has been reported. Nonseminomatous tumors commonly invade adjacent structures, and distant metastases are common.
- Neurogenic tumor. Neurofibroma and schwannoma are benign and rarely undergo malignant degeneration. Malignant tumors can cause local invasion. Neuroblastoma can cause distant metastases.

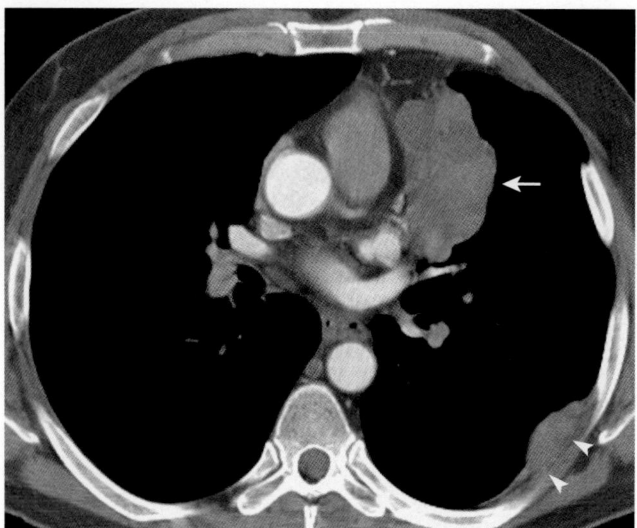

FIGURE 8.2. Thymoma in a 52-year-old man with chest pain. Axial computed tomography image shows a prevascular (anterior) mediastinal mass (*arrow*) and focal pleural thickening (*arrowheads*). Biopsy revealed metastatic pleural disease. Note that dissemination of metastases in the pleural space has been referred to as drop metastases.

IMAGING

Imaging has an important role in the evaluation of a mediastinal neoplasm and establishing relevant differentials in most patients. Specifically, the location of a neoplasm in the mediastinum, together with its morphologic features, is helpful in differentiating a benign from a malignant neoplasm. Although conventional radiography may suggest the presence of a mediastinal mass, CT, MRI, and/or integrated PET/CT are required for further evaluation. CT is frequently performed to evaluate the mediastinum for a suspected mediastinal mass. MRI is usually reserved for clarifying problems encountered on CT or to examine patients who cannot tolerate intravenous administration of iodinated contrast material. Moreover, MRI is better suited for posterior mediastinal tumors and for some thymic masses. PET/CT can be used to detect disease, differentiate benign from malignant masses, and diagnose disease recurrence.

The normal thymus in young children and thymic hyperplasia can mimic a mediastinal mass on chest radiographic assessment. CT and MRI are useful in differentiating normal thymic tissue and the hyperplastic thymus from tumors. Thymic hyperplasia manifesting as diffuse and symmetrical enlargement on CT or MRI is differentiated from a primary mediastinal neoplasm based on preservation of the normal shape of the thymus (see Fig. 8.1). Similar findings may be seen in rebound hyperplasia, which can occur 3 to 8 months after cessation of chemotherapy in approximately 25% of patients.[35] When CT and conventional MRI sequences are not able to differentiate between a normal thymus or thymic hyperplasia and a thymoma, chemical-shift MRI sequences (in-phase and out-of-phase gradient echo sequences) can be helpful in the diagnosis—that is, homogeneous signal decrease occurs in normal and hyperplastic tissue, compared with the absence of a signal decrease in tumors. PET/CT imaging is being increasingly used in oncologic patients. The normal thymus can have mildly increased 2-[^{18}F] fluoro-2-deoxy-D-glucose (FDG), especially in children. In addition, increased FDG uptake in the thymus, mainly related to hyperplasia after chemotherapy, has been reported to occur in 28% of patients, and is more common in younger patients.[36]

Thymic Neoplasms

Thymomas are usually located in the prevascular compartment, but can occasionally occur in the cardiophrenic recesses.[4,37] They typically manifest as a large (mean 5 cm) smooth or lobulated well-marginated mass that characteristically arises from one lobe of the thymus. Although thymomas typically manifest as a unilateral mass, bilateral involvement can also occur.[38] On CT, thymomas are usually of homogeneous soft tissue attenuation (see Fig. 8.2). Calcification, seen in up to 7% of cases, is usually thin, linear, and located in the capsule. Homogeneous enhancement after intravenous contrast administration is common, except in the one-third of thymomas that have necrotic, cystic, or hemorrhagic components. Lobulation or irregular contours, the presence of a cystic or a necrotic portion within the tumor, and multifocal calcification are more suggestive of invasive thymoma (Fig. 8.3).[39] On MRI, thymomas usually exhibit low to intermediate signal intensity (similar to skeletal muscle) on T1-weighted (T1W) images and high signal intensity on T2-weighted (T2W) images. Heterogeneous signal intensity can be present in those tumors that have focal areas of necrosis, hemorrhage, or cystic changes. MRI can depict fibrous septa within the masses. Pleural metastases manifest on CT and MRI as an isolated pleural nodule, multifocal masses, or contiguous pleural involvement, which can be smooth, nodular, or diffuse, mimicking malignant pleural mesothelioma. Pericardial thickening and/or effusion typically are associated with invasive thymomas. The precise role of PET/CT in the evaluation of thymomas is unclear. One difficulty is that FDG uptake in the normal thymus is variable, and increased FDG uptake by the thymus is common, especially in young patients.[36] In our experience, PET/CT is unreliable in distinguishing noninvasive from invasive thymomas or thymic carcinomas. Also, ^{11}C-acetate PET/CT has been used to depict thymomas[40] and, in combination with FDG-PET/CT, may allow differentiation between thymomas of different histologic types, especially A and AB.[41]

Thymic carcinomas commonly manifest as large, poorly marginated prevascular mediastinal masses that are calcified in almost 40% of cases.[39,42,43] Intrathoracic lymphadenopathy is common. On CT, thymic carcinomas are heterogeneous caused by hemorrhage or necrosis, and in general have poorly defined margins. On MRI, they are typically heterogeneous, have intermediate signal intensity (slightly higher than skeletal muscle) on T1W images, and have high signal intensity on T2W images. MRI can be helpful for revealing local soft tissue and vascular invasion. The role of PET/CT in the diagnosis and staging of thymic carcinomas has not been clearly established. Thymic carcinomas typically exhibit increased FDG uptake on

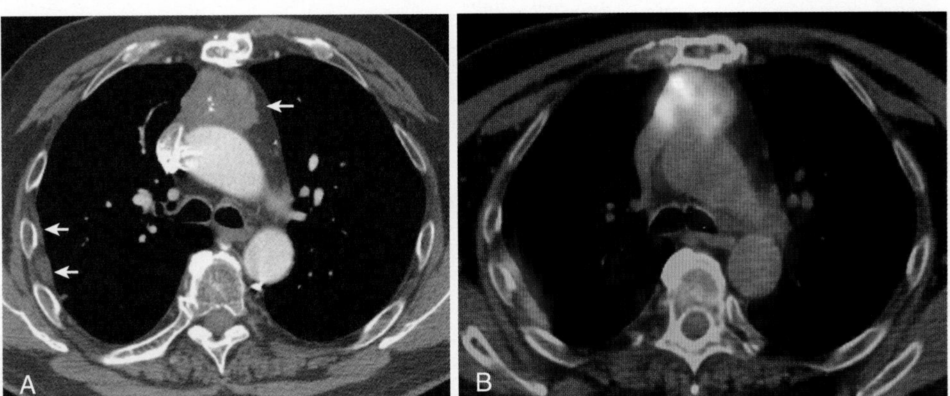

FIGURE 8.3. Invasive thymoma in a 66-year-old man with an incidentally detected mediastinal mass at the time of coronary artery bypass graft surgery. **A,** Axial computed tomography (CT) image shows a prevascular (anterior) mediastinal mass (*large arrow*) with irregular contours and punctate calcification. There is focal pleural thickening (*small arrows*). **B,** Axial positron emission tomography/CT image shows increased 2-[^{18}F] fluoro-2-deoxy-D-glucose uptake in the mass and pleura suspicious for pleural metastasis. Biopsy confirmed pleural metastasis.

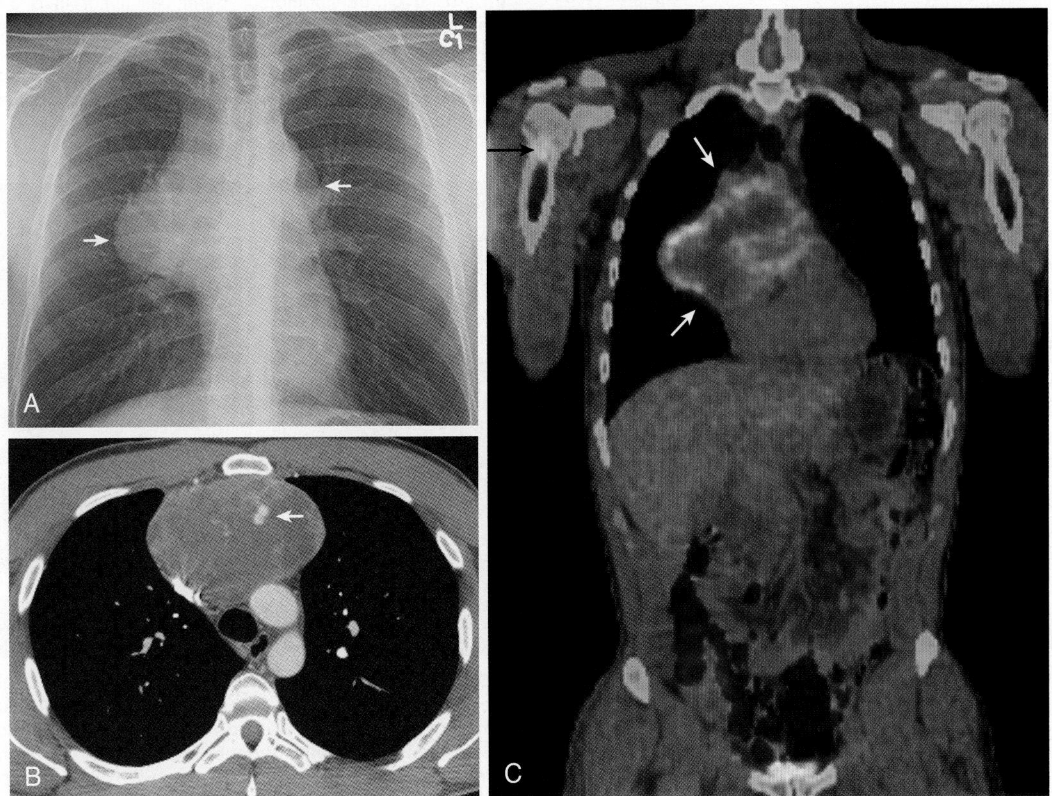

FIGURE 8.4. Small-cell neuroendocrine thymic tumor in a 31-year-old man presenting with hip pain as a result of metastatic disease. **A,** Posteroanterior chest radiograph shows a large prevascular (anterior) mediastinal mass extending into both hemithoraces (*arrows*). **B,** Axial computed tomography (CT) image confirms a large prevascular (anterior) mediastinal mass and shows necrosis and prominent vasculature (*arrow*). **C,** Coronal positron emission tomography/CT image shows 2-[^{18}F] fluoro-2-deoxy-D-glucose (FDG) uptake in the periphery of the mass (*white arrows*) and low FDG activity centrally as a result of of necrosis. Note focal increased FDG uptake in a humeral metastasis (*black arrow*) owing to metastatic bone disease.

PET/CT that is usually higher and more homogeneous than in thymomas and thymic hyperplasia.[44–46] The detection of unexpected nodal and distant metastases is useful in patient management.

Thymic neuroendocrine tumors usually manifest as a large prevascular mediastinal mass with a propensity for local invasion and metastasis (Fig. 8.4). Focal areas of necrosis and calcification may be present.[17] On CT or MRI the masses are usually heterogeneous. Differentiation between thymic neuroendocrine tumors and invasive thymic epithelial tumors may be difficult on the basis of imaging findings alone. Thymic neuroendocrine tumors have a poor prognosis owing to a high prevalence of recurrence and metastasis. For these type of tumors novel PET/CT tracers are being used, most notably ^{68}Ga-DOTATOC, ^{68}Ga-DOTATATE, and ^{68}Ga-DOTANOC.[47] Combined imaging with FDG-PET/CT and ^{111}In-labeled octreotide single-photon emission computed tomography allows differentiation between low-risk and high-risk epithelial tumors and identification of neuroendocrine thymic neoplasias.[48]

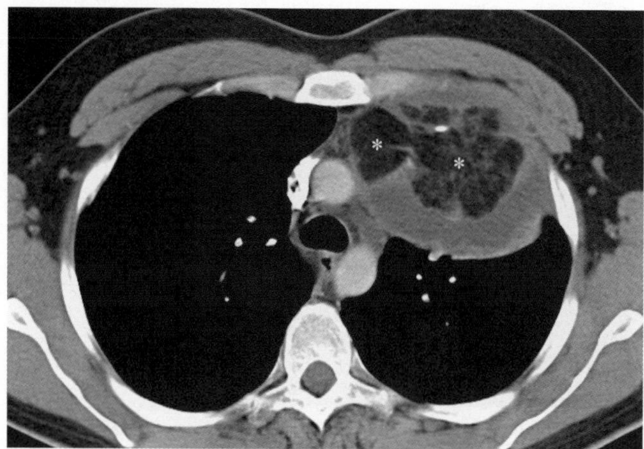

FIGURE 8.5. Teratoma in a 29-year-old man presenting with chest discomfort. Axial computed tomography image shows a mediastinal mass that contains adipose tissue (*) and focal calcification. Note that fat occurs in up to 75% of teratomas. (From S. Rossi, Centro de Diagnostico Dr. Enrique Rossi, Buenos Aires, Argentina.)

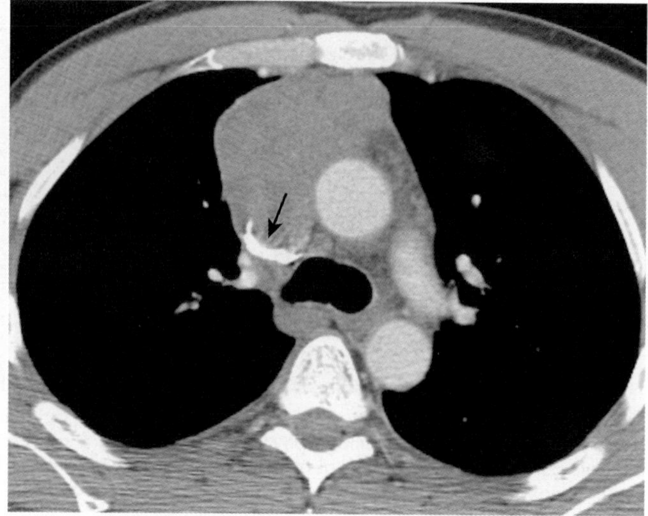

FIGURE 8.6. Seminomatous germ cell tumor in a 37-year-old man presenting with superior vena cava (SVC) syndrome (facial swelling, enlargement of the neck veins). Axial computed tomography image shows homogeneous prevascular (anterior) mediastinal mass and SVC compression (*arrow*). Note that compression of adjacent mediastinal structures is common.

Germ Cell Tumors

These neoplasms have a range of manifestations in the mediastinum. Mature teratomas manifest on CT or MRI as smooth or lobulated mediastinal masses with cystic and solid components, whereas malignant teratomas are usually poorly marginated masses containing areas of necrosis. The combination of fluid, soft tissue, calcium, fat, and/or fat–fluid level is diagnostic of teratomas (Fig. 8.5). Fat occurs in up to 75% of mature teratomas and up to 40% of malignant teratomas. However, only 17% to 39% of mature teratomas will have all tissue components, and approximately 15% of mature teratomas exhibit only a unilocular or multilocular cystic component. In this regard, these masses can mimic mediastinal cysts.

Teratomas can show rim enhancement and enhancement of tissue septa within the mass. Because simple cysts can contain proteinaceous fluid and have high attenuation on CT, MRI can be useful in differentiating these lesions. Teratomas containing fat typically manifest as high signal intensity on T1W images. Fat-saturation MRI techniques can be used to detect and distinguish fat from hemorrhage. Importantly, if a cystic neoplasm is suspected because the CT or MRI findings are atypical or because the mass has increased in size, aspiration and cytologic analysis may be required for diagnosis. Mature teratomas can rupture into lung, the pleural space, and pericardium, and CT or MRI can be useful in detecting fat within these regions if this occurs. In addition, adjacent parenchymal consolidation or atelectasis, pleural effusion, and pericardial effusion are ancillary signs of rupture into the pleural or pericardial space. PET/CT is not useful in the evaluation of mature teratomas, owing to the lack of FDG avidity.

Seminomas manifest as large/bulky, well-marginated masses with lobulated contours and typically have a homogeneous appearance. Cystic or necrotic areas can occur; however, calcification is rare. Seminomas enhance slightly after administration of intravenous contrast. Compression of adjacent mediastinal structures with obliteration of the fat planes is common, but invasion is uncommon (Fig. 8.6).

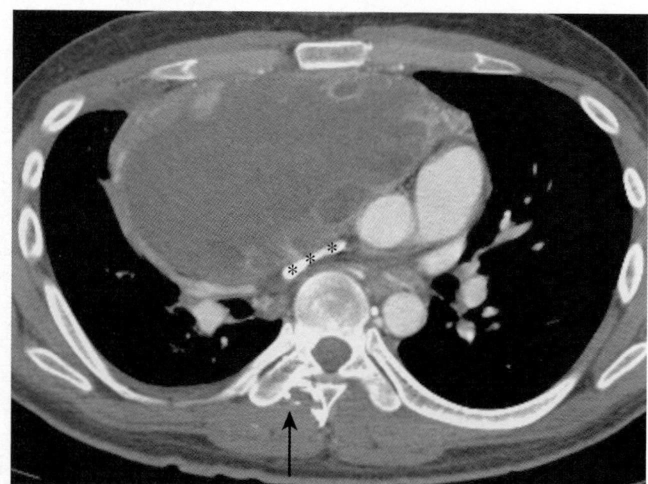

FIGURE 8.7. Nonseminomatous germ cell tumor in a 21-year-old man presenting with shortness of breath and chest pain. Axial computed tomography image shows large heterogeneous prevascular (anterior) mediastinal mass with superior vena cava (*) compression and paravertebral collateral circulation (*arrow*). Mild right pleural effusion is also noted. Note that nonseminomatous tumors tend to exhibit necrosis, and most patients are symptomatic at presentation.

In contradistinction, nonseminomatous tumors are usually large, unencapsulated, heterogeneous soft tissue masses that tend to invade and infiltrate adjacent structures, including the lung and chest wall. The interface between the tumor and the adjacent lung may be irregular and spiculated owing to lung invasion. These tumors can contain large areas of hemorrhage, necrosis, and cyst formation (Fig. 8.7). Associated pleural and pericardial effusions can occur. Metastases to the regional lymph nodes and distant sites such as lung are common. PET/CT can be useful for diagnosing and restaging malignant germ cell tumors, with similar applications in seminomatous and nonseminomatous tumors.[49]

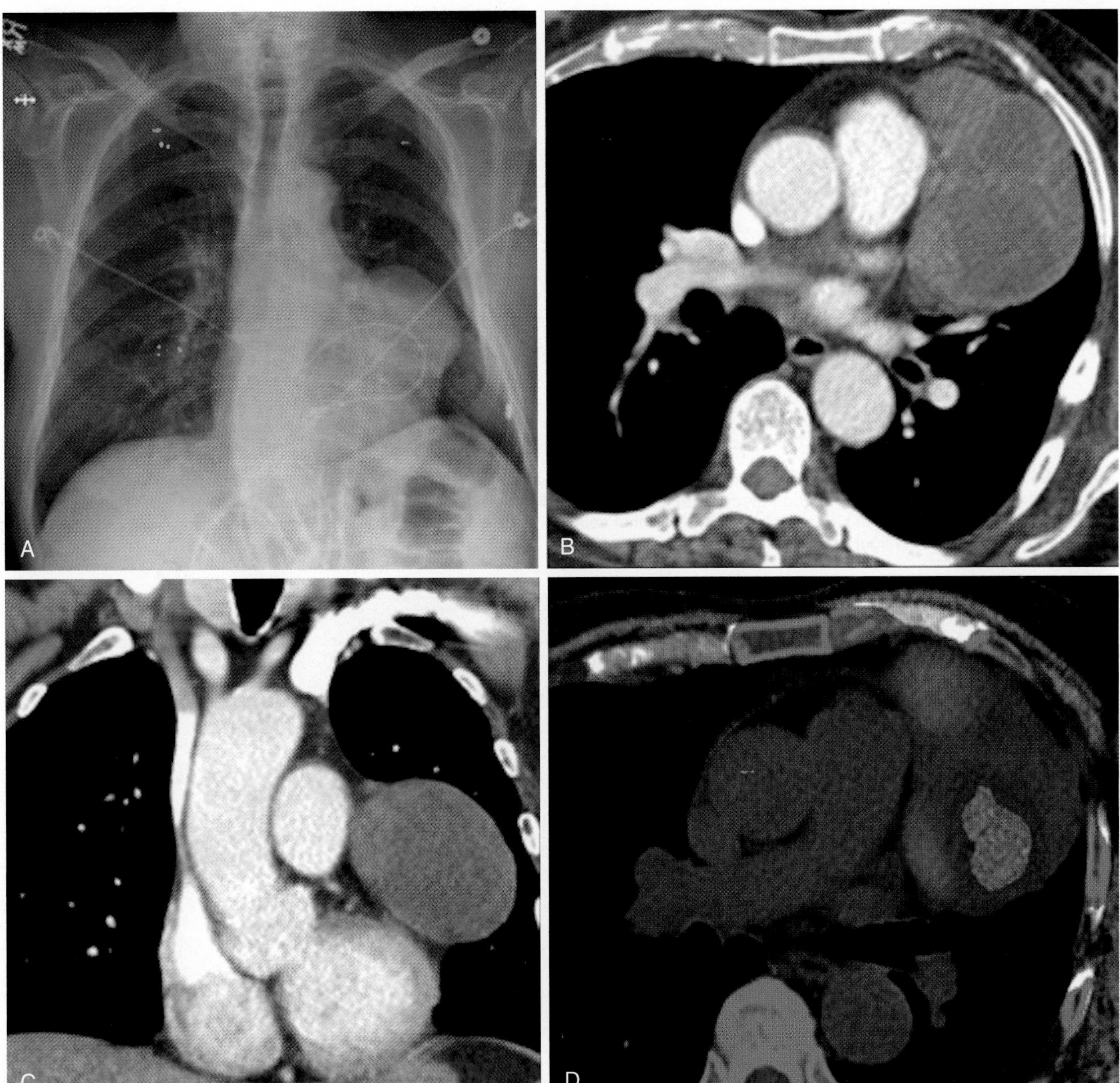

Figure 8.8. Schwannoma in a 60-year-old patient. **A,** Posteroanterior chest radiograph shows a large prevascular (anterior) mediastinal mass. **B,** Axial computed tomography (CT) image and **C,** coronal CT reconstruction shows a heterogeneous solid partially enhancing mass. **D,** Axial positron emission tomography/CT image shows increased 2-[^{18}F] fluoro-2-deoxy-D-glucose uptake in the solid portions of the mass.

Neurogenic Tumors

The benign peripheral nerve tumors (schwannomas and neurofibromas) are slowly growing neoplasms that often are radiologically indistinguishable from each other. Schwannomas and neurofibromas are usually sharply marginated, spherical, and lobulated paravertebral masses (Fig. 8.8). On CT imaging, punctate calcifications and low-attenuation areas caused by the presence of fat, cystic change, or hemorrhage can be seen. Enhancement after intravenous contrast administration is variable and can be homogeneous, heterogeneous,[50] or peripheral.[18] Enlargement of neural foramina with or without extension into the spinal canal and osseous abnormalities, such as rib erosion and splaying of the ribs, can also occur. MRI is the preferred modality for demonstrating intraspinal extension of the tumor or the presence of an associated spinal cord abnormality. On MRI, neurofibromas and schwannomas have variable signal intensity on T1W images, but typically have similar signal intensity to the spinal cord. On T2W images, these neoplasms characteristically have high signal intensity peripherally and low signal intensity centrally (target sign) owing to collagen deposition (Fig. 8.9). This feature helps distinguish neurofibromas from other mediastinal tumors. Areas of cystic degeneration within the mass can result in foci of increased signal intensity on T2W images. Although the high signal intensity of schwannomas and neurofibromas on T2W images can facilitate differentiation of tumors from spinal cord, the tumors can be obscured

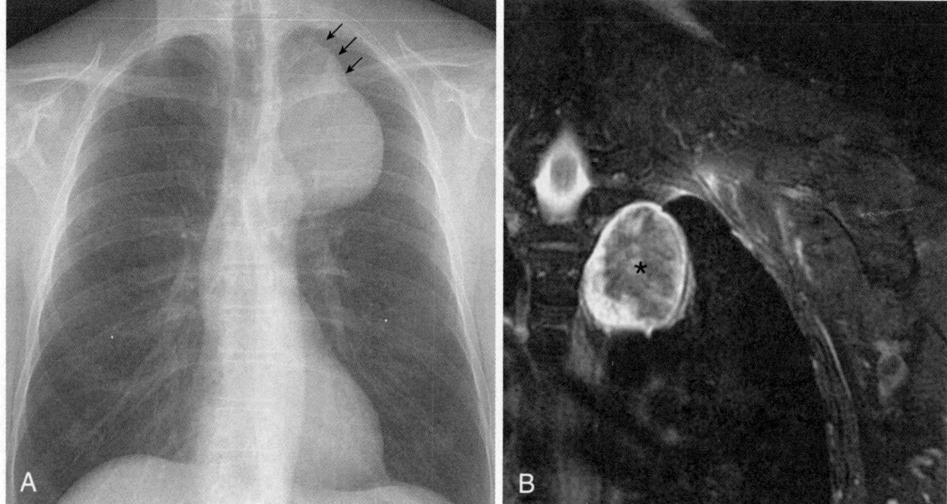

FIGURE 8.9. Neurofibroma in a 35-year-old woman with a history of neurofibromatosis type 1. **A,** Posteroanterior chest radiograph shows a lobulated well-defined paravertebral (posterior) mediastinal mass (*arrows*). **B,** Coronal T2-weighted (T1W) image shows a heterogeneous posterior mediastinal mass (*) with peripheral high signal intensity. Note that neurofibromas characteristically have high signal intensity peripherally and low signal intensity centrally (target sign) on T2W images.

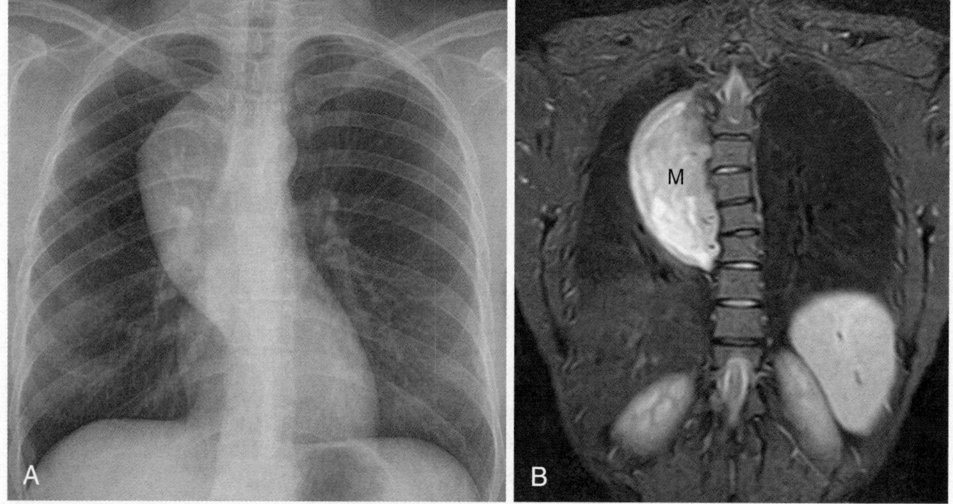

FIGURE 8.10. Ganglioneuroma in a 10-year-old girl. **A,** Posteroanterior chest radiograph shows a large paravertebral (posterior) mediastinal mass. **B,** Coronal T2-weighted image shows a high–signal intensity, well-marginated large right paravertebral mass (M). Note that the elongated elliptical shape that extends vertically over five to six vertebrae is typical of sympathetic ganglia tumors.

by the high signal intensity of cerebrospinal fluid. Schwannomas and neurofibromas enhance with gadolinium, a feature that can be useful in detecting intradural extension of these tumors. Paravertebral neurofibromas and schwannomas that extend into the spinal canal manifest as dumbbell-shaped masses with widening of the affected neural foramen. In several small series, neurofibromas and schwannomas have been reported to be FDG-avid on PET/CT. On CT, plexiform neurofibromas manifest as low-attenuation, poorly marginated masses located along the mediastinal nerves and sympathetic chains. MRI of plexiform neurofibromas can show the infiltrative nature of the tumors, and the masses typically have low signal on both T1W and T2W images, owing to the fibrous nature of the tumors.

Malignant tumors of nerve sheath origin are rare but typically develop from solitary or plexiform neurofibromas. On CT or MRI, malignant tumors of nerve sheath origin typically manifest as paravertebral mediastinal masses larger than 5 cm in diameter. Findings that suggest malignancy include a sudden change in size of a preexisting mass or the development of heterogeneous signal intensity on MRI (caused by necrosis and hemorrhage). The presence of multiple target signs throughout the lesion on MRI favors the diagnosis of a plexiform neurofibroma rather than a malignant tumor of nerve sheath origin. Neurofibrosarcomas are often FDG-avid and have a standardized uptake value greater than 3, and aggressive behavior has been reported. The sympathetic ganglia tumors, ganglioneuromas and ganglioneuroblastomas, usually manifest as well-marginated, elliptical, paravertebral mediastinal masses that extend vertically over three to five vertebral bodies (Fig. 8.10). They are usually located lateral to the spine and can cause pressure erosion on adjacent vertebral bodies. On CT, they are typically heterogeneous, and up to 30% of masses contain stippled or punctate calcification.[51]

On T1W and T2W MRI, they are usually homogeneous and of intermediate signal intensity. Occasionally, these lesions are heterogeneous and of high signal intensity on T2W images.[52] Ganglioneuroblastomas are typically larger and more aggressive, with evidence of local and intraspinal invasion, compared with ganglioneuromas. Neuroblastomas manifest as a paraspinal mass of heterogeneous, predominantly soft tissue, attenuation. The masses usually contain areas of hemorrhage, necrosis, and cystic generation. Calcification occurs in up to 80% of cases and can be coarse, mottled, solid, or ring-shaped.[53] Neuroblastomas often show widespread local invasion and have irregular margins, although many of these lesions are well-marginated on CT or MRI. The primary tumor can also spread through the adjacent neural foramina, resulting in a classic dumbbell-shaped tumor.[12] On CT, discrete lytic or mixed lytic and sclerotic areas or metaphyseal lucencies are typical of metastatic osseous involvement. On MRI, neuroblastomas show homogeneous or heterogeneous signal intensity on all sequences and variable enhancement after contrast administration.[52] Iodine-123-metaiodobenzylguanidine (^{123}I-MIBG) is an essential part of the evaluation for patients with neuroblastomas, improves the detection of the primary malignancy and metastases, and is also useful in the assessment of response to therapy. PET/CT can be useful in ^{123}I-MIBG–negative neuroblastoma patients and is better able to evaluate disease extent in the chest, abdomen, and pelvis. PET/CT is superior in depicting stage 1 and 2 neuroblastoma, although ^{123}I-MIBG is overall superior in the evaluation of stage 4 neuroblastoma, mainly because of the better detection of bone or marrow metastases.[54]

Key Points Imaging

- Thymic neoplasms. Thymoma, a lobulated mass within the prevascular compartment. Mediastinal fat, great vessel invasion, and pleural seeding are suggestive of local invasion. Thymic carcinoma, a large prevascular mediastinal mass with local and distant metastasis.
- Germ cell tumors. Teratoma, a multiloculated cystic mass, can contain adipose tissue. Seminoma is a homogeneous and well-marginated mass. Nonseminomatous germ cell tumors are large masses that are irregular in shape owing to hemorrhage, necrosis, or cystic change.
- Neurogenic tumors. Neurofibroma and schwannoma are paravertebral mediastinal tumors associated with enlargement of neural foramina. The MRI target appearance is high signal intensity in the periphery and intermediate signal intensity in the central zone. Ganglion cell tumors are paraspinal soft tissue masses with vertical elongation. Neuroblastomas are heterogeneous paraspinal masses that exhibit predominantly soft tissue attenuation, with calcification seen in up to 80%.

TREATMENT

Treatment of primary mediastinal tumors is complex. This section provides a brief general outline of the standard therapeutic options. For more detailed therapy guidelines please consult later chapters dedicated to specific tumor types and specific recommendations.

Thymic Tumors

Surgical resection is generally the cornerstone of treatment for patients with thymomas.[55] Postoperative radiotherapy is recommended in patients with incompletely resected thymomas, and chemoradiation should be considered in nonsurgical patients. Treatment recommendations are dependent on stage. In this regard, patients with stage I tumors are treated with surgical resection alone. In patients with Masaoka stage II who undergo complete resection, adjuvant radiation therapy is controversial; however, in high-risk WHO categories such as B2 or B3, adjuvant radiotherapy should be considered. Adjuvant radiotherapy is generally considered an effective treatment in patients with advanced thymomas (Masaoka stages III and IVa). Cisplatin-based chemotherapy is advocated in patients with inoperable or gross residual disease after resection, mainly for Masaoka stage III or IV thymomas.[56] Multimodality therapy has been used to manage patients with unresectable tumors (Masaoka III, IVa, and IVb). In this regard, induction chemoradiotherapy can be used to downstage thymomas to improve surgical resectability.[57–59] In addition, Lucchi and associates have reported reasonable long-term survival in patients with Masaoka stage III and IVa thymomas using neoadjuvant chemotherapy, surgery, and postoperative radiotherapy or primary surgical resection followed by adjuvant chemotherapy, radiation therapy, or both.[60] In view of the complexity of managing thymic tumors, a schematic approach as outlined by the National Comprehensive Cancer Network (NCCN) is included to clarify the management of resectable and advanced disease (Figs. 8.11 and 8.12).

Germ Cell Tumors

The treatment of mature teratomas consists of complete surgical resection. Residual disease can be associated with a risk of malignant transformation. The treatment approach for mediastinal seminomas and nonseminomas is based on recommendations of the International Germ Cell Cancer Collaborative Group.[61] This approach is based on a risk assignment algorithm used in clinical practice that includes the histology of the primary tumor, serum tumor marker levels, and the presence of nonpulmonary visceral metastases. The therapeutic management of seminomas is typically chemoradiation. Surgical resection can be used in patients with bulky or residual tumors. The therapy of choice for nonseminomatous tumor is a cisplatin-based chemotherapy regimen followed by resection of residual tumor.

Neurogenic Tumors

Neurofibromas and schwannomas can be either observed or resected. For malignant transformation, adjuvant chemotherapy and radiation overall has only a limited effect on survival. Neuroblastomas detected in infants by screening or incidentally on sonography before birth can be observed without obtaining a definitive histologic diagnosis and without surgical intervention, owing to the

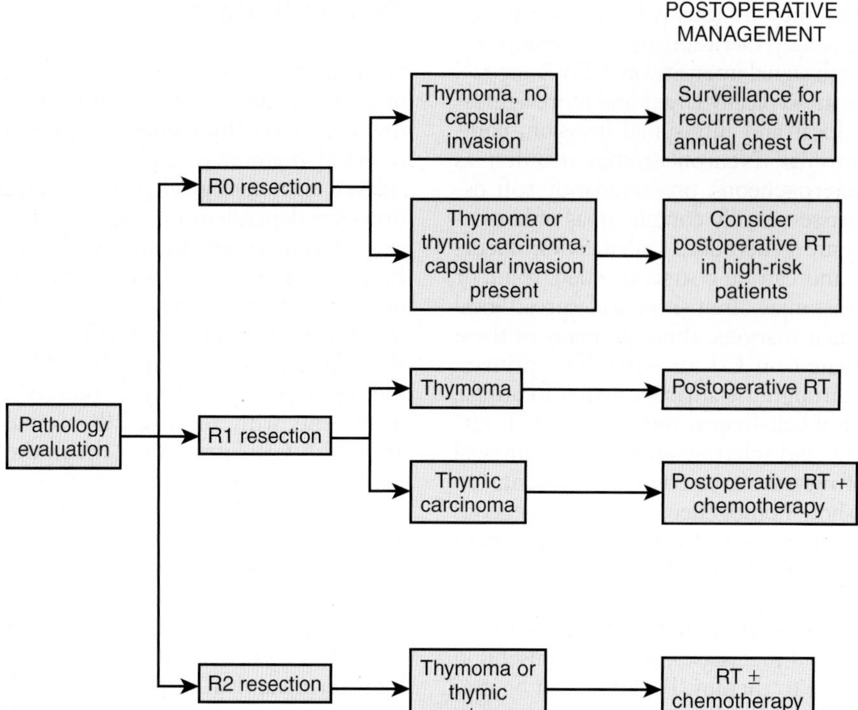

FIGURE 8.11. Treatment of thymic tumors—postoperative management of resectable disease. *CT*, Computed tomography; *RT*, radiotherapy.

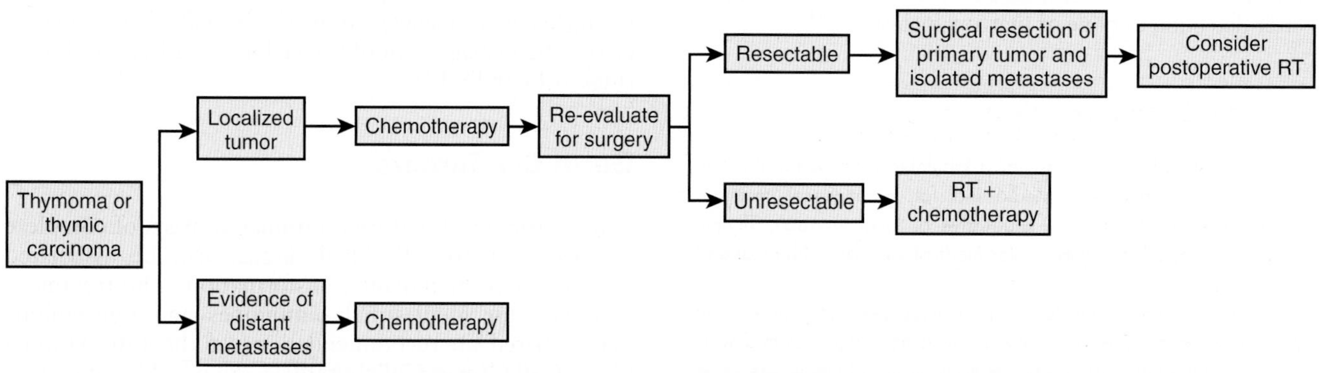

FIGURE 8.12. Treatment of thymic tumors—advanced disease. *RT*, radiotherapy.

likelihood of spontaneous regression. Otherwise, treatment strategies for patients with neuroblastomas depend on a risk stratification that includes multiple factors such as age at diagnosis, staging, histopathology, and genetic abnormalities. Patients are stratified into low-, intermediate-, or high-risk groups (Table 8.3). Patients in the low-risk group are managed by surgery alone; chemotherapy is reserved for symptomatic patients or in stage IVS. Management of the intermediate-risk patient consists of surgical resection and chemotherapy. Patients in the high-risk group receive an intensive combination of induction chemotherapy, radiation therapy, surgery, high-dose chemotherapy with autologous stem cell rescue, and differentiation therapy with retinoic acid. Radiation therapy can be used to treat the residual tumor and metastases.

KEY POINTS Treatment

- Thymic neoplasms. Complete tumor resection is the preferred treatment for localized disease; advanced disease is treated with multimodality therapy.
- Germ cell tumors. Teratoma is treated with surgical excision. Seminoma and nonseminomatous germ cell tumors are treated with cisplatin-based chemotherapy and radiotherapy. Surgical resection is helpful in cases of residual mass.
- Neurogenic tumors. Neurofibroma and schwannoma are treated surgically. Neuroblastoma treatment depends on risk stratification. Low-risk groups are treated with surgery. Intermediate-risk groups are treated with surgery followed by chemotherapy. High-risk groups are treated with chemotherapy, which can be followed by surgery, radiation therapy, and stem cell transplantation.

TABLE 8.3 The International Neuroblastoma Risk Group Classification Scheme

STAGE	AGE (MONTHS)	HISTOLOGIC CATEGORY/ GRADE OF TUMOR DIFFERENTIATION	*MYCN*	11q ABERRATION	PLOIDY	PRETREATMENT RISK GROUP[a]
L1/L2	—	GN maturing, GNB intermixed	—	—	—	A: Very low
L1	—	Any, except GN maturing or GNB intermixed	NA	—	—	B: Very low
			Amp			K: High
L2	<18	Any, except GN maturing or GNB intermixed	NA	No	—	D: Low
				Yes	—	G: Intermediate
	≥18	GNB nodular; differentiating NB, differentiating	NA	No	—	E: Low
		GNB nodular, poorly differentiated, or undifferentiated; NB, poorly undifferentiated, or undifferentiated	NA	Yes	—	H: Intermediate
			Amp	—	—	N: High
M	<18	—	NA	—	Hyperdiploid[b]	F: Low
	<12	—	NA	—	Diploid[c]	I: Intermediate
	12 to <18	—	NA	—	Diploid[c]	J: Intermediate
	<18	—	Amp	—	—	O: High
	≥18	—	—	—	—	P: High
MS	<18	—	NA	No	—	C: Very low
					—	Q: High
			Amp	Yes	—	R: High

[a]Five-year event-free survival according to the International Neuroblastoma Risk Group: very low risk, >85%; low risk, >75% to ≤85%; intermediate risk, ≥50% to ≤75%; high risk, <50%.
[b]DNA index >1.0, includes near-triploid and near-tetraploid tumors.
[c]DNA index ≤1.0.
—Blank field indicates "any."
NA, No amplification; *Amp*, amplified; *GN*, ganglioneuroma; *GNB*, ganglioneuroblastoma; *NB*, neuroblastoma.
(From Cohn SL, Pearson AD, London WB, et al. The International Neuroblastoma Risk Group (INRG) classification system: an INRG Task Force report. *J Clin Oncol.* 2009;27:289-297.)

SURVEILLANCE

Each specific neoplasm discussed has a different approach for evaluation after treatment. A complete explanation is beyond the scope of this chapter, and the reader is referred to the NCCN for more details. In all cases, patients should be managed by an experienced multidisciplinary team. In patients with thymic tumors, annual chest CT can be performed to evaluate for disease recurrence. CT of the abdomen and pelvis, brain MRI, and PET/CT scans can be performed based on sites of metastases and symptomatology. Surveillance for germ cell tumors depends on the type and stage of the tumor. Usually, patients with seminoma are followed after treatment with evaluation of serum markers (AFP, β-hCG, and LDH) and chest CT. In cases of nonseminomatous tumors, surveillance is also achieved by evaluation of serum markers (LDH, β-hCG, and AFP) and chest and abdominal/pelvic CT. PET/CT, brain MRI, and bone scan are obtained when clinically indicated. For malignant nerve sheath tumors, chest CT is performed routinely, and MRI can also be useful in cases with neural foramina or spinal cord invasion. In cases of neuroblastoma, CT is performed routinely to detect relapses, which can occur in a substantial portion of patients. The most reliable test to detect disease progression or recurrence is ^{123}I-MIBG imaging.

KEY POINTS Surveillance

- Thymic tumor: annual chest computed tomography (CT).
- Germ cell tumor: serum tumor markers and chest radiograph/chest CT.
- Neuroblastoma: ^{123}I-MIBG scan is the most reliable test to detect recurrence/progression.

NEW THERAPIES

The increasing understanding of tumor-associated genes/cancer immunotherapy and molecular-targeted therapeutic options has clinical potential in the future treatment of patients. The use of somatostatin analogs (octreotide) in combination with prednisone has demonstrated complete response in 5.3% of patients and partial response in 25% of patients with thymomas, but no response in thymic carcinomas.[62,63] Cyclooxygenase-2, epidermal growth factor receptor, c-KIT inhibitors, and histone deacetylase inhibitors have been used in the treatment of thymomas and in thymic carcinomas.[62] In a phase II study of gefitinib treatment in 26 patients with advanced thymic malignancies, one patient had a partial response, and 14 patients (54%) had stable disease.[64] In a phase II study of the insulin-like growth factor-1 receptor inhibitor cixutumumab, five of 37 patients (14%) achieved partial response.[65]

New antitumoral agents such as bevacizumab combined with oxaliplatin are being assessed in patients with refractory or relapsed germ cell tumors.[66] Pegfilgrastim, a granulocyte colony–stimulating factor, is being used in combination with chemotherapy in patients with untreated germ cell tumors.[67]

Patients with NF-1 and multiple neurofibromas have a high recurrence rate after resection, and patients with large plexiform neurofibromas have a risk of malignant transformation.[68–70] Innovative therapeutic options are being investigated in preclinical and clinical trials. Proposed treatments that target mast cell function, Ras signaling pathways, Ras signaling pathway downstream effectors, PI3K, or c-KIT all have the potential to be effective in the management of patients with neurofibromas.[68,71–75] An additional therapeutic option is to target the mTOR pathway with the mTOR inhibitor rapamycin. which has shown encouraging preclinical results in the treatment of malignant peripheral nerve sheath tumors.[68,76–79]

Some researchers are studying the use of monoclonal antibody therapy with granulocyte-macrophage colony–stimulating factor and interleukin-2 combined with *cis*-retinoic acid after chemotherapy.[80–82] The New Approaches to Neuroblastoma Therapy consortium is evaluating the inclusion of myeloablative doses of ^{131}I-MIBG with chemotherapy before stem cell transplantation in patients with an incomplete response to induction chemotherapy. Readers interested in new treatment options for high-risk neuroblastoma are referred to an article by Wagner and coworkers.[83]

Key Points The Radiology Report

- Describe the mediastinal compartment involved.
- Define the lesion shape, contours, composition (e.g., fluid, fat, soft tissue, calcification), and enhancement.
- Assess for compression, displacement, and invasion of surrounding mediastinal structures.
- Evaluate for locoregional and distant metastatic disease.

SUMMARY

Thymic, germ cell, and neurogenic neoplasms of the mediastinum are uncommon. However, an understanding of their clinical and radiologic manifestations is useful in distinguishing these tumors from one another and from the more commonly encountered benign mediastinal neoplasms. Once a definitive diagnosis has been established, imaging is important in determining the local extent of disease and detecting metastases. Awareness of the patterns of spread and knowledge of the current staging of these neoplasms are essential in patient evaluation and treatment.

ACKNOWLEDGMENT

The authors wish to thank Marcelo F. K. Benveniste, M.D. and Peter E. Zage, M.D., Ph.D. for their valuable contributions to this chapter from the first edition, on which this revision is based.

REFERENCES

1. Hoffman OA, Gillespie DJ, Aughenbaugh GL, et al. Primary mediastinal neoplasms (other than thymoma). *Mayo Clin Proc*. 1993;68:880-891.
2. Davis Jr RD, Oldham Jr HN, Sabiston Jr DC. Primary cysts and neoplasms of the mediastinum: recent changes in clinical presentation, methods of diagnosis, management, and results. *Ann Thorac Surg*. 1987;44:229-237.
3. Strollo DC, Rosado de Christenson ML, Jett JR. Primary mediastinal tumors. Part 1: tumors of the anterior mediastinum. *Chest*. 1997;112:511-522.
4. Rosai J, Levine GD. *Tumors of the thymus*. Washington, DC: Armed Forces Institute of Pathology; 1976.
5. O'Gara RW, Horn Jr. RC, Enterline HT. Tumors of the anterior mediastinum. *Cancer*. 1958;11:562-590.
6. Morgenthaler TI, Brown LR, Colby TV, et al. Thymoma. *Mayo Clin Proc*. 1993;68:1110-1123.
7. Nichols CR. Mediastinal germ cell tumors. Clinical features and biologic correlates. *Chest*. 1991;99:472-479.
8. Davidson KG, Walbaum PR, McCormack RJ. Intrathoracic neural tumours. *Thorax*. 1978;33:359-367.
9. Reed JC, Hallet KK, Feigin DS. Neural tumors of the thorax: subject review from the AFIP. *Radiology*. 1978;126:9-17.
10. Ribet ME, Cardot GR. Neurogenic tumors of the thorax. *Ann Thorac Surg*. 1994;58:1091-1095.
11. Aughenbaugh GL. Thoracic manifestations of neurocutaneous diseases. *Radiol Clin North Am*. 1984;22:741-756.
12. Lonergan GJ, Schwab CM, Suarez ES, et al. Neuroblastoma, ganglioneuroblastoma, and ganglioneuroma: radiologic-pathologic correlation. *Radiographics*. 2002;22:911-934.
13. Carter BW, Benveniste MF, Madan R, et al. ITMIG Classification of mediastinal compartments and multidisciplinary approach to mediastinal masses. *Radiographics*. 2017;37:413-436.
14. Lattes R, Pachter MR. Benign lymphoid masses of probable hamartomatous nature. Analysis of 12 cases. *Cancer*. 1962;15:197-214.
15. Lee JKT, Sagel SS, Stanley RJ. *Computed body tomography with MRI correlation*. New York: Raven Press; 1989.
16. Okumura M, Ohta M, Tateyama H, et al. The World Health Organization histologic classification system reflects the oncologic behavior of thymoma: a clinical study of 273 patients. *Cancer*. 2002;94:624-632.
17. Wick MR, Carney JA, Bernatz PE, et al. Primary mediastinal carcinoid tumors. *Am J Surg Pathol*. 1982;6:195-205.
18. Kumar AJ, Kuhajda FP, Martinez CR, et al. Computed tomography of extracranial nerve sheath tumors with pathological correlation. *J Comput Assist Tomogr*. 1983;7:857-865.
19. Hiorns MP, Owens CM. Radiology of neuroblastoma in children. *Eur Radiol*. 2001;11:2071-2081.
20. Shields TW, Reynolds M. Neurogenic tumors of the thorax. *Surg Clin North Am*. 1988;68:645-668.
21. Page DL, DeLellis RA, Hough AJ. *Atlas of Tumor Pathology: Tumors of the Adrenal*. Washington, DC: Armed Forces Institute of Pathology; 1986:219-260.
22. Lewis JE, Wick MR, Scheithauer BW, et al. Thymoma. A clinicopathologic review. *Cancer*. 1987;60:2727-2743.
23. Osserman KE, Genkins G. Studies in myasthenia gravis: review of a twenty-year experience in over 1200 patients. *Mt Sinai J Med*. 1971;38:497-537.
24. Bukowski RM, Wolf M, Kulander BG, et al. Alternating combination chemotherapy in patients with extragonadal germ cell tumors. A Southwest Oncology Group study. *Cancer*. 1993;71:2631-2638.
25. Gale AW, Jelihovsky T, Grant AF, et al. Neurogenic tumors of the mediastinum. *Ann Thorac Surg*. 1974;17:434-443.
26. Caty MG, Shamberger RC. Abdominal tumors in infancy and childhood. *Pediatr Clin North Am*. 1993;40:1253-1271.
27. Travis WD, Brambilla E, Müller-Hermelink HK, et al. Pathology and genetics of tumours of the lung, pleura, thymus and heart. *World Health Organization Classification of Tumors*. France: IARC Press; 2004.
28. Marx A, Chan JKC, Coindre JM, et al. The 2015 WHO classification of tumors of the thymus: continuity and changes. *J Thorac Oncol*. 2015;10(10):1383-1395.
29. Masaoka A, Monden Y, Nakahara K, et al. Follow-up study of thymomas with special reference to their clinical stages. *Cancer*. 1981;48:2485-2492.

30. Montclaire T, Brodeur GM, Ambos PF, et al. The international Neuroblastoma Risk Group (INRG) Staging System: An INRG Task Force Report. *J Clin Oncol*. 2009;27:298-303.
31. Cohn SL, Pearson ADJ, London WB, et al. The international Neuroblastoma Risk Group (INRG) Classification System: An INRG Task Force Report. *J Clin Oncol*. 2009;27:289-297.
32. Scatarige JC, Fishman EK, Zerhouni EA, et al. Transdiaphragmatic extension of invasive thymoma. *AJR Am J Roentgenol*. 1985;144:31-35.
33. Bokemeyer C, Droz JP, Horwich A, et al. Extragonadal seminoma: an international multicenter analysis of prognostic factors and long term treatment outcome. *Cancer*. 2001;91:1394-1401.
34. Takeda S, Miyoshi S, Ohta M, et al. Primary germ cell tumors in the mediastinum: a 50-year experience at a single Japanese institution. *Cancer*. 2003;97:367-376.
35. Choyke PL, Zeman RK, Gootenberg JE, et al. Thymic atrophy and regrowth in response to chemotherapy: CT evaluation. *AJR Am J Roentgenol*. 1987;149:269-272.
36. Jerushalmi J, Frenkel A, Bar-Shalom R, et al. Physiologic thymic uptake of 18F-FDG in children and young adults: a PET/CT evaluation of incidence, patterns, and relationship to treatment. *J Nucl Med*. 2009;50:849-853.
37. Verstandig AG, Epstein DM, Miller Jr WT, et al. Thymoma—report of 71 cases and a review. *Crit Rev Diagn Imaging*. 1992;33:201-230.
38. Rosado-de-Christenson ML, Galobardes J, Moran CA. Thymoma: radiologic-pathologic correlation. *Radiographics*. 1992;12:151-168.
39. Tomiyama N, Johkoh T, Mihara N, et al. Using the World Health Organization Classification of thymic epithelial neoplasms to describe CT findings. *AJR Am J Roentgenol*. 2002;179:881-886.
40. Grassi I, Nanni C, Allegri V, et al. The clinical use of PET with 11C-acetate. *Am J Nucl Med Mol Imaging*. 2002;2(1):33-47.
41. Shibata H, Nomori H, Uno K, et al. 18F-Fluorodeoxyglucose and 11C-Acetate positron emission tomography are useful modalities for diagnosing the histologic type of thymoma. *Cancer*. 2009;115(11):2531-2538.
42. Sadohara J, Fujimoto K, Muller NL, et al. Thymic epithelial tumors: comparison of CT and MR imaging findings of low-risk thymomas, high-risk thymomas, and thymic carcinomas. *Eur J Radiol*. 2006;60:70-79.
43. Jeong YJ, Lee KS, Kim J, et al. Does CT of thymic epithelial tumors enable us to differentiate histologic subtypes and predict prognosis? *AJR Am J Roentgenol*. 2004;183:283-289.
44. Sung YM, Lee KS, Kim BT, et al. 18F-FDG PET/CT of thymic epithelial tumors: usefulness for distinguishing and staging tumor subgroups. *J Nucl Med*. 2006;47:1628-1634.
45. Endo M, Nakagawa K, Ohde Y, et al. Utility of 18FDG-PET for differentiating the grade of malignancy in thymic epithelial tumors. *Lung Cancer*. 2008;61:350-355.
46. Kumar A, Regmi SK, Dutta R, et al. Characterization of thymic masses using (18)F-FDG PET-CT. *Ann Nucl Med*. 2009;23:569-577.
47. Johnbeck CB, Knigge U, Kjaer A. PET tracers for somatostatin receptor imaging of neuroendocrine tumors: current status and review of the literature. *Future Oncol*. 2004;10(14):2259-2277.
48. De Luca S, Foti R, Palmieri G, et al. Combined imaging with 18F-FDG PET/CT and 111In-Labeled Octreotide SPECT for evaluation of thymic epithelial tumors. *Clin Nucl Med*. 2013;38:354-358.
49. Sharma P, Jain TK, Parida GK, et al. Diagnostic accuracy of integrated 18F-FDG PET/CT for restaging patients with malignant germ cell tumors. *Br J Radio*. 2014;87:20140263.
50. Coleman BG, Arger PH, Dalinka MK, et al. CT of sarcomatous degeneration in neurofibromatosis. *AJR Am J Roentgenol*. 1983;140:383-387.
51. Sofka CM, Semelka RC, Kelekis NL, et al. Magnetic resonance imaging of neuroblastoma using current techniques. *Magn Reson Imaging*. 1999;17:193-198.
52. Sakai F, Sone S, Kiyono K, et al. Intrathoracic neurogenic tumors: MR-pathologic correlation. *AJR Am J Roentgenol*. 1992;159:279-283.
53. Stark DD, Moss AA, Brasch RC, et al. Neuroblastoma: diagnostic imaging and staging. *Radiology*. 1983;148:101-105.
54. Sharp SE, Shulkin BL, Gelfand MJ, et al. 123I-MIBG scintigraphy and 18F-FDG PET in neuroblastoma. *J Nucl Med*. 2009;50:1237-1243.
55. Girard N, Mornex F, Van Houtte P, et al. Thymoma: a focus on current therapeutic management. *J Thorac Oncol*. 2009;4:119-126.
56. Falkson CB, Bezjak A, Darling G, et al. The management of thymoma: a systematic review and practice guideline. *J Thorac Oncol*. 2009;4:911-919.
57. Bretti S, Berruti A, Loddo C, et al. Multimodal management of stages III-IVa malignant thymoma. *Lung Cancer*. 2004;44:69-77.
58. Jacot W, Quantin X, Valette S, et al. Multimodality treatment program in invasive thymic epithelial tumor. *Am J Clin Oncol*. 2005;28:5-7.
59. Tomaszek S, Wigle DA, Keshavjee S, et al. Thymomas: review of current clinical practice. *Ann Thorac Surg*. 2009;87:1973-1980.
60. Lucchi M, Ambrogi MC, Duranti L, et al. Advanced stage thymomas and thymic carcinomas: results of multimodality treatments. *Ann Thorac Surg*. 2005;79:1840-1844.
61. International Germ Cell Consensus Classification: a prognostic factor-based staging system for metastatic germ cell cancers. *J Clin Oncol*. 1997;15:594-603.
62. Chen Y, Gharwan H, Thomas A. Novel biologic therapies for thymic epithelial tumors. *Front Oncol*. 2014;4:103.
63. Loehrer PJ, Wang W, Johnson DH, et al. Octerotide alone or with prednisone in patients with advanced thymoma and thymic carcinoma: An eastern cooperative oncology group phase II trial. *J Clin Oncol*. 2004;22:293-299.
64. Meister M, Schirmacher P, Dienemann H, et al. Mutational status of the epidermal growth factor receptor (EGFR) gene in thymomas and thymic carcinomas. *Cancer Lett*. 2007;248:186-191.
65. Rajan A, Giaccone G. Target therapy for advanced thymic tumors. *J Thorac Oncol*. 2010;5:S361-S364.
66. Jain A, Brames MJ, Vaughn DJ, et al. Phase II clinical trial of oxaliplatin and bevacizumab in refractory germ cell tumors. *Am J Clin Oncol*. 2014;37(5):450-453.
67. Iwamoto H, Izumi K, Natsagdorj A, et al. Effectiveness and safety of pegfilgrastim in BEP treatment for patients with germ cell tumor. *In vivo*. 2018;32:899-903.
68. Gottfried ON, Viskochil DH, Couldwell WT. Neurofibromatosis Type 1 and tumorigenesis: molecular mechanisms and therapeutic implications. *Neurosurg Focus*. 2010;28:E8.
69. Katz D, Lazar A, Lev D. Malignant peripheral nerve sheath tumour (MPNST): the clinical implications of cellular signalling pathways. *Expert Rev Mol Med*. 2009;11:e30.
70. Tucker T, Friedman JM, Friedrich RE, et al. Longitudinal study of neurofibromatosis 1 associated plexiform neurofibromas. *J Med Genet*. 2009;46:81-85.
71. Weiss B, Bollag G, Shannon K. Hyperactive Ras as a therapeutic target in neurofibromatosis type 1. *Am J Med Genet*. 1999;89:14-22.
72. Yang FC, Ingram DA, Chen S, et al. Neurofibromin-deficient Schwann cells secrete a potent migratory stimulus for Nf1± mast cells. *J Clin Invest*. 2003;112:1851-1861.
73. Yang FC, Ingram DA, Chen S, et al. Nf1-dependent tumors require a microenvironment containing Nf1±- and c-kit-dependent bone marrow. *Cell*. 2008;135:437-448.
74. Yan N, Ricca C, Fletcher J, et al. Farnesyltransferase inhibitors block the neurofibromatosis type I (NF1) malignant phenotype. *Cancer Res*. 1995;55:3569-3575.
75. Karajannis M, Ferner RE. Neurofibromatosis-related tumors: emerging biology and therapies. *Curr Opin Pediatr*. 2015;27(1):26-33.
76. Brems H, Beert E, de Ravel T, et al. Mechanisms in the pathogenesis of malignant tumours in neurofibromatosis type 1. *Lancet Oncol*. 2009;10:508-515.
77. Johannessen CM, Johnson BW, Williams SM, et al. TORC1 is essential for NF1-associated malignancies. *Curr Biol*. 2008;18:56-62.
78. Johannessen CM, Reczek EE, James MF, et al. The NF1 tumor suppressor critically regulates TSC2 and mTOR. *Proc Natl Acad Sci U S A*. 2005;102:8573-8578.
79. Bhola P, Banerjee S, Mukherjee J, et al. Preclinical in vivo evaluation of rapamycin in human malignant peripheral nerve sheath explant xenograft. *Int J Cancer*. 2010;126:563-571.
80. Cheung NK, Kushner BH, Cheung IY, et al. Anti-G(D2) antibody treatment of minimal residual stage 4 neuroblastoma diagnosed at more than 1 year of age. *J Clin Oncol*. 1998;16:3053-3060.
81. Simon T, Hero B, Faldum A, et al. Consolidation treatment with chimeric anti-GD2-antibody ch14.18 in children older than 1 year with metastatic neuroblastoma. *J Clin Oncol*. 2004;22:3549-3557.
82. Louis CU, Shohet JM. Neuroblastoma: molecular pathogenesis and therapy. *Annu Rev Med*. 2015;66:49-63.
83. Wagner LM, Danks MK, et al. New therapeutic targets for the treatment of high-risk neuroblastoma. *J Cell Biochem*. 2009;107:46-57.

CHAPTER 9

Pleural Tumors

Jitesh Ahuja, M.D.; Chad D. Strange, M.D.; Joe Y. Chang, M.D.; Reza J. Mehran, M.D.; and Mylene T. Truong, M.D.

INTRODUCTION

Neoplasms of the pleura are a diverse group of benign and malignant pathologic entities that include both primary and secondary malignancies. Most neoplasms of the pleura are metastases, typically from lung cancer, although extrathoracic neoplasms such as breast and ovarian cancer have a predilection for spread to the pleura. This chapter discusses the most common primary malignant neoplasm to arise from the pleura, diffuse malignant pleural mesothelioma (MPM), with a comprehensive review of the imaging, staging evaluation, and treatment considerations for MPM. Imaging findings that are important in establishing the diagnosis are discussed, and computed tomography (CT), magnetic resonance imaging (MRI), and positron emission tomography (PET)/CT findings that need to be emphasized or clarified so that oncologists and surgeons can deliver appropriate care are addressed.

MPM is an uncommon neoplasm arising from mesothelial cells of the pleura. The annual incidence in the United States is 3000 cases. The worldwide figure is expected to increase in the coming decade owing to the patterns of occupational exposure to asbestos and a latency period of up to 50 years.[1] There is currently no universally accepted standard therapy for MPM, and the prognosis is poor, with a median survival of 9 to 17 months after diagnosis.[2] However, important advances in the treatment of patients with MPM have occurred over the past few years, including a unified staging system, novel targeted agents, improved radiation therapy techniques for local control, and decreased morbidity and mortality in patients who undergo curative surgical resection.[1,3] Furthermore, multimodality regimens combining chemotherapy, radiotherapy, and surgery are being used more frequently because of the failure of single-modality therapy. In cases of limited disease, there has been an increasing tendency to perform surgical resection as part of the treatment algorithm. Extrapleural pneumonectomy (EPP), the removal of the visceral and parietal pleura, ipsilateral lung, hemidiaphragm, and part of the pericardium, is the surgical treatment of choice in the 10% to 15% of patients who present with resectable disease and is reported to prolong survival (74% 2-yr survival and 39% 5-yr survival).[4] The greatest survival benefit in patients with MPM after EPP is seen in those with epithelial histology, a primary tumor that is limited in extent, and no nodal metastases. Conversely, patients with sarcomatoid histology and nodal metastases have a poor survival benefit after EPP and are typically primarily treated with palliative chemotherapy.[5]

EPIDEMIOLOGY AND RISK FACTORS

MPM occurs more frequently in men than in women, at a ratio of 4:1; however, the incidence in women is increasing.[6] Peak incidence occurs in the sixth to seventh decades of life and is associated with a history of occupational exposure to asbestos in 40% to 80% of patients.[7] In asbestos workers, the incidence of MPM is 10%.[8] In contrast, the incidence of MPM in the general population is lower, estimated at 0.01% to 0.24%.[7,8]

Asbestos, a collective term for a group of complex hydrated silicates, has varying degrees of carcinogenicity. MPM develops after a latent period of up to 50 years from the time of exposure to asbestos. There are two principal forms of asbestos: long, thin fibers known as amphiboles (amosite and crocidolite) and serpentine fibers known as chrysotile. The exposure-specific risk of MPM from the three principal commercial asbestos types is approximately 1:100:500 for chrysotile, amosite, and crocidolite.[9] Chrysotile accounts for approximately 80% of the asbestos used in the Western world. Occupations at highest risk include insulation work, asbestos production and manufacture, the heating industry, shipyard work, construction, and automotive brake-lining manufacture and repair.[7]

Because 20% of MPM patients have not been exposed to asbestos, alternative factors are presumed to be involved. Simian virus 40 (SV40), a DNA virus, has been implicated as a cofactor in the etiology of MPM. SV40 nucleic acids have been documented in a proportion of MPM cases.[10] This virus blocks tumor suppressor genes and is a potent oncogenic virus in human and rodent cells.

Molecular biologic features of angiogenesis in MPM are important in the development of novel therapeutic strategies. MPM cells produce many growth factors such as epidermal growth factor, platelet-derived growth factor (PDGF), and transforming growth factor–β.[11–13] MPM expresses the highest known levels of vascular endothelial growth factor (VEGF) of any solid tumor. VEGF expression in MPM is associated with poor survival and is now considered to be an independent prognostic factor in MPM. There is a positive correlation between VEGF expression and tumor stage ($P < .05$).[14] VEGF inhibitors have been shown to reduce MPM growth in animal models. Studies on the use of antiangiogenesis agents to target the VEGF pathway are ongoing. These agents include PTK787, an inhibitor of the PDGF/VEGF pathway, and bevacizumab, a recombinant human anti-VEGF monoclonal antibody.[13] Genetic alterations in tumor suppressors such as p16, p14, and NF2 are common, and the activity of the antiapoptosis molecule Bcl-xL is elevated in MPM.[9,15] Furthermore, MPM cells usually express telomerase, enabling them to develop resistance to anticancer drugs. In addition, interleukin-8, a potent chemokine with proangiogenetic activity, has been shown to be an autocrine growth factor in MPM cell lines.[13]

ANATOMY AND PATHOLOGY

The anatomy of the pleura is complex. The inferior margins of the pleura in the posterior costodiaphragmatic recesses of the hemithorax extend considerably lower than the corresponding border of the lung, to the level of the T12 vertebra. Macroscopically, the affected lung is covered by a thick layer of soft, gelatinous, grayish-pink tumor. Microscopically, MPM is classified into three histologic categories that provide a foundation for prognosis and therapy, forming a critical basis for epidemiologic and clinical studies. These categories are epithelial (55%–65%), sarcomatoid (10%–15%), and mixed or biphasic (20%–35%).[16] The desmoplastic variant is considered a subtype of sarcomatous diffuse MPM. The epithelial type consists of cuboidal or polygonal cells with abundant pink cytoplasm and uniform round nuclei forming a tubular and papillary structure. The sarcomatoid or mesenchymal type of MPM consists of sheets of spindle cells of variable size, cellularity, and pleomorphism. The mixed type of MPM contains both epithelial and sarcomatoid patterns. The World Health Organization (WHO) classification requires that 10% or more of each component be present to fit the classification of biphasic.[17] Special features of MPM include positive staining for acid mucopolysaccharide, strong staining for keratin proteins, and, on electron microscopy, the presence of long microvilli and abundant tonofilaments but the absence of microvillous rootlets and lamellar bodies. To differentiate epithelial MPM from adenocarcinoma, immunohistochemistry panels are useful. Epithelial MPM cells are positive for certain keratin proteins (AE1/AE3, CK5/6, CK7), calretinin, WT-1, D2–40, HBMe1, mesothelin, and thrombomodulin and negative for many markers including pCEA, TTF1, CD15(Leu-M1), BerEp4, B72.3, BG-8, and MOC-31.[17] In contrast, immunohistochemistry is less helpful in sarcomatoid diffuse MPM.

Cytologic evaluation of pleural fluid (26% sensitivity) and needle aspiration biopsy (20.7% sensitivity) are inadequate to diagnose MPM.[18] If tumor cells are present, distinguishing MPM from metastatic adenocarcinoma or severe atypia can be difficult. In contrast, image-guided core needle biopsy to obtain larger tissue samples has been shown to improve diagnostic accuracy (77% with ultrasound guidance and 83% with CT guidance).[19] When a larger diagnostic specimen is needed, Cope needle biopsy, video-assisted thoracoscopic surgery (VATS), or open biopsy is performed. VATS has a diagnostic rate of 98% and is becoming the preferred method of diagnosis. However, this procedure has two disadvantages: the visceral and parietal layers of the pleura must not be adherent, and chest wall seeding occurs in up to one-half of patients.[6,18] In contrast, chest wall seeding occurs in 22% of image-guided biopsies.[19] To prevent tumor growth within biopsy sites, trocar ports, thoracoscopic tracts, and chest tube tracts, patients undergoing EPP typically have these tracts resected. In addition, local radiation therapy can be used to prevent chest wall seeding.

Key Points Anatomy and Pathology

- Malignant pleural mesothelioma (MPM) involves parietal and visceral pleural surfaces and extends into the interlobar fissures, along the diaphragm, mediastinum, and pericardium.
- Tumor can invade lung and peritoneum.
- MPM is divided into three histologic categories: epithelial (55%–65%), sarcomatoid (10%–15%), and mixed or biphasic (20%–35%).

CLINICAL PRESENTATION

Patients with MPM typically present with insidious onset of chest pain, shortness of breath, and cough. Invasion of the chest wall can lead to intractable pain. Pleural effusion is present in up to 95% of cases. As the tumor grows, there is complete infiltration of the pleura and encasement of the lung. Mediastinal invasion can lead to dysphagia, phrenic nerve paralysis, cardiac tamponade, and superior vena cava syndrome.

PATTERNS OF TUMOR SPREAD

MPM spreads by contiguity over the parietal and visceral pleural surfaces, along the diaphragm, mediastinum, and pericardium, and possibly into the peritoneum. MPM can involve the interlobar fissures and invade the lung directly or by interstitial and alveolar spread. MPM is usually associated with a pleural effusion and can present with direct invasion of thoracic structures. The initial diagnosis of diffuse MPM requires demonstration of tumor invasion, most often into the parietal pleural fibrous tissue, extrapleural adipose tissue, or soft tissues of the chest wall.

Lymphatic dissemination is common, and mediastinal nodes are involved in 50% of cases. To understand the lymphatic spread of MPM, it is essential to examine the complex lymphatic drainage system of the pleura. The visceral pleural lymphatics follow the same drainage pattern as the lungs. However, the parietal pleural lymphatic drainage system is different. The anterior parietal pleura drains into the internal mammary lymph nodes (Fig. 9.1). The posterior parietal pleura drains into the extrapleural/intercostal lymph nodes, which are located in the paraspinal fat adjacent to the heads of the ribs (Fig. 9.2). The anterior and lateral diaphragmatic lymphatics drain into the internal mammary and anterior diaphragmatic lymph nodes. The posterior diaphragm drains into the paraaortic and posterior mediastinal lymph nodes. There are free anastomoses between lymphatics on both surfaces of the diaphragm, including the retrocrural, inferior phrenic, and gastrohepatic space, and the region of the celiac axis.

Distant hematogeneous metastases are common and can involve the lungs, liver, spleen, adrenals, lymph nodes, bones, and brain (Fig. 9.3). Extrathoracic metastatic disease has been documented at autopsy in 50% to 80% of cases.[20]

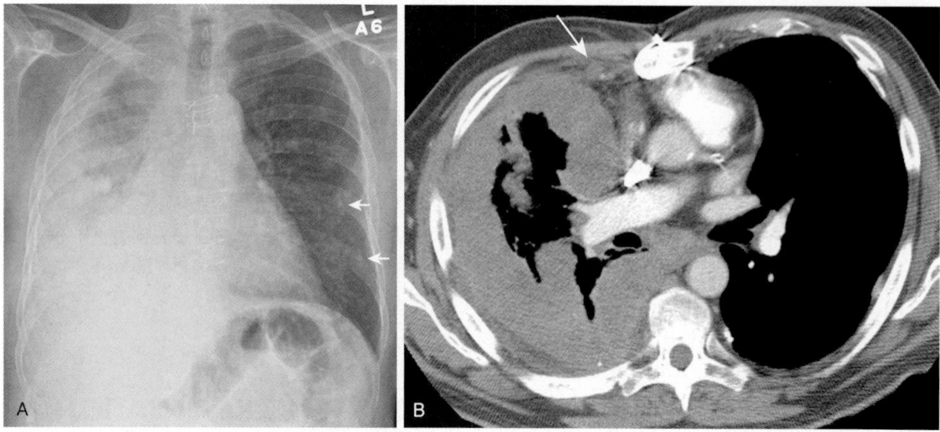

FIGURE 9.1. A 64-year-old man with epithelioid malignant pleural mesothelioma. **A,** Posteroanterior chest radiograph shows nodular pleural thickening forming a rind of tumor encasing the right lung. Note left calcified pleural plaques (*arrows*) from prior exposure to asbestos. **B,** Contrast-enhanced chest computed tomography shows that circumferential nodular right pleural thickening along mediastinal surface is indistinguishable from subcarinal adenopathy. Note adenopathy of the right internal mammary lymph node (*arrow*), a lymphatic drainage pathway for diseases involving the anterior parietal pleura.

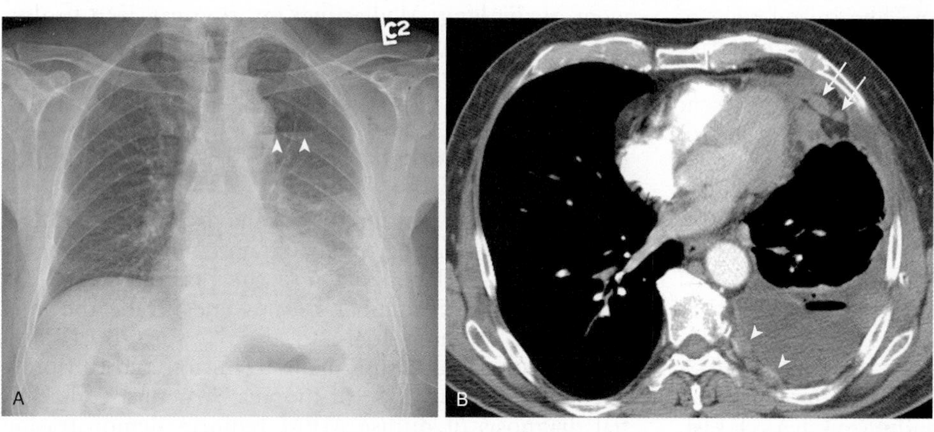

FIGURE 9.2. A 70-year-old man presented with shortness of breath and underwent left thoracentesis. **A,** Posteroanterior chest radiograph shows a left pleural catheter with an air–fluid level (*arrowheads*) in the left pleural space. **B,** Contrast-enhanced computed tomography scan of the chest shows air and fluid in the left pleural space. Nodular left pleural thickening is consistent with malignant pleural mesothelioma. Note that the lymphatic drainage system for the parietal pleura can be via the left anterior diaphragmatic (*arrows*) and left intercostal (*arrowheads*) lymph nodes.

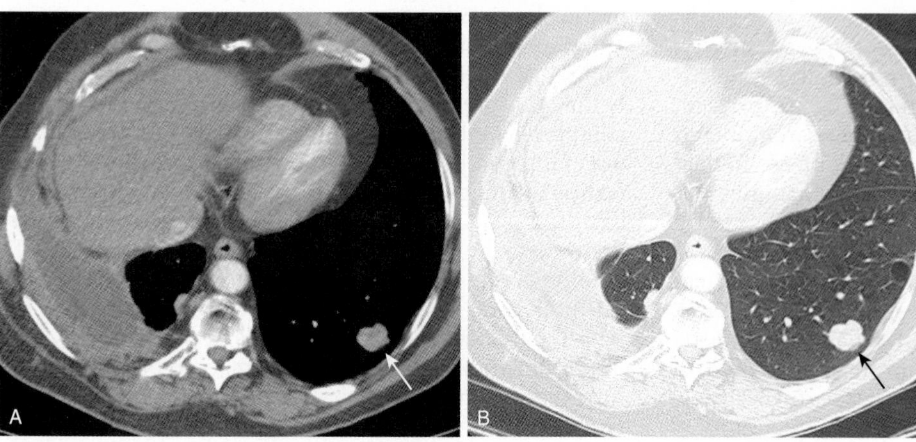

FIGURE 9.3. A 61-year-old man with right epithelioid malignant pleural mesothelioma. Contrast-enhanced computed tomography with mediastinal window (**A**) and lung window (**B**) shows nodular right pleural thickening, small right pleural effusion, and rounded atelectasis in the middle and right lower lobes. Note the well-circumscribed left lower lobe 1.5-cm nodule (*arrows*) consistent with metastasis. The presence of metastatic disease precluded surgery, and the patient was treated with cisplatin and pemetrexed.

Key Points Tumor Spread

- Local spread involves the parietal and visceral pleura and extends to interlobar fissures and along the diaphragm, mediastinum, and pericardium.
- Owing to the complex drainage system of the pleura, evaluation of nodal disease in the extrapleural/intercostal, internal mammary, diaphragmatic, and upper abdominal regions is essential.
- Mediastinal nodal disease is seen in 50% of cases.
- Transdiaphragmatic invasion can result in spread to the peritoneum, liver, and spleen.
- Hematogeneous dissemination is observed in 50% to 80% of cases at autopsy.

STAGING EVALUATION

Multiple staging systems have been proposed for MPM.[21,22] In an attempt to distinguish patients who would benefit from surgical resection from those needing palliative treatment, the International Mesothelioma Interest Group (IMIG) staging system for MPM was proposed and is gaining universal acceptance (Tables 9.1 and 9.2).[23] This system describes the extent of tumor according to a traditional tumor-node-metastasis (TNM) classification: local extent of the primary tumor (T descriptor), the presence and location of lymph node involvement (N descriptor), and the presence or absence of distant metastatic disease (M descriptor) (Figs. 9.4 and 9.5). This system stratifies patients into categories with similar prognoses in an effort to select homogeneous groups of patients for entry into clinical trials to better assess new treatment options. Primarily to identify patients who are potentially resectable, this staging system uses criteria to determine the extent of local tumor and regional lymph node status, two factors that have been shown to be related to overall survival rate.[23,24] The presence of advanced locoregional primary tumor (T4), N2–N3 disease (mediastinal, internal mammary, and supraclavicular lymph nodes), and M1 disease preclude surgery. However, staging using imaging modalities such as CT, MRI, and PET has limitations. This limitation, together with the morbidity and mortality associated with EPP, has resulted in the need for extended surgical staging (ESS) in patients being evaluated for resection. In our institution, cervical mediastinoscopy or endobronchial ultrasound-guided lymph node biopsy, laparoscopy, and peritoneal lavage are routinely performed in MPM patients undergoing preoperative evaluation. Rice and coworkers[25] reported that ESS excluded 15 of the 118 patients (12.7%) assessed by clinical staging alone as candidates for EPP.

T Staging

Accurate T staging is emphasized by the IMIG primarily to determine resectability.[23] In patients with locally advanced tumors, radiologic imaging is usually directed at distinguishing T3 disease (a solitary focus of chest wall involvement, involvement of the endothoracic fascia, mediastinal fat extension, or nontransmural pericardial involvement)

Table 9.1 Tumor-Node-Metastasis International Staging System for Diffuse Malignant Pleural Mesothelioma

T—Primary Tumor	
T1	Tumor involving the ipsilateral parietal pleura (including mediastinal and diaphragmatic pleura) with or without involvement of visceral pleura
T2	Tumor involving each ipsilateral pleural surface with at least one of the following features: • Involvement of diaphragmatic muscle • Confluent visceral pleural tumor (including fissures) or extension of tumor from visceral pleura into underlying pulmonary parenchyma
T3	Locally advanced but potentially resectable tumor. Tumor involving all of ipsilateral pleural surfaces with at least one of the following: • Involvement of endothoracic fascia • Extension into mediastinal fat • Solitary, completely resectable focus of tumor extending into soft tissues of chest wall • Nontransmural involvement of pericardium
T4	Locally advanced, technically unresectable tumor. Tumor involving all of ipsilateral pleural surfaces with at least one of the following: • Diffuse extension or multifocal masses of tumor in chest wall, with or without associated rib destruction • Direct transdiaphragmatic extension of tumor to peritoneum • Direct extension of tumor to contralateral pleura • Direct extension of tumor to one or more mediastinal organs • Direct extension of tumor into spine • Tumor extending through to internal surface of pericardium with or without pericardial effusion, or tumor involving myocardium
N—Lymph Nodes	
NX	Regional lymph nodes not assessable
N0	No regional lymph node metastases
N1	Metastases in ipsilateral bronchopulmonary, hilar, or mediastinal lymph nodes (including the internal mammary, peridiaphragmatic, pericardial fat pad, or intercostal lymph nodes)
N2	Metastases in the contralateral bronchopulmonary, hilar, or mediastinal lymph nodes or ipsilateral or contralateral supraclavicular lymph nodes
M—Metastases	
MX	Distant metastases not assessable
M0	No distant metastases
M1	Distant metastases present

Table 9.2 Staging Classification of Stage by Tumor-Node-Metastasis Description

STAGE	DESCRIPTION
IA	T1N0M0
IB	T2N0M0; T3N0M0
II	T1N1M0; T2N1M0
IIIA	T3N1M0
IIIB	T1N2M0; T2N2M0; T3N2M0 T4N0M0; T4N1M0; T4N2M0
IV	Any T, any N, M1

from nonresectable (T4) disease (diffuse tumor extension or multiple chest wall foci; direct extension to the mediastinal organs, spine, internal pericardial surface, or contralateral pleura; and transdiaphragmatic invasion) (Fig. 9.6). However, the parameters for T staging are pathologic descriptors that are often difficult to determine by CT and MRI.

In locally advanced (T4) disease, the poor accuracy of older CT in assessing transdiaphragmatic extension of MPM is the result of its inability to detect small volume invasion, as well as the inherent limitation of axial imaging to delineate the diaphragm from the primary pleural tumor. With the use of multidetector computed tomography (MDCT), PET/CT imaging allows high-resolution multiplanar reconstruction to better evaluate the diaphragm. However, the accuracy of PET/CT is also suboptimal in detecting subtle transdiaphragmatic extension. Because of the limitations of imaging, preoperative laparoscopy is routinely performed in our institution in patients being evaluated for EPP. In the study by Rice and coworkers,[25] laparoscopy identified 10/109 patients (9%) with transdiaphragmatic invasion or peritoneal metastases compared with 3/109 patients identified by cross-sectional imaging. Importantly, laparoscopy even identified transdiaphragmatic extension in patients with minimal peridiaphragmatic tumor on CT.

N Staging

The N descriptor defines the presence and location of nodal metastases (see Table 9.1). Large retrospective studies have shown that up to 50% of patients with MPM who undergo EPP have intrathoracic nodal metastases.[26] The accurate detection of intrathoracic nodal metastases is important, because survival is poor in patients with mediastinal, supraclavicular, and internal mammary nodal metastases, and the presence of N2 disease would preclude curative resection. CT is almost uniformly used to evaluate for the presence or absence of nodal metastases. However, although CT is accurate in demonstrating enlarged nodes, the specificity for metastases is less than optimal, because metastases can be present in small nodes, and enlarged lymph nodes can

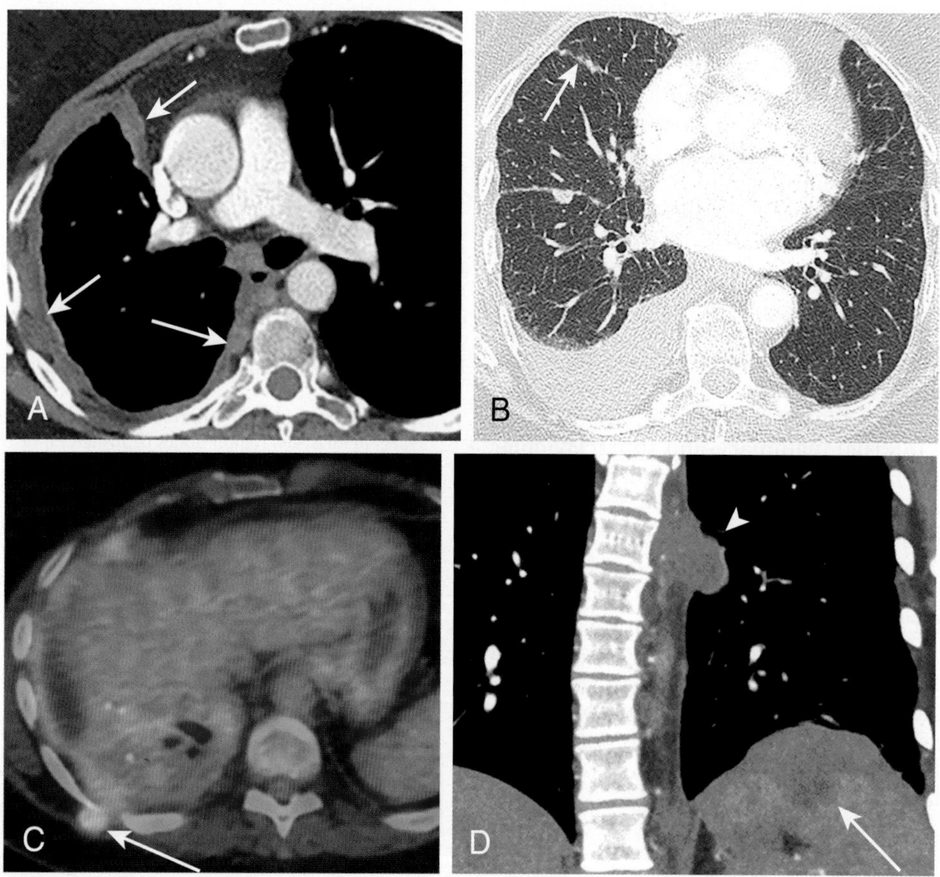

FIGURE 9.4. Cross-section (**A–D**) and illustration (**E–H**) of the local extent of the primary tumor (T descriptor) in the tumor-node-metastasis classification of malignant pleural mesothelioma. Axial computed tomography (CT) with soft tissue window (**A**) and illustration (**E**) of a T1 tumor involving the ipsilateral parietal pleura (including mediastinal and diaphragmatic pleura) with or without involvement of visceral pleura (*arrows*). Axial CT with lung window (**B**) and illustration (**F**) of a T2 tumor involving each ipsilateral pleural surface with confluent visceral pleural tumor including fissures (*arrows*) or extension of tumor from visceral pleura into underlying pulmonary parenchyma or involvement of diaphragmatic muscle. Axial fused 2-[^{18}F] fluoro-2-deoxy-D-glucose positron emission tomography/CT (**C**) and illustration (**G**) of a T3 locally advanced but potentially resectable tumor. Tumor is involving all ipsilateral pleural surfaces with a solitary, completely resectable focus of tumor extending into soft tissues of chest wall (*arrow*). Coronal reformat CT with soft tissue window (**D**) and illustration (**H**) of a T4 locally advanced technically unresectable tumor. Tumor is involving all ipsilateral pleural surfaces with direct transdiaphragmatic extension of tumor to peritoneum (*arrow*) and thoracic spine (*arrowhead*).

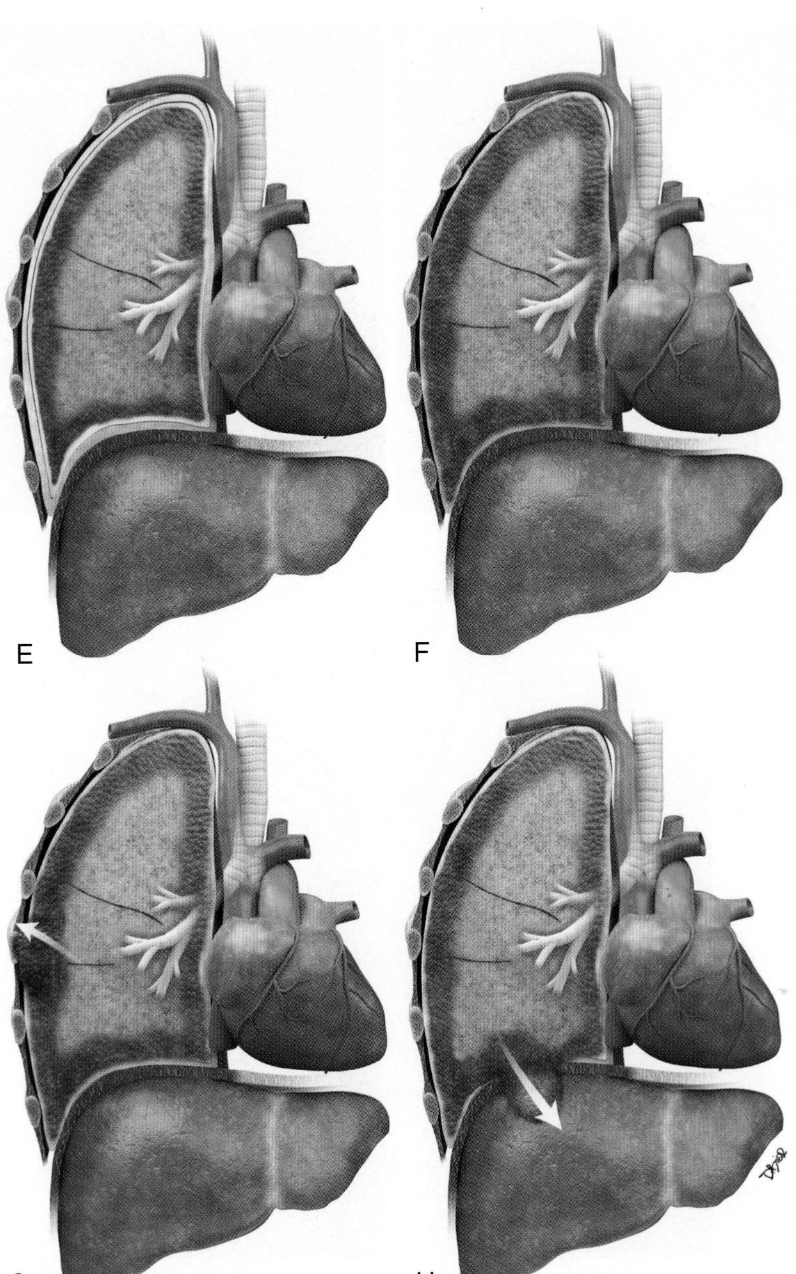

FIGURE 9.4. *(Continued)*

be hyperplastic (Figs. 9.7 and 9.8). In addition, when compared with other intrathoracic malignancies, the lymphatic pattern of spread of MPM is complex, with multiple drainage systems, and detection of nodal metastases is suboptimal. Because the survival of patients with extrapleural nodal involvement has been reported to be poor, assessment by invasive sampling before EPP has been suggested to be important in patient selection.[5] Complete nodal evaluation by mediastinoscopy or endobronchial ultrasound-guided lymph node biopsy, although important, lacks the required sensitivity and specificity to determine appropriate management of MPM. In a study at our institution, mediastinoscopy had a sensitivity of only 36% for intrathoracic (N2) nodal metastases detected at surgery.[25] Schouwink and colleagues[27] performed mediastinoscopy in 43 patients with MPM and compared the staging accuracy with that of CT. Sensitivity, specificity, and accuracy were 80%, 100%, and 93% for mediastinoscopy compared with 60%, 71%, and 67% for CT.

The role of PET in the detection of mediastinal nodal metastases, particularly for nodal stations not accessible by mediastinoscopy, can aid in the preoperative evaluation of patients considered for EPP.[28–30] However, Flores and associates[31] reported a sensitivity of only 11% for PET imaging in the detection of nodal metastases in patients with MPM. The low sensitivity of PET in their study may have been caused in part by PET findings not being correlated with CT. However, in a study at our institution, integrated PET/CT imaging was also found to be inaccurate in the evaluation of nodal MPM metastases. The

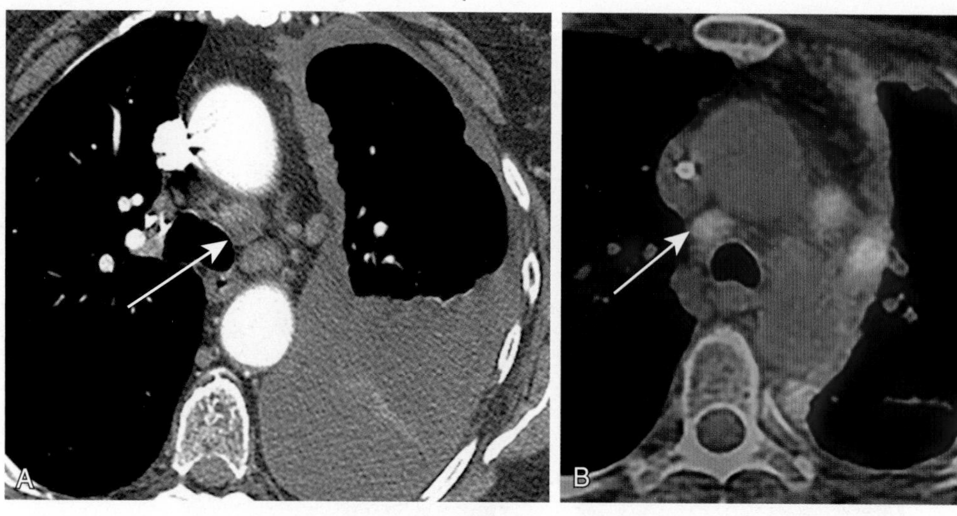

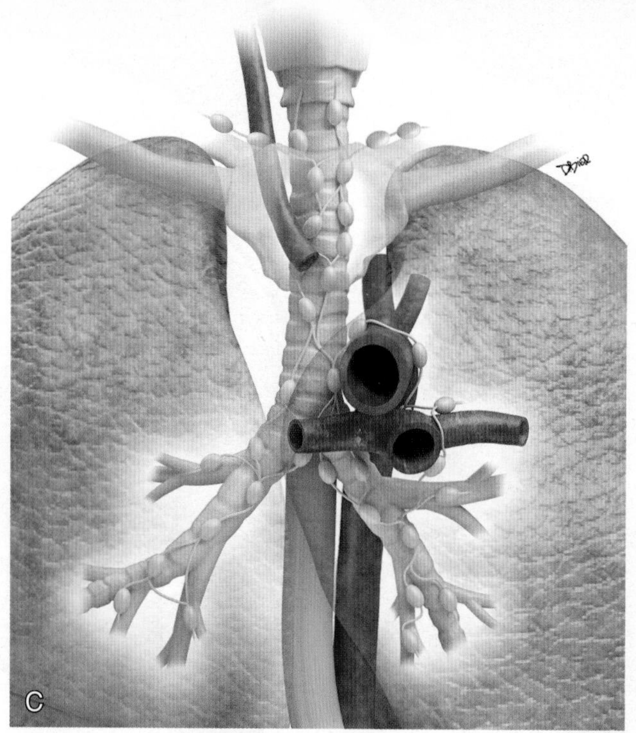

FIGURE 9.5. Cross-section (**A–B**) and illustration (**C**) of nodal disease spread (N descriptor) in the tumor-node-metastasis classification of malignant pleural mesothelioma. Axial computed tomography (CT) with soft tissue window (**A**); N1 denotes metastases in the ipsilateral bronchopulmonary, hilar, or mediastinal (*arrow*) lymph nodes (including the internal mammary, peridiaphragmatic, pericardial fat pad, or intercostal lymph nodes). Axial fused 2-[^{18}F] fluoro-2-deoxy-D-glucose positron emission tomography/CT (**B**); N2 denotes metastases in the contralateral bronchopulmonary, hilar, or mediastinal (*arrow*) lymph nodes or ipsilateral or contralateral supraclavicular lymph nodes.

sensitivity, specificity, positive predictive value, negative predictive value, and accuracy of PET/CT in lymph node staging in patients with N2 disease were 38%, 78%, 60%, 58%, and 59%, respectively.[32]

In the detection of nodal disease, PET/CT is limited not only by the false-negative results in patients with microscopic disease below the resolution of PET, but also by the false-positive results in patients with 2-[^{18}F] fluoro-2-deoxy-D-glucose (FDG)–avid inflammatory/infectious etiologies. These potential pitfalls can lead to misinterpretation and have implications for management. Thus, we advocate sampling of all FDG-avid nodes in patients with MPM being considered for EPP.

M Staging

Distant metastases have historically been considered to be an uncommon late manifestation of MPM.[33] The poor prognosis and rapid demise of patients, together with the lack of an effective medical therapeutic option or potentially curative surgical resection in the past, negated the need for accurate determination of the presence or absence of distant metastases. These distant metastases are now considered to occur more commonly than previously reported and can be solitary or diffuse, with involvement of brain, lung, bone, adrenal, peritoneum, abdominal nodes, and abdominal wall.

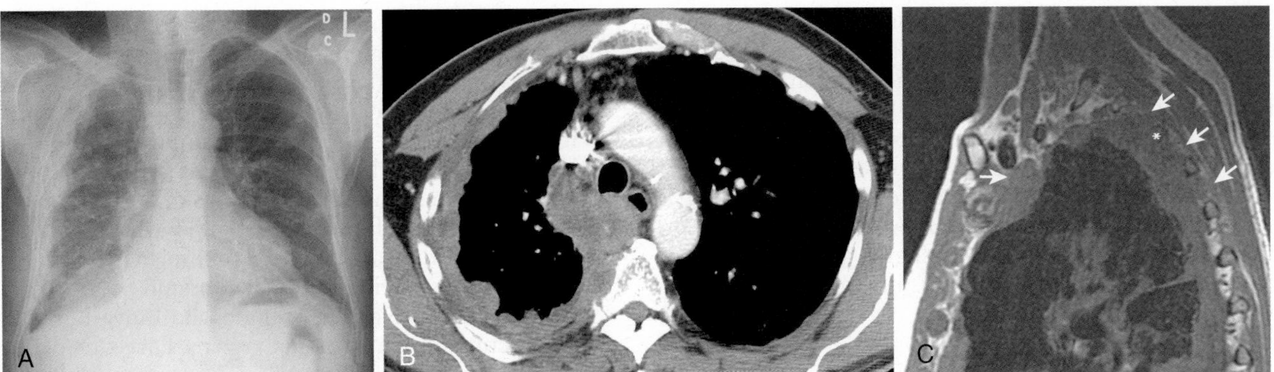

FIGURE 9.6. A 69-year-old man with right chest wall pain and right arm numbness and pain. **A,** Posteroanterior chest radiograph shows nodular right pleural thickening. **B,** Contrast-enhanced computed tomography (CT) shows circumferential right nodular pleural thickening with erosion of the lateral aspect of the T3 vertebra. **C,** Sagittal T1-weighted magnetic resonance imaging (MRI) shows extensive chest wall invasion anteriorly and posteriorly (*arrows*), with abnormal signal intensity in the third rib (*) consistent with tumor infiltration. Note that MRI is superior to CT in evaluating chest wall invasion. This is important for staging, because a single focus of chest wall invasion is resectable, and multifocal disease is unresectable.

FIGURE 9.7. A 62-year-old man with epithelioid malignant pleural mesothelioma (MPM). **A,** Chest radiograph shows right pleural abnormality consistent with an effusion. **B,** Contrast-enhanced computed tomography scan of the chest reveals nodular right pleural thickening consistent with MPM. Note the contralateral mediastinal enlarged lymph node in the left paratracheal region (*). Mediastinoscopy was negative for malignancy, and the patient proceeded to extrapleural pneumonectomy.

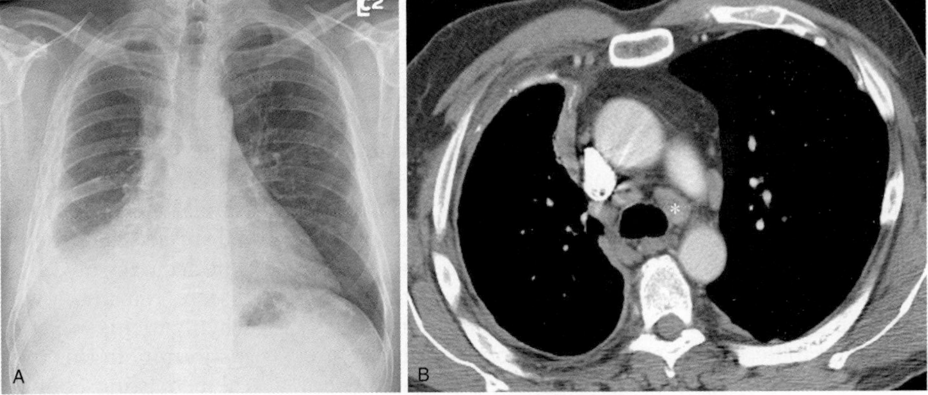

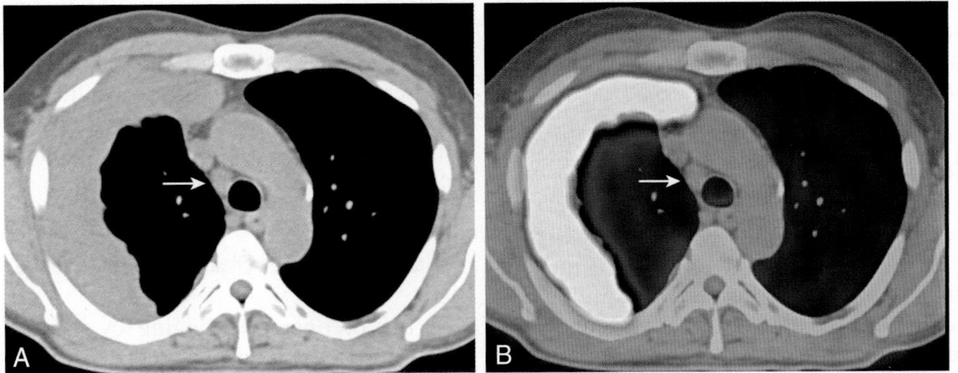

FIGURE 9.8. A 64-year-old man with epithelioid malignant pleural mesothelioma (MPM) is being evaluated for extrapleural pneumonectomy (EPP). **A,** Axial noncontrast-enhanced computed tomography (CT) shows circumferential pleural thickening in the right hemithorax with a 1-cm lymph node in the right paratracheal region (*arrow*). **B,** Axial integrated positron emission tomography/CT shows increased 2-[^{18}F] fluoro-2-deoxy-D-glucose (FDG) uptake in the right MPM. The right paratracheal lymph node (*arrow*) is not FDG-avid. Mediastinoscopy, laparoscopy, and peritoneal lavage, performed as part of extended surgical staging in patients undergoing preoperative evaluation for EPP, showed no evidence of malignancy, and the patient proceeded to surgery.

There are few reports of the use of PET in detecting extrathoracic metastases in patients with MPM.[29,31,32] Improvement in the accuracy of M staging with PET/CT can lead to more appropriate selection of patients for EPP and decrease the number of patients with early recurrence of MPM.

IMAGING

MPM typically manifests radiologically as a unilateral pleural effusion, moderate to large in size, with or without a pleural mass or diffuse pleural thickening. The primary modality in the diagnosis and staging of MPM is CT. CT is readily available and most frequently used in evaluating patients for surgical resection. CT findings that preclude surgery include diffuse chest wall invasion, peritoneal involvement, and distant metastasis. MRI and PET can be used to complement CT in the preoperative evaluation of patients with MPM. MRI can aid in the diagnosis of chest wall invasion or transdiaphragmatic extension. PET/CT is useful in the evaluation for nodal involvement and distant metastasis. Knowledge of the strengths and limitations of each of these imaging modalities is important in performing appropriate staging.

Chest Radiography

Radiographic evaluation of patients with MPM typically shows a unilateral pleural abnormality. A pleural effusion is seen in 30% to 80% of patients with MPM.[34] In 45% to 60% of patients, a smooth lobular pleural mass is demonstrated.[34] Diffuse unilateral pleural thickening occurs in up to 60% of patients with MPM.[34] The pleural thickening can form a rind and grow into the fissures. As the tumor grows, there is encasement of the lung, with signs of volume loss on the affected side, including ipsilateral shift of the mediastinum, elevation of the hemidiaphragm, and narrowing of the intercostal spaces. If the pleural tumor is bulky, there can be contralateral shift of the mediastinum. It is important to be aware that calcified pleural plaques occur in only 20% of patients, and consequently the absence of pleural plaques should not be used to exclude MPM in patients presenting with a pleural abnormality.[35]

Radiographic evaluation of local extent of disease and identification of metastases is not sensitive or specific. For instance, although periosteal reaction along the ribs, rib erosion, or destruction has been described as a manifestation of chest wall invasion, these findings are not common (20%).[34] Because findings in the lungs can be obscured by the pleural disease on chest radiography, CT better evaluates pulmonary metastases.

Computed Tomography

CT is more sensitive than radiography in the detection of early abnormalities in patients with MPM. CT features of MPM include unilateral pleural effusion (74%) and nodular pleural thickening (92%), which can be discrete or diffuse with involvement of the fissures.[36] As the tumor grows to form a pleural rind, circumferential encasement of the lung results in volume loss in the ipsilateral hemithorax in 42% of patients.[36] The signs of volume loss include ipsilateral mediastinal shift, elevation of the ipsilateral hemidiaphragm, and narrowing of the intercostal spaces. However, contralateral shift of the mediastinum has been described in 14% of patients because of bulky disease and/or large pleural effusions.[36]

CT is valuable in evaluating the extent of disease at initial staging. CT can assess for involvement of the chest wall, diaphragm, and mediastinum. CT features of local chest wall invasion include obliteration of extrapleural fat planes, invasion of intercostal muscles, displacement of ribs by tumor, and bone destruction.

Diaphragmatic invasion is suspected when a soft tissue mass encases the hemidiaphragm. Conversely, a clear fat plane between the inferior diaphragmatic surface and the adjacent abdominal organs and a smooth diaphragmatic contour suggest that the disease is limited to the thorax and does not extend through the diaphragm.[37] Scanning in the axial plane has inherent limitations in the assessment of the inferior surface of the diaphragm. However, the advent of MDCT and the capability for multiplanar reformation has improved evaluation of the diaphragm.

Mediastinal involvement includes local invasion of vascular structures and mediastinal organs. Direct mediastinal extension results in obliteration of mediastinal fat planes. CT evidence of invasion of vascular structures and mediastinal organs such as the great vessels, esophagus, and trachea is suggested when a soft tissue mass surrounds more than 50% of the structure.[37] Pericardial invasion is characterized by nodular pericardial thickening with or without a pericardial effusion.

Mediastinal lymph node involvement can be caused by direct invasion or metastatic spread. Intrathoracic nodal disease is reported in 34% to 50% of patients with MPM.[25,38,39] Although CT is the most frequently used modality to evaluate thoracic lymph nodes, it can be difficult or impossible to distinguish hilar or mediastinal lymph nodes as separate structures from the pleural tumor. Similarly, irregular pleural thickening along the mediastinal surface can obscure enlarged mediastinal lymph nodes. The accuracy of CT in the assessment of mediastinal nodal disease remains low,[40] and mediastinoscopy is indicated when patients are considered for surgical resection in our institution. In this regard, the diagnostic accuracy of cervical mediastinoscopy is 93% compared with 67% for CT.[27]

CT is also useful in evaluation of the lungs, often obscured by pleural masses or effusions in patients with MPM on chest radiographs. Hematogenous metastases to the lungs can manifest as nodules, masses, and, rarely, diffuse miliary disease. Lymphangitic spread of tumor presents as focal or diffuse nodular interlobular septal thickening. In addition to revealing pulmonary neoplastic involvement, CT can also demonstrate pulmonary fibrosis caused by prior exposure to asbestos.

Magnetic Resonance Imaging

In the preoperative staging evaluation of patients with MPM, MRI is typically used to answer specific questions raised by CT concerning local extent of tumor. By imaging in multiple planes and using different pulse sequences, MRI can improve differentiation of tumor from normal tissues. Typically, MPM has a slightly increased signal on T1-weighted images compared with muscle, and subtle invasion can be difficult to discern. However, the signal of T2-weighted images is moderately increased and aids in tissue differentiation. In addition, because MPM typically enhances, the use of intravenous contrast can improve detection of tumor and local extension. Additional techniques such as fat suppression can be used to detect tumor invasion of adjacent structures.

MRI has been shown to be superior to CT in staging evaluation of areas of local invasion in two sites: the endothoracic fascia/single chest wall focus (accuracy 69% vs. 46%) and the diaphragm (accuracy 82% vs. 55%).[40] Thus, MRI can be used to assess diaphragmatic involvement when CT findings are equivocal. However, in our institution, patients do not undergo routine MRI evaluation of the diaphragm. This is because the accuracy of MRI is not optimal for diagnosing subtle transdiaphragmatic extension. Instead, laparoscopy is performed in patients considered for EPP to evaluate for transdiaphragmatic extension and peritoneal disease. The rationale for performing laparoscopy is that direct visualization of the undersurface of the diaphragm can detect small-volume disease. In addition, peritoneal lavage performed concurrently can detect unsuspected peritoneal metastases. This is particularly important in view of the significant morbidity and mortality rate of EPP.

Positron Emission Tomography

Another potentially valuable tool in the preoperative assessment of patients with MPM is PET. PET imaging of malignancies is typically performed with the radiopharmaceutical FDG, a D-glucose analog. Increased glucose metabolism by malignant cells results in increased uptake and accumulation of FDG, allowing diagnosis, staging, and assessment of treatment response. However, the role of FDG-PET in the staging of MPM has not been fully elucidated. In our experience, integrated PET/CT (the integration of functional PET data with anatomic CT data) has improved diagnostic accuracy in the staging of patients with MPM. A small study comparing FDG-PET imaging with CT performed in 18 patients with MPM showed that PET detected occult metastases in two patients being considered for surgical resection.[29] In addition, because FDG-PET provides information on metabolically active sites of disease, this modality can be used in conjunction with anatomic imaging to select the most appropriate area for biopsy.[39] Integrated PET/CT allows more precise anatomic localization of disease and is useful in detecting nodal and systemic metastatic disease.[32,41] However, the ability of PET/CT to correctly stage locoregional disease is suboptimal.[41] In a study performed at our institution, T staging was accurately determined in 63% of patients undergoing EPP, and 29% of the patients had understaged T disease secondary to locoregional disease not detected by preoperative imaging.[32] The strength of PET/CT in staging patients with MPM is in the detection of extrathoracic metastases. In one recent study, integrated PET/CT identified occult metastases in 25% of the patients being evaluated for EPP.[32] Importantly, in more than half of these patients, extrathoracic metastases were not identified by routine clinical and conventional radiologic evaluation. In addition, coregistration of PET/CT data allows precise anatomic localization of areas of increased FDG uptake and can be useful in guiding biopsy of these sites.

Novel imaging agents are expected to have an important role in the management of MPM. The use of molecular bioprobes, such as technicium-99m–labeled mAb K1 antibodies that bind the mesothelin antigen, can prove useful for imaging MPM in the posttherapy setting. These bioprobes target tumor based on biochemical and physiologic properties rather than structural properties.[42]

DIFFERENTIAL DIAGNOSIS

MPM typically manifests radiologically as a unilateral pleural effusion, moderate to large in size, with or without a pleural mass, or diffuse pleural thickening with or without a pleural effusion. The differential diagnosis of a unilateral pleural effusion is extensive and includes congestive heart failure, infection, subdiaphragmatic disease, pulmonary embolism, and collagen vascular disease. In contradistinction, the differential diagnosis of diffuse nodular pleural thickening is limited and includes MPM, metastatic disease, and, in cases with a mediastinal mass, thymic malignancy with pleural metastases. CT features that aid in differentiating malignant from benign pleural disease include pleural thickening with a circumferential distribution encasing the lung (sensitivity 100%, specificity 41%), pleural thickening of greater than 1 cm in thickness (sensitivity 94%, specificity 36%), and nodular morphology (sensitivity 94%, specificity 51%).[35]

Occasionally, MPM can manifest as a focal pleural mass, mimicking localized fibrous tumor of the pleura (LFTP). LFTPs arise from mesenchymal cells, can be benign or malignant, and are not related to asbestos exposure. It is important to be able to identify the much rarer LFTP, which is managed differently and has a better prognosis than MPM.

Patients with LFTP range broadly in age from 5 to 87 years, with most being between 45 and 65 years of age, and there is no significant sex predilection. In about half of the cases, patients are asymptomatic, and LFTP is detected incidentally at chest radiography. The most common symptoms are cough, chest pain, and dyspnea. Other symptoms can include chills, fever, weight loss, debility, and a sensation of something flopping around in the chest. Symptomatic hypoglycemia is seen in up to 6% of patients. Hypertrophic osteoarthropathy is seen in 17% to 35% of cases.[43]

Benign and malignant subtypes of LFTP have been described. On histologic examination, the lesion consists of ovoid or spindle-shaped cells with round to oval nuclei, evenly distributed fine chromatin, inconspicuous nucleoli, and bipolar faintly eosinophilic cytoplasm with indistinct cell borders separated by collagen. Based on the presence of more than four mitotic figures per 10 high-power fields, these tumors are classified as malignant. On macroscopic examination, the tumor arises from the visceral pleura. Pedunculation is present in approximately 50%, and, owing to the presence of the stalk, which can be up to 9 cm in length, LFTP can be mobile. Radiologically, LFTPs have classic features of extraparenchymal masses (Fig. 9.9). On cross-sectional imaging, they have a well-defined lobular contour with homogeneous or heterogeneous attenuation. Surgical resection is curative in the majority of patients, although a small number of LFTPs can recur, undergo malignant transformation, or metastasize. The prognosis for patients with LFTP is generally favorable. The majority of lesions behave in a benign manner (88%), but approximately 12% of patients die of extensive intrathoracic tumor growth or unresectable recurrence.[43]

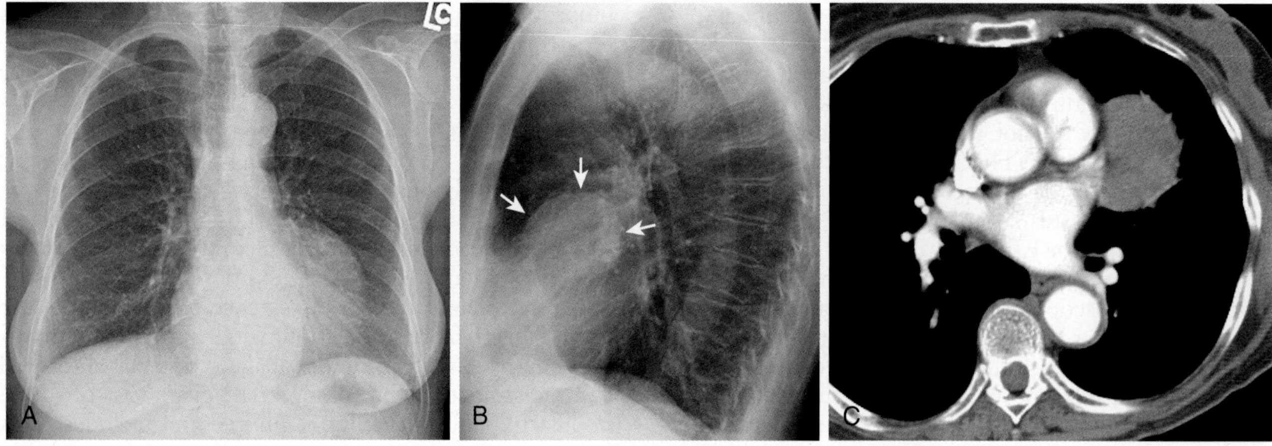

FIGURE 9.9. A 67-year-old woman presents for rectal fissure surgery. Preoperative posteroanterior (**A**) and lateral (**B**) chest radiographs show a lobular mass measuring 6×5×5 cm along the left heart border (*arrows in* **B**). **C,** Contrast-enhanced computed tomography demonstrated a soft tissue mass with a well-circumscribed border forming obtuse angles with the heart border, consistent with extraparenchymal lesion. Biopsy revealed spindle cell proliferation consistent with fibrous tumor of the pleura.

KEY POINTS The Radiology Report

- For resectability, it is important to distinguish T3 disease (a solitary focus of chest wall involvement, involvement of the endothoracic fascia, mediastinal fat extension, or nontransmural pericardial involvement) from nonresectable (T4) disease.
- The presence of N2 disease (contralateral mediastinal, contralateral internal mammary, and supraclavicular lymph nodes) and M1 metastasis precludes surgery.

TREATMENT

Single-modality approaches to treating MPM (i.e., surgery, chemotherapy, or radiation) failed to effectively extend survival.[44] Thus, an aggressive, multimodality treatment strategy has been developed that combines complete macroscopic resection with some form of additional therapy to prevent local recurrence by addressing the microscopic residual disease.[5] This strategy remains the only treatment option for prolonging survival beyond the current median of 7 months without treatment, and the only means of producing long-term survivors among select patients with favorable prognostic factors. Currently, the standard of care for first-line systemic therapy is cisplatin plus pemetrexed. Pemetrexed, a multitargeted antifolate, in combination with cisplatin has been reported in a multicenter phase III study of 448 patients to have an objective response rate of 41% and to improve overall survival by 3 months.[3] In 2016, the addition of bevacizumab to this combination demonstrated a further incremental benefit in overall survival.[45] More recently, immunotherapy has emerged as a possible therapeutic strategy for MPM. Okada et al. reported the results of the single-arm phase II MERIT trial of monotherapy with the immune-checkpoint inhibitor nivolumab as the second or subsequent line of therapy for patients with MPM.[46] In this study, patients with tumors expressing programmed cell death 1 ligand 1 (PD-L1) at levels of 1% or more (based on staining with the Dako 28-8 antibody) were more likely to have a response than those with PD-L1 levels less than 1% (objective response rate 70% vs. 33%).[46] With a median progression-free survival of 6.1 months, duration of response of 11.1 months, and overall survival of 17.3 months, the results from the MERIT study underscore the potential role of immune-checkpoint inhibitors in MPM.[46] In terms of future directions in therapy, researchers are evaluating different multimodality treatment approaches utilizing combinations of surgery, chemotherapy, immunotherapy, and radiation.

Surgical options include EPP and pleurectomy and decortication (P/D). EPP is the radical *en bloc* resection of the lung, pleura, diaphragm, and pericardium. Fusion of the pleura at the central tendon of the diaphragm and the lateral portion of the pericardium mandates resection and subsequent reconstruction with a prosthetic patch. P/D is a lung-sparing operation in which the diseased pleural envelope that encases and traps the lung is mobilized off the chest wall, mediastinum, diaphragm, and pericardium and then meticulously stripped from the surface of the lung. P/D is generally well tolerated, with low morbidity. The mortality rate is approximately 1.8% when the procedure is performed at a high-volume center.[26] Reports of median survival in the literature range from 9 to 20 months. However, the technical challenge of separating tumor and visceral pleura from the lung parenchyma can result in suboptimal cytoreduction.

The relatively low incidence of MPM and, therefore, difficulty in patient accrual for clinical trials, particularly large, randomized, prospective trials, pose a challenge in the establishment of standardized treatment protocols. Given this limitation, it is known that, for patients with MPM of epithelial histology, early-stage disease, negative nodes, and adequate pulmonary function, trimodality therapy with induction systemic therapy, surgery, and ipsilateral postoperative radiation therapy is most likely to prolong survival (68% 2-year survival and 46% 5-year survival).[5] Patients who undergo an EPP or P/D for definitive surgical management of MPM receive radiation therapy to the entire ipsilateral hemithorax for curative intent. All scars and drain sites are delineated at the time of simulation, because these will be targeted in the radiation field as

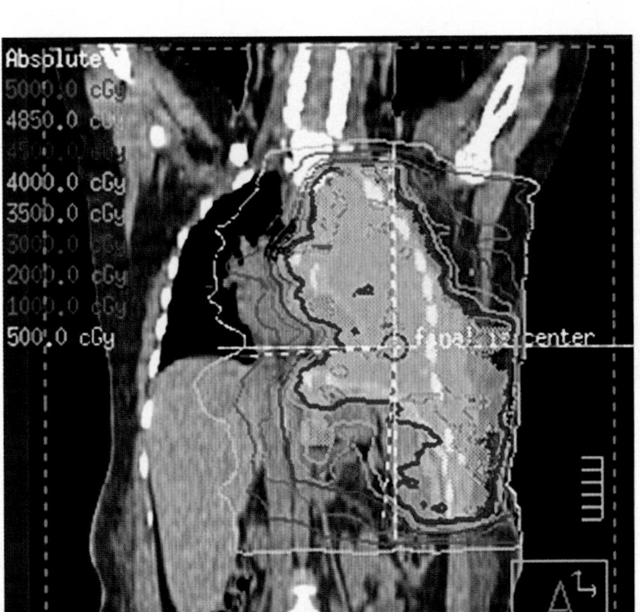

FIGURE 9.10. A 48-year-old woman with left epithelioid malignant pleural mesothelioma had extrapleural pneumonectomy and postoperative intensity-modulated radiation therapy planning. Note that, by using many treatment angles and modulating the beam intensity across apertures, it is possible to achieve a fairly homogeneous dose distribution to the target and shape the high-dose lines around and away from surrounding critical structures such as the heart and right lung.

well. The treatment field is generally defined by the following borders: superiorly, the thoracic inlet; inferiorly, the insertion of the diaphragm (generally, the bottom of L2); laterally, flashing the skin; and medially, the contralateral edge of the vertebral body if no mediastinal disease or 2.0 cm medial to the contralateral edge if mediastinal disease is present.

With these general treatment fields in mind, a novel technique to treat the entire hemithorax after surgery uses intensity-modulated radiation therapy (IMRT), which was developed at MD Anderson Cancer Center, with good outcomes.[47] In this technique, the region of the removed pleura is contoured by the radiation oncologist in consultation with the surgeon to carefully delineate appropriate target volumes, which include all preoperative pleural surfaces, ipsilateral mediastinal lymph nodes, the retrocrural space, and the deep margin of the thoracotomy incision. Multiple beams and inverse planning are then used to treat the region at risk to the same dose of 4500 cGy in 25 fractions while placing dose constraints on normal structures such as the heart, kidney, spinal cord, and stomach (Fig. 9.10). However, caution is warranted to limit the contralateral lung to very low doses to prevent the development of severe pneumonitis, because prior retrospective studies have shown that fatal complications can occur.[48] Typically, the contralateral lung is constrained to a mean lung dose of less than 800 cGy and to restrict the amount of lung receiving 20 Gy or higher to less than 7%.

The P/D surgical procedure has historically been thought to be palliative in nature, but the technique is increasingly used for the treatment of this disease owing to recent studies that have shown similar survival and decreased morbidity compared with EPP in well-selected patients.[26] In the past, the radiation treatment field targeted after P/D consisted of high-risk postoperative regions, as determined by postoperative imaging and discussion with the treating surgeon. However, with the advent of IMRT, the possibility of whole-pleura radiation in this setting is being explored, such that patients who are not candidates for EPP could still be considered for definitive treatment.

KEY POINTS Therapies

- First-line systemic chemotherapy is cisplatin plus pemetrexed.
- Trimodality therapy is most likely to prolong survival in patients with malignant pleural mesothelioma of epithelial histology, early-stage disease, negative nodes, and adequate pulmonary function.
- Intensity-modulated radiation therapy uses multiple beams and inverse planning to treat the region at risk to the same dose of 4500 cGy in 25 fractions while placing dose constraints on normal structures such as the heart, kidney, spinal cord, and stomach.
- There is a potential role for immunotherapy.

TREATMENT RESPONSE AND PROGNOSIS

Surveillance

In terms of anatomic imaging assessment of treatment response, bidimensional measurement of the tumor based on guidelines from WHO has been replaced by unidimensional longest-diameter measurement of the tumor in a single CT slice that shows the greatest tumor extent, based on the Response Evaluation Criteria In Solid Tumors (RECIST) approach.[49] The RECIST response criteria categorize a change in tumor diameter between two CT scans as progressive disease if this change reflects an increase in diameter of at least 20%, partial response if this change reflects a decrease in diameter of at least 30%, and stable disease if the change is between these two threshold values. However, because of the unique morphology of the pleural rind of MPM, shortcomings of this approach have led to the proposal of an alternative measurement protocol.[50,51] "Modified RECIST" has become standard for MPM, with unidimensional tumor thickness measurements perpendicular to the chest wall or mediastinum measured in two sites at three different levels on CT.[52] Axial CT slices used for measurement must be at least 1 cm apart and related to anatomic landmarks in the thorax, preferably above the level of division of the main bronchi. Nodal, subcutaneous, and other measurable lesions are measured unidimensionally as per the RECIST criteria. Unidimensional measurements are added to produce the total tumor measurement, with the sum of six pleural thickness measurements forming one univariate diameter.

Alternatively, volumetric tumor analysis can be done by serial segmentation.[51] Computerized techniques that quantify tumor volume on CT before, during, and after therapy can aid in the evaluation of tumor regression/progression and assessment of therapeutic response using full three-dimensional volumetric tumor analysis.

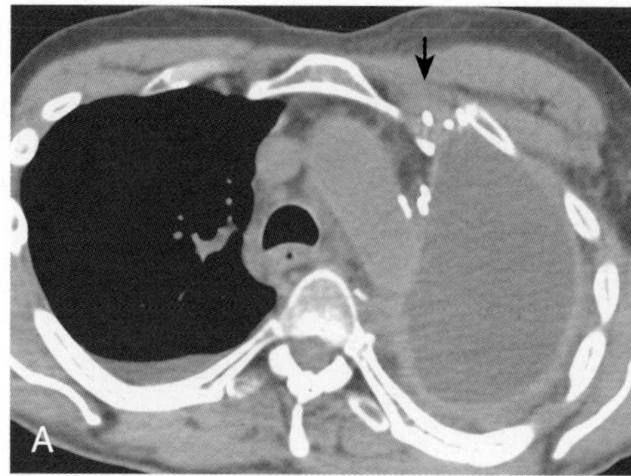

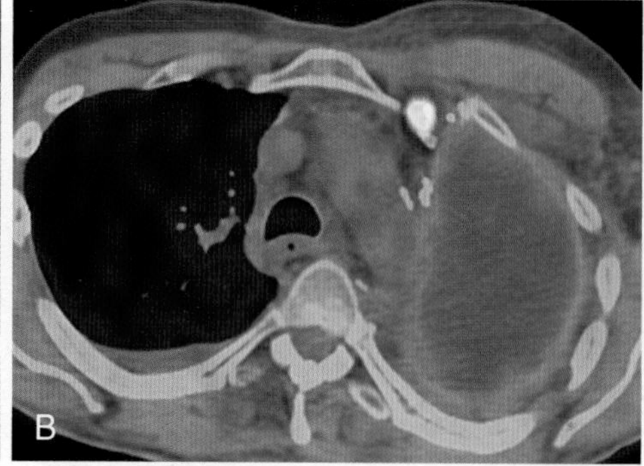

FIGURE 9.11. A 58-year-old asymptomatic man presents for surveillance 8 months after extrapleural pneumonectomy for malignant pleural mesothelioma. **A,** Axial non–contrast-enhanced computed tomography (CT) shows fluid in the left pneumonectomy space and surgical clips in the left hemithorax. **B,** Axial integrated positron emission tomography/CT shows increased 2-[^{18}F] fluoro-2-deoxy-D-glucose uptake in the left parasternal region. Tumor recurrence was confirmed by biopsy.

In terms of functional imaging, the semiquantitative evaluation of FDG uptake on PET as measured by the standardized uptake value (SUV) has been used as an indicator of prognosis and in the assessment of treatment response.[52,53] Low SUV and epithelial histology indicate the best survival, whereas high SUV and nonepithelial histology indicate the worst survival.[53] In a multivariate analysis of 65 patients with MPM, median survival was 14 and 24 months for the high- and low-SUV groups, respectively. High-SUV tumors were associated with a 3.3 times greater risk of death than low-SUV tumors ($P = .03$).[53] Mixed histology carried a 3.2 times greater risk of death than epithelial histology ($P = .03$).[53] Gerbaudo and coworkers[54] reported that the intensity of FDG uptake by the primary malignancy had a poor correlation with histologic grade but a good correlation with surgical stage. Furthermore, in this study, the increment of FDG lesion uptake over time was a better predictor of disease aggressiveness than was the histologic grade. The findings from these two small studies suggest that PET can have a role in the stratification of patients with MPM for treatment and clinical trials.

In the assessment of treatment response, PET using the semiquantitative measurement of FDG uptake has been evaluated with direct comparison between the pretreatment and the posttreatment scans.[55] The predictive value of PET to assess treatment efficacy after two cycles of single-agent pemetrexed or pemetrexed in combination with carboplatin was evaluated in 20 patients with MPM.[55] Ceresoli and colleagues[55] reported a significant correlation ($P < .05$) between early metabolic response and median time-to-tumor progression: 14 months for metabolic responders compared with 7 months for nonresponders. Patients showing metabolic response also had a trend toward longer overall survival. Interestingly, no correlation was found between radiologic response assessed by CT and time to tumor progression.

In terms of surveillance, recurrence and/or progressive metastatic disease are usually evaluated by CT scan. Patterns of recurrence include a soft tissue lesion along the resection margin, pericardial effusion/thickening, ascites, peritoneal fat stranding, new pulmonary nodules, and mediastinal adenopathy (Fig. 9.11). The emerging role for PET/CT is in the restaging of MPM, in evaluating response to therapy, and as an independent metabolic indicator of prognosis.[56,57]

Complications of Therapy

Chest radiographs and CT are typically the modalities used to monitor patients for complications caused by chemotherapy, radiation therapy, and surgery. Chemotherapy-induced toxicity to the lungs is discussed in Chapter 40. In terms of complications of radiation therapy, although IMRT following EPP limits the contralateral lung to very low doses, radiation pneumonitis remains a concern, because fatal complications can occur.[48]

Chest radiographs are usually used to evaluate for complications following surgery for MPM. Typically, the pneumonectomy space begins to fill with fluid, generally at the rate of one intercostal space per week. Whereas a sudden increase in fluid can indicate hemothorax or a chylous leak, a decrease in the amount of fluid in the pneumonectomy space can signify the presence of a bronchopleural fistula or leakage of fluid into the abdomen via the diaphragmatic reconstruction. MDCT with the capability for multiplanar reformats and three-dimensional imaging can help delineate a bronchopleural fistula.

A rare but serious complication after left pneumonectomy is gastric herniation, which can lead to gastric strangulation. This complication can be detected on chest radiographs with the gastric bubble located above the reconstructed left hemidiaphragm. Another rare complication is postpneumonectomy syndrome.[58] This rare syndrome is caused by extreme rotation and shift of the mediastinum after pneumonectomy, resulting in symptomatic central airway compression and obstruction.

Following radical pleurectomy, PET/CT is helpful in differentiating the granulation tissue from recurrent tumor, because both entities can present as irregular and nodular tissue along the resection margins. Using semiquantitative evaluation of tracer uptake, serial PET/CT can distinguish tumor, which manifests as progressive increase in FDG uptake, from granulation tissue, which remains stable or decreases in FDG avidity over time.[59]

KEY POINTS Detecting Recurrence

- Computed tomography (CT) is routinely used to evaluate for local tumor recurrence.
- Positron emission tomography/CT is useful in detecting locoregional recurrence, as well as interval metastases.

Key Points Therapy Complications

- Chest x-ray and computed tomography are typically used to monitor patients for complications that arise because of therapy, including drug toxicity and radiation pneumonitis.
- After extrapleural pneumonectomy, the pneumonectomy space fills with fluid, generally at the rate of one intercostal space per week.
- An increase in fluid can indicate hemothorax or a chylous leak.
- A decrease in fluid can indicate bronchopleural fistula or leakage of fluid into the abdomen via the diaphragmatic reconstruction. Multidetector-row computed tomography can help delineate a bronchopleural fistula.

SUMMARY

MPM is an uncommon neoplasm arising from mesothelial cells of the pleura, with poor prognosis. Multimodality regimens combining chemotherapy, radiotherapy, and surgery are being used more frequently in patient management. Accurate staging is important to distinguish patients who are resectable from those requiring palliative therapy. The primary imaging modality used in the diagnosis, staging, and treatment management of MPM is CT. CT is usually performed to assess the extent of chest wall, mediastinal, and diaphragmatic invasion and the presence or absence of nodal and distant metastases. MRI can be used to complement CT in the evaluation of patients with chest wall invasion and/or transdiaphragmatic extension being considered for resection. Integrated PET/CT has limitations in staging the primary tumor, particularly when tissue planes are invaded, but is useful in detecting nodal and systemic metastatic disease. In addition, PET can have a role in predicting treatment response and prognosis.

REFERENCES

1. Sugarbaker DJ. Multimodality management of malignant pleural mesothelioma: introduction. *Semin Thorac Cardiovasc Surg*. 2009;21:95-96.
2. Tsao AS, Wistuba I, Roth JA, et al. Malignant pleural mesothelioma. *J Clin Oncol*. 2009;27:2081-2090.
3. Vogelzang NJ, Rusthoven JJ, Symanowski J, et al. Phase III study of pemetrexed in combination with cisplatin versus cisplatin alone in patients with malignant pleural mesothelioma. *J Clin Oncol*. 2003;21:2636-2644.
4. Sugarbaker DJ, Garcia JP. Multimodality therapy for malignant pleural mesothelioma. *Chest*. 1997;112:272S-275S.
5. Sugarbaker DJ, Flores RM, Jaklitsch MT, et al. Resection margins, extrapleural nodal status, and cell type determine postoperative long-term survival in trimodality therapy of malignant pleural mesothelioma: results in 183 patients. *J Thorac Cardiovasc Surg*. 1999;117:54-63:discussion 63-65.
6. Pisani RJ, Colby TV, Williams DE. Malignant mesothelioma of the pleura. *Mayo Clin Proc*. 1988;63:1234-1244.
7. McDonald AD, McDonald JC. Malignant mesothelioma in North America. *Cancer*. 1980;46:1650-1656.
8. Ribak J, Lilis R, Suzuki Y, et al. Malignant mesothelioma in a cohort of asbestos insulation workers: clinical presentation, diagnosis, and causes of death. *Br J Ind Med*. 1988;45:182-187.
9. Hodgson JT, Darnton A. The quantitative risks of mesothelioma and lung cancer in relation to asbestos exposure. *Ann Occup Hyg*. 2000;44:565-601.
10. Gazdar AF, Butel JS, Carbone M. SV40 and human tumours: myth, association or causality? *Nat Rev Cancer*. 2002;2:957-964.
11. Dazzi H, Hasleton PS, Thatcher N, et al. Malignant pleural mesothelioma and epidermal growth factor receptor (EGF-R). Relationship of EGF-R with histology and survival using fixed paraffin embedded tissue and the F4, monoclonal antibody. *Br J Cancer*. 1990;61:924-926.
12. Marzo AL, Fitzpatrick DR, Robinson BW, et al. Antisense oligonucleotides specific for transforming growth factor beta2 inhibit the growth of malignant mesothelioma both in vitro and in vivo. *Cancer Res*. 1997;57:3200-3207.
13. Zucali PA, Giaccone G. Biology and management of malignant pleural mesothelioma. *Eur J Cancer*. 2006;42:2706-2714.
14. Demirag F, Unsal E, Yilmaz A, et al. Prognostic significance of vascular endothelial growth factor, tumor necrosis, and mitotic activity index in malignant pleural mesothelioma. *Chest*. 2005;128:3382-3387.
15. Robinson BW, Creaney J, Lake R, et al. Soluble mesothelin-related protein—a blood test for mesothelioma. *Lung Cancer*. 2005;49(Suppl 1):S109-S111.
16. Attanoos RL, Gibbs AR. Pathology of malignant mesothelioma. *Histopathology*. 1997;30:403-418.
17. Chirieac LR, Corson JM. Pathologic evaluation of malignant pleural mesothelioma. *Semin Thorac Cardiovasc Surg*. 2009;21:121-124.
18. Boutin C, Rey F, Gouvernet J, et al. Thoracoscopy in pleural malignant mesothelioma: a prospective study of 188 consecutive patients. Part 2: prognosis and staging. *Cancer*. 1993;72:394-404.
19. Metintas M, Ozdemir N, Isiksoy S, et al. CT-guided pleural needle biopsy in the diagnosis of malignant mesothelioma. *J Comput Assist Tomogr*. 1995;19:370-374.
20. Pass HI, Kranda K, Temeck BK, et al. Surgically debulked malignant pleural mesothelioma: results and prognostic factors. *Ann Surg Oncol*. 1997;4:215-222.
21. Butchart EG, Ashcroft T, Barnsley WC, et al. Pleuropneumonectomy in the management of diffuse malignant mesothelioma of the pleura. Experience with 29 patients. *Thorax*. 1976;31:15-24.
22. Sugarbaker DJ, Strauss GM, Lynch TJ, et al. Node status has prognostic significance in the multimodality therapy of diffuse, malignant mesothelioma. *J Clin Oncol*. 1993;11:1172-1178.
23. Rusch VW. A proposed new international TNM staging system for malignant pleural mesothelioma. From the International Mesothelioma Interest Group. *Chest*. 1995;108:1122-1128.
24. Tammilehto L, Kivisaari L, Salminen US, et al. Evaluation of the clinical TNM staging system for malignant pleural mesothelioma: an assessment in 88 patients. *Lung Cancer*. 1995;12:25-34.
25. Rice DC, Erasmus JJ, Stevens CW, et al. Extended surgical staging for potentially resectable malignant pleural mesothelioma. *Ann Thorac Surg*. 2005;80:1988-1992:discussion 1992-1993.
26. Wolf A, Daniel J, Sugarbaker DJ. Surgical techniques for multimodality treatment of malignant pleural mesothelioma: extrapleural pneumonectomy and pleurectomy/decortication. *Semin Thorac Cardiovasc Surg*. 2009;21:132-148.
27. Schouwink JH, Kool LS, Rutgers EJ, et al. The value of chest computer tomography and cervical mediastinoscopy in the preoperative assessment of patients with malignant pleural mesothelioma. *Ann Thorac Surg*. 2003;75:1715-1718:discussion 1718-1719.
28. Nanni C, Castellucci P, Farsad M, et al. Role of 18F-FDG PET for evaluating malignant pleural mesothelioma. *Cancer Biother Radiopharm*. 2004;19:149-154.
29. Schneider DB, Clary-Macy C, Challa S, et al. Positron emission tomography with F18-fluorodeoxyglucose in the staging and preoperative evaluation of malignant pleural mesothelioma. *J Thorac Cardiovasc Surg*. 2000;120:128-133.
30. Benard F, Sterman D, Smith RJ, et al. Metabolic imaging of malignant pleural mesothelioma with fluorodeoxyglucose positron emission tomography. *Chest*. 1998;114:713-722.
31. Flores RM, Akhurst T, Gonen M, et al. Positron emission tomography defines metastatic disease but not locoregional disease in patients with malignant pleural mesothelioma. *J Thorac Cardiovasc Surg*. 2003;126:11-16.
32. Erasmus JJ, Truong MT, Smythe WR, et al. Integrated computed tomography-positron emission tomography in patients with potentially resectable malignant pleural mesothelioma: staging implications. *J Thorac Cardiovasc Surg*. 2005;129:1364-1370.
33. Antman KH. Natural history and staging of malignant mesothelioma. *Chest*. 1989;96:93S-95S.

34. Wechsler RJ, Rao VM, Steiner RM. The radiology of thoracic malignant mesothelioma. *Crit Rev Diagn Imaging*. 1984;20:283-310.
35. Leung AN, Muller NL, Miller RR. CT in differential diagnosis of diffuse pleural disease. *AJR Am J Roentgenol*. 1990;154:487-492.
36. Kawashima A, Libshitz HI. Malignant pleural mesothelioma: CT manifestations in 50 cases. *AJR Am J Roentgenol*. 1990;155:965-969.
37. Patz Jr EF, Shaffer K, Piwnica-Worms DR, et al. Malignant pleural mesothelioma: value of CT and MR imaging in predicting resectability. *AJR Am J Roentgenol*. 1992;159:961-966.
38. Grondin SC, Sugarbaker DJ. Pleuropneumonectomy in the treatment of malignant pleural mesothelioma. *Chest*. 1999;116:450S-454S.
39. Zubeldia J, Abou-Zied M, Nabi H. Evaluation of patients with known mesothelioma with 18F-fluorodeoxyglucose and PET. Comparison with computed tomography. *Clin Positron Imaging*. 2000;3:165.
40. Heelan RT, Rusch VW, Begg CB, et al. Staging of malignant pleural mesothelioma: comparison of CT and MR imaging. *AJR Am J Roentgenol*. 1999;172:1039-1047.
41. Wilcox BE, Subramaniam RM, Peller PJ, et al. Utility of integrated computed tomography-positron emission tomography for selection of operable malignant pleural mesothelioma. *Clin Lung Cancer*. 2009;10:244-248.
42. Lindmo T, Boven E, Cuttitta F, et al. Determination of the immunoreactive fraction of radiolabeled monoclonal antibodies by linear extrapolation to binding at infinite antigen excess. *J Immunol Methods*. 1984;72:77-89.
43. Rosado-de-Christenson ML, Abbott GF, McAdams HP, et al. From the archives of the AFIP: localized fibrous tumor of the pleura. *Radiographics*. 2003;23:759-783.
44. Boutin C, Schlesser M, Frenay C, et al. Malignant pleural mesothelioma. *Eur Respir J*. 1998;12:972-981.
45. Zalcman G, Mazieres J, Margery J, et al. Bevacizumab for newly diagnosed pleural mesothelioma in the Mesothelioma Avastin Cisplatin Pemetrexed Study (MAPS): a randomised, controlled, open-label, phase 3 trial. *Lancet*. 2016;387:1405-1414.
46. Okada M, Kijima T, Aoe K, et al. Clinical efficacy and safety of nivolumab: results of a multicenter, open-label, single-arm, Japanese phase II study in malignant pleural mesothelioma (MERIT). *Clin Cancer Res*. 2019;25:5485-5492.
47. Rice DC, Stevens CW, Correa AM, et al. Outcomes after extrapleural pneumonectomy and intensity-modulated radiation therapy for malignant pleural mesothelioma. *Ann Thorac Surg*. 2007;84:1685-1692:discussion 1692-1693.
48. Allen AM, Czerminska M, Janne PA, et al. Fatal pneumonitis associated with intensity-modulated radiation therapy for mesothelioma. *Int J Radiat Oncol Biol Phys*. 2006;65:640-645.
49. James K, Eisenhauer E, Christian M, et al. Measuring response in solid tumors: unidimensional versus bidimensional measurement. *J Natl Cancer Inst*. 1999;91:523-528.
50. Byrne MJ, Nowak AK. Modified RECIST criteria for assessment of response in malignant pleural mesothelioma. *Ann Oncol*. 2004;15:257-260.
51. van Klaveren RJ, Aerts JG, de Bruin H, et al. Inadequacy of the RECIST criteria for response evaluation in patients with malignant pleural mesothelioma. *Lung Cancer*. 2004;43:63-69.
52. Steinert HC, Santos Dellea MM, Burger C, et al. Therapy response evaluation in malignant pleural mesothelioma with integrated PET-CT imaging. *Lung Cancer*. 2005;49(Suppl 1):S33-S35.
53. Flores RM. The role of PET in the surgical management of malignant pleural mesothelioma. *Lung Cancer*. 2005;49(Suppl 1):S27-S32.
54. Gerbaudo VH, Britz-Cunningham S, Sugarbaker DJ, et al. Metabolic significance of the pattern, intensity and kinetics of 18F-FDG uptake in malignant pleural mesothelioma. *Thorax*. 2003;58:1077-1082.
55. Ceresoli GL, Chiti A, Zucali PA, et al. Early response evaluation in malignant pleural mesothelioma by positron emission tomography with [18F]fluorodeoxyglucose. *J Clin Oncol*. 2006;24:4587-4593.
56. Gerbaudo VH, Sugarbaker DJ, Britz-Cunningham S, et al. Assessment of malignant pleural mesothelioma with (18)F-FDG dual-head gamma-camera coincidence imaging: comparison with histopathology. *J Nucl Med*. 2002;43:1144-1149.
57. Flores RM, Akhurst T, Gonen M, et al. Positron emission tomography predicts survival in malignant pleural mesothelioma. *J Thorac Cardiovasc Surg*. 2006;132:763-768.
58. Shen KR, Wain JC, Wright CD, et al. Postpneumonectomy syndrome: surgical management and long-term results. *J Thorac Cardiovasc Surg*. 2008;135:1210-1216:discussion 1216-1219.
59. Gill RR, Gerbaudo VH, Sugarbaker DJ, et al. Current trends in radiologic management of malignant pleural mesothelioma. *Semin Thorac Cardiovasc Surg*. 2009;21:111-120.

PART IV LIVER, BILIARY TRACT, AND PANCREAS

CHAPTER 10 Liver Cancer: Hepatocellular and Fibrolamellar Carcinoma

Aaron Coleman, M.D.; Elainea N. Smith, M.D.; Samuel J. Galgano, M.D.; and Kristin K. Porter, M.D., Ph.D.

HEPATOCELLULAR CARCINOMA

Introduction

Hepatocellular carcinoma (HCC) is the most common primary liver cancer and the fifth most common cancer in the world. HCC typically develops in patients with background liver disease. Screening patients at risk with ultrasound (US) and for α-fetoprotein (AFP) levels every 5 months improves early detection rates. HCC can be diagnosed with multiphase computed tomography (CT) or magnetic resonance imaging (MRI) without the need for biopsy if characteristic imaging features are present. The American College of Radiology developed the Liver Imaging Reporting and Data System (LI-RADS) to provide uniform criteria for the diagnosis of HCC.

Transplantation and tumor resection are potentially curative surgical options for HCC. Additional therapies include percutaneous ablation, transarterial chemoembolization (TACE), transarterial radioembolization (TARE), and stereotactic body radiotherapy. These therapies can be used alone or in combination for palliation or as a bridge to liver transplant. HCC is resistant to most chemotherapeutic agents; however, systemic therapy with sorafenib or lenvatinib can be used as first-line therapies in advanced disease. In addition to providing diagnostic criteria, LI-RADS also includes guidelines for assessing posttreatment tumor response.

Epidemiology

HCC is the fifth most common cancer in the world and the most common primary liver cancer.[1–3] It is more common in sub-Saharan Africa and Eastern Asia than in other parts of the world because of the prevalence of hepatitis B (HBV) infection.[4] The incidence of HCC in the United States has markedly increased over the past few decades and is expected to rise until 2030.[1,3] HCC is often diagnosed below the age of 60 years in countries with endemic HBV and above the age of years 60 in countries where HBV is less prevalent.[1] It is more common in men than women, at a ratio as high as 4:1.[1,4] More than 80% of patients diagnosed with HCC have underlying cirrhosis.[1,3] Therefore, etiologies leading to the development of cirrhosis are also risk factors for HCC.[1]

HBV and hepatitis C virus (HCV) are major risk factors for HCC. HBV infection is the most common cause of HCC worldwide and accounts for approximately 50% of all cases; it is estimated to increase the risk of developing HCC by 15- to 20-fold.[3,4] HBV is transmitted through exposure to infected blood, semen, and other body fluids. The virus is typically acquired through vertical and perinatal transmission in endemic areas. Sexual and parenteral transmission are more common in areas with low HBV prevalence.[4] HCV is the most common cause of HCC in the United States, and patients infected with HCV are 17 times more likely to develop HCC.[3] HCV is commonly transmitted through exposure to infected blood. Sexual transmission is also possible, but is less common. Development of HBV vaccinations and treatments for both viruses has helped decrease the incident of HCC.[1]

Nonalcoholic fatty liver disease (NAFLD) is currently the number one cause of chronic liver disease (CLD) in the United States. This is attributed to increasing rates of obesity and metabolic syndrome.[4] NAFLD is a potential HCC risk factor because it can ultimately lead to cirrhosis. A prospective study by Ascha et al. compared the development of HCC in patients with cirrhosis secondary to HCV and NAFLD. Their results showed a 4% incidence in the HCV cohort compared with a 2.6% incidence in the patients with NAFLD.[5] Controlling risk factors for the development of metabolic syndrome could ultimately lead to a decreased incidence of HCC attributed to NAFLD.

Several other etiologies leading to CLD and cirrhosis also contribute to the development of HCC. It is reported that there is a 5-fold increase in HCC in individuals whose alcohol consumption exceeds 80 g/day for 10 years.[6] Exposure to the aflatoxins produced by *Aspergillus* species can cause mutation in the *P53* tumor suppressor gene, which also increases the risk of HCC.[4] Additional causes of cirrhosis such as hemochromatosis, autoimmune hepatitis, primary biliary cirrhosis, and α-1 antitrypsin deficiency can also ultimately lead to the development of HCC.[1]

KEY POINTS Epidemiology of Hepatocellular Carcinoma

- Hepatocellular carcinoma is the most common primary liver cancer.
- Diseases leading to cirrhosis, such as hepatitis C virus, hepatitis virus, and nonalcoholic fatty liver disease, are important risk factors.

Anatomy

The liver has a dual blood supply from the portal venous system and the hepatic artery.

It is divided into the right and left lobes and subdivided into eight anatomic segments (Fig. 10.1). The segments are defined by their portal vein supply and are separated from each other by the hepatic veins. The caudate lobe is considered segment I. The portal supply to the caudate lobe commonly arises from the main portal vein, but may also arise from the left or right portal veins. Segments II and III of the liver are in the left lobe and are supplied by the first and second lateral branches of the left portal vein, respectively. Segment IV is also in the left lobe and is separated from II and III by the left hepatic vein and by the falciform ligament; the medial branches of the left portal vein supply it. The right hepatic vein separates segments in the right lobe: segment VII from VIII and segment VI from V. Segments VII and VI are supplied by the superior and inferior branches, respectively, of the posterior branch of the right portal vein. Segments VIII and V are supplied by the superior and inferior branches, respectively, of the anterior branch of the right portal vein. The middle hepatic vein separates the right and left lobes, segment VIII from IV, and segment V from IV. Segment V is also separated from segment IV by the gallbladder fossa (see Fig. 10.1).

The liver has an assortment of vascular variants. Michel's classification describes ten hepatic arterial anomalies.[7] The most common, type I, describes a common hepatic artery that arises from the celiac artery and bifurcates into the right and left hepatic artery, supplying the right and left lobes. Other common vascular variants include a replaced or accessory right hepatic artery from the superior mesenteric artery and a replaced or accessory left hepatic artery from the left gastric artery. Documentation of the vascular supply of the liver is essential for correct treatment planning.

KEY POINTS Anatomy of Hepatocellular Carcinoma

- Eight liver segments are defined by their portal venous supply.
- Documentation of the segmental distribution of hepatocellular carcinoma is essential for treatment planning.
- Documentation of vascular variants to the liver is essential for treatment planning.

Pathology

HCC carcinogenesis occurs in a stepwise progression from regenerative nodules (RNs), to premalignant dysplastic

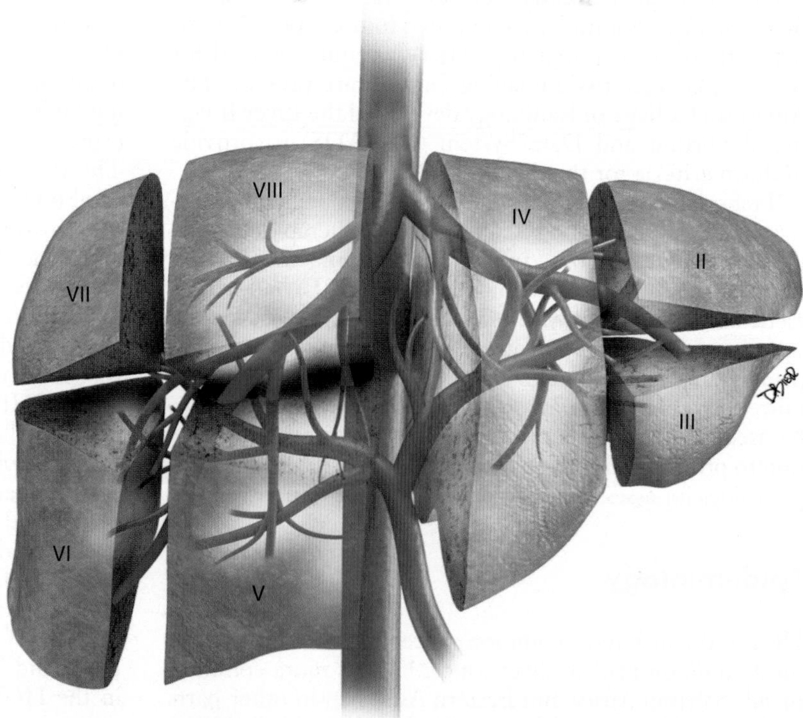

FIGURE 10.1. Segmental anatomy of the liver. The liver is divided into the right and left lobes. There are eight segments: three in the left lobe (II, III, and IV), four in the right lobe (V, VI, VII, VIII), and one in the caudate lobe (I) (not visualized). The segments are divided by the hepatic veins and defined by the portal vein supply.

nodules (DNs), to early or well-differentiated HCC, to advanced or poorly differentiated HCC.[8,9] RNs are surrounded by a fibrous septum. The size of these nodules determines the characterization of the cirrhotic liver as micro-, macro-, or mixed nodular. DNs contain cell atypia and range in size from 0.8 to 1.5 cm; these nodules have a reduced number of portal tracts and an increased number of unpaired arteries. Allelic loss, chromosomal changes, gene mutations, epigenetic alterations, and alterations in molecular cellular pathways play a role in the transformation of RNs to DNs and, ultimately, HCC.[10]

HCC may appear as a solitary mass, multifocal, or diffusely infiltrative. HCC has four main histologic classifications: trabecular, pseudoglandular, compact, and scirrhous. The most common type is the trabecular pattern, and scirrhous is the least common. The trabecular pattern is composed of fibrous stroma separating the tumor cell plates.[11] The histologic grading of HCC ranges from well-differentiated to highly anaplastic tumors. Grade I tumors can mimic hepatocellular adenomas, whereas grade IV tumors may mimic nonhepatocellular malignancies.

KEY POINTS Pathology of Hepatocellular Carcinoma

- Variable presentation: solitary mass, multiple masses, or infiltrative mass.
- Stepwise progression of development: from regenerative nodules to dysplastic nodules to hepatocellular carcinoma.
- Four histologic classifications: trabecular, pseudoglandular, compact, and scirrhous.

Clinical Presentation

The clinical presentation of HCC is nonspecific and is often related to underlying cirrhosis and chronic hepatitis. Symptoms include right upper quadrant pain, weight loss, fullness, anorexia, abdominal swelling, vomiting, fever, fatigue, and jaundice.[11,12] In the setting of cirrhosis, the development of weakness, malaise, and weight loss should raise clinical suspicion for HCC.

An irregular, enlarged, and nodular liver is the most common finding on physical examination. Jaundice, ascites, and enlarged supraclavicular lymph nodes may also be present. In the setting of portal compromise (portal hypertension or tumor extension), splenomegaly or hematemesis resulting from esophageal varices may be present. Tumoral vascular invasion of the hepatic veins may result in Budd–Chiari syndrome. Paraneoplastic manifestations of HCC, seen in fewer than 5% of patients with HCC, include erythrocytosis, hypercholesterolemia, porphyria cutanea tarda, gynecomastia, hypercalcemia, and hyperglycemia.[13]

The most commonly used tumor marker for HCC screening is serum AFP. The normal range is 10 to 20 ng/mL. The positive predictive value (PPV) of AFP in predicting HCC depends on the etiology of the tumor. Elevated AFP is seen more commonly in Asian countries (70%) than in Western countries (50%). AFP in a nonviral-related etiology has a 94% PPV compared with 70% for viral-related HCC.[14] A mass in the liver with an AFP level of more than 200 ng/mL is considered diagnostic of HCC. However, in 20% of cases of HCC, AFP is not elevated. It is also important to note that AFP may be elevated in patients with chronic hepatitis and cirrhosis without HCC.

KEY POINTS Clinical Presentation of Hepatocellular Carcinoma

- Symptoms are nonspecific and can be masked by cirrhosis and chronic hepatitis.
- An elevated α-fetoprotein level is the most common tumor marker, but it is normal in 20% of hepatocellular carcinomas.
- α-fetoprotein may be elevated in chronic hepatitis and cirrhosis without hepatocellular carcinoma.

Staging Classification

HCC staging is more complex compared to other malignancies because the majority of patients also have underlying cirrhosis. Prognosis and treatment options for these patients depend on both tumor burden and the degree of liver dysfunction.[1,15,16] The TNM (tumor, nodes, metastasis) staging system commonly used to stage other malignancies does not address underlying liver dysfunction and patient performance status. Several systems, such as the Barcelona Clinic Liver Cancer (BCLC) system, the Hong Kong Liver Cancer system, the Okuda system, and the Cancer of the Liver Italian Program, have been developed to stage patients based on tumor burden and the degree of liver dysfunction.[17–20] A study comparing seven staging systems showed that the BCLC system was the best at predicting survival.[21] The BCLC system is one of the most common staging systems used and has been adopted by both the American Association for the Study of Liver Diseases (AASLD) and the European Association for the Study of the Liver.[1,15]

The BCLC system classifies patients as very early stage (0), early stage (A), intermediate stage (B), advanced stage (C), and terminal stage (D) according to tumor burden, liver function, and patient performance status (Table 10.1). It also provides a treatment algorithm according to severity of disease.[19,22] Tumor burden is assessed by tumor size, tumor number, portal vein invasion, and extrahepatic

TABLE 10.1 Barcelona Clinic Liver Cancer Staging

Very early stage (0)	• Single tumor ≤2 cm • Preserved liver function • ECOG PS 0
Early stage (A)	• Up to three nodules ≤3 cm • Preserved liver function • ECOG PS 0
Intermediate stage (B)	• Multinodular • Preserved liver function • ECOG PS 0
Advanced stage (C)	• Portal invasion • Extrahepatic spread • Preserved liver function • ECOG PS 1–2
Terminal stage (D)	• End-stage liver disease • ECOG PS 3–4

ECOG PS, Eastern Cooperative Oncology Group performance status.

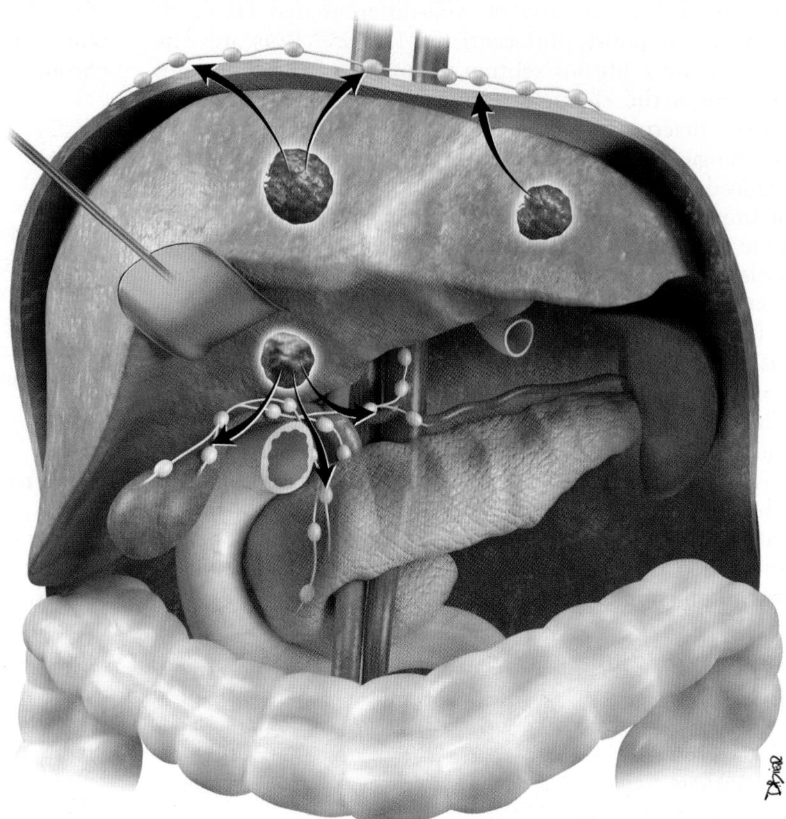

Figure 10.2. Pattern of nodal spread of hepatocellular carcinoma. Tumors in the central liver drain to the hepatoduodenal ligament. Tumors near the dome drain to the diaphragmatic nodal stations. Tumors in the left liver drain to the gastrohepatic nodes.

spread.[22,23] The Child–Pugh score has historically been used to assess liver function. However, recent updates recommend that liver function should be evaluated using both biochemical parameters and the overall compensation status of the patient, since the Child–Pugh score is often not a reliable indicator of liver function status.[22] Patient performance status is typically evaluated using the Eastern Cooperative Oncology Group scale.[23,24]

Key Points Staging of Hepatocellular Carcinoma

- The prognosis of patients with hepatocellular carcinoma depends on tumor burden and severity of cirrhosis.
- The Barcelona Clinic Liver Cancer system stages patients based on tumor burden, liver function, and functional status.

Patterns of Tumor Spread

HCC may present with intrahepatic and extrahepatic tumor spread.[25] The most common type of spread seen in HCC is intrahepatic tumors followed by portal vein tumor thrombosis. Extrahepatic spread is more common with larger tumors (>5 cm). Extrahepatic (hematogenous+lymphatic) spread has been reported in autopsy series in over half of cases, with the lung as the most common site.[13] Hematogenous spread may also be seen to the adrenal glands, bone, pancreas, kidney, and spleen. Lymphatic metastases are commonly found and typically occur at the hepatic hilum (Fig. 10.2).[25] Other commonly involved nodal stations include anterior diaphragmatic, peripancreatic, perigastric, retroperitoneal, paratracheal, carinal, and supraclavicular lymph nodes.

Key Points Tumor Spread of Hepatocellular Carcinoma

- The most common types of tumor spread are intrahepatic and portal vein tumor thrombus.
- Over 50% of patients have extrahepatic spread, based on autopsy series.
- Hepatocellular carcinoma mortality is typically due to liver failure rather than extrahepatic metastases.

Imaging

Liver Imaging Reporting and Data System

The LI-RADS was developed to provide uniform guidelines for the diagnosis of HCC on MRI, CT, and US.[26,27] LI-RADS should only be used in patients older than 18 years who are at high risk for developing HCC. High-risk populations include patients with cirrhosis, chronic HBV, and current or prior HCC. LI-RADS does not apply to children, patients with congenital hepatic fibrosis, or patients with CLD attributed to vascular disorders.[28,29]

According to the LI-RADS guidelines for US, the US report should include a liver visualization score and lesion categorization. Visualization is scored as A (no or minimal limitations), B (moderate limitations), or C (severe limitations). Visualization is affected by liver heterogeneity, US beam attenuation, and shadowing resulting in obscuration of the liver. Lesions seen on US are categorized as US-1 (negative), US-2 (subthreshold), or US-3 (positive).[28,30] US-1 is assigned when there is no observation or when there is an observation that is definitively benign. US-2 is assigned when there is an observation less than 1 cm in diameter. US-3 is assigned for new venous thrombosis and lesions larger than 1.0 cm that are not definitively benign.[28]

The LI-RADS CT/MRI guidelines classify observations as LR-1 (definitely benign), LR-2 (probably benign), LR-3 (intermediate), LR-4 (probably HCC), LR-5 (definitely HCC), LR-TIV (malignancy with tumor in vein), or LR-M (malignant, but not HCC-specific). LR-1 and LR-2 observations include lesions such as cysts, hemangiomas, focal fat deposition, perfusion anomalies, and scarring.[26] LR-3, LR-4, and LR-5 observations are classified by the major imaging features of HCC, which include size, threshold growth, nonrim arterial phase enhancement, washout, and presence of an enhancing capsule.[26,28,29] Table 10.2 outlines the specifics of the LR-3 through LR-5 classifications. The LR-M category includes malignancies such as intrahepatic cholangiocarcinoma, hepatocholangiocarcinoma, and metastasis; however, it does not exclude HCC.[31] A systemic review showed that 36% of lesions classified as LR-M were eventually diagnosed as HCC.[32] The criteria for LR-M are shown in Table 10.3.

In addition to the major imaging features of HCC, LI-RADS recognizes several ancillary features that can help with lesion classification. A list of these features is shown in Table 10.4. Ancillary features can only be used to upgrade or downgrade an observation by one classification (e.g., LR-3 to LR-4). Additionally, a lesion cannot be upgraded to LR-5 based on ancillary features alone.[29,33]

Key Points Liver Imaging Reporting and Data System

- Provides uniform guidelines and criteria for diagnosing hepatocellular carcinoma on computed tomography (CT), magnetic resonance imaging (MRI), ultrasound (US), and contrast-enhanced US.
- Major CT and MRI Liver Imaging Reporting and Data System (LI-RADS) criteria for hepatocellular carcinoma (HCC) include size, nonrim arterial phase enhancement, nonperipheral washout, presence of an enhancing capsule, and threshold growth.
- LI-RADS also includes several ancillary features of HCC that can aid in diagnosis.

Primary Tumor

Ultrasound

US is the most widely accepted modality for HCC screening. The AASLD currently recommends screening with US with or without AFP every 6 months in patients with cirrhosis.[1] The most common sonographic appearance of HCC is a hypoechoic solid mass (Fig. 10.3). This is more common in smaller, well-differentiated tumors. In larger tumors, the sonographic appearance is varied, possibly related to necrosis (hypoechoic), intralesional fat (hyperechoic), fibrosis (hyperechoic), hemorrhage (hyperechoic), or calcium (hyperechoic). As stated earlier, the US report should include a visualization score (A, B, or C) as well as a lesion categorization (US-1, US-2, US-3). The AASLD recommends repeat US with or without AFP in 3 to 6 months in patients with US-2.

Table 10.2 Computed Tomography/Magnetic Resonance Imaging Liver Imaging Reporting and Data System criteria (LR-3 through LR-5)

LR-3: Intermediate probability of malignancy	• <20 mm+nonrim APHE, and no additional major features[a] OR • <20 mm+one major feature other than APHE OR • ≥20 mm and no major features
LR-4: Probably HCC	• <10 mm+nonrim APHE+at least one additional major feature OR • 10–20 mm+nonrim APHE+enhancing "capsule" OR • ≥20 mm+nonrim APHE and no additional major features OR • <20 mm+at least two major features other than APHE OR • ≥20 mm+at least one major feature other than APHE
LR-5: Definitely HCC	• 10–19 mm+nonrim APHE+nonperipheral washout OR • 10–19 mm+nonrim APHE+threshold growth[b] OR • ≥20 mm+at least one major feature

[a]Major features: enhancing "capsule," nonperipheral "washout," threshold growth.
[b]Threshold growth: 50% growth in ≤6 months.
APHE, Arterial phase hyperenhancement; *HCC*, hepatocellular carcinoma.

Table 10.3 Computed Tomography/Magnetic Resonance Imaging Liver Imaging Reporting and Data System LR-M Criteria

LR-M: Probably or definitely malignant, not hepatocellular carcinoma (HCC) specific	• Rim arterial phase hyperenhancement • Peripheral washout • Delayed central enhancement • Targetoid Hepatobiliary phase signal hyperintensity • Targetoid diffusion restriction • Infiltrative appearance • Marked diffusion restriction • Necrosis • Other features of non-HCC malignancy

Patients with US-3 should be evaluated further with multiphase CT or MRI.[1]

Contrast-enhanced ultrasound (CEUS) has emerged as an alternative technique for the evaluation of HCC. In this technique, a microbubble contrast agent is injected intravenously. Following injection, continuous real-time US is performed for up to 5 minutes to assess for lesion arterial phase enhancement and washout. LI-RADS has recently included a diagnostic algorithm for diagnosing HCC with CEUS. Diagnostic criteria are similar to those specified by the LI-RADS CT/MRI guidelines. A unique application

Table 10.4 Computed Tomography/Magnetic Resonance Imaging Liver Imaging Reporting and Data System Ancillary Features Favoring Malignancy

FEATURE	COMPUTED TOMOGRAPHY	MAGNETIC RESONANCE IMAGING EXTRACELLULAR AGENT	MAGNETIC RESONANCE IMAGING HEPATOBILIARY AGENT
Subthreshold growth[a]	+	+	+
Restricted diffusion[a]	–	+	+
Mild/moderate T2 hyperintensity[a]	–	+	+
Corona enhancement[a]	+	+	+
Fat sparing in solid mass[a]	±	+	+
Iron sparing in solid mass[a]	–	+	+
Transitional phase hypointensity[a]	–	–	+
Hepatobiliary phase hypointensity[a]	–	–	+
Nodule-in-nodule architecture[b]	+	+	+
Mosaic architecture[b]	+	+	+
Nonenhancing "capsule"[b]	+	+	+
Fat in mass[b]	±	+	+
Blood products in mass[b]	±	+	+

[a]Features favoring malignancy in general, not specific for hepatocellular carcinoma.
[b]Features more specific for hepatocellular carcinoma.

of CEUS is its ability to distinguish arterioportal shunts accurately (commonly seen on multiphase CT and MRI) from true, arterially enhancing masses.[28,34]

Key Points Ultrasound Imaging of Hepatocellular Carcinoma

- Ultrasound (US) is used for hepatocellular carcinoma screening.
- US Liver Imaging Reporting and Data System evaluation should include a liver visualization score and lesion categorization.
- Lesions categorized as US-3 should be evaluated further with multiphase computed tomography or magnetic resonance imaging.

Computed Tomography

HCC should be evaluated using multidetector CT with eight or more detector rows. Images should be obtained in the late arterial phase, portal venous phase, and delayed phase (Fig. 10.4).[28] Precise timing of the late arterial phase is important, because mistiming can decrease the sensitivity for detecting HCC arterial phase hyperenhancement. An adequate late arterial phase is achieved when the hepatic artery and portal veins are hyperenhancing compared with the hepatic veins.[27]

As previously discussed, major LI-RADS criteria for the diagnosis of HCC include size, nonrim arterial-phase hyperenhancement, nonperipheral washout, an enhancing capsule, and threshold growth (defined as ≥50% size increase in ≤6 months).[28] Note that lesion size should not be measured on the arterial phase, as peritumoral arterial enhancement and mistiming of the arterial phase can lead to inaccurate measurements.[27]

Other imaging appearances of HCC, which are listed as ancillary features in LI-RADS (see Table 10.4), include corona enhancement, nodule-in-nodule architecture, mosaic architecture, intralesional fat, and blood products within a mass.[33,35] Corona enhancement is a rim of peritumoral enhancement seen in more progressed HCC. This finding is seen in the late arterial or early portal venous phase and is caused by aberrant tumor venous drainage into adjacent portal venules and sinusoids.[29,36] When an outer nodule contains an inner nodule that displays an enhancement pattern suggestive of HCC, this is referred to as nodule-in-nodule architecture and is the result of HCC developing within a DN.[33,36] When a lesion contains randomly distributed nodules and compartments that demonstrate varying sizes, shapes, and enhancement patterns, it has mosaic architecture. Intralesional fat and blood products

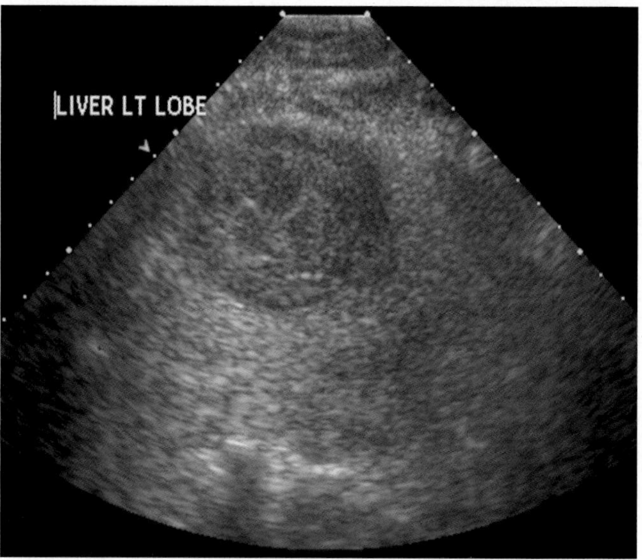

Figure 10.3. Transabdominal ultrasound of the liver shows a hypoechoic solid mass in the left lobe of the liver, consistent with hepatocellular carcinoma.

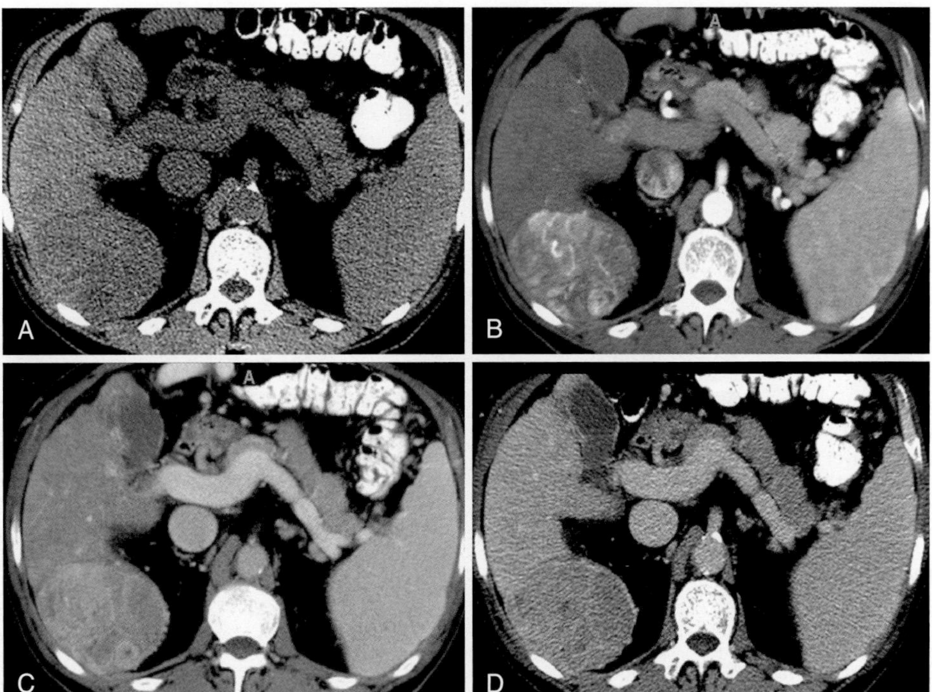

FIGURE 10.4. **A**, Noncontrast computed tomography (CT) scan of the abdomen shows a hypoattenuating mass in segment VI of the liver. **B**, Late arterial–phase CT of the abdomen shows an arterially enhancing mass in segment VI of the liver. **C**, Portal venous–phase CT of the abdomen shows a mostly isoattenuating mass in segment VI of the liver with some areas of washout. **D**, Delayed-phase CT of the abdomen shows a hypointense mass in segment VI of the liver with a late-enhancing pseudocapsule, consistent with hepatocellular carcinoma.

in a lesion manifest on unenhanced CT as areas of hypoattenuation and hyperattenuation, respectively.[29,33,36]

The presence of regenerative, siderotic, and DNs in a cirrhotic liver can complicate the diagnosis of HCC. RNs can be micronodular (<3 mm) or macronodular (≥3 mm).[37] RNs are usually isoattenuating to adjacent liver parenchyma on both unenhanced and enhanced CT. They are occasionally hypoattenuating on the portal venous phase due to enhancement of surrounding liver fibrosis.[38] Siderotic nodules contain iron deposits that result in hyperattenuation on unenhanced CT. These nodules are usually isoattenuating or hypoattenuating on arterial phase and hypoattenuating on portal venous phase.[39] Low-grade DNs are typically hypoattenuating or isoattenuating on arterial and portal venous phases. High-grade DNs can occasionally demonstrate hyperenhancement on arterial phase, as seen in HCC. These nodules can usually be distinguished from HCC by the absence of a pseudocapsule and washout on portal venous and delayed phases.[36–38]

KEY POINTS Computed Tomography of Hepatocellular Carcinoma

- Multiphasic computed tomography (CT) study is required for hepatocellular carcinoma (HCC) diagnosis.
- Major Liver Imaging Reporting and Data System (LI-RADS) criteria include size, nonrim arterial phase enhancement, an enhancing capsule, nonperipheral washout, and threshold growth.
- Other characteristics of HCC on CT are included in LI-RADS ancillary features.

Magnetic Resonance Imaging

HCC can be evaluated using either a 1.5T or a I3T MR system. In- and out-of-phase T1-weighted (T1W) images and T2-weighted (T2W) images with or without fat suppression are required precontrasted sequences. Diffusion-weighted images are often included, but are not required in the LI-RADS technical requirements. T1 fat-saturated pre- and postcontrasted images can be obtained using either extracellular (i.e., Gadoteridol) or hepatobiliary (i.e., gadoxetic acid) contrast agents.[28]

Hepatobiliary contrast agents differ from extracellular agents because, after first distributing to the extracellular space, they are either excreted by the kidneys through glomerular filtration or taken up by hepatocytes. The proportion of contrast excreted by the kidneys versus the hepatocytes depends on the particular agent. Hepatobiliary agents are taken up by hepatocytes via the organic anion transporting polypeptide 1 (OATP1), the same transporter used for bilirubin.[40] Excretion of hepatobiliary agents into the biliary system via the canalicular multispecific organic anion transport results in increased signal within the bile ducts, gallbladder, and, ultimately, the duodenum, on T1Wimaging. Biliary transit time is dependent almost exclusively on liver function. In patients with normal liver function, contrast can appear in the biliary system in as early as 5 minutes after injection.[41]

Late arterial, portal venous, and delayed (2–5 min following injection) phase images should be obtained for extracellular agents. If using a hepatobiliary agent, late arterial phase, portal venous phase, transitional phase (2–5 min

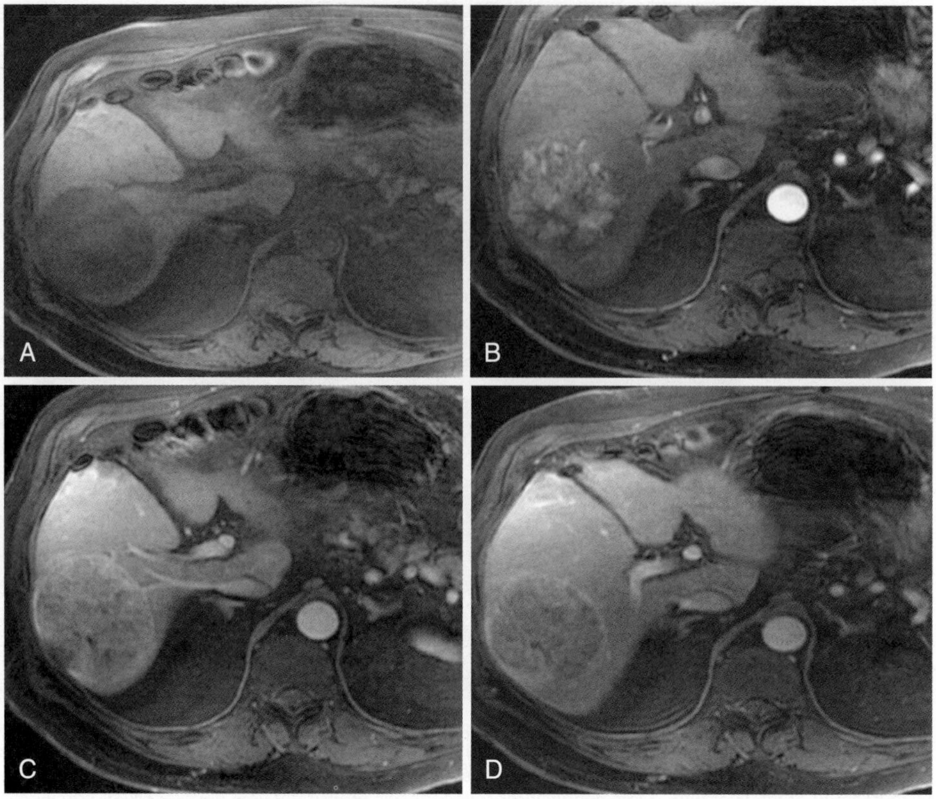

FIGURE 10.5. **A**, Axial precontrast fat-saturated three-dimensional (3D) gradient echo (LAVA) image of the liver shows a hypointense mass in the right lobe of the liver. **B**, Axial late arterial fat-saturated 3D gradient echo (LAVA) image of the liver shows an arterially enhancing mass in the right lobe of the liver. **C**, Axial portal venous fat-saturated 3D gradient (LAVA) echo series of the liver shows an isointense complex mass in the right lobe of the liver. **D**, Axial delayed fat-saturated 3D gradient (LAVA) echo series of the liver shows a hypointense mass with an enhancing pseudocapsule in the right lobe of the liver. *LAVA*, Liver acquisition with volume acceleration.

after injection), and hepatobiliary phase (10–20 min following injection) images should be acquired.[27,28,41] The transitional phase is not equivalent to the delayed phase obtained with extracellular agents. It occurs as contrast enhancement shifts from predominately extracellular to predominately intracellular.[36]

The major LI-RADS criteria for diagnosing HCC are the same as for CT and include size, nonrim arterial-phase hyperenhancement, nonperipheral washout, an enhancing capsule, and threshold growth (defined as ≥50% size increase in ≤6 months) (Fig. 10.5).[28] Similar to CT, lesions should not be measured on the arterial phase. Additionally, lesion measurements should not be made on diffusion-weighted images, since these measurements could be inaccurate because of phase errors and geometric distortion from susceptibility artifacts.[27]

Several additional features of HCC on MRI include corona enhancement, nodule-in-nodule architecture, mosaic architecture, restricted diffusion, mild/moderate T2 hyperintensity, iron sparing in a solid mass, hepatobiliary phase hypointensity, intralesional fat, and intralesional hemorrhage. As with CT, corona enhancement on MRI is defined as peritumoral enhancement seen on the late arterial or early portal venous phase that occurs because of aberrant venous drainage into adjacent portal venules and sinusoids.[29,36] In nodule-in-nodule architecture, the inner nodule will show signal characteristics (i.e., diffusion restriction and T2 hyperintensity) and an enhancement pattern (i.e., arterial enhancement) suggestive of HCC when compared with the outer nodule. Similar to CT, heterogeneous signal characteristics and enhancement patterns are seen in lesions with mosaic architecture; this heterogeneity of signal is due to the varying degree of blood products, fat, and fibrosis. Restricted diffusion and mild/moderate T2 hyperintensity are features suggestive of malignancy in general and are not specific for HCC.[36] Iron sparing within a solid mass appears as a T2 isointense focus (corresponding to HCC) within a T2 hypointense siderotic nodule. This finding occurs because HCC loses the ability to accumulate iron.[29,33,36] Hepatobiliary phase hypointensity is defined as lesion hypointensity compared to the surrounding liver 10 to 20 minutes after the administration of a hepatobiliary contrast agent. This occurs because HCC usually has decreased expression of OATP1, which is responsible for contrast uptake.[29,33,40] However, it is important to note that some well- and moderately differentiated HCCs can display hepatobiliary contrast uptake due to OATP1 expression. These tumors will display hepatobiliary phase isointensity or hyperintensity.[40] Intralesional fat appears as an area of hypointensity on T1 opposed phase images. Intralesional hemorrhage has variable T1 and T2 signal characteristics depending on the age of the blood products.[29]

MRI is also useful in characterizing RNs, siderotic modules, and DNs. RNs are typically isointense on T1-, T2-, and diffusion-weighted images. Following contrast, these nodules are usually isointense on the arterial, portal venous, and hepatobiliary phases. Siderotic nodules

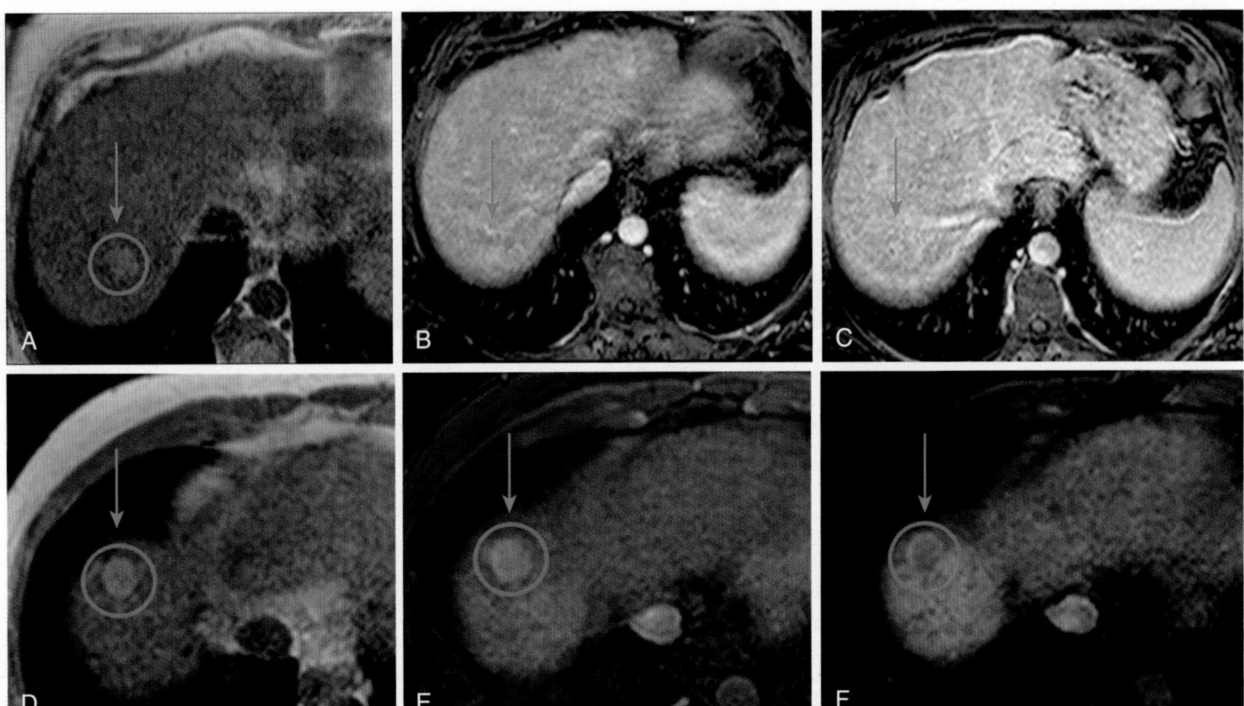

FIGURE 10.6. **A**, Axial T1-weighted (T1W) magnetic resonance (MR) image without fat saturation shows a T1-hyperintense nodule in the posterior right hepatic lobe indicated by green arrow and circle. **B**, This nodule in the posterior right hepatic lobe does not demonstrate nonrim arterial phase hyperenhancement on the axial, postcontrast arterial-phase T1W fat-saturated MR images with expected nodule location indicated by green arrow. **C**, No washout or pseudocapsule is seen on postcontrast portal-venous phase, T1W axial MR images, consistent with a dysplastic nodule. **D**, A different nodule in the posterior right hepatic lobe demonstrates intrinsic T1-signal hyperintensity on axial T1W non–fat-saturated precontrast images indicated by green arrow and circle. **E**, This nodule does demonstrate nonrim arterial phase hyperenhancement on axial T1W images. **F**, This nodule also demonstrates central washout and peripheral pseudocapsule on axial T1W portal-venous phase MR images, consistent with hepatocellular carcinoma, most likely arising within a dysplastic nodule.

are usually hypointense or isointense on T1 in phase images and hypointense on T2W images. These nodules are usually isointense or hypointense on arterial phase and hypointense on the portal venous and hepatobiliary phases. DNs can be hyperintense or isointense on T1 in phase images and are either isointense or hypointense on T2W images. Postcontrasted images usually demonstrate isointensity or hypointensity on the arterial/portal venous phases and isointensity on the hepatobiliary phase (Fig. 10.6). High-grade DNs can occasionally display arterial phase hyperintensity and hepatobiliary phase hypointensity, as seen in HCC.[39]

KEY POINTS Magnetic Resonance Imaging of Hepatocellular Carcinoma

- Multiphasic magnetic resonance imaging (MRI) with extracellular or hepatobiliary contrast agents can be used to evaluate hepatocellular carcinoma (HCC).
- Major Liver Imaging Reporting and Data System criteria include size, nonrim arterial phase enhancement, an enhancing capsule, nonperipheral washout, and threshold growth.
- HCC has many ancillary features on MRI that can aid in diagnosis.
- MRI can help distinguish regenerative, siderotic, and dyplastic nodules from HCC.

Positron Emission Tomography

The role of 2-[^{18}F] fluoro-2-deoxy-D-glucose positron emission tomography (FDG PET) is limited in the evaluation of patients with HCC. The sensitivity of FDG PET for HCC is 50% to 60%.[42–44] It has been suggested that there is an association between the degree of FDG uptake and the histology of the tumors, tumor size, vascular endothelial growth factor (VEGF) expression, and doubling time. Well-differentiated tumors exhibit less uptake, whereas poorly differentiated tumors show more activity (Fig. 10.7).[42–44] In the setting of extrahepatic disease, FDG PET may assist in the detection of metastatic disease. However, a negative FDG PET examination does not exclude metastatic disease.

11C acetate–PET imaging has been evaluated in the characterization of liver lesions. The tracer is short-lived, with a half-life of only 20 minutes (18F has a half-life of 110 min). It has been postulated that the combination of FDG -PET and 11C acetate–PET can provide improved specificity and sensitivity in the detection of HCC. An FDG PET scan and an 11C acetate–PET scan that are both positive makes the diagnosis of HCC very likely. An FDG PET scan that is positive with a negative 11C acetate–PET scan makes the diagnosis of a poorly differentiated HCC or a non-HCC malignancy more likely. In the setting of a negative FDG PET scan and a negative 11C acetate–PET scan, benign lesions are the most common diagnoses.[45]

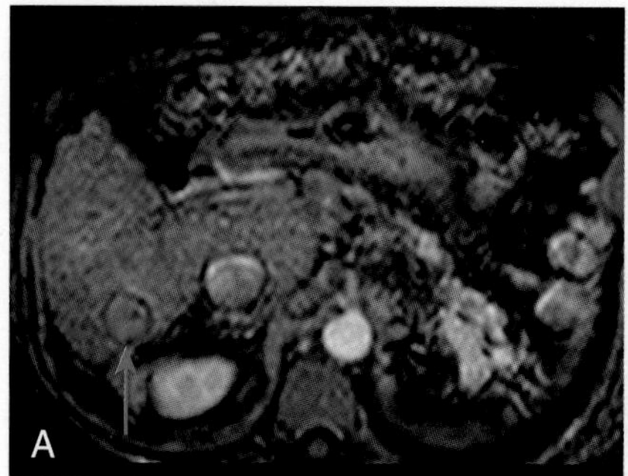

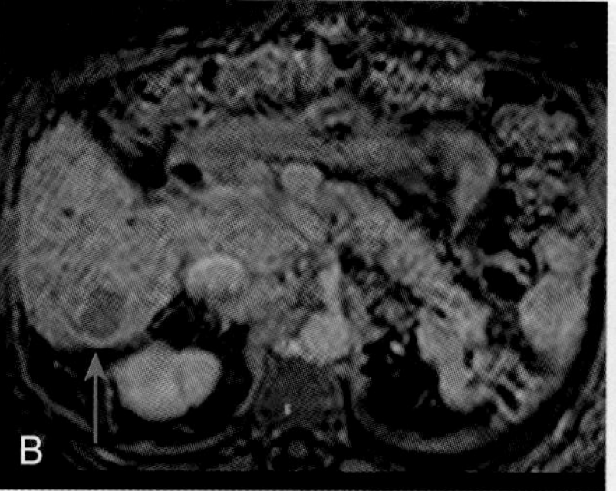

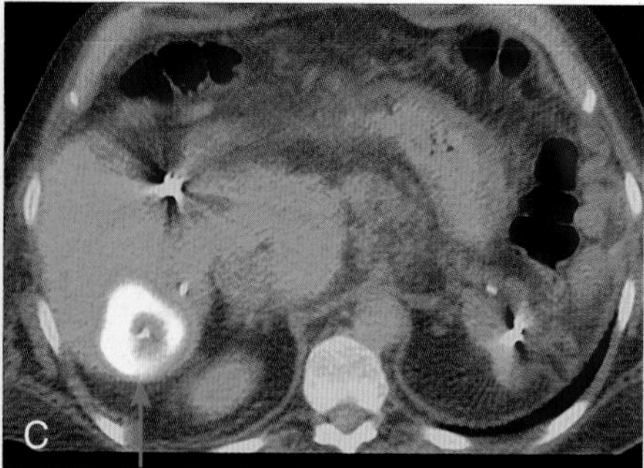

FIGURE 10.7. A, Axial T1-weighted (T1W) postcontrast arterial phase magnetic resonance (MR) image with posterior right hepatic lobe enhancing lesion (*arrow*). **B**, Axial T1W postcontrast portal-venous phase MR image with washout within this posterior right hepatic lobe lesion, consistent with hepatocellular carcinoma. **C**, Axial 2-[^{18}F] fluoro-2-deoxy-D-glucose positron emission tomography/computed tomography fused scan of the abdomen shows metabolic activity in the right hepatic lobe lesion, most consistent with poorly differentiated hepatocellular carcinoma.

KEY POINTS Positron Emission Tomography Imaging of Hepatocellular Carcinoma

- 2-[^{18}F] fluoro-2-deoxy-D-glucose positron emission tomography (FDG PET) has a limited role and may assist in detecting extrahepatic disease.
- A combination of 11C acetate–PET and FDG PET can improve the specificity of PET.

Lymph Nodes

The radiologic evaluation of lymph nodes is based on size, morphology, and location.[46,47] Nodes larger than 1 cm are more likely to be malignant. Nodes located near the primary tumor are also likely to be malignant, even if they measure less than 1 cm in minimum diameter. A round node is also more likely to be malignant than an oval node. In patients with cirrhosis, enlarged nodes (>1.5 cm) are commonly seen in the portocaval nodal station and along the hepatoduodenal ligament. Although these nodes are commonly reactive, the distinction between malignant and benign nodes in this setting is difficult. Imaging features that suggest a malignant node include a pattern of enhancement during the multiphase images that resembles HCC and a necrotic/heterogeneous appearance. Nodal stations that should be carefully examined in a patient with HCC include the anterior, posterior, and middle diaphragmatic; celiac; hepatic artery; left gastric; and retroperitoneal nodal stations.[47,48]

KEY POINTS Imaging of Lymph Nodes of Hepatocellular Carcinoma

- Nodes that are larger than 1 cm, necrotic, or have an HCC image pattern are indicative of malignancy.
- Enlarged lymph nodes may be seen in the periportal region in the setting of cirrhosis and are often benign.
- Diffusion-weighted imaging may be useful in the detection of nodal disease.

Metastatic Disease

As discussed earlier, the pattern of tumor spread for HCC may be extrahepatic or intrahepatic. Intrahepatic spread may include extension of tumor into the portal or hepatic vein. In addition to tumor thrombus, bland thrombus of these vessels may be encountered. The distinction between these two entities is important for staging classification and surgical planning. A portal vein diameter greater than 23 mm is highly suggestive of tumor thrombus.[49] Portal vein tumor will also demonstrate early enhancement during the late arterial phase of contrast administration (Fig. 10.8).[50,51] US evaluation with color Doppler imaging or CEUS may be helpful in detecting tumor extension into the portal or hepatic vein. On CT and MRI examination, early enhancement of the portal vein may not be due to tumor thrombus but rather arterial portal shunting in the tumor. In the setting of a vascular shunt, the delay images will not show thrombus in the portal vein.

Distant metastatic disease can be assessed with a chest radiograph or CT of the chest to evaluate for lung metastases. Evaluating bone windows on CT of the abdomen and pelvis may demonstrate skeletal metastases. Soft tissue nodules in the peritoneum seen on CT may represent metastatic deposits; however, these nodules can also be obscured by extensive ascites. Diffusion-weighted imaging may increase the conspicuity of these nodules because the high signal from ascitic fluid is suppressed.

KEY POINTS Imaging of Metastases of Hepatocellular Carcinoma

- Portal vein tumor thrombus will arterially enhance.
- Chest computed tomography is recommended to evaluate for lung metastases.
- Diffusion-weighted imaging may be useful in the detection of metastatic disease.

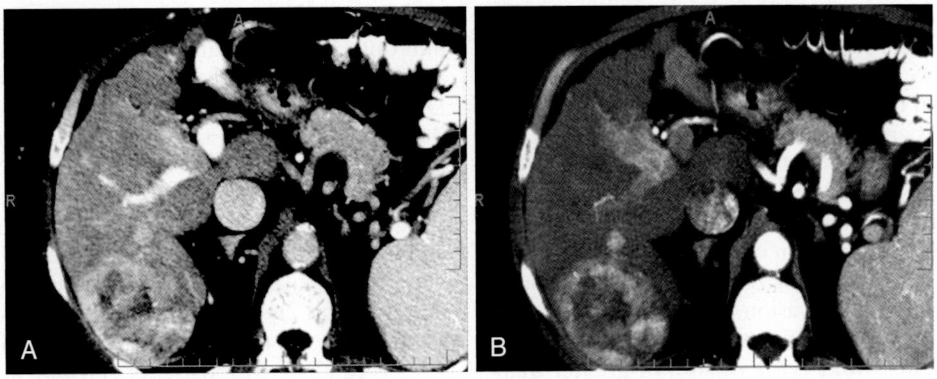

FIGURE 10.8. **A**, Late arterial-phase contrast-enhanced computed tomography (CT) of the abdomen shows early enhancement of the right portal vein, consistent with tumor thrombosis. **B**, Portal venous-phase contrast-enhanced CT of the abdomen shows thrombus in the right portal vein.

TREATMENT

Liver Resection

Pretreatment imaging with CT and/or MRI is essential to stratify the patient as a surgical candidate. Providing detailed anatomic information about the tumor aids the surgeon in patient selection and determining if special resection techniques are needed. Important information includes tumor relationship to adjacent vasculature and bile ducts, arterial supply, nodal disease, segmental involvement, and extrahepatic disease.[52,53] Incidentally, the size of the tumor is not a contraindication to resection, with a 35% 5-year survival reported for patients with masses larger than 10 cm.[54] In addition to anatomic information, knowledge of the patient's underlying liver disease is required. For example, a patient with poor liver function (Child–Pugh C) is a contraindication to liver resection.

For patients considered for resection, volumetric studies are commonly used to assess residual functional liver reserve (FLR). For a noncirrhotic liver, an FLR of 20% is recommended to reduce surgical morbidity.[55] For the cirrhotic patient, a higher FLR of 40% is recommended. In the setting of suboptimal FLR, preoperative portal vein embolization is performed to induce compensatory hypertrophy.[56]

The location and number of the lesions will dictate the surgical approach. Open surgical resection may include extended resection, anatomic resection, and nonanatomic resection.[53,57,58] Extended resection refers to the removal of at least four liver segments with or without biliary and vascular resection, anatomic resection refers to segmental resection, and nonanatomic resection refers to resection of the HCC with a 1-cm margin of normal tissue. Nonanatomic resection is the less favorable technique and has a high risk of recurrence owing to the nonresection of micrometastases.[57] The use of laparoscopic US may assist in the detection of vascular involvement and screening of the nonresected liver.

Overall survival and recurrence free–survival have improved in patients with anatomic (segmental) resection of the liver.[59,60] In addition, the operative mortality rate for partial hepatectomy is less than 5%.[55] The reported overall 5-year survival after resection ranges from 24% to 76%.[61–63] The 5-year survival for tumors less than 5 cm is over 70%.[63,64] *En bloc* resection of primary tumors and vascular tributaries potentially reduces the risk of recurrent disease.

KEY POINTS Liver Resection for Hepatocellular Carcinoma

- Location and number of lesions dictate surgical approach.
- Size is not a contraindication for resection.
- Portal vein embolization improves functional liver reserve.

Liver Transplant

Liver transplant is a potentially curative treatment for HCC, with reported 5-year posttransplant survival rates as high as 80%.[1,15,65] Under the current United Network for Organ Sharing (UNOS) policy, HCC patients must meet Milan criteria and have an AFP less than 1000 to be transplant eligible.[1] The Milan criteria are defined as one lesion less than or equal to 5 cm or up to three lesions of 3 cm or smaller.[66] Both HCC and non-HCC transplant candidates are prioritized on the waiting list using the Model for End-Stage Liver Disease (MELD) score. The MELD score assesses the severity of liver disease and is calculated using international normalized ratio, bilirubin, and creatinine.[67] Mortality in patients with HCC is often due to cancer rather than underlying liver disease.[68] As a result, these patients' MELD scores are generally lower at the time of HCC diagnosis compared with those of non-HCC transplant candidates. In order to allocate liver allografts evenly, the current UNOS policy grants a MELD exception score of 28 to HCC patients who meet transplant criteria 6 months after their initial diagnosis.[1]

Locoregional therapies, such as radiofrequency ablation (RFA) and TACE, are often used to control tumor burden to keep patients within Milan criteria. These therapies are also used to downstage patients who are initially outside of Milan criteria to within acceptable transplant criteria. The University of California San Francisco downstaging protocol was adopted by UNOS in 2017.[1] Eligible patients must have a single lesion 8 cm or smaller, two to three lesions 5 cm or smaller with the sum of maximal tumor diameters 8 cm or smaller, or four to five lesions 3 cm or smaller with the sum of maximal tumor diameters 8 cm or smaller.[69]

The rate of HCC recurrence after transplant is 11% to 18%.[1] The Risk Estimation of Tumor Recurrence After Transplant score has been shown to be a reliable predictor of HCC recurrence after transplant. Variables used in the score calculation are the sum of the largest diameter of viable tumor plus the number of viable tumors on explant, presence of microvascular invasion on explant pathology, and AFP levels at the time of transplant. The 5-year recurrence risks of patients with a score of zero or greater than five are less than 3% and greater than 75%, respectively.[70] The Model of Recurrence After Liver transplantation score is another reliable system to predict recurrence. It estimates recurrence risk using neutrophil-to-lymphocyte ratio at the time of transplant, AFP levels, tumor size, tumor number, tumor pathological grade, and the presence of vascular invasion.[71]

KEY POINTS Liver Transplant for Hepatocellular Carcinoma

- Under United Network for Organ Sharing policy, patients must be with Milan criteria and have α-fetoprotein under 1000 to be considered for transplant.
- Liver allografts are prioritized using the Model for End-Stage Liver Disease score.
- Locoregional therapies can be used as a bridge to transplant or to downstage initially ineligible patients to within Milan criteria.

Transarterial Chemoembolization

TACE induces direct cytotoxicity and ischemia by delivering chemotherapy and embolic material directly to the tumor. It is used for palliation and as a bridge to transplant in patients with intermediate stage disease (BCLB stage B).[1,72,73] Conventional TACE (c-TACE) and drug-eluting bead TACE (DEB-TACE) are the two most commonly used techniques.[73,74]

In c-TACE, a mixture of doxorubicin emulsified in lipiodol and an embolic agent (typically gelfoam) is injected into an artery supplying the tumor. The lipiodol/doxorubicin mixture is taken up by tumor cells and is often retained for months.[75] A systematic review of seven randomized controlled trials that included a total of 545 patients showed improved 2-year survival in patients receiving c-TACE compared with patients receiving supportive care alone.[76] Although there is a clear survival benefit, many patients cannot tolerate c-TACE owing to systemic toxicity.[72,74,77] Another issue is that numerous HCCs demonstrate no lipiodol uptake, resulting in decreased treatment efficacy.[73,75]

In DEB-TACE, doxorubicin-eluting beads are injected into the tumor-supplying artery. The nonbiodegradable polyvinyl alcohol beads typically measure 100 to 300 microns. The beads are loaded with doxorubicin through an ion exchange mechanism.[72,77] Compared with c-TACE, DEB-TACE delivers a higher concentration of chemotherapy agent to the tumor, which results in lower serum levels and less systemic toxicity.[72,74,77,78] Although DEB-TACE has less systemic toxicity, studies are conflicting about which TACE method has superior efficacy.[72] A metaanalysis including seven studies with a total of 700 patients revealed that DEB-TACE was associated with better 1- and 2-year survival rates compared to c-TACE.[79] Conversely, another metaanalysis including seven studies with a total of 693 patients showed no statistically significant difference in tumor response when comparing DEB-TACE with c-TACE.[80]

KEY POINTS Transarterial Chemoembolization for Hepatocellular Carcinoma

- Transarterial chemoembolization (TACE) induces cytotoxicity and ischemia via direct delivery of chemotherapy and embolic agents to the tumor.
- Conventional TACE and drug-eluting bead TACE (DEB-TACE) are the two techniques used.
- Studies are conflicting regarding which method has superior efficacy.
- DEB-TACE typically has less systemic toxicity.

Ablation

Liver ablation is used in patients with very early-stage and early-stage HCC (BCLC stage 0 and A).[1,81] Ablation can be used as a curative therapy or as a bridge to transplant.[82] Heat-based ablation therapies, such as RFA and microwave ablation, are currently favored over chemical ablation with ethanol.

RFA delivers alternating electrical current directly to the tumor through a needle electrode placed under image guidance.[81–83] Resistive heating occurs as the target tissue ions attempt to follow the applied current.[81,83] The target tissue undergoes coagulative necrosis once temperatures reach 60°C to 100°C.[82] A 0.5- to 1-cm margin surrounding the tumor should be ablated to ensure adequate treatment of microscopic tumor extension.[82,83] Ablation has a higher success rate in tumors less than 3 cm that are at least 1 cm away from adjacent vasculature.[82,84] Blood flow from adjacent vasculature decreases ablation temperatures through convective heat loss, which results in decreased treatment efficacy.[85] In single tumors measuring 3 to 5 cm, RFA combined with TACE can improve treatment response.[81,84]

Microwave ablation generates heat by agitating water molecules through a monopolar electrode placed under image guidance.[82,84,85] Similar to RFA, tissue death occurs by coagulation necrosis.[84,85] Microwave ablation is faster and produces a larger ablation zone compared to RFA.[84] In addition, microwave ablation is not limited by convective heat loss from adjacent blood flow.[81,85]

Key Points Radiofrequency Ablation for Hepatocellular Carcinoma

- Radiofrequency ablation (RFA) can be used as a curative treatment or bridge to transplant.
- RFA induces coagulative necrosis by delivering electrical current directly to the tumor.
- RFA achieves optimal results in tumors smaller than 3 cm located more than 1 cm from an adjacent vessel.
- Microwave ablation is faster and achieves a larger ablation zone compared with RFA.

Systemic Therapy

HCCs are relatively chemoresistant tumors. Many chemotherapy regimens have been tested, and have all shown negative results.15 Among the factors responsible for this chemoresistance is the presence of the *P53* mutation, which is the most common mutation in HCC. Since most HCCs have a *P53* mutation, this pathway cannot be used for chemotherapeutic apoptosis, resulting in chemoresistant tumors. Other factors such as the overexpression of DNA topoisomerase II alpha and p-glycoprotein are thought to contribute to the chemoresistance of HCC.[86]

Sorafenib and lenvatinib are U.S. Food and Drug Administration (FDA)–approved first-line treatments for unresectable HCC. Sorafenib is an oral multikinase inhibitor that blocks tumor proliferation by targeting various growth factor pathways and exerts antiangiogenic effects by targeting tyrosine kinase VEGF-2,3 and PDGFR-β.[87] The significant vascularity of HCC reflects intense activation of angiogenic signaling pathways, and sorafenib's antiagiogenic effects target these pathways. The Sorafenib Hepatocarcinoma Assessment Randomized Protocol trial reported a 2.8-month improvement in median overall survival rate, along with increased time to progression and disease control rate, but only a 2.3% response rate as assessed by response evaluation criteria in solid tumors (RECIST) criteria.[87,88] Lenvatinib inhibits VEGF 1–3, PDGFR-α, FGF 1–4, KIT, and RET. A more recent study compared lenvatinib with sorafenib in a cohort of 954 patient with unresectable HCC. The results showed that lenvatinib was noninferior to sorafenib in terms of overall survival.[89]

Current FDA-approved second-line treatments for unresectable HCC include regorafenib and nivolumab.[1,15] Regorafenib is an oral multikinase inhibitor that inhibits several important tumorigenic and angiogenic kinases.[90] A study performed by Bruix et al. demonstrated that regorafenib increased median survival from 7.8 months to 10.6 months in patients with HCC progression despite sorafenib therapy.[77] Nivolumab is a monoclonal antibody that increases the antitumor activity of T cells by inhibiting PD-1 signaling. A recent dose escalation and expansion trial in patients with advanced HCC showed a 15% and 20% objective response rate (using RECIST version 1.1) in the dose-escalation and dose-expansion phase, respectively.[91]

Key Points Systemic Therapy for Hepatocellular Carcinoma

- Hepatocellular carcinoma is relatively chemoresistant, and most agents failed to improve survival.
- Sorafenib and lenvatinib are current U.S. Food and Drug Administration (FDA)–approved first-line agents.
- FDA-approved second-line agents include regofenib and nivolumab.

Radioembolization

HCC is sensitive to radiotherapy; however, external beam radiation is limited, because damage to adjacent liver parenchyma can occur with radiation doses as low as 35 Gy.[92–94] TARE significantly decreases the chance of adjacent liver parenchymal injury by delivering a radioisotope directly into the tumor-supplying artery. The most commonly used radioisotope is yttrium-90 (^{90}Y). ^{90}Y is a pure beta emitter that is loaded onto resin or glass microspheres measuring less than 40 microns.[92–97] Because of their smaller size, these microspheres have minimal embolic effect when compared with TACE. As a result, TARE can be used in the setting of tumor portal vein thrombosis, whereas TACE is contraindicated.[92,94,96,98] Before treatment, a simulation is performed using technetium-99m–labeled macroaggregated albumin particles. Hepatopulmonary shunting and average tumor radiation dose are then calculated using single-photon emission computed tomography and/or planar gamma camera imaging.[92,94]

TACE is the most widely accepted treatment for intermediate-stage disease; however, many studies evaluating ^{90}Y have shown positive results. A metaanalysis of 10 studies revealed similar overall survival rates in patients receiving ^{90}Y and TACE.[96] However, a *post hoc* analysis demonstrated that a randomized control trial with more than 1000 patients would be needed to show a true survival difference.[98] ^{90}Y could play a major role in patients receiving therapy as a bridge to transplantation. A randomized study with 45 patients demonstrated a longer time to progression in the ^{90}Y group (>26 months) compared with the c-TACE group (6.8 months).[99] Similarly, a comparative effectiveness analysis of 463 patients showed a longer time to progression in the ^{90}Y group.[98]

Key Points Radioembolization for Hepatocellular Carcinoma

- Radioembolization delivers radioisotope (yttrium-90) directly to the tumor.
- Minimal embolic effect compared to transarterial chemoembolization (TACE), making it suitable for treating patients with malignant portal vein thrombus.
- More data is needed to prove a clear survival benefit compared to TACE.

Stereotactic Body Radiotherapy

Stereotactic body radiation (SBRT) is a radiation technique in which high doses of radiation are administered in fewer than 10 fractions. The radiation is delivered in a geometrically precise manner that reduces the risk of radiation-induced liver disease.[100–102] SBRT causes tumor cell death by damaging DNA and local vasculature.[100]

SBRT has been shown to be safe and effective. A study of SBRT in 60 patients with a median tumor diameter of 3.1 cm showed favorable local control, decreased time to progression, increased progression-free survival, and increased overall survival.[103] An additional sequential phase I and II study of 102 patients with locally advanced HCC showed that SBRT achieved a local control rate of 87%.[101] SBRT has also been shown to be an effective alternative to other locoregional therapies as a bridge to transplant. An intention-to-treat analysis compared SBRT to both TACE and RFA as a bridge to transplant. The results showed that SBRT has similar safety and efficacy compared to TACE and RFA.[104] SBRT has also been shown to be effective when combined with other therapies. A recent propensity score matched analysis compared 49 patients receiving TACE plus SRBT versus 98 patients receiving TACE alone. The TACE+SBRT group had better 1- and 3-year overall and progression-free survival.[102]

KEY POINTS Stereotactic Body Radiotherapy for Hepatocellular Carcinoma

- High doses of fractionated radiation are administered in a geometrically precise manner.
- Effective alternative therapy as a bridge to transplant.
- Combination with transarterial chemoembolization has been shown to increase survival.

POSTTREATMENT IMAGING

Liver Imaging Reporting and Data System Assessment

A multiphase CT or MRI is typically obtained 3 months after treatment to assess tumor response. LI-RADS version 2017 introduced an algorithm to help assess treatment response and guide further management decisions.[28,105] The algorithm can be used following percutaneous ablation, TACE, surgical resection, radioembolization, and SBRT. Importantly, the algorithm was not developed to be used following systemic chemotherapy or immunologic therapy.[28]

The LI-RADS treatment response (LR-TR) categories are divided into LR-TR nonviable, LR-TR viable, and LR-TR equivocal. The LR-TR nonviable category is assigned when a treated lesion shows either no residual enhancement or expected posttreatment-related enhancement. A treated lesion is categorized as LR-TR viable when it has residual irregular/nodular arterial enhancement and/or washout or an enhancement pattern similar to pretreatment. LR-TR equivocal is reserved for treated lesions not meeting criteria for either LR-TR viable or LR-TR nonviable. The size of LR-TR viable lesions should be reported using the single largest measurement of the enhancing component. Nonenhancing components should not be included in the measurement.[28,105]

KEY POINTS Liver Imaging Reporting and Data System Posttreatment Assessment

- Algorithm cannot be applied following chemotherapy or immunologic therapy.
- Tumors are categorized as nonviable, viable, or equivocal.
- Irregular/nodular enhancement and washout of a treated lesion is worrisome for residual tumor viability.

Imaging Following Radiofrequency Ablation

Imaging obtained shortly after ablation may show small air bubbles in the ablation bed. These usually resolve in 1 month and should not be mistaken for an abscess.[106] At 1- to 3-month follow-up, a thin rim of enhancement surrounding the ablation cavity is often observed. This enhancement is due to reactive tissue hyperemia and/or small iatrogenic arterioportal shunts. This finding should be distinguished from nodular/irregular enhancement, which is observed in residual tumor.[105,106] Central hyperdensity and T1 hyperintensity can be observed on CT and MRI as a result of ablation-induced coagulative necrosis.[106] The ablation cavity is typically larger than the original tumor because a 5- to 10-mm margin of normal liver parenchyma is included in the ablation zone to treat potential microscopic tumor extension.[105,106] On follow-up imaging, the ablation cavity will decrease in size (Fig. 10.9); interval enlargement is suspicious for residual viable disease (Fig. 10.10).

KEY POINTS Imaging Following Radiofrequency Ablation

- Thin rim of enhancement surrounding the ablation zone is expected.
- Nodular/irregular enhancement is worrisome for residual tumor/recurrence.

Imaging Following Transarterial Chemoembolization

A noncontrasted CT obtained shortly after c-TACE should demonstrate tumor hyperdensity from retained lipiodol (Fig. 10.11).[105] The amount of lipiodol uptake correlates with a greater degree of tumor necrosis.[105,107] Poor uptake of lipiodol suggests inadequate treatment of a tumor-supplying artery (Fig. 10.12).[106,107] Similar to RFA, a thin rim of peripheral enhancement surrounding the lesion can be seen on contrasted MRI or CT at

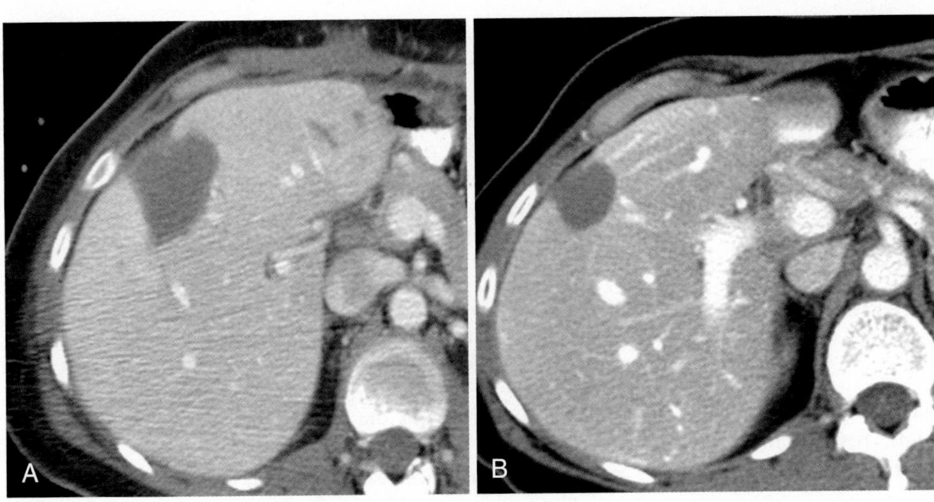

FIGURE 10.9. **A**, Computed tomography (CT) examination of the abdomen at 1 month after radiofrequency ablation (RFA) of a right lobe hepatocellular carcinoma (HCC). There is a homogeneous low-attenuation area. **B**, CT examination of the abdomen at 24 months after RFA of a right lobe HCC. There is decrease in size of the homogeneous low-attenuation area, consistent with successful response to treatment.

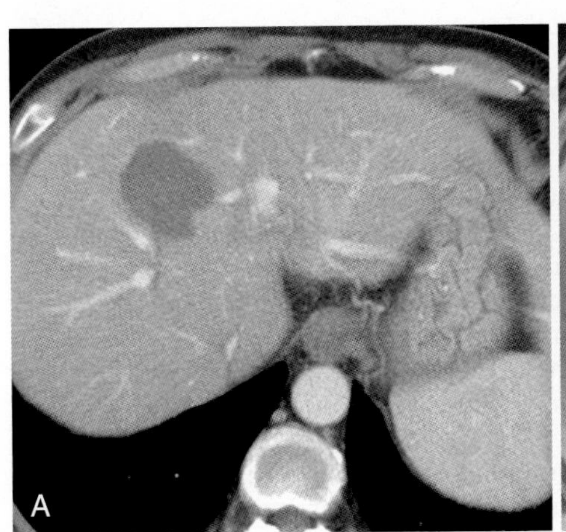

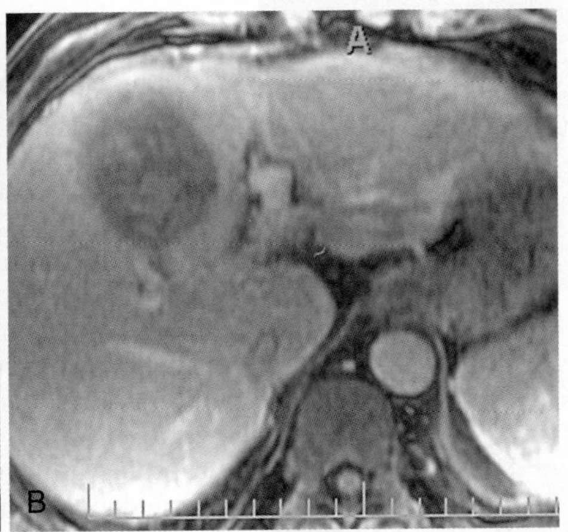

FIGURE 10.10. **A**, Computed tomography examination of the abdomen at 1 month after radiofrequency ablation (RFA) of the hepatocellular carcinoma (HCC) in the left liver shows a hypointense homogeneous mass. **B**, Magnetic resonance imaging postgadolinium image of the abdomen at 11 months after RFA of the HCC in the left lobe of the liver shows enlargement of the treated cavity, consistent with recurrent disease.

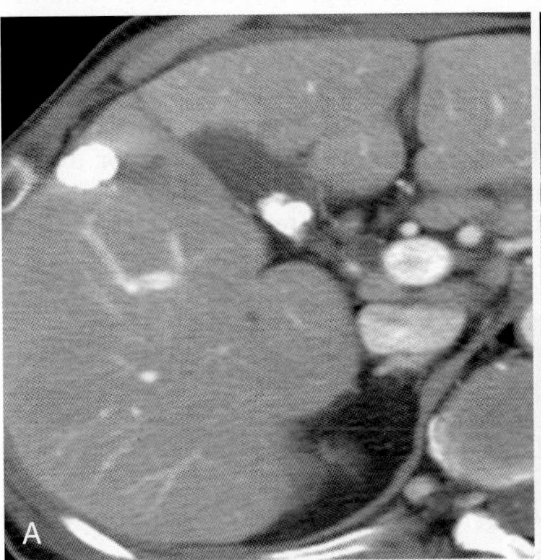

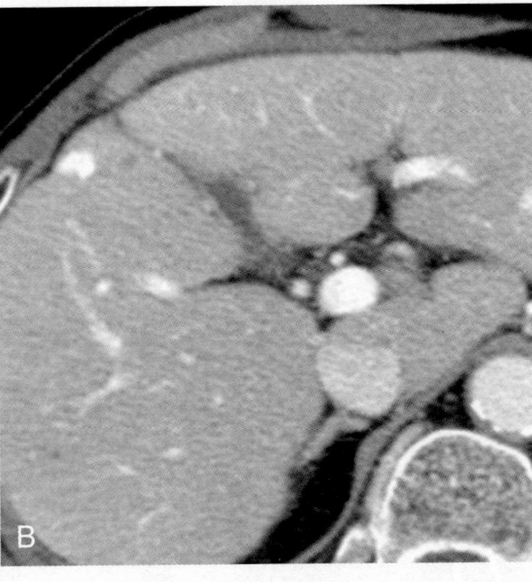

FIGURE 10.11. **A**, Computed tomography (CT) examination of the abdomen at 1 month after transarterial chemoembolization (TACE) of a right-lobe hepatocellular carcinoma (HCC). There is homogeneous uptake of lipiodol. **B**, CT examination of the abdomen at 39 months after TACE of a right-lobe HCC. There is interval decrease in size, homogeneous lipiodol, and no areas on enhancement, consistent with successful treatment.

1- to 3-month follow-up. Nodular arterial enhancement is indicative of residual tumor.[105–107] Tumors treated with c-TACE may have residual lipiodol up to 6 months after treatment, which can obscure areas of arterial phase enhancement on CT.[105,107] MRI is more accurate for detecting enhancement patterns in these cases, because lipiodol has no effect on MRI signal.[106,107] Residual tumor can also manifest as areas of T2 hyperintensity and diffusion restriction; however, these features are currently not used in the LR-TR criteria.[105,106]

KEY POINTS Imaging Following Transarterial Chemoembolization

- Poor tumor uptake of lipiodol suggests inadequate treatment.
- Residual lipiodol may be seen up to 6 mo after treatment.
- Nodular arterial enhancement is worrisome for residual tumor.

Imaging Following Transarterial Radioembolization

The microspheres used in TARE have minimal embolic effect compared with TACE, which results in variable lesion enhancement patterns at follow-up imaging.

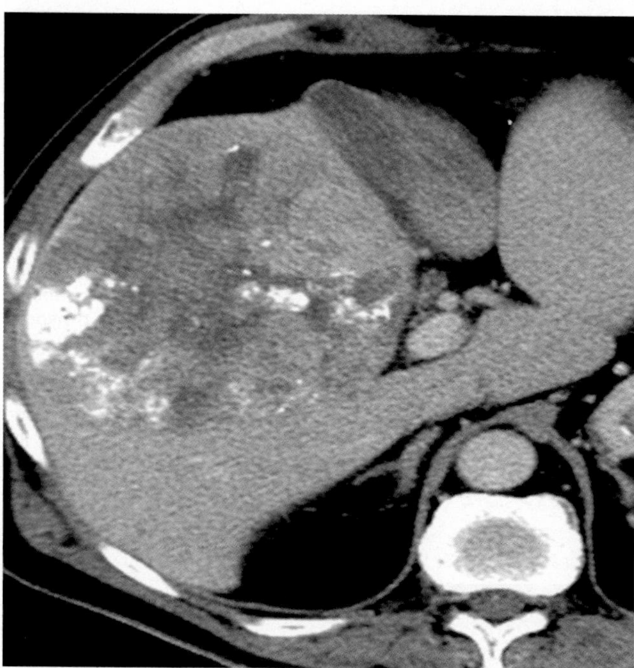

FIGURE 10.12. Computed tomography examination of the abdomen at 1 month after transarterial chemoembolization of a right-lobe hepatocellular carcinoma. There is residual tumor with areas of enhancement and incomplete opacification with lipiodol.

Nodular enhancement observed up to 6 months after treatment is not always indicative of residual tumor with TARE. A study performed by Riaz et al. showed that 38% of lesions with nodular enhancement after TARE had complete pathologic necrosis.[108] Geographic enhancement surrounding the tumor can also be seen for months following treatment and should not be mistaken for infiltrating tumor (Fig. 10.13).[105,107]

KEY POINTS Imaging Following Transarterial Radioembolization

- Enhancement patterns are variable and should be interpreted with caution.
- Geographic enhancement surrounding the treated area should not be mistaken for infiltrating tumor.

The Radiology Report

The selection criteria for each different therapeutic approach for HCC are highly dependent on the radiologic interpretation. Thus, the radiology report should include the relevant information to allow the patient to receive the best therapeutic option. Lesions should be assigned a LI-RADS score based on the degree of suspicion for HCC. The report should include a detailed description of the size, number, and segmental location of the masses. The relationship of the tumor to vessels, bile ducts, and liver capsule, with comments on any evidence of tumor invasion, should be included. Vascular anatomy, including hepatic artery variants, portal vein variants, and accessory hepatic veins, should be examined and documented. In the preoperative liver resection setting, segmental liver volumes should be calculated if the FLR is suspected to be suboptimal. The presence of cirrhosis, ascites, portal hypertension, and a fatty liver should be noted in the report. Complete radiologic staging with evaluation of the regional and distant nodes and the evaluation for intrahepatic or distant metastases should also be included. Recommendation of the appropriate follow-up time interval for indeterminate

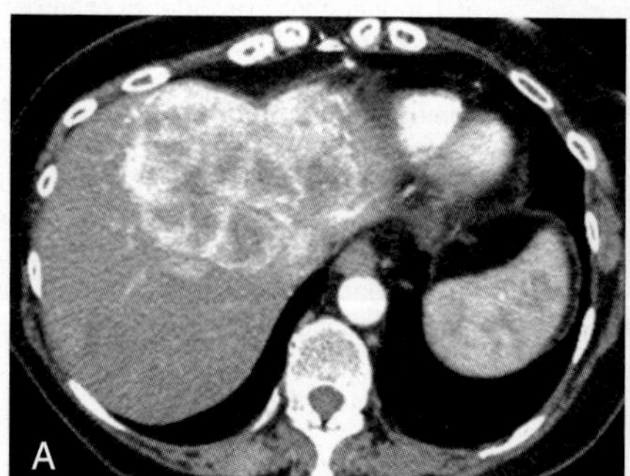

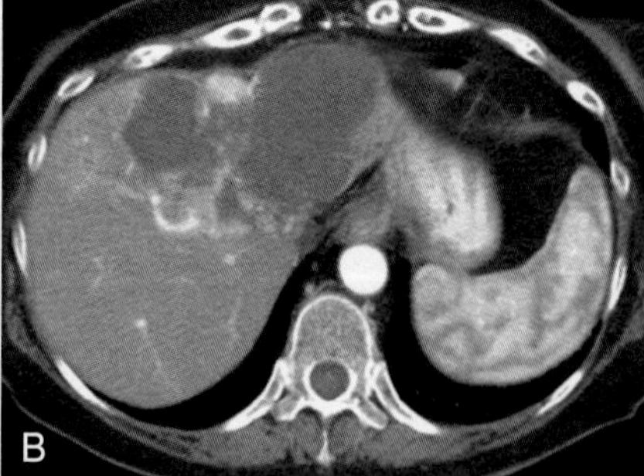

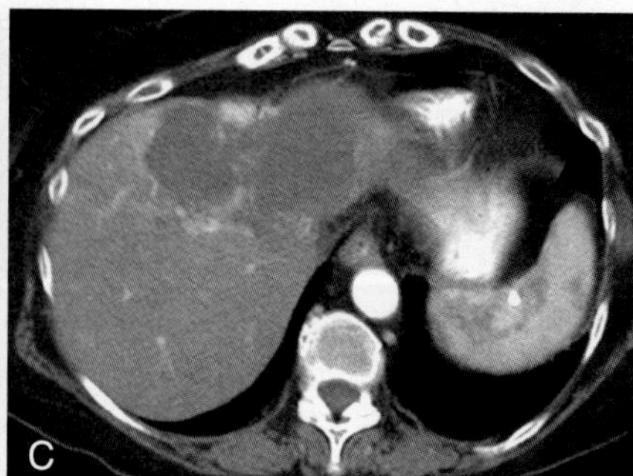

FIGURE 10.13. **A**, Late arterial-phase contrast-enhanced computed tomography (CT) of the abdomen shows a hypervascular lesion in the left liver, consistent with hepatocellular carcinoma (HCC). **B**, Late arterial–phase contrast-enhanced CT of the abdomen at 6 months after treatment with yttrium-90 shows decreased enhancement owing to necrosis of the HCC in the liver, consistent with some response to treatment. **C**, Late arterial–phase contrast-enhanced CT of the abdomen at 12 months after treatment with yttrium-90 shows continued decreased enhancement owing to necrosis of the HCC in the liver, consistent with some response to treatment without any further treatment.

lesions should be included. After therapy, the radiology report should include not only evidence of residual disease but also any evidence of complications from therapy.

Key Points The Radiology Report for Hepatocellular Carcinoma

- Liver Imaging Reporting and Data System score for suspicious lesions.
- Number, size, and segmental distribution of suspicious lesions.
- Vascular evaluation: involvement, relationship to tumor, and variant anatomy.
- Evaluation of functional liver reserve pre– and post–portal vein embolization.
- Evaluation for cirrhosis, portal hypertension, fatty liver, and ascites.
- Regional and distant nodal disease.
- Metastatic implants: liver, organs, or peritoneal disease.

SUMMARY

HCC is a common cancer worldwide. The proper management of HCC requires a multidisciplinary team with input from the radiologist, oncologist, surgeon, interventional radiologist, and pathologist. This team approach helps in patient selection for surgical and nonsurgical treatment. For the nonsurgical approach, both systemic and directed therapy should be considered, and the best option should be tailored to the individual patient.

The diagnosis and management of HCC remain a challenge to the entire team. However, advances in imaging techniques are leading to improved selection of patients for appropriate therapies. Newer nonsurgical therapies are also in development and early implementation. Improvements in these and other therapeutic approaches may permit longer survival or allow patients with downgraded tumors to receive surgical options that would not have been otherwise feasible.

FIBROLAMELLAR HEPATOCELLULAR CARCINOMA

Introduction

Fibrolamellar hepatocellular carcinoma (FLHCC) is an uncommon subtype of HCC that disproportionally affects younger patients. Surgical resection with aggressive resection of the primary tumor, nodal metastases, and distant metastatic disease improves survival and is the best treatment option.

Epidemiology

FLHCC is a rare cancer that accounts for approximately 5% of HCC diagnoses.[109] FLHCC occurs primarily in young patients, with a median age at diagnosis of 21. There is no gender predilection, and the majority of patients do not have underlying liver disease.[110–112] Race and ethnicity are not associated with an increased risk for developing FLHCC.[113] The population-based relative survival rate for FLHCC in the United States is 73% to 90% at 1 year and 32% to 38% at 5 years.[114–116]

Key Points Epidemiology of Fibrolamellar Hepatocellular Carcinoma

- Fibrolamellar hepatocellular carcinoma accounts for less than 10% of all hepatocellular carcinomas.
- Median age of diagnosis is 21.

Pathology

The gross specimen of FLHCC is most commonly a bile-stained, pale or yellow-tan, large, solitary mass. The texture ranges from a soft to a hard mass in the background of a noncirrhotic liver. The mass has a lobular contour and well-defined margins. A central scar and calcifications are often present.

The malignant cells are much larger than normal hepatocytes and contain abundant eosinophilic cytoplasm, vesiculated nuclei, and prominent nucleoli. The cells are arranged in a pattern of nests, sheets, or cords surrounded by dense bands of fibrosis. Fibrosis most commonly occurs in a lamellar type pattern. However, irregular patterns of fibrosis can also be seen. Thick septations and scars occur when the fibrosis coalesces.[117,118]

On immunohistochemistry, FLHCC will stain positive for hepatocyte paraffin 1 (HepPar-1), CK7, and CD68. However, note that CK7 and HepPar-1 staining are not unique to FLHCC. The scirrhous subtype of HCC and cholangiocarcinoma will also both stain positive for CK7. Additionally, the classic form of HCC will often display HepPar-1 staining. CD68 staining has been shown to be 96% sensitive and 80% specific for FLHCC.[117]

Key Points Pathology of Fibrolamellar Hepatocellular Carcinoma

- Central calcifications may be present.
- Central scar is composed of bands of connective tissue.
- Fibrolamellar hepatocellular carcinoma stains positive for HepPar-1, CK7, and CD68.

Clinical Presentation

The most common symptoms are nonspecific and include abdominal pain, weight loss, and malaise.[119] Rare symptoms such as the presence of gynecomastia due to aromatase production by FLHCC have been described. Other rare symptoms include liver failure and pain associated with skeletal metastases. At the time of diagnosis, the tumors are usually large intrahepatic liver masses. Extrahepatic disease, including nodal metastases, is common at presentation. Unlike HCC, patients typically have no history of cirrhosis or CLD.

Abnormal liver function tests with mild elevation of aspartate transaminase and alanine transaminase levels may be detected at presentation. Owing to mass effect on the biliary tree, bilirubin may also be elevated. The level of AFP is usually normal, with less than 10% of patients presenting with an AFP greater than 200 ng/mL.[120] Elevated levels of serum des-carboxy prothrombin and B12 binding capacity can be seen in most patients with FLHCCs.[121,122]

KEY POINTS Clinical Presentation of Fibrolamellar Hepatocellular Carcinoma

- Large liver masses at diagnosis.
- Nonspecific symptoms: abdominal pain, weight loss, and malaise.
- α-fetoprotein level usually normal.

Staging

FLHCC is staged according to the American Joint Committee on Cancer TNM staging system. Staging is based on tumor number, tumor size, and vascular invasion (T); local and distant metastatic adenopathy (N); and the presence of metastatic disease (M).[123,124]

T1 tumor stage classification is for all solitary tumors, regardless of size, without vascular invasion. T2 tumor is defined as solitary tumors with vascular invasion or multiple tumors, none larger than 5 cm. T3 tumors are classified as multiple tumors larger than 5 cm or tumors with major vascular invasion of a major branch of the portal or hepatic veins. T4 tumor stage is reserved for tumors that demonstrate direct invasion to adjacent organs, other than the gallbladder, or in the setting of perforation to the visceral peritoneum.

Regional and distant nodal disease are staged as N1 and N2, respectively. In central cancers, the nodes along the hepatoduodenal ligament are considered N1, and nodes distant to this location are considered N2 (e.g., retroperitoneal nodes). Diaphragmatic nodes in the anterior, posterior, or middle diaphragmatic nodal stations may be considered as N1 nodes for FLHCC that is located near the dome of the liver. Tumors are staged as M1 if there is metastasis to any other organ or bone.[124]

Patterns of Tumor Spread

Metastatic disease is more common at presentation in FLHCC than in HCC. At the time of presentation, up to 70% of patients with FLHCC will have metastatic nodal disease.[125] Lymphadenopathy can be seen in the hepatic hilum, retroperitoneum, pelvis, and mediastinum. Distant metastasis is also common at initial presentation and is seen in up to 30% of patients. Metastases can be observed in the lungs, adrenal gland, peritoneum, bones, ovaries, and skeletal muscles.[126–128]

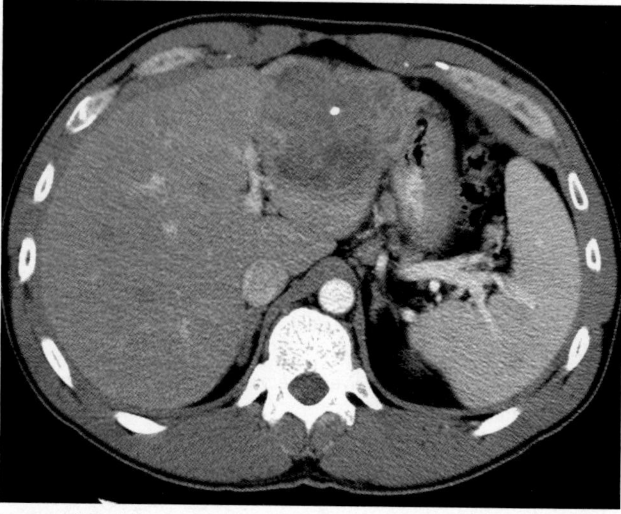

FIGURE 10.14. Portal venous–phase contrast-enhanced computed tomography of the abdomen shows a large fibrolamellar hepatocellular carcinoma in segments II and III, with central calcification.

KEY POINTS Tumor Spread of Fibrolamellar Hepatocellular Carcinoma

- Metastatic disease is more common at presentation of fibrolamellar hepatocellular carcinoma than with hepatocellular carcinoma.
- Distant metastases are seen in up to 30% of patients.

Imaging

US is not typically used to evaluate known FLHCC. However, the clinical presentation of an abdominal mass and right upper quadrant pain may suggest obtaining an US examination. FLHCC appears as a well-defined mass with variable echogenicity. The central scar is usually hyperechoic.[129]

Multiphase CT is commonly used to evaluate patients with FLHCC. On noncontrasted images, FLHCC usually appears as a well-defined low-attenuating mass with lobulated margins.[127] Central calcifications can be seen in up to 68% of tumors (Fig. 10.14).[127,129] A central scar consisting of radiating bands of fibrosis is also a common feature. Following the administration of iodinated contrast, the nonfibrous portions of the tumor demonstrate heterogeneous arterial phase enhancement (Fig. 10.15). The enhancement pattern on the portal venous and delayed phases varies from hypoattenuating to hyperattenuating compared to the adjacent liver parenchyma. If present, the central scar will often enhance on the delayed phase.[127]

FLHCC appears on MRI as a large and lobulated mass that is hypointense on T1W images and hyperintense on T2W images (Fig. 10.16). The central scar usually demonstrates low signal intensity on both T1W and T2W images.[127] During the multiphasic dynamic postcontrast MRI evaluation of the liver, there is early and heterogeneous enhancement of the nonfibrous portion of the tumor. The central scar usually does not enhance, or enhances late.

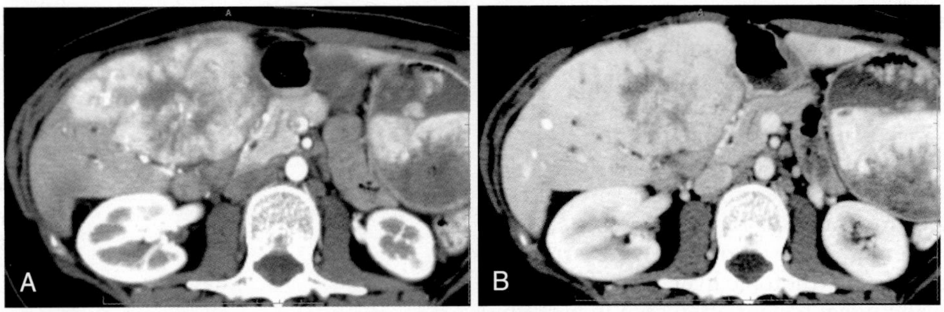

FIGURE 10.15. **A**, Late arterial–phase contrast-enhanced computed tomography (CT) of the abdomen demonstrates a large hypervascular liver mass in the left lobe of the liver, consistent with fibrolamellar hepatocellular carcinoma (FLHCC). There is relative decreased enhancement of the central scar. **B**, Portal venous–phase contrast-enhanced CT of the abdomen demonstrates a relatively isointense liver mass in the left liver, consistent with FLHCC. There is relative decreased enhancement of the central scar.

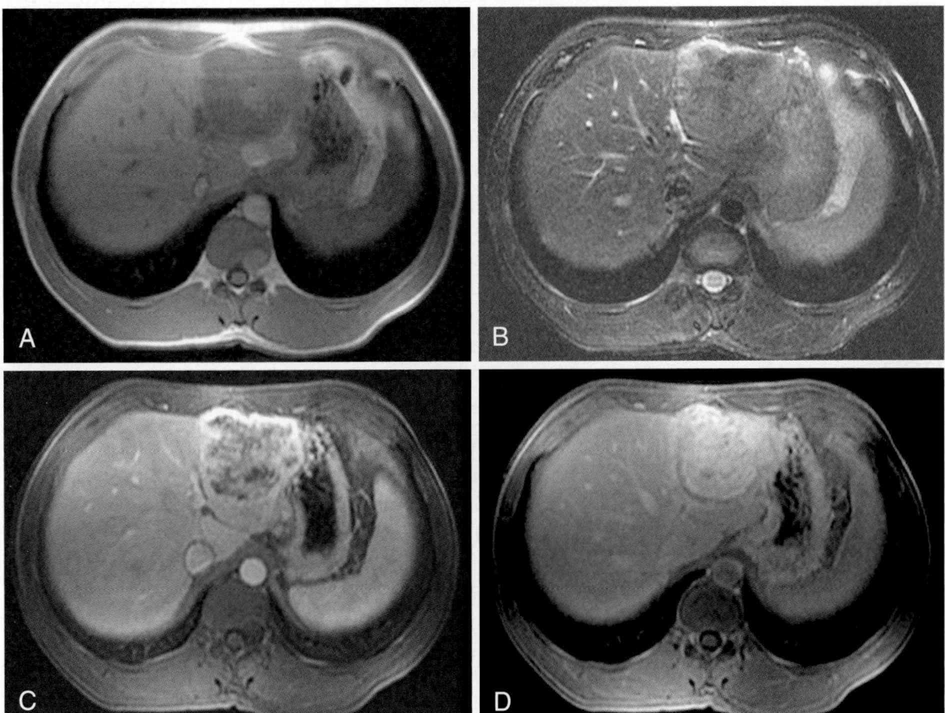

FIGURE 10.16. **A**, Axial T1-weighted imaging of the abdomen shows a hypointense mass, consistent with fibrolamellar hepatocellular carcinoma (FLHCC), occupying segments II and III of the liver. **B**, Axial T2-weighted imaging of the abdomen shows a peripheral hyperintense and centrally mostly hypointense mass, consistent with FLHCC, occupying segments II and III of the liver. **C**, Late arterial–phase postgadolinium image of the abdomen shows a heterogeneous enhancing mass, consistent with FLHCC, occupying segments II and III of the liver. **D**, Portal venous–phase postgadolinium image of the abdomen shows a delayed enhancement of the central portion of the mass, consistent with FLHCC, occupying segments II and III of the liver.

If using a hepatobiliary contrast agent, FLHCC will be hypointense to the background liver parenchyma on the hepatobiliary phase. Hepatobiliary phase hypointensity is helpful in distinguishing FLHCC from other lesions that display a central scar, such as focal nodular hyperplasia.[109,127]

KEY POINTS Imaging of Fibrolamellar Hepatocellular Carcinoma

- Multiphasic dynamic postcontrast protocol (computed tomography and magnetic resonance imaging) is required.
- Appears as a large mass and often has calcification and a central scar.
- Central scar often displays delayed enhancement.
- Hepatobiliary contrast agents are helpful for distinguishing fibrolamellar hepatocellular carcinoma from focal nodular hyperplasia.

TREATMENT

Surgery

Surgical resection provides the best outcome for the treatment of FLHCC. Hepatic resection with or without anatomic resection or liver transplant is available for surgical management. The median survival of the unresected patient is 12 months, with a 0% 5-year survival rate. In contrast to conventional HCC, aggressive approaches to resecting lymph node and lung metastases are associated with increased long-term survival.

FLHCC is treated aggressively because the patient population is younger without underlying cirrhotic liver disease. The 5-year survival rates associated with hepatic resection range from 45% to 80%.[115,116,120] In one series, the most significant prognostic factor was the presence of lymph node metastases. In another series, tumor size, number of lesions, vascular, capsular, or lymph node invasion did not affect the prognosis.[115] In the setting of recurrent disease or lymph node metastases, resection is performed, because surgery remains the best treatment option.[115,120]

Liver transplant has been considered for unresectable FLHCCs. In multiple small series, the 5-year survival for patients receiving orthotopic liver transplant ranges from 35% to 50%.[115,116] Because there is no underlying cirrhosis in the setting of FLHCC, orthotopic liver transplant does not have the same additional benefit often seen in patients with classic HCC of improved liver function and resection of the underlying liver pathology.

Transarterial Chemoembolization/ Chemotherapy Agents

FLHCC has been treated with single and combined agents. A trial of combination 5-fluorouracil and interferon-α-2b demonstrated a 62.5% response rate and an overall survival of 23.1 months. In this trial, FLHCC responded better than HCC (median survival 15.5 mo) and, subsequently, this regimen has gained a wide acceptance among medical oncologists.[130]

FLHCC can be treated with TACE. The main indications for TACE in FLHCC are tumor reduction in preoperative management (downstaging) and in the setting of unresectable disease, although FLHCC is generally considered a "surgical" disease.[131,132]

Radiation Therapy

Radiation therapy has not been useful in the management of FLHCC, except for palliation.

Key Points Treatment of Fibrolamellar Hepatocellular Carcinoma

- Aggressive resection of the primary tumor, nodal, and lung metastases improves survival.
- Reresection of recurrent disease remains the best treatment option.
- Combination chemotherapy improves survival in fibrolamellar hepatocellular carcinoma more than for hepatocellular carcinoma.
- Radiation therapy is indicated for palliation.

Surveillance

CT and MRI evaluation are performed routinely after resection of the tumor. Because FLHCC occurs in a younger population, MRI is the modality of choice to eliminate radiation risks. Close attention should be paid to the regional nodes—diaphragmatic, precaval, periportal, and retroperitoneal—for evidence of recurrence. Because these are younger patients without underlying liver disease, management is aggressive. Repeat surgical intervention with resection of the metastatic adenopathy improves survival.[133]

Key Points Surveillance of Fibrolamellar Hepatocellular Carcinoma

- Close attention for all signs of recurrent or metastatic disease.
- Repeat surgical resection improves survival.
- Magnetic resonance imaging to reduce radiation risk in a younger population.

The Radiology Report

The radiology report for patients with FLHCC should include a detailed description of the size, number, and segmental location of the masses. The relationship of the tumor to vessels, bile ducts, and liver capsule, with comments on any evidence of tumor invasion, is to be included. Vascular anatomy, including hepatic artery variants, portal vein variants, and accessory hepatic veins, should be examined and documented. In the preoperative liver resection setting, segmental liver volumes should be calculated if the FLR is suspected to be suboptimal. Complete radiologic staging with evaluation of the regional and distant nodes and evaluation for intrahepatic or distant metastases should also be included. After therapy, the radiology report should include evidence of all residual disease. A detailed description of any metastatic disease will allow complete metastectomy when reresection is performed.

Key Points The Radiology Report for Fibrolamellar Hepatocellular Carcinoma

- Size, location, and relationship to vessels, bile ducts, and adjacent organs.
- Nodal disease in the regional and distant nodes.
- Evaluation of the functional liver reserve.
- Detailed description of all suspected metastatic sites.

SUMMARY

FLHCC is an uncommon subtype of HCC that primarily occurs in the younger population without CLD. The diagnosis may be suggested by imaging, but it is confirmed by histology. The prognosis for FLHCC is better than that for HCC, which may be related to its high resectability and aggressive management compared with HCC.

REFERENCES

1. Marrero JA, Kulik LM, Sirlin CB, et al. Diagnosis, staging, and management of hepatocellular carcinoma: 2018 Practice guidance by the American Association for the Study of Liver Diseases. *Hepatology*. 2018;68(2):723-750.
2. Clark T, Maximin S, Meier J, et al. Hepatocellular carcinoma: review of epidemiology, screening, imaging diagnosis, response assessment, and treatment. *Curr Prob Diagn Radiol*. 2015;44(6):479-486.
3. Massarweh NN, El-Serag HB. Epidemiology of hepatocellular carcinoma and intrahepatic cholangiocarcinoma. *Cancer Control*. 2017;24(3):1073274817729245.

4. Mittal S, El-Serag HB. Epidemiology of hepatocellular carcinoma: consider the population. *J Clin Gastroenterol*. 2013;47(Suppl):S2-S6.
5. Ascha MS, Hanouneh IA, Lopez R, et al. The incidence and risk factors of hepatocellular carcinoma in patients with nonalcoholic steatohepatitis. *Hepatology*. 2010;51(6):1972-1978.
6. Morgan TR, Mandayam S, Jamal MM. Alcohol and hepatocellular carcinoma. *Gastroenterology*. 2004;127(5 Suppl 1):S87-S96.
7. Michels NA. Newer anatomy of the liver and its variant blood supply and collateral circulation. *Am J Surg*. 1966;112(3):337-347.
8. Kudo M. Multistep human hepatocarcinogenesis: correlation of imaging with pathology. *J Gastroenterol*. 2009;44(Suppl 19):112-118.
9. Kobayashi M, Ikeda K, Hosaka T, et al. Dysplastic nodules frequently develop into hepatocellular carcinoma in patients with chronic viral hepatitis and cirrhosis. *Cancer*. 2006;106(3):636-647.
10. Wong CM, Ng IO. Molecular pathogenesis of hepatocellular carcinoma. *Liver Int*. 2008;28(2):160-174.
11. Trevisani F, D'Intino PE, Caraceni P, et al. Etiologic factors and clinical presentation of hepatocellular carcinoma. Differences between cirrhotic and noncirrhotic Italian patients. *Cancer*. 1995;75(9):2220-2232.
12. Schafer DF, Sorrell MF. Hepatocellular carcinoma. *Lancet*. 1999;353(9160):1253-1257.
13. Kassianides C, Kew MC. The clinical manifestations and natural history of hepatocellular carcinoma. *Gastroenterol Clin North Am*. 1987;16(4):553-562.
14. Soresi M, Magliarisi C, Campagna P, et al. Usefulness of alphafetoprotein in the diagnosis of hepatocellular carcinoma. *Anticancer Res*. 2003;23(2c):1747-1753.
15. European Association for the Study of the Liver. EASL Clinical Practice Guidelines: Management of hepatocellular carcinoma. *J Hepatol*. 2018;69(1):182-236.
16. Li JW, Yun M, Lee JM, et al. Barcelona Clinic Liver Cancer outperforms Hong Kong Liver Cancer staging of hepatocellular carcinoma in multiethnic Asians: Real-world perspective. *World J Gastroenterol*. 2017;23(22):4054-4063.
17. Yau T, Tang VYF, Yao T, et al. Development of Hong Kong Liver Cancer staging system with treatment stratification for patients with hepatocellular carcinoma. *Gastroenterology*. 2014;146(7):1691-1700 e3.
18. Okuda K, Ohtsuki T, Obata H, et al. Natural history of hepatocellular carcinoma and prognosis in relation to treatment. Study of 850 patients. *Cancer*. 1985;56(4):918-928.
19. Llovet JM, Bru C, Bruix J. Prognosis of hepatocellular carcinoma: the BCLC staging classification. *Semin Liver Dis*. 1999;19(3):329-338.
20. A new prognostic system for hepatocellular carcinoma: a retrospective study of 435 patients: the Cancer of the Liver Italian Program (CLIP) investigators. *Hepatology*. 1998;28(3):751-755.
21. Marrero JA, Fontana RJ, Barrat A, et al. Prognosis of hepatocellular carcinoma: Comparison of 7 staging systems in an American cohort. *Hepatology*. 2005;41(4):707-715.
22. Forner A, Reig M, Bruix J. Hepatocellular carcinoma. *The Lancet*. 2018;391(10127):1301-1314.
23. Tellapuri S, Sutphin PD, Beg MS, et al. Staging systems of hepatocellular carcinoma: A review. *Indian J Gastroenterol*. 2018;37(6):481-491.
24. Oken MM, Creech RH, Tormey DC, et al. Toxicity and response criteria of the Eastern Cooperative Oncology Group. *Am J Clin Oncol*. 1982;5(6):649-655.
25. Yuki K, Hirohashi S, Sakamoto M, et al. Growth and spread of hepatocellular carcinoma. A review of 240 consecutive autopsy cases. *Cancer*. 1990;66(10):2174-2179.
26. American College of Radiology (ACR). Liver Reporting & Data System (LI-RADS). 2019. Available from: https://www.acr.org/Clinical-Resources/Reporting-and-Data-Systems/LI-RADS.
27. Elsayes KM, Fowler KJ, Chernyak V, et al. User and system pitfalls in liver imaging with LI-RADS. *J Magn Reson Imaging*. 2019;50(6):1673-1686.
28. Chernyak V, Fowler KJ, Kamaya A, et al. Liver Imaging Reporting and Data System (LI-RADS) Version 2018: Imaging of Hepatocellular Carcinoma in At-Risk Patients. *Radiology*. 2018;289(3):816-830.
29. Cerny M, Chernyak V, Olivie D, et al. LI-RADS Version 2018 Ancillary Features at MRI. *Radiographics*. 2018;38(7):1973-2001.
30. Son JH, Choi SH, Kim SY, et al. Validation of US liver imaging reporting and data system version 2017 in patients at high risk for hepatocellular carcinoma. *Radiology*. 2019;292(2):390-397.
31. Kim Y-Y, Kim M-J, Kim EH, et al. Hepatocellular Carcinoma versus Other Hepatic Malignancy in Cirrhosis: Performance of LI-RADS Version 2018. *Radiology*. 2019;291(1):72-80.
32. van der Pol CB, Kim M-J, Kim EH, et al. Accuracy of the Liver imaging reporting and data system in computed tomography and magnetic resonance image analysis of hepatocellular carcinoma or overall malignancy-a systematic review. *Gastroenterology*. 2019;156(4):976-986.
33. Chernyak V, Tang A, Flusberg M, et al. LI-RADS® ancillary features on CT and MRI. *Abdom Radiol (NY)*. 2018;43(1):82-100.
34. Wilson SR, Lyshchik A, Piscaglia F, et al. CEUS LI-RADS: algorithm, implementation, and key differences from CT/MRI. *Abdom Radiol (NY)*. 2018;43(1):127-142.
35. Alhasan A, Lyshchik A, Piscaglia F, et al. LI-RADS for CT diagnosis of hepatocellular carcinoma: performance of major and ancillary features. *Abdom Radiol (NY)*. 2019;44(2):517-528.
36. Choi JY, Lee JM, Sirlin CB. CT and MR imaging diagnosis and staging of hepatocellular carcinoma: part II. Extracellular agents, hepatobiliary agents, and ancillary imaging features. *Radiology*. 2014;273(1):30-50.
37. Hanna RF, Aguirre DA, Kased N, et al. Cirrhosis-associated hepatocellular nodules: correlation of histopathologic and MR imaging features. *Radiographics*. 2008;28(3):747-769.
38. Park YN, Kim MJ. Hepatocarcinogenesis: imaging-pathologic correlation. *Abdom Imaging*. 2011;36(3):232-243.
39. Choi JY, Lee JM, Sirlin CB. CT and MR imaging diagnosis and staging of hepatocellular carcinoma: part I. Development, growth, and spread: key pathologic and imaging aspects. *Radiology*. 2014;272(3):635-654.
40. Goodwin MD, Aguirre DA, Kased N, et al. Diagnostic challenges and pitfalls in MR imaging with hepatocyte-specific contrast agents. *Radiographics*. 2011;31(6):1547-1568.
41. Schwope RB, May LA, Reiter MJ, et al. Gadoxetic acid: pearls and pitfalls. *Abdom Imag*. 2015;40(6):2012-2029.
42. Torizuka T, Tamaki N, Inokuma T, et al. In vivo assessment of glucose metabolism in hepatocellular carcinoma with FDG-PET. *J Nucl Med*. 1995;36(10):1811-1817.
43. Trojan J, Schroeder O, Raedle J, et al. Fluorine-18 FDG positron emission tomography for imaging of hepatocellular carcinoma. *Am J Gastroenterol*. 1999;94(11):3314-3319.
44. Lee JD, Yun M, Lee JM, et al. Analysis of gene expression profiles of hepatocellular carcinomas with regard to 18F-fluorodeoxyglucose uptake pattern on positron emission tomography. *Eur J Nucl Med Mol Imaging*. 2004;31(12):1621-1630.
45. Ho CL, Yu SC, Yeung DW. 11C-acetate PET imaging in hepatocellular carcinoma and other liver masses. *J Nucl Med*. 2003;44(2):213-221.
46. De Gaetano AM, Vecchioli A, Minordi LM, et al. Role of diagnostic imaging in abdominal lymphadenopathy. *Rays*. 2000; 25(4):463-484.
47. Moron FE, Szklaruk J. Learning the nodal stations in the abdomen. *Br J Radiol*. 2007;80(958):841-848.
48. Efremidis SC, Vougiouklis N, Zafiriadou E, et al. Pathways of lymph node involvement in upper abdominal malignancies: evaluation with high-resolution CT. *Eur Radiol*. 1999;9(5):868-874.
49. Tublin ME, Dodd 3rd GD, Baron RL. Benign and malignant portal vein thrombosis: differentiation by CT characteristics. *AJR Am J Roentgenol*. 1997;168(3):719-723.
50. Tarantino L, Francica G, Sordelli I, et al. Diagnosis of benign and malignant portal vein thrombosis in cirrhotic patients with hepatocellular carcinoma: color Doppler US, contrast-enhanced US, and fine-needle biopsy. *Abdom Imaging*. 2006;31(5):537-544.
51. Catalano OA, Choy G, Zhu A, et al. Differentiation of malignant thrombus from bland thrombus of the portal vein in patients with hepatocellular carcinoma: application of diffusion-weighted MR imaging. *Radiology*. 2010;254(1):154-162.
52. Pawlik TM, Delman KA, Vauthey J-N, et al. Tumor size predicts vascular invasion and histologic grade: Implications for selection of surgical treatment for hepatocellular carcinoma. *Liver Transpl*. 2005;11(9):1086-1092.
53. Pawlik TM, Poon RT, Abdalla EK, et al. Hepatectomy for hepatocellular carcinoma with major portal or hepatic vein invasion: results of a multicenter study. *Surgery*. 2005;137(4):403-410.
54. Yamashita Y, Taketomi A, Shirabe K, et al. Outcomes of hepatic resection for huge hepatocellular carcinoma (≥10 cm in diameter). *J Surg Oncol*. 2011;104(3):292-298.
55. Vauthey JN, Chaoui A, Do KA, et al. Standardized measurement of the future liver remnant prior to extended liver resection: methodology and clinical associations. *Surgery*. 2000;127(5):512-519.

56. Madoff DC, Abdalla EK, Vauthey JN. Portal vein embolization in preparation for major hepatic resection: evolution of a new standard of care. *J Vasc Interv Radiol.* 2005;16(6):779-790.
57. Ueno S, Kubo F, Sakoda M, et al. Efficacy of anatomic resection vs nonanatomic resection for small nodular hepatocellular carcinoma based on gross classification. *J Hepatobiliary Pancreat Surg.* 2008;15(5):493-500.
58. Palavecino M, Chun YS, Madoff DC, et al. Major hepatic resection for hepatocellular carcinoma with or without portal vein embolization: Perioperative outcome and survival. *Surgery.* 2009;145(4):399-405.
59. Imamura H, Matsuyama Y, Tanaka E, et al. Risk factors contributing to early and late phase intrahepatic recurrence of hepatocellular carcinoma after hepatectomy. *J Hepatol.* 2003;38(2):200-207.
60. Yamashita Y, Taketomi A, Itoh S, et al. Longterm favorable results of limited hepatic resections for patients with hepatocellular carcinoma: 20 years of experience. *J Am Coll Surg.* 2007;205(1):19-26.
61. Nuzzo G, Giuliante F, Gauzolino R, et al. Liver resections for hepatocellular carcinoma in chronic liver disease: experience in an Italian centre. *Eur J Surg Oncol.* 2007;33(8):1014-1018.
62. Belghiti J, Cortes A, Abdalla EK, et al. Resection prior to liver transplantation for hepatocellular carcinoma. *Ann Surg.* 2003; 238(6):885-892;discussion 892-893.
63. Lo CM, Liu AL, Chan SC, et al. A randomized, controlled trial of postoperative adjuvant interferon therapy after resection of hepatocellular carcinoma. *Ann Surg.* 2007;245(6):831-842.
64. Ng KK, Vauthey JN, Pawlik TM, et al. Is hepatic resection for large or multinodular hepatocellular carcinoma justified? Results from a multi-institutional database. *Ann Surg Oncol.* 2005;12(5):364-373.
65. Yao FY, Mehta N, Flemming J, et al. Downstaging of hepatocellular cancer before liver transplant: long-term outcome compared to tumors within Milan criteria. *Hepatology.* 2015;61(6):1968-1977.
66. Mazzaferro V, Regalia E, Doci R, et al. Liver transplantation for the treatment of small hepatocellular carcinomas in patients with cirrhosis. *N Engl J Med.* 1996;334(11):693-699.
67. Kamath PS, Kim WR, Advanced Liver Disease Study Group. The model for end-stage liver disease (MELD). *Hepatology.* 2007;45(3):797-805.
68. Washburn K, Edwards E, Harper A, et al. Hepatocellular carcinoma patients are advantaged in the current liver transplant allocation system. *Am J Transplant.* 2010;10(7):1643-1648.
69. Mehta N, Dodge JL, Roberts JP, et al. Validation of the prognostic power of the RETREAT score for hepatocellular carcinoma recurrence using the UNOS database. *Am J Transplant.* 2018;18(5): 1206-1213.
70. Mehta N, Heimbach J, Harnois DM, et al. Validation of a Risk Estimation of Tumor Recurrence After Transplant (RETREAT) score for hepatocellular carcinoma recurrence after liver transplant. *JAMA Oncol.* 2017;3(4):493-500.
71. Halazun KJ, Najjar M, Abdelmessih RM, et al. Recurrence after liver transplantation for hepatocellular carcinoma: a new MORAL to the story. *Ann Surg.* 2017;265(3):557-564.
72. Nouri YM, Kim JH, Yoon H-K, et al. Update on transarterial chemoembolization with drug-eluting microspheres for hepatocellular carcinoma. *Korean J Radiol.* 2019;20(1):34-49.
73. Liu YS, Lin C-Y, Chuang M-T, et al. Five-year outcome of conventional and drug-eluting transcatheter arterial chemoembolization in patients with hepatocellular carcinoma. *BMC Gastroenterol.* 2018;18(1):124.
74. Burrel M, Reig M, Forner A, et al. Survival of patients with hepatocellular carcinoma treated by transarterial chemoembolisation (TACE) using drug eluting beads. Implications for clinical practice and trial design. *J Hepatol.* 2012;56(6):1330-1335.
75. Song JE, Kim DY. Conventional vs drug-eluting beads transarterial chemoembolization for hepatocellular carcinoma. *World J Hepatol.* 2017;9(18):808-814.
76. Llovet JM, Bruix J. Systematic review of randomized trials for unresectable hepatocellular carcinoma: Chemoembolization improves survival. *Hepatology.* 2003;37(2):429-442.
77. Bruix J, Qin S, Merle P, et al. Regorafenib for patients with hepatocellular carcinoma who progressed on sorafenib treatment (RESORCE): a randomised, double-blind, placebo-controlled, phase 3 trial. *Lancet.* 2017;389(10064):56-66.
78. Varela M, Real MI, Burrel M, et al. Chemoembolization of hepatocellular carcinoma with drug eluting beads: efficacy and doxorubicin pharmacokinetics. *J Hepatol.* 2007;46(3):474-481.
79. Huang K, Zhou Q, Wang R, et al. Doxorubicin-eluting beads versus conventional transarterial chemoembolization for the treatment of hepatocellular carcinoma. *J Gastroenterol Hepatol.* 2014;29(5):920-925.
80. Gao S, Yang Z, Zheng Z, et al. Doxorubicin-eluting bead versus conventional TACE for unresectable hepatocellular carcinoma: a meta-analysis. *Hepatogastroenterology.* 2013;60(124):813-820.
81. Wells SA, Hinshaw JL, Lubner MG, et al. Liver ablation: best practice. *Radiol Clin North Am.* 2015;53(5):933-971.
82. Poulou LS, Botsa E, Thanou I, et al. Percutaneous microwave ablation vs radiofrequency ablation in the treatment of hepatocellular carcinoma. *World J Hepatol.* 2015;7(8):1054-1063.
83. Ni Y, Mulier S, Miao Y, et al. A review of the general aspects of radiofrequency ablation. *Abdom Imaging.* 2005;30(4):381-400.
84. Lencioni R, Crocetti L. Local-regional treatment of hepatocellular carcinoma. *Radiology.* 2012;262(1):43-58.
85. Boutros C, Somasundar P, Garrean S, et al. Microwave coagulation therapy for hepatic tumors: review of the literature and critical analysis. *Surg Oncol.* 2010;19(1):e22-32.
86. Ng IO, Liu CL, Fan ST, et al. Expression of P-glycoprotein in hepatocellular carcinoma. A determinant of chemotherapy response. *Am J Clin Pathol.* 2000;113(3):355-363.
87. Wilhelm SM, Carter C, Tang L, et al. BAY 43-9006 exhibits broad spectrum oral antitumor activity and targets the RAF/MEK/ERK pathway and receptor tyrosine kinases involved in tumor progression and angiogenesis. *Cancer Res.* 2004;64(19):7099-7109.
88. Llovet JM, Ricci S, Mazzaferro V, et al. Sorafenib in advanced hepatocellular carcinoma. *N Engl J Med.* 2008;359(4):378-390.
89. Kudo M, Finn RS, Qin S, et al. Lenvatinib versus sorafenib in first-line treatment of patients with unresectable hepatocellular carcinoma: a randomised phase 3 non-inferiority trial. *Lancet.* 2018;391(10126):1163-1173.
90. Wilhelm SM, Dumas J, Adnane L, et al. Regorafenib (BAY 73-4506): a new oral multikinase inhibitor of angiogenic, stromal and oncogenic receptor tyrosine kinases with potent preclinical antitumor activity. *Int J Cancer.* 2011;129(1):245-255.
91. El-Khoueiry AB, Sangro B, Yau T, et al. Nivolumab in patients with advanced hepatocellular carcinoma (CheckMate 040): an open-label, non-comparative, phase 1/2 dose escalation and expansion trial. *Lancet.* 2017;389(10088):2492-2502.
92. Coldwell D, Sangro B, Salem R, et al. Radioembolization in the treatment of unresectable liver tumors: experience across a range of primary cancers. *Am J Clin Oncol.* 2012;35(2):167-177.
93. Taylor AC, Maddirela D, White SB. Role of radioembolization for biliary tract and primary liver cancer. *Surg Oncol Clin N Am.* 2019;28(4):731-743.
94. Salem R, Mazzaferro V, Sangro B. Yttrium 90 radioembolization for the treatment of hepatocellular carcinoma: biological lessons, current challenges, and clinical perspectives. *Hepatology.* 2013;58(6):2188-2197.
95. Sangro B, Bilbao JI, Boan J, et al. Radioembolization using 90Y-resin microspheres for patients with advanced hepatocellular carcinoma. *Int J Radiat Oncol Biol Phys.* 2006;66(3):792-800.
96. Facciorusso A, Serviddio G, Muscatiello N. Transarterial radioembolization vs chemoembolization for hepatocarcinoma patients: A systematic review and meta-analysis. *World J Hepatol.* 2016; 8(18):770-778.
97. Moreno-Luna LE, Yang JD, Sanchez W, et al. Efficacy and safety of transarterial radioembolization versus chemoembolization in patients with hepatocellular carcinoma. *Cardiovasc Intervent Radiol.* 2013;36(3):714-723.
98. Salem R, Lewandowski RJ, Kulik L, et al. Radioembolization results in longer time-to-progression and reduced toxicity compared with chemoembolization in patients with hepatocellular carcinoma. *Gastroenterology.* 2011;140(2):497-507 e2.
99. Salem R, Gordon AC, Mouli S, et al. Y90 Radioembolization significantly prolongs time to progression compared with chemoembolization in patients with hepatocellular carcinoma. *Gastroenterology.* 2016;151(6):1155-1163.e2.
100. Tanguturi SK, Wo JY, Zhu AX, et al. Radiation therapy for liver tumors: ready for inclusion in guidelines? *Oncologist.* 2014;19(8): 868-879.
101. Bujold A, Massey CA, Kim JJ, et al. Sequential phase I and II trials of stereotactic body radiotherapy for locally advanced hepatocellular carcinoma. *J Clin Oncol.* 2013;31(13):1631-1639.

102. Wong TC, Chiang C-L, Lee A-S, et al. Better survival after stereotactic body radiation therapy following transarterial chemoembolization in nonresectable hepatocellular carcinoma: A propensity score matched analysis. *Surg Oncol*. 2019;28:228-235.
103. Andolino DL, Johnson CS, Maluccio M, et al. Stereotactic body radiotherapy for primary hepatocellular carcinoma. *Int J Radiat Oncol Biol Phys*. 2011;81(4):e447-e453.
104. Sapisochin G, Barry A, Doherty M, et al. Stereotactic body radiotherapy vs. TACE or RFA as a bridge to transplant in patients with hepatocellular carcinoma. *An intention-to-treat analysis. J Hepatol*. 2017;67(1):92-99.
105. Kielar A, Fowler KJ, Lewis S, et al. Locoregional therapies for hepatocellular carcinoma and the new LI-RADS treatment response algorithm. *Abdom Radiol (NY)*. 2018;43(1):218-230.
106. Yaghmai V, Besa C, Kim E, et al. Imaging Assessment of hepatocellular carcinoma response to locoregional and systemic therapy. *AJR Am J Roentgenol*. 2013;201(1):80-96.
107. Kallini JR, Miller FH, Gabr A, et al. Hepatic imaging following intra-arterial embolotherapy. *Abdom Radiol (NY)*. 2016;41(4):600-616.
108. Riaz A, Kulik L, Lewandowski RJ, et al. Radiologic-pathologic correlation of hepatocellular carcinoma treated with internal radiation using yttrium-90 microspheres. *Hepatology*. 2009;49(4):1185-1193.
109. Palm V, Sheng R, Mayer P, et al. Imaging features of fibrolamellar hepatocellular carcinoma in gadoxetic acid-enhanced MRI. *Cancer Imaging*. 2018;18(1):9.
110. Do RK, McErlean A, Ang CS, et al. CT and MRI of primary and metastatic fibrolamellar carcinoma: a case series of 37 patients. *Br J Radiol*. 2014;87(1040):20140024.
111. Chaudhari VA, Khobragade K, Bhandare M, et al. Management of fibrolamellar hepatocellular carcinoma. *Chin Clin Oncol*. 2018;7(5):51.
112. Mavros MN, Mayo SC, Hyder O, et al. A systematic review: treatment and prognosis of patients with fibrolamellar hepatocellular carcinoma. *J Am Coll Surg*. 2012;215(6):820-830.
113. Lafaro KJ, Pawlik TM. Fibrolamellar hepatocellular carcinoma: current clinical perspectives. *J Hepatocell Carcinoma*. 2015;2:151-157.
114. El-Serag HB, Davila JA. Is fibrolamellar carcinoma different from hepatocellular carcinoma? A US population-based study. *Hepatology*. 2004;39(3):798-803.
115. El-Gazzaz G, Wong W, El-Hadary MK, et al. Outcome of liver resection and transplantation for fibrolamellar hepatocellular carcinoma. *Transpl Int*. 2000;13(Suppl 1):S406-S409.
116. Pinna AD, Iwatsuki S, Lee RG, et al. Treatment of fibrolamellar hepatoma with subtotal hepatectomy or transplantation. *Hepatology*. 1997;26(4):877-883.
117. Lin CC, Yang HM. Fibrolamellar carcinoma: a concise review. *Arch Pathol Lab Med*. 2018;142(9):1141-1145.
118. Graham RP, Torbenson MS. Fibrolamellar carcinoma: A histologically unique tumor with unique molecular findings. *Semin Diagn Pathol*. 2017;34(2):146-152.
119. Torbenson M. Review of the clinicopathologic features of fibrolamellar carcinoma. *Adv Anat Pathol*. 2007;14(3):217-223.
120. Stipa F, Yoon SS, Liau KH, et al. Outcome of patients with fibrolamellar hepatocellular carcinoma. *Cancer*. 2006;106(6):1331-1338.
121. Meriggi F, Forni E. [Surgical therapy of hepatic fibrolamellar carcinoma]. *Ann Ital Chir*. 2007;78(1):53-58.
122. van Tonder S, Kew MC, Hodkinson J, et al. Serum vitamin B12 binders in South African blacks with hepatocellular carcinoma. *Cancer*. 1985;56(4):789-792.
123. Vauthey JN, Klimstra D, Blumgart LH. A simplified staging system for hepatocellular carcinomas. *Gastroenterology*. 1995;108(2):617-618.
124. Amin MB, Edge S, Greene FL, et al, eds. *AJCC Cancer Staging Manual*. 8th ed. New York: Springer; 2017.
125. Stevens WR, Johnson CD, Stephens DH, et al. Fibrolamellar hepatocellular carcinoma: stage at presentation and results of aggressive surgical management. *AJR Am J Roentgenol*. 1995;164(5):1153-1158.
126. Ganeshan D, Szklaruk J, Kaseb A, et al. Fibrolamellar hepatocellular carcinoma: multiphasic CT features of the primary tumor on pre-therapy CT and pattern of distant metastases. *Abdom Radiol (NY)*. 2018;43(12):3340-3348.
127. Ganeshan D, Szklaruk J, Kundra V, et al. Imaging features of fibrolamellar hepatocellular carcinoma. *AJR Am J Roentgenol*. 2014; 202(3):544-552.
128. Ichikawa T, Federle MP, Grazioli L, et al. Fibrolamellar hepatocellular carcinoma: pre- and posttherapy evaluation with CT and MR imaging. *Radiology*. 2000;217(1):145-151.
129. Smith MT, Blatt ER, Jedlicka P, et al. Best cases from the AFIP: fibrolamellar hepatocellular carcinoma. *Radiographics*. 2008;28(2): 609-613.
130. Patt YZ, Hassan MM, Lozano RD, et al. Phase II trial of systemic continuous fluorouracil and subcutaneous recombinant interferon Alfa-2b for treatment of hepatocellular carcinoma. *J Clin Oncol*. 2003;21(3):421-427.
131. Sitzmann JV. Conversion of unresectable to resectable liver cancer: an approach and follow-up study. *World J Surg*. 1995;19(6):790-794.
132. Soyer P, Roche A, Rougier P, et al. [Nonresectable fibrolamellar hepatocellular carcinoma: outcome of 4 cases treated by intra-arterial chemotherapy]. *J Belge Radiol*. 1992;75(6):463-468.
133. Hemming AW, Langer B, Sheiner P, et al. Aggressive surgical management of fibrolamellar hepatocellular carcinoma. *J Gastrointest Surg*. 1997;1(4):342-346.

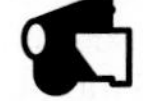

Visit ExpertConsult.com for additional algorithms.

HEPATOCELLULAR CARCINOMA

Note: Consider clinical trials as treatment options for eligible patients.

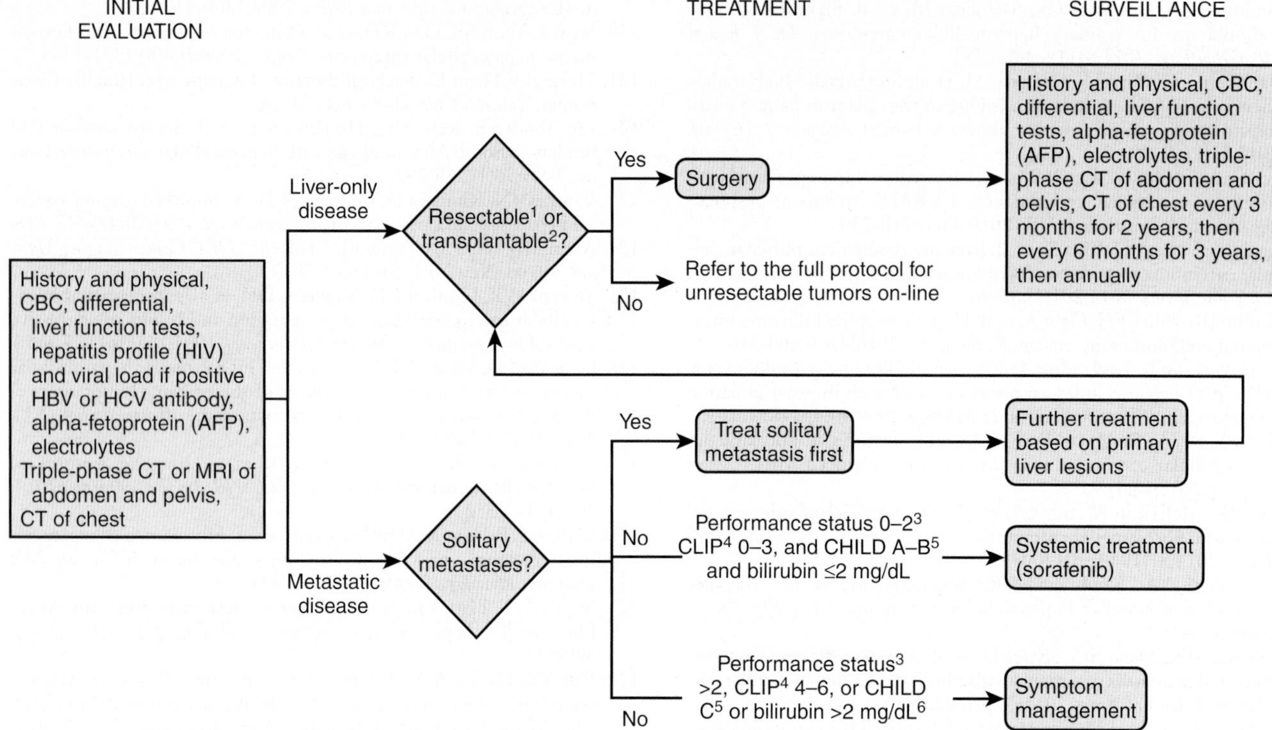

[1] Minor or major resection based on:
* Minor resection: Child A, normal liver function tests (bilirubin ≤1.0 mg%), absence of ascites, and plate count >100,000/mm^3
* Major resection: Idem minor plus absence of portal hypertension, portal vein embolization (PVE) for a small future remnant.

[2] Milan criteria; criteria for eligibility for liver transplantation for patients with hepatocellular carcinoma and cirrhosis: the presence of a tumor 5 cm or less in diameter in patients with single hepatocellular carcinomas, or no more than three tumor nodules, each 3 cm or less in diameter, in patients with multiple tumors, and without macrovascular invasion per imaging studies.

[3] See Appendix A in full protocol on-line for ECOG Performance Status

[4] CLIP – refer to Appendix B in full protocol on-line for determination of CLIP score

[5] CHILD – refer to Appendix C in full protocol on-line for CHILD scores

[6] Treament may be considered in select cases with bilirubin 2–3 mg/dL

This practice algorithm has been specifically developed for M.D. Anderson using a multidisciplinary approach and taking into consideration circumstances particular to M.D. Anderson, including the following: M.D. Anderson's specific patient population; M.D. Anderson's services and structure; and M.D. Anderson's clinical information. Moreover, this algorithm is not intended to replace the independent medical or professional judgment of physicians or other healthcare providers. This algorithm should not be used to treat pregnant women.

CHAPTER

11 Cholangiocarcinoma

Elainea N. Smith, M.D.; Aaron Coleman, M.D.; Samuel J. Galgano, M.D.; Constantine M. Burgan, M.D.; and Kristin K. Porter, M.D., Ph.D.

INTRODUCTION

Cholangiocarcinoma (CCA) refers to cancers that arise from biliary epithelium. These tumors can occur anywhere along the biliary tree and are divided into extrahepatic cholangiocarcinoma (ECC) and intrahepatic cholangiocarcinoma (ICC), with ECC lesions subclassified into perihilar and distal lesions. This practical classification is based on anatomy and surgical management. Cancers of the gallbladder (GB) are part of the CCA family but have a different clinical presentation and therapeutic approach. In this chapter, we present the epidemiology, clinical presentation, anatomy, pathology, staging, pattern of spread, treatment, recommendations for surveillance, and recommendations for a complete radiologic report of patients with CCA. The chapter is divided into sections corresponding to ICC and ECC, and gallbladder cancer (GB CA).

INTRA- AND EXTRAHEPATIC CHOLANGIOCARCINOMA

The clinical presenting symptoms of ICC and ECC are often nonspecific. These tumors are often found incidentally on imaging as a large mass. Because of ICC's similar imaging features to metastatic cancer from a gastrointestinal (GI) source, a search for a primary tumor may be initiated. ECC commonly presents with biliary obstruction. Once the diagnosis is made, management is very similar to that for hepatocellular carcinoma (HCC), with surgery providing the best curative option. Unfortunately, owing to nonspecific symptoms, these tumors typically present late in the disease course, and often exhibit nodal or distant metastases at the time of diagnosis.

Familiarity with the imaging features and patterns of spread of disease is essential for proper diagnosis, staging, and early detection. In this section, we review the epidemiology, clinical presentation, anatomy, spread of disease, therapies, and imaging features of ICC and ECC.

EPIDEMIOLOGY AND RISK FACTORS

CCA is the second most common primary hepatic tumor (second only to HCC), and accounts for approximately 3% of GI cancers diagnosed worldwide.[1] In the United States, CCA accounts for approximately 5000 deaths per year.[2] Approximately 5% to 10% of CCAs are intrahepatic and arise from peripheral bile ducts within the liver parenchyma. ICC is the second most common intrahepatic primary liver cancer (HCC is first), accounting for 10% of primary liver tumors, and occurs most commonly in the sixth and seventh decades. There is a male-to-female predominance of 3:2 for ICC.[3]

The lifetime risk of CCA in a patient with a history of primary sclerosing cholangitis (PSC) is approximately 8% to 40%, with a typically younger age of presentation ranging from 30 to 50 years.[4] Hepatolithiasis is endemic in areas of China, Japan, and Korea and is strongly associated with ICC. It is estimated that up to 10% of patients with hepatolithiasis will go on to develop CCA.[5]

The risk factors for ICC include choledochal cysts, PSC, inflammatory bowel disease, biliary cirrhosis, alcoholic liver disease, thyrotoxicosis, chronic pancreatitis, familial polyposis, congenital hepatic fibrosis, and parasitic infection (*Opisthorchis semensis*). Parasitic infection is the most common cause worldwide.

The risk factors for ECC are similar to those for ICC and include a family history of congenital fibrosis or cysts (Caroli disease, choledochal cyst, polycystic liver, or congenital hepatic fibrosis). Caroli disease and choledochal cysts may carry up to a 15% risk of malignant degeneration after the second decade of life.[6] Also included as risk factors are PSC, ulcerative colitis, certain drugs (oral contraceptives, methyldopa, and isoniazid), chemical exposure (Thorotrast, radionucleides, asbestos, arsenic, and dioxin), and primary biliary cirrhosis.[7] The risk also increases with biliary cirrhosis, cholelithiasis, alcoholic liver disease, diabetes, and chronic pancreatitis.[8] Prior bilioenteric drainage procedures complicated by recurrent bouts of cholangitis may also lead to CCA.[9] Infectious pathogens associated with ECC include liver flukes (*Clonorchis sinensis*).

Likely related to the geographic distribution of various risk factors, incidence rates of CCAs vary widely. The highest rates have been reported in Thailand, China, and other parts of Asia.[10] Recent reports demonstrate a rising incidence, predominantly within the United States and United Kingdom. Over the last 10 to 20 years, the incidence of ICC has risen to become the leading cause of primary liver tumor–related deaths in the United States. This trend is potentially secondary to increased diagnosis and increased prevalence of PSC; however, continued study is required.[1,4]

The majority (60%–70%) of ECCs are perihilar, also known as "Klatskin" tumors, and most commonly involve the hepatic duct bifurcation.[11] The true incidence of ECC is difficult to quantify because historically these tumors have been grouped with GB CA, the incidence of which is

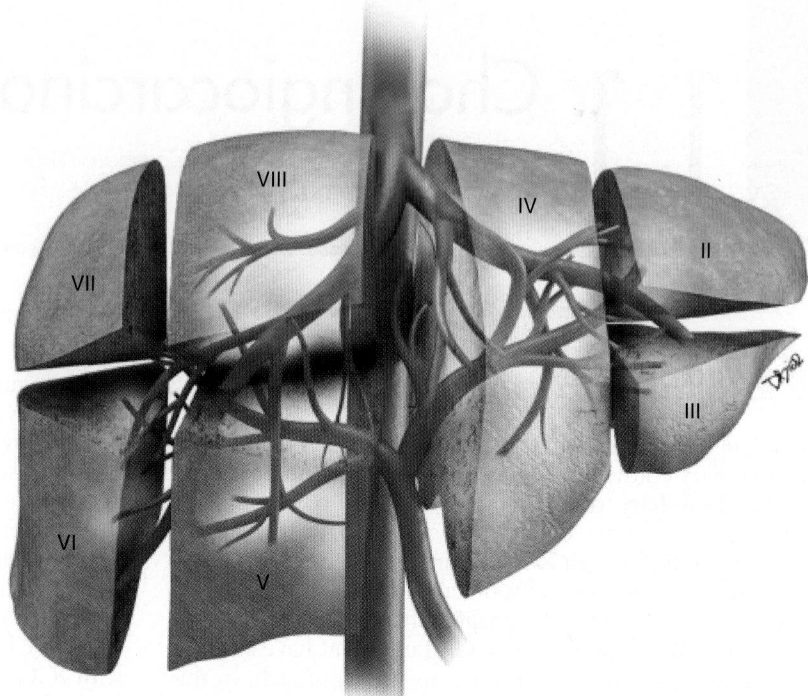

FIGURE 11.1. Segmental anatomy of the liver. The liver is divided into the right and the left lobes. There are eight segments: three in the left lobe (II, III, and IV), four in the right lobe (V, VI, VII, VIII), and one in the caudate lobe (I) (not visualized). The segments are divided by the hepatic veins and defined by the portal vein supply.

falling. Regardless, data suggest that the incidence of and mortality from ECC in the United States and worldwide are declining.[1,12]

> **KEY POINTS Epidemiology and Risk Factors of Cholangiocarcinoma**
>
> - Cholangiocarcinoma is the second most common primary hepatic tumor, accounting for approximately 3% of gastrointestinal cancers diagnosed worldwide.
> - Intrahepatic cholangiocarcinoma accounts for 5% to 10% of primary liver cancers.
> - Risk factors for intrahepatic and extrahepatic cholangiocarcinoma are similar, including choledochal cysts, primary sclerosing cholangitis, inflammatory bowel disease, biliary cirrhosis, alcoholic liver disease, thyrotoxicosis, chronic pancreatitis, familial polyposis, congenital hepatic fibrosis, and parasitic infection.

ANATOMY

There are three main intrahepatic bile ducts, the right, left, and caudate, which come together to form the common hepatic duct. This confluence of the biliary tree is then divided into thirds: the upper third extends from the confluence of the intrahepatic bile ducts to the level of the cystic duct; the middle third extends from the level of the cystic duct to the duodenum; and the distal third extends to the level of the ampulla.

The hepatic ducts and the upper and middle common bile duct (CBD) receive arterial supply mainly via the cystic artery. The middle and distal portions of the duct receive blood supply from the right hepatic and posterosuperior pancreaticoduodenal arcade. The venous drainage of the lower bile duct is through the portal vein. For the upper portion, the venous drainage is through the liver.

The combination of hepatic artery, bile duct, and portal vein is considered the portal triad. These anatomic structures course together to the various segments of the liver (Fig. 11.1) along the portal vein supply. The intimate relationship between these structures can unfortunately lead to a poor prognosis even in the setting of early disease, because a small bile duct tumor can extend to either the portal vein or the hepatic artery and potentially make the tumor inoperable.

The regional nodes in the biliary tree are the nodes in the hepatoduodenal ligament (Fig. 11.2). The lymphatic drainage includes these nodes, as well as the peripancreatic, portacaval, celiac, and hepatic artery nodes. Drainage into the retroperitoneum, including the interaortocaval and paraaortic nodal stations, can portend a worse prognosis because these are not considered regional lymph nodes.

> **KEY POINTS**
>
> - There are three main intrahepatic bile ducts, the right, left, and caudate, which come together to form the common hepatic duct.
> - The biliary tree is divided into thirds, with the cystic duct, duodenum, and ampulla as landmarks.

PATHOLOGY

The majority of CCAs are well-differentiated adenocarcinomas, with other histologic variants compromising less than 5% of cases.[13] There is variety of cellular activity

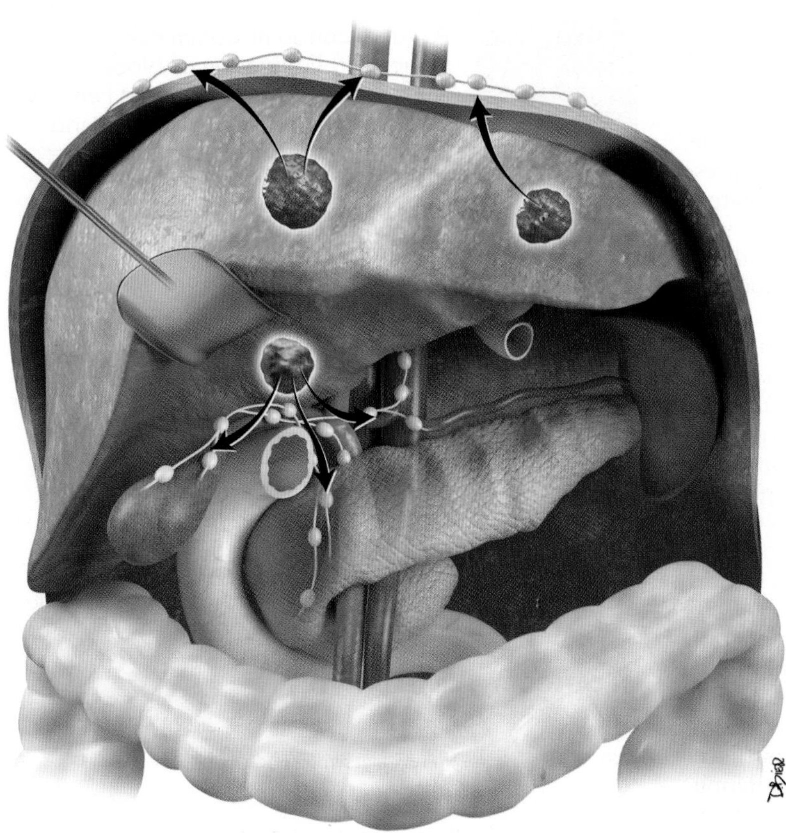

Figure 11.2. Pattern of nodal spread of intrahepatic cholangiocarcinoma. Tumors in the central liver will drain to the hepatoduodenal ligament. Tumors near the dome will drain to the diaphragmatic nodal stations.

in the same tumor, with areas of pleomorphism, atypia, mitotic activity, prominent nucleoli, and hyperchromatic nucleoli. To distinguish ICC from HCC, the detection of mucin and the absence of bile production favor ICC. Immunohistochemical staining for cytokeratin (to distinguish from colon cancer), tissue polypeptide antigen, and epithelial membrane antigen aid in the diagnosis. Additionally, vascular invasion can occur, but is rare compared with HCC.

There are three gross appearances of ECC tumors: sclerosing, nodular, and papillary. The sclerosing (also known as infiltrating) type accounts for 70% of hilar CCAs and causes annular thickening of the bile duct. There is also longitudinal extension of tumor and fibrosis of the periductal structures. The nodular tumors are solid nodules that project into the lumen. The papillary (intraductal) tumors have an intraluminal growth pattern. The most common type is the sclerosing type, with the papillary type being the least common type. The sclerosing type is most commonly seen in the hilar region, whereas the papillary type is more commonly seen in the distal bile duct. The papillary type has a better outcome owing to its association with low-grade histology.

The ECCs are mostly well-differentiated, mucin-producing adenocarcinomas. Histopathology will demonstrate an increased nuclear-cytoplasmic ratio, nucleolar prominence, concentric layering of cellular stroma around neoplastic glands, and a combination of normal-appearing cells with cells having large nuclei with prominent nucleoli.[14]

Key Points Pathology of Cholangiocarcinoma

- Detection of mucin favors intrahepatic cholangiocarcinoma over hepatocellular carcinoma (HCC).
- Vascular invasion can occur, but is rare compared with HCC.
- The sclerosing type is the most common type of hilar tumor. The papillary type is the most common distal extrahepatic cholangiocarcinoma and has the best prognosis.

CLINICAL PRESENTATION

The clinical presentation of CCA depends greatly on the location of the primary tumor. ECC presents with symptoms related to biliary obstruction, such as jaundice, pruritis, clay-colored stools, and dark urine. Later symptoms include weight loss and abdominal pain.[1] Patients with ECC typically present with painless jaundice that is often attributed to a suspected diagnosis of pancreatic cancer. The degree of jaundice is a function of the mechanical obstruction of the biliary tree. In the setting of bilobar or common hepatic duct involvement, the clinical sign of obstructive jaundice may appear early in the disease. In the setting of a unilobar tumor, the tumor typically has to grow and then occlude the contralateral lobe, the cystic duct, or the ipsilateral portal vein to be symptomatic, and therefore often has a different clinical presentation. The cystic duct extension will result in an enlarged GB with a positive Courvoisier sign (palpably enlarged GB that is nontender and accompanied by mild, painless jaundice). Finally, extension to the portal vein will result in lobar or segmental atrophy of the liver.

Other clinical symptoms of ECC at presentation include abdominal pain, weight loss, pruritus, diarrhea, anorexia, and fever. In the setting of chronic obstruction, the presence of the tumor may be complicated by an inflammatory or infectious process of the bile ducts. A biliary stent with percutaneous draining or to reestablish continuity with the bowel is usually required to relieve the obstruction and remove bacterially contaminated bile.

ICCs, unfortunately, are usually asymptomatic, and are usually incidentally discovered during workup for biochemical abnormalities.[15] An enlarged liver may be detected on physical examination. In patients who present with an incidental liver mass, imaging studies or endoscopic evaluation are performed in search of a possible primary GI tumor. In these patients, the diagnosis of ICC is made as a diagnosis of exclusion. In contrast to HCC, the patients do not present with ascites, cirrhosis, or portal hypertension.

Common laboratory studies used to assess liver function such as evaluation of bilirubin levels, alkaline phosphatase, and aminotransferase may be normal at the beginning of the course of the disease in CCA, but become elevated with progression of disease. The bilirubin level may be normal in the setting of unilobar obstruction. This is caused by compensatory biliary drainage of the functional/unobstructed lobe. Laboratory testing may show elevated CA19-9 (median 140 U/mL, with >60% of patients showing a CA19-9 level >100 U/mL) in both ECC and ICC.[16–18] The median carcinoembryonic antigen level is typically elevated, near 2.1 ng/mL, and is not significantly different between intrahepatic and extrahepatic tumors.[18] CA19-9 is not specific, because a portion of the population cannot synthesize the protein; alternatively, its levels may be elevated secondary to inflammation rather than tumor.[19] However, in patients with PSC and a CA19-9 value greater than 100 U/mL, there is a sensitivity and specificity of 89% and 86% for ECC, respectively.[17]

Key Points

- Intrahepatic cholangiocarcinomas are usually incidentally discovered during workup for biochemical abnormalities.
- Jaundice is a common presenting symptom in extrahepatic cholangiocarcinomas.
- Carcinoembryonic antigen and CA19-9 levels are commonly elevated.

STAGING CLASSIFICATION

Recently, the 8th edition of the American Joint Committee on Cancer (AJCC) staging manual was published.[20] In this edition, separate tumor, node, and metastasis (TNM) staging criteria were defined for all CCA subtypes: perihilar and distal ECC, as well as ICC. All differ in their tumor (T) stage and prognostic groupings (Tables 11.1B, 11.2B, 11.3B, and 11.4B).

Table 11.1 A. American Joint Committee on Cancer 8th Edition Tumor Node Metastasis (TNM) Staging for Perihilar Cholangiocarcinoma: TNM Criteria

T CATEGORY	CRITERIA
TX	Primary tumor cannot be assessed
T0	No evidence of primary tumor
Tis	Carcinoma *in situ*/high-grade dysplasia
T1	Tumor confined to bile duct, with extension into muscle layer or fibrous tissue
T2	Tumor invades beyond wall of bile duct – into either:
T2a	⇒ Adjacent adipose tissue
T2b	⇒ Adjacent hepatic parenchyma
T3	Tumor invades unilateral branches of portal vein or hepatic artery
T4	Tumor invades the main portal vein bilaterally, common hepatic artery, or unilateral second-order biliary radicals with contralateral portal vein or hepatic artery
N CATEGORY	**CRITERIA**
NX	Regional nodes cannot be assessed
N0	No regional lymph node metastasis
N1	Positive lymph nodes: 1–3
N2	Positive lymph nodes: ≥4
M CATEGORY	**CRITERIA**
M0	No distant metastasis
M1	Distant metastasis

B. STAGING: PERIHILAR CHOLANGIOCARCINOMA

T	N	M	STAGE
Tis	N0	M0	0
T1	N0	M0	I
T2a-b	N0	M0	II
T3	N0	M0	IIIA
T4	N0	M0	IIIB
Any T	N1	M0	IIIC
Any T	N2	M0	IVA
Any T	Any N	M1	IVB

(From Amin MB, Edge S, Greene F, et al, eds. *AJCC Cancer Staging Manual*. 8th ed. Springer International Publishing: American Joint Commission on Cancer; 2017.)

Perihilar Extrahepatic Cholangiocarcinoma

In perihilar ECC, T1 tumors are classified as a single tumor confined to the bile duct, with extension up to the muscle layer (Table 11.1A, Fig. 11.3). T2 is used to describe lesions that extend beyond the wall of the bile duct: T2a for those that invade surrounding adipose tissue, and T2b when the lesion invades adjacent hepatic parenchyma. T3 is used to describe masses that invade unilateral branches of the hepatic artery or portal vein branches. T4 lesions invade the main portal vein or common hepatic artery.

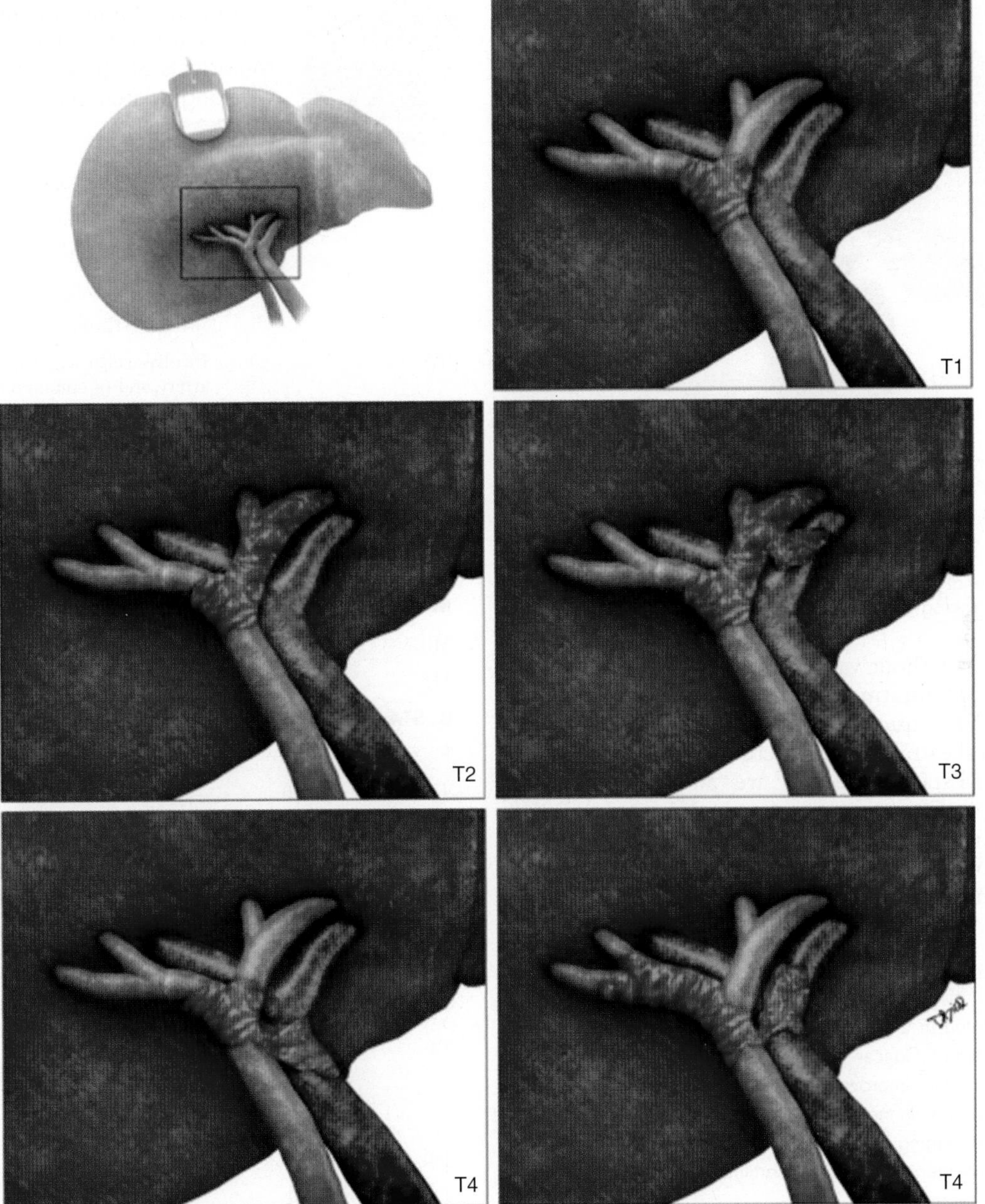

FIGURE 11.3. In perihilar extrahepatic cholangiocarcinoma, T1 tumors are classified as a single tumor confined to the bile duct, with extension up to the muscle layer. T2 is used to describe lesions that extend beyond the wall of the bile duct: T2a for those that invade surrounding adipose tissue, and T2b when the lesion invades adjacent hepatic parenchyma. T3 is used to describe masses that invade unilateral branches of the hepatic artery or portal vein branches. T4 lesions invade the main portal vein or common hepatic artery.

N0 staging is used in the setting of no evidence of nodal metastases. N1 describes one to three pathologic nodes within the hilar, cystic duct, common bile duct, portal vein, or posterior pancreaticoduodenal nodal chains (Fig. 11.4). N2 is used in the setting of more than four pathologic nodes.

M0 staging denotes no evidence of metastatic lesions, whereas M1 staging is used in the setting of any metastasis.[20]

Distal Extrahepatic Cholangiocarcinoma

Distal ECC T staging is slightly different from perihilar ECC staging. In T1 lesions, the tumor invades the bile duct wall to a depth of less than 5 mm (Table 11.2A, Fig. 11.5). T2 describes tumors that invade the bile duct to a depth of 5 to 12 mm. T3 describes any invasion greater than 12 mm. In T4 tumors, invasion of the celiac axis, superior mesenteric artery, and/or common hepatic artery is present.[20]

N and M staging are identical to those of perihilar ECC, as detailed above.

Intrahepatic Cholangiocarcinoma

ICC T staging is subcategorized slightly differently than that of ECC. T1 is used to describe a solitary tumor that is less than 5 cm in size: T1a describes a tumor without vascular invasion, and T1b describes a tumor with vascular invasion present (Table 11.3A). The presence of multiple

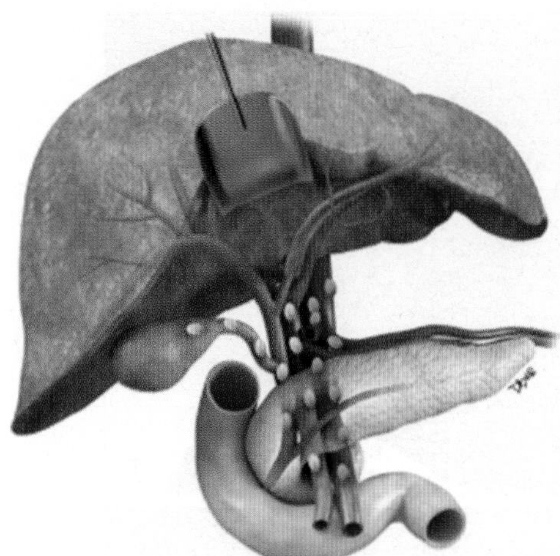

FIGURE 11.4. Pattern of nodal spread of extrahepatic cholangiocarcinoma. N0 staging is used in the setting of no evidence of nodal metastases. N1 describes one to three pathologic nodes within the hilar, cystic duct, common bile duct, portal vein (yellow), or posterior pancreaticoduodenal nodal chains (green). N2 is used in the setting of more than four pathologic nodes.

tumors, with or without vascular invasion, is classified as T2. Any tumor perforating the visceral peritoneum is classified as T3. T4 is used to describe a mass that directly invades the local extrahepatic structures.

The N and M staging for ECC are "all or nothing." N0 represents no nodal metastasis, whereas N1 is used in the setting of any nodes with suspected metastasis. M0 is used in the setting of no metastasis, and M1 is used if any metastases are present.[20]

KEY POINTS Staging of Cholangiocarcinoma

- Staging updated in 2017 with the 8th edition of the American Joint Committee on Cancer staging manual.
- This update contains improved stage-stratified 5-year survival outcomes compared with the previous edition.
- T, N, and M staging are categorized differently for perihilar and distal extrahepatic cholangiocarcinoma, and intrahepatic cholangiocarcinoma.

TABLE 11.2 A. American Joint Committee on Cancer 8th Edition Tumor Node Metastasis Staging for Distal Cholangiocarcinoma: TNM Criteria

T CATEGORY	CRITERIA
TX	Primary tumor cannot be assessed
Tis	Carcinoma *in situ*/high-grade dysplasia
T1	Tumor invades the bile duct wall <5 mm
T2	Invades 5–12 mm
T3	Invades >12 mm
T4	Involves celiac axis, superior mesenteric artery, and/or common hepatic artery
N CATEGORY	**CRITERIA**
NX	Regional nodes cannot be assessed
N0	No regional lymph node metastasis
N1	Positive lymph nodes: 1–3
N2	Positive lymph nodes: ≥4
M CATEGORY	**CRITERIA**
M0	No distant metastasis
M1	Distant metastasis

B. STAGING: DISTAL CHOLANGIOCARCINOMA

T	N	M	STAGE
Tis	N0	M0	0
T1	N0	M0	I
T1	N1	M0	IIA
T1	N2	M0	IIIA
T2	N0	M0	IIA
T2	N1	M0	IIB
T2	N2	M0	IIIA
T3	N0	M0	IIB
T3	N1	M0	IIB
T3	N2	M0	IIIA
T4	N0	M0	IIIB
T4	N1	M0	IIIB
T4	N2	M0	IIIB
Any T	Any N	M1	IV

(From Amin MB, Edge S, Greene F, et al, eds. *AJCC Cancer Staging Manual.* 8th ed. Springer International Publishing: American Joint Commission on Cancer; 2017.)

PATTERNS OF TUMOR SPREAD

ICC may present with intrahepatic or extrahepatic tumor spread. The pattern of tumor spread is very similar to HCC.[21] The most common type of tumor spread is intrahepatic via portal vein invasion. The lymph nodes, skeleton, lung, and peritoneum are common sites of metastases. Nodes along the hepatic hilum are a common site of tumor spread, as well as the paraaortic, retropancreatic, and common hepatic nodes. For tumors in the left lobe of the liver, the left gastric, the paracardiac, and the nodes along the lesser curvature of the stomach may be involved (see Fig. 11.2). Distant lymph node involvement can include mediastinum and paraaortic nodes. For more peripheral tumors, the diaphragmatic nodes may be involved. Invasion through the liver capsule and extension to adjacent sites is more common in ICC than in HCC.[22]

The pattern of tumor spread for ECC is via local extension. The intimate relationship of the bile duct to the hepatic artery and portal vein can make the patient a nonsurgical candidate early in the disease. This is particularly troublesome for the hilar (Klatskin) type tumors. A detailed review of the vascular anatomy is required to assess the surgical options that may be available to the patient. For example, a replaced left hepatic artery from the left gastric artery may provide surgical options that may not be available to patients with a single common hepatic artery.

In upper ECC tumors near the hilum, the nodes in the hepatoduodenal ligament, hilar, and periductal nodal stations are the most commonly involved. For distal ECC

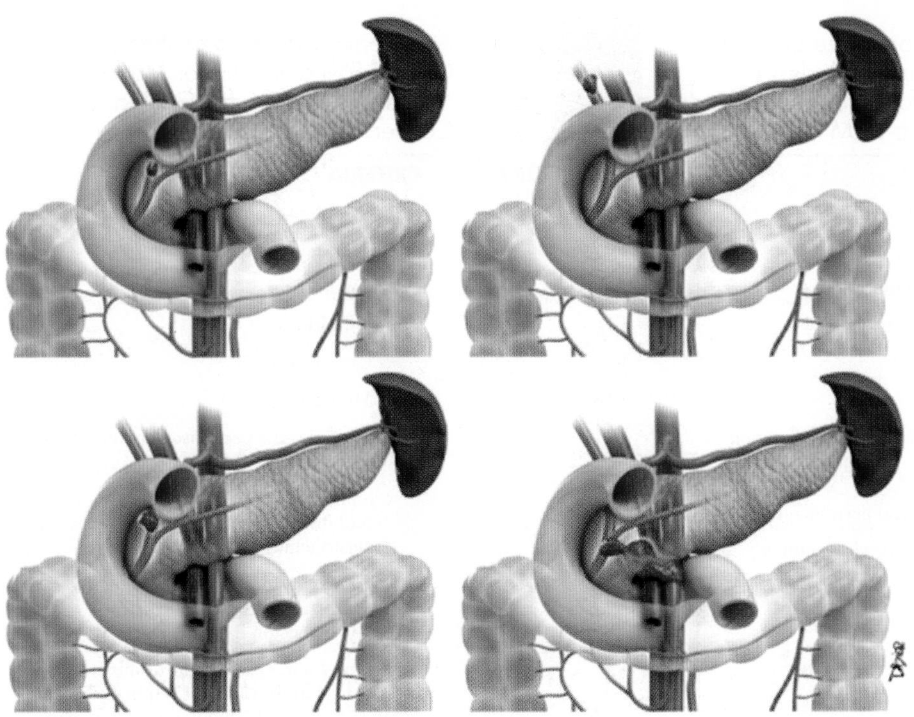

FIGURE 11.5. Distal extrahepatic cholangiocarcinoma (ECC) T staging is slightly different from perihilar ECC staging. In T1 stage lesions, the tumor invades the bile duct wall less than 5 mm in depth. T2 describes tumors that invade the bile duct 5 to 12 mm. T3 describes any invasion greater than 12 mm. In T4 tumors, invasion of the celiac axis, superior mesenteric artery, and/or common hepatic artery is present.

tumors near the ampulla, the regional nodes are the same as for tumors in the head of the pancreas. These include the hepatic artery, CBD, and celiac nodal stations. The anterior and posterior pancreaticoduodenal nodes and superior mesenteric nodes may also be involved. For all types of ECC, evaluation of retroperitoneal nodes is essential because their involvement may make the patient a nonsurgical candidate.

Local extension of the distal ECC near the ampulla may result in tumor extending to regional organs (pancreas, duodenum, stomach, and colon) and arteries (celiac axis and superior mesenteric artery). Hilar ECC tumors will invade the liver via the portal vein. Hilar ECC metastasis to other organs is not common; however, the assessment of hematogenous spread often will require evaluation of the lungs. Similar to ICC, peritoneal/omental disease may be seen.

KEY POINTS Tumor Spread of Cholangiocarcinoma

- Invasion through the liver capsule and extension to adjacent sites is more common in intrahepatic cholangiocarcinoma than in hepatocellular carcinoma.
- Pattern of tumor spread for extrahepatic cholangiocarcinoma is via local extension.
- Detailed vascular anatomy review is required to assess surgical options.

IMAGING

Primary Tumor

Ultrasound

Similar to other abdominal malignancies, ultrasound (US) evaluation is commonly the first imaging modality used to evaluate patients with suspected CCA. US provides a fast and relatively inexpensive evaluation; however, it is dependent on the experience of the operator and quality of the equipment. US may also provide useful guidance for percutaneous biopsy and may be useful for evaluation of vascular invasion with the aid of color Doppler techniques. US is very limited in the assessment of lymph node invasion and metastatic disease.

ICC presents as a mass in the liver with variable echogenicity (Fig. 11.6). In patients with ECC, the goals of the US examination are typically to confirm biliary obstruction, evaluate the extent of obstruction, and identify the cause.[3,23,24] US can detect the level of biliary obstruction in 71% to 100% of cases and the cause of obstruction in 57% to 96% of cases.[25,26] Unfortunately, US has a high percentage of false-positive diagnoses of malignant biliary obstruction, higher than for computed tomography (CT) or magnetic resonance imaging (MRI).[25]

The location of the tumor is inferred from the abrupt change in caliber of the bile ducts (Fig. 11.7). Perihilar ECC can be suggested by dilated intrahepatic ducts with abrupt narrowing or cutoffs at the hepatic duct main bifurcation. Distal ECC presents with dilated intra- and extrahepatic ducts.[27] Signs such as lobar atrophy and crowding of the vessels in addition to the presence of biliary dilatation raise the suspicion that the obstruction is malignant in etiology. Doppler evaluation of the portal vein in search of caliber change or changes in blood flow velocity may suggest vascular involvement.

Endoscopic ultrasound (EUS) is a very useful modality for the diagnosis and staging of ECC. EUS with fine needle aspiration has a reported diagnostic accuracy of 89%. There is the risk of seeding into the peritoneum with EUS, but a reduced risk of biliary contamination compared with brush cytology.[28]

Table 11.3 A. American Joint Committee on Cancer 8th Edition Tumor Node Metastasis Staging for Intrahepatic Cholangiocarcinoma: TNM Criteria

T CATEGORY	CRITERIA
TX	Primary tumor cannot be assessed
T0	No evidence of primary tumor
Tis	Carcinoma *in situ* (intraductal)
T1	Solitary, no vascular invasion –
T1a	⇨ ≤5 cm
T1b	⇨ >5 cm
T2	Solitary with intrahepatic vascular invasion OR Multiple tumors +/– vascular invasion
T3	Tumor perforates visceral peritoneum
T4	Tumor directly invades local structures
N CATEGORY	**CRITERIA**
NX	Regional nodes cannot be assessed
N0	No regional lymph node metastasis
N1	Lymph node metastasis present
M CATEGORY	**CRITERIA**
M0	No distant metastasis
M1	Distant metastasis

B. STAGING: INTRAHEPATIC CHOLANGIOCARCINOMA

T	N	M	STAGE
Tis	N0	M0	0
T1a	N0	M0	IA
T1b	N0	M0	IB
T2	N0	M0	II
T3	N0	M0	IIIA
T4	N1	M0	IIIB
Any T	N1	M0	IIIB
Any T	Any N	M1	IV

(From Amin MB, Edge S, Greene F, et al, eds. *AJCC Cancer Staging Manual.* 8th ed. Springer International Publishing: American Joint Commission on Cancer; 2017.)

Computed Tomography

CT plays a major role in the clinical evaluation of patients with ICC. The CT imaging protocol for a patient with a liver mass is multiphasic examination, the same as one would obtain when evaluating for HCC. The multiphase examination includes the precontrast, late arterial, portal venous, and delayed phases of contrast administration.

ICC will present as a large, hypoattenuating mass on the precontrast images (Fig. 11.8). During the late arterial phase of contrast administration, the enhancement, if present, is minimal and peripheral (see Fig. 11.8). On the portal venous phase, the enhancement will continue in a centripetal fashion and progress on the delayed phase of contrast administration (see Fig. 11.8). The CT findings for ICC are very similar to those for hypovascular metastases, especially from the GI tract. Features that suggest the diagnosis of ICC over metastases include a large single mass and the absence of a primary GI tumor. Other CT findings seen with ICC include calcifications and capsular retraction.

The multiphasic CT evaluation provides key information for surgical planning. This includes hepatic artery, portal vein, and hepatic vein anatomy, which is particularly

Table 11.4 A. American Joint Committee on Cancer 8th Edition Tumor Node Metastasis Staging for Gallbladder Cancer: TNM Criteria

T CATEGORY	CRITERIA
TX	Primary tumor cannot be assessed
T0	No evidence of primary tumor
Tis	Carcinoma *in situ*
T1	Tumor invades –
T1a	⇨ Lamina propria
T1b	⇨ Muscular layer
T2	Tumor invades the perimuscular connective tissue –
T2a	⇨ on the peritoneal side NO involvement of the serosa (visceral peritoneum)
T2b	⇨ Tumor invades the perimuscular connective tissue on the hepatic side NO extension into the liver
T3	Tumor perforates serosa and/or directly invades liver and/or ONE (1) other adjacent organ (i.e., stomach, duodenum, colon, pancreas, omentum, or extrahepatic bile ducts)
T4	Tumor invades main portal vein or hepatic artery, or TWO (2) other adjacent organs or structures
N CATEGORY	**CRITERIA**
NX	Regional nodes cannot be assessed
N0	No regional lymph node metastasis
N1	Positive lymph nodes: 1–3
N2	Positive lymph nodes: ≥4
M CATEGORY	**CRITERIA**
M0	No distant metastasis
M1	Distant metastasis

B. STAGING: GALLBLADDER CANCER

T	N	M	STAGE
Tis	N0	M0	0
T1	N0	M0	I
T2a	N0	M0	IIA
T2b	N0	M0	IIB
T3	N0	M0	IIIA
T1–3	N1	M0	IIIB
T4	N0–1	M0	IVA
Any T	N2	M0	IVB
Any T	Any N	M1	IVB

(From Amin MB, Edge S, Greene F, et al, eds. *AJCC Cancer Staging Manual.* 8th ed. Springer International Publishing: American Joint Commission on Cancer; 2017.)

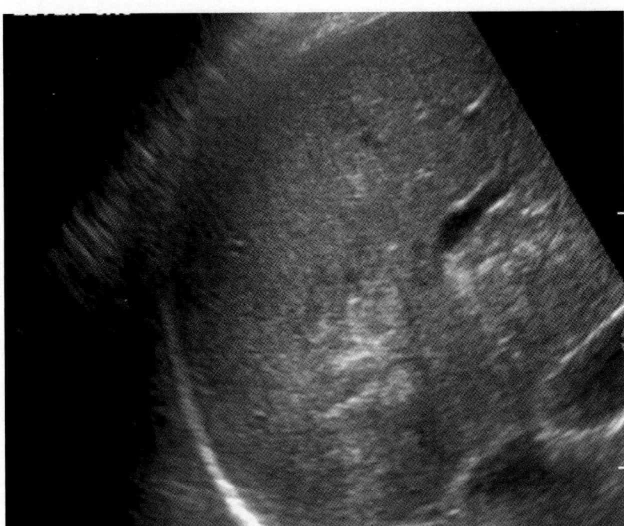

FIGURE 11.6. Transabdominal ultrasound of the liver shows a solid mass with heterogeneous echotexture in the right liver, consistent with intrahepatic cholangiocarcinoma.

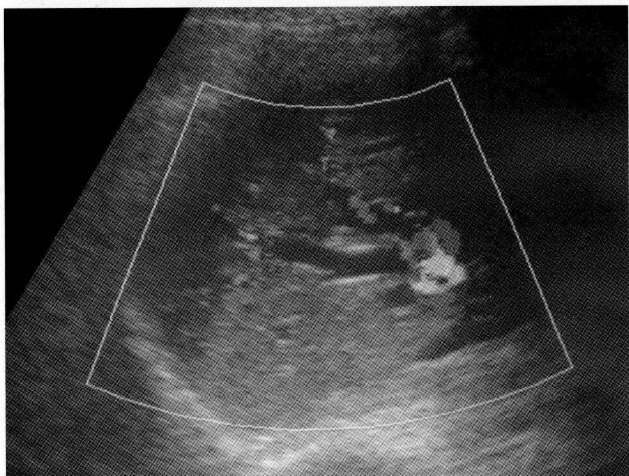

FIGURE 11.7. Transabdominal ultrasound of the liver demonstrates biliary dilatation in a patient with a proximal extrahepatic cholangiocarcinoma near the hilum. The tumor was not well visualized.

important in the setting of variant anatomy. Before surgery, calculations of future liver remnant (FLR) are made (FLR=future liver volume/total expected liver volume). In the setting of an FLR of less than 20% (for a noncirrhotic liver) and less than 40% (for a cirrhotic liver), embolization of the portal vein may be performed, with resultant compensatory hypertrophy and subsequent reduction in postoperative complications.[29]

For evaluation of the biliary tree in suspected ECC, the images are acquired with a pancreas protocol (including parenchyma and delayed phase).[30] The features used to determine tumor extension and location are enhancement of the bile duct wall, abrupt caliber changes in the bile duct, an intraductal mass, and soft tissue attenuation in the bile duct (rather than bile/fluid attenuation) (Figs. 11.9 and 11.10). The detection of bile duct wall enhancement suggests the possibility of malignancy; however, inflammation is also a consideration. The most distinctive feature is irregular circumferential thickening of the bile duct with proximal biliary dilatation and narrowing of the lumen (see Figs. 11.9 and 11.10). The detection of soft tissue attenuation with obliteration of the fat surrounding the bile ducts and vessels in the hepatic hilum is consistent with perivascular spread (Fig. 11.11). Tumor invasion can also extend beyond the regional vessels to adjacent organs (liver, GB, and bowel).

Multidetector computed tomography (MDCT) with thin-slice images can be used to create multiplanar reconstruction of the biliary tree (Fig. 11.12). These three-dimensional (3D) images are helpful in the conceptualization of tumor size, regional extension, and relationship to regional vascular structures, which may be of great assistance in surgical planning.[31,32]

Positron Emission Tomography

Positron emission tomography (PET) has become an important imaging modality in oncologic imaging. The most widely used radiopharmaceutical is 2-[^{18}F] fluoro-2-deoxy-D-glucose (FDG; Fig. 11.13). The benefits of PET/CT over CT include increased accuracy in the detection of distant metastatic disease, particularly nodal staging.[33,34]

For patients with ICC, treatment depends on the surgical resectability of the primary tumor, and the presence of distant metastasis, such as nodal disease beyond the porta hepatis, is usually a contraindication for surgery. In these patients, PET/CT is useful for accurate nodal staging and detection of unexpected metastases, with higher sensitivity than conventional imaging.[34]

The role of FDG PET is limited in the evaluation of patients with ECC distal tumors near the ampulla.[35,36] The detection rates for FDG PET have been reported as 74% for the infiltrating tumor and 96% for the nodular type of ECC. The specificity and sensitivity for nodal metastases were reported as 97% and 33%, respectively, for FDG PET compared with 79% and 57% respectively, for MDCT.[36] FDG PET/CT evaluation for resectability has demonstrated improved accuracy over conventional imaging.[37]

Magnetic Resonance Imaging

MRI examinations typically take longer than CT examinations and may not be as readily available. However, MRI provides superior soft tissue contrast and allows for multiple sequences optimized for evaluation of the biliary tree, hepatic vasculature, and hepatic parenchyma. On noncontrast sequences, ICC will demonstrate low signal relative to the liver on T1-weighted (T1W) imaging high signal on T2-weighted (T2W) imaging, and restricted diffusion on diffusion-weighted imaging (DWI) (Fig. 11.14). On T2W imaging, the signal can be variable as a function of fibrosis (dark), mucous secretions (bright), or necrosis (bright).[22,38] The darker central fibrosis may be a distinctive feature not commonly seen in metastatic disease to the liver.[22] DWI is typically obtained with at least two different B-values (such as 0 and 700 sec/mm^2). The higher B-value allows the suppression of signal from vessels, bile ducts, and other fluids, resulting in an increased contrast between the liver and the lesion. The primary tumor, as well as vascular invasion, will have similar imaging features on DWI, which is useful in the assessment of vascular invasion.

The postcontrast MRI evaluation consists of late arterial, portal venous, delayed, and potentially hepatobiliary phases

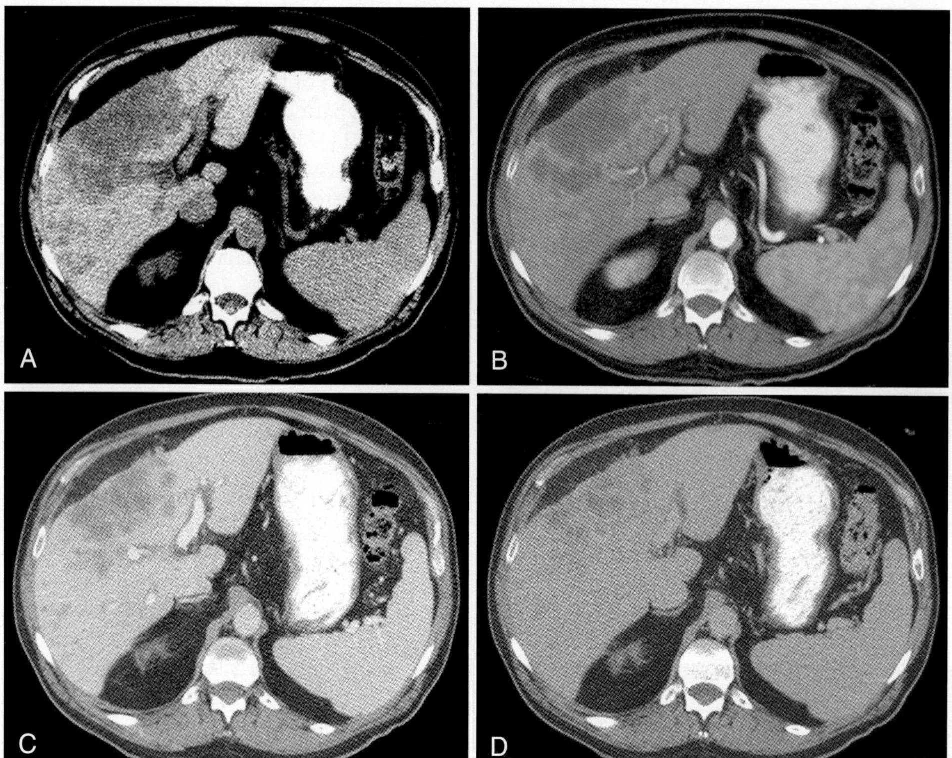

FIGURE 11.8. A, Noncontrast computed tomography (CT) of the abdomen shows a hypoattenuating mass in segment IV of the liver, in keeping with intrahepatic cholangiocarcinoma (ICC). **B,** Late arterial–phase CT of the abdomen shows a mildly peripherally enhancing mass in segment IV of the liver, in keeping with ICC. **C,** Portal venous–phase CT of the abdomen shows an increased enhancement of the mass in segment IV of the liver, in keeping with ICC. **D,** Excretory phase CT of the abdomen shows an almost complete enhancement of the mass in segment IV of the liver, in keeping with ICC.

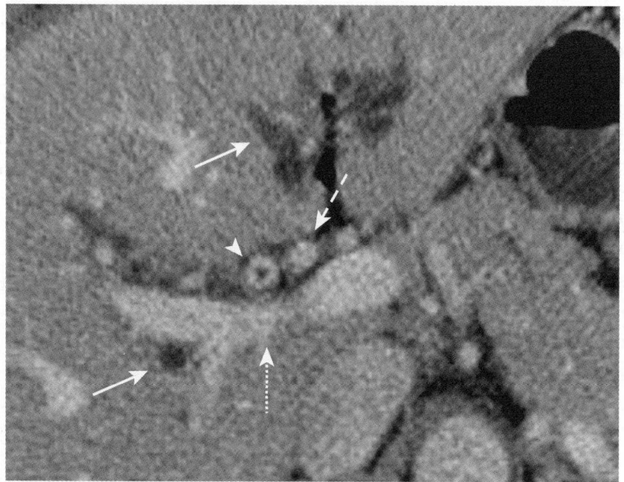

FIGURE 11.9. Portal venous–phase computed tomography examination of the abdomen demonstrates thickening and enhancement of the common hepatic duct (*arrowhead*) in a patient with extrahepatic cholangiocarcinoma. There is biliary dilatation (*solid arrows*). The hepatic artery (*dashed arrow*) and portal vein (*dotted arrow*) are spared, with normal fat attenuation between the tumor and the vessels.

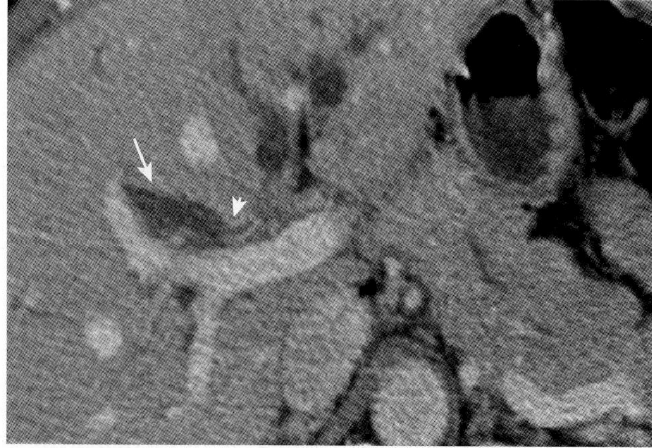

FIGURE 11.10. Delayed-phase computed tomography examination of the abdomen demonstrates enhancement of the right hepatic duct in a patient with extrahepatic cholangiocarcinoma and abrupt caliber change of the bile duct (*arrowhead*). There is biliary dilatation (*solid arrow*).

of contrast administration. The timing of the injection is less critical than in the evaluation of patients with HCC, as the diagnosis of these tumors is not dependent on the identification of arterial phase hyperenhacement. ICC will demonstrate peripheral enhancement with centripetal fill-in (see Fig. 11.14). Metastatic disease from colorectal cancer may show a similar peripheral pattern of enhancement; however, the centripetal fill-in is not seen. The delayed enhancement in ICC may be seen only on the delayed phase or even later in the examination if imaging protocols extend beyond 3 minutes post–contrast injection. In the setting of hepatocyte-specific contrast administration, ICC will not demonstrate uptake of contrast during the hebatobiliary phase and will appear hypointense relative to the liver.[24]

Imaging features of a mass in the liver that suggest malignancy include capsular retraction (can be seen with

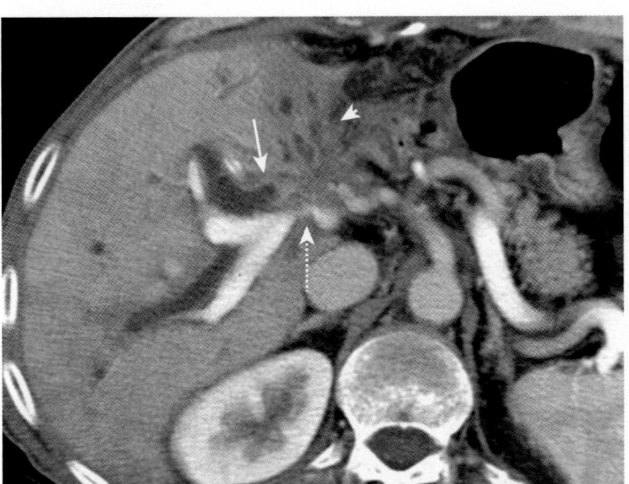

FIGURE 11.11. Portal venous-phase computed tomography examination of the abdomen demonstrates abrupt termination of the bile duct (*solid arrow*), vascular involvement of the portal vein and hepatic artery (*dotted arrow*), and atrophy of the left lobe (*arrowhead*) with nonvisualization of the left portal vein.

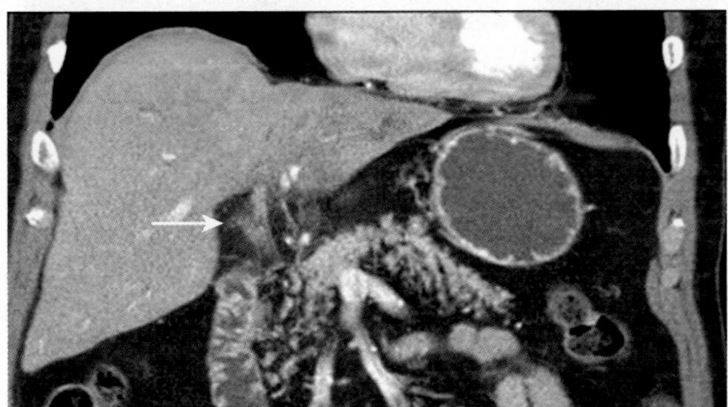

FIGURE 11.12. Multiplanar coronal reconstruction from computed tomography images of the abdomen shows wall thickening and enhancement of the common hepatic duct at the bifurcation (*arrow*), in keeping with type IV Klatzkin tumor.

fibrolamellar HCC, lymphoma, colon cancer metastases, and epithelioid hemangioendothelioma), vascular invasion (can be seen with HCC), and transient hepatic arterial enhancement (can be seen with hilar CCA).

MRI and magnetic resonance cholangiopancreatography (MRCP) are used in combination for the evaluation of patients with suspected ECC. The protocol includes a routine multiphasic MRI of the abdomen. The MRCP images are heavily fluid-weighted and are obtained in either the axial or coronal planes. These thin-slice images can then be used to generate both radial maximum intensity projection (MIP) images and thick-slab MIP images. These are radial images centered on the CBD and can assist in delineation of 3D hepatic ductal anatomy and relationships. The thick-slab images correspond to images obtained during endoscopic retrograde cholangiopancreatography (ERCP). A single-shot fast spin echo or half-Fourier acquisition single shot turbo spin echo (Siemens) sequence is routinely used for the MRCP images. These sequences are fast and have low sensitivity to motion artifacts.

The imaging features of the primary tumor on MRCP are proximal bile duct dilatation with abrupt termination of the bile ducts (shoulder sign) (Fig. 11.15). On post-contrast MRI, features of ECC include thickening and enhancement of the bile duct wall, a mass in the lumen, lobar atrophy, and crowding of the vessels (Fig. 11.16). Similar to CT, some of the imaging features are shared by nonneoplastic inflammatory processes (Fig. 11.17). The tumors are usually hyperintense on T2W imaging and hypointense on T1W imaging and have a heterogeneous enhancement pattern (see Fig. 11.16).[39] In a significant number of patients, the cross-sectional images are obtained after the placement of a biliary stent. This results in interval resolution of biliary dilatation with the loss of the transition site of bile duct caliber attenuation. In addition, a newly placed stent can result in enhancement of the bile duct wall and infiltration of the periductal fat (see Fig. 11.17). This may result in false-positive image interpretations, and careful review of prestent imaging is preferred for the diagnosis of tumoral vascular invasion.

The accuracy of MRI/MRCP for resectability ranges from 80% to 93.3%.[40] MRI/MRCP was comparable with CT in a series evaluating tumor extent and resectability[41]; however, MRI and MRCP still understage up to 20% of patients with perihilar ECC.[42]

Percutaneous Transhepatic Cholangiography and Endoscopic Retrograde Cholangiopancreatography

Percutaneous transhepatic cholangiography (PTC) and ERCP are considered gold standards for imaging the bile ducts. The biliary tree is visualized following opacification with iodinated contrast. Malignancy presents as abrupt termination or irregular narrowing of the bile duct with proximal intrahepatic bile duct dilatation (Fig. 11.18). ERCP provides the additional benefit of intervention, including the ability to place a stent for bile duct decompression and obtain a tissue sample for diagnosis. The major complications of these techniques, which require cannulation of the bile ducts, include sepsis, bile leak, hemorrhage, and even death.[43] Both PTC and ERCP have limited value for the evaluation of extraluminal tumor spread.

KEY POINTS Imaging Cholangiocarcinoma Primary Tumor

- Intrahepatic cholangiocarcinoma (ICC) primary tumor may have variable echogenicity on ultrasound.
- Extrahepatic cholangiocarcinoma (ECC) primary tumor location is inferred from change in caliber of the bile ducts.
- Peripheral pattern of enhancement on computed tomography, magnetic resonance imaging, and positron emission tomography may mimic intrahepatic metastases (e.g., colon cancer); however, centripetal contrast fill-in and dark central fibrosis T2-weighted imaging help distinguish ICC.
- Thickening and enhancement of the bile duct wall is nonspecific and can be seen with ECC and in inflammation (stent placement) or infection.
- Abrupt termination of bile duct (shoulder sign) on magnetic resonance cholangiopancreatography is highly suggestive of ECC.

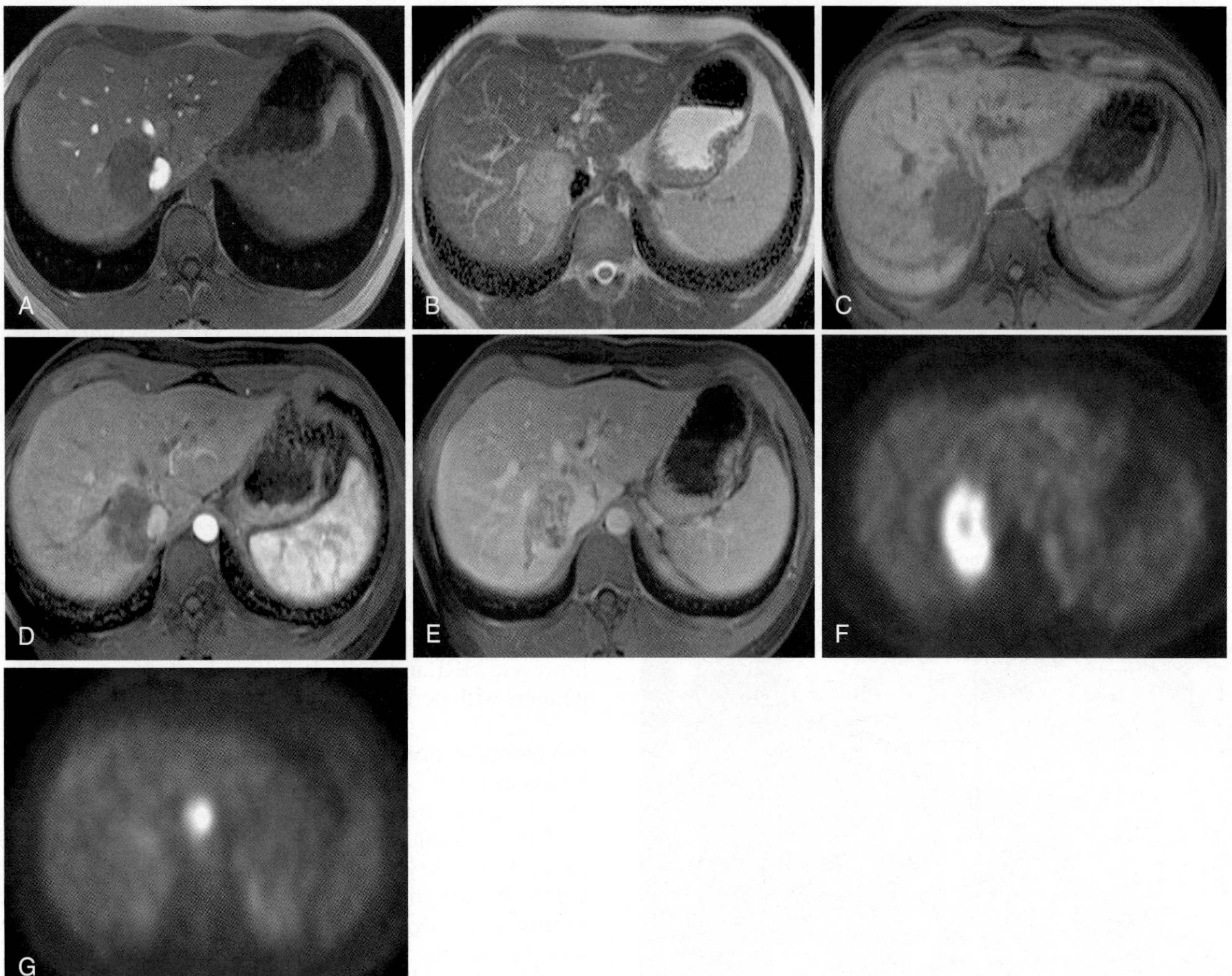

Figure 11.13 **A,** Axial T1-weighted imaging of the liver shows a hypointense mass in the right lobe of the liver, in keeping with intrahepatic cholangiocarcinoma (ICC). **B,** Axial T2-weighted imaging of the liver shows a hyperintense mass in the right lobe of the liver, in keeping with ICC. **C,** Axial precontrast fat-saturated three-dimensional (3D) gradient echo (LAVA) image of the liver shows a hypointense mass in the right lobe of the liver, in keeping with ICC. **D,** Axial late arterial fat-saturated 3D gradient echo (LAVA) image of the liver shows a mildly peripherally enhancing mass in the right lobe of the liver, in keeping with ICC. **E,** Axial delayed fat-saturated 3D gradient (LAVA) echo series of the liver shows an almost complete enhancement of the mass in the right lobe of the liver, in keeping with ICC. **F,** Axial 2-[^{18}F] fluoro-2-deoxy-D-glucose positron emission tomography (FDG PET) image of the abdomen shows metabolic activity in the right lobe of the liver, corresponding to the magnetic resonance imaging studies, in a patient with ICC. **G,** Axial FDG PET image of the abdomen shows metabolic activity in the precaval node, in keeping with metastatic adenopathy in a patient with ICC. *LAVA*, Liver acquisition with volume acceleration.

Lymph Nodes

The imaging evaluation of lymph nodes is based on size, morphology, and location. Nodes located near the primary tumor are likely to be malignant, even if they measure less than 1 cm in minimum diameter. A round node is also more likely to be malignant than a morphologically normal-appearing oval node.

Lymph node metastases are a poor predictor of survival. In various series, the rate of positive lymph nodes found at surgery ranged from 31% to 59%.[44–47] Lymph node metastases have a reported negative effect on survival. In one series, patients with three or more involved nodes had a 0% 3-year survival rate compared with 50% and 60% 3-year survival rates for patients with one/two nodes or no nodes, respectively.[46]

Imaging features that may suggest tumor extension to the lymph nodes include short-axis diameter larger than 1 cm, low-density (necrotic) center, or delayed enhancement. CT has a high negative predictive value but a low positive predictive value for nodal involvement.[48] The accuracy of FDG PET/CT is higher than that of CT alone (75.9% vs. 60.9%).[49] DWI is also very useful in the detection of lymph nodes (Fig. 11.19). In the setting of prior biliary stent placement, reactive periportal nodes may be seen and may mimic metastatic disease.

Key Points Imaging of Lymph Nodes in Cholangiocarcinoma

- Suspicious nodes are necrotic, larger than 1 cm, and located near tumor.
- 2-[^{18}F] fluoro-2-deoxy-D-glucose–positron emission tomography/computed tomography and diffusion-weighted imaging are useful in the detection of nodal disease.

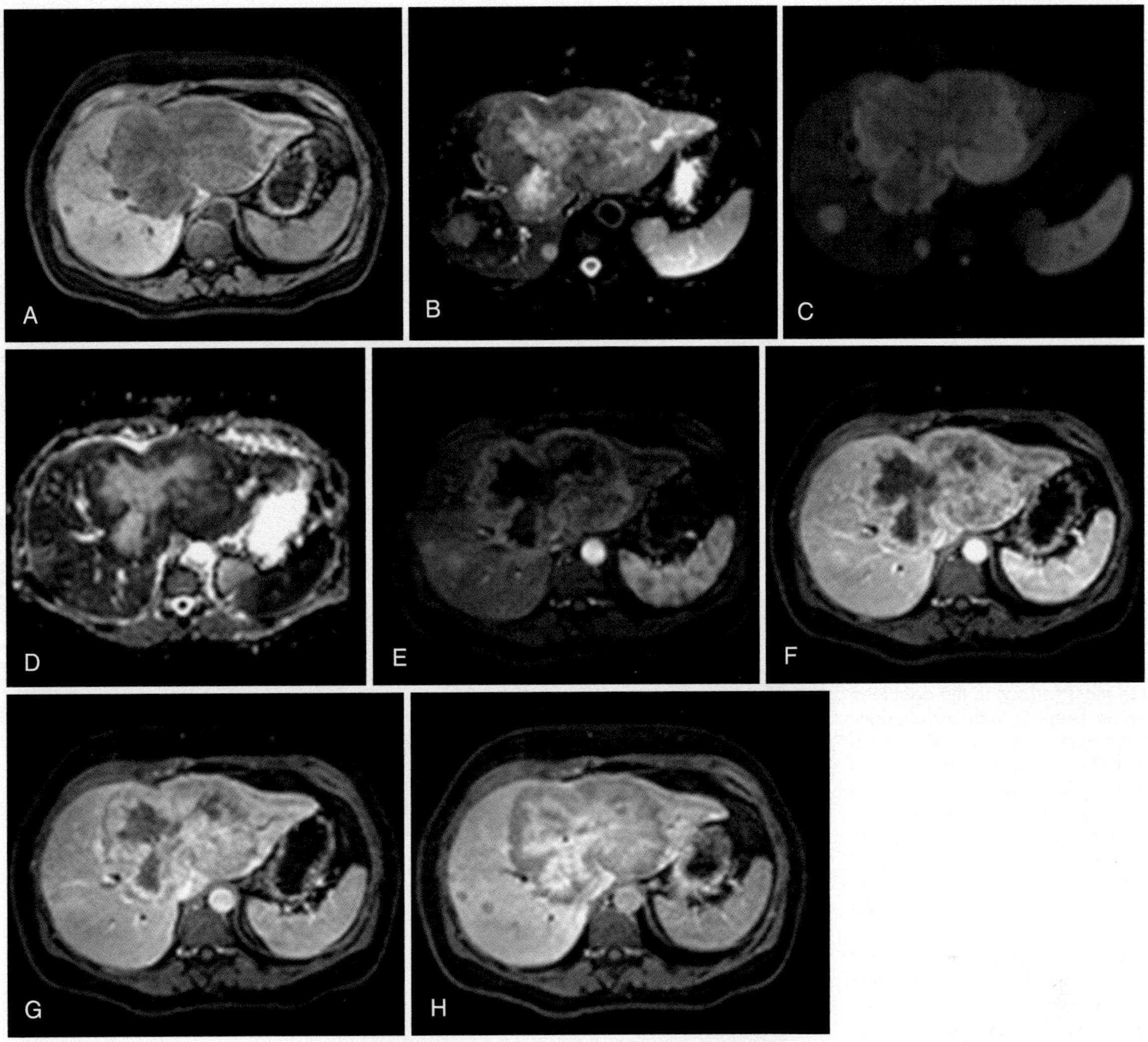

Figure 11.14 A, Axial T1-weighted (T1W) imaging of the liver demonstrates a left hepatic lobe lesion with low signal relative to the liver, consistent with intrahepatic cholangiocarcinoma (ICC). Smaller satellite lesions are also seen in the right hepatic lobe. **B,** On axial T2-weighted (T2W) imaging, this left hepatic lobe lesion demonstrates high signal. **C,** On axial diffusion-weighted imaging, this lesion has peripheral restricted diffusion consistent with abundant tumor cells at the periphery and central fibrous stroma. On postcontrast axial T1W imaging, the large left hepatic lobe lesion demonstrates peripheral arterial enhancement on early arterial phase (**E**) with centripetal fill-in on axial T1W imaging late arterial (**F**), portal venous (**G**), and equilibrium (**H**) phases.

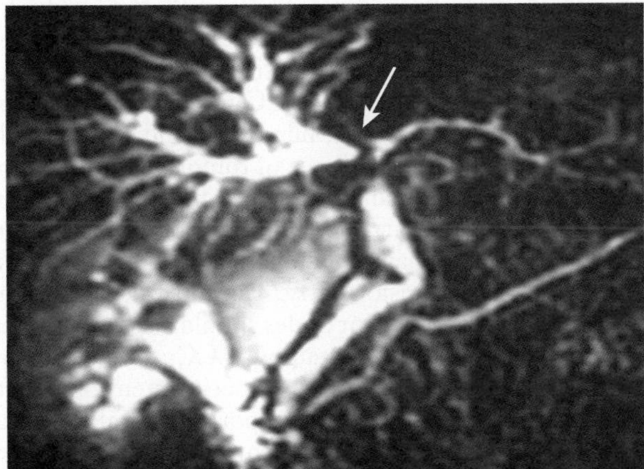

Figure 11.15 Coronal T2-weighted magnetic resonance imaging (40-mm slab) of the abdomen (magnetic resonance cholangiopancreatography) shows bilateral intrahepatic dilatation of the bile duct. There is abrupt termination of the bile duct (*arrow*), in keeping with malignancy (extrahepatic cholangiocarcinoma).

Metastatic Disease

Preoperative imaging should detect satellite nodules in ICC because their presence increases the risk of death by approximately 4- to 11-fold.[45,50] Thus satellite nodules may be considered a relative contraindication to surgery. Distant metastatic disease can be evaluated with a CT of the chest in search of lung metastases, which can be single or multiple. Survey with CT of the abdomen and pelvis may demonstrate skeletal metastases, which are mostly lytic. Adrenal metastases present as large, irregular masses. In the setting of a capsular ICC, soft tissue nodules in the peritoneum or thickening of the omentum are a sign of peritoneal tumor spread. DWI may be useful in the detection of peritoneal disease by suppressing signal from the fluid in the bowel or peritoneum.

Metastatic disease from biliary tract tumors may be detected in the liver, peritoneum, and distant nodal stations. Liver metastases present as low-attenuation lesions

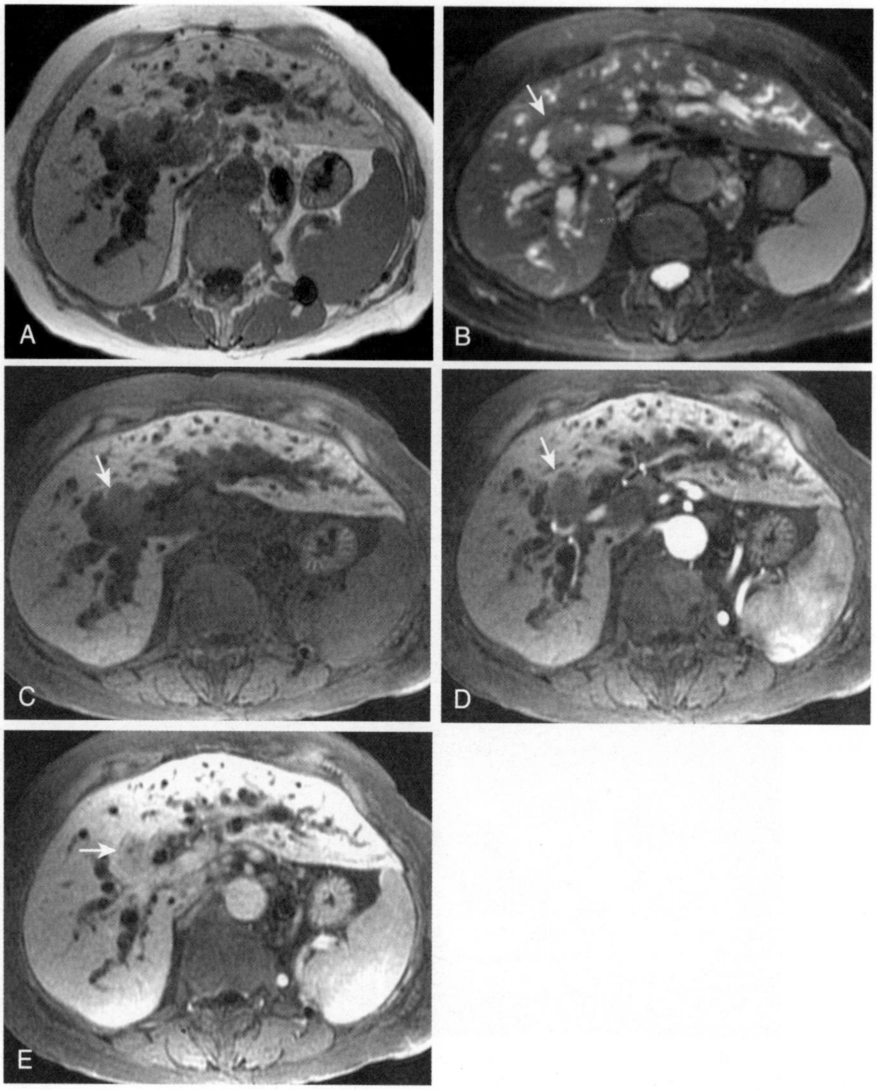

FIGURE 11.16. **A,** Axial T1-weighted imaging of the liver shows a hypointense mass in the right lobe of the liver, in keeping with a proximal ECC. **B,** Axial T2-weighted imaging of the liver shows a hyperintense mass (*arrow*) in the right lobe of the liver, in keeping with extrahepatic cholangiocarcinoma (ECC). **C,** Axial precontrast fat-saturated three-dimensional (3D) gradient echo (LAVA) image of the liver shows a hypointense mass (*arrow*) in the right lobe of the liver, in keeping with ECC. **D,** Axial late arterial fat-saturated 3D gradient echo (LAVA) image of the liver shows a non–early-enhancing mass (*arrow*) in the right lobe of the liver, in keeping with ECC. **E,** Axial delayed fat-saturated 3D gradient (LAVA) echo series of the liver shows an almost complete enhancement of the mass (*arrow*) in the right lobe of the liver, in keeping with ECC. *LAVA*, Liver acquisition with volume acceleration.

on CT and are best seen during the portal venous phase of contrast administration. For MRI, liver metastases are hyperintense on T2W imaging, low-signal on T1W imaging, and demonstrate delayed enhancement. FDG PET liver metastases may be hypermetabolic. In the setting of subcentimeter lesions in the liver, the distinction of benign and malignant disease is difficult with CT, MRI, or PET. In this setting, follow-up imaging at 3-month and 6-month intervals is suggested. Peritoneal disease usually presents as soft tissue nodules and is a common source of error in understaging patients with CCA (Fig. 11.20). These nodules demonstrate restricted diffusion on DWI.

KEY POINTS Imaging of Metastases of Intrahepatic Cholangiocarcinoma

- Detection of satellite nodules in intrahepatic cholangiocarcinoma has important prognostic implications.
- Metastatic disease may be detected in the lungs, bone, adrenals, and peritoneum.
- 2-[^{18}F] fluoro-2-deoxy-D-glucose–positron emission tomography/computed tomography is helpful for detecting distant metastases.

THE RADIOLOGY REPORT

The operative decision for patients with ICC is highly dependent on imaging interpretation. The imaging report should include a detailed description of the size, number, and segmental location of the ICC masses. The relationship of the tumor to vessels, bile ducts, and liver capsule, with comments on any evidence of tumor invasion, should be included. Vascular anatomy including hepatic artery variants, portal vein variants, and accessory hepatic veins should be examined and documented. The presence of ascites, portal hypertension, fatty liver, and especially evaluation of regional and distant nodes should also be included.

The radiology report detailing ECC should include similar details as that of ICC, with special attention paid to any biliary variant anatomy. The report should also include documentation of vascular abutment and encasement.

In the preoperative liver resection setting for both ICC and ECC, segmental liver volumes should be calculated if the FLR is suspected to be suboptimal. Complete imaging staging with evaluation of the regional and distant nodes and the evaluation for intrahepatic or distant metastases

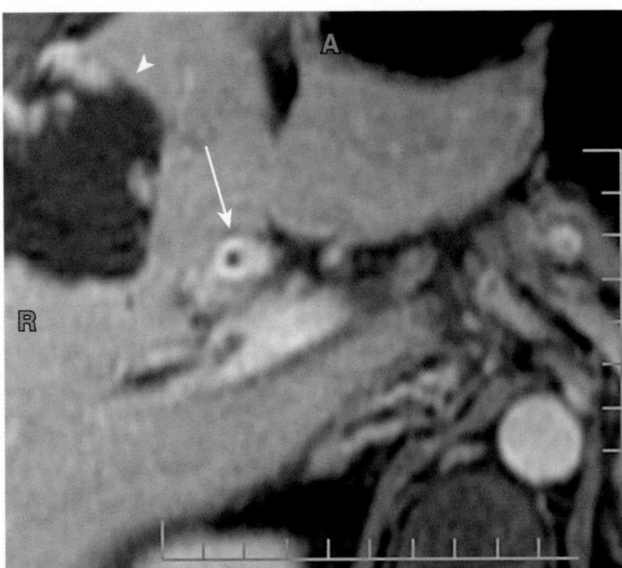

FIGURE 11.17 Axial delayed fat-saturated three-dimensional gradient echo (LAVA) series of the liver shows thickening and enhancement of the bile duct of the liver (*arrow*) in keeping with post–stent placement. An incidental hemangioma (*arrowhead*) is also shown. *LAVA*, Liver acquisition with volume acceleration.

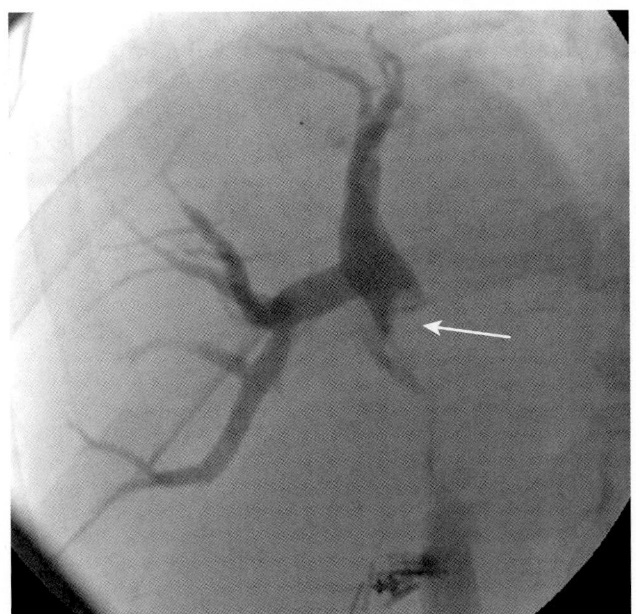

FIGURE 11.18 Endoscopic cholangiopancreatography shows abrupt termination of the bile ducts (*arrow*), in keeping with malignant obstruction in a patient with extrahepatic cholangiocarcinoma.

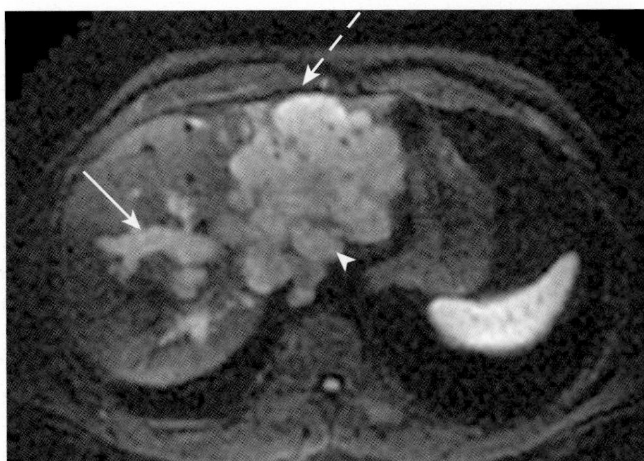

FIGURE 11.19 Axial diffusion-weighted imaging (B=500 sec/mm^2) demonstrates a hyperintense mass in the left liver (*dashed arrow*) and portal vein tumor extension (*solid arrow*) in a patient with intrahepatic cholangiocarcinoma. Enlarged nodes are also visualized (*arrowhead*).

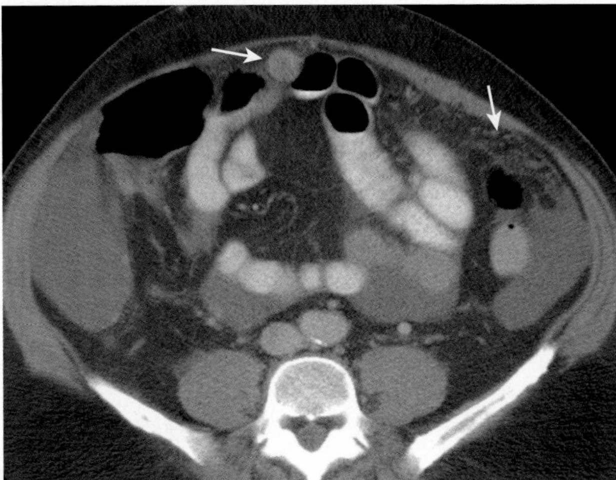

FIGURE 11.20 Delayed post–contrast-enhanced computed tomography image of the abdomen in a patient with extrahepatic cholangiocarcinoma shows omental implants (*arrows*). Ascites is also present.

should also be included. After therapy, the radiology report should include not only evidence of residual disease but also any evidence of complications from therapy.

KEY POINTS The Radiology Report for Cholangiocarcinoma

- Tumor size, number, and vascular involvement.
- Hepatic artery, portal vein, hepatic vein anatomic variants.
- Location of biliary obstruction and extension of tumor in the biliary tree.
- Nodal or metastatic disease.
- Evaluation of residual disease and complications post treatment.

TREATMENT

Surgery

Surgery provides the best outcome for patients with ICC. However, routine intraoperative lymph node dissection is not recommended, because it has limited effect on survival.[47] For the evaluation of disease in the lymph nodes, optimum imaging techniques and attention to detail in preoperative imaging interpretation are essential in correctly identifying surgical candidates. If preoperative imaging is suspicious for nodal metastatic disease, EUS-guided fine needle aspiration or core biopsy can be performed for pathologic evaluation of the periportal lymph nodes.

The primary tumor usually presents as a large mass that invades adjacent structures, requiring extended hepatectomy,[51,52] which may include vascular and biliary resection.[53,54] The 5-year overall survival for resected patients is 23% to 40%.[45,50,53] The resection rate for patients explored for curative intent is 50% to 87%.[3,52,55] Prognostic factors for recurrence include a positive margin, satellite lesions, lymph node metastases, and vascular invasion.[3,45,50,56] Positive margins at surgery have been reported to yield a survival rate equivalent to that of patients who did not undergo surgery.[57]

Surgical resection provides the only curative option for patients with ECC, and high-quality preoperative imaging is essential for presurgical evaluation of potential surgical candidates. The contraindications to surgical resection include advanced disease, inadequate functional liver remnant, and patient factors. Findings of advanced disease that may make a patient unresectable include metastatic disease (N2 nodes, peritoneal disease, or distant metastases), bilateral segmental bile duct tumor extension, contralateral portal vein or hepatic artery involvement, contralateral lobar atrophy, portal vein and bilateral portal vein extension, and tumor extending into the bilateral hepatic artery branches.[58–60] Patient factors such as significant medical comorbidities should be evaluated, and patients with Eastern Cooperative Oncology Group scores of 0, 1, and 2 are potential candidates for surgery.[61]

In the setting of biliary obstruction, biliary drainage (percutaneous or endoluminal) has been suggested for presurgical management.[62,63] This may reverse hepatic dysfunction caused by biliary stasis. In the setting of stenting, preoperative antibiotics are recommended to reduce the risk of postoperative infection.

The surgical approach for hilar or proximal ECC is different from that for distal bile duct tumors near the ampulla. For the hilar tumors, the resection may include cholecystectomy, resection of extrahepatic bile ducts, regional lymphadenectomy, hepatic lobar resection, caudate lobe resection, Roux-en-Y hepaticojejunostomy, and vascular reconstruction or resection. The extent of hepatic resection depends on the Bismuth–Corlette classification of the tumor (Fig. 11.21).[60]

For distal tumors of the bile duct near the ampulla, the surgical approach is similar to the management of ampullary or pancreatic head cancer. The surgical intervention includes pancreaticoduodenectomy and sampling of regional nodes. The median survival after surgery is 2 years, with a 20% to 40% 5-year survival rate.[20]

In the setting of nonsurgical resection of the tumor, palliative surgical intervention may be required to alleviate symptoms of biliary obstruction. This includes jaundice, cholangitis, and liver failure. Surgical bypass is easier for distal bile duct tumors and is not recommended for proximal tumors, because they are technically more challenging and have higher associated procedure-related morbidity.

Endoscopic-guided placement of a stent can be performed to alleviate biliary obstruction. The selection of a plastic versus a metal stent is based on the expected survival, because the plastic stents have to be exchanged every 3 months. Therefore, metallic stents are preferred in patients with an expected survival of more than 6 months.

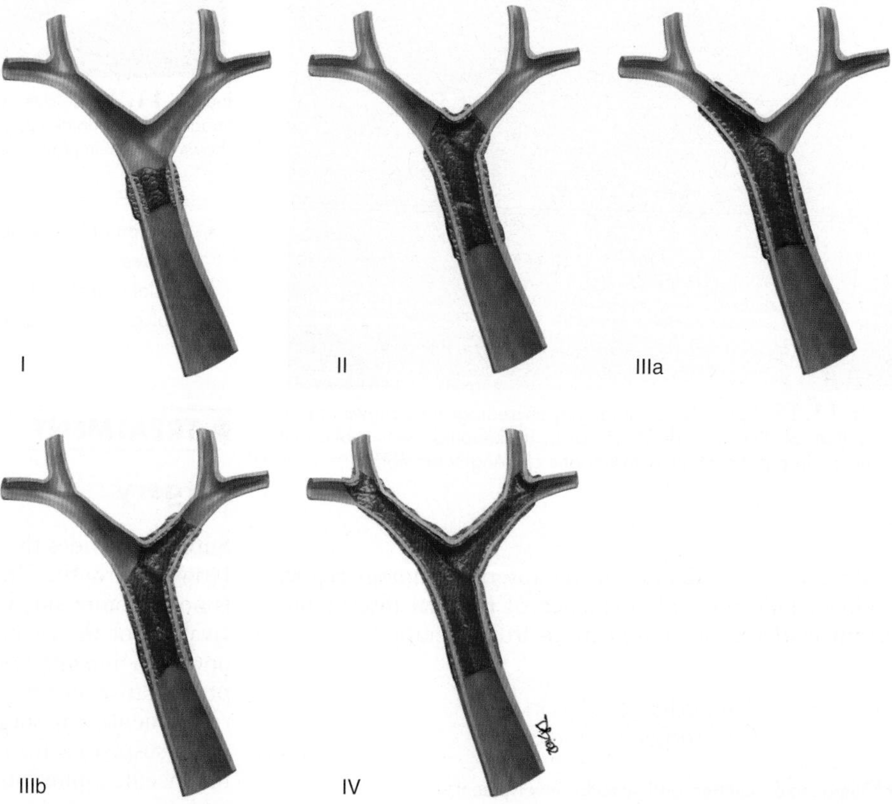

FIGURE 11.21. Bismuth–Corlette classification of hilar tumors. Type I: tumors below the confluence of the left and right hepatic ducts. Type II: tumors at the confluence of the hepatic ducts. Type IIIa: tumors at the confluence and extends into the right hepatic duct. Type IIIb: tumors at the confluence and extends into the left hepatic duct. Type IV: tumors at the confluence and extends into the right and left hepatic ducts.

Stents may need to be placed percutaneously if the endoscopic technique is unsuccessful.

The use of liver transplant for the treatment of ICC has been reported, and this remains a controversial topic. Multiple studies have demonstrated a 20% to 40% overall survival rate at 3 to 5 years after transplant for ICC.[64–66] More recently, a retrospective study demonstrated that liver transplantation in select cirrhotic patients with solitary lesions smaller than 2 cm achieved a 5-year survival rate of 73%.[67] At this time, however, prospective, randomized clinical trials are needed to confirm the benefits of liver transplantation in ICC. It does not currently serve a role in the treatment of ECC.

Key Points Surgery for Cholangiocarcinoma

- Risk factors for recurrence are positive margin, satellite lesions, lymph node metastases, and vascular invasion.
- Surgical approach to perihilar and distal bile duct extrahepatic cholangiocarcinoma tumor resection is different; perihilar tumors will probably include hepatic resection, whereas distal tumors may include pancreaticoduodenectomy.

Transarterial Chemoembolization

Transarterial chemoembolization (TACE) involves selectively injecting embolization beads with a high concentration of chemotherapy into the afferent arteries of the tumor. Several recent studies have examined the use of TACE in patients with unresectable ICC; however, owing to the relatively low numbers of patients diagnosed with ICC yearly, results are still unclear.[68] Additionally, given the relative hypovascularity of ICC, these lesions are not as readily visualized on angiography compared with HCC.

The main contraindications to TACE are portal vein thrombosis, advanced liver disease (Child–Pugh C), active GI bleeding, encephalopathy, refractory ascites, portosystemic shunt, hepatofugal flow, renal failure, clotting disorder, and extrahepatic disease.

Chemotherapy agents used include gemcitabine, mitomycin C, and doxorubicin.[68] Recent improvements in TACE techniques have included the use of new embolics that bind chemical drug molecules electrochemically (such as through ion exchange) and release them in a sustained manner over a prolonged period. This has resulted in greater tumor necrosis with decreased systemic toxicity.

Various publications describe the application of TACE to the management of patients with ICC. Median survival after TACE of unresectable ICC is 11 to 14 months, with overall time to progression of 5.9 to 14.2 months. Additional study is required to determine in which cases TACE is preferred over radiofrequency ablation (RFA; detailed later), or if a combination of TACE and systemic chemotherapy is preferred.[68]

Radiofrequency Ablation

The principle of RFA is to apply a localized thermal treatment, resulting in tumor death. The high temperature (100°C) reached during RFA will result in coagulative necrosis of the tumor and surrounding liver.[69,70] Several case series have demonstrated modest efficacy for ICC, especially in the setting of primary tumors less than 3 cm in size if a patient is not a candidate for resection, but more commonly in the setting of recurrence if the patient is not a candidate for repeat resection.[71]

The imaging description of ICC should indicate the tumor's proximity to major vessels, diaphragm, or other structures that may interfere with the technical success of this procedure. Tumor response to RFA is best evaluated by extent of necrosis rather than the Response Evaluation Criteria in Solid Tumors (RECIST) size criteria.

Chemotherapy

In patients with ICC that is unresectable, either because of advanced invasion or metastatic disease, systemic chemotherapy is the standard treatment. The Advanced Biliary Cancer Trial demonstrated that combination therapy with gemcitabine and cisplatin significantly improved progression-free survival and overall survival compared with treatment with gemcitabine alone.[72] Therefore, this is now the gold standard of care for first-line therapy. In patients who fail to respond to first-line therapy, there is no standard second-line therapy. Several ongoing trials are evaluating potential second-line therapy with multidrug regimens.[73]

Unfortunately, 60% to 70% of patients diagnosed with ECC are not candidates for curative resection. Overall survival in patients with unresectable disease is 2 to 4 months with medical management alone.[74] The current National Comprehensive Cancer Network guidelines recommend multiagent chemotherapy with gemcitabine and cisplatin as first-line chemotherapy for unresected ECC. Chemoradiation with 5-fluorouracil is also an option. However, prospective randomized controlled trials comparing these treatments have not yet been performed, likely because of the rarity of ECC, and further study is warranted.[57]

Multiple ongoing trials are evaluating the role of molecularly-targeted therapies for the treatment of biliary tract cancers as well. These agents include tyrosine kinase inhibitors combined with anti–endothelial growth factor receptor (EGFR) agents such as erlotinib. Cetuximab is an additional anti-EGFR agent. Antiangiogenics such as bevacizumab are also undergoing further investigation.[75]

Radiotherapy

Radiotherapy (RT) has been applied to the management of ECC. The method of radiation delivery is varied, including external-beam irradiation (delivered by either conventional approaches or with conformal treatment planning techniques), brachytherapy with iridium-192, or stereotactic RT.[75] Some patients receive concurrent chemotherapy, and others receive only radiation. In all instances, the proximity of the bowel mucosa often limits the dose of radiation that can be safely given.

Although the role for adjuvant RT in the treatment of distal ECC cannot be conclusively established, locoregional control with chemoradiation seems appropriate to consider in these patients.[26,28] Radiochemotherapy, however, has been reported to have conflicting success rates in several randomized controlled trials.[74]

In the case of hilar CCAs, even with optimal margins after surgery, two in three patients have a recurrence within 2 years, with 60% being locoregional for hilar CCAs.[30] This pattern of locoregional recurrence provides a rationale for adjuvant treatment with a locoregional modality such as RT with or without radiosensitizing chemotherapy. At this time, the optimal radiation dose and standardized treatment protocol of biliary cancers has not yet been defined.[74]

External-beam RT may be used as palliative treatment to relieve pain, maintain biliary patency, and improve survival. Statistics vary among many studies due to small sample size and the frequent administration of palliative chemotherapy in addition to RT. Ghafoori et al. demonstrated a median survival of 14 months with palliative irradiation, with a 2-year survival rate of 22%.[76]

KEY POINTS Nonsurgical Treatment of Cholangiocarcinoma

- There are a limited number of studies in the evaluation of chemotherapy, radiotherapy (RT), and combination therapies for the treatment of extrahepatic cholangiocarcinoma.
- A combination of chemotherapy agents may improve survival and response rates.
- RT as neoadjuvant therapy may improve survival and can also provide pain relief and maintain biliary patency.

SURVEILLANCE

Imaging features of recurrence at the surgical margin after surgical resection and chemotherapy are the same as for the preoperative resection of tumor; for example, on MRI, a mass that enhances on delayed images and demonstrates high signal on T2W imaging. Postsurgical change at the margin after resection owing to edema and/or granulation tissue may be seen on MRI as an enhancing area with high signal on T2W imaging; however, this enhancement is typically not nodular and will resolve at the 6-month follow-up imaging evaluation.

The recommended image protocol after surgery is an imaging study (CT or MRI) three times a year for the first year, two or three times a year for the second year, and then twice a year thereafter. RECIST or the World Health Organization (WHO) criteria are used to assess response to treatment.

After TACE, response to treatment on CT and MRI is confirmed with a decrease in size and no enhancement on the postcontrast images on multiple follow-up studies. In the setting of lipiodol, the evaluation of enhancement on the CT images is limited. A decrease in size on follow-up images is suggestive of response to treatment. Alternatively, MRI may be considered.

After RFA, the ablated tissue will show changes owing to hemorrhage and necrosis (liquefactive and coagulative).[77,78] Hemorrhage will result in high signal on T1W imaging, coagulative necrosis will result in low signal on T2W imaging, and liquefactive necrosis will result in high signal on T2W imaging. Liquefactive necrosis will demonstrate nonrestricted diffusion on DWI (B=500) and an increase in the apparent diffusion coefficient.[79]

Note that the WHO and RECIST criteria are suboptimal in the evaluation of post–RFA-treated ICC. The size of the cavity following RFA treatment will appear larger than the size of the original tumor. In these first scans, the evaluation should be focused on the margin of the RFA cavity. The detection of nodular enhancement, irregular wall, or the distortion of a smooth tumor margin is a sign of an unsuccessful treatment.[78] Subtraction images in MRI using the precontrast as the mask for subtracted images can be very helpful in detecting intracavity residual or recurrent enhancement.

On follow-up studies, successful RFA will demonstrate a subsequent decrease in size of the cavity.[77] An increase in size of the cavity (on CT or MRI) indicates either interval hemorrhage or recurrent disease.[80,81]

The recommended imaging protocol after TACE and RFA is an imaging study (CT or MRI) at 1 month after RFA/TACE to ensure complete treatment, then three times a year in the first year, two or three times a year for the second year, and then twice a year thereafter. To evaluate response to treatment after chemotherapy or RT, the RECIST and the WHO criteria are used.

Imaging features of recurrence at the surgical margin after surgical resection of ECC are similar to those for the preoperative resection of tumor. The detection of biliary obstruction, progression of soft tissue thickening at the surgical bed, abrupt termination of the bile duct, or a mass along the bile duct is considered potential recurrence, and tissue sampling or follow-up imaging should be pursued. For RT and chemotherapy, the signs of recurrence include an increase in soft tissue thickening at the surgical bed. In addition, the detection of masses or biliary obstruction may suggest recurrent disease. Imaging should evaluate for metastatic disease, with particular attention to peritoneal nodules that suggest metastatic implants.

The recommended imaging protocol after surgery for ECC is an imaging study (CT or MRI) three times a year for the first year, two or three times a year for the second year, and twice a year thereafter.

KEY POINTS Surveillance of Cholangiocarcinoma

- Following surgery: three times a year in year 1, two or three times a year in year 2, and twice a year thereafter.
- Response Evaluation Criteria (RECIST)/World Health Organization (WHO) criteria to assess response to treatment with radiotherapy and chemotherapy.
- RECIST/WHO criteria are suboptimal in intrahepatic cholangiocarcinoma evaluation post–radiofrequency ablation, given expected cavity increase in size.

SUMMARY

Management of both ICC and ECC requires a team approach, including the radiologist, oncologist, surgeon, interventional radiologist, and pathologist. This team approach helps in patient selection for surgical and nonsurgical treatment.

Patients with ICC have a very poor prognosis. We have reviewed the clinical, pathologic, imaging, and therapeutic features of this malignancy. The management of this disease is very similar to that of HCC. Although it is a CCA, the clinical presentation usually does not include biliary obstruction. The imaging features mimic liver metastases from the GI tract, and commonly a search for a primary GI tumor is performed. The diagnosis and management of ICC remain a challenge to the entire team. Once the diagnosis is made, the management is very similar to that for HCC. Nonsurgical approaches including both systemic and directed therapies are available.

Advances in imaging, including MDCT with very thin–slice images and MRI in combination with MRCP, have resulted in the ability of a single study to answer all questions in evaluation of biliary obstruction. MRCP and MDCT multiplanar reconstruction images of the biliary tree mimic those of the traditionally used ERCP and allow for assessment of the obstruction and its cause. Angiographic images of the arterial and vascular anatomy in multiple planes facilitate identification of vascular involvement and variant anatomy. Imaging with FDG PET/CT and DWI MRI improve the sensitivity and accuracy of tumor, node, and metastasis staging and help facilitate appropriate treatment selection. Improved image acquisition and processing has facilitated appropriate patient selection for surgery, which, for ECC and ICC, is the only option for cure. Correct image interpretation and patient selection reduce the number of unnecessary surgeries and improve morbidity and survival for these patients.

GALLBLADDER CANCER

Introduction

GB CA is the fifth most common malignancy of the GI tract. The etiology of GB CA is indeterminate, but chronic inflammation secondary to recurrent irritation of the mucosa of the GB is a proposed origin. The symptoms of GB CA are nonspecific and may mimic other, more common, nonmalignant abdominal diseases. In early stages, surgical resection may be curative, as in cases in which the tumor is incidentally found at the time of a cholecystectomy for the diagnosis of acute cholecystitis. Unfortunately, patients commonly present with unresectable disease, and overall outcome is poor, with an overall 5-year survival rate of less than 5%.[82] Familiarity with the imaging features and patterns of spread of disease is essential for proper diagnosis, staging, and early detection. In this section, we review the epidemiology, clinical presentation, anatomy, spread of disease, therapies, and imaging features of GB CA.

EPIDEMIOLOGY

GB CA is part of the CCA family, but behaves differently from ICC or ECC. Since the 1960s, the incidence and mortality of GB CA have decreased. A possible explanation is the increased frequency of cholecystectomy, with a subsequent decrease in the population at risk. GB CA is found in 0.2% to 3% of all cholecystectomies. In those diagnosed, it was suspected in only 30% of patients before surgery.[82]

GB stones, in particular cholesterol stones, are the most common risk factor for GB CA. Gallstones are present in 74% to 92% of patients with GB CA.[83] Gallstones larger than 3 cm are associated with a greater than 10-fold increased risk of cancer compared with smaller stones. Additionally, cholesterol gallstones specifically are associated with a higher risk.[82] Other reported risk factors include congenital biliary cysts, environmental factors (tobacco), infectious factors (*Opisthorchis viverrini*, *Salmonella typhi*), PSC, and genetic factors.[84] Porcelain GB, which was formerly believed to be associated with GB CA, has since been demonstrated to have no definitive association with this malignancy.[85]

GB polyps are present in up to 5% of adults and are important to manage because of their potential for malignant growth. Factors on imaging that are concerning for malignancy include: polyps greater than 10 mm in size, rapid increase in polyp size, solitary or sessile polyps, association with gallstones, and patient age of 50 years or older. Polyps greater than 5 mm in size warrant cholecystectomy in high-risk individuals and sonographic follow-up in low risk patients. Any polyp greater than 1 cm in size warrants cholecystectomy, regardless of risk.[82]

There is a geographic prevalence of GB CAs, with the highest number of cancers found in Chile and Bolivia. Other locations with a higher incidence of GB CA are India, Japan, Israel, and Poland. There is a female preponderance, with an average female-to-male ratio of 3:1. GB CA tends to present in an older population, with the greatest incidence in patients older than 65 years.[86]

Key Points Epidemiology of Gallbladder Cancer

- Gallbladder stones, in particular cholesterol stones, are the most common risk factor.
- Female-to-male ratio is 3:1.
- Median age at presentation is 73 years.

ANATOMY

The GB is part of the biliary system, which is composed of the intrahepatic and extrahepatic bile ducts and the GB. The GB is divided into the fundus, body, and neck (infundibulum or cystic duct). Most of the tumors are located in the fundus (60%), with 30% within the body and 10% within the neck.[87]

Important anatomic considerations in the management of GB CA are the location of the tumor in relation to the portal vein, bile ducts, and hepatic artery. For example, when the tumor extends to the CBD, it may be clinically and radiologically indistinct from primary bile duct tumors. These tumors may also invade the portal vein and hepatic artery. In contrast, tumors in the fundus and body of the GB can readily invade segments IV and V of the liver due to anatomic proximity. The GB is attached to segment IV of the liver. In autopsy series, liver extension was reported in 65% of cases of GB CA.[88] Its propensity to invade the peritoneal cavity and seed wounds (e.g., laparoscopy ports) also affects treatment planning.

KEY POINTS Anatomy of Gallbladder

- The gallbladder (GB) is divided into the fundus, body, and neck.
- Most tumors are located in the fundus.
- The GB is attached to segment IV of the liver, which is often involved in GB cancer.

CLINICAL PRESENTATION

Gallstones are a common finding in GB CA, with copresentation in over 70% of patients. Although there is a high association, the recommendation for prophylactic cholecystectomy is reserved for high-risk populations, given the low incidence of the disease.[89]

Early diagnosis is rare, except in the case of the incidental tumor discovered after a cholecystectomy for suspected cholecystitis. The early clinical presentation of GB CA overlaps with the signs and symptoms of gallstones. The presenting signs and symptoms may vary, and depend on the stage of the disease. Distinctive features are persistent right upper quadrant pain, anorexia, weight loss, and palpable mass. More advanced disease may present with weight loss, hepatomegaly, and jaundice. In the setting of extension to the adjacent bowel, small or large bowel obstruction may be seen, and a fistulous communication to bowel may be seen in advanced cases. Additional findings of advanced GB CA on physical examination may include periumbilical adenopathy (Sister Mary Joseph nodes) and enlarged left supraclavicular nodes (Virchow nodes).

The best serum markers for GB CA are CA19-9 and CA125.[90] However, these markers are nonspecific and may be elevated in other malignancies and benign processes.[91] An elevated serum marker has to be evaluated in combination with clinical history, physical examination, and diagnostic imaging results, and these values should not be interpreted in isolation.

KEY POINTS Clinical Presentation of Gallbladder Cancer

- Gallstones are the most common copresentation.
- Symptoms overlap with acute cholecystitis.
- Distinctive features include weight loss and a palpable mass.
- CA19-9 and CA125 are the best serum markers, but are nonspecific.

PATHOLOGY

Carcinomas, sarcomas, lymphoma, carcinoid, and other malignancies may be found in the GB. The most common malignancy is a primary GB CA, with adenocarcinoma as the most common type of cancer, with an incidence greater than 85%. Other less common GB CA histologies are papillary adenocarcinoma, mucinous carcinoma, and squamous cell carcinoma.[92]

The most widely accepted sequence of GB CA development is a stepwise progression from dysplasia to carcinoma, rather than the adenoma-to-adenocarcinoma model. The rate of progression from dysplasia to invasive carcinoma is estimated at 5 to 15 years.[93]

The gross pathology description of GB CA is either an intraluminal polypoid lesion or, more commonly, a diffusely infiltrating mass. The tumors are commonly described as having one of three patterns: infiltrative (most common), nodular, and papillary (best prognosis) forms.[94]

There are several variants of adenocarcinomas: papillary, intestinal, mucinous, signet-ring cell, and clear cell.[87] The best prognosis is seen with the papillary type, which fill the GB before invading the wall. Most common tumor grades are moderately and poorly differentiated.

KEY POINTS Pathology of Gallbladder Cancer

- Most common type is adenocarcinoma.
- Model is stepwise progression from metaplasia to carcinoma.
- Gallbladder cancer has infiltrative (most common), nodular, and papillary (best prognosis) forms.

STAGING

The AJCC 8th edition staging system for GB CA is based on the TNM classification: tumor depth of invasion (T), nodal disease (N), and metastatic disease (M) (Table 11.4A).

The T classification is based on the thickness of the tumor within the GB wall. It ranges from carcinoma *in situ* (Tis) to T4, depending on the degree of invasion of the lamina propria, muscle layer, connective tissue, serosa, liver, blood vessels, and number of organs involved. T1 and T2 tumors are confined to the GB, and both have a and b subcategorizations. T3 and T4 tumors have extended beyond the GB.

The nodal staging is based on no nodal involvement (N0), involvement of a single node (N1), or involvement of more than one node (N2). M staging is based on the absence or presence of metastatic disease (M0 or M1, respectively).[95]

A stage I tumor is subserosal in location. A stage II tumor is perimuscular in location. Stage III has invaded the liver, and hepatoduodenal metastases may be seen. Stages I to III may be amenable to surgical resection or reresection. For stage IV, distant metastases are detected. Histologic grading of GB CA ranges from G1 to G4 (from well-differentiated to poorly differentiated tumors); this has prognostic significance but is not part of the staging criteria.

KEY POINTS Staging of Gallbladder Cancer

- T classification is based on degree of gallbladder wall involvement.
- Stages I to III may be amenable to surgical resection.

PATTERN OF TUMOR SPREAD

Direct extension to adjacent organs is the most common method of tumor spread. Lymphatic and vascular spread are less common. Other organs most frequently involved, in order

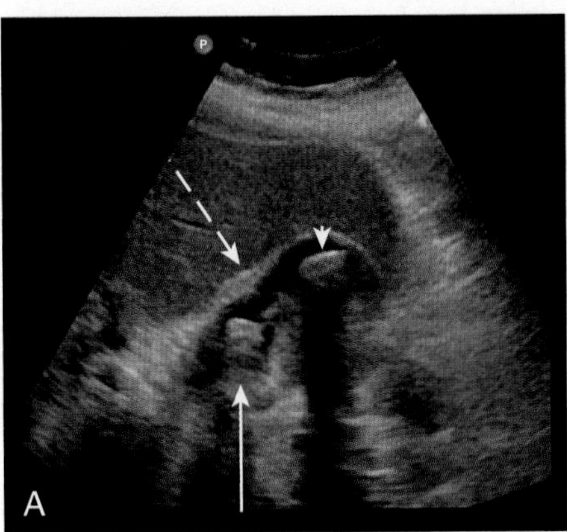

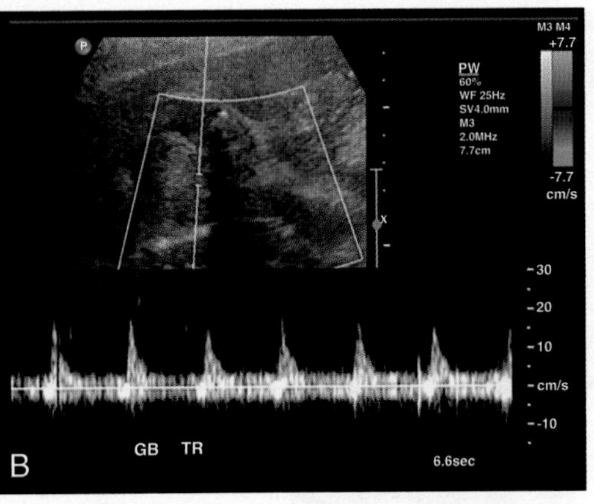

FIGURE 11.22. **A,** Transabdominal ultrasound of the liver shows a solid mass in the gallbladder (GB; *dashed arrow*) and heterogeneous echotexture in a patient with gallbladder cancer (GB CA, *arrow*). A gallstone (*arrowhead*) is also present. **B,** On color and spectral Doppler examination, vascular flow is seen within the heterogeneous in echogenicity GB mass, consistent with GB CA.

of frequency, are liver, colon, duodenum, and pancreas.[88] The most common distant metastatic site is the lungs. Metastatic disease by hematogenous spread can be also be detected in the bones, kidneys, adrenals, and central nervous system. In the setting of prior surgical intervention, wound invasion is a significant problem with GB CA.

The nodal drainage of the GB begins with the cystic and pericholedochal nodes.[96] From these nodes, there is extension to the periportal, hepatic artery, and posterior pancreatic nodal stations. The interaortocaval, celiac, and superior mesenteric nodes are also important routes in the spread of disease.[97]

KEY POINTS Tumor Spread of Gallbladder Cancer

- Direct extension is most common.
- Liver, colon, duodenum, and pancreas are most frequently involved.
- Most common distant metastasis is to the lung.
- Surgical seeding is a significant problem.

IMAGING

As in many other tumors of the abdomen, the nonspecific clinical presentation including right upper quadrant abdominal pain results in the ordering of US evaluation of the abdomen.

The sonographic imaging features of GB CA include wall thickening, gallstones, a mass in the GB, echogenic foci, discontinuous and echogenic mucosa, heterogeneous echogenicity, and a hypoechoic submucosal layer (Fig. 11.22). The detection of echogenic foci may be related to gallstones, calcifications in the wall, or calcifications in the tumor. GB wall thickening and gallstones are more commonly related to acute cholecystitis. Wall thickening of more than 1 cm raises suspicion for GB CA, particularly if focal. The detection of heterogeneous echogenicity may be related to tumor necrosis.

The reported sensitivity of US in the diagnosis of GB ranges from 34% to 85%.[98–100] Color Doppler may assist in the distinction between benign and malignant processes (see Fig. 11.22).[101] Arterial branches showing irregular extensions and tortuous-type vascularity raise suspicion for malignancy.[82] Although US may be useful in the detection of disease, for the detection of the extent of tumor spread, US is suboptimal.[102] CT and MRI are more useful imaging modalities for staging.[103]

A multiphasic CT liver protocol with precontrast, late arterial, portal venous, and delayed phases is recommended for surgical staging. For advanced disease, a single phase suffices to detect a mass that partially replaces the GB, and findings for surgical planning (e.g., vascular involvement) are less pertinent. Thin-slice images are of benefit in evaluating the extent of disease and providing optimal source images for multiplanar reconstruction. A noncontrast CT examination may be useful to detect calcifications within the mass.

The normal GB on the contrast-enhanced CT demonstrates thin (<3 mm) homogeneous mucosal enhancement. The GB wall may appear thickened because of underdistention. Similar to US, the detection of wall thickening (>1 cm) with mural irregularity on CT raises the suspicion for malignancy. Additionally, a highly arterially-enhancing thick inner wall layer or diffuse heterogeneously-enhancing thick layer are both highly suggestive of GB CA. However, adenomyomatosis is a potential mimicker of this enhancement and attenuation. Alternatively, in chronic cholecystitis, the inner GB layer is usually isoattenuating.[82]

Based on gross morphology, the GB CA can be divided into papillary, nodular, flat, filling, and massive. The nodular, papillary, and filling types of tumors share the same imaging feature of a soft tissue–attenuation mass filling the low-attenuation fluid in the GB. Irregular thickening of the GB on the CT examination may be seen in flat tumors. A large mass that replaces the GB and adjacent liver parenchyma is an imaging feature of the massive type. The sensitivity, specificity, and diagnostic accuracy of MDCT in the staging of GBCA are 72.7%, 100%, and 85% respectively.[82]

The mass may be iso- to hypoattenuating relative to the liver on postcontrast CT examination. The mass attenuation after intravenous contrast may be heterogeneous owing to necrosis. The CT examination may detect the presence of metastatic adenopathy, extension to the liver and other organs, or distant metastases that will assist in the staging of these tumors (Fig. 11.23). Biliary dilatation can be seen by CT in over 30% of patients. This may be a result of tumor spread along the cystic duct or extrinsic mass effect from tumor infiltration or enlarged nodes.

Using the CT criteria for nodes larger than 1 cm, for the presence of malignancy, the specificity is 99% for N1 and

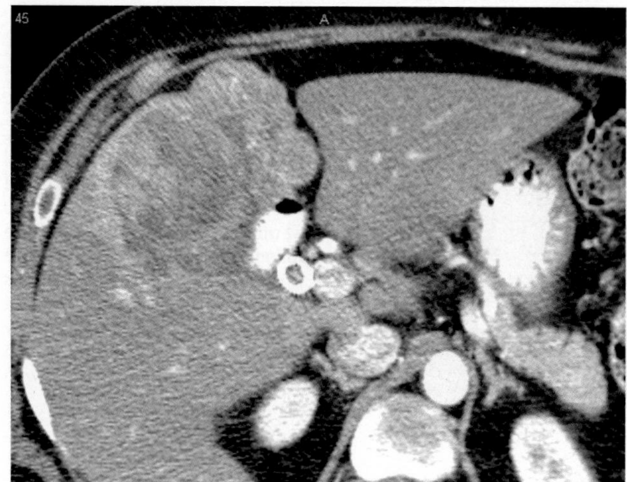

FIGURE 11.23. Delayed-phase postcontrast computed tomography examination of the abdomen demonstrates a mass in the gallbladder fossa with regional extension, consistent with gallbladder cancer.

N2 nodal stations. Another imaging factor that suggests nodal spread of malignancy is the detection of necrotic nodes.[104,105] Hypodense nodes are more suspicious.

GB spread into the peritoneum is common. The imaging features of peritoneal deposits are discrete nodules and fat stranding of the low-attenuation peritoneal fat (see Fig. 11.20). The detection of peritoneal disease is a challenge to the radiologist and may be very difficult. The sensitivity of CT for the detection of peritoneal metastases has been reported to be from 63% to 93%.[104–106]

MRI is a useful modality for the evaluation of patients with GB CA. The image protocol is a liver study with T1W imaging, T2W imaging, DWI, and postcontrast images. MRCP images performed with heavily T2-weighted scans and with thin (≤3 mm) slices are obtained in the axial and coronal planes. For survey of the biliary anatomy, thick (40-mm) slabs can be obtained in radial planes centered on the CBD, with three thick slabs at 45-degree angles from each other.

On T1W imaging, the tumor is hypo- to isointense, and the contents of the GB may be hypo- or hyperintense depending on the fat-to-bile composition ratio of the GB fluid (Fig. 11.24). The higher the fat content, the higher the signal on T1W imaging. On T2W imaging, the tumor is heterogeneous in signal intensity in the background of a fluid-filled (high-signal) GB (see Fig. 11.24). The postcontrast images demonstrate enhancement of the tumor. Similar to CT and US, a GB wall thickness greater than 1 cm with an irregular margin raises suspicion for malignancy. During multiphasic postcontrast evaluation, tumor will enhance early, which is useful for assessing local tumor extension (see Fig. 11.24). In the setting of prior surgical resection for acute cholecystitis, careful review of the wound and laparoscopic ports is essential, with any soft tissue mass suspicious for metastatic implant.

MRI is useful to detect invasion to lymph nodes, portal vein, and hepatoduodenal nodes. The sensitivity and specificity of the combination of MRI and MRCP for the evaluation of GB CA for vascular invasion are 100% and 87%, respectively. For liver invasion, these are 67% and 89%, respectively. For lymph node involvement, these are 56% and 89%, respectively.[107,108] If tumor extends into the cystic duct and CBD, intrahepatic biliary dilatation is best evaluated with MRCP. Additionally, biliary dilatation may result from enlarged metastatic nodes rather than tumor extension, and MRCP would help differentiate these etiologies.

FDG PET is evolving in is applicability for GB CA and has been reported as identifying GB primary, nodal disease, and metastatic disease with sensitivities greater than 75%.[109,110] Specifically, the sensitivity of FDG PET in the detection of metastases is 94.7% (compared with 63.2% for MDCT). There is a significantly higher positive predictive value of 94.1% for the detection of regional lymph node metastases with FDG PET as well.[82]

KEY POINTS Imaging of Gallbladder Cancer

- Multiphasic liver protocol is useful for presurgical planning.
- Focal wall thickening more than 1 cm is suspicious for gallbladder cancer.
- 2-[^{18}F] fluoro-2-deoxy-D-glucose–positron emission tomography improves sensitivity for detection of metastasis and nodal disease.

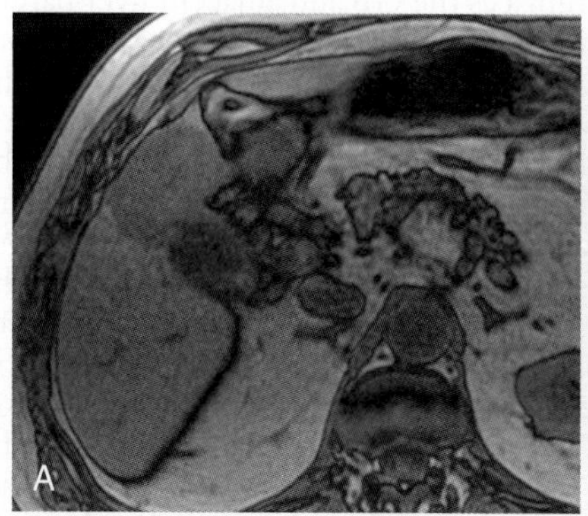

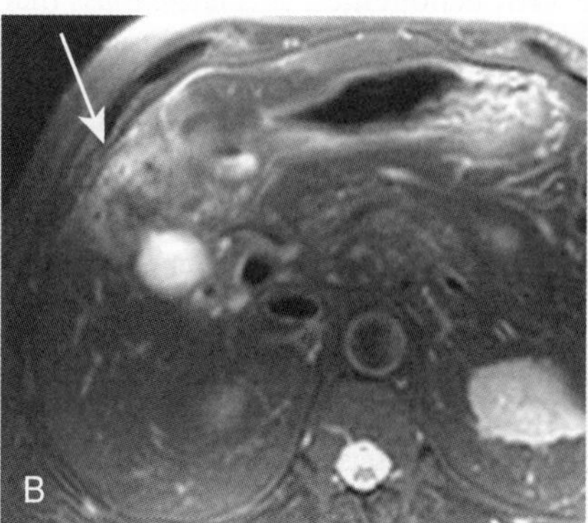

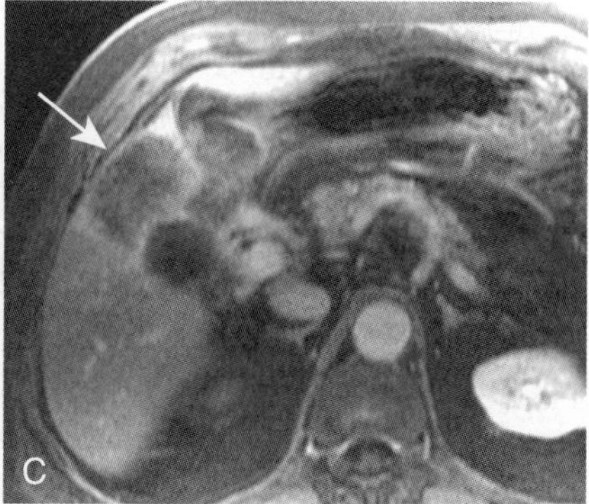

FIGURE 11.24 A, Axial T1-weighted imaging of the liver shows a hypointense mass in the gallbladder (GB) fossa in a patient with gallbladder cancer (GB CA). **B,** Axial T2-weighted imaging of the liver shows a hypointense mass (*arrow*) in the GB fossa in a patient with GB CA. **C,** Axial postcontrast delayed image of the liver shows a mildly enhancing mass (*arrow*) in the GB fossa in a patient with GB CA.

THE RADIOLOGY REPORT

The imaging interpretation of a patient with a diagnosis of GB-related symptoms should include an assessment of signs and complications related to the more commonly encountered acute cholecystitis. This includes evaluation of the GB wall, presence of pericholecystic fluid and/or collections, gallstones, and the relationship of any infiltrative process to adjacent organs. These features are similar to the findings present in GB CA. Distinctive features of GB CA include the presence of a mass, organ invasion, liver metastases, and nodal metastases; documentation of these findings should be included in the report.

In the presurgical patient, the report should include a detailed description of the tumor and its relationship to adjacent organs, vascular structures, and bile ducts. Vascular anatomy including hepatic artery variants, portal vein variants, and accessory hepatic veins should be examined and documented. The presence of cirrhosis, ascites, portal hypertension, and hepatic steatosis should be included in the report. Complete imaging staging with evaluation of the regional and distant nodes and the evaluation for intrahepatic or distant metastases should also be included.

In the postsurgical patient who has had a cholecystectomy for suspected cholecystitis, in addition to the previous description, the radiology report should address the laparoscopic ports or wound site after laparoscopic or open cholecystectomy.

Recommendations on the appropriate follow-up time interval for indeterminate lesions should be included. After therapy, the radiology report should include not only evidence of residual disease but also any evidence of complications from therapy.

KEY POINTS The Radiology Report for Gallbladder Cancer

- Relationship of tumor to vessels, bile ducts, and adjacent organs.
- Nodal description of N1 and N2 nodal stations.
- Evaluation of peritoneum and wound sites for metastatic disease.

THERAPY

Surgery

GB CA is incidentally found in 2% of 70,000 routine cholecystectomies in the United States every year. The procedure carries a small risk of seeding cancer cells at the peritoneal surfaces and the laparoscopic ports. If a patient is suspected of having a GB CA pre- or intraoperatively, he or she should undergo open laparotomy or percutaneous biopsy rather than laparoscopic resection.[111,112]

The goal of surgery in GB CA is complete resection of the tumor, with negative margins. Although prophylactic cholecystectomy has been debated in the management of GB CA, since the incidence of gallstones is so high relative to the incidence of GB CA it is not routinely indicated. Prophylactic cholecystectomy may be pursued in higher-risk populations, such patients with pancreaticobiliary anatomic anomalies, however. Elevated CA19-9 may help select higher-risk patients, too. For the surgical approach for high-risk populations, one should consider an open cholecystectomy rather than laparoscopic intervention, owing to the risk of seeding.

The resection of GB CA is dependent on the tumor stage and prior history of cholecystectomy. If GB CA is detected before cholecystectomy for presumed cholecystitis, it would be best to postpone the cholecystectomy for when a complete resection is possible. An incomplete cholecystectomy does not improve outcome for patients who later have a complete resection.[94] For early-stage tumors (T1a), a simple cholecystectomy with negative margins is adequate. For T1b tumors, a more aggressive approach should be considered. However, extended resection has a mortality rate of 2% to 5% and a postoperative morbidity rate of over 13%.[113,114]

T2 lesions require *en bloc* resection of liver and regional nodes.[115,116] The degree of hepatic resection is dependent on the vascular extension of tumor. Careful review of preoperative images for the vascular anatomy will assist the surgeon in planning the surgical approach. In tumors in which the right portal vein is involved, a right hepatectomy is required.[117] In T2 tumors, there is a higher chance of nodal involvement, and lymphadenectomy is recommended. Patients with celiac and retroperitoneal nodes may not benefit from surgical resection.

T3 lesions, similar to T2 lesions, require aggressive liver and regional node resection. In addition, all involved organs, for example, the stomach, duodenum, pancreas, or colon, are resected *en bloc*.[115] In the setting of T4 disease, surgery has been considered if vascular reconstruction, biliary bypass, and complete *en bloc* resection of the tumor are plausible. The benefit of this procedure is inconclusive at present.

If a T1, T2, or T3 lesion is found incidentally in a laparoscopic specimen, reexploration with excision of the laparoscopic port sites has been recommended.[94,118]

Most patients with GB CA with symptomatic jaundice and gastroduodenal obstruction are diagnosed with advanced disease. Jaundice symptoms can be relieved by palliative procedures such as biliary tract bypass, intrahepatic cholangioenteric anastomosis, and percutaneous transhepatic biliary catheters. Gastroduodenal obstruction can be treated with gastrojejunostomy, intraoperative radiation, decompression gastrostomy, or jejunostomy feeding tube.

KEY POINTS Surgery for Gallbladder Cancer

- Resection of the primary tumor with *en bloc* resection of any adjacent organ invasion.
- Intraoperative survey of pancreaticoduodenal, interaortocaval, and superior mesenteric nodes.
- Biliary bypass or catheters for relief of biliary obstruction.

Chemotherapy/Radiation Therapy

Locally advanced, unresectable, and metastatic GB CA is associated with poor prognosis, and systemic chemotherapy is considered first-line treatment in these patients.

A variety of regimens have been studied in observational and phase II trials. The largest phase III trial ABC-02 established gemcitabine and cisplatin as a standard regimen for GB CA. Additional ongoing studies are evaluating the use of gemcitabine combined with additional agents.[119]

There is a high rate of recurrence and locoregional disease in GB CA patients. Thus adjuvant therapy has been explored. There have been reports of adjuvant RT with external-beam radiation, brachytherapy, and intraoperative RT.[120,121] Complete remission is very rare, and the median survival is 11 months or less.[122] The duration of response is usually 3 to 6 months.

Most studies of reexploration for incidentally diagnosed GB CAs are small and nonrandomized and do not have sufficient power to address the survival benefit of chemoradiation. In contrast to CCAs, because the patterns of failure suggest a predominantly distant pattern of failure for GB CAs, it may be reasonable to establish that there is no unrecognized metastatic disease (over a course of systemic chemotherapy) before consolidating with chemoradiation therapy.

Based on population-based registries such as Surveillance, Epidemiology, and End Results, regionally advanced or hepatic-invasive GB CA is treated with adjuvant radiation in the United States, and this may result in survival improvement.[123] For advanced unresectable tumors, external-beam RT may be used as palliative treatment to relieve pain and maintain biliary patency.

Recent data indicate that EGFR and vascular endothelial growth factor receptor (VEGFR) are important targets in biliary cancer that could potentially be targeted by future therapies, requiring additional study at the time of this publication.[124]

KEY POINTS Chemotherapy/Radiation for Gallbladder Cancer

- ABC-02 showed improved survival with gemcitabine combined with cisplatin.
- Radiotherapy is used as adjuvant therapy or palliative treatment.

SURVEILLANCE

CT and MRI are the most commonly used imaging modalities to follow up patients with GB CA. Imaging features of recurrence at the surgical margin after surgical resection include the detection of a soft tissue nodule or mass in the surgical field. Postoperative change to the liver because of surgical manipulation will present as an early enhancing area on CT or MRI and will resolve within 6 months. This area is isointense to the liver on delayed imaging and demonstrates high signal on T2W imaging; postoperative change is rarely nodular.

In the setting of intrahepatic metastases, the RECIST or WHO criteria are used to assess response to treatment. In the evaluation of EGFR- and VEGFR-targeted therapy, FDG PET scan may show response to treatment that may not be assessed using the RECIST criteria. As in the cases of other antiangiogenic therapies used for liver metastases, response to treatment on CT and MRI may demonstrate increased necrosis rather than a change in size.

Imaging after resection of GB CA is generally recommended three times per year for 2 years, then every 6 to 12 months thereafter.

KEY POINTS Surveillance of Gallbladder Cancer

- Response Evaluation Criteria in Solid Tumors and the World Health Organization criteria are used for response to treatment.
- 2-[^{18}F] fluoro-2-deoxy-D-glucose–positron emission tomography may be useful in the setting of vascular endothelial growth factor receptor– and endothelial growth factor receptor–targeted therapy.
- After resection, follow-up with computed tomography or magnetic resonance imaging three times a year for 2 years and every 6 to 12 months thereafter.

SUMMARY

GB CA is a highly lethal disease, and surgical resection offers the only chance for a cure. We have reviewed the clinical, pathologic, imaging, and therapeutic features of this malignancy. The management of this disease requires a team approach, including input from the radiologist, oncologist, surgeon, and pathologist.

Early diagnosis of GB CA is difficult because the clinical presentation mimics the common diagnosis of acute cholecystitis. The role of MRI and CT in the staging of the presurgical and postsurgical patients is essential for successful outcome. Surgery provides the best outcome, and a detailed description from imaging studies of the primary tumor, regional and distant nodal stations, peritoneum, and adjacent organs for any evidence of metastatic disease is essential. Careful attention to the detection of soft tissue nodules in the surgical bed, wound site, and peritoneum is essential for the detection of residual and recurrent disease. The response to treatment is evaluated with the RECIST and the WHO criteria. Recent advances in targeted therapy show some improved survival, and in these cases the response to treatment may be assessed with functional imaging such as FDG PET.

The GB remains a clinical and radiologic challenge, in part because of the increasing incidence of obesity. Obesity is known to contribute to gallstone formation, and gallstones are the most common risk factor for both acute cholecystitis and GB CA. Hopefully, with improved imaging techniques such as DWI MRI, use of functional and molecular imaging, and increased spatial and temporal resolution, there will be improvement in early diagnosis, accurate staging, and reliable monitoring of response to treatment.

REFERENCES

1. Khan SA, Taylor-Robinson SD, Toledano MB, et al. Changing international trends in mortality rates for liver, biliary and pancreatic tumours. *J Hepatol.* 2002;37(6):806-813.
2. Lazaridis KN, Gores GJ. Cholangiocarcinoma. *Gastroenterology.* 2005;128(6):1655-1667.

3. Nakagohri T, Kinoshita T, Konishi M, et al. Surgical outcome and prognostic factors in intrahepatic cholangiocarcinoma. *World J Surg*. 2008;32(12):2675-2680.
4. Shaib Y, El-Serag HB. The epidemiology of cholangiocarcinoma. *Semin Liver Dis*. 2004;24(2):115-125.
5. Kubo S, Kinoshita H, Hirohashi K, et al. Hepatolithiasis associated with cholangiocarcinoma. *World J Surg*. 1995;19(4):637-641.
6. Chapman RW. Risk factors for biliary tract carcinogenesis. *Ann Oncol*. 1999;10(Suppl 4):308-311.
7. Szendroi M, Nemeth L, Vajta G. Asbestos bodies in a bile duct cancer after occupational exposure. *Environ Res*. 1983;30(2):270-280.
8. Welzel TM, Graubard BI, El-Serag HB, et al. Risk factors for intrahepatic and extrahepatic cholangiocarcinoma in the United States: a population-based case-control study. *Clin G Hepatol*. 2007;5(10):1221-1228.
9. Tocchi A, Mazzoni G, Liotta G, et al. Late development of bile duct cancer in patients who had biliary-enteric drainage for benign disease: a follow-up study of more than 1,000 patients. *Ann Surg*. 2001;234(2):210-214.
10. Lim JH, Park CK. Pathology of cholangiocarcinoma. *Abdom Imaging*. 2004;29(5):540-547.
11. Esnaola NF, Meyer JE, Karachristos A, et al. Evaluation and management of intrahepatic and extrahepatic cholangiocarcinoma. *Cancer*. 2016;122(9):1349-1369.
12. Patel T. Worldwide trends in mortality from biliary tract malignancies. *BMC Cancer*. 2002;2:10.
13. Olnes MJ, Erlich R. A review and update on cholangiocarcinoma. *Oncology*. 2004;66(3):167-179.
14. Weinbren K, Mutum SS. Pathological aspects of cholangiocarcinoma. *J Pathol*. 1983;139(2):217-238.
15. Hammill CW, Wong LL. Intrahepatic cholangiocarcinoma: a malignancy of increasing importance. *J Am Coll Surg*. 2008;207(4):594-603.
16. Nichols JC, Gores GJ, LaRusso NF, et al. Diagnostic role of serum CA 19-9 for cholangiocarcinoma in patients with primary sclerosing cholangitis. *Mayo Clin Proc*. 1993;68(9):874-879.
17. Patel AH, Harnois DM, Klee GG, et al. The utility of CA 19-9 in the diagnoses of cholangiocarcinoma in patients without primary sclerosing cholangitis. *Am J Gastroenterol*. 2000;95(1):204-207.
18. Singal AG, Rakoski MO, Salgia R, et al. The clinical presentation and prognostic factors for intrahepatic and extrahepatic cholangiocarcinoma in a tertiary care centre. *Aliment Pharmacol Ther*. 2010;31(6):625-633.
19. Chintanaboina J, Badari AR, Gopavaram D, et al. Transient marked elevation of serum CA 19-9 levels in a patient with acute cholangitis and biliary stent. *South Med J*. 2008;101(6):661.
20. Amin MB, Edge S, Green F, et al. *AJCC Cancer Staging Manual*. 8th ed. New York, NY: Springer International Publishing; 2017.
21. Kaczynski J, Hansson G, Wallerstedt S. Incidence, etiologic aspects and clinicopathologic features in intrahepatic cholangiocellular carcinoma--a study of 51 cases from a low-endemicity area. *Acta Oncol*. 1998;37(1):77-83.
22. Choi BI, Lee JM, Han JK. Imaging of intrahepatic and hilar cholangiocarcinoma. *Abdom Imaging*. 2004;29(5):548-557.
23. Patel T. Increasing incidence and mortality of primary intrahepatic cholangiocarcinoma in the United States. *Hepatology*. 2001;33(6):1353-1357.
24. Michels NA. Newer anatomy of the liver and its variant blood supply and collateral circulation. *Am J Surg*. 1966;112(3):337-347.
25. Gerhards MF, Vos P, van Gulik TM, et al. Incidence of benign lesions in patients resected for suspicious hilar obstruction. *Br J Surg*. 2001;88(1):48-51.
26. Neumaier CE, Bertolotto M, Perrone R, et al. Staging of hilar cholangiocarcinoma with ultrasound. *JCU*. 1995;23(3):173-178.
27. Saini S. Imaging of the hepatobiliary tract. *N Engl J Med*. 1997;336(26):1889-1894.
28. Fritscher-Ravens A, Broering DC, Knoefel WT, et al. EUS-guided fine-needle aspiration of suspected hilar cholangiocarcinoma in potentially operable patients with negative brush cytology. *The Am J Gastroenterol*. 2004;99(1):45-51.
29. Madoff DC, Abdalla EK, Vauthey JN. Portal vein embolization in preparation for major hepatic resection: evolution of a new standard of care. *JVIR*. 2005;16(6):779-790.
30. Sahani D, Saini S, Pena C, et al. Using multidetector CT for preoperative vascular evaluation of liver neoplasms: technique and results. *AJR Am J Roentgenol*. 2002;179(1):53-59.
31. Uchida M, Ishibashi M, Abe T, et al. Three-dimensional imaging of liver tumors using helical CT during intravenous injection of contrast medium. *JCAT*. 1999;23(3):435-440.
32. Nanashima A, Abo T, Sakamoto I, et al. Three-dimensional cholangiography applying C-arm computed tomography in bile duct carcinoma: a new radiological technique. *Hepatogastroenterology*. 2009;56(91-92):615-618.
33. Breitenstein S, Apestegui C, Clavien PA. Positron emission tomography (PET) for cholangiocarcinoma. *HPB*. 2008;10(2):120-121.
34. Lee Y, Yoo IR, Boo SH, et al. The Role of F-18 FDG PET/CT in Intrahepatic Cholangiocarcinoma. *Nucl Med Mol Imaging*. 2017;51(1):69-78.
35. Li J, Kuehl H, Grabellus F, et al. Preoperative assessment of hilar cholangiocarcinoma by dual-modality PET/CT. *J Surg Oncol*. 2008;98(6):438-443.
36. Furukawa H, Ikuma H, Asakura-Yokoe K, et al. Preoperative staging of biliary carcinoma using 18F-fluorodeoxyglucose PET: prospective comparison with PET+CT, MDCT and histopathology. *Eur Radiol*. 2008;18(12):2841-2847.
37. Kim JH, Yoon HK, Sung KB, et al. Transcatheter arterial chemoembolization or chemoinfusion for unresectable intrahepatic cholangiocarcinoma: clinical efficacy and factors influencing outcomes. *Cancer*. 2008;113(7):1614-1622.
38. Manfredi R, Barbaro B, Masselli G, et al. Magnetic resonance imaging of cholangiocarcinoma. *Semin Liver Dis*. 2004;24(2):155-164.
39. Lee DH, Lee JM, Kim KW, et al. MR imaging findings of early bile duct cancer. *JMRI*. 2008;28(6):1466-1475.
40. Masselli G, Manfredi R, Vecchioli A, et al. MR imaging and MR cholangiopancreatography in the preoperative evaluation of hilar cholangiocarcinoma: correlation with surgical and pathologic findings. *Eur Radiol*. 2008;18(10):2213-2221.
41. Park HS, Lee JM, Choi JY, et al. Preoperative evaluation of bile duct cancer: MRI combined with MR cholangiopancreatography versus MDCT with direct cholangiography. *AJR Am J Roentgenol*. 2008;190(2):396-405.
42. Zidi SH, Prat F, Le Guen O, et al. Performance characteristics of magnetic resonance cholangiography in the staging of malignant hilar strictures. *Gut*. 2000;46(1):103-106.
43. May GR, Bender CE, Williams Jr. HJ. Radiologic approaches to the treatment of benign and malignant biliary tract disease. *Semin Liver Dis*. 1987;7(4):334-342.
44. Yamamoto M, Nakajo S, Tahara E. Dysplasia of the gallbladder. Its histogenesis and correlation to gallbladder adenocarcinoma. *Pathol Res Pract*. 1989;185(4):454-460.
45. Ohtsuka M, Ito H, Kimura F, et al. Results of surgical treatment for intrahepatic cholangiocarcinoma and clinicopathological factors influencing survival. *Br J Surg*. 2002;89(12):1525-1531.
46. Nakagawa T, Kamiyama T, Kurauchi N, et al. Number of lymph node metastases is a significant prognostic factor in intrahepatic cholangiocarcinoma. *World J Surg*. 2005;29(6):728-733.
47. Shimada K, Sano T, Nara S, et al. Therapeutic value of lymph node dissection during hepatectomy in patients with intrahepatic cholangiocellular carcinoma with negative lymph node involvement. *Surgery*. 2009;145(4):411-416.
48. Grobmyer SR, Wang L, Gonen M, et al. Perihepatic lymph node assessment in patients undergoing partial hepatectomy for malignancy. *Ann Surg*. 2006;244(2):260-264.
49. Kim JY, Kim MH, Lee TY, et al. Clinical role of 18F-FDG PET-CT in suspected and potentially operable cholangiocarcinoma: a prospective study compared with conventional imaging. *Am J Gastroenterol*. 2008;103(5):1145-1151.
50. Suzuki S, Sakaguchi T, Yokoi Y, et al. Clinicopathological prognostic factors and impact of surgical treatment of mass-forming intrahepatic cholangiocarcinoma. *World J Surg*. 2002;26(6):687-693.
51. Valverde A, Bonhomme N, Farges O, et al. Resection of intrahepatic cholangiocarcinoma: a Western experience. *J Hepatobiliary Pancreat Surg*. 1999;6(2):122-127.
52. Weber SM, Jarnagin WR, Klimstra D, et al. Intrahepatic cholangiocarcinoma: resectability, recurrence pattern, and outcomes. *J Am Coll Surg*. 2001;193(4):384-391.
53. Weimann A, Varnholt H, Schlitt HJ, et al. Retrospective analysis of prognostic factors after liver resection and transplantation for cholangiocellular carcinoma. *Br J Surg*. 2000;87(9):1182-1187.
54. Madariaga JR, Fung J, Gutierrez J, et al. Liver resection combined with excision of vena cava. *J Am Coll Surg*. 2000;191(3): 244-250.

55. Hanazaki K, Kajikawa S, Shimozawa N, et al. Prognostic factors of intrahepatic cholangiocarcinoma after hepatic resection: univariate and multivariate analysis. *Hepatogastroenterology*. 2002;49(44):311-316.
56. Uenishi T, Hirohashi K, Haba T, et al. Portal thrombosis due to intrahepatic cholangiocarcinoma following successful treatment for hepatocellular carcinoma. *Hepatogastroenterology*. 2003;50(52):1140-1142.
57. Torgeson A, Lloyd S, Boothe D, et al. Chemoradiation therapy for unresected extrahepatic cholangiocarcinoma: a propensity score-matched analysis. *Ann Surg Oncol*. 2017;24(13):4001-4008.
58. Gazzaniga GM, Filauro M, Bagarolo C, Mori L. Surgery for hilar cholangiocarcinoma: an Italian experience. *J Hepatobiliary Pancreat Surg*. 2000;7(2):122-127.
59. Hemming AW, Reed AI, Fujita S, et al. Surgical management of hilar cholangiocarcinoma. *Ann Surg*. 2005;241(5):693-699. discussion 699-702.
60. Hidalgo E, Asthana S, Nishio H, et al. Surgery for hilar cholangiocarcinoma: the Leeds experience. *Eur J Surg Oncol*. 2008;34(7):787-794.
61. di Sebastiano P, Festa L, Buchler MW, et al. Surgical aspects in management of hepato-pancreatico-biliary tumours in the elderly. *Best Pract Res Clin Gastroenterol*. 2009;23(6):919-923.
62. Nagino M, Takada T, Miyazaki M, et al. Preoperative biliary drainage for biliary tract and ampullary carcinomas. *J Hepatobiliary Pancreat Surg*. 2008;15(1):25-30.
63. Coss A, Byrne MF. Preoperative biliary drainage in malignant obstruction: indications, techniques, and the debate over risk. *Curr Gastroenterol Rep*. 2009;11(2):145-149.
64. Becker NS, Rodriguez JA, Barshes NR, et al. Outcomes analysis for 280 patients with cholangiocarcinoma treated with liver transplantation over an 18-year period. *J Gastrointest Surg*. 2008;12(1):117-122.
65. Meyer CG, Penn I, James L. Liver transplantation for cholangiocarcinoma: results in 207 patients. *Transplantation*. 2000;69(8):1633-1637.
66. Shimoda M, Farmer DG, Colquhoun SD, et al. Liver transplantation for cholangiocellular carcinoma: analysis of a single-center experience and review of the literature. *Liver Transpl*. 2001;7(12):1023-1033.
67. Sapisochin G, Rodriguez de Lope C, Gastaca M, et al. "Very early" intrahepatic cholangiocarcinoma in cirrhotic patients: should liver transplantation be reconsidered in these patients? *Am J Transplant*. 2014;14(3):660-667.
68. Aliberti C, Carandina R, Sarti D, et al. Chemoembolization with drug-eluting microspheres loaded with doxorubicin for the treatment of cholangiocarcinoma. *Anticancer Res*. 2017;37(4):1859-1863.
69. Carrafiello G, Lagana D, Cotta E, et al. Radiofrequency ablation of intrahepatic cholangiocarcinoma: preliminary experience. *Cardiovasc Intervent Radiol*. 2010;33(4):835-839.
70. Chiou YY, Hwang JI, Chou YH. Percutaneous ultrasound-guided radiofrequency ablation of intrahepatic cholangiocarcinoma. *Kaohsiung J Med Sci*. 2005;21(7):304-309.
71. Shindoh J. Ablative therapies for intrahepatic cholangiocarcinoma. *Hepatobiliary Surg Nutr*. 2017;6(1):2-6.
72. Valle J, Wasan H, Palmer DH, et al. Cisplatin plus gemcitabine versus gemcitabine for biliary tract cancer. *N Engl J Med*. 2010;362(14):1273-1281.
73. Bupathi M, Ahn DH, Bekaii-Saab T. Therapeutic options for intrahepatic cholangiocarcinoma. *Hepatobiliary Surg Nutr*. 2017;6(2):91-100.
74. Autorino R, Mattiucci GC, Ardito F, et al. Radiochemotherapy with gemcitabine in unresectable extrahepatic cholangiocarcinoma: long-term results of a phase ii study. *Anticancer Res*. 2016;36(2):737-740.
75. Ramirez-Merino N, Aix SP, Cortes-Funes H. Chemotherapy for cholangiocarcinoma: An update. *World J Gastrointest Oncol*. 2013;5(7):171-176.
76. Ghafoori AP, Nelson JW, Willett CG, et al. Radiotherapy in the treatment of patients with unresectable extrahepatic cholangiocarcinoma. *Int J Radiat Oncol Biol Phys*. 2011;81(3):654-659.
77. Dromain C, de Baere T, Elias D, et al. Hepatic tumors treated with percutaneous radio-frequency ablation: CT and MR imaging follow-up. *Radiology*. 2002;223(1):255-262.
78. Kuszyk BS, Boitnott JK, Choti MA, et al. Local tumor recurrence following hepatic cryoablation: radiologic-histopathologic correlation in a rabbit model. *Radiology*. 2000;217(2):477-486.
79. Okuma T, Matsuoka T, Yamamoto A, Hamamoto S, Nakamura K, Inoue Y. Assessment of early treatment response after CT-guided radiofrequency ablation of unresectable lung tumours by diffusion-weighted MRI: a pilot study. *Br J Radiol*. 2009;82(984):989-994.
80. Limanond P, Zimmerman P, Raman SS, et al. Interpretation of CT and MRI after radiofrequency ablation of hepatic malignancies. *AJR Am J Roentgenol*. 2003;181(6):1635-1640.
81. Braga L, Semelka RC. Magnetic resonance imaging features of focal liver lesions after intervention. *TMRI*. 2005;16(1):99-106.
82. Kalra N, Gupta P, Singhal M, et al. Cross-sectional imaging of gallbladder carcinoma: an update. *J Clin Exp Hepatol*. 2019; 9(3):334-344.
83. Nagorney DM, McPherson GA. Carcinoma of the gallbladder and extrahepatic bile ducts. *Semin Oncol*. 1988;15(2):106-115.
84. Chaurasia P, Thakur MK, Shukla HS. What causes cancer gallbladder?: a review. *HPB Surg*. 1999;11(4):217-224.
85. Towfigh S, McFadden DW, Cortina GR, et al. Porcelain gallbladder is not associated with gallbladder carcinoma. *Am Surg*. 2001;67(1):7-10.
86. Henson DE, Albores-Saavedra J, Corle D. Carcinoma of the gallbladder. Histologic types, stage of disease, grade, and survival rates. *Cancer*. 1992;70(6):1493-1497.
87. Albores-Saavedra J, Henson DE, Sobin LH. The WHO histological classification of tumors of the gallbladder and extrahepatic bile ducts. A commentary on the second edition. *Cancer*. 1992;70(2):410-414.
88. Sons HU, Borchard F, Joel BS. Carcinoma of the gallbladder: autopsy findings in 287 cases and review of the literature. *J Surg Oncol*. 1985;28(3):199-206.
89. Wood R, Fraser LA, Brewster DH, et al. Epidemiology of gallbladder cancer and trends in cholecystectomy rates in Scotland, 1968-1998. *Eur J Cancer*. 2003;39(14):2080-2086.
90. Shukla VK, Gurubachan Sharma D, et al. Diagnostic value of serum CA242, CA 19-9, CA 15-3 and CA 125 in patients with carcinoma of the gallbladder. *Trop Gastroenterol*. 2006;27(4):160-165.
91. Murray MD, Burton FR, Di Bisceglie AM. Markedly elevated serum CA 19-9 levels in association with a benign biliary stricture due to primary sclerosing cholangitis. *J Clin Gastroenterol*. 2007;41(1):115-117.
92. Carriaga MT, Henson DE. Liver, gallbladder, extrahepatic bile ducts, and pancreas. *Cancer*. 1995;75(1 Suppl):171-190.
93. Goldin RD, Roa JC. Gallbladder cancer: a morphological and molecular update. *Histopathology*. 2009;55(2):218-229.
94. Fong Y, Heffernan N, Blumgart LH. Gallbladder carcinoma discovered during laparoscopic cholecystectomy: aggressive reresection is beneficial. *Cancer*. 1998;83(3):423-427.
95. Aloia TA, Charnsangavej C, Faria S, et al. High-resolution computed tomography accurately predicts resectability in hilar cholangiocarcinoma. *Am J Surg*. 2007;193(6):702-706.
96. Wang JD, Liu YB, Quan ZW, et al. Role of regional lymphadenectomy in different stage of gallbladder carcinoma. *Hepatogastroenterology*. 2009;56(91-92):593-596.
97. Shirai Y, Yoshida K, Tsukada K, et al. Identification of the regional lymphatic system of the gallbladder by vital staining. *Br J Surg*. 1992;79(7):659-662.
98. Hawkins WG, DeMatteo RP, Jarnagin WR, et al. Jaundice predicts advanced disease and early mortality in patients with gallbladder cancer. *Ann Surg Oncol*. 2004;11(3):310-315.
99. Onoyama H, Yamamoto M, Takada M, et al. Diagnostic imaging of early gallbladder cancer: retrospective study of 53 cases. *World J Surg*. 1999;23(7):708-712.
100. Tsuchiya Y. Early carcinoma of the gallbladder: macroscopic features and US findings. *Radiology*. 1991;179(1):171-175.
101. Komatsuda T, Ishida H, Konno K, et al. Gallbladder carcinoma: color Doppler sonography. *Abdom Imaging*. 2000;25(2):194-197.
102. Bach AM, Loring LA, Hann LE, et al. Gallbladder cancer: can ultrasonography evaluate extent of disease? *J Ultrasound Med*. 1998;17(5):303-309.
103. Kim SJ, Lee JM, Lee JY, et al. Accuracy of preoperative T-staging of gallbladder carcinoma using MDCT. *AJR Am J Roentgenol*. 2008;190(1):74-80.

104. Ohtani T, Shirai Y, Tsukada K, et al. Spread of gallbladder carcinoma: CT evaluation with pathologic correlation. *Abdom Imaging*. 1996;21(3):195-201.
105. Levin B. Gallbladder carcinoma. *Ann Oncol*. 1999;10(Suppl 4):129-130.
106. Kalra N, Suri S, Gupta R, et al. MDCT in the staging of gallbladder carcinoma. *AJR Am J Roentgenol*. 2006;186(3):758-762.
107. Choi JY, Lee JM, Lee JY, et al. Navigator-triggered isotropic three-dimensional magnetic resonance cholangiopancreatography in the diagnosis of malignant biliary obstructions: comparison with direct cholangiography. *JMRI*. 2008;27(1):94-101.
108. Oikarinen H. Diagnostic imaging of carcinomas of the gallbladder and the bile ducts. *Acta Radiol*. 2006;47(4):345-358.
109. Koh T, Taniguchi H, Yamaguchi A, et al. Differential diagnosis of gallbladder cancer using positron emission tomography with fluorine-18-labeled fluoro-deoxyglucose (FDG-PET). *J Surg Oncol*. 2003;84(2):74-81.
110. Anderson CD, Rice MH, Pinson CW, et al. Fluorodeoxyglucose PET imaging in the evaluation of gallbladder carcinoma and cholangiocarcinoma. *J Gastrointest Surg*. 2004;8(1):90-97.
111. Miwa S, Miyagawa S, Kobayashi A, et al. Predictive factors for intrahepatic cholangiocarcinoma recurrence in the liver following surgery. *J Gastroenterol*. 2006;41(9):893-900.
112. Kapoor VK. Incidental gallbladder cancer. *Am J Gastroenterol*. 2001;96(3):627-629.
113. Abdalla EK, Vauthey JN. Extrahepatic bile duct resection: standard treatment for advanced gallbladder cancer? *J Surg Oncol*. 2006;94(4):269-270.
114. D'Amico D, Bassi N, D'Erminio A, et al. Current situation in the treatment of gallbladder cancer. Considerations on the utility of an extended resection. *Hepatogastroenterology*. 1991;38(Suppl 1):16-21.
115. Bartlett DL, Fong Y, Fortner JG, et al. Long-term results after resection for gallbladder cancer. Implications for staging and management. *Ann Surg*. 1996;224(5):639-646.
116. Oertli D, Herzog U, Tondelli P. Primary carcinoma of the gallbladder: operative experience during a 16 year period. *Eur J Surg*. 1993;159(8):415-420.
117. Duffy A, Capanu M, Abou-Alfa GK, et al. Gallbladder cancer (GBC): 10-year experience at Memorial Sloan-Kettering Cancer Centre (MSKCC). *J Surg Oncol*. 2008;98(7):485-489.
118. Hueman MT, Vollmer Jr CM, Pawlik TM. Evolving treatment strategies for gallbladder cancer. *Ann Surg Oncol*. 2009;16(8):2101-2115.
119. Azizi AA, Lamarca A, Valle JW. Systemic therapy of gallbladder cancer: review of first line, maintenance, neoadjuvant and second line therapy specific to gallbladder cancer. *Chin Clin Oncol*. 2019;8(4):43.
120. Oswalt CE, Cruz Jr. AB. Effectiveness of chemotherapy in addition to surgery in treating carcinoma of the gallbladder. *Rev Surg*. 1977;34(6):436-438.
121. Todoroki T, Iwasaki Y, Orii K, et al. Resection combined with intraoperative radiation therapy (IORT) for stage IV (TNM) gallbladder carcinoma. *World J Surg*. 1991;15(3):357-366.
122. de Aretxabala X, Roa I, Berrios M, et al. Chemoradiotherapy in gallbladder cancer. *J Surg Oncol*. 2006;93(8):699-704.
123. Wang SJ, Fuller CD, Kim JS, et al. Prediction model for estimating the survival benefit of adjuvant radiotherapy for gallbladder cancer. *J Clin Oncol*. 2008;26(13):2112-2117.
124. Thomas MB. Targeted therapies for cancer of the gallbladder. *Curr Opin Gastroenterol*. 2008;24(3):372-376.

CHAPTER 12

Pancreatic Ductal Adenocarcinoma

Anushri Parakh, M.D.; Yoshifumi Noda M.D.; Avinash R. Kambadakone M.D.; and Dushant V. Sahani, M.D.

INTRODUCTION

Pancreatic ductal adenocarcinoma (PDAC) has a poor prognosis, with a 5-year survival rate of less than 10%, and accounts for 90% of all pancreatic tumors.[1] It remains one of the most difficult challenges in oncology because patients are typically asymptomatic until the disease is in an advanced stage. It is also not unusual to present with symptomatic metastases in the presence of a small primary tumor. Furthermore, many of its symptoms are nonspecific and overlap with a variety of other diseases such as cholecystitis, pancreatitis, and bowel disorders.

Effective treatment of PDAC requires multidisciplinary cooperation amongst surgeons, oncologists, radiation oncologists, and radiologists. The standard therapy for resectable PDAC is surgery. Neoadjuvant chemotherapy with or without radiation is being increasingly adopted as treatment for borderline resectable tumors to improve the rate of negative resection margins. Chemotherapeutic agents like FOLFIRINOX and gemcitabine plus nanoparticle albumin-bound paclitaxel are approved for patients with distant metastases or locally advanced tumors.

Imaging is critical in the management of these patients, as it has an important role in tumor staging, determining resectability, and predicting patient outcome.

EPIDEMIOLOGY AND RISK FACTORS

PDAC is the fourth leading cause of cancer-related mortality in both males and females. An estimated 45,750 PDAC-related deaths have occurred in the United States thus far in 2019.[1] PDAC is typically seen in the elderly, with a slight predilection for men over women in most countries.[2] Exposure to cigarette smoke is a significant risk factor and is implicated in as many as 20% to 30% of pancreatic cancers.[3] Although excessive alcohol consumption is a common risk factor for chronic pancreatitis, it has not been shown to result in an increased risk of PDAC. However, chronic pancreatitis itself is strongly related to the development of PDAC.[4] PDAC is often diagnosed within 2 years of a diagnosis of chronic pancreatitis.[5] Therefore, close follow-up in the first years following a diagnosis of chronic pancreatitis is necessary.

PDAC itself can induce diabetes mellitus secondary to its destructive effects on the pancreatic parenchyma. Approximately 8% patients with PDAC have comorbid type 3c diabetes.[6] On the other hand, a metaanalysis showed a twofold increase in the pooled relative risk for PDAC in patients suffering from diabetes for 5 years.[7] Although the mechanism of diabetes is complex, the increased risk has been found to be secondary to insulin deficiency, potential immunopathogenesis, reduced incretin effect, peripheral insulin resistance, and hepatic insulin resistance.

Other risk factors include inherited genetic risk, pancreatitis, pancreatic cyst, physical inactivity, and obesity.[8]

A variety of syndromes are also associated with an increased risk of PDAC, including hereditary pancreatitis, Peutz–Jeghers syndrome, Lynch syndrome, familial adenomatous polyposis, familial atypical multiple mole melanoma, and ataxic telangiectasia.

MOLECULAR BIOMARKERS

Activation of oncogenes and inactivation of tumor suppressor genes play a significant role in the manifestation of PDAC.[9,10] Mutations in genes such as *DPC4*, *P53*, and *P16* are present in over half of all cases. Carriers of germline *BRCA2* mutation have up to tenfold higher risk for developing PDAC than the general population. Moreover, several molecular biomarkers, including SMAD4, Ki-67 index, Vimentin, E-cadherin, and TWIST, have been reported as predictive factors for overall survival. Among them, Vimentin, E-cadherin, and Twist are associated with epithelial-to-mesenchymal transition, which is a key step in primary tumor progression to metastasis.[11] E-cadherin–negative PDACs have been shown to have a worse prognosis than positive cases (hazard ratio, 2.21). Irregular tumor margins are more frequently observed in E-cadherin–negative PDACs than in E-cadherin–positive PDACs.[12]

ANATOMY AND PATHOLOGY

The pancreas, measuring between 12 and 15 cm in length, is located deep within the retroperitoneum and lacks a capsule. This allows adjacent fat to extend within the clefts between glandular components.

The pancreas can be divided into five components: the head, uncinate process, neck, body, and tail (Fig. 12.1). The pancreatic head is defined as the portion to the right of the left border of the superior mesenteric vein (SMV). The pancreatic head is bounded on the right by the descending portion of the duodenum and inferiorly by the horizontal portion of the duodenum. To the left of the pancreatic head is a narrow projection called the uncinate process, which lies posterior to the SMV. The neck is a narrow segment

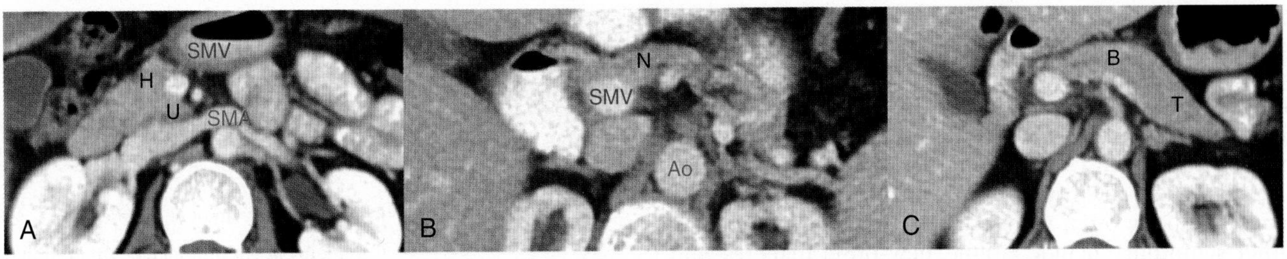

Figure 12.1. Pancreatic anatomy on axial cross-sectional contrast enhanced multidetector row computed tomography. **A**, Inferior pancreas. *H*, Head; *SMA*, superior mesenteric artery; *SMV*, superior mesenteric vein; *U*, uncinate. **B**, Superiorly, the neck (N). **C**, Further cranially, the pancreatic body (B) and tail (T). *Ao*; Aorta.

that joins the pancreatic head to the body. The body is located between the left border of the SMV and the left aortic margin. The pancreatic body is located posterior to the stomach. The tail extends from the left border of the body laterally into the splenic hilum.

Vascular structures also provide important anatomical boundaries to localize the extent of disease. The gastroduodenal artery (GDA), originating from the common hepatic artery (CHA), forms the right lateral and anterior boundary of the pancreatic head. The inferior pancreaticoduodenal artery courses along the posterior border of the pancreatic head, and the SMV, as described previously, is an important landmark. Knowledge of the vascular supply is important because it also provides a pathway for spread of tumor.

The pancreas receives its arterial supply from the GDA from above and the inferior pancreaticoduodenal artery from below. These supply the anterior and posterior pancreaticoduodenal arcades to supply the pancreatic head and the uncinate process. Branches of the dorsal pancreatic artery, which typically arises from the celiac trunk, also provide supply to the pancreatic head and anastomoses with the pancreaticoduodenal arcade and small vascular branches from the GDA and CHA. The pancreatic body is supplied by branches of the dorsal pancreatic artery and the great pancreatic artery, which in turn arises from the splenic artery. Multiple splenic artery branches provide supply to the pancreatic tail.[13]

The venous drainage is via branches that drain into the SMV and splenic veins. These then join to form the portal vein (PV) at the splenoportal confluence posterior to the pancreatic neck. The splenic vein runs along the posterior pancreatic body, and this proximity leads to its frequent occlusion secondary to pancreatic cancer or pancreatitis.

Both sympathetic and parasympathetic innervations of the pancreas are present. The sympathetic supply controls pancreatic blood flow, and the parasympathetic innervations, originating from the posterior vagus nerve and celiac plexus, promote pancreatic secretions. Both the parasympathetic and the sympathetic tracts contain nerve fibers that transmit pain. These nerve fibers provide a means for tumor spread, and their involvement results in debilitating pain. Extrapancreatic neural invasion by PDAC can occur along any of the following four pathways: the plexuses pancreaticus capitalis 1 and 2, anterior pathway along the GDA plexus and CHA plexus, and root of the mesentery pathway.[14–17]

Histologically, the pancreas is composed of both exocrine and endocrine cell types. The exocrine component consists of acinar and ductal cells responsible for a variety of digestive enzymes and bicarbonate that are ultimately emptied into the duodenum at the ampulla of Vater to facilitate digestion. The endocrine cellular types include alpha cells (that produce glucagon), beta cells (that produce insulin), delta cells (that produce somatostatin), and PP cells (that produce pancreatic polypeptides).

PDAC represents an invasive epithelial tumor type that, at least focally, shows sites of ductal or glandular differentiation. Typically, it induces an intense desmoplastic reaction made up of a variety of cellular types, including myofibroblasts, inflammatory cells such as lymphocytes and plasma cells, and dense collagen.[18] Tumor cells, in the well-differentiated type, form well-defined glands with mild pleomorphism. Moderately differentiated forms exhibit poorly defined glands, whereas poorly differentiated forms do not show well-defined glands. The poorly defined forms grow as individual cells or in sheets and with extensive nuclear pleomorphism.[19] Growth tends to be haphazard, and most forms show vascular invasion and lymphatic, as well as perineural, invasion.[19] On gross examination, these tumors form firm but poorly defined masses that are white to yellow in color. They are typically of variable size, and vary from poorly seen small forms to large forms with central regions that can be necrotic, show cystic change, or manifest mucinous features.[19]

Key Points Anatomy and Pathology

Anatomy

- The pancreas is divided into the head, neck, body, tail, and uncinate process.
- Critical vessels are the celiac artery, superior mesenteric artery, common hepatic artery, splenic artery, portal vein, superior mesenteric vein, first jejunal vein, and gastrocolic venous trunk.

Pathology

- Ductal adenocarcinoma is the most common solid malignant neoplasm of the pancreas.
- Tumor induces characteristic desmoplastic changes in the surrounding pancreatic stroma.

CLINICAL PRESENTATION

Because the pancreas is located deep within the retroperitoneum, clinical symptoms typically manifest when the tumor has involved local vessels, caused perineural infiltration, or caused biliary obstruction. Accordingly, patients present with jaundice, weight loss, and/or abdominal pain.[20] Symptomatology depends on tumor location and extent of metastatic disease. Tumors in the pancreatic head, neck, and sometimes body often obstruct the common bile duct and cause jaundice. Pancreatic tail tumors often cause left-sided abdominal pain, whereas those in the pancreatic body often manifest with midepigastric pain.[21] Other symptoms include fatigue, new-onset diabetes, and steatorrhea related to pancreatic insufficiency.[6,21] Physicians should have a high suspicion for PDAC when patients without discernible risk factors present with pancreatitis.[22]

Unfortunately, such nonspecific symptoms often result in a delayed diagnosis, with a median time of 6 months between onset of symptoms and presentation. Uncommon symptoms include nausea and vomiting secondary to gastric outlet obstruction and increasing abdominal distention secondary to accumulation of ascites. Unexplained progressive weight loss is a common symptom and can be related to jaundice, nausea, or catabolic syndrome. It can be seen in patients with resectable as well as advanced tumors. Patients with PDAC are prone to hypercoagulable state, and the initial presentation can be deep venous thrombosis, pulmonary embolism, or, less commonly, aseptic/marantic endocarditis.

Biliary obstruction typically causes elevated serum bilirubin levels and transaminases. Liver function tests can be significantly abnormal, with extensive liver metastases as well. Serum amylase may be normal, but when greater than 300 U/L, advanced disease is typically present. Often, serum glucose levels are mildly to moderately elevated.[23]

A variety of tumor markers have been considered for screening PDAC, such as carcinoembryonic antigen, CA50, and cell adhesion molecule 17-1, but the most useful so far has been carbohydrate antigen (CA)19-9. Although CA19-9 is not specific for PDAC, it serves as a prognostic indicator in some patients. Besides in PDAC, CA19-9 can be elevated in various gastrointestinal tumors, including stomach, colon, and biliary tree tumors, and is often elevated in the setting of biliary obstruction alone.

CLASSIFICATION

Accurate tumor staging is vital to stratify patients correctly to the most appropriate treatment. It is important to balance the need to perform potentially curative surgery on the small percentage of patients who may benefit, at the cost of remaining months of fair to good quality of life, with postoperative morbidity in patients who undergo surgery without potential benefit because of locally advanced or metastatic disease. When patients presenting with all stages were pooled, it was found that the 5-year survival rate overall was only 8%.[24] Importantly, patients who show negative resection margins (R0 resection) have significantly better overall survival than those with positive resection margins (R1 or R2 resections).[25,26]

The staging system most extensively used is from the American Joint Committee on Cancer (AJCC) and the International Union Against Cancer (Table 12.1). This system evaluates the primary tumor (T), the presence or absence of nodal disease (N), and the presence or absence of metastatic disease (M), to come up with TNM grades that are, in turn, used to determine staging. For the 8th edition, staging of exocrine and endocrine pancreatic cancer is separated.

TABLE 12.1 American Joint Committee on Cancer Staging for Pancreatic Ductal Adenocarcinoma

STAGE	CHARACTERISTICS		
Primary Tumor (T)			
Tx	Primary tumor cannot be assessed		
Tis	Carcinoma *in situ* (this includes high-grade pancreatic intraepithelial neoplasia, intraductal papillary mucinous neoplasm with high-grade dysplasia, intraductal tubulopapillary neoplasm with high-grade dysplasia, and mucinous cystic neoplasm with high-grade dysplasia)		
T1	Tumors ≤2 cm in greatest dimension		
T1a	Tumor ≤0.5 cm in greatest dimension		
T1b	Tumor >0.5 and <1 cm in greatest dimension		
T1c	Tumor 1–2 cm in greatest dimension		
T2	Tumor >2 cm and ≤4 cm in greatest dimension		
T3	Tumor >4.1 cm in greatest dimension		
T4	Tumor involves celiac axis, superior mesenteric artery, and/or common hepatic artery		
Regional Lymph Nodes (N)			
NX	Regional lymph nodes cannot be assessed		
N0	No regional node metastasis		
N1	Metastasis in one to three regional lymph nodes		
N2	Metastasis in four or more regional lymph nodes		
Distant Metastasis (M)			
MX	Distant metastasis cannot be assessed		
M0	No distant metastasis		
M1	Distant metastasis		
Stage Grouping			
Stage IA	T1	N0	M0
Stage IB	T2	N0	M0
Stage IIA	T3	N0	M0
Stage IIB	T1, T2, T3	N1	M0
Stage III	T1, T2, T3	N2	
	T4	Any N	M0
Stage IV	Any T	Any N	M1

Primary Tumor (T)

As shown in Table 12.1 and Fig. 12.2, T staging is based on tumor size, tumor confinement within the pancreas, and involvement of major local arterial structures (celiac artery, SMA, and CHA). Tumors that are 2 cm or less in size are identified as T1. T2 is identified if the tumor measures between 2.1 cm and 4 cm in its greatest dimension. Tumors

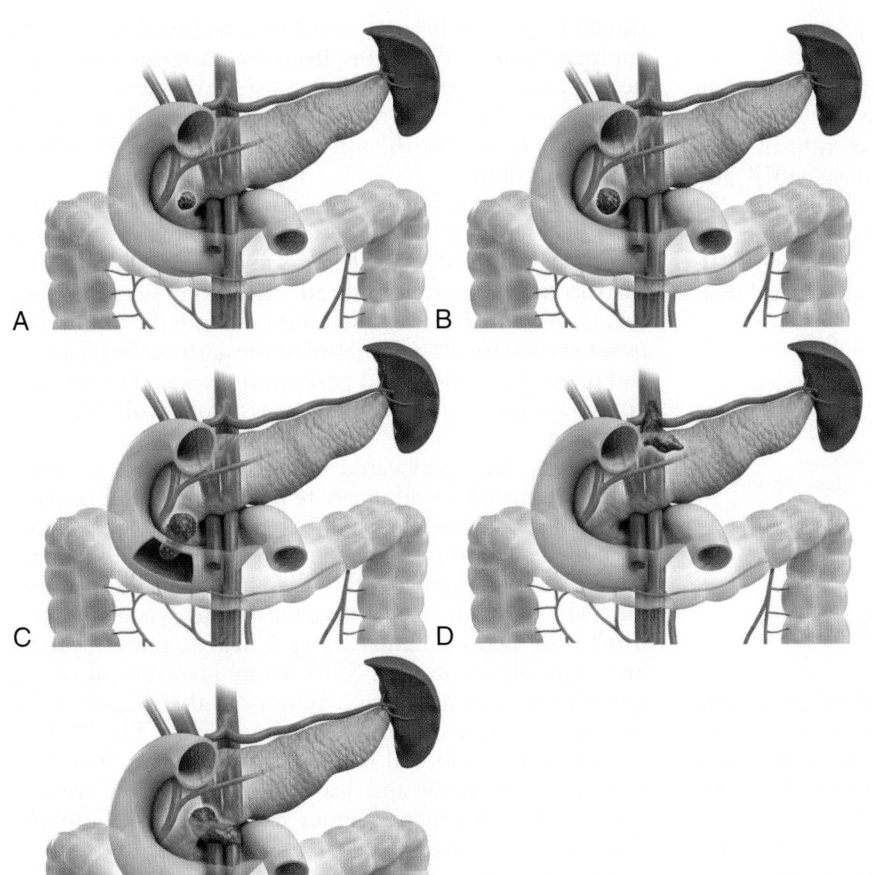

FIGURE 12.2. T staging. **A**, T1, tumors are limited to the pancreas but less than or equal to 2 cm. **B**, T2 is between 2.1 and 4 cm in diameter but still confined to the pancreas. **C**, T3 extends beyond the pancreas without involving the celiac or superior mesenteric arteries. **D** and **E**, T4 tumors involve the celiac axis, superior mesenteric artery, or common hepatic artery.

that are more than 4 cm in greatest dimension are identified as T3. When the extension is such that it involves the celiac axis, SMA and/or CHA, it is identified as T4.

Nodal Disease (N)

The N descriptor in TNM staging refers to regional nodal disease (Fig. 12.3). This criterion is very difficult to assess preoperatively and is further described under "Imaging." It commonly indicates pathologic staging and therefore requires an adequate lymphadenectomy. Typically, the histologic evaluation should include no less than 10 regional nodes located in the celiac, CHA, gastric (pyloric), and splenic regions. Although N stage is more specialized, no significant differences were found in the median overall survival between pN1 and pN2 stages (18.1 vs. 16.9 months).[27]

Metastatic Disease (M)

The prognosis for patients with metastatic pancreatic cancer is poor, and median survival rarely exceeds 6 months.[28] Unfortunately, approximately 40% of patients with PDAC are already suffering from distant metastases at the time of diagnosis.[29] Common sites of metastatic disease are the liver, peritoneum, and lung.

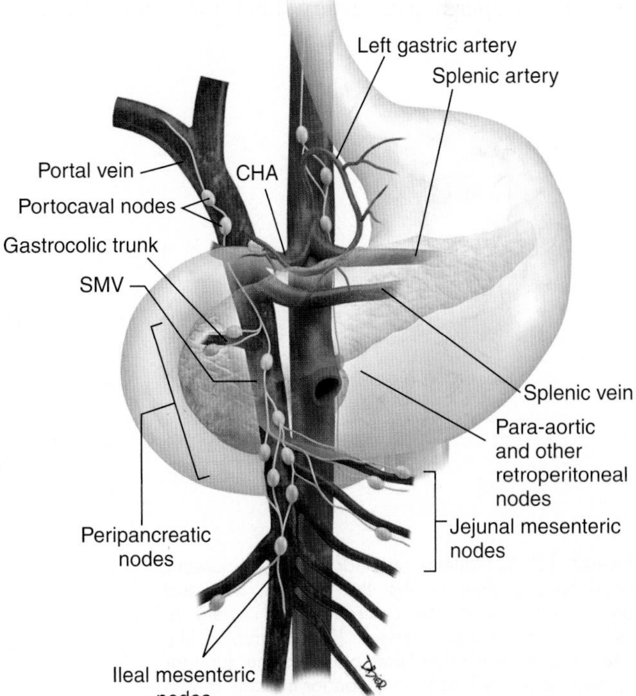

FIGURE 12.3. Nodal sites. Sites of pancreatic adenocarcinoma nodal involvement include near the left gastric artery, common hepatic artery, portal vein (portacaval region), retroperitoneal, periceliac, peripancreatic, along the gastrocolic trunk, and along the jejunal and ileocolic mesenteric regions. *CHA*, Common hepatic artery; *SMV*, superior mesenteric vein.

Stage Grouping

During a median follow-up of 24.5 months, the median overall survival of each stage according to the AJCC 8th edition was 73.5 months in stage IA, 41.9 months in stage IB, 24.2 months in stage IIA, 18.3 months in stage IIB, and 16.8 months in stage III.[27] In the AJCC 8th edition, pN2 patients are classified into stage III regardless of tumor size. Although pT4 and pN2 belong to the same stage III, pN2 had a significantly longer median overall survival than pT4 (16.9 .vs 11.2 months).[27]

Key Points Staging

- Pancreatic cancer is staged using the TNM system.
- T and N categories and stage grouping have changed in the American Joint Committee on Cancer 8th edition.

PATTERNS OF TUMOR SPREAD

The most important factor in the spread of pancreatic tumor is the intrapancreatic tumor location (Fig. 12.4). This is because of the vascular and neural structures that provide a pathway for tumor to spread outwards from the primary tumor.[30,31]

Tumors located within the anterior portion of the pancreatic head extend along the local vasculature, the anterior pancreaticoduodenal arcades superiorly, until reaching their closest supplying vessel, the GDA. Tumors then tend to extend further superiorly along the GDA to its origin from the proper hepatic artery. Therefore, close attention should be paid to this region on cross-sectional imaging. In contrast, tumors originating from the posterior pancreatic head typically grow towards the posterior pancreaticoduodenal veins. These are then used by the tumor to extend superiorly to involve the inferior surface of the PV, where these veins drain.

Tumors that are located superiorly within the pancreatic head/neck grow towards the CHA and often involve this vessel early in the disease. Tumors in close proximity to the gastrocolic trunk often infiltrate early along that structure to its vascular tributaries and ultimately into the base of the transverse mesocolon to extend to the gastrocolic ligament and ultimately widespread peritoneal disease. The splenoportal confluence is commonly at risk for involvement or occlusion.

Tumors that are located in the much more medially and posteriorly located uncinate process and inferior pancreatic head commonly extend along the inferior pancreaticoduodenal arcade to the inferior pancreaticoduodenal artery. Tumors then use this vessel to infiltrate towards the SMA from which this vessel originates, via a common trunk with the first jejunal artery. Uncinate tumors, therefore, typically involve the SMA before involvement of the celiac trunk or its tributaries. Tumor can also spread via the first jejunal artery into the jejunal mesentery. The SMV is frequently involved and is at risk for occlusion. The first jejunal venous branch and ileal branch of the SMV are also at risk for involvement. Tumor can also extend into the ileocolic vasculature.

Tumors that originate in the pancreatic body infiltrate towards the celiac trunk and involve the splenic artery, CHA, left gastric artery, celiac trunk, or any combination of these structures. They can consequently spread along the CHA towards the liver hilum and/or along the left

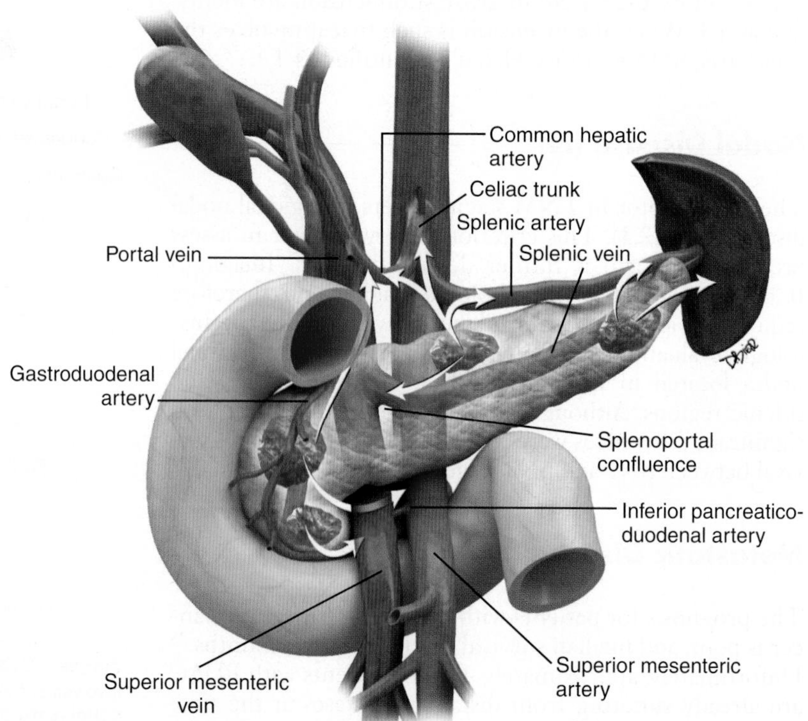

Figure 12.4. Patterns of tumor spread. Pancreatic head lesions often involve the common bile duct and spread along the gastroduodenal artery to the common hepatic artery (CHA) and/or the inferior pancreaticoduodenal artery to the superior mesenteric artery (SMA) and superior mesenteric vein (SMV). Uncinate process tumors similarly spread to the SMA and SMV. Pancreatic body tumors tend to spread towards the CHA, splenic artery, celiac trunk, and splenoportal confluence. Pancreatic tail lesions spread to the splenic hilum and are associated with occlusion of the splenic vein.

gastric artery into the gastrohepatic ligament. The splenoportal confluence and splenic vein are at risk for involvement and occlusion.

Tumors in the pancreatic tail typically extend along the splenic artery and vein and are frequently associated with occlusion of the splenic vein. Those located more medially can extend to the celiac axis, whereas those located more laterally can invade into the splenic hilum. These tumors typically grow large before causing symptoms owing to the lack of biliary occlusion and hence are often associated with metastases. Tail lesions are at a significant risk for direct invasion into the stomach, colon (particularly the splenic flexure), and left adrenal gland.

Typically, the pattern of nodal involvement is that of adjacent regional nodes (Fig. 12.3). Head and body tumors are of concern for left gastric, common hepatic, and portacaval nodes, and subsequently celiac axis nodes. Head and uncinate lesions are also of concern for peripancreatic nodes and jejunal mesenteric nodes. Body tumors are of concern for left gastric and common hepatic nodes. In contrast, tail lesions may be associated with peripancreatic/splenic nodes, although with medial extension they may spread to celiac trunk nodes. Inferior pancreatic head tumors and uncinate tumors can also spread to nodes along the proximal ileocolic vessels. In advanced disease, retroperitoneal nodes can also be involved.

Metastatic disease typically goes initially to the liver and/or peritoneum.[32] Pulmonary metastases typically occur later and can have a varied appearance like small nodules, irregular lesions, small cavitary lesions, and infrequently lymphangitic spread. Osseous lesions are less frequent, as low as 2.2% in one recent study, and usually do not become evident until later in the disease.[32] Rarely, muscle or subcutaneous metastases can be also seen.

Key Points Patterns of Tumor Spread

- The intrapancreatic location of the tumor determines it spread.
- Vessels and neural structures provide critical pathways for tumoral spread.

Imaging

A combination of modalities is crucial for accurate diagnosis and staging of pancreatic cancer. Fig. 12.5 shows a simplified algorithmic approach when PDAC is suspected.

Primary Tumor

Transabdominal ultrasound (US) is often one of the initial studies used to work up patients with abdominal pain and jaundice. US is advantageous because it can provide a comprehensive evaluation of the gallbladder, visualize radiolucent gallstones, gallbladder wall thickening, and pericholecystic fluid, identify the level of biliary obstruction, and localize abdominal tenderness (sonographic Murphy's sign). However, US has limited utility in visualizing the pancreas owing to its retroperitoneal location.

Often, endoscopic retrograde cholangiopancreatography (ERCP) is subsequently performed when common bile duct obstruction is identified on US. On ERCP, malignant strictures are typically irregular, with abrupt cutoff of the duct, whereas benign strictures have a smooth and tapered appearance. However, often these are indiscernible. Brushings of the stricture region are therefore taken to provide tissue

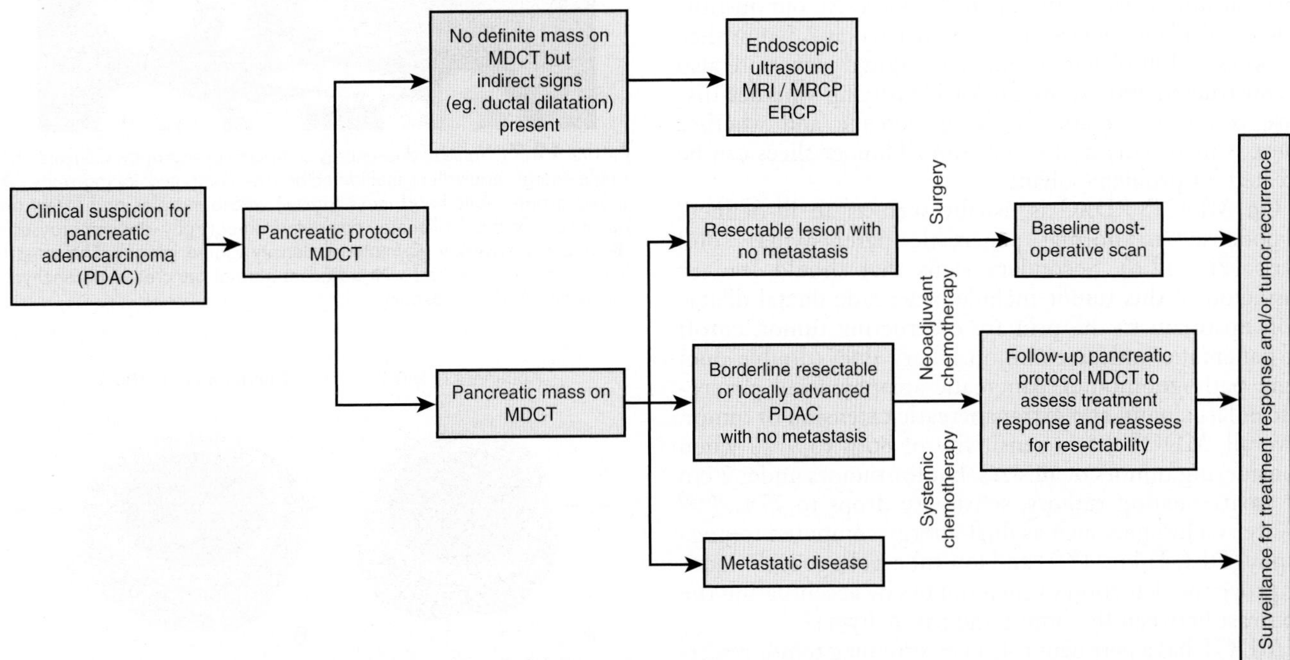

Figure 12.5. Algorithm for working up patients with suspicion of a pancreatic mass. potential pancreatic cancer. *MDCT*, Multidetector row computed tomography; *ERCP*, endoscopic retrograde cholangiopancreatography; *MRI*, magnetic resonance imaging; *MRCP*, magnetic resonance cholangiopancreatography.

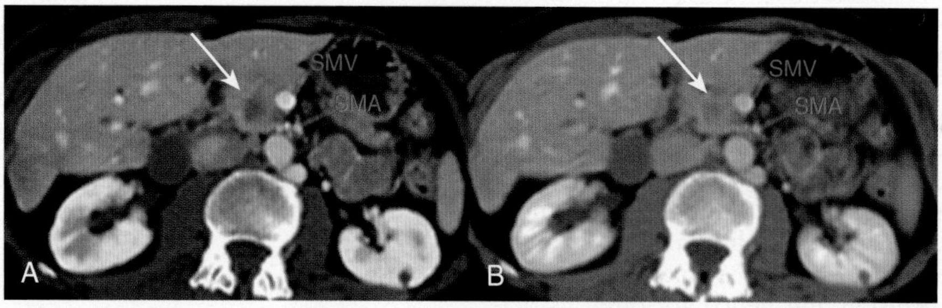

FIGURE 12.6. Importance of pancreatic parenchymal phase on multidetector row computed tomography (MDCT). Dual-phase contrast-enhanced MDCT examination. **A**, Pancreatic parenchymal phase examination shows tumor (*arrow*) in the pancreatic head that is hypodense compared with normal parenchyma. **B**, The tumor is less conspicuous on portal venous phase (*arrow*) because it is closer in density/appearance to the surrounding normal parenchyma. *SMA*, Superior mesenteric artery; *SMV*, superior mesenteric vein.

diagnosis. ERCP is also therapeutic and can guide biliary stent placement. Unfortunately, ERCP-induced pancreatitis degrades subsequent cross-sectional imaging. Therefore, cross-sectional imaging should be performed first in patients who present with suspicion for pancreatic or biliary cancer.

Multidetector computed tomography (MDCT) has become a workhorse for the workup of suspected PDAC. Close attention must be paid to scan technique. Typically, intravenous iodinated contrast medium (>300 mgI/mL) is injected rapidly, approximately 3 to 5 mL/sec, with an injection duration of 30 seconds to improve tumor conspicuity.[33–35] Scans are then obtained during both peak parenchymal (pancreatic phase) and hepatic enhancement (portovenous phase). Pancreatic phase, during a 30-second injection duration, occurs approximately 40 to 50 seconds after the start of contrast enhancement and provides the maximum contrast between tumor and normal pancreatic parenchyma (Fig. 12.6). Portovenous phase images, acquired at 65 to 70 seconds after injection, are useful to assess venous involvement and liver metastases.[36] Thin-section (1–3 mm) imaging is important to evaluate the relationship between tumor and vessels. At our institution, axial-plane images are reconstructed at 2.5-mm slice thickness. Multiplanar coronal and sagittal planes are also reconstructed and are useful for identifying whether disease is intrapancreatic or extrapancreatic and whether there is involvement of vasculature. Thinner slices can be created for problem-solving.

On MDCT, PDAC is usually seen as an ill-defined, hypodense (to normal pancreatic parenchyma) solid mass (Fig. 12.6). Secondary signs that should lead to suspicion of this tumor include pancreatic ductal dilatation upstream to the primary obstructing tumor, cutoff of pancreatic and/or common biliary duct (double duct sign; pathognomonic), pancreatic atrophy, focal pancreatic enlargement, and extrapancreatic extension of tumor. Overall, MDCT has a sensitivity of 86% to 97% when considering tumors of all sizes, but for tumors under 2 cm or isoattenuating tumors, sensitivity drops to 77%.[36–40] Newer techniques such as dual-energy computed tomography (DECT; Fig. 12.7) and low tube-voltage techniques improve the detection of such tumors by accentuating the contrast between the tumor and parenchyma.

MDCT has a pertinent role in determining tumor resectability. Vascular involvement is identified by assessing the degree of the circumferential extent or deformity of the vascular structure (Figs. 12.8 and 12.9). Borderline resectable

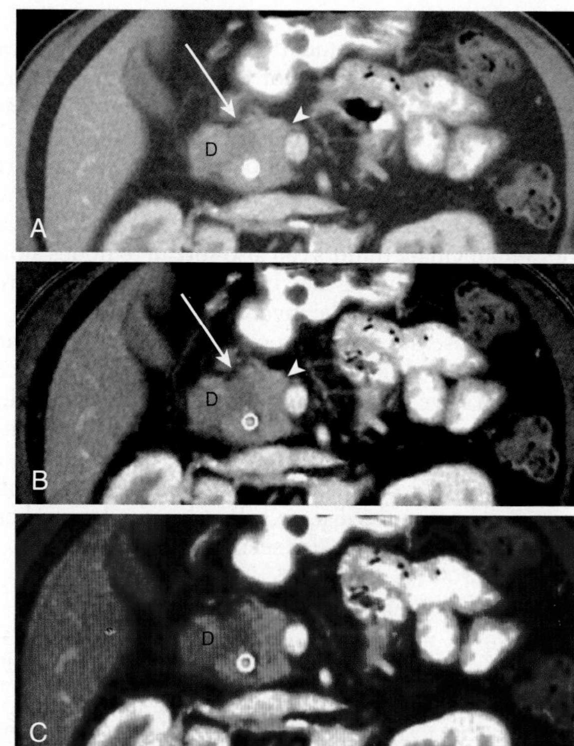

FIGURE 12.7. Value of dual-energy computed tomography. Conventional single-energy equivalent multidetector row computed tomography (**A**) shows a pancreatic head mass (*arrow*) whose margins and extent are better seen on the dual-energy computed tomography–derived grayscale (**B**) and color-overlay (**C**) material density iodine images. The mass is hypovascular compared with adjacent normal pancreatic parenchyma (*arrowhead*). *D*, Duodenum.

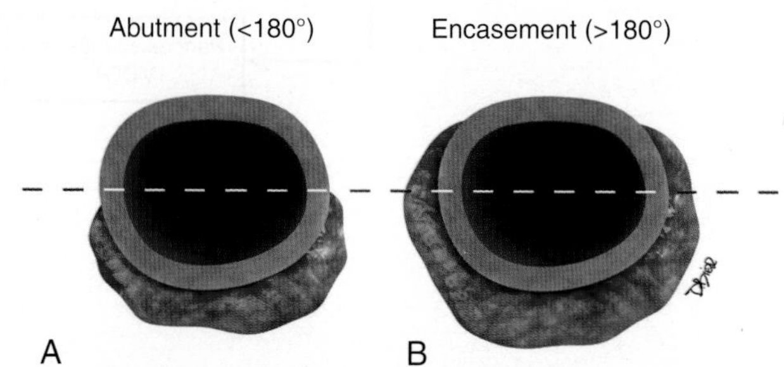

FIGURE 12.8. Criteria for defining vascular involvement. **A**, Less than or **B**, greater than 180-degree involvement is judged by viewing a vessel in cross-section and looking at the extent of circumferential involvement of the opacified lumen.

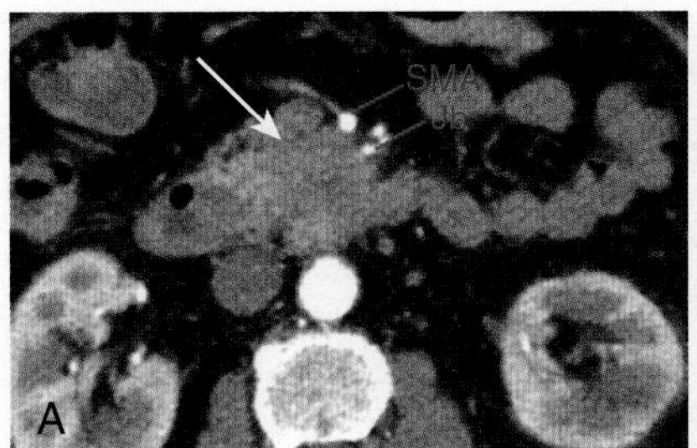

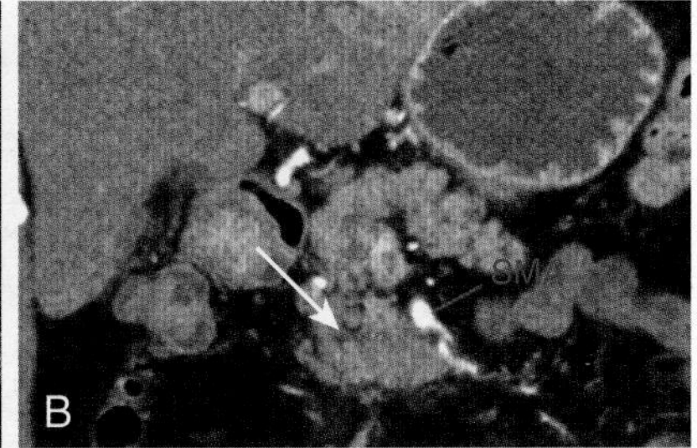

FIGURE 12.9. Resectable tumor. **A**, Axial and **B**, coronal contrast-enhanced computed tomography scan shows tumor (*arrow*) abutting (less than 180 degrees) of the superior mesenteric artery (*SMA*). *Jb*, First jejunal branch.

disease (Fig. 12.10) is defined as less than 180-degree involvement of SMA, short segment abutment (<180 degrees) or encasement (>180 degrees) of CHA (but >1 cm uninvolved segment of CHA at its origin), or short segment venous occlusion with conditional suitable for venous graft placement superiorly and inferiorly. Using greater than 180 degrees of vascular involvement as a criterion for unresectable disease (Fig. 12.11) has shown a sensitivity of 84% and a specificity of 98% for unresectable disease.[41] With the development of venous interposition grafts, the focus for identifying unresectable vascular involvement has shifted to involvement of SMA, celiac artery, and CHA. However, it still remains prudent to identify the extent of venous occlusion (Fig. 12.12), as extension to ileocolic vessels precludes the placement of a bypass graft and renders patients unresectable.

Magnetic resonance imaging (MRI) has a greater soft-tissue contrast than MDCT and is a suitable alternative when patients are allergic to iodinated contrast media or have renal function impairment. Sequences of a typical scan protocol include fat-suppressed T2-weighted, T1-weighted, and fat-suppressed T1-weighted (pre- and postcontrast, and dynamically obtained) images. Dynamically obtained images are typically acquired 20, 60, and 120 seconds from the start of contrast injection and enable pancreatic parenchymal, portal venous, and delayed phase imaging.[42,43] A combination of gradient recalled echo and three-dimensional acquisitions with parallel imaging facilitates rapid, thin-section overlapping dynamic imaging of the entire abdomen in a single breath-hold for each phase.[44,45] A variety of techniques including either respiratory triggered/compensated or breath-hold such as fast-recovery fast spin echo (GE Medical Systems, Milwaukee, WI) allows for either more detailed and/or faster T2-weighted acquisitions.[41]

The typical appearance of a primary tumor is a hypointense mass on the pancreatic parenchymal phase, but, similar to MDCT, it can be isointense on later phases of dynamic imaging.[46] MRCP sequences (Fig. 12.13), in which long echo times suppress soft-tissue signal, cause ductal structures to stand out and demonstrate ductal cutoff with a sensitivity of 84% and specificity of 97%.[47] Both computed tomography (CT) and magnetic resonance angiography have similar accuracy (87%–90%) for determining resectability and local staging.

Positron emission tomography (PET) is typically performed with 2-[^{18}F] fluoro-2-deoxy-D-glucose (FDG) as the radiotracer. Typically, it is fused with CT, and its sensitivity and specificity for depicting primary tumor are 46% to 71% and 63% to 100%, respectively.[48] PET/CT

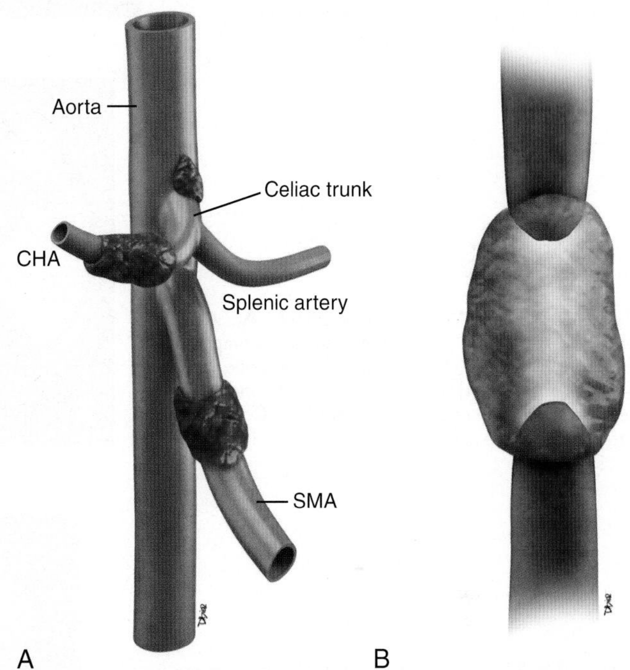

FIGURE 12.10. Borderline resectable tumor. **A**, The criteria for borderline resectable disease include focal short segment encasement of the common hepatic artery (*CHA*) with greater than 1 cm of involved artery between the celiac trunk and the site of CHA involvement, abutment of up to 180 degrees of the celiac artery or the superior mesenteric artery (*SMA*), **B**, and short segment occlusion of the superior mesenteric vein.

is typically reserved for treatment monitoring in patients on chemotherapy, postresection, or to delineate metastatic disease (Fig. 12.14).

Endoscopic US (EUS) has a significant role in detection and histopathological confirmation of PDAC. Using a combination of radial and curvilinear arrays with color Doppler, EUS with fine needle aspiration (FNA) can be used to image and biopsy the tumor in real time without the aid of contrast media. EUS-FNA has been found to be significantly more sensitive (99%) than MDCT (89%–93%).[40] However, the negative predictive value can be as low as 21% in the setting of biliary stents.[40] EUS can also provide locoregional extension of tumor. However, a prospective study of 62 patients showed that helical CT performed better than either MRI or EUS for assessing vascular invasion, with an accuracy of 83% versus 75% for EUS and 74% for MRI. Loss of the echoplane between tumor and surrounding vessels, a sign used to assess

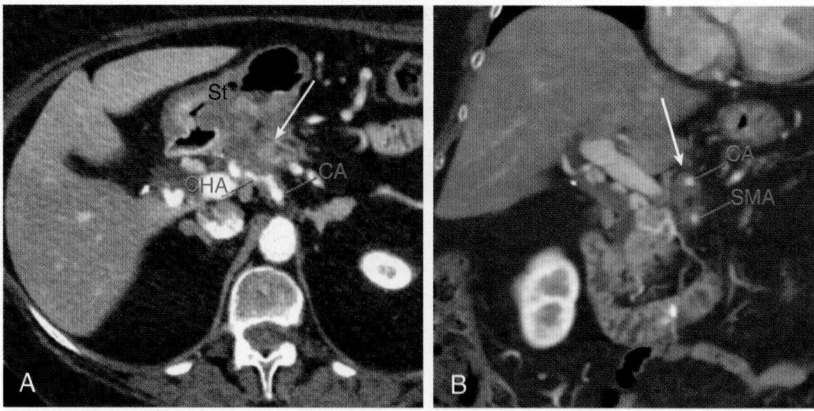

FIGURE 12.11. Unresectable tumor. **A**, Axial and **B**, coronal contrast-enhanced scan shows tumor (*arrow*) encasing over 360 degrees of the celiac trunk up to its bifurcation and the common hepatic artery (*CHA*). Anteriorly it is invading the stomach (St). *CA***MA*, superior mesenteric artery.

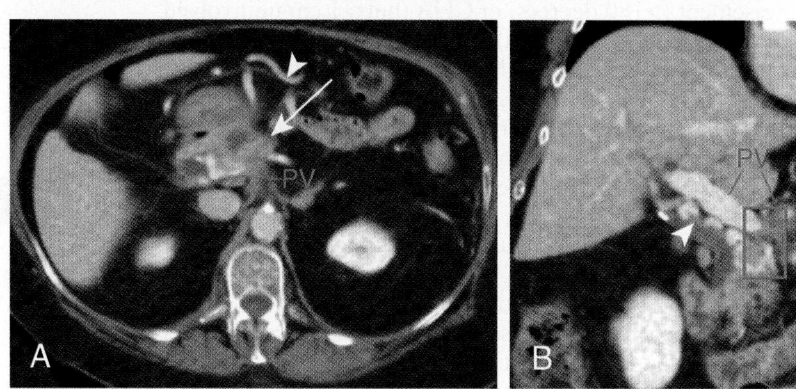

FIGURE 12.12. Venous involvement. **A**, Axial and **B**, coronal contrast-enhanced computed tomography image shows primary pancreatic mass encasement (*arrow*) causing narrowing and short segment occlusion of the portal vein (*PV*). Collaterals (*arrowheads*) are seen in the abdomen and hilum.

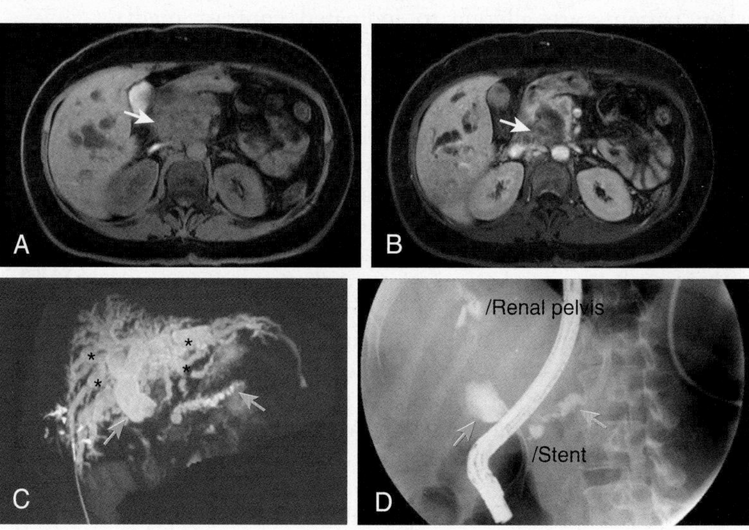

FIGURE 12.13. Pancreatic ductal adenocarcinoma on magnetic resonance imaging. **A**, Precontrast T1-weighted image shows isointense pancreatic head mass (*white arrow*) that shows heterogeneous enhancement (**B**) on contrast administration demonstrating mixed solid and cystic components. **C**, Magnetic resonance cholangiopancreatography (MRCP) shows dilated common bile duct (*green arrow*) with abrupt cutoff in the region of the pancreatic head (tumor), dilated pancreatic duct (*yellow arrow*; "double duct sign") and dilated intrahepatic biliary ducts (*). **D**, Endoscopic retrograde cholangiopancreatography confirms the findings of MRCP with dilated common bile and pancreatic ducts, and a stent was deployed to decompress the biliary system.

vascular involvement, had limited utility, with only 29% of cases with this sign having adherence of tumor to the vessel and none having actual invasion.[49]

Nodal Disease

All modalities show limitations in assessing nodal disease. Typically, a short axis size cutoff of has been used on CT and MRI to differentiate between benign and metastatic nodes, but this is nonspecific. In a study by Valls and coworkers,[50] only three of 18 patients (16.7%) with nodal involvement identified at surgery were detected on CT when using a size criterion of greater than 1.5 cm to define adenopathy. Non–size-based criteria for adenopathy such as hypodensity, ill-defined boundaries, or rounding of nodes improve the specificity at the expense of sensitivity. On EUS, absence of an echogenic center is suggestive of metastatic disease. EUS with FNA improves assessment of metastatic nodes, but it has a limited field of view and is not useful for evaluating paraaortic or mesenteric nodes. The role of PET/CT is still being defined for nodal disease, with reported sensitivities of 46% to 71% and specificities of 63% to 100%.[51–53] Overall, all

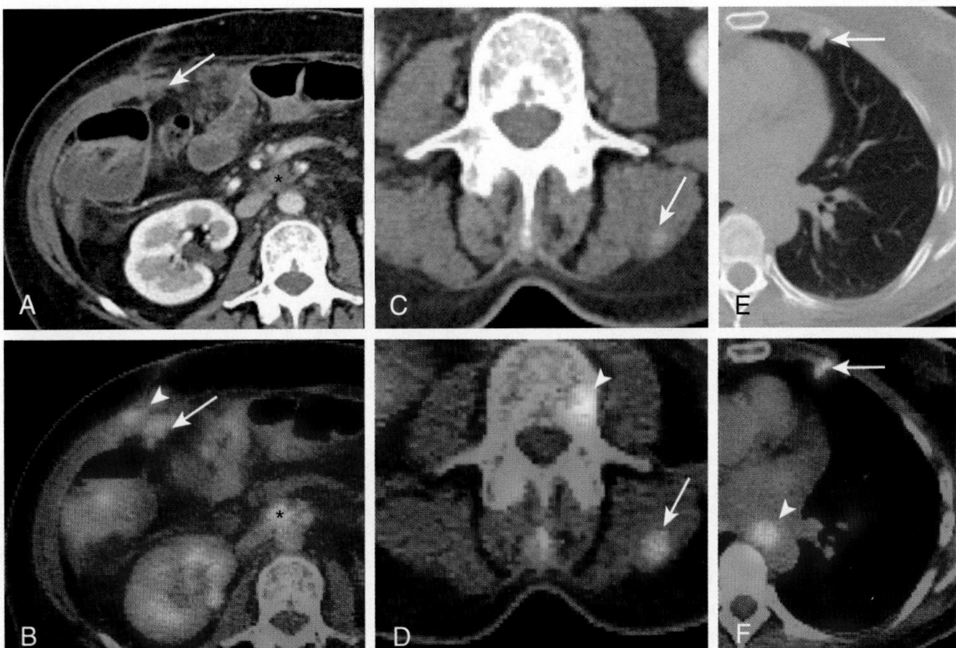

FIGURE 12.14. Role of positron emission tomography in metastatic pancreatic cancer. 2-[^{18}F] fluoro-2-deoxy-D-glucose–avid hypermetabolic metastasis is seen at multiple sites, some of which are not discernable on computed tomography alone. **A** and **B**, Preaortic lymphadenopathy (*), peritoneal (*arrow*) and muscular (*arrowhead*) metastasis. **C** and **D**, Muscular (*arrow*) and skeletal (*arrowhead*) metastasis. **E** and **F**, Pulmonary parenchymal nodule (*arrow*) and mediastinal lymphadenopathy (*arrowhead*) metastasis.

current modalities are unable to detect micrometastases and have difficulty in differentiating inflammatory nodes from malignancy.

Metastatic Disease

The assessment for liver metastases is most commonly made by CT and/or MRI. CT reportedly has a sensitivity of 75% to 87%.[54–56] Gadolinium-ethoxybenzyl-diethylenetriamine pentaacetic acid–enhanced MRI has shown excellent diagnostic performance in detecting liver metastases compared with dynamic contrast-enhanced CT in patients with PDAC (92%–94% vs. 74%–76%).[57,58] Even without contrast media, PET/CT has been shown to have a higher sensitivity than conventional CT (88%–91% vs. 30%–57%).[48,59] It is most impactful in detecting small or distant metastatic disease. However, evaluation of hepatic lesions may be limited because of high FDG uptake of the background hepatic parenchyma.

Currently, all modalities are limited in detecting small peritoneal implants. Some institutions use laparoscopy to improve the detection of peritoneal implants; however, a metaanalysis suggested that laparoscopy may affect management in only 4% to 15% of patients after thin-section CT.[60]

KEY POINTS Imaging

- Radiologists should include the level of certainty regarding metastatic disease and sites of potential metastatic disease.
- A description of arterial and vascular involvement must be made for adequate local (T) staging.

CLINICIAN'S PERSPECTIVE ON IMAGING

Imaging provides a crucial role in PDAC. Noninvasive cross-sectional imaging can identify the primary tumor and detect its local and distant extent.

EUS is the most sensitive for detecting, and EUS-FNA for confirming, small suspected pancreatic primary tumors, especially those that are isodense on CT images. Baseline CT studies are important for localizing, staging, and following indeterminate small liver lesions. If liver lesions are equivocal, they can be further investigated with MRI. MRI is also indicated when patients are allergic to iodinated contrast media or have renal insufficiency/renal failure. It is important to remember that the use of gadolinium is typically precluded in patients with renal failure because of the risk of nephrogenic systemic fibrosis.[61] However, unlike MDCT, MRI's inherently superior soft-tissue contrast provides useful information even without the administration of gadolinium. The role of PET/CT in the initial staging of pancreatic cancer is limited at our institution and is typically ordered for problem-solving.

KEY POINTS Clinician's Perspective on Imaging and Therapy

- Surgeons need to know the relationship of tumor to vessels and the length of venous involvement for planning venous graft placement.
- The oncologist needs to know the size of tumor, extent of liver metastases, and sites of peritoneal disease.
- The radiation oncologist needs to know the extent of disease, both craniocaudally and transversely, degree of tumor spread, and all local sites of disease.

TREATMENT

General Considerations

Only 20% of patients with PDAC have a resectable tumor at the time of diagnosis.[62] Of these, 75% to 80% have locally advanced disease or distant metastases.[62] Structured templates have been published by the Society of Abdominal Radiology and the American Pancreatic Association for reporting PDAC to provide a concise, accurate, and efficient tool for communicating with referring physicians.

Surgery

The resectability of PDAC is based on the National Comprehensive Cancer Network guidelines which is mainly determined by the presence or absence of vascular invasion. According to this guideline, the tumor is classified into one of the three following categories: resectable, borderline resectable, and unresectable (Table 12.2).

The most commonly performed procedure for head, uncinate process, and proximal neck tumors is pancreaticoduodenectomy, with or without preservation of the distal stomach and pylorus. Classically, this procedure, called as Whipple surgery, involves removal of the gastric antrum and establishment of intestinal continuity by creating pancreaticojejunostomy, hepaticojejunostomy, or choledochojejunostomy and gastrojejunostomy. Central pancreatectomy is performed for small neck and body tumors. Tail, body, and distal neck tumors are managed by distal pancreatectomy and splenectomy. For tumors located in the body that involve the celiac axis, a distal pancreatectomy and celiac axis resection, called an Appleby procedure, with or without arterial reconstruction, is performed. Preoperative imaging helps in surgical planning by identifying vascular involvement, variant vascular anatomy like replaced hepatic artery, and collateral circulation.[63]

Follow-up imaging is performed at 3- to 4-month intervals in the first 2 years and 6-monthly afterwards. Postoperative findings depend on the time elapsed since surgery. Knowledge of the normal altered anatomy is important to identify complications and tumor recurrence. For example, collapsed jejunal loops (Fig. 12.15) in the right upper quadrant may mimic tumor recurrence. Common normal postsurgical findings include pneumobilia (67%–80%), perivascular cuffing (60%), and lymphadenopathy simple fluid collections and stranding in the surgical bed (20%–50%).[64] DECT has been shown to improve assessment of the surgical bed by reducing artifacts from clips or stents

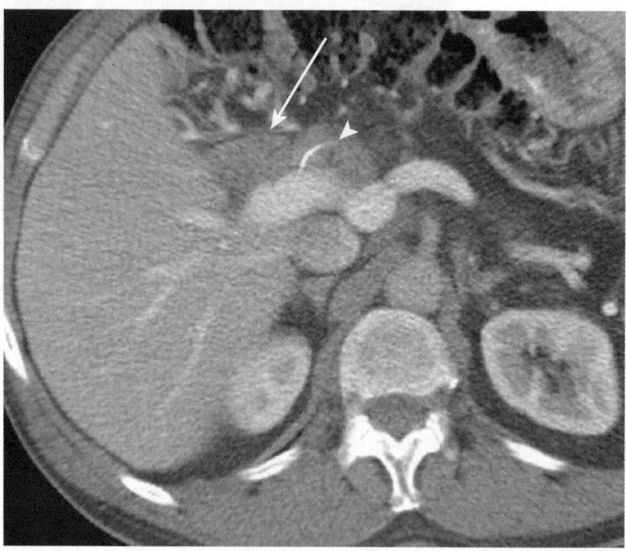

FIGURE 12.15. Importance of normal postoperative anatomy. Apparent soft-tissue density changes (*arrow*) in the surgical bed (post–Whipple procedure) near the hepatic hilum are actually collapsed bowel loops, which can mimic residual or recurrent tumor. Note the pancreatic stent (*arrowhead*) in the residual pancreas.

TABLE 12.2 National Comprehensive Cancer Network Guideline (Pancreatic Adenocarcinoma)

RESECTABILITY STATUS	ARTERIAL	VENOUS
Resectable	No arterial tumor contact (celiac axis [CA], superior mesenteric artery [SMA], or common hepatic artery [CHA])	No tumor contact with the superior mesenteric vein (SMV) or portal vein (PV) or ≤180-degree contact without vein contour irregularity
Borderline resectable	Pancreatic head/uncinate process: • Solid tumor contact with CHA without extension to CA or hepatic artery bifurcation allowing for safe and complete resection and reconstruction • Solid tumor contact with the SMA of ≤180 degrees Pancreatic body/tail: • Solid tumor contact with CA of ≤180 degrees • Solid tumor contact with CA of >180 degrees without involvement of the aorta and with intact and uninvolved gastroduodenal artery	• Solid tumor contact with the SMA or PV of >180 degree, contact of ≤180 degree, with contour irregularity of the vein or thrombosis of the vein but with suitable vessel proximal and distal to the site of involvement allowing for safe and complete resection and vein reconstruction • Solid tumor contact with the inferior vena cava
Unresectable	• Distant metastasis • Pancreatic head/uncinate process: • Solid tumor contact with SMA >180 degrees • Solid tumor contact with the CA >180 degrees • Solid tumor contact with the first jejunal SMA branch Pancreatic body/tail: • Solid tumor contact of >180 degrees with the SMA or CA • Solid tumor contact with the CA and aortic involvement	Pancreatic head/uncinate process: • Unreconstructible SMV/PV because of tumor involvement or occlusion • Solid tumor contact with most proximal draining jejunal branch into SMV Pancreatic body/tail: • Unreconstructible SMV/PV because of tumor involvement or occlusion

From National Comprehensive Cancer Network website. NCCN clinical practice guidelines in oncology: pancreatic adenocarcinoma, version 2.2015.

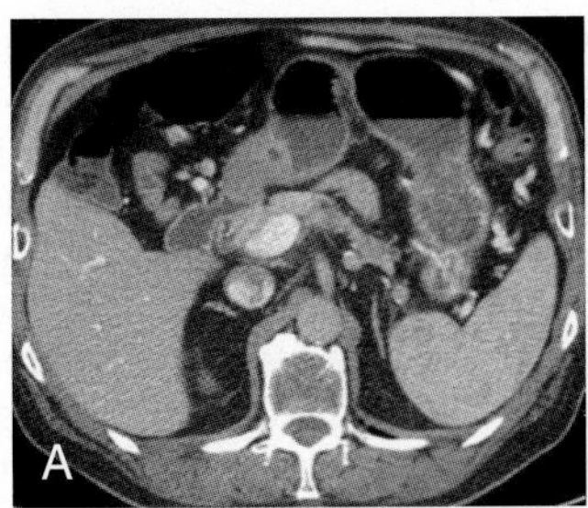

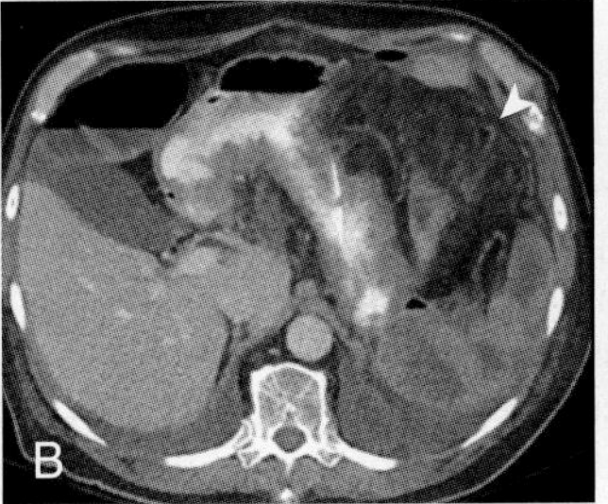

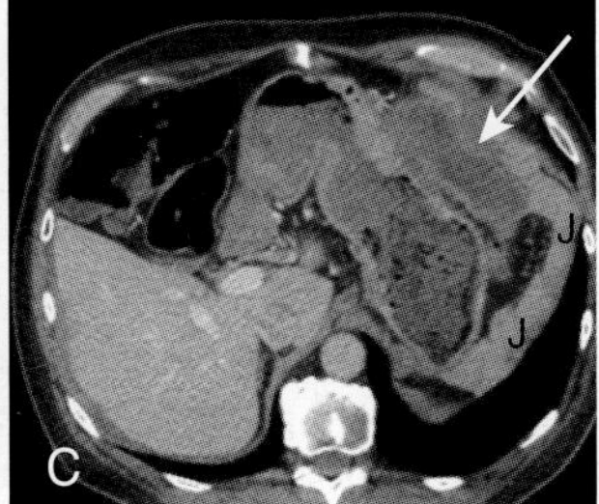

FIGURE 12.16. Fat necrosis. **A**, Preoperative contrast-enhanced multidetector row computed tomography (January 2015) shows no peritoneal soft tissue masses. The first postoperative scan (**B**; February 2015) demonstrates extensive peritoneal stranding (*arrowhead*) that evolved over a year (**C;** May 2016) into fat necrosis seen as a heterogenous density mass anterior to the stomach displacing the jejunal bowel loops (J).

and improving the confidence in discriminating unenhancing versus enhancing tissue.

Early complications include delayed gastric emptying (prevalence 20%–50%) that can be confirmed with nuclear medicine or fluoroscopic studies, bleeding, pancreatitis (incidence 2%–3%), phlegmon, fluid collections, fat necrosis (Fig. 12.16), and abscess (incidence 4%–10%).[64–68] Presence of fluid collections should raise the concern for a pancreatic fistula (10%–30%) or anastomotic leak (Fig. 12.17) from an anastomosis or the jejunal stump. Therefore, close attention must be paid to the gastrojejunostomy, pancreaticojejunostomy, and choledochojejunostomy sites. Fluoroscopic studies or MDCT with water-soluble contrast are often used to confirm leaks from the jejunal stump, gastrojejunostomy, and pancreaticojejunostomy anastomoses, whereas hepatoiminodiacetic acid or ERCP is indicated when a biloma is suspected. Vascular complications include hepatic infarction (1%), which can be identified on MDCT as hypovascular areas in the liver, and portal or superior mesenteric venous thrombosis. The incidence of venous thrombosis is increasing because of advancements in surgical reconstruction techniques and is seen on CT as intraluminal filling defects or secondary signs such as bowel ischemia or ascites. The most common delayed complication is an anastomotic stricture that can affect both the pancreaticojejunostomy and hepaticojejunostomy sites, with an incidence of 4.6% and 8.2% at 5 years, respectively.[64] Diagnosis is made by evaluating the ductal anatomy with MDCT, MRI, or MRCP and identifying dilated ducts and progressive pancreatic parenchymal atrophy. Stenosis of the choledochojejunostomy has an incidence of 8% at 7 years.[69] It can cause jaundice and pruritus and usually is treated by biliary stent placement and/or balloon dilation.

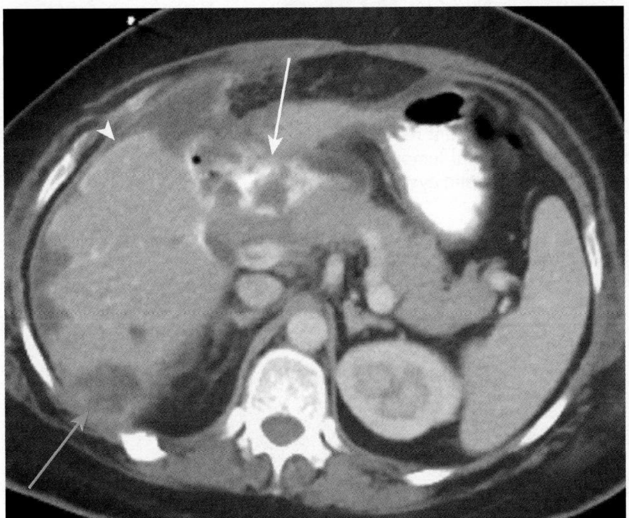

FIGURE 12.17. Anastomotic leak. Axial contrast-enhanced computed tomography scan with water-soluble contrast after a Whipple procedure. Pooling of oral contrast media (*white arrow*) is seen at the pancreatojejunostomy site that is tracking along the hepatic surface (*arrowhead*). Multiple surface collections are also seen along the liver (*green arrow*).

Adjuvant and Neoadjuvant Chemotherapy and Radiation Therapy

Adjuvant and neoadjuvant therapy are the two approaches for chemotherapy and radiation therapy for resectable disease. In the adjuvant approach, patients with resectable PDAC undergo upfront surgery followed by chemotherapy and radiation therapy to reduce the risk of locoregional and metastatic recurrence. It is also favored for R1 resections.[70] For locally advanced PDAC, offering combined chemotherapy and radiation therapy first (neoadjuvant approach) can downstage the disease in approximately 30% of patients and help attain R0 resection.[71] Systemic chemotherapy alone is administered for advanced PDAC to improve long-term outcome and reduce the burden of distant disease. Posttherapy, imaging is performed to assess response and reassess surgical resectability.

Image-Guided Locoregional Therapies

Tumors that are unamenable to surgery are increasingly being managed with image-guided locoregional therapies like irreversible electroporation or NanoKnife. This method employs nonthermal ablation of the tumor with high-energy pulses of electricity and can be used in conjunction with systemic chemotherapy.

SURVEILLANCE

Monitoring Tumor Response

Imaging plays a vital role in identifying treatment response or failure. Early diagnosis is beneficial because patients can be changed to a potentially more effective treatment protocol. Baseline CA19-9 level is measured and may predict recurrence up to 10 months before clinical symptoms or radiological signs manifest. However, care must be taken to identify Lewis-a–/b–negative patients, as CA19-9 is an ineffective tumor marker in this population.[72]

Imaging plays a vital role in monitoring treatment response and involves assessment of changes in the primary pancreatic tumor as well as extrapancreatic metastasis. A baseline scan is obtained before initiating therapy, irrespective of the local stage and treatment plan. Patients are then monitored at defined intervals of the treatment cycle to assess for a change in size of primary tumor and measurable sites of metastatic disease. The intervals are more stringent when a patient is in a clinical trial for novel therapeutic agents.

Size-based assessment is conventionally used to determine therapeutic efficacy. However, there are limitations with morphological criteria because PDACs often have irregular, poorly-defined margins and show a nonuniform pattern of shrinkage. This leads to inter- and intraradiologist variability. Moreover, neoadjuvant therapy results in fibrotic and inflammatory intratumoral changes (Fig. 12.18). This makes distinguishing fibroinflammatory tissue from tumoral tissue difficult on imaging, and CT often underestimates the response to neoadjuvant therapy. Katz et al.[73] found that R0 resection was achieved in 80% patients who had no imaging evidence of treatment response, and only 13% patients met the imaging criteria for response. Functional imaging with MRI diffusion-weighted imaging has been evaluated as an imaging technique for assessing and predicting tumor response, with promising pilot results.[74] Metabolic response with PET/CT has also been associated with a longer survival, and quantitative response from chemotherapy is demonstrated by an interval reduction of standardized uptake value (SUV).[75–77] These changes tend to precede morphological changes. A recent study demonstrated that a greater number of patients showed metabolic response compared with morphological response.[78] Careful evaluation of the liver and peritoneum is mandated, as they are often the first sites of metastases and are challenging to evaluate on PET alone.[79,80] A close comparison with all available prior imaging is therefore recommended.

Detection of Recurrence

CT is the modality that is most commonly performed to evaluate for recurrence, and a similar scan protocol as the baseline scan is used. Imaging earlier than 8 weeks from the surgery is problematic because of postsurgical changes, and comparison with preoperative CT scans may be helpful in differentiating peritoneal disease from inflammatory changes, identifying new small liver metastases (Fig. 12.19), and differentiating pulmonary metastases from benign inflammatory nodules.

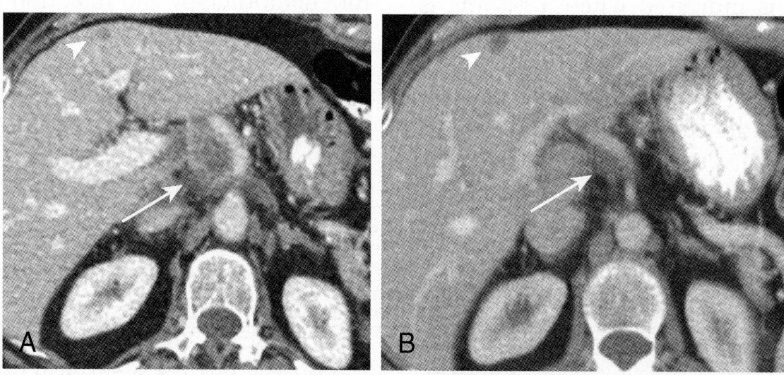

FIGURE 12.18. Effect of neoadjuvant therapy: baseline contrast-enhanced multidetector row computed tomography (MDCT). **A**, A heterogeneous mass (*arrow*) encasing the celiac artery. Postneoadjuvant therapy surveillance scan; **B**, significant reduction in the size, density, and extent of the infiltrative soft tissue (*arrow*). Conventional MDCT scans may be unable to differentiate residual tumor vs. fibrosis. This patient underwent surgery, and pathology of the resected tissue demonstrated no tumor cells. Note the benign stable hepatic cyst (*arrowhead*).

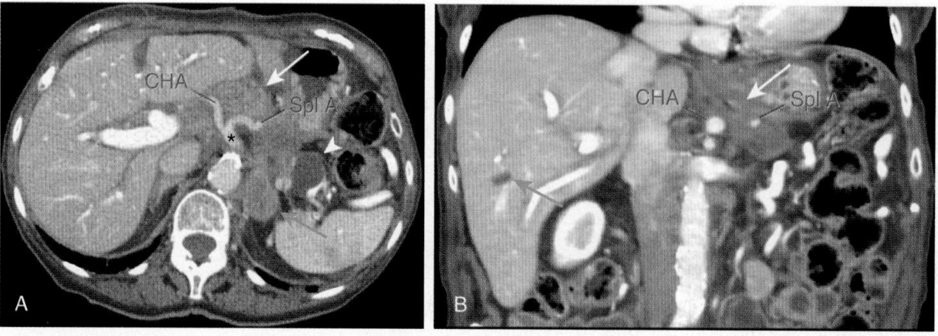

FIGURE 12.19. Tumor recurrence. **A**, Post–Whipple procedure axial contrast-enhanced multidetector row computed tomography shows an infiltrative heterogeneous mass (*white arrow*) with associated tumoral cyst (*arrowhead*) encasing the celiac artery (*) at its bifurcation, common hepatic artery (*CHA*), and splenic artery (*Spl A*). There was interval development of left adrenal metastasis (*orange arrow*). **B**, The coronal image shows interval development of liver metastasis (*orange arrow*).

After surgery, nonspecific regions of soft-tissue thickening, called perivascular cuffing, are common near the CHA, SMA, and SMV. These can mimic or mask locoregional recurrence. Ishigami et al.[81] found that such thickening was present in all 44 postpancreaticoduodenectomy patients they studied and speculated it to be secondary to lymph node dissections. Factors that increase the suspicion for recurrence include lymph node and/or margin positivity.[81] Careful evaluation of the superior mesenteric artery is suggested, as its often the leading site for locoregional recurrence. Recurrent tissue may be also identified with secondary findings such as gastric outlet obstruction because of extrapancreatic extension or dilated biliary ductal system secondary to stent occlusion by recurrent/metastatic tumor.

PET/CT has shown a higher sensitivity for detection of locoregional recurrence than CT or MRI.[82] It may also have a role when no postoperative baseline study is available or when postoperative changes are moderately extensive; however, its utility for detecting hepatic metastasis is limited. Radiologists must be aware of pitfalls when interpreting PET, as biliary stents and pancreatitis can show FDG uptake. In a study of 51 patients, DECT has shown promising results for characterizing soft tissue in the postpancreaticoduodenectomy surgical bed.[83]

KEY POINTS Detection of Recurrence

- Distant recurrence (i.e., liver, lung metastases) is more common than local recurrence.
- Local recurrence is more likely in the setting of positive surgical margin (R1) or positive nodal status.

Screening in Pancreatic Ductal Adenocarcinoma

Because of its low incidence in the general population, population-based screening for PDAC is not warranted. Panels have suggested screening "high-risk individuals" who have a greater than 5% lifetime risk for developing PDAC.[84] These include individuals (1) with two first-degree relatives with PDAC, (2) who are carriers of germline mutations in *BRCA1*, *BRCA2*, *ATM*, *PALB2*, *CDKN2A*, *STK11*, *MLH1*, and *MSH2*, and (3) with hereditary pancreatitis. Annual surveillance is recommended starting between 50 and 55 years of age or 10 years earlier than the youngest relative diagnosed with PDAC. Imaging with MRI, MRCP, and/or EUS is suggested because these methods lack ionizing radiation and have high sensitivity. MDCT is reserved for patients who cannot undergo MRI or EUS. More supporting evidence is still needed to assess the outcome, cost-effectiveness, and risk for PDAC screening programs.

FUTURE DIRECTIONS

Positron Emission Tomography/ Magnetic Resonance

Integrated PET/MR is being increasingly evaluated for PDAC. It is advantageous over PET/CT owing to superior temporal and spatial resolution and can provide quantitative parameters such as SUV and apparent diffusion coefficient values. PET/MR has been shown to have a diagnostic performance similar to PET/CT for staging,[85] but still has low sensitivity for detecting metastatic lymph nodes. A pilot study with 13 patients showed that PET/MR-derived metrics correlated with longer progression-free and overall survival, whereas no morphological differences were observed between responders and nonresponders.[86]

Imaging-Based Biomarkers

Markers of heterogeneity that are derived from radiological images are being increasingly evaluated as noninvasive biomarkers for predicting histology and response. These include histogram, texture, and radiomic analysis, and have been correlated with metabolic activity, intratumoral angiogenesis, and hypoxia. For PDAC, such radiomic signatures obtained from PET, CT, DECT, and MRI images have shown promising results to identify *SMAD4*[87] or *KRAS* mutation status[88] and predict survival in treatment-naïve,[89] postradiation,[90] or postchemotherapy patients.[91,92] However, these still need to be validated in large prospective cohorts.

Deep Learning

Advancements in computational power have led to increasing interest in using deep learning models for clinical applications. However, challenges remain, including sourcing well-annotated, large sets of validated data and dealing with the vast number of mobile structures within the abdomen, particularly the pancreas, which has a variable location and contour. Nevertheless, preliminary studies have shown a mean segmentation accuracy of 87.8%.[93] Researchers have also developed an end-to-end model that detects PDAC with a sensitivity of 94.1% and specificity of 98.5% on CT images.[94]

CONCLUSION

PDAC remains a difficult, challenging disease. Surgical advances and preoperative therapy have increased the pool of surgical candidates, but the prognosis for survival remains dismal. Imaging provides crucial information for accurately staging tumors, assessing treatment response, and detecting tumor recurrence. Growing knowledge of the biology of pancreatic cancer is being used to develop novel approaches to potentially intervene in this disease.

REFERENCES

1. Siegel RL, Miller KD, Jemal A. Cancer statistics, 2019. *CA Cancer J Clin*. 2019;69(1):7–34.
2. Chang KJ, Parasher G, Christie C, et al. Risk of pancreatic adenocarcinoma: disparity between African Americans and other race/ethnic groups. *Cancer*. 2005;103(2):349–357.
3. Lowenfels AB, Maisonneuve P. Epidemiology and risk factors for pancreatic cancer. *Best Pract Res Clin Gastroenterol*. 2006;20(2):197–209.

4. Whitcomb DC, Frulloni L, Garg P, et al. Chronic pancreatitis: An international draft consensus proposal for a new mechanistic definition. *Pancreatology*. 2016;16(2):218–224.
5. Kirkegard J, Mortensen FV, Cronin-Fenton D. Chronic pancreatitis and pancreatic cancer risk: a systematic review and meta-analysis. *Am J Gastroenterol*. 2017;112(9):1366–1372.
6. Hart PA, Bellin MD, Andersen DK, et al. Type 3c (pancreatogenic) diabetes mellitus secondary to chronic pancreatitis and pancreatic cancer. *Lancet Gastroenterol Hepatol*. 2016;1(3):226–237.
7. Everhart J, Wright D. Diabetes mellitus as a risk factor for pancreatic cancer. A meta-analysis. *JAMA*. 1995;273(20):1605–1609.
8. Khalaf N, Wolpin BM. Metabolic alterations as a signpost to early pancreatic cancer. *Gastroenterology*. 2019;156(6):1560–1563.
9. Hruban RH, Petersen GM, Ha PK, et al. Genetics of pancreatic cancer. From genes to families. *Surg Oncol Clin N Am*. 1998;7(1):1–23.
10. Martinez-Useros J, Garcia-Foncillas J. Can molecular biomarkers change the paradigm of pancreatic cancer prognosis? *Biomed Res Int*. 2016;2016:4873089.
11. Boyer B, Valles AM, Edme N. Induction and regulation of epithelial-mesenchymal transitions. *Biochem Pharmacol*. 2000;60(8):1091–1099.
12. Noda Y, Goshima S, Tsuji Y, et al. Prognostic evaluation of pancreatic ductal adenocarcinoma: associations between molecular biomarkers and CT imaging findings. *Pancreatology*. 2019;19(2):331–339.
13. Okahara M, Mori H, Kiyosue H, et al. Arterial supply to the pancreas; variations and cross-sectional anatomy. *Abdom Imaging*. 2010;35(2):134–142.
14. Mochizuki K, Gabata T, Kozaka K, et al. MDCT findings of extrapancreatic nerve plexus invasion by pancreas head carcinoma: correlation with en bloc pathological specimens and diagnostic accuracy. *Eur Radiol*. 2010;20(7):1757–1767.
15. Deshmukh SD, Willmann JK, Jeffrey RB. Pathways of extrapancreatic perineural invasion by pancreatic adenocarcinoma: evaluation with 3D volume-rendered MDCT imaging. *AJR Am J Roentgenol*. 2010;194(3):668–674.
16. Patel BN, Giacomini C, Jeffrey RB, et al. Three-dimensional volume-rendered multidetector CT imaging of the posterior inferior pancreaticoduodenal artery: its anatomy and role in diagnosing extrapancreatic perineural invasion. *Cancer Imaging*. 2013;13(4):580–590.
17. Chang ST, Jeffrey RB, Patel BN, et al. Preoperative multidetector CT diagnosis of extrapancreatic perineural or duodenal invasion is associated with reduced postoperative survival after pancreaticoduodenectomy for pancreatic adenocarcinoma: preliminary experience and implications for patient care. *Radiology*. 2016;281(3):816–825.
18. Iacobuzio-Donahue CA, Ryu B, Hruban RH, et al. Exploring the host desmoplastic response to pancreatic carcinoma: gene expression of stromal and neoplastic cells at the site of primary invasion. *Am J Pathol*. 2002;160(1):91–99.
19. Von Hoff DD, Evans DB, Hruban RH. *Pancreatic Cancer*. 1st ed. Sudbury: Jones and Bartlett Publishers;; 2005.
20. Modolell I, Guarner L, Malagelada JR. Vagaries of clinical presentation of pancreatic and biliary tract cancer. *Ann Oncol*. 1999;10(Suppl 4):82–84.
21. Kelsen DP, Portenoy R, Thaler H, et al. Pain as a predictor of outcome in patients with operable pancreatic carcinoma. *Surgery*. 1997;122(1):53–59.
22. Mujica VR, Barkin JS, Go VL. Acute pancreatitis secondary to pancreatic carcinoma. Study Group Participants. *Pancreas*. 2000;21(4):329–332.
23. Saruc M, Pour PM. Diabetes and its relationship to pancreatic carcinoma. *Pancreas*. 2003;26(4):381–387.
24. Siegel RL, Miller KD, Jemal A. Cancer statistics, 2018. *CA Cancer J Clin*. 2018;68(1):7–30.
25. Ferrone CR, Marchegiani G, Hong TS, et al. Radiological and surgical implications of neoadjuvant treatment with FOLFIRINOX for locally advanced and borderline resectable pancreatic cancer. *Ann Surg*. 2015;261(1):12–17.
26. Heestand GM, Murphy JD, Lowy AM. Approach to patients with pancreatic cancer without detectable metastases. *J Clin Oncol*. 2015;33(16):1770–1778.
27. Shin DW, Lee JC, Kim J, et al. Validation of the American Joint Committee on Cancer 8th edition staging system for the pancreatic ductal adenocarcinoma. *Eur J Surg Oncol*. 2019
28. Kulke MH, Tempero MA, Niedzwiecki D, et al. Randomized phase II study of gemcitabine administered at a fixed dose rate or in combination with cisplatin, docetaxel, or irinotecan in patients with metastatic pancreatic cancer: CALGB 89904. *J Clin Oncol*. 2009;27(33):5506–5512.
29. Pollom EL, Koong AC, Ko AH. Treatment approaches to locally advanced pancreatic adenocarcinoma. *Hematol Oncol Clin North Am*. 2015;29(4):741–759.
30. Tamm EP, Silverman PM, Charnsangavej C, et al. Diagnosis, staging, and surveillance of pancreatic cancer. *AJR Am J Roentgenol*. 2003;180(5):1311–1323.
31. Rozenblum E, Schutte M, Goggins M, et al. Tumor-suppressive pathways in pancreatic carcinoma. *Cancer Res*. 1997;57(9):1731–1734.
32. Borad MJ, Saadati H, Lakshmipathy A, et al. Skeletal metastases in pancreatic cancer: a retrospective study and review of the literature. *Yale J Biol Med*. 2009;82(1):1–6.
33. Kim T, Murakami T, Takahashi S, et al. Pancreatic CT imaging: effects of different injection rates and doses of contrast material. *Radiology*. 1999;212(1):219–225.
34. Schueller G, Schima W, Schueller-Weidekamm C, et al. Multidetector CT of pancreas: effects of contrast material flow rate and individualized scan delay on enhancement of pancreas and tumor contrast. *Radiology*. 2006;241(2):441–448.
35. Tublin ME, Tessler FN, Cheng SL, et al. Effect of injection rate of contrast medium on pancreatic and hepatic helical CT. *Radiology*. 1999;210(1):97–101.
36. Fletcher JG, Wiersema MJ, Farrell MA, et al. Pancreatic malignancy: value of arterial, pancreatic, and hepatic phase imaging with multidetector row CT. *Radiology*. 2003;229(1):81–90.
37. Agarwal B, Abu-Hamda E, Molke KL, et al. Endoscopic ultrasound-guided fine needle aspiration and multidetector spiral CT in the diagnosis of pancreatic cancer. *Am J Gastroenterol*. 2004;99(5):844–850.
38. DeWitt J, Jowell P, Leblanc J, et al. EUS-guided FNA of pancreatic metastases: a multicenter experience. *Gastrointest Endosc*. 2005;61(6):689–696.
39. Bronstein YL, Loyer EM, Kaur H, et al. Detection of small pancreatic tumors with multiphasic helical CT. *AJR Am J Roentgenol*. 2004;182(3):619–623.
40. Tamm EP, Loyer EM, Faria SC, et al. Retrospective analysis of dual-phase MDCT and follow-up EUS/EUS-FNA in the diagnosis of pancreatic cancer. *Abdom Imaging*. 2007;32(5):660–667.
41. Lu DS, Reber HA, Krasny RM, et al. Local staging of pancreatic cancer: criteria for unresectability of major vessels as revealed by pancreatic-phase, thin-section helical CT. *AJR Am J Roentgenol*. 1997;168(6):1439–1443.
42. Fayad LM, Mitchell DG. Magnetic resonance imaging of pancreatic adenocarcinoma. *Int J Gastrointest Cancer*. 2001;30(1-2):19–25.
43. Pamuklar E, Semelka RC. MR imaging of the pancreas. *Magn Reson Imaging Clin N Am*. 2005;13(2):313–330.
44. Schima W, Ba-Ssalamah A, Kolblinger C, et al. Pancreatic adenocarcinoma. *Eur Radiol*. 2007;17(3):638–649.
45. Lall CG, Howard TJ, Skandarajah A, et al. New concepts in staging and treatment of locally advanced pancreatic head cancer. *AJR Am J Roentgenol*. 2007;189(5):1044–1050.
46. Ly JN, Miller FH. MR imaging of the pancreas: a practical approach. *Radiol Clin North Am*. 2002;40(6):1289–1306.
47. Adamek HE, Albert J, Breer H, et al. Pancreatic cancer detection with magnetic resonance cholangiopancreatography and endoscopic retrograde cholangiopancreatography: a prospective controlled study. *Lancet*. 2000;356(9225):190–193.
48. Kauhanen SP, Komar G, Seppanen MP, et al. A prospective diagnostic accuracy study of 18F-fluorodeoxyglucose positron emission tomography/computed tomography, multidetector row computed tomography, and magnetic resonance imaging in primary diagnosis and staging of pancreatic cancer. *Ann Surg*. 2009;250(6):957–963.
49. Aslanian H, Salem R, Lee J, et al. EUS diagnosis of vascular invasion in pancreatic cancer: surgical and histologic correlates. *Am J Gastroenterol*. 2005;100(6):1381–1385.
50. Valls C, Andia E, Sanchez A, et al. Dual-phase helical CT of pancreatic adenocarcinoma: assessment of resectability before surgery. *AJR Am J Roentgenol*. 2002;178(4):821–826.
51. Pakzad F, Groves AM, Ell PJ. The role of positron emission tomography in the management of pancreatic cancer. *Semin Nucl Med*. 2006;36(3):248–256.
52. Bares R, Klever P, Hauptmann S, et al. F-18 fluorodeoxyglucose PET in vivo evaluation of pancreatic glucose metabolism for detection of pancreatic cancer. *Radiology*. 1994;192(1):79–86.

53. Bares R, Dohmen BM, Cremerius U, et al. [Results of positron emission tomography with fluorine-18 labeled fluorodeoxyglucose in differential diagnosis and staging of pancreatic carcinoma]. *Radiologe*. 1996;36(5):435–440.
54. Richter GM, Simon C, Hoffmann V, et al. [Hydrospiral CT of the pancreas in thin section technique]. *Radiologe*. 1996;36(5):397–405.
55. Trede M, Rumstadt B, Wendl K, et al. Ultrafast magnetic resonance imaging improves the staging of pancreatic tumors. *Ann Surg*. 1997;226(4):393–405. discussion 405-397.
56. Calculli L, Casadei R, Diacono D, et al. [Role of spiral computerized tomography in the staging of pancreatic carcinoma]. *Radiol Med*. 1998;95(4):344–348.
57. Motosugi U, Ichikawa T, Morisaka H, et al. Detection of pancreatic carcinoma and liver metastases with gadoxetic acid-enhanced MR imaging: comparison with contrast-enhanced multi-detector row CT. *Radiology*. 2011;260(2):446–453.
58. Ito T, Sugiura T, Okamura Y, et al. The diagnostic advantage of EOB-MR imaging over CT in the detection of liver metastasis in patients with potentially resectable pancreatic cancer. *Pancreatology*. 2017;17(3):451–456.
59. Heinrich S, Goerres GW, Schafer M, et al. Positron emission tomography/computed tomography influences on the management of resectable pancreatic cancer and its cost-effectiveness. *Ann Surg*. 2005;242(2):235–243.
60. Pisters PW, Lee JE, Vauthey JN, et al. Laparoscopy in the staging of pancreatic cancer. *Br J Surg*. 2001;88(3):325–337.
61. Perez-Rodriguez J, Lai S, Ehst BD, et al. Nephrogenic systemic fibrosis: incidence, associations, and effect of risk factor assessment--report of 33 cases. *Radiology*. 2009;250(2):371–377.
62. Valle JW, Palmer D, Jackson R, et al. Optimal duration and timing of adjuvant chemotherapy after definitive surgery for ductal adenocarcinoma of the pancreas: ongoing lessons from the ESPAC-3 study. *J Clin Oncol*. 2014;32(6):504–512.
63. Cannella R, Borhani AA, Zureikat AH, et al. Appleby procedure (distal pancreatectomy with celiac artery resection) for locally advanced pancreatic carcinoma: indications, outcomes, and imaging. *AJR Am J Roentgenol*. 2019:1–10.
64. Chincarini M, Zamboni GA, Pozzi Mucelli R. Major pancreatic resections: normal postoperative findings and complications. *Insights Imaging*. 2018;9(2):173–187.
65. Grobmyer SR, Pieracci FM, Allen PJ, et al. Defining morbidity after pancreaticoduodenectomy: use of a prospective complication grading system. *J Am Coll Surg*. 2007;204(3):356–364.
66. Scialpi M, Scaglione M, Volterrani L, et al. Imaging evaluation of post pancreatic surgery. *Eur J Radiol*. 2005;53(3):417–424.
67. Schulick RD. Complications after pancreaticoduodenectomy: intraabdominal abscess. *J Hepatobiliary Pancreat Surg*. 2008; 15(3):252–256.
68. DeOliveira ML, Winter JM, Schafer M, et al. Assessment of complications after pancreatic surgery: A novel grading system applied to 633 patients undergoing pancreaticoduodenectomy. *Ann Surg*. 2006;244(6):931–937. discussion 937-939.
69. Reid-Lombardo KM, Ramos-De la Medina A, Thomsen K, et al. Long-term anastomotic complications after pancreaticoduodenectomy for benign diseases. *J Gastrointest Surg*. 2007;11(12):1704–1711.
70. Westerdahl J, Andren-Sandberg A, Ihse I. Recurrence of exocrine pancreatic cancer--local or hepatic? *Hepatogastroenterology*. 1993;40(4):384–387.
71. Gillen S, Schuster T. Meyer Zum Buschenfelde C, et al. Preoperative/neoadjuvant therapy in pancreatic cancer: a systematic review and meta-analysis of response and resection percentages. *PLoS Med*. 2010;7(4):e1000267.
72. Tempero MA, Uchida E, Takasaki H, et al. Relationship of carbohydrate antigen 19-9 and Lewis antigens in pancreatic cancer. *Cancer Res*. 1987;47(20):5501–5503.
73. Katz MH, Fleming JB, Bhosale P, et al. Response of borderline resectable pancreatic cancer to neoadjuvant therapy is not reflected by radiographic indicators. *Cancer*. 2012;118(23):5749–5756.
74. Cuneo KC, Chenevert TL, Ben-Josef E, et al. A pilot study of diffusion-weighted MRI in patients undergoing neoadjuvant chemoradiation for pancreatic cancer. *Transl Oncol*. 2014;7(5):644–649.
75. Heinrich S, Schafer M, Weber A, et al. Neoadjuvant chemotherapy generates a significant tumor response in resectable pancreatic cancer without increasing morbidity: results of a prospective phase II trial. *Ann Surg*. 2008;248(6):1014–1022.
76. Maisey NR, Webb A, Flux GD, et al. FDG-PET in the prediction of survival of patients with cancer of the pancreas: a pilot study. *Br J Cancer*. 2000;83(3):287–293.
77. Nakata B, Chung YS, Nishimura S, et al. 18F-fluorodeoxyglucose positron emission tomography and the prognosis of patients with pancreatic adenocarcinoma. *Cancer*. 1997;79(4):695–699.
78. Ramanathan RK, Goldstein D, Korn RL, et al. Positron emission tomography response evaluation from a randomized phase III trial of weekly nab-paclitaxel plus gemcitabine versus gemcitabine alone for patients with metastatic adenocarcinoma of the pancreas. *Ann Oncol*. 2016;27(4):648–653.
79. Evans DB, Varadhachary GR, Crane CH, et al. Preoperative gemcitabine-based chemoradiation for patients with resectable adenocarcinoma of the pancreatic head. *J Clin Oncol*. 2008;26(21):3496–3502.
80. Van den Broeck A, Sergeant G, Ectors N, et al. Patterns of recurrence after curative resection of pancreatic ductal adenocarcinoma. *Eur J Surg Oncol*. 2009;35(6):600–604.
81. Ishigami K, Yoshimitsu K, Irie H, et al. Significance of perivascular soft tissue around the common hepatic and proximal superior mesenteric arteries arising after pancreaticoduodenectomy: evaluation with serial MDCT studies. *Abdom Imaging*. 2008;33(6):654–661.
82. Ruf J, Lopez Hanninen E, Oettle H, et al. Detection of recurrent pancreatic cancer: comparison of FDG-PET with CT/MRI. *Pancreatology*. 2005;5(2-3):266–272.
83. Parakh A, Patino M, Muenzel D, et al. Role of rapid kV-switching dual-energy CT in assessment of post-surgical local recurrence of pancreatic adenocarcinoma. *Abdom Radiol (NY)*. 2018;43(2):497–504.
84. Goggins M, Overbeek KA, Brand R, et al. Management of patients with increased risk for familial pancreatic cancer: updated recommendations from the International Cancer of the Pancreas Screening (CAPS) Consortium. *Gut*. 2020;69(1):7–17.
85. Joo I, Lee JM, Lee DH, et al. Preoperative assessment of pancreatic cancer with FDG PET/MR imaging versus FDG PET/CT plus contrast-enhanced multidetector CT: a prospective preliminary study. *Radiology*. 2017;282(1):149–159.
86. Wang ZJ, Behr S, Consunji MV, et al. early response assessment in pancreatic ductal adenocarcinoma through integrated PET/MRI. *AJR Am J Roentgenol*. 2018;211(5):1010–1019.
87. Attiyeh MA, Chakraborty J, McIntyre CA, et al. CT radiomics associations with genotype and stromal content in pancreatic ductal adenocarcinoma. *Abdom Radiol (NY)*. 2019;44(9):3148–3157.
88. Lim CH, Cho YS, Choi JY, et al. Imaging phenotype using (18)F-fluorodeoxyglucose positron emission tomography-based radiomics and genetic alterations of pancreatic ductal adenocarcinoma. *Eur J Nucl Med Mol Imaging*. 2020;47(9):2113–2122.
89. Attiyeh MA, Chakraborty J, Doussot A, et al. Survival prediction in pancreatic ductal adenocarcinoma by quantitative computed tomography image analysis. *Ann Surg Oncol*. 2018;25(4):1034–1042.
90. Cozzi L, Comito T, Fogliata A, et al. Computed tomography based radiomic signature as predictive of survival and local control after stereotactic body radiation therapy in pancreatic carcinoma. *PLoS One*. 2019;14(1):e0210758.
91. Noda Y, Goshima S, Miyoshi T, et al. Assessing chemotherapeutic response in pancreatic ductal adenocarcinoma: histogram analysis of iodine concentration and CT number in single-source dual-energy CT. *AJR Am J Roentgenol*. 2018;211(6):1221–1226.
92. Kaissis G, Ziegelmayer S, Lohofer F, et al. A machine learning model for the prediction of survival and tumor subtype in pancreatic ductal adenocarcinoma from preoperative diffusion-weighted imaging. *Eur Radiol Exp*. 2019;3(1):41.
93. Wang Y, Zhou Y, Shen W, et al. Abdominal multi-organ segmentation with organ-attention networks and statistical fusion. *Med Image Anal*. 2019;55:88–102.
94. Zhu Z, Xia Y, Xie L, et al. Multi-scale coarse-to-fine segmentation for screening pancreatic ductal adenocarcinoma. *InInter Conf Medi Img Com Compu-Ass Inter*. 2019;13:3–12.

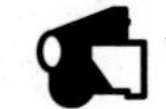
Visit ExpertConsult.com for additional algorithms.

PANCREATIC ADENOCARCINOMA

Notes: Consider clinical trials as treatment options for eligible patients.

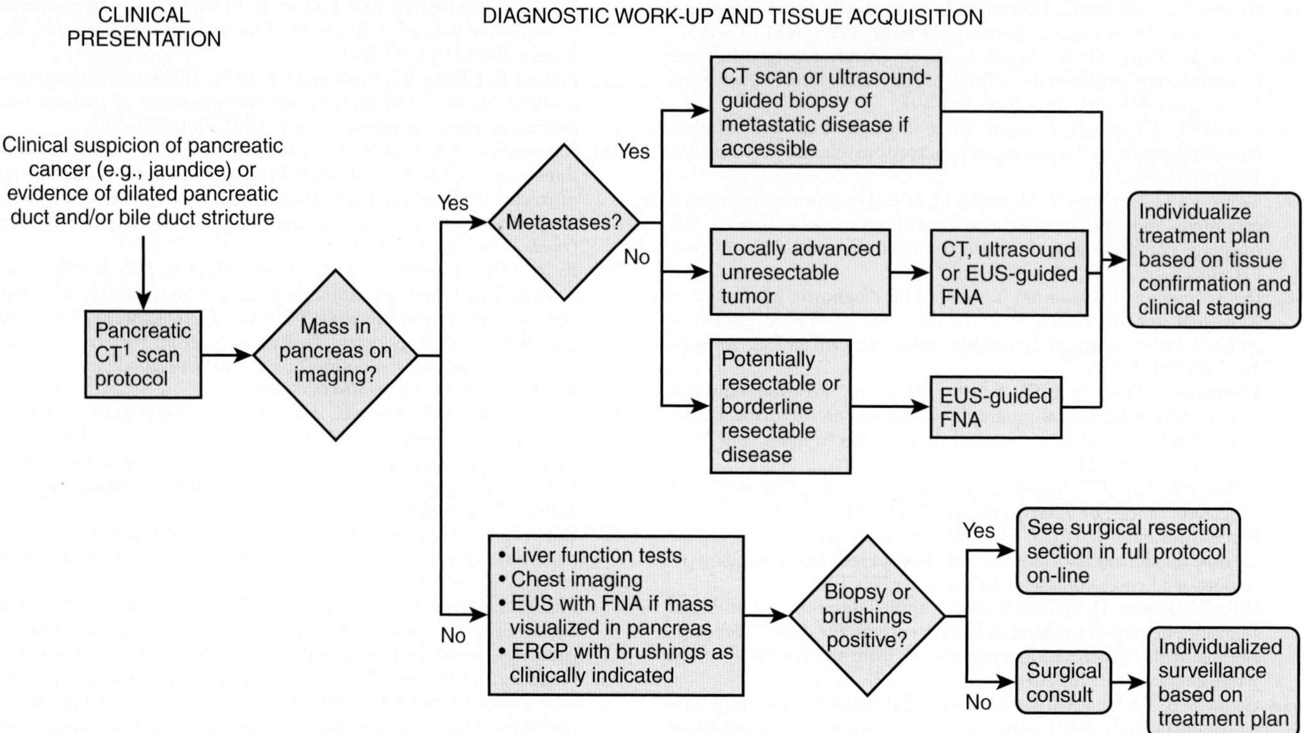

[1] Pancreatic protocol CT: triphasic cross sectional imaging and thin slices; consider PET scan if CT results are equivocal

ERCP, endoscopic retrograde cholangiopancreatography
EUS, endoscopic ultrasound

This practice algorithm has been specifically developed for M.D. Anderson using a multidisciplinary approach and taking into consideration circumstances particular to M.D. Anderson, including the following: M.D. Anderson's specific patient population; M.D. Anderson's services and structure; and M.D. Anderson's clinical information. Moreover, this algorithm is not intended to replace the independent medical or professional judgment of physicians or other health care providers. This algorithm should not be used to treat pregnant women.

CHAPTER 13

Cystic Pancreatic Lesions

Sanaz Javadi, M.D.; Jason B. Fleming, M.D.; Milind Javle, M.D.; Jeffrey H. Lee, M.D.; and Priya R. Bhosale, M.D.

INTRODUCTION

Cystic lesions of the pancreas include malignant and benign processes and may or may not cause clinical symptoms. The risk of malignancy in symptomatic cyst can be high, whereas asymptomatic cysts can be benign, malignant, or premalignant. Pancreatic cystic neoplasms account for 10% to 15% of pancreatic cysts, and less than 1% of primary pancreatic malignancies.[1]

Currently, CT and magnetic resonance imaging (MRI) are used in the assessment of pancreatic cystic lesions. CT is widely available, requires less scan time, and is the most accessible. MRI is able to identify communication of the cystic lesion with the main pancreatic duct, although, with currently available thin-section imaging, CT has a similar capacity.[2] 2-[^{18}F] fluoro-2-deoxy-D-glucose-positron emission tomography (PET)/CT has been used to differentiate malignant from benign cystic lesions based on metabolic activity.[3]

Cross-sectional imaging can characterize a cystic lesion based on the imaging findings. Currently, the available imaging modalities for detecting and diagnosing cystic lesions are contrast-enhanced CT (CECT), ultrasound (US), MRI, and PET/CT.

CECT and MRI are not operator-dependent, and can visualize the entire pancreas without difficulty. Endoscopic US (EUS) is operator- and patient-dependent, and EUS-guided fine needle aspiration (EUS-FNA) plays a complementary role in accomplishing this difficult task by providing additional real-time assessment and cystic content for further analysis. In combination with a Doppler device, this approach allows tissue sampling by FNA, avoiding the major vessels. PET/CT is an evolving modality for detecting malignancy in cystic pancreatic lesions. It has been shown to detect invasive cancer in cystic lesions; however, it cannot identify carcinoma *in situ*.[3] This modality can help detect distant metastases in the setting of invasive cancer.[4] Pancreatic cystic lesions may be identified by transabdominal US. However, this approach is limited in patients with a large body habitus, and overlying bowel gas may obscure lesions. Calcifications within the lesion are better seen on CECT; septations may or may not be seen, depending on the size of the lesion and the thickness of the septations. MRI can better identify septations and hemorrhagic contents of the cystic lesions; however, detection of mucin is equivocal. EUS can be used to evaluate the cyst, and concomitant cytological analysis of cyst fluid can be obtained by EUS-FNA. The pancreatic cyst fluid analysis should include staining for mucin, and measurement of the levels of amylase, lipase, and various tumor markers such as carcinoembryonic antigen (CEA) in the cyst fluid.

Cystic lesions of the pancreas can be divided into two categories: primary cystic lesions, which include pseudocysts, serous cystadenomas, various mucin-containing cysts (mucinous nonneoplastic cysts [MNCs], mucinous cystic neoplasm [MCNs], mucinous cystadenocarcinomas, and intraductal papillary mucinous neoplasms), pseudopapillary tumors of the pancreas and lymphoepithelial cysts, and secondary cystic lesions, which comprise various solid neoplasms undergoing cystic changes (ductal adenocarcinoma with cystic features and cystic neuroendocrine tumors). In this chapter we will discuss primary cystic lesions of the pancreas.

Pseudocysts make up the majority of all cystic lesions of the pancreas, whereas the rest are cystic tumors and true cysts. Hydatid cysts of the pancreas are rare, and should be considered as a differential diagnosis of a cystic pancreatic lesion in countries where hydatid disease is endemic.[5] Pancreatic primary cystic tumors fall into one of three major groups: serous tumors (including serous cystadenoma and cystadenocarcinoma), mucinous tumors (including MCNs, mucinous cystadenocarcinomas, intraductal papillary adenomas, and intraductal papillary adenocarcinoma), and solid pseudopapillary tumors (SPTs). The majority of cystic pancreatic tumors are asymptomatic and slow-growing. When patients are symptomatic, the symptoms are due to mass effect, and are usually vague and poorly localized. Intraductal papillary mucinous neoplasms (IPMNs) may present with pain that can mimic chronic pancreatitis.[6] On cross-sectional imaging, they can be characterized as simple (containing no internal nodularity) or complex (containing internal septations or mural nodules). They can also be classified as unilocular or multilocular, depending on the number of locules present.

PANCREATIC PSEUDOCYSTS

Epidemiology and Risk Factors

The majority of cystic lesions found in the pancreas are pseudocysts, which comprise 70% of all cystic lesions.[7]

They lack an epithelial lining and have a fibrous capsule. Pancreatic pseudocysts occur after an episode of pancreatitis and are caused by leakage of pancreatic enzymes, such as amylase and lipase, which cause fat necrosis and hemorrhage because of erosion of adjacent vessels.

Clinical Presentation

Patients with pancreatitis may present with nausea, vomiting, abdominal pain, or sepsis because of infection or obstructive jaundice.[8] Because there is leakage of pancreatic enzymes, fistulation into nearby structures, such as the common bile duct, esophagus,[9,10] and pleura,[11] can occur. Pancreatic pseudocysts seldom demonstrate internal hemorrhage, but this finding is associated with increased mortality. Pseudocysts can erode adjacent vessels and cause pseudoaneurysms, which may rupture, leading to hemorrhage. The most common arteries involved are the splenic, gastroduodenal, and superior pancreaticoduodenal arteries.[12] Pseudocysts are commonly seen in males, are usually are seen in alcoholics, and can be associated abdominal trauma.[13]

Imaging

On cross-sectional imaging (Figs. 13.1 and 13.2), pseudocysts usually appear as unilocular lesions without internal septations or mural nodules. They do communicate with the main pancreatic duct.[7] These cysts on imaging have an irregular wall in the early stages, but tend to evolve and become well-marginated.[14] On CECT, pseudocysts look like a fluid collection, which may have an imperceptible or a thick wall that may or may not enhance in the delayed phase images, as it is fibrous.[14] Pseudocysts may have a high signal on T1-weighted (T1W) MRI attributed to blood products. On magnetic resonance cholangiopancreatography (MRCP), they may show communication with the main pancreatic duct. On US, they may appear as thin-walled, unilocular, anechoic masses with increased through transmission. Complicated cysts may have low-level internal echoes with a fluid-debris level, or can have internal septations. If calcification is present within the cyst wall, this may obscure the cyst. Cysts do not have enhancing nodules; if nodules are present, one must consider a mucinous cystic neoplasm in the differential. One clue that can be seen on CT or MRI is peripancreatic stranding, which is considered the hallmark of pancreatitis, and, when associated with a cystic lesion, is suggestive of a pseudocyst.

Treatment

Treatment is usually conservative if the patient is asymptomatic. These cysts may be drained via a transperitoneal, retroperitoneal, transgastric, or transduodenal route if they are larger than 4 to 5 cm or if the patient is symptomatic. Sometimes cystogastrostomy or cystojejunostomy can be performed.

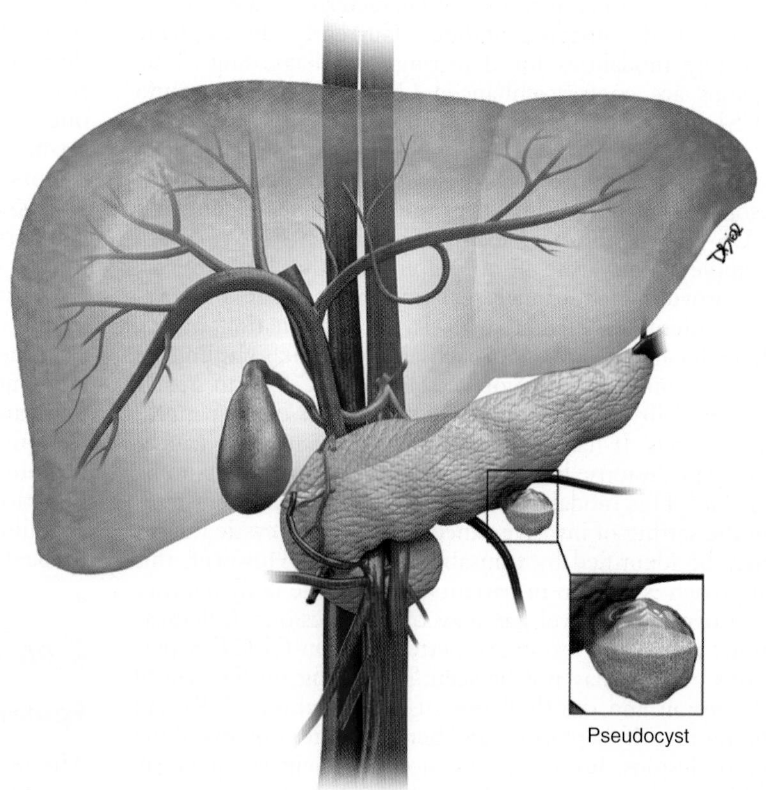

Figure 13.1. A cystic mass in the pancreatic tail contains debris representing a pseudocyst.

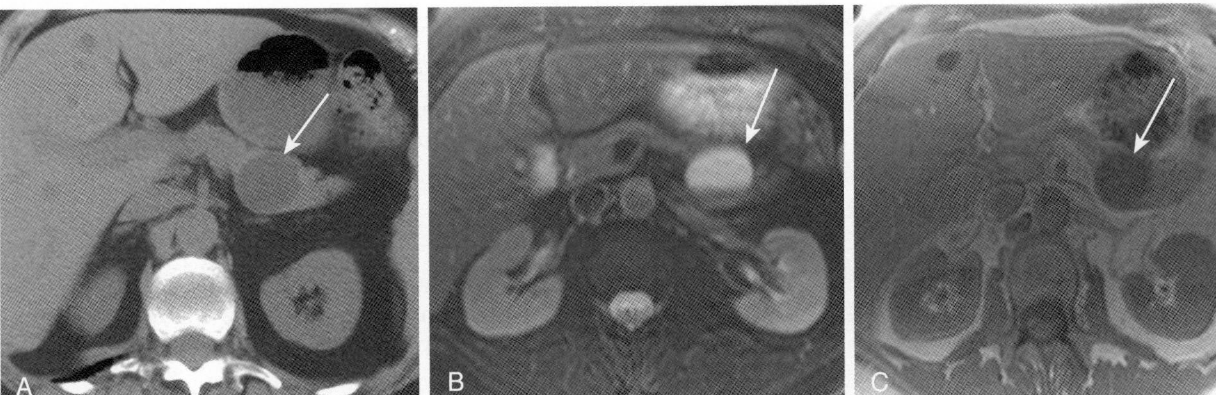

FIGURE 13.2. A 63-year-old woman with abdominal pain. **A**, Axial noncontrast computed tomography scan shows a cystic lesion in the pancreatic tail (*arrow*) without any internal septations. **B**, Axial T2-weighted magnetic resonance imaging (MRI) shows a high-signal intensity cystic lesion (*arrow*) in the pancreatic tail, containing debris. **C**, Axial T1-weighted MRI shows a low-signal intensity cystic lesion (*arrow*) in the pancreatic tail indicating the presence of a pseudocyst.

Surveillance

Depending on the suspicion, these tumors can be followed over a period of time, because a pseudocyst will resolve, and a cystic neoplasm may persist without change or growth. Although pseudocysts have no known malignant potential, many cystic neoplasms of the pancreas may mimic pseudocysts. The differential diagnosis of the cyst is mucinous cystic neoplasm, and if communication to the pancreatic duct is present one may consider an IPMN. To clinch the diagnosis of a pseudocyst, age, gender, and history of pancreatitis can help.

> **KEY POINTS Pseudocysts**
>
> - Pseudocysts are a sequela of pancreatitis, and are not lined by epithelium.
> - There is a known association with alcohol abuse.
> - On endoscopic ultrasound-guided fine needle aspiration the cyst fluid has high amylase and low carcinoembryonic antigen levels.

SIMPLE CYSTS

Epidemiology and Risk Factors

True cystic lesions of the pancreas are common,[4,15] are lined by epithelium, and can be seen in patients with von Hippel-Lindau (vHL) disease,[16] cystic fibrosis, or polycystic kidney disease. These cysts have a similar imaging appearance to the simple cysts seen in the liver and the kidneys.[15]

Clinical Presentation

Most simple cysts are found incidentally.

Imaging

On CT simply cysts have Hounsfield unit (HU) values consistent with fluid. On MRI, they have a high signal on T2-weighted (T2W) imaging and a low signal on T1W imaging and do not show enhancement. They do not have mural nodules. On US, they are anechoic with posterior acoustic enhancement. The differential of these cysts includes MCN because there is no distinguishing radiological feature between the two. When these cysts are larger than 3 cm, EUS can be performed, and a biopsy can be obtained to exclude a mucinous neoplasm. These cysts are not usually resected.

Treatment

These cysts require no treatment unless they are symptomatic.

Surveillance

No follow-up is needed.

> **KEY POINTS Simple Cysts**
>
> - Simple cysts are associated with von Hippel-Lindau disease, cystic fibrosis, and polycystic kidney disease.
> - They have a thin, imperceptible wall on computed tomography and appear as cysts on ultrasound.
> - On endoscopic ultrasound-guided fine needle aspiration they have low carcinoembryonic antigen and low amylase.

MUCINOUS NONNEOPLASTIC CYST

Epidemiology and Risk Factors

MNCs are common cystic tumors of the pancreas.[17] It is speculated that they are caused by a developmental defect of the pancreas resulting in a focal cystic transformation of the duct system.

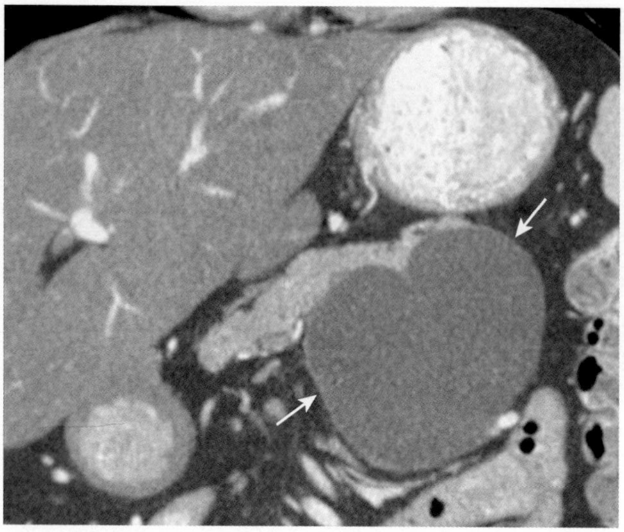

Figure 13.3. A 60-year-old woman in whom a cystic lesion was found incidentally on computed tomography (CT) colonography. Coronal reformatted CT scan of the abdomen shows a cyst (*arrows*) within the pancreatic tail, without internal septations or mural nodules, and represents a mucinous nonneoplastic cyst.

Pathology

MNCs are lined by tall columnar epithelium that secretes mucin.[18] Their maximum diameter ranges from 3 to 12 cm, they may be either unilocular or multilocular, and they may be filled with turbid or bloody fluid.[17] These tumors do not have an ovarian stroma, which is a characteristic of MCNs. These cysts do not communicate with the main pancreatic duct, do not show cellularity, do not have papillary projections as seen in IPMNs, and are believed to be benign.[17]

Clinical Presentation

Clinical symptoms may include epigastric discomfort and pain. Obstructive jaundice can be caused by compression of the common bile duct by the cystic lesion when it occurs in the pancreatic head.

Imaging

On imaging, MNCs (Fig. 13.3) are usually small and unilocular, with thin septa. On MRI they have a signal intensity consistent with simple fluid, and on CECT their HU is less than 20. On imaging, MNCs cannot be easily differentiated from MCNs, especially if the mucinous cyst is large or has a thick wall. One of the important distinguishing factors is that MCNs are commonly seen in females, whereas MNCs have no sex predilection.[19] If these cysts are larger than 2 cm, then EUS-FNA can be performed, and the cyst contents can be differentiated from those of other MCNs by immunohistochemical staining (Table 13.1).

Treatment

Usually MNCs do not require treatment unless they become symptomatic because of internal hemorrhage or cause biliary obstruction, which is rare.[17]

Surveillance

If an MNC occurs in the head of the pancreas, it can cause ductal obstruction, and should be followed at different time intervals depending on its size.

Key Points Mucinous Nonneoplastic Cysts

- These tumors secrete mucin but do not have the ovarian stroma.
- They do not communicate with the main pancreatic duct, but may cause biliary obstruction when in a critical location.

MUCINOUS CYSTADENOMAS

Epidemiology and Risk Factors

MCNs account for approximately 10% of pancreatic cystic neoplasms.[11]

Anatomy and Pathology

MCNs (Fig. 13.4) are generally found in the body and tail of the pancreas; they are usually solitary, and their size ranges from 6 to 35 cm.[20] They are lined with an inner layer of cells that secrete mucin and an outer layer of cells that resemble the ovarian stroma.[4,21] They have several locules and a thick wall.[6] These tumors do not communicate with the main pancreatic duct unless they erode into the duct, causing a fistula.[6,22] They have fewer than six locules, and the size of the locules is generally greater than 2 cm. They may contain watery fluid or hemorrhagic, necrotic, or mucinous material. These tumors usually have intramural nodules, which histologically may range from high-grade dysplasia to invasive carcinoma.[22] Pancreatic MCNs resemble ovarian MCNs, are seen almost exclusively in women of reproductive age (>95%; mean age 45 years), and are typically present in the body or tail of the pancreas.[19,20,22,23] The malignancy rate in MCNs with ovarian stroma is reported to be as low as 10% to 17%.[24,25] Curvilinear calcifications may be noted in the periphery of the tumor and/or capsule in 10% to 25% of cases.[14]

Clinical Presentation

Patients with MCNs may present with vague abdominal discomfort and have symptoms such as weight loss and anorexia.

TABLE 13.1 Clinical and Demographic Features of Pancreatic Cyst

	SCA	MCN	IPMN	SPT	PSEUDO
Prevalent age	Elderly women	Middle age	Elderly men	Young	Variable
Sex	Female > male	Female	Male > female	Female	Male > female
Alcohol abuse	No	No	No	No	Yes
Pancreatitis	No	No	Not uncommon	No	Yes
Location	Evenly	Body/tail	Head and tail	Evenly	Evenly
Malignant potential	Rare	Moderate/high	Low/high	Low	None

SCA, Serous cystadenoma; *MCN*, mucinous cystic neoplasm; *IPMN*, intraductal papillary mucinous neoplasm; *SPT*, solid pseudopapillary tumor; *PSEUDO*, pseudocyst.

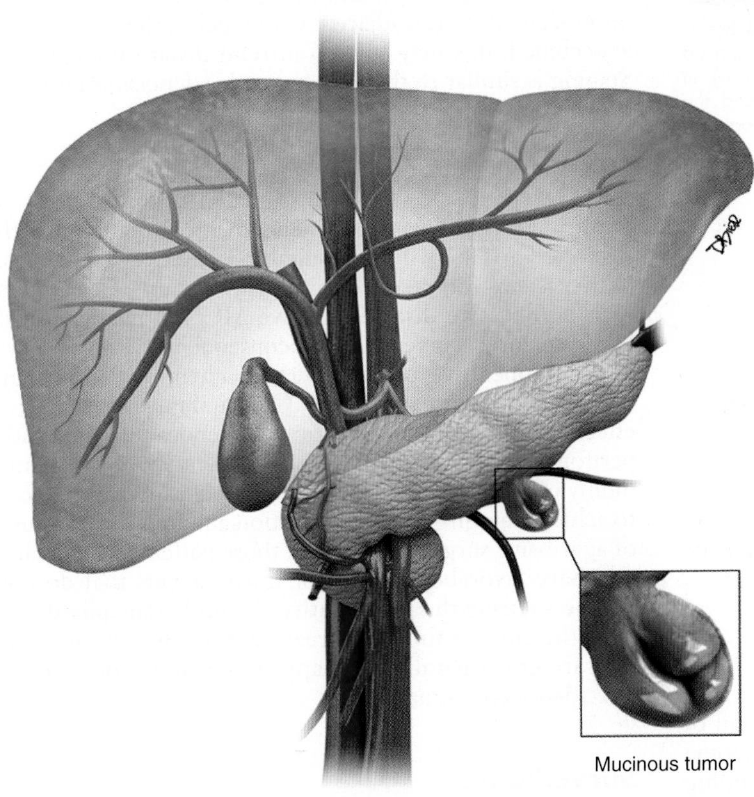

FIGURE 13.4. A cystic lesion in the pancreatic tail with septations, indicating a mucinous cystic lesion.

Imaging

On cross-sectional imaging, these tumors may appear as a single large cyst or as a large cyst with multiple locules, a thick outer wall, thick septations, and enhancing intramural nodules. Sometimes calcification of the outer wall can be seen,[6] and the outer wall of the cyst may enhance on the delayed phase, a finding that correlates with the observation of a fibrotic capsule on histopathology. On MRI, the fluid within the cyst may have a low signal on T1W imaging and a high signal on T2W imaging; the increased signal on T1W imaging is owing to presence of mucin,[26] but unfortunately this is an unreliable test for definitively diagnosing MCN. The presence of enhancing nodules should raise suspicion for malignancy.[23]

On US, MCNs (Fig. 13.5) can appear as well-demarcated, anechoic, thick-walled cystic masses and may have echogenic thick septa, internal nodularity, or mural calcification. Differential diagnosis of these lesions includes pseudocyst; these can be differentiated on serial follow-up imaging, in which the pseudocyst may decrease in size, whereas the mucinous neoplasm usually persists.

Treatment

These tumors are resected, as cystadenoma and carcinoma cannot be differentiated by imaging, and these tumors have malignant potential.

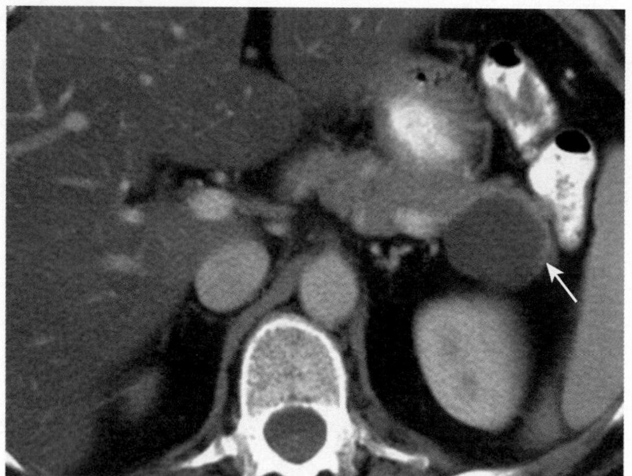

Figure 13.5. A 45-year-old woman with a history of right breast cancer presented with abdominal pain. Axial contrast-enhanced computed tomography shows a unilocular cystic lesion (*arrow*) in the pancreatic tail. The imaging findings are nonspecific, and the differential here would be pseudocyst and mucinous cystic neoplasm. However, the lack of a history of pancreatitis strongly suggests that this is a mucinous cystic neoplasm.

Surveillance

Following surgical resection, no follow-up is necessary.

MUCINOUS CYSTADENOCARCINOMAS

Epidemiology and Risk Factors

When invasive carcinoma is present in the mucinous cyst, it is called as mucinous cystadenocarcinoma, although the rate of invasive carcinoma is low at 12%.[20]

Anatomy and Pathology

These masses are usually seen in the body and the tail of the pancreas. Patients with invasive mucinous carcinoma are older than those with noninvasive MCN; this finding is suggestive of a progression from cystadenoma to cystadenocarcinoma.[20] The earliest genetic change seen within MCNs is mutation of the *KRAS2* oncogene located on chromosome 12p,[27] which is present in 90% of MCNs with carcinoma *in situ*.[27] MCNs progress toward malignancy, similar to pancreatic intraepithelial neoplasia.[27]

Clinical Presentation

These patients may present with vague abdominal pain and discomfort. Rarely, mucinous cystadenocarcinoma can cause pancreatitis.

Staging Evaluation

Staging is according to the American Joint Committee on Cancer (AJCC) classification of pancreatic cancer.

Imaging

Although the presence of enhancing nodules and septations correlates with malignancy, absence of these findings does not preclude malignancy. On imaging, mucinous cystadenocarcinomas (Fig. 13.6) appear as large, complex, cystic pancreatic masses that can be distinguished from MCNs by the presence of intracystic enhancing soft tissue. These tumors are usually large (>6 cm), and tumors smaller than 4 cm are usually not malignant unless intramural nodules are present.[20] Hence, any enhancing soft tissue within a cystic neoplasm detected on CECT or MRI is considered an indication for resection; however, all mucinous lesions are considered premalignant and are generally resected because, in the majority of cases, radiological discrimination between benign and malignant MCN is currently impossible. When an adjacent vessel such as the splenic vein is occluded, this may suggest a trend toward malignancy. Staging is similar to that of pancreatic adenocarcinoma.

Treatment

Surgical resection is recommended for all patients with suspected MCN who are suitable operative candidates. Whereas surgical resection is usually curative in patients with noninvasive disease, invasive MCN is characterized by frequent recurrence, and consequently poorer survival; preoperative or postoperative chemoradiation may be useful in these patients.[28,29] Gemcitabine appears to be effective in cases of pancreatic cystadenocarcinomas with peritoneal metastases.[30,31] This treatment strategy is commonly offered to patients with resectable pancreatic cancer to achieve margin-negative resection and to reduce the use of aggressive surgical therapy in those patients whose cancers have favorable biology (or those cancers that do not progress during the preoperative chemotherapy phase).[32]

At the current time, the treatment of advanced cystadenocarcinoma parallels the approaches used for pancreatic adenocarcinoma.

Surveillance

At MD Anderson Cancer Center, we typically evaluate these patients annually for the first few years after resection. In contrast, if analysis of surgical specimens shows invasive adenocarcinoma, patients should be monitored closely for the presence of local recurrence and distant metastasis, with periodic physical examination and cross-sectional imaging. Our schedule for these patients is similar to that for patients with resected pancreatic adenocarcinoma, and includes one visit every 4 months for 2 years, then biannually until year 5, and then yearly thereafter. At each follow-up visit, the patient undergoes staging CECT and tumor marker evaluation if he or she was antigen-positive before surgical resection.

Key Points Mucinous Cystic Neoplasms

- Mucinous cystadenomas and carcinomas have ovarian stroma.
- They are unilocular and may have papillary projections.

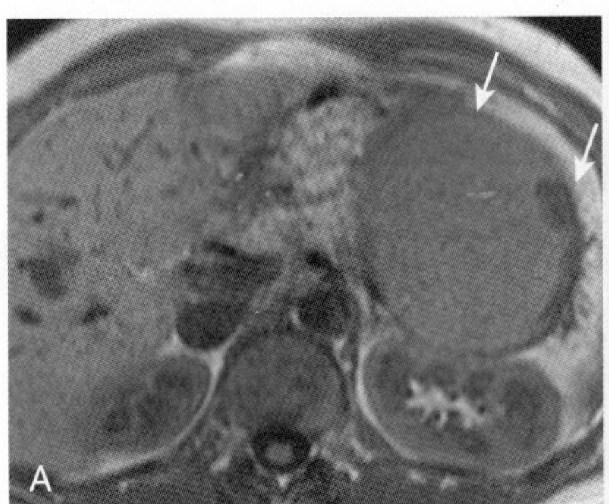

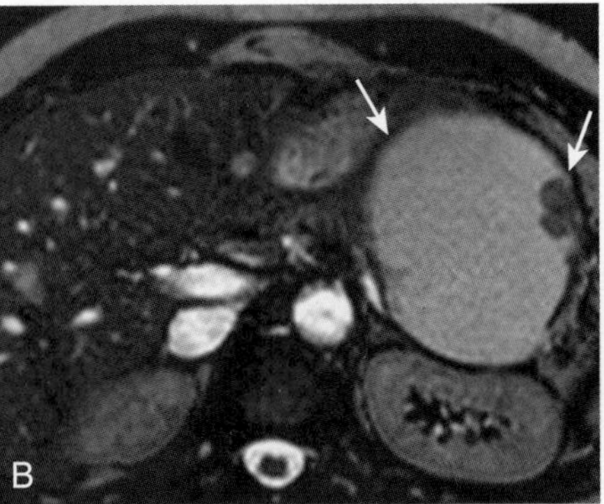

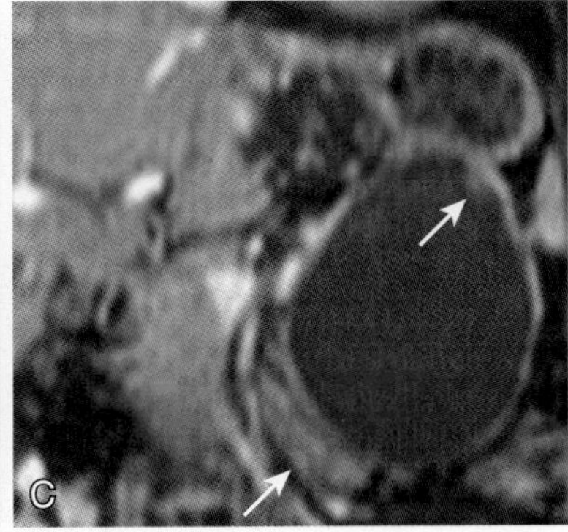

FIGURE 13.6 A 48-year-old woman with abdominal pain. **A**, Axial T1-weighted magnetic resonance imaging (MRI) shows a high-signal intensity mass (*arrow*) in the pancreatic tail and a low-signal intensity mural nodule (*arrow*). **B**, Axial T2-weighted MRI shows a cystic mass (*arrow*) in the pancreatic tail with intramural nodules (*arrow*). **C**, Coronal contrast-enhanced T1-weighted MRI shows a mass (*bottom arrow*) in the pancreatic tail with enhancing tumor nodules (*top arrow*), suggesting a mucinous cystic neoplasm. Given the age and sex of the patient and the location of the cyst, a diagnosis of mucinous cystic neoplasm was suggested.

- They commonly do not communicate with the main pancreatic duct.
- They are exclusively seen in menstruating females.
- On endoscopic ultrasound-guided fine needle aspiration, carcinoembryonic antigen levels can be high as 200 to 500 ng/mL, and amylase is low.

INTRADUCTAL PAPILLARY MUCINOUS NEOPLASM

Introduction

There are three main types of IPMNs, classified based on their location: the main duct type, the branch-duct type (BD-IPMN), and the combined type.[33] These tumors produce mucin, which accumulates in the ducts and results in cystic dilatation of the duct. Most commonly, IPMNs involve the main pancreatic duct, but they may also affect the side branches.[32] Depending on their size and type they can be premalignant or malignant. They may exhibit a spectrum of dysplasia ranging from minimal mucinous hyperplasia to invasive carcinoma.[34] The main duct-type and combined-type IPMNs have similar malignancy rates of 38% to 68% and 38% to 65%, respectively, whereas the malignancy rate of BD-IPMNs is lower, at approximately 12% to 47%.[35] The differential diagnosis of BD-IPMNs may include pseudocyst.

Epidemiology and Risk Factors

IPMNs arise from the columnar epithelium of the pancreatic duct. The cells become dysplastic and form papillary projections that extend into the pancreatic ducts and secrete mucin. These tumors are more commonly seen in males, with a male-to-female ratio of 2:1. These patients typically present in the seventh to eighth decades of life. Initially IPMNs were thought to represent only 5% of all cystic lesions, but they are being increasingly reported, likely owing to increased awareness of the disease and the use of cross-sectional imaging modalities. According to the World Health Organization (WHO), IPMNs are classified based on the degree of epithelial dysplasia as adenoma, borderline tumor, or carcinoma (either *in situ* or invasive).[36]

Anatomy and Pathology

IPMNs can be classified depending on whether they involve the main pancreatic duct (Fig. 13.7) or isolated side branches. They may be also characterized by whether they exhibit a diffuse pattern of ductal dilatation or a segmental cystic appearance.[37] The location of the tumor is an important factor for prognosis.[33] Some 20% to 30% are multifocal, and 5% to 10% involve the entire pancreas.[22,38]

Clinical Presentation

These patients may be asymptomatic or may present with pancreatitis, and sometimes with jaundice.

Main Duct-Type Intraductal Papillary Mucinous Neoplasm

Anatomy and Pathology

These are different from the mucinous cystic tumors because they lack an associated ovarian-type stroma. There are two types of main duct IPMN histologically: the intestinal or gastric type and the pancreaticobiliary type.[27,39] The intestinal subtype produces abundant extracellular mucin as it progresses toward invasive malignancy, and is associated with the good survival after surgical resection that is typical of IPMNs.[27] The pancreaticobiliary subtypes evolve into ductal adenocarcinoma and have the associated poor survival that characterizes invasive ductal adenocarcinoma of pancreatic origin.[27] Predictors of malignancy are main duct type with mucin leakage from the ampulla of Vater, main pancreatic duct dilatation, large tumor size, jaundice, and diabetes.[40-42] The pancreaticobiliary type of IPMN has a higher malignant potential compared with the other types.[39] Mucin extruding from the ampulla of Vater is a pathognomic feature of a main duct IPMN, seen

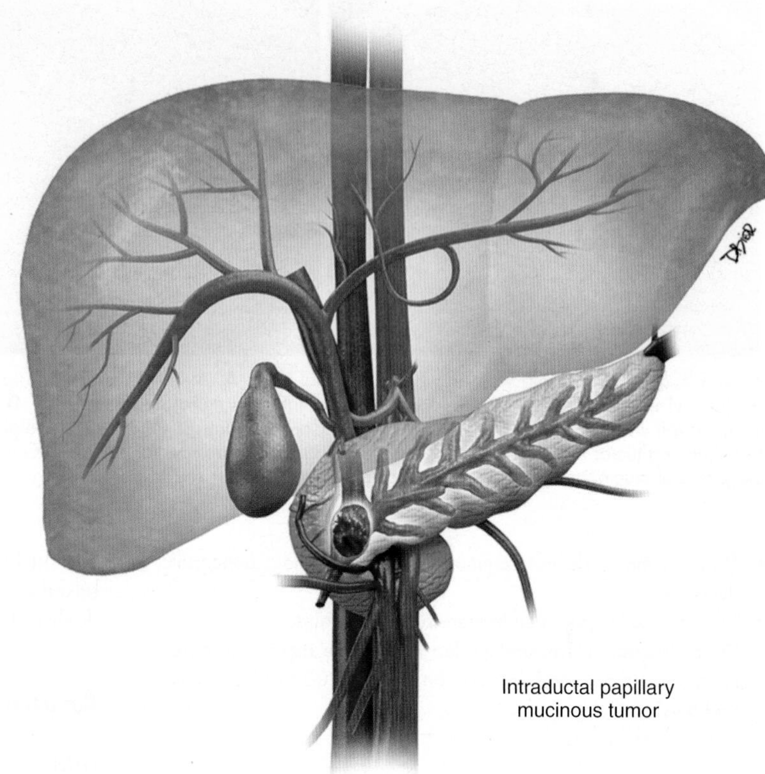

FIGURE 13.7. A mass (*red*) in the pancreatic head causes pancreatic ductal dilatation owing to mucin production.

on cholangiopancreatography, and is caused by excessive mucin production by the neoplastic cells.[13,21] The tumors have a papillary or polypoid appearance and arise from mucinous cells, which are transformed pancreatic ductal epithelium.[37,43] When the size of the main duct increases to 1 cm, the tumor nodule may show cell atypia, ranging from slight dysplasia to frank invasive carcinoma. In addition, these cell types may coexist within the same lesion. The spectrum of IPMNs ranges from noninvasive neoplasms with varying degrees of epithelial dysplasia to foci of carcinoma *in situ* and frank invasive adenocarcinoma. The precise rate of progression from benign to malignant status is unknown, but is estimated to range is from 5 to 7 years.[6,12,38,44] Malignancy is more common in main duct IPMNs, and approximately 60% to 92% of cases demonstrate invasive carcinoma.[43,45] The prevalence of invasive carcinoma is higher in main duct IPMN (23%-57%).[4,36]

Clinical Presentation

Theses tumors occur most frequently in men with a mean age of 65 years.[22] Most patients with main duct IPMNs are symptomatic, and patients present with epigastric abdominal pain that is frequently exacerbated by food. The pain is likely caused by mucin production that blocks the pancreatic duct and can result in pancreatitis, leading to ductal strictures. Patients frequently complain of pain, often epigastric pain that radiates to the back.[6] Therefore, many patients may be misdiagnosed as having chronic pancreatitis, rather than IPMN; other symptoms and signs include weight loss, fever, and jaundice.[42]

Patterns of Tumor Spread

Patients with invasive carcinoma can develop metastases to the liver or lung or can have local recurrence.[46]

Staging

Staging is similar to pancreatic ductal adenocarcinoma.

Imaging

Several imaging modalities can be used to image IPMNs, such as CT, MRI, MRCP, EUS, and PET/CT. Any one of these, or any combinations of these modalities, has the ability to characterize these lesions. MRI may provide better depiction of ductal communication than CT.[47,48] The appearance of IPMNs on CT depends on their type and location. The main pancreatic duct is dilated in the setting of a main duct IPMN (Figs. 13.8 and 13.9); sometimes the entire duct can be dilated if the tumor is present in the head, and there may be segmental dilation of the duct if the tumor is present in the body. However, eventually the entire duct becomes dilated as the disease progresses.[21,22]

Because these tumors result in pancreatitis, changes in the pancreatic parenchyma may be visible on CT and MRI, such as loss of T1 signal on the noncontrast images and delayed uptake of contrast material, which are indicative of chronic fibrosis.[49] On CT, US, and MRI, the main duct may be markedly dilated and tortuous. In some cases, mural nodules can be identified that show enhancement following administration of intravenous contrast. The gland may become atrophic, and dysmorphic calcifications may be present, mimicking

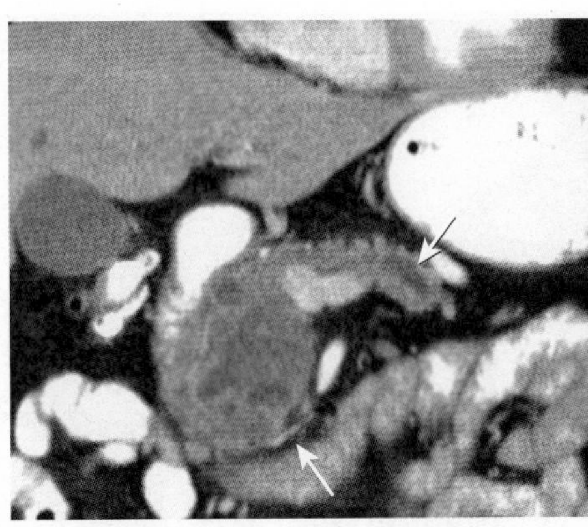
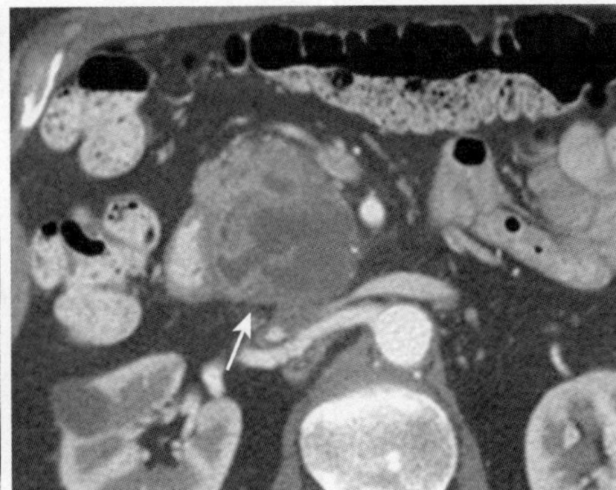

Figure 13.8. A 65-year-old man with a cystic mass in the pancreas. **Left**, Coronal contrast-enhanced computed tomography scan shows a cystic mass in the pancreatic head arising from the main pancreatic duct (*white arrow*) and causing dilatation of the main pancreatic duct because of mucin accumulation (*shadowed arrow*). Right, Axial CT scan shows a heterogenous mass (*arrow*) in the pancreatic head due to an intraductal papillary mucinous neoplasm (IPMN) extruding mucin.

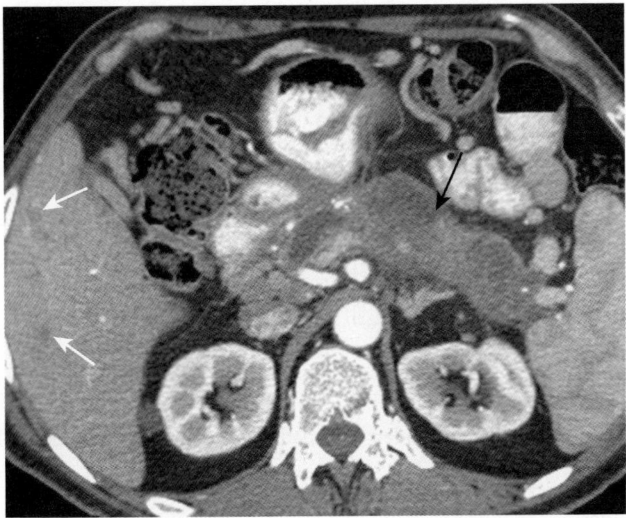

Figure 13.9. A 67-year-old man who presented with abdominal pain. Axial contrast-enhanced computed tomography of the abdomen shows a low-attenuation mass (*black arrow*) in the pancreatic tail, representing an intraductal papillary mucinous neoplasm with metastases (*white arrows*) in the liver.

findings of chronic pancreatitis. However, patients with main duct IPMN present at a later age compared with those with chronic pancreatitis, and may have a bulging papilla on imaging owing to mucin production. The features of malignancy or invasive carcinoma on imaging in main duct IPMN include main duct dilation to greater than 1.5 cm in diameter, enhancing nodules or excrescences, diffuse or multifocal involvement of the pancreatic duct, presence of a focal hypovascular soft tissue mass, or bile duct obstruction.[50] All main duct lesions are considered premalignant and should be considered for surgical resection.[4,15]

Branch-Duct Intraductal Papillary Mucinous Neoplasms

Anatomy and Pathology

BD-IPMNs follow a more clinically indolent course than duct type or combined type IPMNs. These tumors are located mostly in the head of the pancreas (usually the uncinate process). Histologically, the BD-IPMNs display a distinct architecture, known as gastric foveolar-type epithelium, which rarely progresses toward frank malignancy.[27] The prevalence of cancer in BD-IPMN ranges from 6% to 46%.[4,36,46] These IPMNs usually occur in the uncinate process of the pancreas and appear as a small cystic mass described on imaging as a "bunch of grapes." On US, they are well-defined, hypoechoic cystic lesions with internal septations. This tumor secretes a large amount of mucin, which may extrude into the main pancreatic duct and cause main pancreatic ductal dilation downstream from the site of communication of the side branch with the main pancreatic duct. Usually the side branch communication is larger in the setting of malignancy than in a benign lesion. BD-IPMNs can be multifocal because all pancreatic ductal epithelium may be at risk for developing malignancy.[46]

Clinical Presentation

BD-IPMNs are found in younger patients and have a low potential for malignancy.[51]

Patterns of Tumor Spread

The pattern of spread is similar to that of main duct IPMNs.

Imaging

On cross-sectional imaging, BD-IPMNs are characterized by cystic dilatation of the ductal side branches. Sometimes, papillary projections or intramural nodules can be seen with the dilated side branch on endoscopic retrograde cholangiopancreatography, MRCP, or CECT. The previously mentioned imaging modalities can also show communication of the dilated side branch to the main pancreatic duct, which confirms the diagnosis. BD-IPMNs show dilatation of multiple side branches on T2W MRI, and these lesions are most commonly seen in the pancreatic head.[52] These tumors may mimic a serous cystadenoma (SCA); however, BD-IPMNs (Fig. 13.10) show communication with the main pancreatic duct, which helps differentiate between these two entities. The imaging features suggestive of malignancy include enhancing soft tissue nodularity and a size of greater than 3 cm.[38,46,53-55]

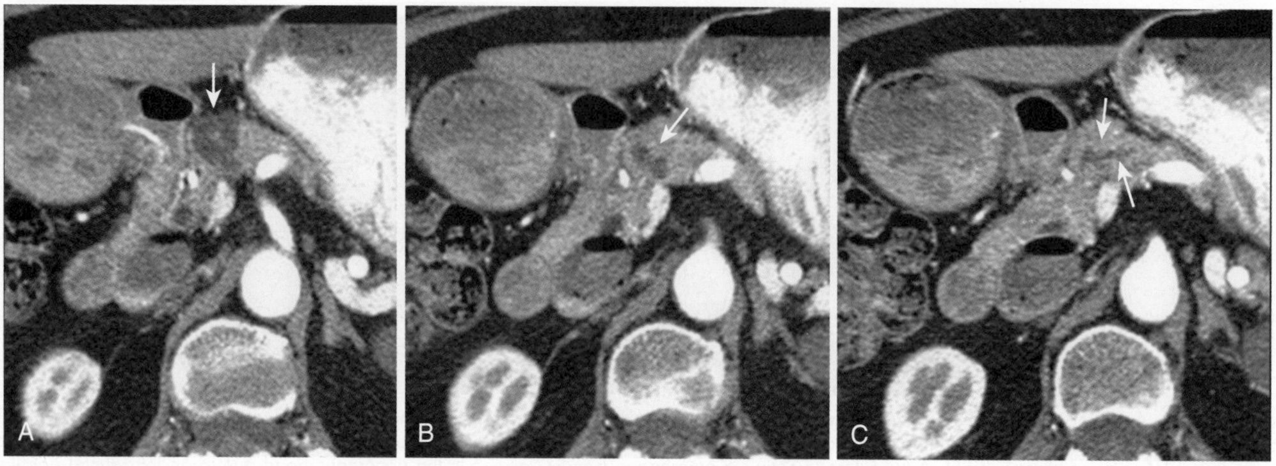

FIGURE 13.10. A 71-year-old woman with epigastric and upper abdominal pain. **A**, Axial contrast-enhanced computed tomography scan shows a cystic lesion (*arrow*) in the pancreatic neck. **B**, A lower image shows that the cystic lesion (*arrow*) is tubular. **C**, A lower image shows that this dilated duct (*arrows*) communicates with the main pancreatic duct, which is suggestive of a branch-duct intraductal papillary mucinous neoplasm.

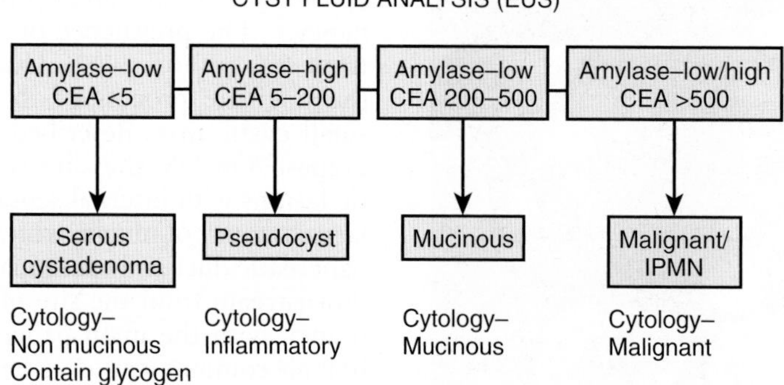

FIGURE 13.11. Analysis of the cystic fluid in different cystic lesions after endoscopic ultrasound-guided fine needle aspiration. *IPMN*, Intraductal papillary mucinous neoplasm.

In the absence of these features, some groups have advocated conservative management with regular follow-up imaging evaluations of localized BD-IPMNs in asymptomatic patients.[38]

Combined Intraductal Papillary Mucinous Neoplasms

When the main pancreatic duct and the side branches are dilated, this is called a combined IPMN; in this case, the tumor is present in the side branches as well as in the main pancreatic duct. The presence of malignancy within an IPMN is confirmed via biopsy, usually performed by EUS-FNA. EUS can further characterize IPMN by visualizing papillary growth along the pancreatic duct. FNA can be used to obtain tissue from this papillary growth and aspirate ductal content to evaluate for the presence of mucin and perform other studies.

The aspirated fluid is sent for cytology (Fig. 13.11), cyst fluid tumor markers, and amylase. Cyst fluid viscosity has been described to be higher in mucinous cysts.[56] The use of cyst fluid tumor markers such as CEA, carbohydrate antigen 19-9, carbohydrate antigen 72-4, carbohydrate antigen 125, and carbohydrate antigen 15-3 has been proposed, but these markers have limitations.[56-58]

In a study performed by Brugge and colleagues, CEA was found to be the most specific marker for pancreatic cysts malignancy.[59] Using the CEA value of 192 ng/mL, the sensitivity for diagnosis of a mucinous cyst was 75%, with a specificity of 84% and an accuracy of 79%. In comparison, the accuracy of EUS morphology was 51%, and for cytology was 59%.[60] For cytological examination, specimens are analyzed for the presence of mucinous epithelium, the extent of cytologic atypia, and the presence of malignant cells. Having a cytologist available on-site reduces the number of FNA passes needed to establish the final diagnosis, thus reducing procedure time and complications.

Treatment

Whereas cross-sectional imaging can be used to diagnose IPMN with reasonable accuracy, no combination of imaging techniques, serum tumor markers, or tumor biopsies can reliably distinguish invasive from noninvasive disease. Because of the high rates of invasive disease associated with main duct lesions, international consensus guidelines for the management of patients with MCN and IPMN suggest that resection be considered for all patients with main duct IPMN who have good functional status and a reasonable life expectancy.[4] Surgical resection is recommended in patients with symptomatic or large (>3 cm) branch-duct lesions. In contrast, a period of observation is reasonable for asymptomatic patients with a BD-IPMN less than 3 cm in diameter and no radiographic features suggestive of malignancy. These lesions are associated with a favorable survival rate despite nonoperative management.[53,61,62] In this group, close follow-up with cross-sectional imaging should be used to detect an increase in tumor size, a change in radiographic characteristics, or the development of symptoms, any of which would suggest the need to reevaluate the need for surgical resection. Importantly, small BD-IPMNs in patients of advanced age do not need immediate surgery.

Adjuvant chemoradiation is offered for patients with invasive adenocarcinoma, and this improves survival, as indicated by several prospective studies.[63,64] At MD Anderson Cancer Center, preoperative therapy is commonly offered to patients with resectable pancreatic cancer, with intent to (1) achieve margin-negative resection and (2) restrict the use of aggressive surgical therapy in those patients whose cancers have a favorable biology (or those cancers that do not progress during the preoperative chemotherapy phase).[32] Such a strategy can also be applied to cystic pancreatic tumors that have an invasive component, because these can grow to significant dimensions before detection, and the likelihood of margin-negative resection can be improved with the preoperative approach. Gemcitabine, either as a single agent or in combination with erlotinib, is considered the standard of care for the treatment of advanced pancreatic adenocarcinoma; however, the resultant clinical benefit is modest.[65,66]

Adjuvant chemoradiation can improve the median survival in patients with IPMN with an invasive component.[67] Adjuvant chemoradiation in patients with IPMN with an invasive component is associated with a significantly higher overall survival rate among node-positive patients and those with positive margins. Anatomic partial pancreatectomy represents the standard surgical treatment for patients with IPMN. Surgical margins should be assessed intraoperatively by frozen section analysis.

Surveillance

Patients with residual noninvasive IPMN at the pancreatic transection margin have a very low likelihood of developing recurrent disease.[68] We elect to follow these patients annually after the initial postoperative period with repeat imaging of the pancreatic remnant. In contrast, we believe that an attempt should be made to achieve margins clear of invasive IPMN in patients with good performance status. Postoperative survival of patients with IPMN is related primarily to the presence of invasive adenocarcinoma. In rare instances, this may require total pancreatectomy. The high rates of recurrence after resection for invasive disease mandate closer follow-up; we follow these patients as we would patients with pancreatic adenocarcinoma and use cross-sectional imaging at each visit to detect locoregional or distant recurrence.

Key Points Intraductal Papillary Mucinous Neoplasms

- A cystic lesion that communicates with the main pancreatic duct is a branch-duct intraductal papillary mucinous neoplasm (IPMN).
- A main pancreatic duct dilated to greater than 15 mm is suggestive of a main duct IPMN.
- The presence of nodules in main duct IPMN or branch-duct IPMN is suggestive of malignancy.
- IPMN can transform into an invasive carcinoma that is difficult to differentiate from ductal adenocarcinoma.
- Endoscopic ultrasound-guided fine needle aspiration may show high levels of carcinoembryonic antigen and mucin.

SEROUS CYSTADENOMA

Introduction

SCAs are the most common cystic neoplasms, accounting for 1% of pancreatic exocrine neoplasms and 30% of cystic neoplasms. They can arise from any part of the pancreas, but are commonly seen in the body and tail.

Epidemiology and Risk Factors

SCAs more commonly occur in women than in men; in women they occur in the sixth decade of life, and in men in the seventh decade.[22,69] These cystic lesions present with nonspecific symptoms such as epigastric abdominal pain and weight loss. They are categorized into microcystic serous SCAs (mutilocular) and oligocystic lesions (unilocular). Unilocular/macrocystic SCAs, also known as oligocystic serous cystadenomas (OSCs), may have a single locule, making them difficult to distinguish from an MCN[6] or even a pseudocyst.

These tumors do not produce mucin, have a lobulated, well-defined border, and have a histologically have clear or eosinophil-rich cytoplasm. SCAs are usually less than 5 cm in diameter, with a median size of 25 to 30 mm. These tumors can be seen in VHL syndrome,[21,70] which consists of retinal and central nervous system hemangioblastomas and pheochromocytomas. Mutation of the VHL gene is also seen in sporadic cases of SCA. These tumors are benign, and the risk of malignancy is low, at approximately 3% (Fig. 13.12).[71]

Microcystic Serous Cystadenomas

Anatomy and Pathology

Microcystic SCAs (glycogen-rich adenomas) are usually composed of more than six locules that range in size from 0.1 to 2 cm but are typically less than 1 cm, resemble a sponge, and may have a calcified stellate scar,[2,21] although this is only seen in approximately 10% to 30% of cases.

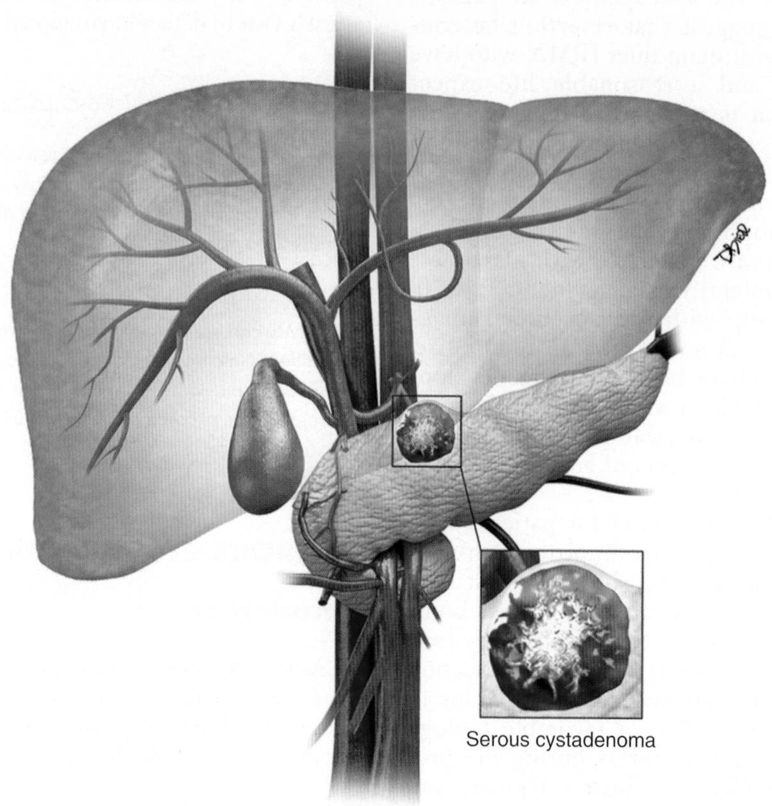

FIGURE 13.12. A cystic mass (*red*) in the pancreatic body has a central stellate scar (*white*), indicating a serous cystadenoma.

Clinical Presentation

Most tumors are found incidentally, but large tumors can cause symptoms owing to mass effect. For example, a mass in the pancreatic head can cause jaundice by obstructing the common bile duct.[70]

On cross-sectional imaging, these are purely cystic masses and have a "honeycomb" appearance. On noncontrast examination, they have CT attenuation of less than 20 HU (Fig. 13.13); and they do enhance owing to the central fibrovascular scar.[2,21] Enhancement in this lesion may be misleading in cases in which the tiny locules are not visible, leading this cystic neoplasm to be misdiagnosed as a solid mass such as a pancreatic neuroendocrine tumor.

In these situations, MRI (Fig. 13.15) is the most appropriate modality to definitively characterize these tumors, because they have a characteristic high T2 signal because of the presence of fluid, and the thin fibrous septa enhance on the delayed phase of contrast. On US, these tumors can appear as echogenic masses or as a partly solid mass with cystic and anechoic areas. On color Doppler, the peripheral areas and the central areas show flow. These tumors do not communicate with the main pancreatic duct, unlike BD-IPMNs.[72] If large dystrophic calcification is present in the central scar, a corresponding signal void may be seen on any MRI sequence, and posterior acoustic shadowing may be seen on US. The echo features of SCA on EUS include sunburst calcification with numerous microcysts; this is pathognomic for SCA.

Treatment

Treatment of SCAs is discussed at the end of this section.

Oligocystic Serous Cystadenoma

Anatomy and Pathology

These tumors are larger, have fewer locules, and may mimic an MCN on imaging.[73] The individual cysts may be larger than 2 cm, and rarely, only one locule may be seen.

Imaging

The imaging features of this tumor overlap with those of MCNs (Fig. 13.14). When a unilocular lesion is seen in the head of the pancreas containing no papillary projections or intramural nodularity, one should consider a diagnosis of OSC.[14] On US, these tumors may appear as solid echogenic masses because of the many interfaces produced by the numerous cysts, or may be completely anechoic and cystic if they comprise a single locule.

Treatment

Decisions regarding operative intervention for presumed SCA should be made on the basis of symptoms, tumor size, and the certainty of the diagnosis. We generally recommend resection to symptomatic patients with good performance status, regardless of the size of the tumor.

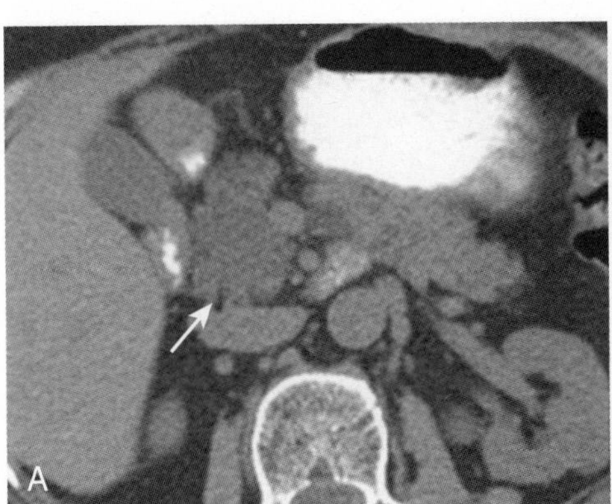

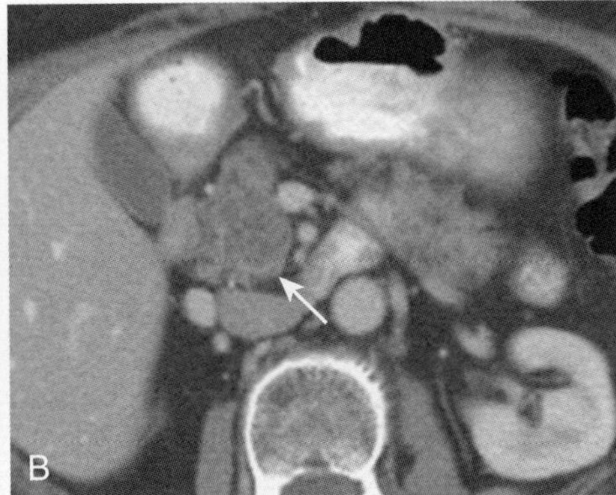

Figure 13.13. A 69-year-old woman with a history of B-cell non-Hodgkin lymphoma had an incidentally discovered mass in the pancreatic head. **A**, Noncontrast computed tomography scan of the abdomen shows a mass (*arrow*) in the pancreatic head, which has low attenuation consistent with fluid. **B**, Axial contrast-enhanced computed tomography scan of the abdomen shows a multilocular mass (*arrow*) in the head of the pancreas with enhancing septa and the characteristic "honeycomb" appearance suggestive of a microcystic serous cystadenoma.

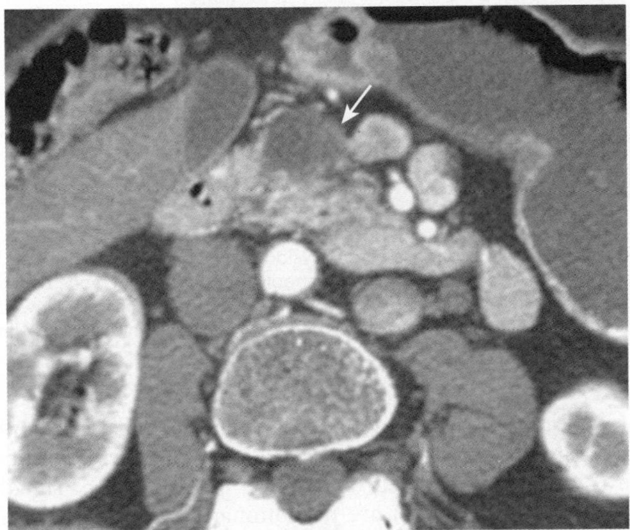

Figure 13.14. An 82-year-old woman with an incidentally discovered cystic lesion in the pancreatic head. Axial computed tomography scan of the abdomen shows a unilocular mass (*arrow*) in the pancreatic head, indicating an oligocystic serous cystadenoma. This imaging pattern is nonspecific, but when one takes into account the age and sex of the patient, a diagnosis of a serous cystadenoma is likely.

Surveillance

Patients with incidentally discovered slow-growing tumors less than 4 cm in diameter may be observed initially with semiannual/annual cross-sectional imaging to evaluate the presence or absence of tumor growth. It is reasonable to consider surgical resection for incidentally discovered tumors greater than 4 cm in diameter (although this number is somewhat arbitrary) or those that exhibit rapid growth or a significant change in radiographic appearance during observation, particularly in younger patients. Resection is also recommended when a definitive diagnosis cannot be established. It is our opinion that surgery is applied too early and too often for patients with this disease, particularly for those of advanced age with asymptomatic tumors less than 4 to 5 cm in size. For patients selected for surgery, complete anatomic resection by pancreaticoduodenectomy or distal pancreatectomy is generally curative. The reported 5-year survival rate is high, at greater than 81%.[74,75] Therefore, postoperative surveillance is probably unnecessary; we follow these patients after the initial postoperative period only to screen for the presence of gastrointestinal or metabolic complications after pancreatectomy.

Key Points Serous Cystadenoma

- These tumors are more common in elderly women.
- Oligocystic serous cystadenomas are unilocular.
- Microcystic serous cystadenomas are multilocular and have fibrovascular septa and central stellate calcification.

SOLID PSEUDOPAPILLARY TUMOR

Introduction

Previously known as "solid and cystic papillary epithelial neoplasms of the pancreas," "papillary cystic neoplasms," or "Hamoudi" or "Frantz" tumors, these neoplasms were named solid pseudopapillary tumors of the pancreas by the WHO in 1996.[37]

Epidemiology and Risk Factors

These tumors are less common than IPMNs, SCAs, and MCNs. The histogenesis of these tumors is unknown; however, ultrastructural and immunohistochemical studies have suggested that they have both epithelial and neuroendocrine differentiation.[76]

Anatomy and Pathology

On pathology, necrotic debris, blood, and foamy macrophages can be seen in these cystic areas.[14,21] These tumors are usually large at presentation (>10 cm), can occur anywhere within the pancreas, and can have calcification.[77] SPTs are usually seen in young women in the second to

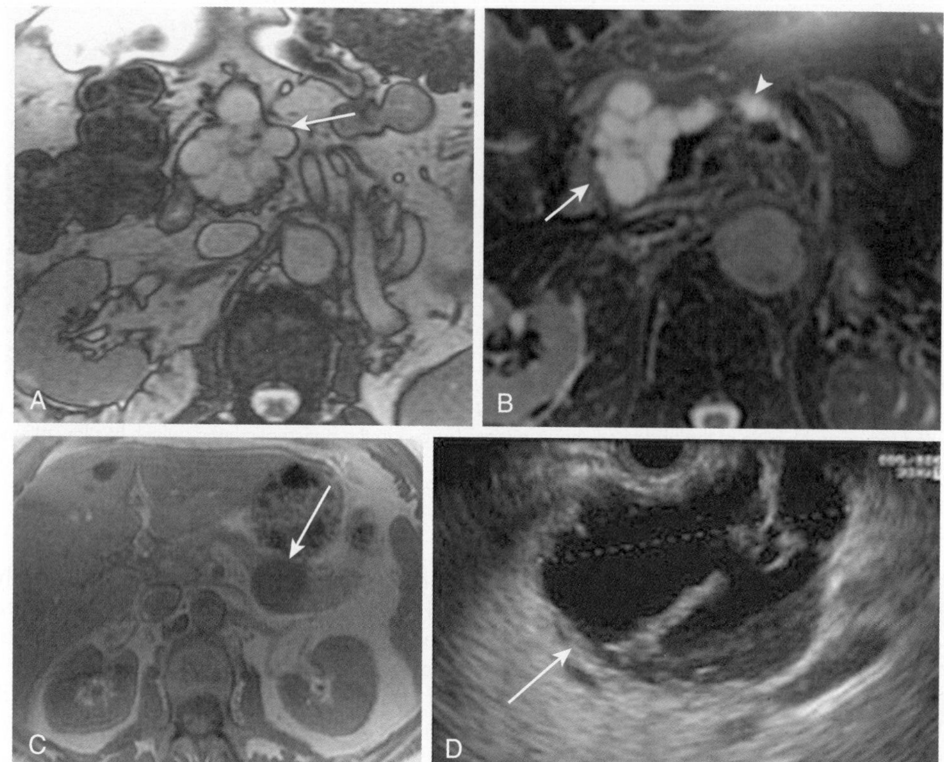

FIGURE 13.15. A 74-year-old man with a recent diagnosis of left renal mass and a pancreatic mass. **A**, Axial fast imaging employing steady state acquisition shows a high-signal intensity multicystic mass (*arrow*) in the pancreatic head, indicating a serous cystadenoma. **B**, Axial fat-saturated T2-weighted magnetic resonance imaging (MRI) shows a high-signal intensity multicystic mass (*arrow*) in the pancreatic head and pancreatic ductal dilatation (*arrowhead*), indicating a serous cystadenoma. **C**, Axial fat-saturated T1-weighted gradient MRI shows a low-signal intensity multicystic mass (*arrow*) in the pancreatic head, indicating a serous cystadenoma. **D**, Endoscopic ultrasound shows a hypoechoic multicystic mass (*arrow*) in the pancreatic head, indicating a serous cystadenoma.

third decade of life, with an age range of 7 to 79 years.[78,79] The tumors can have both epithelial and neuroendocrine components. The tumors occur exclusively in the pancreas. SPTs are tumors of low malignant potential. These tumors are predominantly solid, develop cystic spaces when they degenerate, and vary in both size and morphology.[80]

Clinical Presentation

Clinical manifestations include abdominal pain, sensation of plenitude or early satiety, abdominal mass, nausea, and vomiting.

Staging

SPTs are staged according to the AJCC staging system, similar to pancreatic ductal cancer.

Patterns of Tumor Spread

Metastatic disease is present in up to 15% of cases, us usually synchronous, and is confined to the liver or peritoneum. Lymphatic disease is not a feature.

Imaging

On CT (Fig. 13.16), SPTs appear as solid masses that enhance avidly on the arterial phase and plateau on the portal venous and delayed phases of contrast. They may have a central scar, may have eccentric calcifications, and may show hemorrhage. On T2W imaging, these tumors are well-circumscribed and have slightly high signal intensity. Tumors that are predominantly cystic will have a high T2 signal intensity similar to that of fluid. These tumors enhance progressively, which can help differentiate them from neuroendocrine neoplasms, which commonly have arterial phase enhancement. On noncontrast T1W imaging, hemorrhage within the tumor has high signal intensity. On US, they may show fluid-debris levels and posterior acoustic enhancement. Benign SPTs are smoothly lobulated and encapsulated; sometimes, they can be completely cystic and contain rim calcifications.[77] The features of malignancy include discontinuity of the capsule or eccentric lobulated margin, focal nodular calcification, and amorphous/scattered calcifications; upstream main pancreatic duct dilatation may be present.[77] Peritoneal, cutaneous, and hepatic metastases have all been reported after excision of SPT; however, nodal metastases appear to be rare.[80]

Treatment

Surgery is offered in these patients to prevent local tumor growth and distant metastases and to palliate symptoms. Although locoregional tumor extension and metastasis may be identified in up to 20% of patients, surgical resection can lead to favorable survival even in the face of advanced

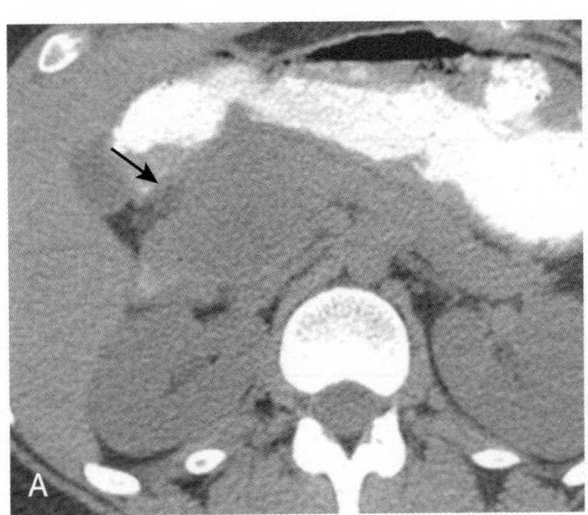

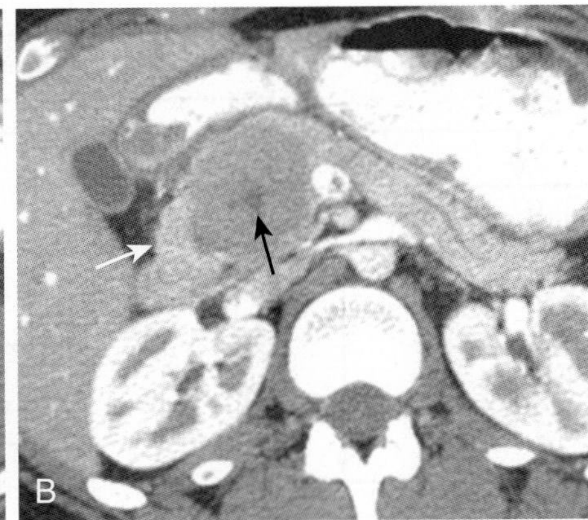

FIGURE 13.16. A 17-year-old girl with abdominal pain. **A**, Axial noncontrast computed tomography of the abdomen shows a soft tissue mass (*arrow*) in the pancreatic head with central necrosis. **B**, Axial contrast-enhanced computed tomography shows an enhancing mass (*white arrow*) with central necrosis (*black arrow*) in the pancreatic head abutting the superior mesenteric vein, indicating a solid papillary neoplasm. Given the patient's age and sex, a diagnosis of solid papillary neoplasm was suggested.

disease. Pancreaticoduodenectomy or distal pancreatectomy are usually required to achieve a complete *en bloc* resection, owing to the large size of these tumors. Enucleation and central pancreatectomy may be possible in some cases, because lymph node metastases are rare, making formal lymphadenectomy relatively unimportant.[81] Overall, aggressive surgical resection is associated with a 5-year survival rate exceeding 95%.[82]

Surveillance

Postoperative follow-up need not to be aggressive in patients with this low-grade malignancy. Annual examination with cross-sectional imaging is used in our practice.

KEY POINTS Solid Pseudopapillary Tumor

- Solid tumors with central necrosis.
- Usually seen in young females.
- Potential for malignancy.

GUIDELINES FOR IMAGING SURVEILLANCE

A 2013 study published by the National Cancer Institute reported an overall pancreatic cyst prevalence of 2.5% in the United States in individuals between 40 and 84 years old.[83] In another study, the prevalence of pancreatic cysts identified incidentally during EUS was reported to be as high as 21.5%.[84] There is increased prevalence of pancreatic cystic neoplasms in patients with a family history or genetic predisposition to pancreatic cancer[85]; however, an increased risk of malignancy in cystic lesions in these populations has not been proven. The rate of progression of IPMN to pancreatic cancer in a study of 300 patients with IPMN and a first-degree relative with pancreatic cancer was similar to that of patients without a family history of pancreatic cancer.[86] In this study, the rate of malignant transformation of IPMNs of 3 cm or more was significantly higher than that of IPMNs less than 3 cm in size.[86] Recently, the American College of Radiology published a white paper providing guidelines and recommendations for follow-up and management of cystic pancreatic lesions (Figs. 13.17, 13.18, 13.19, and 13.20).[87] The new recommendation for most patients is 9- to 10-year follow-up until the age of 80 years. For patients older than 80 years at the time of initial diagnosis, a different follow-up is recommended (Fig. 13.21, p. 18)[87]. The new guidelines also recommend reporting some elements, including cyst morphology, location, and size, the presence of communication with the main pancreatic duct, the presence of worrisome features, interval growth, and multiplicity. All incidental cysts should be presumed mucinous unless there are features of a different etiology. Comparison with prior imaging exams is important to document stability and the lack of development of worrisome features. The guidelines also recommend using a multidisciplinary approach and engaging in team-based decision-making in the follow-up and management of cystic pancreatic lesions.

KEY POINTS Follow-Up

- Cysts should be followed up for 9 to 10 years until the patient is 80 years old.
- For patients older than 80 years at the time of diagnosis, the follow-up recommendation is different.
- The new follow-up recommendation is based on cyst morphology, location, and size, possible communication with main pancreatic duct, the presence of worrisome features, growth, and multiplicity.
- Cysts should be considered mucinous unless proven otherwise.

SUMMARY

When a cystic lesion of the pancreas is discovered incidentally on imaging, correlation with clinical history is important, as a prior history of acute pancreatitis may suggest a pseudocyst. If the cystic lesion communicates with the

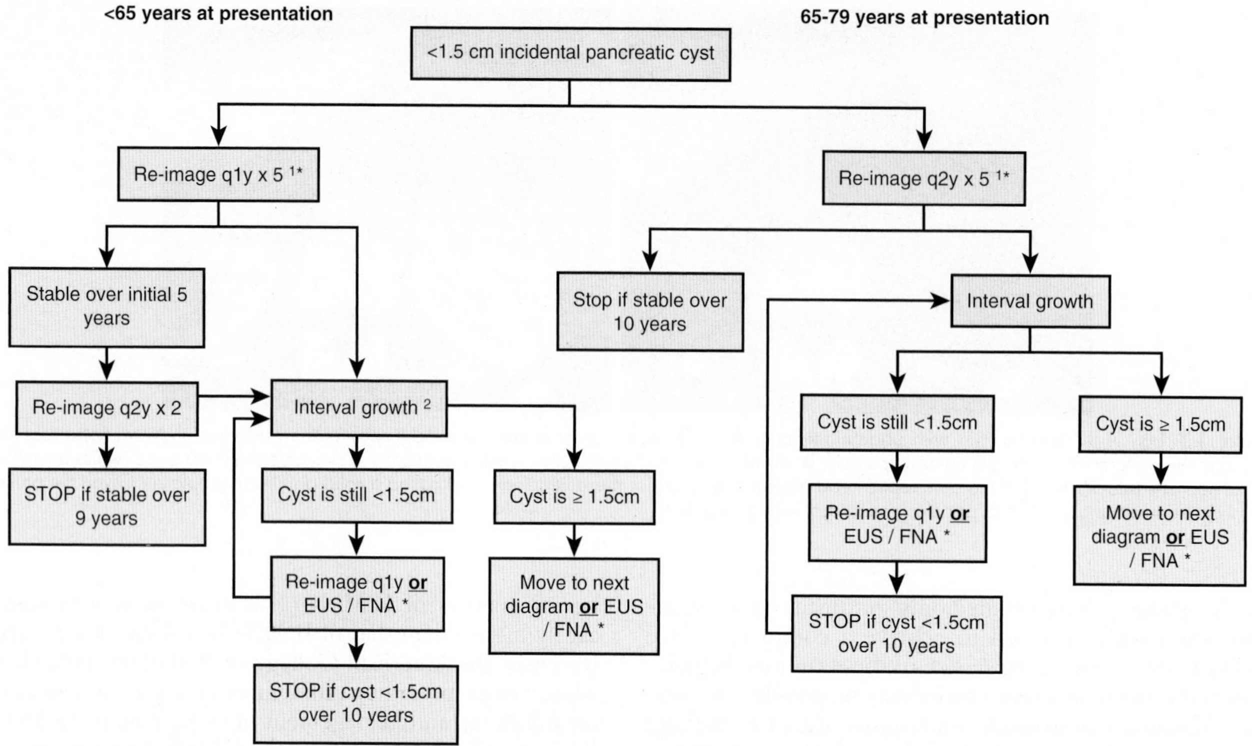

FIGURE 13.17. Management of incidental pancreatic cysts under 1.5 cm. *EUS, FNA* Megibow AJ, et al. Management of incidental pancreatic cysts: a white paper of the ACR incidental findings committee. *J Am Coll Radiol.* 2017;14(7):911-923.

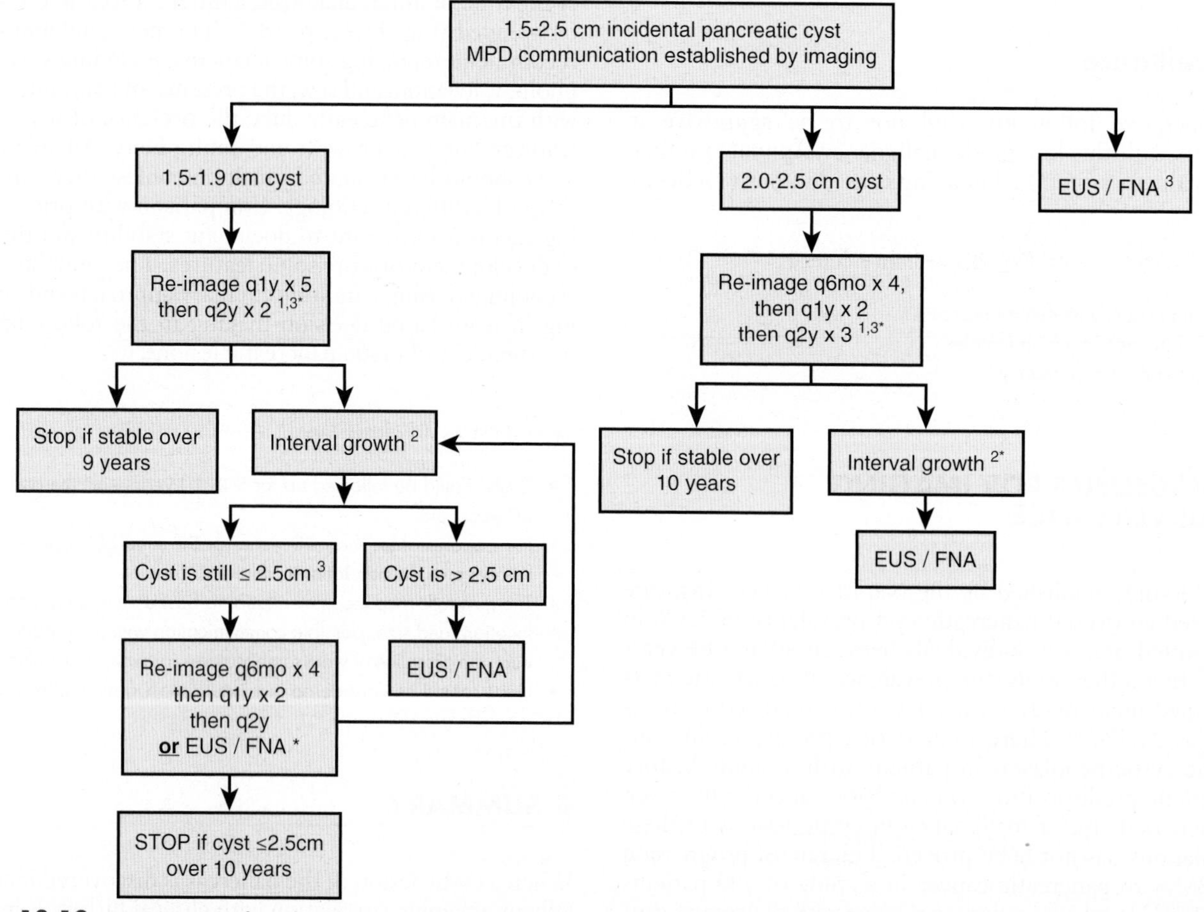

FIGURE 13.18. Management of incidental pancreatic cysts 1.5-2.5 cm when main pancreatic duct communication can be established. *EUS, FNA, MPD* Megibow AJ, et al. Management of incidental pancreatic cysts: a white paper of the ACR incidental findings committee. *J Am Coll Radiol.* 2017;14(7):911-923.

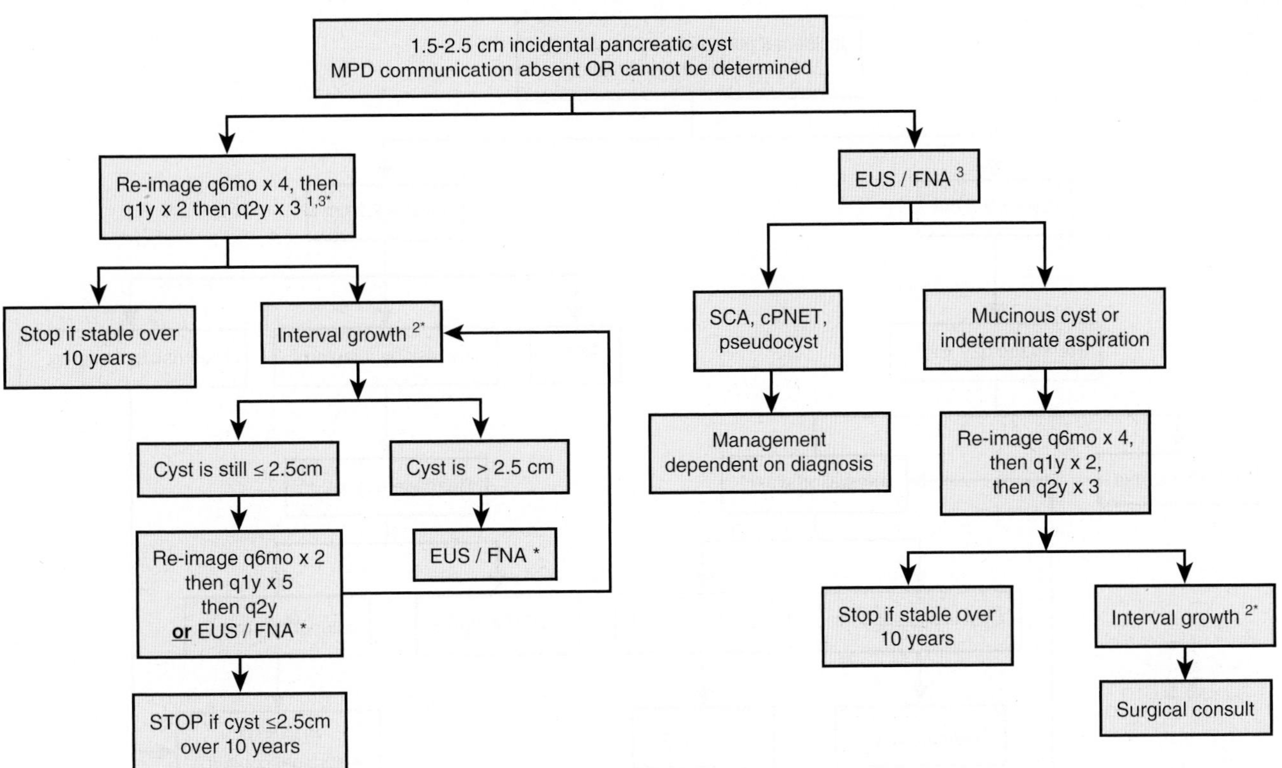

FIGURE 13.19. Management of incidental pancreatic cysts 1.5 to 2.5 cm when main pancreatic duct communication is absent or cannot be established. *EUS, FNA, cPNET, MPD* Megibow AJ, et al. Management of incidental pancreatic cysts: a white paper of the ACR incidental findings committee. *J Am Coll Radiol.* 2017;14(7):911-923.

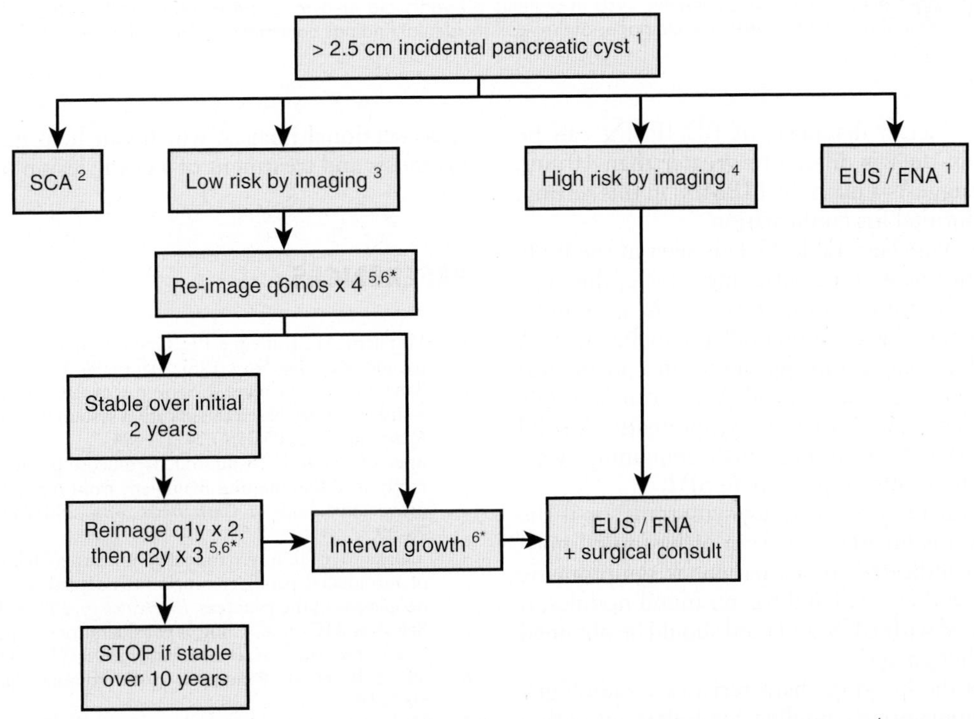

FIGURE 13.20. Management of incidental pancreatic cysts > 2.5 cm when main pancreatic duct communication is absent or cannot be established. *EUS, FNA, SCA* Megibow AJ, et al. Management of incidental pancreatic cysts: a white paper of the ACR incidental findings committee. *J Am Coll Radiol.* 2017;14(7):911-923.

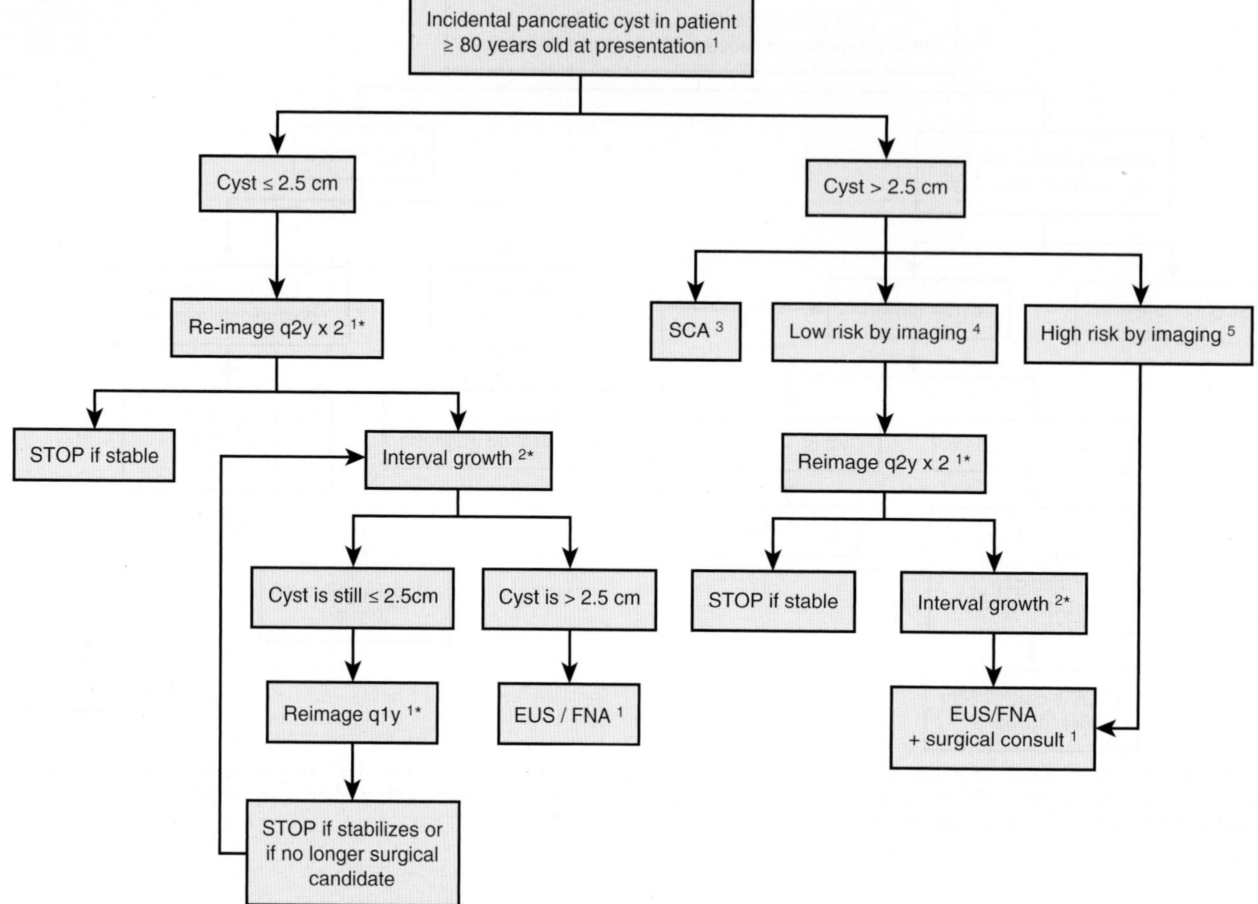

FIGURE 13.21. Management of incidental pancreatic cysts in patients 80 years old or over at presentation. *EUS, FNA, SCA.* Megibow AJ, et al. Management of incidental pancreatic cysts: a white paper of the ACR incidental findings committee. *J Am Coll Radiol.* 2017;14(7):911-923.

main pancreatic duct, a diagnosis of BD-IPMN can be made. If the main duct is dilated to greater than 10 mm, this most likely suggests a main duct IPMN; in this setting, EUS can be performed for confirmation.

When a cystic mass (see Table 13.1) is seen in the body or tail of the pancreas in a menstruating female, this suggests an MCN; in these cases, resection is warranted, because these lesions have a potential for malignancy. A cystic lesion with a honeycomb appearance in a postmenopausal female likely represents an SCA and can be safely followed if it is less than 4 cm and asymptomatic. A solid mass within the pancreas in young female containing cystic and solid components may represent an SPT.

If an indeterminate cyst is causing symptoms, or if the asymptomatic cyst is greater than 3 cm or has mural nodules, resection is indicated. If the patient is symptomatic and the cyst is less than 3 cm and has no mural nodules, it should be evaluated with EUS, and fluid should be obtained by FNA for further analysis.

Depending on the imaging characteristics, a radiologist can suggest an appropriate timeline for follow-up with a modality such as MRI, which will provide the most information about the cystic lesion without exposing the patient to radiation.

In conclusion, radiologists should take into account the patient's presentation, age, and sex when interpreting cross-sectional images, which can help guide appropriate diagnosis and treatment of a cystic lesion of the pancreas.

REFERENCES

1. Warshaw AL, Rutledge PL. Cystic tumors mistaken for pancreatic pseudocysts. *Ann Surg*. 1987;205(4):393-398.
2. Sahani DV, Kadavigere R, Saokar A, et al. Cystic pancreatic lesions: a simple imaging-based classification system for guiding management. *Radiographics*. 2005;25(6):1471-1484.
3. Sperti C, et al. F-18-fluorodeoxyglucose positron emission tomography in differentiating malignant from benign pancreatic cysts: a prospective study. *J Gastrointest Surg*. 2005;9(1):22-28. discussion 28-29.
4. Tanaka M, et al. International consensus guidelines for management of intraductal papillary mucinous neoplasms and mucinous cystic neoplasms of the pancreas. *Pancreatology*. 2006;6(1-2):17-32.
5. Safioleas MC, et al. Clinical considerations of primary hydatid disease of the pancreas. *Pancreatology*. 2005;5(4-5):457-461.
6. Salvia R, et al. Pancreatic cystic tumors. *Minerva Chir*. 2004;59(2):185-207.
7. Singhal D, et al. Issues in management of pancreatic pseudocysts. *JOP*. 2006;7(5):502-507.
8. Baron TH, Morgan DE. The diagnosis and management of fluid collections associated with pancreatitis. *Am J Med*. 1997;102(6):555-563.
9. Tanaka A, et al. Severe complications of mediastinal pancreatic pseudocyst: report of esophagobronchial fistula and hemothorax. *J Hepatobiliary Pancreat Surg*. 2000;7(1):86-91.

10. Boulanger S, et al. Pancreatic pseudocyst with biliary fistula: treatment with endoscopic internal drainage. *South Med J.* 2001;94(3):347-349.
11. Goh BK, Tan YM, Chung YF, Chow PK, Cheow PC, Wong WK, et al. A review of mucinous cystic neoplasms of the pancreas defined by ovarian-type stroma: clinicopathological features of 344 patients. *World J of Surg. 2006*; Dec;30(12):2236–2245.
12. Flati G, et al. Severe hemorrhagic complications in pancreatitis. *Ann Ital Chir*. 1995;66(2):233-237.
13. Grace PA, Williamson RC. Modern management of pancreatic pseudocysts. *Br J Surg*. 1993;80(5):573-581.
14. Kim YH, et al. Imaging diagnosis of cystic pancreatic lesions: pseudocyst versus nonpseudocyst. *Radiographics*. 2005;25(3):671-685.
15. Katz DS, et al. Relative accuracy of CT and MRI for characterization of cystic pancreatic masses. *AJR Am J Roentgenol.* 2007;189(3):657-661.
16. Leung RS, et al. Imaging features of von Hippel-Lindau disease. *Radiographics*. 2008;28(1):65-79. quiz 323.
17. Kosmahl M, et al. Mucinous nonneoplastic cyst of the pancreas: a novel nonneoplastic cystic change? *Mod Pathol*. 2002;15(2):154-158.
18. Hruban RH, et al. In: Hahn KS, ed. *AFIP Atlas of tumor pathology, series 4*. Washington, DC: American Registry of Pathology; 2007:358-360.
19. Goh BK, et al. A review of mucinous cystic neoplasms of the pancreas defined by ovarian-type stroma: clinicopathological features of 344 patients. *World J Surg*. 2006;30(12):2236-2245.
20. Crippa S, et al. Mucinous cystic neoplasm of the pancreas is not an aggressive entity: lessons from 163 resected patients. *Ann Surg*. 2008;247(4):571-579.
21. Adsay NV. Cystic neoplasia of the pancreas: pathology and biology. *J Gastrointest Surg*. 2008;12(3):401-404.
22. Campbell F, Azadeh B. Cystic neoplasms of the exocrine pancreas. *Histopathology*. 2008;52(5):539-551.
23. Goh BK, et al. Pancreatic serous oligocystic adenomas: clinicopathologic features and a comparison with serous microcystic adenomas and mucinous cystic neoplasms. *World J Surg*. 2006;30(8):1553-1559.
24. Park JW, et al. Mucinous cystic neoplasm of the pancreas: is surgical resection recommended for all surgically fit patients? *Pancreatology*. 2014;14(2):131-136.
25. Yamao K, et al. Clinicopathological features and prognosis of mucinous cystic neoplasm with ovarian-type stroma: a multi-institutional study of the Japan pancreas society. *Pancreas*. 2011;40(1):67-71.
26. Nishihara K, et al. The differential diagnosis of pancreatic cysts by MR imaging. *Hepatogastroenterology*. 1996;43(9):714-720.
27. Singh M, Maitra A. Precursor lesions of pancreatic cancer: molecular pathology and clinical implications. *Pancreatology*. 2007;7(1):9-19.
28. Doberstein C, et al. Cystic neoplasms of the pancreas. *Mt Sinai J Med*. 1990;57(2):102-105.
29. Wood D, et al. Cystadenocarcinoma of the pancreas: neo-adjuvant therapy and CEA monitoring. *J Surg Oncol*. 1990;43(1):56-60.
30. Mizuta Y, et al. Pseudomyxoma peritonei accompanied by intraductal papillary mucinous neoplasm of the pancreas. *Pancreatology*. 2005;5(4-5):470-474.
31. Shimada K, et al. A case of advanced mucinous cystadenocarcinoma of the pancreas with peritoneal dissemination responding to gemcitabine. *Gan To Kagaku Ryoho*. 2009;36(6):995-998.
32. Evans DB, et al. Preoperative gemcitabine-based chemoradiation for patients with resectable adenocarcinoma of the pancreatic head. *J Clin Oncol*. 2008;26(21):3496-3502.
33. Terris B, et al. Intraductal papillary mucinous tumors of the pancreas confined to secondary ducts show less aggressive pathologic features as compared with those involving the main pancreatic duct. *Am J Surg Pathol*. 2000;24(10):1372-1377.
34. D'Angelica M, et al. Intraductal papillary mucinous neoplasms of the pancreas: an analysis of clinicopathologic features and outcome. *Ann Surg*. 2004;239(3):400-408.
35. Stark A, et al. Pancreatic Cyst Disease: A Review. *JAMA*. 2016;315(17):1882-1893.
36. Pelaez-Luna M, et al. Do consensus indications for resection in branch duct intraductal papillary mucinous neoplasm predict malignancy? A study of 147 patients. *Am J Gastroenterol*. 2007;102(8):1759-1764.
37. Lack E. *Pathology of the pancreas, gallbladder, extrahepatic biliary tract and ampullary region*. New York, NY: Oxford University Press; 2003.
38. Salvia R, et al. Branch-duct intraductal papillary mucinous neoplasms of the pancreas: to operate or not to operate? *Gut*. 2007;56(8):1086-1090.
39. Takasu N, et al. Intraductal papillary-mucinous neoplasms of the gastric and intestinal types may have less malignant potential than the pancreatobiliary type. *Pancreas*. 2010;39(5):604-610.
40. Shima Y, et al. Diagnosis and management of cystic pancreatic tumours with mucin production. *Br J Surg*. 2000;87(8):1041-1047.
41. Yamaguchi K, et al. Mucin-hypersecreting tumors of the pancreas: assessing the grade of malignancy preoperatively. *Am J Surg*. 1996;171(4):427-431.
42. Traverso LW, et al. Intraductal neoplasms of the pancreas. *Am J Surg*. 1998;175(5):426-432.
43. Balzano G, Zerbi A, Di Carlo V. Intraductal papillary mucinous tumors of the pancreas: incidence, clinical findings and natural history. *JOP*. 2005;6(1 Suppl):108-111.
44. Sohn TA, et al. Intraductal papillary mucinous neoplasms of the pancreas: an updated experience. *Ann Surg*. 2004;239(6):788-797. discussion 797-799.
45. Salvia R, et al. Main-duct intraductal papillary mucinous neoplasms of the pancreas: clinical predictors of malignancy and long-term survival following resection. *Ann Surg*. 2004;239(5):678-685. discussion 685-687.
46. Rodriguez JR, et al. Branch-duct intraductal papillary mucinous neoplasms: observations in 145 patients who underwent resection. *Gastroenterology*. 2007;133(1):72-79. quiz 309-310.
47. Song SJ, et al. Differentiation of intraductal papillary mucinous neoplasms from other pancreatic cystic masses: comparison of multirow-detector CT and MR imaging using ROC analysis. *J Magn Reson Imaging*. 2007;26(1):86-93.
48. Waters JA, et al. CT vs MRCP: optimal classification of IPMN type and extent. *J Gastrointest Surg*. 2008;12(1):101-109.
49. Zhang XM, et al. Suspected early or mild chronic pancreatitis: enhancement patterns on gadolinium chelate dynamic MRI. Magnetic resonance imaging. *J Magn Reson Imaging*. 2003;17(1):86-94.
50. Manfredi R, et al. Main pancreatic duct intraductal papillary mucinous neoplasms: accuracy of MR imaging in differentiation between benign and malignant tumors compared with histopathologic analysis. *Radiology*. 2009;253(1):106-115.
51. Tanaka M. Intraductal papillary mucinous neoplasm of the pancreas: diagnosis and treatment. *Pancreas*. 2004;28(3):282-288.
52. Procacci C, et al. Intraductal papillary mucinous tumor of the pancreas: a pictorial essay. *Radiographics*. 1999;19(6):1447-1463.
53. Matsumoto T, et al. Optimal management of the branch duct type intraductal papillary mucinous neoplasms of the pancreas. *J Clin Gastroenterol*. 2003;36(3):261-265.
54. Sugiyama M, et al. Endoscopic pancreatic stent insertion for treatment of pseudocyst after distal pancreatectomy. *Gastrointest Endosc*. 2001;53(4):538-539.
55. Irie H, et al. MR cholangiopancreatographic differentiation of benign and malignant intraductal mucin-producing tumors of the pancreas. *AJR Am J Roentgenol*. 2000;174(5):1403-1408.
56. Lewandrowski KB, et al. Cyst fluid analysis in the differential diagnosis of pancreatic cysts. A comparison of pseudocysts, serous cystadenomas, mucinous cystic neoplasms, and mucinous cystadenocarcinoma. *Ann Surg*. 1993;217(1):41-47.
57. Ryu JK, et al. Cyst fluid analysis for the differential diagnosis of pancreatic cysts. *Diagn Cytopathol*. 2004;31(2):100-105.
58. van der Waaij LA, van Dullemen HM, Porte RJ. Cyst fluid analysis in the differential diagnosis of pancreatic cystic lesions: a pooled analysis. *Gastrointest Endosc*. 2005;62(3):383-389.
59. Song MH, et al. EUS in the evaluation of pancreatic cystic lesions. *Gastrointest Endosc*. 2003;57(7):891-896.
60. Brugge WR, et al. Diagnosis of pancreatic cystic neoplasms: a report of the cooperative pancreatic cyst study. *Gastroenterology*. 2004;126(5):1330-1336.
61. Serikawa M, et al. Management of intraductal papillary-mucinous neoplasm of the pancreas: treatment strategy based on morphologic classification. *J Clin Gastroenterol*. 2006;40(9):856-862.
62. Sugiyama M, et al. Predictive factors for malignancy in intraductal papillary-mucinous tumours of the pancreas. *Br J Surg*. 2003;90(10):1244-1249.
63. Chu QD, et al. Should adjuvant therapy remain the standard of care for patients with resected adenocarcinoma of the pancreas? *Ann Surg Oncol*. 2003;10(5):539-545.
64. Neoptolemos JP, et al. Adjuvant chemoradiotherapy and chemotherapy in resectable pancreatic cancer: a randomised controlled trial. *Lancet*. 2001;358(9293):1576-1585.

65. Burris 3rd HA, et al. Improvements in survival and clinical benefit with gemcitabine as first-line therapy for patients with advanced pancreas cancer: a randomized trial. *J Clin Oncol*. 1997;15(6):2403-2413.
66. Moore MJ, et al. Erlotinib plus gemcitabine compared with gemcitabine alone in patients with advanced pancreatic cancer: a phase III trial of the National Cancer Institute of Canada Clinical Trials Group. *J Clin Oncol*. 2007;25(15):1960-1966.
67. Swartz MJ, et al. Adjuvant chemoradiotherapy after pancreatic resection for invasive carcinoma associated with intraductal papillary mucinous neoplasm of the pancreas. *Int J Radiat Oncol Biol Phys*. 2010;76(3):839-844.
68. Raut CP, et al. Intraductal papillary mucinous neoplasms of the pancreas: effect of invasion and pancreatic margin status on recurrence and survival. *Ann Surg Oncol*. 2006;13(4):582-594.
69. Wargo JA, Fernandez-del-Castillo C, Warshaw AL. Management of pancreatic serous cystadenomas. *Adv Surg*. 2009;43:23-34.
70. Mohr VH, et al. Histopathology and molecular genetics of multiple cysts and microcystic (serous) adenomas of the pancreas in von Hippel-Lindau patients. *Am J Pathol*. 2000;157(5):1615-1621.
71. Strobel O, et al. Risk of malignancy in serous cystic neoplasms of the pancreas. *Digestion*. 2003;68(1):24-33.
72. Martin DR, Semelka RC. MR imaging of pancreatic masses. *Magn Reson Imaging Clin N Am*. 2000;8(4):787-812.
73. Tseng JF. Management of serous cystadenoma of the pancreas. *J Gastrointest Surg*. 2008;12(3):408-410.
74. Bassi C, et al. Management of 100 consecutive cases of pancreatic serous cystadenoma: wait for symptoms and see at imaging or vice versa? *World J Surg*. 2003;27(3):319-323.
75. Pyke CM, et al. The spectrum of serous cystadenoma of the pancreas. Clinical, pathologic, and surgical aspects. *Ann Surg*. 1992;215(2):132-139.
76. Adams AL, Siegal GP, Jhala NC. Solid pseudopapillary tumor of the pancreas: a review of salient clinical and pathologic features. *Adv Anat Pathol*. 2008;15(1):39-45.
77. Chung YE, et al. Differentiation of benign and malignant solid pseudopapillary neoplasms of the pancreas. *J Comput Assist Tomogr*. 2009;33(5):689-694.
78. Faraj W, et al. Solid pseudopapillary neoplasm of the pancreas in a 12-year-old female: case report and review of the literature. *Eur J Pediatr Surg*. 2006;16(5):358-361.
79. Choi SH, et al. Solid pseudopapillary tumor of the pancreas: a multicenter study of 23 pediatric cases. *J Pediatr Surg*. 2006;41(12):1992-1995.
80. Tipton SG, et al. Malignant potential of solid pseudopapillary neoplasm of the pancreas. *Br J Surg*. 2006;93(6):733-737.
81. Goh BK, et al. Solid pseudopapillary neoplasms of the pancreas: an updated experience. *J Surg Oncol*. 2007;95(8):640-644.
82. Papavramidis T, Papavramidis S. Solid pseudopapillary tumors of the pancreas: review of 718 patients reported in English literature. *J Am Coll Surg*. 2005;200(6):965-972.
83. Gardner TB, et al. Pancreatic cyst prevalence and the risk of mucin-producing adenocarcinoma in US adults. *Am J Gastroenterol*. 2013;108(10):1546-1550.
84. Martinez B, Martinez JF, Aparicio JR. Prevalence of incidental pancreatic cyst on upper endoscopic ultrasound. *Ann Gastroenterol*. 2018;31(1):90-95.
85. Canto MI, et al. Frequent detection of pancreatic lesions in asymptomatic high-risk individuals. *Gastroenterology*. 2012;142(4):796-804. quiz e14-15.
86. Mandai K, Uno K, Yasuda K. Does a family history of pancreatic ductal adenocarcinoma and cyst size influence the follow-up strategy for intraductal papillary mucinous neoplasms of the pancreas? *Pancreas*. 2014;43(6):917-921.
87. Megibow AJ, et al. Management of incidental pancreatic cysts: a white paper of the acr incidental findings committee. *J Am Coll Radiol*. 2017;14(7):911-923.

CHAPTER 14

Pancreatic Neuroendocrine Tumors

Leonardo P. Marcal, M.D.; Hubert H. Chuang, M.D., Ph.D.; Hop S. Tran Cao, M.D.; and Daniel M. Halperin, M.D.

INTRODUCTION

Pancreatic neuroendocrine tumors (PNETs) are a heterogeneous subgroup of gastroenteropancreatic neuroendocrine tumors (NETs). The term neuroendocrine is derived from the similarity to neural cells in the expression of proteins such as synaptophysin, neuron-specific enolase, and chromogranin A.[1] PNETs are thought to arise from a common precursor neuroendocrine cell that shares features with similar cells throughout the body that constitute the "neuroendocrine system." The embryologic origin of this common precursor cell is controversial. Masson and coworkers suggested that the neuroendocrine cell was an endocrine cell derived from the gastrointestinal epithelium, suggesting an endodermal origin.[2] However, in 1968, Pearse showed that all neuroendocrine cells throughout the body share various features, including amine precursor uptake and decarboxylation (APUD) capacity, and postulated that the neural crest was the common origin for these cells, called the APUD cells.[3] These cells have pluripotential capabilities, including differentiation into various types of NETs.[4] More recently, an endodermal origin for these pluripotent cells has been favored.[5]

The World Health Organization (WHO) categorizes PNETS based on cell morphology into two groups: well-differentiated PNETs and poorly-differentiated neuroendocrine carcinomas (NECs). As a general rule, well-differentiated PNETs tend to have an indolent course, while poorly-differentiated NECs exhibit aggressive behavior and have a poor prognosis. However, some well-differentiated PNETS have a mitotic count and Ki-67 labeling in the high-grade range (G3), and, despite being more aggressive than low-grade PNETs (G1), their prognosis is better than that of poorly-differentiated carcinomas. This important distinction in biologic behavior is addressed in the current WHO classification.[6–9]

PNETs have the ability to induce clinical syndromes secondary to their secretion of functional hormones. The tumors can therefore be divided into functional and nonfunctional tumors based on whether they are associated with such clinical syndromes. This chapter discusses PNETs such as insulinomas, gastrinomas, vasoactive intestinal polypeptidomas (VIPomas), glucagonomas, and nonfunctional PNETs.

EPIDEMIOLOGY AND RISK FACTORS

According to large, comprehensive, population-based studies analyzing data from the National Cancer Institute's Surveillance, Epidemiology, and End Results (SEER) Program, the incidence and prevalence of NETs in the United States has been steadily rising since 1973. This increase was observed across all tumor sites, grades, and stages. The annual incidence of PNETs is reported to be only between 2.5 and 5 per 100,000 per year. Despite the increase in incidence, they still account for only 2% of all pancreatic neoplasms, and although they may occur at any age, they are more common after the fourth decade of life.[10,11]

Four syndromes have been associated with a higher incidence of PNETs: multiple endocrine neoplasia type I (MEN I or Wermer syndrome); von Hippel–Lindau (vHL) syndrome; neurofibromatosis-1 (NF-1 or von Recklinghausen syndrome), and tuberous sclerosis (TS).[12] The relative frequency with which patients with these disorders develop PNETs is MEN I > vHL > NF-1 > TS.

MEN I is a syndrome characterized by tumors/hyperplasia of endocrine glands. This is inherited as an autosomal dominant trait. MEN I gene mutations can be identified in 78% to 93% of MEN I patients.[13] MEN I patients usually have a family history of MEN I. The syndrome is characterized primarily by tumors of the parathyroid glands, endocrine components of the gastrointestinal and pancreatic systems, and the pituitary gland (Fig. 14.1). The different incidences of PNETs in patients with MEN I are nonfunctional tumors (80%–100%), gastrinomas (20%–61%), insulinomas (7%–31%), and other functional PNETs (<5%). With increasing control of symptoms of excess hormone production, PNETs have become an important factor in determining survival in patients with MEN I. Patients with MEN I syndrome have a higher incidence of premature death, and this is owing in part to the development of PNETs.[14,15] Thus, identifying and treating PNETs in this subgroup of patients may have a significant impact on survival.

vHL is a syndrome characterized by autosomal dominant inheritance. vHL patients develop hemangioblastomas of the central nervous system (prevalence 44%–72%), including retinal hemangioblastomas, cerebellar hemangioblastomas, renal cysts, and renal cell carcinomas (25%–60%), endolymphatic sac tumors (10%), and pheochromocytomas (10%–20%).[16] Pancreatic tumors or cysts develop in 35% to 70% of patients (Fig. 14.2). Pancreatic cysts or serous cystadenomas develop in 17% to 56% of patients, and PNETs occur in 8% to 17% of patients.[17] The majority of the PNETs are nonfunctional.

NF-1 is more common than MEN I and vHL syndromes. Duodenal somatostatinomas (0%–10%) and ampullary carcinoid tumors can occur in NF-1 patients. Pancreatic somatostatinomas (functional PNET) occur in

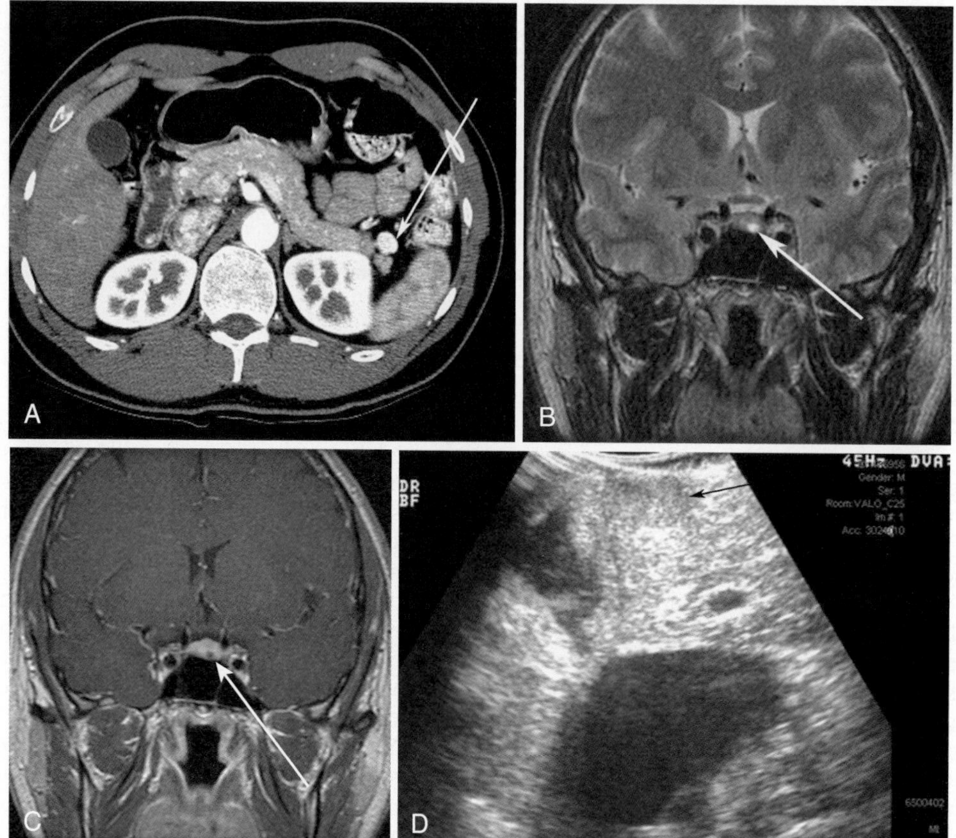

FIGURE 14.1. A 28-year-old patient with dizziness and confusion. **A**, Cross-sectional computed tomography scan during the arterial phase of imaging. The *arrow* shows a small hypervascular primary tumor in the pancreatic tail. This was staged as a T1 tumor. **B**, T2-weighted coronal magnetic resonance imaging (MRI) of the pituitary. The *arrow* points to a T2 hyperintense focus in the left pituitary. **C**, T1-weighted postcontrast coronal MRI of the pituitary. The *arrow* points to a nonenhancing focus in the left pituitary consistent with an adenoma. **D**, Intraoperative ultrasound of the pancreas. The *arrow* points to a slightly hypoechoic nodule consistent with an insulinoma. This patient had genetic testing confirming multiple endocrine neoplasia type 1 syndrome.

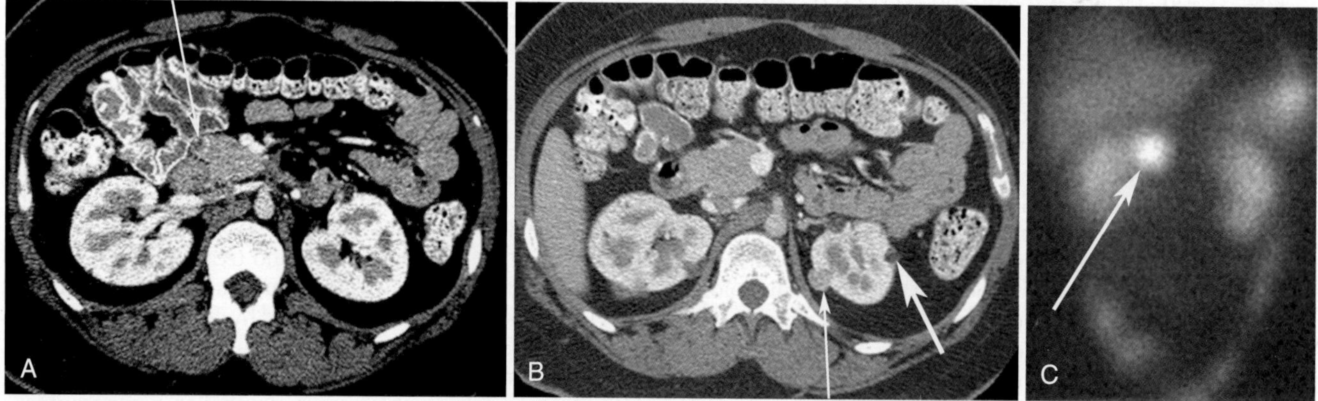

FIGURE 14.2. A 45-year-old woman with known tuberous sclerosis. **A**, Cross-sectional computed tomography scan during arterial phase of imaging. The *arrow* points to a subtle rim-enhancing lesion in the pancreatic head. **B**, Two renal lesions. The *thin arrow* points to a hypervascular nodule in the left upper kidney with a small component of fat inferiorly, and the *thick arrow* points to a predominantly fat-containing renal lesion in the left upper kidney. Both renal lesions were stable and presumed to represent angiomyolipoma. **C**, Coronal octreotide scan. The *arrow* points to increased activity corresponding to the primary pancreatic neuroendocrine tumor in the head of the pancreas.

patients with NF-1 at a much lower prevalence than do duodenal somatostatinomas.[18] Insulinomas and nonfunctional PNETs are less common but can also be present in patients with NF-1.[19]

TS also has autosomal dominant inheritance. Patients with TS have been reported to have both functional and nonfunctional PNETs (<1%), especially patients with the *TSC-2* gene mutation.[12]

ANATOMY

The pancreas is an elongated organ varying from 12.5 to 15 cm in length with a weight ranging from 60 to 100 g. It is composed of both exocrine portions and endocrine portions. Multiple fat lobulations are seen on the surface because of invaginating adipose tissue.[20,21] The portion of the pancreas located to the right side of the abdomen is recognized as the head and lies within the curve of the duodenum. A narrow neck, anterior to the superior mesenteric vein (SMV), connects the head to an elongated body that tapers in the left upper quadrant to form the tail. The pancreas is located in the retroperitoneum, except for a portion of the tail, which may be intraperitoneal along the gastrosplenic ligament.

The main pancreatic duct lies to the left of the common bile duct and opens into the medial aspect of the second portion of the duodenum. A smaller additional duct from the pancreatic duct in the neck of the pancreas, the accessory pancreatic duct, opens into the duodenum about 2.5 cm above the major papilla and receives ductules from the lower part of the head of the pancreas.

The arterial supply for the pancreas is from the pancreaticoduodenal arteries and the splenic artery. The celiac trunk gives rise to the common hepatic artery, the splenic artery, and the left gastric artery. The common hepatic artery gives off the gastroduodenal artery (GDA) and becomes the proper hepatic artery. The GDA divides into the superior pancreaticoduodenal arteries (anterior and posterior) and the right gastroepiploic artery. The anterior and posterior superior pancreaticoduodenal arteries supply the cranial aspect of the pancreas and descend between the duodenum and the pancreas, supplying both these organs. These arteries anastomose with the anterior and posterior inferior pancreaticoduodenal arteries and the pancreatic branches of the splenic artery. The anterior and posterior inferior pancreaticoduodenal arteries are branches of the inferior pancreaticoduodenal artery arising from the superior mesenteric artery (SMA). The splenic artery gives rise to numerous small branches that supply the body and tail of the pancreas. One branch, the pancreatica magna artery, runs along the body of the pancreas. The dorsal pancreatic artery is usually another branch of the splenic artery but can have a variable origin. It is usually located posterior to the portal venous confluence, passing behind the splenic vein.[22] This artery divides into two terminal bifurcating branches.

The venous drainage of the pancreas parallels the arterial supply. Four major pancreaticoduodenal veins drain the pancreas, in addition to multiple smaller pancreatic veins that drain the pancreas and enter the splenic vein directly.[23] The inferior pancreaticoduodenal veins drain the inferior portion of the pancreas and enter the first jejunal vein, which drains into the SMV. The posterior superior pancreaticoduodenal vein drains directly into the caudal portion of the portal vein. The anterior superior pancreaticoduodenal vein runs horizontally and drains into either the gastrocolic branch of the SMV or the right gastroepiploic vein, which drains into the SMV. The SMV and the splenic veins join posterior to the neck of the pancreas to form the portal vein. The inferior mesenteric vein enters at this confluence in one-third of patients, enters the splenic vein close to this confluence in one-third of patients, and enters the SMV in one-third of patients.

KEY POINTS

Anatomy

- Arterial supply for the pancreas is from the pancreaticoduodenal arteries and splenic artery.
- Venous drainage is from the pancreaticoduodenal veins and splenic vein.
- Pancreatic neuroendocrine tumors generally arise from the pancreas, peripancreatic area, and gastrinoma triangle.

TUMOR TYPES AND CLINICAL PRESENTATION

PNETs can be divided into the functional and nonfunctional, based on the presence or absence of a specific clinical syndrome. Given that PNETs can harbor or secrete granules of active or inert forms of hormones, clinical evidence of biochemical activity is required to diagnose a functional tumor, rather than pathological or biochemical evidence. The main functional PNETs include insulinomas, gastrinomas, glucagonomas, somatostatinomas, and VIPomas.[1] The majority (~70%) of PNETS are nonfunctional. Nonfunctional PNETs, although capable of secreting a number of substances, including pancreatic polypeptide, chromogranins, ghrelin, and neuron-specific enolase, do not produce a clinical hormonal syndrome. For this reason, they tend to be clinically silent as they grow and present later along the course of the disease, or may be found incidentally on imaging.

KEY POINTS

Tumor Types

Functional pancreatic neuroendocrine tumors

- Insulinoma
- Gastrinoma
- Vasoactive intestinal polypeptidoma
- Glucagonoma
- Somatostatinoma

Nonfunctional pancreatic neuroendocrine tumors

PATHOLOGY

PNETs are typically well-circumscribed, solitary masses within the pancreas.[24] They can vary in size from less than 1 cm to large tumors greater than 15 cm. They can be white to yellow or pink-brown in color. To definitively diagnose the neuroendocrine features of the specimen, immunostaining for synaptophysin and chromogranin A should be performed. Synaptophysin is a membrane protein present on the surface of small, clear vesicles (within the cytoplasm) that occur in all neuroendocrine cells. Chromogranin A is a protein located within large secretory granules, and the expression of this protein can be variable depending on the differentiation of the tumor.

The first classification of PNETs based on criteria with prognostic significance appeared in 1995, and included degree of histological differentiation, size, functional status (presence or absence of hormonal clinical syndrome), and presence of metastatic spread, among other criteria. The 2000, 2004, and 2010 WHO classifications largely followed this paradigm, emphasizing proliferative activity as the best criterion to assess tumor growth.[6,8,9] The 2010 WHO classification adopted the European Society of Neuroendocrine Tumors (ENETS) grading system, utilizing defined Ki-67 labeling cutoffs for prognostic stratification into three separate tiers. Ki-67 grading was shown to be a strong predictor of survival in subsequent years and has been validated in several large studies.[25–27]

The 2017 WHO classification has refined the previous versions and divides PNETs into two separate groups: well-differentiated PNETs and poorly-differentiated NECs. The well-differentiated tumors are further subdivided into low-grade (G1) PNETs (<2 mitoses/10 high-power fields [HPF] or Ki-67 <2%), intermediate-grade (2–20 mitoses/10 HPF or Ki-67 2%–20%), and high-grade (>20 mitoses/10 HPF or >20% Ki-67). The main change to the 2017 WHO classification was the addition of the G3 high-grade PNET category to recognize the fact that, even though some well-differentiated tumors have mitotic rate and Ki-67 labeling in the high histologic grade range, their prognosis is different from that of poorly-differentiated NECs, which are defined by their histology.[9,27]

Key Points

Pathology

Pancreatic neuroendocrine tumors are divided in two groups:

- Well-differentiated tumors (neuroendocrine tumors [NETs])
- Poorly-differentiated carcinomas

Well-differentiated NETs are further subdivided into three groups:

- Low-grade (G1) NETs
- Intermediate-grade (G2) NETs
- High-grade (G3) NETs

Well-differentiated tumors are characterized by monomorphic tumor cells with abundant cytoplasm and low mitotic index. They tend to have a well-developed stroma with well-formed blood vessels and may exhibit a trabecular, glandular, or acinar pattern. Poorly differentiated carcinomas are characterized by a solid appearance with large areas of necrosis, and round, small tumor cells with a high mitotic index and cellular atypia.[25]

STAGING

The staging systems for PNETs have been evolving alongside progress in scientific knowledge and better understanding of tumor biology, behavior, and prognostic factors. The most commonly used staging systems in the management of PNETs are the ENETS the American Joint Committee on Cancer (AJCC) staging systems.[28] Based on analysis of the ENETS and AJCC staging systems using the SEER registry (*n*=2529 patients) and validated by a large multicentric series (*n*=1,143 patients), a modified ENETS system was proposed, and was found to be more suitable for PNETs than either of the previous AJCC or ENETS versions.[28] The modified ENETS system maintained the original ENETS tumor, node, and metastasis (TNM) definitions and adopted the AJCC staging definitions.

The recently revised 8th edition of the AJCC staging system organizes the anatomic extent of disease and provides information on prognosis and treatment strategies. It has incorporated the classification criteria asserted by ENETs and applies to well-differentiated PNETs (ENETS/WHO grades 1, 2, and 3), excluding poorly-differentiated NECs.[29] One of the most important goals of the initial staging evaluation is to accurately distinguish between resectable and nonresectable disease, as this distinction determines the potential for cure. It is important to note that resectability criteria are based on data from pancreatic adenocarcinoma and extrapolated to PNETs. Important aspects of the TNM staging system are summarized in Fig. 14.3.

Key Points

Staging

- The most widely accepted stating systems are the modified European Society of Neuroendocrine Tumors system and the American Joint Committee on Cancer system (8th edition).
- T stage is based on size (2 cm, 2–4 cm, >4 cm), involvement of adjacent organs (duodenum, bile duct), and vascular involvement (portal vein/superior mesenteric vein, celiac axis, superior mesenteric artery).
- N stage is based involvement of regional lymph nodes (0, 1–3, >4 regional lymph nodes).
- M stage is based on the presence or absence of metastases.
- To distinguish between resectable and nonresectable disease is the main goal of the initial staging evaluation.

IMAGING

There is great variability in the size, morphology, and imaging appearances of PNETs, ranging from small homogenously hypervascular nodules to large heterogeneous solid masses with central necrosis and calcifications, and cystic lesions with varying degrees of solid and cystic components.[30,31] Imaging plays a significant role in the multidisciplinary care of PNETs, providing critical information from the initial diagnosis, staging, and delineation of disease extent and patterns of spread to treatment selection, monitoring response to treatment, and surveillance. It is comprised of anatomic cross-sectional imaging with ultrasound (US), endoscopic US (EUS), multidetector computed tomography (MDCT), magnetic resonance imaging (MRI), and functional imaging.

Anatomic Imaging

Ultrasound

Transabdominal US is a noninvasive, relatively inexpensive, and widely available modality that could be used in the

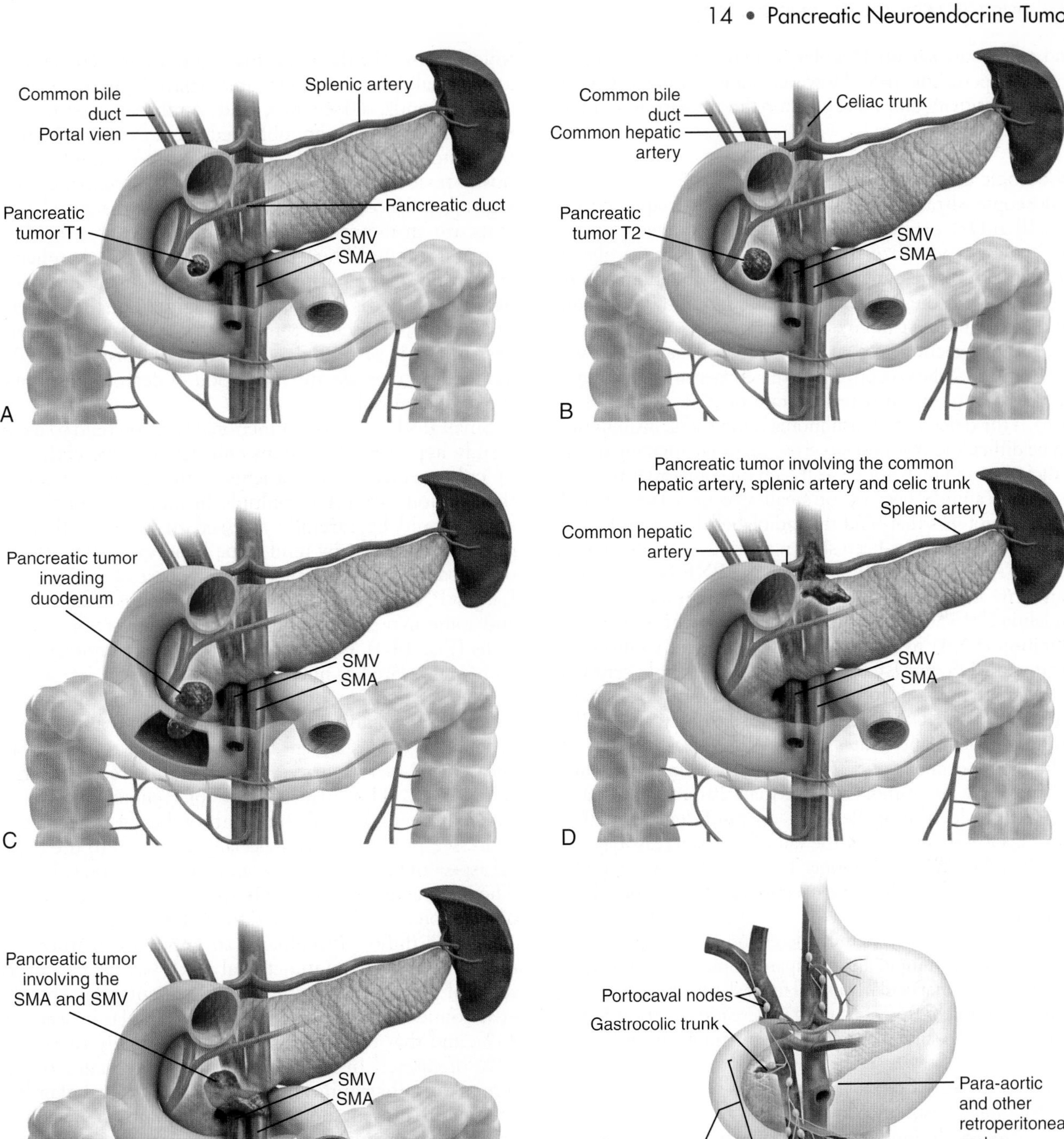

FIGURE 14.3. Tumor-node-metastasis staging. **A**, T1 is a primary tumor confined to the pancreas and less than 2 cm in size. *SMA*, Superior mesenteric artery; *SMV*, superior mesenteric vein. **B**, T2 is a primary tumor confined to the pancreas and between 2 and 4 cm in size. **C**, T3 is a primary tumor greater than 4 cm that invades the duodenum. **D**, T4 is a primary tumor of any size that involves (>180-degree contact) the celiac trunk. **E**, T4 is a tumor of any size that involves (>180-degree contact) the SMA. **F**, Nodal staging demonstrates the different nodal groups that could be involved.

evaluation of thin patients with nonfunctional PNETs who present with symptoms related to mass effect. For optimal detection of PNETs, the patient should be asked to drink water before the US to provide a good window through the stomach for evaluation of the pancreas. The patient can be positioned in the supine, left lateral decubitus, or standing position. The PNET is typically a well-defined hypoechoic mass when compared with the rest of the pancreas. PNETs tend to be vascular on Doppler imaging and may demonstrate a hyperechoic halo. However, transabdominal US has limited sensitivity and detection for the primary lesion and nodal metastases.[31,32]

Endoscopic Ultrasound

Endoscopic ultrasound (EUS) uses a high-frequency US (7.5–10 mHz) probe placed within the stomach or the duodenum to visualize the pancreas. With the probe in the duodenum, the pancreatic head and duodenum can be evaluated; with the probe in the duodenum, the body and tail of the pancreas can be evaluated.

A mean detection rate of 90% (range 77%–100%) was shown in 10 studies according to the consensus statement.[33] EUS also had a mean detection rate of 92% (range 88%–94%) in the detection of insulinomas alone. The insulinomas can be difficult to diagnose on cross-sectional imaging owing to their size and may not be well seen on somatostatin (SST) receptor scanning because of small size or a lack of SST receptor subtypes that bind the radiolabeled octreotide with high affinity. EUS has been shown to have a role in patients with MEN I and also vHL, in which the PNETs may be less than 1 cm and can be difficult to detect by other imaging modalities.[16,32,34,35] EUS can be used along with fine needle aspiration (FNA) to obtain tissue samples and confirm the diagnosis. EUS and EUS-guided FNA are highly sensitive and accurate methods for diagnosis PNETs. EUS sensitivity was 96.7%, and EUS-FNA diagnostic sensitivity was 89.2%, yielding concordance rates with WHO classification of pathologic specimens of 87.5% for tumors less than 20 mm and of 57.1% for tumors greater than 20 mm.[36] However, EUS is not widely available and is operator dependent. The entire liver and portions of the tail of the pancreas may not be well evaluated by EUS alone. The role of EUS is complementary to that of other cross-sectional imaging modalities in evaluation of PNETs.

Intraoperative US has similar detection rates as EUS and is an important technique during laparoscopic or open pancreatic surgery. It is particularly useful for real-time localization of small and multiple PNETs during pancreatic resection, lesion enucleation, and surveillance of the remnant pancreas.[37]

Multidetector Row Computed Tomography and Magnetic Resonance Imaging

Multiphasic technique is required when imaging PNETs, as the pattern and degree of contrast enhancement can be drastically different among tumors and unpredictable for any given tumor. Multiphasic technique improves the chances of achieving maximum tumor conspicuity on at least one of the phases and detecting all sites of disease involvement.

Multidetector Row Computed Tomography

MDCT is readily available, nonoperator dependent, and easy to perform, and is useful for initial diagnosis, staging-restaging evaluation, and surveillance. The accuracy of MDCT for staging PNETs has been confirmed in a recent study, being in the range of 85% to 88% for T stage and 83% to 89% for nodal metastasis.[38]

Our pancreas MDCT protocol includes a precontrast series of the abdomen, followed by rapid intravenous injection of contrast (150 mL of Omnipaque 350 at 4–5 mL/sec followed by 50 mL of normal saline) and acquisition of an arterial, portal venous, and delayed phases, typically at 40 seconds, 60 seconds, and 2 minutes postinjection, respectively. Images are obtained with 2.5-mm slice thickness/pitch 0.984, reconstructed at 2.5 mm (standard diagnostic review) and 0.625 mm (multiplanar reformations in sagittal and coronal planes). Coronal and sagittal reformats are an important adjunct to axial images for detection and staging. The technique provides a comprehensive evaluation of the peripancreatic vessels, liver, and peritoneal cavity that is necessary for staging. For the detection of small hypervascular tumor with MDCT, particularly if gastrinoma is suspected, we use water to distend the duodenum and increase the likelihood of detecting tumors in the duodenal wall.

Small PNETs (usually functional tumors) tend to be uniformly hypervascular lesions enhancing in the early phase of enhancement.[39] In patients with MEN I syndrome, these lesions are often multiple in number, and the pancreas should be carefully assessed to localize all tumors present. They usually tend to be hypervascular to the rest of the pancreas on the portal venous phase of enhancement. Larger PNETs tend to have heterogeneous enhancement, and some may show central areas of necrosis or calcifications (Fig. 14.4). One study showed that tumor enhancement was related to microvascular density.[40]

The relationship of these tumors to the surrounding vasculature should be carefully assessed to conform to the proposed TNM staging. The presence of celiac or SMA encasement (>180-degree contact) can preclude surgery (Fig. 14.5). The management of venous involvement with narrowing or with tumor thrombus also needs to be addressed preoperatively, especially as related to the technical aspect of venous resection and reconstruction (Fig. 14.6). The resectability criteria are borrowed from pancreatic adenocarcinoma and extrapolated to PNETs.[41]

Venous tumor thrombus is an important feature commonly seen with nonfunctional PNETs that can impact surgical planning. In a study of 88 patients, Balachandran et al. found that the incidence of intravascular invasion was 33%, and that this finding was not accurately reported in 62% of cases.[42] In 18% of patients the presence of large tumor thrombi significantly altered the surgical plan.[42]

Atypical presentations are not uncommon, which can compound the diagnosis. The primary tumors can be hypovascular in up to 49% of cases.[40,43–46] PNETs may also be infiltrative and heterogeneous, creating a diagnostic dilemma with pancreatic ductal adenocarcinoma (PDAC).[45] Less commonly, primary tumors can be cystic (5%–17%).

Liver metastases can have a variable appearance. In hypervascular PNETs, the liver metastases are typically hypervascular and are better seen in the arterial phase of images (Fig. 14.7A). However, like the hypovascular primary tumors, the liver metastases are frequently hypovascular and are seen better in the portal venous phase of enhancement. These metastases may have areas of central necrosis. Some cystic primary tumors can have cystic liver metastases with a fluid-fluid level (Fig. 14.7B).[30]

Nodal metastases may show heterogeneous enhancement (Fig. 14.8). They are typically located in the peripancreatic, periportal, and retroperitoneal areas.

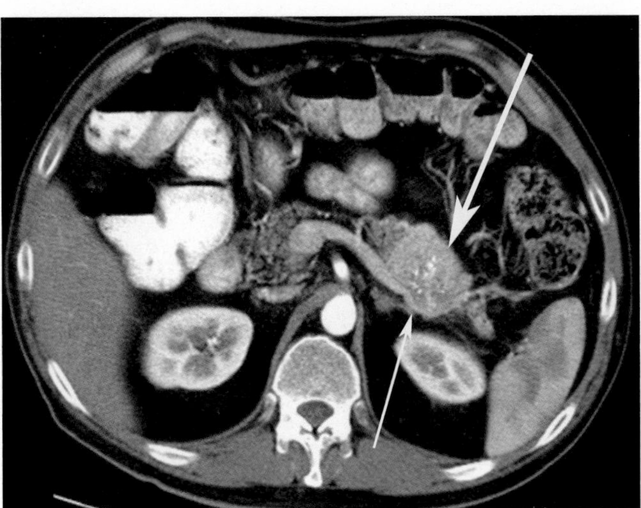

FIGURE 14.4. T3 tumor. Cross-sectional computed tomography scan during the arterial phase of imaging. The *thick arrow* points to a greater than 4 cm hypervascular pancreatic tail mass containing central calcifications. The mass narrowed the splenic vein (*thin arrow*) but does not involve adjacent organs, celiac trunk, or the superior mesenteric artery and was staged as a T3 tumor.

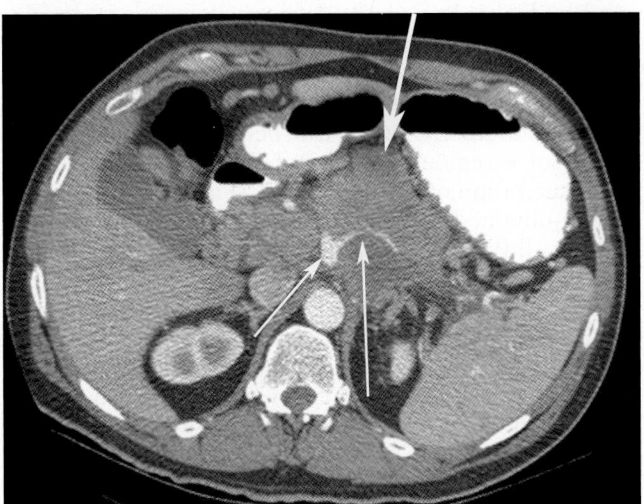

FIGURE 14.5. T4 nonfunctional pancreatic neuroendocrine tumor (PNET). Cross-sectional computed tomography image in the portal venous phase of enhancement. The *thick arrow* points to the heterogeneously enhancing nonfunctional PNET. The *thin arrows* point to the encasement of the splenic artery and the celiac trunk. The tumor was staged T4.

Magnetic Resonance Imaging

MRI is preferred over computed tomography (CT) in the assessment of patients with a history of allergy to iodinated contrast material or in those with renal insufficiency. Even in patients with more pronounced renal insufficiency in whom use of gadolinium contrast is contraindicated (owing to the risk of nephrogenic systemic fibrosis), MRI may be of help based on the T2-weighted (T2W) sequences.

Both 1.5- and 3-T magnets are used at our institution with the cardiac eight-channel coil or the upper body eight-channel coil. All patients are asked to complete a general MRI questionnaire to rule out those with contraindications for MRI. The most recent serum blood urea nitrogen, creatinine, and glomerular filtration rate (GFR) values are also checked. In the absence of acute renal failure

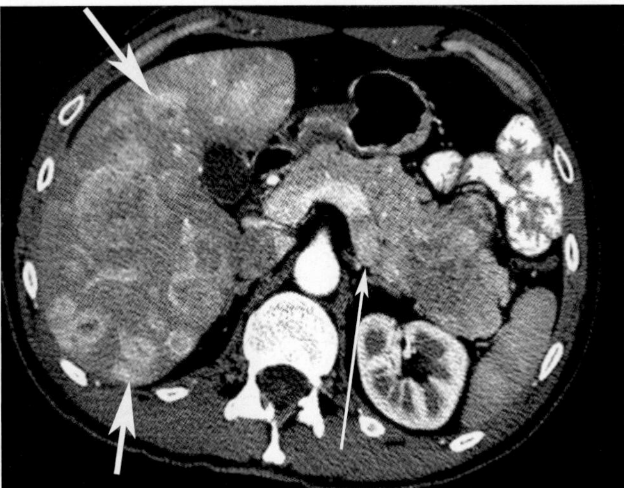

FIGURE 14.6. Cross-sectional computed tomography scan during the arterial phase of imaging in a patient with a nonfunctional pancreatic neuroendocrine tumor (PNET). The *thin arrow* points to a tumor thrombus in the splenic vein growing from a pancreatic tail PNET. The *thick arrows* point to hypervascular liver metastases.

and a GFR over 30 mL/min, gadolinium is used. Acute renal failure is a contraindication to gadolinium use at our institution. In patients with GFR levels below 30 mL/min, a separate consent is required so that the patient may be informed of the possibility of nephrogenic systemic fibrosis and the benefits of the gadolinium administration and have an opportunity to discuss this with the radiologist.

The routine sequences used are coronal fat-saturated fast imaging employing steady-state acquisition (at 5-mm slice thickness with a 0-mm skip), axial respiratory-triggered T2W fat-saturated fast spin echo (FSE) sequence (at 6-mm slice thickness with a 0-mm skip), axial T1-weighted spoiled gradient (SPGR) pre- and postcontrast (at 5-mm slice thickness with a 0-mm skip), dynamic multiphasic axial fat-saturated SPGR sequence before contrast administration and at 20, 60, and 120 seconds postcontrast injection (at 4-mm slice thickness with a 2- to 2.5-mm thickness overlap), and a delayed fat-saturated axial SPGR sequence at 5 minutes postcontrast administration (at 4-mm slice thickness with a 2- to 2.5-mm thickness overlap). An additional axial T2 FSE sequence just through the region of the pancreas can be performed to assess the vascular structures and perivascular involvement (at 3-mm slice thickness with a 0-mm skip). Multiphasic three-dimensional (3D) SPGR fat-saturated liver acquisition with volume acceleration dynamic evaluation (3D SPGR FATSAT LAVA precontrast, multiphasic arterial – portal venous phase axial 3D SPGR FATSAT LAVA, axial SPGR FT 3D LAVA obtained 5 minutes postinjection) may be performed with extracellular agent (GADAVIST – Gadobutrol, injection 1 mmoL/mL. 0.1 mmoL/kg of body weight, given at a rate of 2 mL/s followed by a saline flush) or hepatobiliary agent EOVIST (gadoxetate disodium) at a dose of 0.025 mmol/kg at a rate of 2 mL/s, followed by saline flush), with the addition of an axial 3D GRE FT 3D LAVA phase 20 minute postinjection acquisition with hepatobiliary agent.

A mean sensitivity of 93% and a specificity of 88%[40] have been reported in two studies.[47,48] MRI may also be more sensitive than CT for the detection of liver metastases.[49,50]

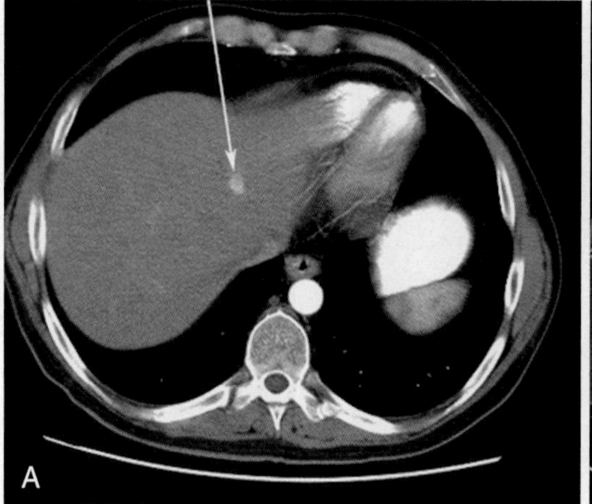

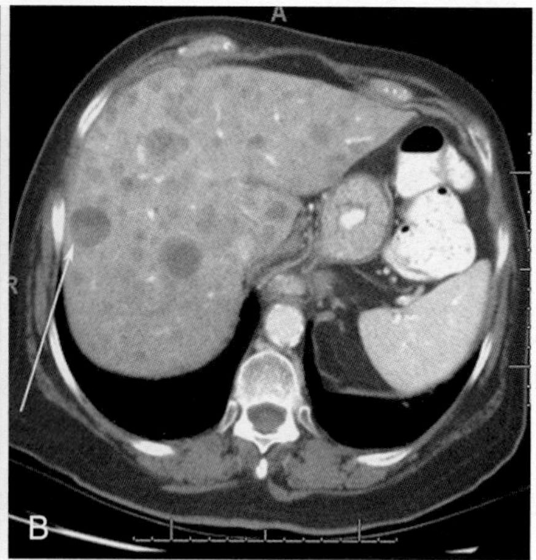

FIGURE 14.7. Different appearances of liver metastases in different patients. **A**, Cross-sectional computed tomography (CT) scan during the arterial phase of imaging. The *arrow* points to a typical hypervascular liver metastasis. **B**, Cross-sectional CT scan during the portal venous phase of imaging in another patient. The *arrow* points to an infrequently seen cystic liver metastasis with a fluid level.

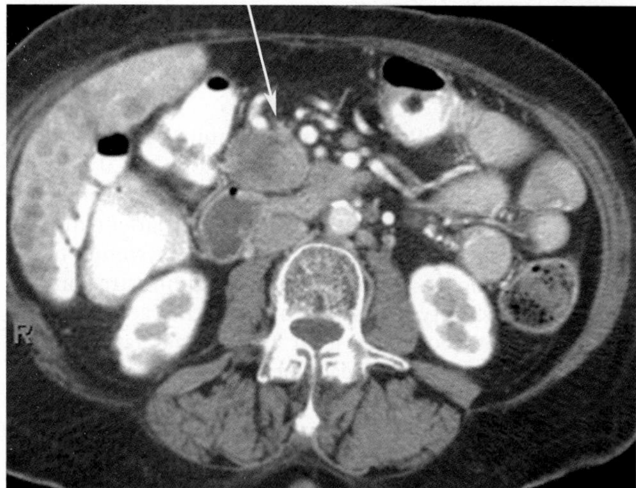

FIGURE 14.8. Cross-sectional computed tomography image in the portal venous phase of enhancement. The *arrow* points to metastatic adenopathy in the small bowel mesentery.

PNETs are of low T1 and high T2 signal intensity. Small PNETs may demonstrate uniform hypervascular enhancement. Larger PNETs can demonstrate heterogeneous enhancement similar to CT enhancement characteristics (Fig. 14.9). Common bile duct and pancreatic ductal dilatation can be well evaluated by MRI on the T2W sequences. Liver metastases are of low T1 signal intensity and can be of high T2 signal intensity. The enhancement of the nodes is similar to that on CT, demonstrating significant enhancement.

Vascular involvement should be carefully assessed as described in the earlier section on multidetector computed tomography.

Functional Imaging

SST is a 14–amino acid peptide hormone that binds to receptors commonly expressed on NETs, including those arising from the pancreas.[51,52] Synthetic analogs of SST have been used to treat PNETs, but can also be used for imaging. SST receptor scintigraphy (SRS) is commonly performed with an ^{111}In-pentretreotide.[53,54]

With SRS, whole-body planar images are obtained at 4 to 6 hours and at 24 hours. Higher lesion conspicuity can be obtained on delayed images because of physiologic clearance of unbound radiotracer; however, bowel excretion is more prominent on delayed images and can complicate interpretation. Single-photon emission CT (SPECT) or SPECT/CT can be used to generate 3D images of a region that allow better identification and characterization of sites of activity (Fig. 14.10); these are usually obtained at 24 hours. It is important to mention that not all PNETs have SST receptors, and that the sensitivity for insulinomas is reported to be around 60% to 70%.[54,55] Furthermore, SST receptors are not specific to PNETs, and other tumors such as nonsmall cell lung cancer, breast cancer, lymphoma, and meningioma, as well as nonspecific inflammatory cells, may also express these receptors, potentially creating false-positive results on SRS.

More recently, SST analogs linked to positron-emitting radionuclides have been developed, allowing for SST receptor positron emission tomography (PET)/CT imaging (SR-PET/CT). ^{68}Ga-DOTATATE is one of these. SR-PET/CT identifies many more lesions compared with SRS. It also offers several advantages over SRS, in that it can be performed more quickly (in about 2 hours instead of 2 days), exposes the patient to less radiation, and provides tomographic images of the whole body instead of a single region.[56,57] Similar to SRS, false positives may be encountered with other tumors and inflammatory processes. Of note, increased activity in the head and uncinate process of the pancreas has been reported as a common false-positive finding.[58,59]

2-[18 F] fluoro-2-deoxy-D-glucose (FDG)-PET/CT is commonly used for many malignant tumors, but is more limited in use for PNETs, likely because these tumors tend to be slow growing. Nevertheless, PNETs with high proliferation (measured by Ki-67 staining) tend to have lower sensitivity on SST imaging and higher detection on FDG-PET/CT. In contrast, tumors with low proliferation tend to be better detected by SST imaging and are often falsely negative on FDG-PET/CT.[60]

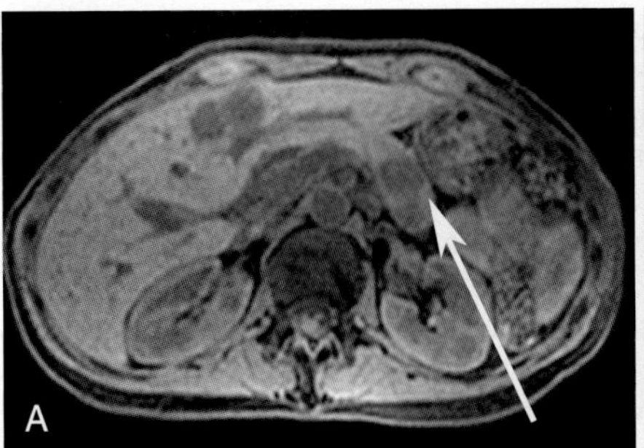

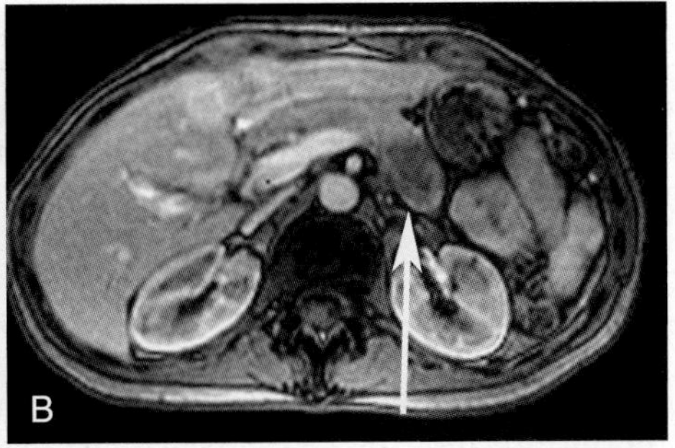

FIGURE 14.9. Magnetic resonance imaging of pancreatic neuroendocrine tumor (PNET). **A**, Precontrast T1-weighted (T1W) gradient echo sequence demonstrates a T1 hypointense PNET (*arrow*) in the pancreatic tail. **B**, Postcontrast T1W gradient echo sequence demonstrates a heterogeneously enhancing PNET (*arrow*) in the pancreatic tail.

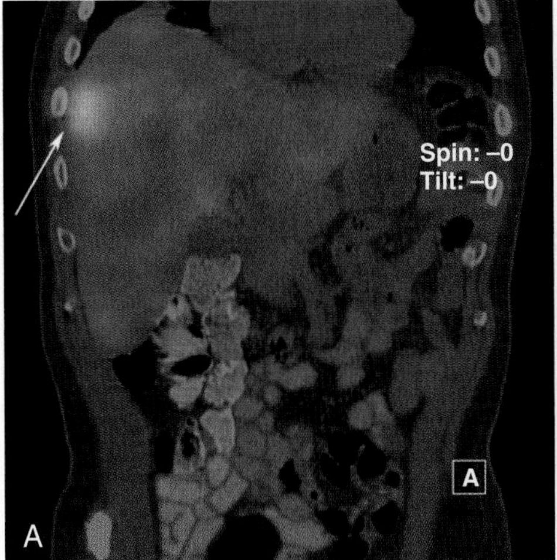

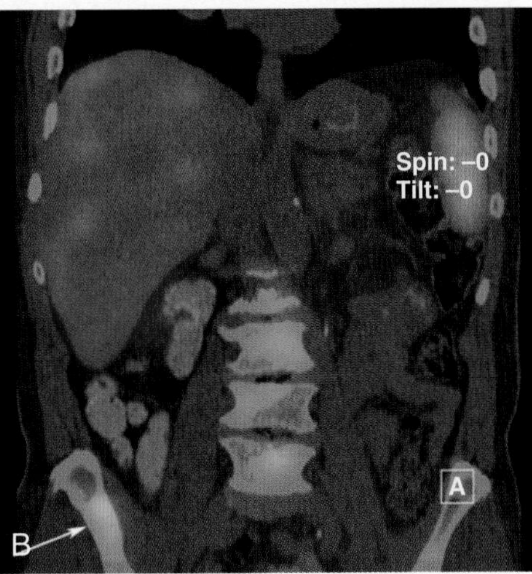

FIGURE 14.10. Octreotide scanning in distant metastases. **A**, Coronal image from SRS single-photon emission computed tomography (SPECT) computer tomography (CT) shows increased activity in a liver metastasis (*arrow*). **B**, Coronal SRS SPECT/CT image demonstrates increased activity in a bone metastasis involving the right ilium (*arrow*).

Angiography

Angiography is invasive, uses ionizing radiation and contrast, and is reserved for patients with findings of functional tumors without detection of the tumor on anatomic cross-sectional and functional imaging. This procedure include arterial stimulation with hepatic venous sampling and percutaneous transhepatic portal venous sampling.

For arterial stimulation, calcium gluconate is administered via the catheter placed in either the splenic artery, the GDA, or the SMA.[61] Venous sampling from the hepatic veins is performed to document a greater than twofold increase in the level of the hormone produced by the tumor. A sensitivity of greater than 90% in the detection of functional tumors such as insulinomas has been reported.[62]

Percutaneous transhepatic portal venous sampling involves the placement of a catheter into the intrahepatic portal vein with subsequent positioning into the main portal, superior mesenteric, and splenic veins for venous sampling and assessment of hormone levels.

KEY POINTS

Imaging

- Imaging of pancreatic neuroendocrine tumors is performed with anatomic imaging modalities combined with functional imaging with somatostatin analogs.
- Anatomic imaging is performed by computed tomography (CT), magnetic resonance imaging (MRI), endoscopic ultrasound, and intraoperative ultrasound. Multiphasic technique is required for CT and MRI, regardless of the primary tumor.
- Functional imaging uses somatostatin receptor scintigraphy (SRS) and positron emission tomography (PET)/CT. Somatostatin receptor PET/CT is faster, uses less radiation, and is more sensitive than SRS.
- Imaging is critical to accurately define extent of disease, provide the essential information for determining resectability, and carry out adequate patient staging and stratification.

TREATMENT

For all PNETs, the primary method of treatment, if feasible, is surgery, as complete resection of localized disease determines the potential for cure. A number of possible surgical procedures exist, including simple enucleation, distal pancreatectomy with and without splenectomy, central pancreatectomy, pancreaticoduodenectomy, and total pancreatectomy. Available surgical options for each type of tumor are discussed under the specific tumor. Systemic treatment options are selected to control symptoms of hormone secretion and tumor bulk, maximize progression-free survival (PFS) and overall survival (OS), and minimize toxicity.

Systemic Therapy

In recent years, major scientific advances have been achieved in our understanding of PNET biology, resulting in broader options and newer drug therapies for PNETs.

Somatostatin Analogs

SST receptors are expressed by approximately 80% of well-differentiated NETs, and this led to the investigation of the therapeutic role of the synthetic somatostatin analogs (SSAs) octreotide and lanreotide. SSAs have an established role in the treatment of hormone hypersecretory symptoms. More recently, octreotide was demonstrated to significantly prolong PFS in patients with midgut NET, and lanreotide was proven to be similarly effective. Patients without symptoms from hormone hypersecretion can also be considered for SSA therapy if they have uptake on somatostatin imaging (SRS or SR-PET/CT) (Fig. 14.11). Given their biological similarity, the National Comprehensive Cancer Network guidelines currently recommend either octreotide or lanreotide as first-line choices for symptom control and/or tumor cytostatic control.[63–65] Of note, SSA therapy for insulinomas should be approached cautiously, as these tumors may not express SST receptors, and therapy can also suppress counterregulatory hormones, resulting in paradoxical precipitous worsening of hypoglycemia, and even death.[66]

Targeted Drugs

Sunitinib, a multitargeted receptor tyrosine kinase inhibitor, and everolimus, an mTOR inhibitor, have been investigated in clinical trials as single agents or combination therapy. A phase III trial of patients with advanced and progressive well-differentiated PNETs showed a significant PFS benefit of sunitinib compared with placebo.[65,67] The phase III RADIANT-3 study of everolimus has also been completed, demonstrating a significant improvement in PFS.[68] The US Food and Drug Administration (FDA) approved everolimus for the treatment of PNETs based on these results.[65] Subsequently, based upon the results of the RADIANT-4 trial, which demonstrated a significant improvement in PFS with everolimus versus placebo in patients with advanced nonfunctional NETs of gastrointestinal or lung origin, the FDA approved everolimus for the treatment of these tumors.[65]

Cytotoxic Chemotherapy

Cytotoxic chemotherapy has different roles in the care of patients with pancreatic neuroendocrine carcinomas (PNECs) and PNETs. For patients with poorly-differentiated PNECs, systemic cytotoxic chemotherapy is the primary treatment modality, generally consisting of platinum-based combination regimens extrapolated from small-cell lung cancer approaches. For well-differentiated PNETs, regardless of Ki-67 labeling, alkylating chemotherapy can be used in situations of substantial tumor burden or aggressive clinical course. Because single agents have shown only modest clinical activity, combination chemotherapy regimens have been investigated, with the oldest backbone agent being streptozocin. In a study of 84 consecutive patients with PNET treated with fluorouracil, doxorubicin and streptozocin, a response rate of 39% based on Response Evaluation Criteria for Solid Tumors (RECIST) was observed. For this regimen, the 2-year PFS rate was 41%, and the 2-year OS rate was 74%.[69] However, because of the toxicities of this multiagent intravenous regimen, including cytopenias and high emetogenic risk, it is generally reserved for extenuating circumstances in the modern era.

More recently, studies of the oral alkylating agent temozolomide have demonstrated substantial improvements in PFS, specifically in combination with capecitabine, the oral prodrug of 5-fluorouracil.[70] Given the modest side-effect profile of this oral regimen, it has largely replaced streptozocin-based regimens in routine clinical practice.

Peptide Receptor Radionuclide Therapy

The development of SSAs conjugated to therapeutic radionuclides, known as peptide receptor radionuclide therapy (PRRT), is perhaps one of the most dramatic advancements in nuclear medicine in recent years. Although SSAs remain the first-line treatment option for most patients with unresectable, advanced PNETs, PRRT has been shown to be a safe and effective option for patients with tumors expressing SST receptors. The multicenter phase III NETTER-1 trial concluded that treatment with ^{177}Lu-DOTATATE resulted in improved PFS and likely OS compared with high-dose SSA therapy in patients with midgut NETs that had previously progressed on standard-dose SSA therapy.[71] Both the European Medicines Agency and the US FDA have approved ^{177}Lu-DOTATATE for the treatment of advanced gastroenteropancreatic NETs, likely based on the combination of randomized data from NETTER-1 and the significant volume of real-world evidence generated from decades of European experience with PRRT administered as four fixed doses every 8 weeks.[72] Therapy is generally well tolerated, although severe nausea and vomiting have been associated with some amino acid solutions administered during therapy for renal protection. Blood counts and liver enzymes should be monitored during therapy, and treatment can be delayed to allow for count recovery/normalization; there are rare reports of carcinoid crisis with infusion, delayed renal toxicity, or marrow failure/secondary leukemia.

Treatment Sequencing

Treatment strategies for advanced PNETs are often best determined in multidisciplinary rounds and include a whole host of systemic therapies, liver-directed therapies (i.e., transarterial chemoembolization, radiofrequency ablation [RFA], radioembolization, targeted radiation therapy, etc.), and surgical resection. Several factors must be considered when determining the beast treatment strategy, including tumor pathologic grade, overall burden of disease, biologic

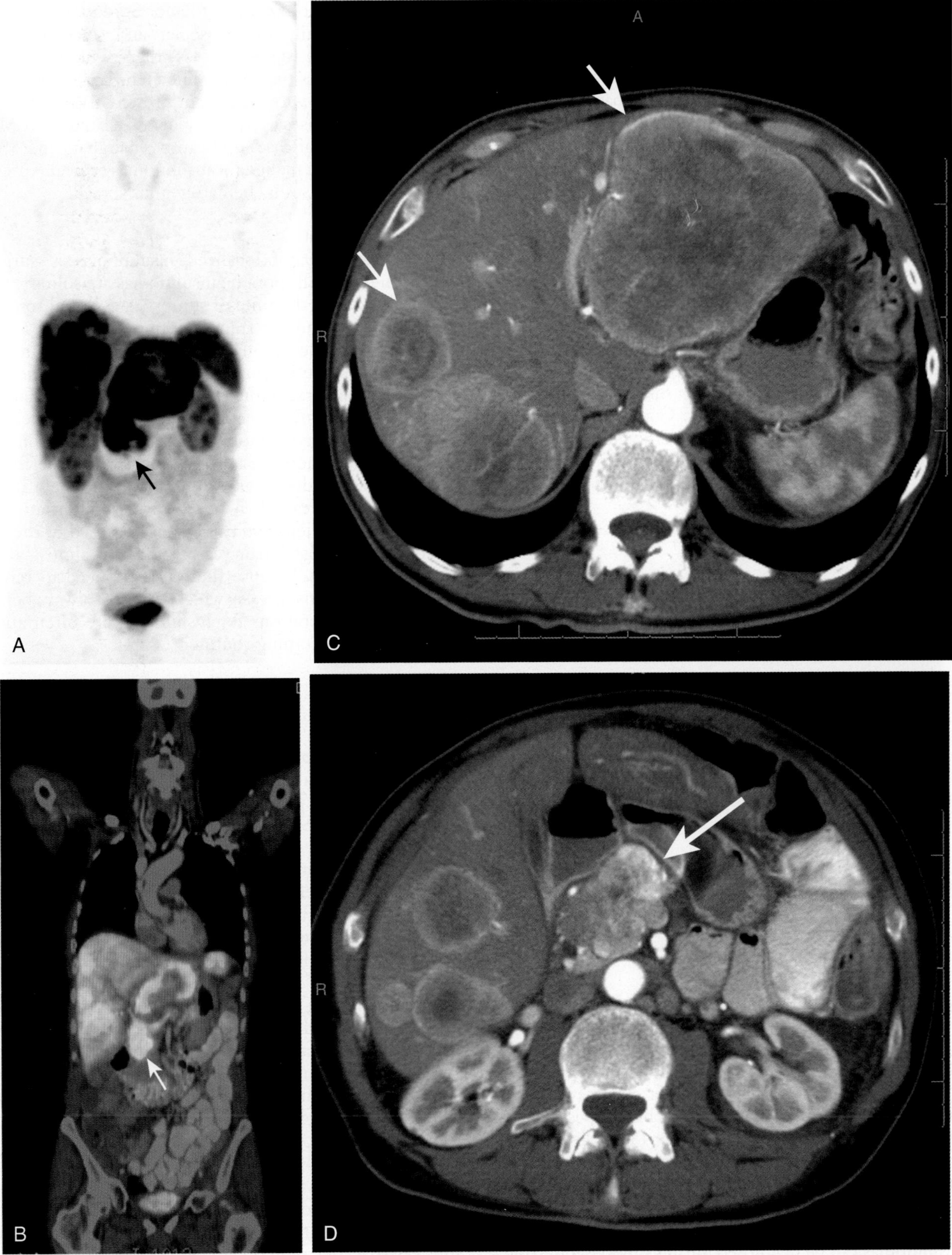

FIGURE 14.11. A 66-year-old male with metastatic well-differentiated pancreatic neuroendocrine tumor (PNET) with intense uptake on somatostatin receptor imaging. Maximum intensity projection coronal image (**A**) and fused positron emission tomography (PET)/computed tomography (CT) coronal image (**B**) of ^{68}Ga-DOTATATE PET/CT shows intense uptake in multifocal hepatic metastases and primary pancreatic head mass neuroendocrine tumor (arrow), making the patient a candidate for somatostatin analog therapy. Axial CT images (**C** and **D**) show large hypervascular hepatic metastases (*arrows*) and an arterially-hyperenhancing mass in the head of the pancreas (*long arrow*), typical of well-differentiated PNETs. Biopsy revealed an intermediate-grade (G2) PNET.

behavior, tumor functional status, activity on SST receptor imaging, and presence of metastatic disease limited to the liver or liver and extrahepatic metastases.

Functional tumors, particularly those secreting serotonin (carcinoid syndrome), glucagon, and vasoactive intestinal peptide, are usually initiated on SSAs as the first line of treatment to offer control of both hormonal production and tumor progression. For insulin and gastrin-secreting tumors, octreotide and lanreotide have a more limited role, as worsening of hypoglycemia may occur because of unopposed SST receptor-2 and -5 activation in insulinomas, and proton pump inhibitors (PPIs) are usually the choice for gastrin-secreting tumors. Options for biochemical control of functional PNETs that have progressed on SSAs include dose escalation of long-acting SSAs, use of short-acting SSAs, and tumor debulking (surgical resection and liver-directed therapies). A number of systemic treatments are available for control of PNETs that have progressed on SSAs, including sunitinib, everolimus, cytotoxic chemotherapy, and PRRT. Combination chemotherapy regimens incorporating platinum agents should be the primary treatment modality for patients with PNECs.[65]

> **KEY POINTS**
>
> **Treatment**
>
> - Surgery is the primary method of treatment, as complete surgical resection determines the potential for cure.
> - Several surgical procedures exist, including pancreaticoduodenectomy, total, central, or distal pancreatectomy with or without splenectomy, and simple enucleation.
> - Systemic treatment encompasses a large host of options, including somatostatin analogs (octreotide or lanreotide), targeted drugs (sunitinib, everolimus), cytotoxic chemotherapy (temozolomide with capecitabine), and peptide radionuclide therapy.
> - Treatment strategies for advanced pancreatic neuroendocrine tumors are best determined in multidisciplinary rounds.

SPECIFIC TUMOR TYPES

Insulinoma

Clinical Presentation

Insulinomas are PNETs that release inappropriately high amounts of insulin, resulting in a hyperinsulinemic hypoglycemic state.[35] Insulinomas are the most common functional PNETs and occur mainly in the pancreas. The patients typically present with fasting hypoglycemia and may present with neuroglycopenic symptoms such as blurred vision, diplopia, confusion, and abnormal behavior (Table 14.1). This can progress to loss of consciousness, coma, or even permanent brain damage. Symptoms related to release of catecholamines following hypoglycemia such as weakness, sweating, hunger, tremors, and palpitations may also occur.

Insulinomas can be diagnosed during supervised fasting. A serum glucose level less than 45 mg/dL associated with a plasma insulin level of greater than or equal to 3 μU/mL is found.[35,73] For patients who are symptomatic during supervised fasting, 1 mg of glucagon can be administered intravenously to reverse the hypoglycemia.

Primary Tumor and Patterns of Tumor Spread

These are typically hypervascular and solitary tumors. Some 90% of the tumors are less than 2 cm, and 30% of the tumors are less than 1 cm. They tend to be benign in a majority of cases, with malignant presentation in approximately 10% of cases. They may be associated with MEN I in 7% to 31% of cases and can be malignant in 25% of these cases.[74] The malignant insulinomas typically present with liver metastases by hematogenous spread.

Surgical Treatment

The management of localized insulinomas is surgical. Although nearly all sporadic insulinomas are solitary, careful exploration at the time of surgery is essential to detect the presence of multiple tumors; intraoperative US is often a valuable tool. Ideal management of insulinomas involves enucleation of the tumor. However, tumors that lie close to the main pancreatic duct may be more safely managed by formal pancreatic resection (pancreaticoduodenectomy for pancreatic head tumors or distal pancreatectomy for tumors in the pancreatic tail). If enucleation is performed and a pancreatic duct leak is identified intraoperatively, a formal resection can then be performed; alternatively, a Roux limb of the jejunum can be anastomosed to the pancreatic defect. Distal pancreatectomy can almost always be spleen-sparing, because there is little need to remove lymph nodes in this disease, which is almost always benign. Laparoscopic operations for insulinoma are often appropriate and are becoming routine.[75,76]

Gastrinoma

Clinical Presentation

Gastrinomas are functional PNETs characterized by high levels of gastrin production leading to Zollinger–Ellison syndrome (ZES). The classic triad of ZES consists of severe peptic ulcer disease, gastric acid hypersecretion, and non-β islet cell tumors of the pancreas. Gastrinomas can occur in the duodenum (more common) or within the pancreas (especially in the head/uncinate process). The most common symptoms, which include abdominal pain and peptic ulcers, are found in 90% to 95% of these patients (see Table 14.1).

Often, a fasting serum gastrin level is the first test to be requested for these patients. However, other causes of hypergastrinemia are present, including the routine use of PPI therapy. PPI use causes hypo- or achlorhydria, resulting in hypergastrinemia. In patients on PPI therapy, these medications should be stopped for at least 1 week before testing for gastrinomas.

The upper limit of normal serum gastrin levels is 100 pg/mL. A serum gastrin level of 1000 pg/mL or greater and a gastric pH of 2 or less is diagnostic of a gastrinoma.[77] In patients with serum gastrin levels between 100 and 1000 pg/mL and a gastric pH of 2 or less, a secretin stimulation test can be performed. A positive secretin test is performed by administering 0.4 μg/kg of secretin by subcutaneous injection. A postinjection serum gastrin level increase of greater than 120 pg/mL has been shown to have a sensitivity of 94% and a specificity of 100%.[78]

Table 14.1 Clinical Findings

TUMOR	HORMONE	SYNDROME	% MEN I	SITE OF ORIGIN	% MALIGNANT	OPERATION
Gastrinoma	Gastrin	Peptic ulcer disease, abdominal pain, esophagitis, diarrhea	20	75% gastrinoma triangle 25% duodenum	>50	Resection with regional lymph node dissection; include duodenotomy with careful search for additional tumors
Insulinoma	Insulin	Hypoglycemia, weight gain	<10	Anywhere throughout the pancreas	<10	Enucleation or resection; usually no regional lymph node dissection
Glucagonoma	Glucagon	Diabetes, necrolytic migratory erythema	Rare	Pancreas; 90% in body and tail	>70	Distal pancreatectomy, splenectomy, regional lymph node dissection
Vasoactive intestinal polypeptidoma	Vasoactive intestinal peptide	Watery diarrhea, hypokalemia, achlorhydria	Rare	75% pancreas, 20% neurogenic, 5% duodenum	>50	Resection with regional lymph node dissection (usually distal pancreatectomy and splenectomy)
Somatostatinoma	Somatostatin	Steatorrhea, diabetes, hypochlorhydria	Rare	66% pancreas, 33% duodenum	>70	Resection with regional lymph node dissection (usually pancreaticoduodenectomy)
Nonfunctional pancreatic neuroendocrine tumor	Pancreatic polypeptide, other, none	None	>15	60% pancreatic head	>60	Resection with regional lymph node dissection; no role for incomplete debulking

Primary Tumor and Patterns of Tumor Spread

These tumors often occur in the gastrinoma triangle, the area between the confluence of the cystic and common bile duct, the junction of the second and third portions of the duodenum, and the junction of the neck and body of the pancreas. Overall, duodenal tumors are three to 10 times more common than pancreatic tumors. In contrast to insulinomas, the majority of gastrinomas tend to be malignant. They can present with lymph node (nodal spread) and liver metastases (hematogenous spread) at the time of diagnosis in 75% to 80% of cases and with bone metastases in 12% of cases.[79] The presence of liver metastases at the time of diagnosis is the most important determinant of survival and is found more often in patients with pancreatic than with duodenal gastrinomas. The presence of lymph node metastases does not appear to have a significant impact on survival.[80]

They are associated with MEN I syndrome in 20% to 60% of cases. These tumors tend to be predominantly small and difficult to visualize by imaging. They also tend to present earlier in life and can be multiple. The OS of patients with MEN I–associated gastrinomas is similar to that of patients with the sporadic form and is determined by the presence of liver metastases.[81]

Surgical Treatment

There is evidence to support routine surgical management of gastrinoma in sporadic cases; surgery is associated with little morbidity and can provide a postoperative cure rate of 60%, with a third of patients achieving long-term cure (10 years).[82,83] The goal of surgery is to perform a complete resection of disease and preserve the maximal amount of pancreas. Tumors in the tail of the pancreas can be managed by distal pancreatectomy. Tumors in the head of the pancreas can often be managed by enucleation. Duodenal tumors can be managed by full-thickness excision. Duodenotomy with careful palpation of the duodenum or endoscopic transillumination should be performed routinely, even for patients who do not have a diagnosed duodenal primary, because duodenal tumors in patients with gastrinoma are extremely common and can be multiple and very small. Routine peripancreatic lymph node dissection should also be performed because of the high incidence of lymph node metastasis at the time of diagnosis.[84] There is growing evidence to support more extensive surgery (pancreaticoduodenectomy) in certain cases: the presence of a large duodenal or pancreatic head tumor that is not amenable to enucleation; the presence of multiple duodenal tumors or multiple enlarged lymph nodes; and failure of cure after routine surgical management.[85] Minimally invasive options, such as endoscopic resection of duodenal tumors, or laparoscopic pancreatic procedures can also play a role in selected cases.

Vasoactive Intestinal Polypeptidoma

Clinical Presentation

VIPomas occur because of vasoactive intestinal polypeptide (VIP) overproduction by PNETs. The classic triad in Verner–Morrison syndrome is watery diarrhea, hypokalemia, and achlorhydria. These patients experience dehydration, hyperglycemia, and flushing.[86] The large-volume diarrhea seen is at least 700 mL/day, with 70% to 80% of patients having more than 3 L/day. Most VIPomas arise from the pancreas in adults but can be extrapancreatic in children, arising in ganglioneuromas, ganglioneuroblastomas, and neurofibromas involving the retroperitoneum and mediastinum. Fluid and electrolyte replacement is often needed at the time of diagnosis.

An elevated VIP level (>500 pg/mL) in the presence of a secretory diarrhea is highly suggestive of a VIPoma.[87]

Primary Tumor and Patterns of Tumor Spread

These tumors are of pancreatic origin in over 80% of all cases. The rest of the cases are of neural origin. The pancreatic tumors present as larger masses and tend to be malignant. They metastasize to the liver (hematogenous spread) and lymph nodes (nodal spread) in the majority of cases.[88]

Surgical Treatment

Approximately half of pancreatic VIPomas are malignant, with metastases most commonly to regional lymph nodes and the liver. Neurogenic VIPomas are mostly benign. Pancreatic VIPomas are located in the body and tail of the pancreas 75% of the time, and formal resection (usually distal pancreatectomy and splenectomy) with regional lymph node dissection is the ideal management strategy.

Glucagonoma

Clinical Presentation

Glucagonomas cause hypersecretion of glucagon. Glucagonomas can cause glucose intolerance, weight loss, diarrhea, migratory necrolytic erythema, glossitis, deep vein thrombi, and stomatitis (see Table 14.1). Migratory necrolytic erythema is a skin condition characterized by erythematous macules, which become papules and heal with necrosis and pigmented scarring.[89] Serum glucagon levels of 500 to 1000 pg/mL are diagnostic of glucagonomas.

Primary Tumor and Patterns of Tumor Spread

Glucagonomas are typically sporadic and are pancreatic in origin. Glucagonomas can be large and are typically malignant. The majority of cases tend to have liver metastases (hematogenous spread) at the time of diagnosis.[90] They may be associated with MEN I syndrome in about 5% of cases. Patients with MEN I syndrome and glucagonomas tend to present earlier than the patients with sporadic cases.

Surgical Treatment

More than 80% of glucagonomas ultimately display malignant behavior; over 50% of patients have regional or distant metastatic disease at the time of diagnosis.[91] Glucagonomas are always located in the pancreas, and 90% are located in the body and tail. They are often very large tumors that are best managed by distal pancreatectomy and splenectomy, with regional lymph node dissection.

Nonfunctional Pancreatic Neuroendocrine Tumors

Clinical Presentation

These are PNETs not associated with any syndrome. They are usually found because of symptoms related to mass effect caused by the pancreatic tumor on adjacent organs or, less often, are found incidentally. They typically present with larger primary tumors and advanced disease.[92] The most common symptoms include nonspecific abdominal pain (40%–60%), weight loss (25%–50%), or jaundice (30%–40%). The diagnosis for a nonfunctional PNET is based on biopsy of the tumor.

Primary Tumor and Patterns of Tumor Spread

These tend to be large and solitary pancreatic masses and present from symptoms of local mass effect. The majority of tumors are malignant.[92] They can present with lymph node (nodal spread) and liver (hematogenous spread) metastases at the time of diagnosis.

They can be associated with MEN I syndrome in 80% to 100% of cases. In these patients, the tumors tend to be multiple (Fig. 14.12).

Surgical Treatment

Nonfunctional PNETs are usually diagnosed because of the mechanical effects from local growth or metastatic disease (e.g., pain, jaundice). Thus, most nonfunctioning PNETs are diagnosed when the primary tumor is large or has already metastasized; only 25% of patients are candidates for a potentially curative resection at the time of diagnosis.[93] These tumors are malignant in more than 60% of cases, with metastasis most commonly to lymph nodes and liver.

Approximately 60% of nonfunctioning PNETs are located in the pancreatic head.[94] Surgical resection (pancreaticoduodenectomy or distal pancreatectomy) with lymph node dissection is indicated for localized resectable tumors. However, only approximately 50% of those patients experience long-term cure.[93] There is no survival benefit to incomplete resection of a primary tumor (cytoreduction or debulking), and patients experience considerable morbidity and mortality.[95]

The surgical management of patients who present with a localized but unresectable tumor is controversial. Because the majority of nonfunctioning PNETs are located in the pancreatic head, local growth will eventually result in bile duct and duodenal obstruction. Although endoscopic stents can be used to manage these situations in patients with localized but unresectable tumors, we prefer surgical biliary and gastric bypass. Such patients typically have a median survival of 5 years, and surgical bypass provides a much more durable response than endoscopic stenting.[93]

The management of an intact primary tumor in the setting of metastatic disease is also controversial. A small number of patients (<5%) will be candidates for complete resection of the primary tumor and all metastatic disease and may experience a survival benefit.[93] There is no evidence that surgical resection of the primary tumor without complete resection of all metastatic disease results in increased survival.[94] The only indication for surgery in this subpopulation of patients is symptom palliation. In the case of tumors in the body and tail of the pancreas, symptoms are unusual, even with tumors that become very large. However, surgical resection may be considered for symptom palliation of tumors in the pancreatic head, especially in the setting of biliary and duodenal obstruction or gastrointestinal hemorrhage from erosion into the duodenum; these symptoms may be managed

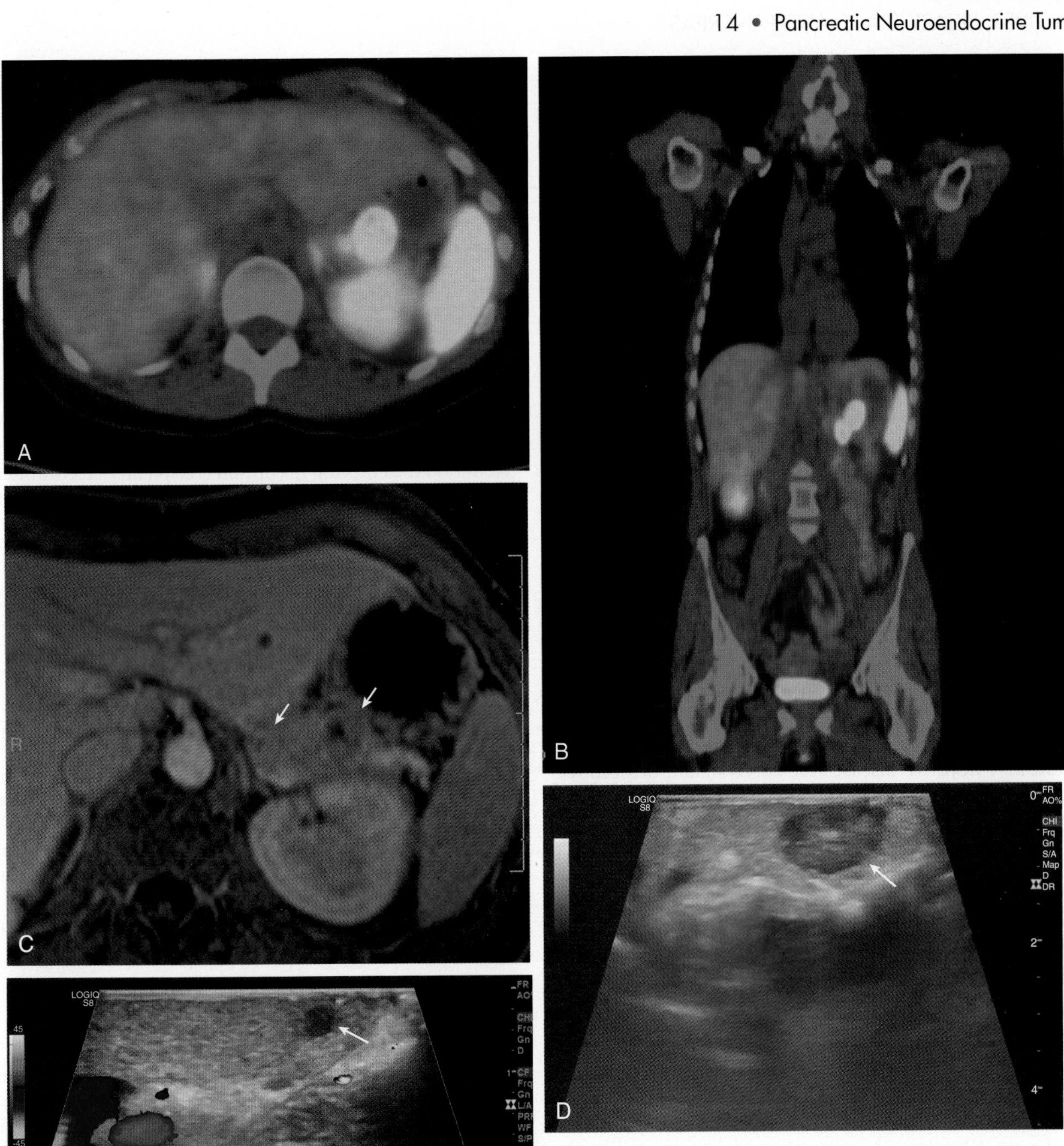

Figure 14.12. A 35-year-old female with multiple endocrine neoplasia type I syndrome and nonfunctional pancreatic neuroendocrine tumors (PNETs). Axial (**A**) and coronal (**B**) fused ^{68}Ga-DOTATATE positron emission tomography (PET)/computed tomography (CT) show two ^{68}Ga-DOTATATE-avid masses in the pancreatic tail consistent with PNETs. Axial magnetic resonance imaging (**C**) shows subtle heterogenously-enhancing masses in the pancreatic tail, correlating with the PET/CT findings. In addition, intraoperative ultrasound (IOS) confirmed the pancreatic tail masses, one of which is shown in **D**, as well as a 4-mm nodule not previously seen by any imaging modality (**E**). A distal pancreatectomy with *en bloc* splenectomy and gastric artery lymph nodes was performed. Pathology revealed well-differentiated tumor, grade 2, forming two masses (1.7 cm and 1.4 cm), and four microadenomas ranging in size from 1 to 4 mm.

better by pancreaticoduodenectomy than by palliative bypass alone.[76]

According to a recent, large, population-based study analyzing SEER data of 709 patients from 2007 to 2015, the resection rate for patients presenting with stage I PNETs remains high.[96] This study showed superior OS for surgically resected stage I PNETs (92% in the surgical cohort vs. 56% in the nonsurgical cohort, $P < .001$), but the cancer-specific survival was not improved (98% in the surgical cohort vs. 94% in the nonsurgical cohort; $P=.207$). These data raises the possibility of selection bias in favor of surgery in studies analyzing all-cause mortality of patients with localized PNETs and emphasize the need for careful selection of endpoints in observational data and rigorous assessment of potential bias in survival analyses. The data also support a surveillance strategy with close follow-up for well-differentiated stage I PNETs.[96]

Surgical resection of highly aggressive, poorly-differentiated PNECs should only be attempted if an R0 resection seems feasible, and currently there is no role for cytoreductive surgery in these highly aggressive malignancies.[76,97]

The decision on surgical management of syndromic PNETs, especially those associated with the MEN I syndrome, differs slightly from that of sporadic PNETs. Whereas current guideline recommendations call for surgical resection of sporadic PNETs greater than 2 cm in size, timing of surgical intervention for MEN I–associated PNETs should take into consideration the high likelihood of multifocal and metachronous tumors. Moreover, even in the setting of metastatic disease, the clinical course tends to be more indolent, and disease progression slower, with MEN I syndrome. For these reasons, nonfunctional indolent tumors can be observed unless they begin to grow or become refractory to medical management.[98]

In summary, PNETs are a heterogeneous group of tumors with varied biological behaviors and a considerably different course from PDAC. Surgical resection is the only potential for cure, and parenchymal-preserving surgery, including enucleations and laparoscopic approaches, should be pursued whenever possible. Lymph node dissection may improve disease-free survival, and cytoreductive surgery or palliative debulking of liver metastases may extend survival and be an option for patients with locally advanced and metastatic disease.

Radiation Therapy

Wherever possible, surgical resection is the preferred and only potentially curative therapy for PNETs.[76] Given their relatively indolent natural history and better prognosis than exocrine adenocarcinomas of the pancreas, surgical resection is advocated as a reasonable strategy, even for patients with metastatic disease. Nevertheless, a majority of patients do not undergo surgical resection, as documented by an analysis of the National Cancer Database.[99]

Potential scenarios in which external beam radiation may be an attractive therapeutic modality are palliative therapy of symptomatic primary or metastatic disease, primary tumor-directed therapy of unresectable disease (with or without metastatic disease), and consolidation therapy after systemic chemotherapy. Palliation of pain, gastric outlet/duodenal obstruction, and bleeding at the primary site or similar pain, compressive symptoms, and bleeding at a site of metastasis may be achieved using fewer fractions of large doses administered with or without concurrent chemotherapy.[100,101]

IMAGING METASTATIC DISEASE

The incidence of metastatic disease is directly related to the histological grade of the tumor, and distant metastases at presentation are seen in 21% of G1, 30% of G2, and 50% of G3 tumors.[10,11] Lymph nodes, liver, peritoneal cavity, and bones are frequent sites of metastatic involvement. The lymphatic drainage of the primary tumor should be carefully surveyed for nodal metastases. Important predictors of nodal involvement in PNETs are size of the primary tumor greater than 4 cm and short-axis diameter of lymph nodes exceeding 5 mm.[102]

The liver is the most common site of metastatic disease.[103] Liver metastases have varied morphologic appearances and patterns of enhancement on CT and MRI, and may be solid, cystic, hypervascular, hypovascular, isodense, or isointense to the hepatic parenchyma, or any combination of the above.[30] Some metastases are seen only in the arterial phase, whereas others, owing to subtle internal enhancement, may be better appreciated on noncontrast CT or T2W MRI (Fig. 14.13). Similarly to the primary tumor, imaging liver metastases requires multiphasic technique, to increase the likelihood of achieving maximum conspicuity. According to a study of 44 patients, a hypovascular pattern of hepatic metastases was associated with early progression.[104] The presence of hepatic metastatic disease may not be symptomatic, even when significant tumor burden is present. However, the implication of liver metastases demands careful consideration because approximately 80% of patients will succumb to the disease in 5 years if untreated.

A systematic search of the peritoneal cavity must be undertaken if small peritoneal deposits are to be detected on imaging before they become clinically evident, causing symptoms, most commonly bowel obstruction.

SST imaging can identify distant metastases that are difficult to identify by conventional anatomic imaging. This difficulty can be caused by small size, such as metastases within the peritoneal cavity or in small lymph nodes, or distant sites, such as metastases outside of the abdomen and pelvis or in the bone marrow. SR-PET/CT is becoming the preferred functional imaging study for these tumors and can change management in a significant number of cases.[57]

Tumor Response

Assessing response to treatment in an objective and reproducible way is of utmost importance in oncologic imaging, both for individual patient management in daily clinical practice and in the context of randomized and nonrandomized clinical trials. Tumor response is based on careful analysis of objective and subjective parameters.

Objective Criteria Based on Tumor Size

The revised RECIST version 1.1 is the mainstay for response evaluation in a wide variety of tumors, including PNETs, both for the primary and metastatic sites of disease involvement with focus on the liver.[105] RECIST 1.1 is based on careful assessment of percent changes in tumor measurements at baseline and across multiple endpoints, as well as identification of new sites of disease. There are specific criteria to define measureable and nonmeasureable disease in solid organs, lymph nodes, peritoneum, and bone, and what lesions should be selected as target and nontarget. To determine response or progression, it is necessary

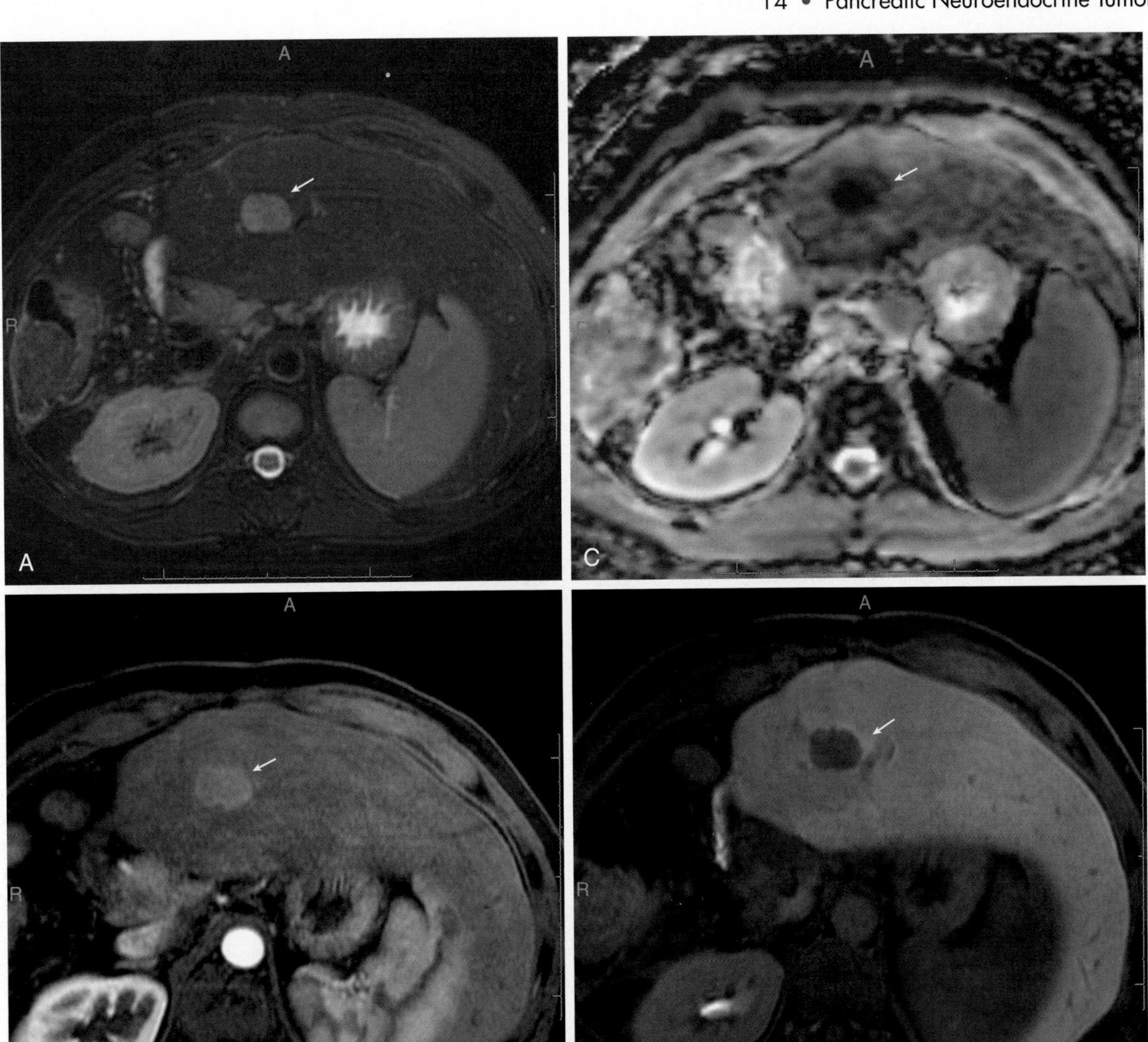

FIGURE 14.13. A 43-year-old male with metastatic well-differentiated pancreatic neuroendocrine tumor, grade 2. There are postoperative changes of extended right hepatectomy with hypertrophy of the liver remnant (segments II and IIII). Axial T2-weighted image shows a hypertense metastasis in the liver remnant (**A**). The metastasis shows homogenous enhancement during the arterial phase (*arrow* in **B**), and there is evidence of diffusion restriction in the apparent diffusion coefficient map (*arrow* in **C**). The 20 minute delayed hepatobiliary phase shows the lesion with great conspicuity (*arrow* in **D**). This sequence is it is not affected by the quality of intravenous bolus, making it ideally suited for tumor measurements, reducing the chances of interobserver variability that can be caused by technical differences between scans.

to estimate the overall tumor burden at baseline and use it as a comparator on subsequent endpoint assessments. If more than one site of measurable disease is present, up to five target lesions may be selected (two per organ), and the radiologist should select those that would allow reproducible measurements on subsequent examinations. Four distinct groups are defined based on percent changes in size of the lesions. Complete response is defined as disappearance of all target lesions. Partial response is defined as 30% decrease in the sum of longest diameters (SLD) of all target lesions in relation to baseline measurements. Progressive disease is defined as at least 20% increase in the SLD of target lesions from nadir (in addition to 20% increase, an absolute increase of at least 5 mm must be documented) or the appearance of new lesions. Stable disease is defined as neither sufficient decrease to qualify as partial response nor sufficient increase to qualify for progressive disease.[105] Measurements are to be obtained in the axial plane on contrast-enhanced CT or MRI. The 20minute delayed series of MRI performed with hepatocyte-specific contrast agents provides a simple, reliable way to reproducibly measure hepatic metastases.

Size criteria are objective and reproducible, and have been proven useful with cytotoxic chemotherapy in advanced PNETs.[106] However, RECIST 1.1 is not ideal to assess response with targeted therapies, or for tumors with slow growth rate.[107] Response rates by RECIST 1.1 tend to be low with long-acting SST analogs and PRRT, and response is inferred from improved PFS or time to progression.[108,109]

Morphologic Changes Unrelated to Size

With the advent of targeted therapy, new response criteria unrelated to tumor size, but based on tumor morphology, focusing on texture and attenuation, have emerged and been found to be useful in several tumors.[110–113]

These studies underscore the importance of assessing not only size, but also morphological and textural changes such as lesion margins, internal attenuation, presence, or absence of internal enhancement, and so on, to evaluate response. Evaluating response in hepatic metastases from PNETs following bland-embolization, chemoembolization, or radioembolization is similar to what has been reported in the literature with hepatocellular carcinoma. Response is based not only on a decrease in size, but also, and perhaps more importantly, on a decrease in internal solid components judged by loss of internal vascularity/enhancing components in comparison to baseline. With radioembolization, a decrease in size may be delayed by 6 months, but tumor viability or response can be assessed sooner by carefully checking for the persistence, decrease, and/or disappearance of internal enhancement within the lesion.[112,114,115]

Evaluation after radiofrequency ablation requires meticulous assessment of the size of the ablation zone and its margins, systematically comparing pre- and postprocedure examinations.[116]

Response by Functional Imaging

SST imaging may reveal disease sites that are difficult to identify on conventional anatomic imaging studies. SRS may provide a qualitative assessment of disease and may identify new sites when compared with an appropriate baseline study. SR-PET/CT can identify many more sites of disease than can SRS, so comparison between these two types of studies should be done very cautiously. Although standardized uptake values (SUVs), a semiquantative measurement, can be obtained on SR-PET/CT, it is unclear how much change in SUV indicates a relevant clinical change, and superimposed SST therapy may also affect SUV measurements. SR-PET/CT may most useful when there is clinical suspicion for recurrent or progressive disease and anatomic imaging studies are unrevealing or considered stable.[117]

KEY POINTS

Image Response

- Tumor response is based on careful evaluation of objective and subjective criteria such as size (change in size and detection of new lesions), morphology (morphological changes unrelated to size/internal attenuation and enhancement) and functional imaging (standard uptake value on positron emission tomography/computed tomography).
- Response Evaluation Criteria for Solid Tumors 1.1 is the mainstay for objective response evaluation in pancreatic neuroendocrine tumors and dominates the context of clinical trials.

SUMMARY

PNETs are a group of relatively uncommon pancreatic tumors that are increasing in incidence and prevalence, so they are likely to be encountered at some frequency in any oncology or radiology practice. There is great variability in their imaging appearances, morphologic characteristics, and biological behavior, ranging from extremely indolent lesions to highly aggressive high-grade malignancies with dismal prognosis. Nonfunctional PNETs account for the majority of PNETs. MDCT and MRI with multiphasic technique are necessary to optimize conspicuity of the primary lesion, as well as potential sites of metastatic disease (lymph nodes and liver). A multidisciplinary approach to patient care is important to incorporate evolving advances in pathological classification, imaging techniques for diagnosis and staging, and therapeutic options and interventions. This chapter presents a review of the pathology, clinical presentation, proposed TNM staging, imaging findings, and treatment options.

REFERENCES

1. Ehehalt F, Saeger HD, Schmidt CM, et al. Neuroendocrine tumors of the pancreas. *Oncologist*. 2009;14:456–467.
2. Thompson M, Fleming KA, Evans DJ, et al. Gastric endocrine cells share a clonal origin with other gut cell lineages. *Development*. 1990;110:477–481.
3. Pearse AG. The cytochemistry and ultrastructure of polypeptide hormone-producing cells of the APUD series and the embryologic, physiologic and pathologic implications of the concept. *J Histochem Cytochem*. 1969;17:303–313.
4. Heitz PU, Kasper M, Polak JM, et al. Pancreatic endocrine tumors. *Hum Pathol*. 1982;13:263–271.
5. Andrew A, Kramer B, Rawdon BB. The origin of gut and pancreatic neuroendocrine (APUD) cells--the last word? *J Pathol*. 1998;186:117–118.
6. Klimstra DS, Modlin IR, Coppola D, et al. The pathologic classification of neuroendocrine tumors: a review of nomenclature, grading, and staging systems. *Pancreas*. 2010;39:707–712.
7. Basturk O, Yang Z, Tang LH, et al. The high-grade (WHO G3) pancreatic neuroendocrine tumor category is morphologically and biologically heterogenous and includes both well differentiated and poorly differentiated neoplasms. *Am J Surg Pathol*. 2015;39:683–690.
8. Bosman F, Carneiro F, Hruban RH, et al. *WHO classification of tumours of the digestive system*. 4th ed. Lyon: International Agency for Research on Cancer; 2010.
9. Kloppel G, Klimstra DS, Hruban R, et al. Pancreatic neuroendocrine tumors: update on the new World Health Organization classification. *AJSP: Reviews & Reports*. 2017;22:233–239.

10. Yao JC, Hassan M, Phan A, et al. One hundred years after "carcinoid": epidemiology of and prognostic factors for neuroendocrine tumors in 35,825 cases in the United States. *J Clin Oncol*. 2008;26:3063–3072.
11. Dasari A, Shen C, Halperin D, et al. Trends in the incidence, prevalence, and survival outcomes in patients with neuroendocrine tumors in the United States. *JAMA Oncol*. 2017;3:1335–1342.
12. Jensen RT, Berna MJ, Bingham DB, et al. Inherited pancreatic endocrine tumor syndromes: advances in molecular pathogenesis, diagnosis, management, and controversies. *Cancer*. 2008;113:1807–1843.
13. Lemos MC, Thakker RV. Multiple endocrine neoplasia type 1 (MEN1): analysis of 1336 mutations reported in the first decade following identification of the gene. *Hum Mutat*. 2008;29:22–32.
14. Wilkinson S, Teh BT, Davey KR, et al. Cause of death in multiple endocrine neoplasia type 1. *Arch Surg*. 1993;128:683–690.
15. Dean PG, van Heerden JA, Farley DR, et al. Are patients with multiple endocrine neoplasia type I prone to premature death? *World J Surg*. 2000;24:1437–1441.
16. Lonser RR, Glenn GM, Walther M, et al. von Hippel-Lindau disease. *Lancet*. 2003;361:2059–2067.
17. Libutti SK, Choyke PL, Bartlett DL, et al. Pancreatic neuroendocrine tumors associated with von Hippel Lindau disease: diagnostic and management recommendations. *Surgery*. 1998;124:1153–1159.
18. Mao C, Shah A, Hanson DJ, et al. Von Recklinghausen's disease associated with duodenal somatostatinoma: contrast of duodenal versus pancreatic somatostatinomas. *J Surg Oncol*. 1995;59:67–73.
19. Fujisawa T, Osuga T, Maeda M, et al. Malignant endocrine tumor of the pancreas associated with von Recklinghausen's disease. *J Gastroenterol*. 2002;37:59–67.
20. Kadir S, Lundell C, Saeed M. Celiac, superior and inferior mesenteric arteries. In: *Atlas of Normal and Variant Angiographic Anatomy*. 1st ed. Philadephia, PA: Saunders; 1991:297–364.
21. Kadir S, Lundell C. The portal venous system and hepatic veins. In: *Atlas of Normal and Variant Angiographic Anatomy*. Philadephia, PA: Saunders; 1991:365–385.
22. Witte B, Frober R, Linss W. Unusual blood supply to the pancreas by a dorsal pancreatic artery. *Surg Radiol Anat*. 2001;23:197–200.
23. Crabo LG, Conley DM, Graney DO, et al. Venous anatomy of the pancreatic head: normal CT appearance in cadavers and patients. *AJR Am J Roentgenol*. 1993;160:1039–1045.
24. Frankel WL. Update on pancreatic endocrine tumors. *Arch Pathol Lab Med*. 2006;130:963–966.
25. Kloppel G, Couvelard A, Perren A, et al. ENETS Consensus Guidelines for the Standards of Care in Neuroendocrine Tumors: towards a standardized approach to the diagnosis of gastroenteropancreatic neuroendocrine tumors and their prognostic stratification. *Neuroendocrinology*. 2009;90:162–166.
26. Kloppel G, Rindi G, Perren A, et al. The ENETS and AJCC/UICC TNM classifications of the neuroendocrine tumors of the gastrointestinal tract and the pancreas: a statement. *Virchows Arch*. 2010;456:595–597.
27. Leung HHW, Chan AWH. Updates of pancreatic neuroendocrine neoplasm in the 2017 World Health Organization classification. *Surg Pract*. 2019:42–47.
28. Luo G, Javed A, Strosberg JR, et al. Modified staging classification for pancreatic neuroendocrine tumors on the basis of the American Joint Committee on Cancer and European Neuroendocrine Tumor Society systems. *J Clin Oncol*. 2017;35:274–280.
29. Bergsland EK, Woltering EA, Rindi G, et al. Neuroendocrine tumors of the pancreas. In: *AJCC Cancer Staging Manual*. 8th ed. Chicago, IL: Springer; 2017:407–419.
30. Marcal LP, Patnana M, Yedururi S, et al. Abdominal manifestations of neuroendocrine tumors. *Dig Dis Interv*. 2019;03:14–29.
31. Sahani DV, Bonaffini PA, Fernandez-Del Castillo C, et al. Gastroenteropancreatic neuroendocrine tumors: role of imaging in diagnosis and management. *Radiology*. 2013;266:38–61.
32. Langer P, Kann PH, Fendrich V, et al. Prospective evaluation of imaging procedures for the detection of pancreaticoduodenal endocrine tumors in patients with multiple endocrine neoplasia type 1. *World J Surg*. 2004;28:1317–1322.
33. Sundin A, Vullierme MP, Kaltsas G, et al. ENETS consensus guidelines for the standards of care in neuroendocrine tumors: radiological examinations. *Neuroendocrinology*. 2009;90:167–183.
34. Wamsteker EJ, Gauger PG, Thompson NW, et al. EUS detection of pancreatic endocrine tumors in asymptomatic patients with type 1 multiple endocrine neoplasia. *Gastrointest Endosc*. 2003;58:531–535.
35. Metz DC, Jensen RT. Gastrointestinal neuroendocrine tumors: pancreatic endocrine tumors. *Gastroenterology*. 2008;135:1469–1492.
36. Fujimori N, Osoegawa T, Lee L, et al. Efficacy of endoscopic ultrasonography and endoscopic ultrasonography-guided fine-needle aspiration for the diagnosis and grading of pancreatic neuroendocrine tumors. *Scand J Gastroenterol*. 2016;51:245–252.
37. Sun MR, Brennan DD, Kruskal JB, et al. Intraoperative ultrasonography of the pancreas. *Radiographics*. 2010;30:1935–1953.
38. Kim JH, Eun HW, Kim YJ, et al. Pancreatic neuroendocrine tumour (PNET): Staging accuracy of MDCT and its diagnostic performance for the differentiation of PNET with uncommon CT findings from pancreatic adenocarcinoma. *Eur Radiol*. 2016;26:1338–1347.
39. Buetow PC, Parrino TV, Buck JL, et al. Islet cell tumors of the pancreas: pathologic-imaging correlation among size, necrosis and cysts, calcification, malignant behavior, and functional status. *AJR Am J Roentgenol*. 1995;165:1175–1179.
40. Rodallec M, Vilgrain V, Couvelard A, et al. Endocrine pancreatic tumours and helical CT: contrast enhancement is correlated with microvascular density, histoprognostic factors and survival. *Pancreatology*. 2006;6:77–85.
41. Tempero MA, Malafa MP, Al-Hawary M, et al. Pancreatic Adenocarcinoma, Version 2.2017, NCCN Clinical Practice Guidelines in Oncology. *J Natl Compr Canc Netw*. 2017;15:1028–1061.
42. Balachandran A, Tamm EP, Bhosale PR, et al. Venous tumor thrombus in nonfunctional pancreatic neuroendocrine tumors. *AJR Am J Roentgenol*. 2012;199:602–608.
43. Manfredi R, Bonatti M, Mantovani W, et al. Non-hyperfunctioning neuroendocrine tumours of the pancreas: MR imaging appearance and correlation with their biological behaviour. *Eur Radiol*. 2013;23:3029–3039.
44. Humphrey PE, Alessandrino F, Bellizzi AM, et al. Non-hyperfunctioning pancreatic endocrine tumors: multimodality imaging features with histopathological correlation. *Abdom Imaging*. 2015;40:2398–2410.
45. Jeon SK, Lee JM, Joo I, et al. Nonhypervascular pancreatic neuroendocrine tumors: differential diagnosis from pancreatic ductal adenocarcinomas at MR imaging-retrospective cross-sectional study. *Radiology*. 2017;284:77–87.
46. Procacci C, Carbognin G, Accordini S, et al. Nonfunctioning endocrine tumors of the pancreas: possibilities of spiral CT characterization. *Eur Radiol*. 2001;11:1175–1183.
47. Thoeni RF, Mueller-Lisse UG, Chan R, et al. Detection of small, functional islet cell tumors in the pancreas: selection of MR imaging sequences for optimal sensitivity. *Radiology*. 2000;214:483–490.
48. Semelka RC, Custodio CM, Cem Balci N, et al. Neuroendocrine tumors of the pancreas: spectrum of appearances on MRI. *J Magn Reson Imaging*. 2000;11:141–148.
49. Dromain C, de Baere T, Baudin E, et al. MR imaging of hepatic metastases caused by neuroendocrine tumors: comparing four techniques. *AJR Am J Roentgenol*. 2003;180:121–128.
50. Debray MP, Geoffroy O, Laissy JP, et al. Imaging appearances of metastases from neuroendocrine tumours of the pancreas. *Br J Radiol*. 2001;74:1065–1070.
51. Krenning EP, Bakker WH, Breeman WA, et al. Localisation of endocrine-related tumours with radioiodinated analogue of somatostatin. *Lancet*. 1989;1:242–244.
52. Tamm EP, Kim EE, Ng CS. Imaging of neuroendocrine tumors. *Hematol Oncol Clin North Am*. 2007;21:409–432; vii.
53. Krenning EP, Bakker WH, Kooij PP, et al. Somatostatin receptor scintigraphy with indium-111-DTPA-D-Phe-1-octreotide in man: metabolism, dosimetry and comparison with iodine-123-Tyr-3-octreotide. *J Nucl Med*. 1992;33:652–658.
54. Balon HR. Updated practice guideline for somatostatin receptor scintigraphy. *J Nucl Med*. 2011;52:1838.
55. Krenning EP, Kwekkeboom DJ, Bakker WH, et al. Somatostatin receptor scintigraphy with [111In-DTPA-D-Phe1]- and [123I-Tyr3]-octreotide: the Rotterdam experience with more than 1000 patients. *Eur J Nucl Med*. 1993;20:716–731.
56. Gabriel M, Decristoforo C, Kendler D, et al. 68Ga-DOTA-Tyr3-octreotide PET in neuroendocrine tumors: comparison with somatostatin receptor scintigraphy and CT. *J Nucl Med*. 2007;48:508–518.
57. Deppen SA, Blume J, Bobbey AJ, et al. 68Ga-DOTATATE Compared with 111In-DTPA-Octreotide and conventional imaging for pulmonary and gastroenteropancreatic neuroendocrine tumors:

a systematic review and meta-analysis. *J Nucl Med*. 2016;57: 872–878.
58. Hofman MS, Lau WF, Hicks RJ. Somatostatin receptor imaging with 68Ga DOTATATE PET/CT: clinical utility, normal patterns, pearls, and pitfalls in interpretation. *Radiographics*. 2015;35:500–516.
59. Shastry M, Kayani I, Wild D, et al. Distribution pattern of 68Ga-DOTATATE in disease-free patients. *Nucl Med Commun*. 2010;31:1025–1032.
60. Binderup T, Knigge U, Loft A, et al. Functional imaging of neuroendocrine tumors: a head-to-head comparison of somatostatin receptor scintigraphy, 123I-MIBG scintigraphy, and 18F-FDG PET. *J Nucl Med*. 2010;51:704–712.
61. Aoki T, Sakon M, Ohzato H, et al. Evaluation of preoperative and intraoperative arterial stimulation and venous sampling for diagnosis and surgical resection of insulinoma. *Surgery*. 1999;126:968–973.
62. Brandle M, Pfammatter T, Spinas GA, et al. Assessment of selective arterial calcium stimulation and hepatic venous sampling to localize insulin-secreting tumours. *Clin Endocrinol (Oxf)*. 2001;55:357–362.
63. Rinke A, Muller HH, Schade-Brittinger C, et al. Placebo-controlled, double-blind, prospective, randomized study on the effect of octreotide LAR in the control of tumor growth in patients with metastatic neuroendocrine midgut tumors: a report from the PROMID Study Group. *J Clin Oncol*. 2009;27:4656–4663.
64. Clark OH, Benson 3rd AB, Berlin JD, et al. NCCN Clinical Practice Guidelines in Oncology: neuroendocrine tumors. *J Natl Compr Canc Netw*. 2009;7:712–747.
65. Raj N, Fazio N, Strosberg J. Biology and systemic treatment of advanced gastroenteropancreatic neuroendocrine tumors. *Am Soc Clin Oncol Educ Book*. 2018:292–299.
66. NCC Network. About the NCCN Clinical Practive Guidelines in Oncology (NCCN Guidelines). Available at: https://www.nccn.org/professionals/.
67. Raymond E, Borbath I, Raoul J, et al. Phase III, randomized, double-blind trial of sunitinib versus placebo in patients with progressive, well-differentiated pancreatic islet cell tumours. *Annals of Oncology*. 2009;20:11–11.
68. Yao JC, Shah MH, Ito T, et al. Everolimus for advanced pancreatic neuroendocrine tumors. *N Engl J Med*. 2011;364:514–523.
69. Kouvaraki MA, Ajani JA, Hoff P, et al. Fluorouracil, doxorubicin, and streptozocin in the treatment of patients with locally advanced and metastatic pancreatic endocrine carcinomas. *J Clin Oncol*. 2004;22:4762–4771.
70. Kunz PL, Catalano PJ, Nimeiri H, et al. A randomized study of temozolomide or temozolomide and capecitabine in patients with advanced pancreatic neuroendocrine tumors: A trial of the ECOG-ACRIN Cancer Research Group (E2211). *J Clin Oncol*. 2018;36 4004-4004.
71. Strosberg J, Krenning E. 177Lu-Dotatate for Midgut Neuroendocrine Tumors. *N Engl J Med*. 2017;376:1391–1392.
72. Brabander T, van der Zwan WA, Teunissen JJM, et al. Long-term efficacy, survival, and safety of [(177)Lu-DOTA(0),Tyr(3)]octreotate in patients with gastroenteropancreatic and bronchial neuroendocrine tumors. *Clin Cancer Res*. 2017;23:4617–4624.
73. Grant CS. Insulinoma. *Best Pract Res Clin Gastroenterol*. 2005;19: 783–798.
74. Service FJ, McMahon MM, O'Brien PC, et al. Functioning insulinoma--incidence, recurrence, and long-term survival of patients: a 60-year study. *Mayo Clin Proc*. 1991;66:711–719.
75. Fernandez-Cruz L, Saenz A, Astudillo E, et al. Outcome of laparoscopic pancreatic surgery: endocrine and nonendocrine tumors. *World J Surg*. 2002;26:1057–1065.
76. D'Haese JG, Tosolini C, Ceyhan GO, et al. Update on surgical treatment of pancreatic neuroendocrine neoplasms. *World J Gastroenterol*. 2014;20:13893–13898.
77. Berna MJ, Hoffmann KM, Serrano J, et al. Serum gastrin in Zollinger-Ellison syndrome: I. Prospective study of fasting serum gastrin in 309 patients from the National Institutes of Health and comparison with 2229 cases from the literature. *Medicine (Baltimore)*. 2006;85:295–330.
78. Frucht H, Howard JM, Slaff JI, et al. Secretin and calcium provocative tests in the Zollinger-Ellison syndrome. A prospective study. *Ann Intern Med*. 1989;111:713–722.
79. Tomassetti P, Migliori M, Lalli S, et al. Epidemiology, clinical features and diagnosis of gastroenteropancreatic endocrine tumours. *Ann Oncol*. 2001;12(Suppl 2):S95–S99.
80. Weber HC, Venzon DJ, Lin JT, et al. Determinants of metastatic rate and survival in patients with Zollinger-Ellison syndrome: a prospective long-term study. *Gastroenterology*. 1995;108:1637–1649.
81. Skogseid B, Eriksson B, Lundqvist G, et al. Multiple endocrine neoplasia type 1: a 10-year prospective screening study in four kindreds. *J Clin Endocrinol Metab*. 1991;73:281–287.
82. Fraker DL, Norton JA, Alexander HR, et al. Surgery in Zollinger-Ellison syndrome alters the natural history of gastrinoma. *Ann Surg*. 1994;220:320–328; discussion 328-330.
83. Norton JA, Fraker DL, Alexander HR, et al. Surgery to cure the Zollinger-Ellison syndrome. *N Engl J Med*. 1999;341:635–644.
84. Dickson PV, Rich TA, Xing Y, et al. Achieving eugastrinemia in MEN1 patients: both duodenal inspection and formal lymph node dissection are important. *Surgery*. 2011;150:1143–1152.
85. Norton JA, Jensen RT. Resolved and unresolved controversies in the surgical management of patients with Zollinger-Ellison syndrome. *Ann Surg*. 2004;240:757–773.
86. Nikou GC, Toubanakis C, Nikolaou P, et al. VIPomas: an update in diagnosis and management in a series of 11 patients. *Hepatogastroenterology*. 2005;52:1259–1265.
87. Ghaferi AA, Chojnacki KA, Long WD, et al. Pancreatic VIPomas: subject review and one institutional experience. *J Gastrointest Surg*. 2008;12:382–393.
88. Soga J, Yakuwa Y. Vipoma/diarrheogenic syndrome: a statistical evaluation of 241 reported cases. *J Exp Clin Cancer Res*. 1998;17:389–400.
89. van Beek AP, de Haas ER, van Vloten WA, et al. The glucagonoma syndrome and necrolytic migratory erythema: a clinical review. *Eur J Endocrinol*. 2004;151:531–537.
90. Wermers RA, Fatourechi V, Wynne AG, et al. The glucagonoma syndrome. Clinical and pathologic features in 21 patients. *Medicine (Baltimore)*. 1996;75:53–63.
91. Soga J, Yakuwa Y. Glucagonomas/diabetico-dermatogenic syndrome (DDS): a statistical evaluation of 407 reported cases. *J Hepatobiliary Pancreat Surg*. 1998;5:312–319.
92. Falconi M, Plockinger U, Kwekkeboom DJ, et al. Well-differentiated pancreatic nonfunctioning tumors/carcinoma. *Neuroendocrinology*. 2006;84:196–211.
93. Solorzano CC, Lee JE, Pisters PW, et al. Nonfunctioning islet cell carcinoma of the pancreas: survival results in a contemporary series of 163 patients. *Surgery*. 2001;130:1078–1085.
94. Evans DB, Skibber JM, Lee JE, et al. Nonfunctioning islet cell carcinoma of the pancreas. *Surgery*. 1993;114:1175–1181; discussion 1181-1172.
95. Bloomston M, Muscarella P, Shah MH, et al. Cytoreduction results in high perioperative mortality and decreased survival in patients undergoing pancreatectomy for neuroendocrine tumors of the pancreas. *J Gastrointest Surg*. 2006;10:1361–1370.
96. Powers BD, Rothermel LD, Fleming JB, et al. A survival analysis of patients with localized, asymptomatic pancreatic neuroendocrine tumors: no surgical survival benefit when examining appropriately selected outcomes. *J Gastrointest Surg*. 2019;24(12):1773–1779.
97. Falconi M, Bartsch DK, Eriksson B, et al. ENETS Consensus Guidelines for the management of patients with digestive neuroendocrine neoplasms of the digestive system: well-differentiated pancreatic non-functioning tumors. *Neuroendocrinology*. 2012;95:120–134.
98. Kamilaris CDC, Stratakis CA. Multiple endocrine neoplasia type 1 (MEN1): An update and the significance of early genetic and clinical diagnosis. *Front Endocrinol (Lausanne)*. 2019;10:339.
99. Bilimoria KY, Tomlinson JS, Merkow RP, et al. Clinicopathologic features and treatment trends of pancreatic neuroendocrine tumors: analysis of 9,821 patients. *J Gastrointest Surg*. 2007;11:1460–1467; discussion 1467-1469.
100. Modlin IM, Oberg K, Chung DC, et al. Gastroenteropancreatic neuroendocrine tumours. *Lancet Oncol*. 2008;9:61–72.
101. Chan DL, Thompson R, Lam M, et al. External beam radiotherapy in the treatment of gastroenteropancreatic neuroendocrine tumours: a systematic review. *Clin Oncol (R Coll Radiol)*. 2018;30:400–408.
102. Partelli S, Gaujoux S, Boninsegna L, et al. Pattern and clinical predictors of lymph node involvement in nonfunctioning pancreatic neuroendocrine tumors (NF-PanNETs). *JAMA Surg*. 2013;148:932–939.
103. Riihimaki M, Hemminki A, Sundquist K, et al. The epidemiology of metastases in neuroendocrine tumors. *Int J Cancer*. 2016;139:2679–2686.
104. Denecke T, Baur AD, Ihm C, et al. Evaluation of radiological prognostic factors of hepatic metastases in patients with non-functional pancreatic neuroendocrine tumors. *Eur J Radiol*. 2013;82:e550–e555.

105. Eisenhauer EA, Therasse P, Bogaerts J, et al. New response evaluation criteria in solid tumours: revised RECIST guideline (version 1.1). *Eur J Cancer*. 2009;45:228–247.
106. Krug S, Gress TM, Michl P, et al. The role of cytotoxic chemotherapy in advanced pancreatic neuroendocrine tumors. *Digestion*. 2017;96:67–75.
107. de Mestier L, Dromain C, d'Assignies G, et al. Evaluating digestive neuroendocrine tumor progression and therapeutic responses in the era of targeted therapies: state of the art. *Endocr Relat Cancer*. 2014;21:R105–R120.
108. Strosberg J, El-Haddad G, Wolin E, et al. Phase 3 trial of (177) Lu-Dotatate for midgut neuroendocrine tumors. *N Engl J Med*. 2017;376:125–135.
109. Enzler T, Fojo T. Long-acting somatostatin analogues in the treatment of unresectable/metastatic neuroendocrine tumors. *Semin Oncol*. 2017;44:141–156.
110. Choi H. Response evaluation of gastrointestinal stromal tumors. *Oncologist*. 2008;13(Suppl 2):4–7.
111. Chun YS, Vauthey JN, Boonsirikamchai P, et al. Association of computed tomography morphologic criteria with pathologic response and survival in patients treated with bevacizumab for colorectal liver metastases. *JAMA*. 2009;302:2338–2344.
112. Lencioni R, Llovet JM. Modified RECIST (mRECIST) assessment for hepatocellular carcinoma. *Semin Liver Dis*. 2010;30:52–60.
113. Smith AD, Shah SN, Rini BI, et al. Morphology, attenuation, size, and structure (MASS) criteria: assessing response and predicting clinical outcome in metastatic renal cell carcinoma on antiangiogenic targeted therapy. *AJR Am J Roentgenol*. 2010;194:1470–1478.
114. Joo I, Kim HC, Kim GM, et al. Imaging evaluation following (90) Y radioembolization of liver tumors: what radiologists should know. *Korean J Radiol*. 2018;19:209–222.
115. Faivre S, Ronot M, Dreyer C, et al. Imaging response in neuroendocrine tumors treated with targeted therapies: the experience of sunitinib. *Target Oncol*. 2012;7:127–133.
116. Yedururi S, Terpenning S, Gupta S, et al. Radiofrequency ablation of hepatic tumor: subjective assessment of the perilesional vascular network on contrast-enhanced computed tomography before and after ablation can reliably predict the risk of local recurrence. *J Comput Assist Tomogr*. 2017;41:607–613.
117. Hope TA, Bergsland EK, Bozkurt MF, et al. Appropriate use criteria for somatostatin receptor PET imaging in neuroendocrine tumors. *J Nucl Med*. 2018;59:66–74.

PART V

GASTROINTESTINAL TRACT

CHAPTER 15

Esophageal Cancer

Sonia L. Betancourt-Cuellar, M.D.; Marcelo F. Kuperman Benveniste, M.D.; Diana P. Palacio, M.D.; Wayne L. Hofstetter, M.D.; and Edith M. Marom, M.D.

INTRODUCTION

Esophageal cancer (EC) is a devastating diagnosis with a high morbidity and mortality. The overall 5-year survival rate for all combined stages remains dismally low, at approximately 17%.[1] Although it is a relatively uncommon malignancy, accounting for less than 1% of all malignancies, it has been steadily increasing in incidence since the 1980s. Approximately 17,650 new cases were reported in the United States in 2019 with an estimated 16,080 deaths.[2] At the time of presentation, 20% of patients have a localized stage suitable for curative resection, nearly 30% have a locally advanced stage, and more than 30% have metastatic disease.[1] However, during the last few years a greater understanding of the biology of the disease has led to significant improvements in both staging and therapeutic options.

Optimal management depends on effective multidisciplinary care that includes multimodality staging and combined modality treatment, incorporating chemotherapy, radiation therapy, and surgery. For the radiologist, appropriate imaging requires a full understanding of the behavior and staging of EC in addition to a familiarity with the available treatment options.

For the surgeon and clinician, recognition of the limitations and pitfalls of each imaging modality is important to appropriately use the information obtained from imaging during the initial evaluation and follow-up.

Epidemiology and Risk Factors

EC is a worldwide disease with an incidence that varies according to geographic location. In the United States, EC accounts for less than 1% of all cancers, but has a high mortality rate and is responsible for 3% of all cancer deaths.[2]

The two most common histologic types of EC are squamous cell carcinoma (SCC) and adenocarcinoma (AC). SCC accounts for over 80% of all cases of EC worldwide and is the predominant type in less developed countries (e.g., Central and Southeast Asia). The incidence of SCC in men has decreased globally since the early 1980s; in contrast, the incidence in women has decreased slightly or stabilized.[3]

During the last four decades there has been an increasing incidence of AC in Europe, Northern America, and Australia. The incidence of AC has exceeded that of SCC in many Western countries.[3,4] AC has a male predominance, with a worldwide male to female ratio of 6 to 8:1 in the United States; in addition, the incidence of AC is markedly higher in White people than in other races in the United States.[3,4]

Risk factors for the development of SCC of the esophagus include alcohol intake, smoking, and lower socioeconomic status. Multiple studies have reported an increased risk of SCC associated with low consumption of fresh vegetables and fruit and high intake of pickled vegetables, but there is a lack of prospective studies confirming this factor.[3]

Risk factors for AC of the esophagus include Barrett's esophagus (epithelial metaplasia) related to chronic gastroesophageal reflux, and increased body mass index; alcohol does not appear to be a significant risk factor for AC.[5]

There is not a clear explanation for the rising incidence of AC of the esophagus and its striking male predominance (7:1). Epidemiologic data do not support direct correlations with the increased incidence of AC and gastroesophageal reflux, the greater incidence of obesity, or the decreased incidence of *Helicobacter pylori* infection.[1] Tobacco use among males has decreased in recent years, which may partly account for the decreasing incidence in SCC of the esophagus but does not explain the increasing incidence of AC.

Currently there is not enough evidence to implement a mass-screening program in the United States, because of the low incidence of EC in the country. In areas of China with high-risk populations, it has been found that screening and subsequent early diagnosis and treatment provide great cost savings because of the much lower cost of screening compared with the cost of multimodality treatment of invasive esophageal carcinoma.[6,7]

KEY POINTS

Epidemiology and Risk Factors

- In the United States, esophageal cancers accounts for less than 1% of all cancers, but has high mortality, accounting for 3% of cancer deaths.
- Risk factors: gastroesophageal reflux, obesity, lower socioeconomic state, alcohol, smoking.
- There is male predominance and a rising incidence of esophageal adenocarcinoma.

Anatomy and Pathology

SCC and AC are both epithelial in origin but otherwise differ greatly in anatomic proclivity, risk factors, pathologic behavior, and prognosis. For staging and clinical purposes, they can be considered separate diseases. SCC is a disease of nicotine and alcohol abuse, risk factors that affect the entire esophagus and partly explain why SCC arises in the mid- and upper thoracic esophagus above the level of the carina in up to 65% of cases. AC, conversely, is strongly linked to gastroesophageal reflux disease and Barrett's esophagus, and is most often located below the level of the carina. SCC of the esophagus is also associated with a significantly worse prognosis than AC.

Because the behavior of and surgical options for EC vary according to its location, the esophagus is divided into four distinct anatomic regions for EC classification; but for the purposes of staging, the location of the tumor is defined by taking endoscopic measurements of each region from the incisors.[8] The cervical esophagus extends from the cricopharyngeus muscle to the suprasternal notch, and the typical endoscopic measurement places it at 15 to 20 cm from the incisors; the upper thoracic esophagus extends from the suprasternal notch to the lower border of the azygos vein, at 20 to 25 cm from the incisors; the midthoracic esophagus extends from the lower border of the azygos vein to the inferior pulmonary veins, at 25 to 30 cm from the incisors; and the lower thoracic esophagus extends from the inferior pulmonary veins to the stomach and includes the intraabdominal esophagus and the gastroesophageal junction, at 30 to 40 cm from the incisors[8] (Fig. 15.1).

According to the 8th edition of the American Joint Commission on Cancer (AJCC), cancers involving the gastroesophageal junction that have their epicenter within the proximal 2 cm of the cardia are to be staged as ECs, whereas those with a epicenter more than 2 cm distal from the gastroesophageal junction, even is the junction is involved, will be staged as stomach cancers.[8,9].

Histologically, the esophageal wall comprises the mucosa, the submucosa, the muscularis propria, and the adventitia. Local tumor invasion is determined according to the involvement of each of these histologic layers. There is no serosa surrounding the esophagus, facilitating local tumor invasion into pleura, pericardium, diaphragm, or peritoneum.

A rich lymphatic network drains the esophagus, with channels running both radially and longitudinally, facilitating early dissemination of lymphatic and distant metastases. Most of the lymphatics are concentrated in the submucosa, but they are also present in the lamina propria of the mucosa and connect to periesophageal lymph node stations and with the thoracic duct. The longitudinal lymphatic plexus in the submucosa facilitates orthogonal drainage both cranially and caudally, with the result that nodal disease may be located distant to the primary tumor without involvement of adjacent lymph nodes ("skip" metastases).[10]

Regional lymph nodes are defined as any periesophageal lymph node from the upper esophageal sphincter to the celiac axis. These include lower cervical periesophageal lymph nodes; intrathoracic lymph nodes in the periesophageal region, bilateral paratracheal nodes, and subcarinal nodes; diaphragmatic lymph nodes adjacent to the crura; left gastric and pericardial lymph nodes; and common hepatic, splenic, and celiac lymph nodes. Lymph node involvement outside these regions is considered distant metastatic disease.[8]

KEY POINTS

Anatomy and Pathology

- Squamous cell carcinoma of the esophagus is more commonly located above the level of the carina and is associated with a significantly worse prognosis than adenocarcinoma.
- The esophagus does not have a serosa, thereby facilitating adjacent organ invasion by tumor.
- The extensive submucosal lymphatic plexus facilitates both orthogonal and radial spread of metastatic disease in the lymphatics.

Clinical Presentation

Most ECs, particularly ACs, arise in the distal esophagus or at the gastroesophageal junction. Given the distensibility of the esophagus, patients in early stage typically do not exhibit recognizable symptoms. Early-stage patients are discovered on Barrett's surveillance, incidentally, or when being worked up for anemia. The majority of patients with EC present with locally advanced to advanced stages, and the most common symptoms are dysphagia and odynophagia, which are often attributed to underlying chronic gastroesophageal reflux. Weight loss, dysphagia, and odynophagia occur later on when the tumor is locally advanced.[11] Tumors in the more proximal cervical esophagus may also present with dysphagia or signs of local tumor extension, such as dysphonia or sympathetic nerve dysfunction.[11]

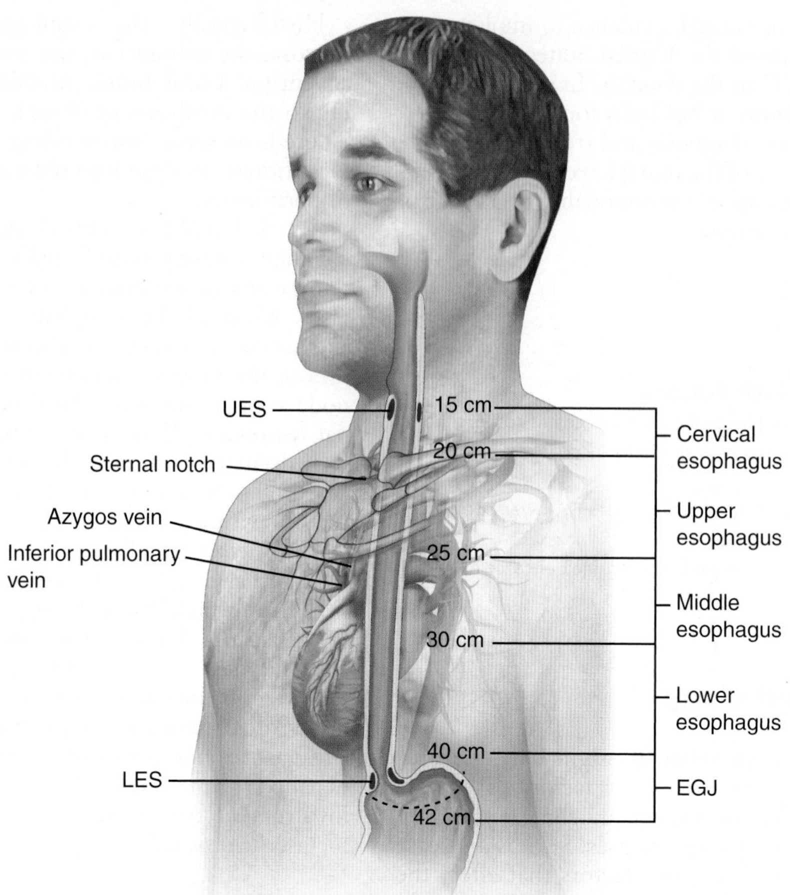

FIGURE 15.1. Schematic illustration of esophageal divisions. The cervical esophagus starts 15 cm from the incisors at the level of the cricopharyngeus muscle and ends at the level of the sternal notch. The upper thoracic esophagus starts 20 cm from the incisors and extends from the level of the sternal notch to the azygos arch. The middle thoracic esophagus starts 25 cm from the incisors and extends from the level of the azygos arch to the level of the inferior pulmonary vein. The lower thoracic esophagus is 30 cm from the incisors and extends from the level of the inferior pulmonary vein to the lower esophageal sphincter. Cancers involving the esophagogastric junction with epicenters 2 cm or less into the gastric cardia are staged as esophageal carcinoma, whereas those greater than 2 cm into the cardia are staged as gastric carcinoma. *EGJ*, Esophagogatric junction; *UES*, Upper esophageal sphincter; *LES*, Lower esophageal sphincter.

Staging Evaluation

The most commonly used international staging system for EC is the tumor-node-metastasis (TNM) classification published by the AJCC, currently in its 8th edition.[8,12] According to this system, tumor categories are assigned based on the extent of local tumor invasion (T), nodal involvement (N), presence of distant metastases (M), grade (G), and location (L) (Table 15.1, Fig. 15.2). Stages are formulated according to combinations of categories that are associated with similar prognoses, and are intended as a guide to disease management and prognosis.

The 8th edition of the AJCC staging classification presents separate classifications for the clinical stage (cTNM), based on imaging studies with minimal histologic information (Tables 15.2 and 15.3) and pathologic stage (pTNM), after resection and examination of surgical specimen (Tables 15.4 and 15.5). There is a new stage, postneoadjuvant pathologic (ypTNM), for patients who have undergone neoadjuvant therapy and had pathologic review of the resected specimen. ypTNM stage groups are identical for both histopathological cell types (Table 15.6), unlike those for cTNM and pTNM or AC.[8,12] In this edition, pTNM stage I has been subcategorized into pT1a and pT1b, undifferentiated histologic grade (G4) has been eliminated, and location has been removed as a category for pT2N0MO SCC.[8]

The T category ranges from Tis (high-grade dysplasia) to T4 (tumor invades into adjacent structures) (see Fig. 15.2). Malignant cells confined to the epithelium are categorized as Tis, and T1 is subdivided into T1a and T1b, depending on whether tumors are confined to the mucosa (T1a) or whether there is invasion of the submucosa (T1b). T2 is cancer that invades into but through the muscularis propria, and T3 is cancer that invades the adventitia. T4 indicates local invasion into surrounding structures and is subcategorized as T4a (potentially resectable invasion of the pleura, pericardium or diaphragm) and T4b (typically unresectable invasion of adjacent structures, such as the aorta, vertebral body, or

TABLE 15.1 Tumor-Node-Metastasis Descriptors

Primary Tumor (T)	
TX	Primary tumor cannot be assessed
T0	No evidence of primary tumor
Tis	High-grade dysplasia
T1a	Tumor invades lamina propria or muscularis mucosae
T1b	Tumor invades submucosa
T2	Tumor invades muscularis propria
T3	Tumor invades adventitia
T4a	Resectable tumor invading pleura, pericardium, diaphragm, or peritoneum
T4b	Tumor invading other adjacent structures such as aorta, vertebral body, or trachea
Regional Lymph Nodes (N)	
NX	Regional lymph nodes cannot be assessed
N0	No regional lymph node metastasis
N1	Metastasis in one or two regional lymph nodes
N2	Metastasis in three to six regional lymph nodes
N3	Metastasis in seven or more regional lymph nodes
Distant Metastasis (M)	
M0	No distant metastasis
M1	Distant metastasis
Histologic Grade (G)	
GX	Grade cannot be assessed—stage grouping as G1
G1	Well differentiated
G2	Moderately differentiated
G3	Poorly differentiated

trachea) (see Fig. 15.2). According to the National Comprehensive Cancer Network (NCCN) clinical practice guidelines, T1a or T1b tumors without nodal metastases are amenable to surgical monotherapy (endoscopic resection or esophagectomy), but more advanced tumors will require combined modality treatment involving chemotherapy, radiotherapy, and surgery, and T4b tumors are often unresectable.[13]

The N category includes the number of involved regional lymph nodes found from the upper esophageal sphincter to the celiac artery. These include lower cervical and supraclavicular lymph nodes; intrathoracic lymph nodes in the periesophageal region, mediastinum, and hilar regions; diaphragmatic lymph nodes adjacent to the crura; left gastric and paracardial lymph nodes; and common hepatic, splenic, and celiac lymph nodes. The number of involved lymph nodes has been shown to have an important influence on survival, and this is reflected in the subdivision of the N category into N1 (one or two lymph nodes involved), N2 (three to six lymph nodes involved), and N3 (more than six lymph nodes involved) (see Fig. 15.2). These subcategories also imply that an adequate lymph node dissection must be performed to ensure adequate pathologic staging and optimize survival. A recommended number of lymph nodes that should be removed has not been universally determined, but based on worldwide data the number or lymph nodes that should be dissected depends on pT category (≥10 for T1; ≥20 for T2; and >30 for T3 and T4).[9,14]

Sites of distant metastases are those not in direct continuity with the esophagus, and include visceral metastases and nonregional lymph nodes (M1).[9]

> **KEY POINTS**
>
> **Staging**
> - Different staging systems for squamous cell carcinoma and adenocarcinoma.
> - T1 category subdivided into T1a (tumor confined to mucosa) and T1b (extension of tumor into submucosa).
> - T4 category subdivided into T4a (limited invasion of pleura, pericardium, or diaphragm) and T4b (invasion into other adjacent structures).
> - N category subdivided into N1 (one to two lymph node metastases), N2 (three to six lymph node metastases), and N3 (more than six lymph node metastases).
> - The M1 category includes both distant visceral metastases and nonregional lymph node metastases.

Patterns Of Tumor Spread

As with most gastrointestinal malignancies, tumor spread can occur by direct local extension, by spread along lymphatic channels, or by dissemination via blood stream to distant sites. The esophageal submucosa contains a rich plexus of lymphatics, and lymphatic dissemination of malignancy occurs early, with the likelihood of both lymphatic and vascular spread increasing with more advanced local tumor invasion.[15]

Local Extension

Most esophageal carcinomas are epithelial in origin (i.e., SCC and AC) and normally progress in a radial fashion from involvement of the mucosa, to breach of the muscularis mucosae with extension into the submucosa, to invasion of the muscularis propria and involvement of adjacent organs. The absence of a serosa means that there is no anatomic barrier to prevent tumor invasion of adjacent organs.[16]

Lymphatic Dissemination

Lymph node metastases occur via the submucosal lymphatic plexus, with radial and longitudinal spread to adjacent periesophageal lymph nodes. Tumor dissemination via the thoracic duct leads to more distant lymph node stations and systemic disease.[15] Longitudinal lymphatic spread occurs in a roughly predictable fashion: tumors located in the cervical and upper thoracic esophagus drain preferentially in a cranial direction to cervical lymph nodes; tumors in the distal esophagus and gastroesophageal junction drain caudally to intraabdominal lymph nodes; and tumors in the midthoracic esophagus may drain in either direction.[10,17] However, lymphatic spread is not limited to these trends; lymph node metastases along the recurrent laryngeal nerves in the neck can still occur with distal esophageal tumors. Furthermore, because of the rich submucosal lymphatic plexus, "skip" metastases to distant lymph node stations may occur that bypass regional lymph nodes. Such skip metastases are found in 10% to 20% of patients undergoing tumor resection, an important argument for extended lymph node dissection in surgery performed with curative intent.[17] Although lymphatic spread of EC occurs early, the probability of lymph node metastases increases

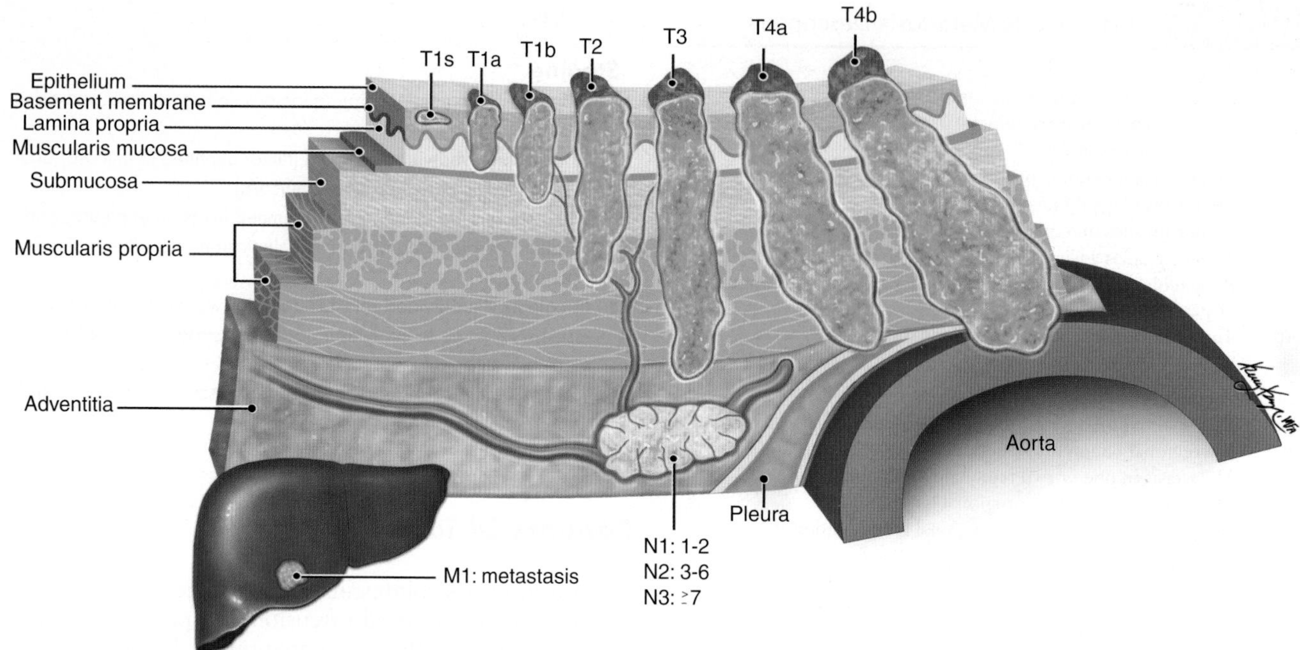

FIGURE 15.2. Schematic illustration of the 8th edition of the tumor-node-metastasis (TNM) staging system. Depth of invasion is categorized as: Tis, high-grade dysplasia; T1 is disease limited to the mucosal layers, subcategorized into T1a (cancer that invades the lamina propria or muscularis mucosae) and T1b (cancer that invades the submucosa); T2 cancer invades the muscularis propria; T3 tumors invade the adventitia; T4 is subcategorized as T4a (cancer that invades adjacent structures such as the pleura, pericardium, azygos vein, diaphragm, or peritoneum) and T4b (cancer that invades the major adjacent structures, such as the aorta, vertebral body, or trachea). Regional nodal disease is categorized by number of involved nodes: N0 (no regional lymph node metastasis), N1 (regional lymph node metastases involving one to two nodes), N2 (regional lymph node metastases involving three to six nodes), and N3 (regional lymph node metastases involving 7 or more nodes). M is categorized as M0 (no distant metastasis) and M1 (distant metastasis).

TABLE 15.2 Clinical Stage Groupings: Squamous Cell Carcinoma

STAGE	T	N	M
0	Tis	N0	M0
I	T1	N0–N1	M0
II	T2	N0–N1	M0
	T3	N0	M0
III	T3	N1	M0
	T1–3	N2	M0
IV	T4	N0–N2	M0
IIIA	T1–T2	N2	M0
	T1–T4	N3	M0
IVA	T4	N0–N2	M0
IVB	Any T	Any N	M1

TABLE 15.3 Clinical Stage Groupings: Adenocarcinoma

STAGE	T	N	M
0	Tis	N0	M0
I	T1	N0	M0
IIA	T1	N1	M0
IIB	T2	N0	M0
III	**T2–T3**	**N1**	**M0**
	T3–T4a	N0–N1	M0
IVA	T1–T4a	N2	M0
	T4b	N0–N2	M0
	T1–T4	N3	M0
IVB	Any T	Any N	M1

with greater local tumor invasion. For instance, lymph node metastases occurs in up to 35% of T1b patients and up to 80% of T3 patients.[18,19]

Dissemination of metastases to lymph nodes beyond the regional stations to the mid and upper neck and to the retroperitoneum below the celiac axis is considered distant metastatic disease. Consequently, these stations are typically treated with systemic therapy and are a contraindication to upfront surgery.

Hematogenous Dissemination

Hematogenous metastases to distant organ sites are common and are estimated to be present in up to 18% to 30% of patients at the time of presentation.[20] The risk of hematogenous tumor spread increases with more advanced local tumor invasion and nodal involvement, but can also occur early with small primary tumors and no apparent nodal metastases. The most common sites of distant metastases include the liver, bones, lungs, and adrenal glands, but they may also occur in more unusual sites (brain, skeletal muscle, subcutaneous fat, and thyroid gland), with a reported prevalence of 7.7%.[21,22]

Table 15.4 Pathologic Stage Groupings: Squamous Cell Carcinoma

STAGE	T	N	M	G	LOCATION
0	Tis	N0	M0	1, X	Any
IA	T1a	N0	M0	G1, X	Any
IB	T1b	N0	M0	G1, X	Any
	T1	N0	M0	G2-3	Any
	T2	N0	M0	G1	Any
IIA	T2	N0	M0	G2–G3, X	Any
	T3	N0	M0	G1	Upper/middle
IIB	T3	N0	M0	G2–G3	Upper/middle
	T3	N0	M0	X	Any
	T3	N1	M0	Any	X
	T1	N1	M0	Any	Any
IIIA	T1	N2	M0	Any	Any
	T2	N1	M0	Any	Any
IIIB	T4a	N0–N1	M0	Any	Any
	T3	N1	M0	Any	Any
	T2–T3	N2	M1	Any	Any
IVA	T4a	N2	M0	Any	Any
	T4b	N0–N2	M0	Any	Any
	T1–T4	N3	M0	Any	Any
IVB	T1–T4	N0–N3	M1	Any	Any

Table 15.5 Pathologic Stage Groupings: Adenocarcinoma

STAGE	T	N	M	G
0	Tis	N0	M0	N/A
IA	T1a	N0	M0	G, X
IB	T1a	N0	M0	G2
	T1b	N0	M0	G1–G2, X
IC	T1	N0	M0	G3
	T2	N0	M0	G1–G2
IIA	T2	N0	M0	G3, X
IIB	T1	N1	M0	Any
	T3	N1	M0	Any
IIIA	T1	N2	M0	Any
	T2	N0–N1	M0	Any
IIIB	T4a	N1–N2	M0	Any
	T3	N1	M0	Any
	T2–T3	N2	M0	Any
IVA	T4a	N2	M0	Any
	T4b	N0–N2	M0	Any
	T1–T4	N3	M0	Any
	T1–T4	N0–N3	M1	Any

TABLE 15.6 Post Neoadjuvant Therapy Groupings

STAGE	T	N	M
I	T0–T2	N0	M0
II	T3	N0	M0
IIIA	T0–T2	N1	M0
IIIB	T4a	N0	M0
III	T3	N1–N2	M0
	T0–T3	N2	M0
IVA	T4a	N1–N2, X	M0
	T4b	N0–N2	M0
	T1–T4	N3	M0
IVB	T1–T4	N0–N3	M1

KEY POINTS

Tumor Spread

- Lymphatic and hematogenous metastases occur early, and their probability increases with locally advanced tumor.
- "Skip" nodal metastases are found in 10% to 20% of patients undergoing tumor resection.
- Hematogenous metastases are present in up to 30% of patients at the time of initial presentation.

IMAGING

Currently, staging of patients with EC includes multimodality evaluation using a combination of esophagogastroduodenoscopy/endoscopic ultrasound (EGD/EUS), computed tomography (CT), and positron emission tomography (PET)/CT.

EGD is critical for initial diagnosis, and EUS is an extremely useful tool in determining the depth of invasion of the primary tumor and the presence of regional nodal disease. Standard radiologic baseline staging also includes contrast-enhanced CT and, for patients with potentially resectable tumor, PET/CT.

PET/CT imaging with 2-[^{18}F] fluoro-2-deoxy-D-glucose (FDG) is considered an indispensable imaging modality for baseline staging and therapeutic response evaluation. It provides both functional and anatomic information that is of great use for guiding clinical decision-making. Conventional contrast-enhanced CT provides better-quality images of the soft tissues, and particularly of the lungs; therefore, both CT and PET/CT are complementary modalities for the evaluation of EC.

Primary Tumor

Computed Tomography and Endoscopic Ultrasound

On axial CT scans, the primary tumor may be visualized as a focal or diffuse area of esophageal wall thickening (Fig. 15.3). An esophageal wall thickness greater than 5 mm has been described as abnormal[23]; however, in practice, it is difficult to accurately measure the esophageal wall thickness, because it is frequently nondistended and often cannot be accurately differentiated from adjacent structures such as the thoracic duct and small periesophageal lymph nodes. EUS is the preferred method of evaluating the T category of TNM staging, with a reported sensitivity and specificity of 82% and 91%, respectively.[24] EUS provides a detailed examination of the esophageal wall and is the most accurate modality for assessing the depth of tumor invasion. The performance index to distinguish T1 or T2 cancer from T3 or T4 by EUS is approximately 89% to 91%; however, it is difficult to confidently differentiate between cT1a and cT1b tumors. In such cases, endoscopic mucosal resection and endoscopic submucosal dissection are effective in differentiating cT1a from cT1b.

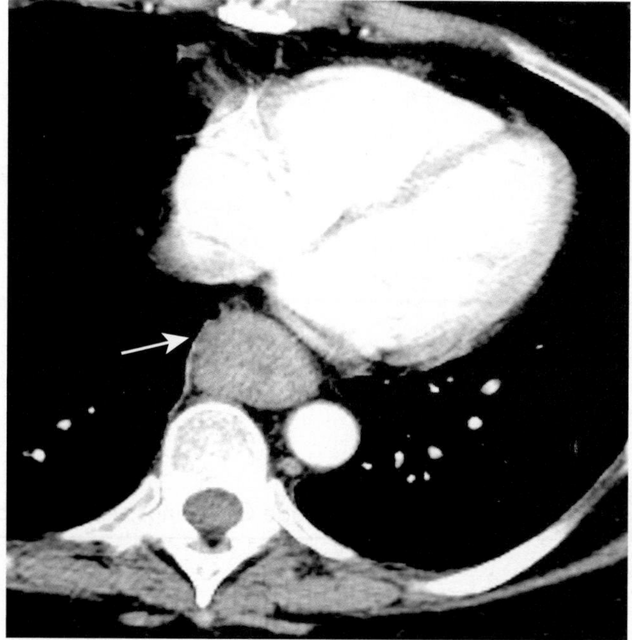

FIGURE 15.3. A 62-year-old man with adenocarcinoma of the distal esophagus. Axial computed tomography (CT) scans at the level of the left ventricle show diffuse esophageal wall thickening (*arrow*). The fat planes around the esophagus are preserved, and there is no evidence of invasion into adjacent structures, indicating that the primary tumor is technically resectable; however, the exact depth of tumor infiltration into the esophageal wall cannot be determined on CT. Endoscopic ultrasound is considered to be the most accurate imaging modality available for evaluating the depth of primary tumor invasion (T category).

Compared with EUS, CT has a relatively poor sensitivity for depiction of the primary mass (~67%), and cannot resolve invasion of the different histologic layers of the esophageal wall.[25]

Invasion into adjacent structures (T4 disease) may be suggested on CT by contiguity between the esophagus and the adjacent organs and by loss of the normal periesophageal fat planes. Aortic invasion is suggested by encasement greater than 90 degrees, and diaphragmatic invasion by loss of the retrocrural fat planes (see Fig. 15.3). In practice, however, the fat planes are often absent without invasive disease, and periesophageal fat stranding may also occur secondary to fibrosis or inflammation incited by the primary tumor. In the absence of evidence of obvious invasion into surrounding structures, a T4 status is often difficult to determine with certainty by any modality, and this diagnosis most often made at the time of attempted resection.

Positron Emission Tomography/Computed Tomography

Most, but not all, esophageal malignancies are FDG-avid. Although there is some evidence to suggest that the metabolic activity of the primary tumor (as measured by the maximum standard uptake value [SUVmax] or metabolic tumor volume) is of prognostic value, there are conflicting reports as to the reliability of this correlation.[26–28]

Although PET/CT does provide functional information concerning the primary malignancy and may be able to localize tumors that are not evident on CT images, its utility in determining the T status is limited by its poor spatial resolution. Invasion through the esophageal wall layers or into adjacent structures cannot be diagnosed with any greater accuracy than with conventional CT.

In patients with EC, FDG uptake in the esophagus is most often secondary to activity in the primary tumor itself, but can also occur secondary to multiple additional factors that may confound the apparent longitudinal extent of the tumor. Esophagitis or mucosal ulceration secondary to acid reflux is a common cause of false-positive FDG uptake, appearing as linear or focal areas of high activity in the distal esophagus.[29] Another frequent cause of false-positive FDG uptake in the esophagus is inflammation after endoscopic biopsy of the mucosa.[30] For these reasons, evaluation of the apparent metabolic activity of the primary esophageal tumor should be correlated with the recent clinical history and findings at endoscopy.

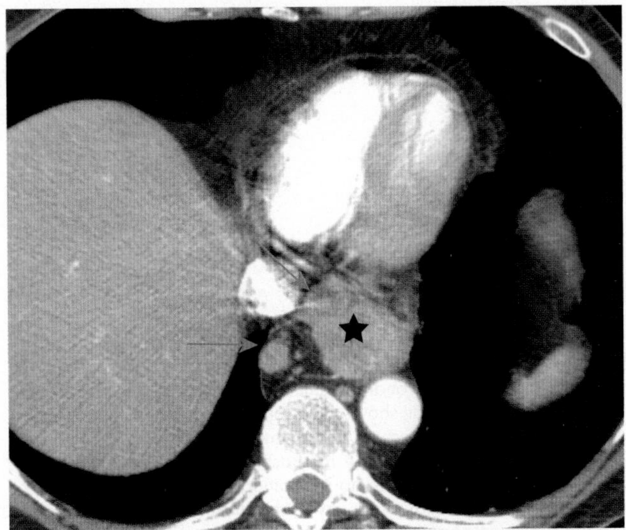

FIGURE 15.4. A 55-year-old man with adenocarcinoma of the distal esophagus. Axial computed tomography (CT) scan at the level of the left ventricle shows concentric thickening of the esophagus consistent with the primary malignancy (*star*). There are adjacent enlarged lymph nodes suspicious for nodal disease (*arrows*) that were confirmed to be positive by endoscopic ultrasound–guided fine needle aspiration. Because the detection of metastatic lymph nodes on CT depends primarily on size criteria (>1 cm on the short axis), CT lacks sensitivity for detecting lymph node metastases, because a normal-sized lymph node might contain microscopic metastatic foci. In addition, the presence of benign enlarged and inflammatory lymph nodes in esophageal cancer reduces the specificity of CT for detecting lymph node metastases.

Nodal Disease

Computed Tomography

CT has a relatively poor diagnostic accuracy for the diagnosis of nodal metastases, depending entirely on size criteria that are neither sensitive nor specific. As a general rule, lymph nodes that are greater than 1 cm on the short axis are considered suspicious for malignancy; however, smaller lymph nodes may still harbor metastatic disease, and large lymph nodes may simply be reactive (Fig. 15.4). The lymph node status is best determined by EGD/EUS and fine-needle aspiration (FNA). The reported diagnostic accuracy of CT varies considerably from study to study, depending on the gold standard used; in one study of 75 patients in which tissue confirmation was used as the gold standard, CT had a sensitivity and specificity of 84% and 67%, respectively.[31] It is important to remember that the presence of regional nodal metastases is not a contraindication to surgery, because the lymph nodes will normally be resected with the primary tumor. The main objective of CT is to identify suspicious lymph nodes that are not immediately adjacent to the esophagus and that may not be dissected out at the time of surgery. This is particularly important in patients for whom transhiatal esophagectomy, rather than transthoracic or three-field esophagectomy, is planned, and who would normally undergo a more limited mediastinal lymph node dissection.

Positron Emission Tomography/Computed Tomography

Compared with CT, PET/CT has a similar sensitivity (46%–82%) and greater specificity (49%–98%) for the detection of nodal metastases in patients with EC.[31–34] Evaluation of the presence of nodal metastases by PET/CT is limited by its inability to detect micrometastases and by its difficulty in resolving FDG-avid lymph nodes that are located close to the primary tumor, owing to the "bloom" effect from activity in the primary mass.

PET/CT does have greater specificity than CT in identifying nodal metastases, which is useful for directing EUS-guided FNA of specific lymph nodes and for alerting the surgeon to possible nodal metastases in atypical locations. A combination of EUS and PET/CT is the optimal method for prospectively evaluating the N status of EC. As discussed previously, the main objective of PET/CT is the identification of celiac or other lymph nodes that lie outside the locoregional nodal field, the presence of which will have

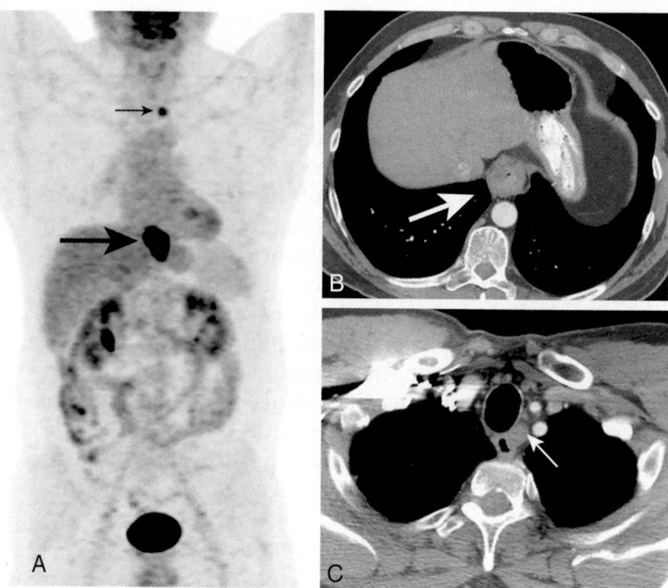

FIGURE 15.5. A 62-year-old man with adenocarcinoma of the distal esophagus. **A**, Coronal maximum intensity projection positron emission tomography scan shows metabolic activity within the primary tumor in the distal esophagus (*long arrow*) and focal 2-[18F] fluoro-2-deoxy-D-glucose uptake in the mediastinum (*short arrow*). **B** and **C**, Axial contrast-enhanced computed tomography scan confirms the location of the primary malignancy in the distal esophagus (*arrow*) and the presence of an enlarged node suspicious for nodal disease (*arrow*). cN1 was confirmed by endoscopic ultrasound–guided fine needle aspiration.

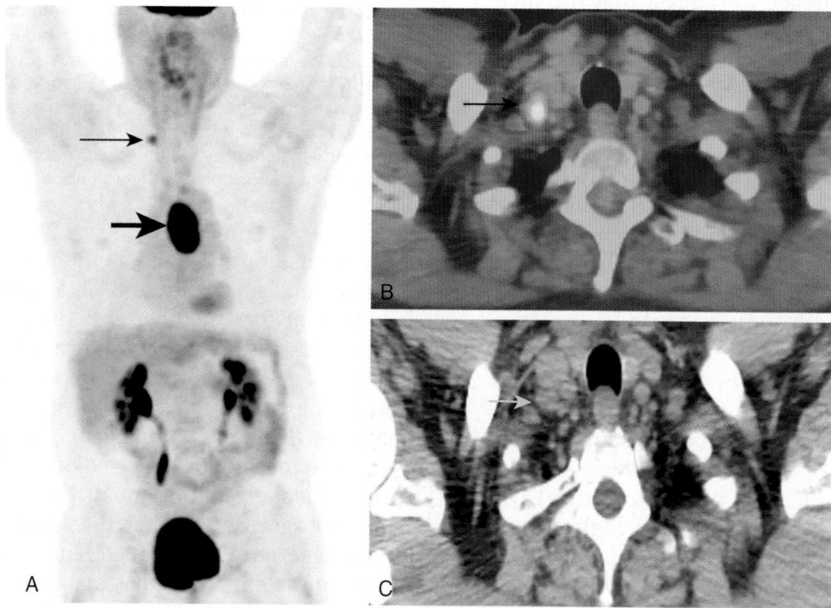

FIGURE 15.6. A 72-year-old man with a new diagnosis of squamous cell carcinoma of the midthoracic esophagus. **A**, Coronal maximum intensity projection positron emission tomography (PET) scan shows increased 2-[18F] fluoro-2-deoxy-D-glucose (FDG) uptake in the mediastinum (*short arrow*) and right supraclavicular region (*long arrow*), consistent with the esophageal malignancy and nodal metastasis. **B**, Axial fused PET/computed tomography (CT) scan shows a FDG-avid node in the supraclavicular region arrow that is not adjacent to the esophagus and is considered to represent nonregional metastatic adenopathy (M1 disease). **C**, Axial CT scan confirms the presence of an enlarged node that lies outside the definition of a regional node (*arrow*).

a great influence on surgical decision-making (Fig. 15.5). Accuracy of PET in diagnosis of regional nodal disease is also stage-dependent. In patients with early disease, false-positive and false-negative readings limit the utility of FDG-PET and may lead to inappropriate therapy.[30] In those cases, it is important to confirm the diagnosis histologically.

Metastases

Computed Tomography

Metastases from EC most commonly occur in the liver, lungs, and bones.[20] Most of these metastases are readily detectable by CT, with a sensitivity of approximately 66% to 81%,[31,35] particularly when multiphasic imaging of the liver is included as part of the baseline CT scanning protocol. CT is also the ideal imaging modality for detection of pulmonary metastases and has greater sensitivity in this regard than PET/CT, in which images of the lungs are not acquired in full inspiration and in which pulmonary metastases may be too small for resolution by PET scanning.

Importantly, 7% to 17% of EC metastases are occult or are difficult to prospectively diagnose by CT alone[22,36] (Fig. 15.6). A combination of CT and PET/CT is the optimal method for detection of metastatic disease from EC.

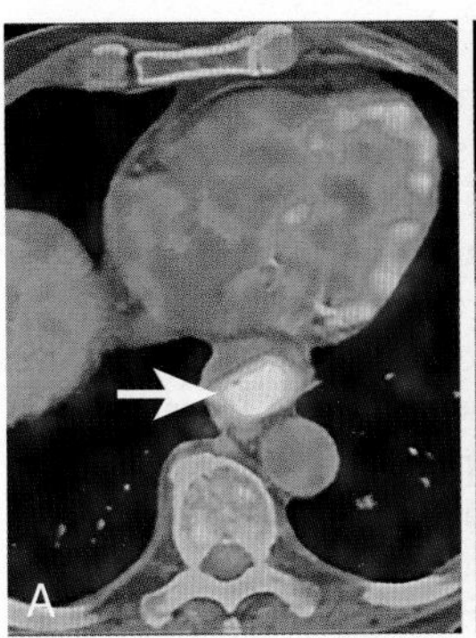

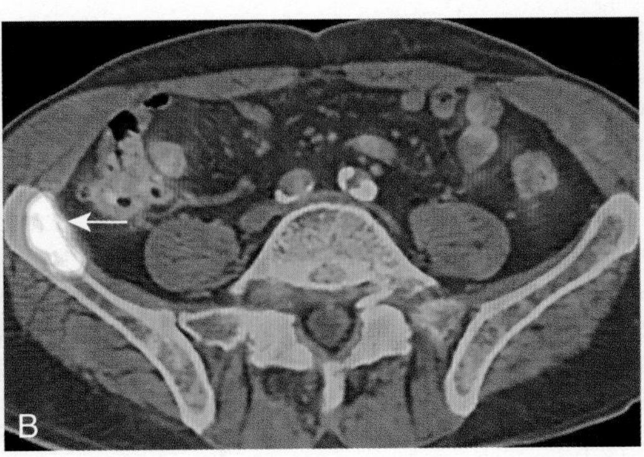

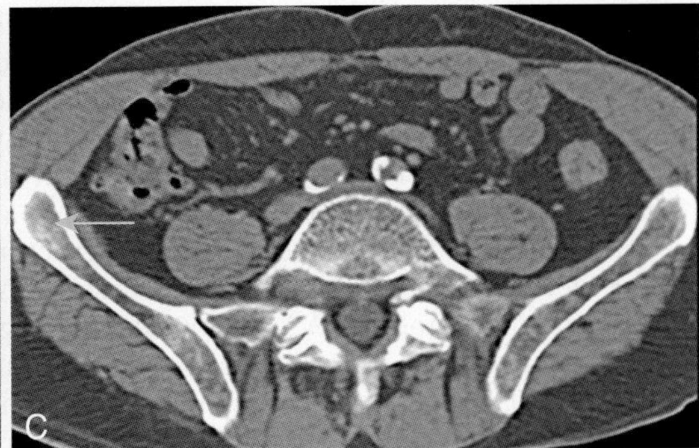

Figure 15.7. A 70-year-old man with adenocarcinoma of the distal esophagus. **A** and **B**, Axial fused positron emission tomography (PET)/computed tomography (CT) scans show intense 2-[^{18}F] fluoro-2-deoxy-D-glucose uptake in the primary tumor (*arrow*) and increased metabolic activity in the right iliac bone (*arrow*). **C**, Axial CT scan at the level of the iliac bone demonstrates subtle area of sclerosis (*arrow*) suspicious for metastasis (M1 disease) that was confirmed by percutaneous biopsy. PET/CT is the imaging modality with the highest sensitivity and specificity for the detection of distant metastases.

Positron Emission Tomography/Computed Tomography

PET/CT is the imaging modality with the highest sensitivity and specificity for the detection of distant metastases (83.3% and 98.4%, respectively).[37] PET/CT improves baseline staging over CT and EUS and can obviate futile surgery.[37] The increased sensitivity and specificity of PET/CT over other imaging modalities for the detection of distant metastases makes it an indispensable tool in the evaluation of patients with newly diagnosed EC (Fig. 15.7, see Fig. 15.6). The detection of metastatic disease by PET/CT will have a profound influence on subsequent clinical decision-making, and consideration should always be given to biopsy of the abnormal lesions to confirm the presence of malignancy.

Key Points

What the Treating Clinician Needs to Know from the Radiology Report

- Location and longitudinal extent of primary esophageal tumor.
- Potentially involved lymph node stations.
- Involvement of adjacent organs.
- Presence of distant metastases.

TREATMENT

Esophagectomy remains the primary treatment for early superficial cancer (cT1N0), although its role in superficial (T1a) cancer is in debate since the development of endoscopic mucosal treatment. There is a general agreement that smaller cT2N0 tumors proceed to surgical resection. These patients would be reevaluated after surgery, and patients who are discovered to be understaged would be considered for adjuvant therapy.[38]

For patients with locally advanced cancer (large cT2N0, cT3-4aN0, any cN+), multimodal treatment with neoadjuvant chemotherapy or combined chemoradiotherapy followed by surgery is the recommended treatment.[38] Systemic therapy is the most effective treatment modality for patients with metastatic disease.[38]

Neoadjuvant Chemoradiation Therapy

Concurrent neoadjuvant chemoradiation therapy (CRT) combining platinum-based chemotherapy and 5-fluorouracil or taxanes with radiation therapy to the primary tumor are the most commonly used regimens in most U.S. institutions. Accumulating evidence supports the role of CRT in improving resectability and survival in patients with locally advanced disease.[39] The ChemoRadiotherapy for Oesophageal cancer followed by Surgery Study, which included 366 patients with esophageal carcinoma (25% SCC, 75% AC), demonstrated that CRT followed by surgery resulted in a significant improvement of overall survival (OS) compared with surgery alone (median: 49 vs. 24 months). Postoperative complications were similar in the two groups, and the mortality rate was 4% in both.[40]

There are several trials comparing definitive CRT (dCRT) and neoadjuvant CRT (nCRT) in esophageal SCC that have shown similar OS in the surgery and nonsurgery groups, although surgery seems to provide a better control of the tumors, but without a better long-term outcome; however, this continues to be a topic of discussion.[38]

Radiation Therapy

The goal of radiation therapy in the management of EC as part of either preoperative or definitive treatment with concurrent systemic therapy is to improve locoregional disease control by delivering a sufficient tumoricidal radiation dose while minimizing adjacent normal tissue radiation exposure. To achieve this end, it is critical for the radiation oncologist to be able to identify the areas with gross tumor involvement, as well as those areas at risk for microscopic disease extension.[41] Currently, CT and/or PET/CT is used in localizing the gross tumor volume (GTV) of the primary tumor, as well as the involved lymph nodes. However, information from EGD should also be reviewed and incorporated in GTV delineation, particularly in cases where delineation of tumor may not be entirely clear secondary to factors such as overlap with adjacent structures or low FDG-avidity of the tumor.[41] The advantage of CT-based planning is the ability to better visualize the target and contour the adjacent critical normal tissue structures. A more conformal treatment plan can be developed using three-dimensional (3D) reconstruction of the target and structures to avoid. From the 3D information, it is possible to estimate the radiation dose to be delivered to any given percent volume of the target or avoidance structure.[42]

The determination of microscopic disease extent, or clinical target volume (CTV), is more complex, given the intricate network of submucosal lymphatic drainage of the esophagus that allows microscopic dissemination to occur. The superior border of the CTV includes an expansion of 3 to 4 cm above the gross tumor or 1 cm above any grossly involved paraesophageal lymph node, whichever is more superior. The inferior border is defined as either 3 to 4 cm below the gross disease or at least 2 cm along clinically uninvolved gastric mucosa if the tumor was distally located, to reduce radiation dose to normal stomach. Radially, a 1- to 1.5-cm margin is recommended to include the periesophageal lymph nodes, with the exception of smaller margins of 0.5 cm in areas that interface with uninvolved cardiac and hepatic tissue.[42]

The current standard of care for EC treatment is 3D conformal radiation therapy, that allows delivery of an optimal dose covering the target volumes while minimizing radiation dose to the normal soft tissues.[42] In the neoadjuvant setting, radiation doses range from 41.4 to 50.4 Gy,[43] whereas the dose for definitive radiation is more controversial, ranging from 50.4 Gy to over 60 Gy.[44]

Another approach that modulates the dose intensity of the radiation beam to minimize dose to the adjacent critical normal tissues while providing full tumor target coverage is aptly called intensity-modulated radiation therapy (IMRT). IMRT has been shown to significantly reduce dose to the lungs and heart, and has been associated with a lower risk of grade 3 or higher nonhematologic toxicities. Although IMRT has not been established as a standard of care for EC, it has been favored for cervical EC treatment because of the close proximity of the esophagus to radiosensitive normal structures in the head and neck. In cervical EC, IMRT has shown improved coverage of the target volume with decreased dose to the normal structures.[42]

Proton therapy is an emerging treatment technique in EC. In contrast to 3D conformal radiation therapy and IMRT, proton beams are composed of charged particles that deliver most of their energy at a specific tissue depth, limiting the dose to the surrounding organs. The volume and/or dose to the surrounding organs is reduced compared to that of IMRT and 3D conformal radiation therapy without sacrificing coverage of the target volumes.[42] This technique is expected to provide clinically meaningful benefit in patients with mid- and distal esophageal tumors because these tumors are surrounded by the lungs, heart, and spine.[45]

Surgery

Esophageal resection may be performed using a transhiatal approach, a combined transthoracic and abdominal approach, a three-field approach (incorporating cervical, thoracic, and abdominal incisions), or minimally invasive techniques. The choice of which technique to use often depends on individual factors such as surgeon preference, patient performance status, cancer stage, or tumor location. Despite the numerous options, the one critical principle of EC surgery is to achieve a complete resection.

Lower esophageal tumors located at the distal esophagus or gastroesophageal junction can be managed by subtotal esophagectomy, esophagogastrectomy, or segmental esophagectomy with bowel interposition. The extent of gastric involvement, as well as the stage of the primary tumor, will guide the surgeon to determine the necessity for partial or complete removal of the stomach and extent of esophageal resection.

Approaching a subtotal esophagectomy through a right thoracotomy and laparotomy (Ivor Lewis esophagectomy) allows for resection of the stomach and abdominal lymph nodes followed by an intrathoracic esophageal resection and reconstruction combined with a complete two-field lymph node dissection.[46] Because the reconstruction takes place in the chest, locally advanced tumors with involvement of the distal esophagus and proximal stomach lend themselves to this approach, because a two-field lymphadenectomy and negative margins can be obtained with less worry of gastric necrosis compared with stretching the stomach to a cervical reconstruction.[47]

Early-stage distal tumors with minimal risk for lymph node involvement (stage I, T1a lesions) can be treated with segmental esophagectomy and small bowel interposition (Merendino procedure) or vagal-sparing esophagectomy with gastric or bowel interposition. Alternatively, a transhiatal esophagectomy can be performed with mobilization of the intrathoracic esophagus from the esophageal hiatus to the thoracic inlet without the need for thoracotomy. The advantage of the transhiatal technique is that it avoids thoracotomy while achieving a complete removal of the esophagus.[48] The more conservative transhiatal approach preserves chest wall function and decreases perioperative morbidity. The potential disadvantages of this technique include a limited periesophageal and mediastinal lymphadenectomy, the risk of causing intrathoracic injury to surrounding structures during blunt dissection of the esophagus, and higher locoregional recurrence rates. In comparison, more radical resections involving thoracotomy provide excellent local control but can be associated with increased morbidity.[49]

Proximally located (e.g., mid- and upper esophageal) tumors often require a total esophagectomy with a cervical anastomosis, because it is difficult to achieve negative margins with subtotal resections (e.g., Ivor Lewis esophagectomy). A three-field (McKeown) approach uses a right thoracotomy or thoracoscopy combined with laparotomy and left cervicotomy for esophageal resection, and (typically) a two-field, abdominal, and thoracic lymphadenectomy.[50] Patients who present with cervical esophageal carcinomas have several treatment options. The vast majority of these tumors are SCCs and are sensitive to chemoradiotherapy; therefore, efforts at organ preservation have relegated resection of cervical lesions to salvage procedures when there is locoregional failure after definitive medical therapy.[38]

Although it is generally agreed that surgical resection is the primary form of therapy for local and locoregional disease, there is controversy over the value and extent of lymphadenectomy. Some believe that certain patients with affected lymph nodes can be successfully cured with an aggressive surgical approach that focuses on wide peritumoral soft tissue excision and extended lymphadenectomy using a transthoracic approach with *en bloc* lymphadenectomy. The downside to this approach is an increase in perioperative morbidity associated with the more extensive resection. Unfortunately, it is unclear whether more extensive dissection actually leads to improved survival.[15]

THERAPEUTIC RESPONSE EVALUATION

Surgical series have consistently shown that patients who have a good pathologic response to neoadjuvant treatment have an improved survival after complete esophagectomy compared with those who do not demonstrate a pathologic response, of the order of 34.9% to 53% 5-year survival for responders and 0% to 10.7% for nonresponders.[51,52] It has therefore been suggested that esophagectomy may not be appropriate for all patients, and that a selective approach to surgery may be considered. The difficulty in preoperatively identifying which patients will benefit from surgery, as well as the limited alternative treatment options available, remain obstacles to the adoption of such a selection process into standard treatment protocols.

Conventional practice is to evaluate treatment response by repeat EGD/EUS and PET or CT scanning after neoadjuvant therapy and, in patients without new metastatic disease, to proceed directly to surgery. However, EGD/EUS in some cases is not technically feasible, owing to luminal stenosis, and is susceptible to overstaging residual disease.[53] The sensitivity of EUS-directed FNA is also limited by the often extensive necrosis and fibrosis that occur after CRT.[54] Similarly, CT cannot accurately evaluate the esophageal wall and is unable to differentiate esophageal wall thickening because of viable tumor from that because of treatment-related inflammation and fibrosis.[21]

Because PET/CT provides functional, rather than pure morphologic, information, there has been much interest in its use for the evaluation of therapeutic response to neoadjuvant therapy and for the detection of residual viable malignancy. Multiple studies have shown that therapeutic response, as measured either by a percentage decrease in SUVmax or by a single posttreatment SUVmax, correlates with histological response in resected specimens and may be used to select pathologic responders who are most likely to benefit from esophagectomy.[53] Conversely, persistent FDG uptake in the tumor above a certain threshold has been shown to correlate with persistent viable macroscopic malignancy and a poor clinical outcome.[53] However, this is not a consistent finding, and definitions of a "metabolic" response vary considerably from institution to institution, most often being derived from analysis of receiver-operating curves. Furthermore, the overlap between perceived responders and nonresponders has made it difficult to incorporate posttreatment PET findings into clinical decision-making.

Interpretative difficulties that may be encountered when using PET/CT for the assessment of therapeutic response include FDG uptake secondary to biopsy or chemoradiotherapy-induced esophagitis or ulceration that may be confused with malignancy. Thus, most investigators recommend that PET/CT be performed no earlier than 3 weeks after the completion of chemoradiation therapy if it is to be used for local tumor response assessment. In addition, PET/CT cannot detect residual microscopic disease, and for this reason esophagectomy or definitive chemoradiation therapy should still be offered to patients who have had an apparent complete metabolic response to neoadjuvant therapy.

Whole-body PET/CT performed after neoadjuvant therapy is also useful for detecting new interval metastases that were not present at baseline evaluation, which occur in 8% of cases.[55] Such metastases may occur even when there has been an apparent complete local metabolic response to therapy, and they may be occasionally occult on CT scanning or lie outside the usual range of restaging scans. Although the incidence of interval metastases is relatively rare, repeat PET/CT after neoadjuvant therapy and before surgery should be considered in patients who have locally advanced tumors at baseline and in those who may not be ideally fit for surgery (Fig. 15.8).

In the context of therapeutic response assessment earlier during the course of neoadjuvant therapy (e.g., after one to two cycles of induction chemotherapy rather than at the completion of neoadjuvant therapy), there is convincing early evidence to suggest that PET/CT can predict the response of the primary tumor. In patients with FDG-avid tumors at baseline who undergo repeat PET/CT after one or two cycles of chemotherapy, a failure of metabolic activity (as measured by SUVmax) to decrease by 30% to 35% is predictive of a poor pathologic response and a worse 3-year survival after esophagectomy.[56]

Other imaging modalities may be better suited to predict treatment response. Diffusion-weighted magnetic resonance imaging (DW-MRI) is an emerging technique that has been evaluated in predicting treatment response after CRT. This technique reflects the microscopic diffusion motion of water molecules in tissues.[57] Highly cellular tissues or those with cellular swelling present lower diffusion coefficients. An apparent diffusion coefficient (ADC) map can be derived from the DW-MRI images to quantify the diffusion restriction. ADC is inversely proportional to tissue cellularity, and, as CRT can result in the loss of cell membrane integrity, tumor response can be detected as an increase in tumor ADC.[57]

Van Rossum et al. evaluated the predictive value of initial tumor ADC and change in ADC (ΔADC) during and after treatment for the identification of pathologic complete response (pathCR) and good response. Good response was defined as pathCR or near-pathCR. The authors found that a low ΔADC of less than 29% predicted residual cancer (e.g., no pathCR) with a sensitivity of 100% and a specificity of 75%.[58] Another study aimed to determine the diagnostic performance of visual response assessment of the primary tumor after nCRT on T2-weighted (T2W) and DW-MRI. This study reported a sensitivity and specificity for T2W + DW-MRI for detection of residual tumor ranging from 90% to 97% and 42% to 50%, respectively, indicating a high rate of false-positive results that may be explained by the fact that normal stomach wall shows increased signal

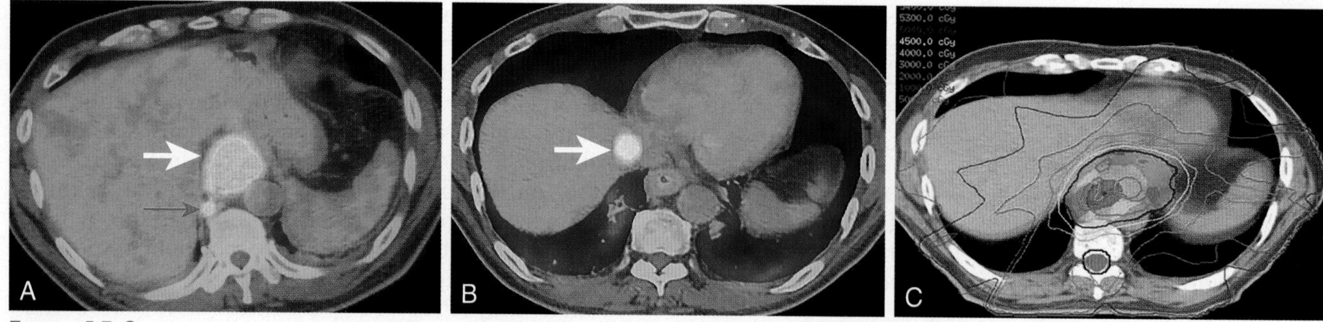

FIGURE 15.8. A 68-year-old man with adenocarcinoma of the distal esophagus. **A**, Axial fused positron emission tomography (PET)/computed tomography (CT) scan shows the primary malignancy in the distal esophagus (*white arrow*) and an adjacent 2-[^{18}F] fluoro-2-deoxy-D-glucose (FDG)-avid node (*arrow*) consistent with nodal disease. **B**, Axial fused PET/CT at the same level, 12 weeks after the patient completed chemoradiation, shows a FDG-avid liver lesion (*arrow*) outside the radiation treatment plan (**C**) consistent with metastasis. PET/CT performed after neoadjuvant therapy is useful for detecting new metastases that were not present at baseline evaluation, which occur in up to 8% of cases.

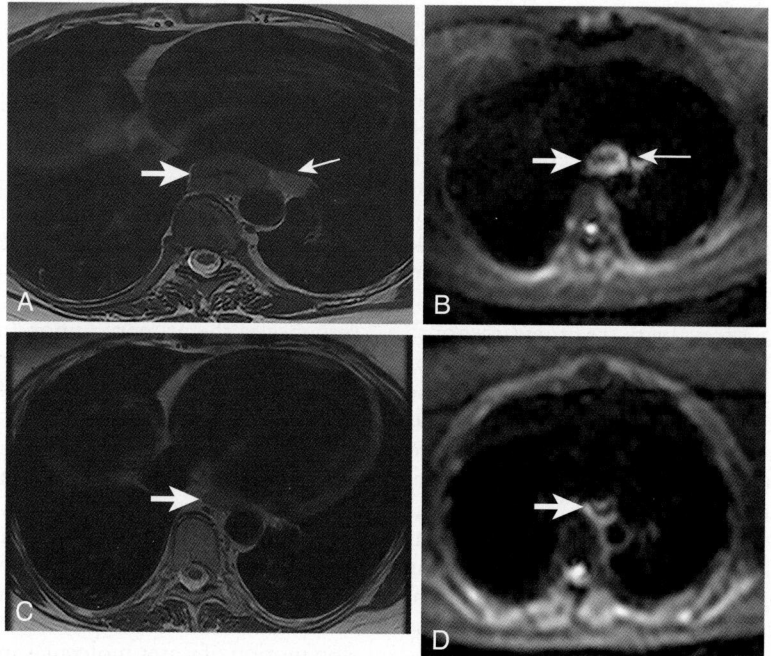

FIGURE 15.9. A 68-year-old woman with adenocarcinoma of the distal esophagus. **A**, T2-weighted (T2W) axial image shows diffuse thickening of the distal esophagus, consistent with the primary tumor (*thick arrow*). There is an adjacent enlarged lymph node (*arrow*) suspicious for nodal disease. **B**, Axial diffusion-weighted (DW) image at the same level demonstrates a clear, high signal intensity within the esophageal wall in addition to wall thickening (*thick arrow*). The adjacent adenopathy (*arrow*) also shows high signal intensity. **C**, T2W axial image, 12 weeks after the patient completed neoadjuvant therapy, demonstrates decrease in thickness of the esophageal wall (*arrow*). The previously identified adenopathy is no longer seen. **D**, Axial DW image shows residual hyperintense signal within the esophageal wall (*arrow*) suspicious for residual tumor that was confirmed by endoscopy and biopsy.

on DW-MRI and/or by the presence radiation-induced inflammation (Fig. 15.9).[59]

An important area in which DW-MRI may have additional diagnostic difficulties is the evaluation of residual nodal disease. On DW-MRI, normal and pathologic lymph node signals may overlap, limiting the evaluation of residual nodal disease. In addition, lymph nodes outside the field of view cannot be assessed. The presence of susceptibility artifact, low spatial resolution, and the partial volume averaging effect also contribute to unreliable evaluation of normal-sized lymph nodes.[60] Technique improvements and larger studies are needed to validate MRI as a useful tool in the identification of residual disease after nCRT.

KEY POINTS

Treatment and Therapeutic Response Assessment

- In surgically fit patients, neoadjuvant chemoradiation therapy (followed by esophagectomy or definitive chemoradiation therapy) represents a standard of care for any tumor that has invaded beyond the submucosa or that is associated with nodal metastases.
- A survival benefit from esophagectomy is seen only in patients who have a pathologic response to neoadjuvant therapy.
- Whole-body positron emission tomography/computed tomography performed after neoadjuvant therapy is also useful for detecting new interval metastases that were not present at baseline evaluation.
- Diffusion-weighted magnetic resonance imaging is an emerging technique that may be useful in the evaluation of response to treatment after neoadjuvant chemoradiation therapy.

SURVEILLANCE

Following definitive treatment by esophagectomy or combined modality treatment, tumor recurrence presents in approximately 50% of cases and most often occurs in the form of distant metastases rather than local recurrence.[43] Over 50% of recurrence occurs during the first 2 years after treatment.[61] Local tumor recurrence may manifest clinically as dysphagia or unexplained weight loss.

On CT, local tumor recurrence should be suspected if there is new soft-tissue thickening adjacent to the surgical anastomosis or new regional lymphadenopathy. It is important to keep in mind that the anastomotic site is a region that may be inflamed at the time of imaging owing to surgery, recent endoscopic biopsy, or neoadjuvant therapy, as radiation-induced inflammation may take many months to completely resolve. Consequently, on PET/CT a focal increase in metabolic activity at the anastomosis is commonly secondary to inflammation rather than tumor (Fig. 15.10).[61]

For recurrent regional nodal disease, PET/CT is useful for detection and to guide biopsy for confirmation of recurrence, as this often occurs in areas that are not visualized by EUS and that are often overlooked by conventional CT, such as the supraclavicular region.[61] Distant metastatic disease may occur in the peritoneum, nonregional lymph nodes, or distant visceral sites (lungs, brain, bones, or muscle). PET/CT has a reported sensitivity and specificity in the identification of recurrence in the form of distant metastases ranged from 97% to 100% and 94% to 96%, respectively.[61,62]

Posttreatment surveillance strategies remain controversial. Clinical thresholds for repeat imaging (CT or PET/CT) are likely to be governed by local resources, patient-specific factors, and remaining treatment options.

The NCCN recommendations for follow-up in patients with Tis or T1a treated with endoscopic resection/ablation or esophagectomy are upper gastrointestinal endoscopy (GIE) every 3 months for the first year, then every 6 months for 2 years, and then every year indefinitely. For patients with T1b and any N treated with chemotherapy, CT of the chest and abdomen with contrast every 6 to 9 months is recommended for the first 2 years, and then annually up to 5 years, in addition to upper GIE every 3 to 6 months for 2 years and annually for 3 years. Follow-up recommendations for patients with T1b and any N treated with esophagectomy include CT of the chest and abdomen with contrast starting at 6 to 12 months for up to 3 years, then as clinically indicated, and upper GIE as needed. For patients treated with dCRT or nCRT+ esophagectomy, imaging follow-up with CT of the chest and abdomen with contrast is recommended every 4 to 6 months for the first year and less frequently for the next 2 years. Upper GIE every 3 to 6 months for the first 2 years and every 6 months for the third year is recommended for patients treated with definitive CRT without surgery, but endoscopy is not recommended as a surveillance tool for patients treated with nCRT and esophagectomy, given very low rates of local recurrence.[13]

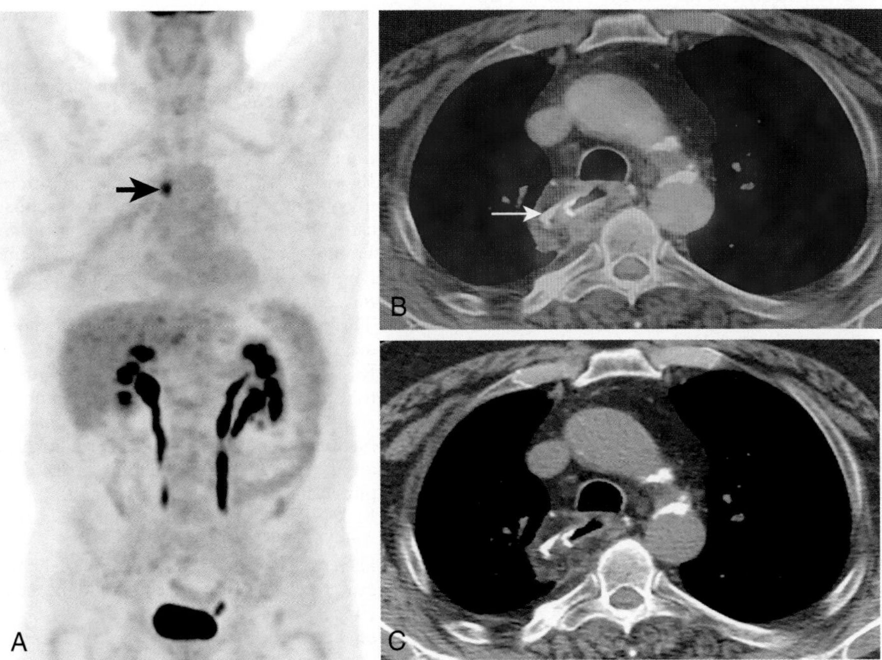

FIGURE 15.10. A 61-year-old man, status post transhiatal esophagectomy and gastric pull-up. **A**, Coronal maximum intensity projection positron emission tomography (PET) scan shows 2-[^{18}F] fluoro-2-deoxy-D-glucose (FDG) uptake in the mediastinum (*arrow*). **B**, Axial fused PET/computed tomography (CT) scans at the level of the aortic arch demonstrates focal metabolic activity at the proximal anastomosis (*arrow*). **C**, Axial CT scan at the same level shows normal appearance of the anastomosis. Endoscopy with biopsy demonstrated inflammatory changes and was negative for recurrent disease. The anastomotic site is a region that may be FDG-avid secondary to inflammation related to the surgery or recent endoscopic biopsy, as well as radiation-induced inflammation that may take months to completely resolve.

NEW THERAPIES

Treatment options for patients with locally advanced and metastatic esophageal carcinoma are limited, and their efficacy is restricted by the development of resistance after first- and second-line treatment.[63] Immunotherapy is a novel treatment option that may improve outcomes by targeting the immune system in tumors that are resistant to conventional systemic treatments. In patients with esophageal carcinoma the immune system is activated by an intrinsic, increased mutational burden that escape immune surveillance.[64–66] In patients with EC, expression of programmed death ligand 1 (PD-L1) on tumor cells has been reported in up to 40% of patients with SCC, although expression is lower on tumor cells in patients with AC. PD-L1 expression is reported to be present on infiltrating myeloid cells at the invasive margin of the tumor in AC, and may also have clinical relevance.[63]

Two PD-L1 inhibitors, pembrolizumab and nivolumab, have shown potential efficacy in EC. In a multicohort that included patients with PD-L1–positive SCC or AC, pembrolizumab demonstrated manageable toxicity and durable antitumor action. A decrease in the size of target lesions was reported in more than 50% of patients, and the reported median OS was 7.0 months (95% confidence interval [CI], 4.3–17.7 months).[67] Nivolumab was also evaluated in a multicenter study that included 65 SCC patients who were intolerant or refractory to conventional chemotherapy. Target lesion and tumor burden decreased in 45% of patients, with a median OS of 10.8 months (95% CI, 7.4–13.3 months).[68]

An alternative approach to improving patient outcomes includes the addition of immunotherapy to the adjuvant or neoadjuvant setting in stage II or III disease. It is known that CRT induces immunogenic cell death, which suggests that a tumor might respond favorably to immune therapy added to CRT.[63,64] There are different ongoing studies evaluating the synergistic effect of radiation or chemoradiation and anti–PD-L1. For instance, an ongoing trial (NCT02998268) compares the concomitant versus sequential use of pembrolizumab as part of induction CRT before surgery for locally advance AC, followed by adjuvant use of pembrolizumab after surgery.[64] There are additional studies that are currently assessing the efficacy of nivolumab and durvalumab in the neoadjuvant setting.[64] This new generation of clinical trials may help to develop immunotherapy as a more effective EC treatment.

Other strategies such as the use of tumor-specific neoantigen vaccines and adoptive T-cell therapy are the subject of active investigation. In adoptive T-cell therapy, T cells that have been previously manipulated to deliver an enhanced response against specific tumor cells antigens are administered to the patient with the goal of improving a specific immune response against the tumor cells.[64]

CONCLUSION

EC is challenging to treat and requires a multidisciplinary approach to improve outcomes. Esophagectomy remains the primary treatment for early stages. Currently, multimodality treatment with nCRT followed by surgery is recommended for patients with locally advanced disease.

Chemotherapy based on platinum agents and 5-fluorouracil or a taxane is the standard chemotherapy doublet for EC, but there is inherent resistance to systemic therapy because of histological, molecular, and etiological heterogeneity in EC patients, with reported limited responses seen after first- and second-line therapy. Immunotherapy is a promising field that is currently in development. Ongoing clinical trials evaluating combined strategies such as immunotherapy and radiation or immunochemotherapy may help to establish a new treatment paradigm for EC.

From an imaging perspective, it is important for the radiologist to be familiar with the current staging system and the anatomy and patterns of spread of malignancy. Radiologists should have an understanding of the influence of imaging on clinical decision-making. PET/CT is currently a well-established imaging tool that is valuable in the initial staging, evaluation of treatment response, and follow-up of patients with EC. DW-MRI is an emerging imaging modality whose potential in the evaluation of treatment response is the current subject of active research.

REFERENCES

1. Zhang Y. Epidemiology of esophageal cancer. *World J Gastroenterol*. 2013;19:5598–5606.
2. American Cancer Society. *Esophagus cancer*. 2019. Available at: https://www.cancer.org/cancer/esophagus-cancer.html.
3. Xie SH, Lagergren J. Risk factors for oesophageal cancer. *Best Pract Res Clin Gastroenterol*. 2018;36-37:3–8.
4. Coleman HG, Xie SH, Lagergren J. The epidemiology of esophageal adenocarcinoma. *Gastroenterology*.. 2018;154:390–405.
5. Lao-Sirieix P, Fitzgerald RC. Screening for oesophageal cancer. *Nat Rev Clin Oncol*. 2012;9:278–287.
6. Ro TH, Mathew MA, Misra S. Value of screening endoscopy in evaluation of esophageal, gastric and colon cancers. *World J Gastroenterol*. 2015;21:9693–9706.
7. Yang J, et al. Estimating the costs of esophageal cancer screening, early diagnosis and treatment in three high risk areas in china. *Asian Pac J Cancer Prev*. 2011;12:1245–1250.
8. Rice TW, et al. Cancer of the esophagus and esophagogastric junction: An eighth edition staging primer. *J Thorac Oncol*. 2017;12:36–42.
9. Rice TW, Patil DT, Blackstone EH. 8th edition AJCC/UICC staging of cancers of the esophagus and esophagogastric junction: Application to clinical practice. *Ann Cardiothorac Surg*.. 2017;6:119–130.
10. Wang Y, et al. Anatomy of lymphatic drainage of the esophagus and lymph node metastasis of thoracic esophageal cancer. *Cancer Manag Res*.. 2018;10:6295–6303.
11. Thrumurthy SG, et al. Oesophageal cancer: Risks, prevention, and diagnosis. *BMJ*.. 2019;366:l4373.
12. Rice TW, et al. Cancer of the esophagus and esophagogastric junction-major changes in the american joint committee on cancer eighth edition cancer staging manual. *CA Cancer J Clin*. 2017;67:304–317.
13. National Comprehensive Cancer Network. *Clinical practice guidelines in oncology*. 2019. Available at: http://www.nccn.org/professionals/physician_gls/f_guidelines.asp.
14. Rizk NP, et al. Optimum lymphadenectomy for esophageal cancer. *Ann Surg*. 2010;251:46–50.
15. Hagens ERC, et al. The extent of lymphadenectomy in esophageal resection for cancer should be standardized. *J Thorac Dis*.. 2017;9:S713–S723.
16. Shaheen O, Ghibour A, Alsaid B. Esophageal cancer metastases to unexpected sites: A systematic review. *Gastroenterol Res Pract*.. 2017;2017:1657310.
17. Prenzel KL, et al. Prognostic relevance of skip metastases in esophageal cancer. *Ann Thorac Surg*. 2010;90:1662–1667.
18. Lerut T, et al. Three-field lymphadenectomy for carcinoma of the esophagus and gastroesophageal junction in 174 r0 resections: Impact on staging, disease-free survival, and outcome: A plea for

adaptation of TNM classification in upper-half esophageal carcinoma. *Ann Surg*. 2004;240:962–972. discussion 972-964.
19. Hagen JA, et al. Curative resection for esophageal adenocarcinoma: Analysis of 100 en bloc esophagectomies. *Ann Surg*. 2001;234:520–530. discussion 530-521.
20. Quint LE, et al. Incidence and distribution of distant metastases from newly diagnosed esophageal carcinoma. *Cancer*.. 1995;76:1120–1125.
21. Kim TJ, et al. Multimodality assessment of esophageal cancer: Preoperative staging and monitoring of response to therapy. *Radiographics*.. 2009;29:403–421.
22. Bruzzi JF, et al. Integrated CT-PET imaging of esophageal cancer: Unexpected and unusual distribution of distant organ metastases. *Curr Probl Diagn Radiol*. 2007;36:21–29.
23. Reinig JW, Stanley JH, Schabel SI. CT evaluation of thickened esophageal walls. *AJR Am J Roentgenol*. 1983;140:931–934.
24. Pech O, et al. Accuracy of endoscopic ultrasound in preoperative staging of esophageal cancer: Results from a referral center for early esophageal cancer. *Endoscopy*.. 2010;42:456–461.
25. Rasanen JV, et al. Prospective analysis of accuracy of positron emission tomography, computed tomography, and endoscopic ultrasonography in staging of adenocarcinoma of the esophagus and the esophagogastric junction. *Ann Surg Oncol*. 2003;10:954–960.
26. Tamandl D, et al. Prognostic value of volumetric PET parameters in unresectable and metastatic esophageal cancer. *Eur J Radiol*. 2016;85:540–545.
27. Hatt M, et al. Prognostic value of 18F-FDG PET image-based parameters in oesophageal cancer and impact of tumour delineation methodology. *Eur J Nucl Med Mol Imaging*. 2011;38:1191–1202.
28. Tan TH, Boey CY, Lee BN. Role of pre-therapeutic (18)F-FDG PET/CT in guiding the treatment strategy and predicting prognosis in patients with esophageal carcinoma. *Asia Ocean J Nucl Med Biol*. 2016;4:59–65.
29. Jo K, et al. A comparison study of esophageal findings on (18)F-FDG PET/CT and esophagogastroduodenoscopy. *Nucl Med Mol Imaging*. 2016;50:123–129.
30. Cuellar SL, et al. Clinical staging of patients with early esophageal adenocarcinoma: Does FDG-PET/CT have a role? *J Thorac Oncol*. 2014;9:1202–1206.
31. Lowe VJ, et al. Comparison of positron emission tomography, computed tomography, and endoscopic ultrasound in the initial staging of patients with esophageal cancer. *Mol Imaging Biol*. 2005;7:422–430.
32. van Westreenen HL, et al. Positron emission tomography with f-18-fluorodeoxyglucose in a combined staging strategy of esophageal cancer prevents unnecessary surgical explorations. *J Gastrointest Surg*. 2005;9:54–61.
33. Flamen P, et al. The utility of positron emission tomography for the diagnosis and staging of recurrent esophageal cancer. *J Thorac Cardiovasc Surg*. 2000;120:1085–1092.
34. Bille A, et al. Preoperative intrathoracic lymph node staging in patients with non-small-cell lung cancer: Accuracy of integrated positron emission tomography and computed tomography. *Eur J Cardiothorac Surg*. 2009;36:440–445.
35. van Vliet EP, et al. Detection of distant metastases in patients with oesophageal or gastric cardia cancer: A diagnostic decision analysis. *Br J Cancer*. 2007;97:868–876.
36. Nguyen NC, Chaar BT, Osman MM. Prevalence and patterns of soft tissue metastasis: Detection with true whole-body F-18 FDG PET/CT. *BMC Med Imaging*. 2007;7:8.
37. Purandare NC, et al. Incremental value of 18F-FDG PET/CT in therapeutic decision-making of potentially curable esophageal adenocarcinoma. *Nucl Med Commun*. 2014;35:864–869.
38. D'Journo XB, Thomas PA. Current management of esophageal cancer. *J Thorac Dis*. 2014;6(Suppl 2):S253–264.
39. Fokas E, Rodel C. Definitive, preoperative, and palliative radiation therapy of esophageal cancer. *Viszeralmedizin*.. 2015;31:347–353.
40. van Hagen P, et al. Preoperative chemoradiotherapy for esophageal or junctional cancer. *N Engl J Med*. 2012;366:2074–2084.
41. Tai P, Yu E. Esophageal cancer management controversies: Radiation oncology point of view. *World J Gastrointest Oncol*. 2014;6:263–274.
42. Wu AJ, et al. Expert consensus contouring guidelines for intensity modulated radiation therapy in esophageal and gastroesophageal junction cancer. *Int J Radiat Oncol Biol Phys*. 2015;92:911–920.
43. Shapiro J, et al. Neoadjuvant chemoradiotherapy plus surgery versus surgery alone for oesophageal or junctional cancer (cross): Long-term results of a randomised controlled trial. *Lancet Oncol*. 2015;16:1090–1098.
44. Minsky BD, et al. Int 0123 (radiation therapy oncology group 94-05) phase III trial of combined-modality therapy for esophageal cancer: High-dose versus standard-dose radiation therapy. *J Clin Oncol*. 2002;20:1167–1174.
45. Lin SH, Hallemeier CL, Chuong M. Proton beam therapy for the treatment of esophageal cancer. *Chin Clin Oncol*. 2016;5:53.
46. Kent MS, et al. Revisional surgery after esophagectomy: An analysis of 43 patients. *Ann Thorac Surg*. 2008;86:975–983. discussion 967-974.
47. Chen L, et al. Minimally invasive esophagectomy for esophageal cancer according to the location of the tumor: Experience of 251 patients. *Ann Med Surg (Lond)*. 2017;17:54–60.
48. Orringer MB. Transhiatal esophagectomy: How I teach it. *Ann Thorac Surg*. 2016;102:1432–1437.
49. Orringer MB, et al. Two thousand transhiatal esophagectomies: Changing trends, lessons learned. *Ann Surg*. 2007;246:363–372. discussion 372-364.
50. Chen B, et al. Modified mckeown minimally invasive esophagectomy for esophageal cancer: A 5-year retrospective study of 142 patients in a single institution. *PLoS One*. 2013;8:e82428.
51. Laterza E, et al. Induction chemo-radiotherapy for squamous cell carcinoma of the thoracic esophagus: Long-term results of a phase II study. *Ann Surg Oncol*. 1999;6:777–784.
52. Adham M, et al. Combined chemotherapy and radiotherapy followed by surgery in the treatment of patients with squamous cell carcinoma of the esophagus. *Cancer*.. 2000;89:946–954.
53. Huang JW, et al. To evaluate the treatment response of locally advanced esophageal cancer after preoperative chemoradiotherapy by FDG-PET/CT scan. *J Chin Med Assoc*. 2015;78:229–234.
54. Valero M, Robles-Medranda C. Endoscopic ultrasound in oncology: An update of clinical applications in the gastrointestinal tract. *World J Gastrointest Endosc*. 2017;9:243–254.
55. Stiekema J, et al. Detecting interval metastases and response assessment using 18F-FDG PET/CT after neoadjuvant chemoradiotherapy for esophageal cancer. *Clin Nucl Med*. 2014;39:862–867.
56. Schroer-Gunther M, et al. The role of PET and PET-CT scanning in assessing response to neoadjuvant therapy in esophageal carcinoma. *Dtsch Arztebl Int*.. 2015;112:545–552.
57. Guo L, Zhang L, Zhao J. CT scan and magnetic resonance diffusion-weighted imaging in the diagnosis and treatment of esophageal cancer. *Oncol Lett*.. 2018;16:7117–7122.
58. van Rossum PS, et al. Diffusion-weighted magnetic resonance imaging for the prediction of pathologic response to neoadjuvant chemoradiotherapy in esophageal cancer. *Radiother Oncol*. 2015;115:163–170.
59. Vollenbrock SE, et al. Diagnostic performance of MRI for assessment of response to neoadjuvant chemoradiotherapy in oesophageal cancer. *Br J Surg*. 2019;106:596–605.
60. Kwee TC, et al. Complementary roles of whole-body diffusion-weighted MRI and 18F-FDG PET: The state of the art and potential applications. *J Nucl Med*. 2010;51:1549–1558.
61. Betancourt Cuellar SL, et al. (18)FDG-PET/CT is useful in the follow-up of surgically treated patients with oesophageal adenocarcinoma. *Br J Radiol*. 2018;91:20170341.
62. Kim SJ, et al. Diagnostic value of surveillance (18)f-fluorodeoxyglucose PET/CT for detecting recurrent esophageal carcinoma after curative treatment. *Eur J Nucl Med Mol Imaging*. 2019;46:1850–1858.
63. Kelly RJ. Immunotherapy for esophageal and gastric cancer. *Am Soc Clin Oncol Educ Book*. 2017;37:292–300.
64. Alsina M, Moehler M, Lorenzen S. Immunotherapy of esophageal cancer: Current status, many trials and innovative strategies. *Oncol Res Treat*.. 2018;41:266–271.
65. Vogelstein B, et al. Cancer genome landscapes. *Science*.. 2013;339:1546–1558.
66. Yarchoan M, Hopkins A, Jaffee EM. Tumor mutational burden and response rate to PD-1 inhibition. *N Engl J Med*. 2017;377:2500–2501.
67. Doi T, et al. Safety and antitumor activity of the anti-programmed death-1 antibody pembrolizumab in patients with advanced esophageal carcinoma. *J Clin Oncol*. 2018;36:61–67.
68. Kudo T, et al. Nivolumab treatment for oesophageal squamous-cell carcinoma: An open-label, multicentre, phase 2 trial. *Lancet Oncol*. 2017;18:631–639.

CHAPTER

16 Gastric Carcinoma

Raghunandan Vikram, M.D.; Naruhiko Ikoma, M.D.; Madhavi Patnana, M.D.; Catherine Devine, M.D.; Paul Mansfield, M.D.; and Alexandria Phan, M.D.

INTRODUCTION

Over the past several decades, the incidence of gastric carcinoma in the world has been on a decline, but it remains the second most common cause of cancer-related death worldwide. There are differences in the geographic distribution, epidemiologic trends, presentation, and location of gastric carcinoma that have been studied in detail recently. Gastric carcinoma tends to be diagnosed at an advanced stage, particularly in the West, and generally has a poor prognosis. Japan has the highest incidence of gastric carcinoma, but it also has a national gastric carcinoma screening program, allowing for more patients to be diagnosed at an early stage. For localized gastric carcinoma, the best chance for durable disease control and survival is with curative surgery. Unfortunately, surgery alone is not enough when the 5-year overall survival (OS) rate is 23% to 25%.[1,2] Multimodality therapy has become common practice for resectable gastric carcinoma to improve the rate of disease control and minimize recurrence. Postoperative chemoradiotherapy is the standard of practice in the United States and other parts of North and South America, and perioperative chemotherapy is adopted by most European countries. Regional differences in outcomes are probably the result of many different factors, most importantly early disease detection in countries with a screening program, such as Japan, and also difficulty in accurate staging with currently available imaging and staging modalities.

Radiologic and endoscopic ultrasound (EUS) staging are crucial in the management of patients with gastric carcinoma. Various imaging techniques, including double-contrast upper gastrointestinal (UGI) barium examinations, multidetector computed tomography (MDCT), magnetic resonance imaging (MRI), positron emission tomography/computed tomography (PET/CT), and EUS, are all used in the diagnosis and staging of gastric carcinoma to varying degrees.

EPIDEMIOLOGY AND RISK FACTORS

Epidemiology

Although the incidence of gastric carcinoma is decreasing in Western countries, it remains the fourth most frequent cancer diagnosed and the second most lethal cancer worldwide, behind only lung cancer. The number of new cases of gastric carcinoma per year worldwide was recently estimated as over 683,000 in males and 349,000 in females.[3,4] It is the third most common cancer in males and the fifth most common cancer in females worldwide.[5] Some 60% of cases occur in developing countries.[6] The areas with the highest incidence rates are Eastern Asia, South America, and Eastern Europe. Regions in which gastric carcinoma is least frequent are North America, Western Europe, and parts of Africa. There is approximately a 20-fold difference in the incidence rates between Japan and some White populations in the United States.[6] In the United States, approximately 27,600 new cases of gastric carcinoma were expected to be diagnosed during 2020, with 11,010 estimated deaths from the disease during the same period.[7,8]

Of the several classification systems that have been proposed to describe gastric carcinoma, the Lauren classification is the most widely used. The Lauren classification describes tumors based on the microscopic configuration and growth pattern into intestinal and diffuse types.[9,10] Diffuse cancers are noncohesive and diffusely infiltrate the stomach. These often exhibit deep infiltration of the gastric wall and show little or no gland formation. These tumors are often associated with marked desmoplasia and inflammation, with relative sparing of the overlying mucosa. The intestinal type, conversely, shows recognizable gland formation similar in microscopic appearance to the colonic mucosa. The glandular formation ranges from well to poorly differentiated tumors and grows in expanding rather than infiltrative patterns.[6] Intestinal cancers are believed to be related to environmental factors and are thought to arise from precancerous lesions such as gastric atrophy, and intestinal metaplasia. These are also associated with *Helicobacter pylori* infection and are considered an "epidemic" form of cancer. The intestinal type is gradually declining in the United States but still remains a common cause of gastric carcinoma worldwide. The diffuse cancers, conversely, are less related to environmental factors and occur more often in young patients.[6] The relative incidence of diffuse cancers is believed to have increased mainly owing to the decrease in the incidence of intestinal type cancers.[11]

There are regional differences in the pathology and anatomic location of gastric carcinoma. A predominance of the Lauren intestinal type of adenocarcinoma occurs in high-risk areas, whereas the Lauren diffuse type is relatively more common in low-risk areas. Proximal gastric carcinomas and cancers of the gastroesophageal junction are more common in the West, and distal gastric carcinoma is more common in high-risk regions. At the MD Anderson Cancer Center, 41% of all UGI cancers involve the gastroesophageal junction.[12] A steady decline in the incidence and mortality rates of gastric carcinoma has been observed worldwide over the past several decades. This is mainly attributed to a decrease in the intestinal variety of gastric carcinoma, with the incidence of diffuse cancer being relatively stable.[6]

Etiology and Risk Factors

Because gastric carcinoma is more common in Asia than in Western countries, ethnic origin was thought to be an important contributory factor for the observed difference.[13] Although first-generation Asian immigrants to Western countries carry the same high susceptibility for gastric carcinoma as their counterparts in their native country, subsequent generations acquire risk levels approaching that of the population of their adopted countries. This epidemiologic pattern underlines the importance of environmental factors in the pathogenesis of gastric carcinoma.[14] Diets poor in fruits and vegetables and rich in smoked or poorly preserved food, salt, nitrates, and nitrites, infection with *H. pylori*, and smoking have all been implicated as significant risk factors in the development of gastric carcinoma in several studies.[15–17] Chronic atrophic gastritis, previous gastric surgery, gastric polyps, and obesity, as well as low socioeconomic status, are also associated with an increased risk of gastric carcinoma.[18,19]

Gastric carcinoma is also seen as a part of the hereditary nonpolyposis colon cancer syndrome and other gastrointestinal (GI) polyposis syndromes such as Peutz–Jeghers syndrome and familial adenomatous polyposis.[19] Mutations in the gene encoding E-cadherin are a well-recognized cause of hereditary diffuse gastric cancer.[20]

Key Points Epidemiology and Risk Factors

- More common in Asia than in Western countries.
- Important environmental factors: smoked or poorly preserved food, chemicals, *Helicobacter pylori* infection.
- Additional risk factors: smoking, obesity, low economic status.
- Predisposing factors: genetic mutation or polyposis syndromes.

Clinical Presentation

The symptoms of patients with gastric carcinoma are nonspecific. As a result, diagnosis is often delayed, and patients will have advanced disease at the time of diagnosis. Frequent symptoms associated with gastric carcinoma include dysphagia, early satiety, nausea, vomiting, and other symptoms attributable to gastric outlet obstruction or anemia. However, the most common symptoms at the time of diagnosis are upper abdominal pain and weight loss.[21]

ANATOMY AND PATHOLOGY

Anatomy

Being a derivative of the foregut, the blood supply to the stomach is provided almost entirely by the branches of the celiac trunk (Fig. 16.1). The left gastric artery, arising from the celiac axis, and the right gastric artery, a branch of the hepatic artery, supply the lesser curvature in the gastrohepatic ligament and form an anastomotic arcade along the lesser curvature. The left and right gastroepiploic arteries, branches of the splenic artery and the gastroduodenal artery, supply the greater curvature of the stomach and traverse the gastrosplenic ligament and the gastrocolic ligament, respectively. The gastrocolic ligament is the supracolic part of the greater omentum. Numerous short gastric arteries, branches of the splenic artery, also supply the greater curvature. A rich lymphatic network accompanies these vessels, creating a conduit for lymphatic drainage, and traverses these complex ligamentous structures. The various ligamentous attachments can be identified by noting vascular landmarks on cross-sectional imaging (Table 16.1).[22] These ligamentous structures are important to understand, because they represent the critical conduits for local extension of primary gastric carcinoma.

The stomach is divided for descriptive purposes into the fundus, body, pyloric antrum, and pylorus by imaginary lines drawn on its external surface (Fig. 16.2). The fundus is dome shaped, immediately under the left dome of the diaphragm, and is superior to the cardiac orifice. It lies above an imaginary line drawn horizontally at the level of the cardia (incisura cardia) to the greater curvature. At the lower end of the lesser curvature is a constant external notch (incisura angularis). The body extends from the cardia to the incisura angularis. A slight groove, the sulcus intermedius on the greater curvature of the stomach, separates the body from the pyloric antrum. The antrum extends from an imaginary line drawn from the incisura angularis to the sulcus intermedius. The pylorus is the narrowest part of the stomach, measuring only approximately 1 to 2 cm in length, and terminates into the duodenum (see Fig. 16.2).[23]

Key Points Anatomy

- The stomach is divided into the fundus, body, pyloric antrum, and pylorus by imaginary lines drawn on its external surface.
- The stomach is almost entirely supplied by the branches of the celiac artery.
- Complex ligamentous attachments of the stomach provide conduits for direct spread of malignancies to the adjoining structures and the peritoneum.

Pathology

Malignant tumors of the stomach can be divided into four major subtypes based on cells of origin: epithelial, mesenchymal, and neuroendocrine tumors, and lymphoma. Leiomyosarcomas, neurofibrosarcomas, and malignant GI stromal tumors are mesenchymal in origin. The World Health Organization classification of gastric tumors takes into consideration the morphologic and molecular characteristics of the tumors and is shown in Table 16.2.[6]

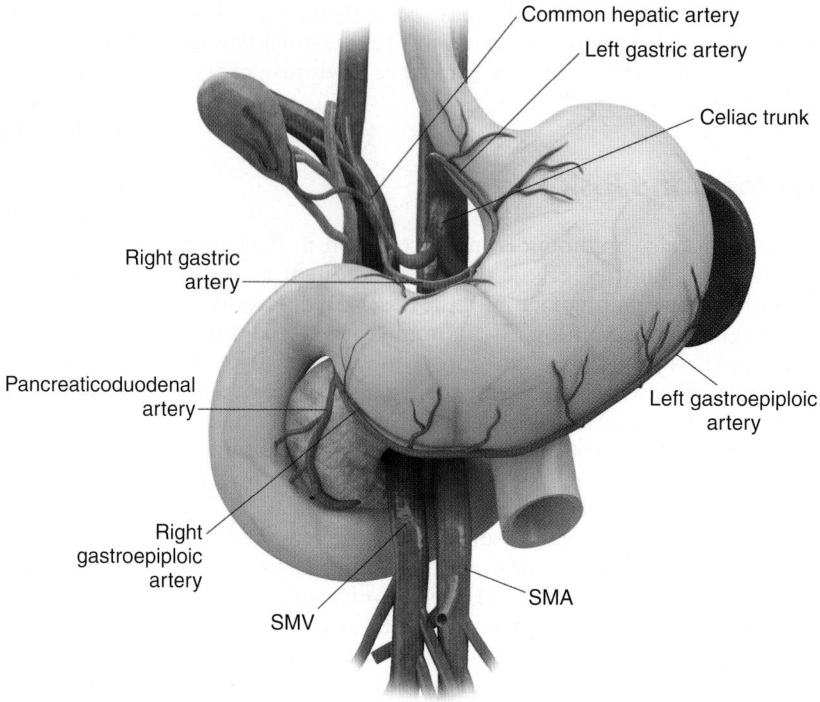

Figure 16.1. The blood supply of the stomach. The stomach is predominantly supplied by the branches of the celiac artery, being a derivative of the foregut. The greater curvature is supplied by the left and right gastroepiploic arteries, which are branches of the splenic and pancreaticoduodenal arteries. The lesser curvature is supplied by the left and right gastric arteries, which are branches of the celiac and common hepatic artery. In addition, several short gastric arteries (not shown) from the splenic artery supply the posterior wall of the stomach and the fundus. *SMA*, Superior mesenteric artery; *SMV*, superior mesenteric vein.

Table 16.1 The Various Ligamentous Attachments of the Stomach Can Be Identified by Identifying Vascular Landmarks on Cross-Sectional Imaging

PERITONEAL LIGAMENTS AND FOLD	RELATION TO ORGANS	VASCULAR LANDMARK
Gastrohepatic ligament	Lesser curvature of the stomach to the liver	Left and right gastric arteries
Hepatoduodenal ligament	From the duodenum to the hepatic fissure	Proper hepatic artery, portal vein
Gastrocolic ligament	Greater curvature of the stomach to the transverse colon	Left and right gastroepiploic arteries and vein
Gastrosplenic ligament	From the left side of the greater curvature of the stomach to the splenic hilum	Left gastroepiploic vessels

(From Vikram R, et al. Pancreas: peritoneal reflections, ligamentous connections, and pathways of disease spread. Radiographics. 2009;29:e34.)

Malignant epithelial tumors constitute the majority of gastric neoplasias, and nearly 90% of them are adenocarcinomas. Several classification systems are used for describing adenocarcinomas. Based on histology, they are subdivided into tubular, papillary, mucinous, and signet-ring cell carcinomas.[6] Usually, one of the subtypes predominates in adenocarcinomas. Based on gross appearance, tumors are classified into four types: type I is a polypoid and fungating variety; type II is a polypoid tumor with central ulceration; type III is an ulcerated tumor with infiltrative margins; and type IV is linitis plastica.[10,24] This method of classification is called the *Borrmann classification* and is generally reserved for advanced cancers. However, the simplest and the most widely accepted classification is the *Lauren classification*, in which the gastric carcinomas are divided into two types: intestinal and diffuse.[9,10] The intestinal type is associated with various degrees of glandular formation and intestinal metaplasia. The diffuse type is infiltrative, presents as a plaque or linitis plastica, and tends to be poorly differentiated or of a signet-ring variety.[6] Those cancers having features of both intestinal and diffuse types are considered *mixed*.

Key Points Pathology

- Some 90% of malignant epithelial tumors of the stomach are adenocarcinomas.
- Several histologic classification systems are used, but the simplest and most widely accepted is the Lauren classification, in which gastric carcinomas are divided into two types: intestinal and diffuse.
- Intestinal cancers show an expansile growth pattern with recognizable gland formation similar in microscopic appearance to the colonic mucosa. Diffuse cancers are noncohesive, diffusely infiltrate the gastric wall, and are associated with desmoplasia and inflammation.

Patterns of Tumor Spread

Gastric carcinoma shows a propensity to spread through direct contiguous invasion of adjacent peritoneal reflections, and also to adjacent organs. In addition, dissemination via lymphatic and hematogenous routes also occurs. Both

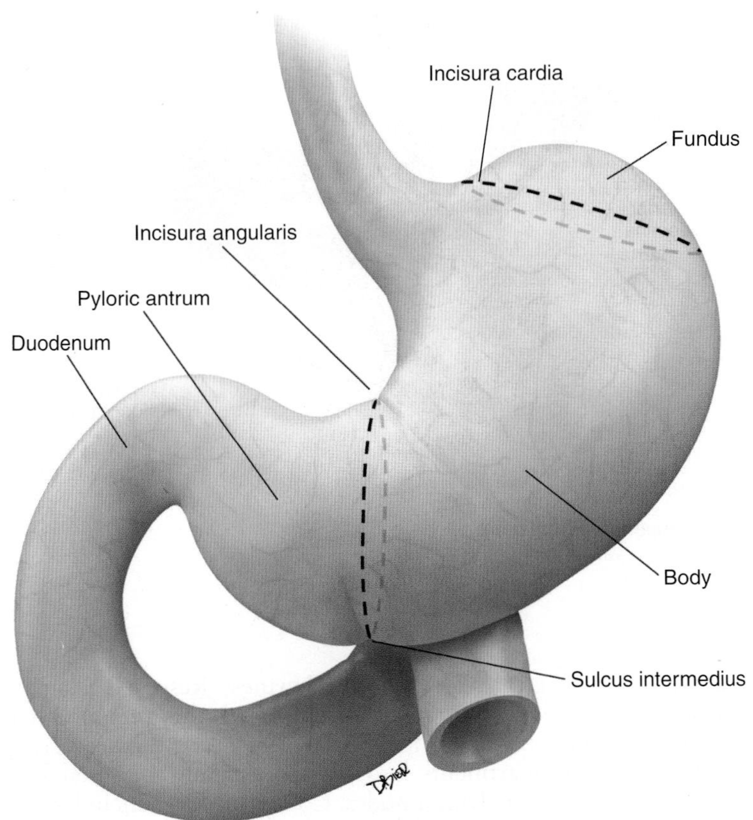

Figure 16.2. The different parts of the stomach. The incisura cardia, sulcus intermedius, and incisura angularis are the landmarks used to divide the stomach into the fundus, body, and pyloric antrum.

Table 16.2 The World Health Organization Classification of Tumors of the Stomach

EPITHELIAL TUMORS	NONEPITHELIAL TUMORS
Intraepithelial neoplasia—adenoma	Leiomyoma
Carcinoma	Schwannoma
Adenocarcinoma	Granular cell tumor
Papillary adenocarcinoma	Glomus tumor
Tubular adenocarcinoma	Leiomyosarcoma
Mucinous adenocarcinoma	Gastrointestinal stromal tumor
Signet-ring cell carcinoma	Kaposi sarcoma
Adenosquamous carcinoma	
Squamous cell carcinoma	
Small cell carcinoma	
Undifferentiated carcinoma	
Carcinoid (well-differentiated endocrine neoplasm)	

(Modified from Hamilton SR, Aaltonen LA, eds. World Health Organization Classification of Tumours. Pathology and Genetics of Tumours of the Digestive System. Lyon: IARC Press; 2000.)

Lauren intestinal and diffuse varieties show a propensity for direct contiguous spread, but it is more commonly seen in the diffuse type of cancer. The gastrocolic, gastrohepatic, gastrosplenic, and hepatoduodenal ligaments all serve as conduits for tumor dissemination. Once the integrity of the peritoneal lining is breached, the tumor can seed into the peritoneal cavity, likely in the greater omentum, the paracolic gutters, and the pelvic floor. It is not uncommon to encounter tumor deposits in the ovaries and the rectovesicle pouch.

Periserosal implants into adjacent and distant organs are not infrequent, particularly with diffuse cancers, producing an appearance similar to linitis plastica, commonly in the colon.[25,26]

Lymphatic spread is seen commonly in advanced and not infrequently in early gastric carcinomas. Several nodal stations drain the stomach. These generally run parallel to the gastric blood supply: lymphatics along the lesser curve drain to the left gastric and celiac nodes; lymphatics along the pylorus and lesser curvature run parallel to the right gastric artery and drain into the hepatic and celiac nodes; a third group of lymphatics drain the proximal greater curvature of the stomach into the pancreaticosplenic nodes; and the fourth group parallels the right gastroepiploic vessels along the greater curvature and drain into the infrapyloric nodes and the nodes in the transverse mesocolon (Fig. 16.3).

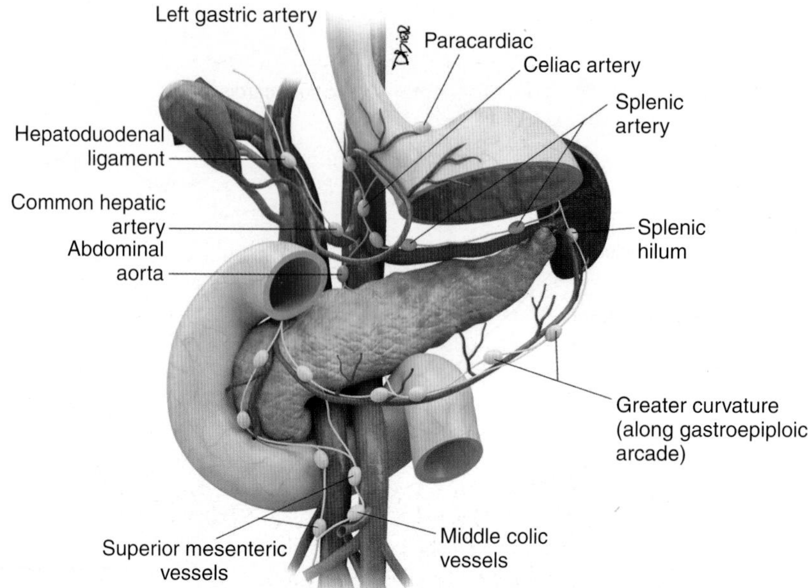

FIGURE 16.3. The major nodal stations draining the stomach. These generally parallel the gastric blood supply.

Hematogenous metastasis is common to the liver owing to the predominant portal venous drainage of the stomach. Metastases to the lungs, bones, and other soft tissues are also documented. Peritoneal dissemination leads to direct spread of tumors to the organs in the abdominal cavity. Direct seeding along the laparoscopic tract and percutaneous biopsy tract is also seen.

KEY POINTS Pattern of Tumor Spread

- Direct contiguous spread occurs via the various ligamentous connections of the stomach, such as the gastrocolic, gastrohepatic, gastrosplenic, and hepatoduodenal ligaments.
- Peritoneal dissemination and seeding are common in advanced gastric carcinoma. Transperitoneal seeding of tumor to other abdominal organs is also seen.
- Lymphatic spread is to the perigastric and regional lymph nodes running parallel to the branches of the celiac artery.
- Hematogenous spread occurs to the liver, lungs, bones, and other soft tissues.

Staging

The tumor-node-metastasis (TNM) staging system is the most widely accepted method for staging gastric carcinomas.[27] Radiologic investigations such as CT, MRI, and ultrasound are used for preoperative staging. Pathologic staging is considered the gold standard, particularly in specimens not subject to preoperative chemo- or radiotherapy.

Depth of invasion, or T stage, is an important independent prognostic factor for both survival and local recurrence. T1 cancers have a 10-year survival rate of approximately 80%, T2 lesions 55%, and T3 and T4 lesions only 30%.[28–31]

Knowledge of nodal anatomy is very important in staging lymph nodes in gastric carcinoma because this is useful in surgical planning. The Japanese Research Society for Gastric Carcinoma has classified the regional lymph nodes based on location.[32] These are further classified as compartments 1 to 4. Compartment 1 consists of the perigastric lymph nodes. Compartment 2 includes lymph nodes along the left gastric artery, common hepatic artery, celiac axis, and splenic artery. Compartment 3 includes lymph nodes along the hepatoduodenal ligament, at the posterior head of the pancreas, and at the root of the mesentery. In cancers of the antrum, the lymph nodes along the splenic artery are classified as compartment III. Paraaortic lymph nodes constitute compartment 4. These are useful in describing the extent of lymph node dissection in surgery. D1 dissection includes compartment 1; D2 dissection compartments 1 and 2; D3 dissection compartments 1, 2, and 3; and D4 dissection includes all four compartments.

Although compartmental dissection is methodologically sound, the International Committee on Gastric Carcinoma has recommended that, for accurate staging and predicting prognosis, a minimum of 16 lymph nodes must be included in the surgical specimen before an N stage can be determined.[33] N stage is an independent variable for survival: N0 disease has a 10-year survival rate of 70%; N1, 41%; and N2 or N3 less than 20%.[34]

KEY POINTS Staging

- The tumor-mode-metastasis system is the most commonly used staging system and is provides important prognostic information.
- Nodal stations are classified into different compartments based on the distance from the primary tumor. These compartments are used to guide surgery.
- At least 16 nodes should be harvested at surgery and pathologically evaluated to complete pathologic staging for gastric carcinoma.

IMAGING EVALUATION

Imaging modalities used to evaluate the extent of gastric carcinoma include conventional fluoroscopic barium studies, esophagoduodenoscopy (EGD) with EUS, MDCT, MRI, and PET.

Tumor Detection and Staging

EGD has replaced UGI double-contrast barium study as the modality of choice to detect and diagnose gastric carcinoma, owing to its specificity and the advantage of obtaining a tissue biopsy, as well as the ability to perform EUS, which offers a reliable way to T stage the tumor.[35] However, some reports indicate that endoscopy and UGI barium studies are equally sensitive in the detection of primary gastric carcinoma.[36,37] Gastric carcinoma has various appearances on GI barium studies. These include plaque-like lesions, sessile or pedunculated polypoid lesions, ulcerated lesions, and nondistention of the stomach, as in the scirrhous type of carcinoma or linitis plastica with diffuse loss of mucosal detail (Fig. 16.4).

EUS is superior to all other modalities in visualizing the different layers of the gastric wall and thus is most accurate in preoperative local (T) staging of gastric tumors, with an accuracy rate of 78% to 94%.[38,39] Despite this, it is not uncommon (particularly for T2 tumors) for there to be discordance with the actual pathologic specimen. The gastric wall layers appear as a five-layered structure on EUS with alternating hyperechoic and hypoechoic bands: serosa, muscularis propria, submucosa, deep mucosa, and superficial mucosa.[40] Tumors generally are hypoechoic or hyperechoic and are seen disrupting this regular pattern. EUS is also valuable in assessing smaller perigastric lymph nodes (Fig. 16.5). EUS is of little to no benefit after preoperative therapy.

CT is generally less accurate than EUS for T staging of gastric tumors. However, with the latest development in multidetector scanners, optimization of gastric distention, negative oral contrast, and dynamic contrast-enhanced CT with multiplanar reconstructions, the accuracy of CT in T staging appears to have improved.[41] The normal gastric wall shows a two- to three-layered structure: an inner, markedly enhancing mucosal layer; a submucosal layer with low attenuation; and an outer muscular-serosal layer with moderate enhancement (Fig. 16.6).[42] T staging is assessed by studying the integrity of these layers. On CT, T1 and T2 lesions are limited to the gastric wall. T3 lesions, however, may show slight blurring of the serosal contour, with associated stranding of perigastric fat.[43] T4 lesions spread via ligamentous attachments and peritoneal reflections in T4 lesions (Figs. 16.7 and 16.8). The early phase of the multiphase dynamic CT study after intravenous contrast is considered optimal in determining the depth of tumor invasion, as well as defining the vascular anatomy of the stomach.[44] Takao and coworkers,[45] in a study of 108 patients with gastric carcinoma using a multiphasic protocol CT, reported a tumor detection rate and T staging accuracy of 98% and 82%, respectively, for advanced gastric carcinomas. However, the detection and accuracy of T staging in early gastric carcinomas was significantly low, at 23% and 15%, respectively. Use of multiplanar reformatting in coronal and sagittal planes appears to improve detection and T staging.[41,46] To improve the quality of three-dimensional

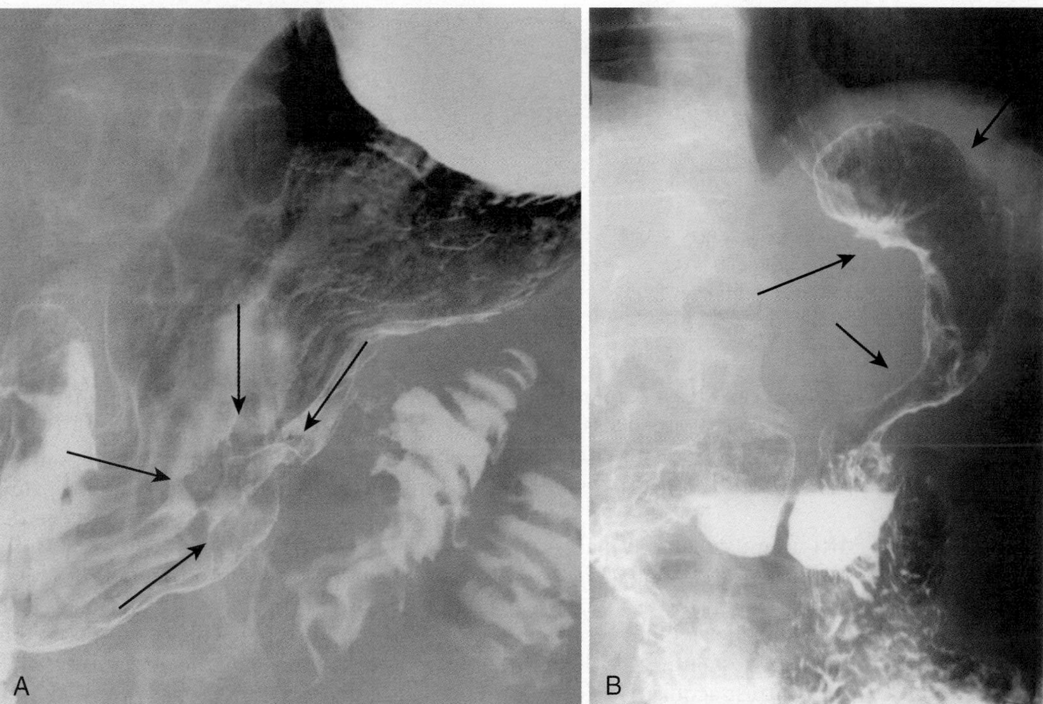

Fig. 16.4 A, Double-contrast barium meal study in a 54-year-old patient shows a mucosal mass (*arrows*) owing to adenocarcinoma at the greater curvature. **B,** Linitis plastica seen on double-contrast barium study. The body of the stomach fails to distend (*arrows*). Irregularity of the mucosa is also seen because of the diffuse infiltrative process.

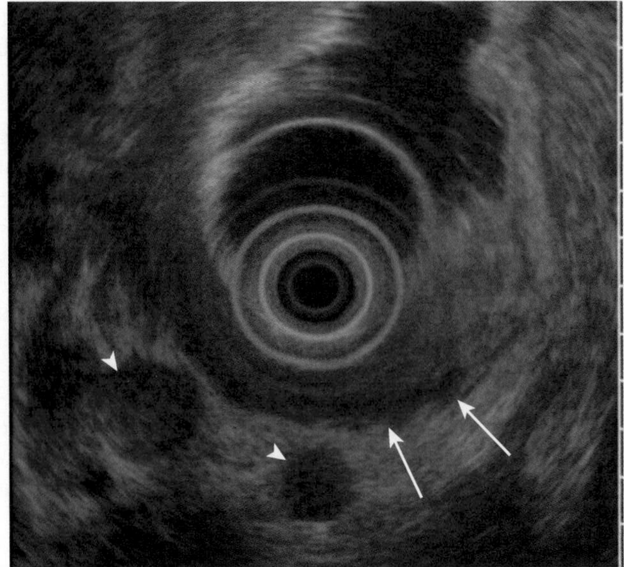

FIGURE 16.5. Endoscopic ultrasound shows the loss of the normal alternating hyper- and hypoechoic bands caused by the gastric carcinoma. Here, the tumor is seen infiltrating through the serosa (*arrows*). Enlarged perigastric lymph nodes (*arrowheads*) are also visualized.

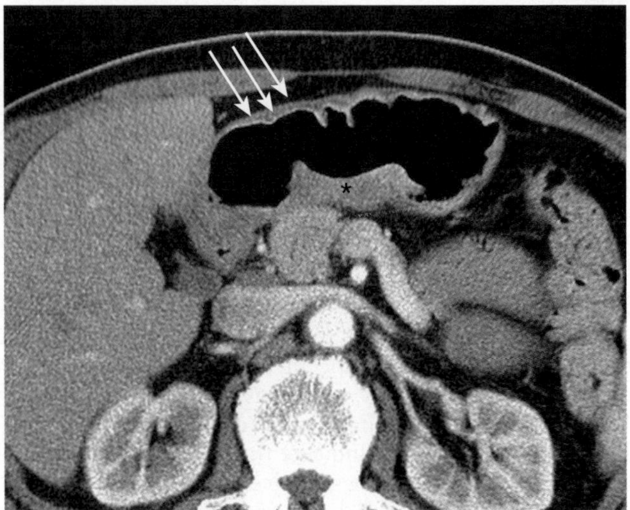

FIGURE 16.6. Axial computed tomography scan with intravenous contrast. The normal stomach shows three layers: an enhancing mucosa, a low-attenuation stripe of muscularis, and an outer enhancing serosa (*white arrows*). A tumor in the lesser curve (*black asterisk*) shows loss of anatomic detail, indicating involvement of the submucosa and muscularis.

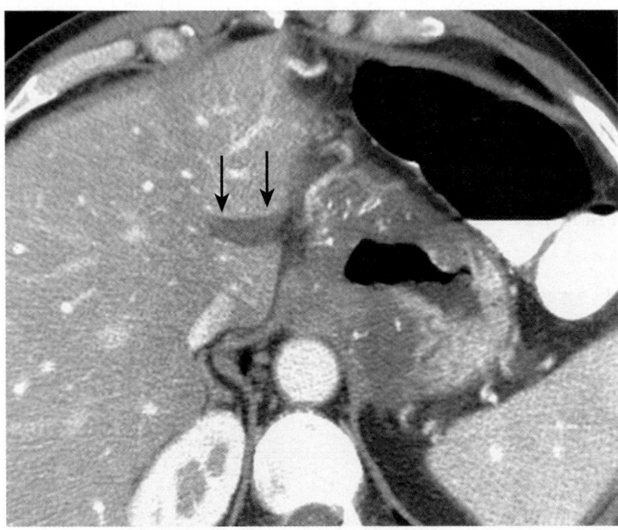

FIGURE 16.7. Diffuse thickening of the cardia and lesser curve of the stomach because of adenocarcinoma shows soft tissue infiltration of the gastrohepatic ligament and extending into the hepatic fissure (*arrows*).

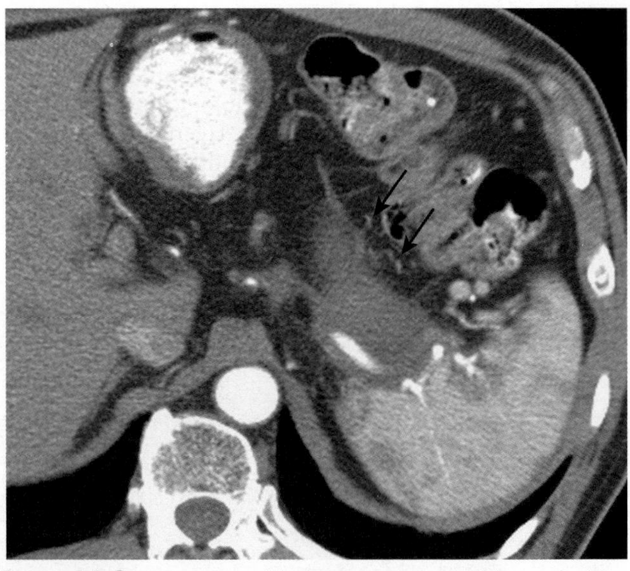

FIGURE 16.8. Carcinoma of the greater curvature of the stomach (not shown) with tumor extension along the gastrosplenic ligament (*arrows*).

(3D) imaging, however, thinner slices of at least 1.25-mm slice thickness are required. Advanced postprocessing techniques with volume rendering to produce an endoscopic-type image (virtual gastroscopy) have also been described.[47]

The major advantage of MRI is multiplanar capability and better tissue contrast. However, the use of MRI in staging gastric carcinoma is limited, owing to respiratory and cardiac motion, although some smaller studies report that MRI is comparable with CT for T staging.[48–50] Fat-suppressed 3D T1-weighted postcontrast acquisitions can demonstrate the mucosal lesion in the arterial phase.[51] Loss of rugae and diffuse thickening and enhancement of the gastric mucosa and wall represent diffuse scirrhous tumors or linitis plastica (Fig. 16.9). Overall, the accuracy of MRI is similar when compared with CT in the evaluation of T staging. However, its limited availably and higher cost limits its routine use, and it should primarily be used as an alternative when CT is contraindicated.[52]

PET/CT and 2-[^{18}F] fluoro-2-deoxy-D-glucose (FDG)-PET perform inconsistently in detection of gastric carcinoma and are not useful in the T staging of gastric carcinomas because of the normal background uptake of FDG in the gastric mucosa and also the variability in FDG uptake depending on the tumor's histologic type. Signet-ring carcinoma (diffuse type) and poorly differentiated adenocarcinoma show little to no uptake (Fig. 16.10).[53,54] The use of water to distend the stomach appears to improve

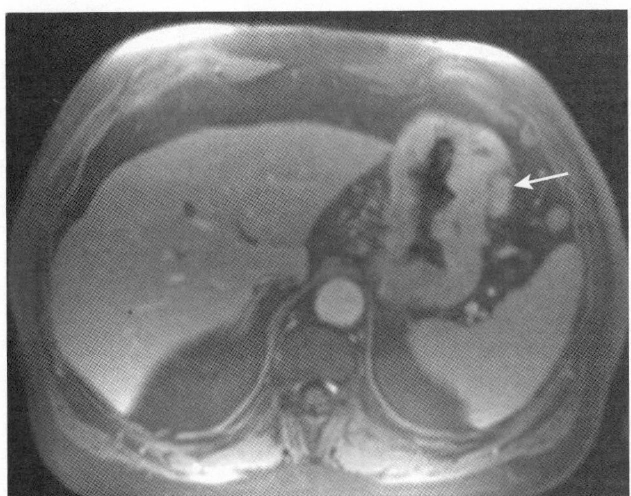

FIGURE 16.9. Fat-suppressed three-dimensional T1-weighted postcontrast magnetic resonance imaging acquisition shows loss of rugae and diffuse thickening and enhancement of the gastric mucosa and wall representing diffuse scirrhous tumor or linitis plastica. An enlarged gastroepiploic node (*arrow*) is also seen.

the specificity of PET/CT for diagnosis to a modest degree.[55] However, owing to its poor performance, the role of PET/CT in diagnosis and T staging of gastric carcinoma is uncertain.

Lymph Node Staging

Nodal staging is challenging, even with the current advances in imaging technology, owing to significant limitations in detecting microscopic metastases by currently available imaging modalities. Owing to the lack of any reliable indicator to detect metastatic lymph nodes on cross-sectional imaging, size is the major criterion used, with a presumed upper limit of 8 to 10 mm in short-axis diameter (Fig. 16.11; see also Fig. 16.9).This parameter has significant shortcomings.[56] In a prospective study of patients with gastric carcinoma, Monig and colleagues reported that 80% of lymph nodes less than 5 mm in size were benign, but 55% of metastatic lymph nodes were also less than 5 mm in diameter, clearly demonstrating the

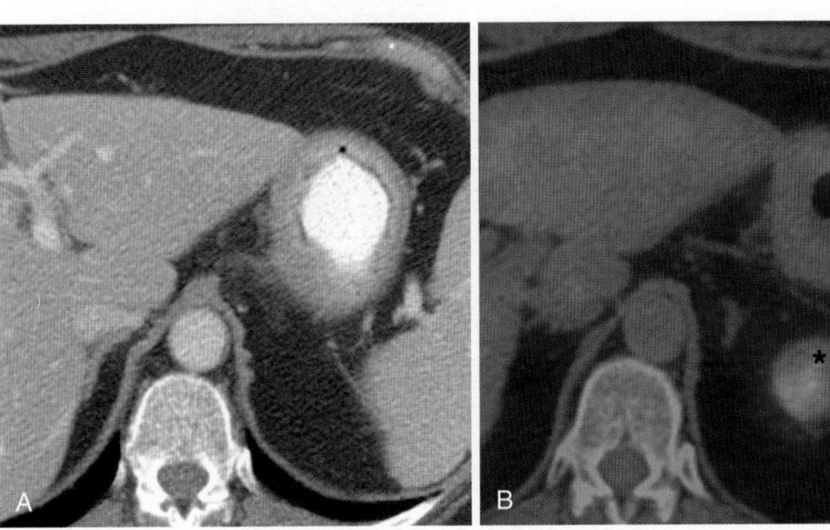

FIGURE 16.10. A, Axial computed tomography (CT) scan with intravenous and oral contrast shows diffuse thickening of the stomach because of infiltrating carcinoma, signet-cell variety (linitis plastica). **B,** A fused positron emission tomography (PET)/CT scan shows poor uptake of 2-[^{18}F] fluoro-2-deoxy-D-glucose. Left, Increased activity in the kidney (*asterisk*) is also noted on PET/CT.

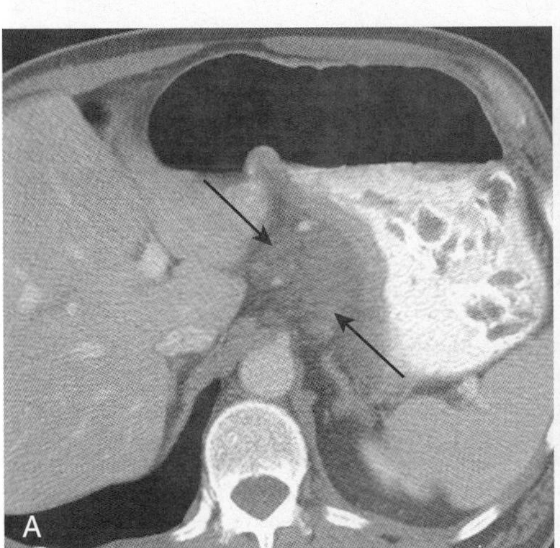

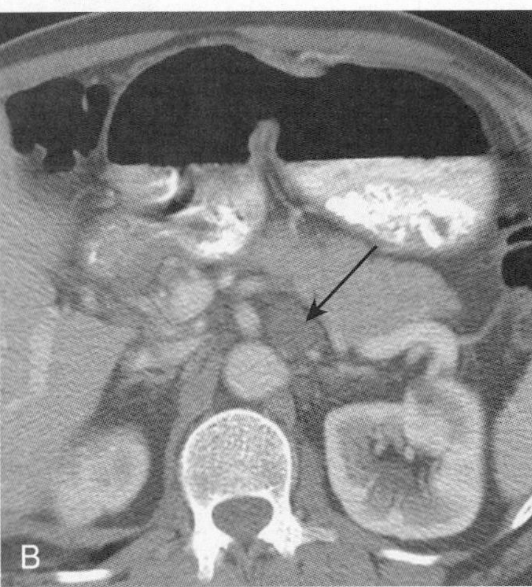

FIGURE 16.11. A, Enlarged left gastric lymph nodes (*arrows*). There is thickening of the lesser curvature caused by infiltrative gastric adenocarcinoma of the proximal stomach. **B,** Enlarged celiac lymph node (*arrow*) in a patient with gastric adenocarcinoma of the proximal stomach.

weakness of any size criterion as a parameter on imaging modalities.[48,57] CT sensitivity ranges from 62.5% to 91.9% (median 80.0%) and specificity from 50.0% to 87.9% (median 77.8%), based on a systematic review including 10 studies.[58]

In addition to the challenges faced by CT regarding the staging of lymph nodes, MRI also suffers owing to movement artifact because of peristalsis and breathing.[51] Use of diffusion-weighted imaging sequences increases the sensitivity for detecting nodes, which offers a significant advantage over CT. A few small studies have found that MRI is comparable to CT in detection of lymph node metastases.[48–50,59,60] Use of lymphotrophic ultrasmall superparamagnetic iron oxide (USPIO) particles (ferumoxtran-10) for detecting metastatic lymph nodes showed some promise in staging distant lymph nodes, such as those in the retroperitoneal and paraaortic regions. Owing to movement artifact, the nodes in the perigastric region are not clearly assessed. Tatsumi and associates[61] demonstrated a sensitivity of 100% and a specificity of 92.6% in detecting metastatic lymph nodes using lymphotrophic USPIO particles in MRI. Currently, the USPIO is not commercially available in the United States, which limits its clinical application.

Morphology and echo texture are used to identify metastatic lymph nodes by EUS. Because of the proximity to the probe, this is an excellent modality to detect nodes in the immediate vicinity of the stomach, such as the perigastric lymph nodes. For surgical planning, however, the important stations (station III and station IV nodes) are not adequately staged by this modality, because they are beyond the focal zone of the transducer.

FDG-avid nodes on PET/CT are likely malignant, and, hence, PET/CT enjoys a higher specificity than CT or MRI. However, PET/CT suffers from inherently poor resolution and, hence, poor sensitivity.[62] In addition, the previously mentioned lack of FDG avidity for diffuse type cancers is a severe limitation (see Fig. 16.10). Therefore, the likelihood of this modality improving nodal staging is remote, unless there is technologic innovation with widespread availability of high-resolution PET/CT scanners.

Metastatic Gastric Carcinoma

Involvement of distant lymph nodes such as the right supraclavicular lymph node (Virchow node) is considered distant metastasis, and curative surgery is not feasible in such patients (Fig. 16.12). According to the American Joint Committee on Cancer staging, the presence of cancer in the hepatoduodenal, retropancreatic, mesenteric, or paraaortic region is classified as distant metastasis.[27]

Gastric carcinoma frequently metastasizes to the liver, owing to its portal venous drainage. The metastatic deposits most often are hypovascular, with or without a rim of enhancement. Hence, a routine scan during portal venous phase is adequate.

CT scan of the chest is considered essential in patients to stage gastric carcinoma and to look for pulmonary metastases. Even though postmortem studies have put the incidence of pulmonary metastasis in gastric carcinoma as high as 25%, such a picture is not commonly seen in the clinical setting.[42]

Advanced gastric carcinoma metastasizes much more frequently into the peritoneum, typically to the omentum (Fig. 16.13), ovaries (Krukenberg tumor, usually bilateral) (Fig. 16.14), or rectovesicular pouch (Blumer shelf tumor).[42] Ascites in gastric carcinoma was shown in one

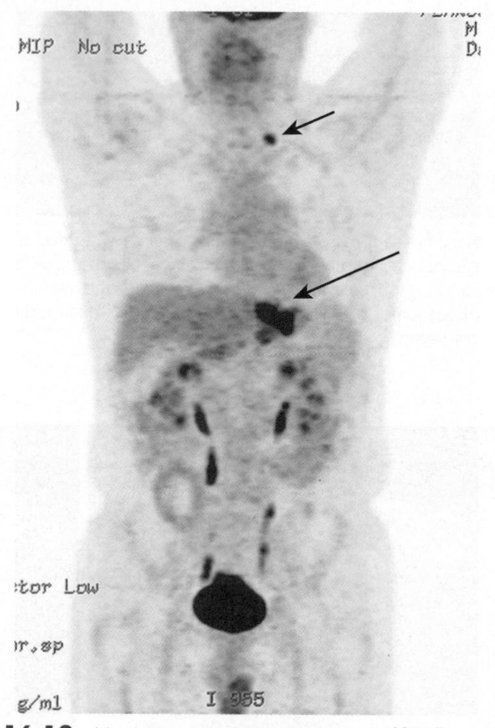

FIGURE 16.12. Maximum intensity projection 2-[^{18}F] fluoro-2-deoxy-D-glucose–positron emission tomography/computed tomography study in a patient with gastric carcinoma. There is intense uptake in the primary tumor (*long arrow*) and a metastatic left supraclavicular node (*short arrow*).

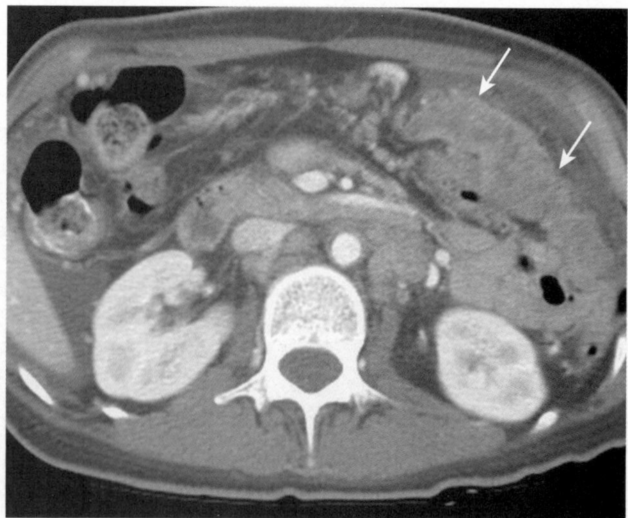

FIGURE 16.13. Soft tissue masses (*arrows*) in the greater omentum in a patient with gastric carcinoma form extensive peritoneal metastases (omental cake).

study to be associated with positive free tumor cells (40% sensitivity and 97% specificity) and peritoneal metastasis (51% sensitivity and 97% specificity).[63]

Although laparoscopy predates CT in staging peritoneal disease, it remains superior to all other imaging modalities in small-volume peritoneal disease. Its sensitivity for detecting peritoneal disease is quoted as 96%.[64] Various factors are likely to affect the ability of CT to detect peritoneal metastasis, including size, location, and morphology of the deposits and the presence or paucity of intraabdominal fat.[13,65] On CT, peritoneal metastasis can be seen as a nodular mass, peritoneal plaque, or infiltrative soft tissue mass lesion.[43] A diffusely thickened and enhancing peritoneal lining can be a manifestation of diffuse peritoneal carcinomatosis.

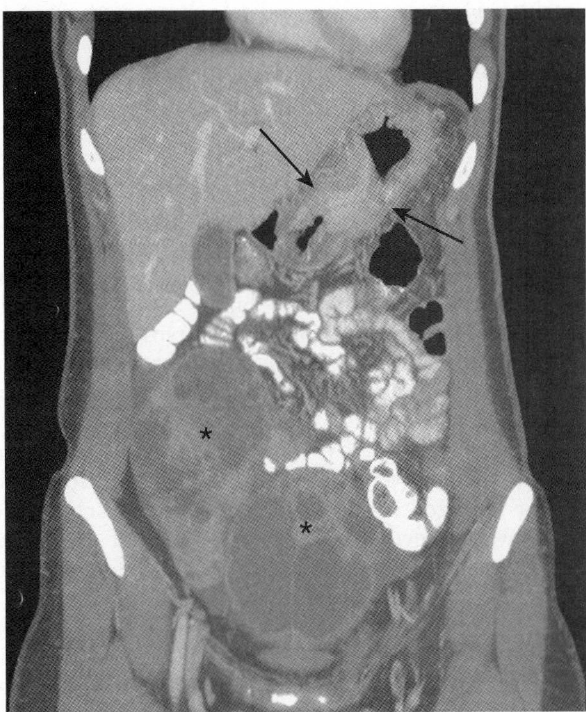

FIGURE 16.14. Coronal reconstruction of a computed tomography scan performed with intravenous contrast. Diffuse thickening of the stomach from infiltrative gastric adenocarcinoma (*arrows*). There are bilateral predominantly cystic ovarian masses (*asterisks*) from secondary deposits.

MRI is considered superior to CT scan by some authors in detecting extragastric metastasis.[51,66] Owing to factors such as greater soft-tissue resolution and greater sensitivity to contrast enhancement, as well as the recent development of hepatobiliary contrast agents, MRI can be superior to CT in detecting hepatic metastases (Fig. 16.15).[66] Its multiplanar capabilities make it useful in detecting peritoneal metastasis, but laparoscopic staging has been proved to be superior to both CT and MRI in detecting peritoneal involvement.

The value of PET/CT is limited by the poor FDG avidity of some subtypes, notably the signet-ring cell variety. However, in some instances it may be useful in detecting distant metastasis that may not be seen on conventional imaging. In fact, there are a few authors reporting that use of PET/CT changed management by detecting unsuspected metastasis.[67,68] However, there are currently no data to support the widespread use of PET/CT in routine use.

PET may be useful in detecting peritoneal metastases in some instances. Some studies have shown that PET has greater sensitivity than CT in detecting peritoneal metastasis.[69,70] There are two distinct patterns described in peritoneal metastasis in PET.[43] One is a diffuse increase in uptake in which the silhouette of the abdominal organs such as the liver and spleen is obscured, indicating diffuse peritoneal carcinomatosis. The second is nodular increase in uptake in areas not corresponding to the normal anatomic locations of nodes or other solid organs (Fig. 16.16). The detectability of metastasis has benefited considerably from combined PET/CT because of its ability to distinguish abnormal uptake from bowel activity.[70] It should be remembered, however, that certain histologic types of gastric tumors, such as signet-cell carcinoma and poorly differentiated adenocarcinoma (the most common type of gastric carcinoma to spread to the peritoneum), have little to no FDG uptake, and therefore their metastatic deposits may not be picked up on PET.[53]

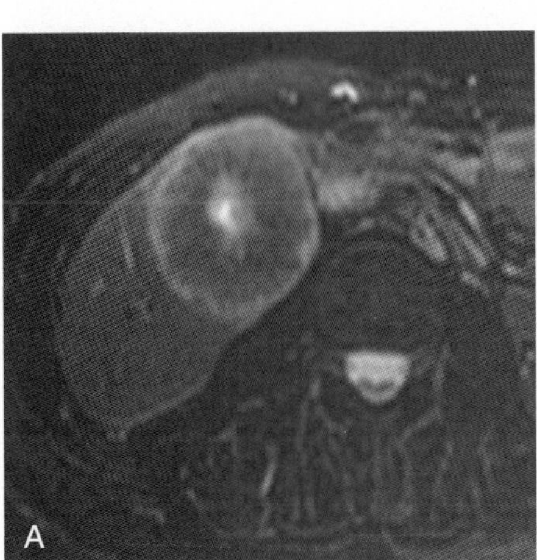

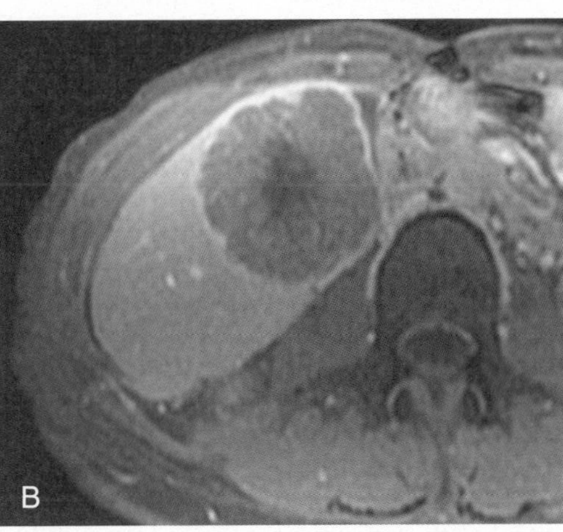

FIGURE 16.15. Large metastatic mass in the right lobe of the liver with central area of necrosis and rim enhancement. **A,** Axial fat-suppressed T2-weighted magnetic resonance imaging (MRI). **B,** Axial fat-suppressed T1-weighted MRI with intravenous contrast.

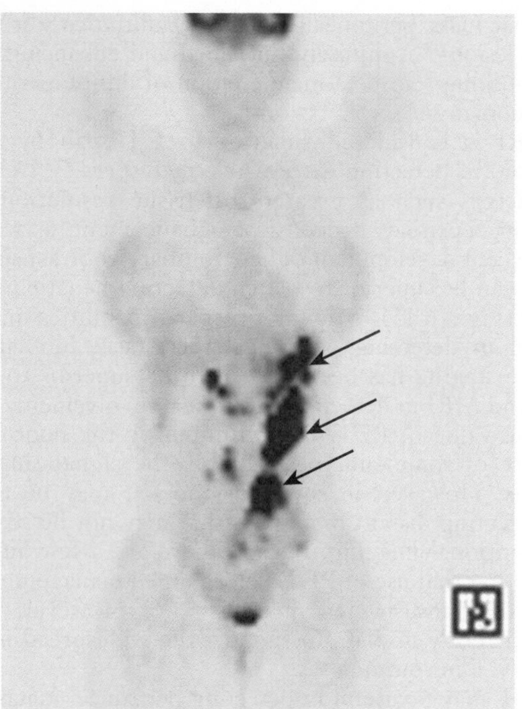

FIGURE 16.16. Coronal positron emission tomography scan of a patient with gastric carcinoma with multiple nodular 2-[^{18}F] fluoro-2-deoxy-D-glucose–avid peritoneal deposits (*arrows*).

KEY POINTS Imaging Radiology

Primary tumor (T)
- Lesion: polypoidal, ulcerated, or diffuse.
- Location: cardia, fundus, body, antrum, pylorus, greater curvature, lesser curvature.
- Local extent: presence of any extraluminal extension into the adjoining ligaments, direct invasion of adjoining organs.

Lymph node (N)
- Number of nodes visible in the expected nodal basins draining the site of primary.
- Presence, size, location.

Metastases (M)
- Liver metastases.
- Peritoneal deposits (ascites has a high positive predictive value for peritoneal involvement).
- Special attention to nodes in the posterior to the head of pancreas, in the paraaortic region, and in the supraclavicular region. These are considered distant metastases.

Treatment

The treatment modality of gastric carcinoma offering the best chance of cure is complete surgical resection (R0). Unfortunately, because most patients will present with advance gastric carcinoma, and because of inaccuracy of clinical staging, the 5-year survival rate with surgery alone is approximately 25%.[1,2] In individuals with a high risk of recurrence, locoregional control with concurrent chemoradiotherapy and perioperative chemotherapy is the current standard of care in Western countries.

Japanese investigators report promising results with curative surgery, with a 5-year survival rate of over 90% in stage 0 and stage 1 disease, 70% in stage 2 disease, and more than 40% in stage 3 disease. These results are significantly better than the survival figures in Western patients. Several factors contribute to this disparity. For a start, the intestinal variety of gastric carcinoma is seen more commonly in Japan, with a significantly higher number of patients with diffuse gastric carcinoma in the West. Proximal tumors, which portend a poorer prognosis, are more common in Western patients, and distal gastric carcinomas are more common in Asian countries. Moreover, a more radical surgery with extended lymphadenectomy is practiced in Japan, which can upstage many patients (stage migration) who would have otherwise been wrongly staged in the West.

Surgery

Surgeons dealing with gastric carcinoma will have to make a series of choices in designing the most appropriate surgery for a particular patient by taking into consideration the location of the cancer (proximal versus distal), type of cancer (intestinal versus diffuse), stage of the cancer, reconstruction options, and lastly, patient factors such as overall fitness and surgical risk.[71]

After staging, all newly diagnosed gastric carcinoma will need to be grouped as localized or metastatic disease. For localized disease, surgery is the only chance for cure. However, several caveats are important to remember, especially among patients with localized disease, which are for all practical purposes divided into three groups: (1) early disease, (2) localized resectable, and (3) localized but unresectable.

For early gastric carcinoma, endoscopic mucosal resection (EMR) or limited resections may be used. EMR is a technique developed and popularized for use in select patients with early gastric carcinoma. These cancers are generally T1a tumors less than 2 cm, either flat or protuberant, and have no ulceration or involvement of the submucosa.[72,73] In the United States, because early gastric carcinoma is not common, expertise with EMR is limited.

Resection of small T1b tumors with only a cuff of surrounding stomach tissue with limited dissection of lymph nodes can be considered with sentinel lymphatic mapping and biopsy, although this approach is still under investigation.[74] Minimally invasive (laparoscopic and robotic) gastrectomies have been increasingly performed for select patients in high-volume centers, with improved postoperative morbidity.[75] Most recently, the Korean Laparoscopic Gastrointestinal Surgery Study (KLASS)-2 randomized controlled trial comparing laparoscopic and open distal gastrectomy for advanced (cT2–4a) gastric cancer showed improved complication rate, faster recovery, and less pain in the laparoscopic group compared with open group. Long-term (3-year) follow up is the primary outcome of the KLASS-2 trial and is expected to be reported in the near future.[76] The majority of studies investigating efficacy of minimally-invasive gastrectomy were conducted in Asian countries; thus, generalizability to Western population should be carefully considered.

Aggressive gastric surgery has been practiced for many decades in the East and is followed by many surgeons who see large numbers of gastric carcinoma patients in the West. This includes an extended lymph node dissection, along with appropriate luminal resection. The extent of lymphadenectomy is a subject of considerable debate.[71,77] D1 lymphadenectomy and D2 lymphadenectomy are commonly followed. A metaanalysis of several trials found no significant difference in the mean 5-year survival of patients who underwent gastrectomy with D1 and D2 dissection (mean weighted 5-year survival of 41% and 42.6%, respectively).[78] However, with T3 and T4 lesions, patients with a D2 lymphadenectomy had a slightly better outcome (although this was not statistically significant). In two large, prospective, randomized trials of D2 versus D1 dissection in Western patients, D2 lymphadenectomy clearly resulted in a significant increase in mortality, but a subgroup analysis showed that there was a very strong and independent association between postoperative mortality and splenectomy.[78] These studies have substantial issues that limit the applicability of their conclusions. At high-volume centers in the United States and elsewhere, D2 dissection is routinely performed with mortality rates that are lower than that for D1 dissection reported in randomized trials. At the authors' institute, spleen-sparing D2 lymphadenectomy is routinely performed, with an operative mortality rate of 2% or less (in patients who are usually receiving neoadjuvant therapy).[21]

More radical dissections with D3 and D4 lymphadenectomy that include paraaortic nodes are less commonly performed even in Asian countries, particularly after the publication of the results from the Japan Clinical Oncology Group 95-01 randomized trial, which demonstrated no benefit and increased morbidity.[77,79]

Surgery is also sometimes used for palliation of intractable symptoms not responding to conservative management. The symptoms of advanced gastric carcinoma include pain, vomiting, GI bleeding, and anorexia. Although anorexia is not relieved by palliative surgery, intractable nausea and vomiting caused by gastric obstruction may be helped by either inserting a duodenal stent or performing gastric bypass surgery.[80] These procedures, however, are fraught with potential problems and should be considered only in extenuating circumstances. However, the use of palliative surgery for gastric carcinoma has decreased over the past few decades with development and improvement of the nonsurgical techniques as well as recognition of the severely limited prognosis for patients with stage IV disease and this degree of symptoms.

Key Points Role of Surgery

- Primary curative treatment of gastric carcinoma is complete curative resection.
- Early gastric carcinoma: limited procedures such as endoscopic mucosal resection and limited local excision of cancer may be used in appropriately selected cases.
- Gastrectomy with lymph node dissection is commonly performed; the extent of lymphadenectomy is a subject of ongoing debate.
- D1 dissection includes perigastric nodes; D2, perigastric plus along the hepatic, splenic, left gastric, and celiac arteries; D3, dissection as the other forms plus paraaortic nodes.
- Surgery is also sometimes used for palliation of intractable symptoms not responding to conservative management.

Chemotherapy and Radiation Therapy

Traditionally, the universally accepted standard treatment for patients with potentially resectable disease was surgery alone. In those patients, in whom curative surgery is not possible, the treatment is often time-limited to chemotherapy with or without definitive chemoradiotherapy. The use of chemoradiotherapy is extrapolated from results of earlier unresectable localized esophageal cancer studies, most notably the Radiation Therapy Oncology Group 85-01 trial, in which the relapse-free survival and OS rates were improved with concurrent chemoradiotherapy.[81] The Intergroup 123 trial, in which patients with localized but unresectable esophageal cancer were treated with either standard-dose (50.4 Gy) or higher-dose (64.8 Gy) radiotherapy while concurrently on a chemotherapy regimen of weekly cisplatin and 5-fluorouracil (5-FU) once every other week, yielded some surprising results, indicating that combining standard-dose radiotherapy with chemotherapy results in similar survival outcomes without adding significant toxicity. Currently, many physicians consider concurrent chemoradiotherapy as standard therapy where possible.

Although surgery remains the modality with the best chance for durable survival, the survival figures, particularly in the Western countries, are not satisfactory. Hence, many clinical trials have been performed to assess the additional survival advantage of adjuvant multimodality therapy in patients with localized resectable disease. Many of the older studies were inadequately designed to answer this question, and their results were inconsistent. Results from more recent clinical trials performed during the 2000s have firmly established that adding adjuvant therapy to surgery improves survival outcomes. Another confounding factor that has not been completely resolved regards the timing of adjuvant therapy (pre-, post-, or perioperative). Results from many clinical studies had shown variable results regarding the benefit of postoperative chemotherapy. Several metaanalyses suggest a benefit with postoperative chemotherapy. However, subgroup analysis demonstrates that the benefit is restricted to patients in Asian countries. Whereas postoperative chemotherapy with S1 is the standard of care for Japanese and Asian patients with resectable gastric carcinoma, management of resectable gastric carcinoma in Western countries is predominantly guided by two positive randomized phase III studies.[1,2,82–85]

In the United States, the Intergroup 116 conducted a phase III randomized adjuvant therapy trial.[86] Gastric carcinoma patients after R0 resection were randomized to receive either observation or postoperative therapy. Postoperative therapy consisted of one cycle of chemotherapy with bolus 5-FU and leucovorin, followed by 4 to 5 weeks of concurrent chemoradiotherapy, then two more cycles of chemotherapy. Macdonald and coworkers[1] reported their results in the 2001 issue of the *New England Journal of Medicine*, showing that postoperative chemotherapy plus chemoradiotherapy improved the 3-year survival rates from 41% to 50%. Although applauded for being the first adjuvant trial that was completed and demonstrated statistically significant results, Intergroup 116 was also criticized on several points. First, only approximately 10% of patients had D2 lymph node dissection, and 50% had D1 lymph node dissection.[84] Most would argue that the additional therapy after surgery may not have been necessary if patients had optimal resection. Second, it was found that many patients' radiotherapy fields had to be revised when their treatment plans were centrally reviewed, prompting some critics to suggest that community practice is not the best place to practice multimodality therapy. Third, only those patients who did well after surgery were enrolled in and randomized as part of the study, introducing a selection bias and arguably limiting the applicability of the results to other subgroups of patients. It is also important to note that only 64% of the patients completed the full postoperative course, highlighting the difficulty in patient compliance with multimodality, intense, postoperative therapy. Overall, despite the criticisms, the results from the Intergroup 116 study established that additional postoperative therapy with chemotherapy-chemoradiotherapy improves survival outcome after surgery.

The Medical Research Council Adjuvant Gastric Infusional Chemotherapy (MAGIC) trial performed by Cunningham and colleagues[2] showed an improvement in survival with the addition of perioperative chemotherapy using epirubicin, cisplatin, and infusional 5-FU (ECF); three cycles were given before and after surgery. Patients on the perioperative chemotherapy arm compared with those on the surgery only arm had better median OS (30 months vs. 18 months), and more were able to have curative surgery (74% vs. 68%).[2] These results offer another option in the management of patients with resectable gastric carcinoma. Unfortunately, because there has been no head-to-head comparison of the American postoperative chemoradiotherapy protocol and the UK perioperative chemotherapy protocol, it is not clear which option is superior. Several observations can be made when the results of Intergroup 116 and MAGIC are combined. It is clear that surgery alone for patients with locally advanced gastric carcinoma is not adequate. Survival can be improved with additive therapy, and the improvement may be similar with either approach. Therapy given preoperatively potentially can downstage the tumor and improve the surgical cure rate. Therapy given postoperatively is associated with less tolerance and compliance, with more patients unable to finish therapy. For patients to get the maximum amount of effective therapy, it is apparent that therapy has to be given before surgery. It may not be as important to know which one is better as to be able to have options for patients before going into their curative surgery.

The question of which therapy should be given with surgery for patients with resectable gastric carcinoma remains unanswered. Therefore, treatment options for patients are both perioperative chemotherapy and postoperative chemotherapy-chemoradiotherapy. Postoperative (adjuvant) chemotherapy may be more appropriate for patients in Asian countries.

Ongoing phase III studies may clarify the role of multimodality therapy added to surgery. Cancer and Leukemia Group B 80101 and MAGIC 2 are ongoing studies in the United States and the United Kingdom, respectively. In Asian countries, ongoing phase III studies are also accruing to determine more effective chemotherapy in the postoperative settings. These and other ongoing studies hopefully will clarify the optimal additive therapy to surgery.

ADVANCED OR METASTATIC GASTRIC CARCINOMA

Patients with advanced unresectable or metastatic gastric carcinoma may benefit from systemic chemotherapy to palliate symptoms and possibly improve survival outcome.[87,88] Patient selection is important, and those with intact performance status tend to have a more meaningful benefit with chemotherapy.

The chemotherapy regimens used are variable and are regionally dependent. Cisplatin plus 5-FU (CF) and ECF were the standard regimens used in the United States and Europe. More recently, docitoxen in combination with CF has been found to be superior. Use of capecitabine or oxaliplatin in combination with cisplatin or 5-FU has been found to be of comparable efficacy.[89–92]

In the interest of improving efficacy without increasing toxicity, recent studies have focused on the use of bevacizumab, a monoclonal antibody against vascular endothelial growth factor (VEGF). Use of bevacizumab in combination with cisplatin and irinotecan has been shown to improve time to progression compared with historical control (8.4 mo vs. 5.8 mo).[93] Results from a more recent international phase III randomized study, Avastin in Gastric Cancer (AVAGAST), performed in 774 therapy-naïve patients with advanced or metastatic gastric carcinoma randomized to receive capecitabine plus cisplatin (XP) or infusional 5-FU plus cisplatin (FP) with or without bevacizumab, are available. The data, presented during American Society of Clinical Oncology 2010, show that progression-free survival (PFS) is better with bevacizumab, but OS is not different with the addition of bevacizumab to chemotherapy.[94] However, subgroup analysis suggested that OS was improved in the bevacizumab plus chemotherapy arm among patients from the West. The role of bevacizumab remains open because more studies are ongoing. Investigations are under way to evaluate other monoclonal antibodies such as cetuximab and panitumumab to address the role of antiepidermal growth factor receptor (EGFR) therapy in gastric carcinoma.[95,96]

Perhaps the most exciting and practice-changing study in the past 18 months is the Trastuzumab for Gastric Cancer (ToGA) study.[97] *HER2* gene amplification and HER2 protein overexpression occur in approximately 20% to 30% of patients with gastric carcinomas and are associated with poorer survival. In fact, *HER2* amplification occurs more frequently in Lauren intestinal than in diffuse-type gastric carcinoma.[98] Among 3807 patients screened, only 810 were HER2-positive, and, out of those, 584 had advanced or metastatic disease, and were therefore eligible to enroll in ToGA. Patients were randomized to receive FP/XP with or without trastuzumab. The benefit of trastuzumab was true in all measure of outcomes. Overall response rate (ORR) (47% vs. 35%, $P = .0017$), median PFS (6.7 months vs. 5.5 months; hazard ratio [HR] 0.71; 95% confidence interval [CI] 0.59–0.85, $P = .0002$), and OS (13.8 months vs. 11.1 months, HR 0.74, 95% CI 0.60–0.91, $P = .0046$) were all greatest with trastuzumab plus chemotherapy. The strongest benefit was seen in patients who were fluorescence *in situ* hybridization–positive for HER2 expression and immunohistochemical grade 3+ or 2+. For the first-time patients, gastric carcinoma has a molecular predictor of response that can be easily evaluated. The role of anti-HER2 therapy is still being studied, but it had been suggested to bring trastuzumab into adjuvant therapy for patients with resectable disease.

In summary, the goals of therapy for patients diagnosed with advanced or metastatic gastric carcinoma are to palliate symptoms and improve survival. However, survival improvement is modest. Patients with the potential to obtain this modest benefit are usually those with intact performance status. Meaningful benefit of chemotherapy can be obtained only if side effects of therapy are tolerable to patients. Currently, there are many first-line chemotherapy regimens available. However, since 2006, three cytotoxic agents have been introduced to patients. Docetaxel, capecitabine, and oxaliplatin in phase III randomized studies became recognized as active agents for patients with gastric carcinoma. Targeted therapeutic agents evaluated in gastric carcinoma include inhibitors of VEGF/VEGF receptor, EGF/EGF receptor, and HER2. Although PFS was improved, AVAGAST did not demonstrate OS benefit when bevacizumab was added to chemotherapy. Patients with *HER2* amplification had improved outcomes—PFS, OS, ORR—when trastuzumab was added to chemotherapy in the ToGA study. Ongoing studies, including Erbitux in combination with Xeloda and Cisplatin in advanced esophago-gastric cancer and Revised European American Classification of Lymphoid Neoplasms-3, are designed to evaluate the role of cetuximab and panitumumab in patients with advanced gastric carcinoma. Recognizing the need to achieve improved outcomes for patients with advanced disease, many more studies are under way to assess other targeted agents with or without chemotherapy.

SURVEILLANCE AND RECURRENCE

Ikeda and associates[99] found that nearly 42% of patients with gastric carcinoma who undergo curative surgical resection face disease recurrence, and that most of these recurrences are identified within the first 2 years. The cancer recurs locally in 54%, at a distant metastatic site in 51%, and in the peritoneum in 29%. Lymph node metastasis and old age were found to be risk factors for recurrence. There are no reliable tumor markers that can be used to detect recurrence early.

Follow-up after curative resection is generally performed to detect recurrent disease early, with the hope that this will lead to improved outcomes. There is a lack of recommendations or national protocols in follow-up of these patients owing to the paucity of high-quality evidence. Hence, many surgical centers have adopted widely disparate regimes, with the only constant being visits to the outpatient department. Recurrent disease is rarely curable, and therefore some argue that there is no benefit from follow-up.[100,101]

CT scan is the standard modality used in most centers to screen for recurrence and is typically performed biannually for 5 years. Distinguishing postsurgical and postradiotherapy changes from tumor recurrence remains a problem in CT. Improperly distended bowel, surgical placation, postoperative adhesions, or hypertrophic gastritis at the stoma can all be mistaken for local recurrence (Fig. 16.17).[102] PET can sometimes help in differentiating posttreatment changes from recurrence when CT findings are equivocal.

Most centers perform routine endoscopy to diagnose anastomotic recurrence. MRI can be slightly superior to CT in detecting liver metastases owing to its superior contrast resolution. However, the most specific test in diagnosing metastases is FDG-PET/CT (>85% specificity, 90% sensitivity), followed by MRI (76%) and CT (72%).[103] It is likely that use of PET/CT may increase in these patients in the near future owing to its increased specificity.

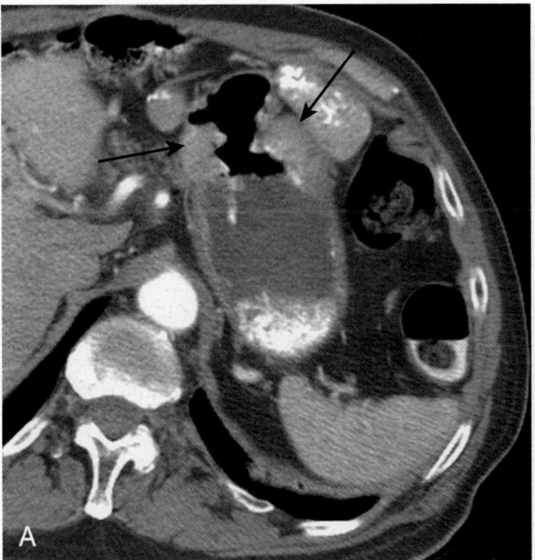

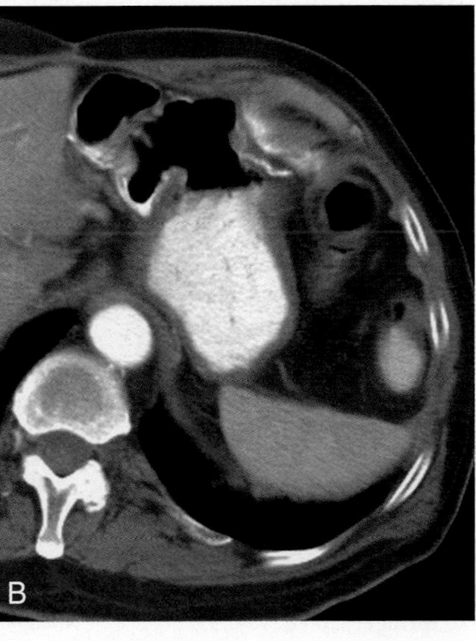

FIGURE 16.17. A, Circumferential thickening at the site of gastrojejunal anastomosis (*arrows*) in a patient who underwent partial gastrectomy and gastrojejunostomy for carcinoma of the stomach. **B,** Same patient imaged on another occasion with a better distention of the stomach. Improper distention can be erroneously interpreted as recurrence.

Key Points Surveillance and Recurrence

- Nearly 42% of patients with gastric carcinoma who undergo curative surgical resection face disease recurrence, and most of these recurrences occur within the first 2 years postsurgery.
- Cancer recurs locally in 54%, at a distant metastatic site in 51%, and in the peritoneum in 29%.
- There are no reliable tumor markers that can be used to detect recurrence early.
- Computed tomography scan is the modality of choice in detecting for recurrence.

REFERENCES

1. Macdonald JS, et al. Chemoradiotherapy after surgery compared with surgery alone for adenocarcinoma of the stomach or gastroesophageal junction. *N Engl J Med*. 2001;345:725–730.
2. Cunningham D, et al. Perioperative chemotherapy versus surgery alone for resectable gastroesophageal cancer. *N Engl J Med*. 2006;355:11–20.
3. Ferlay J, Bray F, Pisani P, et al. GLOBOCAN 2002: Cancer Incidence, Mortality and Prevalence Worldwide, Version 2.0. *IARC CancerBase*. 2004:5.
4. Stomach–cancer fact sheet 2018. International agency for Research on Cancer. WHO. https://gco.iarc.fr/today/data/factsheets/cancers/7-Stomach-fact-sheet.pdf. Accessed 5/8/2020.
5. Ferlay J, et al. Estimates of the cancer incidence and mortality in Europe in 2006. *Ann Oncol*. 2007;18:581–592.
6. Pathology and genetics of tumours of the digestive system. In: Hamilton S, Aaltonen L, eds. *World Health Organization Classification of Tumours*. Lyon: IARC Press; 2000.
7. American Cancer Society. *Cancer Facts & Figures 2011*. Atlanta: American Cancer Society; 2011.
8. American Cancer Society. *Cancer Facts & Figures 2020*. Atlanta: American Cancer Society; 2020. changes: American Joint Committee on Cancer. Stomach. In: Edge SB, et al, eds. *AJCC Cancer Staging Manual*. New York: Springer-Verlag; 2017:203–220.
9. Lauren P. The two histological main types of gastric carcinoma: diffuse and so-called intestinal-type carcinoma. an attempt at a histo-clinical classification. *Acta Pathol Microbiol Scand*. 1965;64:1–49.
10. Kuan S-F. Pathology of gastric neoplasms. In: Posner MC, Vokes EE, Weichselbaum RR, eds. *Cancer of the Upper Gastrointestinal Tract*. Hamilton and London: BC Decker Inc; 2002:218–236.
11. Dicken J, et al. Gastric adenocarcinoma: review and considerations for future directions. *Ann Surg*. 2005;241:27–39.
12. Ajani JA, Curley SA, Janjan NA, et al. *Gastrointestinal Cancer*. New York: Springer; 2005.
13. Davis PA, Sano T. The difference in gastric cancer between Japan, USA and Europe: What are the facts? What are the suggestions? *Crit Rev Oncol Hematol*. 2001;40:77–94.
14. Gore RM, et al. Gastric cancer. Radiologic diagnosis. *Radiol Clin North Am*. 1997;35:311–329.
15. Huang XE, et al. Effects of dietary, drinking, and smoking habits on the prognosis of gastric cancer. *Nutr Cancer*. 2000;38:30–36.
16. Ramon JM, et al. Dietary factors and gastric cancer risk. A case-control study in Spain. *Cancer*. 1993;71:1731–1735.
17. Devesa SS, Blot WJ, Fraumeni Jr. JF. Changing patterns in the incidence of esophageal and gastric carcinoma in the United States. *Cancer*. 1998;83:2049–2053.
18. Gore RM. Gastric cancer. Clinical and pathologic features. *Radiol Clin North Am*. 1997;35:295–310.
19. Fenogilo-Preiser C, Carneiro F, Correa P, et al. Gastric carcinoma. In: Hamilton S, Aaltonin L, eds. *Pathology and Genetics. Tumors of the Digestive System*. Lyon: IARC Press; 2000:37–52.
20. Brooks-Wilson AR, et al. Germline E-cadherin mutations in hereditary diffuse gastric cancer: assessment of 42 new families and review of genetic screening criteria. *J Med Genet*. 2004; 41:508–517.
21. Yao JC, et al. Gastric cancer. In: Jaffer SAC, Ajani A, Janjan NA, eds. *Gastrointestinal Cancer*. New York: Springer; 2004:219–231.
22. Vikram R, et al. Pancreas: peritoneal reflections, ligamentous connections, and pathways of disease spread. *Radiographics*. 2009;29:e34.
23. Gray H. Stomach. In: Lewis WH, ed. *Anatomy of the Human Body*. Philadelphia: Lea & Febiger; 1918.
24. Borrman R. Geschwulste des Magens und Duodenums. In: Henke F, Lubarsch O, eds. *Handbuch der speziellen pathologischen Anatomie und Histologie*. Berlin: Springer; 1926:864–871.
25. Jang HJ, et al. Intestinal metastases from gastric adenocarcinoma: helical CT findings. *J Comput Assist Tomogr*. 2001;25:61–67.
26. Tanakaya K, et al. Metastatic carcinoma of the colon similar to Crohn's disease: a case report. *Acta Med Okayama*. 2004;58:217–220.
27. American Joint Committee on Cancer Stomach. In: Edge SB, ed. *AJCC Cancer Staging Manual*. New York: Springer-Verlag; 2017:203–220.
28. Siewert JR, et al. Relevant prognostic factors in gastric cancer: ten-year results of the German Gastric Cancer Study. *Ann Surg*. 1998;228:449–461.
29. Roder JD, et al. Classification of regional lymph node metastasis from gastric carcinoma. German Gastric Cancer Study Group. *Cancer*. 1998;82:621–631.
30. Yokota T, et al. Significant prognostic factors in patients with early gastric cancer. *Int Surg*. 2000;85:286–290.
31. Adachi Y, et al. Most important lymph node information in gastric cancer: multivariate prognostic study. *Ann Surg Oncol*. 2000;7:503–507.
32. Japanese Gastric Cancer Association. Japanese Classification of Gastric Carcinoma—2nd English Edition. *Gastric Cancer*. 1998;1:10–24.
33. Sobin L, Wittekind C. *UICC TNM classification of malignant tumors*. New York: Wiley; 2002.
34. Brennan MF. Current status of surgery for gastric cancer: a review. *Gastric Cancer*. 2005;8:64–70.
35. Karpeh Jr MS, Brennan MF. Gastric carcinoma. *Ann Surg Oncol*. 1998;5:650–656.
36. Halvorsen Jr RA, Yee J, McCormick VD. Diagnosis and staging of gastric cancer. *Semin Oncol*. 1996;23:325–335.
37. Kunisaki C, et al. Outcomes of mass screening for gastric carcinoma. *Ann Surg Oncol*. 2006;13:221–228.
38. Bhandari S, et al. Usefulness of three-dimensional, multidetector row CT (virtual gastroscopy and multiplanar reconstruction) in the evaluation of gastric cancer: a comparison with conventional endoscopy, EUS, and histopathology. *Gastrointest Endosc*. 2004;59:619–626.
39. Kelly S, et al. A systematic review of the staging performance of endoscopic ultrasound in gastro-oesophageal carcinoma. *Gut*. 2001;49:534–539.
40. Hargunani R, et al. Cross-sectional imaging of gastric neoplasia. *Clin Radiol*. 2009;64:420–429.
41. Chen CY, et al. Gastric cancer: preoperative local staging with 3D multi-detector row CT—correlation with surgical and histopathologic results. *Radiology*. 2007;242:472–482.
42. Meyers MA, ed. *Dynamic Radiology of the Abdomen*. New York: Springer-Verlag; 2000.
43. Lim JS, et al. CT and PET in stomach cancer: preoperative staging and monitoring of response to therapy. *Radiographics*. 2006;26:143–156.
44. Mani NB, et al. Two-phase dynamic contrast-enhanced computed tomography with water-filling method for staging of gastric carcinoma. *Clin Imaging*. 2001;25:38–43.
45. Takao M, et al. Gastric cancer: evaluation of triphasic spiral CT and radiologic-pathologic correlation. *J Comput Assist Tomogr*. 1998;22:288–294.
46. Kim YH, et al. Staging of T3 and T4 gastric carcinoma with multidetector CT: added value of multiplanar reformations for prediction of adjacent organ invasion. *Radiology*. 2009;250:767–775.
47. Horton KM, Fishman EK. Current role of CT in imaging of the stomach. *Radiographics*. 2003;23:75–87.
48. Sohn KM, et al. Comparing MR imaging and CT in the staging of gastric carcinoma. *AJR Am J Roentgenol*. 2000;174:1551–1557.
49. Giganti F, Orsenigo E, Arcidiacono PG, et al. Preoperative locoregional staging of gastric cancer: is there a place for magnetic resonance imaging? prospective comparison with EUS and multidetector computed tomography. *Gastric Cancer*. 2016;19:216–225.
50. Kim AY, Han JK, Seong CK, et al. MRI in staging advanced gastric cancer: is it useful compared with spiral CT? *J Comput Assist Tomogr*. 2000;24:389–394.
51. Motohara T, Semelka RC. MRI in staging of gastric cancer. *Abdom Imaging*. 2002;27:376–383.

52. Borggreve AS, Goense L, Brenkman HJF, et al. Imaging strategies in the management of gastric cancer: current role and future potential of MRI. PMID: 30789792 PMCID: PMC6580902 DOI: 10.1259/bjr.20181044
53. Yoshioka T, et al. Evaluation of 18F-FDG PET in patients with advanced, metastatic, or recurrent gastric cancer. *J Nucl Med.* 2003;44:690–699.
54. Stahl A, et al. FDG PET imaging of locally advanced gastric carcinomas: correlation with endoscopic and histopathological findings. *Eur J Nucl Med Mol Imaging*. 2003;30:288–295.
55. Kamimura K, et al. Role of gastric distention with additional water in differentiating locally advanced gastric carcinomas from physiological uptake in the stomach on 18F-fluoro-2–deoxy-d-glucose PET. *Nucl Med Commun*. 2009;30:431–439.
56. Noda N, Sasako M, Yamaguchi N, et al. Ignoring small lymph nodes can be a major cause of staging error in gastric cancer. *Br J Surg.* 1998;85:831–834.
57. Monig SP, et al. Staging of gastric cancer: correlation of lymph node size and metastatic infiltration. *AJR Am J Roentgenol.* 1999;173:365–367.
58. Kwee RM, Kwee TC. Imaging in assessing lymph node status in gastric cancer. *Gastric Cancer*. 2009;12:6–22.
59. Arslan H, Fatih Özbay M, Çallı İ, et al. Contribution of diffusion weighted MRI to diagnosis and staging in gastric tumors and comparison with multi-detector computed tomography. *Radiol Oncol.* 2017;51(1):23–29.
60. Joo I, Lee JM, Kim JH, et al. Prospective comparison of 3T MRI with diffusion-weighted imaging cof gastric cancer. *J Magn Reson Imaging*. 2015;41:814–821.
61. Tatsumi Y, et al. Preoperative diagnosis of lymph node metastases in gastric cancer by magnetic resonance imaging with ferumoxtran-10. *Gastric Cancer*. 2006;9:120–128.
62. Mawlawi O, et al. Performance characteristics of a newly developed PET/CT scanner using NEMA standards in 2D and 3D modes. *J Nucl Med*. 2004;45:1734–1742.
63. Yajima K, et al. Clinical and diagnostic significance of preoperative computed tomography findings of ascites in patients with advanced gastric cancer. *Am J Surg*. 2006;192:185–190.
64. Ozmen MM, et al. Staging laparoscopy for gastric cancer. *Surg Laparosc Endosc Percutan Tech*. 2003;13:241–244.
65. Dux M, et al. Helical hydro-CT for diagnosis and staging of gastric carcinoma. *J Comput Assist Tomogr*. 1999;23:913–922.
66. Semelka RC, et al. Focal liver lesions: comparison of dual-phase CT and multisequence multiplanar MR imaging including dynamic gadolinium enhancement. *J Magn Reson Imaging*. 2001;13:397–401.
67. Chen J, et al. Improvement in preoperative staging of gastric adenocarcinoma with positron emission tomography. *Cancer*. 2005;103:2383–2390.
68. Tian J, et al. The value of vesicant 18F-fluorodeoxyglucose positron emission tomography (18F-FDG PET) in gastric malignancies. *Nucl Med Commun*. 2004;25:825–831.
69. Tanaka T, et al. Usefulness of FDG-positron emission tomography in diagnosing peritoneal recurrence of colorectal cancer. *Am J Surg*. 2002;184:433–436.
70. Turlakow A, et al. Peritoneal carcinomatosis: role of (18)F-FDG PET. *J Nucl Med*. 2003;44:1407–1412.
71. Misra N, Harwick R, McCulloch P. Role of surgery in stomach cancer. In: McCulloch P, ed. *Gastrointestinal Oncology*. New York: Informa Healthcare; 2007:73–84.
72. Miyata M, et al. What are the appropriate indications for endoscopic mucosal resection for early gastric cancer? Analysis of 256 endoscopically resected lesions. *Endoscopy*. 2000;32:773–778.
73. Wang YP, Bennett C, Pan T. Endoscopic mucosal resection for early gastric cancer. *Cochrane Database Syst Rev*. 2006;1:CD004276.
74. *Gastric Cancer*. 2017; 20(Suppl 1):53–59.
75. *Gastric Cancer*. 2019;22(5):909–919; *Ann Surg*. 2016;263:28–35; *Ann Surg*. 2019; 270(6):983–991; *Ann Surg*. 2016; 263(1):103–109.
76. Lee H-J, Jin Hyung W, Yang H-K, et at., Korean Laparo-endoscopic Gastrointestinal Surgery Study (KLASS) Group Short-term Outcomes of a Multicenter Randomized Controlled Trial Comparing Laparoscopic Distal Gastrectomy With D2 Lymphadenectomy to Open Distal Gastrectomy for Locally Advanced Gastric Cancer (KLASS-02-RCT)
77. Yang SH, et al. An evidence-based medicine review of lymphadenectomy extent for gastric cancer. *Am J Surg*. 2009;197:246–251.
78. McCulloch P, Nita ME, Gama-Rodrigues J, et al. Extended versus limited lymph nodes dissection technique for adenocarcinoma of the stomach. *Cochrane Database Syst Rev*. 2004;4:CD001964.
79. Sasako M, et al. D2 lymphadenectomy alone or with para-aortic nodal dissection for gastric cancer. *N Engl J Med.* 2008;359:453–462.
80. Fiori E, et al. Palliative management of malignant antro-pyloric strictures. Gastroenterostomy vs. endoscopic stenting. A randomized prospective trial. *Anticancer Res*. 2004;24:269–271.
81. Cooper JS, et al. Chemoradiotherapy of locally advanced esophageal cancer: long-term follow-up of a prospective randomized trial (RTOG 85-01). Radiation Therapy Oncology Group. *JAMA*. 1999;281:1623–1627.
82. Earle CC, Maroun JA. Adjuvant chemotherapy after curative resection for gastric cancer in non-Asian patients: revisiting a meta-analysis of randomised trials. *Eur J Cancer*. 1999;35:1059–1064.
83. Janunger KG, Hafstrom L, Glimelius B. Chemotherapy in gastric cancer: a review and updated meta-analysis. *Eur J Surg.* 2002;168:597–608.
84. Cunningham D, Chua YJ. East meets west in the treatment of gastric cancer. *N Engl J Med*. 2007;357:1863–1865.
85. Sakuramoto S, et al. Adjuvant chemotherapy for gastric cancer with S-1, an oral fluoropyrimidine. *N Engl J Med*. 2007;357:1810–1820.
86. Kelsen DP. Postoperative adjuvant chemoradiation therapy for patients with resected gastric cancer: intergroup 116. *J Clin Oncol.* 2000;18(Suppl 21):32S–34S.
87. Murad AM, et al. Modified therapy with 5-fluorouracil, doxorubicin, and methotrexate in advanced gastric cancer. *Cancer*. 1993;72:37–41.
88. Pyrhonen S, et al. Randomised comparison of fluorouracil, epidoxorubicin and methotrexate (FEMTX) plus supportive care with supportive care alone in patients with non-resectable gastric cancer. *Br J Cancer*. 1995;71:587–591.
89. Vanhoefer U, et al. Final results of a randomized phase III trial of sequential high-dose methotrexate, fluorouracil, and doxorubicin versus etoposide, leucovorin, and fluorouracil versus infusional fluorouracil and cisplatin in advanced gastric cancer: a trial of the European Organization rfor Research and Treatment of Cancer Gastrointestinal Tract Cancer Cooperative Group. *J Clin Oncol*. 2000;18:2648–2657.
90. Waters JS, et al. Long-term survival after epirubicin, cisplatin and fluorouracil for gastric cancer: results of a randomized trial. *Br J Cancer*. 1999;80:269–272.
91. Kang YK, et al. Capecitabine/cisplatin versus 5-fluorouracil/cisplatin as first-line therapy in patients with advanced gastric cancer: a randomised phase III noninferiority trial. *Ann Oncol*. 2009;20:666–673.
92. Cunningham D, et al. Capecitabine and oxaliplatin for advanced esophagogastric cancer. *N Engl J Med*. 2008;358:36–46.
93. Shah MA, et al. Multicenter phase II study of irinotecan, cisplatin, and bevacizumab in patients with metastatic gastric or gastroesophageal junction adenocarcinoma. *J Clin Oncol*. 2006;24:5201–5206.
94. Kang Y, et al. AVAGAST: A randomized, double-blind, placebo-controlled, phase III study of first-line capecitabine and cisplatin plus bevacizumab or placebo in patients with advanced gastric cancer (AGC). *J Clin Oncol*. 2010;28:18s.
95. Pinto C, et al. Phase II study of cetuximab in combination with FOLFIRI in patients with untreated advanced gastric or gastroesophageal junction adenocarcinoma (FOLCETUX study). *Ann Oncol*. 2007;18:510–517.
96. Lordick F, et al. Cetuximab plus oxaliplatin/leucovorin/5-fluorouracil in first-line metastatic gastric cancer: a phase II study of the Arbeitsgemeinschaft Internistische Onkologie (AIO). *Br J Cancer*. 2010;102:500–505.
97. VanCutsem E, et al. Efficacy results from the ToGA trial: a phase III study of trastuzumab added to standard chemotherapy (CT) in first-line human epidermal growth factor receptor 2 (HER2)-positive advanced gastric cancer (GC). *J Clin Oncol*. 2009;27:18s.
98. Bang Y, et al. HER2-positivity rates in advanced gastric cancer (GC): results from a large international phase III trial. *J Clin Oncol*. 2008;26
99. Ikeda Y, et al. Effective follow-up for recurrence or a second primary cancer in patients with early gastric cancer. *Br J Surg*. 2005;92:235–239.
100. Tan IT, So BY. Value of intensive follow-up of patients after curative surgery for gastric carcinoma. *J Surg Oncol*. 2007;96:503–506.
101. Whiting J, et al. Follow-up of gastric cancer: a review. *Gastric Cancer*. 2006;9:74–81.
102. Ha HK, et al. Local recurrence after surgery for gastric carcinoma: CT findings. *AJR Am J Roentgenol*. 1993;161:975–977.
103. Kinkel K, et al. Detection of hepatic metastases from cancers of the gastrointestinal tract by using noninvasive imaging methods (US, CT, MR imaging, PET): a meta-analysis. *Radiology*. 2002;224:748–756.

CHAPTER 17

Small Bowel Malignant Tumors

Yulia Bronstein, M.D.; Michael J. Overman, M.D.; Hubert H. Chuang, M.D., Ph.D.; Bharat Raval, M.B.; and Paul M. Silverman, M.D.

INTRODUCTION

Small bowel (SB) malignancies account for only 3% of all gastrointestinal (GI) neoplasms and 0.6% of all cancers in the United States.[1] Common primary malignant tumors include carcinoid (40%), adenocarcinoma (31%), lymphoma (17%), and sarcoma (9%).[2] The risk of a specific SB tumor type depends on the exact location in the SB, with adenocarcinomas the most common duodenal tumor and carcinoids the most common ileal tumor; both sarcoma and lymphoma more equally distributed throughout the entire SB. The clinical presentation of SB tumors is nonspecific, with abdominal pain, weight loss, nausea, vomiting, GI bleeding, and SB obstruction being the most common symptoms.[3] Endoscopic evaluation of the SB has been hampered by the long length of the SB, at approximately 5 to 6m. Novel endoscopic technologies, such as video capsule endoscopy, and device-assisted enteroscopy have allowed evaluation of the entire SB.[4,5]

The heterogeneous biology of SB tumors is reflected in survival rates, which are lowest for adenocarcinoma and highest for carcinoid (Fig. 17.1). The most common malignancies of the SB are discussed in this chapter as separate entities.

I CARCINOID

INTRODUCTION

Carcinoid is the most common SB malignancy, representing 39% to 44% of all primary SB tumors, more commonly affecting Black males in United States, with rising incidence since 2000.[2,6]

Epidemiology

The vast majority of these tumors are sporadic. A small subset is associated with the inherited syndrome MEN I (multiple endocrine neoplasia type I).

Anatomy and Pathology

Carcinoid tumor is a well-differentiated low grade malignant neuroendocrine tumor (NET) originating from the Kulchitsky cell, an enterochromaffin cell located in the crypts of Lieberkuhn of the GI tract. Microscopically, carcinoid is composed of uniform small cells containing neurosecretory granules with bioactive products such as serotonin, somatostatin, glucagon, histamine, or gastrin. Macroscopically, carcinoid tumors are present as small submucosal nodules, often subcentimeter in size, not causing obstruction of the lumen *per se*, with intense desmoplastic response within the adjacent mesentery resulting in shortening and thickening of mesentery and retraction and kinking of nearby vessels. Some 30% of patients with SB carcinoids have multicentric disease at diagnosis.[7] Although much rarer than carcinoid tumors, intermediate- and high-grade NET, characterized by both a higher rate of mitotic activity and tumor necrosis, can also arise in the SB. These tumors have a more aggressive biology, with high-grade NET of the SB behaving like small cell carcinomas of the lung.

KEY POINTS

Anatomy and Pathology of Carcinoid

- Carcinoid is a well-differentiated neuroendocrine tumor.
- Microscopically, carcinoid is composed of uniform small cells containing neurosecretory granules, with bioactive products such as serotonin, somatostatin, glucagon, histamine, or gastrin.
- Macroscopically, carcinoid tumors are often small submucosal nodules, multifocal in 30% of cases, with intense desmoplastic response within the adjacent mesentery.

Clinical Presentation

Because of their indolent growth, most SB carcinoids are asymptomatic and identified incidentally. One-third of carcinoids present with abdominal pain or bowel obstruction, and only 10% are associated with carcinoid syndrome because of serotonin hypersecretion. The carcinoid syndrome is primarily seen in the context of liver metastases, in which the release of serotonin gains access to the systemic circulation without undergoing hepatic metabolism.[8] Carcinoid syndrome consists of secretory diarrhea, bouts of cutaneous flushing, wheezing, and dyspnea because of bronchospasm. Longstanding carcinoid syndrome may cause fibrotic changes in the cardiac valves predominantly affecting the right heart, typically leading to tricuspid regurgitation and pulmonic stenosis.

A 24-hour urinary collection for the serotonin metabolite 5-hydroxyindole acetic acid (5-HIAA) has both good sensitivity and good specificity for the diagnosis of carcinoid syndrome.

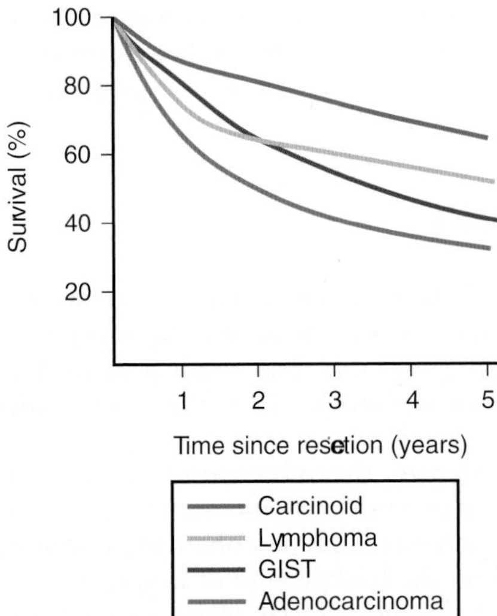

FIGURE 17.1. Five-year survival rates by histologic subtype for patients who underwent resection (Data from National Cancer Data Base, 1985–2000). *GIST*, Gastrointestinal stromal tumor. (Modified from Bilimoria KY, Bentrem DJ, Wayne JD, et al. Small bowel cancer in the United States: changes in epidemiology, treatment, and survival over the last 20 years. *Ann Surg*. 2009;249:63-71. With permission.)

Patterns of Tumor Spread

Tumorous spread via lymphatics into the mesenteric lymph nodes induces extensive desmoplastic reaction, leading to retraction of the mesentery, kinking and obstruction of the mesenteric veins, and retraction and mechanical obstruction of the surrounding SB loops (Fig. 17.2). This mesenteric nodal metastasis produces a typical mesenteric mass detectable by computed tomography (CT), as opposed to the small primary tumor that is commonly too small to detect by imaging.

Hematogenous spread to the liver is very common. Liver metastases allow development of carcinoid syndrome. Spread to the bones is rare, producing osteoblastic metastases.

Peritoneal spread is usually a late development in the course of the disease. Peritoneal metastases commonly remain discrete nodular lesions without ascites, as opposed to peritoneal spread of adenocarcinoma, which causes massive ascites.

KEY POINTS

Patterns of Tumor Spread of Carcinoid

- Lymphatic spread to mesenteric lymph nodes is associated with desmoplastic reaction causing retraction of the mesentery, potentially leading to bowel obstruction.
- Hematogenous spread to the liver may be associated with the development of carcinoid syndrome.
- Peritoneal metastases are commonly small and rarely cause ascites.
- Bone metastases of carcinoid are osteoblastic.

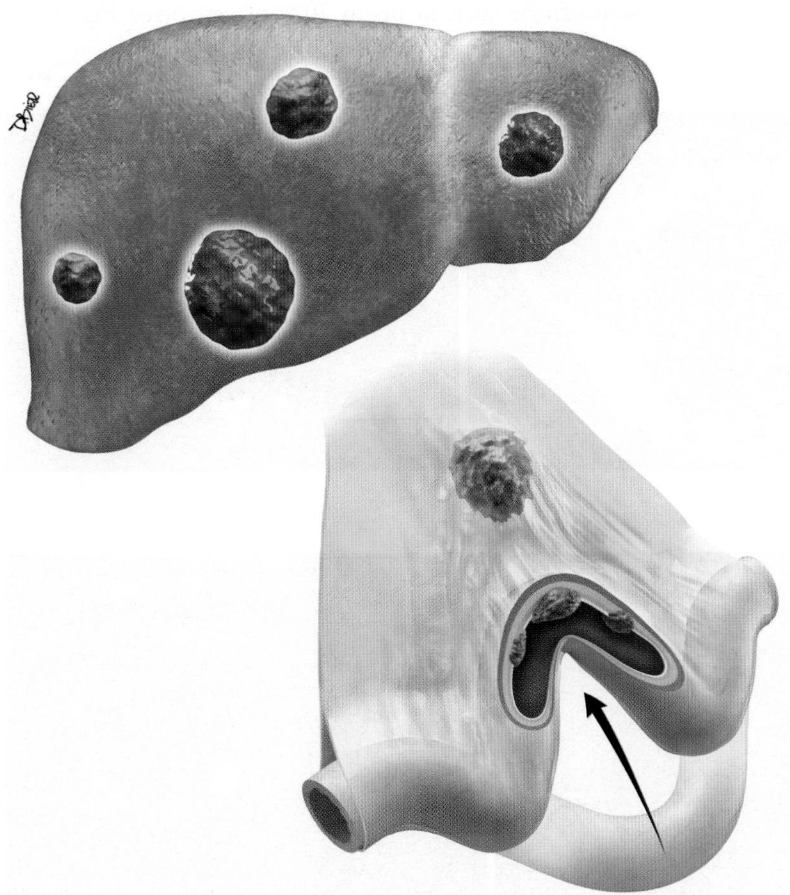

FIGURE 17.2. Small bowel (SB) carcinoid metastatic pathway into the mesentery and the liver. Desmoplastic reaction causes thickening and shortening of the mesentery and tethering of the SB loop (*arrow*).

Staging Evaluation

A revised TNM (tumor, node, metastasis) staging for carcinoid tumors, which is slightly different from the TNM staging of SB adenocarcinoma, has been proposed[9] (Table 17.1).

Table 17.1 Proposed Staging System for Small Bowel Carcinoid Tumors

STAGE	CHARACTERISTICS OF TUMOR-NODE-METASTASIS CLASSIFICATION SYSTEM
T	Primary Tumor
T1	<2 cm up to the muscularis propria
T2	>2 cm up to the muscularis propria or <2 cm propria beyond muscularis propria
T3	>2 cm beyond muscularis propria
N	Regional Lymph Nodes
N0	No regional lymph node metastasis present
N1	Regional lymph node metastasis
M	Distant Metastases
M0	No distant metastasis present
M1	Distant metastasis
STAGE	**GROUPING**
I	T1, N0–N1, M0
II	T2, any N, M0
III	T3, any N, M0
IV	Any T, any N, M1

(From Landry CS, Brock G, Scoggins CR, et al. A proposed staging system for small bowel carcinoid tumors based on an analysis of 6,380 patients. *Am J Surg*. 2008;196:896-903; discussion 903.)

Key Point

Staging of Carcinoid

- The TNM (tumor, nodes, metastasis) staging of carcinoid is similar to that of adenocarcinoma, with the exception of T staging including not only the depth of invasion into the bowel wall, but also a size as a separate criterion. Two centimeters serves as a threshold, with tumors larger than 2 cm upstaged to T3 and having a worse prognosis.

IMAGING

Mesenteric nodal metastases and liver metastases are usually larger, more easily detectable by imaging, and cause more clinical symptoms than small primary tumors. The primary tumor within the SB is the most challenging for detection by imaging.

CT may identify the submucosal carcinoid tumor as a small mural mass with early intense contrast enhancement owing to hyperemia.[10] Hyperenhancing tumor can be best appreciated on the background of negative contrast in the bowel lumen in the arterial phase of contrast injection (Figs. 17.3 and 17.4). Classic mesenteric nodal metastasis of carcinoid has a nearly pathognomonic CT pattern as a spiculated soft tissue density mesenteric mass because of desmoplastic reaction[10] (Figs. 17.5 and 17.6). Sometimes, a longer segment of adjacent SB has a thickened edematous wall because of mesenteric venous engorgement (see Fig. 17.6). Calcification within the mesenteric extension can be seen in up to 70% of cases (see Fig. 17.5).

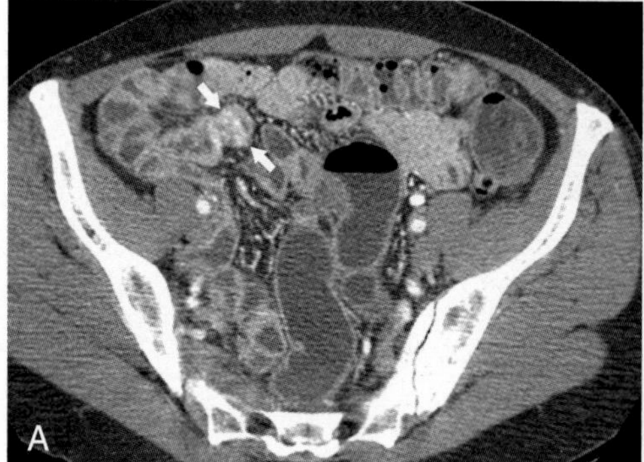

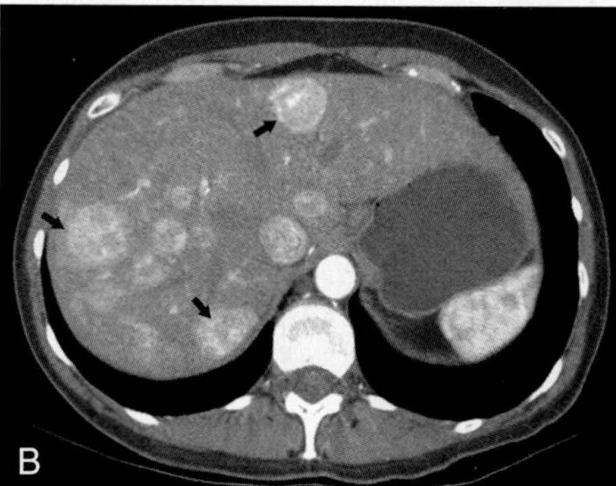

Figure 17.3. A 54-year-old woman with liver metastases found incidentally on a workup for renal colic. **A**, Computed tomography (CT) scan through the pelvis shows a subtle, very small hyperenhancing segment (*arrows*) in the ileum. On surgery, five carcinoids were found in this segment, ranging from 0.5 to 1.1 cm. **B**, An arterial phase of multiphase staging CT of the liver demonstrates multiple hyperenhancing liver metastases of a well-differentiated neuroendocrine carcinoma (carcinoid) (*arrows*).

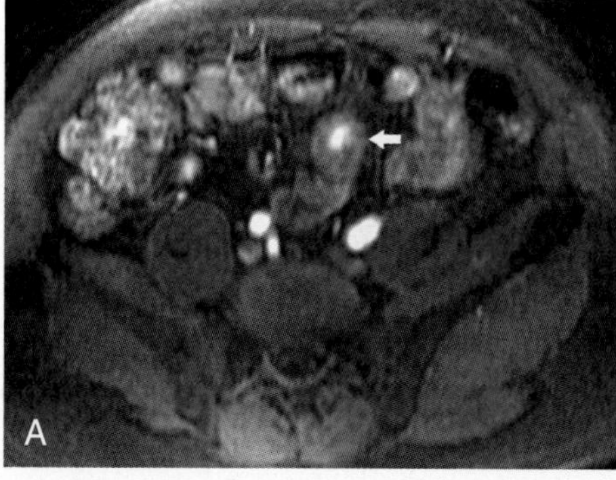

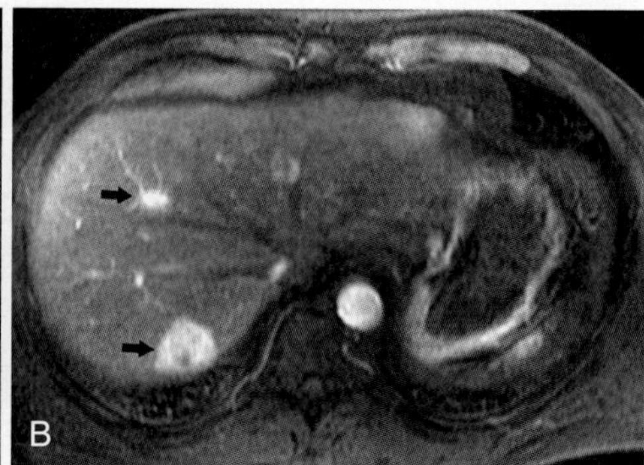

Figure 17.4. A 66-year-old man with multiple liver metastases of carcinoid incidentally found on the routine staging computed tomography scan for treated prostate cancer. **A**, Fat-suppressed magnetic resonance imaging (MRI) liver acquisition with volume acquisition (LAVA) with gadolinium shows a small hyperenhancing focus in the ileum representing the primary carcinoid (*arrow*). **B**, Fat-suppressed MRI LAVA with gadolinium shows two hyperenhancing liver metastases (*arrows*).

Differential diagnostic considerations for the mesenteric component include sclerosing mesenteritis and treated lymphoma. A minority of mesenteric nodal metastases demonstrate a nonspecific pattern of well-circumscribed ovoid or round masses.

Liver metastases are hypervascular and best detected as hyperenhancing lesions on the late arterial phase of CT (see Figs. 17.3 and 17.4) and as hypoenhancing lesions on the delayed venous phase of CT. Lesions may become isodense and least conspicuous in the portal phase. Dual-phase contrast-enhanced CT of the liver should always be performed to detect carcinoid liver metastasis. Noncontrast CT is very helpful for liver metastases detection, unless limited by fatty liver changes. Small carcinoid metastases can be mistaken for benign hypervascular lesions such as hemangiomas or small foci of focal nodular hyperplasia, especially in the absence of a baseline scan. Rarely, liver metastases have a cystic appearance (Fig. 17.7).

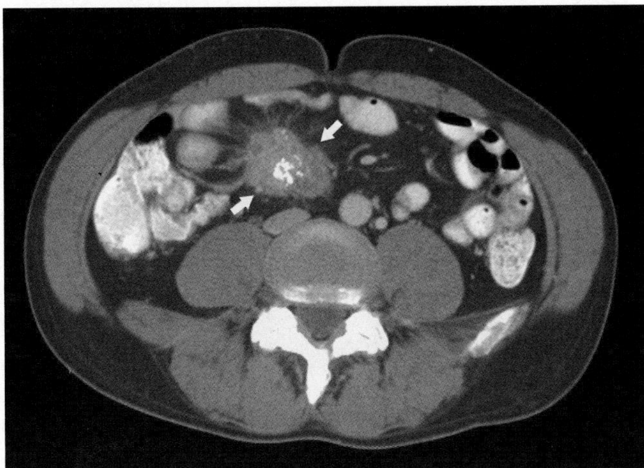

FIGURE 17.5. Computed tomography scan at the level of the umbilicus demonstrates a spiculated soft tissue mass (*arrows*) with calcifications and retraction of the mesentery, representing mesenteric nodal metastasis from carcinoid.

Magnetic resonance imaging (MRI) with gadolinium can demonstrate the primary hyperenhancing carcinoid in the bowel on fast dynamic sequences with T1 contrast (see Fig. 17.4). Owing to increased sensitivity to gadolinium enhancement, MRI can detect more liver metastases than can CT.[11] MRI is a preferred modality when there are no extrahepatic metastases. Unlike CT, MRI evaluation of liver metastases is not limited by fatty liver. Whereas gadolinium is necessary for initial characterization of liver lesions in a patient with carcinoid, follow-up MRI examinations maintain diagnostic quality even in the absence of contrast, so they can be used in patients with severely impaired renal function or lack of intravenous access.

Carcinoid tumors tend to express somatostatin receptors (SSTR), allowing for imaging with radiolabeled somatostatin analogues. Somatostatin scintigraphy using ^{111}indium-DPTA-D-Phe-1-octreotide (Octreoscan) allows whole-body planar images and single photon emission computed tomography (SPECT) or SPECT/CT images. More recently, SSTR positron emission tomography (PET)/CT with ^{68}Ga-DOTATATE (Netspot) has come into use. In addition to identifying more

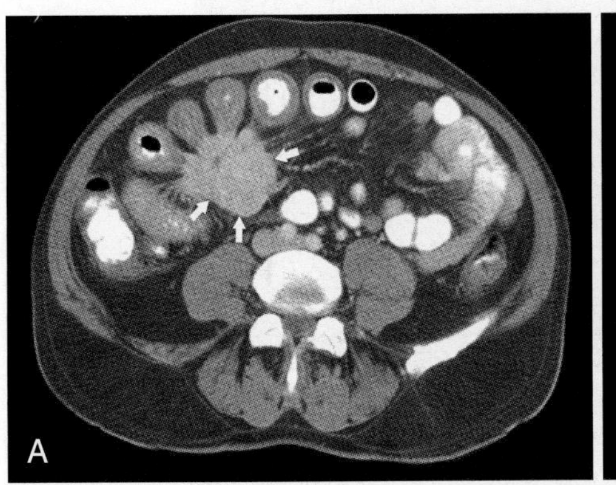

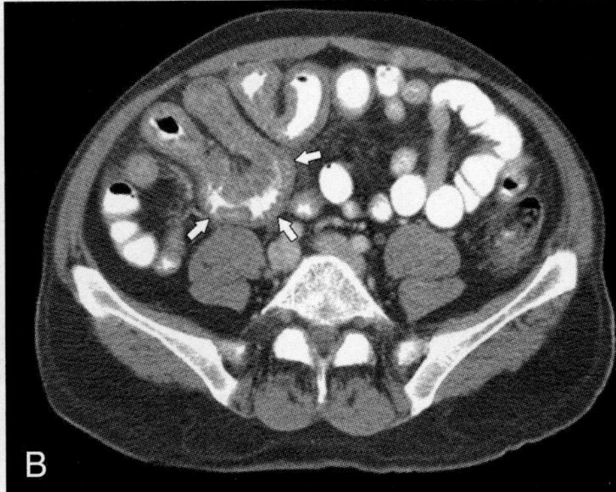

FIGURE 17.6. A 44-year-old man with carcinoid syndrome. **A**, Computed tomography (CT) shows a mesenteric mass (*arrows*) with tethering of small bowel (SB) loops because of desmoplastic reaction, representing mesenteric nodal metastasis. **B**, CT shows a long segment of thickened SB around the mesenteric metastasis, characteristic of carcinoid (*arrows*). On other slices, liver metastases were noted, accounting for carcinoid syndrome.

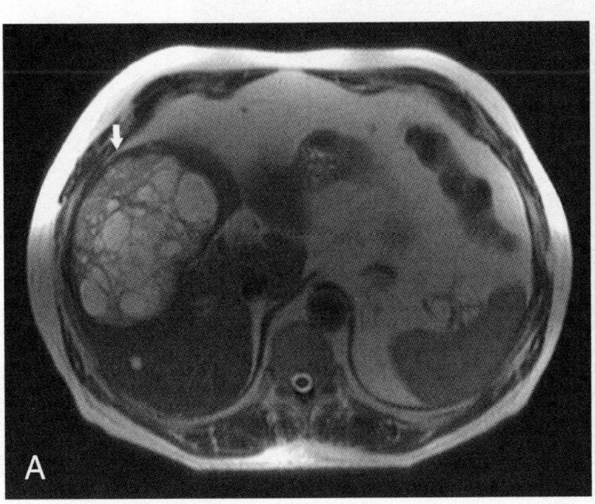

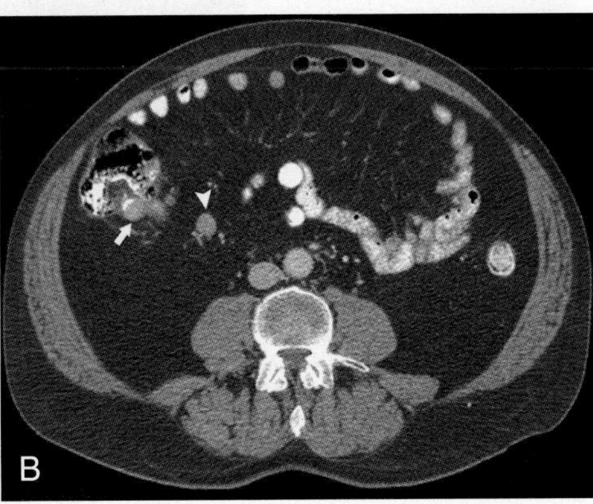

FIGURE 17.7. A 67-year-old man with acute onset of right upper quadrant pain. **A**, Single-shot fast spin echo T2-weighted magnetic resonance imaging shows predominantly cystic low-grade neuroendocrine carcinoma liver metastasis (*arrow*). **B**, Computed tomography shows a small tumor in the terminal ileum (*arrow*) and a small mesenteric nodal metastasis (*arrowhead*).

lesions than somatostatin scintigraphy, these scans are better for the patient as they can be done faster (in a few hours rather than 2–3 days) and therefore expose the patient to less radiation.[12,13] SSTR PET/CT has a complementary role to CT and MRI not only in identifying occult primary SB carcinoid, but also in detecting mesenteric nodal metastasis and distant metastases (Fig. 17.8). Although SSTR PET/CT performance in the detection of liver metastasis is inferior to that of CT and MRI owing to decreased spatial resolution,[14] it can help characterize indeterminate hypervascular lesions. Moreover, it may provide valuable information for predicting the efficacy of somatostatin analog (octreotide) treatment.

Key Points

The Imaging Report for Carcinoid Tumor

- Location of primary small bowel carcinoid if possible (rarely visualized on computed tomography [CT] or magnetic resonance imaging [MRI] as a hyperenhancing mural nodule).
- Description of mesenteric nodal metastasis that may have the pathognomonic CT pattern of a spiculated soft tissue density mesenteric mass because of desmoplastic reaction, with a 70% calcification rate.
- Evaluation of the liver for presence of hypervascular metastases best seen on the late arterial phase of CT or MRI. Small liver metastasis is difficult to distinguish from hemangioma by either CT or MRI.

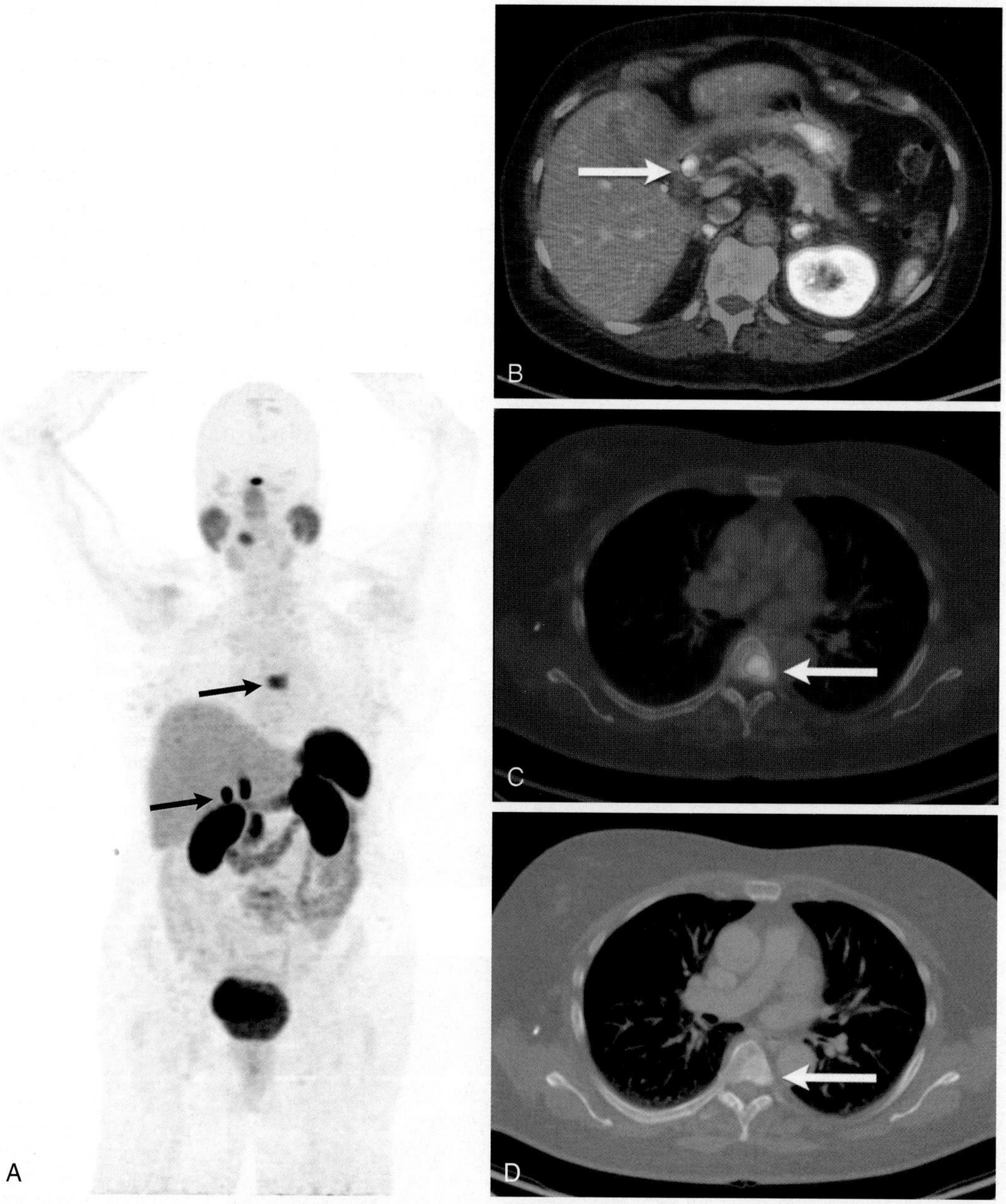

Figure 17.8. A 68-year old woman with duodenal carcinoid tumor identified on endoscopy. **A**, Maximum intensity projection image from Ga-DOTATATE positron emission tomography/computed tomography (CT) scan showing expected uptake in the known duodenal primary tumor, and an unexpected focus in the spine (*arrows*). Normal uptake is noted incidentally at other sites, including the pituitary, salivary glands, liver, spleen, adrenals, and genitourinary system, and along the bowel. **B**, Axial fused image showing focal intense uptake in the known duodenal primary (*arrow*). **C** and **D**, Axial fused and CT images show a somatostatin-avid sclerotic osseous metastasis (*arrows*).

Imaging Algorithm for Carcinoid

1. CT (most commonly the first modality to lead to detection of mesenteric and liver metastases).
2. SSTR PET/CT (for identification of occult SB primary or distant metastases, also for SSTR expression before some therapies).
3. MRI of the liver for follow-up when no significant extrahepatic disease is present (advantage of sparing radiation dose for long-term survivors).

TREATMENT

Localized disease requires treatment with wide *en bloc* surgical resection that includes the adjacent mesentery and lymph nodes.[15] Resection of a primary tumor should also be considered in patients with liver metastases, to prevent the development of fibrosing mesenteritis and possible mechanical obstruction, bleeding, and perforation.

Liver metastases are the most common site of metastatic disease and can become symptomatic owing to hormone secretion or pain. Local modalities addressing the liver metastases have been shown to result in improved overall survival.[16] Therefore, in patients with resectable liver disease, metastasectomy should be favored. When resection is either not feasible or incomplete, other local ablative techniques such as chemoembolization, radiofrequency ablation, and cryotherapy should be considered.[17]

Owing to the slow-growing nature of carcinoid tumors, systemic chemotherapy is not effective in the treatment of this malignancy. The primary medical therapy for metastatic carcinoid tumors is with an analog of the potent inhibitory GI hormone somatostatin, such as octreotide or lanreotide. Their use is extremely effective in controlling the symptoms of carcinoid syndrome, slowing the growth of carcinoid tumors, and inducing biochemical marker responses in approximately 50% of patients. Actually, tumor shrinkage from octreotide treatment is extremely rare.[18] Octreotide-resistant disease can be addressed by treatment with the radiolabeled somatostatin analogue ^{177}Lu-Dotatate[19] or by molecular targeting therapy with the mTOR kinase inhibitor everolimus.[20] SSTR PET/CT is required before ^{177}Lu-Dotatate treatment to confirm that the tumor activity is greater than that of the liver.

KEY POINTS

Therapies for Carcinoid Syndrome

- Resection of the primary tumor is indicated, regardless of the presence of liver metastases, to prevent bowel obstruction.
- Local modalities such as resection or ablation for the treatment of liver metastases improve disease-free survival.
- The somatostatin analog octreotide is of value in symptomatic relief from carcinoid syndrome, although actual tumor responses are extremely rare.

SURVEILLANCE

Two effective markers are available for monitoring patients with metastatic carcinoid tumors:

1. Serotonin metabolite 5-HIAA (in 24-hour urine collections).
2. Plasma chromogranin A.

Imaging monitoring of tumor response to treatment is usually performed by CT, allowing detection of both liver metastasis and peritoneal metastasis, as well as evaluation of potential risk for an SB obstruction. MRI is preferred over CT for monitoring of intrahepatic target lesions. SSTR PET/CT is helpful for problem-solving in cases of clinical or laboratory progressive disease with no evidence of progression on CT or MRI, and for characterization of new lesions of indeterminate significance.

KEY POINTS

Detecting Recurrence of Carcinoid

- Metabolic markers (5-hydroxyindole acetic acid in 24-hr urine collection and plasma chromogranin A).
- Imaging by periodic computed tomography, magnetic resonance imaging, or ^{68}Ga-DOTATATE positron emission tomography/computed tomography scan.

CONCLUSION

SB carcinoid is the most common SB malignancy of neuroendocrine origin, commonly with indolent clinical course, often requiring long-term follow-up by imaging. The hypervascular nature of this tumor requires late arterial-phase cross-sectional imaging to detect metastatic disease. The small primary tumors commonly remain undetected by preoperative imaging. Surgery or ablative therapy of this tumor is the preferred treatment.

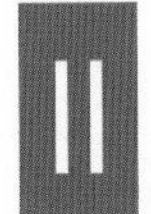

II ADENOCARCINOMA

INTRODUCTION

Adenocarcinoma is the second most common primary malignancy of the SB (31% of all primary SB tumors). One of the more interesting aspects of small intestine adenocarcinoma is its rarity in comparison with large intestine adenocarcinoma. Despite the small intestine representing approximately 70% to 80% of the length and over 90% of the surface area of the alimentary tract, the incidence of SB adenocarcinoma is 30-fold less than that of colon adenocarcinoma.[1]

Epidemiology and Risk Factors

Most cases of adenocarcinoma are sporadic, with a male predominance and peak incidence in the seventh and eighth decades. An increased incidence is associated with the genetic cancer syndromes of hereditary nonpolyposis colorectal cancer, Peutz–Jeghers, familial adenomatous polyposis, and Lynch syndrome. Inflammatory bowel disease, and in particular Crohn's disease, is a risk factor, with risk correlated with both the extent and the duration of SB involvement.

Anatomy and Pathology

Most frequently, the tumor occurs within the duodenum (49%), particularly around the papilla of Vater, and with decreasing frequency in the jejunum (21%) and ileum (15%).[21] In Crohn's disease–associated cases, 70% of tumors present in the distal ileum.

There are four histologic types of adenocarcinoma: well, moderately, and poorly differentiated, and undifferentiated.[22] Prognostic factors consistently associated with poor outcome include the presence of metastatic disease, noncurative surgical resection, poor differentiation, and advanced age.[6] In patients who have had surgical resection, the pathologic factors associated with increased risk of relapse include lymph node involvement, positive surgical margins, poor tumor differentiation, T4 tumor stage, and lymphovascular spread.[23] The genomic profiles of SB adenocarcinomas show common mutations in the *KRAS* oncogene.[24]

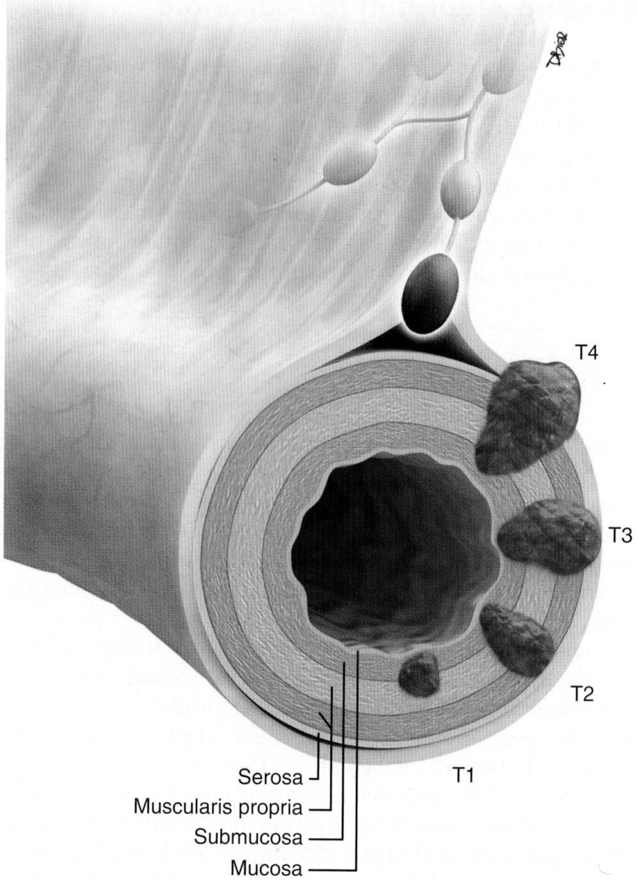

FIGURE 17.9. This diagram illustrates T (tumor) and N (node) components of TNM staging for small bowel adenocarcinoma.

> KEY POINTS
>
> **Anatomy and Pathology of Small Bowel Adenocarcinoma**
> - Sporadic adenocarcinoma is most common in duodenum.
> - Crohn's disease–associated adenocarcinoma is most common in the distal ileum.

Clinical Presentation

Symptoms of SB adenocarcinoma are nonspecific and frequently do not occur until advanced disease is present. The most commonly reported symptoms are abdominal pain, nausea, vomiting, weight loss, and GI bleeding. Adenocarcinoma of the proximal duodenum involving the ampulla of Vater may present with obstructive jaundice.

Patterns of Tumor Spread

Adenocarcinomas spread via lymphatics to the regional mesenteric lymph nodes; the most common sites of hematogenous spread are the liver and lung. Owing to the advanced stage of presentation for most patients, peritoneal carcinomatosis is also common. After a curative resection, the pattern of failure for SB adenocarcinoma is predominantly systemic, with the most common sites being liver, lung, retroperitoneum, and peritoneal carcinomatosis.[23] See Fig. 17.9 for staging evaluation.

> KEY POINTS
>
> **Patterns of Tumor Spread of Small Bowel Adenocarcinoma**
> - Lymphogenic spread to regional mesenteric lymph nodes.
> - Hematogenous spread to liver and lungs.
> - Common early peritoneal spread with diffuse carcinomatosis.

> KEY POINTS
>
> **Staging of Small Bowel Adenocarcinoma**
> - T staging: based on depth of tumor penetration into and beyond the SB wall. Imaging is contributory for T3 and T4 tumors.
> - N staging by imaging: limited by an overlap in appearance of benign reactive and metastatic mesenteric lymph nodes.
> - M staging: liver and lung metastases best appreciated on cross-sectional imaging. Peritoneal carcinomatosis is commonly unmeasurable by imaging.

IMAGING

Tumor Detection

Duodenal adenocarcinoma is usually diagnosed by an esophagogastroduodenoscopy. Tumors distal to the duodenum are accessible to endoscopic evaluation by capsule endoscopy and device-assisted enteroscopy.

A routine multidetector computed tomography (MDCT) scan, commonly ordered for nonspecific abdominal symptoms, may demonstrate SB adenocarcinoma as a focal area of wall thickening causing luminal narrowing (Fig. 17.10). These tumors are often rigid and fibrotic and, therefore, result in early obstruction, although infiltrative lesions without narrowing have also been reported (Fig. 17.11). Adenocarcinomas complicating longstanding Crohn's disease generally arise in the distal ileum. These tumors are difficult to detect because of a preexisting abnormality causing thickening and retraction of the bowel, deforming normal anatomy and masking early diagnosis.

Enteroclysis has been a standard invasive imaging modality performed with nasojejunal cannulation before the introduction of video capsule endoscopy to evaluate SB loops.[23] On barium studies such as standard SB series and enteroclysis, the tumor is seen as a short, circumferentially narrowed segment with overhanging borders, an "apple core" lesion (Fig. 17.12).

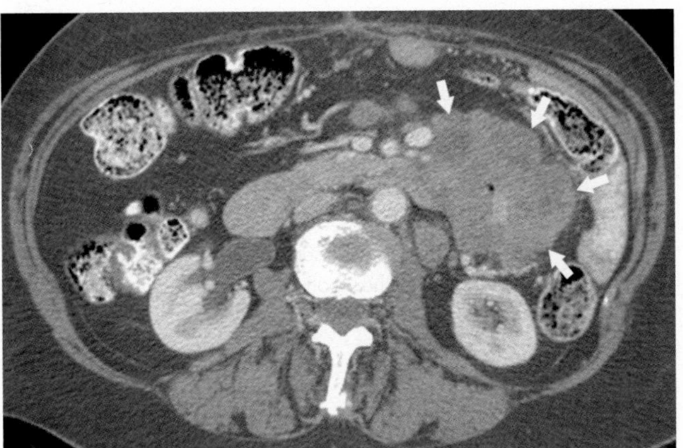

FIGURE 17.10. A 70-year-old woman with jejunal adenocarcinoma. Computed tomography shows a bulky, lobulated mass (*arrows*).

MDCT and MRI can scan the entire SB, but can be limited by lack of optimal opacification of the GI tract. MDCT enterography and MDCT enteroclysis share the advantages and disadvantages of both conventional enteroclysis and cross-sectional imaging, with accurate detection of SB tumors (84% sensitivity and 96% specificity).[26] Lesions as small as 5 mm can be identified.[27]

MRI enteroclysis is capable of demonstrating an SB abnormality, with a reported sensitivity of 91% and sensitivity of 95%.[28,29]

Primary Tumor (T)

T staging is based on the depth of tumorous involvement of the bowel wall. Both CT and MRI have little role in the evaluation of T status for T1 and T2 tumors, owing to limited spatial and contrast resolution in assessment of

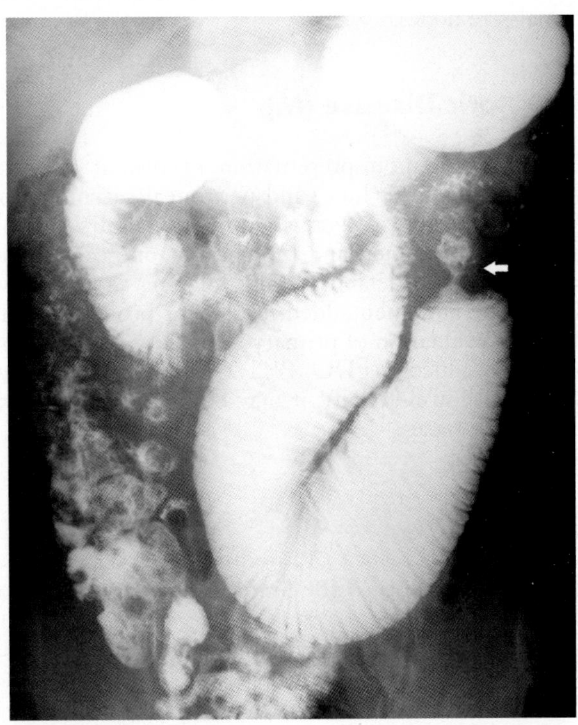

FIGURE 17.12. A 38-year-old man with jejunal adenocarcinoma. Small bowel follow-through shows an "apple core" stricture (*arrow*).

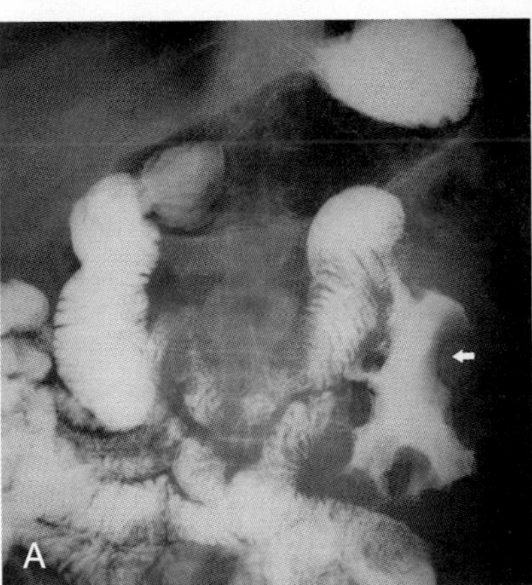

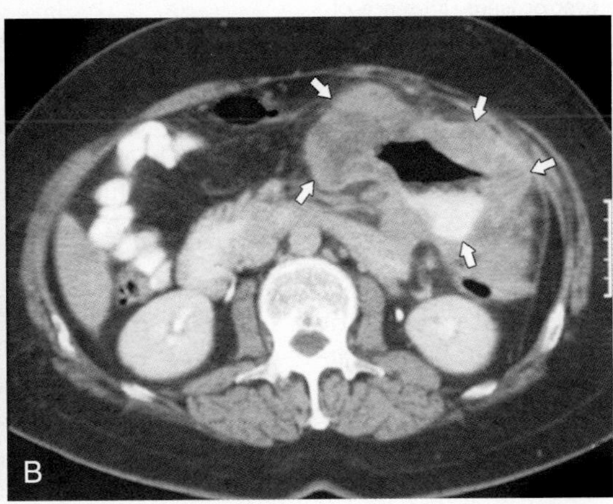

FIGURE 17.11. A 49-year-old man with moderately differentiated adenocarcinoma of the jejunum. **A**, Small bowel follow-through shows an irregular large necrotic mass (*arrow*) in the proximal jejunum. **B**, Computed tomography confirms a nonobstructive tumor (*arrows*) in the proximal jejunum.

thin layers of the SB wall. Cross-sectional modalities can be valuable in advanced T3 and T4 lesions when tumor extends beyond the bowel wall. Endoscopic ultrasound, known for an excellent T staging ability in esophageal and gastric cancers, is technically not applicable to the SB beyond the duodenum.

Nodal Disease (N)

Regional nodal metastases (N1) most commonly occur within the mesentery adjacent to the SB tumor. Mesenteric lymph nodes are considered abnormal when they measure more than 1 cm in the short axis. CT and MRI are equally accurate for nodal status because both are based on size criteria. However, the status of the regional nodes is most accurately established by microscopic pathology of the resection specimen, because the reactive nodes may become enlarged, and small tumor foci can exist within normal-size nodes.

Metastatic Disease (M)

The most common presentation of distant metastasis (M1) includes liver, lung, and peritoneal carcinomatosis. CT has an advantage over MRI in that it allows screening of both the abdomen and the chest at one examination. CT is used as a default staging imaging modality, with MRI of the abdomen added mostly for problem-solving. Although evaluation of primary tumors by 2-[^{18}F] fluoro-2-deoxy-D-glucose (FDG) PET/CT may be complicated by normal bowel activity, it may be useful in identifying distant metastases.

KEY POINTS

The Imaging Report for Small Bowel Adenocarcinoma

- Location and size of the primary tumor, if detectable by imaging.
- Tumorous involvement of adjacent vascular structures, which may preclude resection. This is particularly critical for duodenal adenocarcinoma, potentially involving superior mesenteric vessels and the portal vein.
- Presence of enlarged regional mesenteric lymph nodes.
- Presence of distant metastases in the liver or lungs. Presence of ascites is suspicious for peritoneal carcinomatosis until proved otherwise. Peritoneal spread commonly presents as ascites rather than measurable, discrete omental implants.

TREATMENT

Wide segmental resection with regional mesenteric lymphadenectomy is the standard approach for both treatment and staging purposes. In the case of adenocarcinoma involving the proximal duodenum, pancreaticoduodenectomy may be required. Curative radical surgery is the most important prognostic factor.[28]

After curatively resecting adenocarcinoma, adjuvant chemoradiation based on 5-fluorouracil (5-FU) is used in patients at high risk for relapse, although no definite survival benefit for adjuvant therapy after curative resection was found.[30–32] Patients with locally advanced unresectable tumors and metastatic tumors are treated with chemotherapy, most commonly 5-FU combined with oxaliplatin.[31] The overall survival for SB adenocarcinoma remains poor, with a median survival for patients with metastatic disease of 12 to 18 months.[32,34]

KEY POINTS

Treatment of Small Bowel Adenocarcinoma

- Radical curative surgery is the most desired approach, when achievable. Duodenal adenocarcinoma requires pancreaticoduodenectomy (Whipple's surgery). Limited detection of peritoneal spread and military liver metastases by imaging sometimes leads to the need for diagnostic laparoscopy as the first step before attempted curative resection.
- 5-fluorouracil–based chemotherapy for unresectable disease has a low response rate with poor survival.

SURVEILLANCE

CT is the main modality for imaging surveillance after curative resection of adenocarcinoma. PET/CT can be used for patients with rising carcinoembryonic antigen posttreatment and nondiagnostic CT.

KEY POINT

Detecting Recurrence of Small Bowel Adenocarcinoma

- Recurrent disease commonly presents as peritoneal carcinomatosis or liver metastases, rather than as local recurrence within the resection bed.

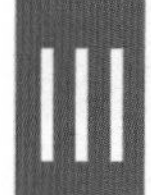

III LYMPHOMA

INTRODUCTION

Primary GI lymphoma is the most common extranodal form. The sites of involvement include the stomach (75%), the SB including the duodenum (9%), and the ileocecal region (7%).

Epidemiology

Non-Hodgkin lymphoma (NHL) is the third most common SB malignancy, representing about 17% of all SB malignancies. Involvement of the SB by Hodgkin lymphoma is extremely rare.

In the United States, SB lymphoma occurs predominantly in adults, peaking in the 7th decade. Patients at increased risk for SB lymphoma are those with autoimmune diseases, immunodeficiency syndromes such as acquired immunodeficiency syndrome, longstanding immunosuppressive therapy such as posttransplantation, celiac disease, and prior radiation therapy. Mucosa-associated lymphoid tissue (MALT) lymphomas are most commonly found in the stomach, where they have a strong association with *Helicobacter pylori*.

Anatomy and Pathology

Lymphomas most often involving the GI tract consist of the extranodal marginal zone B-cell lymphoma of MALT type, diffuse large B-cell lymphoma, mantle cell lymphoma, enteropathy-associated T-cell intestinal lymphoma, and Burkitt lymphoma.[35] The distribution of lymphoma in the SB follows the distribution of lymphoid follicles in the SB, with the lymphoid-rich distal ileum the most common site of SB lymphoma.[35] Owing to the submucosal origin of lymphoma involving the SB, SB lymphomas tend not to result in early luminal occlusion and, thus, often present with large, bulky tumors.

> **Key Points**
>
> **Anatomy and Pathology of Lymphoma**
>
> - Only non-Hodgkin lymphoma involves the small bowel (SB). The five most common types include extranodal marginal zone B-cell lymphoma of mucosa associated lymphoid tissue (MALT), diffuse large B-cell lymphoma, mantle cell lymphoma, enteropathy-associated T-cell intestinal lymphoma, and Burkitt lymphoma.
> - SB lymphoma originates from the submucosal layer and may present with a large mass without obstruction of the lumen.

Patterns of Tumor Spread

NHL predominantly spreads hematogenously. However, regional mesenteric lymphadenopathy is commonly associated and is inseparable from the involved segment of the SB, reflecting the component of lymphatic spread.

Staging Evaluation

The modified Ann Arbor staging system and the International Prognostic Index, which are used for staging and prognostication of NHL, are discussed in detail in Chapter "Hematologic Malignancy: The Lymphomas".

IMAGING

Four major patterns of SB lymphoma have been identified on radiographic studies:[36]

1. Infiltrating pattern that appears as wall thickening with destruction of the normal SB folds. Because the tumor infiltrates the muscular layer of the wall, it can inhibit peristalsis and, therefore, result in aneurysmal dilatation of the affected bowel loop. As a result, the lumen is dilated, with focal excentric bulging of the wall. On CT, this mass appears homogeneously hypodense with minimal contrast enhancement (Fig. 17.13).
2. Exophytic mass, which can ulcerate. This pattern can simulate an adenocarcinoma or gastrointestinal stromal tumor (GIST). Ulceration may result in localized perforation.
3. Single mass lesion, which can lead to intussusception (Fig. 17.14) but rarely will result in obstruction, because the masses are typically pliable and soft.

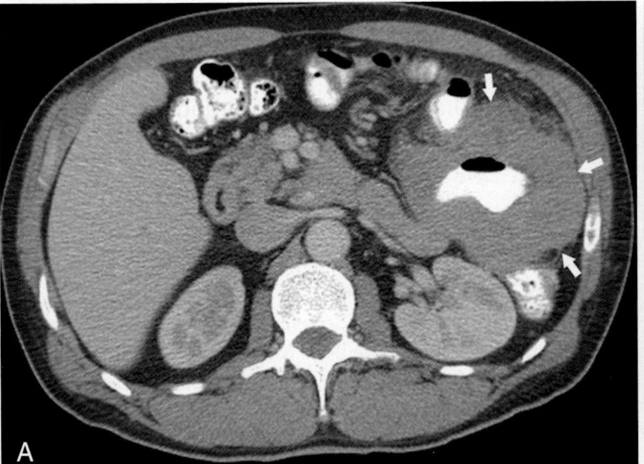

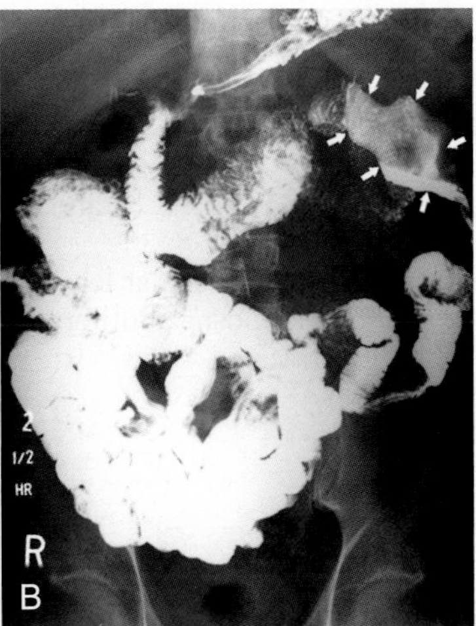

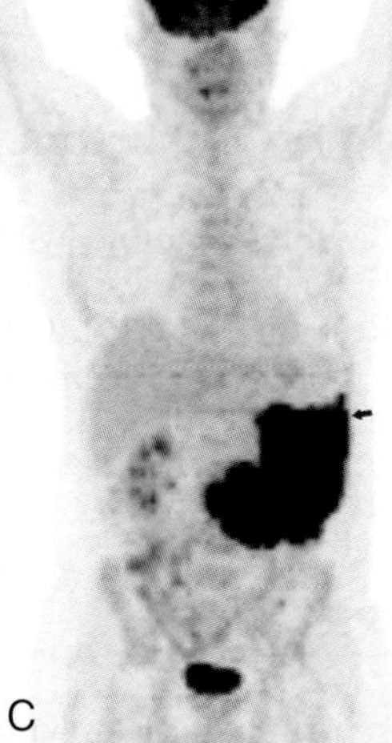

Figure 17.13. A 50-year-old man with follicular and diffuse large B-cell lymphoma in the jejunum. **A**, Computed tomography shows a bulky concentric mass with expansion of the lumen (*arrows*). **B**, Small bowel follow-through shows an irregular nonobstructive lesion (*arrows*) in the jejunum. **C**, Positron emission tomography scan shows highly 2-[^{18}F] fluoro-2-deoxy-D-glucose–avid jejunal mass (*arrow*).

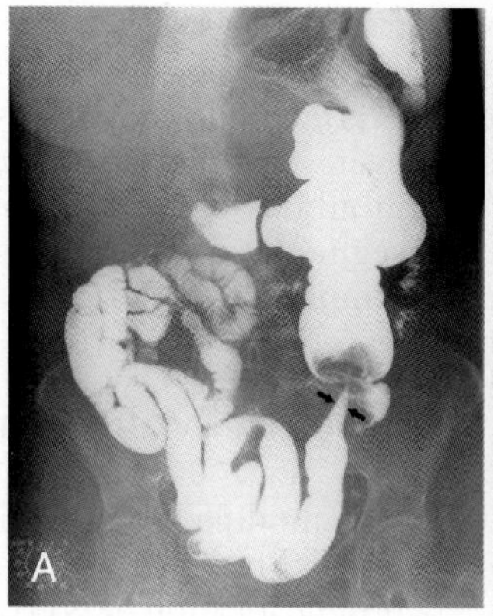

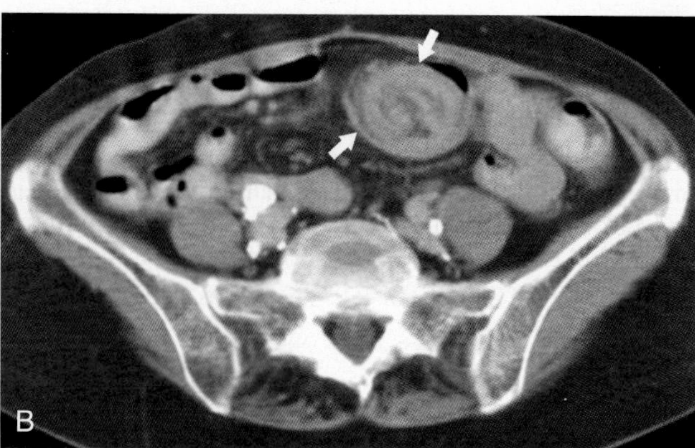

FIGURE 17.14. A 74-year-old woman with diffuse large B-cell lymphoma in the small bowel. **A**, Small bowel follow-through shows intussusception (*arrows*). **B**, Computed tomography shows the characteristic swirling appearance of the jejunum consistent with the intussusception (*arrows*).

4. Multifocal submucosal nodules within the SB. This appearance is often better appreciated on an SB series or enteroclysis as "bull's eye" or "target" lesions because the nodules can be very small. Small-volume lymphomatous implants in the bowel are not well resolved by CT or PET/CT.

FDG-PET/CT is a gold standard for the baseline staging imaging for most NHLs.[37] PET/CT evaluation of the bowel lymphoma may be limited by incidental physiologic increased background activity within the bowel, occasionally in the SB, and even more commonly in the colon, but can be useful in identifying nodal sites of involvement and other focal extranodal sites, such as in the bone marrow.

> KEY POINTS
>
> **The Imaging Report for Lymphoma**
>
> - Location and extent of small bowel (SB) involvement. When characterizing an undiagnosed SB mass, aneurysmal dilatation of the involved segment of the bowel and lack of bowel obstruction despite the large tumor are features suggestive of lymphoma.
> - Presence of lymphadenopathy or other extranodal sites of lymphomatous involvement.

Imaging Algorithm for Lymphoma

1. Baseline staging with contrast-enhanced CT and FDG-PET/CT.
2. Restaging by PET/CT 2 months post surgery, at least 2 months post chemotherapy, and as far post radiotherapy as possible.

TREATMENT

As in lymphomas of lymph node origin, chemotherapy is the primary therapeutic modality. In general, patients should be assumed to have systemic disease and be treated with systemic chemotherapy, even if a complete surgical resection has been performed. Treatment options based on histologic subtype are described in Chapter "The Lymphomas". Radiation therapy is rarely used for the management of SB lymphoma. The prognosis for SB lymphomas is overall better than that for adenocarcinoma, with 20% to 50% 5-year survival for aggressive advanced-stage lymphoma, and up to 90% 5-year survival for localized, less aggressive subtypes.[35]

Close monitoring by CT during the initial course of chemotherapy is recommended for aggressive types of lymphoma, owing to the risk of perforation with the rapid response to therapy and shrinking of the lymphomatous mass involving the SB wall.

PET/CT scan plays a crucial role in monitoring response to treatment. A positive FDG PET scan after the completion of chemotherapy is a strong predictor of relapse and lower disease-free survival.[38] Five-point scale visual evaluation of posttreatment PET/CT imaging based on the residual tumor uptake compared with physiologic activity in the mediastinum and in the liver is used to assess metabolic response.[37,39] A score of 1 or 2 (residual uptake that is undetectable or equal to or lower than that of mediastinum) indicates complete metabolic response, even if there is a residual soft tissue abnormality. A score of 3 (residual uptake exceeding that of mediastinum but equal to or lower than liver activity) also indicates metabolic response, especially at the end of therapy, but may be considered inadequate in clinical trials assessing early response. A score of 4 or 5 (residual uptake moderately greater than liver uptake) is suspicious for residual active lymphoma.

> KEY POINTS
>
> **Therapy for Lymphoma**
>
> - Histologic type– and stage-dependent systemic chemotherapy is administered. Diffuse large B-cell lymphoma is commonly treated with an RCHOP (rituximab, cyclophosphamide, hydroxydaunorubicin, Oncovin, prednisone) regimen.
> - Small bowel resection may contribute to disease-free survival, but is rarely curative without chemotherapy.
> - A 5-point scale is used for interpretation of posttreatment PET/CT imaging to define metabolic response.

SURVEILLANCE

CT is the standard imaging modality used for surveillance of lymphoma survivors, including neck, chest, abdomen, and pelvis, because this systemic malignancy commonly recurs away from the primary presentation within the SB. With high-grade lymphomas, the risk of recurrence decreases after the first 1 to 2 years posttreatment, whereas the risk of recurrence of low-grade lymphomas persist throughout patient's life. PET/CT is more sensitive than CT alone in early detection of relapse.[40]

CONCLUSION

Lymphoma of the SB is a heterogeneous group of diseases in terms of histologic grade and biologic aggressiveness. Radiographic manifestations of lymphoma vary from large masses with perforation to multifocal disease undetectable by any imaging modality. PET/CT posttreatment is required to evaluate for metabolic response, which correlates well with clinical outcome.

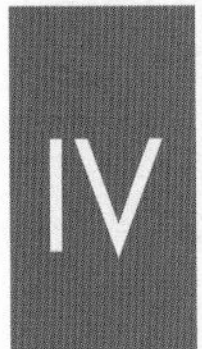

IV Gastrointestinal Stromal Tumor

INTRODUCTION

GIST is a sarcoma subtype, accounting for 67% of SB sarcomas.[2] Sarcomas are rare sporadic tumors found anywhere within the GI tract, with the most common location being the stomach (51%), followed by the SB.[38,41]

Epidemiology and Risk Factors

GIST is the most common sarcoma subtype, representing the fourth most common form of malignant SB tumors (9%). Most cases of GIST are sporadic. There are reports of increased incidence of both benign and malignant GISTs in patients with neurofibromatosis type 1.[42]

Anatomy and Pathology

GISTs derive from CD34-positive stem cells differentiating into the interstitial cells of Cajal lineage. These differentiated cells have features of both smooth muscle and neuronal cells and serve as GI "pacemaker cells" regulating peristalsis. The cellular morphology of GISTs ranges from predominantly spindle-shaped (70%) to epithelioid (20%), with 10% mixed type.

By light microscopy alone, it can be difficult to distinguish among GISTs and other tumors (leiomyosarcoma, leiomyoma, malignant melanoma, schwannoma, malignant peripheral nerve sheath tumor, or desmoid tumor), because histologic findings do not reliably relate to the immunophenotype or the molecular genetics of the lesions. More than 80% of GIST cells, however, express the CD117 antigen, part of the KIT transmembrane receptor tyrosine kinase that is the product of the *KIT* protooncogene.[43,44]

KEY POINTS

Anatomy and Pathology of Gastrointestinal Stromal Tumor

- Gastrointestinal stromal tumors (GISTs) arise from the interstitial cells of Cajal, exhibiting features of both smooth muscle and neuronal differentiation.
- By light microscopy, GIST is indistinguishable from leiomyosarcoma and other mesenchymal tumors.
- Some 80% of GISTs express mutated forms of the *KIT* protooncogene.

Clinical Presentation

GISTs usually do not cause bowel obstruction, and commonly present as very large masses. Nearly 50% of patients with GISTs present with metastasis. Benign GIST masses may present as an incidental finding on cross-sectional imaging performed for other reasons.

Patterns of Tumor Spread

As with other sarcomas, GIST spreads hematogenously, most commonly to the liver. Peritoneal sarcomatosis is common with GIST, commonly without significant ascites. Nodal metastases of GIST are uncommon.

KEY POINT

Patterns of Tumor Spread of Gastrointestinal Stromal Tumor

- Hematogenous spread to the liver and peritoneal sarcomatosis.

Staging Evaluation

TNM staging of GIST is similar to adenocarcinoma staging by the American Joint Committee on Cancer.[45]

IMAGING

Because of the exophytic growth, CT is the imaging modality of choice. Small tumors tend to appear homogeneous on CT, although larger tumors (>6 cm) frequently show central areas of necrosis or hemorrhage.[46] These tumors may be so large that it is difficult to appreciate the communication of the tumor with the intestinal wall (Fig. 17.15). If intraluminal contrast is seen in the tumor, bowel origin is confirmed (Fig. 17.16). Large size, significant necrosis, and cavitation are signs suggestive of malignancy. It is difficult to distinguish benign from malignant GIST unless obvious metastases are present. GISTs tend to demonstrate an early contrast enhancement owing to their hypervascular nature (Fig. 17.17).

Liver metastases appear isodense or hypodense to normal liver parenchyma on noncontrast images and usually are hypodense on the postcontrast images. They can appear cystic and can be difficult to differentiate from other cystic hepatic lesions, but this appearance is more commonly seen posttreatment (Fig. 17.18). Stable, treated, cystic-appearing GIST metastases should not be mistaken for benign hepatic cysts. Growing enhancing nodules within these cystic lesions indicate reactivation of tumor growth. Peritoneal metastasis may be seen as separate nodules (sarcomatous pattern of peritoneal spread), but ascites is rarely seen.

MRI can show liver metastases with equal or higher accuracy than CT, but it has the disadvantage of poorer resolution of extrahepatic disease.

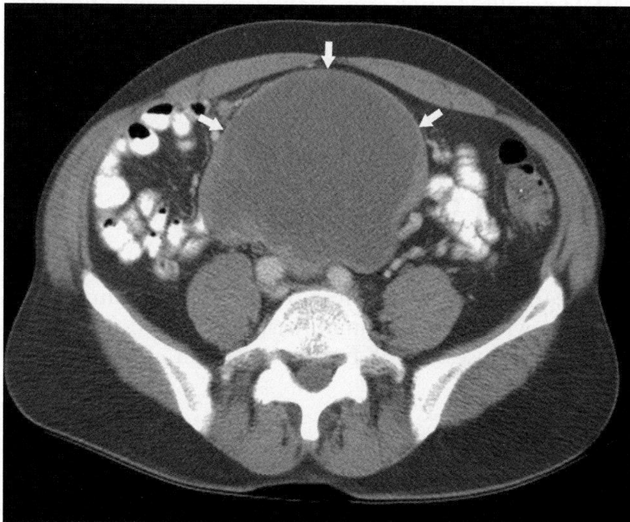

FIGURE 17.15. A 56-year-old man with small bowel (SB) gastrointestinal stromal tumor metastatic to the liver. Computed tomography shows a large low-attenuation mesenteric mass (*arrows*) without obvious communication with the SB.

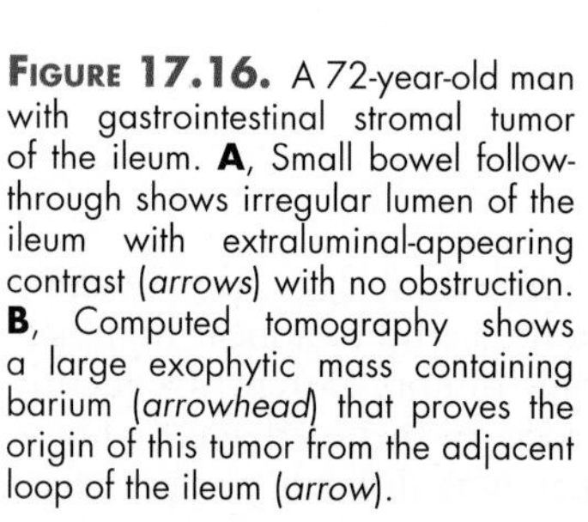
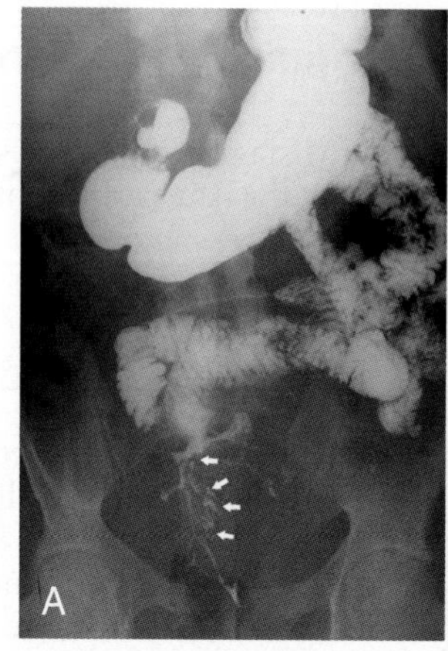

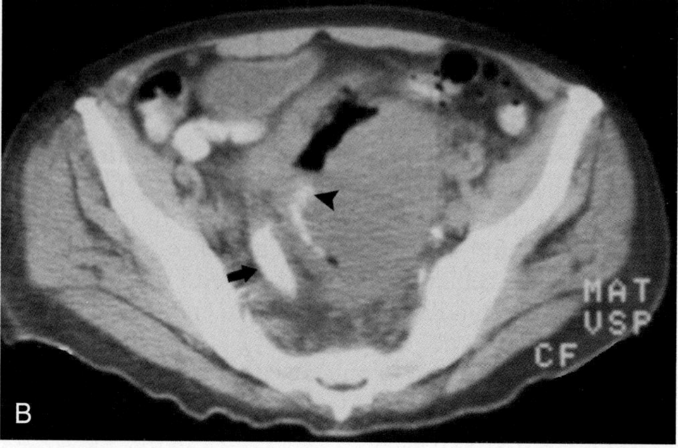

FIGURE 17.16. A 72-year-old man with gastrointestinal stromal tumor of the ileum. **A**, Small bowel follow-through shows irregular lumen of the ileum with extraluminal-appearing contrast (*arrows*) with no obstruction. **B**, Computed tomography shows a large exophytic mass containing barium (*arrowhead*) that proves the origin of this tumor from the adjacent loop of the ileum (*arrow*).

Key Points

The Imaging Report for Gastrointestinal Stromal Tumor

- Location of the primary mass in relation to the bowel (sometimes difficult to trace the tumor origin to any of the surrounding parts of gastrointestinal tract). If intraluminal contrast is seen in the necrotic tumor, bowel origin is confirmed.
- Presence of liver metastases and peritoneal sarcomatosis.

TREATMENT

Surgical resection is the treatment of choice. Unlike adenocarcinoma and carcinoid, which spread through lymphatics, GISTs metastasize hematogenously, obviating

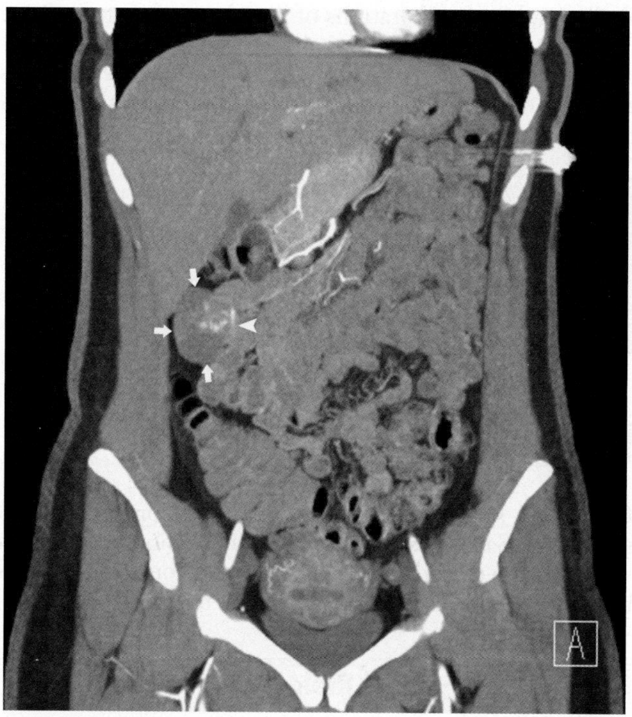

FIGURE 17.17. A 31-year-old woman with gastrointestinal stromal tumor of the small bowel (SB). Coronal reformatted image of computed tomography angiogram shows an approximately 4.5-cm mass exophytic from the SB (*arrows*) with intense early contrast enhancement (*arrowhead*).

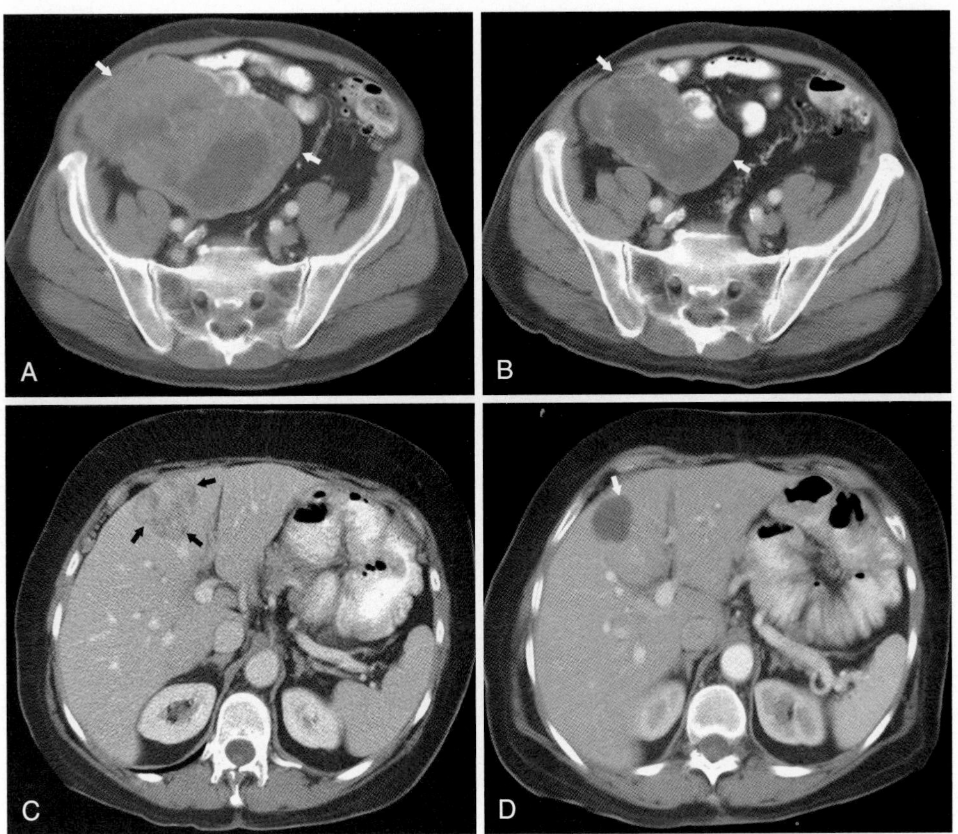

FIGURE 17.18. A 67-year-old man with prostate cancer. Small bowel (SB) gastrointestinal stromal tumor with liver metastases was incidentally found on workup of elevated prostate-specific antigen. **A**, Computed tomography (CT) shows a large mass (*arrows*) exophytic from the ileum. **B**, After 1 year of imatinib therapy, CT shows a decrease in size and a mild decrease in density of the primary SB tumor (*arrows*). **C**, CT shows an intensely enhancing liver metastasis (*arrows*). **D**, After 1 year of imatinib therapy, CT shows a decrease in size and density of the liver metastasis (*arrow*), mimicking a cystic lesion.

the need for more complete surgery with removal of the lymphatic drainage in the mesentery. This may be significant in the duodenal tumor, allowing the surgeon to avoid a major procedure such as pancreaticoduodenectomy. Although GISTs may present as very large masses, the "pushing" rather than the invasive nature of tumor growth may sometimes allow for the development of a safe plane of resection. GISTs smaller than 2 cm are generally considered benign, with a very low risk of recurrence.

KIT-positive GISTs can be targeted therapeutically with orally active tyrosine kinase inhibitors (TKIs) such as imatinib and sunitinib. These agents can be used in both the neoadjuvant setting to downstage borderline surgical candidates and in the adjuvant setting, and have been shown to be highly effective.[47] These agents are used to enable patients with metastatic unresectable disease to achieve long-term survival.[48] With prolonged treatment, resistance develops because of secondary *KIT* mutations. Dose escalation can be attempted initially. Newer TKIs can be used for broader target profiles.[49] A potential role for immunotherapy is under investigation.[50]

KEY POINTS

Therapies for Gastrointestinal Stromal Tumor

- Radical resection is the treatment of choice.
- Unresectable KIT-positive gastrointestinal stromal tumor is successfully treated by the tyrosine kinase inhibitors imatinib and sunitinib. The same agents can be used in the adjuvant and neoadjuvant settings for surgical candidates.
- Resistance to imatinib develops after prolonged treatment.

SURVEILLANCE

Follow-up of GIST patients treated with imatinib showed that tumor size alone was a poor indicator of a positive response. In 75% of the patients, the tumor was stable, as determined by usual size-based Response Evaluation Criteria In Solid Tumors (RECIST) criteria, despite the favorable clinical outcome. Decrease in tumor density after treatment indicated radiographic response because of myxoid degeneration and necrosis within the tumor (Fig. 17.19; see Fig. 17.18). Successfully treated GISTs sometimes became so uniformly hypodense that they could mimic benign cysts and vice versa. Tumor progression may be manifested not only as an enlarging mass or new masses, but also as a partial to complete filling-in of a previously hypodense lesion, or as a hyperdense "nodule-within-a-mass" pattern.[51]

According to RECIST, a partial response is defined as a 30% decrease in the longest dimension of measurable tumor. To address the discrepancy between the standard RECIST criteria and GIST behavior, an alternative set of Choi criteria were developed that define a partial response as a 10% decrease in unidimensional tumor size or a 15% decrease in tumor density on contrast-enhanced CT scans.[51]

FDG-PET/CT is more effective than CT in monitoring tumor response to chemotherapy.[52,53] A dramatic decrease in FDG uptake within initially hypermetabolic GIST tumors is noted within a short interval after initiation of imatinib therapy (see Fig. 17.19). Reemergence of activity on PET/CT may indicate the development of resistance to TKI therapy.[54]

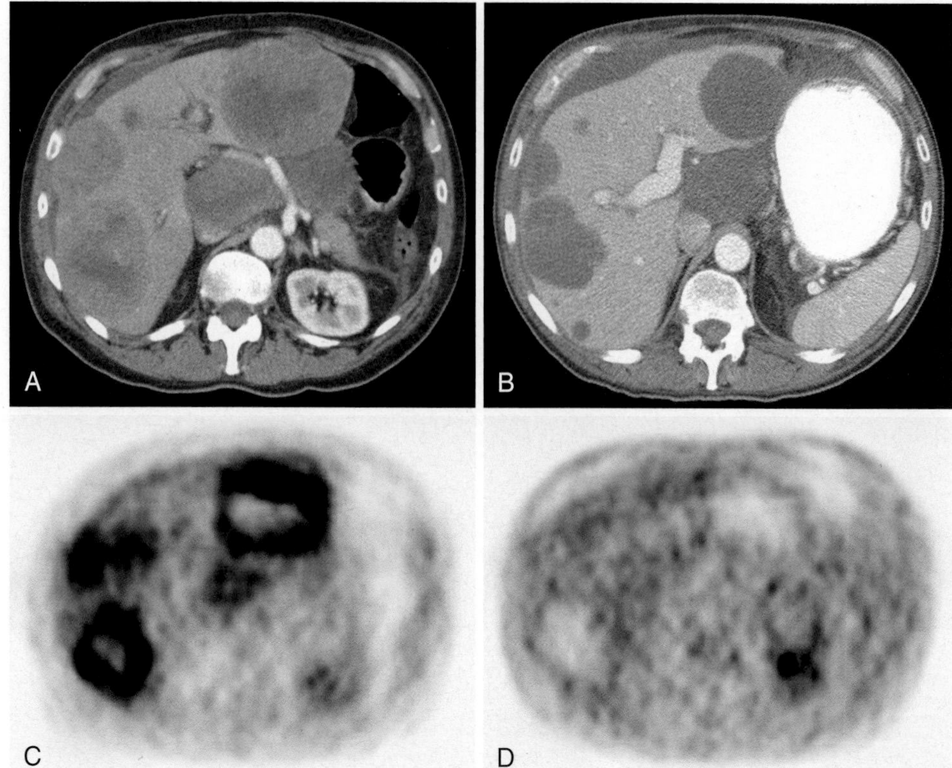

FIGURE 17.19. A 65-year-old man with Small bowel gastrointestinal stromal tumor metastatic to the liver. Multiple heterogeneously enhancing liver metastases on contrast-enhanced computed tomography (CT) (**A**) are hypermetabolic on positron emission tomography (PET) scan (**B**). After 2 months' therapy with imatinib (Gleevec), liver metastases decreased in size and became very homogeneously hypodense on CT (**C**) and hypometabolic on PET scan (**D**).

KEY POINTS

Detecting Recurrence of Gastrointestinal Stromal Tumor

- Clinical response to imatinib does not follow Response Evaluation Criteria In Solid Tumors criteria. The alternative Choi criteria are based not only on tumor size but also on the degree of enhancement.
- Tumor progression may be manifested not only as an enlarging mass but also as a new hyperdense nodule within a previously uniformly hypodense mass.
- 2-[^{18}F] fluoro-2-deoxy-D-glucose positron emission tomography/computed tomography may be helpful in identifying response to tyrosine kinase inhibitor therapy or the development of resistance.

V METASTASES TO THE SMALL BOWEL

Epidemiology and Risk Factors

The most common primary malignancies to spread into the SB include colon, lung, and breast cancer and melanoma. The SB is commonly involved by peritoneal metastases from GI and ovarian-uterine cancers causing diffuse peritoneal carcinomatosis.

Anatomy and Pathology

Depending on the pathway of spread, SB can be involved on the serosal surface from the peritoneum or arise from the mucosal layer.

Clinical Presentation

As with other SB masses, metastases may cause bowel obstruction and GI bleeding.

Patterns of Tumor Spread

There are three pathways of secondary involvement of the SB:

1. Intraperitoneal spread: commonly from GI and ovarian-uterine cancers. The areas most prone to involvement are the ileocecal valve and ileal loops in the cul-de-sac. Mesenteric metastases generally involve the mesenteric margin of the bowel. Desmoplastic reaction of these tumors may cause obstruction.
2. Hematogenous dissemination. Melanoma is the most common solid tumor metastatic to the SB, followed by lung cancer and breast cancer.[55] Although SB metastases in lung cancer are usually concomitant with overall progressive disease and often clinically obscure, the situation may be different with melanoma (Fig. 17.20), in which metastases may appear years after the diagnosis of the primary tumor as the only site of recurrence.[56] Hematogenous metastases are usually

multiple and commonly involve the antimesenteric border of the bowel.

3. Extension from an adjacent tumor either directly or via lymphatics. The most common primary tumor accounting for this appearance is colon cancer.

KEY POINTS

Patterns of Tumor Spread of Small Bowel Metastases

- Intraperitoneal spread is common from gastrointestinal and ovarian-uterine cancers. Dependent areas of the peritoneal cavity are most likely to be involved, including the ileocecal valve and ileal loops in the cul-de-sac. The mesenteric margin of the SB is usually involved. Desmoplastic reaction of these tumors may cause obstruction.
- Hematogenous spread is most common from melanoma and lung and breast cancer, usually with multiple lesions involving the antimesenteric border of the bowel.
- Extension from an adjacent tumor either directly or via lymphatics is most commonly from colon cancer.

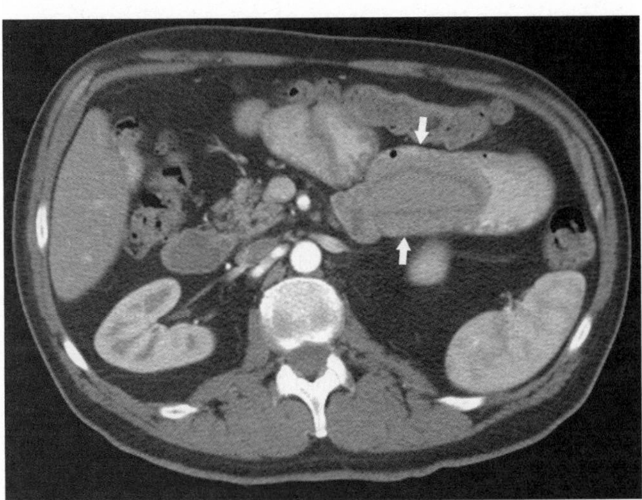

FIGURE 17.20. A 55-year-old man 8 years after resection of melanoma from his back presenting with abdominal pain. Computed tomography shows an ovoid mass (*arrows*) expanding the jejunum, representing metastatic melanoma with intussusception.

Staging Evaluation

Metastasis in the SB indicates stage IV of known malignancy.

IMAGING

Neither SB follow-through nor CT seems to be reliable in demonstrating melanoma metastases to the SB.[57] Focal wall thickening and polypoid filling defects are seen with the advanced cases. PET/CT is more sensitive and specific for the detection of early SB metastases.[58] (Figs. 17.21 and 17.22).

KEY POINTS

The Imaging Report for Small Bowel Metastases

- Description of the suspicious areas of focal wall thickening.
- Presence or imminent danger of bowel obstruction.
- Areas of focal highly increased 2-[^{18}F] fluoro-2-deoxy-D-glucose uptake in the small bowel should be considered suspicious for metastases even when not associated with computed tomography abnormality. Capsule endoscopy may be suggested for further evaluation.

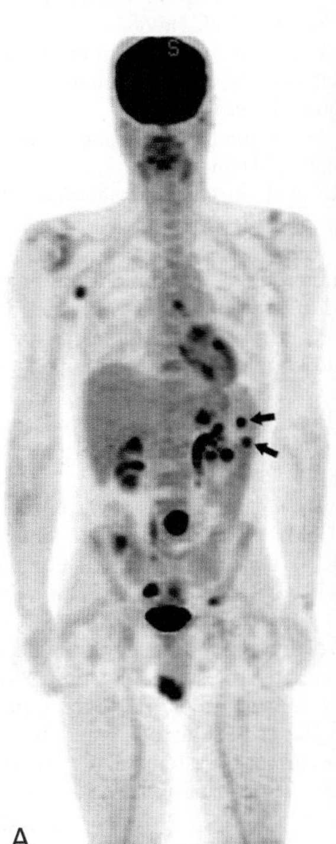

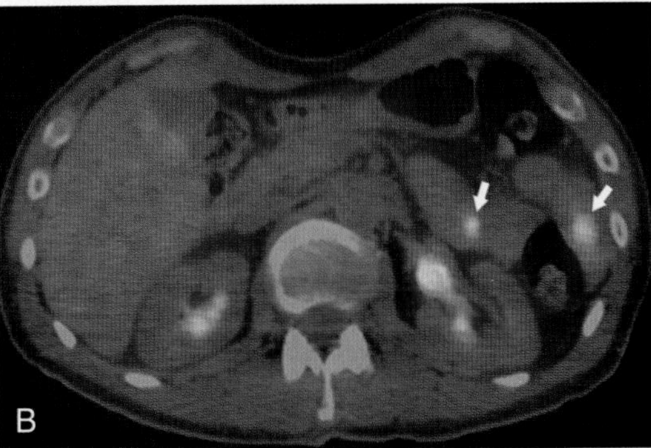

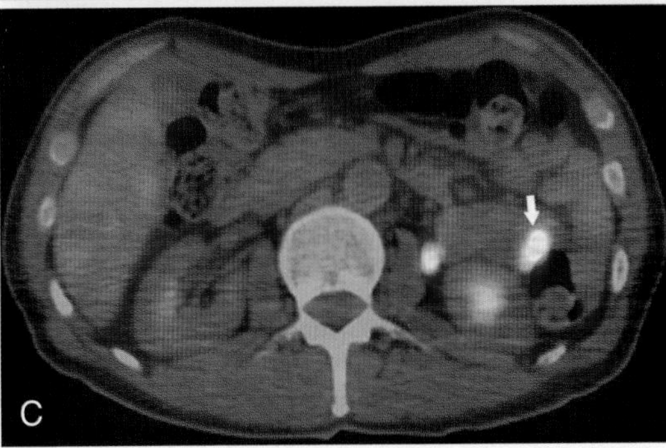

FIGURE 17.21. A–C, A 53-year-old man with disseminated metastatic melanoma (*arrows* in **B** and **C**). **A**, Position emission tomography/computed tomography shows numerous foci of 2-[^{18}F] fluoro-2-deoxy-D-glucose uptake in the jejunum (*arrows*), representing melanoma metastases.

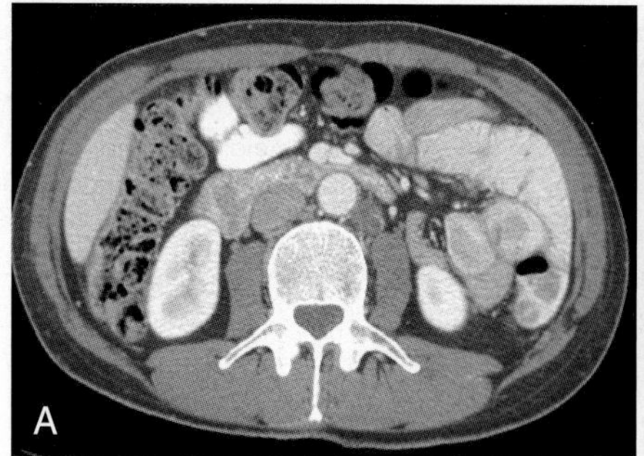

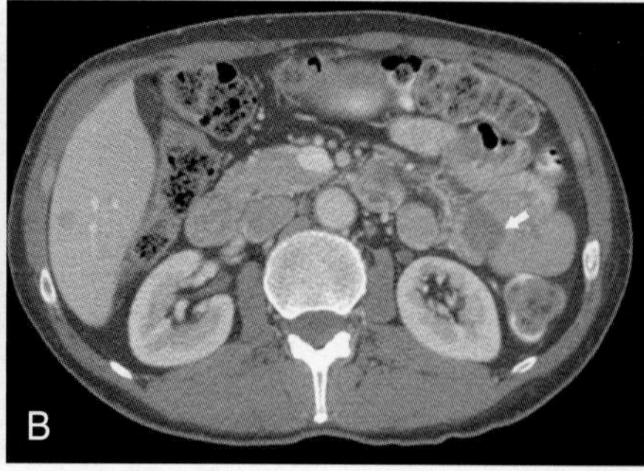

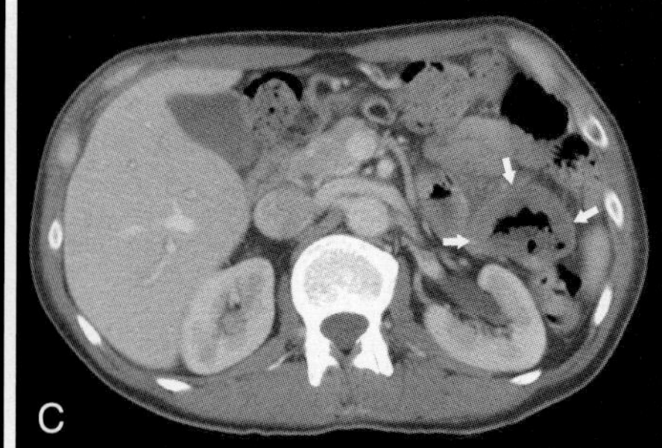

FIGURE 17.22. A 53-year-old man with disseminated metastatic melanoma. **A**, Contrast-enhanced computed tomography (CT) performed at the same time as position emission tomography/CT shows no obvious abnormality in the jejunum. **B**, Contrast-enhanced CT 1 month later shows a small metastasis (*arrow*) in the jejunum. **C**, Contrast-enhanced CT 3 months later shows a now obvious and progressive metastasis (*arrows*) in the jejunum.

TREATMENT

SB metastases indicate poor prognosis with less than 12 months' survival. Resection of melanoma metastases is indicated when possible for palliation and to increase symptom-free survival.[56]

CONCLUSION

A heterogeneous group of tumors involving the SB shares the clinical presentation of occult blood loss with anemia or bowel obstruction. Detection of early small tumors is challenging for all imaging modalities. Imaging plays an important role in staging and surveillance for metastatic disease.

REFERENCES

1. Siegel RL, Miller KD, Jemal A. Cancer statistics, 2019. *CA Cancer J Clin*. 2019;69(1):7–34.
2. Goodman MT, Matsuno RK, Shvetsov YB, et al. Racial and ethnic variation in the incidence of small-bowel cancer subtypes in the United States 1995-2008. *Dis Colon Rectum*. 2013;56(4):441–448.
3. Minardi Jr AJ, Zibari GB, Aultman DF, et al. Small bowel tumors. *J Am Coll Surg*. 1998;186:664–668.
4. Eliakim E. Video capsule endoscopy of the small bowel. *Curr Opin Gastroenterol*. 2008;24(2):159–163.
5. Law JK. New developments in small bowel enteroscopy. *Curr Opin Gastroeneterol*. 2016;32(5):387–391.
6. Bilimoria KY, Bentrem DJ, Wayne JD, et al. Small bowel cancer in the United States: changes in epidemiology, treatment, and survival over the last 20 years. *Ann Surg*. 2009;249:63–71.
7. Caplin ME, Buscombe JR, Hilson AJ, et al. Carcinoid tumor. *Lancet*. 1998;352:799–805.
8. Modlin IM, Champaneria MC, Chan AK, et al. A three-decade analysis of 3,911 small intestinal neuroendocrine tumors: the rapid pace of no progress. *Am L Gastroenterol*. 2007;102:1464–1473.
9. Landry CS, Brock G, Scoggins CR, et al. A proposed staging system for small bowel carcinoid tumors based on an analysis of 6,380 patients. *Am J Surg*. 2008;196:896–903.
10. Horton KM, Kamel I, Hofmann L, et al. Carcinoid tumors of the small bowel: a multitechnique imaging approach. *Am J Roentgenol*. 2004;182:559–567.
11. Dromain C, de Baere T, Lumbroso J, et al. Detection of liver metastases from endocrine tumors: a prospective comparison of somatostatin receptor scintigraphy, computed tomography, and magnetic resonance imaging. *J Clin Oncol*. 2005;23:70–78.
12. Gabriel M, Decristoforo C, Kendler D, et al. 68Ga-DOTA-Tyr3-octreotide PET in neuroendocrine tumors: comparison with somatostatin receptor scintigraphy and CT. *J Nucl Med*. 2007;48:508–518.
13. Hope TA, Bergsland EK, Bozkurt MF, et al. Appropriate Use Criteria for Somatostatin Receptor PET Imaging in Neuroendocrine Tumors. *J Nucl Med*, 2018;59:66–74.
14. Srirajaskanthan R, Kayani I, Quigley AM, et al. The role of 68Ga-DOTATATE PET in patients with neuroendocrine tumors and negative or equivocal findings on 111In-DTPA-octreotide scintigraphy. *J Nucl Med*. 2010;51:875–882.
15. Farley HA, Pommier RF. Surgical treatment of small bowel neuroendocrine tumors. *Hematol/Oncol Clin North Am*. 2016;30(1):49–61.
16. Sarmiento JM, Heywood G, Rubin J, et al. Surgical treatment of neuroendocrine metastases to the liver: a plea for resection to increase survival. *J Am Coll Surg*. 2003;197(1):29.
17. Fairweather M, Swanson R, Wang J. Management of neuroendocrine tumor liver metastases: long-term outcomes and prognostic factors from a large prospective database. *Ann Surg Oncol*. 2017;24(8):2319.
18. Sidéris L, Pierre D, Rinke A. Antitumor effects of somatostatin analogs in neuroendocrine tumors. *Oncologist*. 2012;17(6):747–755.
19. Strosberg J, El-Haddad G, Wolin E, et al. Phase 3 trial of (177) lu-dotatate for midgut neuroendocrine tumors. *N Engl J Med*. 2017;376(2):125.
20. Yao JC, Fazio N, Singh S, Buzzoni R, et al. Everolimus for the treatment of advanced, non-functional neuroendocrine tumours of the lung or gastrointestinal tract (RADIANT-4): a randomised, placebo-controlled, phase 3 study. *Lancet*. 2016;387(10022):968.
21. Abrahams NA, Halverson A, Fazio VW, et al. Adenocarcinoma of the small bowel: a study of 37 cases with emphasis on histologic prognostic factors. *Dis Colon Rectum*. 2002;45:1496–1502.
22. Weiss NS, Yang CP. Incidence of histologic types of cancer of the small intestine. *J Natl Cancer Inst*. 1987;78:653–656.
23. Agrawal S, McCarron EC, Gibbs JF, et al. Surgical management and outcome in primary adenocarcinoma of the small bowel. *Ann Surg Oncol*. 2007;14:2263–2269.
24. Schrock AB, Devoe CE, McWilliams R, et al. Genomic profiling of small-bowel adenocarcinoma. *JAMA Oncol*. 2017;3(11):1546–1553.
25. Hara AK, Leighton JA, Sharma VK, et al. Imaging of small bowel disease: comparison of capsule endoscopy, standard endoscopy, barium examination, and CT. *Radiographics*. 2005;25:697–711.
26. Pilleul F, Penigaud M, Milot L. Possible small bowel neoplasms: contrast-enhanced and water-enhanced multidetector CT enteroclysis. *Radiology*. 2006;241(3):796–801.
27. Lappas J, Heitkamp DE, Maglinte DD. Current status of CT enteroclysis. *Crit Rev Comput Tomogr*. 2003;44:145–175.
28. Van Weyenberg SJ, Meijerink MR, Jacobs MA, et al. MR enteroclysis in the diagnosis of small-bowel neoplasms. *Radiology*. 2010;254(3):765.
29. Pappalardo G, Gianfranco G, Nunziale A, et al. Impact of magnetic resonance in the preoperative staging and the surgical planning for treating small bowel neoplasms. *Surg Today*. 2013;43(6):613–619. Jun.
30. Meijer LL, Alberga A, de Bakker JK, et al. Outcomes and treatment options for duodenal adenocarcinoma: a systematic review and meta-analysis. *Ann Surg Oncol*. 2018;25(9):2681–2692.

31. Ecker BL, McMillan MT, Datta J, et al. Lymph node evaluation and survival after curative-intent resection of duodenal adenocarcinoma: A matched cohort study. *Eur J Cancer*. 2016;69:135–141.
32. Dabaja BS, Suki D, Pro B, et al. Adenocarcinoma of the small bowel: presentation, prognostic factors, and outcome of 217 patients. *Cancer*. 2004;101:518–526.
33. Locher C, Malka D, Boige V, et al. Combination chemotherapy in advanced small bowel adenocarcinoma. *Oncology*. 2005;69:290–294.
34. Young JI, Mongoue-Tchokote S, Wieghard N, et al. Treatment and survival of small-bowel adenocarcinoma in the united states: a comparison with colon cancer. *Dis Colon Rectum*. 2016;59(4):306–315.
35. Koch P, del Valle F, Berdel WE, et al. Primary gastrointestinal non-Hodgkin's lymphoma: I. Anatomic and histologic distribution, clinical features, and survival data of 371 patients registered in the German Multicenter Study GIT NHL 01/92. *J Clin Oncol*. 2001;19:3861–3873.
36. Horton KM, Fishman EK. Multidetector-row computed tomography and 3-dimensional computed tomography imaging of small bowel neoplasms: current concept in diagnosis. *J Comput Assist Tomogr*. 2004;28:106–116.
37. Cheson BD, Fisher R, Barrington SF, et al. Recommendations for initial evaluation, staging, and response assessment of Hodgkin and non-Hodgkin lymphoma: the Lugano classification. *J Clin Oncol*. 2014;32(27):3059–3068.
38. Barrington SF, Mikhaeel NG, Kostakoglu L, et al. Role of imaging in the staging and response assessment of lymphoma: Consensus of the International Conference on Malignant Lymphomas Imaging Working Group. *J Clin Oncol*. 2014;32(27):3048–3058.
39. Van Heertum RL, Scarimbolo R, Wolodzko JG, et al. Lugano 2014 criteria for assessing FDG-PET/CT in lymphoma: an operational approach for clinical trials. *Drug Des Devel Ther*. 2017;11: 1719–1728.
40. Zinzani PL, Stefoni V, Tani M, et al. Role of [18F]fluorodeoxyglucose positron emission tomography scan in the follow-up of lymphoma. 2009;27(11):1781-1787.
41. Tran T, Davila JA, El-Serag HB. The epidemiology of malignant gastrointestinal stromal tumors: an analysis of 1,458 cases from 1992 to 2000. *Am J Gastroenterol*. 2005;100:62–68.
42. Miettinen M, Fetsch J, Sobin LH, et al. Gastrointestinal stromal tumors in patients with neurofibromatosis 1: a clinicopathologic and molecular genetic study of 45 cases. *Am J Surg Pathol*. 2006;30(1):90.
43. Emile JF, Theou N, Tabone S, et al. Clinicopathologic, phenotypic, and genotypic characteristics of gastrointestinal mesenchymal tumors. *Clin Gastroenterol Hepatol*. 2004;2(7):597.
44. Miettinen M, Kopczynski J, Makhlouf HR, et al. Gastrointestinal stromal tumors, intramural leiomyomas, and leiomyosarcomas in the duodenum: a clinicopathologic, immunohistochemical, and molecular genetic study of 167 cases. *J Surg Pathol*. 2003;27:625–641.
45. Amin MB, Edge S, Greene F, et al. eds. *AJCC Cancer Staging Manual. 8th ed.*: Springer International Publishing: American Joint Commission on Cancer; 2017.
46. Horton KM, Juluru K, Montgomery E, et al. Computed tomography imaging of gastrointestinal stromal tumors with pathology correlation. *J Comput Assist Tomogr*. 2004;28:811–817.
47. Blanke CD, Rankin C, Demetri GD, et al. Phase III randomized, intergroup trial assessing imatinib mesylate at two dose levels in patients with unresectable or metastatic gastrointestinal stromal tumors expressing the kit receptor tyrosine kinase: S0033. *J Clin Oncol*. 2008;26:626–632.
48. Heinrich MC, Rankin C, Blanke CD, et al. Correlation of long-term results of imatinib in advanced gastrointestinal stromal tumors with next-generation sequencing results: Analysis of Phase 3 SWOG Intergroup Trial S0033. *JAMA Oncol*. 2017;3(7):944.
49. Serrano C, Marino-Enriquez A, Tao DL, et al. Complementary activity of tyrosine kinase inhibitors against secondary kit mutations in imatinib-resistant gastrointestinal stromal tumours. *Br J Cancer*. 2019;120(6):612.
50. Singh AS, Chmielowski B, Hecht R, et al. A randomized phase 2 study of nivolumab monotherapy versus nivolumab combined with ipilimumab in patients with metastatic or unresectable gastrointestinal stromal tumor (GIST). *J Clin Oncol*. 2018;36(4):55.
51. Choi H, Chamsangavej C, Faria SC, et al. Correlation of computed tomography and positron emission tomography in patients with metastatic gastrointestinal stromal tumor treated at a single institution with imatinib mesylate: proposal of new computed tomography response criteria. *J Clin Oncol*. 2007;25:1753–1759.
52. Choi H, Chamsangavej C, de Castro Faria S, et al. CT evaluation of the response of gastrointestinal stromal tumors after imatinib mesylate treatment: a quantitative analysis correlated with FDG PET findings. *AJR Am J Roentgenol*. 2004;182:1619–1628.
53. Gayed I, Vu T, Iyer R, et al. The role of 18F-FDG PET in staging and early prediction of response to therapy of recurrent gastrointestinal stromal tumors. *J Nucl Med*. 2004;45:17–21.
54. Abbeele DVdA. The lessons of GIST-PET and PET/CT: a new paradigm for imaging. *Oncologist*. 2008;13(Suppl 2):8.
55. Farmer RG, Hawk WA. Metastatic tumors of the small bowel. *Gastroeneterology*. 1964;47:496–504.
56. Schuchter LM, Green R, Fraker D. Primary and metastatic diseases in malignant melanoma of the gastrointestinal tract. *Curr Opin Oncol*. 2000;12:181–185.
57. Bender GN, Maglinte DD, McLamey JH, et al. Malignant melanoma: patterns of metastasis to the small bowel, reliability of imaging studies, and clinical relevance. *Am J Gastroenterol*. 2001;96:2392–2400.
58. Swetter SM, Carroll LA, Johnson DL, et al. Positron emission tomography is superior to computed tomography for metastatic detection in melanoma patients. *Ann Surg Oncol*. 2002;9:646–653.

CHAPTER 18

Colorectal Cancer

Cher Heng Tan M.D.; Van K. Morris M.D.; Prajnan Das M.D.; Miguel Rodriguez-Bigas M.D.; and Revathy B. Iyer M.D.

INTRODUCTION

Colorectal cancer (CRC) is one of the most common adult cancers.[1] Imaging plays an important role in the management of CRC, including screening, staging, and surveillance. Understanding the anatomy of the colon and rectum is important when interpreting radiologic examinations pertaining to CRC. This especially applies when evaluating for the pattern and extent of disease spread.

Computed tomographic colonography (CTC) is one of the recommended imaging screening tests for CRC.[2] Staging involves accurate depiction of disease based on the tumor-node-metastasis (TNM) classification system. Endoscopic ultrasound (EUS) can play a role in the staging of rectal cancer.[3] Computed tomography (CT) remains the mainstay for CRC imaging owing to its widespread availability. Its value lies more in the assessment of nodal and distant disease rather than of the primary tumor itself. Magnetic resonance imaging (MRI), with its superior soft tissue resolution capability, is the preferred modality for staging primary rectal cancer, and it also has a role in the assessment of distant metastatic disease in the liver.[4] Positron emission tomography (PET)/CT provides both functional and anatomic information. It allows for whole-body assessment in a single examination, making it valuable for detection of unsuspected sites of disease.

Surveillance by imaging is usually carried out in tandem with serum carcinoembryonic antigen (CEA) assays. In the appropriate setting, surgical resection of locally recurrent disease in the pelvis and metastatic disease in the liver and lungs has been shown to improve survival.[5,6] Therefore, when CEA levels show a rise during postoperative surveillance, it is important to identify the presence and location of recurrent and distant disease to allow for prompt treatment. PET/CT has emerged as an indispensable modality in this regard, and its use has increased tremendously since its introduction.

In this chapter, we briefly discuss the relevant anatomy, staging, and treatment options in CRC and how imaging may play a role in its current management.

EPIDEMIOLOGY AND RISK FACTORS

In the United States, CRC is the fourth most commonly diagnosed malignancy and the second leading cause of mortality from cancer, with an estimated 50,000 deaths annually.[1] The majority of CRC patients are older than age 50 years, with slight male predominance.[1] The incidence and mortality rates are variable across racial groups, with the highest rates of disease and mortality occurring in African Americans and Native Americans.[1] Recent declines in CRC incidence and mortality are attributable to reduced risk factor exposure, early detection and prevention through colonoscopy and polypectomy, and improved medical and surgical treatment.[7,8]

Most CRCs develop from adenomatous polyps through a process known as the adenoma-carcinoma sequence. Malignant potential of a polyp increases with size. Polyps smaller than 0.5 cm have virtually no risk, whereas those greater than 2 cm have a 40% risk for invasive carcinoma.[9] Although previously thought to be benign, the serrated form of hyperplastic colonic polyps have been shown to be associated with malignant transformation.[10]

The most common form of hereditary CRC is hereditary nonpolyposis CRC (Lynch syndrome), accounting for approximately 3% of CRCs.[11] Others include familial adenomatous polyposis, juvenile polyposis, and Peutz–Jeghers. Mutations in *P53*, *APC*, and *KRAS* have been linked to CRC.[12] With inflammatory bowel disease (ulcerative colitis or Crohn disease), the risk of CRC increases with duration and anatomic extent of colitis, degree of inflammation, and concomitant family history of CRC.[13] Dietary and lifestyle factors that have been implicated as risk factors include obesity, hyperglycemia, consumption of red and processed meat and animal fat, and high alcohol intake.[14,15]

Key Points Epidemiology and Risk Factors

- Most colorectal cancers develop from adenomatous polyps through a process known as the adenoma-carcinoma sequence.
- Mutations in *P53*, *APC*, and *KRAS* have been linked to colorectal cancer[12].

ANATOMY AND PATHOLOGY

The large intestine is about 1.5 m long, being one-fifth of the whole extent of the intestinal canal. The large intestine is divided into the cecum, colon, rectum, and anal canal. It is generally accepted that tumors with epicenters located more than 2 cm proximal to the dentate line are rectal, whereas those that are distal to this are considered anal.[16] This distinction is important for staging. Based on the American Joint Committee on Cancer (AJCC) staging system, the T stage of CRC is determined by degree of involvement of the bowel wall, whereas that of the anus is determined by the size of the primary tumor. Also, the N stage of CRC is defined by the number of involved nodes, as opposed to the location of nodes in anal cancer.

The mucous membrane of the colon and rectum is formed by columnar epithelium, which explains the predominance of adenocarcinoma. The muscular layer of the colon consists of an external longitudinal and an internal circular layer of nonstriated muscular fibers. The longitudinal fibers form the tenia coli, which are lost in the rectum. The circular fibers are thin in the cecum and colon and become thick in the rectum and anal canal.

The serous layer of the colon is derived from the peritoneum. The mid and distal rectum have no serosal layer. The ascending colon, descending colon, and inferior rectum are retroperitoneal, whereas the rest of the colon, including the cecum, transverse colon, sigmoid colon, and superior rectum, are intraperitoneal.

The arteries supplying the colon are derived from the superior and inferior mesenteric arteries, namely the ileocolic and right colic (cecum and ascending colon), middle colic (transverse colon), left colic (descending colon), and sigmoid arteries (sigmoid colon).

The superior rectum is supplied by the superior hemorrhoidal (branch of inferior mesenteric), the middle rectum by the middle hemorrhoidal (branch of hypogastric), and the inferior rectum by the inferior hemorrhoidal (branch of internal pudendal) arteries. The veins of the colon and rectum parallel the arteries. The veins of the rectum form the hemorrhoidal plexus and, therefore, provide a communication between the systemic and the portal circulations. The nerves are derived from the sympathetic plexuses around the branches of the superior and inferior mesenteric arteries.

The lymphatics of the colon and rectum follow their vascular supply (see "Patterns of Tumor Spread"). The cecum and appendix (ileocolic) and ascending and transverse colon (right colic) eventually drain to the superior mesenteric nodes. The descending (left colic), sigmoid colon (sigmoid), and superior rectum eventually drain to the inferior mesenteric nodes. The middle and inferior rectum drain to the iliac nodes. The lymphatics from the anal verge pass into the superficial inguinal glands.

Tumor size has not been shown to carry prognostic significance in CRC.[17,18] Other than the prognostic indicators defined by the AJCC staging system (which are discussed in "Staging"), histologic subtype, tumor grade, lymphovascular involvement, tumor border invasion, and host lymphoid response to tumor also affect prognosis.

The World Health Organization classifies the CRCs into the following: adenocarcinoma, medullary, mucinous (colloid) adenocarcinoma (>50% mucinous), signet-ring cell carcinoma (>50% signet-ring cells), squamous cell (epidermoid) carcinoma, adenosquamous carcinoma, small-cell (oat-cell) carcinoma, undifferentiated carcinoma, and others (e.g., papillary carcinoma). Adenocarcinomas make up more than 95% of colorectal primaries. Of the remaining primaries, neuroendocrine (1.8%), lymphoma (0.6%), squamous cell carcinoma (0.3%), and sarcoma (<0.1%) are considered rare. Among the histologic subtypes of CRC, carcinoid and neuroendocrine carcinoma show the best and the worst relative 5-year survival rates, respectively. Also, both malignant lymphoma and squamous cell carcinoma patients have significantly worse overall 5-year and early-stage (localized and regional) survival rates than adenocarcinoma patients.[19] The signet-ring cell type of adenocarcinoma and small-cell (oat-cell) carcinoma are the only histologic types of colonic carcinoma that consistently have been found to have a stage-independent adverse effect on prognosis. The prognostic significance of mucinous carcinoma remains controversial. Conversely, medullary carcinoma is prognostically favorable.[20]

In terms of tumor grade, a two-tier system of low- (well- and moderately differentiated) and high- (poorly and undifferentiated) grade tumors has been proposed to reduce interobserver variability.[17] Multivariate analysis has also shown the presence of lymphovascular invasion to be an adverse prognostic indicator.[17,18,20] The configuration of the tumor at the advancing edge (irregular and infiltrating pattern) has been shown to be an independent adverse prognostic factor as well. In contrast, the presence of lymphocytic infiltration of tumor or peritumoral tissue at pathology implies a host immunologic response to the tumor and, therefore, is a favorable prognostic factor. Use of molecular markers as prognostic indicators is still the subject of research. Microsatellite instability or defective mismatch repair, as well as *BRAF* mutations, are prognostic factors in CRC.[21] With advances in genomics, CRCs have been classified into four consensus molecular subtypes (CMSs): CMS1 microsatellite instability immune, hypermutated microsatellite unstable, strong immune activation; CMS2 (canonical, epithelial, chromosomal unstable, marked WNT and MYC signaling activation); CMS3 (metabolic), epithelial, evident metabolic dysregulation; and CMS4 (mesenchymal), prominent transforming growth factor β activation, stromal invasion, and angiogenesis.[22] The CMS grouping correlates with prognosis.[22]

Key Points Anatomy

- The lymphatics of the colon and rectum follow their vascular supply.
- Tumor size is not a significant prognosticator.
- Signet-ring cell type and small-cell carcinoma have consistently poorer stage-independent prognoses.
- Adenocarcinoma accounts for more than 95% of colorectal primaries.
- The consensus molecular subtype classification system for colorectal cancer correlates molecular pathways and tumor biology.

PATTERNS OF TUMOR SPREAD

Local Spread

Locally, tumor can spread either intramurally or transmurally. Intramural spread of tumor can occur longitudinally along the bowel wall or superficially toward the serosa. Tumor preferentially grows circumferentially, resulting in luminal narrowing. Longitudinal spread is not common and is generally approximately 2 cm from the primary site of disease. This supports the practice of a 5-cm surgical margin.[23] Transmural spread is present in more advanced tumors. The depth of invasion within the bowel wall determines prognosis, as detailed in standard staging classification systems (see "Staging"). The ascending colon, descending colon, and rectum, which are primarily retroperitoneal in location, can directly invade the adjacent retroperitoneal organs such as the ureters, duodenum, and pancreas via this mode of spread. Locally advanced rectal cancer often involves the pelvic viscera, including the bladder base, prostate gland, uterus, and vagina.[24] These may present with rectovaginal or rectovesical fistulas. Invasion of adjacent organs depends upon the site of primary tumor and mandates *en bloc* resection to achieve curative surgery.[25]

Disease can also spread along the neurovascular structures. Extramural venous invasion is associated with increased metastatic burden and poorer overall prognosis. This has been shown in multiple studies (see "Imaging"). Perineural spread in rectal cancer can result in tumor deposits along the perineural spaces more than 10 cm from the primary tumor. This has been reported in as many as 35% of cases.[26]

Nodal

Distant spread of disease most commonly occurs in the liver, followed by the lymph nodes.[27] The nodal pathways of spread for CRC are illustrated in Fig. 18.1.[28] Lymph node spread from carcinomas of the right colon follow along the marginal vessels of the cecum and ascending colon and then along the ileocolic vessels to the root of the superior mesenteric artery. Tumors of the proximal transverse colon tend to spread along the marginal vessels on the mesocolic side of the colon. These marginal vessels in turn drain to the right or middle colic vessels and to the root of the mesocolon, anterior to the head of the pancreas. Lymphatics from the distal transverse colon and splenic flexure follow the left middle colic vessels to the inferior mesenteric vein just caudal to the body and tail of the pancreas. Cancers of the descending colon and sigmoid colon will spread to nodes along the left ascending colic and sigmoidal vessels that can then be followed to the origin of the inferior mesenteric artery.[29] Proximal rectal tumors spread cranially via the superior hemorrhoidal nodes, antegrade to the inferior mesenteric lymph nodes. The more distal rectal tumors spread laterally along the internal iliac lymph nodes, antegrade to the common iliac and retroperitoneal chains. Those located at the rectosigmoid junction tend to spread to the perirectal lymph nodes rather than along the sigmoid mesenteric chain.[30]

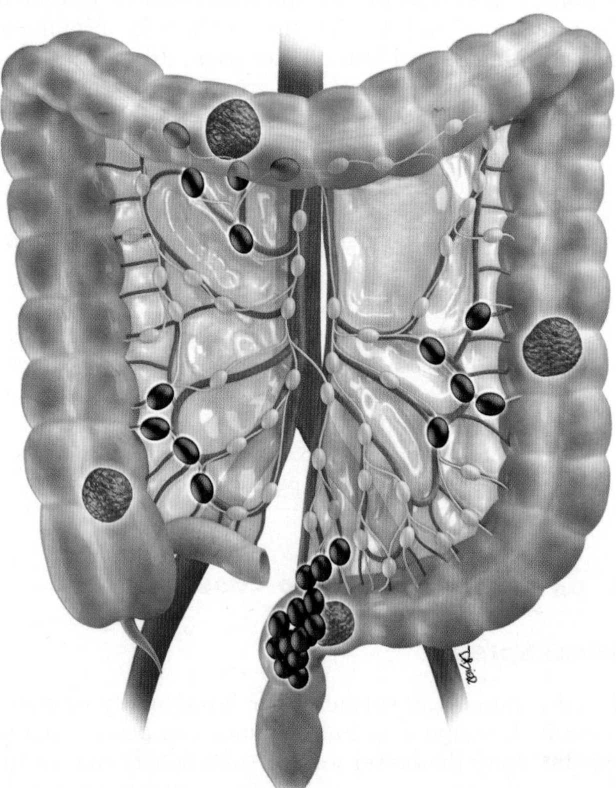

FIGURE 18.1. Pathways of nodal spread for cancers arising from different parts of the colon and rectum.

Peritoneal

Peritoneal spread of disease is seen in up to 43% of patients.[24] Tumor cells can spread throughout the peritoneal cavity and implant on the omentum and peritoneal surfaces. This pattern of spread is seen more commonly in the intraperitoneal portions of the colon, including the cecum and transverse and sigmoid colon.[24] The ovaries are a common site of involvement by peritoneal dissemination. In animal models, injection of neoplastic cells into the mesenteric border tends to give rise to nodal metastases, whereas injection into the antimesenteric border gives rise to peritoneal metastases, alluding to the role of tumor location to the method of dissemination.[31] The presence of peritoneal involvement predicts a higher rate of local recurrence and is strongly associated with a mucinous tumor phenotype (signet-ring feature).[32]

Hematogenous

Some 10% to 25% of patients harbor detectable metastases at the time of initial diagnosis.[33] Hematogeneous spread of colonic and upper rectal tumors initially occurs via the portal circulation. The liver is often the first site of metastatic disease and may be the only site of spread in as many as 30% to 40% of patients with advanced disease.[34] In addition, 20% to 25% of patients will have clinically detectable liver metastases at the time of the initial diagnosis, and a further 40% to 50% of patients will eventually develop liver metastases after resection of the primary. Approximately 20% to 30% of patients with metastatic CRC have disease that is confined to the liver and is potentially resectable.[35] In low rectal tumors, venous drainage occurs through the systemic circulation via the iliac vessels. This may explain the higher propensity of pulmonary metastases in low rectal cancers compared with tumors from the more proximal parts of the colon and rectum.[24] In the appropriate clinical setting, aggressive surgical resection of distant metastases (including the liver and lung, and on occasion at isolated sites such as the adrenal gland, and spleen) has been shown to confer survival benefit.[36] Therefore, early detection of metastatic disease by imaging is important.

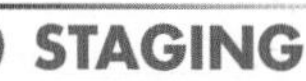

Key Points Tumor Spread

- Colorectal cancers (CRCs) can spread locally or through lymphatic, peritoneal, and hematogenous routes.
- Nodal disease has predictable spread.
- Peritoneal disease occurs in up to 43% in patients and is a predictor of local recurrence and mucinous histology. There is 10% to 25% hematogenous spread at diagnosis.
- CRCs can spread locally or through lymphatic, peritoneal, and hematogenous routes.
- Resection of distant metastases can be curative in some patients.

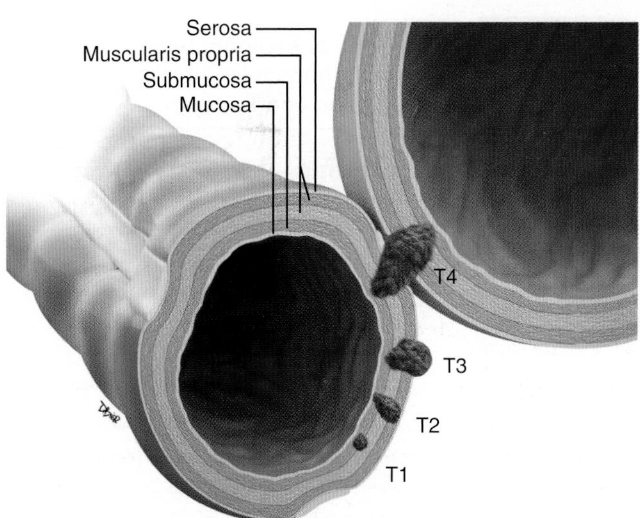

Figure 18.2. T staging of primary carcinomas of the colon and rectum.

STAGING

The TNM staging system of the AJCC and the International Union Against Cancer is currently the standard for CRC staging recommended by the National Cancer Institute and tumor registries worldwide.[37,38]

Clinical classification (cTNM) is based on clinical and radiologic information. Pathologic classification (pTNM) is based on the surgical specimen. cTNM, once assigned, is not changed on the basis of subsequent information, even when pTNM becomes available and may be considered more accurate.[37] In the case of recurrent cancers, the TNM classification should be prefixed by r (rTNM). The posttreatment status of the tumor (yTNM) carries prognostic importance as well. A patient with recurrent cancer who has received previous chemotherapy and/or radiation should be staged with the prefix ry (rycTNM or rypTNM). For multiple synchronous tumors, the lesion with the highest T category determines the stage.

Because TNM staging is applicable only to primary carcinomas of the colon and rectum, other tumors such as colorectal lymphomas, carcinoid tumors, and metastases are excluded.[39] The staging classification is summarized in Fig. 18.2.

T Stage

Tis (carcinoma *in situ*) refers to disease that is superficial to the muscularis mucosa. Penetration of the muscularis mucosa and invasion of the submucosa is classified as T1. CRC that has penetrated into, but not completely through, the muscularis propria is classified as T2.

T3 disease includes all transmurally invasive tumors confined to the perimuscular soft tissue (i.e., that have neither violated the serosal surface nor infiltrated an adjacent structure).[40] Extramural tumor nodules discontinuous from the primary tumor mass that are irregular in shape are also included.[40] Nodules with smooth contours are regarded as lymph nodes.

Direct invasion of the visceral peritoneum or invasion/attachment to adjacent organs or structures or other segments of the colorectum by way of the serosa or mesocolon (e.g., invasion of the sigmoid colon by carcinoma of the cecum) is classified as T4 disease. Intramural (longitudinal) extension of tumor from one subsite (segment) of the large intestine into an adjacent subsite (either the terminal ileum or the anal canal) does not affect the T classification.[40] Invasion of the visceral peritoneum or perforation is classified as T4a disease, whereas tumor invasion to other organs or structures is considered T4b.

N Stage

The definition of regional nodes is covered in Table 18.1. Because it has been shown that many nodal metastases in CRC are found in small lymph nodes (<5 mm in diameter), a minimum of 12 lymph nodes is considered adequate for curative surgical resection.[17,41,42] Regional nodal involvement is classified as N disease (see Table 18.1), whereas all other nodal metastases are classified as M1. As mentioned, extramural tumor nodules with smooth contours are regarded as replaced regional lymph nodes.[37,38,40] The number of pericolonic tumor deposits has been shown to correlate inversely with disease-free survival.[43]

In rare cases, the regional nodes of the primary tumor site are free of malignancy, but the nodes in the drainage area of an organ directly invaded by the primary tumor contain metastases. When this occurs, the lymph nodes of the invaded site are considered as those of the primary site and are also classified under the N category.[40]

Isolated tumor cells (ITCs) are defined as tumor cells measuring 0.2 mm or less. According to current recommendations, ITCs are classified as N0 or M0, as appropriate.[37,40,44] The biologic significance of ITCs is unknown.[18] In contrast, metastatic tumors that measure greater than 0.2 mm but less than 2.0 mm are defined as micrometastases and classified as N1 or M1.

TABLE 18.1 Definitions of Regional Lymph Node Groups in Anatomic Subsites of the Colon and Rectum

COLON AND RECTUM SUBSITE	DEFINITION
Cecum	Anterior cecal, posterior cecal, ileocolic, right colic
Ascending colon	Ileocolic, right colic, middle colic
Hepatic flexure	Middle colic, right colic
Transverse colon	Middle colic
Splenic flexure	Middle colic, left colic, inferior mesenteric
Descending colon	Left colic, inferior mesenteric, sigmoid
Sigmoid colon	Inferior mesenteric, superior rectal sigmoidal, sigmoid mesenteric[a]
Rectosigmoid colon	Perirectal,[b] left colic, sigmoid mesenteric, sigmoidal, inferior mesenteric, superior rectal, middle rectal
Rectum	Perirectal,[b] sigmoid mesenteric, inferior mesenteric, lateral sacral, presacral, internal iliac, sacral promontory, superior rectal, middle rectal, inferior rectal

[a]Lymph nodes along the sigmoid arteries are considered pericolic nodes, and their involvement is classified as pN1 or pN2 according to the number involved.
[b]Perirectal lymph nodes include the mesorectal (paraproctal), lateral sacral, presacral, sacral promontory (Gerota), middle rectal (hemorrhoidal), and inferior rectal (hemorrhoidal) nodes. Metastasis in the external iliac or common iliac nodes is classified as pM1.
(Modified from Compton CC, Greene FL. The staging of colorectal cancer: 2004 and beyond. *CA Cancer J Clin.* 2004;54:295-308.)

M Stage

Positive peritoneal fluid cytology and tumor present (only) in lymphatic vessels of a distant site are also considered pM1 disease. Excluded from the pM1 designation are tumor foci in the mucosa or submucosa of adjacent bowel (also known as satellite lesions or skip metastasis); these must be distinguished from synchronous primary tumors.

Surgical Resection Margin

The pertinent margins of a CRC resection specimen include the proximal and distal transverse margins, the mesenteric margin, and, in rectal tumors, the circumferential margin. When the distance between the tumor and the nearest transverse margin is 5 cm or more, anastomotic recurrences are very rare.[45] For rectal tumors in which sphincter preservation is an important consideration, a mucosal margin of 2 cm is accepted as adequate, especially for T1 and T2 tumors. Ideally, the mesorectum should be resected up to 4 to 5 cm below the level of the tumor, as lymphatic spread can occur at this level; this approach is referred to as tumor-specific mesorectal excision.

The circumferential resection margin (CRM) is defined by the distance between the retroperitoneal or the peritoneal adventitial soft tissue margin closest to the furthest advancing edge of the tumor. This applies to all segments of the large intestine that are either incompletely encased (ascending colon, descending colon, upper rectum) or not encased (lower rectum) by peritoneum. Multivariate analyses have suggested that tumor involvement of the CRM is the most critical factor in predicting local recurrence in rectal cancer.[46,47] Emerging data on CRM involvement in the colon suggest likewise.[46]

Based on published data from clinical trials, the risk of local recurrence is strongly increased if the CRM is less than 1 mm.[47] Thus, the current recommendation is for a clearance of 2 mm or less to be considered a positive CRM.[48] Remnant disease after primary surgical resection is categorized by a separate system (R classification), where RX means presence of residual tumor cannot be assessed; R0 indicates no residual tumor; R1 is microscopic residual tumor; and R2 is macroscopic residual tumor. This classification carries stage-independent prognostic significance.

Lymphovascular Invasion

Venous invasion by tumor has been demonstrated repeatedly to be a stage-independent adverse prognostic factor, by both multivariate and univariate analyses.[49–52] Mixed results have also been reported for lymphatic invasion, although the general consensus is that lymphovascular invasion is a negative prognostic factor.[52–54] The presence of tumor cells within the lymphatics or veins does not affect the T stage. Intravascular spread via lymphatic or venous vessels is classified as L1 and V1, respectively. Tumor within the lymphatics of a distant organ is classified as M1 disease.

KEY POINTS Staging

- The circumferential resection margin is defined by the distance between the retroperitoneal or the peritoneal adventitial soft tissue margin closest to the furthest advancing edge of the tumor.
- Serosal penetration (T4b) is associated with short survival times.
- Metastases are not uncommon, even in small lymph nodes; at least 12 lymph nodes should be removed during curative surgical resection for colorectal cancer. Fewer lymph nodes may be cleared in rectal surgery in patients treated with neoadjuvant chemoradiation.

IMAGING

Screening

Computed Tomography Colonography

CTC (also known as virtual colonoscopy [VC]) allows minimally invasive imaging examination of the entire colon and rectum. Multidetector CT permits high-resolution image acquisition of the entire large intestine in a single breathhold. Integrated three-dimensional (3D) and two-dimensional (2D) analysis allows for ease of polyp detection, characterization of lesion, and location. Unlike colonoscopy, extracolonic structures can also be evaluated. Adequate bowel preparation and gaseous distention of the colon are essential. Fecal tagging may reduce need for vigorous bowel preparation.

The American College of Radiology Imaging Network National CT Colonography Trial, which studied 2500 patients across 15 institutions in the United States, has shown comparable accuracy between CTC and standard colonoscopy.[55] Using fecal tagging and primary 3D polyp detection in asymptomatic adults, Pickhardt and coworkers[56] reported a sensitivity of 89% for adenomas 6 mm or larger. For invasive CRC, the pooled CTC sensitivity was higher, at 96%. As with other screening techniques, CTC accuracy improves with lesion size. Other than detection, consistent polyp size measurement is important because it will influence referrals for polypectomy. Use of 3D reconstructed images or 2D assessment in the lung window is recommended for accurate polyp size measurement.[57] All patients with polyps 6 mm or larger should be referred for colonoscopy. The management of patients with fewer polyps (<3) in which the largest is 6 to 9 mm or smaller remains controversial.[58,59] CTC is an acceptable screening tool for CRC (see Box 18.1). Use of CTC for screening has been shown to be a cost-effective strategy, and possibly more so than optical colonoscopy.[60] The main drawback of CTC is radiation exposure. One CTC study in a 50-year-old patient resulted in an estimated organ dose to the colon of 7 to 13 mSv, which adds 0.044% to the lifetime risk of colon cancer.[61] More efficient low-dose protocols have demonstrated decreased estimated organ dose ranges of 1 to less than 5 mSv.[62] The risk for colonic perforation during screening is extremely low, at 0.005% for asymptomatic patients and higher for symptomatic patients (0.03%–0.06%), and may be safer with carbon dioxide delivery than with room air.[63,64]

Key Points Imaging

- Computed tomographic colonography, or virtual colonoscopy (VC), allows minimally invasive imaging examination of the entire colon and rectum.
- The drawback of VC is the cumulative radiation dose.
- Radiation doses with VC are decreasing using some newer protocols.

Box 18.1 Testing Options for the Early Detection of Colorectal Cancer and Adenomatous Polyps for Asymptomatic Adults Aged 50 Years and Older

Tests that Detect Adenomatous Polyps and Cancer

Flexible sigmoidoscopy every 5 years **or** colonoscopy every 10 years **or** computed tomographic colonography every 5 years

Tests that Primarily Detect Cancer

Annual guaiac-based fecal occult blood test with high test sensitivity for cancer **or** Annual fecal immunochemical test with high test sensitivity for cancer **or** Stool DNA test with high sensitivity for cancer, every 3 years

(Modified from Wolf AMD, Fontham ETH, Church TR, et al. Colorectal cancer screening for average-risk adults: 2018 guideline update from the American Cancer Society. *CA Cancer J Clin.* 2018;68(4):250–281.)

Cancer Staging

Patients with CRC should be clinically staged before surgery. Current imaging guidelines for invasive colon cancer include chest, abdomen, and pelvic CT scans to evaluate local extent of the tumor, potential lymphadenopathy, and distant disease. In patients with rectal cancer, in addition to CT scans, high resolution MRI is used as the preferred modality for staging the primary tumor, although at times EUS is used.

Endoscopic Ultrasound

The role of Endoscopic Ultrasound (EUS) is largely confined to local staging for rectal cancer because more proximal tumors are difficult to assess.

EUS provides accurate depiction of the rectal wall layers. Most practices use a 7.5- or 10-MHz rigid transducer with a saline-filled balloon tip, allowing a 360-degree field of view. Tumor most commonly appears as a hypoechoic mass disrupting the rectal wall layers.[3] Early rectal cancer is demonstrated by tumor ingrowth into the superficial layers of the rectal wall, with staging accuracy ranging from 69% to 97%.[65,66] A metaanalysis by Bipat and colleagues[67] comparing CT, EUS, and MRI showed that endorectal ultrasound may be the imaging modality of choice for rectal cancer.

Owing to the similar appearances between peritumoral inflammatory changes and extramural extension, overstaging T2 tumors as T3 tumors is common.[68] Perirectal nodal involvement is also limited. This is related to its limited acoustic window, depth of penetration, and small field of view, which also limits evaluation of the distance between the tumor and the mesorectal fascia. Operator dependence, need for bowel preparation, and intraprocedural pain because of stenotic lesions are other limitations.

Patients with early tumors considered for local excision may benefit from additional referral for endorectal ultrasound, given its superior diagnostic performance for differentiating T1 from T2 tumors.[67]

Computed Tomography

Clinical use of CT for rectal cancer staging is limited, owing to the lack of contrast resolution to discriminate between tumor and normal visceral soft tissue, with an accuracy of approximately 70%.[69] In a study by O'Neil and associates,[70] CT consistently overestimated tumor volume and underestimated distance from the anal verge compared with MRI. It is also poor for assessment of levator ani invasion in low rectal lesions.[71] For the more proximal colon, however, CT may be the modality of choice, given its high temporal resolution.

In general, CT is more useful for nodal and metastasis staging than it is for local tumor staging. However, the optimal strategy for the elective distant staging of CRC is controversial. For instance, in patients with CRC, chest CT often detects indeterminate lung lesions, of which only a small proportion develops into definite metastases.[72] Similarly, in rectal cancer, if pelvic MRI has already been performed, CT including the pelvis does not provide additional value.[73] Therefore, further studies are required to define optimal preoperative imaging.

Novel techniques such as perfusion CT and combined perfusion CT–PET/CT show promise but require further validation.[74-76] In the posttreatment phase of CRC, in patients who demonstrate a rise in CEA, PET/CT carries high sensitivity and specificity rates (94.1% and 77.2%, respectively) in detecting tumor recurrence.[77]

Magnetic Resonance Imaging

The advent of high-resolution phased array coils in combination with improvements in MRI sequences has led to significant improvements in rectal cancer staging. The Magnetic Resonance Imaging and Rectal Cancer European Equivalence study, which recruited 679 patients, showed that MRI is accurate in preoperative evaluation of rectal cancer.[4] Currently, MRI allows for accurate detection of extramural extension, venous invasion, nodal involvement, and, at times, peritoneal dissemination. High-resolution T2-weighted (T2W) fast spin echo imaging using an external phased array coil is the sequence of choice owing to superior discrimination between hyperintense mesorectal fat, hypointense rectal wall and mesorectal fascia, and intermediate tumor signal.[78] Use of endorectal coil MRI is not recommended.[78] MRI accurately predicts T stage and CRM status. It predicts histopathologic involvement of the CRM to within 0.5 mm.[4] Using 1 mm as a cutoff to determine clear margins from the mesorectal fascia, the authors of one study showed that MRI has a specificity of 92%.[79] It may also demonstrate the presence of extramural venous invasion, an important indicator of poor prognosis. Furthermore, MRI has been shown to be superior to CT in the assessment of pelvic floor muscle, as well as sacral bone, invasion.[80] Diffusion-weighted imaging (DWI) is a useful adjunct to T2W MRI for assessment of response to neoadjuvant chemoradiation. Beyond rectal imaging, DWI may improve liver metastasis detection with greater sensitivity compared with CT.[81]

MRI is limited in nodal evaluation, for which it is no better than CT.[82] Using a short-axis diameter cutoff of 5 mm, the nodal status accuracy rate of MRI lies between 59% and 85%.[83,84] For nodes that are between 5 and 8 mm in size, presence of spiculation, indistinct margins, round configuration, and mixed signal intensity on T2W imaging are suspicious features that can increase specificity of diagnosis.[85] Ultrasmall superparamagnetic iron oxide (USPIO) has not gained acceptance in routine practice. Whole-body MRI is a promising "one-stop" method for examining colon cancer patients for recurrence and metastatic disease but cannot displace the present role of PET/CT, for reasons such as cost and availability.[86]

KEY POINTS Endoscopic Ultrasound, Computed Tomography, and Magnetic Resonance Imaging

- Endoscopic ultrasound provides an accurate depiction of the rectal wall layers. Tumor most commonly appears as a hypoechoic mass disrupting the rectal wall layers.
- Computed tomography is most useful for nodal and metastasis staging.
- Preoperative positron emission tomography/computed tomographic colonography may yield information in synchronous tumor but is not recommended for staging of the primary tumor.
- Radiology report should include location and size of tumor, presence and distribution of nodes, and presence or absence of metastases.
- Magnetic resonance imaging (MRI) accurately predicts T stage and circumferential resection margin status and is regarded as the first-choice technique for both primary staging and restaging of rectal cancer.
- Morphological and signal assessment increases specificity of nodal disease detection by MRI.

Positron Emission Tomography

2-[^{18}F] fluoro-2-deoxy-D-glucose (FDG) is the most widely used substrate for PET imaging. Fusion PET/CT combines the functional evaluation by PET with the anatomic detail provided by CT. Contrast-enhanced PET/CT and PET/CTC show promise for improving accuracy.[87,88]

For local disease, PET/CT can improve preoperative target volume delineation by CT for conformal radiation therapy in rectal cancer.[89] However, by far the greatest value of PET in CRC lies in whole-body lesion detection. It can reveal unsuspected disease and modify the scope of surgery in approximately 10% of patients.[90] In one study, FDG-PET/CT altered treatment plans in 38% of patients, largely through the detection of unsuspected lymphadenopathy.[91] PET/CT also shows high accuracy in detection of liver metastases, with reported accuracy up to 99%, sensitivity up to 100%, and specificity up to 98%. It resulted in a change of management in approximately 30% of cases.[92,93]

Physiologic uptake in the gastrointestinal tract (because of lymphoid, glandular, and muscular tissues), infection, and inflammation can result in false positives. Benign colonic adenomas may also not be distinguished from FDG-avid carcinomas.[94] PET/CT is relatively insensitive to mucinous colorectal tumors, owing to paucicellularity.[95] Urinary excretion of tracer can potentially be confused with tumor spread or recurrence in the retroperitoneum or pelvis. Most current PET scanners have a spatial resolution of 5 mm, which is below that of other imaging modalities. Even with fusion PET/CT, the various layers of the colonic wall are not distinguishable, limiting ability for T staging. Furthermore, small nodal metastases in the vicinity of the primary lesion may be missed.[96] Despite these limitations, PET/CT has become an indispensable imaging tool in CRC management.

KEY POINTS Positron Emission Tomography/Computed Tomography

- The greatest value of positron emission tomography in colorectal cancer lies in whole-body lesion detection.
- Infection and inflammation may result in false positives.
- Urinary excretion can potentially be mistaken for spread in the retroperitoneum.
- Layers of colonic wall are not distinguishable.

THERAPIES AND CLINICAL PERSPECTIVES

Surgery

Surgical technique influences local recurrence and survival in the treatment of CRC; hence, a standardized operative technique is important. Strict adherence to the principles of *en bloc* resection and complete surgical removal of tumor along with the regional lymphatics is the best prevention strategy against local recurrence and affords the best prognosis.[97] Proximal and distal margins of 5 cm are the standard of care for colonic tumors.[98] For rectal tumors, a distal margin of 2 cm is adequate.[99]

The extent of colonic resection and location of the anastomosis are based on the tumor location and corresponding colonic blood supply. Ligation of the vascular pedicles at their origin is important. Cecal and ascending colonic tumors require right hemicolectomy with ligation of the ileocolic and right colic vessels. Hepatic flexure tumors require an extended right hemicolectomy with additional ligation of the middle colic artery. Transverse colonic tumors will require either subtotal colectomy or extended right hemicolectomy with preservation of the left colic vessels.[98,100] Splenic flexure tumors require either subtotal colectomy or extended left hemicolectomy with ligation of the inferior mesenteric vessels. Descending or sigmoid colonic tumors require extended left hemicolectomy with ligation of the inferior mesenteric vessels.

Rectal tumors require either anterior or abdominoperineal resection, depending on the proximity to the sphincter.[101] Sharp dissection along the mesorectal fascia with *en bloc* resection of the tumor and its draining lymph nodes (total mesorectal excision [TME]) is currently the gold-standard technique in rectal surgery.[101] An adequate CRM of more than 2 mm is important.[102] Preservation of anal sphincter, bladder, and sexual function is important but must not compromise adequate resection margins, unless performed for palliation. For those with impaired preoperative anorectal function, radical resection and permanent colostomy may be preferred. Less invasive procedures such as transanal excision for T1 tumors and laparoscopic-assisted TME surgery are feasible in select patients.[103–105] For T3 disease, a negative CRM after TME is associated with a lower risk of local recurrence.[106] The more conservative approaches of transanal excision or observation for patients with a complete biochemical response to neoadjuvant therapy are not favored, owing to the difficulty in precisely determining tumor response to chemoradiation and assessing residual mesorectal lymph node involvement. Currently, there are no data to support the routine use of transanal excision in these patients, and therefore TME remains to be the definitive treatment.

Lymph node status is one of the most important prognostic factors in CRC. Inconsistencies in the number of nodes harvested can affect staging accuracy. Accurate nodal staging allows upstaging of patients and consideration for adjuvant treatment. Therefore, a minimum of 12 lymph nodes is advocated.[107] Interestingly, long-term survival increases along with the number of harvested nodes, independent of the proportion of involved nodes.[108]

Hepatic and pulmonary metastectomy in selected patients improves survival.[109] The presence of extrahepatic disease, such as in the spleen and adrenal glands, is no longer considered a contraindication to hepatic metastastectomy.[36] For liver metastases, patients with unilobar disease, with fewer than four lesions, and requiring limited resection fare better.[110] Portal vein embolization and two-stage resections may be considered in select cases to optimize outcome. Conversely, increased size and number of lesions, margins, extrahepatic disease, poorly differentiated tumor, and high CEA levels negatively affect prognosis.[111] Underlying disease such as decompensated liver cirrhosis would, however, preclude liver resection. Criteria for resection of pulmonary metastases from CRC include fewer than three lesions in either lung, absence of extrapulmonary disease (other than resectable hepatic metastases), and adequate cardiorespiratory reserve. Size of metastases has been shown to correlate inversely with mean survival time.[112]

Radiofrequency ablation (RFA) has been reserved for cases in which complete resection is not possible, either alone or in combination with surgery. However, it does not provide survival comparable with that of resection and provides survival slightly superior to that of nonsurgical treatment.[113]

Role of Radiation Therapy in the Treatment of Colorectal Cancer

Multiple randomized trials have established the role of postoperative radiation therapy for stage II and III rectal cancer.[114–116] A randomized trial from Germany showed that preoperative chemoradiation leads to higher rates of locoregional control and sphincter preservation and lower rates of acute and long-term toxicity compared with postoperative chemoradiation.[117] Preoperative chemoradiation has therefore been widely accepted as a standard of care for stage II and III rectal cancer. Preoperative chemoradiation is typically delivered with a dose of 45 to 54 Gy, delivered in 1.8- to 2-Gy fractions, over 5 to 6 weeks. An alternative to preoperative chemoradiation is preoperative short-course radiotherapy alone, with a dose of 25 Gy, delivered in 5-Gy fractions, in a single week. Recent randomized trials have shown that short-course radiotherapy leads to similar outcomes compared with long-course chemoradiation.[118] Hence, preoperative short-course radiotherapy is also considered a standard of care for rectal cancer. In addition to the role of radiotherapy in the preoperative treatment of rectal cancer, radiation therapy can also play a role in selected colon and rectal cancer patients with recurrences or oligometastases. Finally, radiation therapy plays an important role in the palliation of symptoms in many colon and rectal cancer patients with metastatic disease.

Chemotherapy

The decision regarding use of systemic therapies for CRC centers around the patient's presenting stage of disease and personalized molecular profiling, which in the metastatic setting may inform on the underlying driving tumor biology. In the nonmetastatic setting, most patients with node-negative disease do not require adjuvant chemotherapy, owing to a lack of definitive evidence for survival benefit.[120] However, in this population, patients may be considered for adjuvant chemotherapy at the discretion of the treating medical oncologist if clinical and/or pathologic risk factors for the CRC are deemed at high risk for recurrence. Those with node-positive, nonmetastatic CRC are generally recommended a 6-month course of a 5-fluorouracil/oxaliplatin combination following surgical resection. Here, patients may be considered for a shorter duration of adjuvant therapy (3 months) should they have neither a T4 primary tumor nor N2 nodal disease on the corresponding pathology.[121]

Patients with metastatic CRC are most frequently treated with combinations of cytotoxic chemotherapy and biologic agents targeting the tumor. Bevacizumab is a monoclonal antibody against vascular endothelial growth factor that has demonstrated improvements in survival outcomes for patients with metastatic disease.[122] Monoclonal antibodies against epidermal growth factor receptor (EGFR) have antitumor activity for patients whose CRCs are wild-type for the *KRAS* and *NRAS* oncogenes, with better activity specifically in those with left-sided primary tumors.[123,124] BRAFV600E mutations occur in approximately 10% of CRC cases,[125] and a triple combination of targeted therapies against BRAF, MEK, and EGFR have demonstrated improvements in overall survival for this population of patients.[126] Immune checkpoint blockade agents against PD-1 with or without CTLA-4 have revolutionized not only the treatment paradigm but also (favorably) the prognostic outlook for the 3% to 5% of patients with metastatic CRC characterized by microsatellite instability.[127–129]

Key Points Therapies

- Use a standardized operative technique; *en bloc* resection is critical.
- Optional minimal surgery is the best prevention against local recurrence.
- Adequate sampling of nodes is critical for prognostic assessment.
- Hepatic and pulmonary "metastectomy" in selected patients affects survival.
- Preoperative chemoradiation has been widely accepted as a standard of care for stage II and III rectal cancer.
- Patients with metastatic colorectal cancer are most frequently treated with combinations of cytotoxic chemotherapy and biologic agents targeting the tumor.

SURVEILLANCE

Monitoring Tumor Response

Owing to its ability to depict the rectal wall, EUS has high accuracy (93%) in detecting residual early-stage (T1 and T2) disease, although high positive rates occur owing to overlap with scar and edema. Therefore, the decision to limit surgical intervention after neoadjuvant therapy cannot be based upon EUS findings.[130,131] As with pretreatment assessment, EUS is limited by its small field of view for distant disease. For both local and nodal assessment of rectal cancer after neoadjuvant chemoradiotherapy (CRT), CT is not able to reliably predict pathologic response, with a tendency to overstage disease.[132]

MRI in rectal cancer (performed ≤12 weeks after CRT) correlates well with histopathology, with accuracies of 82% for local tumor staging and 88% for nodal staging.[133] Advanced techniques such as USPIO and dynamic contrast-enhanced MRI have been reported to improve detection of residual disease after treatment.[134,135] Mesorectal fascia invasion post-CRT is determined by the presence of diffuse iso- or hyperintense tissue in the treated region. Conversely, the development of a fat pad larger than 2 mm is associated with treated disease.[136] For CRM involvement, post-CRT restaging MRI had an accuracy of 81% and a high negative predictive value of 91%.[137] High-resolution T2W MRI, together with diffusionW MRI, is used to assess response to neoadjuvant chemoradiation. Nevertheless, MRI still cannot reliably discriminate residual tumor from posttreatment fibrosis, because they both appear as hypointense soft tissue thickening on T2W images.[138] Therefore, if R0 resection is the goal, pretreatment MRI is preferred to determine the extent of surgical resection. Imaging should be combined with digital rectal examination and endoscopy to identify complete responders who may elect for organ preservation.[139]

PET/CT provides both functional and anatomic information. In a study by Capirci and coworkers,[140] using a decrease in standardized uptake value (SUV) of more than 65% to define metabolic response, the accuracy of PET for detection of residual rectal cancer after neoadjuvant CRT was 81%. Furthermore, FDG-PET can aid prognostication.[141] Guillem and colleagues showed that rectal cancer patients who remained disease free at a median follow-up of 42 months showed a greater reduction in maximum SUV after neoadjuvant treatment than patients who eventually developed recurrence.[142] Quantitative assessment based on tumor volume and SUV (PET metabolic volume) are significantly correlated with CEA levels after surgery.[143] It may also enable titration of treatment based on individual response.[144]

In one study, PET/CT correctly assessed response of liver metastases to bevacizumab-based therapy in 70% of cases compared with 35% by CT.[145] For evaluating liver metastases after RFA, MRI and PET/CT are comparable. In the study by Keuhl and associates,[146] the accuracy and sensitivity for detection of liver metastases were 91% and 83% for PET/CT and 92% and 75% for MRI, respectively. After treatment of liver metastases with yttrium-90 microspheres, metabolic response on PET/CT correlates better with CEA levels than anatomic response with both CT and MRI.[147] Nevertheless, it must be noted that complete metabolic response on FDG-PET after neoadjuvant chemotherapy may not necessarily imply complete pathologic response. Therefore, currently, curative resection of liver metastases should not be deferred solely on the basis of FDG-PET findings.[148,149]

Detection of Recurrence

Nearly 85% of recurrences occur within the first 3 years after surgery and none after 5 years. Therefore, most surveillance strategies focus resources on the first 3 years. A metaanalysis by Bruinvels and coworkers[150] involving 3923 patients showed that, in patients with intensive follow-up that included CEA assays, there were more asymptomatic recurrences that were amenable to surgery, leading to 9% better 5-year survival rates, than those with minimal or no follow-up. For routine surveillance, the American Society of Clinical Oncology currently recommends CEA assays every 3 months for the first 3 years; CT scan of the chest, abdomen, and pelvis annually for the first 3 years; and colonoscopy at 3 years in patients with stage 2 and stage 3 CRC.[151]

As a result of its superior soft-tissue resolution, MRI is better than CT at detecting local disease recurrence in rectal cancer, and especially in differentiating normal pelvic soft tissue structures from recurrent tumor.[80,152] For the more proximal colon, CT is probably better than MRI because of its higher temporal resolution. On CT, recurrence is demonstrated by serial progression of a mass, nodular configuration, and invasion of adjacent structures.[153] MRI also relies on anatomic evaluation, although tumor tissue can be differentiated from fibrous tissue when it shows hyperintense signal on T2W images.

PET/CT is increasingly shown to be superior to the other imaging modalities in demonstrating recurrent disease activity and has become an integral part of the surveillance strategy. It has the potential to replace CT as the first-line diagnostic tool for restaging patients for recurrent CRC.[154] PET/CT can distinguish between tumor recurrence and postsurgical scar, as well as pinpoint the site of recurrence in cases of unexplained rise in serum CEA.[144] It is recommended for evaluation of equivocal findings on serial CT and MRI.[155] For recurrent nodal disease, PET/CT is superior to MRI, with a sensitivity of 93%.[156] PET/CT is superior to contrast-enhanced CT in detecting local recurrences at the colorectal anastomosis, intrahepatic recurrences, and extrahepatic disease, with sensitivity rates close to or exceeding 90%.[157] Quantitative measurements of SUV and tumor volume may be used as a marker of tumor burden in cases of tumor recurrence.[143] Note that PET/CT should be performed more than 6 weeks after surgery, because inflammatory changes can result in false positives.

KEY POINTS Surveillance

- Routine surveillance: the American Society of Clinical Oncology currently recommends carcinoembryonic antigen assays every 3 months for the first 3 years; computed tomography scan of the chest, abdomen, and pelvis annually for the first 3 years; and colonoscopy at 3 years in patients with stage 2 and stage 3 colorectal cancer.
- Positron emission tomography/computed tomography is increasingly shown to be superior to the other imaging modalities in demonstrating recurrent disease activity and has become an integral part of the surveillance strategy.

CONCLUSION

Established indications for imaging include screening, staging, and surveillance of disease. High-resolution EUS, CT, and MRI, along with PET/CT, are able to provide important information for disease detection and treatment planning. As the management of CRC continues to evolve with time, so too will the imaging techniques and strategies. To tailor specific therapies based on treatment response, increased demand for more and accurate functional imaging at the cellular and molecular levels is foreseeable in the future.

REFERENCES

1. Siegel RL, Miller KD, Fedewa SA, et al. Colorectal cancer statistics, 2017. *CA Cancer J Clin*. 2017;67:177–193.
2. Wolf A, Fontham ETH, Church TR, et al. Colorectal cancer screening for average-risk adults: 2018 guideline update from the American Cancer Society. *CA Cancer J Clin*. 2018;68:250–281.
3. Uberoi AS, Bhutani MS. Has the role of EUS in rectal cancer staging changed in the last decade? *Endosc Ultrasound*. 2018;7(6):366–370.
4. MERCURY Study Group Extramural depth of tumor invasion at thin-section MR in patients with rectal cancer: results of the MERCURY study. *Radiology*. 2007;243:132–139.
5. Adam R. The importance of visceral metastasectomy in colorectal cancer. *Ann Oncol*. 2000;11(Suppl 3):29–36.
6. Goldberg RM, Fleming TR, Tangen CM, et al. Surgery for recurrent colon cancer: strategies for identifying resectable recurrence and success rates after resection. Eastern Cooperative Oncology Group, the North Central Cancer Treatment Group, and the Southwest Oncology Group. *Ann Intern Med*. 1998;129:27–35.
7. Edwards BK, Ward E, Kohler BA, et al. Annual report to the nation on the status of cancer, 1975-2006, featuring colorectal cancer trends and impact of interventions (risk factors, screening, and treatment) to reduce future rates. *Cancer*. 2010;116:544–573.
8. Espey DK, Wu XC, Swan J, et al. Annual report to the nation on the status of cancer, 1975-2004, featuring cancer in American Indians and Alaska Natives. *Cancer*. 2007;110:2119–2152.
9. Nusko G, Mansmann U, Partzsch U, et al. Invasive carcinoma in colorectal adenomas: multivariate analysis of patient and adenoma characteristics. *Endoscopy*. 1997;29:626–631.
10. Higuchi T, Jass JR. My approach to serrated polyps of the colorectum. *J Clin Pathol*. 2004;57:682–686.
11. Hampel H, Frankel WL, Martin E, et al. Feasibility for screening for Lynch syndrome among patients with colorectal cancer. *J Clin Oncol*. 2008;26:5783–5788.
12. Conlin A, Smith G, Carey FA, et al. The prognostic significance of K-ras, p53, and APC mutations in colorectal carcinoma. *Gut*. 2005;54:1283–1286.
13. Triantafillidis JK, Nasioulas G, Kosmidis PA. Colorectal cancer and inflammatory bowel disease: epidemiology, risk factors, mechanisms of carcinogenesis and prevention strategies. *Anticancer Res*. 2009;29:2727–2737.
14. Chung YW, Han DS, Park YK, et al. Association of obesity, serum glucose and lipids with the risk of advanced colorectal adenoma and cancer: a case-control study in Korea. *Dig Liver Dis*. 2006;38:668–672.
15. Gonzalez CA. Nutrition and cancer: the current epidemiological evidence. *Br J Nutr*. 2006;96(Suppl 1):S42–S45.
16. Compton CC. Colorectal carcinoma: diagnostic, prognostic, and molecular features. *Mod Pathol*. 2003;16:376–388.
17. Compton CC, Fielding LP, Burgart LJ, et al. Prognostic factors in colorectal cancer. College of American Pathologists Consensus Statement 1999. *Arch Pathol Lab Med*. 2000;124:979–994.
18. Compton C, Fenoglio-Preiser CM, Pettigrew N, et al. American Joint Committee on Cancer Prognostic Factors Consensus Conference: Colorectal Working Group. *Cancer*. 2000;88:1739–1757.
19. Kang H, O'Connell JB, Leonardi MJ, et al. Rare tumors of the colon and rectum: a national review. *Int J Colorectal Dis*. 2007;22:183–189.
20. Compton CC. Pathology report in colon cancer: what is prognostically important? *Dig Dis*. 1999;17:67–79.
21. Sinicrope FA, Shi Q, Smyrk TC, et al. Molecular markers identify subtypes of stage III colon cancer associated with patient outcomes. *Gastroenterol*. 2015;148:88–99.
22. Guinney J, Dientsmann R, Wang X, et al. The consensus molecular subtypes of colorectal cancer. *Nat Med*. 2015;21:1350–1356.
23. Sarela A, O'Riordain DS. Rectal adenocarcinoma with liver metastases: management of the primary tumour. *Br J Surg*. 2001;88:163–164.

24. Niederhuber JE. Colon and rectum cancer. Patterns of spread and implications for workup. *Cancer*. 1993;71(Suppl 12):4187–4192.
25. Weiss EG, Laverly I, et al. Colon cancer evaluation and staging. In: Wolff BG, Fleshman JW, Beck DE, eds. *The ASCRS Textbook of Colon and Rectal Surgery*. New York: Springer Science + Business Media; 2007:388–389.
26. Knudsen JB, Nilsson T, Sprechler M, et al. Venous and nerve invasion as prognostic factors in postoperative survival of patients with resectable cancer of the rectum. *Dis Colon Rectum*. 1983;26:613–617.
27. Giess CS, Schwartz LH, Bach AM, et al. Patterns of neoplastic spread in colorectal cancer: implications for surveillance CT studies. *AJR Am J Roentgenol*. 1998;170:987–991.
28. Iyer RB, Silverman PM, DuBrow RA, et al. Imaging in the diagnosis, staging and follow-up of colorectal cancer. *AJR Am J Roentgenol*. 2002;179:3–13.
29. Charnsangavej C. Pathways of lymph node metastases in cancer of the gastrointestinal and hepatobiliary tracts. In: Myers MA, ed. *Dynamic Radiology of the Abdomen*. New York: Springer-Verlag; 2000:287–308.
30. Park IJ, Choi GS, Lim KH, et al. Different patterns of lymphatic spread of sigmoid, rectosigmoid, and rectal cancers. *Ann Surg Oncol*. 2008;15:3478–3483.
31. Boni L, Benevento A, Dionigi G, et al. Injection of colorectal cancer cells in mesenteric and antimesenteric sides of the colon results in different patterns of metastatic diffusion: an experimental study in rats. *World J Surg Oncol*. 2005;3:69.
32. Shepherd NA, Baxter KJ, Love SB. The prognostic importance of peritoneal involvement in colonic cancer: a prospective evaluation. *Gastroenterology*. 1997;112:1096–1102.
33. Kemeny N. Systemic and regional chemotherapy in advanced colorectal carcinoma. In: MacDonald JS, ed. *Gastrointestinal Oncology: Basic and Clinical Aspects*. Boston: Martin Nijhoff; 1987:235–251.
34. Weiss L, Grundmann E, Torhorst J, et al. Haematogenous metastatic patterns in colonic carcinoma: an analysis of 1541 necropsies. *J Pathol*. 1986;150:195–203.
35. Stangl R, Altendorf-Hofmann A, Charnley RM, et al. Factors influencing the natural history of colorectal liver metastases. *Lancet*. 1994;343:1405–1410.
36. Garden OJ, Rees M, Poston GJ, et al. Guidelines for resection of colorectal cancer liver metastases. *Gut*. 2006;55(Suppl 3):iii1–iii8.
37. Jessup JM, Goldberg RM, Asare EA, et al. *AJCC Cancer Staging Manual*. 8th ed. New York: Springer-Verlag; 2017:251–274.
38. Colon and rectumSobin LH, Wittekind C, eds. *TNM: Classification of Malignant Tumors*. New York: Wiley-Liss; 2002:72–76.
39. Compton CC, Greene FL. The staging of colorectal cancer: 2004 and beyond. *CA Cancer J Clin*. 2004;54:295–308.
40. Jessup JM, Goldberg RM, Asare EA, et al. Colon and Rectum. In: Amin MB, ed. *AJCC Cancer Staging Manual*. 8th ed. : Springer International Publishing; 2017.
41. Herrera-Ornelas L, Justiniano J, Castillo N, et al. Metastases in small lymph nodes from colon cancer. *Arch Surg*. 1987;122:1253–1256.
42. Brown HG, Luckasevic TM, Medich DS, et al. Efficacy of manual dissection of lymph nodes in colon cancer resections. *Mod Pathol*. 2004;17:402–406.
43. Goldstein NS, Turner JR. Pericolonic tumor deposits in patients with T3N+M0 colon adenocarcinomas. Markers of reduced disease free survival and intra-abdominal metastases and their implications for TNM classification. *Cancer*. 2000;88:2228–2238.
44. Singletary SE, Greene FL, Sobin LH. Classification of isolated tumor cells: clarification of the 6th edition of the American Joint Committee on Cancer Staging Manual. *Cancer*. 2003;98:2740–2741.
45. Sloane JP. *Minimum dataset for colorectal cancer histopathology reports. Standards and Minimum Datasets for Reporting Common Cancers. Minimum Datasets for Reporting Common Cancers*. London: The Royal College of Pathologists; 1998:1–10.
46. Petersen VC, Baxter KJ, Love SB, et al. Identification of objective pathologic prognostic determinants and models of prognosis in Dukes' B colon cancer. *Gut*. 2002;51:65–69.
47. Stocchi L, Nelson H, Sargent DJ, et al. Impact of surgical and pathological variables in rectal cancer: a United States community and cooperative group report. *J Clin Oncol*. 2001;19:3895–3902.
48. Mulcahy HE, Skelly MM, Husain A, et al. Long-term outcome following curative surgery for malignant large bowel obstruction. *Br J Surg*. 1996;83:46–50.
49. Chapuis PH, Dent OF, Fisher R, et al. A multivariate analysis of clinical and pathological variables in prognosis after resection of large bowel cancer. *Br J Surg*. 1985;72:698–702.
50. Newland R, Dent O, Lyttle M, et al. Pathologic determinants of survival associated with CRC with lymph node metastases. A multivariate analysis of 579 patients. *Cancer*. 1994;73:2076–2082.
51. Talbot I, Ritchie S, Leighton MH, et al. The clinical significance of invasion of veins by rectal cancer. *Br J Surg*. 1980;67:439–442.
52. Horn A, Dahl O, Morild I. Venous and neural invasion as predictors of recurrence in rectal adenocarcinoma. *Dis Colon Rectum*. 1991;34:798–804.
53. Takahashi Y, Tucker S, Kitadai Y, et al. Vessel counts and expression of vascular endothelial growth factor as prognostic factors in node-negative colon cancer. *Arch Surg*. 1997;132:541–546.
54. Minsky B, Mies C, Recht A, et al. Resectable adenocarcinoma of the rectosigmoid and rectum. II. The influence of blood vessel invasion. *Cancer*. 1988;61:1417–1424.
55. Johnson CD, Chen MH, Toledano AY, et al. Accuracy of CT colonography in the detection of large adenomas and cancers. *N Engl J Med*. 2008;359:1207–1217. erratum in *N Engl J Med*. 2008;359:2853.
56. Pickhardt PJ, Choi JR, Hwang I, et al. Computed tomographic virtual colonoscopy to screen for colorectal neoplasia in asymptomatic adults. *N Engl J Med*. 2003;349:2191–2200.
57. Young BM, Fletcher JG, Paulsen SR, et al. Polyp measurement with CT colonography: multiple-reader, multiple-workstation comparison. *AJR Am J Roentgenol*. 2007;188:122–129.
58. ACR–SAR–SCBT-MR Practice Parameter for the Performance of Computed Tomography (CT) Colonography. The American College of Radiology (2019) ACR–SAR–SCBT-MR practice parameter for the performance of computed tomography (CT) colonography in adults. *The American College of Radiology*, Virginia, United States. Available via https://www.acr.org/-/media/ACR/Files/Practice-Parameters/ct-colonog.pdf.
59. Neri E, Halligan S, Hellström M, et al. ESGAR CT Colonography Working Group. The second ESGAR consensus statement on CT colonography. *Eur Radiol*. 2013;23(3):720–729.
60. van der Meulen MP, Lansdorp-Vogelaar I, Goede SL, et al. Colorectal cancer: cost-effectiveness of colonoscopy versus CT colonography screening with participation rates and costs. *Radiology*. 2018; 287(3):901–911.
61. Brenner DJ, Georgsson MA. Mass screening with CT colonography: should the radiation exposure be of concern? *Gastroenterology*. 2005;129:328–337.
62. An S, Lee KH, Kim YH, et al. Screening CT colonography in an asymptomatic average-risk Asian population: a 2-year experience in a single institution. *AJR Am J Roentgenol*. 2008;191(3):W100–W106.
63. Pickhardt PJ. Incidence of colonic perforation at CT colonography: review of existing data and implications for screening of asymptomatic adults. *Radiology*. 2006;239:313–316.
64. Burling D, Halligan S, Slater A, et al. Potentially serious adverse events at CT colonography in symptomatic patients: national survey of the United Kingdom. *Radiology*. 2006;239:464–471.
65. Akasu T, Kondo H, Moriya Y, et al. Endorectal ultrasonography and treatment of early stage rectal cancer. *World J Surg*. 2000;24:1061.
66. Beets-Tan RG, Beets GL. Rectal cancer: review with emphasis on MR imaging. *Radiology*. 2004;232:335.
67. Bipat S, Glas AS, Slors FJ, et al. Rectal cancer: local staging and assessment of lymph node involvement with endoluminal US, CT, and MR imaging-a metaanalysis. *Radiology*. 2014;232:773–783.
68. Heriot AG, Grundy A, Kumar D. Preoperative staging of rectal carcinoma. *Br J Surg*. 1999;86:17.
69. Kwok H, Bissett IP, Hill GL. Preoperative staging of rectal cancer. *Int J Colorectal Dis*. 2000;15:9.
70. O'Neill BD, Salerno G, Thomas K, et al. MR vs CT imaging: low rectal cancer tumour delineation for three-dimensional conformal radiotherapy. *Br J Radiol*. 2009;82:509–513.
71. Wolberink SV, Beets-Tan RG, de Haas-Kock DF, et al. Multislice CT as a primary screening tool for the prediction of an involved mesorectal fascia and distant metastases in primary rectal cancer: a multicenter study. *Dis Colon Rectum*. 2009;52:928–934.
72. Brent A, Talbot R, Coyne J, Nash G. Should indeterminate lung lesions reported on staging CT scans influence the management of patients with colorectal cancer? *Colorectal Dis*. 2007;9:816–818.
73. Adeyemo D, Hutchinson R. Preoperative staging of rectal cancer: pelvic MRI plus abdomen and pelvic CT. Does extrahepatic

abdomen imaging matter? A case for routine thoracic CT. *Colorectal Dis*. 2009;11:259–263.
74. Wu GY, Ghimire P. Perfusion computed tomography in colorectal cancer: protocols, clinical applications and emerging trends. *World J Gastroenterol*. 2009;15:3228–3231.
75. Goh V, Halligan S, Wellsted DM, et al. Can perfusion CT assessment of primary colorectal adenocarcinoma blood flow at staging predict for subsequent metastatic disease? A pilot study. *Eur Radiol*. 2009;19:79–89.
76. Veit-Haibach P, Treyer V, Strobel K, et al. Feasibility of integrated CT-liver perfusion in routine FDG-PET-CT. *Abdom Imaging*. 2010;35:528–536.
77. Lu YY, Chen JH, Chien CR, et al. Use of FDG-PET or PET/CT to detect recurrent colorectal cancer in patients with elevated CEA: a systematic review and meta-analysis. *Int J Colorectal Dis*. 2013;28(8):1039–1047.
78. Brown G, Daniels IR, Richardson C, et al. Techniques and trouble-shooting in high spatial resolution thin slice MRI for rectal cancer. *Br J Radiol*. 2005;78:24.
79. MERCURY Study Group Diagnostic accuracy of preoperative magnetic resonance imaging in predicting curative resection of rectal cancer: prospective observational study. *BMJ*. 2006;333:779.
80. Beets-Tan RG, Beets GL, Borstlap AC, et al. Preoperative assessment of local tumor extent in advanced rectal cancer: CT or high-resolution MRI? *Abdom Imaging*. 2000;25:533–541.
81. Shinya S, Sasaki T, Nakagawa Y, et al. The efficacy of diffusion-weighted imaging for the detection of colorectal cancer. *Hepatogastroenterology*. 2009;56:128–132.
82. Lahaye MJ, Engelen SM, Nelemans PJ, et al. Imaging for predicting the risk factors—the circumferential resection margin and nodal disease—of local recurrence in rectal cancer: a meta-analysis. *Semin Ultrasound CT MR*. 2005;26:259–268.
83. Ferri M, Laghi A, Mingazzini P, et al. Pre-operative assessment of extramural invasion and sphincteral involvement in rectal cancer by magnetic resonance imaging with phased-array coil. *Colorectal Dis*. 2005;7:387.
84. Brown G, Radcliffe AG, Newcombe RG, et al. Preoperative assessment of prognostic factors in rectal cancer using high-resolution magnetic resonance imaging. *Br J Surg*. 2003;90:355.
85. Brown G, Richards CJ, Bourne MW, et al. Morphologic predictors of lymph node status in rectal cancer with use of high-spatial-resolution MR imaging with histopathologic comparison. *Radiology*. 2003;227:371–377.
86. Squillaci E, Manenti G, Mancino S, et al. Staging of colon cancer: whole-body MRI vs. whole-body PET-CT—initial clinical experience. *Abdom Imaging*. 2008;33:676–688.
87. Badiee S, Franc BL, Webb EM, et al. Role of IV iodinated contrast material in 18F-FDG PET-CT of liver metastases. *AJR Am J Roentgenol*. 2008;191:1436–1439.
88. Veit-Haibach P, Kuehle CA, Beyer T, et al. Diagnostic accuracy of colorectal cancer staging with whole-body PET-CT colonography. *JAMA*. 2006;296:2590–2600.
89. Bassi MC, Turri L, Sacchetti G, et al. FDG-PET-CT imaging for staging and target volume delineation in preoperative conformal radiotherapy of rectal cancer. *Int J Radiat Oncol Biol Phys*. 2008;70:1423–1426.
90. Llamas-Elvira JM, Rodríguez-Fernández A, Gutiérrez-Sáinz J, et al. Fluorine-18 fluorodeoxyglucose PET in the preoperative staging of colorectal cancer. *Eur J Nucl Med Mol Imaging*. 2007;34:859–867.
91. Gearhart SL, Frassica D, Rosen R, et al. Improved staging with pretreatment positron emission tomography/computed tomography in low rectal cancer. *Ann Surg Oncol*. 2006;13:397–404.
92. Nahas CSR, Akhurst T, Yeung H, et al. Positron emission tomography detection of distant metastatic or synchronous disease in patients with locally advanced rectal cancer receiving preoperative chemoradiation. *Ann Surg Oncol*. 2007;15:704–711.
93. Wiering B, Krabbe PF, Jager GJ, et al. The impact of fluoro-18-deoxyglucose-positron emission tomography in the management of colorectal liver metastases. *Cancer*. 2005;104:2658–2670.
94. Yasuda S, Fujii H, Nakahara T, et al. 18F-FDG-PET detection of colonic adenomas. *J Nucl Med*. 2001;42:989–992.
95. Berger KL, Nicholson SA, Dehadashti F, et al. FDG-PET evaluation of mucinous neoplasms: correlation of FDG uptake with histopathologic features. *AJR Am J Roentgenol*. 2000;174:1005–1008.
96. Kosugi C, Saito N, Murakami K, et al. Positron emission tomography for preoperative staging in patients with locally advanced or metastatic colorectal adenocarcinoma in lymph node metastasis. *Hepatogastroenterology*. 2008;55:398–402.
97. Bokey EL, Chapuis PH, Dent OF, et al. Surgical technique and survival in patients having a curative resection for colon cancer. *Dis Colon Rectum*. 2003;46:860–866.
98. Fengler SA, Pearl RK. Technical considerations in the surgical treatment of colon and rectal cancer. *Semin Surg Oncol*. 1994;10:200–207.
99. Pollett WG, Nicholls RJ. The relationship between the extent of distal clearance and survival and local recurrence rates after curative anterior resection for carcinoma of the rectum. *Ann Surg*. 1983;198:159–163.
100. Ruo L, Guillem JG. Surgical management of primary CRC. *Surg Oncol*. 1998;7:153–163.
101. Lange MM, Rutten HJ, van de Velde CJ. One hundred years of curative surgery for rectal cancer: 1908-2008. *Eur J Surg Oncol*. 2009;35:456–463.
102. Bernstein TE, Endreseth BH, Romundstad P, et al. Norwegian CRC Group. Circumferential resection margin as a prognostic factor in rectal cancer. *Br J Surg*. 2009;96:1348–1357.
103. Doornebosch PG, Tollenaar RA, De Graaf EJ. Is the increasing role of transanal endoscopic microsurgery in curation for T1 rectal cancer justified? A systematic review. *Acta Oncol*. 2009;48:343–353.
104. Leroy J, Jamali F, Forbes L, et al. Laparoscopic total mesorectal excision (TME) for rectal cancer surgery: long-term outcomes. *Surg Endosc*. 2004;18:281–289.
105. Clinical Outcomes of Surgical Therapy Study Group A comparison of laparoscopically assisted and open colectomy for colon cancer. *N Engl J Med*. 2004;350:2050–2059.
106. Nagtegaal ID, Quirke P. What is the role for the circumferential margin in the modern treatment of rectal cancer? *J Clin Oncol*. 2008;26:303–312.
107. Compton CC. Updated protocol for the examination of specimens from patients with carcinomas of the colon and rectum, excluding carcinoid tumors, lymphomas, sarcomas, and tumors of the vermiform appendix: a basis for checklists. Cancer Committee. *Arch Pathol Lab Med*. 2000;124:1016–1025.
108. Chang GJ, Rodriguez-Bigas MA, Skibber JM, et al. Lymph node evaluation and survival after curative resection of colon cancer: systematic review. *J Natl Cancer Inst*. 2007;99:433–441.
109. Neeff H, Hörth W, Makowiec F, et al. Outcome after resection of hepatic and pulmonary metastases of CRC. *J Gastrointest Surg*. 2009;13:1813–1820.
110. Wanebo HJ, Chu QD, Vezeridis MP, Soderberg C. Patient selection for hepatic resection of colorectal metastases. *Arch Surg*. 1996;131:322–329.
111. Rees M, Tekkis PP, Welsh FK, et al. Evaluation of long-term survival after hepatic resection for metastatic CRC: a multifactorial model of 929 patients. *Ann Surg*. 2008;247:125–135.
112. Vogelsang H, Haas S, Hierholzer C, et al. Factors influencing survival after resection of pulmonary metastases from CRC. *Br J Surg*. 2004;91:1066–1071.
113. Abdalla EK, Vauthey JN, Ellis LM, et al. Recurrence and outcomes following hepatic resection, radiofrequency ablation, and combined resection/ablation for colorectal liver metastases. *Ann Surg*. 2004;239:818–825.
114. Prolongation of the disease-free interval in surgically treated rectal carcinoma. Gastrointestinal Tumor Study Group. *N Engl J Med*. 1985;312:1465-1472.
115. Douglass Jr. HO, Moertel CG, Mayer RJ, et al. Survival after postoperative combination treatment of rectal cancer [letter]. *N Engl J Med*. 1986;315:1294–1295.
116. Wolmark N, Wieand HS, Hyams DM, et al. Randomized trial of postoperative adjuvant chemotherapy with or without radiotherapy for carcinoma of the rectum: National Surgical Adjuvant Breast and Bowel Project Protocol R-02. *J Natl Cancer Inst*. 2000;92:388–396.
117. Sauer R, Becker H, Hohenberger W, et al. Preoperative versus postoperative chemoradiotherapy for rectal cancer. *N Engl J Med*. 2004;351:1731–1740.
118. Ngan SY, Burmeister B, Fisher RJ, et al. Randomized trial of short-course radiotherapy versus long-course chemoradiation comparing rates of local recurrence in patients with T3 rectal cancer: Trans-Tasman Radiation Oncology Group trial 01.04. *J Clin Oncol*. 2012;30(31):3827–3833.

119. Bujko K, Wyrwicz L, Rutkowski A, et al. Long-course oxaliplatin-based preoperative chemoradiation versus 5×5 Gy and consolidation chemotherapy for cT4 or fixed cT3 rectal cancer: results of a randomized phase III study. *Ann Oncol*. 2016;27(5):834–842.
120. Wolmark N, Rockette H, Fisher B, et al. The benefit of leucovorin-modulated fluorouracil as postoperative adjuvant therapy for primary colon cancer: results from National Surgical Adjuvant Breast and Bowel Project protocol C-03. *J Clin Oncol*. 1993;11(10):1879–1887.
121. Grothey A, Sobrero AF, Shields AF, et al. Duration of adjuvant chemotherapy for stage iii colon cancer. *N Engl J Med*. 2018;378(13):1177–1188.
122. Giantonio BJ, Catalano PJ, Meropol NJ, et al. Bevacizumab in combination with oxaliplatin, fluorouracil, and leucovorin (FOLFOX4) for previously treated metastatic colorectal cancer: results from the Eastern Cooperative Oncology Group Study E3200. *J Clin Oncol*. 2007;25(12):1539–1544.
123. Di Nicolantonio F, Martini M, Molinari F, et al. Wild-type BRAF is required for response to panitumumab or cetuximab in metastatic colorectal cancer. *J Clin Oncol*. 2008;26(35):5705–5712.
124. Van Cutsem E, Kohne CH, Lang I, et al. Cetuximab plus irinotecan, fluorouracil, and leucovorin as first-line treatment for metastatic colorectal cancer: updated analysis of overall survival according to tumor KRAS and BRAF mutation status. *J Clin Oncol*. 2011;29(15):2011–2019.
125. Tol J, Nagtegaal ID, Punt CJ. BRAF mutation in metastatic colorectal cancer. *N Engl J Med*. 2009;361(1):98–99.
126. Cutsem EV, Cuyle P-J, Huijberts S, et al. BEACON CRC study safety lead-in (SLI) in patients with BRAFV600E metastatic colorectal cancer (mCRC): efficacy and tumor markers. *J Clin Oncol*. 2018;36(4 Suppl). 627-627.
127. Le DT, Uram JN, Wang H, et al. PD-1 blockade in tumors with mismatch-repair deficiency. *N Engl J Med*. 2015;372(26):2509–2520.
128. Overman MJ, McDermott R, Leach JL, et al. Nivolumab in patients with metastatic DNA mismatch repair-deficient or microsatellite instability-high colorectal cancer (CheckMate 142): an open-label, multicentre, phase 2 study. *Lancet Oncol*. 2017;18(9):1182–1191.
129. Overman MJ, Lonardi S, Wong KYM, et al. Durable clinical benefit with nivolumab plus ipilimumab in DNA mismatch repair-deficient/microsatellite instability-high metastatic colorectal cancer. *J Clin Oncol*. 2018;36(8):773–779.
130. Meyenberger C, Huch Böni RA, Bertschinger P, et al. Endoscopic ultrasound and endorectal magnetic resonance imaging: a prospective, comparative study for preoperative staging and follow-up of rectal cancer. *Endoscopy*. 1995;27:469–479.
131. Maor Y, Nadler M, Barshack I, et al. Endoscopic ultrasound staging of rectal cancer: diagnostic value before and following chemoradiation. *J Gastroenterol Hepatol*. 2006;21:454–458.
132. Huh JW, Park YA, Jung EJ, et al. Accuracy of endorectal ultrasonography and computed tomography for restaging rectal cancer after preoperative chemoradiation. *J Am Coll Surg*. 2008;207:7–12.
133. Johnston DF, Lawrence KM, Sizer BF, et al. Locally advanced rectal cancer: histopathological correlation and predictive accuracy of serial MRI after neoadjuvant chemotherapy. *Br J Radiol*. 2009;82:332–336.
134. Lahaye MJ, Beets GL, Engelen SM, et al. Locally advanced rectal cancer: MR imaging for restaging after neoadjuvant radiation therapy with concomitant chemotherapy. Part II. What are the criteria to predict involved lymph nodes? *Radiology*. 2009;252:81–91.
135. de Lussanet QG, Backes WH, Griffioen AW, et al. Dynamic contrast-enhanced magnetic resonance imaging of radiation therapy-induced microcirculation changes in rectal cancer. *Int J Radiat Oncol Biol Phys*. 2005;63:1309–1315.
136. Vliegen RF, Beets GL, Lammering G, et al. Mesorectal fascia invasion after neoadjuvant chemotherapy and radiation therapy for locally advanced rectal cancer: accuracy of MR imaging for prediction. *Radiology*. 2008;246:454–462.
137. Kulkarni T, Gollins S, Maw A, et al. Magnetic resonance imaging in rectal cancer downstaged using neoadjuvant chemoradiation: accuracy of prediction of tumour stage and circumferential resection margin status. *Colorectal Dis*. 2008;10:479–489.
138. Suppiah A, Hunter IA, Cowley J, et al. Magnetic resonance imaging accuracy in assessing tumour down-staging following chemoradiation in rectal cancer. *Colorectal Dis*. 2009;11:249–253.
139. Maas M, Lambregts DM, Nelemans PJ, et al. Assessment of clinical complete response after chemoradiation for rectal cancer with digital rectal examination, endoscopy, and MRI: selection for organ-saving treatment. *Ann Surg Oncol*. 2015;22:3873–3880.
140. Capirci C, Rubello D, Pasini F, et al. The role of dual-time combined 18-fluorodeoxyglucose positron emission tomography and computed tomography in the staging and restaging workup of locally advanced rectal cancer, treated with preoperative chemoradiation therapy and radical surgery. *Int J Radiat Oncol Biol Phys*. 2009;74:1461–1469.
141. Dirisamer A, Halpern BS, Flöry D, et al. Performance of integrated FDG-PET/contrast-enhanced CT in the staging and restaging of colorectal cancer: comparison with PET and enhanced CT. *Eur J Radiol*. 2010;73:324–328.
142. Guillem JG, Moore HG, Akhuurst T, et al. Sequential preoperative fluorodeoxyglucose-positron emission tomography assessment of response to preoperative chemoradiation: a means for determining long term outcomes of rectal cancer. *J Am Coll Surg*. 2004;199:1–7.
143. Choi MY, Lee KM, Chung JK, et al. Correlation between serum CEA level and metabolic volume as determined by FDG PET in postoperative patients with recurrent colorectal cancer. *Ann Nucl Med*. 2005;19:123–129.
144. Vriens D, de Geus-Oei LF, van der Graaf WT, et al. Tailoring therapy in colorectal cancer by PET-CT. *Q J Nucl Med Mol Imaging*. 2009;53:224–244.
145. Goshen E, Davidson T, Zwas ST, et al. PET/CT in the evaluation of response to treatment of liver metastases from colorectal cancer with bevacizumab and irinotecan. *Technol Cancer Res Treat*. 2006;5:37–43.
146. Kuehl H, Antoch G, Stergar H, et al. Comparison of FDG-PET, PET/CT and MRI for follow-up of colorectal liver metastases treated with radiofrequency ablation: initial results. *Eur J Radiol*. 2008;67:362–371.
147. Wong CY, Salem R, Raman S, et al. Evaluating 90Y-glass microsphere treatment response of unresectable colorectal liver metastases by [18F]FDG PET: a comparison with CT or MRI. *Eur J Nucl Med Mol Imaging*. 2002;29:815–820.
148. Tan MC, Linehan DC, Hawkins WG, et al. Chemotherapy-induced normalization of FDG uptake by colorectal liver metastases does not usually indicate complete pathologic response. *J Gastrointest Surg*. 2007;11:1112–1119.
149. Lubezky N, Metser U, Geva R, et al. The role and limitations of 18-fluoro-2-deoxy-d-glucose positron emission tomography (FDG-PET) scan and computerized tomography (CT) in restaging patients with hepatic colorectal metastases following neoadjuvant chemotherapy: comparison with operative and pathological findings. *J Gastrointest Surg*. 2007;11:472–478.
150. Bruinvels DJ, Stiggelbout AM, Kievit J, et al. Follow-up of patients with colorectal cancer. A meta-analysis. *Ann Surg*. 1994;219:174–182.
151. Desch CE, Benson 3rd AB, Somerfield MR, et al. Colorectal cancer surveillance: 2005 update of an American Society of Clinical Oncology practice guideline. *J Clin Oncol*. 2005;23:8512–8519.
152. Pema PJ, Bennett WF, Bova JG, et al. CT vs MRI in diagnosis of recurrent rectosigmoid carcinoma. *J Comput Assist Tomogr*. 1994;18:256–261.
153. McCarthy SM, Barnes D, Deveney K, et al. Detection of recurrent rectosigmoid carcinoma: prospective evaluation of CT and clinical factors. *AJR Am J Roentgenol*. 1985;144:577–579.
154. Soyka JD, Veit-Haibach P, Strobel K, et al. Staging pathways in recurrent colorectal carcinoma: is contrast-enhanced 18F-FDG PET-CT the diagnostic tool of choice? *J Nucl Med*. 2008;49:354–361.
155. Potter KC, Husband JE, Houghton SL, et al. Diagnostic accuracy of serial CT/magnetic resonance imaging review vs. positron emission tomography/CT in colorectal cancer patients with suspected and known recurrence. *Dis Colon Rectum*. 2009;52:253–259.
156. Schmidt GP, Baur-Melnyk A, Haug A, et al. Whole-body MRI at 1.5 T and 3 T compared with FDG-PET-CT for the detection of tumour recurrence in patients with colorectal cancer. *Eur Radiol*. 2009;19:1366–1378.
157. Selzner M, Hany TF, Wildbrett P, et al. Does the novel PET/CT imaging modality impact on the treatment of patients with metastatic colorectal cancer of the liver? *Ann Surg*. 2004;240:1027–1034.

Visit ExpertConsult.com for additional algorithms.

COLORECTAL CANCER SCREENING - AVERAGE RISK

Note: Screening for adults age 76 to 85 should be evaluated on an individual basis by their health care provider to assess the risks and benefits of screening. Colorectal cancer screening is not recommended over age 85.

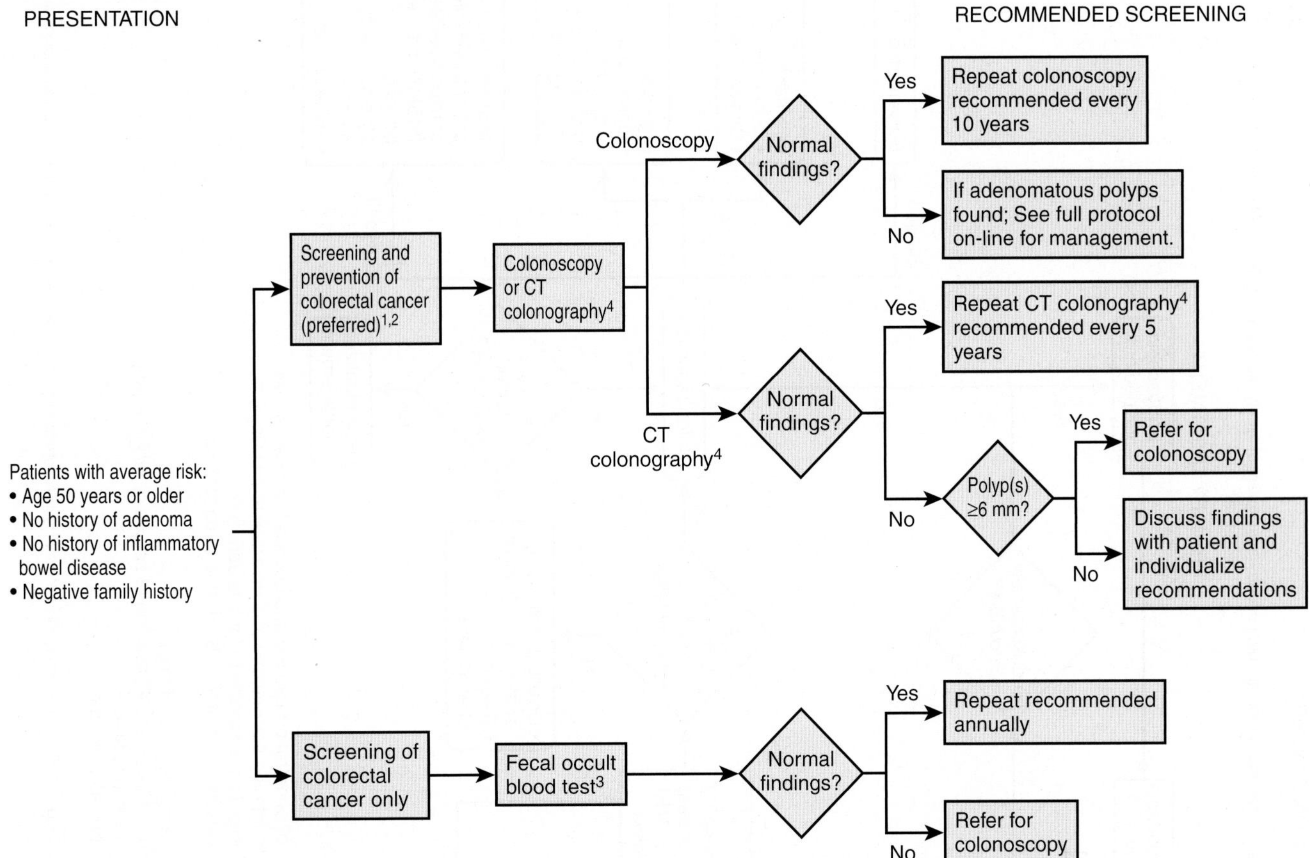

[1]While there is good evidence to support fecal occult blood testing, tests that both screen for and prevent colon cancer are the preferred screening modality. Annual fecal occult blood tests should not be performed if colonoscopy or CT colonography is used as the screening measure in an average-risk patient.

[2]Flexible sigmoidoscopy is an alternate option, but is not the preferred endoscopic modality as the entire colon is not visualized.

[3]High sensitivity fecal occult blood test (guaic-based or immunochemical).

[4]Preauthorization with one's insurance carrier is always advised.

This practice algorithm has been specifically developed for M.D. Anderson using a multidisciplinary approach and taking into consideration circumstances particular to M.D. Anderson, including the following: M.D. Anderson's specific patient population; M.D. Anderson's services and structure; and M.D. Anderson's clinical information. Moreover, this algorithm is not intended to replace the independent medical or professional judgment of physicians or other health care providers. This algorithm should not be used to treat pregnant women.

COLON CANCER

Note: If available, clinical trials should be considered as preferred treatment options for eligible patients. Initial evaluation should include assessment of family history for HNPCC, FAP, or other less-common germline mutations associated with colorectal cancer.

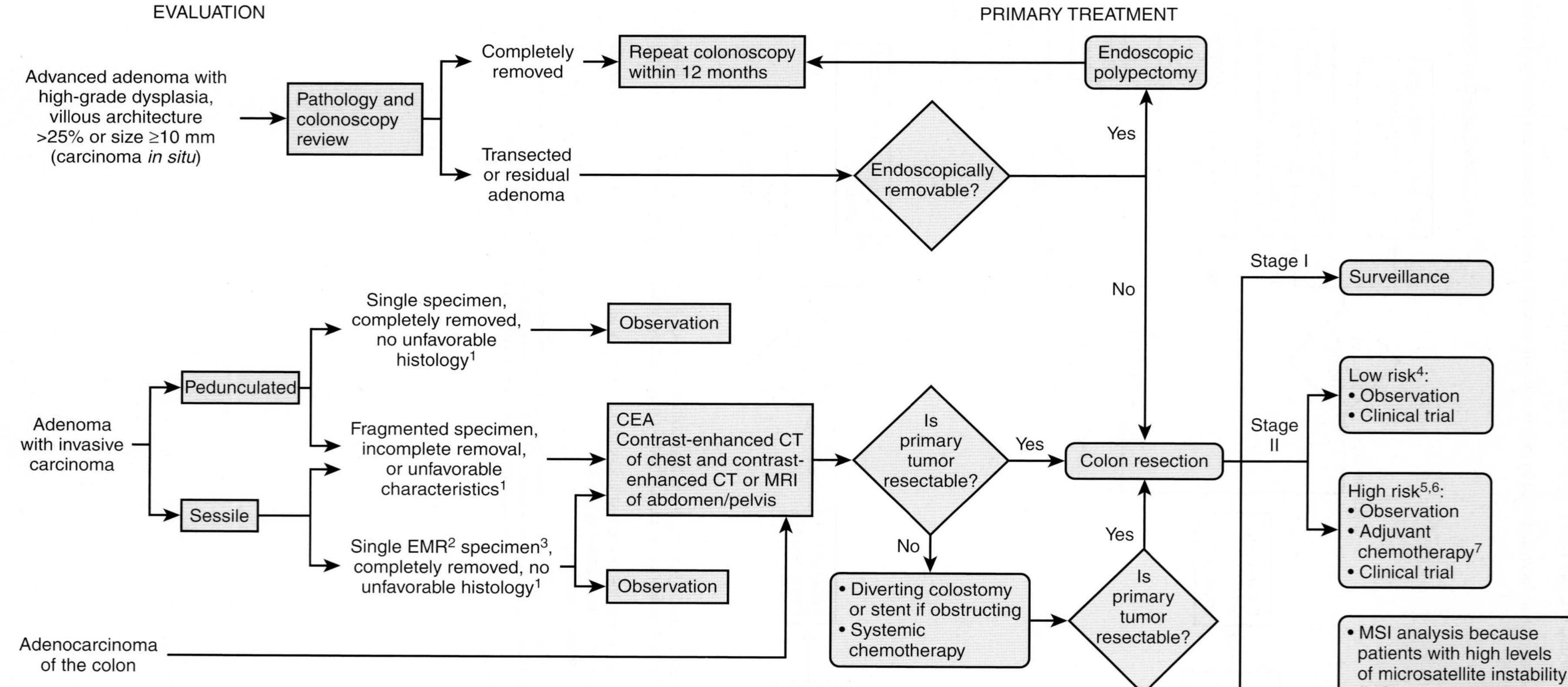

[1]Unfavorable pathology characteristics:
- Poor differentiation
- Lymphatic, vascular or perineural invasion
- Transection of carcinoma or resection margin <3 mm
- Sessile configuration of lesion

[2]EMR, endoscopic mucosal resection with submucosal elevation

[3]There is controversy regarding endoscopic management of malignant polyps. The depth of penetration into the submucosa has been shown to be associated with the risk of metastasis or recurrence. Those with minimal penetration into the submucosa and no adverse histologic features, may be candidates for EMR followed by observation. Careful histopathologic review is a prerequisite for this approach.

[4]Low-risk defined by absence of high-risk features (see footnote 5) or high levels of microsatellite instability (MSI-H) due to hazard ratio of 0.67.

[5]High-risk features for Stage II colon cancer:
- Poor differentiation
- Inadequate nodal sampling (<12 nodes)
- Lymphatic, vascular or perineural invasion
- T4 disease (invasion of serosa or other organ)

[6]In cases of tumor perforation, combination chemoradiation therapy to the tumor bed may be considered.

[7]Capecitabine or 5-fluorouracil/leucovorin or 5-fluorouracil/leucovorin/oxaliplatin or capecitabine/oxaliplatin

This practice consensus algorithm is not intended to replace the independent medical or professional judgment of physicians or other health care providers. Without specific instructions from an M.D. Anderson health care provider about individual patient care, this algorithm should be used for informational purposes only.

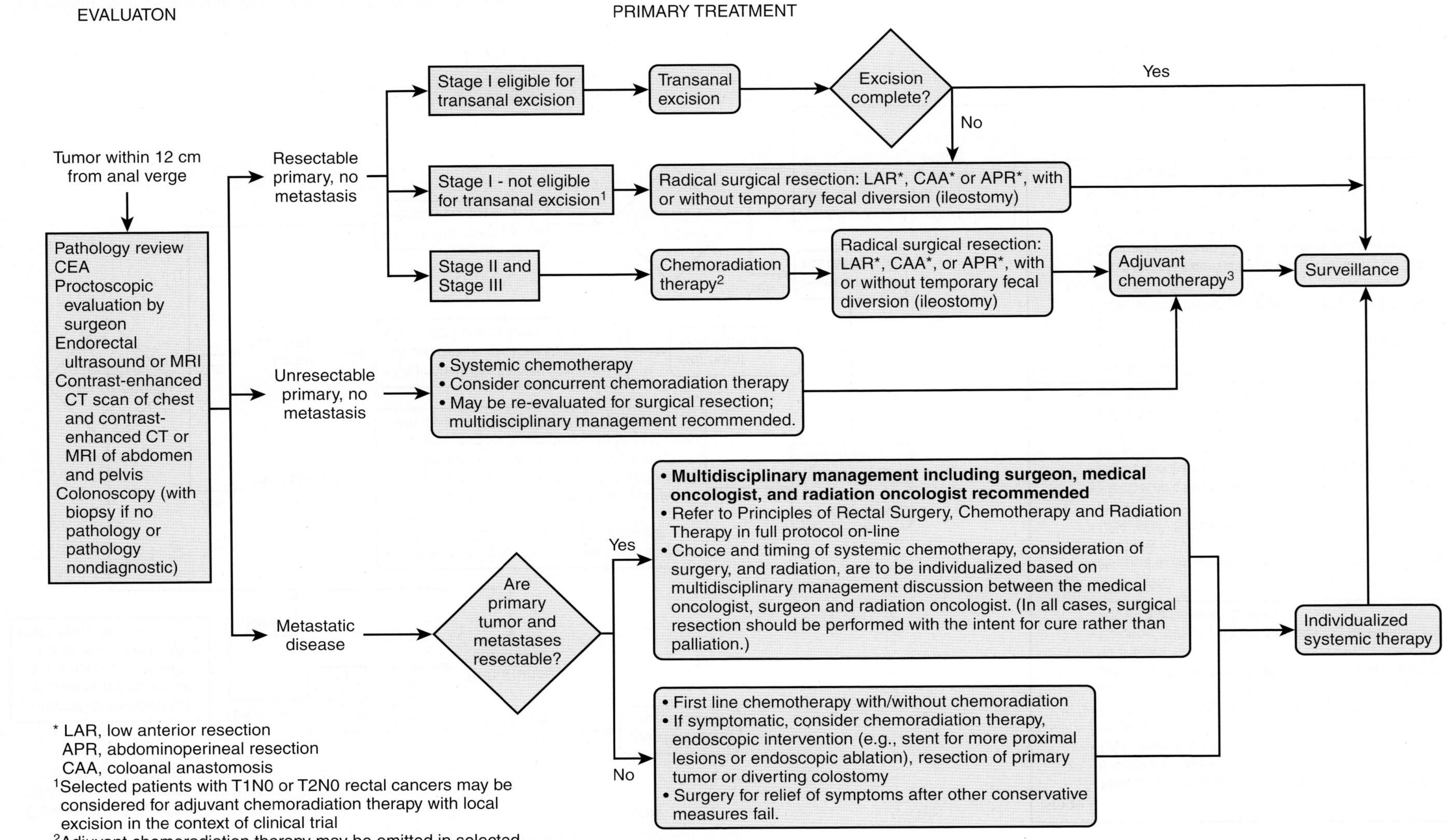

This practice consensus algorithm is not intended to replace the independent medical or professional judgment of physicians or other health care providers. Without specific instructions from an M.D. Anderson health care provider about individua patient care, this algorithm should be used for informational purposes only.

RECTAL CANCER

Note: If available, clinical trials should be considered as preferred treatment options for eligible patients. For adenomatous polyp with high-grade dysplasia, recommendations are the same as for colon cancer. Refer to Colon consensus algorithm.

EVALUATION AND MANAGEMENT OF SUSPECTED OR RECURRENT RECTAL CANCER

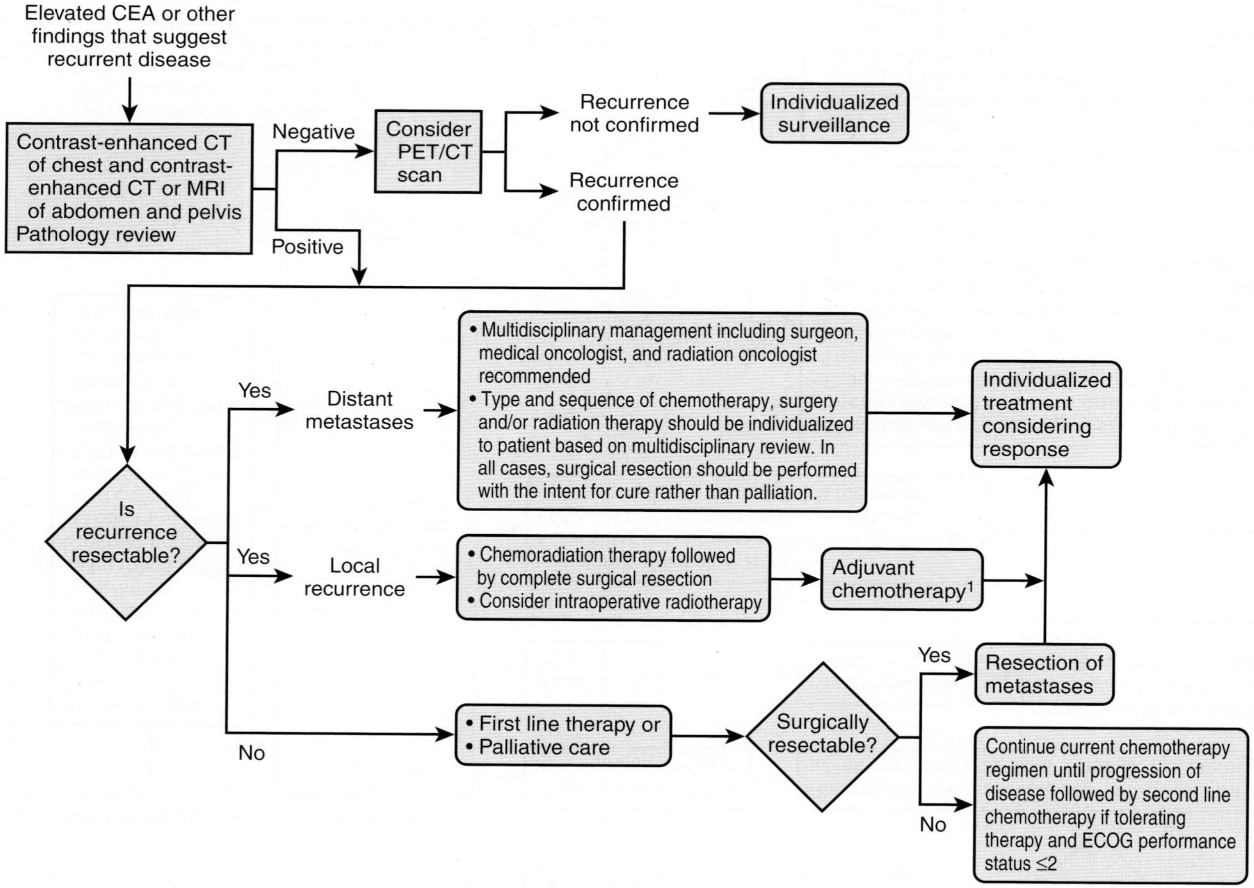

Elevated CEA or other findings that suggest recurrent disease
→ Contrast-enhanced CT of chest and contrast-enhanced CT or MRI of abdomen and pelvis
Pathology review

- Negative → Consider PET/CT scan
  - Recurrence not confirmed → Individualized surveillance
  - Recurrence confirmed → Is recurrence resectable?
- Positive → Is recurrence resectable?

Is recurrence resectable?

- Yes → Distant metastases →
  - Multidisciplinary management including surgeon, medical oncologist, and radiation oncologist recommended
  - Type and sequence of chemotherapy, surgery and/or radiation therapy should be individualized to patient based on multidisciplinary review. In all cases, surgical resection should be performed with the intent for cure rather than palliation.

  → Individualized treatment considering response
- Yes → Local recurrence →
  - Chemoradiation therapy followed by complete surgical resection
  - Consider intraoperative radiotherapy

  → Adjuvant chemotherapy[1] → Individualized treatment considering response
- No →
  - First line therapy or
  - Palliative care

  → Surgically resectable?
  - Yes → Resection of metastases → Individualized treatment considering response
  - No → Continue current chemotherapy regimen until progression of disease followed by second line chemotherapy if tolerating therapy and ECOG performance status ≤2

OBSERVATION/SURVEILLANCE*

Stage I:	• Physical exam: every 3–6 months for 3 years, then every 6 months for years 4–5 • CEA: every 3 months for 3 years, then every 6 months for years 4–5 • Proctoscopic examination every 6 months for 5 years • Contrast-enhanced CT scan of chest and contrast-enhanced CT of abdomen/pelvis or MRI every 12 months for 5 years • Colonoscopy: at one year then after 3 years (if normal) and then once every 5 years.
Stage II (low risk):	• Physical exam: every 3–6 months for 3 years, then every 6 months for years 4–5 • CEA: every 3 months for 3 years, then every 6 months for years 4–5 • Proctoscopic examination every 6 months for 5 years • Contrast-enhanced CT scan of chest and contrast-enhanced CT of abdomen/pelvis or MRI every 12 months for 5 years • Colonoscopy: at one year then after 3 years (if normal) and then once every 5 years.
Stage II (high risk) and Stage III:	• Physical exam: every 3 months for 3 years, then every 6 months for years 4–5 • CEA: every 3 months for 3 years, then every 6 months for years 4–5 • Proctoscopic examination every 6 months for 5 years • Contrast-enhanced CT scan of chest and contrast-enhanced CT of abdomen/pelvis or MRI every 12 months for at least 3 years • Colonoscopy: at one year then after 3 years (if normal) and then once every 5 years.

*NOTES:

- For patients who have not been irradiated, it is recommended that a flexible sigmoidoscopy be completed every 6 months for 5 years.
- Surveillance imaging with PET/CT alone is not recommended as primary imaging modality.

[1]Capecitabine or 5-fluorouracil/leucovorin or 5-fluorouracil/leucovorin/oxaliplatin

This practice consensus algorithm is not intended to replace the independent medical or professional judgment of physicians or other health care providers. Without specific instructions from an M.D. Anderson health care provider about individual patient care, this algorithm should be used for informational purposes only.

PART VI GENITOURINARY

CHAPTER 19 Renal Tumors

Raghunandan Vikram, M.D., and Eric Jonasch, M.D.

INTRODUCTION

Cancer of the kidneys constitutes nearly 2% of the total human cancer burden worldwide, with a slightly increased incidence in developed countries. Renal neoplasms represent several histologic subtypes that show a characteristic pattern of somatic mutations, which, along with histopathology, constitute the major criteria for their classification. The 2016 World Health Organization (WHO) classification of adult renal neoplasms[1] is based on cytologic, architectural, genetic, and molecular features and recognizes several newer subtypes. The increasing use of partial nephrectomy and other nephron-sparing techniques has generated an increasingly important role for pretreatment staging of renal cell carcinoma (RCC), in which factors such as perinephric and renal sinus fat and calyceal involvement are important in surgical planning for these patients. Moreover, the introduction of newer biologic therapeutic agents such as tyrosine kinase inhibitors, monoclonal antibodies, and checkpoint inhibitors has shown promise in treatment of metastatic RCC (mRCC). These agents bring about unique changes in the appearance of the target lesions of interest and may be valuable in guiding therapy and future research.

EPIDEMIOLOGY AND RISK FACTORS

RCC constitutes over 90% of all malignancies occurring in the kidney in adults. Overall, it is the twelfth most common site of cancer in men and 17th in women and represents 2% of all solid cancers in adults worldwide.[2] In males living in industrialized countries, including Japan, it is more common, ranking sixth along with non-Hodgkin lymphoma, whereas in less developed countries it ranks sixteenth. In the United States, it is the seventh most common site in males and the eighth most common site in females, with 14,830 deaths and 73,750 new cancers of the kidney and renal pelvis expected in the United States in 2020.[3,4]

The incidence of RCCs has been gradually increasing in both the United States and Europe over the past few decades. This is not entirely accounted for by increased detection of incidental carcinomas owing to frequent use of imaging studies, because the incidence of advanced RCC has also increased over time.[5] However, there has been a decreasing trend in incidence over the past few years. RCC is nearly twice as common in men as in women and in White people as in Black people. However, over the past few decades, there has been a rapid increase in incidence in women and also in Black people, thereby tilting these ratios. Age-adjusted incidence rates of RCC among White men, White women, Black men, and Black women in the United States from 1992 to 2002 were 13.8, 6.6, 16.8, and 8.0 per 100,000 person years, respectively.[3,5] In contrast to incidence trends, mortality from RCC has been declining in the recent decades. Between 2008 and 2017, the death rate decreased by 1% per year.[6]

Rates of RCC vary considerably internationally, sometimes by up to a factor of 10, with increased incidence in several Western countries including Australia/New Zealand and the lowest rates in Asia and Africa. These demographic trends highlight the significant role of exogenous risk factors.[2,7]

RCC can be familial or sporadic. The kidney is also associated with several inherited cancer syndromes. The familial RCC syndromes are briefly described later in this chapter.

Several exogenous and endogenous factors appear to contribute to the development of RCC (Table 19.1). Cigarette smoking is an established causal risk factor for developing RCC and is estimated to account for nearly 20% to 30% of cancers in men and 10% to 20% cancers in women. A metaanalysis including more than 20,000 patients reported estimated relative risks of developing

TABLE 19.1 Risk Factors for Developing Sporadic Renal Cell Carcinoma

Cigarette smoking
Obesity
Dietary factors
Hypertension and antihypertensive medications
Analgesics
Hormonal and reproductive factors
Kidney transplantation and dialysis
Radiation

RCC of 2.0 and 1.6 among heavy smokers for males and females, respectively, with a slow decline in risk with several years of cessation.[8]

Several studies have now provided compelling evidence that links obesity to an excess risk of RCC. It is estimated that the relative risk of RCC is increased by 1.07 per unit increase in body mass index.[9] Obesity is considered to be a causal factor in nearly 30% to 40% of all RCCs in the Western world.[5] The mechanism underlying the association between obesity and RCC is not clear, but several metabolic factors such as increased levels of peptide hormones, steroid hormones, or estrogen, and signaling pathways such as increased activation of the insulin-like growth factor-1 and interleukin-6 pathways have been hypothesized to be involved.

The differences in RCC incidence between Asia and the West suggest that diet may have an important role in its etiology. In general, diets low in fat and rich in fruits and vegetables have a protective effect.[10] There is an increased incidence of RCC in patients with hypertension, and the odds ratio is calculated by many authors to be 1.3 to 2.0. It is now thought that hypertension-induced renal injury is the risk factor, although the exact mechanism is unknown.[5,10] Although historically the use of analgesics, especially phenacetin, was linked to the risk of RCC, this has not been proven. Ionizing radiation is weakly linked to the development of RCC, and this increased incidence has been recorded in patients who received treatment for ankylosing spondylitis and cervical cancer.[5]

ANATOMY

The kidneys are paired structures situated in the retroperitoneum on either side of the vertebral bodies. Whereas most individuals have single renal arteries, multiple renal arteries are the most common anatomic variant, seen in up to 30% of normal individuals.[11,12]

Bilateral multiple renal arteries occur in approximately 10% to 15% of the population. Accessory renal arteries most commonly arise from the abdominal aorta and are classified as polar (supplying one of the poles) and hilar (running along with the main renal artery). The polar accessory renal arteries are usually slender, but the hilar renal artery is not always smaller than the main renal artery. Rarely, the accessory renal arteries arise from the celiac, mesenteric, lumbar, middle colic, or middle sacral artery.[13]

The left renal vein receives the gonadal and lumbar veins before draining into the inferior vena cava (IVC) anterior to the aorta and posterior to the superior mesenteric artery. The right renal vein, usually shorter than the left, directly drains into the IVC. Renal veins usually lie anterior to the arteries at the hilum. Multiple renal veins are the most common anatomic variant, seen in 15% to 30% of the population, and are more common on the right side. The most common anomaly of the left renal vein is the circumaortic renal vein, seen in 2% to 17% of the population, in which the left renal vein divides into ventral and dorsal limbs that encircle the aorta. A rarer anatomic variant, the retroaortic renal vein, is seen in 2% to 3% of the population.[13]

PATHOLOGY

It is now well understood that RCC is actually a family of related tumors with different histologies, prognoses, and therapies. The 2016 WHO classification describes various categories and entities based on pathologic and genetic analyses and builds upon previous classifications, including the Heidelberg classification. The classification system is based on the predominant cell type (clear-cell and chromophobe RCC), architectural feature (e.g., papillary RCC), anatomic location (such as collecting duct and medullary RCC), correlation with background renal disease (e.g., acquired cystic disease–associated RCCs), newly revealed and validated molecular alterations pathognomonic for RCC subtypes (MiT family translocation carcinomas and succinate dehydrogenase–deficient renal carcinomas) and familial predisposition syndromes (e.g., hereditary leiomyomatosis and RCC syndrome–associated RCC). Subtypes seen in some familial syndromes that are also seen as sporadic RCCs, such as clear-cell RCC in patients with von Hippel-Lindau syndrome or chromophobe RCC in patients with Birt–Hogg–Dubé syndrome.

Histologic subtypes include clear-cell ("conventional") adenocarcinoma (80%), papillary (15%), chromophobe (5%), collecting duct (1%), and unclassified (4%).[1,14,15] Major changes in the 2016 WHO classification include an emphasis on clarifying subtypes of RCCs according to familial inheritance and renaming multilocular cystic RCC as multilocular cystic renal neoplasm of low malignant potential, based on multiple reports that have shown no evidence of metastases. Papillary RCCs were classified as type 1 or type 2 RCC in the 2004 WHO system. It is now recognized that papillary type 2 RCC is not a homogenous entity, but rather a subgroup of tumors with different molecular backgrounds. Furthermore, adult cystic nephromas are now considered a variant of mixed epithelial and stromal tumors. The new classification system also discourages the use of the term "renal carcinoid" for neuroendocrine tumors of the kidney. An adapted version of classification is presented in Table 19.2.

Clear-cell carcinoma is the most common subtype, accounting for nearly 80% of all RCCs. Papillary RCC (15%) and chromophobe (5%) are the second and third most common subtypes. Each of these subtypes has

TABLE 19.2 World Health Organization Classification of Renal Tumors

Clear-cell renal cell carcinoma (RCC)
Multilocular cystic renal neoplasm of low malignant potential
Papillary RCC
Chromophobe RCC
Collecting duct carcinoma
Renal medullary carcinoma
MiT family translocation carcinoma
Tubulocystic renal cell carcinoma
Mucinous tubular and spindle cell carcinoma

(From Eble JM, Sauter G, Epstein JI, et al. *Pathology and genetics of tumors of the urinary system and male genital organs. World Health Organization Classification of Tumors.* Lyon: IARC Press; 2004.)

differing cytogenetic and immunohistochemical profiles, and each is thought to arise from a different part of the nephron. Histopathologic grading of the tumor nuclei divides them into the four-tier Fuhrman nuclear classification,[16] with grade I being the best-differentiated and grade IV the most anaplastic. There is a separate category of spindle-shaped cells with ominous prognostic significance seen in all histologic subtypes, referred to as a sarcomatoid variant. Clear-cell carcinoma displays large, uniform cells with abundant clear cytoplasm rich in glycogen and lipid (Fig. 19.1). All clear-cell kidney tumors of any size are considered malignant. Most clear-cell RCCs are solitary cortical neoplasms. They may be multicentric in up to 4% and bilateral in 0.5% to 3%. The term granular cell carcinoma, indicating acidophilic cytoplasm, was an entity in the 1998 WHO classification and is now considered to be clear-cell RCC based on clinical and pathologic similarities. Clear-cell RCC is typically highly vascular. Defects in the *VHL* suppressor gene are reported in over 60% of sporadic cases of clear-cell RCC.[17] The *VHL* gene is found on the short arm of chromosome 3, at 3p25. vHL protein, the product of this gene, is a potent tumor suppressor. Its loss, mutation, or inactivation in turn leads to higher expression levels of the hypoxia-inducible factor (HIF) family of transcription factors which are produced constitutively but bound to and degraded by a functional VHL protein under normoxic conditions. Under hypoxic conditions, or in absence of functional *VHL*, high levels of HIF will result in the transcription and translation of several proteins involved in tumor angiogenesis, including vascular endothelial growth factor.

Multilocular cystic renal neoplasm of low malignant potential is a tumor composed entirely of numerous cysts with low-grade tumor cells (grade 1 or 2). The cysts are lined by a single layer of tumor cells with abundant clear cytoplasm, similar to clear-cell carcinoma. (Figs. 19.2 and 19.3).[18,19] These tumors tend to be indolent and have a very low metastatic potential.

Papillary RCCs are characterized by abnormalities of chromosomes 7 and 17 and loss of chromosome Y. They typically have a papillary growth pattern and exhibit a frond-like appearance on histologic examination (Fig. 19.4). There is a 5:1 male predominance.

Hereditary papillary RCC is an autosomal dominant form of the disease associated with multifocal papillary RCC.[20] Papillary RCCs may have a less aggressive course than clear-cell RCC and are subdivided into cellular type 1 and type II. These tumors have cells arranged over a fibrovascular core and a papillary growth pattern. These terminologies are preferred over the terms "basophilic" (type 1 papillary) and "eosinophilic" (type 2 papillary) RCC, which were used in previous classifications. Type 2 papillary RCC is a heterogeneous entity, and the classification of this subtype is evolving. These are typically higher grade and more aggressive than type 1. Once metastatic, patients with papillary RCC fare more poorly than patients with clear cell histologies, owing to the absence of effective systemic therapies.

Chromophobe RCCs (Fig. 19.5) are a less aggressive subtype, with 86% of tumors being T1 or T2 at diagnosis. The relationship between oncocytoma and chromophobe RCC is still under investigation, and both are considered

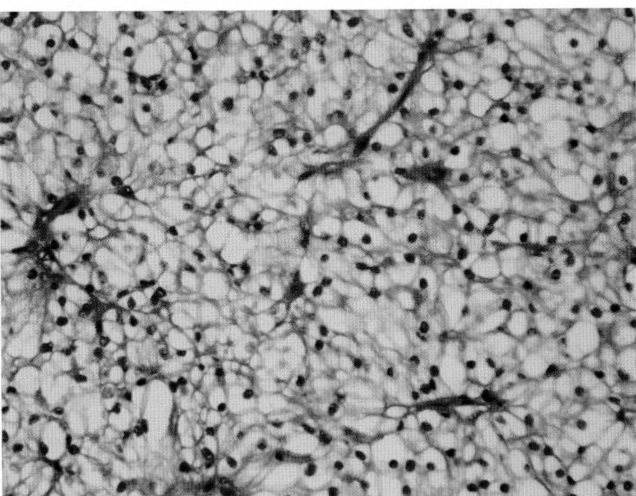

FIGURE 19.1. Clear-cell carcinoma. Histology image (×100 magnification) shows abundant clear cells filled with glycogen.

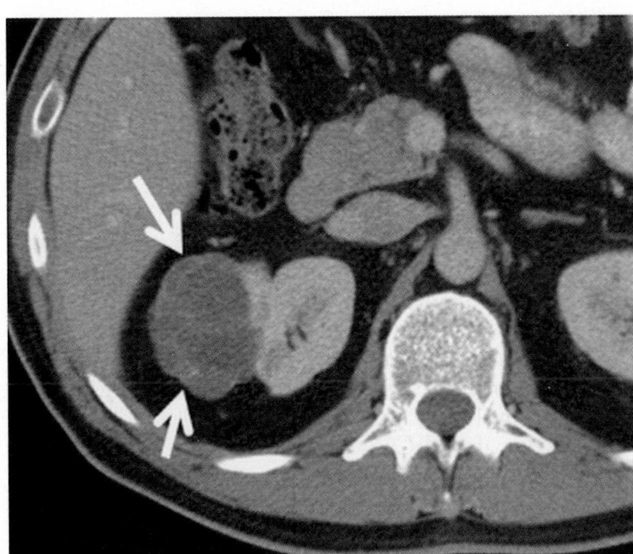

FIGURE 19.2. Multilocular cystic renal cell carcinoma. Contrast-enhanced computed tomography scan of the abdomen shows a multiloculated cystic mass in the right kidney with thin enhancing septa (*arrows*). There are no nodular solid components.

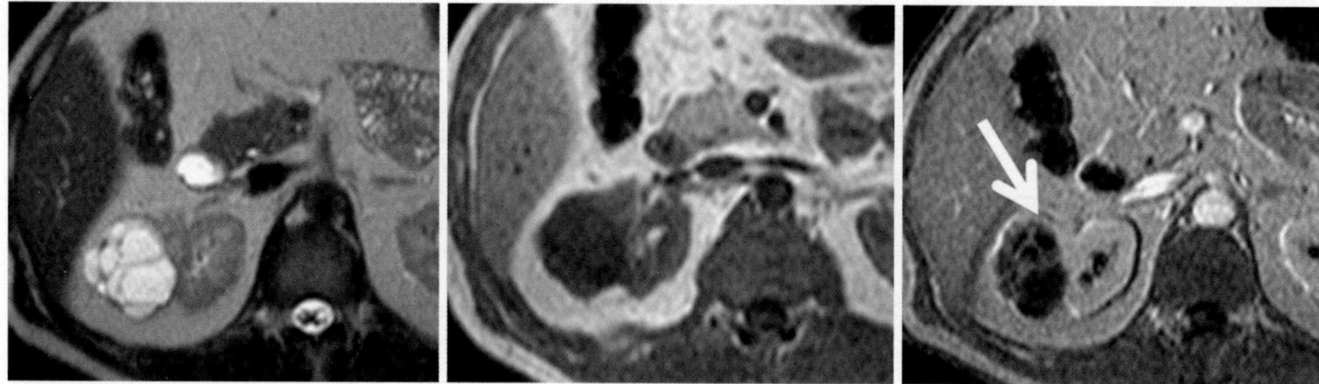

FIGURE 19.3. Multilocular cystic renal cell carcinoma. Axial T2-weighted (left) and axial T1-weighted pre- (center) and postcontrast (right) images of the abdomen show a multiloculated cystic mass with thin septa (*arrow*), which enhances on postcontrast images. No nodular solid component.

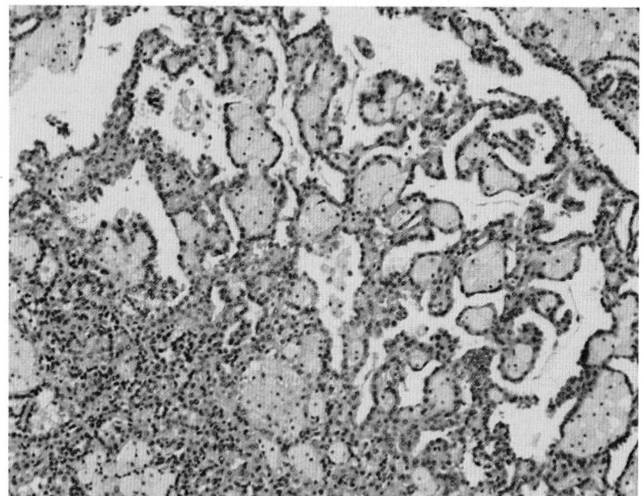

FIGURE 19.4. Papillary carcinoma. Histology image (×100 magnification) show the frond-like architecture typical of papillary tumors.

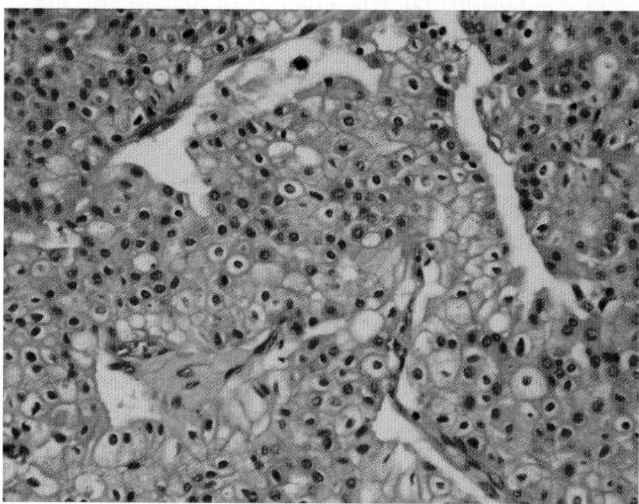

FIGURE 19.5. Chromophobe renal cell carcinoma. Histology specimen shows prominent pale cytoplasm with perinuclear halos.

to be derived from the intercalated cells of the collecting duct. The Birt–Hogg–Dubé syndrome is a form of inherited RCC also characterized by hair follicle hamartomas. Patients with this syndrome often have chromophobe tumors or mixed chromophobe tumors and oncocytomas.[21]

Oncocytomas are benign tumors that have a male predilection and a mean age of presentation in the 7th decade. They account for approximately 5% of renal tumors. Oncocytomas most often are detected as an incidental finding and average more than 7 cm in diameter. Occasionally, patients may complain of a flank mass, pain, or hematuria.

Sporadic oncocytomas are relatively common and are considered benign but indistinguishable from RCCs on imaging (Fig. 19.6).

Collecting duct RCCs, which arise from the medullary collecting duct, often occur in younger patients and frequently present with advanced disease at the time of diagnosis. Renal medullary carcinoma is a rare subtype, closely related to collecting duct carcinoma, with a very poor prognosis, that occurs in young patients with sickle cell trait.[22,23]

RCC has a propensity for extending, as a tumor thrombus, into the tributaries of the renal veins and subsequently to the main renal vein, IVC, hepatic veins, and potentially the right atrium. Rarely, the tumor may extend directly into the ipsilateral adrenal gland or adjacent musculature, liver, spleen, pancreas, and colon. Hematogenous metastases are more common and occur earlier than lymphatic dissemination, the former most commonly to the lungs and bone, but essentially to any organ, including the subcutaneous tissues and skeletal muscle. Lymphatic dissemination, however, can involve regional nodes and spread to the chest via the cisterna chylii with mediastinal nodal involvement.

KEY POINTS

Histologic Classification

- Clear-cell (conventional) renal cell carcinoma is the most common histologic subtype.
- Papillary tumors have a less aggressive course, except when metastatic.
- Chromophobe tumor is less aggressive and mostly T1 or T2 at diagnosis.
- Collecting duct tumor generally occurs in younger patients.

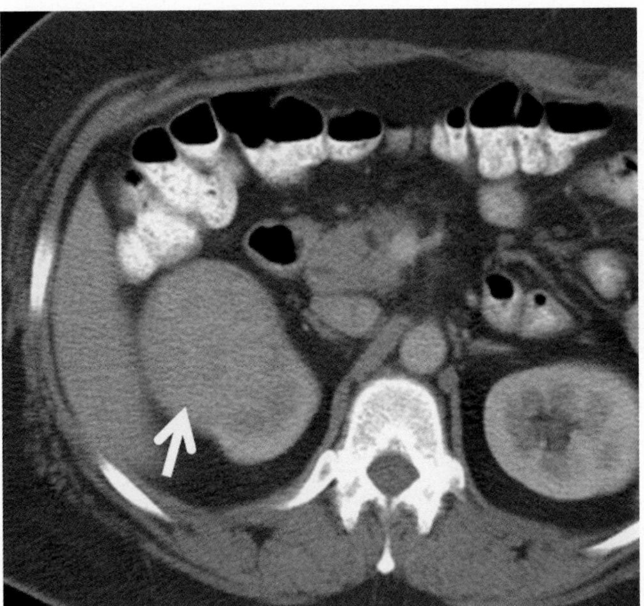

Figure 19.6. Axial computed tomography scan of the abdomen with intravenous contrast shows an enhancing mass (*arrow*) in the upper pole of the right kidney, histologically proven to be an oncocytoma. Oncocytomas are very similar and often indistinguishable from clear-cell renal cell carcinoma on imaging.

STAGING

Staging systems are designed to reflect the modes of spread (Fig. 19.7) and are used to stratify treatment options and prognoses and assess survival characteristics. The current version of the tumor-node-metastasis (TNM) staging of the American Joint Committee on Cancer and the Union for International Cancer Control was revised in 2017.[3,24,25]

The major changes from the previous version is clarification of the definition of T3a disease: the word "grossly" was eliminated from the description of renal vein involvement, and "muscle containing" was changed to "segmental veins." Another change to the classification system is the addition of invasion of the pelvicalyceal system to T3a disease. The Robson classification is an alternative staging system that no longer used but that is still referred to in some of the older literature.

Prognosis is generally reflected in staging severity, with lower-stage disease associated with longer survival rates. For example, a patient with a T1a N0 M0 lesion has a 90% to 100% probability of 5-year survival, whereas the probability of survival for a patient with a T3b-c N0 M0 lesion in this timeframe decreases to 40% to 65%. Systemic metastases at the time of presentation were previously associated with only 0% to 20% 5-year survival, although these estimates are increasing with improvements in therapy.[26–28] The histologic type of tumor is an important consideration not included in the TNM system. For example, the time from nephrectomy to metastasis is twice as long for patients with chromophobe tumors than for those with clear-cell or papillary subtypes.[29]

Key Points

Staging

- Prognosis is generally reflected by staging severity.
- Histology is an important consideration, but is not included in the tumor-node-metastasis system.

IMAGING EVALUATION

The goals of radiologic imaging are to detect and stage the primary tumor. In most institutions, computed tomography (CT) is the main imaging modality used for the evaluation of the intraabdominal component of renal tumors. In some specific instances, such as allergy to iodinated contrast medium or in patients with depressed renal function, magnetic resonance imaging (MRI) and ultrasound can provide complementary information.

A risk-adapted approach is generally used for workup of possible sites of metastases. Chest CT should be performed if the primary tumor is large or locally aggressive, because metastases are more common in these patients.[30] Plain chest radiography without CT should be reserved for patients with a very low risk of metastatic disease or for those in long-term follow-up. Brain MRIs and nuclear medicine bone scans are generally only justified if there are symptoms and signs to suggest disease at these sites, or if the tumor is large and locally aggressive (although even the latter is debated).[31] Technetium-99m methylene diphosphate bone scans, however, may have limitations in detecting the typical osteolytic bone metastases from RCC. The value of pelvic CT in staging is limited.[32]

Calcification, which can be detected on an abdominal radiograph in as many as 20% of renal adenocarcinomas, is even easier to detect on an unenhanced CT examination (Fig. 19.8). However, calcification also may be seen in other renal masses, including common lesions such as benign cysts. In all but very large tumors, renal function is preserved. In fact, diminished renal function suggests tumor thrombus in the renal vein. The tumor is identified as a mass with mottled density that causes a focal bulge in the renal contour. Such tumors are termed exophytic (Fig. 19.9). Tumors that do not deform the renal contour are termed intrarenal or central (Fig. 19.10). Tumors that have both an exophytic and a central component are referred to as mixed. Involvement of the collecting system is seen as irregularity of the urothelial surface or complete occlusion of a calyx or infundibulum. A filling defect within the collecting system may represent a blood clot or tumor invasion but is relatively uncommon with renal parenchymal tumors. In fact, if a mass is present in the collecting system, the lesion is more likely to represent a transitional cell carcinoma that has invaded the renal parenchyma, rather than an RCC that invades the collecting system. Some tumors, particularly those with sarcomatoid features, have an infiltrative appearance in which the reniform shape of the kidney is preserved (Fig. 19.11).

Occasionally, the tumor can be found arising in the wall of a simple renal cyst (Fig. 19.12). In some cases, the tumor

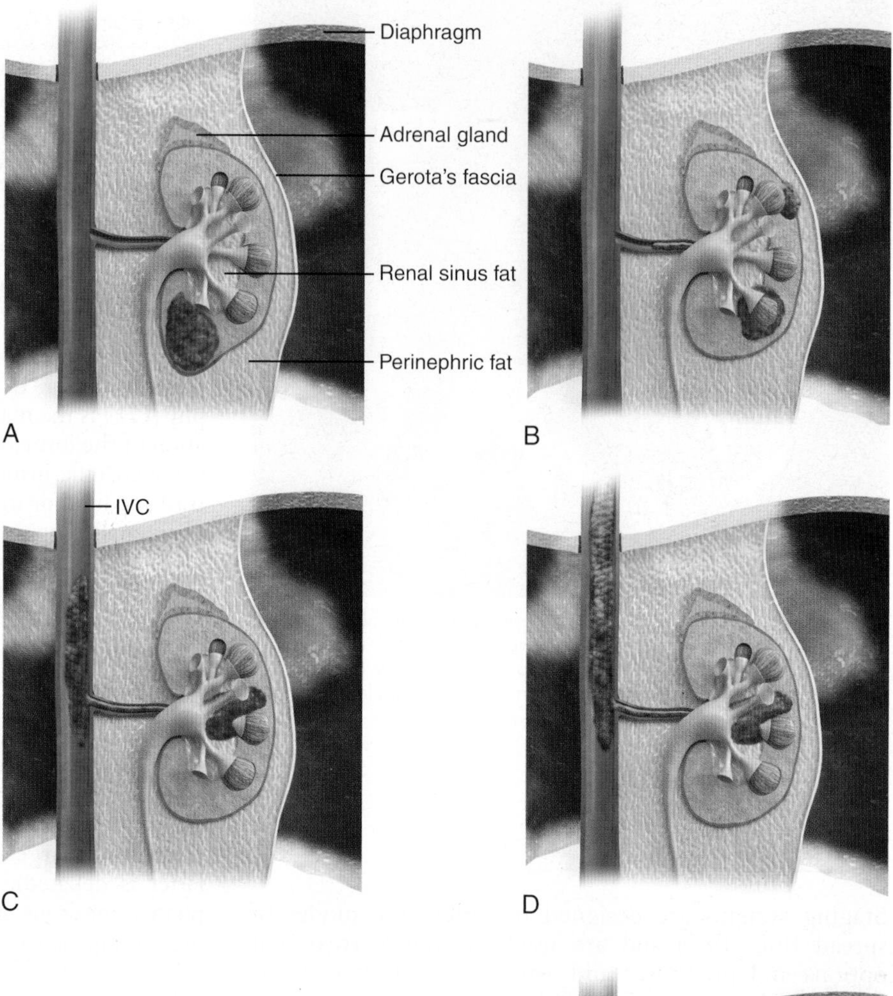

FIGURE 19.7. A-E, T staging according to the American Joint Committee on Cancer tumor-node-metastasis (TNM) staging system for renal cell carcinoma. Tumors confined to the kidney are staged as T1 when smaller than 7 cm and as T2 when larger than 7 cm. Tumors invading the renal sinus fat or perinephric fat are staged as T3a, and tumors involving Gerota's fascia and adrenal gland are staged T4. *IVC*, Inferior vena cava.

itself has a cystic appearance and may be difficult to distinguish from a complex but benign renal cyst. Hartman[33] estimates that 15% of cases of RCC are cystic on radiologic and pathologic examination. The clinical features of cystic RCC are similar to those that are completely solid. The majority will have clear-cell histology, but some may also be papillary.

Computed Tomography Evaluation

Suggested protocols for preoperative evaluation and follow-up using multislice CT (MSCT) are discussed. In addition to assessing tumor staging, preoperative evaluation focuses on delineating the tumor, paying particular attention to the relationship of the tumor to adjacent structures, including vascular relationships. In comparison, follow-up evaluation is directed toward surveillance for residual or recurrent disease. In general, 100 to 150 mL of iodinated intravenous (IV) contrast medium is used, with a flow rate of 2 to 3 mL/s.

Preoperative Computed Tomography Evaluation

The protocol for MSCT is to obtain noncontrast images of the liver and kidneys with 5-mm collimation in 5-mm

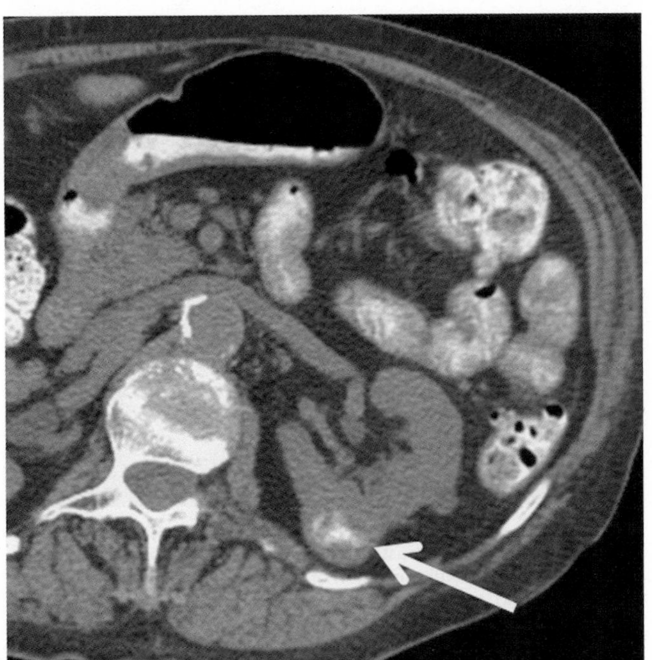

FIGURE 19.8. Axial computed tomography scan of the abdomen without intravenous contrast. Dystrophic calcification is seen in a exophytic mass (*arrow*), proven to be a renal cell carcinoma in the left kidney.

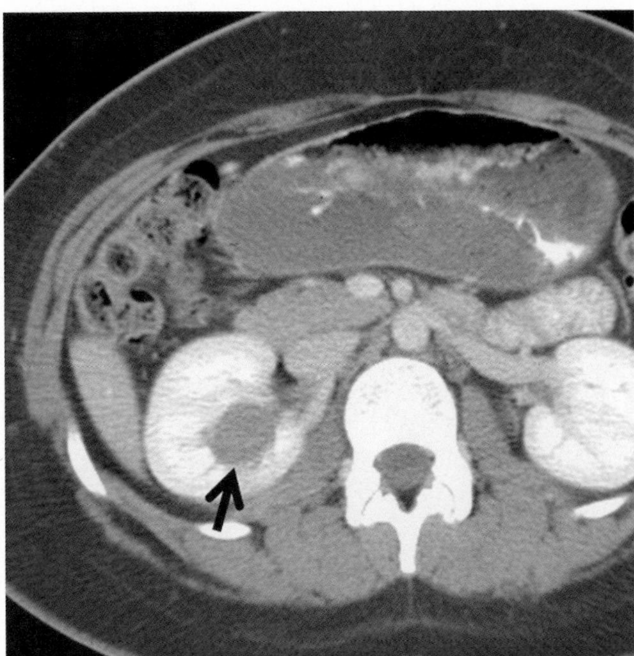

FIGURE 19.10. Axial computed tomography scan of the abdomen with intravenous contrast shows a central tumor (*arrow*) in the right kidney.

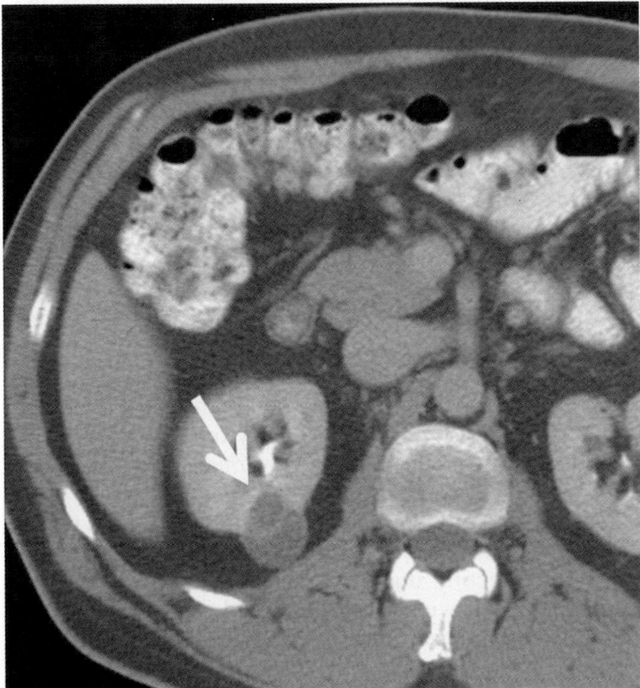

FIGURE 19.9. Axial computed tomography scan of the abdomen with contrast shows a partially enhancing exophytic mass (*arrow*) arising from the dorsal aspect of the right kidney.

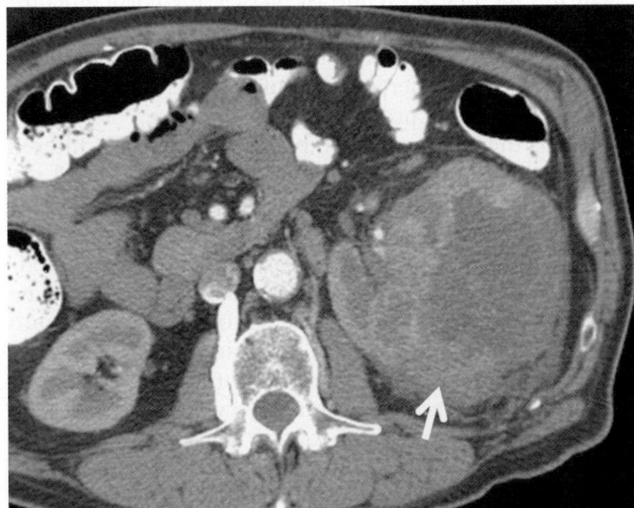

FIGURE 19.11. Axial computed tomography scan of the abdomen with intravenous contrast show an infiltrative-appearing renal tumor (*arrow*) in the left kidney. Note that the reniform shape of the kidney is maintained.

increments. Unenhanced images of the kidneys allow detection of calcification or fat within the kidney and assessment of postcontrast enhancement, and assist in characterizing the lesion. Postcontrast images targeted on the kidneys are obtained in the arterial, late arterial (corticomedullary/portal venous), nephrographic, and excretory phases at 45 to 60, 80 to 90, and 180 seconds after commencement of the IV infusion, respectively. Some 100 to 150 milliliters of contrast is injected at 2 to 4 mL/s using a power injector.

Imaging of the remaining abdominal structures is obtained in the portal venous phase. Excretory phase images from the kidneys through the bladder are generally obtained to complete the evaluation of the entire urinary tract when requested by the referring clinician.

Images are then obtained using IV contrast in the corticomedullary (15–30 s postinjection), nephrographic (60–90 s postinjection), and excretory (180–300 s postinjection) phases.

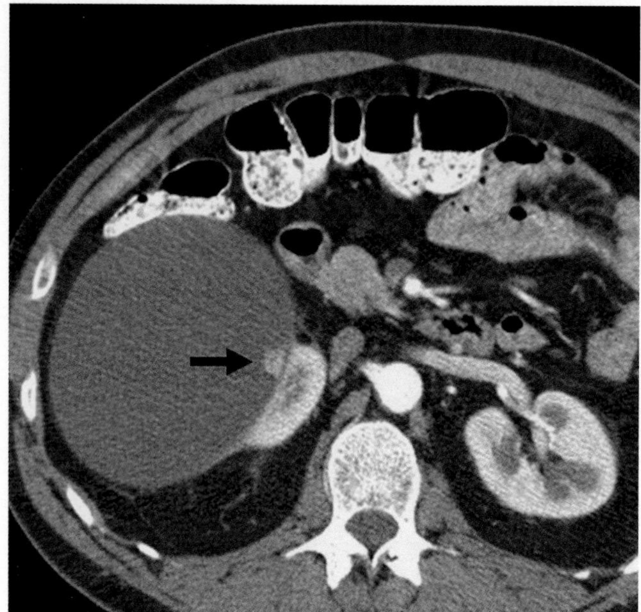

FIGURE 19.12. Axial computed tomography scan of the abdomen with intravenous contrast shows an enhancing tumor nodule (*arrow*) in the wall of a large renal cyst.

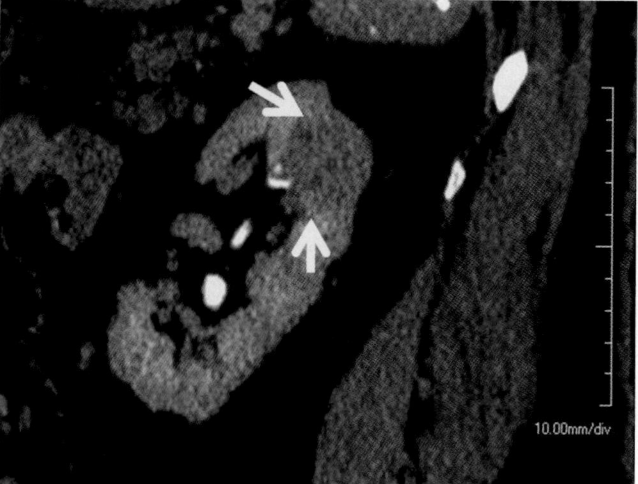

FIGURE 19.13. Sagittal reconstruction of computed tomography scan of the left kidney with contrast in the excretory phase shows a mass in the upper pole (*arrows*) with distortion of the upper pole calyx. Multiplanar reformatted and three-dimensional volume-rendered presentations of the renal phase images are helpful in allowing appreciation of the relationships of structures.

During the first postcontrast phase—the corticomedullary phase—much of the contrast resides in the renal cortical capillaries. The cortex enhances markedly in contrast to the medulla. The differences in enhancement of the cortex and the medulla are pronounced in this phase.

During the nephrographic phase, the contrast, filtered through the glomeruli, enters the loop of Henle and the collecting ducts. It is to be noted that the nephrographic phase can occur earlier in patients injected with contrast at a rapid rate. During the nephrographic phase, renal medullary enhancement is similar to that of the cortex. The excretory phase begins when the contrast is excreted into the calyces at approximately 3 to 5 minutes. Although the nephrograms remain homogeneous in the excretory phase, the attenuation decreases uniformly, owing to a decrease in the plasma concentration of contrast and continued excretion from the kidneys.[34] The corticomedullary phase and all the subsequent phases can last longer in patients with renal dysfunction and in those with diminished cardiac output.

Multiplanar reformatted and three-dimensional (3D) volume-rendered presentations of the renal phase images are helpful in allowing appreciation of the relationships of structures, particularly for surgeons (Fig. 19.13). Such reformations are best obtained with the thinnest possible collimation and some degree of reconstruction interval overlap (typically a <1.5-mm interval and 10%–50% overlap) and transferred to a workstation for the purpose of creating multiplanar reformatted images, 3D volume rendering, and maximum intensity projection images. The late-arterial phase provides a useful angiographic image of arterial and venous supply to the kidney, but it has limited additional utility for lesion detection and characterization when a nephrographic phase is employed. The combination of excretory and nephrographic phases has been shown to improve lesion detection and staging.[35,36]

It has been shown by several investigators that clear-cell RCC enhances to a greater extent and is more heterogeneous in appearance than other histologic subtypes of RCC (Fig. 19.14). Kim and coworkers[37] showed that an increase in attenuation of 84 Hounsfield units in the corticomedullary phase differentiated clear-cell RCC from nonclear-cell tumors, with a sensitivity of 74% and a specificity of 100%. Herts and colleagues[38] showed that papillary tumors were more homogeneous and had a much lower tumor-to-parenchyma enhancement ratio than was present in nonpapillary subtypes, particularly with tumors less than 3 cm in diameter (Fig. 19.15). Chromophobe tumors also are less hypervascular than clear-cell tumors and tend to have a more peripheral pattern of enhancement; their appearance, however, is not sufficiently characteristic to allow them to be reliably differentiated from papillary lesions (Fig. 19.16). Oncocytomas cannot be reliably differentiated from RCCs by imaging and thus are also considered to be surgical lesions (see Fig. 19.15). The well-known prominent central scar that can be used to suggest the diagnosis may also be present in necrotic clear-cell tumors. Collecting duct and medullary RCC tumors are located centrally within the kidney and show variable, typically limited, postcontrast enhancement (Figs. 19.17 and 19.18). They cannot be reliably distinguished from other RCCs or urothelial tumors, but a medullary tumor can be suggested when an aggressive tumor in a young patient with sickle cell disease or trait is encountered.

Extension of tumor into the renal veins has been reported to occur in 20% to 35% of patients and into the IVC in 4% to 10%. Invasion can be seen in all three segments of the IVC (infrahepatic 50%, intrahepatic IVC 40%, and intraatrial 10%).[42,43]

Identification of thrombus within the venous system, especially the IVC, is particularly important because it affects surgical management, typically necessitating an anterior abdominal approach. Furthermore, if thrombus

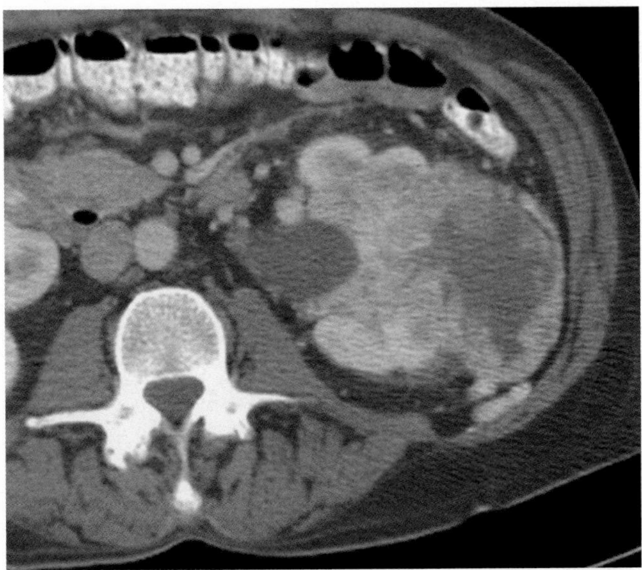

FIGURE 19.14. Large heterogeneous-enhancing mass in the left kidney revealed clear cell carcinoma on excision.

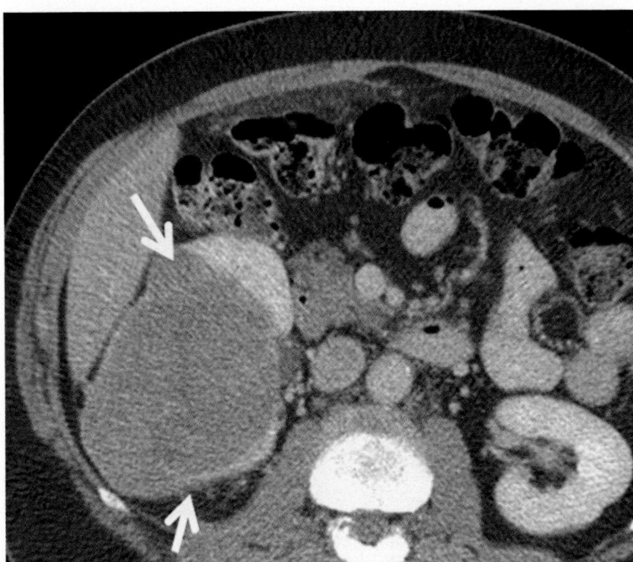

FIGURE 19.16. Chromophobe renal cell carcinoma. Relatively hypovascular, homogeneous expansile mass (*arrows*) arises from the right kidney.

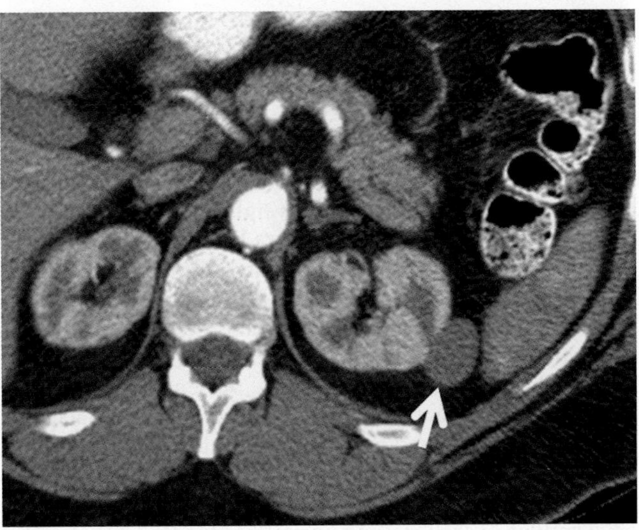

FIGURE 19.15. Papillary renal cell carcinoma. A small, poorly enhancing mass (*arrow*) arises from the lateral aspect of the left kidney.

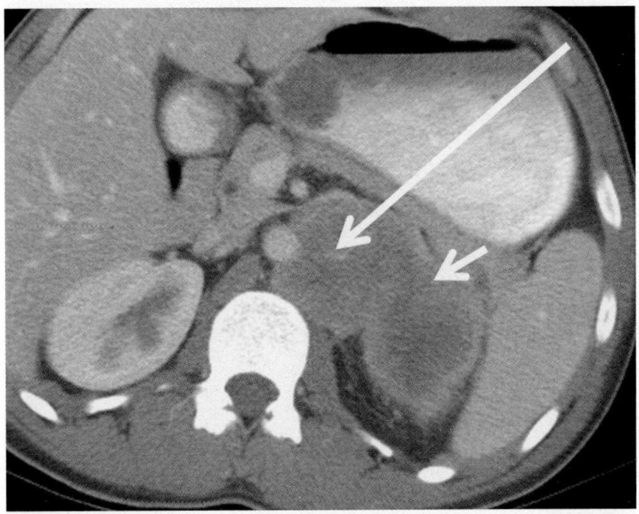

FIGURE 19.17. Axial computed tomography scan with intravenous contrast in a young patient with sickle cell trait shows an infiltrating mass (*short arrow*) of the left kidney with paraaortic adenopathy (*long arrow*). This proved to be a medullary carcinoma.

extends into the heart, a combined thoracic and intracardiac approach with cardiac bypass may be required. Current CT techniques have reported sensitivities and specificities for detecting renal vein thrombus of 85% and 98%, respectively.[44] Color Doppler ultrasonography has reported sensitivities and specificities for detecting thrombus in the renal veins of 75% and 96%, respectively, with 100% accuracy for detection of thrombus in the IVC.[45] MRI has similar reported sensitivity and specificity for detecting thrombus in the renal vein, at 86% to 94% and 75% to 100%, respectively, and also has 100% accuracy for detecting IVC thrombus.[46,47] MRI, with its multiplanar capability, is probably the best modality for identifying the superior extent of IVC involvement (Fig. 19.19).[48,49]

Fortunately, prognosis is not adversely affected by tumor within the venous system, nor its level within the IVC, provided the tumor is free-floating and can be successfully removed (5-year survival rates of 50%–69% in the absence of metastatic disease). It is, however, severely impaired if the tumor invades into the wall of the IVC (5-year survival 25%), although this can improve if the involved IVC can be resected completely (5-year survival rate 57%).[50–52] Unfortunately, current imaging modalities have some limitations in distinguishing bland from tumor thrombus and in distinguishing invasive from noninvasive tumor with respect to the vessel wall.[52] Intravascular tissue that enhances after IV contrast administration or that contains neovascularization ("thread-and-streak" sign) is good evidence of tumor, rather than bland, thrombus (Fig. 19.20).

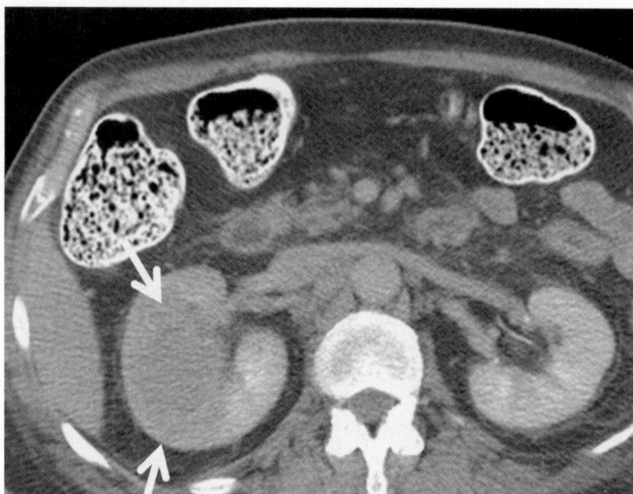

FIGURE 19.18. Axial computed tomography scan with intravenous contrast shows a large, relatively poorly enhancing mass (*arrows*) in the right kidney, proven to be a collecting duct tumor.

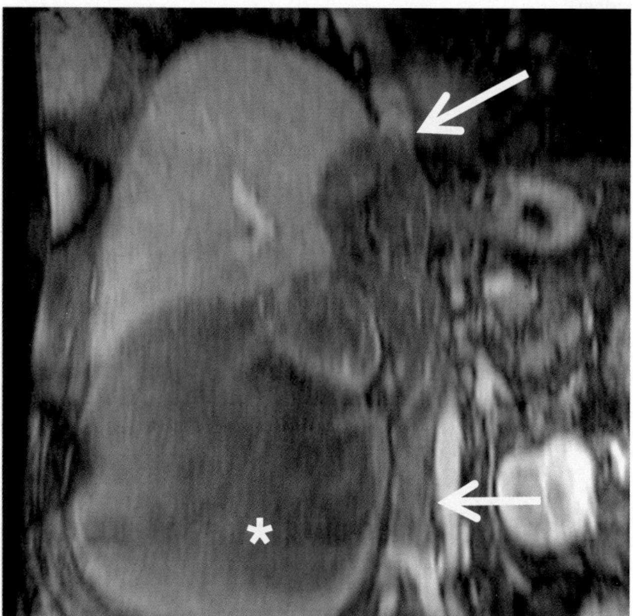

FIGURE 19.19. Coronal postcontrast fat-suppressed T1-weighted magnetic resonance imaging acquisition in a patient with a large right renal cell carcinoma (*asterisk*) with extension into the inferior vena cava (IVC). Note fine tumor vasculature in the tumor thrombus (*arrows*) in the IVC.

Magnetic Resonance Imaging Evaluation

MRI is generally used when optimal CT cannot be performed, as in the case of severe allergy to iodinated contrast medium or pregnancy. MRI also finds application in instances in which there is equivocal contrast enhancement on CT or in instances of hemorrhagic lesions. MRI has similar reported overall staging accuracies compared with CT. Its multiplanar capability, however, is particularly useful for delineating the superior extent of tumor within the IVC.[52–54]

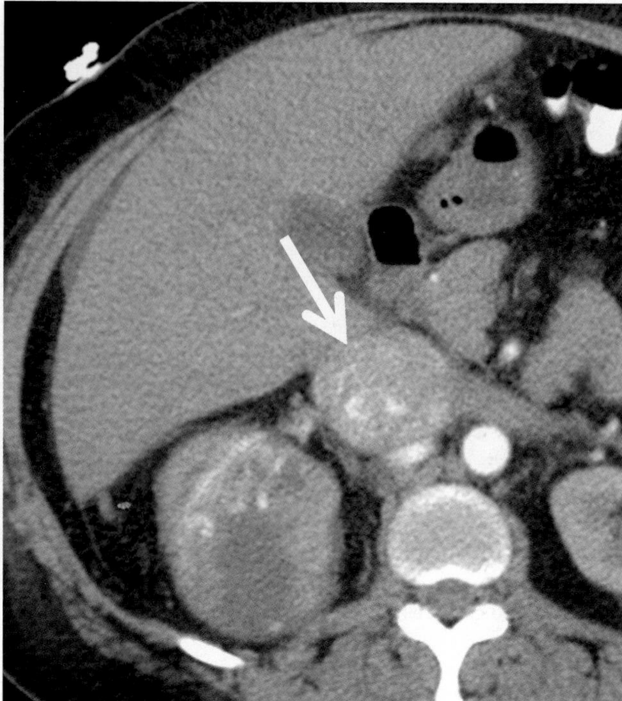

FIGURE 19.20. Renal cell carcinoma with tumor extension to inferior vena cava (*arrow*). Neovascular tumor thrombus shows the "thread-and-streak" sign.

Coronal and axial conventional T1-weighted (T1W) and axial fast spin echo T2-weighted (T2W) fat-suppressed images of the abdomen are generally used. Images are supplemented by dynamic contrast-enhanced 3D fast spoiled gradient echo sequences to further delineate the primary tumor and/or liver lesions and to evaluate any vascular thrombus identified; in particular, tumor (rather than bland) thrombus is indicated by the presence of enhancing vessels within the thrombus. Multiple dynamic acquisitions can be employed to obtain arterial, nephrogenic, and pyelographic-like images.[49,55–57]

Multidetector row CT with 3D reformations and MRI have similar overall staging accuracies for RCC.[58]

Ultrasound Evaluation

Ultrasound can be useful to assessing the presence and extent of venous thrombus. It can also be helpful in distinguishing cysts from hypovascular solid tumors seen on CT (e.g., papillary RCC). Ultrasound is able to see the septations better, owing to complex interfaces to the ultrasound beam. Ultrasound has reported accuracies for T staging of 77% to 85% and detection of venous thrombus of 87%.[43,45,59] However, it has limitations in visualizing the retroperitoneum and perinephric tissues, although some proponents argue otherwise.[30,43,45,60]

Partial nephrectomy has seen an increased use of image guidance during the operative procedure. Of the potential intraoperative modalities that can be used, ultrasound is the best, based on its portability, real-time capabilities, and access. Use of ultrasound at the time of operation allows

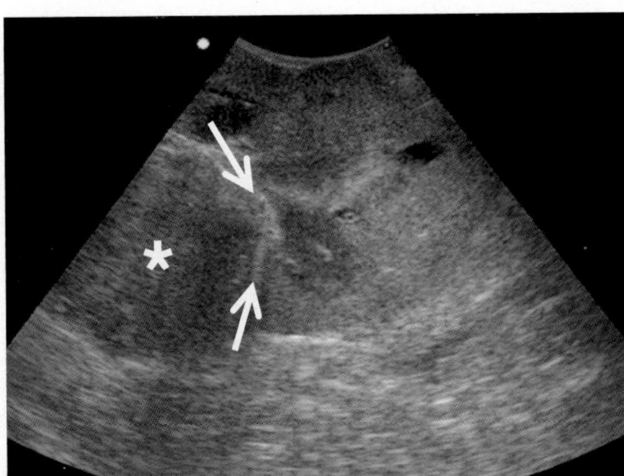

FIGURE 19.21. Intraoperative ultrasound shows a solid mass (*asterisk*) in the upper pole of the kidney abutting and distorting the renal sinus fat (*arrows*).

high-resolution imaging of the tumor and the kidney, because it allows for use of a high-frequency probe that can be applied directly on the surface of the kidney. Intraoperative ultrasound guidance offers multiple advantages to the surgeon (Fig. 19.21).[61]

Small tumors that are completely below the surface of the kidney can be identified by intraoperative ultrasound guidance, thereby allowing the surgeon to "see" before placing an incision on the surface of the kidney.[62] Moreover, the accurate depiction of the relationship of the tumor to the vascular structures and the calyces allows the surgeon to avoid injuries to these structures and still achieve negative margins. Intraoperative ultrasound frequently identifies occult lesions that are not seen on conventional imaging modalities such as contrast-enhanced CT or MRI. Such lesions can also be characterized. Purely cystic lesions are benign and can be ignored. Partially cystic and solid lesions are suspicious and can be excised. This modality can be used for both open and laparoscopic approaches. Intraoperative ultrasound can also be used to monitor radiofrequency ablation (RFA) or cryotherapy of a tumor during laparoscopy.[63]

PERCUTANEOUS BIOPSY

Attitudes toward biopsy have undergone some refinement in the past 20 years. In the past, biopsy was discouraged or even thought to be potentially dangerous, but this is no longer the case, and biopsy is now recognized as a valuable adjunct to management in selected patients. Preoperative percutaneous biopsy of the renal lesion is still not routinely undertaken in the nonmetastatic setting or before cytoreductive nephrectomy in the metastatic setting, because the results usually do not affect what therapy will be recommended, except in patients with multiple tumors or occasionally in patients with an underlying predisposing condition. Percutaneous biopsies may be considered in selected cases; for example, when abscesses or metastatic disease from a known primary is suspected, especially from lymphoma or melanoma.[53,64] It is also generally performed in patients who will undergo ablative or thermal therapy to determine the underlying histologic subtype of the tumor or the need for retreatment in patients who have undergone ablative therapy in whom imaging studies are equivocal. Biopsy is also mandated in the presence of central lesions that could arise from the renal collecting system to differentiate between a transitional cell carcinoma and an RCC.

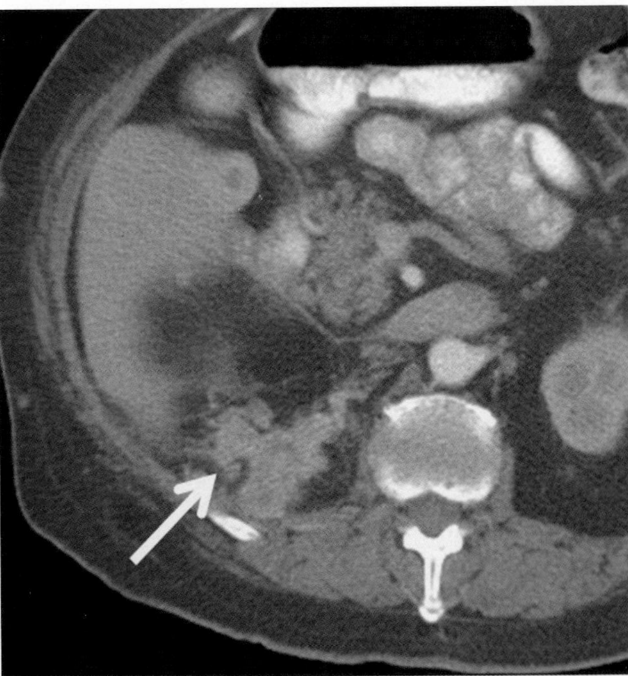

FIGURE 19.22. Recurrent renal cell carcinoma (*arrow*) in the surgical bed on the right kidney 18 months postradical nephrectomy for a clear-cell renal cell carcinoma.

PATTERNS OF METASTASIS

RCC metastasizes both hematogenously and by lymphatic spread. Hematogenous spread occurs via the renal vein and into the lungs; when tumor cells invade the systemic circulation, bloodborne metastases ensue. Metastasis to regional lymph nodes in the perinephric space is the initial manifestation of lymphatic spread. Tumor cells may then travel via the thoracic duct to involve nodal groups elsewhere in the body. In addition, RCC may recur in the surgical bed (Fig. 19.22). In a comprehensive review of patterns of tumor recurrence and spread, Chae and associates[65] concluded that 83% of recurrences occurred within the first 2 years after surgery; nonetheless, late recurrences, sometimes as long as 10 years after initial surgery, have been reported. Lung and bone metastases most commonly manifest within 1 to 2 years after initial surgery. Recurrence in the nephrectomy site, however, occurred at varying times between 1 and 3 years after surgery. As expected, there was a significant correlation between tumor size and stage and the occurrence of metastatic disease and the nuclear (Fuhrman) grade of the tumor. The most frequent sites of distant metastasis are, in decreasing order of frequency, lung (38%–71%), bone (17%–37%), lymph nodes (12%–63%), and liver (15%–23%), followed by adrenal gland, contralateral kidney, retroperitoneum, and brain with approximately 5% each.[66]

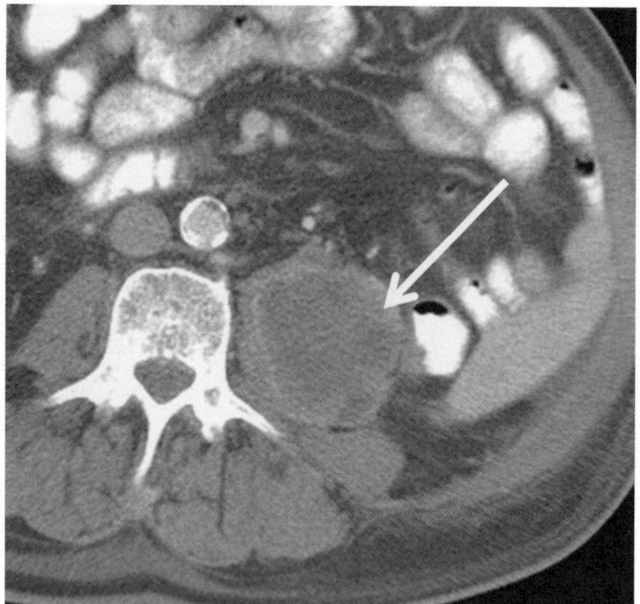

FIGURE 19.23. Axial computed tomography scan of the abdomen with intravenous contrast in a patient after left radical nephrectomy shows psoas muscle metastasis (*arrow*).

Metastasis to almost any organ or muscle (Fig. 19.23), however, can occur.

KEY POINTS

Metastasis

Most frequent sites of metastasis from renal cell carcinoma

- Lung
- Bone
- Retroperitoneal and mediastinal lymph nodes
- Nephrectomy site
- Brain
- Liver

The pancreas (Fig. 19.24) is an uncommon, but well-recognized, site for metastasis from RCC. These metastases tend to occur with a long lead time after initial diagnosis; Ghavamian and coworkers[67] reported a mean of 10 years after initial presentation. Typically, pancreatic metastases are well-defined single or multiple hypervascular masses found anywhere in the pancreas. Surgical resection of the metastases is feasible, and in one report mean survival after resection was more than 4 years. Because the majority of such lesions are hypervascular, Ng and colleagues emphasized the value of early-phase images for their detection.[68]

KEY POINTS

Suggested Radiology Report of a patient with newly diagnosed carcinoma of the kidney should include:

- Describe size and location of tumor within the kidney.
- Describe tumor as exophytic, central, or mixed.
- Describe the relationship of the tumor to the central renal sinus.

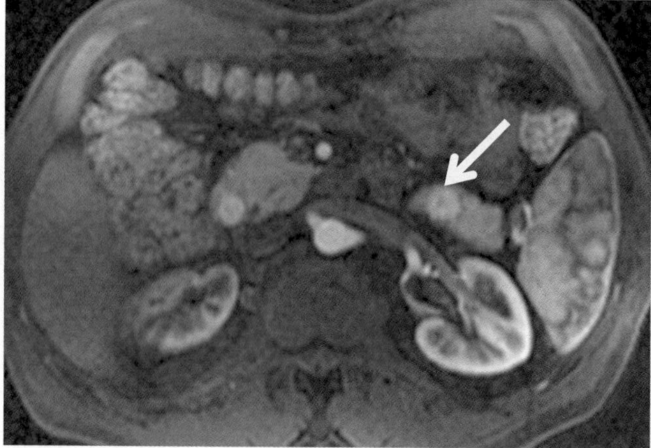

FIGURE 19.24. Axial T1-weighted postcontrast magnetic resonance imaging shows an enhancing metastatic renal cell carcinoma (*arrow*) in the tail of the pancreas.

- Describe the status of the renal vein and regional nodes.
- Describe any visible metastatic lesions.

Staging

- Venous invasion is important to detect because it affects surgical management.
- Prognosis is not advertently affected by venal vein invasion if the tumor is free-floating and resectable.
- High-quality imaging is important for accurate staging.
- Imaging is critical to staging metastases.

THERAPY

Surgical Therapy

Radical Nephrectomy

Survival after the surgical treatment of RCC markedly improved after the 1960s when Robson and associates[69] showed that radical nephrectomy had a superior survival advantage over other forms of surgery performed at the time. Other studies soon followed and corroborated Robson and associates' initial reports.[70,71] Radical nephrectomy, as initially defined by Robson and associates, included early vascular ligation, extrafascial (outside Gerota's fascia) dissection of the kidney, *en bloc* resection of the adrenal gland, and extensive lymphadenectomy from the crus of the diaphragm to the aortic bifurcation. Since then, these associated procedures have been shown to be unnecessary in most cases. For example, the overall incidence of adrenal metastasis is quite low, generally less than 5%. The possibility of adrenal involvement seems to increase with left-sided, large, upper pole, and high-stage tumors, as well as when multiple metastatic sites are present.[72] Contemporary radiographic imaging has been found to be a very sensitive tool for detection of adrenal metastasis, but it may not be specific enough in all cases, because benign lesions may be confused for malignancy.[73] A 99.4% negative predictive value of preoperative CT scans has been reported.[74] The stage is dependent, with T1 to T2 disease associated with a 0.6% rate of adrenal involvement, T3 with 7.8%, and T4 disease with 40%. Therefore, resection of the adrenal gland during radical nephrectomy is not always necessary, particularly if it appears normal on axial imaging, and especially for clinical T1 tumor that does not abut or involve the adrenal gland.

As another example of the shifting trend toward "less radical" radical nephrectomy, lymphadenectomy is not frequently performed for the typical case of RCC because of the lack of a meaningful survival benefit. It is primarily used for staging in select cases only.[75–77] The incidence of lymph node metastases can range from 3% to 15%, varying based on the number of lymph nodes removed, as well as tumor stage, the presence of a sarcomatoid component, necrosis, and tumor grade.[77–81] In addition, lymph node enlargement measuring less than 2 cm on axial imaging is not always attributed to malignant causes.[82] Thus, in these cases, although resection may be reasonable to perform for diagnostic purposes, the therapeutic benefit for most patients is unclear.[83] Interestingly, during the cytokine era, it was shown that patients with metastatic disease but without lymph node involvement (N0 M1) were more likely to respond to systemic interleukin-2 (IL-2) therapy than patients with N+ M1 disease.[76,84] It should be noted also that these data exclusively apply to the conventional, or clear-cell, form of RCC. For papillary RCC, lymphadenectomy can actually provide a survival advantage for those with N+ M0 disease, because this variant represents a distinctly different biology.[85] Such patients may experience a significant increase in recurrence-free survival after complete surgical resection.

As a further example of shifting trends, the gold standard of radical nephrectomy is being supplanted by nephron-sparing surgery (NSS) for nearly all tumors less than 4 cm in size and for many that are 4 to 7 cm in size. Several long-term studies have shown equivalent survival of patients undergoing NSS versus radical nephrectomy for a unilateral renal tumor less than 4 cm in size, with equivalent recurrence-free survival, higher overall survival (OS)[86] and improved quality of life.[86–89] The increasing call to perform NSS more frequently was highlighted in the recent publication of the American Urological Association Guideline for the Treatment of the Clinical Stage 1 Renal Mass.[90–93]

Laparoscopic Radical Nephrectomy

Although the first laparoscopic radical nephrectomy (LRN) was reported in 1991, laparoscopic surgery for kidney cancer was not fully accepted until over 10 years later, owing to various oncologic concerns including dissemination of cancer cells, port site seeding, and other issues.[94] These concerns have been assuaged with several long-term follow-up studies showing equivalent survival of patients undergoing LRN versus open radical nephrectomy.[95] The laparoscopic approach is associated with reduced blood loss, less pain, less narcotic usage, a shorter hospitalization, and generally a quicker recovery. General contraindications to LRN include tumor size larger than 13 cm, prior partial nephrectomy, presence of IVC tumor thrombus, extensive locoregional disease extension (clinical T4 disease), and the presence of bulky adenopathy. There are no differences in complication rates, and some would argue that there is a better adverse event profile with laparoscopic surgery, but no prospective, randomized data exist. Retrospective comparative studies indicate an overall average of approximately 12% to 15% rate of adverse events, as well as operative time, which is equivalent to open surgery in experienced hands, and with lower cost.[96–98] In cases of cytoreduction for metastatic disease, LRN can also be done with the same tumor guidelines as those without metastatic disease.[99,100] There are some who propose to morcellate the specimen during LRN to prevent having to make a small extraction incision and, thus, improve the cosmetic results, even though this has never been shown to cause less pain. Specimen morcellation is not performed at our center, because of the desire for a good pathologic evaluation of the intact specimen. Upward of 26% of patients with clinical T1 to T2 tumors have been found to harbor high-risk disease on pathologic evaluation, warranting a more intensive follow-up regimen or enrollment into an adjuvant trial.[101]

Management of Metastatic Renal Cell Carcinoma: Role of Cytoreductive Nephrectomy

In the era of immunotherapy, cytoreductive nephrectomy before the administration of systemic therapy was an important part of a multidisciplinary approach in properly selected patients. Initially, several retrospective studies demonstrated the safety and potential efficacy of this approach, citing that cytoreductive surgery, before the administration of interferon or IL-2, may improve responses to systemic therapy and survival in appropriately selected patients.[102–105] What was clear from these retrospective studies was that optimal patient selection was paramount to success, defined as minimal perioperative morbidity and the timely administration of systemic immunotherapy postoperatively. Proper patient selection included those with clear-cell histology; good performance status; the absence of brain, liver, or extensive bone metastases; few if any comorbid conditions that could preclude surgery; the absence of sarcomatoid dedifferentiation; and the ability to resect greater than 75% of overall tumor burden.[103] Subsequently, the Southwest Oncology Group and the European Organization for Research and Treatment of Cancer independently conducted phase III randomized trials that demonstrated an improved survival for patients who underwent cytoreductive nephrectomy before systemic interferon therapy.

More recent studies have cast doubt on the role of cytoreductive nephrectomy in the upfront treatment of metastatic RCC. The CARMENA study demonstrated no survival advantage for patients who underwent cytoreductive nephrectomy followed by sunitinib treatment, versus those who received sunitinib treatment alone.[106] The SURTIME study, which assessed timing of cytoreductive nephrectomy in sunitinib-treated patients, found that delayed and selective cytroreductive nephrectomy showed a trend toward benefit over upfront nephrectomy in previously untreated, newly diagnosed patients with metastatic RCC.[107]

The concept of neoadjuvant or presurgical therapy for patients with metastatic RCC has also been explored. In this treatment paradigm, patients are given a defined course of systemic therapy, and those who demonstrate stable disease or evidence of a response would be offered surgery, whereas those who progress through therapy would be spared from a potentially morbid surgery that they are unlikely to benefit from. Several phase II studies have investigated this treatment paradigm using antiangiogenic therapy and shown it to be safe.[108–114] Further study will be required to determine whether this approach provides an advantage in patients treated with immunomodulatory checkpoint antibody therapy, and whether cytoreductive nephrectomy itself still plays an important role in the overall management of patients with metastatic RCC.

Nephron-Sparing Surgery: Open, Laparoscopic, and Robotic Partial Nephrectomy

Contemporary elective indications for NSS include a single renal tumor less than 4 cm in size, as well as selective tumors 4 to 7 cm in size, when a normal contralateral kidney is present.

Imperative indications for NSS include the presence of bilateral renal tumors, a systemic condition threatening renal function (such as severe hypertension or diabetes mellitus), a local condition threatening the contralateral kidney (such as stone disease or chronic pyelonephritis), chronic kidney disease, and a solitary functioning kidney. The basic principles of open partial nephrectomy include a flank approach, allowing the surgeon to operate on the kidney at skin level. The salient steps include hilar clamping, allowing resection in a bloodless, well-visualized field to allow sharp dissection of the renal tumor with a negative margin, followed by suture ligation of any collecting system entry, transection of the renal vessels, and finally renorrhaphy. Although resection with a negative margin is performed, and as long as an actual margin is present, it is not necessary to take wide margins, so maximal renal preservation can be achieved.[115–117] It should be noted that nearly all data on surgical treatments are not based on randomized, controlled studies, although studies from multiple international centers have independently corroborated the advantages of NSS.

Publications on minimally invasive technologies likewise are based on retrospective data, which are still evolving and growing. Laparoscopic partial nephrectomy (LPN) was developed as a way to perform NSS without the flank incision and to reduce the morbidity of open surgery. It has since been shown to be an effective approach for select small renal tumors, adhering to the principles of open surgery detailed previously.[118] Nevertheless, LPN is one of the most complex laparoscopic procedures performed by any surgical specialty, given the requirement for expedient and flawless tumor resection and renal reconstruction under the duress of renal ischemia, requiring extensive laparoscopic experience and careful patient selection. With the availability of a robotic surgery platform (daVinci, Intuitive Corp., Sunnyvale, CA), the laparoscopic approach to NSS has been facilitated. Robot-assisted partial nephrectomy (RAPN) has the potential to improve the results of LPN and allow a larger cadre of urologists to offer minimally invasive NSS. The most recent data, which are still early and growing, suggest that RAPN is associated with shorter warm ischemia time and a shorter operation than LPN, advantages that are seen even in surgeons experienced with LPN.[119]

Cryoablation and Radiofrequency Ablation

Laparoscopic or percutaneous energy-ablative therapies such as cryoablation and RFA are generally reserved for small (<3.5 cm) tumors and patients at higher operative risk. Percutaneous renal cryoablation or RFA may be employed under MRI or CT guidance, respectively, for tumors that are safely accessible percutaneously. Laparoscopic approaches can be used for lesions that are anterior or in close approximation to the ureter, bowel, or other critical structures. Alternatively, several adjunct percutaneous procedures such as hydrodissection and balloon displacement may be used to allow a percutaneous route. Small exophytic tumors are probably treated just as well with either approach, whereas larger (>3.5 cm) and more central lesions have a higher rate of failure with either therapy. Both cryoablation and RFA have a favorable adverse outcome profile and oncologic efficacy ranges in the 90% range, which, although not unfavorable, is less than surgical excision, which has an efficacy of over 98%.[93] Whether cryoablation or RFA is used, two other important factors must be considered. Taking a biopsy to obtain a tissue diagnosis is imperative, and intensive postoperative follow-up imaging is needed to document effective treatment, given the lack of any confirmation of pathologic cure and sparse long-term data. Current recommendations include obtaining a renal mass protocol CT or MRI within the first 3 months after therapy, then at 6, 12, 18, and 24 months and semiannually or annually thereafter.[120] Several centers, including ours, have additionally started to biopsy the zones of ablation 6 months or more after treatment if there has not been satisfactory involution, to confirm adequate treatment, because data exist showing that absence of enhancement by itself may not be a fully reliable finding, as well as the possibility of other causes of false-positive and false-negative imaging findings.[121,122]

Medical Therapy

Systemic therapy for RCC has changed substantially in the past two decades. Up until the early 1980s, no consistently useful therapy existed for this disease. With the cloning of the genes encoding interferon-alpha (IFN-α) and IL-2 and the recognition that an immune reaction may be mounted against some individuals with RCC, IL-2 and IFN-α agents were assessed in clinical trials and found to have some utility. In 1992, IL-2 was approved by the US Food and Drug Administration (FDA) for mRCC on the basis of outcomes in 255 patients.[123]

The discovery of the *VHL* gene in 1993 expanded our understanding of the molecular biology of RCC and led to the assessment of antiangiogenic agents in this disease.[124,125] Numerous antiangiogenic agents have been approved for use in advanced RCC by the FDA. The most commonly used include sunitinib, pazopanib, axitinib, cabozantinib, and lenvatinib in combination with everolimus.[126–133] More recently, immune checkpoint inhibitory (ICI) antibodies have become mainstays of therapy for patients with metastatic RCC. An important consideration for patients being assessed for treatment is their prognostic risk stratum, which is usually defined by either the Memorial Sloan Kettering[134] or the International Metastatic RCC Database Consortium algorithm,[26] which use clinical and laboratory features to categorize individuals into favorable (no risk factors), intermediate (one to two risk factors), or unfavorable (three or more factors) risk groups. These criteria factor into decision-making for the agents summarized in the following paragraphs and provide important prognostic information for patients.

Sunitinib (Sutent, Pfizer Inc.), a small-molecule VEGF receptor inhibitor, was evaluated in a 750-patient study that randomized individuals with clear-cell mRCC to the study drug or IFN-α.[135] A doubling of PFS from 5.0 to 11.0 months was seen in the sunitinib arm ($P < .001$). A borderline improvement in OS was observed, from 21.8 months in the IFN-α arm to 26.4 months in the sunitinib arm ($P = .051$).[136] Pazopanib (Votrient, Novartis Inc.), a small-molecule VEGF receptor inhibitor, was assessed in a study that randomized 435 patients with clear-cell mRCC to pazopanib or placebo, with crossover permitted in the placebo arm at the time of progression. Roughly half the patients were treatment-naïve, and the balance had received prior immunotherapy. The PFS in the pazopanib arm was 9.2 months versus 4.2 months in the placebo arm ($P <.0001$).[130] Frontline treatment with pazopanib was subsequently found to be noninferior to sunitinib in an 1110-patient, randomized study.[137] Axitinib (Inlyta, Pfizer Inc.) was compared with sorafenib in randomized phase 3 study enrolling previously treated patients who progressed on either targeted therapy or a cytokine.[131] The PFS for axitinib was 6.7 months versus 4.7 months for sorafenib-treated patients (hazard ratio [HR] 0.665; 95% confidence interval [CI] 0.544-0.812; one-sided $P <.0001$). There was no difference in OS. Cabozantinib (Cabometyx, Exelixis Inc.) was compared with everolimus (Afinitor, Novartis Inc.) in a 658-patient study enrolling patients who had progressed on a frontline antiangiogenic agent. In this study, cabozantinib showed a PFS of 7.4 months versus 3.8 months for everolimus (HR 0.58; 95% CI 0.45 to 0.75; $P <.001$).[133] Follow-up results demonstrated persistence of improved PFS, as well as improved overall response rate (ORR) and improved OS for cabozantinib.[138] A frontline 157-patient study comparing cabozantinib to sunitinib in previously untreated patients with intermediate and poor risk features demonstrated a PFS of 8.2 versus 5.6 months in favor of cabozantinib (adjusted HR 0.66; 95% CI, 0.46-0.95; one-sided $P = .012$).[139] Lenvatinib (Lenvima, Eisai Inc.) plus everolimus was compared with lenvatinib monotherapy and everolimus monotherapy in a randomized, 153-patient phase II study enrolling patients with previously treated metastatic RCC.[132] The combination of lenvatinib plus everolimus demonstrated a 14.6 month PFS versus 5.5 months for everolimus alone by investigator assessment (HR 0.40, 95% CI 0.24-0.68; $P = .0005$), and showed superior ORR and OS.

Treatment with ICI monotherapy, combination therapy with ICI plus antiangiogenic therapy, and treatment with ICI doublets have recently been incorporated into the RCC treatment algorithm. Nivolumab (Opdivo, Bristol Myers-Squibb Inc.) was compared with everolimus in previously treated patients with metastatic RCC in a randomized, 821-patient phase 3 study.[140] The primary endpoint of OS was met, with 25.0-month survival for nivolumab-treated patients versus 19.6 months for individuals treated with everolimus (HR 0.73; 98.5% CI, 0.57-0.93; P=.002).[140] Subsequently the combination of ipilimumab (Yervoy, Bristol Myers Squibb Inc.) plus nivolumab was compared with sunitinib in a 1096-patient, randomized phase 3 study of patients with previously untreated metastatic RCC,[141] with coprimary endpoints of OS, ORR, and PFS in the intermediate and poor risk groups. The median OS was not reached in the combination arm, and was 26.0 months in the sunitinib-treated patients with intermediate and poor risk features (HR, 0.63; $P <.001$). ORR was 42% versus 27% ($P <.001$), and the complete response rate was 9% versus 1%. Median PFS was numerically higher in the combination arm but did not reach statistical significance.

The combination of axitinib plus pembrolizumab was tested against sunitinib in previously untreated patients with metastatic RCC in a randomized, 861-patient phase 3 trial.[27] The primary endpoints were OS and PFS in the intent-to-treat population. The initial HR for death was 0.53 (95% CI, 0.38-0.74; $P <.0001$) in favor of the combination arm, and median PFS was 15.1 months in the combination arm versus 11.1 months in the sunitinib arm (HR 0.69; 95% CI, 0.57-0.84; $P <.001$). ORR was 59.3% in the combination arm and 35.7% in the sunitinib arm ($P <.001$).

In the frontline setting, patients are frequently treated with either pembrolizumab plus axitinib, or ipilimumab plus nivolumab. Individuals who have contraindications to receiving ICI, typically those with severe autoimmune disease, may receive upfront antiangiogenic monotherapy. Second- and subsequent line agents that are commonly used include cabozantinib and the combination of lenvatinib plus everolimus. There is also still a role for antiangiogenic agents in the previously untreated patient with good risk features.

All of the studies mentioned so far have been in individuals with predominant clear-cell RCC histology. There are data that show benefit from sunitinib or everolimus in the broad and heterogeneous category of nonclear-cell RCC.[142,143] Ongoing and recently reported studies suggest benefit from ICI in this patient population as well,[144] with additional prospective data presented in abstract form at various congresses.

Key Points

Therapy

- Most effective therapies for renal cell carcinoma include immune checkpoint inhibitory (ICI) and antiangiogenic agents.
- Frontline therapy now includes either combination ICI, or the combination of an antiangiogenic agent plus an ICI agent.
- Single-agent antiangiogenic agents still play a role in subsequent line therapy, in frontline treatment for good-risk patients, and in individuals who are not able to receive ICI agents.

OTHER RENAL TUMORS

Wilms Tumor

Wilms tumor (nephroblastoma) arises from metanephric blastema and is most commonly found in young children: 50% of cases are diagnosed in patients younger than 2 years, and 75% of cases are diagnosed in patients younger than 5 years. Because pediatric tumors are beyond the framework of this chapter, this tumor is not discussed further.

MESENCHYMAL TUMORS

Angiomyolipoma

These hamartomatous tumors are composed of mature adipose tissue, thick-walled blood vessels, and sheets of smooth muscle. The amount of each component varies in each tumor. Approximately 5% of angiomyolipomas have insufficient fat to be recognized on CT and cannot be distinguished from RCC.

Angiomyolipomas more often are found in women than in men, and the mean age at presentation is 41 years. Most patients are asymptomatic; however, intra- or perirenal hemorrhage may cause flank pain. Hematuria and hypertension are occasionally reported.

A strong association exists between angiomyolipomas and tuberous sclerosis.[145] However, sporadic angiomyolipomas are being recognized with increasing frequency on cross-sectional imaging examinations. Although 80% of patients with tuberous sclerosis have an angiomyolipoma, less than 40% of patients with an angiomyolipoma have an element of the tuberous sclerosis complex.

Tuberous sclerosis, or Bourneville disease (Fig. 19.25), is caused by an autosomal dominant gene with variable expressivity. Only approximately 50% of patients with tuberous sclerosis have family members with one or more manifestations of the disease. The tuberous sclerosis syndrome includes epilepsy, mental retardation, and various hamartomas. In addition to renal angiomyolipomas and multiple renal cysts, patients often develop retinal phakomas and cerebral hamartomas. Adenoma sebaceum may be seen in the malar areas of the face. In some patients, the clinical syndrome is incompletely manifest. Among patients with tuberous sclerosis, the angiomyolipomas are usually multiple and bilateral. In patients without tuberous sclerosis, the tumors are usually solitary. The female predilection seen in sporadic angiomyolipomas does not occur in patients with tuberous sclerosis. The angiomyolipomas associated with tuberous sclerosis occur at a younger age and tend to be larger in size than the sporadic lesions. As the spatial resolution of CT and ultrasound continues to improve, tiny angiomyolipomas are being detected in asymptomatic patients as incidental findings.

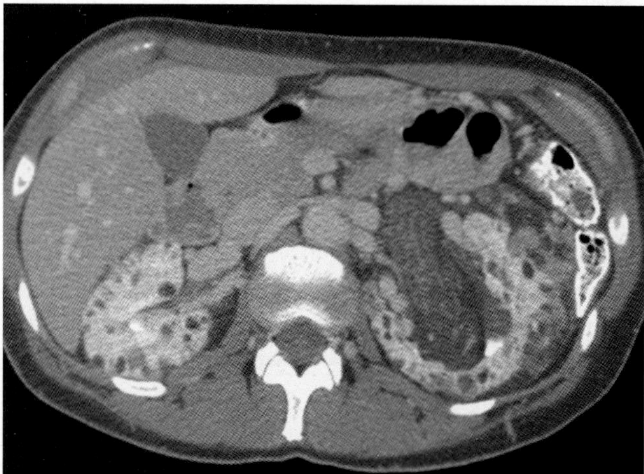

FIGURE 19.25. Axial computed tomography scan in a patient with tuberous sclerosis shows multiple bilateral fat-containing angiomyolipomas.

The typical ultrasonographic finding of a highly echogenic renal mass depends on the fat content of the tumor.[146] If there is relatively little fat, the ultrasonographic pattern will be indistinguishable from other renal masses. Even the very echogenic appearance can occasionally be mimicked by renal adenocarcinoma. If there has been hemorrhage, sonolucent areas may be seen.

The most reliable imaging modality for angiomyolipoma is CT.[147] The detection of a renal mass of fat density makes the diagnosis of angiomyolipoma highly likely. Although Wilms tumor, oncocytoma, metastasis, and renal adenocarcinoma have all been reported with macroscopic fat demonstrable in the tumor mass, these are rare occurrences. When fat is seen with renal carcinoma, it is because either of a large tumor that engulfs perinephric fat or to osseous metaplasia in which calcifications are present. Because angiomyolipomas do not calcify, the presence of calcification should suggest RCC, even when fat is identified. Both lipomas and liposarcomas also may be fat-dense and, thus, are indistinguishable from an angiomyolipoma by imaging techniques; however, they are very rare renal tumors. Because some angiomyolipomas contain little or no fat, the absence of fat does not exclude the diagnosis of angiomyolipoma. These tumors are sometimes referred to as "lipid-poor." Angiomyolipomas without detectable fat are homogeneous tumors with attenuation higher than normal renal parenchyma. They demonstrate homogeneous enhancement after the IV administration of contrast material.

MRI also can detect fat within an angiomyolipoma (Fig. 19.26). A high signal intensity is seen on both T1W and T2W images. When clearly imaged, MRI should have the same accuracy as CT in diagnosing an angiomyolipoma. However, MRI is probably not as sensitive as CT in detecting fat in small tumors.[148,149]

Other Rare Renal Mesenchymal Tumors

A variety of rare mesenchymal tumors may be encountered that cannot be diagnosed with any specificity by imaging studies. These include fibromas and fibrosarcomas; lipoma and liposarcomas; leiomyomas and leiomyosarcomas; and hemangiomas and juxtaglomerular tumors.

Lymphoma

Because the kidneys do not contain lymphoid tissue, primary renal lymphoma is rare. However, the kidneys may become involved by hematogenous dissemination or direct extension from adjacent retroperitoneal disease. Thus, renal lymphoma is usually part of a generalized process involving multiple sites. Renal involvement is much more common in non-Hodgkin lymphomas than in Hodgkin

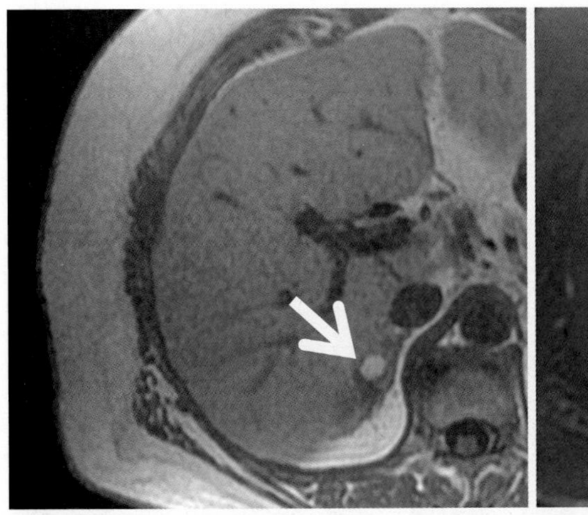
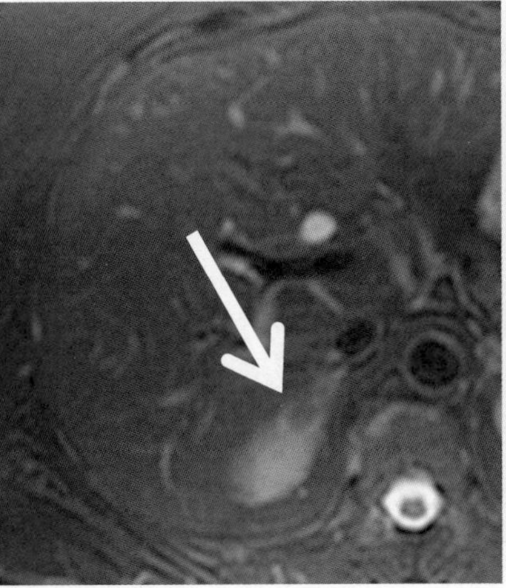
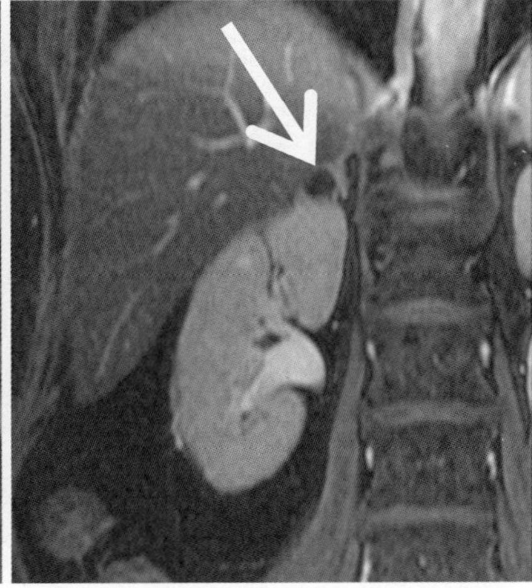

FIGURE 19.26. Axial T1-weighted (left), fat-suppressed axial T2-weighted (center), and coronal fat-suppressed gradient echo T2 (fast imaging employing steady state acquisition; right). Magnetic resonance imaging shows a fat-containing lesion in the upper pole of the kidney (claw sign on the coronal image). The lesion is bright on T1 and suppressed on fat-suppressed T2 sequences (*arrows*), compatible with angiomyolipoma.

disease. When present, involvement is more often bilateral than unilateral. At presentation, involvement of the kidneys by non-Hodgkin lymphoma is seen in 5.8% of cases; at autopsy, the frequency of renal involvement increases to 41.6%. Renal involvement is more frequent among certain subgroups of non-Hodgkin lymphoma. Poorly differentiated Burkitt lymphoma is often described as an extranodal tumor, and the kidneys are affected in approximately 10% of cases at presentation. Acquired immunodeficiency syndrome (AIDS)–related lymphomas were found by CT to involve the kidneys in 11% of patients.

Renal lymphoma is more common among patients with immune deficiencies, including those with AIDS. The incidence of renal lymphoma has increased among patients with graft-versus-host disease, iatrogenic immunosuppression, and renal transplantation, in whom it is 350 times more frequent than in the general population.

Most patients with renal lymphoma have disease in other locations that dominates the clinical presentation. Fever, weight loss, and palpable adenopathy are common complaints. Occasionally, diffuse involvement of both kidneys or ureteral obstruction by adenopathy may compromise renal function. Renal lymphoma is usually clinically silent and occurs late in the course of the disease.

Renal lymphoma may have several different appearances. Multiple lymphomatous masses are the most common and are seen in more than 50% of cases of renal lymphoma. A solitary mass or diffuse infiltration of the kidney by lymphoma also may be seen. Although most renal lymphoma has spread by hematogenous dissemination, CT may demonstrate local extension from paraaortic disease in some cases. Bulky lymphadenopathy often will displace the ureters. Because the proximal ureters lie lateral to the paraaortic lymph nodes, they are displaced laterally. The distal ureters are pushed medially, because the external iliac lymph nodes are lateral to the ureters. On ultrasound, lymphoma is usually hypoechoic, reflecting the homogeneous nature of the tumor. However, a lymphomatous mass shows little sound through transmission, which helps to distinguish it from a cyst. Ultrasound is often helpful in identifying hydronephrosis and is the examination of choice in patients with renal failure or other contraindications to IV contrast media.

CT is routinely used to stage and monitor patients with malignant lymphoma and is an excellent method of detecting renal involvement. Lymphomatous masses are homogeneous and rounded. Renal lymphoma is difficult to detect on unenhanced examinations unless the masses are large. After IV contrast administration, lymphoma is usually well-demarcated from the normal parenchyma by its diminished enhancement. The CT pattern reflects the pathologic involvement as a solitary mass, multiple nodules, or diffuse involvement. Adjacent lymphadenopathy and direct tumor extension to the kidney also are well depicted with CT. Renal or perirenal involvement (Fig. 19.27) without evidence on CT of other retroperitoneal disease is common. Positron emission tomography/CT is also very useful in detecting and characterizing renal involvement.

Solid Tumor Metastases

Metastatic disease involving the kidneys is relatively common in autopsy series, where it may be seen in as many as 20% of patients. The most common primary tumors are carcinomas of the lung, breast, colon, and melanoma. Approximately 50% of these patients have metastases to both kidneys, and the remaining 50% have involvement of only one kidney. The patient's symptoms are usually dominated by manifestations of the primary tumor, but hematuria and proteinuria are common. Tumors that are especially vascular may cause significant renal hemorrhage, resulting in gross hematuria or a perinephric hematoma. Unless extensive metastases involve both kidneys, the renal function is normal. Occasionally, urine cytology may be positive.

Although renal metastases are common in autopsy series, where they outnumber primary renal malignancy 4:1, they are not commonly seen clinically. Most patients

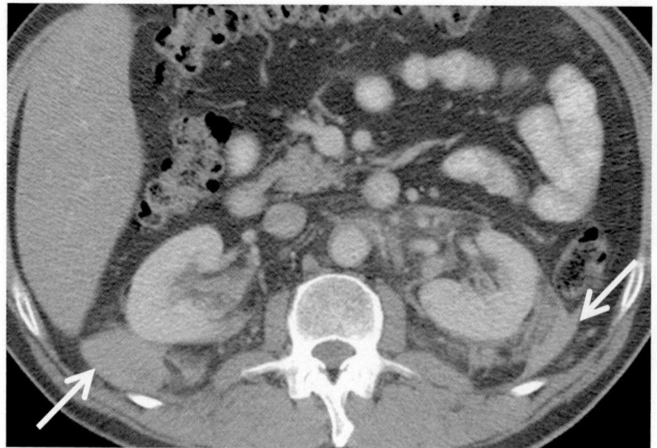

FIGURE 19.27. Perirenal lymphoma. Axial computed tomography scan shows bilateral perirenal soft tissue masses (*arrows*) in a patient with lymphoma.

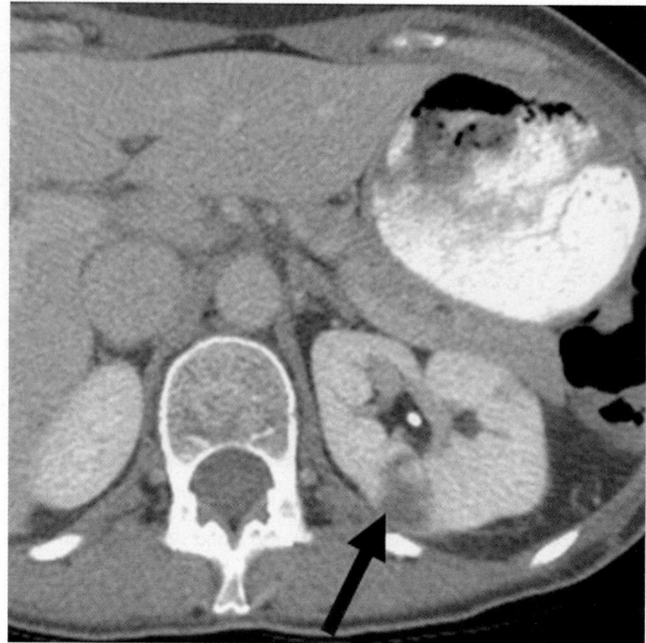

FIGURE 19.28. Mass in the left kidney in a patient with breast cancer shows heterogeneous enhancement (*arrow*). This was biopsy-proven to be metastatic breast carcinoma.

with renal metastases have widespread metastatic disease, and imaging studies are not needed to demonstrate renal involvement as well. In the series reported by Choyke and coworkers,[55] more than 50% of patients died within 3 months of the demonstration of renal metastases.

More recent use of CT to stage and monitor patients with an underlying malignancy has made detection of metastases more common. In a patient with extensive metastases, a renal mass is most likely another metastasis. However, among patients whose disease is in remission, a new renal mass is more likely to be a primary renal tumor. Perirenal metastases are readily detected by CT, because the soft tissue density mass is easy to see within the perirenal fat. Such metastases have been reported in patients with underlying lung cancer, melanoma, and lymphoma. Lymphatic connections may be responsible for this pattern of spread.

Renal metastases are most commonly detected by CT, because this modality is most frequently used to stage and monitor oncology patients (Fig. 19.28). Unenhanced scans are seldom useful in detecting metastases but may be helpful in excluding renal calculi. Metastases often are small and multiple, but certain primary tumors such as colonic carcinomas may produce a solitary, large renal metastasis. These may be indistinguishable from primary renal adenocarcinomas. Renal biopsy may be required to make this distinction. Tumor invasion of the renal vein and extension into the IVC are commonly seen in renal adenocarcinoma but are rare in renal metastases. Although vascular lesions may enhance as much as the normal renal parenchyma during the early vascular phase, they later become hypodense. Small lesions may resemble cysts but can be differentiated by their higher density.

Renal metastases demonstrate high signal intensity on T2W images. However, MRI is seldom useful, because other entities such as primary renal malignancy or an inflammatory process may have similar signal characteristics.

ACKNOWLEDGEMENTS

The authors wish to thank Carl M. Sandler, M.D., Surena F. Matin, M.D., and Christopher Wood, M.D. for their work on this chapter in the first edition of the text, which served as a strong foundation for this revision.

REFERENCES

1. Lopez-Beltran A, et al. WHO classification of the renal tumors of the adults. *Eur Urol*. 2004;2006(49):798–805.
2. Parkin DM, Whelan SL, Ferlay J, et al. eds. *Cancer Incidence in Five Continents*. Lyon: IARC Press; 2002.
3. American Cancer Society. *Cancer Facts and Figures*. Atlanta: ACS; 2011.
4. Rebecca LS, Kimberly DM, Ahmedin J. Cancer statistics, 2020. *CA Cancer J Clin*. 2020;70(1):7–30.
5. McLaughlin JK, Lipworth L, Tarone RE. Epidemiologic aspects of renal cell carcinoma. *Semin Oncol*. 2006;33:527–533.
6. American Cancer Society. *Cancer Facts & Figures*. Atlanta: American Cancer Society; 2020:2020.
7. Eble JM, Sauter G, Epstein JI, et al. *Pathology and genetics of tumors of the urinary system and male genital organs. World Health Organization Classification of Tumors*. Lyon: IARC Press; 2004.
8. Hunt JD, et al. Renal cell carcinoma in relation to cigarette smoking: meta-analysis of 24 studies. *Int J Cancer*. 2005;114:101–108.
9. Bergstrom A, et al. Obesity and renal cell cancer—a quantitative review. *Br J Cancer*. 2001;85:984–990.
10. Murai M, Oya M. Renal cell carcinoma: etiology, incidence and epidemiology. *Curr Opin Urol*. 2004;14:229–233.
11. Geyer JR, Poutasse EF. Incidence of multiple renal arteries on aortography. Report of a series of 400 patients, 381 of whom had arterial hypertension. *JAMA*. 1962;182:120–125.
12. Williams PL, Warwick R, Dyson M, et al. *The urinary organs. Gray's Anatomy*. New York: Churchill Livingstone; 1989:1397–1416.
13. Turkvatan A, et al. Multidetector CT angiography of renal vasculature: normal anatomy and variants. *Eur Radiol*. 2009;19:236–244.
14. Shanks JH. Pathology of renal cell carcinoma: recent developments. *Clin Oncol (R Coll Radiol)*. 1999;11:263–268.
15. Kovacs G, et al. The Heidelberg classification of renal cell tumours. *J Pathol*. 1997;183:131–133.
16. Fuhrman SA, Lasky LC, Limas C. Prognostic significance of morphologic parameters in renal cell carcinoma. *Am J Surg Pathol*. 1982;6:655–663.
17. Cohen HT, McGovern FJ. Renal-cell carcinoma. *N Engl J Med*. 2005;353:2477–2490.
18. Suzigan S, et al. Multilocular cystic renal cell carcinoma: a report of 45 cases of a kidney tumor of low malignant potential. *Am J Clin Pathol*. 2006;125:217–222.

19. Nassir A, et al. Multilocular cystic renal cell carcinoma: a series of 12 cases and review of the literature. *Urology*. 2002;60:421–427.
20. Zbar B, Linehan WM. Hereditary papillary renal cell carcinoma: clinical studies in 10 families. *J Urol*. 1781;1996:156.
21. Fahmy W, et al. Multiple/bilateral renal tumors in patients with Birt-Hogg-Dubé syndrome. *Int Urol Nephrol*. 2007;39:995–999.
22. Yoon SK, et al. Collecting duct carcinoma of the kidney: CT and pathologic correlation. *Eur J Radiol*. 2006;57:453–460.
23. Blitman NM, et al. Renal medullary carcinoma: CT and MRI features. *AJR Am J Roentgenol*. 2005;185:268–272.
24. Choyke PL, et al. von Hippel-Lindau disease: genetic, clinical, and imaging features. *Radiology*. 1995;194:629–642.
25. Amin MB, ed. *AJCC Cancer Staging Manual*. : Springer International Publishing; 2017.
26. Daniel YCH, Wanling X, Meredith MR, et al. Prognostic factors for overall survival in patients with metastatic renal cell carcinoma treated with vascular endothelial growth factor-targeted agents: results from a large, multicenter study. *J Clin Oncol*. 2009;27(34):5794–5799.
27. Brian IR, Elizabeth RP, Viktor S, et al. Pembrolizumab plus Axitinib versus Sunitinib for Advanced Renal-Cell Carcinoma. *N Engl J Med*. 2019;380(12):1116–1127.
28. Robert JM, Brian IR, David FM, et al. Nivolumab plus ipilimumab versus sunitinib in first-line treatment for advanced renal cell carcinoma: extended follow-up of efficacy and safety results from a randomised, controlled, phase 3 trial. *Lancet Oncol*. 2019;20(10):1370–1385.
29. Crotty TB, Farrow GM, Lieber MM. Chromophobe cell renal carcinoma: clinicopathological features of 50 cases. *J Urol*. 1995;154:964–967.
30. Choyke PL, et al. Renal cell carcinoma staging. American College of Radiology. ACR Appropriateness Criteria. *Radiology*. 2000;215(Suppl):721–725.
31. Staudenherz A, et al. Is there a diagnostic role for bone scanning of patients with a high pretest probability for metastatic renal cell carcinoma? *Cancer*. 1999;85:153–155.
32. Fielding JR, et al. Staging of 119 patients with renal cell carcinoma: the yield and cost-effectiveness of pelvic CT. *AJR Am J Roentgenol*. 1999;172:23–25.
33. Hartman DS. Cysts and cystic neoplasms. *Urol Radiol*. 1990;12:7–10.
34. Yuh BI, Cohan RH. Different phases of renal enhancement: role in detecting and characterizing renal masses during helical CT. *AJR Am J Roentgenol*. 1999;173:747–755.
35. Cohan RH, et al. Renal masses: assessment of corticomedullary-phase and nephrographic-phase CT scans. *Radiology*. 1995;196:445–451.
36. Kopka L, et al. Dual-phase helical CT of the kidney: value of the corticomedullary and nephrographic phase for evaluation of renal lesions and preoperative staging of renal cell carcinoma. *AJR Am J Roentgenol*. 1997;169:1573–1578.
37. Kim JK, et al. Differentiation of subtypes of renal cell carcinoma on helical CT scans. *AJR Am J Roentgenol*. 2002;178:1499–1506.
38. Herts BR, et al. Enhancement characteristics of papillary renal neoplasms revealed on triphasic helical CT of the kidneys. *AJR Am J Roentgenol*. 2002;178:367–372.
39. Kearney GP, et al. Results of inferior vena cava resection for renal cell carcinoma. *J Urol*. 1981;125:769–773.
40. Davits RJ, Blom JH, Schroder FH. Surgical management of renal carcinoma with extensive involvement of the vena cava and right atrium. *Br J Urol*. 1992;70:591–593.
41. Kallman DA, et al. Renal vein and inferior vena cava tumor thrombus in renal cell carcinoma: CT, US, MRI and venacavography. *J Comput Assist Tomogr*. 1992;16:240–247.
42. Oto A, et al. Inferior vena cava tumor thrombus in renal cell carcinoma: staging by MR imaging and impact on surgical treatment. *AJR Am J Roentgenol*. 1998;171:1619–1624.
43. Bos SD, Mensink HJ. Can duplex Doppler ultrasound replace computerized tomography in staging patients with renal cell carcinoma? *Scand J Urol Nephrol*. 1998;32:87–91.
44. Welch TJ, LeRoy AJ. Helical and electron beam CT scanning in the evaluation of renal vein involvement in patients with renal cell carcinoma. *J Comput Assist Tomogr*. 1997;21:467–471.
45. Habboub HK, et al. Accuracy of color Doppler sonography in assessing venous thrombus extension in renal cell carcinoma. *AJR Am J Roentgenol*. 1997;168:267–271.
46. Hricak H, et al. Detection and staging of renal neoplasms: a reassessment of MR imaging. *Radiology*. 1988;166:643–649.
47. Roubidoux MA, et al. Renal carcinoma: detection of venous extension with gradient-echo MR imaging. *Radiology*. 1992;182:269–272.
48. Goldfarb DA, et al. Magnetic resonance imaging for assessment of vena caval tumor thrombi: a comparative study with venacavography and computerized tomography scanning. *J Urol*. 1990;144:1100–1103. discussion 1103-1104.
49. Hallscheidt PJ, et al. Preoperative staging of renal cell carcinoma with inferior vena cava thrombus using multidetector CT and MRI: prospective study with histopathological correlation. *J Comput Assist Tomogr*. 2005;29:64–68.
50. Hatcher PA, et al. Surgical management and prognosis of renal cell carcinoma invading the vena cava. *J Urol*. 1991;145:20–23. discussion 23-24.
51. Giberti C, et al. Radical nephrectomy for renal cell carcinoma: long-term results and prognostic factors on a series of 328 cases. *Eur Urol*. 1997;31:40–48.
52. Choyke P, et al. *ACR appropriateness criteria: renal cell carcinoma staging*. Available at:
53. Hilton S. Imaging of renal cell carcinoma. *Semin Oncol*. 2000;27:150–159.
54. Pretorius ES, Wickstrom ML, Siegelman ES. MR imaging of renal neoplasms. *Magn Reson Imaging Clin North Am*. 2000;8:813–836.
55. Choyke PL. Detection and staging of renal cancer. *Magn Reson Imaging Clin North Am*. 1997;5:29–47.
56. Zhang J, et al. Masses and pseudomasses of the kidney: imaging spectrum on MR. *J Comput Assist Tomogr*. 2004;28:588–595.
57. Tuite DJ, et al. Three-dimensional gadolinium-enhanced magnetic resonance breath-hold FLASH imaging in the diagnosis and staging of renal cell carcinoma. *Clin Radiol*. 2006;61:23–30.
58. Hallscheidt PJ, et al. Diagnostic accuracy of staging renal cell carcinomas using multidetector-row computed tomography and magnetic resonance imaging: a prospective study with histopathologic correlation. *J Comput Assist Tomogr*. 2004;28:333–339.
59. Frohmuller HG, Grups JW, Heller V. Comparative value of ultrasonography, computerized tomography, angiography and excretory urography in the staging of renal cell carcinoma. *J Urol*. 1987;138:482–484.
60. Fritzsche PJ, Millar C. Multimodality approach to staging renal cell carcinoma. *Urol Radiol*. 1992;14:3–7.
61. Choyke PL, Daryanani K. Intraoperative ultrasound of the kidney. *Ultrasound Q*. 2001;17:245–253.
62. Campbell SC, et al. Intraoperative evaluation of renal cell carcinoma: a prospective study of the role of ultrasonography and histopathological frozen sections. *J Urol*. 1996;155:1191–1195.
63. Gill IS, et al. Laparoscopic renal cryoablation in 32 patients. *Urology*. 2000;56:748–753.
64. Russo P. Renal cell carcinoma: presentation, staging, and surgical treatment. *Semin Oncol*. 2000;27:160–176.
65. Chae EJ, et al. Renal cell carcinoma: analysis of postoperative recurrence patterns. *Radiology*. 2005;234:189–196.
66. Griffin N, Gore ME, Sohaib SA. Imaging in metastatic renal cell carcinoma. *AJR Am J Roentgenol*. 2007;189:360–370.
67. Ghavamian R, et al. Renal cell carcinoma metastatic to the pancreas: clinical and radiological features. *Mayo Clin Proc*. 2000;75:581–585.
68. Ng CS, et al. Metastases to the pancreas from renal cell carcinoma: findings on three-phase contrast-enhanced helical CT. *AJR Am J Roentgenol*. 1999;172:1555–1559.
69. Robson CJ, Churchill BM, Anderson W. The results of radical nephrectomy for renal cell carcinoma. *Trans Am Assoc Genitourin Surg*. 1968;60:122–129.
70. Skinner DG, Vermillion CD, Colvin RB. The surgical management of renal cell carcinoma. *J Urol*. 1972;107:705–710.
71. Robson CJ, Churchill BM, Anderson W. The results of radical nephrectomy for renal cell carcinoma. *J Urol*. 1969;101:297–301.
72. Sagalowsky AI, et al. Factors influencing adrenal metastasis in renal cell carcinoma. *J Urol*. 1994;151:1181–1184.
73. Kletscher BA, et al. Prospective analysis of the incidence of ipsilateral adrenal metastasis in localized renal cell carcinoma. *J Urol*. 1996;155:1844–1846.
74. Tsui KH, et al. Is adrenalectomy a necessary component of radical nephrectomy? UCLA experience with 511 radical nephrectomies. *J Urol*. 2000;163:437–441.
75. Blom JH, et al. Radical nephrectomy with and without lymph node dissection: preliminary results of the EORTC randomized phase III protocol 30881. EORTC Genitourinary Group. *Eur Urol*. 1999;36:570–575.

76. Vasselli JR, et al. Lack of retroperitoneal lymphadenopathy predicts survival of patients with metastatic renal cell carcinoma. *J Urol.* 2001;166:68–72.
77. Pizzocaro G, Piva L, Salvioni R. Lymph node dissection in radical nephrectomy for renal cell carcinoma: is it necessary? *Eur Urol.* 1983;9:10–12.
78. Tsukamoto T, et al. Regional lymph node metastasis in renal cell carcinoma: incidence, distribution and its relation to other pathological findings. *Eur Urol.* 1990;18:88–93.
79. Terrone C, et al. The number of lymph nodes examined and staging accuracy in renal cell carcinoma. *BJU Int.* 2003;91:37–40.
80. Ditonno P, et al. Role of lymphadenectomy in renal cell carcinoma. *Prog Clin Biol Res.* 1992;378:169–174.
81. Blute ML, et al. A protocol for performing extended lymph node dissection using primary tumor pathological features for patients treated with radical nephrectomy for clear cell renal cell carcinoma. *J Urol.* 2004;172:465–469.
82. Studer UE, et al. Enlargement of regional lymph nodes in renal cell carcinoma is often not due to metastases. *J Urol.* 1990;144:243–245.
83. Minervini A, et al. Regional lymph node dissection in the treatment of renal cell carcinoma: is it useful in patients with no suspected adenopathy before or during surgery? *BJU Int.* 2001;88:169–172.
84. Pantuck AJ, et al. Renal cell carcinoma with retroperitoneal lymph nodes: role of lymph node dissection. *J Urol.* 2003;169:2076–2083.
85. Margulis V, et al. Analysis of clinicopathologic predictors of oncologic outcome provides insight into the natural history of surgically managed papillary renal cell carcinoma. *Cancer.* 2008;112:1480–1488.
86. Lau W, Zincke H. Matched comparison of radical nephrectomy versus elective nephron-sparing surgery for renal cell carcinoma (RCC): evidence for increased renal failure rate on long term follow-up (>10 years). *J Urol.* 2000;163:S153.
87. Novick AC, et al. Long-term follow-up after partial removal of a solitary kidney. *N Engl J Med.* 1991;325:1058–1062.
88. Belldegrun A, et al. Efficacy of nephron-sparing surgery for renal cell carcinoma: analysis based on the new 1997 tumor-node-metastasis staging system. *J Clin Oncol.* 1999;17:2868–2875.
89. Herr HW. Partial nephrectomy for unilateral renal carcinoma and a normal contralateral kidney: 10-year follow-up. *J Urol.* 1999;161:33–34. discussion 34-35.
90. Clark PE, et al. Quality of life and psychological adaptation after surgical treatment for localized renal cell carcinoma: impact of the amount of remaining renal tissue. *Urology.* 2001;57:252–256.
91. Ficarra V, et al. Psycho-social well-being and general health status after surgical treatment for localized renal cell carcinoma. *Int Urol Nephrol.* 2002;34:441–446.
92. Shinohara N, et al. Impact of nephron-sparing surgery on quality of life in patients with localized renal cell carcinoma. *Eur Urol.* 2001;39:114–119.
93. American Urological Association. *Guideline for Management of the Clinical Stage 1 Renal Mass.* Available at: http://www.auanet.org.
94. Clayman RV, et al. Laparoscopic nephroureterectomy: initial clinical case report. *J Laparoendosc Surg.* 1991;1:343–349.
95. Permpongkosol S, et al. Long-term survival analysis after laparoscopic radical nephrectomy. *J Urol.* 2005;174:1222–1225.
96. Matin SF, et al. Evaluation of age and comorbidity as risk factors after laparoscopic urological surgery. *J Urol.* 2003;170:1115–1120.
97. Fazeli-Matin S, et al. Laparoscopic renal and adrenal surgery in obese patients: comparison to open surgery. *J Urol.* 1999;162:665–669.
98. Meraney AM, Gill IS. Financial analysis of open versus laparoscopic radical nephrectomy and nephroureterectomy. *J Urol.* 2002;167:1757–1762.
99. Matin SF, Madsen LT, Wood CG. Laparoscopic cytoreductive nephrectomy: the M. D. Anderson Cancer Center experience. *Urology.* 2006;68:528–532.
100. Walther MM, et al. Laparoscopic cytoreductive nephrectomy as preparation for administration of systemic interleukin-2 in the treatment of metastatic renal cell carcinoma: a pilot study. *Urology.* 1999;53:496–501.
101. Cohen DD, et al. Evaluation of the intact specimen after laparoscopic radical nephrectomy for clinically localized renal cell carcinoma identifies a subset of patients at increased risk for recurrence. *J Urol.* 2005;173:1487–1490. discussion 1490-1491.
102. Levy DA, et al. Timely delivery of biological therapy after cytoreductive nephrectomy in carefully selected patients with metastatic renal cell carcinoma. *J Urol.* 1998;159:1168–1173.
103. Fallick ML, et al. Nephrectomy before interleukin-2 therapy for patients with metastatic renal cell carcinoma. *J Urol.* 1997;158:1691–1695.
104. Rackley R, et al. The impact of adjuvant nephrectomy on multimodality treatment of metastatic renal cell carcinoma. *J Urol.* 1994;152:1399–1403.
105. Wood CG. The role of cytoreductive nephrectomy in the management of metastatic renal cell carcinoma. *Urol Clin North Am.* 2003;30:581–588.
106. Arnaud M, Alain R, Simon T, et al. Sunitinib alone or after nephrectomy in metastatic renal-cell carcinoma. *N Engl J Med.* 2018;379(5):417–427.
107. Roderick de B, Akhila W, Bernadett S, et al. Deferred cytoreductive nephrectomy following presurgical vascular endothelial growth factor receptor-targeted therapy in patients with primary metastatic clear cell renal cell carcinoma: a pooled analysis of prospective trial data. *Eur Urol Oncol.* 2020;3(2):168–173.
108. Thomas AA, et al. Response of the primary tumor to neoadjuvant sunitinib in patients with advanced renal cell carcinoma. *J Urol.* 2009;181:518–523. discussion 523.
109. Jonasch E, et al. Phase II presurgical feasibility study of bevacizumab in untreated patients with metastatic renal cell carcinoma. *J Clin Oncol.* 2009;27:4076–4081.
110. Thomas AA, et al. Surgical resection of renal cell carcinoma after targeted therapy. *J Urol.* 2009;182:881–886.
111. Amin C, et al. Preoperative tyrosine kinase inhibition as an adjunct to debulking nephrectomy. *Urology.* 2008;72:864–868.
112. Margulis V, et al. Surgical morbidity associated with administration of targeted molecular therapies before cytoreductive nephrectomy or resection of locally recurrent renal cell carcinoma. *J Urol.* 2008;180:94–98.
113. Bex A, et al. Neoadjuvant sunitinib for surgically complex advanced renal cell cancer of doubtful resectability: initial experience with downsizing to reconsider cytoreductive surgery. *World J Urol.* 2009;27:533–539.
114. Wood CG, Margulis V. Neoadjuvant (presurgical) therapy for renal cell carcinoma: a new treatment paradigm for locally advanced and metastatic disease. *Cancer.* 2009;115(Suppl 10):2355–2360.
115. Castilla EA, et al. Prognostic importance of resection margin width after nephron-sparing surgery for renal cell carcinoma. *Urology.* 2002;60:993–997.
116. Sutherland SE, et al. Does the size of the surgical margin in partial nephrectomy for renal cell cancer really matter? *J Urol.* 2002;167:61–64.
117. Piper NY, et al. Is a 1-cm margin necessary during nephron-sparing surgery for renal cell carcinoma? *Urology.* 2001;58:849–852.
118. Gill IS, et al. Comparative analysis of laparoscopic versus open partial nephrectomy for renal tumors in 200 patients. *J Urol.* 2003;170:64–68.
119. Benway BM, et al. Robot assisted partial nephrectomy versus laparoscopic partial nephrectomy for renal tumors: a multi-institutional analysis of perioperative outcomes. *J Urol.* 2009;182:866–872.
120. Matin SF, et al. Residual and recurrent disease following renal energy ablative therapy: a multi-institutional study. *J Urol.* 2006;176:1973–1977.
121. Weight CJ, et al. Correlation of radiographic imaging and histopathology following cryoablation and radio frequency ablation for renal tumors. *J Urol.* 2008;179:1277–1281. discussion 1281–1283.
122. Matin S. Determining failure after renal ablative therapy for renal cell carcinoma: false-negative and false-positive imaging findings. *Urology.* 2010;75:1254–1257.
123. Fyfe G, et al. Results of treatment of 255 patients with metastatic renal cell carcinoma who received high-dose recombinant interleukin-2 therapy. *J Clin Oncol.* 1995;13:688–696.
124. Latif F, et al. Identification of the von Hippel-Lindau disease tumor suppressor gene. *Science.* 1993;260:1317–1320.
125. Maxwell PH, et al. The tumour suppressor protein VHL targets hypoxia-inducible factors for oxygen-dependent proteolysis. *Nature.* 1999;399:271–275.
126. Escudier B, et al. Sorafenib in advanced clear-cell renal-cell carcinoma. *N Engl J Med.* 2007;356:125–134.
127. Motzer RJ, et al. Sunitinib versus interferon alfa in metastatic renal-cell carcinoma. *N Engl J Med.* 2007;356:115–124.
128. Escudier B, et al. Bevacizumab plus interferon alfa-2a for treatment of metastatic renal cell carcinoma: a randomised, double-blind phase III trial. *Lancet.* 2007;370:2103–2111.

129. Rini BI, et al. Bevacizumab plus interferon alfa compared with interferon alfa monotherapy in patients with metastatic renal cell carcinoma: CALGB 90206. *J Clin Oncol*. 2008;26:5422–5428.
130. Sternberg CN, et al. Pazopanib in locally advanced or metastatic renal cell carcinoma: results of a randomized phase III trial. *J Clin Oncol*. 2010;28:1061–1068.
131. Brian IR, Bernard E, Piotr T, et al. Comparative effectiveness of axitinib versus sorafenib in advanced renal cell carcinoma (AXIS): a randomised phase 3 trial. *Lancet*. 2011;378(9807):1931–1939.
132. Robert JM, Thomas EH, Hilary G, et al. Lenvatinib, everolimus, and the combination in patients with metastatic renal cell carcinoma: a randomised, phase 2, open-label, multicentre trial. *Lancet Oncol*. 2015;16(15):1473–1482.
133. Toni KC, Bernard E, Thomas P, et al. Cabozantinib versus everolimus in advanced renal-cell carcinoma. *N Engl J Med*. 2015;373(19):1814–1823.
134. Robert JM, Jennifer B, Barbara AM, et al. Interferon-alfa as a comparative treatment for clinical trials of new therapies against advanced renal cell carcinoma. *J Clin Oncol*. 2002;20(1):289–296.
135. Motzer RJ, Figlin RA, Hutson TE, et al. Sunitinib versus interferon alfa (IFN-α) as first-line treatment of metastatic renal carcinoma (mRCC): updated results and analysis of prognostic factors. *J Clin Oncol*. 2007;18S:5024.
136. Motzer RJ, et al. Overall survival and updated results for sunitinib compared with interferon alfa in patients with metastatic renal cell carcinoma. *J Clin Oncol*. 2009;27:3584–3590.
137. Robert JM, Thomas EH, David C, et al. Pazopanib versus sunitinib in metastatic renal-cell carcinoma. *N Engl J Med*. 2013;369(8):722–731.
138. Toni KC, Bernard E, Thomas P. Cabozantinib versus everolimus in advanced renal cell carcinoma (METEOR): final results from a randomised, open-label, phase 3 trial. *Lancet Oncol*. 2016 Jul;17(7):917–927.
139. Toni KC, Susan H, Ben LS, et al. Cabozantinib versus sunitinib as initial targeted therapy for patients with metastatic renal cell carcinoma of poor or intermediate risk: The alliance A031203 CABOSUN trial. *J Clin Oncol*. 2017;35(6):591–597.
140. Robert JM, Bernard E, David FM, et al. Nivolumab versus everolimus in advanced renal-cell carcinoma. *N Engl J Med*. 2015;373(19):1803–1813.
141. Robert JM, Nizar MT, David FM, et al. Nivolumab plus ipilimumab versus sunitinib in advanced renal-cell carcinoma. *N Engl J Med*. 2018;378(14):1277–1290.
142. Nizar MT, Eric J, Laurence A, et al. Everolimus versus sunitinib prospective evaluation in metastatic non-clear cell renal cell carcinoma (ESPN): A randomized multicenter phase 2 trial. *Eur Urol*. 2016;69(5):866–874.
143. Andrew JA, Susan H, Tim E, et al. Everolimus versus sunitinib for patients with metastatic non-clear cell renal cell carcinoma (ASPEN): a multicentre, open-label, randomised phase 2 trial. *Lancet Oncol*. 2016;17(3):378–388.
144. Chahoud J, Msaouel P, Campbell MT, et al. Nivolumab for the treatment of patients with metastatic non-clear cell renal cell carcinoma (nccRCC): A single-institutional experience and literature meta-analysis. *The Oncologist*. 2019;25(3):252–258.
145. Bissler JJ, Kingswood JC. Renal angiomyolipomata. *Kidney Int*. 2004;66:924–934.
146. Lemaitre L, et al. Imaging of angiomyolipomas. *Semin Ultrasound CT MR*. 1997;18:100–114.
147. Bosniak MA, et al. CT diagnosis of renal angiomyolipoma: the importance of detecting small amounts of fat. *AJR Am J Roentgenol*. 1988;151:497–501.
148. Kim JY, et al. CT histogram analysis: differentiation of angiomyolipoma without visible fat from renal cell carcinoma at CT imaging. *Radiology*. 2008;246:472–479.
149. Catalano OA, et al. Pixel distribution analysis: can it be used to distinguish clear cell carcinomas from angiomyolipomas with minimal fat? *Radiology*. 2008;247:738–746.

Visit ExpertConsult.com for additional algorithms.

RENAL CELL CARCINOMA - INITIAL EVALUATION

Note: Consider clinical trials as treatment options for eligible patients.

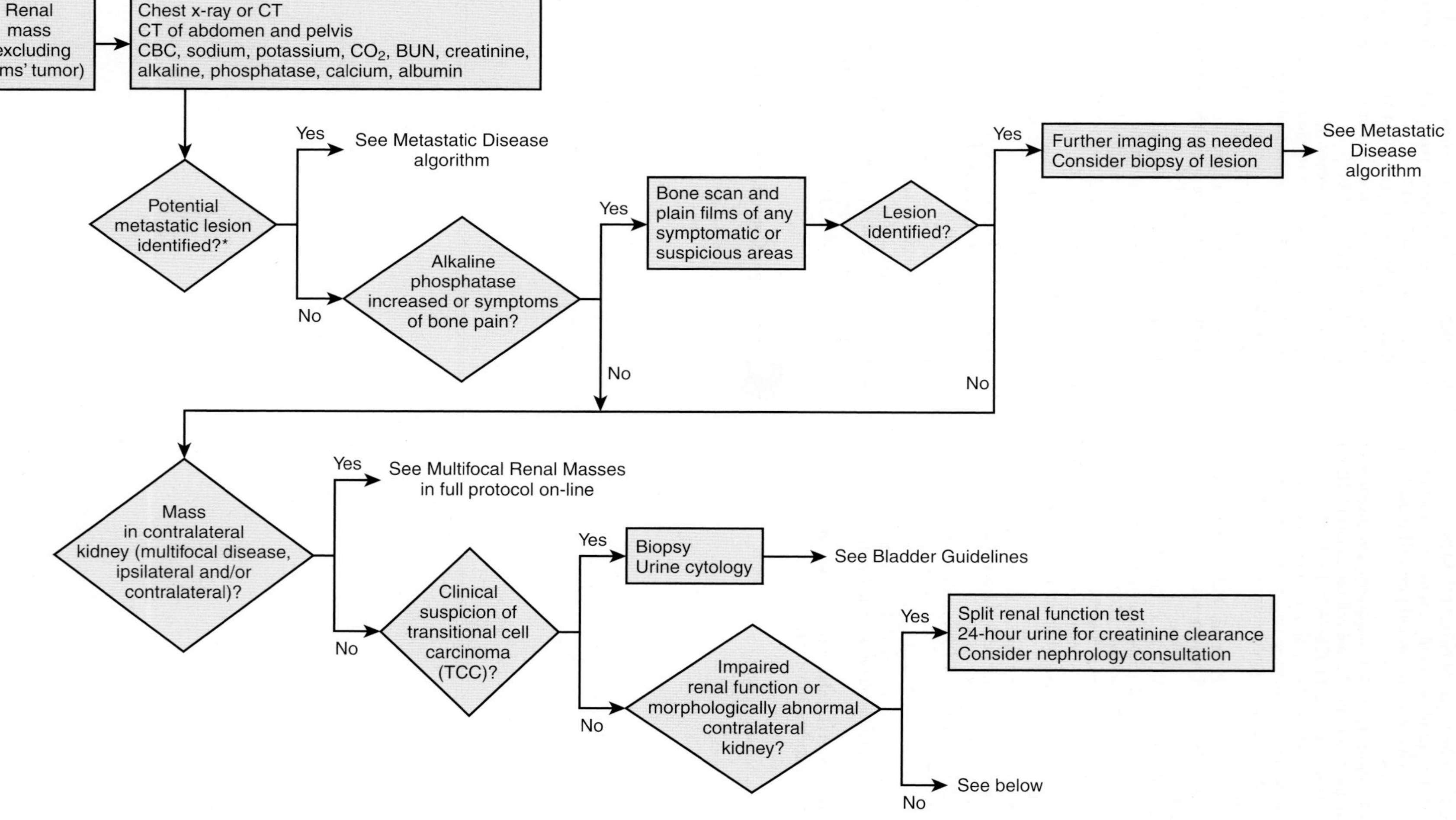

*Note: Retroperitoneal lymph nodes up to 3 cm do not imply unresectable disease. Lymph node biopsy not indicated.

This practice consensus algorithm is not intended to replace the independent medical or professional judgment of physicians or other health care providers. Without specific instructions from an M.D. Anderson health care provider about individual patient care, this algorithm should be used for informational purposes only. This algorithm should not be used to treat pregnant women.

RENAL CELL CARCINOMA

Note: Consider clinical trials as treatment options for eligible patients.

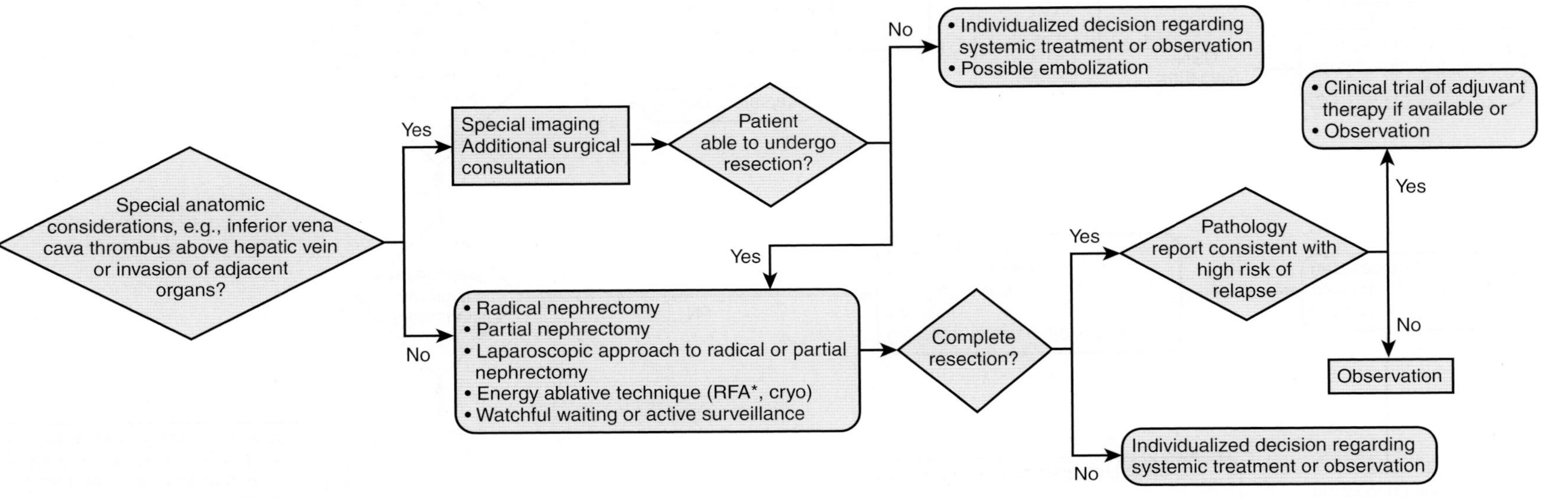

*RFA, radiofrequency ablation

This practice consensus algorithm is not intended to replace the independent medical or professional judgment of physicians or other health care providers. Without specific instructions from an M.D. Anderson health care provider about individual patient care, this algorithm should be used for informational purposes only. This algorithm should not be used to treat pregnant women.

RENAL CELL CARCINOMA: METASTATIC DISEASE AT PRESENTATION OR RECURRENCE

Note: Consider clinical trials as treatment options for eligible patients.

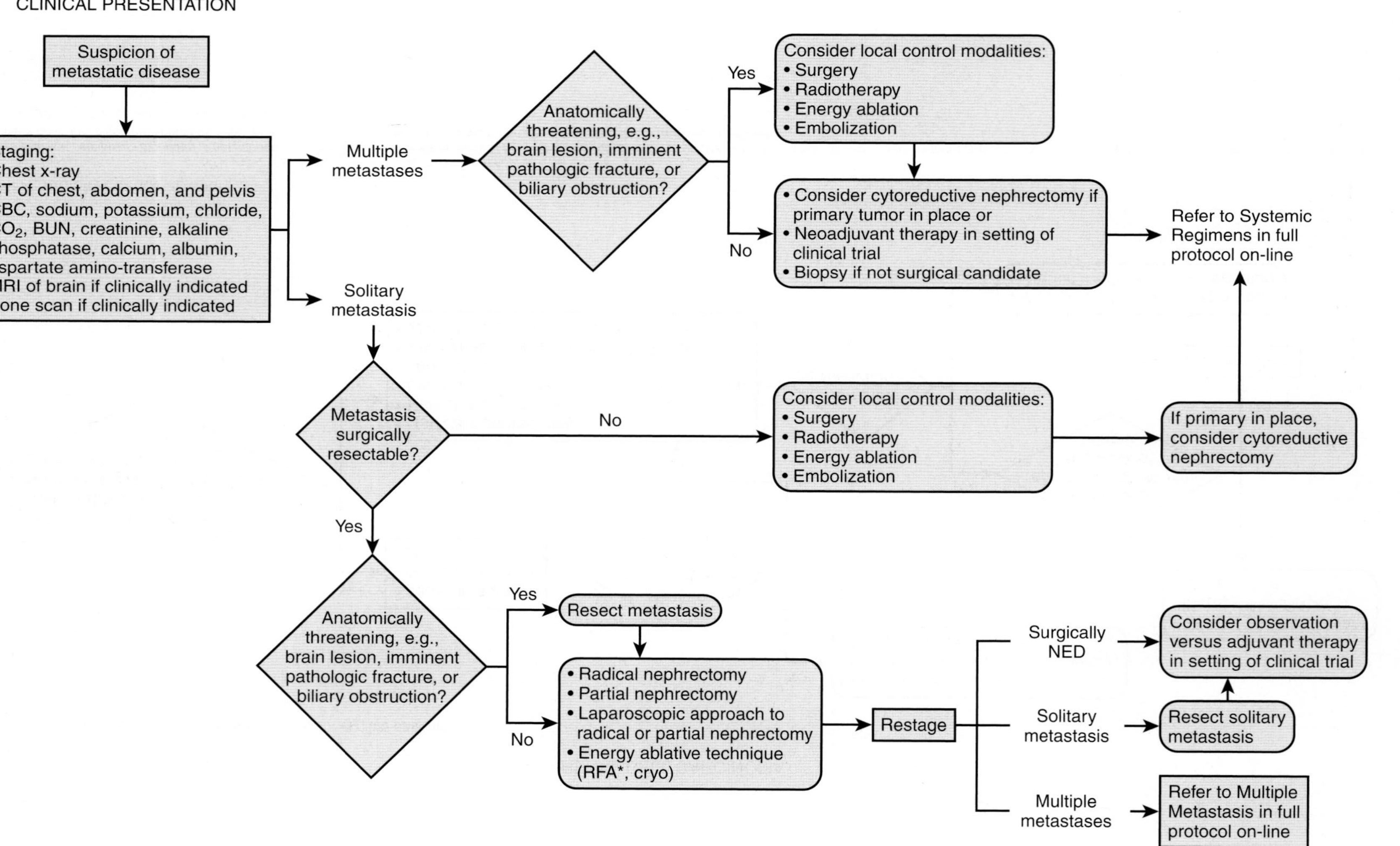

*RFA, radiofrequency ablation

This practice consensus algorithm is not intended to replace the independent medical or professional judgment of physicians or other health care providers. Without specific instructions from an M.D. Anderson health care provider about individual patient care, this algorithm should be used for informational purposes only. This algorithm should not be used to treat pregnant women.

CHAPTER 20

Urothelial Carcinoma (Bladder Cancer and Upper Tracts)

Juan J. Ibarra Rovira, M.D.; Ashish Kamat, M.D.; Arlene O. Siefker-Radtke, M.D.; and Vikas Kundra, M.D., Ph.D.

INTRODUCTION

Carcinoma of the urothelium is 'one of the most common tumor to affect the genitourinary system in the United States. The urothelium is the normal epithelium that lines the entire urinary collecting system from the calyces to the prostatic urethra. We will divide the urinary tract into a lower tract (bladder and prostatic urethra) and upper tract (pyelocaliceal system and ureters).

Urothelial cancer is considered a "field defect," where tumors can develop synchronously or metachronously at multiple sites along the urothelium. If a tumor is found, there is increased propensity to develop further urothelial tumors. It is, therefore, important to consider and evaluate the entire urothelium as a single pathologic landscape. Imaging is fundamental in the staging of lower tract tumors and in the staging and detection of upper tract tumors.

EPIDEMIOLOGY

Urothelial carcinoma of the bladder is the most common tumor of the urinary tract. In the United States, it is the fourth most common malignancy in males, accounting for 7% of all male malignancies and 4% of deaths. The incidence is 4:1 men:women and 2:1 White:Black American. The lifetime risk is 3.8% for men and 1.2% for women.[1] There will be approximately 83,700 new cases and 17,000 deaths from bladder cancer in the United States in 2021.[1,2]

The incidence of upper tract urothelial carcinoma is difficult to estimate, because cancer registries tend to include primary pyelocaliceal system tumors as "renal" cancers.[1,2] Statistical assumptions calculate that 5% of all renal pelvis tumors correspond to urothelial carcinomas; therefore, we can add approximately 4000 new cases and 883 deaths from upper tract renal pelvis carcinomas.[2]

Additionally, there will be an estimated 4200 new cases and 960 deaths from ureteric cancer in the United States in 2021.[1] Ureteral urothelial cancer, like bladder cancer, is more common in men than in women (ratio 2:1), with the incidence peaking in the eighth decade of life. It is estimated that 6.4% of bladder cancer patients will develop upper tract tumors,[3,4] and approximately 40% of patients with upper tract malignancy will develop lower tract disease.[5]

RISK FACTORS

Reported risk factors for urothelial tumors include exposure to aniline dyes, aromatic amines, a high fat diet, radiation, cyclophosphamide, arsenic in drinking water, exposure to diesel fumes, phenacetin abuse, living in urban areas, and substances that are used in the dye, rubber, leather, and aluminum industries. The most important factor remains cigarette smoking. Heavy smokers (>40 pack-years) are four to five times more prone to developing urothelial tumors than nonsmokers.[6]

Balkan nephropathy, an endemic interstitial nephropathy in Eastern Europe that originates with consumption of phytotoxin aristolochic acid, which is contained in a common plant growing in wheat fields, is associated with 100 to 200 times the risk of upper tract urothelial carcinomas that are typically multifocal, but low grade.[7–9]

Coffee drinking and artificial sweeteners have been considered possible risk factors but are unsubstantiated causes of bladder malignancy.[10]

Genetic factors in the etiology of urothelial tumors are constantly being evaluated, and they may be associated with aggressiveness, such as tumor grade, stage, and propensity for vascular invasion.[11]

Histologically, squamous cell carcinoma is the most common type of bladder cancer worldwide and is associated with chronic inflammation, for example, from infections such as schistosomiasis (*Schistosoma haematobium*) or calculi. Squamous cell carcinomas are the most common type of cancers affecting the urethra in both males and females.

Adenocarcinoma of the bladder can arise from the urachal remnant or occur in the setting of cystitis glandularis (which is also associated with bladder extrophy).[12] In addition, micropapillary and small-cell tumors have been reported and are signs of an aggressive histology associated with worse outcomes, likely as a result of early micrometastases.[13,14]

ANATOMY AND PATHOLOGY

The bladder develops from the primitive urogenital sinus that *in utero* communicates with the umbilicus via the allantois. The urogenital sinus normally involutes by birth into a thick fibrous cord, the urachus, that connects the dome of the bladder with the umbilicus.

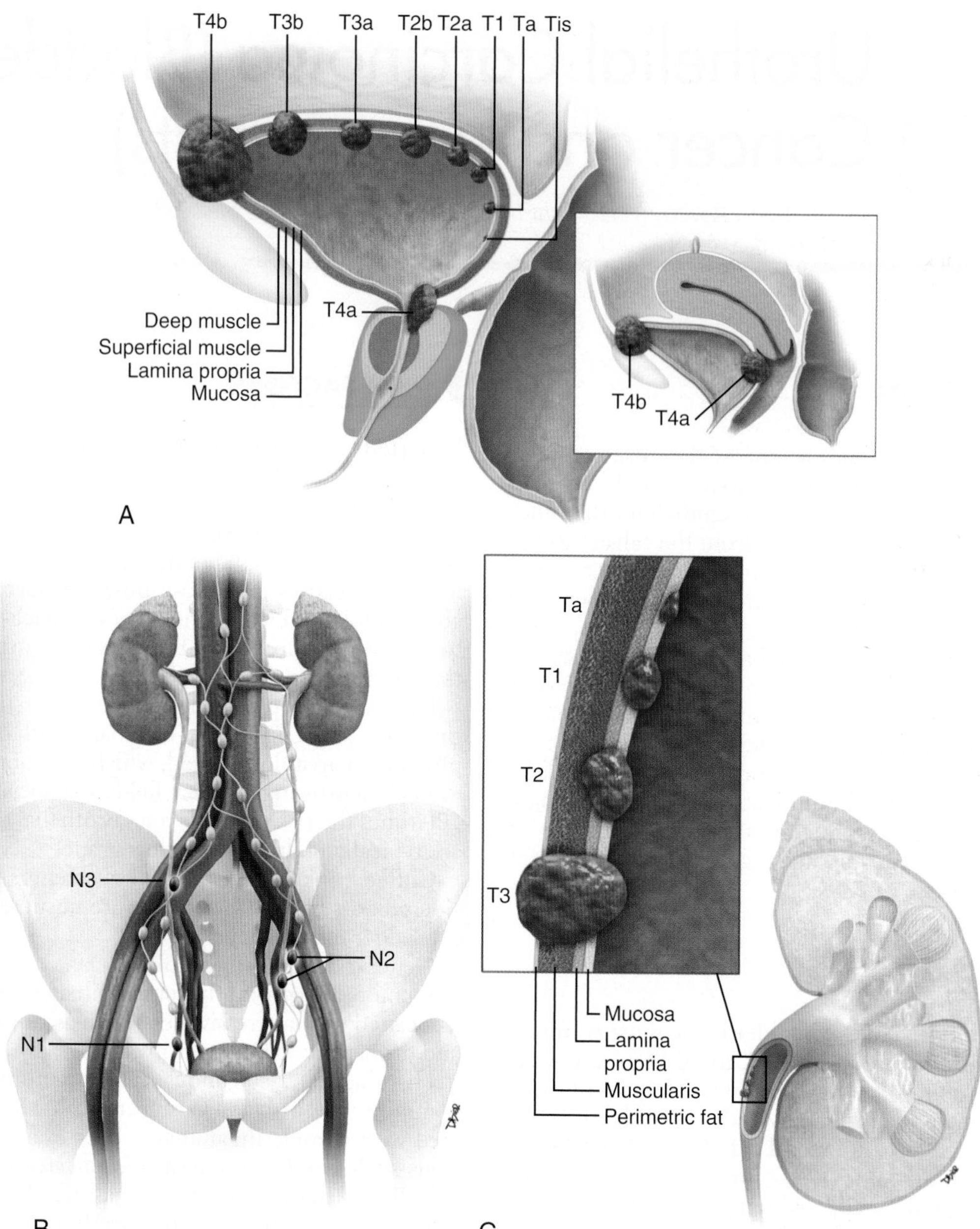

FIGURE 20.1. Bladder staging. Schematic of **A,** T stage and **B,** N stage (**B**). **C,** Upper tract staging: schematic of T stage.

The urothelial system collects, temporarily stores, and excretes urine. It includes the renal calyces, renal pelvis, ureters, bladder urethra. The epithelium of the collecting system to the level of the prostatic urethra, the urothelium, consists of the same cell type: transition cells. Deep to the urothelium is a layer of connective tissue with irregular smooth muscle fibers called the submucosa (although this term is incorrect because there is no true muscularis mucosae) or lamina propria. Deep to it, there are three layers of muscle (internal or superficial longitudinal, middle circular, and external or deep longitudinal). Deep to these is the serosa, and then the perivesical or periureteral fat and, at the dome of the bladder, the peritoneum (Fig. 20.1).

In adult males, chronic bladder outflow obstruction from prostatic hypertrophy commonly leads to hypertrophy of the bladder wall musculature and trabeculation. Outpouchings of mucosa, or diverticula, may also develop.

The vast majority of tumors involving the urothelium are of transitional cell origin (>90%), called urothelial cancer; other subtypes are squamous cell (5%–10%), adenocarcinoma (2%–3%), and small cell carcinoma (<1%).[12] Pure adenocarcinomas can be mucin-secreting tumors, they can form chunky calcifications, and they are most commonly found along the urachal ligament; however, adenocarcinomas mixed with transitional cell histology can be found anywhere along the urothelium.

Other extremely rare tumors include leiomyoma, hemangioma, granular cell tumors, neurofibroma, paraganglioma, pheochromocytoma, leiomyosarcoma, rhabdomyosarcoma, hematopoietic and lymphoid tumors (e.g., non-Hodgkin's lymphoma), carcinosarcoma, malignant melanoma, metastases, and direct invasion from other primary tumors from adjacent organs.[12]

Bladder

Bladder tumors fall biologically into two specific groups: superficial or not muscle-invasive, accounting for approximately 70% to 80%; and invasive, accounting for approximately 20% to 30%.

Superficial tumors are limited to the mucosa or lamina propria and tend to be papillary (i.e., projecting into the lumen) and of low histologic grade. They usually have a good prognosis, but have a propensity to recur (70% at 3 years), and 10% to 20% may progress to invasive disease (although this can be as high as 46% in patients with T1 disease).[15] Some 70% of patients with superficial tumors have low-grade papillary tumors, and 30% have higher-grade, flat, carcinomas *in situ*. The latter carry a higher risk of progression and invasion.[16]

Invasive tumors, which involve the muscle layers, tend to be solid, infiltrating, and of high histologic grade. These typically have a poorer prognosis.

Upper Tracts

In the ureter, the frequency distribution of urothelial tumors is distal (73%), mid (24%), and proximal (3%). Bilateral disease may occur in 2% to 5% of cases. The tumors are histologically similar to those in the bladder.[17] As with urothelial tumors in the bladder, upper tract tumors may be superficial (85%) or infiltrating (15%).

Several histopathologic grading systems relate to the epithelial tumors. The most commonly used is a three-grade system: low-grade (grade I), moderate (grade II), and high-grade or poorly differentiated (grade III).

KEY POINTS Anatomy and Pathology

- The urothelium is lined by transitional cells and extends from the calyces to the prostatic urethra.
- The "upper" urinary collecting tract includes the calyces, renal pelvis, and ureters; the "lower tract" includes the bladder and urethra.
- The entire urothelium is at risk of tumor development once a tumor is found in any location.
- The most common tumor of the collecting system is urothelial carcinoma, previously referred to as transitional cell carcinoma (>90%).
- Urothelial tumors may be superficial (70%) or invasive (30%).
- Muscle invasive tumors are generally of higher histologic grade and more aggressive, with poorer prognosis.

CLINICAL PRESENTATION

The majority of patients with urothelial tumors present with painless macro- or microscopic hematuria. Other symptoms include frequency, dysuria, urgency, and pyrexia. Pain may be a feature if the tumor or blood clots cause ureteric or bladder outflow obstruction or as a sign of advanced disease. Tumors at the vesicoureteral junction may cause ureteric obstruction resulting in hydronephrosis.

Hematuria can be associated with multiple other conditions such as renal parenchymal tumors or medical renal disease (e.g., nephritis), urinary tract inflammatory conditions (e.g., infections, chemotherapy, radiation), calculi (often associated with pain), endometriosis, prostatic disease, coagulopathy, and trauma or instrumentation.

PATTERNS OF TUMOR SPREAD

Bladder Cancer

Bladder urothelial tumors invade progressively through the bladder wall (i.e., lamina propria, muscle, serosa) and eventually to extravesical structures. In advanced local disease, tumor may extend to involve adjacent structures, such as the rectum, anterior abdominal wall, pelvic side wall muscles (e.g., the obturator internus muscle) and bones (e.g., the iliac and pubic bones). The bladder is extraperitoneal but is partially covered by peritoneum superiorly. If disease extends into the peritoneal layer, dissemination can occur within the peritoneal cavity, resulting in peritoneal implants and ascites.

Disease may spread through lymphatics, typically in a contiguous fashion from pelvic (internal iliac, obturator, and external iliac) to common iliac to retroperitoneal nodes. In advanced disease, lymphatic spread may extend above the diaphragm to mediastinal, hilar, and cervical nodes. The incidence of nodal metastasis is approximately 30% in tumors that involve the bladder wall and approximately 60% in those with extravesical invasion.[18] Nodal staging has a very important impact on prognosis. The tumor may also metastasize hematogenously, with the liver being the most common site for metastatic disease, followed by bones and lungs.[19]

The risk for lymphatic and/or hematogenous spread increases with increasing tumor size and stage, and the incidence of distant metastases increases with increasing tumor (T) and node (N) stages.

Urothelial disease in the bladder neck may extend into the urethra. Urethral disease may also involve adjacent structures such as the vaginal wall and the corpora of the penis. In males, urothelial cancer involving the urethra is commonly found in the prostatic urethra, where it may invade locally into the prostate gland itself.

Urachal adenocarcinomas, because they arise from the remnant urachus, have a propensity to spread within the peritoneal cavity and the anterior abdominal wall.

Upper Tracts

Primary urothelial tumors in the upper tracts spread locally to involve periureteral and peripelvic fat. In the renal pelvis, urothelial tumors can infiltrate into the renal parenchyma, where, unlike primary renal tumors, they tend to preserve the contour of the kidney. Infiltrating tumors of the ureters tend to be more aggressive than those in the bladder, probably because of the thinner wall of the ureter.[20,21]

Lymphatic spread is to locoregional periureteral (retroperitoneal, common iliac, and internal iliac) nodes.

Local invasion and lymphatic spread are more common with upper tract tumors than hematogenous spread, likely because of the relatively thin wall and rich lymphatic drainage of the ureters and upper tracts. The sites of hematogenous spread are similar to those of bladder tumors (liver, bones, and lungs).

KEY POINTS Patterns of Tumor Spread

- Tumor typically spreads by lymphatics before using the hematogenous pathway.
- Risk of metastatic disease increases with higher tumor and node stages and the histologic grade of the tumor.
- Distant metastases are less common and may involve liver, bones, and lungs in order of frequency.

STAGING EVALUATION

Bladder

The two main staging classification systems for tumors are (1) the tumor-node-metastasis (TNM) and (2) Jewett-Strong-Marshall classifications (Table 20.1). The TNM system is widely used and very comprehensive. *T stage* mainly describes the depth of local bladder wall invasion of the tumor in relation to normal bladder wall layers. N stage is based on the size and number of nodes involved by metastatic disease. M stage describes whether there are disseminated metastases or not. Retroperitoneal adenopathy is classified as M-stage disease.

T staging is presented in Fig. 20.1A and B. Superficial tumors are considered Tis, Ta, and T1; infiltrative tumors are T2, T3, and T4.[22,23]

Prognosis worsens with increasing T, N, and M stage and higher classes of Jewett-Strong-Marshall staging. The overall 5-year survival rate is 95.8% for *in situ*, 69.5% localized, 36.3% regional, and 4.6% distant disease.[24] Nodal status and organ confinement remain independent predictors of survival.[25]

Urothelial tumors may develop in bladder diverticula and may also arise or involve the prostatic urethra. Both of these have a poorer prognosis, the former because there is no muscle layer to act as a barrier to tumor spread.

Prognosis is also affected by tumor grade, the presence of vascular and lymphatic invasion, and diffuse carcinoma *in situ*. Of note, these latter factors are not currently reflected in staging classifications.[26]

Treatment options are influenced by tumor stage. Cystoscopy and biopsy are critical in the primary staging evaluation of bladder cancer, particularly for wall invasion. Clinical staging can underestimate the extent of disease in up to 50% of cases as compared with pathology, thus the importance of adequate use of imaging modalities according to the area of involvement to reduce error.[26]

TABLE 20.1 Comparison of American Joint Committee on Cancer and Jewett–Strong–Marshall Staging Systems

STAGE	DISEASE EXTENT	TNM CLOSEST EQUIVALENT
0	Limited to mucosa, flat *in situ* or papillary	Tis or Ta
A	Lamina propria invaded	T1
B1	< halfway through muscularis	T2a
B2	> halfway through muscularis	T2b
C	Perivesical fat,prostate, uterus or vagina, pelvic wall or abdominal wall	T3, T4a, T4b
D1	Pelvic lymph node(s) involved	N1-N3
D2	Distant metastases	M1

TNM, Tumor-node-metastasis.
(From National Cancer Institute. Surveillance, Epidemiology, and End Results Program. Staging: Comparison of AJCC & Jewell-Strong-Marshall Staging Systems. Available at https://training.seer.cancer.gov/bladder/abstract-code-stage/staging.html. Accessed May 23 2019.)

Upper Tracts

As with bladder staging, T staging of the upper tracts is assessed in relation to depth of invasion into the various layers of the wall of the ureter (see Fig. 20.1C).

KEY POINTS Staging

- T staging reflects the depth of bladder wall and perivesicle invasion.
- Cystoscopy and biopsy are critical in the primary staging evaluation of bladder cancer.
- Treatment options are directly influenced by tumor stage.
- Clinical staging can underestimate the extent of disease in up to 50% of cases.
- Imaging aids appropriate staging.

IMAGING

There are no established primary screening programs for detecting urothelial tumors. The majority of tumors are detected while investigating hematuria. Primary lower tract tumors are detected and evaluated by cystoscopy, and primary upper tract tumors are detected by imaging, most frequently computed tomography (CT) of the abdomen or CT urogram.

Primary Tumor (T)

Bladder

In early, low–T stage disease (Tis–T1), cystoscopy and deep biopsy with histologic evaluation is the standard of care. For more deeply invasive tumors (T2–T4), clinical staging, which includes bimanual examination under anesthesia to assess the bladder mass and fixation to adjacent organs, has reported rates of both under- and overstaging of 25% to 50%.[27–30] Imaging plays a fundamental role in the evaluation of such tumors, especially for nodal and hematogenous metastasis.

Tumor in a narrow neck diverticulum may escape cystoscopic detection, for which imaging can help. CT is the standard for staging these tumors, but magnetic resonance imaging (MRI) has proven to have additional advantages, such as better tissue contrast resolution and functional imaging that can aid local staging, including bladder wall and adjacent organ involvement, particularly of bladder tumors.[31]

The American College of Radiology (ACR) advocates the use of the ACR Appropriateness Criteria, which categorize the modalities as: (a) favorable, (b) may be appropriate (agreement and disagreement components), and (c) usually not appropriate. Their most recent expert panel consensus in 2018 advises that CT or MRI of the abdomen and pelvis without and with intravenous (IV) contrast, plain film of the chest, and CT or MRI of the pelvis with contrast are usually appropriate for collecting system tumors.[32]

Computed Tomography

Technique. Scanning in the portal venous phase at 60 to 80 seconds after initiation of IV contrast medium (100–150 mL at 2.5–3.0 mL/sec) allows detection of tumor enhancement in the bladder wall, during the corticomedullary phase of the kidneys, before excreted IV contrast medium reaches the bladder. Delayed images (180–300 seconds) allow detection of soft tissue density masses/filling defects against the background of IV contrast within the bladder lumen. Thin-slice (0.625 mm) isovoxel acquisition aids multiplanar reformations. Oral and rectal contrast may assist in delineation of adjacent organs in the pelvis. The bladder should be moderately distended. If a urinary catheter is in place, it should be clamped for a period of time before and during the examination.

Confounders that may limit the evaluation of the bladder and interpretation on CT or MRI include underdistention of the bladder, inflammation, infectious or radiation cystitis, postbiopsy changes, or ureteral jets.

Overall, accuracy for staging is between 55% and 95%, with optimal detection when scanned during corticomedullary phase with a full bladder. CT urogram can have a sensitivity of up to 93% and a specificity of up to 99%.[33,34] CT is most useful for tumors that are stage T3b or higher.

Findings. Urothelial tumors in the bladder may appear as foci of thickening in the wall (Fig. 20.2), (i.e., flat tumors), or as enhancing filling defects, (i.e., papillary tumors) (Fig. 20.3). Fine calcification can be seen on the mucosal surface. The lesions most commonly demonstrate early enhancement after IV contrast, which is thought reflect

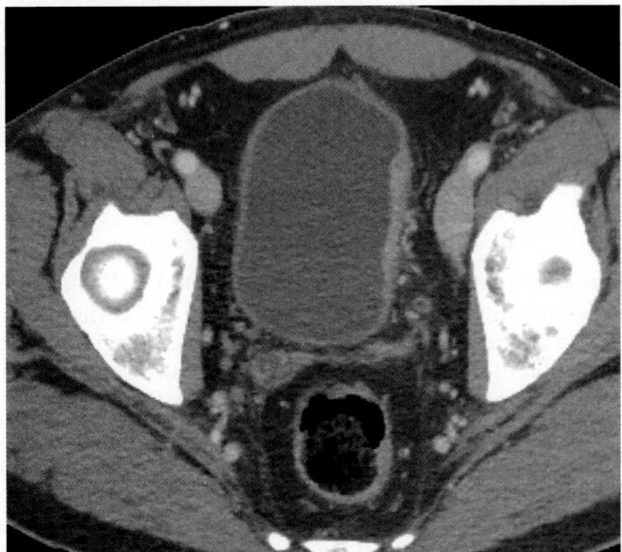

FIGURE 20.2. Urothelial tumor in the bladder. Enhancing thickening in the left lateral wall of the bladder.

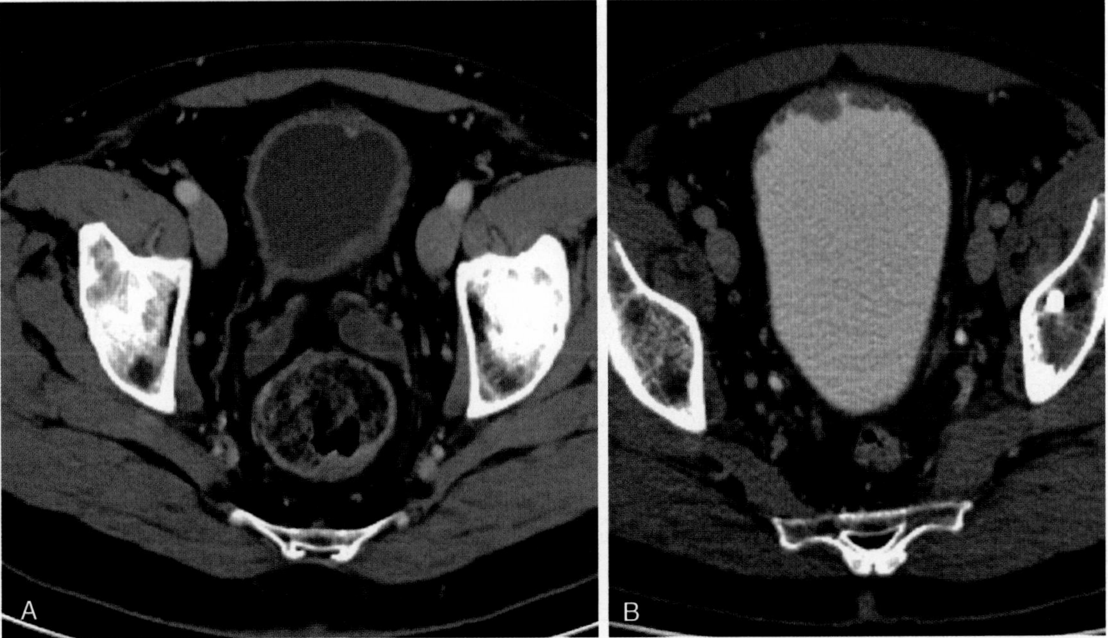

FIGURE 20.3. Urothelial tumor in the bladder. **A,** Enhancing small polypoidal anterior wall nodule and **B,** multifocal filling defects in fully opacified bladder.

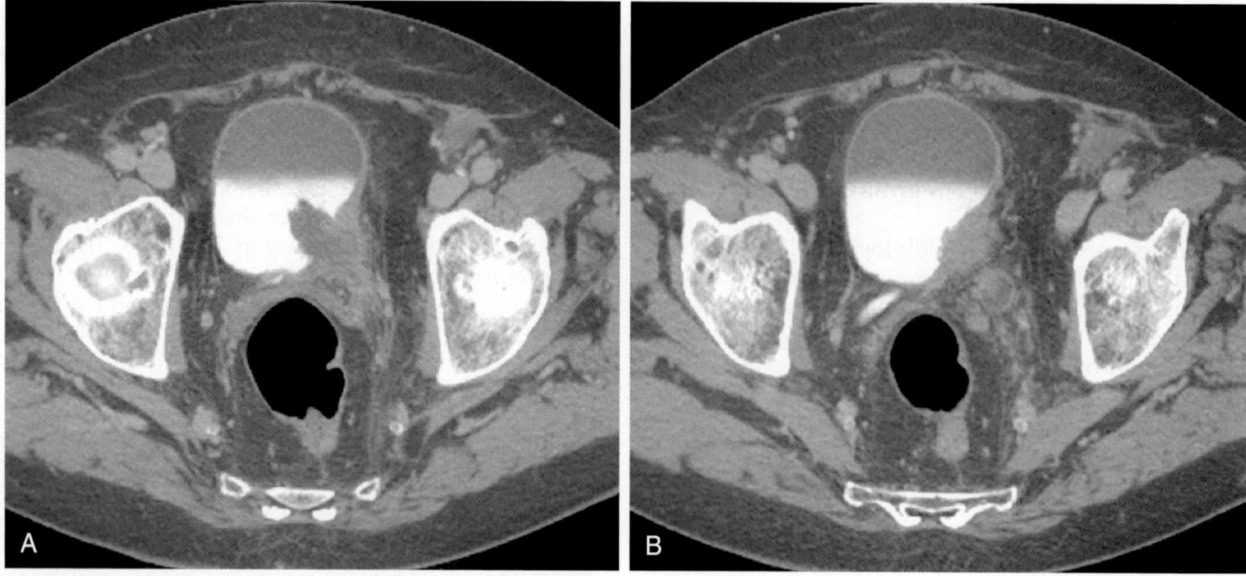

FIGURE 20.4. Urothelial tumor in the bladder. **A,** Large mass in the left posterolateral wall of the bladder causing vesicoureteral obstruction. **B,** Note the presence of the left ureteral dilatation compared to the normally opacified right ureter.

angiogenic activity of the tumor (Fig. 20.3). CT is unable to resolve the various bladder wall layers and is therefore, unable to resolve less than T3b-stage disease. However, retraction of the outer bladder wall at the site of the tumor is suggestive of deep muscle involvement (stage T2b).

Stage T3b representing gross disease beyond the bladder wall is suggested by irregularity and loss of definition of the outer bladder wall and/or nodules and stranding in the perivesical fat. T3a (microscopic perivesical) disease cannot be detected. Evaluation of stage T4 disease, with adjacent organ involvement, is often better undertaken by MRI than by CT because of better soft tissue contract of pelvic organs by MRI.

Tumors close to the vesicoureteral junction may cause ureteral obstruction, which may be a presenting feature of the disease (Fig. 20.4). Tumors may also be detected in bladder diverticula (Fig. 20.5), which importantly may not be visible on cystoscopy.

Magnetic Resonance Imaging.

Technique. The use of either 1.5T or 3T magnets with dedicated multiplanar thin (3- to 4-mm) T2-weighted (T2W) images, diffusion-weighted imaging (DWI)/apparent diffusion coefficient (ADC) and dynamic contrast-enhanced (DCE) imaging can deliver a high-quality MRI that provides not only anatomic but also functional information. Combinations of at least two planes with T2W images without fat suppression and an additional plane are usually obtained with two-dimensional fast spin echo (FSE) or turbo spin echo (TSE).

Protocols commonly include:

- Sagittal and coronal T2 sequence (FSE or TSE) without fat suppression
- Axial T2 fat-suppressed
- Axial T1 dual echo
- Three-dimensional (3D) heavily T2W sequence or single-shot FSE from kidneys to bladder

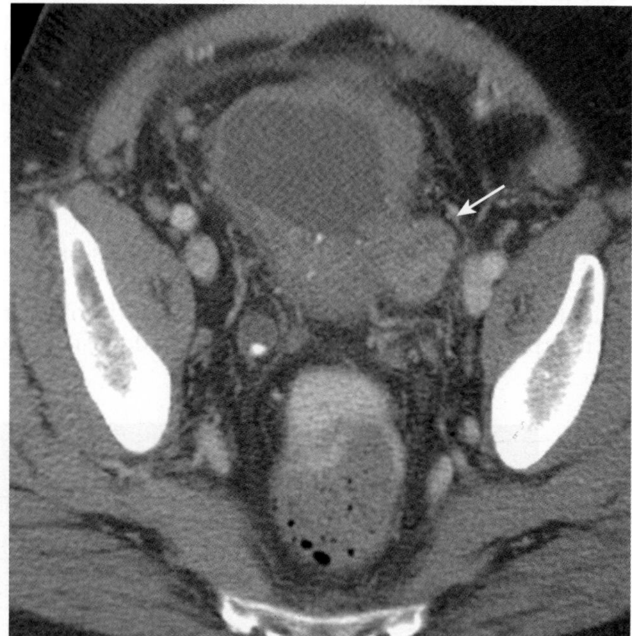

FIGURE 20.5. Urothelial tumor (*arrow*) arising in a bladder diverticulum.

- Coronal or sagittal T1 fat-saturated dynamic (DCE) pre- and postcontrast runs

IV glucagon can be administered to reduce bowel motion artifacts. Saturation bands along the anterior and posterior pelvis may also decrease motion and wrap artifacts. The bladder should be moderately distended because overdistention can cause patient discomfort and restlessness, which may contribute to motion and suboptimal imaging.

The consensus proposal Vesical Imaging-Reporting and Data System has been suggested as a way to stage bladder wall invasion.[35,36] In theory, intrinsic staging errors,

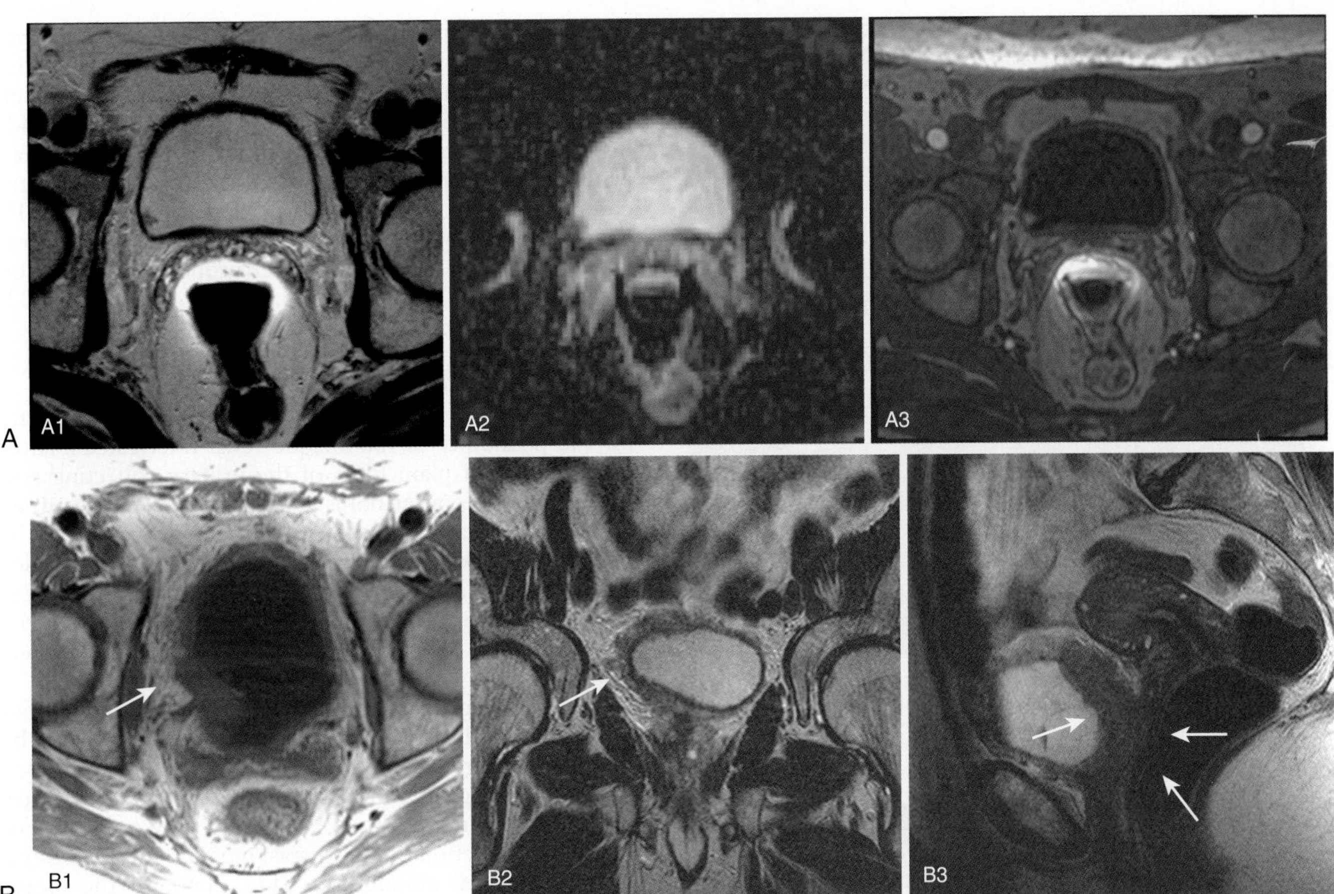

FIGURE 20.6. A small, enhancing bladder nodule on T2 with restriction and enhancement on early stages. **A1** Bladder tumor on axial T1-weighted and **A2**, coronal T2-weighted magnetic resonance imaging (MRI) shows irregular thickening (*arrows*) in the right lateral wall of the bladder. Note stranding and nodularity in the perivesical fat, which in this case was attributed to T3b disease. **B,** Sagittal MRI shows the posterior bladder tumor (*arrows*) closely abutting the vagina. The rectum is posterior to the vagina.

especially understaging, and disagreements between radiologists should be reduced through scripted evaluation of the bladder wall.[37,38] Preliminary early validation and interobserver agreement data are favorable.[35,36,39] There are also reports of quantitative/semiquantitative measurement of tumor characteristics such as ADC and enhancement curves corresponding to histological grading; these remains investigational. [37]

Findings. Tumors are usually hyperintense to muscle on T2W images. The combination of T2W, DWI/ADC, and contrast-enhanced T1 DCE can show early-stage tumors (Fig. 20.6A) and is superior to CT for evaluation of and discrimination between T1 and T2 tumors by evaluating for violation of bladder muscle that normally appears hypointense on T2W imaging and enhances; furthermore, MRI can also identify early perivesicle fat invasion (T3b).[40] DCE differentiation between T1 and T2 stages can approach a sensitivity of 90%, a specificity of 87%, and an accuracy of 84% to 87%.[41–44] Differentiating between T2a and T2b is not very important, as survival/outcomes are similar.[45]

Tumors have predominantly higher signals on DWI than normal bladder. Assessment of DWI may be confused by confounders such as inflammation, infection, or blood products; however, the sensitivity of 88% and specificity of 85% support its use.[46,47] T3b disease appears as hypointense nodules or stranding within the perivesicle fat on T1- and non–fat-suppressed T2W sequences (see Fig. 20.6B).

Overall, for staging, studies suggest that MRI is more accurate than CT, with accuracies ranging from 73% to 96% for MRI compared with 40% to 95% for CT. This is largely because of the superior ability to assess bladder wall involvement. It should be noted that most reported MRI evaluations have been undertaken with body, and not pelvic phase, array coils, and accuracy should improve further with higher-resolution coils.[18,48–66]

Confounders mimicking tumor include inflammation, edema, or fibrosis, for example, following biopsy, transurethral resection of bladder tumor (TURBT), or radiation therapy (Fig. 20.7). Imaging for local staging is best undertaken before biopsy or resection when feasible.[29]

Ultrasonography. A number of ultrasonographic techniques, such as transabdominal, transurethral, transvaginal, and transrectal, have been investigated to evaluate bladder tumors. Ultrasound can distinguish bladder wall layers, that is, inner hyperechoic mucosa, hypoechoic muscularis propria and outer hyperecogenicity from the serosa superiorly and extravesical tissue in the retroperitoneum (Fig. 20.8).[31] However, transabdominal ultrasound has low accuracy for bladder tumor staging. Intravesical ultrasound has been

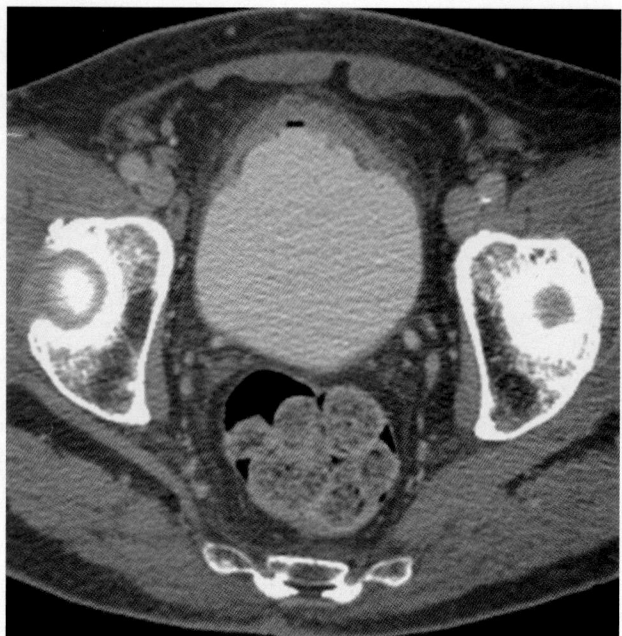

FIGURE 20.7. Perivesical fat stranding after cystoscopic biopsy, which confounds interpretation of extravesical extension of disease. Note gas in the bladder.

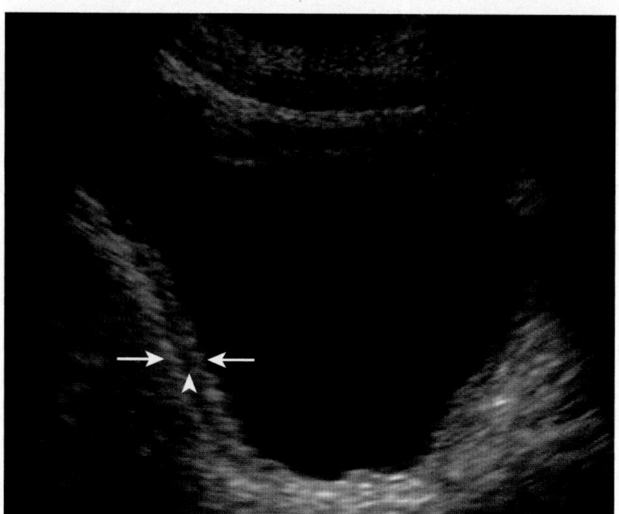

FIGURE 20.8. Layers of bladder wall showing the hypoechoic muscularis propria (*arrowhead*), hyperechoic mucosa (*arrow pointing left*), and hyperechoic serosa (*arrow pointing right*).

reported to have accuracy for T staging ranging from 62% to 92%.[67,68] Unfortunately, it has limited utility because of the poor visualization of extravesical structures.[69]

Upper Tracts

Unlike the lower tract, detection and evaluation of upper tract tumors rely heavily on imaging, because they are relatively inaccessible to direct visualization without more aggressive and invasive instrumentation.

IV urography (IVU) has limited use for detection or staging. In addition to the lumen, CT and MRI can enable evaluation of the bladder wall and adjacent organs. Direct pyelography is more invasive but also allows for cytologic sampling in the same procedure. CT urography (CTU) has a variety of advantages, the most important of which is excellent spatial resolution of the ureters and surrounding tissue. Magnetic resonance urography (MRU) is an evolving technique that has some potential advantages compared with CTU and can be performed without IV contrast use in patients with contraindications for intravenous contrast. MRU has greater propensity for motion artifact and can have worse spatial resolution than CT, depending on technique.

Intravenous Urography.

Technique. A single precontrast film is obtained to evaluate for the possibility of radiopaque renal tract calculi. After that, a series of plain films of the urinary collecting system are obtained after bolus administration of IV contrast medium. Frontal radiographs of the upper tracts may be supplemented with tomographic radiographs of the pyelocaliceal system and prone and oblique films of the ureters with and without abdominal compression to distend the upper tracts to allow better visualization of pyelocaliceal system.

Imaging Findings. Signs of urothelial tumors in the upper tract include filling defects and strictures, which may be smooth or irregular. In the pyelocaliceal system, a stippled appearance suggests contrast medium trapped in papillary fronds of the tumor. Tumors in a calyx may cause lack of or delayed excretion of IV contrast medium into that calyx, termed "calyceal amputation" (Fig. 20.9). In the ureter or region of the vesicoureteral orifice, tumors may cause ureteric obstruction and hydronephrosis, which may also be associated with delayed or absent excretion of contrast medium. IVU may fail to detect upper tract tumors in as many as 50% to 90% of cases.[70,71]

Direct Pyelography.

Technique. Direct access to the upper tracts can be obtained through invasive procedures. Retrograde access requires cystoscopy and cannulation of each vesicoureteral orifice. Antegrade access requires percutaneous puncture of the pyelocaliceal system via percutaneous nephrostomy. It requires traversing the kidney, but it may be indicated if retrograde access is not possible, for example, with a distal obstructing lesion in the ureter or a distorted bladder secondary to tumor or surgery.

Both techniques offer the opportunity to radiographically visualize the relevant upper tract after administration of contrast and to sample urine for cytology. In principle, after direct access, ureteroscopic evaluation and biopsy can also be performed.

Computed Tomography Urography.

Technique. Specific protocols are well documented and very effective; however, the fundamental requirements are (1) high-resolution scans to allow detection of small filling defects, urothelial wall thickening, and 3D reformations and (2) ureteric distention. Current 64- or higher row multidetector CT scanners have the potential for isovoxel submillimeter acquisitions covering the entire urinary collecting system with a single breathhold. These can be reconstructed in different planes at greater slice

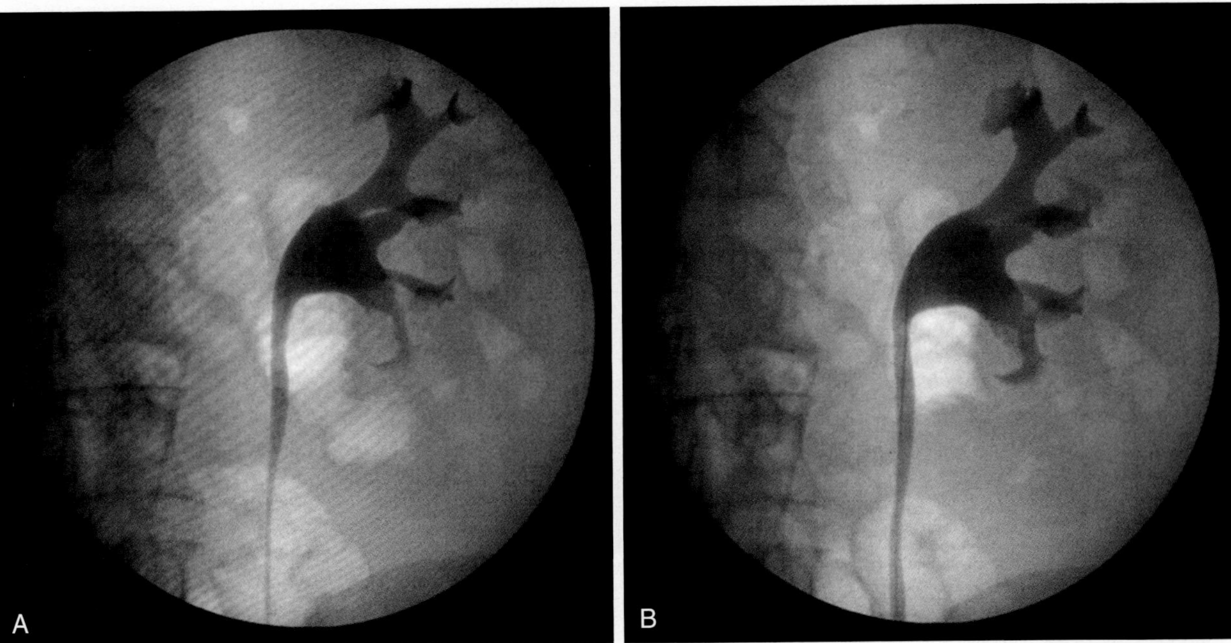

FIGURE 20.9. Urothelial tumor in upper tracts. Retrograde pyelogram findings are of inferior renal collecting system irregularity/near amputation, which should be compared to the rest of normal calyceal systems.

thickness (usually 2.5 mm) for reading to decrease noise and radiation dose.

A precontrast scan of the abdomen and pelvis is usually obtained for presence of radiopaque stones or hyperdense clots. IV fluids and/or furosemide are used to distend the ureters. One technique employs two separate administrations of IV contrast ("split bolus"), with initial infusion of 70 to 120 cc of contrast at 3 cc/sec for initial imaging before urinary excretion followed 10 to 15 minutes later by infusion of normal saline with or without furosemide and a second 50- to 80-cc injection of IV contrast at 3 cc/sec for delayed imaging with contrast in the ureters and bladder.[31,72] The latter imaging results in nephrographic phase of the kidneys from the second IV contrast injection and excretory phase of the pyelocaliceal system from the first IV contrast injection.

With current dose-saving techniques and increase use of dual-energy CT scanners, the amount of contrast injected can be reduced, with some protocols injecting a total of only 100 cc or less. Unlike many other CT applications in oncology, positive gastrointestinal contrast media should be avoided, because it may complicate subsequent evaluation, especially during 3D image reformation and in evaluation of urinary diversions.

Findings. Urothelial lesions may be detected as filling defects or strictures in the upper tracts. However, because of its intrinsic cross-sectional acquisition, CTU also has the capability to visualize urothelial wall thickening (Fig. 20.10).[73] Urothelial cancer can rarely appear as fine encrusted calcifications mimicking renal calculi.

In the pyelocaliceal system, T1 or T2 disease can be suggested by the presence of a fat plane or contrast medium between the lesion and the renal parenchyma. T3 tumors are suggested by the loss of renal sinus fat and abnormal enhancement of the adjacent parenchyma. T4 tumors show invasion of adjacent organs.

Urothelial tumors in the pyelocaliceal system can be difficult to differentiate from primary renal tumors; the former, however, are typically infiltrative and tend to preserve the contour of the kidney.[74] The CT equivalent of calyceal amputation can occasionally be observed (Fig. 20.11).

CTU has higher sensitivity for detecting upper tract disease than IVU, with a reported pooled sensitivity on metaanalysis of 96%, compared with sensitivities for IVU of 50% to 60%.[75–79]

CTU is also able to assess for nodal and metastatic disease, thus offering a comprehensive overall evaluation in one examination. An important consideration in the utilization of CTU is its relatively high radiation dose, which may be up to 40 mSv depending on technique used.[78]

Magnetic Resonance Urography. MRU has several advantages over CTU, including lack of ionizing radiation, lack of iodinated contrast media (and associated allergy and nephrotoxicity), higher contrast resolution, and direct multiplanar imaging. Its disadvantages include commonly relatively poor spatial resolution, relatively prolonged acquisition times, and motion artifacts.

Technique. Techniques keep evolving, and as explained in the bladder segment, unenhanced 3D heavily T2W sequence of the entire pyelocaliceal system ureters and bladder, as well as contrast enhanced coronal T1 dynamic sequence with similar field of view, are suggested for evaluation of the upper tracts (Fig. 20.12). In techniques relying on intravenously administered MRI contrast agents, additional images are acquired when contrast is excreted into the collecting systems, using angiographic-type sequences.

Advantages of the noncontrast techniques are that the collecting systems can be visualized without employing IV contrast and when the system(s) are obstructed or

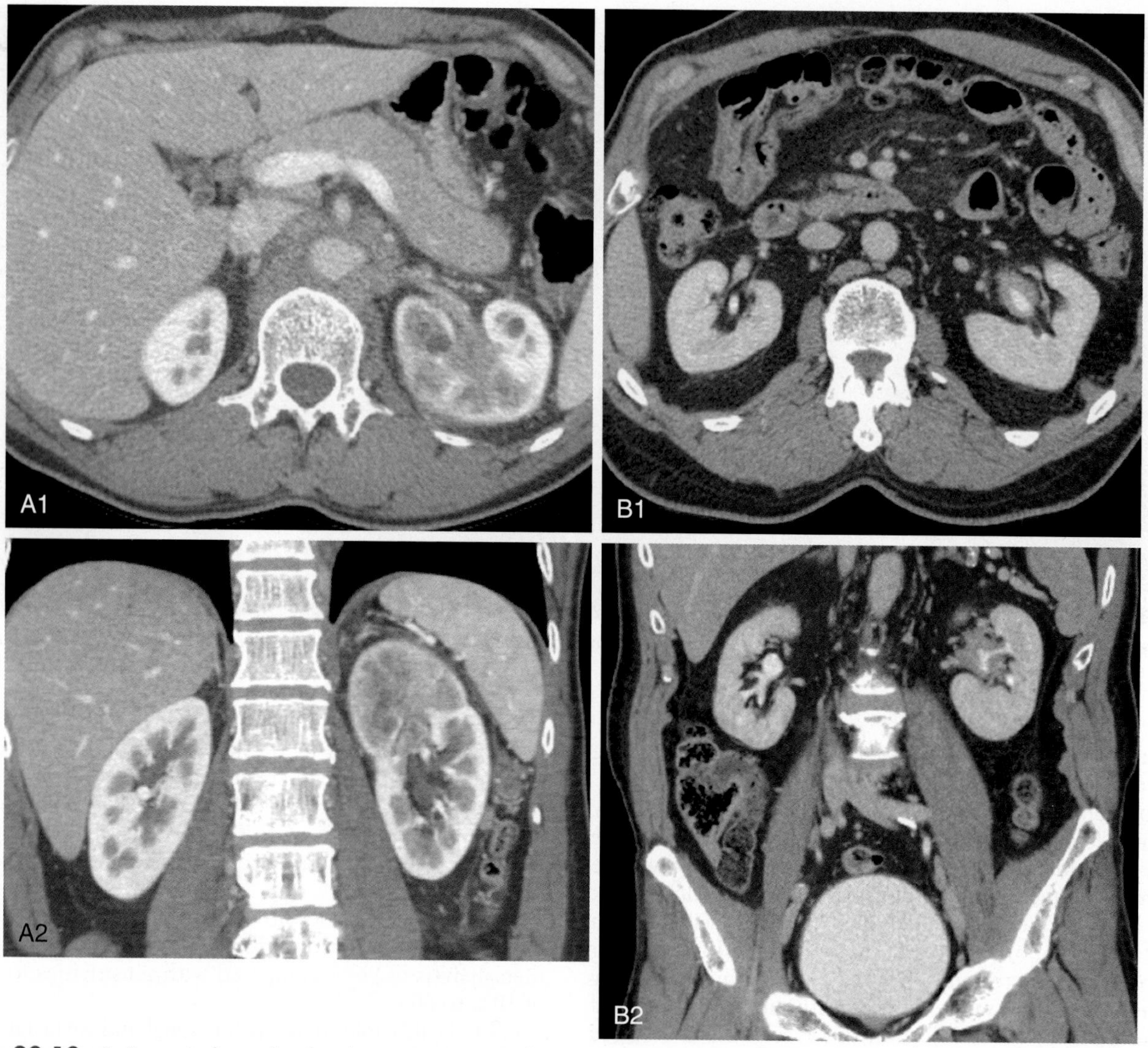

FIGURE 20.10. **A**, Tumor in the pyelocaliceal system on computed tomography urography (CTU). Axial and coronal images of CTU during the nephrographic phase showing the infiltrative nature of the tumor. Note is made of retroperitoneal metastasis on axial image. **B**, Tumor on CTU excretory phase showing filling defect in the left renal pelvis.

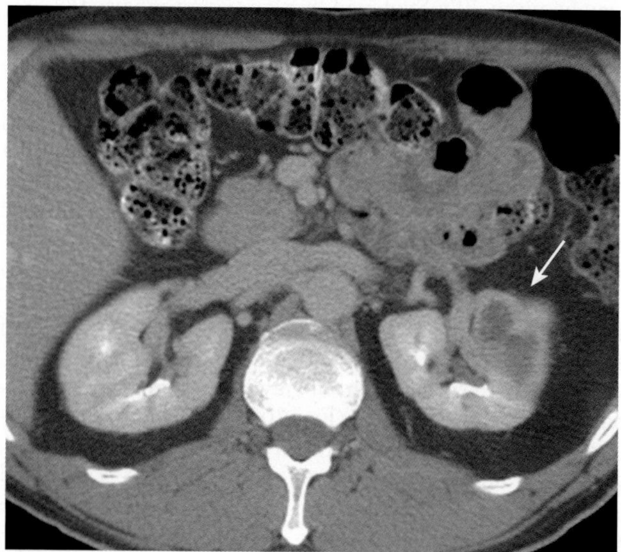

FIGURE 20.11. Urothelial tumor in the upper tracts. Focal dilatation of the calyces in the upper pole of the left kidney (*arrow*; "calyceal amputation") because of tumor in the calyceal orifice.

nonfunctioning. Thus, one can visualize luminal features as well as urothelial wall thickening.

Confounders of urothelial wall thickening and/or periureteric stranding can be attributed to surgery, biopsy, or inflammatory conditions (e.g., radiation or stents).

Ultrasonography. Ultrasonography has a very limited role in the detection and evaluation of upper tract tumors. Urothelial tumors in the renal pelvis may appear as an intraluminal echogenic focus within the renal pelvis or a mass in the echogenic renal sinus, withsout or with hydronephrosis. Infundibular tumors may cause focal calyceal dilatation (the equivalent of the amputated calyx on IVU).[20] Following the entire length of the ureters is very often not possible.

Nodal Disease (N)

Nodal disease from primary bladder tumors involves pelvic nodes and progresses superiorly toward retroperitoneal

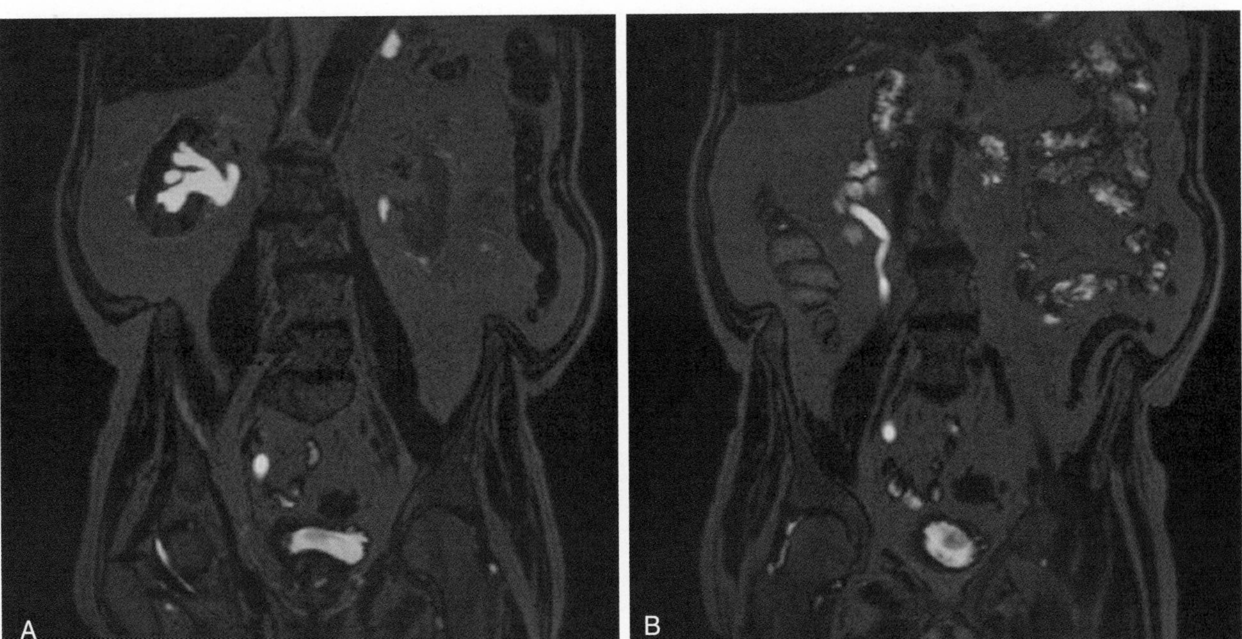

FIGURE 20.12. Magnetic resonance urography using a heavily T2-weighted sequence with fat suppression shows the right pyelocaliceal system and ureter dilated because of right bladder mass.

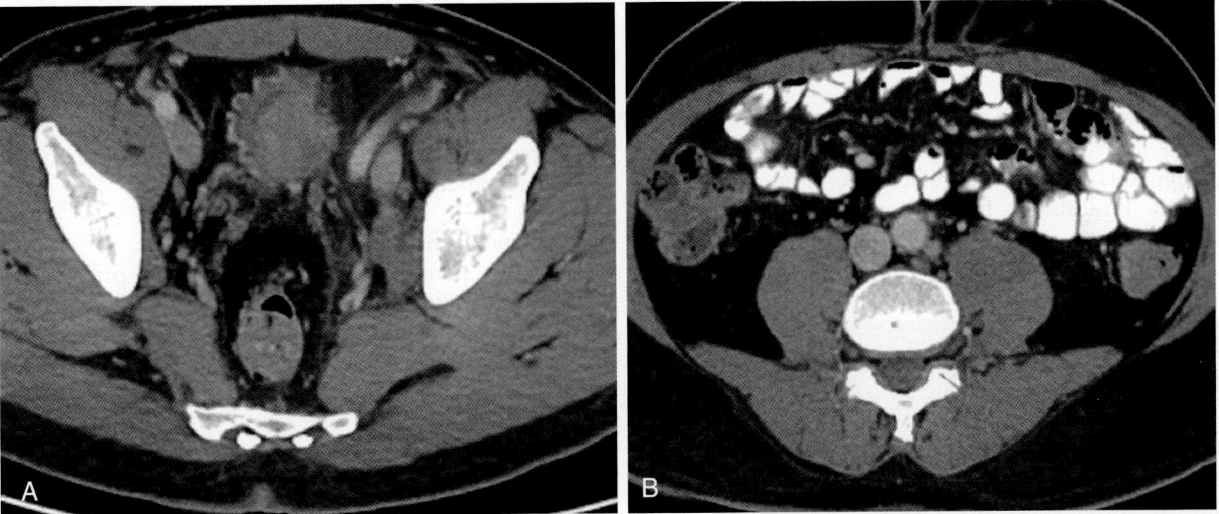

FIGURE 20.13. Nodal metastases. **A**, Left enlarged external iliac adenopathy (note the bladder dome tumor) and **B**, single paraaortic adenopathy.

nodes. In advanced disease, metastatic adenopathy can involve mediastinal, hilar, and cervical nodes. Nodal metastases from upper tract tumors first involves adjacent nodes in the retroperitoneum.

Computed Tomography

Lymph node size is the main criterion for assessing nodal involvement by CT (Fig. 20.13) or MRI. Unfortunately, small nodes can contain tumor, leading to false-negative results, and enlarged nodes may be reactive and may not contain tumor, resulting in false-positive findings. The challenge of detecting lymph node metastases is compounded by the fact that urothelial cancers frequently cause little nodal enlargement.[79]

Magnetic Resonance Imaging

Standard axial (two-dimensional) CT and MRI have very similar nodal staging accuracies for pelvic tumors in general: reported accuracies for assessing nodal disease in pelvic cancers for CT range from 70% to 97% and for MRI from 73% to 98%.[65,80,81] Sensitivities and specificities vary according to the nodal cutoff size, with sensitivities increasing and specificities reducing with smaller cutoff dimensions, and vice versa.

There is a suggestion that volumetric and architectural appearance, rather than planar assessment of the morphology of lymph nodes, may improve accuracy, with rounded nodes being more suspicious than oval nodes. Size cutoff values of 8 mm minimal axial diameter for rounded nodes and 10 mm for flat or oval nodes have reported accuracies of 90%, with positive predictive value of 94% and negative predictive value of 89%.[82] Identification of abnormal clusters of nodes can also be made.

Approaches currently being explored include DCE by MRI using temporal resolutions of 2 seconds or better based on the observation that most metastases, like the primary tumor, enhance more rapidly than normal[82,83] an, lymphographic MRI contrast agents using ultra-small superparamagnetic iron oxide (USPIO; 20 nm). USPIO has a reported sensitivity and specificity of 87% and 92%, respectively; however, this is lymph node size–dependent, and USPIO is not currently available for clinical use.[82–85]

2-[^{18}F] Fluoro-2-Deoxy-D-Glucose Positron Emission Tomography

The role of 2-[^{18}F] fluoro-2-deoxy-D-glucose (FDG)–positron emission tomography (PET) in urothelial cancers is under evaluation. FDG-PET is of limited value in assessing the primary tumor because of excretion of activity into the entire urinary tract. Metastatic lymph nodes may demonstrate increased FDG avidity (Fig. 20.14); however, the combination of the poor spatial resolution of PET and the frequency of small nodes containing metastatic disease limits its utility in general staging.[80,86] Even so, FDG-PET may be able to predict response and assist in treatment evaluation and the differentiation of tumor recurrence from posttreatment (radiation) fibrosis.[87] Other PET tracers are under investigation.[88]

Metastatic Disease (M)

Hematogenous metastases are less common than nodal metastases. Typical sites for the former include the liver, lungs, and bones.

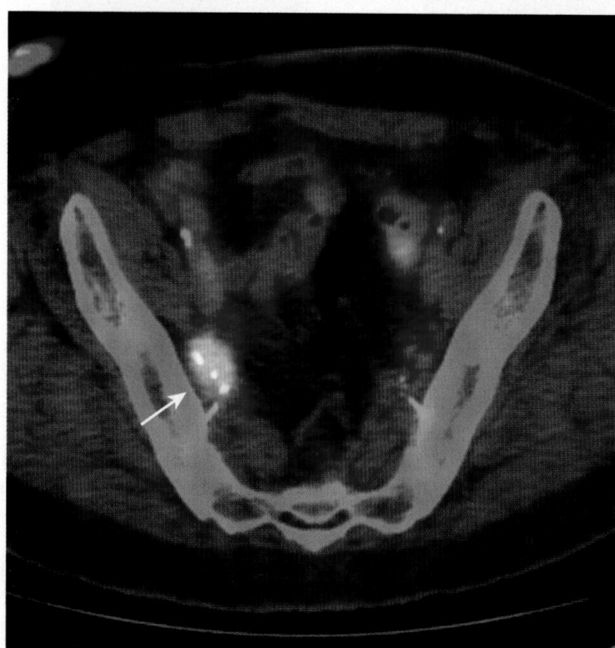

FIGURE 20.14. Pelvic adenopathy on 2-[^{18}F] fluoro-2-deoxy-D-glucose positron emission tomography/computed tomography. Recurrent disease after cystectomy. Hypermetabolic node (*arrow*) in right internal iliac territory.

Computed Tomography

Although CT has its limitations in staging of the primary bladder tumor, it is commonly used for screening and staging nodal and hematogenous metastatic disease from urothelial tumors (Figs. 20.15 and 20.16). If more detailed characterization of lesions, for example, in the liver, is required, or if contrast-enhanced CT cannot be undertaken, then MRI may be considered.

Magnetic Resonance Imaging

MRI is typically employed to solve specific problems, for example, in the evaluation of indeterminate liver lesions. Brain metastases are extremely uncommon in urothelial tumors; one exception is small-cell urothelial cancer, where there has been a reported 50% incidence in stage 3 or greater tumors.[89]

Nuclear Medicine

Skeletal metastases are relatively uncommon in urothelial tumors, and bone scintigraphy is not generally indicated unless there are relevant symptoms such as bone pain. Bone scintigraphy can be supplemented with plain radiography, CT and/or MRI (Fig. 20.17) for lesion characterization. The role of PET/CT is limited. It has shown promising results in predicting treatment efficacy and may be useful in evaluating residual or recurrent disease.

Plain Film Radiography

In most instances, chest radiography suffices for evaluation of the thorax for larger lesions. CT is superior for smaller lesions. Abdominal plain films have little role in asymptomatic patients with urothelial tumors.

Percutaneous Biopsy

Although percutaneous biopsy of the primary tumor is rarely indicated, guided biopsy of abnormal nodes or possible metastatic foci can have an important role in management.

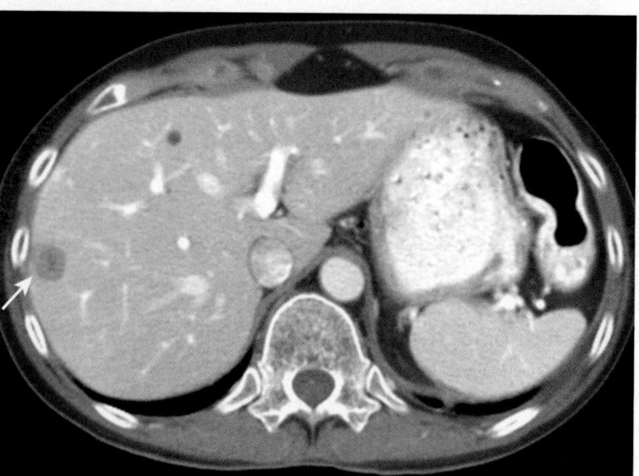

FIGURE 20.15. Liver metastasis from primary urothelial tumor in bladder. Contrast-enhanced computed tomography with a hypodense lesion (*arrow*) in the right lobe of the liver. The other smaller, hypodense lesion is a cyst.

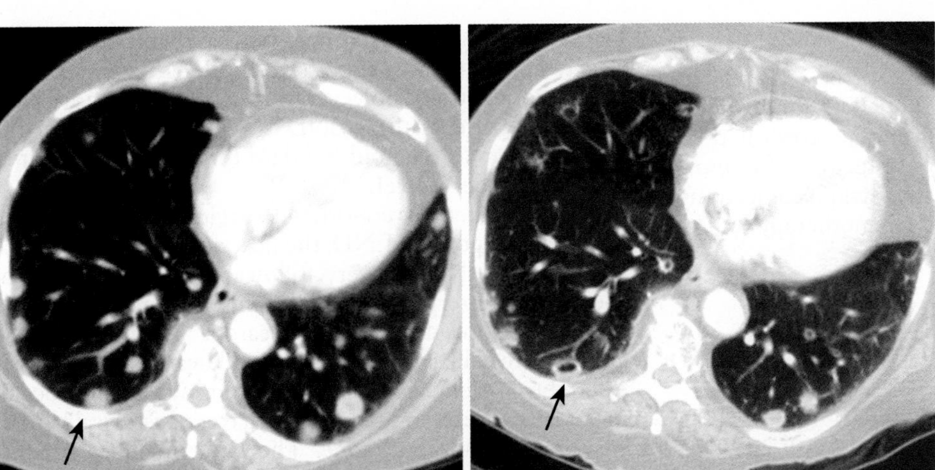

Figure 20.16. **A** and **B**, Metastatic disease to the lungs. Multiple pulmonary nodules. Note cavitation of some nodules with chemotherapy as a sign of treatment response (*arrow*).

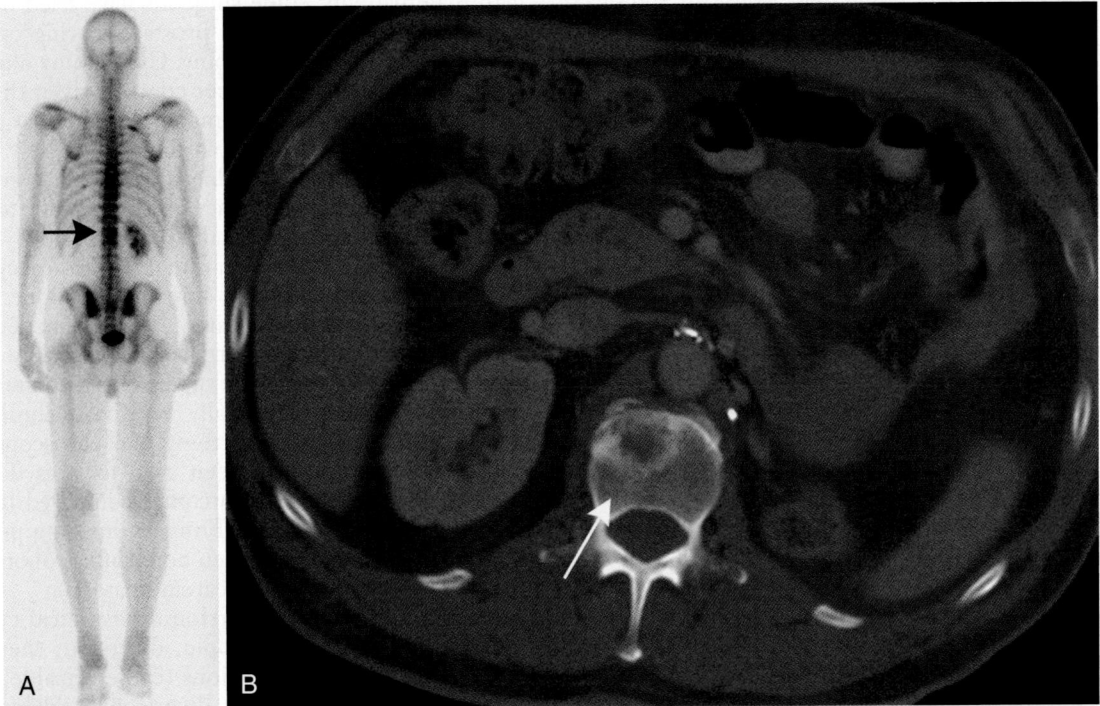

Figure 20.17. Metastatic disease to bone. **A**, Bone scintigram shows activity in the L1 vertebral body, with **B**, lucency on associated computed tomography (*arrow*).

Key Points Imaging

- Magnetic resonance imaging (MRI) is superior to computed tomography (CT) in <T3b-stage bladder cancer.
- CT and MRI have comparable staging accuracies of nodal and hematogenous metastatic disease, although CT is superior for lung metastasis, and MRI can be more sensitive for bone metastases.
- The role of positron emission tomography/CT is limited. It has shown promising results in predicting treatment efficacy and may be useful in evaluating residual or recurrent disease.
- Evaluation and screening for upper tract disease by percutaneous imaging is better undertaken by CT urography.

Key Points The Radiology Report

- Describe the tumor location and depth of invasion, if possible, and the presence of adjacent organ involvement.
- Note the presence of additional urothelial tumors.
- Indicate the size and location of suspicious locoregional and nonlocoregional lymph nodes.
- Identify potential metastases.
- Convey the overall level of confidence of the findings and offer suggestions for other imaging or investigations if needed.
- Quantify the extent of progression or response to therapy.

TREATMENT

Therapeutic measures include TURBT for superficial tumors, with or without adjuvant intravesical therapy, radical cystectomy or cystoprostatectomy for more advanced cases, with or without pelvic lymphadenectomy, and, in inoperable cases, palliative chemotherapy and/or radiotherapy.

Surgery

Initial diagnosis of urothelial carcinoma of the bladder involves cystoscopy with visual identification of an intravesical tumor. This was traditionally done with regular light ("white light"), but recently "blue light cystoscopy," which capitalizes on the fluorescent property of urothelial cancers for better visualization and detection, was approved in the United States. After initial cystoscopy, the tumor is resected via the transurethral route (TURBT). Initial transurethral resection (TUR) should result in complete resection of all visible tumors and be extensive enough that the specimens should include muscularis propria, with a minimum of cautery artifact. In patients who have high-grade tumors resected but no muscle present in the specimen, a repeat resection is recommended. For patients diagnosed with high-risk noninvasive tumors (see definitions later), a second restaging TUR is recommended because upstaging occurs in 49% to 64% of patients with initial apparent T1 lesions. The authors routinely perform the restaging TUR at 4 to 6 weeks to ensure more confident staging and a more accurate gauge of the biology of the disease by identifying tumors with rapid growth potential. This timing also avoids the typical delay of 12 weeks to identify T2 disease; upstaging of many muscle-invasive tumors has been shown with delays greater than 12 weeks.[90]

Treatment for non–muscle-invasive urothelial carcinoma of the bladder is complete TUR of all visible lesions; however, up to 70% of bladder tumors recur even with aggressive resection, and as many as 10% to 30% progress. Certain subgroups of patients with bladder cancer are at higher risk for recurrence and progression and should be considered for intravesical therapy after TUR, including patients with high-grade tumors (which are associated with a 45% risk of progression at 3 years and the greater risk of cancer-related death) and carcinoma *in situ* (Tis, which is associated with a 54% rate of progression to muscle-invasive disease). Irrespective of grade, patients with large lesions (>3 cm), multifocal tumors, evidence of lamina propria invasion, or early recurrence (within 2 years) are at increased risk; in such cases, aggressive intervention with intravesical immunotherapy leads to response rates of up to 85%. However, because even solitary, low-grade, Ta lesions can recur, these must also be considered for adjunctive intravesical therapy of lesser intensity—here, a single perioperative dose of chemotherapy usually suffices.[91]

For patients with muscle-invasive urothelial carcinoma of the bladder with no clinical evidence of metastasis, the first decision required in treatment planning is whether to pursue radical cystectomy plus lymph node dissection (RC+LND) or a bladder-sparing approach. The bladder-sparing approach may be reasonable in carefully selected patients (with aggressive TUR, partial cystectomy, or chemoradiation); however, it is used only in very select groups of patients. RC+LND is widely regarded in the United States as the gold standard for the management of invasive bladder cancer.[92]

Once a patient is considered surgically resectable and able to undergo RC+LND, the next decision is whether to proceed directly to surgery followed by adjuvant chemotherapy or surgery with neoadjuvant chemotherapy, which are subjects of continuing research. An individualized approach may be adopted, with neoadjuvant chemotherapy offered to patients considered to be at high risk for occult metastatic disease or those who have a historically poor survival with surgery alone. The latter includes patients with cT3 disease, preoperative hydronephrosis, or presence of features on TUR specimen such as lymphovascular invasion or variant histology (e.g., small-cell carcinoma or micropapillary cancer).[92–95]

In male patients, some surgeons have tried performing cystectomy alone (so-called prostate-sparing cystectomy) instead of a cystoprostatectomy. Cystectomy alone carries significant risk of poor cancer control, given the inability to exclude prostatic involvement by urothelial carcinoma or prostatic adenocarcinoma before surgery. Furthermore, for patients with bladder cancer, this leaves behind the prostatic urothelial surface as a potential site of occult recurrence, which can be fatal.

Although chemotherapy can augment radical cystectomy, it must be emphasized that surgical technique is critical. Data demonstrate that the extent of lymphadenectomy and the incidence of positive margins, both critically important in determining outcome, are superior in the hands of experienced surgeons.[96] Minimally invasive techniques (e.g., robot-assisted radical cystectomy or laparoscopic-assisted radical cystectomy) have been used for this disease, but there is no difference in outcomes compared to open or robotic radical cystectomy. From an imaging perspective, unusual recurrences have been noted after robotic-assisted procedures (e.g., peritoneal carcinomatosis).

Options for urinary diversion after radical cystectomy include continent orthotopic diversion (neobladder), continent cutaneous diversions (catheterizable pouches), or noncontinent cutaneous diversion (ileal loop stoma) (Fig. 20.18).

Intravesical Therapy

Whereas some non–muscle-invasive urothelial carcinomas can have an indolent course, a large subset of patients presents with disease associated with an increased risk of recurrence or progression. Several intravesical therapies can decrease these risks, and proper selection of patients for intravesical therapy is important to improve prognosis and save the patient's bladder.

For patients with non–muscle-invasive bladder cancer, we recommend complete TUR of all visible disease, followed by intravesical single-dose chemotherapy. The most commonly used intravesical agent in this setting is mitomycin C; however, data suggest that most chemotherapeutic agents have similar efficacy, and gemcitabine has

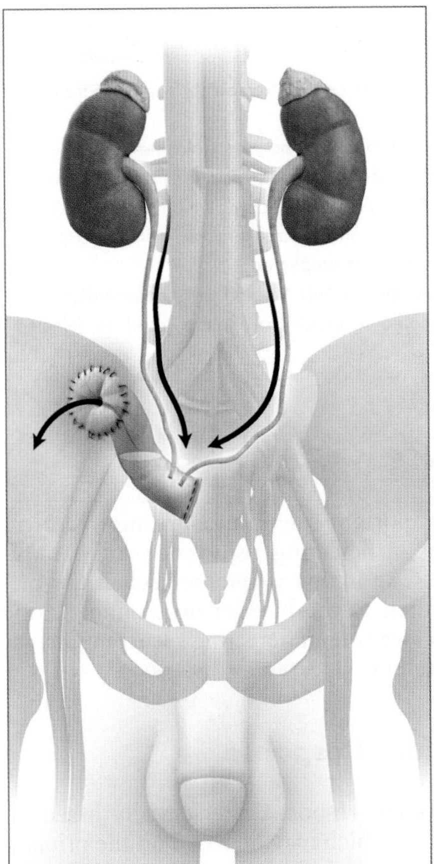
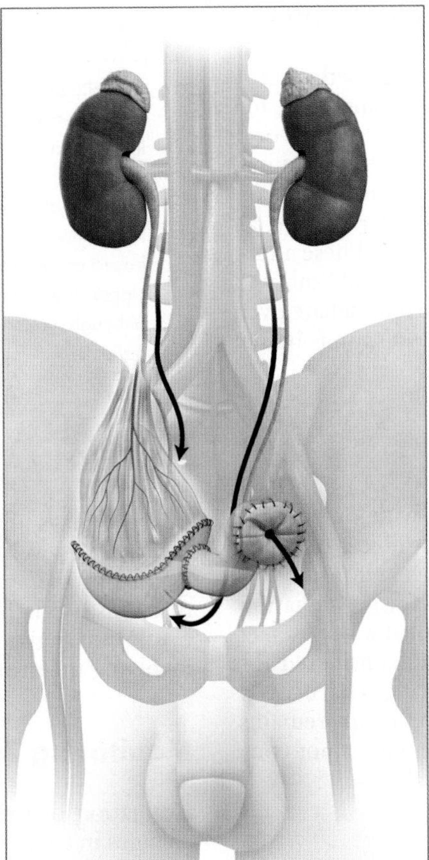
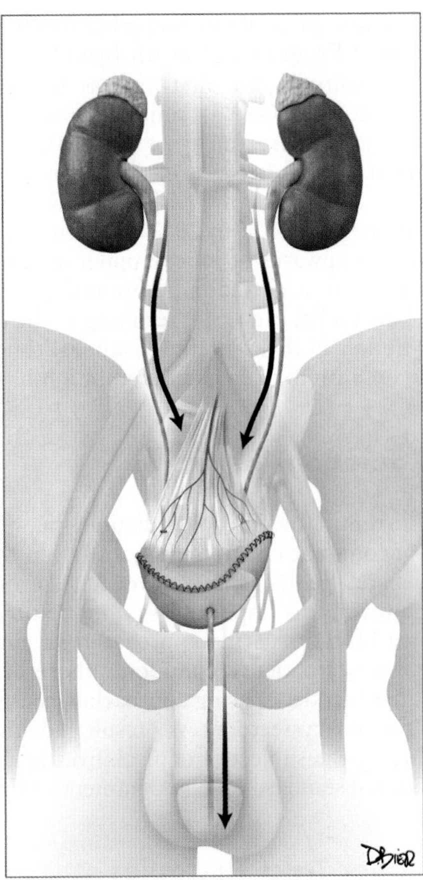

FIGURE 20.18. Schematics of surgical bladder reconstructions. Ileal pouch, catheterizable continent cutaneous diversion, neobladder.

recently replaced mitomycin C. This therapy may be the only treatment necessary for patients with Ta lesions, in whom chemotherapy is associated with a 39% decrease in recurrence. Patients with high-grade or T1 tumors must undergo re-resection as noted previously, following which they are selected for either intravesical therapy or radical cystectomy based on various parameters.

Intravesical bacillus Calmette–Guérin (BCG) has been the benchmark against which all other intravesical therapies are compared since its approval by the U.S. Food and Drug Administration in 1990 for treating carcinoma *in situ* of the bladder. The exact mechanism of action is unknown. BCG attaches to the bladder epithelium, where it is incorporated into the cell, leaving behind surface glycoproteins that are thought to stimulate a nonspecific immune response that includes macrophages, T- and B- lymphocytes, natural killer cells, and a variety of cytokines. Recently, tumor necrosis factor–related apoptosis-inducing ligand has been implicated as having a role in BCG's mechanism of action. Intravesical therapy with BCG is performed on an outpatient basis; it is instilled weekly into the bladder of patients via a Foley catheter. The course of therapy is one 6-week induction course followed by maintenance therapy with 3 weeks of BCG at 3 months, 6 months, and then every 6 months for up to 3 years (the Southwest Oncology Group protocol).[97] If further recurrence is noted, salvage therapies are available; however, operative intervention with cystectomy should be considered.

Chemotherapy

The combination of methotrexate, vinblastine, doxorubicin (adriamycin), and cisplatin, known collectively as M-VAC, was the gold standard to which other chemotherapy was compared and has level 1 evidence showing benefit in the neoadjuvant setting.[95,98–102]

Gemcitabine plus cisplatin has been largely adopted as the standard in the metastatic setting after randomized data suggested equivalent survival but an improved toxicity profile compared with M-VAC.[103] A dose-dense modification of M-VAC (DDMVAC), in which treatment was given every 2 weeks with growth factor support, showed an improved toxicity profile and improved complete response rate compared with classic M-VAC.[104] Although there was no difference in median survival, there was an intriguing improvement in 5-year survival. Use of DDMVAC in the neoadjuvant setting showed similar downstaging as seen with M-VAC, with a 5-year survival rate of approximately 63%.[95] Given its lower toxicity, DDMVAC is now an accepted standard-of-care therapy.

Immune checkpoint inhibitors have now been approved for second-line treatment of metastatic urothelial cancer.[105–109] Currently, only pembrolizumab has level 1 evidence proving benefit over single-agent taxanes in patients treated with prior platinum, showing improved response rate, toxicity profile, and overall survival.[105] Pembrolizumab and atezolizumab may also be used first-line in cisplatin-ineligible patients with overexpression of Programmed death-ligand 1.[110,111]

Erdafitinib, the first-in-class fibroblast growth factor receptor 3 (FGFR3) inhibitor, was recently approved for second-line treatment of urothelial cancer.[112] This oral agent is now being used in patients with selected mutations and fusion of FGFR3. FGFR3 alterations have been observed in 15% to 20% of urothelial bladder tumors, as well as upwards of 35% of upper tract tumors. These alterations are enriched in an immunologically "cold" subtype of urothelial cancer,[113] resulting in the current debate over whether FGFR3-altered urothelial cancer responds better to erdafitinib or to a checkpoint inhibitor.

Radiation Therapy

Currently, the use of radiation therapy with or without concomitant chemotherapy has been the subject of much debate. Some groups advocate aggressively for its use; however, it is important to note that trials using radiation as a bladder-sparing approach have enrolled a very select cohort of patients, commonly those being considered for other bladder-sparing approaches, such as aggressive TUR or partial cystectomy. As a result, radiation therapy remains largely the subject of clinical investigation and is not considered standard for the treatment of this disease.

Upper Tract Therapies

Upper tract urothelial carcinoma of the renal pelvis and ureters is relatively rare. These tumors may arise as primary tumors without a history of bladder tumors or as metachronous lesions in patients with a history of bladder cancer. Radiologic survey of the upper tracts remains an important part of the surveillance of patients with bladder cancer, although the optimal interval and modality are debated.

The optimal method of confirming a diagnosis of upper tract urothelial carcinoma is via ureteroscopy. A biopsy does help in decision-making regarding the type of therapy to use.[114] The main treatment for patients with upper tract urothelial carcinoma and a normal contralateral kidney is a complete nephroureterectomy (open or laparoscopic) with removal of a cuff of urinary bladder and regional node dissection. In situations in which there is suspicion of locally advanced disease, we have advocated for neoadjuvant chemotherapy, similar to that used in bladder cancer, with clinical outcomes in small numbers of patients better than one would anticipate with surgery alone.[95]

In specific situations such as compromised renal function or medical comorbidities, renal-sparing therapy may be considered. In these cases, the tumor is ablated, or segmental resection is undertaken, and then topical chemotherapies or BCG are used as adjuvant treatments. The problem with studies assessing minimally invasive techniques is that the durability of response thus far lacks long-term follow-up. If endoscopic management has been performed, a strict follow-up protocol with imaging and endoscopy is necessary.

KEY POINTS Therapies

- Superficial bladder tumors can be treated surgically by transurethral resection of bladder tumor.
- Intravesical immunotherapy with bacillus Calmette–Guérin is the best therapy for local treatment of early-stage bladder cancer.
- Radical cystectomy typically includes pelvic lymph node dissection.
- Neoadjuvant and adjuvant chemotherapies with a cisplatin-based combination may be employed.
- Upper tract tumors are usually treated by nephroureterectomy, although ureteroscopic resections are being used in selected patients.

SURVEILLANCE

Imaging plays an important role in monitoring treatment response, as well as in detecting recurrence and complications of therapy. Cystoscopy is required when the primary disease is limited to the bladder urothelium. Urine cytology can also play a role in detecting recurrent disease involving the urothelium.

Monitoring Tumor Response

Evaluation of treatment response is essentially based on changes in tumor size, which may be based on the primary tumor or metastatic disease. This can be undertaken by some form of cross-sectional imaging, most commonly CT. For disease limited to the bladder urothelium, cystoscopy is the traditional tool for assessing treatment response.

Detection of Recurrence

Urothelial carcinoma may recur at the primary tumor resection site, or potentially present as nodal or hematogenous metastases. Because of the "field defect," it may recur at any part of the urothelium and at any time, which requires lifelong surveillance of the urothelium. Surveillance of the lower collecting system is best undertaken by cystoscopy and/or urine cytology. Upper tract surveillance, however, primarily uses percutaneous imaging, and most commonly CT urogram.

Detection of recurrent disease at nodal or visceral sites is best undertaken by cross-sectional imaging, most commonly CT. Prior imaging is probably the most helpful adjunct, because increase in size or change in morphology of a node or lesion is the most reliable indicator of new or recurrent disease (Fig. 20.19). Following dissection or irradiation of nodal beds, recurrent disease can appear to "skip" nodal stations (Fig. 20.20) superior to the treated site. In case of an indeterminate lesion, percutaneous fine-needle aspiration or core needle biopsy should be considered.

The role for FDG-PET in surveillance for recurrent disease is limited and is being explored. Limitations can arise because of the typical small size of nodes that contain metastases and the presence of FDG activity in excreted urine.

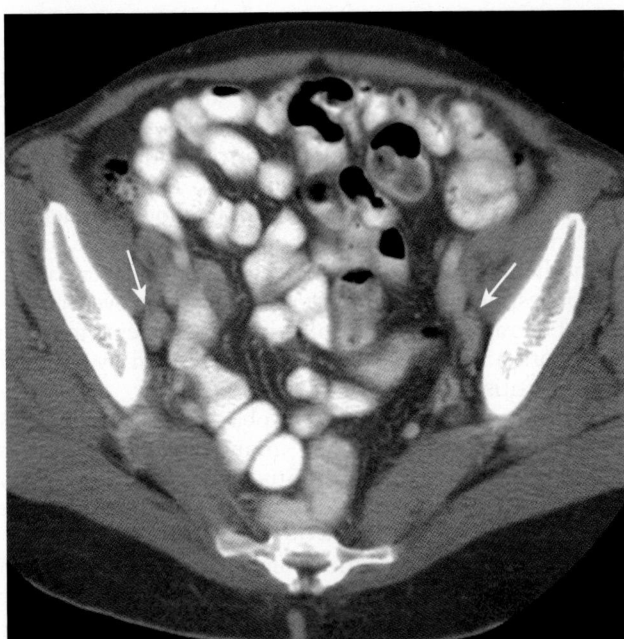

FIGURE 20.19. Pelvic lymph node recurrence after cystectomy. Right external iliac node (*arrow*).

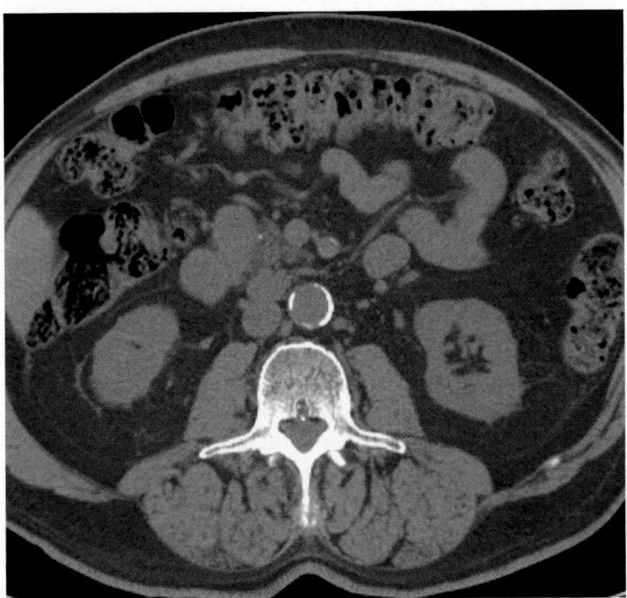

FIGURE 20.20. Retroperitoneal precaval lymph node recurrence after cystectomy and no adenopathy inferior to this location.

Non–Muscle-Invasive Disease

For non–muscle-invasive tumors (the majority of patients in the United States) that are being managed by bladder-conservation protocols, surveillance includes monitoring the bladder for recurrent tumor, as well as monitoring the rest of the urothelial tract (renal pelvis, ureters, and prostatic urethra). Monitoring of the visible urothelium is undertaken by direct visual endoscopy (cystoscopy).

All patients are recommended to undergo a cystoscopy at 3 months after TURBT because cystoscopic findings at 3 months are a prognostic factor of recurrence and progression. Most guidelines for surveillance recommend a follow-up cystoscopy, with or without urine markers, every 3 to 4 months for 2 years, then every 6 months for the second 2 years, then yearly. Patients with a primary, solitary, low-grade Ta tumor may have less frequent cystoscopic examination.

Presently, several urinary markers are available for detecting urothelial tumors. The one most frequently used is urinary cytology; however, overall sensitivity for diagnosis is not optimal and is highly dependent on tumor grade and stage. The UroVysion test is a multitarget fluorescence *in situ* hybridization assay for detection of aneuploidy in chromosomes 3, 7, and 17, as well as loss of the 9p21 locus in exfoliated cells from voided urine. Sensitivities and specificities range from 69% to 87% and 85% to 97%, respectively; however, a high false-positive rate can result in unnecessary, invasive patient workup. Dimashkieh H, Wolff DJ, Smith TM, Houser PM, Nietert PJ, Yang J. Evaluation of urovysion and cytology for bladder cancer detection: a study of 1835 paired urine samples with clinical and histologic correlation. Cancer Cytopathol. 2013;121(10):591-597. doi:10.1002/cncy.21327 Other urinary markers include the BladderCheck NMP22 test, which is a simple, point-of-care, inexpensive assay using antibodies to detect a nuclear matrix protein involved in maintenance of nuclear architecture, DNA transcription, and RNA synthesis. Its median sensitivity and specificity are 71% (range 47%–100%) and 73% (range 5%–98%), respectively. A recent study suggests that the NMP22 BladderCheck assay may detect tumors not seen initially on cystoscopy and may significantly increase the sensitivity of cystoscopy.[115]

Urothelial Surveillance

Although risk-adapted strategies are used to survey the upper urinary tracts, there is no consensus. For low-risk tumors, upper tract imaging can be performed every 2 to 3 years. Annual upper tract imaging is recommended for patients with intermediate- and high-risk non–muscle-invasive tumors. If abnormalities are noted on the imaging test, or if urinary markers are abnormal, bladder visualization is normal, and bladder biopsies are negative, then upper urinary tract endoscopy with small-caliber scopes (ureteroscopy) is performed with the patient under general anesthesia.

Muscle-Invasive Disease

Once the urinary bladder has been removed, sites to be monitored include the remainder of the urinary tract, for example, by CTU. Patients at risk for distant disease are also monitored with cross-sectional imaging (e.g., abdomino-pelvic CT and chest radiographs or CT). The interval prescribed varies from every 3 to 4 months in patients at high risk of recurrence to annually for those who are at low risk of recurrence. Urinary markers have not been studied extensively in this population, although our experience (unpublished data) suggests that invasive investigation does not appear to be indicated simply on the basis of an abnormal urine test without radiologic confirmation of an abnormality.

Metastatic Disease

Although initial response rates are high (typically 50%–70%), relapse is expected, with the majority of patients relapsing within 6 to 9 months of therapy. Patients are typically followed by radiographic imaging with CT or MRI of the chest, abdomen, and pelvis at approximately 3-month intervals.

If a bone scan was previously negative, we typically do not repeat it unless the patient has an elevated alkaline phosphatase or calcium level or has bone pain or other symptoms suggestive of metastases to the bone. A "flare" response, in which the bone scan shows apparent progression, has been observed in patients with urothelial cancer after the first few cycles of treatment (i.e., 6–8 weeks). If the patient is responding clinically (e.g., improved bone pain, urinary symptoms), without progressive symptoms or progression in other areas, we would not alter chemotherapy in the setting of a flare on bone scan.[116]

Key Points Detecting Recurrence

- Lower tract recurrences are best detected by cystoscopy.
- Upper tract screening is best obtained by computed tomography (CT) urography.
- Urothelial disease can also be screened for by urine cytology/markers.
- Nodal and hematogenous recurrence is often better surveyed by CT.
- Increase in size or change in morphology is the most reliable sign of recurrent or residual disease, for which prior imaging is of utmost importance.
- Lifelong surveillance is required.

COMPLICATIONS OF THERAPY

Post-TURBT complications include intra- or extraperitoneal perforation. After surgery, there can be the usual range of postoperative complications of hemorrhage and infection. However, there is also the potential for anastomotic leaks. These can be assessed by direct cystography or CT cystography, or indirectly via CTU. The latter requires delayed images to ensure complete filling of the collecting system, but is less frequently performed in this setting.

Urinary conduits and neobladders can sometimes mimic postoperative collections or even enlarged nodes on CT. Delayed scans with excreted contrast within the entire collecting system can help avoid this potential pitfall.

Radiation therapy and chemotherapy can sometimes cause cystitis, which on cross-sectional imaging can manifest as bladder wall thickening, thereby mimicking a tumor. However, cystitis is usually diffuse, and tumor more focal.

Key Points Complications

- Post–transurethral resection of bladder tumor complications include intra- or extraperitoneal perforation.
- Postsurgical complications include anastomotic leaks and ureteric obstruction.

NEW THERAPIES

Novel therapies for bladder cancer are constantly being developed. For non–muscle-invasive disease, these include photodynamic therapy, electromotive administration of chemotherapy to facilitate penetration, and development of newer chemotherapeutic and immunologic agents and combination therapies. As an example, to mirror systemic chemotherapy regimens, combinations and sequential use of intravesical agents may synergistically improve the efficacy of therapy. Trials for evaluating which agents to use in combination and sequence have been limited by toxicity/severe cystitis.

In the immunologic arena, mycobacterial cell wall–DNA complex may generate similar immunologic responses as BCG to treat bladder cancer. Studies have shown activity in patients with bladder cancer, with a favorable tolerance profile, and long-term follow-up is needed.

Many chemotherapeutic combinations have shown promise in the treatment of muscle-invasive and metastatic urothelial cancer. These include an ifosfamide-based combination developed at Memorial Sloan-Kettering Cancer Center[116] and MD Anderson Cancer Center[117,118]; however, use of these in the community may be limited by the typically poor general health and renal function frequently observed in this frail, elderly population of patients. As a result, modified cisplatin[119,120] and nephron-sparing combinations are currently under investigation. Our front-line combination in the setting of renal insufficiency is gemcitabine, Taxol, and doxorubicin, and is the subject of a currently accruing phase II clinical trial. Novel targeted agents are also a source of active research,[89] but their efficacy in the treatment of urothelial cancer has not yet been definitively proved.

CONCLUSION

Urothelial tumors have a propensity to develop multifocally anywhere along the urothelium from the kidneys to the prostatic urethra. Thorough surveillance of the upper and lower tracts is required at staging and follow-up. Although the lower tract is best evaluated by cystoscopy, cross-sectional imaging provides information about nodal and hematogenous dissemination, for which CT is the workhorse. MRI is helpful in evaluating the extent of disease thanks to its great contrast resolution. The upper tracts are traditionally evaluated by CTU, which has high sensitivity for lesion detection.

REFERENCES

1. Siegel RL, Miller KD, Jemal A. Cancer statistics. *CA Cancer J Clin.* 2019;69(1):7–34.
2. American Cancer Society, Cancer Facts & FIgures https://www.cancer.org/content/dam/cancer-org/research/cancer-facts-and-statistics/annual-cancer-facts-and-figures/2021/cancer-facts-and-figures-2021.pdf *Cancer Facts & Figures*. 2019.

3. Skinner DG, et al. The clinical significance of carcinoma in situ of the bladder and its association with overt carcinoma. *J Urol.* 1974;112(1):68–71.
4. Lindell O, Lehtonen T. Upper urinary tract transitional cell carcinoma after total cystectomy for bladder cancer. *Ann Chir Gynaecol.* 1985;74(6):288–293.
5. Williams CB, Mitchell JP. Carcinoma of the renal pelvis: a review of 43 cases. *Br J Urol.* 1973;45(4):370–376.
6. Fleshner NKF. *Demographics and epidemiology of urothelial cancer of the urinary bladder. Urothelial tumors.* Ontario: Decker, Inc; 2004.
7. Radovanović Z, Janković S, Jevremović I. Incidence of tumors of urinary organs in a focus of Balkan endemic nephropathy. Kidney Int Suppl. 1991 Nov;34:S75-6. PMID: 1762339.
8. Stefanovic V, Radovanovic Z. Balkan endemic nephropathy and associated urothelial cancer. *Nat Clin Pract Urol.* 2008;5(2):105–112.
9. Jelakovic B, et al. Balkan endemic nephropathy and the causative role of aristolochic acid. *Semin Nephrol.* 2019;39(3):284–296.
10. Yu Y, Hu J, Wang PP, Zou Y, Qi Y, Zhao P, Xe R. Risk factors for bladder cancer: a case-control study in northeast China. Eur J Cancer Prev. 1997 Aug;6(4):363-9. doi: 10.1097/00008469-199708000-00008. Erratum in: Eur J Cancer Prev 1998 Apr;7(2):171. PMID: 9370099.
11. Tsai YC, et al. Allelic losses of chromosomes 9, 11, and 17 in human bladder cancer. *Cancer Res.* 1990;50(1):44–47.
12. Mostofi FK, Davis Jr CJ, Sesterhenn IA, Sobin LH. Histological Typing of Urinary Bladder Tumours. International Histological Classification of Tumours. Springer, Berlin, Heidelberg. https://doi.org/10.1007/978-3-642-59871-5_2
13. Siefker-Radtke AO, Dinney CP, Abrahams NA, et al. Evidence supporting preoperative chemotherapy for small cell carcinoma of the bladder: a retrospective review of the MD Anderson cancer experience. *J Urol.* 2004;172:481–484.
14. Arlene O. Siefker-Radtke, Ashish M. Kamat, H. Barton Grossman, et. al. Phase II clinical trial of neoadjuvant alternating doublet chemotherapy with ifosfamide/doxorubicin and etoposide/cisplatin in small-cell urothelial cancer. Journal of Clinical Oncology. 2009;27(16):2592–2597.
15. Bostwick DG, Ramnani D, Cheng L. Diagnosis and grading of bladder cancer and associated lesions. *Urol Clin North Am.* 1999;26(3):493–507.
16. Pashos CL, Botteman MF, Laskin BJ, Redaelli A. Bladder cancer: epidemiology, diagnosis, and management. *Cancer Pract.* 2002;10(6):311–322.
17. Melamed MR, Reuter VE. Pathology and staging of urothelial tumors of the kidney and ureter. *Urol Clin North Am.* 1993;20(2):333–347.
18. MacVicar AD. Bladder cancer staging. *BJU Int.* 2000;86(Suppl 1): 111–122.
19. Knap MM, Lundbeck F, Overgaard J. Prognostic factors, pattern of recurrence and survival in a Danish bladder cancer cohort treated with radical cystectomy. *Acta Oncol.* 2003;42(2):160–168.
20. Browne RF, et al. Transitional cell carcinoma of the upper urinary tract: spectrum of imaging findings. *Radiographics.* 2005;25(6): 1609–1627.
21. Buckley JA, et al. Transitional cell carcinoma of the renal pelvis: a retrospective look at CT staging with pathologic correlation. *Radiology.* 1996;201(1):194–198.
22. Husband J. *Bladder Cancer.* Oxford: Isis Medical Media; 1998.
23. Oosterlinck W, et al. Guidelines on bladder cancer. *Eur Urol.* 2002;41(2):105–112.
24. NIH NCI Surveillance, Epidemiology and End Results Program. Bladder Cancer 2021. https://seer.cancer.gov/statfacts/html/urinb.html Accessed on 9/22/2021
25. Gschwend JE, Dahm P, Fair WR. Disease specific survival as endpoint of outcome for bladder cancer patients following radical cystectomy. *Eur Urol.* 2002;41(4):440–448.
26. Kantoff PWZA, Wishnow K. Bladder cancer. Hamilton, ON: Decker, 2000:1543–1558. https://www.ajronline.org/doi/full/10.2214/AJR.08.1318?mobileUi=0
27. Jewett HJ, Strong GH. Infiltrating carcinoma of the bladder; relation of depth of penetration of the bladder wall to incidence of local extension and metastases. *J Urol.* 1946;55:366–372.
28. Marshall VF. The relation of the preoperative estimate to the pathologic demonstration of the extent of vesical neoplasms. *J Urol.* 1952;68(4):714–723.
29. Levy DA, Grossman HB. Staging and prognosis of T3b bladder cancer. *Semin Urol Oncol.* 1996;14(2):56–61.
30. Whitmore Jr. WF. Assessment and management of deeply invasive and metastatic lesions. *Cancer Res.* 1977;37(8 Pt 2):2756–2758.
31. Lee CH, Tan CH, Faria SC, Kundra V. Role of Imaging in the Local Staging of Urothelial Carcinoma of the Bladder. AJR Am J Roentgenol. 2017 Jun;208(6):1193-1205. doi: 10.2214/AJR.16.17114. Epub 2017 Feb 22. PMID: 28225635.
32. Expert Panel on Urologic I, et al. ACR Appropriateness riteria pretreatment staging of muscle-invasive bladder cancer. *J Am Coll Radiol.* 2018;15(5S):S150–S159.
33. Raman SP, Fishman EK. Bladder malignancies on CT: the underrated role of CT in diagnosis. *AJR Am J Roentgenol.* 2014; 203(2):347–354.
34. Oz II, et al. The role of computerized tomography in the assessment of perivesical invasion in bladder cancer. *Pol J Radiol.* 2016;81:281–287.
35. Ueno Y, Takeuchi M, Tamada T, et al. Diagnostic accuracy and interobserver agreement for the vesical imaging-reporting and data system for muscle-invasive bladder cancer: a multireader validation study. *Eur Urol.* 2019;76(1):54–56.
36. Barchetti G, et al. Multiparametric MRI of the bladder: inter-observer agreement and accuracy with the Vesical Imaging-Reporting and Data System (VI-RADS) at a single reference center. *Eur Radiol.* 2019;29(10):5498–5506.
37. Panebianco V, et al. Multiparametric magnetic resonance imaging for bladder cancer: development of VI-RADS (Vesical Imaging-Reporting And Data System). *Eur Urol.* 2018;74(3):294–306.
38. Panebianco V, et al. Improving staging in bladder cancer: the increasing role of multiparametric magnetic resonance imaging. *Eur Urol Focus.* 2016;2(2):113–121.
39. Wang H, et al. Multiparametric MRI for bladder cancer: validation of VI-RADS for the detection of detrusor muscle invasion. *Radiology.* 2019;291(3):668–674.
40. Barentz JO. Primary staging of urinary bladder carcinoma: the role of MRI and a comparison with CT. *Euro Radiol.* 1996:129–133.
41. Scattoni V, et al. Dynamic gadolinium-enhanced magnetic resonance imaging in staging of superficial bladder cancer. *J Urol.* 1996;155(5):1594–1599.
42. Hayashi N, et al. A new staging criterion for bladder carcinoma using gadolinium-enhanced magnetic resonance imaging with an endorectal surface coil: a comparison with ultrasonography. *BJU Int.* 2000;85(1):32–36.
43. El-Assmy A, et al. Bladder tumour staging: comparison of diffusion- and T2-weighted MR imaging. *Eur Radiol.* 2009;19(7):1575–1581.
44. Stojovska-Jovanovska E, et al. Computed tomography or magnetic resonance imaging - our experiences in determining preoperative TNM staging of bladder cancer. *Pril (Makedon Akad Nauk Umet Odd Med Nauki).* 2013;34(3):63–70.
45. Boudreaux Jr KJ, et al. Comparison of American Joint Committee on Cancer pathologic stage T3a versus T3b urothelial carcinoma: analysis of patient outcomes. *Cancer.* 2009;115(4):770–775.
46. Watanabe H, et al. Preoperative T staging of urinary bladder cancer: does diffusion-weighted MRI have supplementary value? *AJR Am J Roentgenol.* 2009;192(5):1361–1366.
47. Kobayashi S, et al. Diagnostic performance of diffusion-weighted magnetic resonance imaging in bladder cancer: potential utility of apparent diffusion coefficient values as a biomarker to predict clinical aggressiveness. *Eur Radiol.* 2011;21(10):2178–2186.
48. Vock P, et al. Computed tomography in staging of carcinoma of the urinary bladder. *Br J Urol.* 1982;54(2):158–163.
49. Sager EM, et al. The role of CT in demonstrating perivesical tumor growth in the preoperative staging of carcinoma of the urinary bladder. *Radiology.* 1983;146(2):443–446.
50. Fisher MR, Hricak H, Crooks LE. Urinary bladder MR imaging. Part I. Normal and benign conditions. *Radiology.* 1985;157(2):467–470.
51. Fisher MR, Hricak H, Tanagho EA. Urinary bladder MR imaging. Part II. Neoplasm. *Radiology.* 1985;157(2):471–477.
52. Amendola MA, et al. Staging of bladder carcinoma: MRI-CT-surgical correlation. *AJR Am J Roentgenol.* 1986;146(6):1179–1183.
53. Rholl KS, et al. Primary bladder carcinoma: evaluation with MR imaging. *Radiology.* 1987;163(1):117–121.
54. Buy JN, et al. MR staging of bladder carcinoma: correlation with pathologic findings. *Radiology.* 1988;169(3):695–700.
55. Koelbel G, et al. MR imaging of urinary bladder neoplasms. *J Comput Assist Tomogr.* 1988;12(1):98–103.
56. Husband JE, et al. Bladder cancer: staging with CT and MR imaging. *Radiology.* 1989;173(2):435–440.

57. Neuerburg JM, et al. Urinary bladder neoplasms: evaluation with contrast-enhanced MR imaging. *Radiology*. 1989;172(3):739–743.
58. Tavares NJ, Demas BE, Hricak H. MR imaging of bladder neoplasms: correlation with pathologic staging. *Urol Radiol*. 1990; 12(1):27–33.
59. Tachibana M, et al. Efficacy of gadolinium-diethylenetriaminepentaacetic acid-enhanced magnetic resonance imaging for differentiation between superficial and muscle-invasive tumor of the bladder: a comparative study with computerized tomography and transurethral ultrasonography. *J Urol*. 1991;145(6):1169–1173.
60. Tanimoto A, et al. Bladder tumor staging: comparison of conventional and gadolinium-enhanced dynamic MR imaging and CT. *Radiology*. 1992;185(3):741–747.
61. Doringer E. Computerized tomography of colonic diverticulitis. *Crit Rev Diagn Imaging*. 1992;33(5):421–435.
62. Kim B, et al. Bladder tumor staging: comparison of contrast-enhanced CT, T1- and T2-weighted MR imaging, dynamic gadolinium-enhanced imaging, and late gadolinium-enhanced imaging. *Radiology*. 1994;193(1):239–245.
63. Barentsz JO, et al. Staging urinary bladder cancer: value of T1-weighted three-dimensional magnetization prepared-rapid gradient-echo and two-dimensional spin-echo sequences. *AJR Am J Roentgenol*. 1995;164(1):109–115.
64. Barentsz JO, et al. Staging urinary bladder cancer after transurethral biopsy: value of fast dynamic contrast-enhanced MR imaging. *Radiology*. 1996;201(1):185–193.
65. Barentsz JO, Witjes JA, Ruijs JH. What is new in bladder cancer imaging. *Urol Clin North Am*. 1997;24(3):583–602.
66. Caterino M, et al. Bladder cancer within a direct inguinal hernia: CT demonstration. *Abdom Imaging*. 2001;26(6):664–666.
67. Schuller J, et al. Intravesical ultrasound tomography in staging bladder carcinoma. *J Urol*. 1982;128(2):264–266.
68. Abu-Yousef MM, et al. Urinary bladder tumors studied by cystosonography. Part II: Staging. *Radiology*. 1984;153(1):227–231.
69. Dershaw DD, Scher HI. Sonography in evaluation of carcinoma of bladder. *Urology*. 1987;29(4):454–457.
70. Meissner C, et al. The efficiency of excretory urography to detect upper urinary tract tumors after cystectomy for urothelial cancer. *J Urol*. 2007;178(6):2287–2290.
71. Miyake H, et al. Limited significance of routine excretory urography in the follow-up of patients with superficial bladder cancer after transurethral resection. *BJU Int*. 2006;97(4):720–723.
72. Chow LC, et al. Split-bolus MDCT urography with synchronous nephrographic and excretory phase enhancement. *AJR Am J Roentgenol*. 2007;189(2):314–322.
73. Caoili EM, et al. MDCT urography of upper tract urothelial neoplasms. *AJR Am J Roentgenol*. 2005;184(6):1873–1881.
74. Wong-You-Cheong JJ, Wagner BJ, Davis Jr. CJ. Transitional cell carcinoma of the urinary tract: radiologic-pathologic correlation. *Radiographics*. 1998;18(1):123–142. quiz 148.
75. Chlapoutakis K, et al. Performance of computed tomographic urography in diagnosis of upper urinary tract urothelial carcinoma, in patients presenting with hematuria: Systematic review and meta-analysis. *Eur J Radiol*. 2010;73(2):334–338.
76. Albani JM, et al. The role of computerized tomographic urography in the initial evaluation of hematuria. *J Urol*. 2007;177(2): 644–648.
77. Gray Sears CL, et al. Prospective comparison of computerized tomography and excretory urography in the initial evaluation of asymptomatic microhematuria. *J Urol*. 2002;168(6):2457–2460.
78. Cowan NC, et al. Multidetector computed tomography urography for diagnosing upper urinary tract urothelial tumour. *BJU Int*. 2007;99(6):1363–1370.
79. Koss JC, et al. CT staging of bladder carcinoma. *AJR Am J Roentgenol*. 1981;137(2):359–362.
80. Hofer C, et al. Diagnosis and monitoring of urological tumors using positron emission tomography. *Eur Urol*. 2001;40(5):481–487.
81. Husband JE. Computer tomography and magnetic resonance imaging in the evaluation of bladder cancer. *J Belge Radiol*. 1995;78(6):350–355.
82. Jager GJ, et al. Pelvic adenopathy in prostatic and urinary bladder carcinoma: MR imaging with a three-dimensional TI-weighted magnetization-prepared-rapid gradient-echo sequence. *AJR Am J Roentgenol*. 1996;167(6):1503–1507.
83. Barentsz JO, Jager GJ, Witjes JA. MR imaging of the urinary bladder. *Magn Reson Imaging Clin N Am*. 2000;8(4):853–867.
84. Deserno WM, et al. Urinary bladder cancer: preoperative nodal staging with ferumoxtran-10-enhanced MR imaging. *Radiology*. 2004;233(2):449–456.
85. Neuwelt EA, et al. Ultrasmall superparamagnetic iron oxides (USPIOs): a future alternative magnetic resonance (MR) contrast agent for patients at risk for nephrogenic systemic fibrosis (NSF)? *Kidney Int*. 2009;75(5):465–474.
86. Uttam M, et al. Is [F-18]-fluorodeoxyglucose FDG-PET/CT better than CT alone for the preoperative lymph node staging of muscle invasive bladder cancer? *Int Braz J Urol*. 2016;42(2):234–241.
87. Mertens LS, et al. 18F-fluorodeoxyglucose--positron emission tomography/computed tomography aids staging and predicts mortality in patients with muscle-invasive bladder cancer. *Urology*. 2014;83(2):393–398.
88. Hain SF, Maisey MN. Positron emission tomography for urological tumours. *BJU Int*. 2003;92(2):159–164.
89. Siefker-Radtke AO, et al. Phase II clinical trial of neoadjuvant alternating doublet chemotherapy with ifosfamide/doxorubicin and etoposide/cisplatin in small-cell urothelial cancer. *J Clin Oncol*. 2009;27(16):2592–2597.
90. Gore JL, et al. Mortality increases when radical cystectomy is delayed more than 12 weeks: results from a Surveillance, Epidemiology, and End Results-Medicare analysis. *Cancer*. 2009;115(5):988–996.
91. Brassell SA, Kamat AM. Contemporary intravesical treatment options for urothelial carcinoma of the bladder. *J Natl Compr Canc Netw*. 2006;4(10):1027–1036.
92. Herring JC, Kamat AM. Treatment of muscle-invasive bladder cancer: progress and new challenges. *Expert Rev Anticancer Ther*. 2004;4(6):1047–1056.
93. Kamat AM, et al. Micropapillary bladder cancer: a review of the University of Texas M. D. Anderson Cancer Center experience with 100 consecutive patients. *Cancer*. 2007;110(1):62–67.
94. Lynch S, Shen Y, Kamat A, et al. Neoadjuvant Chemotherapy in Small Cell Urothelial Cancer Improves Pathologic Down-staging and Long-term Outcomes: Results from a Retrospective Study at the M. D. Anderson Cancer Center. *European Urology*. 2013;64(2):307–313.
95. McConkey DCW, Shen Y, Lee I, et al. A prognostic gene expression signature in the molecular classification of chemotherapy-naive urothelial cancer is predictive of clinical outcomes from neoadjuvant chemotherapy: a phase 2 trial of dose-dense methotrexate, vinblastine, doxorubicin, and cisplatin with bevacizumab in urothelial cancer. *European Eurology*. 2016;69:855–862.
96. Kamat AM, Fisher MB. Lymph node density: surrogate marker for quality of resection in bladder cancer? *Expert Rev Anticancer Ther*. 2007;7(6):777–779.
97. Lamm DL, et al. Maintenance bacillus Calmette-Guerin immunotherapy for recurrent TA, T1 and carcinoma in situ transitional cell carcinoma of the bladder: a randomized Southwest Oncology Group Study. *J Urol*. 2000;163(4):1124–1129.
98. Sternberg CN, et al. Preliminary results of M-VAC (methotrexate, vinblastine, doxorubicin and cisplatin) for transitional cell carcinoma of the urothelium. *J Urol*. 1985;133(3):403–407.
99. Logothetis CJ, et al. A prospective randomized trial comparing MVAC and CISCA chemotherapy for patients with metastatic urothelial tumors. *J Clin Oncol*. 1990;8(6):1050–1055.
100. Siefker-Radtke AO, et al. Phase III trial of fluorouracil, interferon alpha-2b, and cisplatin versus methotrexate, vinblastine, doxorubicin, and cisplatin in metastatic or unresectable urothelial cancer. *J Clin Oncol*. 2002;20(5):1361–1367.
101. Bamias A, et al. Docetaxel and cisplatin with granulocyte colony-stimulating factor (G-CSF) versus MVAC with G-CSF in advanced urothelial carcinoma: a multicenter, randomized, phase III study from the Hellenic Cooperative Oncology Group. *J Clin Oncol*. 2004;22(2):220–228.
102. Grossman HB, et al. Neoadjuvant chemotherapy plus cystectomy compared with cystectomy alone for locally advanced bladder cancer. *N Engl J Med*. 2003;349(9):859–866.
103. von der Maase H, et al. Gemcitabine and cisplatin versus methotrexate, vinblastine, doxorubicin, and cisplatin in advanced or metastatic bladder cancer: results of a large, randomized, multinational, multicenter, phase III study. *J Clin Oncol*. 2000;18(17):3068–3077.
104. Sternberg CN, et al. Randomized phase III trial of high-dose-intensity methotrexate, vinblastine, doxorubicin, and cisplatin (MVAC) chemotherapy and recombinant human granulocyte colony-stimulating factor versus classic MVAC in advanced urothelial tract

tumors: European Organization for Research and Treatment of Cancer Protocol no. 30924. *J Clin Oncol*. 2001;19(10):2638–2646.
105. Bellmunt K, de Wit R, et al. Pembrolizumab as second-line therapy for advanced urothelial carcinoma. *NEJM*. 2017;376:1015–1026.
106. Sharma P, Retz M, Siefker-Radtke A, et al. Nivolumab in metastatic urothelial carcinoma after platinum therapy (CheckMate 275): a multicentre, single-arm, phase 2 trial. *Lancet Oncol*. 2017;18(3):312–322.
107. Rosenberg JE, et al. Atezolizumab in patients with locally advanced and metastatic urothelial carcinoma who have progressed following treatment with platinum-based chemotherapy: a single-arm, multicentre, phase 2 trial. *Lancet*. 2016;387(10031):1909–1920.
108. Powles T, et al. Efficacy and safety of durvalumab in locally advanced or metastatic urothelial carcinoma: updated results from a phase 1/2 open-label study. *JAMA Oncol*. 2017:e172411.
109. Apolo AB, et al. Avelumab, an anti-programmed death-ligand 1 antibody, in patients with refractory metastatic urothelial carcinoma: results from a multicenter, phase ib study. *J Clin Oncol*. 2017;35(19):2117–2124.
110. Balar AV, et al. Atezolizumab as first-line treatment in cisplatin-ineligible patients with locally advanced and metastatic urothelial carcinoma: a single-arm, multicentre, phase 2 trial. *Lancet*. 2017;389(10064):67–76.
111. Balar AV, et al. First-line pembrolizumab in cisplatin-ineligible patients with locally advanced and unresectable or metastatic urothelial cancer (KEYNOTE-052): a multicentre, single-arm, phase 2 study. *Lancet Oncol*. 2017;18(11):1483–1492.
112. Loriot Y NS, Park J, Garcia-Donas R, et al. Erdafitinib in locally advanced of metastatic urothelial carcinoma. *NEJM*. 2019;381:338–348.
113. McConkey D, Choi W, Ochoa A, et al. Therapeutic opportunities in the intrinsic subtypes of muscle-invasive bladder cancer. *Hematol Oncol Clin North Am*. 2015;29:377–394.
114. Brown GA, et al. Ability of clinical grade to predict final pathologic stage in upper urinary tract transitional cell carcinoma: implications for therapy. *Urology*. 2007;70(2):252–256.
115. Grossman HB, et al. Surveillance for recurrent bladder cancer using a point-of-care proteomic assay. *JAMA*. 2006;295(3):299–305.
116. Bajorin DF, et al. Ifosfamide, paclitaxel, and cisplatin for patients with advanced transitional cell carcinoma of the urothelial tract: final report of a phase II trial evaluating two dosing schedules. *Cancer*. 2000;88(7):1671–1678.
117. Siefker-Radtke AO, et al. A phase 2 clinical trial of sequential neoadjuvant chemotherapy with ifosfamide, doxorubicin, and gemcitabine followed by cisplatin, gemcitabine, and ifosfamide in locally advanced urothelial cancer: final results. *Cancer*. 2013;119(3):540–547.
118. Siefker-Radtke AO, et al. Phase II clinical trial of neoadjuvant alternating doublet chemotherapy with ifosfamide/doxorubicin and etoposide/cisplatin in small-cell urothelial cancer. *J Clin Oncol*. 2009;27(16):2592–2597.
119. Pagliaro LC, et al. Cisplatin, gemcitabine, and ifosfamide as weekly therapy: a feasibility and phase II study of salvage treatment for advanced transitional-cell carcinoma. *J Clin Oncol*. 2002;20(13):2965–2970.
120. Tu SM, et al. Paclitaxel, cisplatin and methotrexate combination chemotherapy is active in the treatment of refractory urothelial malignancies. *J Urol*. 1995;154(5):1719–1722.

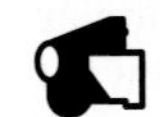
Visit ExpertConsult.com for additional algorithms.

CHAPTER

21 Testicular Germ Cell Tumors

Brinda Rao Korivi, M.D., and Lance C. Pagliaro, M.D.

INTRODUCTION

Testicular cancer is the most common malignancy in males ranging from puberty to the fourth decade of life.[1]

The vast majority of testicular cancers (95%) are gonadal germ cell tumors (GCTs). The remaining 5% of GCTs in males are extragonadal germ cell tumors (EGGCTs). Female gonadal GCTs of the ovary, which account for 30% of ovarian tumors, are not discussed in this chapter.

Although the focus of this chapter is on testicular GCTs, it is important to provide an initial overview of GCTs, which include EGGCTs. The most common sites of EGGCTs are the mediastinum and retroperitoneum; less common sites include the pineal gland and the sacrococcygeal area. EGGCTs stem from primordial germ cells that failed to migrate properly during embryogenesis. Retroperitoneal GCTs are rarely EGGCTs, because most are metastases from a primary testicular tumor. Primary retroperitoneal EGGCTs may be the result of an occult gonadal GCT or metachronous primary retroperitoneal and testicular tumors. Both GCTs and EGGCTs share common histopathology and are divided into seminomatous and nonseminomatous types. Both GCTs and EGGCTs also share a similar pattern of age distribution in the third decade.[2,3]

Testicular GCTs are highly curable, with a 5-year survival rate of more than 95%.[1] The death rate from testicular cancer in the United States is less than 400 per year.[1,4]

Once the diagnosis is made, ultrasound (US), computed tomography (CT), and sometimes magnetic resonance imaging (MRI) and 2-[^{18}F] fluoro-2-deoxy-D-glucose (FDG)–positron emission tomography (PET) examinations are useful for defining the extent of disease and monitoring response to therapy.

EPIDEMIOLOGY

The incidence of testicular germ cell cancer is highest in males from 15 to 44 years old, with a median age of 34 years at initial diagnosis.

The incidence of GCTs in the United States from 2001 to 2005 was 11.8 per 100,000.[1] Approximately 8400 new cases of testicular GCT are diagnosed in the United States each year.[1] The incidence is age-dependent: it is rare before age 5 years, most common at ages 20 to 39 years, then declining at age 40 years and onward.[5] When the tumors occur in childhood, they predominantly occur in the 4 years and younger age groups.

The incidence in the 20- to 40-year-old age group has doubled over the last three decades.[6] From 1976 to 2005, there was an increase of unknown etiology in the incidence in testicular cancer of 1.5% to 2.3%.[7–9] Although testicular cancer is common in young males, it still is a rare tumor, estimated at 1% of male malignancies.[6] Testicular cancer is the most common solid malignancy in males between 15 and 40 years of age. Therefore, if a man in his late 40s presents with a testicular mass, other diagnoses such as lymphoma or metastases should be considered. Most testicular cancers are unilateral, with approximately 1% to 5% presenting with synchronous or metachronous bilateral tumors.[10,11]

Testicular cancer is presumed to have a genetic basis. It has a low incidence in Black Americans, with a 4.5 times higher prevalence in White Americans.[12] The highest rates are in western and northern Europe and New Zealand.[13] Intermediate rates are in the United States.[8,14]

RISK FACTORS

Virtually all histopathologic types of GCT have an abnormality in chromosome 12. Postpubertal tumors contain aneuploid abnormalities associated with a gain of the short arm of chromosome arm 12p, which is labeled as i(12p).[15] Tumors that stem from prepubertal gonads tend to contain diploid abnormalities.[5,15–17]

Associated risks of developing testicular cancer include intratubular germ cell neoplasia (ITGCN), which is testicular carcinoma *in situ*. If not diagnosed and treated, approximately half of all cases will progress to an invasive malignancy.[11,18]

Testicular microlithiasis can be a risk factor and is further discussed in the "Ultrasound" section.

Cryptorchidism is a major risk factor, increasing the risk of germ cell neoplasia five to 10 times.[19] It is one of the main risk factors that predicts disease occurrence in the testis. The higher the location of the undescended testes, the higher the risk; an abdominal undescended testis has a higher risk than an inguinal undescended testis[20] (Fig. 21.1). Therefore, it is important to follow up postorchidopexy patients with a scrotal US. Seminoma accounts for 60% of GCTs with cryptorchidism. The risk factor of developing cancer from cryptorchidism also depends on genetic, environmental, and hormonal factors.[19]

Another important risk factor is personal history. Presence of GCT in one testis increases the risk of involvement of the other testis. The 15-year risk of developing a contralateral testicular cancer in affected patients is

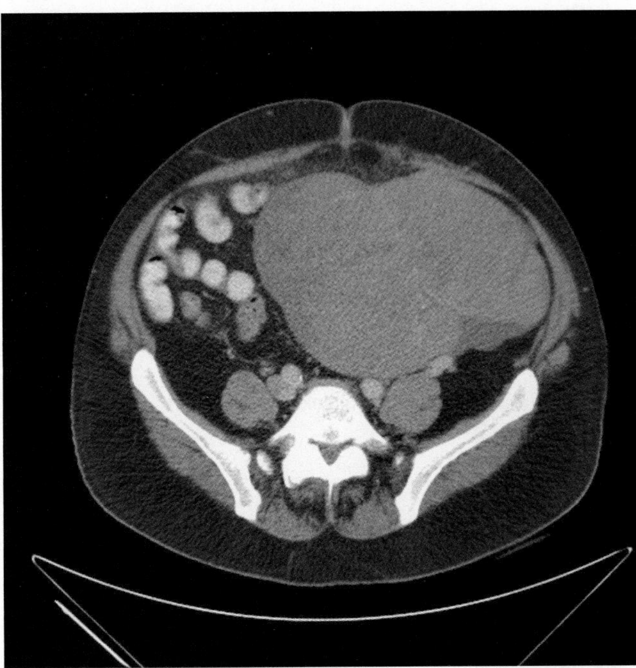

Figure 21.1. Axial computed tomography scan of the abdomen. A large left pelvic mass is a pathologically proven seminoma arising from an undescended left testicle. (Courtesy Dr. Chitra Vishwanathan, Dept of Radiology, MD Anderson Hospital, Houston, Texas.)

approximately 1.2%. The incidence of simultaneous bilateral tumors is 1% to 5%.[10]

Familial history of testicular cancer is a risk factor. Approximately 2% of affected males have a family history, with siblings having up to a tenfold risk and sons having up to a sixfold increased risk.[21,22]

Other associated risk factors are testicular dysgenesis syndromes, which include hypospadias, testicular atrophy, and hypogonadism. Fetal-origin testicular cancer is associated with urogenital congenital anomaly, hypospadias, cryptorchidism, and low fetal birthweight.[8]

Some environmental agents are thought to be associated, including exposure to diethylstilbestrol during maternal pregnancy, increased estrogen levels *in utero*,[23] and pesticides.[24] Other studies have associated increased risk with dietary factors, such as maternal smoking, high cheese diet, and body mass index.[17,24]

Human immunodeficiency virus infection is another risk factor for testicular cancer.[23] Others include Klinefelter syndrome, dysplastic nevus syndrome, inguinal hernias, and EGGCTs.[5]

> **Key Points**
>
> **Epidemiology and Risk Factors**
>
> - Highest incidence is in males 15 to 44 years old.
> - Incidence in patients 20 to 40 years old has doubled over the past three decades.
> - Common abnormality is in chromosome 12.
> - Cryptorchidism is a major risk factor.
> - Other risk factors include environment, personal and family history, and human immunodeficiency virus/acquired immunodeficiency syndrome.

Anatomy and Pathology of the Scrotum and Testes

Anatomy

The testes are a component of the scrotum, a pouch that contains the testes, epididymis, and portions of the spermatic cord. Each testis is surrounded by the tunica vaginalis. Surrounding the tunica are fascial layers that compose the scrotal wall. From internally outward, the scrotal wall components are the internal spermatic fascia, the cremasteric muscle, the external spermatic fascia, and the dartos muscle[25–27] (Fig. 21.2).

Each testis is an elliptical structure containing approximately 400 lobules, which are divided by septa. The septa converge to the mediastum testes, which is contiguous with the tunica albuguinea, a fibrous, dense outer covering of the testis. Each lobule contains two seminiferous tubules, which are lined with germ cells. The seminiferous tubules form a network of ducts known as the rete testis. The ductules connect the rete testis to the head of the epididymis.[25–27]

The epididymis is composed of a head, body, and tail, from superior to inferior. The body and tail are composed of a single tubule. The tubule joins the vas deferens. The vas deferens courses through the inguinal canal and joins the seminal vesicles to form the ejaculatory duct.[25–27]

There are several cell types in the testes:[28]

- Germ cells (in seminiferous tubules): The precursors at the beginning of the spermatogenesis process (Fig. 21.3).
- Sertoli cells (in seminiferous tubules): Play an important role in germ cell development into spermatozoa.
- Leydig cells (in between seminiferous tubules): Important for puberty; produce testosterone and other androgens.
- Other cells: Immature Leydig cells, epithelial cells, and interstitial macrophages.

Pathology

Tumor Types

The vast majority of testicular tumors are GCTs (95%). GCTs originate from spermatogenic cells. GCTs are believed to originate from tissue stem cells and arise from the germinal epithelium of the seminiferous tubules owing to atypical cell proliferation known as testicular ITGCNU.[5,29,30] It is believed that the ITGCNU cells multiply abnormally during puberty, possibly caused by an altered hormonal environment. The tumors retain stem cell properties, which enable self-renewal that leads to tumorigenesis and differentiation into either seminomatous or nonseminomatous cells, which leads to a varied cellular tumor composition and possible resistance to treatments.[17]

Typically, germ cells arise from the yolk sac during the fourth gestation week and migrate to the gonadal ridge, the iliac fossa, and then the scrotum. When there are abnormalities in the migration of these cells, the various types of GCTs arise. Undifferentiated stem cells give rise to embryonal carcinoma. If the cells continue to progress

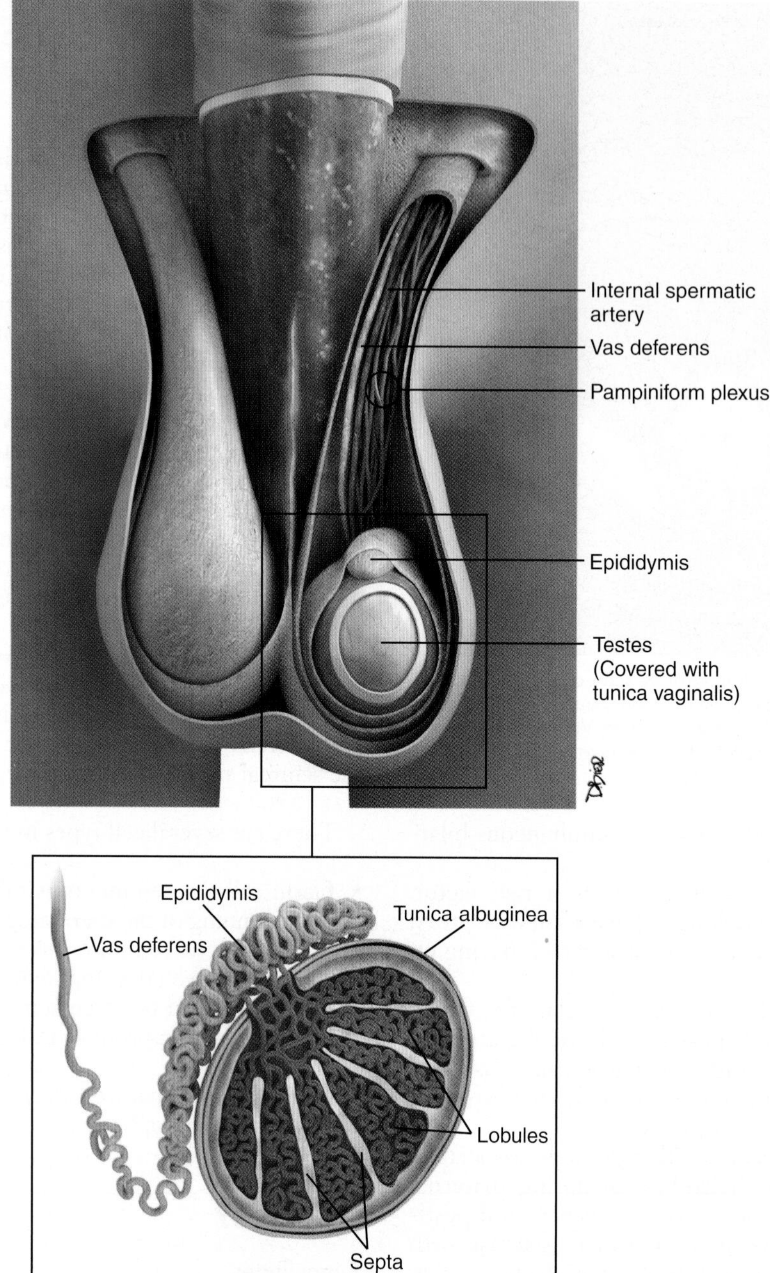

Figure 21.2. Diagram of the testes. (Courtesy David Bier, Houston, Texas.)

toward an embryonic pathway, they become teratomas. If they progress to the extraembryonic pathway, they become choriocarcinomas or yolk sac tumors.[31] Fig. 21.4 describes the histogenesis of GCTs.[17]

There are two main classifications of GCTs: seminomas and nonseminomas, which comprise approximately 95% of malignant testicular tumors. The remainder are lymphomas, which account for 4%; 1% are rare tumors (e.g., interstitial tumors, embryonal sarcomas, and Sertoli cell tumors).[13,32]

Seminomatous tumors most frequently occur in the fourth decade of life and are generally indolent. Pure seminomas are commonly localized to the testes at initial diagnosis, which is stage I. In approximately 25% of cases, seminomas may present with metastatic bulky adenopathy.

Nonseminomatous germ cell tumors (NSGCTs) occur more commonly in the third decade of life. The most common NSGCT is the mixed GCT, which accounts for approximately 32% to 60% of a varied combination of germ cell types; embryonal carcinoma is the most common type.

Gross and Microscopic Features

Seminoma. The gross appearance is a homogeneous firm mass with single or multiple nodules. The tumor cells are homogeneous, with large round cells with clear cytoplasm in bundles outlined by fibrovascular trabeculae. The bands contain an abundance of plasma cells and T lymphocytes. Granulomatous reaction is common, and hemorrhage and necrosis are rare[17,33–35] (Fig. 21.5A).

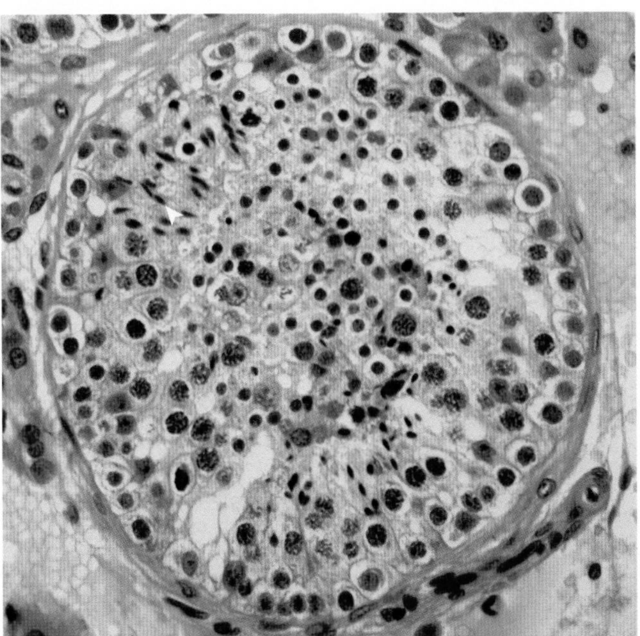

FIGURE 21.3. Normal seminiferous tubule shows intact spermatogenesis with maturation of precursors to spermatozoa (*arrowhead*). (Courtesy Dr. Kanishka Sircar, Pathology Department, MD Anderson Hospital, Houstan, Texas.)

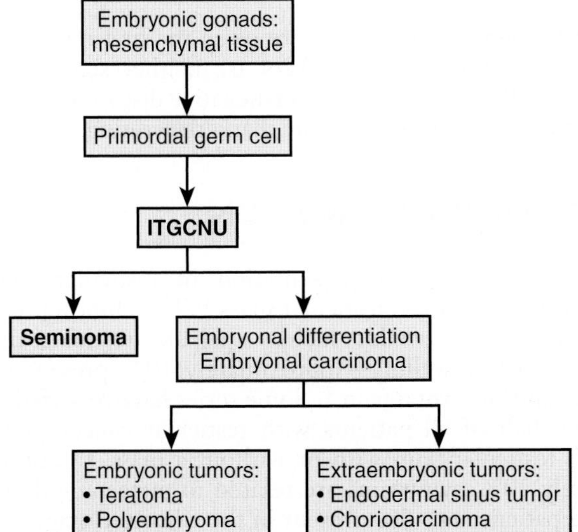

FIGURE 21.4. Diagram of histogenesis of germ cell tumors. (Modified from Cushing B, Perlman E. Germ cell tumors. In: Pizzo PA, Poplack DG, eds. *Principles and Practice of Pediatric Oncology*. 5th ed. Philadelphia: Lippincott-Raven; 2006.)

Note that the spermatocytic seminoma is a histologically distinct subtype of seminoma, which is virtually always cured by an orchiectomy, and usually requires no other treatment because it rarely metastasizes.[5]

Nonseminomatous Germ Cell Tumors. The NSGCTs include a large group of histologically diverse neoplasms such as embryonal tumors, yolk sac tumors, choriocarcinomas, and teratomas. When one or more tumor components are present, they are mixed. The NSGCTs generally are more ill-defined than seminomas and have hemorrhage and necrosis[33,34] (Fig. 21.5B).

- Teratoma: Composed of endoderm, or combined layers of each. Grossly, this tumor is more cystic and multiloculated, sometimes with cartilage. Sebaceous fat and calcifications are typical findings. Immature teratomas have larger solid components with scattered fat and calcification. Different teratomas contain components of nerve, epithelium, and cartilage. The more mature tumors feature differentiated tissue, and the immature teratomas have fetal-based tissues. Histologically, teratomas are predominantly composed of cystic components, with an epithelial lining similar to the epidermis with some appendages. Approximately 85% contain a solid histologically varied element called Rokitansky's protuberance.[17,33,34,36]
- Embryonal carcinoma: Gross appearance is that of an ill-defined mass with hemorrhage and necrosis. Vascular invasion can be present. Histologically, the malignant cells are composed of undifferentiated cells with an indistinct border and an anaplastic epithelial and embryonic appearance. The cells are polygonal, with atypia and an elevated mitotic rate, proliferating in a tubular, acinar, solid, or papillary manner.[17,33,34]
- Yolk sac tumor: Gross appearance is that of a multilobulated solid mass with a mucinous covering, with possible hemorrhage and necrosis. Histologically, it is composed of primitive tumor cells in a loose reticular pattern. Each cell has hyperchromatic nuclei. A distinguishing feature is a Schiller–Duval body, a fibrovascular core containing single vessels.[33,34]
- Choriocarcinoma: Grossly a heterogeneous mass, commonly identified with hemorrhage and necrosis. Histologically, it is composed of syncytiotrophoblastic and cytotrophoblastic cells.[33,34,36,37]
- Mixed tumor: A widely varied composition of histologic subtypes; accounts for up to 60% of testicular GCTs.[33,34]

Note that the presence of yolk sac elements and undifferentiated cells is an important predictor of tumor relapse.[38]

There are two main classifications for germ tumors: the World Health Organization (WHO), commonly used in North America and Europe, and the British Testicular Tumour Panel (BTTP), used in the United Kingdom and Australia. The WHO classification is more common and divides tumor categories into seminomatous and nonseminomatous types. The BTTP divides nonseminomatous tumors into different types of teratomas. Table 21.1 differentiates the WHO and BTTP classifications.[17,39]

KEY POINTS

Pathology

- Seminomatous germ cell tumors and nonseminomatous germ cell tumors (NSGCTs) together are equally divided in prevalence, and together comprise approximately 95% of malignant testicular tumors.
- Seminomas are composed of one histologic type and typically are a homogeneous mass with little necrosis or hemorrhage.
- NSGCTs are composed of one or more histologic type with a more heterogeneous appearance, typically with necrosis and hemorrhage.

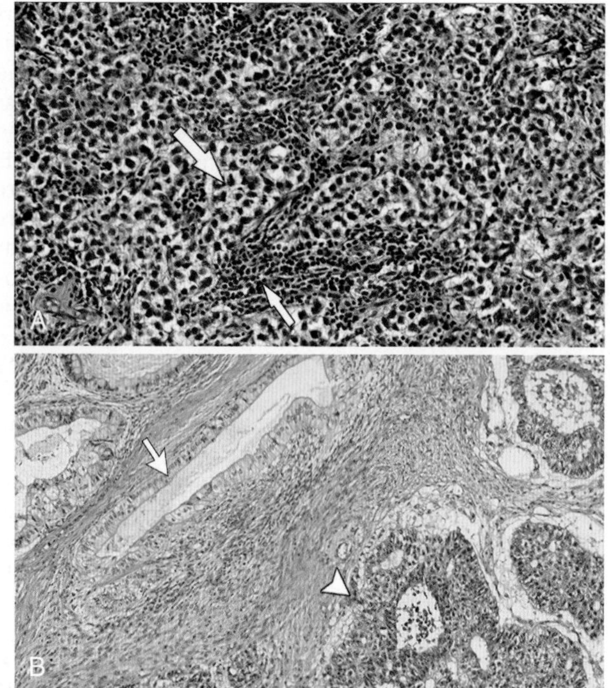

FIGURE 21.5. **A**, Seminoma, classic type, with neoplastic cells (*large arrow*) and the typical accompanying chronic inflammatory infiltrate (*small arrow*). **B**, Mixed nonseminomatous germ cell tumor composed of teratoma (*arrow*) and embryonal carcinoma (*arrowhead*). (Courtesy Dr. Kanishka Sircar, Pathology Department, MD Anderson Hospital, Houston, Texas.)

TABLE 21.1 Comparison of the British Testicular Tumour Panel (BTTP) and World Health Organization Classifications of Testicular Germ Cell Tumors

BRITISH TESTICULAR TUMOUR PANEL (BTTP)	WORLD HEALTH ORGANIZATION
Seminoma	Seminoma
Spermatocytic seminoma	Spermatocytic seminoma
Teratoma • TD (teratoma differentiated) • MTI (malignant teratoma intermediate) • MTU (malignant teratoma undifferentiated) • YST (yolk sac tumour) • Malignant teratoma trophoblastic	Nonseminomatous germ cell tumor • Mature teratoma • Embryonal carcinoma with teratoma (teratocarcinoma) • Embryonal carcinoma • YST • Choriocarcinoma

(From Chieffi P, Franco R, Portella G. Molecular and cell biology of testicular germ cell tumors. *Int Rev Cell Mol Biol.* 2009;278:277–308.)

Tumor Markers. Tumor markers help in the characterization of testicular tumors (Table 21.2).

- α-fetoprotein (AFP): Produced by the fetal yolk sac, gastrointestinal tract, and liver. This tumor marker is elevated in 50% to 60% of patients with NSGCTs, such as yolk sac tumors and mixed GCTs containing yolk sac elements.[17,40,41]
- Human chorionic gonadotropin (hCG): A glycoprotein produced by syncytiotrophoblastic giant cells. It is elevated in 60% of patients with advanced NSCGTs and in 10% to 20% with stage I disease. Advanced seminomatous disease is associated with elevated β-hCG in up to 25% of patients. Choriocarcinomas (pure trophoblastic teratomas) are associated with very high levels of β-hCG and metastasize widely.[17,40,41]
- Lactate dehydrogenase (LDH): A less specific marker because it is produced by multiple organs. It is elevated in greater than 80% of NSCGT cases at the time of initial presentation and is elevated in patients with advanced seminoma. Its levels correlate with disease bulk.[17,40,41]

TABLE 21.2 Testicular Tumors and Their Associated Serum Tumor Markers

	AFP	β-HCG	LDH
Seminoma	0	+	++
Yolk sac tumor	+++	+	+
Choriocarcinoma	0	+++	+
Embryonal carcinoma	+	+	++
Teratoma	0	0	0

AFP, α-fetoprotein; *β-hCG*, β–human chorionic gonadotropin; *LDH*, lactate dehydogenase.

Although rising markers are often the first indicator of recurrent disease, the markers are neither sensitive nor specific. Recurrence of marker-negative disease may occur even if the tumor was initially marker-secreting.

CLINICAL PRESENTATION

The most common presentation of testicular cancer patients is a painless testicular mass.[42] The clinical presentation is highly variable, such as a palpable testicular mass, pain, and/or swelling. Approximately 10% present with fever and/or scrotal pain.[43] Some series have reported that about half of all patients with testicular cancer present with testicular pain with or without a mass. In approximately 20%, symptoms are related to metastatic disease. The patient may also present in the advanced stages with backache from retroperitoneal adenopathy, which should be differentiated from musculoskeletal pain. Other symptoms include neck mass from adenopathy, dyspnea, and hemoptysis from lung metastases or nodal disease in the lungs. Approximately 5% present with gynecomastia. Approximately one in three to four patients presents with abdominal and back pain, headache, malaise, or hemoptysis. The testicular tumor may be an incidental finding secondary to recent trauma in the region, which reveals the finding on further evaluation with imaging or examination.[44]

If retroperitoneal adenopathy or, less commonly, cervical, supraclavicular, or axillary adenopathy is palpated or detected by US or CT in a male patient, particularly between 15 and 35 years old, a testicular examination and US should be performed to evaluate for an underlying primary tumor.

PATTERNS OF TUMOR SPREAD

It is important to know the normal lymphatic drainage and blood supply of the testes to understand how the tumor spreads.

Lymphatic Drainage of Testes

The lymphatics deep to the testes and tunica albuginea follow the lymphatic channels alongside the spermatic cord and testicular vessels to the lateral and periaortic nodes, and then to the retroperitoneum.

Blood Supply of Testes

The pair of testicular arteries arises from the aorta. The right testicular artery originates from the abdominal aorta. The left testicular artery originates from the left renal artery. The testicular arteries course through the inguinal canal. The testis features a dual blood supply. These are the cremasteric artery, which is an inferior epigastric artery branch of the external iliac artery, and the artery of the ductus deferens, an inferior vesicle artery branch of the internal iliac artery. The right testicular vein drains into the inferior vena cava (IVC), and the left testicular vein drains into the left renal vein. The lymph node drainage pattern, therefore, predominantly first involves the aortocaval nodes on the right and paraaortic lymph nodes below the renal vasculature on the left.[13]

Testicular neoplasms spread by the lymphatic system most commonly, followed by hematogenous spread, and least commonly by direct spread. The most common site of metastases is the retroperitoneum, followed by the lungs.

Lymphatic Spread

The pattern originates in the mediastinum of the testes, continues to the internal inguinal ring along the spermatic cords, alongside the lymphatic channels adjacent to the testicular vessels, and to the retroperitoneal lymph nodes.[45] This route is based on the embryologic origin of the testes in the retroperitoneum.[44]

Right-sided nodes have more variability in spread pattern, with preferential spread inferior to the right renal hilum, to the right paracaval, interaortocaval, preaortic, precaval, and retrocaval nodes. Right-sided tumor spreads to right-sided nodes 85% of the time and to contralateral and ipsilateral nodes 13% of the time.[13,46,47]

Left-sided nodes tend to spread inferior to the left renal vessels to the left paraaortic nodes and preaortic nodes. Left-sided tumor spreads to left-sided nodes 80% of the time and to both contralateral and ipsilateral nodes 20% of the time.[13,46,47]

The right and left infrarenal periaortic nodes spread to the renal suprahilar nodes and then to the retrocrural nodes. Direct spread can occur through the retroperitoneum to the diaphragm and then to the posterior mediastinal and subcarinal nodes. Indirect spread can occur through the thoracic duct to the prevascular and supraclavicular nodes[13,46] (Fig. 21.6).

Lymphatic spread can also occur lateral to the aortocaval group to the echelon node, situated between the first and third lumbar vertebral bodies on the right and anterior to the left iliopsoas muscle on the left.[13,48]

It is rare to have contralateral nodal metastases without ipsilateral metastatic or primary disease. It is also rare to have direct spread to iliac or inguinal nodes. In the presence of advanced disease, previous scrotal surgery, or cryptorchidism, or at relapse of tumor, pelvic spread and contralateral nodal spread can occur.[46] Direct spread to inguinal nodes can occur when there are skin metastases.

Nodal disease that spreads cranial to the renal hila follows the direct spread pattern. Seminomatous tumor can spread by the thoracic duct into the posterior mediastinum. NSCGT spread is more of a random pattern, to the anterior mediastinum, neck, supraclavicular, and hilar nodes.

Hematogenous Spread

The primary site of hematogenous spread is the lungs.[48] Other sites include the brain, which is common with choriocarcinoma. Additional sites include the osseous structures and liver. Rare sites of hematogenous spread include pleura, pericardium, muscle, skin, spleen, kidneys, adrenal glands, and peritoneum.[49] Although hematogenous spread is generally associated with synchronous lymph node metastases, it does occasionally "skip" the retroperitoneum in cases of embryonal carcinoma.

KEY POINTS

Tumor Spread

- Predominant form of tumor spread is through the lymphatics.
- Most common site of metastases is the retroperitoneum, followed by the lungs.
- Direct spread can occur through the retroperitoneum to the diaphragm, then to the posterior mediastinal and subcarinal nodes.
- Indirect spread can occur through the thoracic duct to the prevascular and supraclavicular nodes.
- Hematogenous spread is less common, most often to the lungs.

STAGING

Staging is based on several parameters, including histopathology, serum blood markers, radiologic examinations, and clinical examination.

The tumor-node-metastasis-serum (TNMS) marker system is used for staging (Fig. 21.7):

- Stage I: Disease is confined to the testes with no nodal disease or metastases; consists of IA and IB. Stage IS denotes persisting elevated tumor markers after orchiectomy.

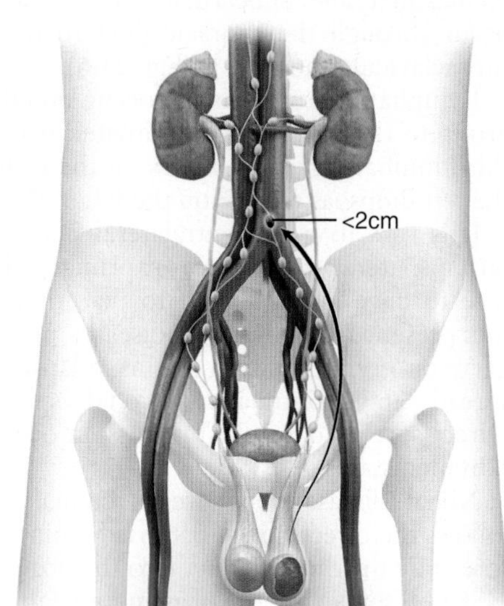

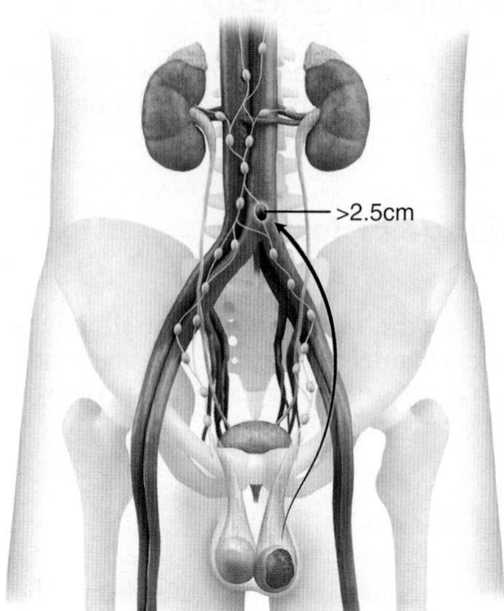

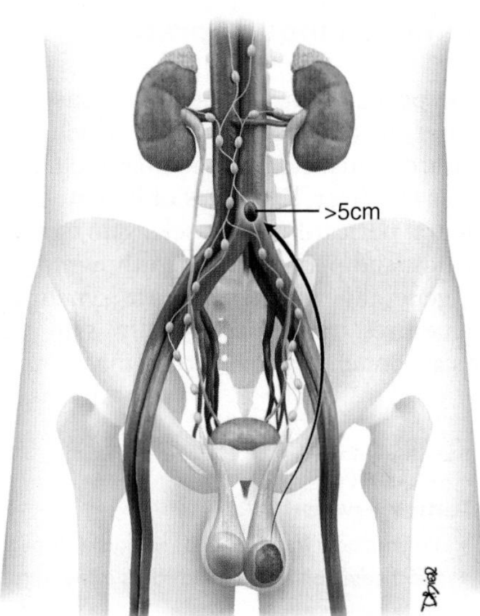

FIGURE 21.6. Staging diagram.

- Stage II: Disease in the retroperitoneum is confined to lymph nodes. Stage IIA has lymph nodes smaller than 2 cm, stage IIB nodes are 2 to 5 cm, and stage IIC nodes are larger than 5 cm.
- Stage III: Regional nodal metastases with moderately elevated tumor markers or visceral or distal sites.

The American Joint Committee on Cancer Staging Manual, 8th edition, describes the TNMS classification and staging criteria for GCTs.[50]

Once the tumor is staged, the European Germ Cell Cancer Consensus Group (EGCCCG) recommends that patient risk be determined using the International Germ Cell Cancer Consensus Group (IGCCCG) guidelines, which is divided into good, intermediate, and poor categories.[51,52] The classification is based on tumor location, metastases, tumor markers, and histology. Table 21.3 lists the IGCCCG guidelines.[51,52]

Patients with pure seminomas are divided into good and intermediate risk groups; there is no poor risk group. Patients with NSCGT or mixed histology are divided into good, intermediate, and poor risk groups.

The poor risk of NSCGT group includes patients with any one of the following: nonpulmonary visceral metastases such as liver and brain metastases, markedly elevated serum markers (AFP >10,000 ng/mL or β-hCG >50,000 IU/L or LDH >10 times the upper limit of normal), or mediastinal primary site.[53,54]

KEY POINTS

Staging

- The tumor-node-metastasis-serum marker system is widely used to stage testicular tumors. After staging, the International Germ Cell Cancer Consensus Group guidelines place the patient into good-, intermediate-, and poor-risk categories.

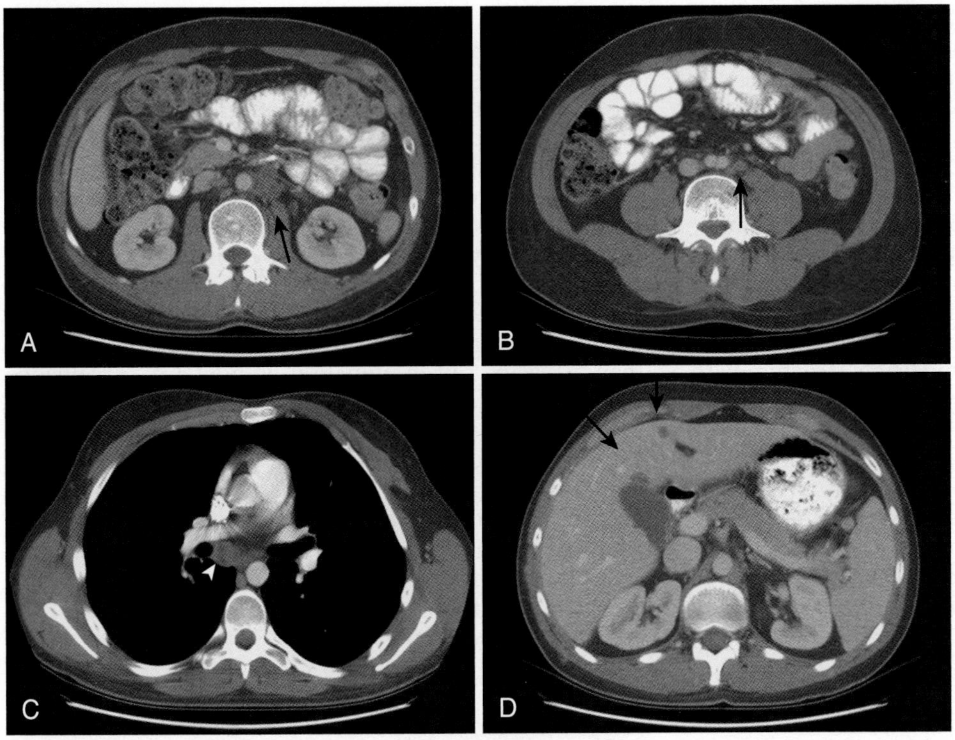

A B C D

Figure 21.7. Axial computed tomography scan of the abdomen. A patient with known left testicular nonseminomatous germ cell tumor has left-sided adenopathy at the left paraaortic space (**A**, *arrow*) and aortic bifurcation (**B**, *arrow*), which has spread to the posterior mediastinum (**C**, *arrow*). The patient also has left liver metastases (**D**, *arrows*).

- Stage I is confined to the testis with no nodal disease or metastases.
- Stage II has disease in the retroperitoneum confined to lymph nodes.
- Stage III has metastases that spread beyond the retroperitoneum or to extranodal sites, or involve regional nodes with moderately elevated tumor markers.

IMAGING

The diagnosis of testicular carcinoma is usually made after an inguinal orchiectomy and is based on the histopathology.[55] Percutaneous biopsy of the testicle can lead to seeding along the biopsy tract, so it is never performed if germ cell malignancy is suspected.[56]

Imaging studies are crucial to the diagnosis, in conjunction with tumor serum markers, and are used to assess the extent of disease and treatment response. At the time of initial staging, approximately 25% of seminomatous cases and 40% to 60% of NSGCT cases have metastases.

When interpreting radiologic examinations, it is important to note that important predictors of tumor relapse are lymphatic invasion and vascular invasion.[38]

Follow-up imaging varies according to the staging of the tumor, but typically involves CT and chest x-rays in conjunction with serum markers and clinic visits.

Table 21.3 International Germ Cell Consensus and Prognosis Classification

SEMINOMA
Good prognosis: all of the following • No nonpulmonary visceral metastases • Any primary site • Normal AFP, any β-hCG, any LDH
Intermediate prognosis: all of the following • Nonpulmonary visceral metastases • Any primary site • Normal AFP, any β-hCG, any LDH
NONSEMINOMA
Good prognosis: all of the following • Testis/retroperitoneal primary • No nonpulmonary visceral metastases • AFP <1000 ng/mL, β-hCG <5000 IU/L (1000 ng/mL), and LDH <1.5 × N
Intermediate prognosis: all of the following • Testis/retroperitoneal primary • No nonpulmonary visceral metastases • AFP 1000–10000 ng/mL, or β-hCG 5000–50000 IU/L, or LDH 1.5–10 × N
Poor prognosis: any of the following • AFP >10,000 ng/mL, β-hCG >50,000 IU/L, or LDH >10×N **or** • Mediastinal primary site or • Nonpulmonary visceral metastases

AFP, α-fetoprotein; *β-hCG*, β–human chorionic gonadotropin; *LDH*, lactate dehydogenase.
Modified from International Germ Cell Cancer Collaborative Group. International Germ Cell Consensus Classification: a prognostic factor-based staging system for metastatic germ cell cancers. *J Clin Oncol.* 1997;15:594–603.

Ultrasound

US is the primary modality for assessing the testes, with a greater than 95% sensitivity and specificity for detecting testicular lesions. It can be easily performed and is cost-effective. It is used to screen for associated abnormalities such as contralateral disease and microlithiasis. Typically, a high-frequency linear transducer from 7 to 10 MHz is used with imaging in at least two planes.[52]

When a patient presents for US evaluation of a scrotal mass, it is important to note whether it is solid or cystic and to differentiate an extratesticular mass, which is generally benign (>90% of the time), from an intratesticular mass, which is almost always malignant.

Generally, seminomas have a homogeneous hypoechoic echotexture, and nonseminomas have a more heterogeneous appearance with calcifications and cystic components (Fig. 21.8). Some tumors exhibit relatively increased vascularity, although this sign is nonspecific.[57] In tumors smaller than 2 cm, it may be difficult to detect vascularity. It is important to distinguish a mass from focal orchitis, which can also present as a hypoechoic structure with increased vascularity; however, orchitis tends to be more ill-defined than tumors.

A burned-out or regressed GCT is clinically not palpable and is believed to represent a tumor that outgrows its blood supply. It typically presents as a scar at the primary site with metastatic disease. Sonographically, the testes features small hypoechoic or hyperechoic nodules.[44] If one suspects a burned-out tumor, notify the surgeon, because patients may not always need to have an orchiectomy if they have a nonviable tumor (Fig. 21.9).

Testicular microlithiasis has benign calcifications within the lumen of the seminiferous tubules and is well-visualized on US. It is defined as five or more punctate calcifications in the US transducer field (Fig. 21.10). Testicular microlithiasis might be the only indication of ITGCN, because it is more frequent in patients with ITGCN than in those without. The risk of ITGCN is approximately 20% with bilateral microlithiasis and 0.5% in patients without testicular microlithiasis.[58] Testicular microlithiasis is associated with infertility, cryptorchidism, and Down syndrome, among other entities. In patients with known testicular cancer, there is a strong association with microlithiasis.[21,59–61] A study found a 48% prevalence of microlithiasis in patients with testicular germ cell cancer, with a 24% prevalence of microlithiasis in family members of an affected patient.[21] Some studies cite the prevalence of microlithiasis in the general population to be approximately 0.6% to 9%.[21,62–64] If incidentally detected without any other associated risk factors, microlithiasis in and of itself does not predict the subsequent development of testicular cancer. It affects approximately 2.4% to 14.1% of asymptomatic adult males. In the pediatric population, it is estimated at 1% to 2% in the asymptomatic population. There have been mixed recommendations for how testicular microlithiasis should be followed, because serial US examinations are not cost-effective. A new follow-up algorithm suggests that, once testicular microlithiasis is detected, the patient should be assessed for other risk factors (e.g., cryptorchidism, infertility). If the patient is younger than 50 years, a testicular biopsy or US might be performed, because the risk of ITGCN is higher in this population.[18,65,66] If no other risk factors are present, and the patient is older than 50 years, self-examination without US surveillance is suggested. If a biopsy is performed and is negative, no further follow-up is advised.[67]

Others suggest that screening US is not recommended for the population with incidental testicular microlithiasis, because it is not cost effective. Instead, they recommend educating men about self-examination.[68] US follow-up is recommended for patients with microlithiasis who cannot proactively perform self-examinations, including the pediatric and adolescent populations.[69]

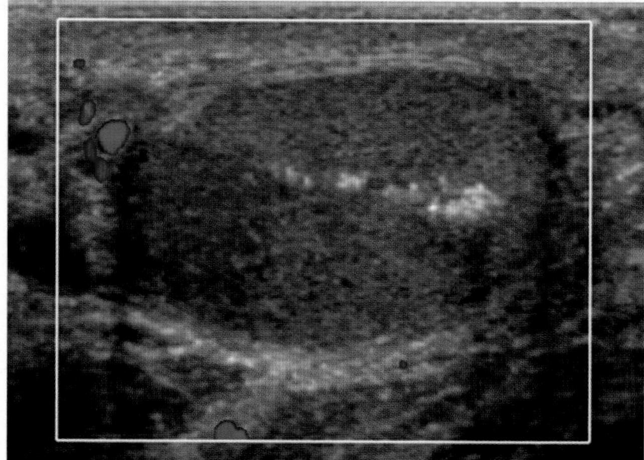

FIGURE 21.9. Transverse ultrasound image of a testes with a "burnt-out" germ cell tumor demonstrates a dystrophic band of calcifications with no discrete mass. Pathology from subsequent orchiectomy reveals a fibrous scar consistent with a regressed, "burnt-out" germ cell tumor.

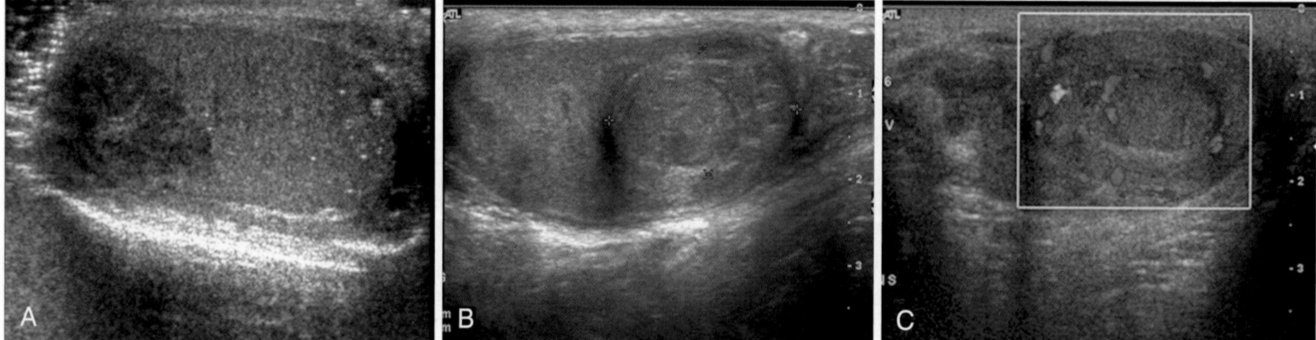

FIGURE 21.8. **A**, Gray-scale image of a testis demonstrates a hypoechoic relatively well-circumscribed mass, pathologically proven to be seminoma. Note the microlithiasis, which is not as diffuse as in Fig. 21.10. Testicular microlithiasis can be an associated risk for developing a testicular malignancy. **B** and **C**, Ultrasound, gray-scale, and color Doppler images of the testes. A primary nonseminomatous germ cell tumor measures 2.5 cm in size, with heterogeneous hemorrhage, necrosis, and some vascularity. Pathology reveals 50% choriocarcinoma, 30% yolk sac, and 20% embryonal carcinoma. (A, Courtesy Dr. F. Eftekhari, Department of Radiology, MD Anderson Hospital, Houston, Texas.)

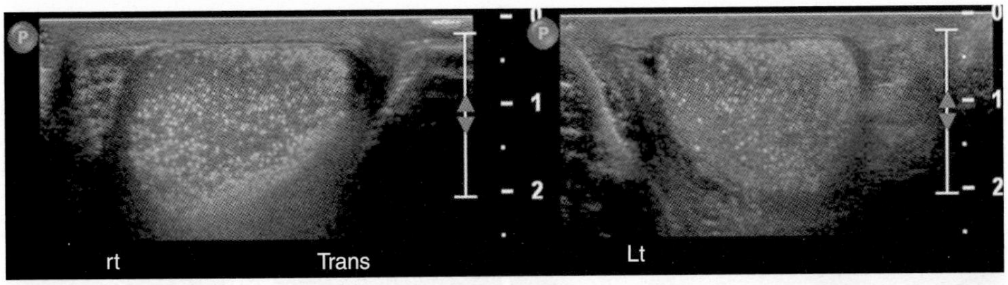

FIGURE 21.10. Transverse ultrasound (US) of the right and left testes. Bilateral diffuse testicular microlithiasis with no testicular mass. Patient has a history of a mediastinal yolk sac tumor and is undergoing routine US surveillance examinations of the testes.

Although there are several suggestions for managing microlithiasis, no definite guideline for their management exists.[58,70]

A US is performed to evaluate for a testicular tumor when a 15- to 40-year-old male presents with retroperitoneal or mediastinal adenopathy or lung metastases. Another useful purpose is to evaluate the contralateral testes for contralateral tumor involvement in a patient with known testicular cancer, which is important because the highest risk of a second malignancy is development of a second primary in the contralateral testes (Fig. 21.11).

Aside from evaluating the testes, US can be used to evaluate liver lesions. It can also be used to biopsy liver or retroperitoneal lesions, which can sometimes be limited owing to overlying bowel gas. The retroperitoneum is frequently not visualized well on US owing to overlying bowel gas and fat. Therefore, a CT-guided biopsy may be alternatively used for liver, retroperitoneal, or other soft tissue biopsies.

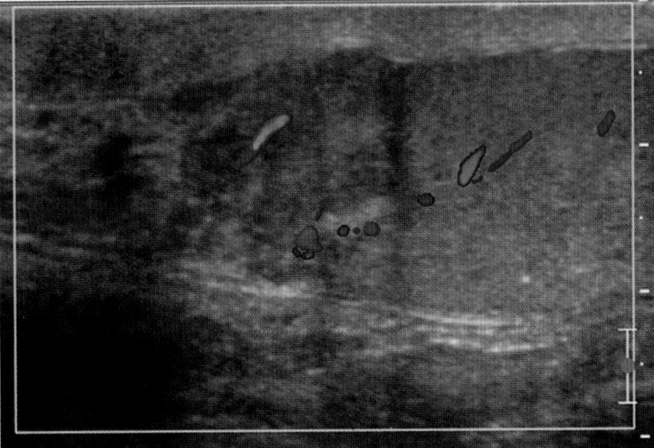

FIGURE 21.11. Transverse color ultrasound image of the left testis. Patient has a history of right testicular cancer and had a right orchiectomy 5 years earlier. This image demonstrates a new heterogeneous mass in the left testis. Pathology reveals a mixed germ cell tumor composed of embryonal and yolk sac tumor.

Computed Tomography

CT is the primary imaging modality for disease staging in testicular cancer patients for disease in the neck, thorax, abdomen, and pelvis, with accuracy close to 80%.[71] Approximately 38% of testicular cancer patients present with retroperitoneal metastases at the time of initial diagnosis, and CT is a sensitive modality for detecting the adenopathy.

According to the EGCCCG, patients should have a contrast-enhanced CT of the chest, abdomen, and pelvis.[72,73] Within the chest, CT is sensitive for detecting mediastinal and supraclavicular adenopathy, pleural disease, and pleural effusions. Nodal dimensions greater than 10 mm are suspicious based on correlative findings, such as interval enlargement and elevating tumor markers. CT does have limitations, because nodal measurements between metastatic and nonmetastatic nodes do overlap. Tumor infiltration into normal-sized nodes is difficult to detect on CT. Finding metastatic nodes is important in the staging of patients, because stage I patients undergo surveillance and stage II patients start chemotherapy. Using a 10- to 15-mm short axis as a criteria for metastatic nodes has been shown to yield false-negative rates ranging from 29% to 44%. If smaller nodes less than 4 mm are used, sensitivity improves but specificity decreases. CT is not able to identify low-volume nodal disease in approximately 30% of GCT patients.[74] Several papers have cited false-negative rates approaching 59% on CT, because disease involvement is based on nodal measurement. The false-positive rate of CT has been reported to be as high as 40%, in which nodes greater than 1 cm short axis may also represent benign reactive nodes from inflammation or hyperplasia.[52] An important point to consider is that nodes in the lower retroperitoneum tend to be slightly larger than those in the upper retroperitoneum.[75] Although it is difficult to determine malignant nodal disease, as a general consensus nodes greater than 1 cm on the short axis are abnormal, and those 8 to 10 mm in size are suspicious.[13,52] The size should be correlated with prior examinations, size measurements, tumor markers, and histologic diagnosis.

Lymph node metastases range in size and typically exhibit the same density as soft tissue, with seminomatous disease and occasional sites of necrosis. Larger nodal masses and NSCGTs are typically heterogeneous, containing soft tissue components with mixed components.

Nodal size is important in postchemotherapy NSGCT patients, because nodes greater than 1 cm are at higher risk for containing mature teratoma or residual cancer. Nodal measurement is also important, because a decrease in posttreatment nodes indicates response to therapy and possible residual teratoma.

Detection of low-volume retroperitoneal disease is low on CT, which may affect management. Based on the size of detectable residual masses, CT is useful in predicting whether a patient should have a retroperitoneal lymphadenectomy or be monitored. Typically, postchemotherapy residual masses greater than 1 cm on the short axis have a higher rate of relapse and are resected.

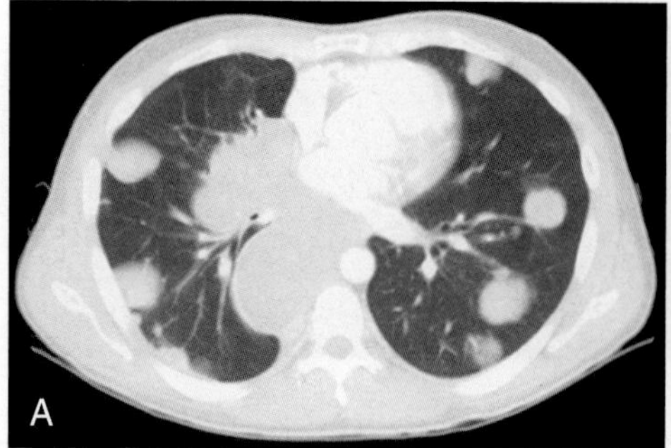

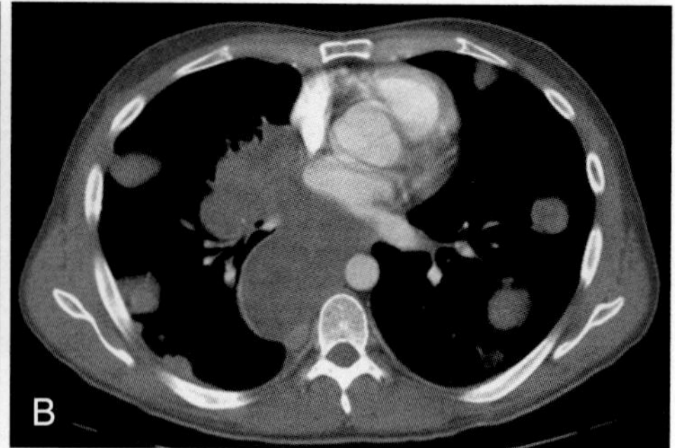

FIGURE 21.12. Computed tomography scan of the chest in a patient with mixed germ cell tumor composed of mature and immature teratoma, focal seminoma, embryonal carcinoma, and choriocarcinoma. **A**, Lung windows demonstrate extensive bilateral metastases. **B**, Mediastinal windows demonstrate extensive right perihilar and posterior mediastinal adenopathy.

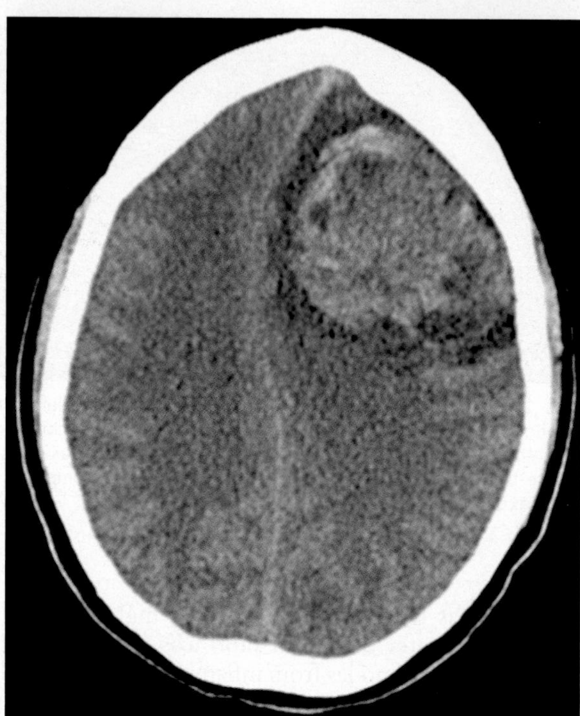

FIGURE 21.13. Noncontrast head computed tomography. A large left frontal hemorrhagic nonseminomatous germ cell tumor metastasis has surrounding edema and rightward midline shift.

Vascular anomalies must be differentiated from retroperitoneal disease. Such vascular anomalies include retroaortic renal vein, circumaortic renal vein, IVC variants such as a duplicated IVC or left-sided IVC, or enlarged gonadal veins. In addition, unopacified loops of bowel in the retroperitoneum may simulate soft tissue attenuation retroperitoneal adenopathy. Using the correct CT scanning technique is important in enabling differentiation. Intravenous contrast will delineate vasculature from nodes. Gastrointestinal contrast will opacify loops of bowel and differentiate them from lower-attenuation nodes. The development of spiral CT with thinner sections with up to 5-mm-thick slices has been able to detect smaller nodes that can be easily missed with thicker slices. The ability to scan in or reconstruct thinner slices in questionable regions can increase the sensitivity for detection.[13]

It is debated whether a CT of the pelvis is useful in patients with testicular cancer. Typically, iliac and inguinal nodes are not involved in stage I cases. Pelvic adenopathy may occur in the presence of bulky retroperitoneal disease or when there has been previous surgery such as inguinal or scrotal surgery, retroperitoneal surgery, or correction of an undescended testis or congenital anomaly.[76] Many clinicians do not scan the pelvis in routine surveillance examinations if the patient does not have any of the previous conditions, to avoid exposing the patient to unnecessary radiation.[13,38,77]

CT of the chest is well recognized as an important examination to perform to evaluate for nodal disease, lung nodules, pleural effusions, or pleural disease (Fig. 21.12). It is common for seminomas to present with pleural disease or pleural effusions.[78] In seminomatous disease, there may be direct spread through the diaphragmatic hiatus and into the posterior mediastinum.[78] Lung metastases may vary according to histology: seminoma metastases tend to be larger, and NSGCT metastases more commonly appear as smaller multiple peripheral nodules.[52] In nonseminotomatous disease, spread tends to be in a more random distribution.[78,79] Nodal disease in the anterior mediastum, hila, neck, and supraclavicular fossa is more common with NSCGT than with seminomatous disease. Chest nodes rarely occur in the absence of retroperitoneal disease.

CT of the chest may also be useful in identifying and managing bleomycin-related toxicity. Pulmonary toxicity related to bleomycin can be self-limiting, but may develop into pneumonitis or fibrosis, and in some cases may be fatal.[80]

CT of the brain is obtained in high-risk patients to evaluate for hemorrhagic metastases, which manifest as high-attenuation foci on noncontrast scans (Fig. 21.13). Alternatively, an MRI may be performed to evaluate the brain.

Cases arise in which patients cannot have intravenous contrast owing to renal compromise or severe allergy, or if they cannot take in gastrointestinal contrast. MRI and PET/CT examinations may be useful in these cases to detect adenopathy and other sites of disease involvement.

Plain Chest Radiographs

Chest radiographs provide a baseline for evaluating for mediastinal disease, lung nodules greater than 1 cm, and the presence of pleural effusions or pleural tumor (Fig. 21.14). It is a considerably less expensive modality than chest CT, can be used for monitoring patients in between serial CT examinations, and can reduce the radiation dose for a patient receiving multiple CT scans. Chest x-rays are typically used in patients with a lower risk, such as patients with seminoma with no retroperitoneal disease, as a screening for lung metastases.[81]

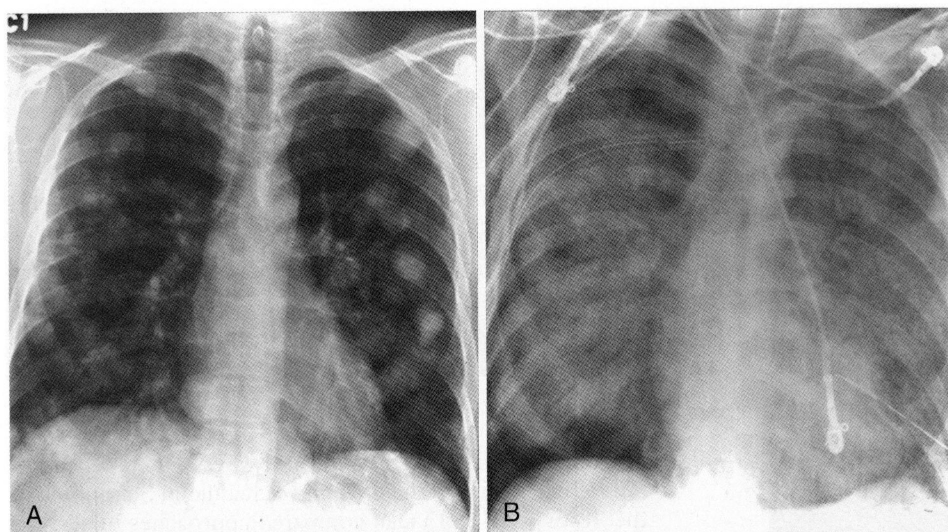

FIGURE 21.14. Chest x-rays, frontal view. **A**, Multiple metastases are present in a patient with metastatic choriocarcinoma. **B**, Short-term follow-up chest x-ray demonstrates pulmonary edema and hemorrhage from the vascular metastases, which bled. (**A** and **B**, Courtesy Dr. F. Eftekhari, Department of Radiology, MD Anderson Hospital, Houston, Texas.)

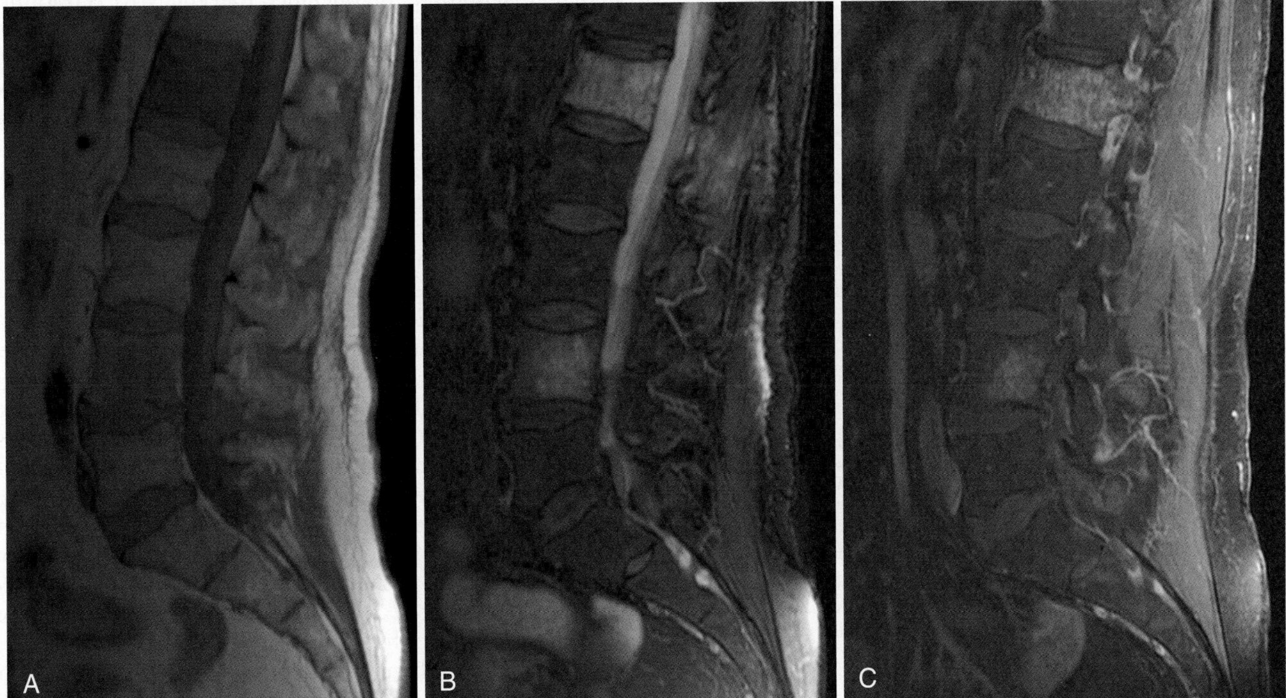

FIGURE 21.15. Magnetic resonance imaging of the lumbar spine. Patient has a history of metastatic seminoma. Axial T1-weighted (**A**) and axial T2-weighted fat-saturated (**B**) images demonstrate low-T1, high-T2 metastatic lesions occupying the L1 and L4 vertebral bodies. **C**, Postcontrast image demonstrates enhancement of L1 and L4, which are suggestive of active metastases.

Magnetic Resonance Imaging

MRI is an important problem-solving tool. It is a particularly good modality to assess for metastatic disease in patients who cannot receive a contrast-enhanced CT, because it has superior contrast resolution to CT. It is also used in patients who have equivocal findings on CT such as indeterminate liver lesions or osseous lesions that need further characterization.

- MRI is superior to CT in assessing the presence of marrow disease.[82] Diffusion-weighted (DW) imaging MRI is particularly useful for differentiating osseous metastases from pathologic compression fractures or spondylitis, which is important for clinical management of a patient who may present with back pain[73] (Fig. 21.15).
- MRI can delineate vascular invasion. With its multiplanar technique and superior contrast resolution to CT, it is good for delineating vascular anatomy, which is beneficial before retroperitoneal nodal dissection, or to evaluate for tumor invasion of the IVC or upper extremity vessels[83] (Fig. 21.16).
- MRI is used for assessing neurologic metastatic disease in patients. This includes detection of brain, meningeal, and spinal cord involvement.[84] A brain MRI is performed as an initial staging device in patients with a high-risk profile. Brain metastases are most common in choriocarcinomas. Central nervous system metastases

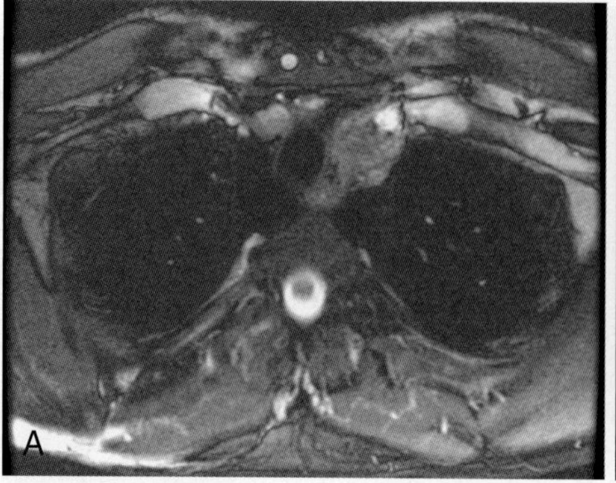

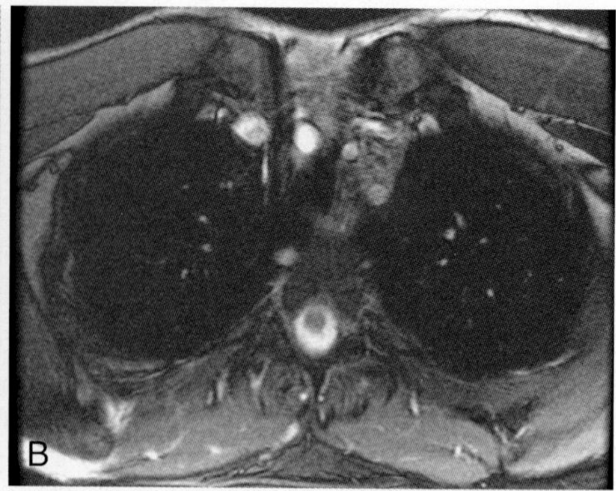

Figure 21.16. Noncontrast magnetic resonance imaging (MRI) of the chest. **A** and **B**, Axial T2-weighted fat-saturated images in a patient who cannot receive intravenous contrast owing to elevated creatinine. A left nodal mass surrounds the left subclavian artery and common carotid artery. It abuts the posterior left brachiocephalic vein. There is no vessel occlusion. Patient has metastatic teratocarcinoma. This is an example of how MRI can be used to delineate vessel involvement without administering intravenous contrast.

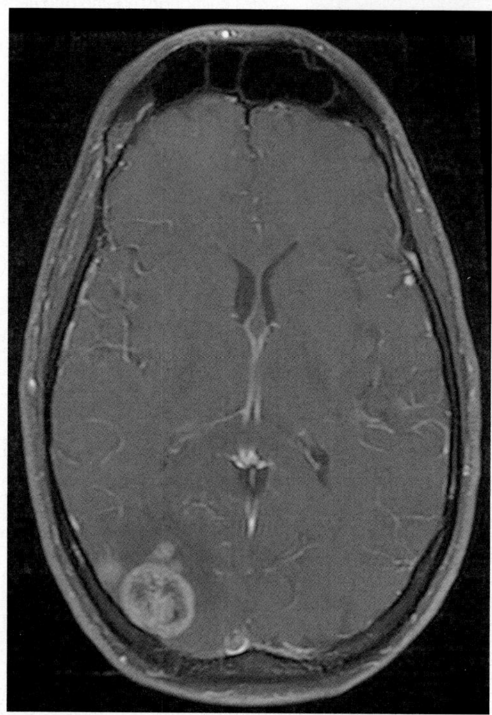

Figure 21.17. Magnetic resonance imaging of the brain. Axial postcontrast fat-saturated image demonstrates a right occipital peripherally enhancing metastasis with satellite nodules in a patient with mixed germ cell tumor.

are found in fewer than 5% of initially staged patients (Fig. 21.17).

MRI is used in evaluating for muscular and soft tissue invasion by delineating soft tissue and intramuscular metastases and their relationship to adjacent organs, which is important for radiation and presurgical planning.

Another problem-solving function for MRI is to assess for some complications that CT may not visualize, such as the presence of a fistula between a retroperitoneal mass and adjacent bowel or skin.[13]

MRI is useful in decreasing the radiation dose of patients who need multiple CT scans for surveillance.[85] The radiation risk of a CT chest, abdomen, and pelvis single combined examination for developing a second cancer is 1 in 2000; with multiple surveillance scans, this may increase the risk to 1 in 300.[85] One study of experienced image readers found that MRI had similar sensitivity to CT, detecting nodal disease greater than 1 cm in 95% of cases. The prospective, randomized Trial of Imaging and Schedule in Seminoma of the Testis (TRISST) trial compared approaches to surveillance imaging of CT and MRI after treatment of stage 1 testicular seminoma. It concluded that the MRI is not inferior to CT, and should be recommended to reduce excessive irradiation for surveillance imaging.[85a] Imaging modality and frequency in surveillance of stage I seminoma testicular cancer: Results from a randomized, phase III, factorial trial (TRISST).[85]

Magnetic Resonance Imaging Sequences

MRI T2-weighted sequences have been of use in differentiating benign from malignant nodes. Benign nodes typically have a high T1-weighted fatty hilum signal and a homogeneous T2 signal. Malignant nodes typically have loss of high T1 fatty hilum signal and exhibit heterogeneous signal.

MRI with lymphotropic nanoparticles is being investigated for differentiating malignant from benign nodes. Some studies indicate that it increases the sensitivity and specificity for differentiating between malignant nodes less than 1 cm from benign nodes greater than 1 cm. The mechanism of lymphatic targeting is based on slow extravasation of nanoparticles into the interstitial space that are transported to lymph nodes and taken up by lymph node macrophages, causing intracellular trapping and MRI signal change, which enables nodal detection. Some studies have demonstrated a sensitivity of 88% and a specificity of 92% for detecting nodal metastases in contrast to regular T1 and T2 sequences alone, which have a sensitivity of 71% and a specificity of 68%. Limitations of the studies include a small sample size, few evaluated nodes, and percutaneous biopsy for pathology evaluation.[44,86–88]

Another application of MRI sequences in oncologic imaging is using the DW imaging functional sequence for imaging the abdomen and pelvis. DW imaging sequences measure the amount of random diffusion of water molecules within tissues. Generally, malignant tissue and malignant nodes have restricted diffusion manifested by high signal because of restricted random water molecule motion owing to higher density of cells in malignant tissue. The DW imaging technique is useful for patients who require a short scan time, because it can be acquired rapidly. This sequence has been used for many years in neurologic imaging. Its function in oncologic body imaging is currently being investigated, with promising initial findings.[89] Several studies have demonstrated that malignant tumors tend to have a lower apparent diffusion coefficient than benign tumors. Also, variations in enhancement patterns may exist between germ cell tumors and Leydig tumors.[90–93]

Although there have been advances in MRI with faster acquisition techniques, MRI continues to not as be used as commonly as CT, owing to longer scan times and higher cost. In addition, this modality is not as readily available as CT. MRI is also not sensitive in the detection of pulmonary metastases.

Magnetic Resonance Imaging of the Scrotum

MRI can readily differentiate a benign simple fluid structure such as a hydrocele or cyst from a complex mass, although US is a quicker and less expensive modality to differentiate these entities.

When performing an MRI of the scrotum, a 3- to 5-cm surface coil is ideal to visualize the scrotum and contents. The testes can be elevated with draping placed between the thighs. A normal testis has intermediate T1 signal and high T2 signal relative to muscle, with the interdigitating fibrous septa that divide the testes into lobules exhibiting low signal (Fig. 21.18). Intratesticular lesions have lower T2 signal than the surrounding parenchyma.[25–27,94]

MRI advantages over US imaging of the testes include multiplanar capability and wide field of view. MRI also has higher resolution than US, enabling visualization of septations that are not seen on US, and therefore may help visualize a small tumor not seen on US. When US findings are indeterminate, an MRI may be performed. An example would be in cases in which sonography or clinical examination cannot adequately differentiate between an intratesticular mass, which is malignant most of the time, and an extratesticular mass, which is rarely malignant.

MRI features of testicular tumors correlate with histologic features. MRI can be used in certain cases to distinguish seminomas from NSCGTs preoperatively. Seminomas typically exhibit a homogeneous signal that is isointense to testes on T1 and hypointense on T2. Lower T2-signal band-like structures correspond to the fibrous septa, which enhance more than the surrounding tumor after gadolinium administration. The presence of a tumor capsule is not useful in differentiating seminomatous from nonseminomatous lesions.[32,94–97]

Nonseminomas typically have mixed signal, generally iso- to hyperintense on T1 and hypointense on T2. They contain areas of hemorrhage and necrosis and demonstrate heterogeneous enhancement.[32,94–97]

Although MRI is helpful in differentiating testicular GCTs, it is not consistently reliable for histologic diagnosis, and surgical biopsy is often recommended to histologically characterize the lesion.[44] MRI findings in tumor characterization currently do not play a significant role in clinical management, because the management protocol mandates an orchiectomy with detailed pathology for tumor classification and initial treatment.

When performing MRI and US imaging, it is important to differentiate testicular tumors from benign entities such as focal testicular infarction or focal orchitis. Intratesticular tumor and inflammation typically exhibit lower signal in comparison with the relatively higher signal of the testes. If there is doubt in differentiation by MRI or US, a short-term follow-up examination to assess for resolution and correlation with serum markers would be useful.

Positron Emission Tomography/ Computed Tomography

PET has become a more sensitive modality with PET/CT fusion examinations, which combine the functional imaging of PET with the anatomic imaging of CT. PET's fusion with CT has shown increased accuracy of metastases detection than CT, except small-volume metastases, which are difficult to detect on PET. One study demonstrated that PET sensitivity and specificity were 80% and 100%, in comparison with CT alone, for which the sensitivity was 70% and the specificity was 74%.[98,99] PET imaging can alter patient management.

FDG-PET uses FDG; malignant cells demonstrate higher uptake of this agent owing to their accelerated metabolism compared with normal cells. Most testicular tumors, including seminomatous tumors, exhibit high metabolism. Mature, well-differentiated teratomas and

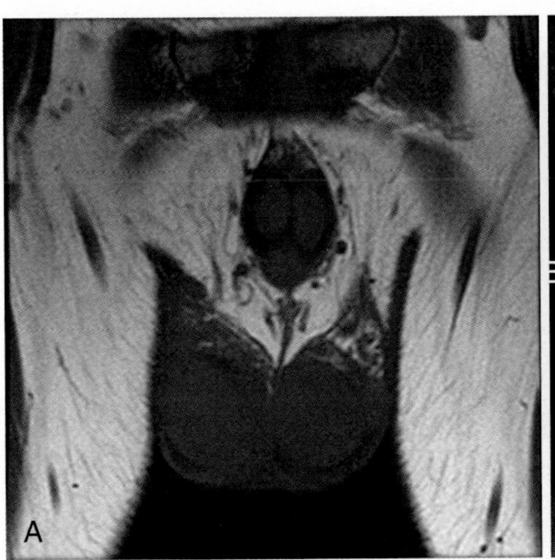

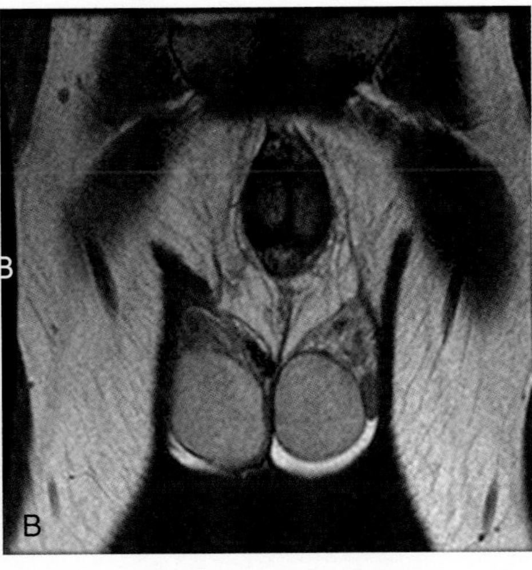

Figure 21.18. Magnetic resonance imaging of the pelvis, including the scrotum. Normal examination. Coronal T1-weighted (**A**) and coronal T2-weighted (**B**) images. A normal study, in which the testes have homogeneous low T1 and high T2 signal.

nonseminomatous metastases typically have less FDG activity (Fig. 21.19).

FDG-PET is a promising modality to detect residual disease in postchemotherapy patients, particularly for seminomas, which generally have higher uptake than NSGCTs.[98,100,101] Typically, it is recommended to perform FDG-PET after about 2 weeks of therapy. Patients with metastatic nodal disease tend to run a long course with residual masses. PET is of use to reassess for potential recurrence by detecting the metabolic activity in the residual mass (Figs. 21.20, 21.21, and 21.22).

FDG-PET has shown some use with seminoma postchemotherapy masses greater than 3 cm. The SEMPET trial prospectively reported results stratified by residual mass size, and correlated the PET-CT results to histologic or clinical outcomes. The study demonstrated that disease could be detected in in small and large residual tumors with a sensitivity of 89% and a specificity of 100%. Not all studies were able to reproduce this. Therefore, current recommendations suggest that FDG-PET is beneficial for postseminoma patients with postchemotherapy masses greater than 3 cm in size.[98,101]

PET imaging is not as useful in NSCGT patients, because mature teratoma does not demonstrate significant uptake on PET. It is difficult to differentiate teratoma from posttreatment necrosis. In NSGCT posttreatment residual masses, approximately 55% are residual carcinoma or mature teratoma.[99,102] The remainder are only posttreatment necrosis. Mature teratomas need to be surgically excised, because they can undergo malignant transformation.[103]

In seminoma, several studies are in agreement that a negative FDG-PET scan reveals a low likelihood of disease, but false-positive scans can occur. An Indiana University study of postchemotherapy seminoma patients with residual masses demonstrated that a negative PET examination is associated with a low likelihood of recurrence, but a positive PET examination does not always indicate residual tumor, and may represent fibrosis, necrosis, or inflammation.[104,105] The current guidelines of the National Comprehensive Cancer Network recommend obtaining a PET/CT scan in seminoma patients with a residual mass on CT with normal-range tumor serum markers. FDG-avid lesions can then be investigated further with biopsy, and negative lesions can be observed.[106]

PET may also be of benefit when a patient with seminoma or NSGCT has a raised tumor marker level and no

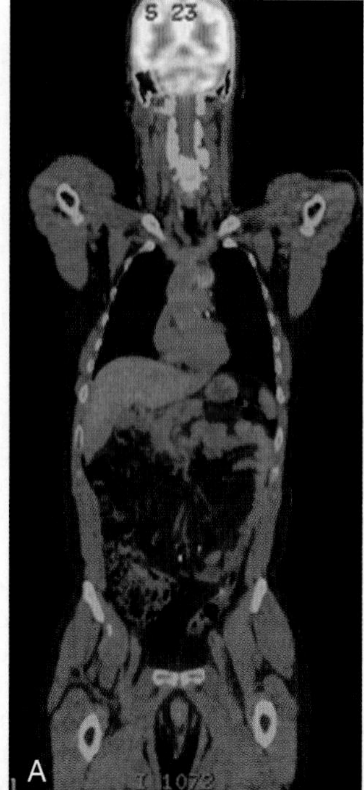

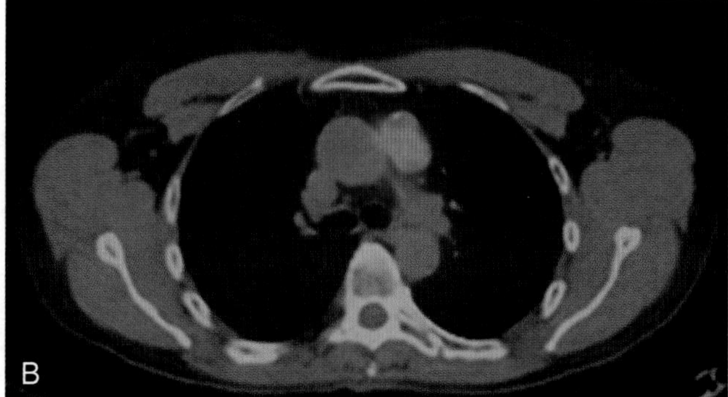

FIGURE 21.19. Positron emission tomography (PET)/computed tomography (CT) examination of an anterior mediastinal metastasis. Patient has recurrent embryonal carcinoma presenting as metastasis to the anterior mediastinum. Coronal (**A**) and axial (**B**) fused images. A PET/CT examination demonstrates an anterior mediastinum metabolically active 3.3-cm mass with peripheral coarse calcification with a standardized uptake value of 4.3. Pathology correlation reveals an anterior cystic teratoma with mature elements and areas of adenocarcinoma growing along a cystic wall.

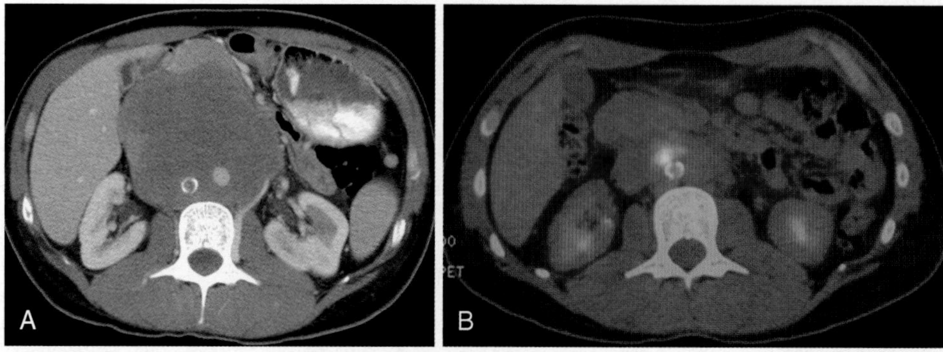

FIGURE 21.20. Computed tomography of the abdomen. **A**, Postcontrast axial image demonstrates a retroperitoneal metastasis surrounding the aorta and inferior vena cava. Patient received radiation and chemotherapy. **B**, A follow-up positron emission tomography/computed tomography axial image 3 months later demonstrates significant decrease in the mass with residual internal hypermetabolic activity representing foci of active disease in a treated mass.

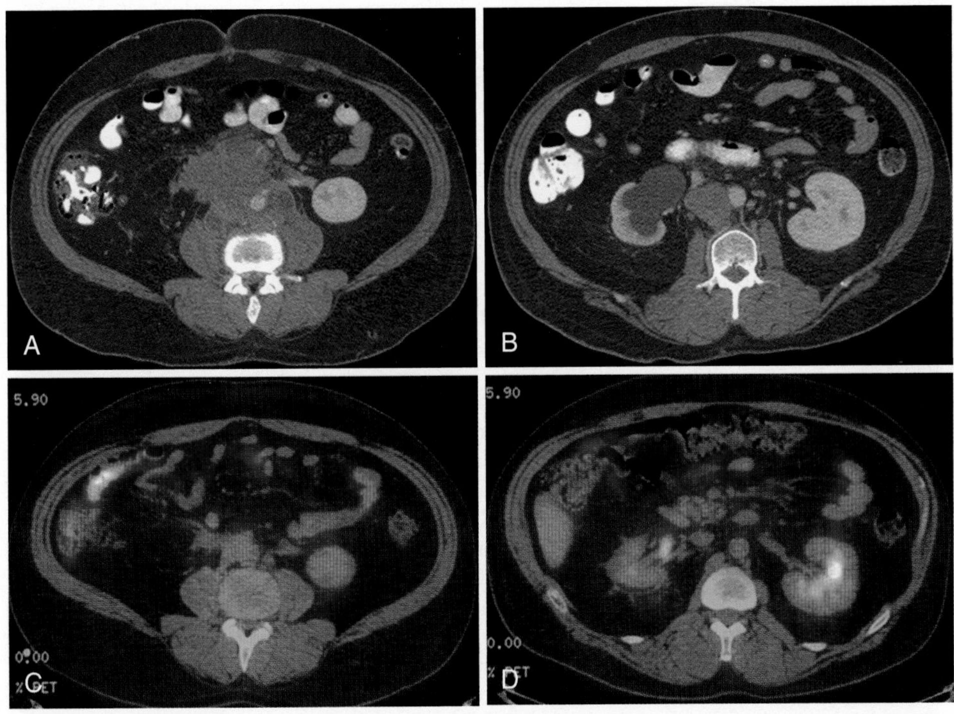

FIGURE 21.21. Computed tomography of the abdomen. **A** and **B**, Axial postcontrast images. Patient has metastatic pure seminoma. A large circumferential metastasis encompasses the aorta and inferior vena cava, with associated right hydronephrosis. **C** and **D**, Follow-up axial positron emission tomography/computed tomography scans after a course of treatment demonstrate a significant decrease in the retroperitoneal mass with no significant internal activity, representing treated disease. Because the mass effect on the right ureter has decreased, the right hydronephrosis has resolved.

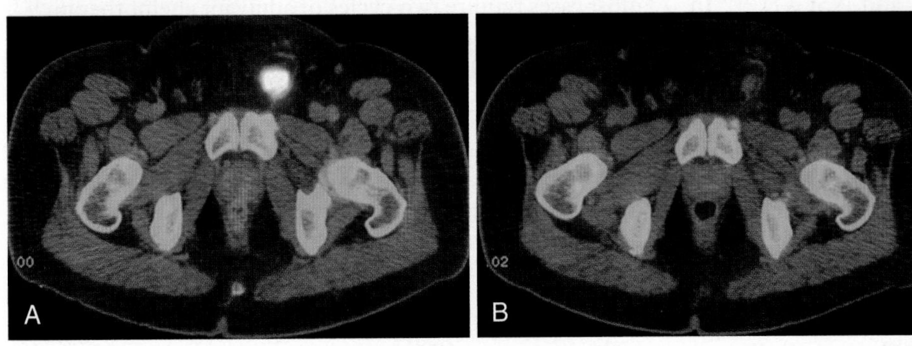

FIGURE 21.22. A, Axial positron emission tomography (PET)/computed tomography (CT) scan. Patient with a history of mixed germ cell tumor composed of seminoma with syncytiotrophoblastic giant cells has a recurrence in the left inguinal canal. **B**, A follow-up PET/CT axial image 2 months later demonstrates that the mass has significantly decreased with scant residual tissue and no metabolic activity, consistent with treated disease.

detectable metastases by CT or MRI. A study that supports this identified the site of disease in most positive cases.[107] False-negative PET scans were present, which later turned positive on subsequent imaging in three out of five cases. These findings indicate that, when a patient has raised tumor serum markers, a negative CT, and a prior negative FDG-PET, a follow-up FDG-PET still may be useful. Another study questioning the importance of PET in patients with raised tumor levels and no detectable disease was published by the Medical Research Council,[108] who reported that, although PET did identify some patients with disease not visible on CT, there was a high false-negative rate. It was concluded from this study that FDG-PET does not eliminate the need for continued close surveillance for these patients.

PET is generally not used for initial staging or routine surveillance in patients, because some studies have demonstrated that it does not detect an sufficient amount of relapsed cases to be used. A large, prospective, multicenter study demonstrated a high rate of tumor relapse in patients with negative FDG-PET findings.[108,109]

Despite the marked advances in imaging for tumor detection, further investigation still remains to be done, because about half of all patients are understaged, and one-quarter of patients are overstaged, by PET. Another limitation of PET is that it cannot detect small nodes, including subcentimeter retroperitoneal nodal metastases. Despite remarkable advancements in PET imaging, the role of FDG-PET is still being evaluated.

Bone Scan

Bone scan, a radionuclide examination, is not commonly performed, because bone metastases are not common. A bone scan may be of use when patients have advanced metastatic disease (stage IIIC).[55,110]

KEY POINTS

Radiology Report

Scrotal Imaging: Ultrasound and Magnetic Resonance Imaging (MRI)

- Evaluate whether the tumor is intratesticular (highly suspicious for malignancy) or extratesticular (less commonly malignant). Also evaluate whether the lesion is solid or cystic.
- Evaluate mass if homogeneous or heterogeneous, and if there is microlithiasis (if ultrasound) or vascularity. Detect other associated findings (e.g., hydrocele).

Abdomen and Pelvic Imaging (computed tomography [CT], MRI, positron emission tomography/CT)

- Evaluate lymph nodes in the retroperitoneum; those greater than10 mm on the short axis are more suspicious.
- Evaluate tumor invasion of inferior vena cava and visceral metastases, particularly in liver and sometimes bone.
- Pelvic metastases are generally uncommon, unless the patient has advanced bulky disease elsewhere or prior surgery.

Chest Imaging (CT or Chest X-ray)

- Evaluate for adenopathy in the mediastinum, hila, and supraclavicular sites.
- Detect lung metastases, malignant pleural effusion, pleural spread of disease, or bleomycin-related toxicity.
- Brain metastases may manifest in advanced cases and may be hemorrhagic.
- Bone metastases may present in advanced cases.

TREATMENT

The curative treatment of testicular GCTs frequently involves coordination of effort between the surgeon, medical oncologist, and radiotherapist. Radical inguinal orchiectomy is the standard surgical treatment for control of the primary tumor in cases of seminoma and NSGCT.[106] In fact, the final diagnosis of pure seminoma versus NSGCT or mixed histology is rarely made before the final histopathology study after orchiectomy. Adjuvant chemotherapy is an established option for patients with clinical stage I NSGCT and lymphovascular invasion, who are otherwise at a high risk of recurrence (~50%).[111–113] One cycle of adjuvant chemotherapy significantly reduces the recurrence rate for men with clinical stage I GCTs, both seminoma and nonseminoma.[114–116] This treatment consists of a single injection of carboplatin for patients with pure seminoma and a single cycle of bleomycin, etoposide, and cisplatin (BEP) for patients with NSGCT. The use of adjuvant radiotherapy for stage I seminoma has declined because of an association with second malignant neoplasms later in life. Active surveillance is also acceptable and is standard for clinical stage I GCTs without high-risk features.

The overall survival rate for patients with clinical stage I testicular GCTs is 98% to 99%.[111,112] The survival rate for patients managed with orchiectomy alone (followed by surveillance) is the same as for those receiving adjuvant treatment,[117] but the outcome requires patient compliance and continuous access to healthcare services. Surveillance also entails a greater burden of therapy for the subset of patients who ultimately experience a recurrence.

As with stage I GCTs, patients presenting with metastatic GCTs (stage II or III) also have a high cure rate. As discussed previously, patients can be classified as having a good prognosis, intermediate prognosis, or poor prognosis, according to their clinical features and degree of tumor marker elevation before chemotherapy.[51] These prognostic groups have corresponding long-term survival rates of approximately 85%, 75%, and 45%, respectively. Some of these patients are cured with combination chemotherapy alone, but such cure rates would not be possible without the routine and standard use of combined modality treatment: chemotherapy plus surgical consolidation for NSGCT[118,119] and chemotherapy plus consolidative radiotherapy for seminoma.[120] Surgery is seldom necessary for metastatic sites in pure seminoma because of its exquisite sensitivity to chemotherapy and radiation, and post-chemotherapy surgery is specifically avoided in seminoma, because the residual tissue is densely fibrotic.

Please refer to the MD Anderson practice consensus algorithm on expertconsult.com

Retroperitoneal Lymph Node Dissection

Retroperitoneal lymph node dissection (RPLND) is surgical removal of "landing zone" lymph nodes. Its role in primary prevention of recurrence in patients with clinical stage I NSGCT is controversial.[112,121,122] An advantage of prophylactic RPLND is that it results in excellent local control for teratoma, which is insensitive to chemotherapy or radiotherapy.[122,123] However, the morbidity of RPLND includes sympathetic nerve damage that may lead to retrograde ejaculation and infertility. Use of a modified surgical template is nerve-sparing and potency-preserving in 90% or more of patients.[101,114] Patients who are found to have metastatic GCT in lymph nodes (pathologic stage II) in most cases require two cycles of adjuvant chemotherapy[124]; hence, they are exposed to "double therapy."[125]

Patients with metastatic NSGCT and a residual mass after definitive chemotherapy treatment require post-chemotherapy RPLND.[126] The purpose is severalfold: (1) to detect persistent germ cell malignancy, (2) to prevent malignant transformation of teratoma, and (3) to remove metastatic teratoma and prevent growing teratoma syndrome. Patients who do not undergo RPLND, either in the adjuvant setting or following complete response to chemotherapy, must undergo periodic CT scanning of the abdomen as surveillance for growing teratoma in the retroperitoneum.[112,122]

Growing teratoma syndrome is the development of a mature enlarging teratoma in patients after treatment for an NSGCT. Typically, the serum tumor markers β-hCG and AFP are within normal ranges. The treatment of choice is complete resection, which has a better outcome than radiation and chemotherapy, which are ineffective. A known complication of RPLND is injury to the thoracic duct resulting in chylous ascites.[127] Abdominal ascites detected by CT scan in the immediate postoperative period should prompt suspicion of chylous ascites. This condition is rarely fatal and requires a period of bowel rest with total parenteral alimentation.

Chemotherapy

The standard chemotherapy for NSGCT is BEP.[106] Bleomycin is associated with a risk of pulmonary toxicity.[128,129] Acute and reversible toxicity is common and has the features of pneumonitis.[130] Serious and fatal toxicity has the features of progressive pulmonary fibrosis, for which there is no effective treatment other than a lung transplant. Bleomycin continues to be used because of its valuable contribution to the overall outcome in patients with NSGCT, although this is less true for seminoma. In NSGCT, bleomycin is a highly effective drug that does not have the neurotoxicity and bone marrow suppression of cisplatin. Combining bleomycin with cisplatin (and etoposide) achieves greater antitumor effect with manageable toxicity. It is possible to treat metastatic NSGCT without bleomycin, but then it is necessary to use additional drugs that have their own toxicities or to lengthen the duration of chemotherapy (from three courses of BEP to four courses of etoposide and cisplatin, in the case of good-prognosis NSGCT).[106] The actual risk of serious, life-threatening pulmonary toxicity after three courses of BEP is approximately 1%.[80] Accordingly, this drug is routinely used in the treatment of metastatic GCTs and for adjuvant treatment of clinical stage I NSGCT. For the appearance of pulmonary nodules or infiltrates on a postchemotherapy CT scan, bleomycin toxicity should be included in the differential diagnosis. The risk of bleomycin toxicity increases with age, smoking, preexisting lung disease, and cumulative dose of drug received.

KEY POINTS

Chemotherapy Treatment for Testicular Germ Cell Tumors

Adjuvant Chemotherapy for High-risk Clinical Stage I Testicular Cancer

- Seminoma: Carboplatin (one dose); alternative is radiotherapy.
- Nonseminomatous germ cell tumors (NSGCTs): bleomycin, etoposide, and platinum (BEP), one or two courses.

Treatment of Stage II or III Metastatic Germ Cell Tumors

- Seminoma: BEP or etoposide and cisplatin for bulky disease or recurrence after adjuvant treatment.
- Primary radiotherapy is standard for stage IIA (small-volume) seminoma.
- NSGCTs: BEP (three or four courses).

SURVEILLANCE

Monitoring Tumor Response

Patients receiving first- or second-line chemotherapy for metastatic GCTs almost always show significant tumor shrinkage.[131,132] The notable exception is teratoma, which can appear to be stable or to enlarge despite chemotherapy.[133] The small percentage of patients who go on to experience a recurrence of chemotherapy-refractory disease can actually show progression of germ cell malignancy during chemotherapy, usually accompanied by an increase in serum tumor markers.

For patients with stage II or III NSGCT undergoing initial chemotherapy, the first follow-up scan is routinely done after the second or third cycle. The finding of tumor shrinkage on this CT scan is confirmatory because it is expected to occur, and, in most cases, it is already reflected in the declining concentration of serum tumor markers (β-hCG and AFP). The presence or absence of a residual mass (partial response or complete response) in the retroperitoneum, lungs, or any other metastatic site at this timepoint helps the medical oncologist and surgeon begin planning for postchemotherapy surgery. The second follow-up scan is done after the completion of chemotherapy, in most cases, where the total duration of chemotherapy is three or four courses, and this scan confirms whether there is a residual mass in the retroperitoneum (or elsewhere). Patients with seminoma and bulky metastases also show a brisk response to chemotherapy, but a residual mass is common.[120] Radiotherapy for consolidation is done only in selected patients and is usually reserved for those with a residual mass greater than 3 cm.[106] Smaller masses can be observed, and the vast majority of these represent scar tissue. Some investigators recommend PET/CT in such cases to determine whether viable tumor is still present.

KEY POINTS

Surveillance

- Recommended frequency of follow-up imaging decreases with time elapsed since the completion of treatment.
- Minimum duration of follow-up is 5 years for nonseminomatous germ cell tumors (NSGCTs) and 10 years for seminoma.
- Continued annual or every-2-year surveillance is recommended indefinitely for detection of late recurrences, growing teratoma, second primary malignancies, and other late effects of treatment.
- Imaging tests for seminoma
  - Computed tomography (CT) scan of abdomen: For detection of retroperitoneal lymph node (landing zone) metastases. It is not necessary for patients who have undergone radiotherapy.
  - CT scan of pelvis: For detection of pelvic lymph node metastases. It is important for patients who have undergone radiotherapy, because they remain at risk of recurrence in pelvic lymph nodes (below the field of radiation).
  - Chest x-ray: For detection of hematogenous (lung) metastases.
- Imaging tests for NSGCTs
  - CT scan of abdomen: For detection of retroperitoneal lymph node (landing zone) metastases. A baseline postoperative study is sufficient for patients who have undergone retroperitoneal lymph node dissection (RPLND). Patients who have undergone chemotherapy (adjuvant or treatment) without RPLND must have continued CT surveillance for teratoma.
  - CT scan of pelvis: Not strictly required, but will detect progression in lymph nodes of the lower retroperitoneum in some cases.
  - Chest x-ray: For detection of hematogenous (lung) metastases.

Detection of Recurrence

The majority of patients with metastatic GCTs who undergo treatment are eventually rendered free of disease. For patients with stage II or III disease, the probability of recurrence can be estimated using the clinical features at presentation and the IGCCC system (see Table 21.3).[51] Most NSGCT recurrences are detected within 2 to 3 years, and those that are detected more than 2 years after chemotherapy are called late relapse and carry a worse prognosis for salvage.[134] Seminoma recurrences can occur up to 10 years after treatment and have similar response to treatment regardless of the time interval.[106,112,114,135]

Follow-up CT scans are very important for patients with stage II or III seminoma treated with chemotherapy because (1) there is often a residual mass, (2) they do not always receive postchemotherapy radiation or surgery, and (3) recurrences are not usually accompanied by elevated serum tumor markers, as they often are in NSGCT. Conversely, patients with stage II seminoma treated with radiotherapy to the retroperitoneum as the primary treatment have almost no risk of recurrence in the treated field. For these patients, the chest x-ray is especially important for detecting pulmonary recurrence and CT scan of the pelvis for detection of pelvic lymphadenopathy (below the treatment field).[114]

Complications of Therapy

As noted previously, seminoma does not recur in the radiated field. There is a risk of second malignancy, however, which can be seen more than 25 years after treatment.[136] In a long-term follow-up study of 2707 testicular cancer survivors, the most common second malignancies were stomach, pancreas, urinary bladder, and kidney; the risk was greatest when both radiotherapy and chemotherapy had been given.[136]

Chemotherapy has a number of long-term risks that are unlikely to show radiographic manifestations. These include cardiovascular disease, infertility, treatment-related leukemia, neurotoxicity, ototoxicity, Reynaud phenomenon, and nephrotoxicity.[112] Bleomycin-induced lung injury can produce radiographic findings, as noted previously.[130] Bleomycin is more commonly used for NSGCT, but published guidelines do include BEP as a treatment for advanced seminoma.[106] In addition, clinical stage I NSGCT patients are increasingly regarded as candidates for BEP chemotherapy, so the radiologist should be aware that any patient with a diagnosis of testicular GCT could potentially have received bleomycin.[113,115,116]

Complications of RPLND include chylous ascites, as noted previously.[127] In addition, hydronephrosis can occur on the basis of surgical injury to the ureter or postoperative retroperitoneal fibrosis, and requires the placement of a ureteral stent. Occasional patients have the ipsilateral kidney resected at the time of RPLND owing to encasement of the kidney or ureter by fibrosis, necrotic tumor, or teratoma.

Key Points

Complications of Treatment

Direct Effects

- Bleomycin: Pulmonary toxicity, Reynaud phenomenon.
- Etoposide: Treatment-induced leukemia.
- Cisplatin: Nephrotoxicity, ototoxicity, peripheral neuropathy.

Long-Term Effects of Chemotherapy and Radiotherapy

- Increased risk of cardiovascular disease.
- Increased frequency of second malignancies.
- Infertility.

NEW THERAPIES

There is not yet a consensus on the question of surveillance versus adjuvant chemotherapy for patients with clinical stage I GCTs at highest risk of recurrence. Adjuvant treatment does mean that some patients are treated unnecessarily, and their corresponding life expectancy would be just as good with surveillance and treatment at the time of recurrence.[113,135] The use of adjuvant radiotherapy for clinical stage I seminoma has already declined, however, owing to the rising acceptance of surveillance as an option and also the availability of adjuvant carboplatin as an alternative. Consequently, there will be a greater need for abdominal CT in patients with seminoma. Those who are on surveillance remain at risk for retroperitoneal recurrence, and the risk continues for 10 years. Patients who have received adjuvant carboplatin have a less than 5% risk of recurrence, but, unlike in patients treated with radiotherapy, tumors can still recur in the retroperitoneum.

High-dose chemotherapy and autologous stem cell transplantation (HDC-SCT) has been studied as a definitive treatment for advanced metastatic GCTs. A phase III study of HDC-SCT versus the standard four courses of BEP in patients with poor- or intermediate-prognosis GCTs showed no significant difference in overall survival, so HDC-SCT is currently used only in the salvage setting.[137] A retrospective study from Indiana University suggested that HDC-SCT can be curative as second- or third-line therapy in selected poor-risk patients, but its optimal role still remains controversial.[138]

CONCLUSION

Testicular tumors that are predominantly germ cell in origin tend to have an excellent long-term prognosis, because the majority can be curable, depending on their tumor type. Radiologic imaging continues to play a vital role in the diagnosis, treatment, and surveillance of these tumors. Although a vast amount is known about this tumor, much remains to be learned about its imaging and treatment, with ongoing investigational studies.

REFERENCES

1. Jemal A, Siegel R, Ward E, et al. Cancer statistics, 2009. *CA Cancer J Clin*. 2009;59:225–249.
2. Choyke PL, Hayes WS, Sesterhenn IA. Primary extragonadal germ cell tumors of the retroperitoneum: differentiation of primary and secondary tumors. *Radiographics*. 1993;13:1365–1375. quiz 1377–1378.
3. Schmoll HJ. Extragonadal germ cell tumors. *Ann Oncol*. 2002;13(Suppl 4):265–272.
4. Carver BS, Serio AM, Bajorin D, et al. Improved clinical outcome in recent years for men with metastatic nonseminomatous germ cell tumors. *J Clin Oncol*. 2007;25:5603–5608.
5. Hayes-Lattin B, Nichols CR. Testicular cancer: a prototypic tumor of young adults. *Semin Oncol*. 2009;36:432–438.
6. Cooper DE, L'Esperance JO, Christman MS, Auge BK. Testis cancer: a 20-year epidemiological review of the experience at a regional military medical facility. *J Urol*. 2008;180:577–581. discussion 581–582.

7. Bray F, Richiardi L, Ekbom A, et al. Trends in testicular cancer incidence and mortality in 22 European countries: continuing increases in incidence and declines in mortality. *Int J Cancer.* 2006;118:3099–3111.
8. Manecksha RP, Fitzpatrick JM. Epidemiology of testicular cancer. *BJU Int.* 2009;104:1329–1333.
9. Huyghe E, Matsuda T, Thonneau P. Increasing incidence of testicular cancer worldwide: a review. *J Urol.* 2003;170:5–11.
10. Tabernero J, Paz-Ares L, Salazar R, et al. Incidence of contralateral germ cell testicular tumors in South Europe: report of the experience at 2 Spanish university hospitals and review of the literature. *J Urol.* 2004;171:164–167.
11. Sonneveld DJ, Schraffordt Koops H, Sleijfer DT, et al. Bilateral testicular germ cell tumours in patients with initial stage I disease: prevalence and prognosis—a single centre's 30 years' experience. *Eur J Cancer.* 1998;34:1363–1367.
12. Gajendran VK, Nguyen M, Ellison LM. Testicular cancer patterns in African-American men. *Urology.* 2005;66:602–605.
13. Husband JE, Kow DM. Testicular germ cell tumors. In: Husband JE, Reznek R, eds. *Imaging in Oncology*. London: Taylor and Francis; 2004:401–427.
14. McGlynn KA, Cook MB. Etiologic factors in testicular germ-cell tumors. *Future Oncol.* 2009;5:1389–1402.
15. van Echten J, Oosterhuis JW, Looijenga LH, et al. No recurrent structural abnormalities apart from i(12p) in primary germ cell tumors of the adult testis. *Genes Chromosomes Cancer.* 1995;14:133–144.
16. Bosl GJ, Ilson DH, Rodriguez E, et al. Clinical relevance of the i(12p) marker chromosome in germ cell tumors. *J Natl Cancer Inst.* 1994;86:349–355.
17. Chieffi P, Franco R, Portella G. Molecular and cell biology of testicular germ cell tumors. *Int Rev Cell Mol Biol.* 2009;278:277–308.
18. Hoei-Hansen CE, Rajpert-De Meyts E, Daugaard G, Skakkebaek NE. Carcinoma in situ testis, the progenitor of testicular germ cell tumours: a clinical review. *Ann Oncol.* 2005;16:863–868.
19. La Vignera S, Calogero AE, Condorelli R, et al. Cryptorchidism and its long-term complications. *Eur Rev Med Pharmacol Sci.* 2009;13:351–356.
20. Giwercman A, Bruun E, Frimodt-Moller C, et al. Prevalence of carcinoma in situ and other histopathological abnormalities in testes of men with a history of cryptorchidism. *J Urol.* 1989;142:998–1001. discussion 1001-1002.
21. Korde LA, Premkumar A, Mueller C, et al. Increased prevalence of testicular microlithiasis in men with familial testicular cancer and their relatives. *Br J Cancer.* 2008;99:1748–1753.
22. Hemminki K, Li X. Familial risk in testicular cancer as a clue to a heritable and environmental aetiology. *Br J Cancer.* 2004;90:1765–1770.
23. Hentrich MU, Brack NG, Schmid P, et al. Testicular germ cell tumors in patients with human immunodeficiency virus infection. *Cancer.* 1996;77:2109–2116.
24. Dieckmann KP, Hartmann JT, Classen J, et al. Is increased body mass index associated with the incidence of testicular germ cell cancer? *J Cancer Res Clin Oncol.* 2009;135:731–738.
25. Fritzsche PJ, Wilbur MJ. The male pelvis. *Semin Ultrasound CT MR.* 1989;10:11–28.
26. Banson ML. Normal MR anatomy and techniques for imaging of the male pelvis. *Magn Reson Imaging Clin North Am.* 1996;4:481–496.
27. Schnall M. Magnetic resonance imaging of the scrotum. *Semin Roentgenol.* 1993;28:19–30.
28. McCarrey JR. Development of the germ cell. In: Desjardins C, Ewing E, eds. *Cell and Molecular Biology of the Testis*. New York: Oxford University Press; 1993:58–89.
29. Skakkebaek NE, Berthelsen JG, Giwercman A, Muller J. Carcinoma-in-situ of the testis: possible origin from gonocytes and precursor of all types of germ cell tumours except spermatocytoma. *Int J Androl.* 1987;10:19–28.
30. Wicha MS, Liu S, Dontu G. Cancer stem cells: an old idea–a paradigm shift. *Cancer Res.* 2006;66:1883–1890. discussion 1895–1896.
31. Urogenital systemMoore K, ed. *The Developing Human*. Philadelphia: WB Saunders; 1998:287–328.
32. Johnson JO, Mattrey RF, Phillipson J. Differentiation of seminomatous from nonseminomatous testicular tumors with MR imaging. *AJR Am J Roentgenol.* 1990;154:539–543.
33. Tumors of germ cell origin. In: Mostofi FK, Price EB, eds. *Atlas of Tumor Pathology: Tumors of the Male Genital System*. Vol. 8. Washington, DC: Armed Forces Institute of Pathology; 1973.
34. Ueno T, Tanaka YO, Nagata M, et al. Spectrum of germ cell tumors: from head to toe. *Radiographics.* 2004;24:387–404.
35. Ulbricht TM. Testicular and paratesticular tumors. In: Carter D, Greenson JK, eds. *Sternberg's Diagnostic Surgical Pathology*. Philadelphia: Lippincott Williams & Williams; 2004:2132–2167.
36. Ulbright TM. Germ cell tumors of the gonads: a selective review emphasizing problems in differential diagnosis, newly appreciated, and controversial issues. *Mod Pathol.* 2005;18(Suppl 2):S61–S79.
37. Bahrami A, Ro JY, Ayala AG. An overview of testicular germ cell tumors. *Arch Pathol Lab Med.* 2007;131:1267–1280.
38. Sohaib SA, Husband J. Surveillance in testicular cancer: who, when, what and how? *Cancer Imaging.* 72007145–147.
39. Theaker JM, Mead GM. Diagnostic pitfalls in the histopathological diagnosis of testicular germ cell tumours. *Curr Diagn Pathol.* 2004;10:220–228.
40. von Eyben FE. Laboratory markers and germ cell tumors. *Crit Rev Clin Lab Sci.* 2003;40:377–427.
41. Mason MD. Tumour markers. In: Horwich A, ed. *Testicular Cancer: Investigation and Management*. London: Chapman and Hall; 1996:33–43.
42. Carver BS, Sheinfeld J. Germ cell tumors of the testis. *Ann Surg Oncol.* 2005;12:871–880.
43. Guthrie JA, Fowler RC. Ultrasound diagnosis of testicular tumours presenting as epididymal disease. *Clin Radiol.* 1992;46:397–400.
44. Hilton S. Contemporary radiological imaging of testicular cancer. *BJU Int.* 2009;104:1339–1345.
45. Sohaib SA, Koh DM, Husband JE. The role of imaging in the diagnosis, staging, and management of testicular cancer. *AJR Am J Roentgenol.* 2008;191:387–395.
46. McMahon CJ, Rofsky NM, Pedrosa I. Lymphatic metastases from pelvic tumors: anatomic classification, characterization, and staging. *Radiology.* 2010;254:31–46.
47. Dixon AK, Ellis M, Sikora K. Computed tomography of testicular tumours: distribution of abdominal lymphadenopathy. *Clin Radiol.* 1986;37:519–523.
48. Williams MP, Cook JV, Duchesne GM. Psoas nodes—an overlooked site of metastasis from testicular tumours. *Clin Radiol.* 1989;40:607–609.
49. Husband JE, Bellamy EA. Unusual thoracoabdominal sites of metastases in testicular tumors. *AJR Am J Roentgenol.* 1985; 145:1165–1171.
50. Edge SB, Byrd DR, Compton CC, eds. *AJCC Cancer Staging Manual*. New York: Springer; 2010.
51. International Germ Cell Cancer Collaborative Group International Germ Cell Consensus Classification: a prognostic factor-based staging system for metastatic germ cell cancers. *J Clin Oncol.* 1997;15:594–603.
52. Dalal PU, Sohaib SA, Huddart R. Imaging of testicular germ cell tumours. *Cancer Imaging.* 2006;6:124–134.
53. Bokemeyer C, Nowak P, Haupt A, et al. Treatment of brain metastases in patients with testicular cancer. *J Clin Oncol.* 1997;15: 1449–1454.
54. Bajorin D, Katz A, Chan E, et al. Comparison of criteria for assigning germ cell tumor patients to "good risk" and "poor risk" studies. *J Clin Oncol.* 1988;6:786–792.
55. Huddart R, Kataja V. Mixed or non-seminomatous germ-cell tumors: ESMO clinical recommendations for diagnosis, treatment and follow-up. *Ann Oncol.* 2008;19(Suppl 2):ii52–ii54.
56. Coakley FV, Hricak H, Presti Jr JC. Imaging and management of atypical testicular masses. *Urol Clin North Am.* 1998;25:375–388.
57. Horstman WG, Melson GL, Middleton WD, et al. Testicular tumors: findings with color Doppler US. *Radiology.* 1992;185:733–737.
58. Meissner A, Mamoulakis C, de la Rosette JJ, Pes MP. Clinical update on testicular microlithiasis. *Curr Opin Urol.* 2009;19:615–618.
59. Yagci C, Ozcan H, Aytac S, et al. Testicular microlithiasis associated with seminoma: gray-scale and color Doppler ultrasound findings. *Urol Int.* 1996;57:255–258.
60. Miller FN, Sidhu PS. Does testicular microlithiasis matter? A review. *Clin Radiol.* 2002;57:883–890.
61. Coffey J, Huddart RA, Elliott F, et al. Testicular microlithiasis as a familial risk factor for testicular germ cell tumour. *Br J Cancer.* 2007;97:1701–1706.
62. Serter S, Gumus B, Unlu M, et al. Prevalence of testicular microlithiasis in an asymptomatic population. *Scand J Urol Nephrol.* 2006;40:212–214.

63. Peterson AC, Bauman JM, Light DE, et al. The prevalence of testicular microlithiasis in an asymptomatic population of men 18 to 35 years old. *J Urol*. 2001;166:2061–2064.
64. Bach AM, Hann LE, Hadar O, et al. Testicular microlithiasis: what is its association with testicular cancer? *Radiology*. 2001;220:70–75.
65. Dieckmann KP, Skakkebaek NE. Carcinoma in situ of the testis: review of biological and clinical features. *Int J Cancer*. 1999;83:815–822.
66. Krege S, Beyer J, Souchon R, et al. European consensus conference on diagnosis and treatment of germ cell cancer: a report of the second meeting of the European Germ Cell Cancer Consensus group (EGCCCG): part I. *Eur Urol*. 2008;53:478–496.
67. Elzinga-Tinke JE, Sirre ME, Looijenga LH, et al. The predictive value of testicular ultrasound abnormalities for carcinoma in situ of the testis in men at risk for testicular cancer. *Int J Androl*. 2010;33:597–603.
68. DeCastro BJ, Peterson AC, Costabile RA. A 5-year follow-up study of asymptomatic men with testicular microlithiasis. *J Urol*. 2008;179:1420–1423. discussion 1423.
69. Slaughenhoupt B, Kadlec A, Schrepferman C. Testicular microlithiasis preceding metastatic mixed germ cell tumor—first pediatric report and recommended management of testicular microlithiasis in the pediatric population. *Urology*. 2009;73:1029–1031.
70. Albrecht W. Words of wisdom. Re: a 5-year follow-up study of asymptomatic men with testicular microlithiasis. *Eur Urol*. 2008;54:1199.
71. Fernandez EB, Moul JW, Foley JP, et al. Retroperitoneal imaging with third and fourth generation computed axial tomography in clinical stage I nonseminomatous germ cell tumors. *Urology*. 1994;44:548–552.
72. Schmoll HJ, Souchon R, Krege S, et al. European consensus on diagnosis and treatment of germ cell cancer: a report of the European Germ Cell Cancer Consensus Group (EGCCCG). *Ann Oncol*. 2004;15:1377–1399.
73. Ozan E, Oztekin O, Kozacioglu Z, et al. Metastatic testicular germ cell tumor presenting with abdominal pain: CT and MRI findings. *JBR-BTR*. 2009;92:256–258.
74. Freedman LS, Parkinson MC, Jones WG, et al. Histopathology in the prediction of relapse of patients with stage I testicular teratoma treated by orchidectomy alone. *Lancet*. 1987;2:294–298.
75. Dorfman RE, Alpern MB, Gross BH, et al. Upper abdominal lymph nodes: criteria for normal size determined with CT. *Radiology*. 1991;180:319–322.
76. Mason MD, Featherstone T, Olliff J, et al. Inguinal and iliac lymph node involvement in germ cell tumours of the testis: implications for radiological investigation and for therapy. *Clin Oncol (R Coll Radiol)*. 1991;3:147–150.
77. White PM, Howard GC, Best JJ, et al. The role of computed tomographic examination of the pelvis in the management of testicular germ cell tumours. *Clin Radiol*. 1997;52:124–129.
78. Williams MP, Husband JE, Heron CW. Intrathoracic manifestations of metastatic testicular seminoma: a comparison of chest radiographic and CT findings. *AJR Am J Roentgenol*. 1987;149:473–475.
79. Wood A, Robson N, Tung K, et al. Patterns of supradiaphragmatic metastases in testicular germ cell tumours. *Clin Radiol*. 1996;51:273–276.
80. O'Sullivan JM, et al. Predicting the risk of bleomycin lung toxicity in patients with germ-cell tumours. *Ann Oncol*. 2003;14(1):91–96.
81. Steinfeld AD. Testicular germ cell tumors: review of contemporary evaluation and management. *Radiology*. 1990;175:603–606.
82. Daffner RH, Lupetin AR, Dash N, et al. MRI in the detection of malignant infiltration of bone marrow. *AJR Am J Roentgenol*. 1986;146:353–358.
83. Ng CS, Husband JE, Padhani AR, et al. Evaluation by magnetic resonance imaging of the inferior vena cava in patients with non-seminomatous germ cell tumours of the testis metastatic to the retroperitoneum. *Br J Urol*. 1997;79:942–951.
84. Arnold PM, Morgan CJ, Morantz RA, et al. Metastatic testicular cancer presenting as spinal cord compression: report of two cases. *Surg Neurol*. 2000;54:27–33.
85. Sohaib SA, Koh DM, Barbachano Y, et al. Prospective assessment of MRI for imaging retroperitoneal metastases from testicular germ cell tumours. *Clin Radiol*. 2009;64:362–367.
85a. Johnathan K Joffe, Fay Helen Cafferty, Laura Murphy, et al. *Journal of Clinical Oncology*. 2021;39:6_suppl:374–374.
86. Harisinghani MG, Saini S, Weissleder R, et al. MR lymphangiography using ultrasmall superparamagnetic iron oxide in patients with primary abdominal and pelvic malignancies: radiographic-pathologic correlation. *AJR Am J Roentgenol*. 1999;172:1347–1351.
87. Pandharipande PV, Mora JT, Uppot RN, et al. Lymphotropic nanoparticle-enhanced MRI for independent prediction of lymph node malignancy: a logistic regression model. *AJR Am J Roentgenol*. 2009;193:W230–W237.
88. Harisinghani MG, Saksena M, Ross RW, et al. A pilot study of lymphotrophic nanoparticle-enhanced magnetic resonance imaging technique in early stage testicular cancer: a new method for noninvasive lymph node evaluation. *Urology*. 2005;66:1066–1071.
89. Alibek S, Cavallaro A, Aplas A, et al. Diffusion weighted imaging of pediatric and adolescent malignancies with regard to detection and delineation: initial experience. *Acad Radiol*. 2009;16:866–871.
90. Manganaro L, et al. Dynamic contrast-enhanced and diffusion-weighted MR imaging in the characterisation of small, non-palpable solid testicular tumours. *Eur Radiol*. 2018;28(2):554–564.
91. Tsili AC, Ntorkou A, Astrakas L, Boukali E, Giannakis D, Maliakas V, Sofikitis N, Argyropoulou MI. Magnetic resonance diffusion tensor imaging of the testis: Preliminary observations. *Eur J Radiol*. 2017;95:265–270. http://dx.doi.org/10.1016/j.ejrad.2017.08.037. Epub 2017 Aug 31. PMID: 28987678.
92. Algebally AM, Tantawy HI, Yousef RR, Szmigielski W, Darweesh A. Advantage of adding diffusion weighted imaging to routine mri examinations in the diagnostics of scrotal lesions. *Pol J Radiol*. 2015;80:442–449. http://dx.doi.org/10.12659/pjr.894399.
93. Imane El Sanharawi, Jean-Michel Correas, Ludivine Glas, Sophie Ferlicot, Vincent Izard, Béatrice Ducot, Marie-France Bellin, Gérard Benoît, Laurence Rocher. Non-palpable incidentally found testicular tumors: Differentiation between benign, malignant, and burned-out tumors using dynamic contrast-enhanced MRI. *Eur J Radiol*. 2016;85(11):2072–2082.
94. Schultz-Lampel D, Bogaert G, Thuroff JW, Schlegel E, Cramer B. MRI for evaluation of scrotal pathology. *Urol Res*. 1991;19:289–292. http://dx.doi.org/10.1007/BF00299060. PMID: 1659016.
95. Rholl KS, Lee JK, Ling D, et al. MR imaging of the scrotum with a high-resolution surface coil. *Radiology*. 1987;163:99–103.
96. Seidenwurm D, Smathers RL, Lo RK, et al. Testes and scrotum: MR imaging at 1.5 T. *Radiology*. 1987;164:393–398.
97. Tsili AC, Tsampoulas C, Giannakopoulos X, et al. MRI in the histologic characterization of testicular neoplasms. *AJR Am J Roentgenol*. 2007;189:W331–W337.
98. DeSantis M, Becherer A, Bokemeyer C, Stoiber F, Oechsle K, Sellner F, et al. 2-18fluoro-deoxy-D-glucose positron emission tomography is a reliable predictor for viable tumor in postchemotherapy seminoma: an update of the prospective multicentric SEMPET trial. *J Clin Oncol*. 2004;22(6):1034–1039.
99. Basu S, Rubello D. PET imaging in the management of tumors of testis and ovary: current thinking and future directions. *Minerva Endocrinol*. 2008;33:229–256.
100. Cremerius U, Effert PJ, Adam G, et al. FDG PET for detection and therapy control of metastatic germ cell tumor. *J Nucl Med*. 1998;39:815–822.
101. Becherer A, De Santis M, Karanikas G, et al. FDG PET is superior to CT in the prediction of viable tumour in post-chemotherapy seminoma residuals. *Eur J Radiol*. 2005;54(2):284–288.
102. Oechsle K, Hartmann M, Brenner W, et al. [18F]Fluorodeoxyglucose positron emission tomography in nonseminomatous germ cell tumors after chemotherapy: the German multicenter positron emission tomography study group. *J Clin Oncol*. 2008;26:5930–5935.
103. Hartmann JT, Schmoll HJ, Kuczyk MA, et al. Postchemotherapy resections of residual masses from metastatic non-seminomatous testicular germ cell tumors. *Ann Oncol*. 1997;8:531–538.
104. Ganjoo KN, Chan RJ, Sharma M, et al. Positron emission tomography scans in the evaluation of postchemotherapy residual masses in patients with seminoma. *J Clin Oncol*. 1999;17:3457–3460.
105. Lewis DA, Tann M, Kesler K, et al. Positron emission tomography scans in postchemotherapy seminoma patients with residual masses: a retrospective review from Indiana University Hospital. *J Clin Oncol*. 2006;24:e54–e55.
106. Motzer RJ, Agarwal N, Beard C, et al. NCCN clinical practice guidelines in oncology: testicular cancer. *J Natl Compr Canc Netw*. 2009;7:672–693.

107. Hain SF, Maisey MN. Positron emission tomography for urological tumours. *BJU Int*. 2003;92:159–164.
108. Huddart RA, O'Doherty MJ, Padhani A, et al. 18Fluorodeoxyglucose positron emission tomography in the prediction of relapse in patients with high-risk, clinical stage I nonseminomatous germ cell tumors: preliminary report of MRC Trial TE22—the NCRI Testis Tumour Clinical Study Group. *J Clin Oncol*. 2007;25:3090–3095.
109. de Wit M, Brenner W, Hartmann M, et al. [18F]-FDG-PET in clinical stage I/II non-seminomatous germ cell tumours: results of the German multicentre trial. *Ann Oncol*. 2008;19:1619–1623.
110. Braga FJ, Arbex MA, Haddad J, Maes A. Bone scintigraphy in testicular tumors. *Clin Nucl Med*. 2001;26:117–118.
111. Swanson DA. Two courses of chemotherapy after orchidectomy for high-risk clinical stage I nonseminomatous testicular tumours. *BJU Int*. 2005;95:477–478.
112. de Wit R, Fizazi K. Controversies in the management of clinical stage I testis cancer. *J Clin Oncol*. 2006;24:5482–5492.
113. Tandstad T, Dahl O, Cohn-Cedermark G, et al. Risk-adapted treatment in clinical stage I nonseminomatous germ cell testicular cancer: the SWENOTECA management program. *J Clin Oncol*. 2009;27:2122–2128.
114. Oliver RT, Mason MD, Mead GM, et al. Radiotherapy versus single-dose carboplatin in adjuvant treatment of stage I seminoma: a randomised trial. *Lancet*. 2005;366:293–300.
115. Westermann DH, Schefer H, Thalmann GN, et al. Long-term follow-up results of 1 cycle of adjuvant bleomycin, etoposide and cisplatin chemotherapy for high risk clinical stage I nonseminomatous germ cell tumors of the testis. *J Urol*. 2008;179:163–166.
116. Albers P, Siener R, Krege S, et al. Randomized phase III trial comparing retroperitoneal lymph node dissection with one course of bleomycin and etoposide plus cisplatin chemotherapy in the adjuvant treatment of clinical stage I nonseminomatous testicular germ cell tumors: AUO trial AH 01/94 by the German Testicular Cancer Study Group. *J Clin Oncol*. 2008;26:2966–2972.
117. Bohlen D, Borner M, Sonntag RW, et al. Long-term results following adjuvant chemotherapy in patients with clinical stage I testicular nonseminomatous malignant germ cell tumors with high risk factors. *J Urol*. 1999;161:1148–1152.
118. Spiess PE, Brown GA, Liu P, et al. Recurrence pattern and proposed surveillance protocol following post-chemotherapy retroperitoneal lymph node dissection. *J Urol*. 2007;177:131–138.
119. Spiess PE, Brown GA, Liu P, et al. Predictors of outcome in patients undergoing postchemotherapy retroperitoneal lymph node dissection for testicular cancer. *Cancer*. 2006;107:1483–1490.
120. Loehrer Sr PJ, Birch R, Williams SD, et al. Chemotherapy of metastatic seminoma: the Southeastern Cancer Study Group experience. *J Clin Oncol*. 1987;5:1212–1220.
121. Donohue JP, Foster RS, Rowland RG, et al. Nerve-sparing retroperitoneal lymphadenectomy with preservation of ejaculation. *J Urol*. 1990;144:287–291. discussion 291-292.
122. Stephenson AJ, Bosl GJ, Bajorin DF, et al. Retroperitoneal lymph node dissection in patients with low stage testicular cancer with embryonal carcinoma predominance and/or lymphovascular invasion. *J Urol*. 2005;174:557–560. discussion 560.
123. Spiess PE, Kassouf W, Brown GA, et al. Surgical management of growing teratoma syndrome: the M. D. Anderson cancer center experience. *J Urol*. 2007;177:1330–1334. discussion 1334.
124. Williams SD, Stablein DM, Einhorn LH, et al. Immediate adjuvant chemotherapy versus observation with treatment at relapse in pathological stage II testicular cancer. *N Engl J Med*. 1987;317(23):1433–1438.
125. Al-Tourah AJ, Murray N, Coppin C, et al. Minimizing treatment without compromising cure with primary surveillance for clinical stage I embryonal predominant nonseminomatous testicular cancer: a population based analysis from British Columbia. *J Urol*. 2005;174:2209–2213. discussion 2213.
126. Spiess PE, Brown GA, Pisters LL, et al. Viable malignant germ cell tumor in the postchemotherapy retroperitoneal lymph node dissection specimen: can it be predicted using clinical parameters? *Cancer*. 2006;107:1503–1510.
127. Evans JG, Spiess PE, Kamat AM, et al. Chylous ascites after postchemotherapy retroperitoneal lymph node dissection: review of the M. D. Anderson experience. *J Urol*. 2006;176:1463–1467.
128. Yagoda A, Mukherji B, Young C, et al. Bleomycin, an antitumor antibiotic. Clinical experience in 274 patients. *Ann Intern Med*. 1972;77:861–870.
129. Kawai K, Akaza H. Bleomycin-induced pulmonary toxicity in chemotherapy for testicular cancer. *Expert Opin Drug Saf*. 2003;2:587–596.
130. Sleijfer S. Bleomycin-induced pneumonitis. *Chest*. 2001;120:617–624.
131. Kondagunta GV, Bacik J, Donadio A, et al. Combination of paclitaxel, ifosfamide, and cisplatin is an effective second-line therapy for patients with relapsed testicular germ cell tumors. *J Clin Oncol*. 2005;23:6549–6555.
132. Motzer RJ, Sheinfeld J, Mazumdar M, et al. Paclitaxel, ifosfamide, and cisplatin second-line therapy for patients with relapsed testicular germ cell cancer. *J Clin Oncol*. 2000;18:2413–2418.
133. Logothetis CJ, Samuels ML, Trindade A, et al. The growing teratoma syndrome. *Cancer*. 1982;50:1629–1635.
134. Baniel J, Foster RS, Gonin R, et al. Late relapse of testicular cancer. *J Clin Oncol*. 1995;13:1170–1176.
135. Aparicio J, Germa JR, Garcia del Muro X, et al. Risk-adapted management for patients with clinical stage I seminoma: the Second Spanish Germ Cell Cancer Cooperative Group study. *J Clin Oncol*. 2005;23:8717–8723.
136. van den Belt-Dusebout AW, de Wit R, Gietema JA, et al. Treatment-specific risks of second malignancies and cardiovascular disease in 5-year survivors of testicular cancer. *J Clin Oncol*. 2007;25:4370–4378.
137. Motzer RJ, Nichols CJ, Margolin KA, et al. Phase III randomized trial of conventional-dose chemotherapy with or without high-dose chemotherapy and autologous hematopoietic stem-cell rescue as first-line treatment for patients with poor-prognosis metastatic germ cell tumors. *J Clin Oncol*. 2007;25:247–256.
138. Adra N, Abonour R, Althouse SK, et al. High-dose chemotherapy and autologous peripheral-blood stem-cell transplantation for relapsed metastatic germ cell tumors: The Indiana University experience. *J Clin Oncol*. 2017;35(10):1096–1102.

CHAPTER

22 Primary Adrenal Malignancy

Dhakshinamoorthy Ganeshan, M.D.; Chitra Viswanathan, M.D.; and Tara Sagebiel, M.D.

INTRODUCTION

Adrenal masses are found in 2% to 9% of adults.[1] In patients with a known history of malignancy, incidentally detected adrenal masses may be either benign or metastastic (the incidence of metastasis in this scenario varies from 25% to 72%, depending upon the type of primary tumor).[2]

In patients with no history of malignancy, the vast majority of adrenal masses tend to be benign adenomas, followed by other benign lesions such as myelolipomas, hematomas, cysts, and granulomatous lesions. The primary adrenal neoplasms, adrenal cortical carcinoma (ACC) and malignant pheochromocytoma, are relatively rare cancers discussed separately in this chapter. Both are usually diagnosed at advanced stages of disease and are associated with relatively poor survival rates.

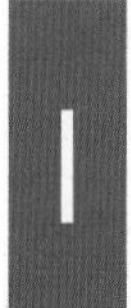

ADRENAL CORTICAL CARCINOMA

EPIDEMIOLOGY AND RISK FACTORS

ACC has a population incidence of 0.5 to 2 per million, with an annual incidence of 0.78 per million.[3–6] The age distribution is bimodal, with the first peak in children before the age of 5 years and a second peak in adults in the fifth to sixth decades. The mean age at diagnosis in adults is approximately 45 years.[7] ACC is more common in female adults than in male adults, with a ratio of 1.5:1, and is slightly more common on the left side.[8] Bilateral tumors are uncommon.

Most cases of ACC are sporadic, with no clear etiology. Smoking and oral contraceptives may be risk factors.[9,10] ACC is associated with complex hereditary syndromes in some patients, including Li–Fraumeni syndrome, Carney complex, Beckwith–Weidmann syndrome, multiple endocrine neoplasia type I, and Gardner syndrome. Sporadic cases are associated with mutations of the tumor suppressor gene *P53*.[11]

ANATOMY AND PATHOLOGY

Anatomy

The adrenal glands are located in the retroperitoneum in the superior aspect of the perirenal space and are bounded by the perirenal fascia. The glands are composed of medial and lateral limbs that converge upon a central ridge. The right adrenal gland is usually the more superiorly located, lying just above the right kidney, posterior to the liver and inferior vena cava (IVC) and lateral to the right diaphragmatic crus. The left gland lies anteromedial to the superior pole of the left kidney, posterior to the pancreatic tail and splenic vessels, and lateral to the left diaphragmatic crus.[12,13]

Arterial supply to the glands is provided by superior, middle, and inferior adrenal arteries. The superior adrenal arteries arise from inferior phrenic arteries, the middle adrenal arteries arise from the aorta, and the inferior adrenal arteries arise from the renal arteries. The right adrenal vein usually drains directly into the IVC, but in 8% to 21% of people it forms a common trunk with an accessory hepatic vein before draining into the IVC.[14,15] The left adrenal vein drains into the left renal vein. Both glands have lymphatic drainage via the retrocrural, upper caval, and aortic lymph nodes.[13]

The adrenals have an outer cortex that accounts for 90% of the volume of the adult adrenal gland. The cortex is derived from the mesoderm and is part of the endocrine system, secreting androgens and the corticosteroids cortisol and aldosterone (Fig. 22.1). ACC arises from the cortex.

> KEY POINTS
>
> **Anatomy of Adrenal Cortical Carcinoma**
> - Paired adrenal glands are retroperitoneal organs.
> - The adrenal glands are supplied by superior, middle, and inferior adrenal arteries.
> - The right adrenal vein can have a variable course.
> - Lymphatic drainage is to the retrocrural, high caval, and paraaortic nodes.

Pathology

On gross pathology, ACC is usually a bulky, coarsely lobulated, yellow to tan tumor with an average weight range of 510 to 1210 g.[16,17] Areas of necrosis and hemorrhage cause a variegated appearance.

ACC is most commonly diagnosed histopathologically using the Weiss criteria. The nine criteria are (1) nuclear grades 3 to 4, (2) mitotic rate greater than five per 50 high-power fields, (3) atypical mitoses, (4) tumors

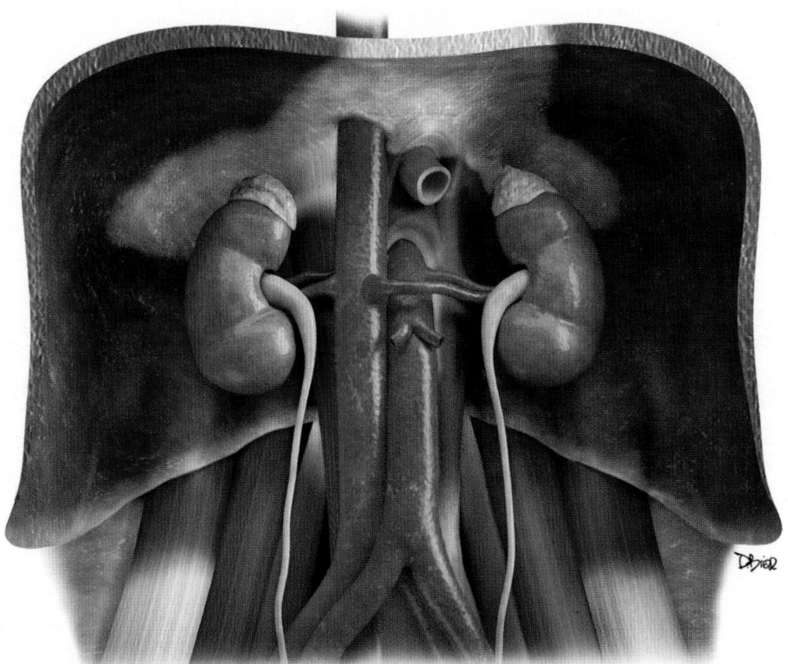

FIGURE 22.1. Anatomy of the adrenal glands.

with 25% or fewer clear cells, (5) diffuse architecture, (6) microscopic necrosis, (7) venous invasion, (8) sinusoidal invasion, and (9) capsular invasion. An adrenal mass is considered malignant if it is positive for three or more of these criteria.[16]

Pathologic features with prognostic significance for ACC include tumor size, the presence of intratumoral hemorrhage, and the number of mitotic figures. Primary tumors larger than 12 cm have a 5-year survival rate of 22% versus 53% for smaller tumors. Intratumoral hemorrhage is a negative prognostic factor compared with tumors without hemorrhage.[18] Patients with a mitotic rate of greater than 20 per 50 high-power fields have a median survival time of 14 months compared with 58 months for mitotic rates lower than 20.[19]

ACCs do not have pathognomonic immunohistochemical findings, although they frequently stain positive for vimentin and negative for cytokeratin. At a molecular level, over 85% of ACCs may demonstrate loss of heterozygosity in 17p13, whereas overexpression of insulin-like growth factor can be seen in 90% of ACCs.[20]

> **KEY POINTS**
>
> **Pathology of Adrenal Cortical Carcinoma**
>
> - Arises from the adrenal cortex.
> - Usually a large tumor with internal hemorrhage and necrosis.
> - Weiss criteria used for histopathologic diagnosis.
> - Large size, internal hemorrhage, and mitotic rate greater than 20 per 50 high-power fields are associated with poorer outcomes.

CLINICAL PRESENTATION

The presenting symptoms of ACC depend on tumor size, the presence of metastases, and functional status. Functional tumors account for 50% to 79% of ACCs, and they can secrete cortisol, estrogens, androgens, or aldosterone. Cortisol hypersecretion is the most common and presents as Cushing syndrome with weight gain, proximal muscle weakness, hyperglycemia, hypertension, and hypokalemia.[21,22] Aldosterone hypersecretion causes hypertension and hypokalemia, but these symptoms are more commonly seen with cortisol excess. Virilization can be seen in women with androgen-secreting tumors, whereas men with estrogen-secreting tumors may develop symptoms of feminization.

Nonfunctional tumors can produce symptoms related to mass effect, including abdominal or back pain, early satiety, nausea, vomiting, and/or a palpable mass. They can also present with fever and weight loss. Nonfunctional tumors tend to present in older patients, with a male predominance.[23] Nonfunctional masses can be discovered incidentally in patients who are undergoing imaging for other reasons. Finally, patients can present with symptoms related to metastatic disease.

> **KEY POINTS**
>
> **Clinical Presentation of Adrenal Cortical Carcinoma**
>
> - The majority of adrenal cortical carcinomas are hormonally functional.
> - Cortisol hypersecretion is most common, producing Cushing syndrome.
> - Nonfunctional tumors are more common in men and can produce symptoms related to mass effect.

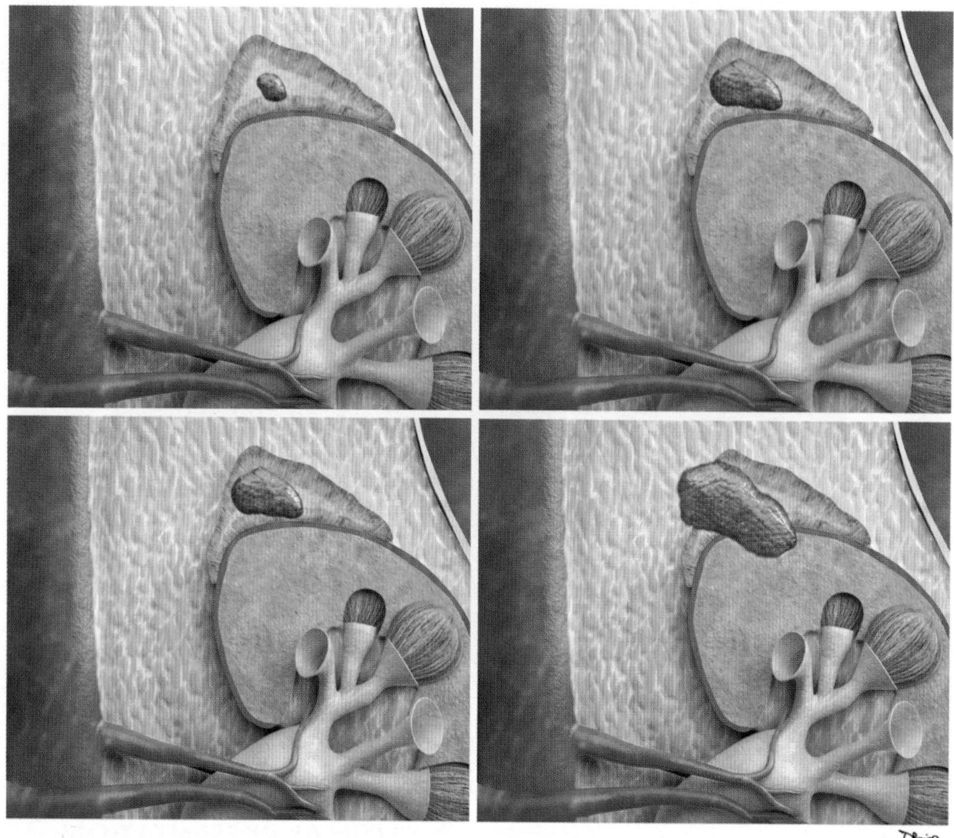

FIGURE 22.2. Staging of adrenocortical carcinoma.

STAGING CLASSIFICATION

The tumor-node-metastasis (TNM) staging system for adrenal tumors was established in 2004 by the Union for International Cancer Control and the World Health Organization.

The TNM classification system is based on the primary tumor size and local invasion (T), regional lymph node involvement (N), and the presence or absence of metastatic disease (M).[24] Table 22.1, Table 22.2 (on p. 366).

Stage I and stage II disease are localized to the adrenal gland. Stage III disease is locally invasive or has regional nodal metastasis. Stage IV disease is locally invasive with regional nodal involvement, invades adjacent organs, or is metastatic (Fig. 22.2).

ACC has a grim survival rate, with a 5-year overall survival rate of only 32% to 48%. This is because approximately 70% of ACCs present at stages III and IV. Stage I and stage II disease have a 5-year survival rate of 62% compared with 7% for stage IV disease.[25]

KEY POINTS

Staging of Adrenal Cortical Carcinoma

- Adrenal cortical carcinoma has poor survival rates because most patients present at advanced stages of disease.
- Stage I, 3% at presentation
- Stage II, 29%
- Stage III, 20%
- Stage IV, 49%

PATTERNS OF TUMOR SPREAD

ACCs can spread by direct extension, first into the surrounding fat and then into adjacent structures such as the liver and kidneys (Fig. 22.3). Tumor thrombus can involve the adrenal and renal veins and IVC (Fig. 22.4). Metastases from hematogenous dissemination most commonly involve the bones, liver, and lungs (Fig. 22.5).[26] ACC also spreads through the lymphatic system to involve the retrocrural, upper caval, and aortic nodes (Fig. 22.6). Simultaneous hematogenous and lymphatic dissemination frequently occurs (Fig. 22.7).

KEY POINTS

Patterns of Tumor Spread of Adrenal Cortical Carcinoma

- Adrenal cortical carcinoma can directly invade adjacent organs.
- Regional nodal metastases involve the upper paraaortic, caval, and retrocrural nodes.
- Distant metastases involve the lungs, liver, and bones.

IMAGING

Tumor

Computed Tomography

Computed tomography (CT) is commonly used for evaluation of adrenal masses. Malignant adrenal masses need to be differentiated from benign lesions.[27,28] The presence of

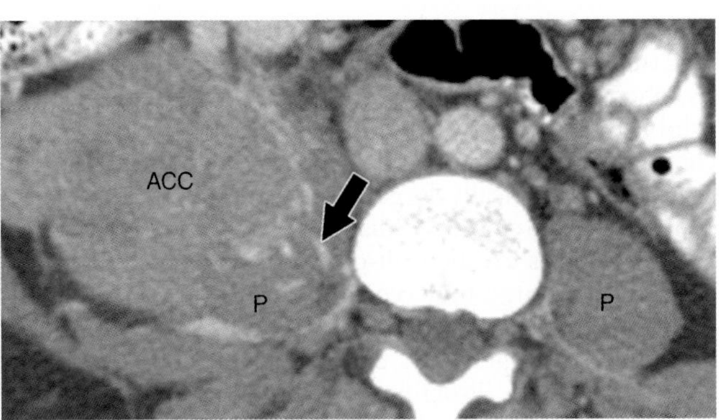

Figure 22.3. A 39-year-old man with a right adrenal cortical carcinoma (*ACC*) with direct extension (*arrow*) into the right psoas muscle (*P*).

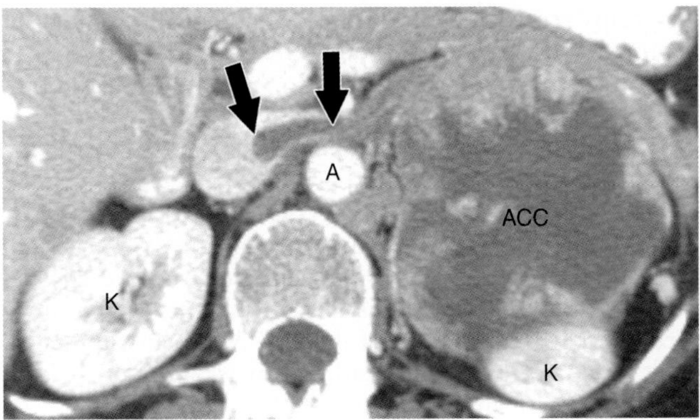

Figure 22.4. A 38-year-old man with a left adrenal cortical carcinoma (*ACC*) with tumor extension into the left renal vein and inferior vena cava (IVC). Axial contrast-enhanced computed tomography scan shows the left ACC with tumor thrombus in the left renal vein and IVC (*arrows*). *A*, Aorta; *K*, kidney.

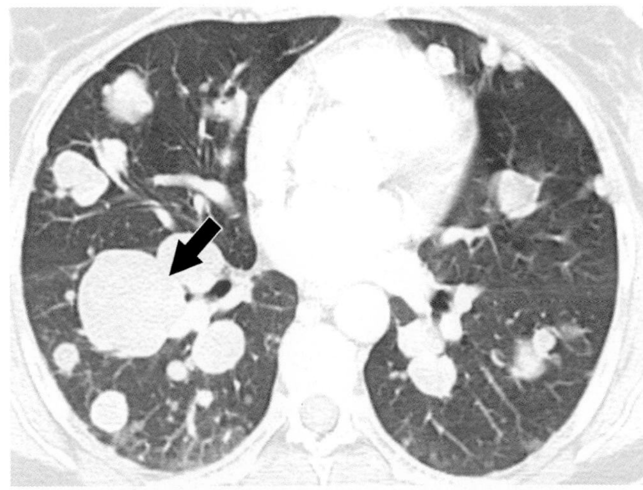

Figure 22.5. A 65-year-old man with metastatic adrenal cortical carcinoma. Axial chest computed tomography scan shows bilateral pulmonary metastases with the largest metastasis (*arrow*) in the right lower lobe.

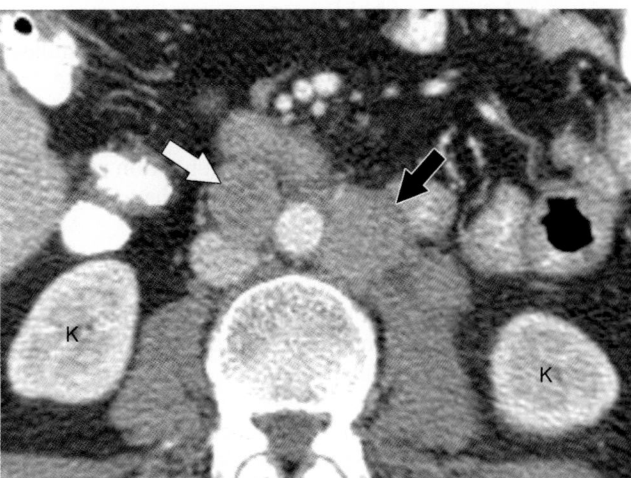

Figure 22.6. A 56-year-old woman with metastatic adrenal cortical carcinoma. Axial contrast-enhanced computed tomography scan shows left paraaortic (*black arrow*) and aortocaval (*white arrow*) adenopathy. *K*, Kidney.

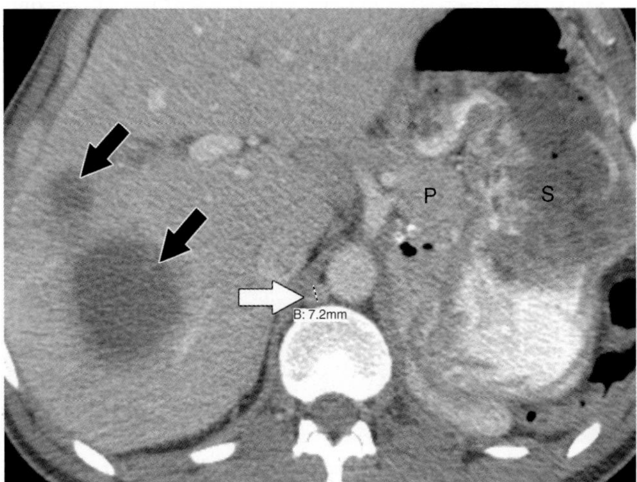

Figure 22.7. A 53-year-old woman with metastatic adrenal cortical carcinoma. Axial contrast-enhanced computed tomography scan shows hepatic metastases (*black arrows*) and right retrocrural adenopathy (*white arrow*). *P*, Pancreas; *S*, stomach.

macroscopic fat within an adrenal mass is a characteristic feature of adrenal myelolipoma, although very rarely other adrenal tumors may demonstrate this feature. A homogenous nonenhancing cystic lesion would be consistent with simple adrenal cyst. Adrenal adenomas are the most common adrenal masses and usually have abundant intracellular lipid, causing them to measure less than 10 Hounsfield units (HUs) on unenhanced CT images (Fig. 22.8).[28] However, up to a third of adenomas are lipid-poor and have higher attenuation on unenhanced images, ranging from 20 to 25 HU.[28–30] An adrenal CT protocol is typically used to evaluate adrenal masses. This would include a precontrast scan, followed by contrast enhanced scan obtained in the portal venous (60 seconds postcontrast injection), and delayed (15 minute) phases. On the noncontrast CT, the HU are calculated by placing a region of interest (ROI) that includes at least two-thirds of the mass. Areas of calcification or necrosis should not be included. If the adrenal mass measures 10 or fewer HU, it is presumed to be an adenoma. For masses measuring greater than 10 HU, further assessment is required to differentiate lipid poor adenoma from malignant lesions. Using the noncontrast and contrast-enhanced study, the absolute and relative percentage washouts are calculated using the following formulas:

Absolute percentage washout = [Attenuation value at enhanced computed tomography (CT) – attenuation value at delayed enhanced CT] / [Attenuation value at enhanced CT = attenuation value at unenhanced CT] × 100

Relative percentage washout = [Attenuation value at enhanced computed tomography (CT) – attenuation value at delayed enhanced CT] / Attenuation value at enhanced CT

Both lipid-rich and lipid-poor adenomas demonstrate rapid washout of contrast and should have greater than 60% absolute washout or greater than 40% relative washout on delayed images (Figs. 22.9 and 22.10).[30–32] A study by Caoili et al.[30] found a sensitivity of 98% and a specificity of 92% for characterizing adrenal masses as adenomas using a protocol that combined the HU of unenhanced scans with delayed contrast-enhanced washout values.

Although findings of absolute washout of less than 60% or relative washout less than 40% in the adrenal mass should make one consider malignancy, it should be noted that this is not pathognomonic for ACC; adrenal metastasis, pheochromocytoma, and adrenal lymphoma may also exhibit this finding, and a comprehensive clinical and biochemical workup may help in further evaluation.

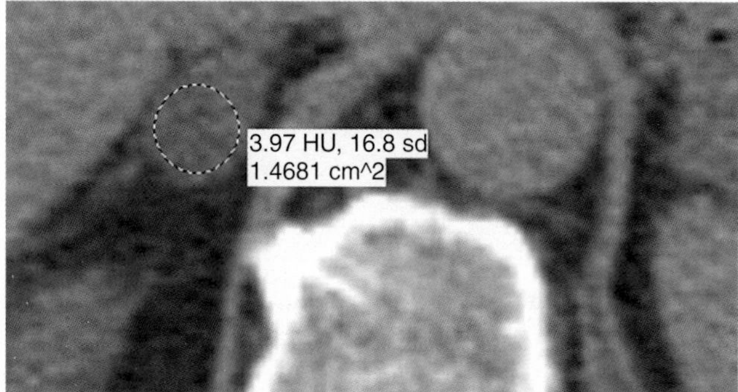

FIGURE 22.8. A 79-year-old man with nonsmall cell lung cancer with a lipid-rich adrenal adenoma. Axial noncontrast computed tomography scan shows a right adrenal adenoma (*circle*) measuring 3.97 Hounsfield units (*HU*).

ACCs are typically large at presentation, with a mean diameter of 9.8 cm and a diameter range of 4 to 25 cm.[33] Smaller tumors can be well-defined homogeneous masses, but as they enlarge they typically develop areas of necrosis that leads to a heterogeneous appearance on both pre- and postcontrast images (Fig. 22.11). ACCs tend to enhance peripherally, with ill-defined margins. Calcification can be present in up to a third, and is usually central.[34] Because most tumors present at an advanced stage, it is common to see local invasion of the surrounding fat and adjacent organs.

If adrenalectomy is to be performed, the adrenal arteries and veins are evaluated with a CT angiogram/venogram protocol. The angiogram/venogram protocol is also used to evaluate the superior extension of tumor thrombus, which alters surgical management.

Magnetic Resonance Imaging

Magnetic resonance imaging (MRI) plays a complementary role to CT in evaluating adrenal masses. It should be the initial imaging modality used to evaluate adrenal masses in pregnant patients and in patients who cannot receive iodinated contrast. Like CT, MRI can simultaneously evaluate the primary adrenal mass and detect local regional disease and metastases.

At our institution, phased array surface coils are used when possible for adrenal imaging, because they offer improved visualization and a better signal-to-noise ratio than body coils. Breathhold gradient echo and fast spin echo sequences are used to minimize motion artifact.

T1-weighted (T1W) images are obtained to assess the adrenal mass size and morphology. T2-weighted (T2W) images are used for tissue characterization.

Chemical shift imaging exploits the different proton resonance frequency rates in fat and water molecules to identify lipid-rich adenomas, and is currently considered the most sensitive modality for distinguishing between

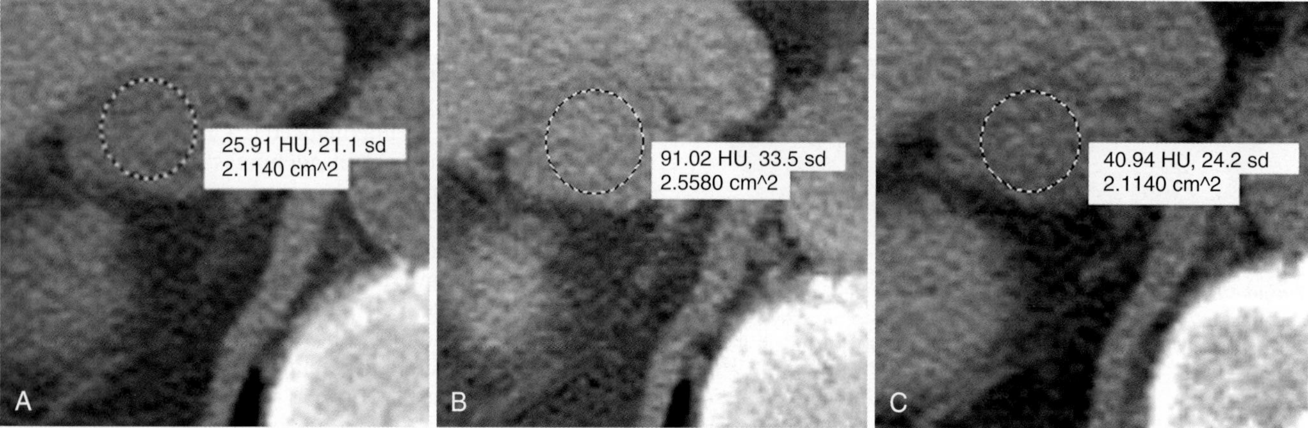

FIGURE 22.9. A 72-year-old women with small cell lung cancer with a lipid-poor adrenal adenoma. **A**, Axial noncontrast computed tomography (CT) scan shows a right adrenal mass (*circle*) measuring 25.91 Hounsfield units (*HU*). **B**, Axial contrast-enhanced CT scan shows the right adrenal mass (*circle*) measuring 91.02 HU. **C**, Axial delayed contrast-enhanced CT scan shows the right adrenal mass (*circle*) measuring 40.94 HU, which equals greater than 60% absolute washout and greater than 40% relative washout.

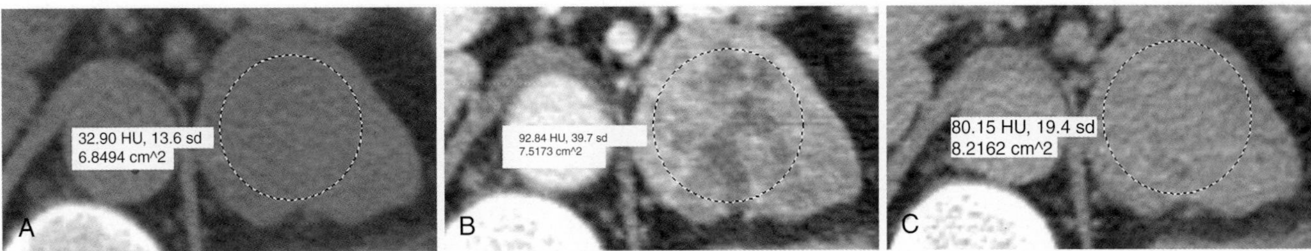

FIGURE 22.10. A 42-year-old woman with a left adrenal cortical carcinoma. **A**, Axial noncontrast computed tomography (CT) scan shows a left adrenal mass (*circle*) measuring 32.90 Hounsfield units (*HU*). **B**, Axial contrast-enhanced CT scan shows the left adrenal mass (*circle*) measuring 92.84 HU. **C**, Axial delayed contrast-enhanced CT scan shows the left adrenal mass (*circle*) measuring 80.15 HU, which does not equal greater than 60% absolute washout or greater than 40% relative washout, consistent with a malignant mass.

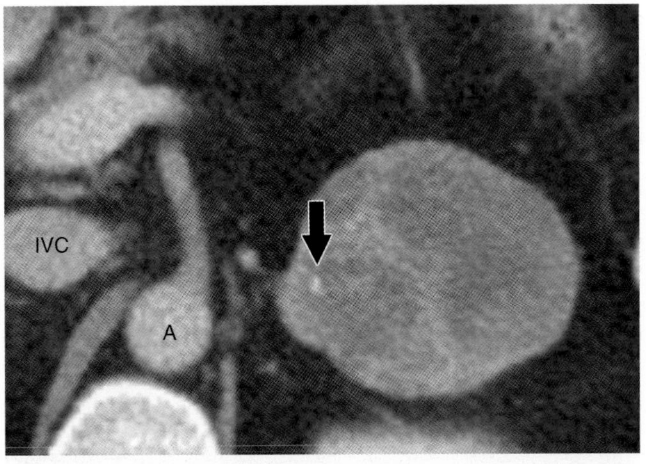

FIGURE 22.11. A 44-year-old man with a left adrenal cortical carcinoma (ACC). Axial contrast-enhanced computed tomography scan shows the ACC has heterogeneous enhancement and contains calcification (*arrow*). *A*, Aorta; *IVC*, inferior vena cava.

benign and malignant adrenal masses, with a sensitivity of 79% to 100% and a specificity of 82% to 100%.[35–40] Sensitivity increases to 91% and specificity to 94% when chemical shift and dynamic gadolinium-enhanced imaging are combined.[41]

For chemical shift imaging, a dual-phase acquisition is performed, in which both in-phase and out-of-phase (OOP) images are acquired during a single breathhold. The adrenal mass signal intensity is analyzed visually against the splenic signal intensity. An adrenal adenoma will show greater signal loss than the spleen on the OOP sequence (Fig. 22.12), whereas a malignant mass will not (Fig. 22.13). The signal intensity percentage decrease can also be calculated, using the formula:

Signal intensity percentage decrease = [Signal intensity in-phase (IP) – signal intensity OP] / Signal intensity IP

The percentage of decrease is proportional to the amount of lipid in the tissue.[37,42,43] The spleen or kidney

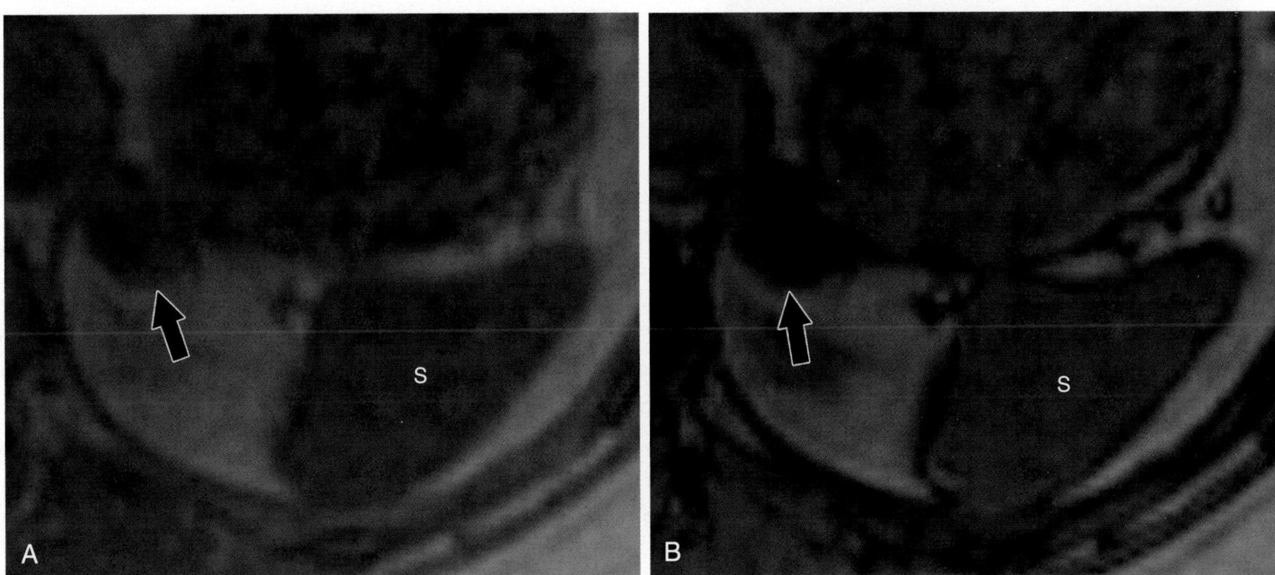

FIGURE 22.12. A 68-year-old woman with a left adrenal adenoma. **A**, Axial in-phase magnetic resonance imaging (MRI) study shows the left adrenal mass (*arrow*). **B**, Axial out-of-phase MRI study shows that the left adrenal mass (*arrow*) drops in signal relative to the spleen (*S*), consistent with an adenoma.

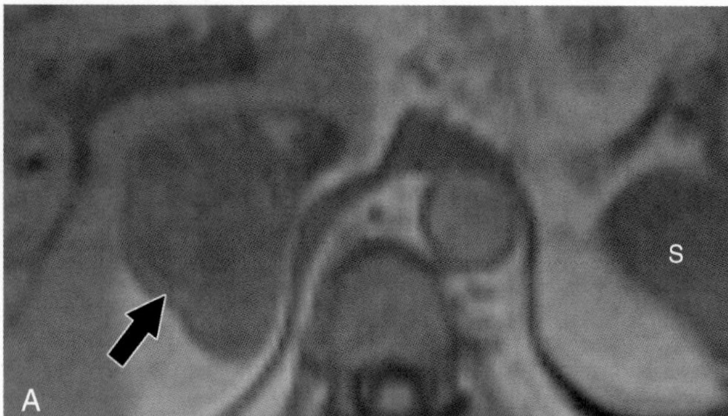

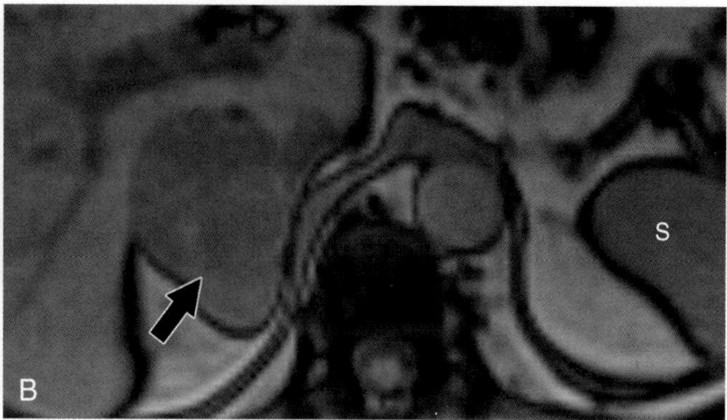

FIGURE 22.13. A 49-year-old woman with a right adrenal cortical carcinoma. **A**, Axial in-phase magnetic resonance imaging (MRI) study shows that the right adrenal mass (*arrow*) has a signal intensity similar to that of the spleen (*S*). **B**, Axial out-of-phase MRI study shows that the right adrenal mass (*arrow*) does not lose signal intensity relative to the spleen.

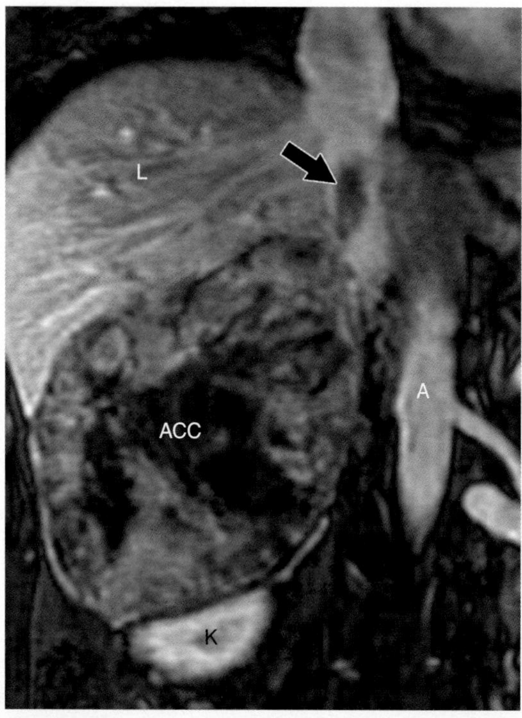

FIGURE 22.14. A 51-year-old man with a right adrenal cortical carcinoma (*ACC*). Coronal magnetic resonance imaging venogram shows a right ACC with tumor thrombus (*arrow*) extending into the intrahepatic inferior vena cava. *A*, Aorta; *K*, right kidney; *L*, liver.

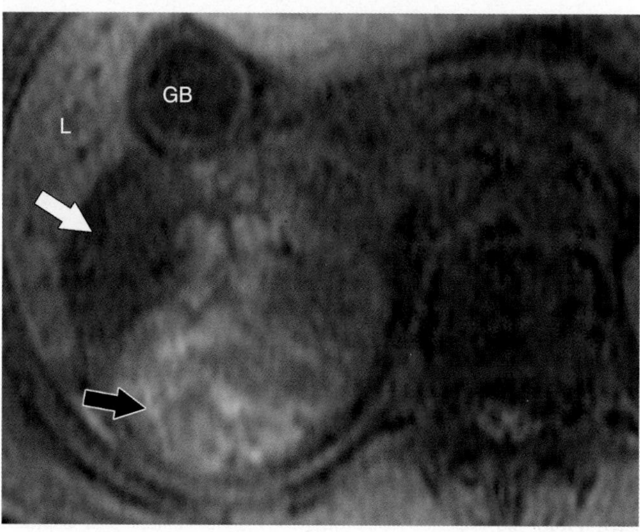

FIGURE 22.15. A 44-year-old man with a right adrenal cortical carcinoma. Axial noncontrast T1-weighted image shows the low T1 signal intensity (*white arrow*) of the right adrenal mass relative to the liver (*L*). The mass also contains areas of high signal (*black arrow*) from internal hemorrhage. *GB*, Gallbladder.

serves as a baseline comparison to normalize the value. Adenomas will have a decrease in signal intensity of more than 20%, whereas malignant masses will decrease by less than 20%.[36,38,42]

Contrast-enhanced images are used for further characterization of the mass and to evaluate for vascular involvement and metastases. MRI is the best test for assessing venous involvement.[44] It can accurately distinguish tumor thrombus from bland thrombus, and detect venous wall invasion. MRI is also the most accurate test for delineating the superior extent of venous involvement (Fig. 22.14).[45,46]

Findings that suggest a mass is an ACC are the same as they are in CT, including size greater than 4 cm, irregular margins, heterogeneous enhancement, and evidence of metastases, lymphadenopathy, or local invasion. ACCs are usually isointense to hypointense compared with the liver on T1W images. Areas of hemorrhage will be hyperintense on T1 (Fig. 22.15). On T2W images, ACC is hyperintense relative to the liver (Fig. 22.16), with areas of heterogeneity related to necrosis or hemorrhage.[47] Occasionally an ACC will contain foci of intracytoplasmic lipid, causing it to lose signal on OOP images, mimicking an adenoma.[47]

If an incidental adrenal mass measuring between 1 and 4 cm remains indeterminate even after CT and MRI evaluation, it can be monitored with follow-up imaging at 6-month intervals or evaluated with positron emission tomography (PET)/CT or biopsy per clinical concern. However, surgical resection is recommended for masses 4 cm or larger, given the higher incidence of malignancy in tumors larger than 4 cm.

Ultrasound

Ultrasound is not typically used to evaluate adrenal masses, given its low sensitivity when evaluating obese patients or patients with little retroperitoneal fat.[48,49]

Both ACCs and pheochromocytomas tend to be larger and have a more heterogeneous echotexture than nonmalignant adrenal masses (Fig. 22.17). However, there is significant overlap between the gray-scale and the duplex Doppler findings of malignant and nonmalignant lesions, and differentiation is not possible using these two parameters.

A recent study by Friedrich-Rust and colleagues[49] found contrast-enhanced sonography to have a sensitivity and specificity similar to those of CT and MRI in differentiating adenomas from nonadenomatous lesions, but this modality is not in widespread use in the United States.

Positron Emission Tomography/Computed Tomography

PET/CT combines functional with anatomic imaging. 2-[^{18}F] fluoro-2-deoxy-D-glucose (FDG)-PET/CT has a sensitivity of 93% to 100% and a specificity of 90% to 96% for distinguishing malignant from benign adrenal masses.[50–53] Although not commonly used to evaluate isolated adrenal masses, PET/CT may be useful for lesions that remain indeterminate after CT and MRI evaluation.[54]

Patients should fast for at least 6 hours before PET/CT. Blood glucose is measured before injection and should be less than 150 mg/dL. After an acceptable blood glucose level is confirmed, the patient is given an intravenous dose of 8 to 10 mCi of FDG per 1.7 m^2 of body surface area. For the next 45 to 60 minutes, the patient is kept in a quiet room with instructions not to talk or move, to prevent muscular uptake.

Images are obtained on a combined PET/CT scanner. The CT is performed according to a standardized protocol and is used for attenuation correction and anatomic localization.

A maximum standard uptake value (SUVmax) is calculated, using an ROI that includes at least two-thirds of the adrenal mass. If the adrenal mass has equal or higher FDG uptake than the liver, the mass is considered positive for malignancy (Fig. 22.18). Although Metser and coworkers[55] have suggested using an SUVmax of 3.1 to identify malignant adrenal masses, subsequent studies have shown that use of an internal control, most commonly the liver, is more accurate.[56,57] This is because a small percentage of benign adrenal masses exhibit low-grade FDG avidity.[58]

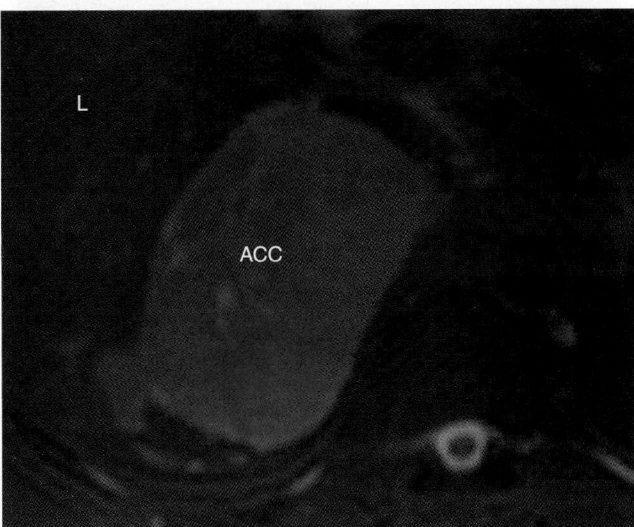

FIGURE 22.16. A 56-year-old woman with a right adrenal cortical carcinoma (*ACC*). Axial noncontrast T2-weighted image shows the ACC has high signal intensity relative to the liver (*L*).

Radionuclide Imaging

^{131}I-6-B-iodomethylnorcholesterol (NP-59) scintigraphy can also be used to evaluate indeterminate adrenal masses. Scintigraphic anterior, lateral, and posterior static images are obtained 5 and 7 days after intravenous administration of 37 MBq. Patients must be initially prepared with a thyroid blockade agent. A laxative is also given to reduce bowel ^{131}I radioactivity, which may interfere with the examination.

NP-59 is specifically accumulated by functional adrenal cortical tissues.[59] Absent or decreased NP-59 uptake is suspicious for a malignant lesion, which may be a primary adrenal cancer or metastasis. Gross and colleagues[60] found NP-59 scintigraphy to be 71% sensitive, 100% specific, and 93% accurate for distinguishing between benign and malignant adrenal lesions.

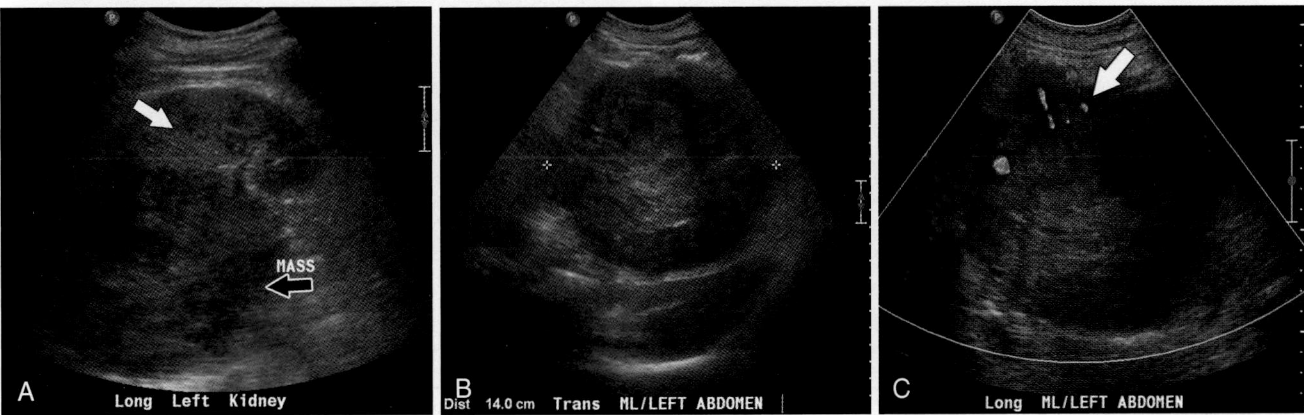

FIGURE 22.17. A 62-year-old man with a left adrenal cortical carcinoma. **A**, Longitudinal gray-scale ultrasound image shows the left adrenal mass (*black arrow*) is inseparable from the left kidney (*white arrow*). **B**, Transverse gray-scale ultrasound image shows a 14-cm left adrenal mass with a heterogeneous internal echotexture. **C**, Color Doppler ultrasound image shows flow in the periphery of the mass (*arrow*).

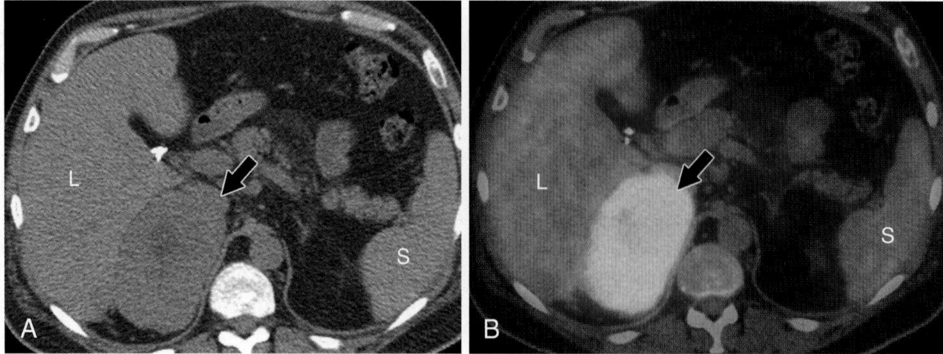

FIGURE 22.18. A 42-year-old woman with a right adrenal cortical carcinoma. **A**, Axial nonenhanced computed tomography (CT) scan from a positron emission tomography (PET)/CT scan shows the right adrenal mass (*arrow*). *S*, Spleen. **B**, Axial fused PET/CT image shows that the mass (*arrow*) is hypermetabolic with more 2-[^{18}F] fluoro-2-deoxy-D-glucose uptake relative to the liver (*L*).

Nodal Disease

CT and MRI primarily use size criteria to differentiate benign from malignant nodes, with retroperitoneal nodes measuring 10 mm or greater on the short axis and retrocrural nodes larger than 6 mm (Fig. 22.19) being suspicious for malignant involvement.[61] Unfortunately, nodes may be enlarged secondary to benign processes, whereas normal-sized nodes can have microscopic metastatic involvement, which limits the accuracy of using lymph node size for staging to approximately 69%.[62,63] Using only size criteria, CT and MRI have similar accuracies for detecting malignant nodal involvement.[64] Lymph node morphology and internal architecture should also be assessed. Normal lymph nodes have a reniform shape with a smooth outline. Nodes with a higher short axis–to–long-axis ratio, which gives them a more rounded appearance, are suspicious, regardless of size. Nodes with irregular borders or central necrosis are also more likely to harbor tumor.[65,66] Finally, nodes that have heterogeneous signal intensity on T2W MRI are suspicious.[67]

PET/CT is useful for evaluation of nodal involvement. Nodes with FDG uptake higher than background activity are considered positive for metastatic involvement (Fig. 22.20). Studies have shown that PET/CT is more

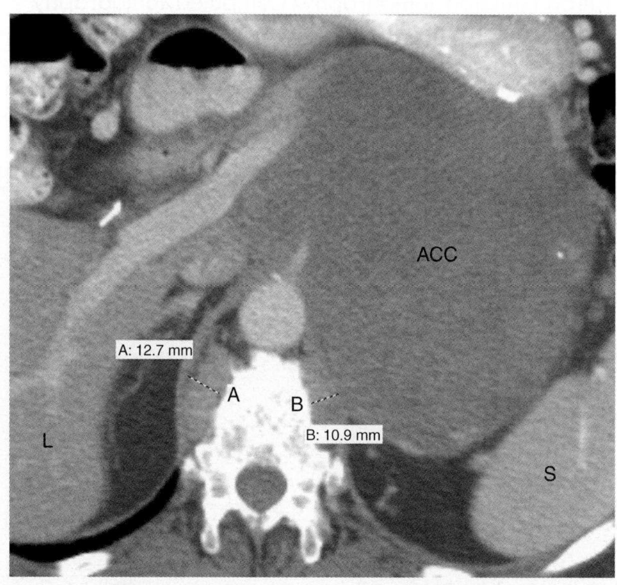

FIGURE 22.19. A 68-year-old man with a left adrenal cortical carcinoma (*ACC*). Axial contrast-enhanced computed tomography scan shows the left ACC with bilateral metastatic retrocrural lymph nodes measuring greater than 6 mm. *L*, Liver; *S*, spleen. *A*, right retrocrural lymph node; *B*, Left retrocrural lymph nodes.

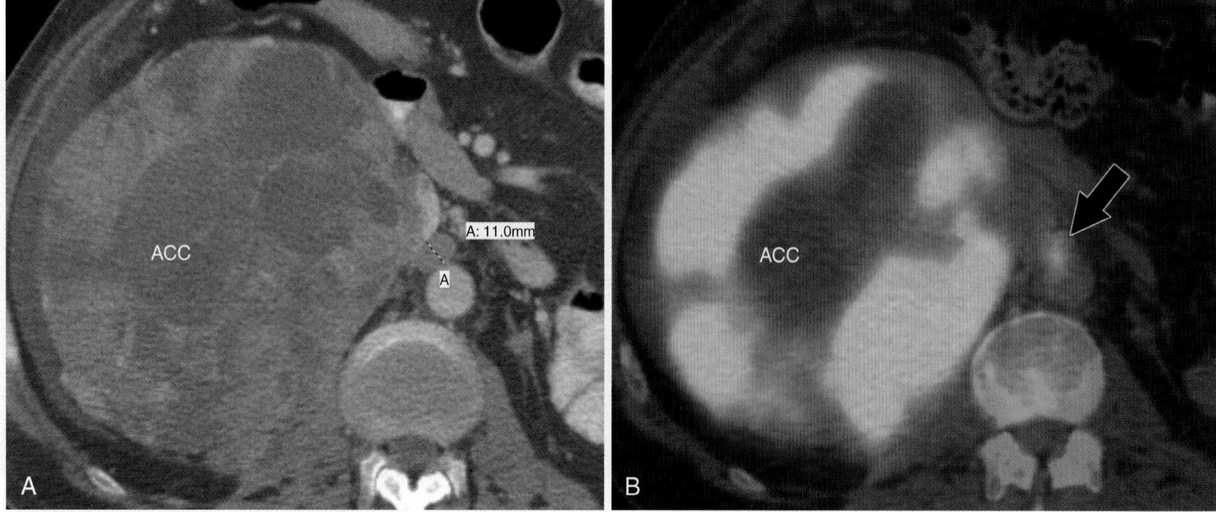

FIGURE 22.20. A 54-year-old woman with a right adrenal cortical carcinoma (*ACC*). *A*, Axial contrast-enhanced computed tomography (CT) scan shows the right ACC and a metastatic aortocaval lymph node measuring 11 mm. *B*, Axial fused positron emission tomography/CT scan shows both the ACC and the node (*arrow*) are hypermetabolic.

sensitive and specific for identifying malignant nodal disease than both CT and MRI.[68–70] Unfortunately, metastatic nodes smaller than 10 mm may not be positive, secondary to PET/CT spatial resolution limitations.

Metastatic Disease

Patients diagnosed with ACC should be staged radiologically using CT chest, CT abdomen and pelvis (or MRI abdomen and pelvis) for detecting metastases.[71–73] PET/CT may be helpful, especially in those being considered for potential curative resection.

CT is superior to PET/CT for detecting lung, abdominal lymph node, and peritoneal metastases, especially those measuring less 1 cm (Fig. 22.21).[74] PET/CT is limited by spatial resolution, becoming more accurate once lesions reach 10 mm, which helps explain this discrepancy.

PET/CT is better at detecting bone metastases (Fig. 22.22), especially those that might not be included in the field of view on conventional CT and MRI scans. A study by Becherer and associates[75] evaluated the use of FDG-PET specifically for ACC and found it to be 100% sensitive and 95% specific for detecting metastases, whereas CT was 89% sensitive and 100% specific.

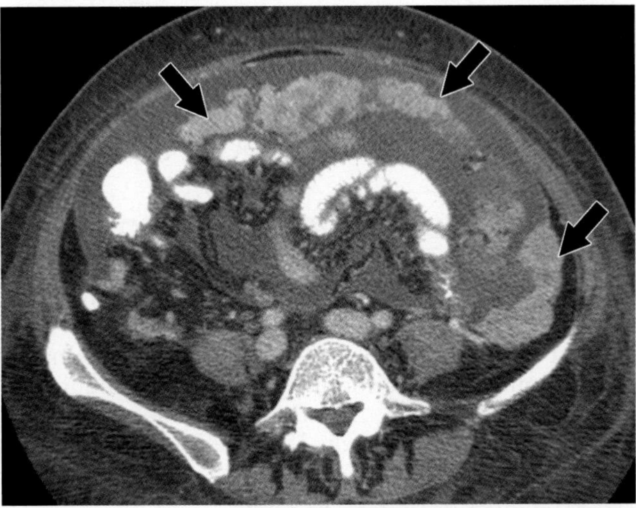

FIGURE 22.21. A 72-year-old man with metastatic adrenal cortical carcinoma involving the peritoneum. Axial contrast-enhanced computed tomography scan shows peritoneal metastases (*arrows*) and ascites.

KEY POINTS

The Radiology Report for Adrenal Cortical Carcinoma: What to Include

- Does mass meet the criteria for benign adenoma? If indeterminate, can another modality clarify?
- Size and location of mass.
- Does the mass extend outside of the gland, and what adjacent organs are involved?
- Venous involvement and what is the superior extent.
- Regional or distal lymphadenopathy.
- Are distal metastases present, and where are they located?
- If adrenalectomy is planned, identify the arterial and venous supply.

TREATMENT

ACC is a highly aggressive tumor, and survival depends on tumor size, stage of disease, patient age, and extent of surgical excision. Radical surgical excision is the only curative option, and is the first step of treatment, except in patients with metastatic disease. Open resections are performed for suspected malignant adrenal masses to reduce the chance of tumor seeding. The excision should include the surrounding retroperitoneal fat, fascia, regional lymph nodes, and all adjacent organs that have been invaded. Tumor thrombus within the IVC or renal vein should be extracted. Patients with liver or pulmonary oligometastases may be considered for wedge resections in carefully selected cases.

Patients with complete resection of ACC have 5-year survival rates of up to 50%.[76–79] Complete resection of the adrenal mass and gland is the goal, because subtotal resection increases the likelihood of local recurrence. Unfortunately, recurrence rates after apparent complete resections still remain high, ranging from 35% to 85%.[80,81] Repeat resection of locally recurrent disease has been shown to prolong survival compared with treatment with chemotherapy alone.[76,82]

Adjuvant radiation of the surgical field is controversial, with studies showing conflicting response rates.[83–85] Radiation is not recommended after the initial surgery, because its effects could make subsequent surgeries more technically difficult, but it may be considered after repeat resections.

Adjuvant use of mitotane may be considered in those patients without macroscopic residual tumor after surgery

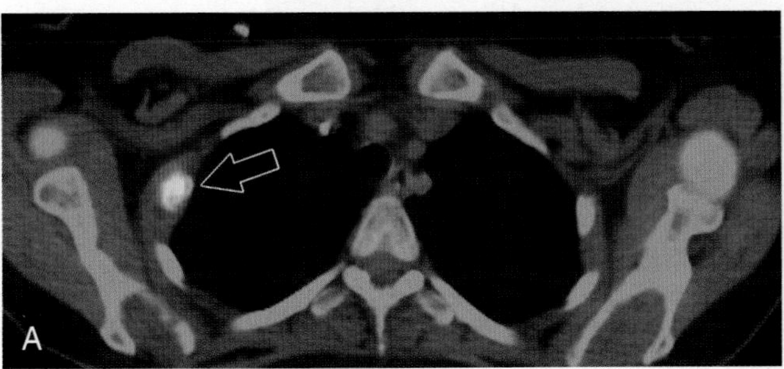

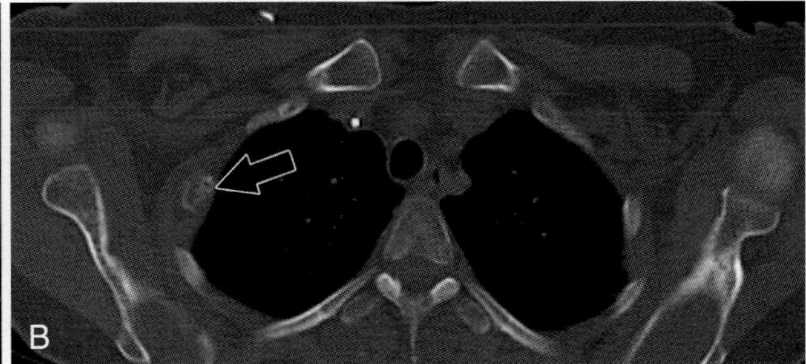

FIGURE 22.22. A 37-year-old woman with metastatic adrenal cortical carcinoma. **A**, Axial fused positron emission tomography (PET)/ computed tomography (CT) scan shows a hypermetabolic right rib metastasis (*arrow*). **B**, Axial nonenhanced CT scan from the PET/CT shows the right rib destruction (*arrow*).

but who have a perceived high risk of recurrence.[73] Mitotane is also used for treating advanced (stages III and IV) tumors. It has a specific cytotoxic effect on adrenocortical cells. Unfortunately, only 20% to 25% of patients respond to mitotane treatment, and several studies have not shown increased survival time for these responders.[24,86–88] However, in some patients, mitotane can lead to long-term survival, even if they have stage IV disease.[89–91]

Combining mitotane with cytotoxic agents such as cisplatin has had limited success.[8,92] Mitotane has also been used in combination with streptozocin, with a median survival time of 16 months for patients with advanced disease, versus a median survival time of 3 months for untreated disease.[26]

Combination therapy using etoposide, doxorubicin, and cisplatin plus mitotane may be used in the treatment of advanced adrenocortical carcinoma.[93] However, it should be noted that mitotane and combination chemotherapy use is complicated by a variety of adverse effects and toxicities, which should be carefully monitored for.[88,91,93] Debulking surgery may be performed in patients with functional metastatic disease to help palliate symptoms related to hyperfunction. Palliative radiation therapy may be considered for symptomatic osseous metastases.

KEY POINTS

Treatment of Adrenal Cortical Carcinoma

- Complete surgical resection is the only curative treatment for adrenal cortical carcinoma (ACC).
- Recurrent and metastatic disease should also be resected if deemed feasible.
  Mitotane may be useful either as a single drug or in combination with other chemotherapeutic drugs, for advanced and recurrent ACC.

SURVEILLANCE

Follow-up is essential in patients after adrenalectomy for ACC because of its high recurrence rate. Hormonal markers can be monitored in patients with functional ACC to detect recurrence, but approximately one-half of these patients have tumor recurrences that produce inactive hormonal precursors, limiting marker use.[94] In addition, nonfunctional tumors will not produce hormonal markers. Therefore, radiologic studies are the mainstay for postsurgical follow-up. Imaging is also used to evaluate patients with metastatic disease to determine whether the disease is progressing or responding to therapy. At our institution, PET/CT and contrast-enhanced CT are commonly alternated at 4- to 6-month intervals. This combination of modalities is used, because PET/CT has been shown to be superior to CT for detecting locally recurrent disease (Fig. 22.23), whereas, as mentioned previously, CT is more accurate for pulmonary, nodal, and peritoneal disease.[74]

KEY POINTS

Surveillance for Adrenal Cortical Carcinoma

- Imaging is the mainstay for surveillance.
- Patients are imaged every 4 to 6 months, alternating computed tomography (CT) with positron emission tomography (PET)/CT.
- PET/CT is superior for detecting local recurrence.
- CT is superior for detecting pulmonary, nodal, and peritoneal metastases.

II MALIGNANT PHEOCHROMOCYTOMA

EPIDEMIOLOGY AND RISK FACTORS

Pheochromocytomas are neuroendocrine tumors that arise from the adrenal medulla's chromaffin cells.[95] They account for approximately 4% of adrenal incidentalomas, with an annual population incidence of 8 per million in the United States.[96,97] Most pheochromocytomas are sporadic, but approximately 25% to 40% are associated

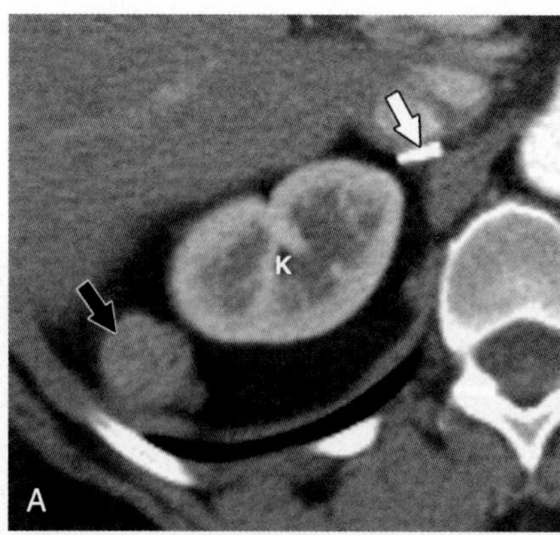

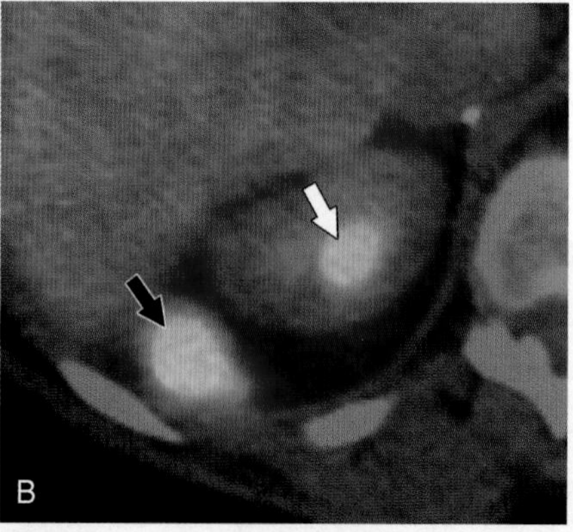

FIGURE 22.23. A 42-year-old woman with recurrent adrenal cortical carcinoma. **A**, Axial contrast-enhanced computed tomography (CT) scan shows a recurrent tumor nodule (*black arrow*) in the perinephric fat. Surgical clip (*white arrow*) from a prior right adrenalectomy is present. *K*, Right kidney. **B**, Axial fused positron emission tomography/CT scan shows that the recurrent tumor (*black arrow*) is hypermetabolic. Physiologic activity is seen in the right kidney (*white arrow*).

with germline genetic mutations that include the von Hippel–Lindau, rearranged during transection (*RET*), neurofibromatosis type 1, and succinate dehydrogenase subunits B (*SDHB*), C (*SDHC*), and D (*SDHD*) genes.[95,98–100] Hereditary pheochromocytoma, seen in patients with multiple endocrine neoplasia type 2, von Hippel–Lindau syndrome, neurofibromatosis type 1, and the familial paragangliomas, are usually diagnosed earlier (before 40 years of age), compared with the sporadic counterparts. Up to 14% of pheochromocytomas are malignant, and there is a higher risk for malignancy in pheochromocytomas caused by mutations in the *SDHB* gene.[99]

Paragangliomas are pheochromocytomas located outside of the adrenal gland, and account for approximately 20% of pheochromocytomas.[101] Paragangliomas have a higher prevalence of malignancy than pheochromocytomas, with approximately one-third being malignant.[102,103]

ANATOMY AND PATHOLOGY

Malignant pheochromocytomas arise from the adrenal gland's inner medulla. The medulla is derived from neural crest cells and is part of the sympathetic autonomic nervous system. It secretes the catecholamines epinephrine and norepinephrine.

No histopathologic markers reliably distinguish benign from malignant pheochromocytomas, including capsular or vascular invasion and cellular atypia. Only the presence of metastases establishes malignancy.[104] In total, 11% to 31% of the patients may present metastases at the time of initial diagnosis. Pheochromocytomas larger than 5 cm do have a greater rate of malignancy than smaller tumors, at 76% versus 24%.[105]

KEY POINTS

Anatomy and Pathology of Malignant Pheochromocytoma

- Malignant pheochromocytoma arises from the inner adrenal medulla.
- No reliable histopathologic markers distinguish between benign and malignant pheochromocytomas.
- The presence of metastases is the only criterion to establish malignancy.
- Pheochromocytomas larger than 5 cm have a higher rate of malignancy.

PATTERNS OF TUMOR SPREAD

Similar to ACC, malignant pheochromocytoma spreads by direct extension into the surrounding fat and adjacent organs. Lymphatic spread is to the regional upper retroperitoneal and retrocrural nodes. The most common sites for hematogenously disseminated metastases are the bones (72%), liver (50%), and lung (50%).[106]

KEY POINTS

Patterns of Tumor Spread of Malignant Pheochromocytoma

- Malignant pheochromocytoma can directly invade adjacent organs.
- Regional nodal metastases involve the upper paraaortic, caval, and retrocrural nodes.
- Distant metastases most commonly involve the bones, liver, and lungs.

CLINICAL PRESENTATION

Functioning malignant pheochromocytomas produce clinical symptoms related to catecholamine excess. These symptoms include paroxysmal hypertension, palpitations, headaches, sweating, and dyspnea.[107] Biochemical investigations typically show elevated plasma and urinary metanephrine levels. Elevated normetanephrine levels may also occur, particularly in the presence of paraganglioma or metastatic pheochromocytoma. Some 10% of pheochromocytomas are nonfunctional and can present with symptoms related to mass effect or metastases or be discovered incidentally.

KEY POINTS

Clinical Presentation of Malignant Pheochromocytoma

- Most patients have symptoms from excess catecholamines.
- Symptoms include hypertension, sweating, and palpitations.
- Nonfunctional tumors may present with symptoms related to mass effect or be discovered incidentally.

STAGING CLASSIFICATION

The staging classification for malignant pheochromocytoma and ACC is the same.

IMAGING

Tumor

Computed Tomography

Malignant pheochromocytomas are usually large, irregular, heterogeneously-enhancing masses that contain areas of necrosis.[108,109] The average size is 5 cm, and approximately 12% contain calcifications (Fig. 22.24).[110] On noncontrast images, pheochromocytomas typically have a density of 40 to 50 HU (Fig. 22.25).[111] Pheochromocytomas may demonstrate delayed contrast washout or rapid washout, similar to adenomas, but they tend to have more avid enhancement on the early phase of the examination, measuring greater than 110 to 130 HU (Fig. 22.26).[112] Rarely, necrotic pheochromocytomas can

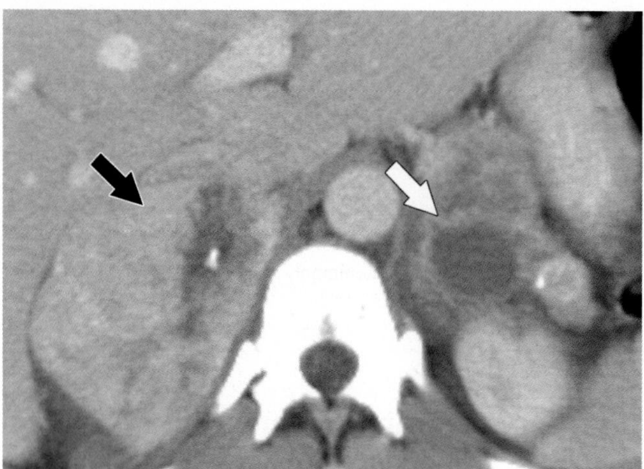

FIGURE 22.24. A 33-year-old woman with von Hippel–Lindau syndrome and a right malignant pheochromocytoma. Axial contrast-enhanced computed tomography scan shows that the right pheochromocytoma (*black arrow*) has areas of necrosis and contains a central calcification. Islet cell tumors are also seen in the pancreas (*white arrow*).

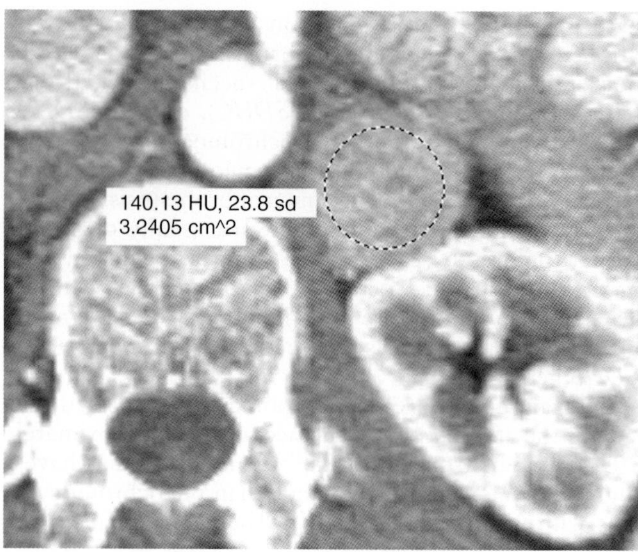

FIGURE 22.26. A 37-year-old woman with a left malignant pheochromocytoma. Axial contrast-enhanced computed tomography scan shows the left adrenal mass (*circle*) measuring 140.13 Hounsfield units (*HU*).

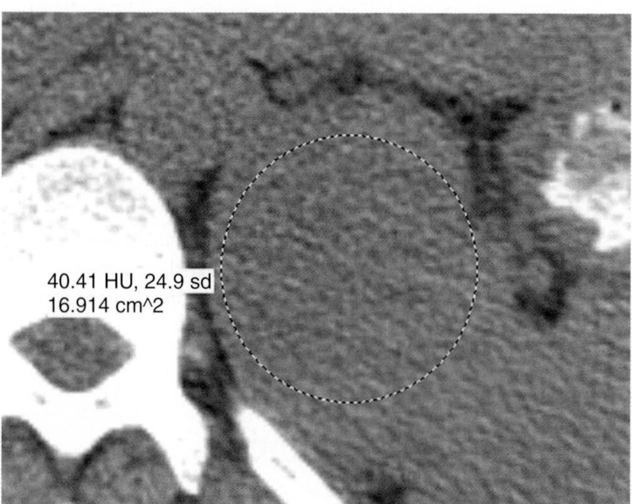

FIGURE 22.25. A 51-year-old man with a left malignant pheochromocytoma. Axial nonenhanced computed tomography scan shows the left adrenal mass (*circle*) measuring 40.41 Hounsfield units (*HU*).

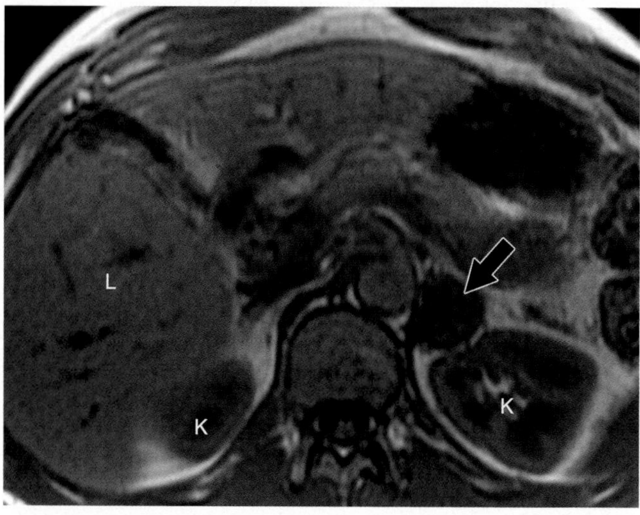

FIGURE 22.27. A 37-year-old woman with a left malignant pheochromocytoma. Axial T1-weighted magnetic resonance imaging shows that the left adrenal mass (*arrow*) is hypointense relative to the liver (*L*). *K*, Kidneys.

mimic a simple adrenal cyst.[113] CT has a sensitivity of 93% to 100% for detecting pheochromocytomas larger than 1 cm.

Magnetic Resonance Imaging

Pheochromocytomas are isointense to hypointense to the liver on T1W images (Fig. 22.27). They usually have intense contrast enhancement (Fig. 22.28). Although initially pheochromocytomas were described as being pathognomonically "light bulb" bright on T2W images, subsequent studies have shown that a significant proportion are heterogeneous, with only moderately high T2 signal (Fig. 22.29).[114,115] MRI and CT have similar sensitivities for detecting adrenal pheochromocytoma.

Radionuclide Imaging

^{123}I-metaiodobenzylguanidine (MIBG) is a type of functional imaging that is useful for evaluating pheochromocytomas, because it can detect the primary mass, along with recurrent and metastatic disease. MIBG is a norepinephrine analog that binds to the human norepinephrine transporter, which transports catecholamines into chromaffin cells.[(116)] ^{123}I-MIBG is the preferred radionuclide for imaging pheochromocytomas because of its specific uptake into the sympathetic nervous system. It has a sensitivity of 90% and a specificity of 92% to 99% for detecting functional pheochromocytomas.[117–120]

^{123}I-MIBG plays a complementary role to anatomic imaging. It can specifically identify an adrenal mass

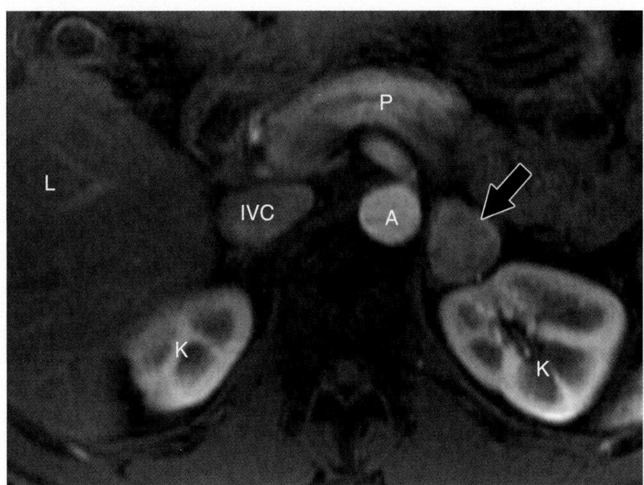

FIGURE 22.28. A 37-year-old woman with a left malignant pheochromocytoma. Axial contrast-enhanced magnetic resonance imaging study shows the enhancing left adrenal mass (*arrow*). *A*, Aorta; *IVC*, inferior vena cava; *K*, kidneys; *L*, liver; *P*, pancreas.

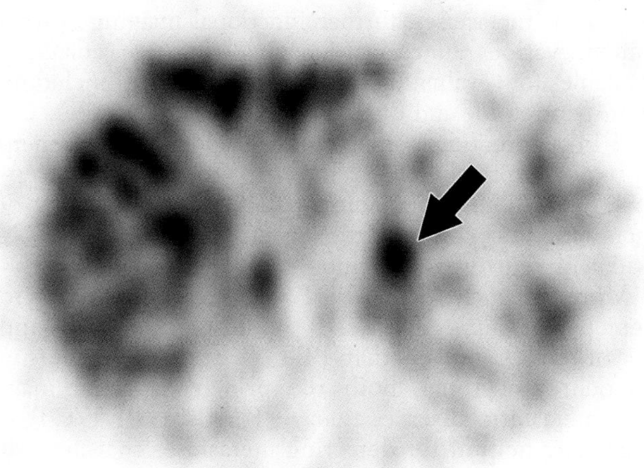

FIGURE 22.30. A 37-year-old woman with a left malignant pheochromocytoma. Axial ^{123}I-metaiodobenzylguanidine scan shows positive tracer uptake in the left adrenal mass (*arrow*).

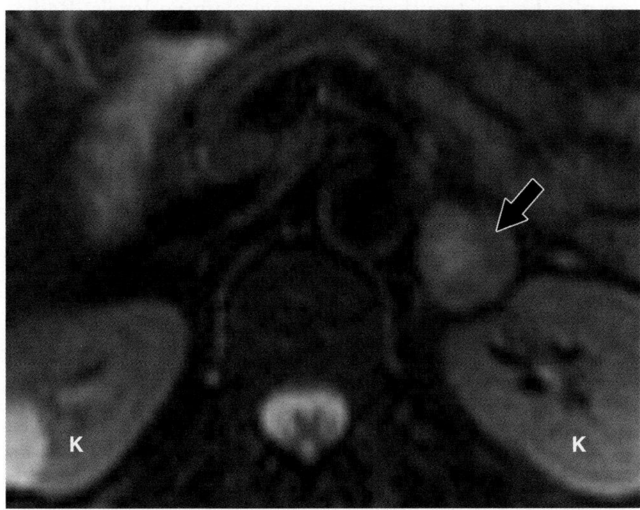

FIGURE 22.29. A 37-year-old woman with a left malignant pheochromocytoma. Axial T2-weighted magnetic resonance imaging study shows the heterogeneous signal in the left adrenal mass (*arrow*). *K*, Kidneys.

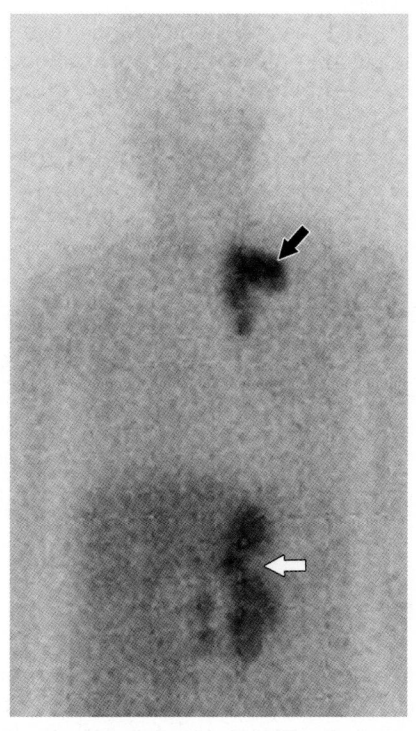

FIGURE 22.31. A 48-year-old man with recurrent, metastatic malignant pheochromocytoma. Frontal static ^{123}I-metaiodobenzylguanidine scan shows uptake in metastatic left supraclavicular (*black arrow*) and retroperitoneal (*white arrow*) adenopathy.

as a pheochromocytoma, whereas CT and MRI cannot. It should also be used when clinical suspicion is strong for the presence of a pheochromocytoma or metastatic disease that is not detected by anatomic imaging.

The initial step in ^{123}I-MIBG imaging is to administer a thyroid blockade agent such as potassium perchlorate, potassium iodate of Lugol solution. Next, 10 mCi of ^{123}I-MIBG is given intravenously. Twenty-four and 48 or 72 hours after administration total body planar imaging is obtained from the head to below the knees, followed by single-photon emission CT. The scan is considered positive when adrenal uptake is greater than hepatic activity and no similar uptake is seen on the contralateral side (Fig. 22.30).[121]

Nodal and Distant Metastases in Malignant Pheochromocytoma

The CT and MRI criteria used to identify suspicious nodes in malignant pheochromocytoma are similar to those in ACC.

Classically, ^{123}I-MIBG has been used to screen for malignant pheochromocytoma metastases, with a sensitivity of 83% to 100% (Fig. 22.31).[122] However, not all metastases are ^{123}I-MIBG–avid, so if there is clinical suspicion for metastases, further functional imaging is warranted. Various functional imaging tests are currently available for evaluating pheochromocytoma, including ^{111}In-pentreotide and PET using various radiotracers.

^{111}In-pentreotide is an octreotide analog that is taken up by tumors expressing type 2 and type 5 somatostatin receptors. It can be used for nonspecific functional imaging of metastatic pheochromocytomas that are not ^{123}I-MIBG–avid, with sensitivities reaching 97%.[119,120]

More recently, FDG-PET/CT has been used to detect metastatic disease.[123] A study by Mann and coworkers[124] showed that PET is better at detecting pheochromocytoma, both the primary adrenal mass and metastatic disease, than ^{123}I-MIBG. PET/CT is especially helpful for detecting metastases that are not ^{123}I-MIBG–avid.[124] PET/CT using the radioisotopes 6–^{18}F-fluorodopamine, 6–^{18}F-fluoroDOPA, and ^{68}Ga-DOTATATE has also been shown to be superior to ^{123}I-MIBG for detecting disease.[125]

Standard bone scintigraphy using technetium-99m methyl diphosphonate is useful for detecting bony metastases.[126]

CT and MRI are less successful than functional imaging at detecting metastatic pheochromocytoma, with both having a sensitivity of approximately 90%.[127–130]

Key Points

The Radiology Report for Malignant Pheochromocytoma: What to Include

- Size and location of mass.
- Does the mass extend outside of the gland, and what adjacent organs are involved?
- Is there venous involvement, and what is the superior extent?
- Regional or distal lymphadenopathy.
- Are distal metastases present, and where are they located?
- If adrenalectomy is planned, identify the arterial and venous supply.

TREATMENT

The prognosis for malignant pheochromocytoma is difficult to predict, but outcomes are worse for patients with liver and lung metastases and for patients with larger tumors.[105,107] The average 5-year survival rate for patients with metastatic disease is approximately 50%.[104]

Surgical resection is the only curative treatment for malignant pheochromocytoma, and patients with locally recurrent disease should undergo repeat surgical resection.[131]

For unresectable tumors, ^{131}I-MIBG is used. It works by providing local radiation therapy through the emission of β particles and induces a predominantly partial tumor response in 24% to 45% of patients, with most experiencing disease progression after 2 years of treatment.[132,133] ^{131}I-MIBG appears to be more effective against soft tissue metastases than skeletal metastases.[131] Thrombocytopenia from bone marrow suppression is the most common side effect. Therapy using radiopharmaceuticals such as peptide receptor radionuclide therapy with ^{177}Lu-DOTATATE have also been reported.[123]

Cytotoxic chemotherapy is used in patients with tumors that do not take up ^{131}I-MIBG. The most common protocol uses a combination of cyclophosphamide, vincristine, and dacarbazine. As with ^{131}I-MIBG, most patients only partially respond to treatment and have progressive disease within 2 years.[134–136] Side effects include bone marrow suppression, paresthesias, nausea, and vomiting. Use of temozolamide and tyrosine kinase inhibitors have also been reported in management of progressive malignant pheochromocytoma. Novel targeted therapies can also be a consideration for rapidly progressive disease. α-adrenergic blockers, calcium channel blockers, and α-methyl paratyrosine are used to provide symptomatic relief from elevated catecholamine levels. Surgery, cryoablation, radiofrequency ablation, and/or embolization for tumor debulking can also be used to decrease catecholamine levels. Radiation can help alleviate symptoms from skeletal metastases.

Key Points

Treatment of Malignant Pheochromocytoma

- Complete surgical resection is the only curative treatment.
- ^{131}I-metaiodobenzylguanidine (MIBG) provides local radiation therapy for metastatic disease, but can be used only in ^{131}I-MIBG–avid tumors
- Cyclophosphamide, vincristine, and dacarbazine cytotoxic chemotherapy is used for non–^{131}I-MIBG–avid tumors.
- Most patients have progressive disease within 2 years with either treatment.

SURVEILLANCE

Patients with completely resected malignant pheochromocytomas are followed indefinitely with annual biochemical screening. Patients are also screened for recurrence at 4- to 6-month intervals, alternating between anatomic (CT or MRI) and functional (^{131}I-MIBG or PET/CT) imaging.

Key Points

Surveillance of Malignant Pheochromocytoma

- Biochemical markers are surveyed annually.
- Patients are imaged every 4 to 6 months, alternating computed tomography (CT) or magnetic resonance imaging with positron emission tomography/CT or ^{131}I-metaiodobenzylguanidine.

TABLE 22.1 Tumor-Node-Metastasis Staging of Adrenal Cortical Carcinoma[24]

T1	Tumor ≤5 cm, no invasion
T2	Tumor >5 cm, no invasion
T3	Tumor extends outside of adrenal gland into the surrounding fat
T4	Tumor invades adjacent organs
N0	No involvement of regional lymph nodes
N1	Positive regional lymph node(s)
M0	No distant metastases
M1	Distant metastases

From Adrenal Cortical Carcinoma. In: Amin MB, Edge SB, Greene FL, et al, eds. AJCC Cancer Staging Manual. 8th ed. New York: Springer; 2017:911–918.

TABLE 22.2 Staging of Adrenal Cortical Carcinoma[24]

Stage I	T1, N0, M0
Stage II	T2, N0, M0
Stage III	T1, N1, M0
	T2, N1, M0
	T3, N0, M0
Stage IV	T3, N1, M0
	T4, N0–N1, M0
	Any T, any N, M1

From Adrenal Cortical Carcinoma. In: Amin MB, Edge SB, Greene FL, et al, eds. AJCC Cancer Staging Manual. 8th ed. New York: Springer; 2017:911–918.

REFERENCES

1. Copeland PM. The incidentally discovered adrenal mass. *Ann Intern Med*. 1983;98:940–945.
2. Choyke PL. ACR Committee on Appropriateness Criteria. ACR Appropriateness Criteria on incidentally discovered adrenal mass. *J Am Coll Radiol*. 2006 Jul;3(7):498–504.
3. Norton JA. Adrenal tumors. In: DeVita VT, Hellman S, Rosenberg SA, eds. *Cancer, Principles and Practice of Oncology*. Philadelphia: Lippincott-Raven; 1997:1659–1674.
4. Vaughan Jr. ED. Diseases of the adrenal gland. *Med Clin North Am*. 2004;88:443–466.
5. Roman S. Adrenocortical carcinoma. *Curr Opin Oncol*. 2006;18:36–42.
6. Kebebew E, Reiff E, Duh QY, et al. Extent of disease at presentation and outcome for adrenocortical carcinoma: have we made progress? *World J Surg*. 2006;30:872–878.
7. Wajchenberg BL, et al. Adrenocortical carcinoma: clinical and laboratory observations. *Cancer*. 2000;88:711–736.
8. Wooten MD, King DK. Adrenal cortical carcinoma. Epidemiology and treatment with mitotane and a review of the literature. *Cancer*. 1993;72:3145–3155.
9. Chow WH, et al. Smoking and adrenal cancer mortality among United States veterans. *Cancer Epidemiol Biomarkers Prev*. 1996;5:79–80.
10. Hsing AW, et al. Risk factors for adrenal cancer: an exploratory study. *Int J Cancer*. 1996;65:432–436.
11. McNicol AM, et al. Expression of p53 in adrenocortical tumours: clinicopathological correlations. *J Pathol*. 1997;181:146–152.
12. Goldman SM, Kenney PJ. The adrenal glands. In: Lee JKT, ed. *Computed Body Tomography with MRI Correlation*. Philadelphia: Lippincott Williams & Wilkins; 2006:1326–1330.
13. Federle MP. Adrenal. In: Federle MP, ed. *Diagnostic and Surgical Imaging Anatomy. Chest, Abdomen, Pelvis*. Salt Lake City: Amirsys; 2006:424–445.
14. Matsuura T, et al. Radiologic anatomy of the right adrenal vein: preliminary experience with MDCT. *AJR Am J Roentgenol*. 2008;191:402–408.
15. McLachlan MS, Roberts EE. Demonstration of the normal adrenal gland by venography and gas insufflation. *Br J Radiol*. 1971;44:664–671.
16. Weiss LM. Comparative histologic study of 43 metastasizing and nonmetastasizing adrenocortical tumors. *Am J Surg Pathol*. 1984;8:163–169.
17. van Slooten H, et al. Morphologic characteristics of benign and malignant adrenocortical tumors. *Cancer*. 1985;55:766–773.
18. Harrison LE, Gaudin PB, Brennan MF. Pathologic features of prognostic significance for adrenocortical carcinoma after curative resection. *Arch Surg*. 1999;134:181–185.
19. Weiss LM, Medeiros LJ, Vickery Jr AL. Pathologic features of prognostic significance in adrenocortical carcinoma. *Am J Surg Pathol*. 1989;13:202–206.
20. Yano T, Linehan M, Anglard P, et al. Genetic changes in human adrenocortical carcinomas. *J Natl Cancer Inst*. 1989;81:518–523.
21. Abiven G, et al. Clinical and biological features in the prognosis of adrenocortical cancer: poor outcome of cortisol-secreting tumors in a series of 202 consecutive patients. *J Clin Endocrinol Metab*. 2006;91:2650–2655.
22. Fassnacht M, Allolio B. Clinical management of adrenocortical carcinoma. *Best Pract Res Clin Endocrinol Metab*. 2009;23:273–289.
23. Venkatesh S, et al. Adrenal cortical carcinoma. *Cancer*. 1989;64:765–769.
24. Phan AT, Perrier ND, et al. Adrenal Cortical Carcinoma. In: Amin MB, Edge SB, Greene FL, et al. (Eds.) *AJCC Cancer Staging Manual*. 8th Ed. New York: Springer; 2017:911–918.
25. Paton BL, et al. Outcomes of adrenal cortical carcinoma in the United States. *Surgery*. 2006;140:914–920. discussion 919–920.
26. Khan TS, et al. Streptozocin and o,p'DDD in the treatment of adrenocortical cancer patients: long-term survival in its adjuvant use. *Ann Oncol*. 2000;11:1281–1287.
27. Kloos RT, et al. Incidentally discovered adrenal masses. *Endocr Rev*. 1995;16:460–484.
28. Park SH, et al. Differentiation of adrenal adenoma and nonadenoma in unenhanced CT: new optimal threshold value and the usefulness of size criteria for differentiation. *Korean J Radiol*. 2007;8:328–335.
29. Lee MJ, et al. Benign and malignant adrenal masses: CT distinction with attenuation coefficients, size, and observer analysis. *Radiology*. 1991;179:415–418.
30. Caoili EM, et al. Adrenal masses: characterization with combined unenhanced and delayed enhanced CT. *Radiology*. 2002;222:629–633.
31. Jhaveri KS, Lad SV, Haider MA. Computed tomographic histogram analysis in the diagnosis of lipid-poor adenomas: comparison to adrenal washout computed tomography. *J Comput Assist Tomogr*. 2007;31:513–518.
32. Hamrahian AH, et al. Clinical utility of noncontrast computed tomography attenuation value (Hounsfield units) to differentiate adrenal adenomas/hyperplasias from nonadenomas: Cleveland Clinic experience. *J Clin Endocrinol Metab*. 2005;90:871–877.
33. Ng L, Libertino JM. Adrenocortical carcinoma: diagnosis, evaluation and treatment. *J Urol*. 2003;169:5–11.
34. Fishman EK, Deutch BM, Hartman DS, et al. Primary adrenal cortical carcinoma: CT evaluation with clinical correlation. *AJR Am J Roentgenol*. 1987;148:531–535.
35. Tsushima Y, Ishizaka H, Matsumoto M. Adrenal masses: differentiation with chemical shift, fast low-angle shot MR imaging. *Radiology*. 1993;186:705–709.
36. Mayo-Smith WW, et al. Characterization of adrenal masses (<5 cm) by use of chemical shift MR imaging: observer performance versus quantitative measures. *AJR Am J Roentgenol*. 1995;165:91–95.
37. Korobkin M, et al. Characterization of adrenal masses with chemical shift and gadolinium-enhanced MR imaging. *Radiology*. 1995;197:411–418.
38. Namimoto T, et al. Adrenal masses: quantification of fat content with double-echo chemical shift in-phase and opposed-phase FLASH MR images for differentiation of adrenal adenomas. *Radiology*. 2001;218:642–646.

39. Sasai N, et al. Differential diagnosis of adrenal masses by chemical shift and dynamic gadolinium enhanced MR imaging. *Acta Med Okayama*. 2003;57:163–170.
40. Fujiyoshi F, et al. Characterization of adrenal tumors by chemical shift fast low-angle shot MR imaging: comparison of four methods of quantitative evaluation. *AJR Am J Roentgenol*. 2003;180:1649–1657.
41. Heinz-Peer G, et al. Characterization of adrenal masses using MR imaging with histopathologic correlation. *AJR Am J Roentgenol*. 1999;173:15–22.
42. Outwater EK, et al. Adrenal masses: correlation between CT attenuation value and chemical shift ratio at MR imaging with in-phase and opposed-phase sequences. *Radiology*. 1996;200:749–752.
43. Outwater E, Siegelman ES, Radecki PD, et al. Distinction between benign and malignant adrenal masses: value of T1–weighted chemical-shift MR imaging. *AJR Am J Roentgenol*. 1995;165:579–583.
44. Goldfarb DA, et al. Magnetic resonance imaging for assessment of vena caval tumor thrombi: a comparative study with venacavography and computerized tomography scanning. *J Urol*. 1990;144: 1100–1103. discussion 1103–1104.
45. Fein AB, et al. Diagnosis and staging of renal cell carcinoma: a comparison of MR imaging and CT. *AJR Am J Roentgenol*. 1987;148:749–753.
46. Soler R, et al. MR imaging in inferior vena cava thrombosis. *Eur J Radiol*. 1995;19:101–107.
47. Schlund JF, et al. Adrenocortical carcinoma: MR imaging appearance with current techniques. *J Magn Reson Imaging*. 1995;5:171–174.
48. Trojan J, Schwarz W, Sarrazin C, et al. Role of ultrasonography in the detection of small adrenal masses. *Ultraschall Med*. 2002;23:96–100.
49. Friedrich-Rust M, et al. Contrast-enhanced sonography of adrenal masses: differentiation of adenomas and nonadenomatous lesions. *AJR Am J Roentgenol*. 2008;191:1852–1860.
50. Yun M, et al. ^{18}F-FDG PET in characterizing adrenal lesions detected on CT or MRI. *J Nucl Med*. 2001;42:1795–1799.
51. Gupta NC, et al. Clinical utility of PET-FDG imaging in differentiation of benign from malignant adrenal masses in lung cancer. *Clin Lung Cancer*. 2001;3:59–64.
52. Kumar R, et al. ^{18}F-FDG PET in evaluation of adrenal lesions in patients with lung cancer. *J Nucl Med*. 2004;45:2058–2062.
53. Jana S, et al. FDG-PET and CT characterization of adrenal lesions in cancer patients. *Eur J Nucl Med Mol Imaging*. 2006;33:29–35.
54. Guerin C, Pattou F, Brunaud L, et al. Performance of ^{18}F-FDG PET/CT in the Characterization of Adrenal Masses in Noncancer Patients: A Prospective Study. *J Clin Endocrinol Metab*. 2017 Jul 1;102(7):2465–2472.
55. Metser U, et al. ^{18}F-FDG PET/CT in the evaluation of adrenal masses. *J Nucl Med*. 2006;47:32–37.
56. Vikram R, et al. Utility of PET/CT in differentiating benign from malignant adrenal nodules in patients with cancer. *AJR Am J Roentgenol*. 2008;191:1545–1551.
57. Blake MA, et al. Adrenal lesions: characterization with fused PET/CT image in patients with proved or suspected malignancy–initial experience. *Radiology*. 2006;238:970–977.
58. Erasmus JJ, et al. Evaluation of adrenal masses in patients with bronchogenic carcinoma using ^{18}F-fluorodeoxyglucose positron emission tomography. *AJR Am J Roentgenol*. 1997;168:1357–1360.
59. Gross MD, et al. The scintigraphic imaging of endocrine organs. *Endocr Rev*. 1984;5:221–281.
60. Gross MD, et al. Scintigraphic evaluation of clinically silent adrenal masses. *J Nucl Med*. 1994;35:1145–1152.
61. Koh DM, Hughes M, Husband JE. Cross-sectional imaging of nodal metastases in the abdomen and pelvis. *Abdom Imaging*. 2006;31:632–643.
62. Gagliardi G, et al. Preoperative staging of rectal cancer using magnetic resonance imaging with external phase-arrayed coils. *Arch Surg*. 2002;137:447–451.
63. Anzai Y, et al. Evaluation of neck and body metastases to nodes with ferumoxtran 10–enhanced MR imaging: phase III safety and efficacy study. *Radiology*. 2003;228:777–788.
64. Sohn KM, et al. Comparing MR imaging and CT in the staging of gastric carcinoma. *AJR Am J Roentgenol*. 2000;174:1551–1557.
65. McMahon CJ, Rofsky NM, Pedrosa I. Lymphatic metastases from pelvic tumors: anatomic classification, characterization, and staging. *Radiology*. 2010;254:31–46.
66. Yang WT, et al. Comparison of dynamic helical CT and dynamic MR imaging in the evaluation of pelvic lymph nodes in cervical carcinoma. *AJR Am J Roentgenol*. 2000;175:759–766.
67. Brown G, et al. Morphologic predictors of lymph node status in rectal cancer with use of high-spatial-resolution MR imaging with histopathologic comparison. *Radiology*. 2003;227:371–377.
68. Veit P, et al. Lymph node staging with dual-modality PET/CT: enhancing the diagnostic accuracy in oncology. *Eur J Radiol*. 2006;58:383–389.
69. Antoch G, et al. Whole-body dual-modality PET/CT and whole-body MRI for tumor staging in oncology. *JAMA*. 2003;290:3199–3206.
70. Schmidt GP, et al. Comparison of high resolution whole-body MRI using parallel imaging and PET-CT. First experiences with a 32-channel MRI system [in German]. *Radiologe*. 2004;44:889–898.
71. Dickson PV, Kim L, Yen TWF, et al. Evaluation, staging, and surgical management for adrenocortical carcinoma: An update from the SSO Endocrine and Head and Neck Disease Site Working Group. *Ann Surg Oncol*. 2018;25(12):3460–3468.
72. Varghese J, Habra MA. Update on adrenocortical carcinoma management and future directions. *Curr Opin Endocrinol Diabetes Obes*. 2017;24(3):208–214.
73. Fassnacht M, Dekkers OM, Else T, et al. European Society of Endocrinology Clinical Practice Guidelines on the management of adrenocortical carcinoma in adults, in collaboration with the European Network for the Study of Adrenal Tumors. *Eur J Endocrinol*. 2018;179(4):G1–G46.
74. Leboulleux S, et al. Diagnostic and prognostic value of 18-fluorodeoxyglucose positron emission tomography in adrenocortical carcinoma: a prospective comparison with computed tomography. *J Clin Endocrinol Metab*. 2006;91:920–925.
75. Becherer A, et al. FDG-PET in adrenocortical carcinoma. *Cancer Biother Radiopharm*. 2001;16:289–295.
76. Pommier RF, Brennan MF. An eleven-year experience with adrenocortical carcinoma. *Surgery*. 1992;112:963–970. discussion 970-971.
77. Icard P, et al. Adrenocortical carcinoma in surgically treated patients: a retrospective study on 156 cases by the French Association of Endocrine Surgery. *Surgery*. 1992;112:972–979. discussion 979-980.
78. Crucitti F, et al. The Italian Registry for Adrenal Cortical Carcinoma: analysis of a multi-institutional series of 129 patients. The ACC Italian Registry Study Group. *Surgery*. 1996;119:161–170.
79. Lee JE, et al. Surgical management, DNA content, and patient survival in adrenal cortical carcinoma. *Surgery*. 1995;118:1090–1098.
80. Third national cancer survey. incidence data. *Natl Cancer Inst Monogr*. 1975;41:i-x-1,454.
81. Schulick RD, Brennan MF. Long-term survival after complete resection and repeat resection in patients with adrenocortical carcinoma. *Ann Surg Oncol*. 1999;6:719–726.
82. Grondal S, et al. Adrenocortical carcinoma. A retrospective study of a rare tumor with a poor prognosis. *Eur J Surg Oncol*. 1990;16:500–506.
83. Fassnacht M, et al. Efficacy of adjuvant radiotherapy of the tumor bed on local recurrence of adrenocortical carcinoma. *J Clin Endocrinol Metab*. 2006;91:4501–4504.
84. Hutter Jr AM, Kayhoe DE. Adrenal cortical carcinoma. Clinical features of 138 patients. *Am J Med*. 1966;41:572–580.
85. Markoe AM, et al. Radiation therapy for adjunctive treatment of adrenal cortical carcinoma. *Am J Clin Oncol*. 1991;14:170–174.
86. Barzon L, et al. Adrenocortical carcinoma: experience in 45 patients. *Oncology*. 1997;54:490–496.
87. Hoffman DL, Mattox VR. Treatment of adrenocortical carcinoma with o, p'-DDD. *Med Clin North Am*. 1972;56:999–1012.
88. Hutter Jr AM, Kayhoe DE. Adrenal cortical carcinoma. Results of treatment with o, p'DDD in 138 patients. *Am J Med*. 1966;41:581–592.
89. Favia G, et al. Adrenocortical carcinoma. *Our experience. Minerva Endocrinol*. 1995;20:95–99.
90. Khorram-Manesh A, et al. Adrenocortical carcinoma: surgery and mitotane for treatment and steroid profiles for follow-up. *World J Surg*. 1998;22:605–611. discussion 611-612.
91. van Slooten H, et al. The treatment of adrenocortical carcinoma with o, p'-DDD: prognostic implications of serum level monitoring. *Eur J Cancer Clin Oncol*. 1984;20:47–53.
92. Brennan MF. Adrenocortical carcinoma. *CA Cancer J Clin*. 1987;37:348–365.

93. Fassnacht M, Terzolo M, Allolio B, et al. Combination chemotherapy in advanced adrenocortical carcinoma. *N Engl J Med.* 2012;366(23):2189–2197.
94. Gicquel C, et al. Adrenocortical carcinoma. *Ann Oncol.* 1997;8:423–427.
95. Favier J, Amar L, Gimenez-Roqueplo AP. Paraganglioma and phaeochromocytoma: from genetics to personalized medicine. *Nat Rev Endocrinol.* 2015;11(2):101–111.
96. Beard CM, Scheps SG, Kurland LT, et al. Occurrence of pheochromocytoma in Rochester, Minnesota, 1950–1979. *Mayo Clin Proc.* 1983;58:802–804.
97. Kasperlik-Zaluska AA, et al. 1,111 patients with adrenal incidentalomas observed at a single endocrinological center: incidence of chromaffin tumors. *Ann N Y Acad Sci.* 2006;1073:38–46.
98. Neumann HP, et al. Germ-line mutations in nonsyndromic pheochromocytoma. *N Engl J Med.* 2002;346:1459–1466.
99. Amar L, et al. Genetic testing in pheochromocytoma or functional paraganglioma. *J Clin Oncol.* 2005;23:8812–8818.
100. Gimm O, et al. The genetic basis of pheochromocytoma. *Front Horm Res.* 2004;31:45–60.
101. Lenders JW, et al. Phaeochromocytoma. *Lancet.* 2005;366:665–675.
102. Whalen RK, Althausen AF, Daniels GH. Extra-adrenal pheochromocytoma. *J Urol.* 1992;147:1–10.
103. John H, et al. Pheochromocytomas: can malignant potential be predicted? *Urology.* 1999;53:679–683.
104. Eisenhofer G, et al. Malignant pheochromocytoma: current status and initiatives for future progress. *Endocr Relat Cancer.* 2004;11:423–436.
105. Kuruba R, Gallagher SF. Current management of adrenal tumors. *Curr Opin Oncol.* 2008;20:34–46.
106. Jimenez P, Tatsui C, Jessop A, et al. Treatment for malignant pheochromocytomas and paragangliomas: 5 years of progress. *Curr Oncol Rep.* 2017;19:83.
107. Goldstein RE, et al. Clinical experience over 48 years with pheochromocytoma. *Ann Surg.* 1999;229:755–764. discussion 764-766.
108. Zarnegar R, et al. Malignant pheochromocytoma. *Surg Oncol Clin North Am.* 2006;15:555–571.
109. Ilias I, et al. The optimal imaging of adrenal tumours: a comparison of different methods. *Endocr Relat Cancer.* 2007;14:587–599.
110. Mukherjee JJ, et al. Pheochromocytoma: effect of nonionic contrast medium in CT on circulating catecholamine levels. *Radiology.* 1997;202:227–231.
111. Sahdev A, Reznek RH. Imaging evaluation of the non-functioning indeterminate adrenal mass. *Trends Endocrinol Metab.* 2004;15:271–276.
112. Horton KM, Johnson PT, Fishman EK. MDCT of the abdomen: common misdiagnoses at a busy academic center. *AJR Am J Roentgenol.* 2010;194:660–667.
113. Bush WH, et al. Cystic pheochromocytoma. *Urology.* 1985;25:332–334.
114. Rha SE, et al. Neurogenic tumors in the abdomen: tumor types and imaging characteristics. *Radiographics.* 2003;23:29–43.
115. Francis IR, Korobkin M. Pheochromocytoma. *Radiol Clin North Am.* 1996;34:1101–1112.
116. Shulkin B, et al. Current trends in functional imaging of pheochromocytomas and paragangliomas. *Ann N Y Acad Sci.* 2006;1073:374–382.
117. Velchik MG, et al. Localization of pheochromocytoma: MIBG [correction of MIGB], CT, and MRI correlation. *J Nucl Med.* 1989;30:328–336.
118. Quint LE, et al. Pheochromocytoma and paraganglioma: comparison of MR imaging with CT and I-131 MIBG scintigraphy. *Radiology.* 1987;165:89–93.
119. Lauriero F, et al. I-131 MIBG scintigraphy of neuroectodermal tumors. Comparison between I-131 MIBG and In-111 DTPA-octreotide. *Clin Nucl Med.* 1995;20:243–249.
120. Hoefnagel CA. Metaiodobenzylguanidine and somatostatin in oncology: role in the management of neural crest tumours. *Eur J Nucl Med.* 1994;21:561–581.
121. Cecchin D, et al. A meta-iodobenzylguanidine scintigraphic scoring system increases accuracy in the diagnostic management of pheochromocytoma. *Endocr Relat Cancer.* 2006;13:525–533.
122. Ilias I, et al. Comparison of $^{6\text{-}18}$F-fluorodopamine PET with ^{123}I-metaiodobenzylguanidine and ^{111}In-pentetreotide scintigraphy in localization of nonmetastatic and metastatic pheochromocytoma. *J Nucl Med.* 2008;49:1613–1619.
123. Taïeb D, Hicks RJ, Hindié E, et al. European Association of Nuclear Medicine Practice Guideline/Society of Nuclear Medicine and Molecular Imaging Procedure Standard 2019 for radionuclide imaging of phaeochromocytoma and paraganglioma. *Eur J Nucl Med Mol Imaging.* 2019;46(10):2112–2137.
124. Mann GN, et al. [11C]metahydroxyephedrine and [18F]fluorodeoxyglucose positron emission tomography improve clinical decision making in suspected pheochromocytoma. *Ann Surg Oncol.* 2006;13:187–197.
125. Hoegerle S, et al. Pheochromocytomas: detection with 18F DOPA whole body PET—initial results. *Radiology.* 2002;222:507–512.
126. Lynn MD, et al. Bone metastases in pheochromocytoma: comparative studies of efficacy of imaging. *Radiology.* 1986;160:701–706.
127. Bravo EL. Evolving concepts in the pathophysiology, diagnosis, and treatment of pheochromocytoma. *Endocr Rev.* 1994;15:356–368.
128. Mannelli M, et al. Pheochromocytoma in Italy: a multicentric retrospective study. *Eur J Endocrinol.* 1999;141:619–624.
129. Maurea S, et al. Diagnostic imaging in patients with paragangliomas. Computed tomography, magnetic resonance and MIBG scintigraphy comparison. *Q J Nucl Med.* 1996;40:365–371.
130. Schmedtje Jr JF, et al. Localization of ectopic pheochromocytomas by magnetic resonance imaging. *Am J Med.* 1987;83:770–772.
131. Kopf D, Goretzki PE, Lehnert H. Clinical management of malignant adrenal tumors. *J Cancer Res Clin Oncol.* 2001;127:143–155.
132. Sisson JC. Radiopharmaceutical treatment of pheochromocytomas. *Ann N Y Acad Sci.* 2002;970:54–60.
133. Troncone L, Rufini V. Nuclear medicine therapy of pheochromocytoma and paraganglioma. *Q J Nucl Med.* 1999;43:344–355.
134. Tato A, et al. Malignant pheochromocytoma, still a therapeutic challenge. *Am J Hypertens.* 1997;10:479–481.
135. Noshiro T, et al. Two cases of malignant pheochromocytoma treated with cyclophosphamide, vincristine and dacarbazine in a combined chemotherapy. *Endocr J.* 1996;43:279–284.
136. Scholz T, et al. Clinical review: current treatment of malignant pheochromocytoma. *J Clin Endocrinol Metab.* 2007;92:1217–1225.
137. Benn DE, et al. Clinical presentation and penetrance of pheochromocytoma/paraganglioma syndromes. *J Clin Endocrinol Metab.* 2006;91:827–836.

CHAPTER

23 Prostate Cancer

Vikas Kundra, M.D., Ph.D.; Lisly J Chery, M.D.; and Karen Hoffman, M.D.

INTRODUCTION

Prostate cancer is the most commonly diagnosed cancer among American men. For prostate cancer, imaging is crucial in assessing both primary disease and metastasis. Imaging is used in diagnosis, staging, pretreatment planning, disease surveillance, and monitoring response to treatment. Imaging is playing an increasing role in disease detection, including location within the gland, and guiding biopsies. Traditional roles continue to include defining intra- versus extraprostatic tumor for local staging and assessing metastatic disease, which most commonly affects lymph nodes and the skeleton. Monitoring therapeutic response and recurrence are also essential functions. For the latter, clinical features such as prostate-specific antigen (PSA) velocity can help guide whether to search for recurrence locally or at distant sites. Most radiologic methods are applied in prostate cancer. The choice of modality depends on the clinical question being addressed. For example, ultrasound is commonly used for guiding biopsies; magnetic resonance imaging (MRI) can be applied for most clinical questions including for evaluating the primary tumor, metastasis, and recurrence; and computed tomography (CT) and nuclear medicine methods are most commonly used in the setting of metastatic disease. Nuclear medicine positron emission tomography (PET) imaging is beginning to play an increasing role in evaluating recurrence.

Epidemiology and Risk Factors

Prostate cancer has the highest incidence and is the second most common cause of cancer death among American men.[1] Risk factors for prostate cancer include age, race, and family history. The majority of cases are diagnosed in men older than 65 years.[2] The disease is more common in men of African descent, with 60% higher incidence compared to White people.[1] The introduction of PSA screening led to a dramatic increase in prostate cancer diagnosis in the late 1980s and early 1990s. Owing to a change in the recommendation for PSA screening in 2012, PSA testing and prostate cancer diagnosis has declined in recent years.[1] The 51% decrease in prostate cancer mortality between 1993 and 2016 is caused by a combination of increased screening and advances in treatment options.[1] Family history, particularly in first-degree relatives, has been shown to be a risk factor in several studies.[3,4] Patients with Lynch syndrome or *BRCA1/2* mutations also have an increased risk of developing prostate cancer.[5,6]

Anatomy and Histology

The prostate gland is bounded superiorly at its base by the urinary bladder and inferiorly by the urogenital membrane. It is encircled by the levator ani bilaterally, the symphysis pubis anteriorly, and the rectum posteriorly. In the model by McNeal and coworkers,[7] the prostate gland is divided into four zones—the transition zone (TZ), the central zone, the peripheral zone (PZ), and the nonglandular anterior fibromuscular stroma (Fig. 23.1)—that contain 5%, 20%, 70% to 80%, and 0% of glandular tissue and 25%, 5%, 70%, and 0% of prostate cancers, respectively. Cancers resolvable by conventional imaging are primarily within the PZ. The TZ is most susceptible to age-related benign prostatic hyperplasia (BPH). Normally, it composes only 5% to 10% of the total glandular tissue of the prostate, but in older men with BPH it can compose the majority of prostate tissue. The TZ is often difficult to separate from the central zone by imaging, and on images the two together are often referred to as the central gland or zone. The central zone is cone-shaped, with its widest portion at the base of the bladder and its apex at the verumontanum. The seminal vesicles are located posterior and superior to the prostate gland and give off the ejaculatory ducts, which traverse the central zone, providing a conduit for seminal fluid from the seminal vesicles to the urethra. The relative amount of PZ to central zone increases from the base of the gland to the apex of the gland. Inferiorly, the PZ comprises all of the prostatic glandular tissue at the apex, and superiorly it invests the posterior and lateral portions of the central zone.

The prostate encases the majority of the posterior urethra termed the prostatic urethra. Voiding is controlled by two sphincters, one at the base of the bladder (a functional but not anatomically distinct sphincter) and the other located at the level of the urogenital diaphragm (the external striated sphincter) that surrounds the membranous urethra, located just beyond the apex of the prostate. The former is under autonomic control and provides the majority of continence in unoperated men. The external striated sphincter is largely under voluntary control. After prostatectomy, the external striated sphincter becomes the primary control mechanism of continence unless preservation of the bladder neck was possible during surgery.

The prostate gland is partially invested by a coalition of fibrous tissue, historically called the "capsule," that is most apparent posteriorly and posterolaterally. The capsule is an important landmark for assessing extraprostatic tumor

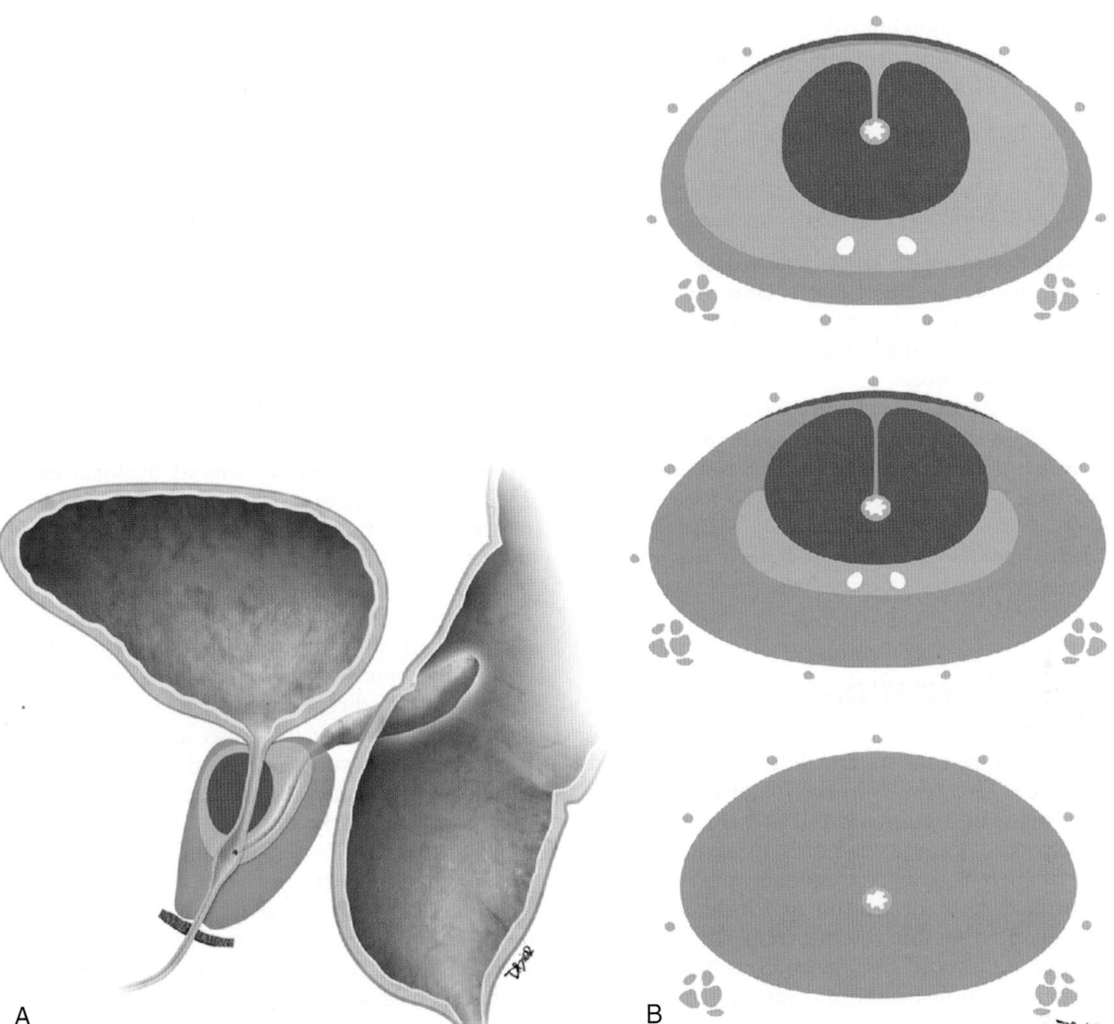

FIGURE 23.1. Prostate gland anatomy. **A**, Sagittal view. **B**, Axial view: top, base; middle, midgland; bottom, apex.

extension (EPE). The neurovascular bundles course posterolateral to the prostate capsule and are seen more prominently bilaterally at 5 and 7 o'clock (see Fig. 23.1). At the apex and the base, the bundles send penetrating branches through the capsule, providing a route for EPE. The normal fat plane between the prostate gland and the neurovascular bundles seen on imaging is lost when there is neurovascular involvement by prostate carcinoma. Whereas perineural invasion by prostate cancer on biopsies does not seem to correlate with positive margins or poorer survival, it may be indicative of EPE.[8,9] Identifying tumor involvement of the neurovascular bundles is important when planning for nerve-sparing prostatectomy. The neurovascular bundles run within the substance of the parietal pelvic fascia, also termed the lateral prostatic fascia. During nerve-sparing radical prostatectomy, this fascia is incised anterior to the bundles and reflected off the prostate capsule.

Histologically, 95% of prostate cancers are adenocarcinomas that develop from the acini of the prostatic ducts. Other histologic types include small-cell carcinoma (the most common variant); mucinous, ductal, squamous, sarcomatoid, and transitional cell carcinomas; adenoid basal cell tumors; and malignant mesenchymal tumors.[10]

In the United States, histologic evaluation of prostate adenocarcinomas is performed using the Gleason grading system. Tumors are assigned a primary grade on the basis of the predominant pattern of differentiation and a secondary grade on the basis of the second most common pattern. The two numbers are added to produce a Gleason score. For example, a tumor described as "Gleason grade 3 + 4 or 4 + 3" will have a Gleason score of "7."[1] The biologic behavior of a Gleason score 4 + 3 is more aggressive than 3 + 4, regardless of the number of cores.[12]

Cancers with Gleason scores of 6 or lower are considered well-differentiated and are associated with a good prognosis. Those with a Gleason score of 8 to 10 have the worst prognosis and the highest risk for recurrence.[11] Tumors with Gleason scores of 7 have a variable prognosis and an intermediate risk of recurrence. Serum PSA is not useful in uncommon high-grade tumors that do not produce PSA.[11] Prostate cancer tends to be multifocal, and the Gleason score at biopsy may differ from that obtained at surgery.[12]

In 2014, the International Society of Urologic Pathology released a Grade Group system that is derived from the Gleason score.[13] The Grade Group system is an attempt to simplify the reporting system for patients and to better convey risk stratification of tumors. It has been validated in a large cohort study, showing risk of 5-year biochemical recurrence-free progression dropping from 96% in Grade Group 1 to 26% in Grade Group 5.[14]

KEY POINTS Anatomy and Histology

- The prostate is divided into the central zone and the peripheral zone. By imaging, the peripheral zone is better evaluable for tumor.
- The base of the gland is near the bladder neck, and the apex is near the urogenital diaphragm.
- The neurovascular bundles are at 5 and 7 o'clock.
- Histology is defined by the Gleason score, which consists of two numbers added. The predominant type goes first, for example, 4 + 3 indicates a Gleason score of 7, with the predominant type being 4.
- The histologic Grade Group system is predictive of recurrence.

CLINICAL PRESENTATION

Over 90% of prostate cancers are detected at the local or regional stage.[2] This results in the majority of cancers being asymptomatic at presentation. If present, symptoms are often nonspecific. Patients can present with local urinary symptoms such as urinary frequency, urgency, hesitancy, slow urinary flow, or painful urination. However, these are usually attributable to coexistent BPH. Distant symptoms from metastatic disease such as pelvic bone pain or back pain are nonspecific and can be attributed to benign causes.

The prostate cancer is often detected as a result of elevated PSA, abnormal digital rectal examination (DRE), or abnormal imaging finding. PSA is produced by both malignant and benign prostate cells and is not specific for prostate cancer. Risk of prostate cancer increases with PSA level, but there is not an absolute number that signifies a lack of cancer.[15,16] In recent years, several serum-based tests have been developed to help determine indications for biopsy. The 4K score uses total PSA, free PSA, intact PSA, and kallikrein-related peptidase 2 levels to determine prostate cancer risk,[17] the Prostate Health index uses [-2] pro-PSA, total PSA, and free PSA,[18] ExoDx uses urine exosome RNA levels of the *ERG*, *PCA3*, and *SPDEF* genes,[19] and SelectMDx uses urine RNA levels of the *HOXC4*, *HOXC6*, *TDRD1*, *DLX1*, *KLK3*, and *PCA3* genes.[20] There is no consensus on which tests to use, and there are few data comparing these tests against one another.

Regarding early detection of prostate cancer, universal PSA screening is no longer recommended. Informed decision making is the preferred recommendation of the American Cancer Society[21], the American Urological Association,[22] and the United States Preventative Services Task Force.[23] This entails an individual patient weighing the risks and benefits of prostate cancer screening. These guidelines only recommend screening for men aged 55 to 69 years at normal risk for prostate cancer, with a life expectancy greater than 10 years.

KEY POINTS Clinical Presentation

- The patient is often asymptomatic or may have nonspecific symptoms such as pain related to voiding for local disease or bone pain for metastatic disease.
- Men aged 55 to 69 years should partake in shared decision-making regarding prostate cancer screening.
- Protein-specific antigen is the most common screening evaluation, but several new tests are available for use.

PATTERNS OF TUMOR SPREAD

Prostate cancer tends to spread by local extension (Fig. 23.2). EPE tends to be seen at 5 and 7 o'clock, where the neurovascular bundles send penetrating branches through the capsule. This also provides a route for neurovascular bundle involvement. Further lateral growth may involve the levator ani and then the pelvic sidewalls. Tumor may also spread superiorly to involve the seminal vesicles (either by direct extension or via the ejaculatory ducts) or the bladder, by direct extension or via the urethra. Superior and inferior growth may also involve the two sphincters for micturation, superiorly at the base of the bladder and inferiorly at the urogenital diaphragm. Rarely, the tumor may grow inferiorly along the urethra beyond the membranous urethra. Posteriorly and uncommonly, the tumor may involve the rectum.

Metastases to regional lymph nodes (Fig. 23.3) occurs most commonly along the obturator chain (medial to external iliac area) but also occurs along other regional nodes such as along the internal iliac, external iliac, and presacral chains.[24] Lymph node metastases may also occur along nonregional lymph nodes such as the common iliac and retroperitoneum chains. Skip metastases to the retroperitoneum may occur in the absence of pelvic lymphatic metastasis. After lymph node resection or radiation therapy to the pelvis, recurrence may occur, particularly in retroperitoneal nodes outside the treated field. Hematogenous metastases (see Fig. 23.3) tend to occur primarily to the skeleton and are usually blastic. Lytic lesions may be seen with advanced disease. Occasionally, spinal metastases may cause cord compression. Metastases to other organs are associated with advanced disease and are rare; if found, such metastases may suggest less differentiated forms of prostate cancer or another primary cancer.

KEY POINTS Tumor Spread

- EPE most commonly occurs at 5 and 7 o'clock; therefore, it can involve the neurovascular bundles.
- Seminal vesicles or other adjacent organs such as bladder and rectum are less commonly involved.
- Lymphatic metastases are usually to intrapelvic lymph nodes, but skip metastases to retroperitoneal lymph nodes may occur.
- Hematogenous metastases are most commonly to bone, and these are most commonly sclerotic.

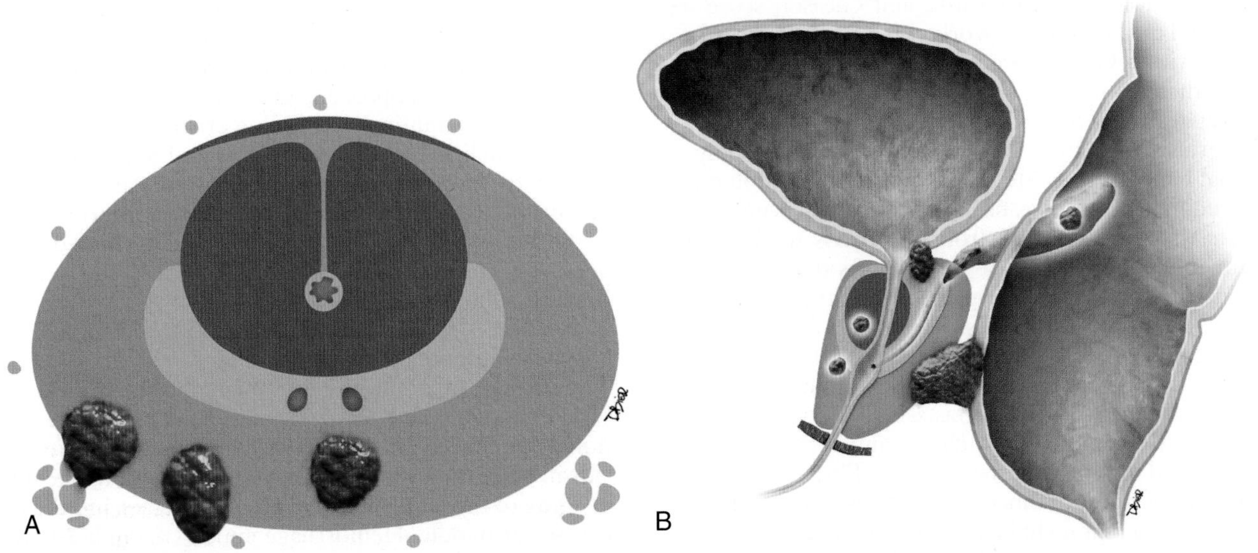

FIGURE 23.2. Prostate cancer local extension. **A**, Axial view. Prostate cancer may be organ-confined (T1 and T2) or may spread via extracapsular extension (T3a). Local extension tends to occur at 5 or 7 o'clock, where the neurovascular bundles are located. Thus, with extraprostatic extension, one may also see neurovascular bundle invasion (T3a). **B**, Sagittal view. Tumors may be within the peripheral zone, the central zone, or both. Standard T2-weighted magnetic imaging tends to visualize tumors in the peripheral zone, where approximately 70% of prostate cancers reside. New functional sequences show promise for evaluating tumors in the imaging central zone (anatomic transitional and central zone). With more advanced disease, spread occurs to adjacent organs such as the seminal vesicles (T3b) or other adjacent structures such as the bladder, rectum, external sphincter, levator muscles, or pelvic wall (T4).

STAGING

The primary goals of staging are, in general, to allow for risk stratification and allocation to reasonable treatment strategies. Specifically, this involves distinguishing patients with organ-confined, locally invasive, or metastatic disease and assessing risk of treatment failure. Risk-stratification guides therapy and integrates PSA; tumor-node-metastasis (TNM) clinical staging; and biopsy data including Gleason score, number of positive cores, and amount of cancer in each core.

Local Staging (T)

Although local tumor staging (see Fig. 23.2) is based upon findings from DRE, imaging can be beneficial. Stage T1 describes incidental detection of cancer. For example, stages T1a and T1b may be noted in specimens from transurethral resection of the prostate performed for BPH. Stage T1c describes prostate cancer detected by elevated PSA, but not palpable by DRE. Cancer palpable by DRE but confined within the prostatic capsule is considered T2. Cancer extending beyond the capsule is considered T3. This latter group includes EPE, periprostatic neurovascular involvement, and/or seminal vesicle involvement. Stage T4 describes tumor extending to other adjacent structures.[25]

Metastatic Disease (N and M Staging)

Prostate cancer may metastasize by lymphatic or hematogenous routes. The incidence of metastatic disease is extremely low in patients with stage T1 to T2 disease,

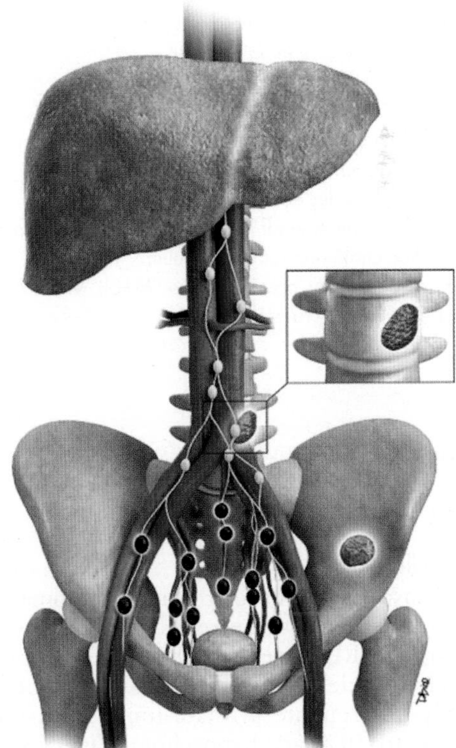

FIGURE 23.3. Metastatic disease. Prostate cancer metastasizes primarily to lymph nodes and bone. Metastasis to regional lymph nodes along the obturator, internal iliac, external iliac, and presacral chains is considered N1 disease (*black lymph nodes*). Metastasis to nonregional lymph nodes such as common illiac or retroperitoneum chains is considered M1a disease (*yellow lymph nodes*). Metastasis to bone is considered M1b disease. Metastases to the viscera (with or without bone metastasis) is rare and is considered M1c.

serum PSA less than 20 ng/mL, and Gleason score less than 8.[26] Thus, metastatic workup is usually reserved for patients with a Gleason score greater than 7, serum PSA greater than 20 ng/mL, stage greater than T2, or symptoms suggestive of metastasis.[26]

Metastasis (see Fig. 23.3) occurs most commonly to regional lymph nodes. Metastasis to inguinal lymph nodes is exceedingly rare. It has been suggested that lymph node metastasis occurs stepwise from the pelvis to the retroperitoneum[27]; however, there are reports that up to 50% of nodal metastases can be paraaortic without a concurrent pelvic nodal metastasis, suggesting hematogenous rather than lymphatic spread,[28] likely via Bateson's plexus. Importantly, at staging, nodal disease within the pelvis is considered regional nodal metastasis (N1), whereas nodal disease in the common iliac chains and retroperitoneum is considered distant metastasis (M1a). This, as well as the propensity of prostate cancer to metastasize to the lumbar spine, suggests that including the abdomen may be helpful when performing prostate MRI, or this area may be evaluated by CT.[29]

Hematogenous metastasis to bone occurs most frequently to the lumbar spine, pelvis, ribs, and femoral heads (M1b). In advanced disease (M1c), viscera more commonly involved include the liver, adrenal glands, and lungs.[25,26]

Key Points Staging

- T2 and T3 lesions may be visualized by imaging, most commonly by magnetic resonance imaging (MRI).
- T4 disease may be visualized by computed tomography and MRI.
- T3 includes extraprostatic tumor extension and microscopic invasion of the bladder neck and seminal vesicles.
- Regional lymph nodes encompass N1.
- M1a includes nonregional lymph nodes, including along the common iliac chain and retroperitoneum.
- Metastases commonly occur to bone (M1b), whereas visceral metastases (M1c) are rare.

IMAGING

Imaging in Local Staging

Transrectal Ultrasound

In patients suspected to have prostate carcinoma, diagnosis is generally made by transrectal ultrasound (TRUS)-guided biopsy. TRUS uses a high-frequency transducer (7–10 MHz) to delineate zonal anatomy, but it cannot reliably differentiate prostate tumors,[30] as approximately 40% to 50% are hypoechoic (Figs. 23.4), 40% are isoechoic, and others are hyperechoic.[31] Random biopsies are used. Traditionally, this employed a systemic sextant (six-site) approach in which a parasagittal plane guided three cores of each lobe (base, midgland, and apex), yielding an approximately 25% cancer detection rate when serum PSA was between 4 and 20 ng/mL.[32] Repeat biopsy demonstrated cancer in approximately 20% of men with persistently elevated serum PSA and negative initial biopsy.[33,34] Thus, more cores were tried. Presti and colleagues[35] achieved approximately 40% yield using a 10-core approach; even more cores have been advocated[36] to minimize sampling errors. Adding vascular imaging such as Doppler was not found to improve upon systematic biopsy in diagnosing prostate cancer.[37] Intravenous sonographic contrast agents can improve sensitivity; however, their role is yet to be determined. It has been reported that TRUS can detect EPE, but accuracy remains suboptimal.[38,39]

Magnetic Resonance Imaging

The prostate anatomically is evaluated using T1-weighted (T1W) imaging and T2-weighted (T2W) imaging. Functional sequences aid in tumor detection. T1W imaging aids in evaluation of the margins of the prostate, including imaging of the fat plane between the prostate and the neurovascular bundle. Hemorrhage appears as high T1 signal and can confound interpretation such as on T2W and diffusion-weighted imaging (DWI). Underlying hemorrhage secondary to biopsy, prostatitis, atrophy, or posttreatment change can present with low T2 signal intensity. Although there is variability, most centers wait to image approximately 5 to 6 weeks postbiopsy to allow hemorrhage to subside. Unlike T1W imaging, T2W imaging separates the low-signal TZ from the normally high–T2-signal PZ (Fig. 23.5). Often, the anatomic central and transitional zones cannot be distinguished by imaging; thus, this area is often referred to as the MRI central zone or TZ, with the latter now more commonly used. The TZ commonly contains heterogeneous, nodular areas of BPH. Collagen fibers may result in linear, low–T1-signal areas in the PZ. Tumors are more apparent on T2W imaging, and present as round or lenticular areas in the PZ and as smudges in the central zone. MRI has greater sensitivity and specificity for tumor in the PZ than in the central zone. The neurovascular bundles appear as linear low signal structures at 5 and 7 o'clock on T1W and T2W imaging. The seminal vesicles have low signal on T1- and high signal on T2W imaging, unless there is hemorrhage, which can increase T1 signal and confound T2 signal. To calculate prostate volume, the formula for a prolate ellipse is commonly used (anteroposterior × transverse × cephalocaudal × 0.52).

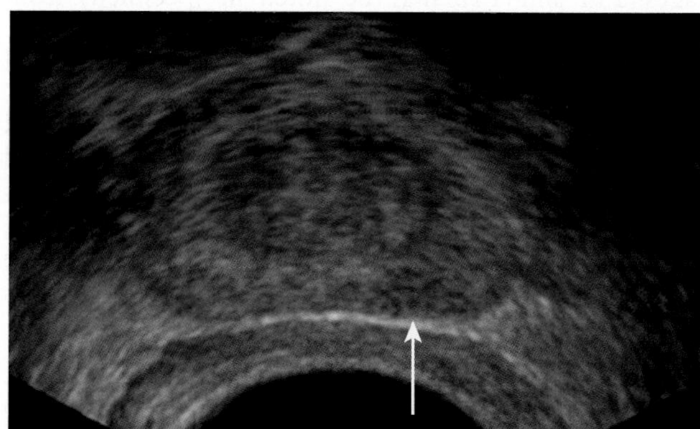

Figure 23.4. Axial prostate ultrasound demonstrates a hypoechoic area (*arrow*) in the peripheral zone suspicious for prostate cancer.

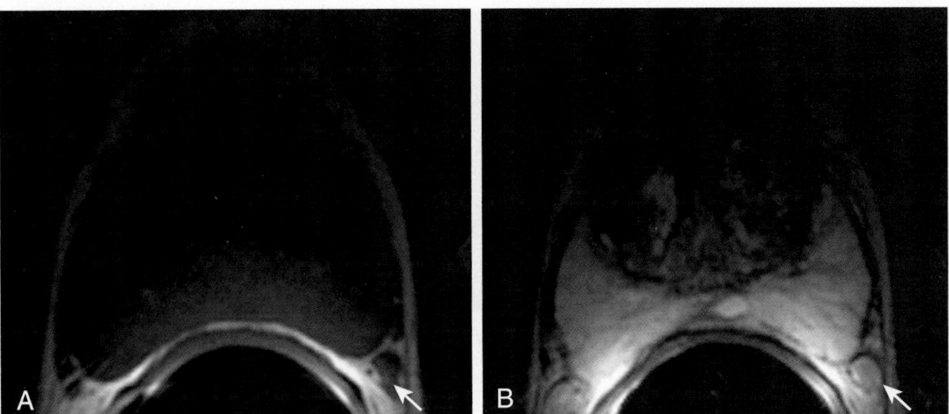

FIGURE 23.5. Normal prostate anatomy by axial magnetic resonance imaging. The peripheral zone and central zone are not distinguishable by T1-weighted (T1W) imaging (**A**) but are by T2-weighted imaging (**B**). The neurovascular bundles are seen at 5 and 7 o'clock. The fat plane between the neurovascular bundle (*arrow*) and the prostate is commonly better seen on T1W images.

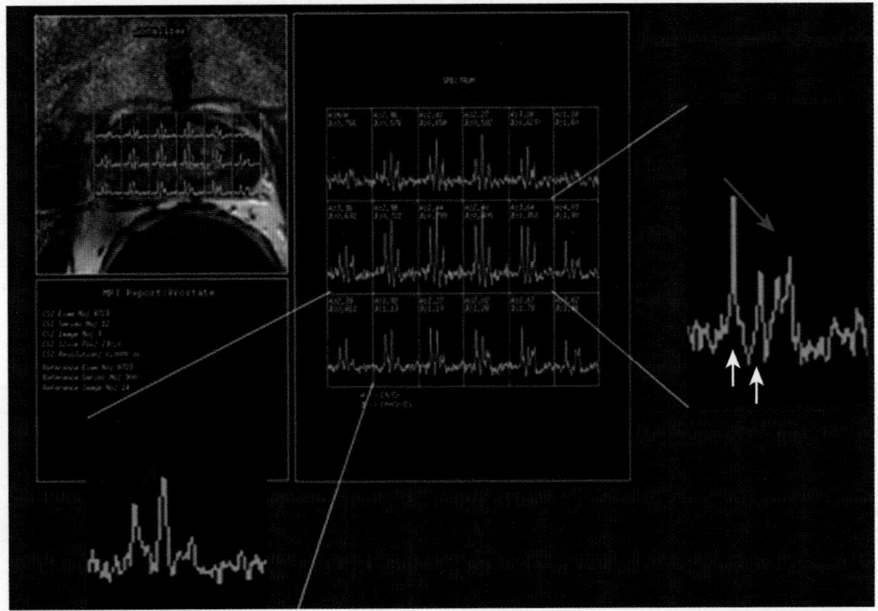

FIGURE 23.6. Magnetic resonance imaging spectroscopy. Choline, creatine, and citrate peaks are commonly used to distinguish prostate cancer. **Right**, Choline and creatine peak is elevated relative to citrate peak, implying prostate cancer. **Left**, Choline and creatine peak is low relative to citrate peak, implying normal prostate tissue.

Detection

Multiparametric MRI (mpMRI) is used for detecting prostate cancer. The primary sequences used for detecting tumor in the prostate are DWI,[40] T2WI, and dynamic contrast-enhanced (DCE) imaging. Apparent diffusion coefficient (ADC) is a quantitative measure of diffusion derived from DWI. Spectroscopy (Fig. 23.6) was for a short time US Food and Drug Administration (FDA)-approved for this application, but is no longer used, although studies using this technique continue. T1W axial images are employed to screen the pelvic nodes and bones for metastasis and to identify hemorrhage (Fig. 23.7) in the prostate gland. Performing axial T1W and T2W images with the same slice thickness and field of view allows alignment of the two sequences, which can aid in distinguishing tumor from hemorrhage. Typically, the central gland is heterogeneous on T2W imaging owing to BPH and is isointense on T1W imaging. In the central zone, it is difficult to separate cancer from the BPH that invariably occurs in this age group. In comparison, the PZ is relatively homogeneous and hyperintense on T2W imaging and isointense on T1W imaging. In the PZ, prostate tumors appear hypointense on T2W imaging and isointense on T1W imaging (Fig. 23.8). However, low T2W signal is not specific for cancer. Prostatitis can lead to decreased signal on T2W imaging but tends to be diffuse and not focal as in tumor.

Metaanalyses suggest that all three methods, and primarily two, have similar performance, as assessed by (ROC) analysis.[41,42] Both DWI and DCE had high specificity. Sensitivity increased by combining two sequences, but adding a third sequence did not increase sensitivity, and a combination of DWI and T2W imaging was favored.[27,28] DCE can be evaluated visually or semiquantitatively to derive parameters such as k_{trans}; no significant

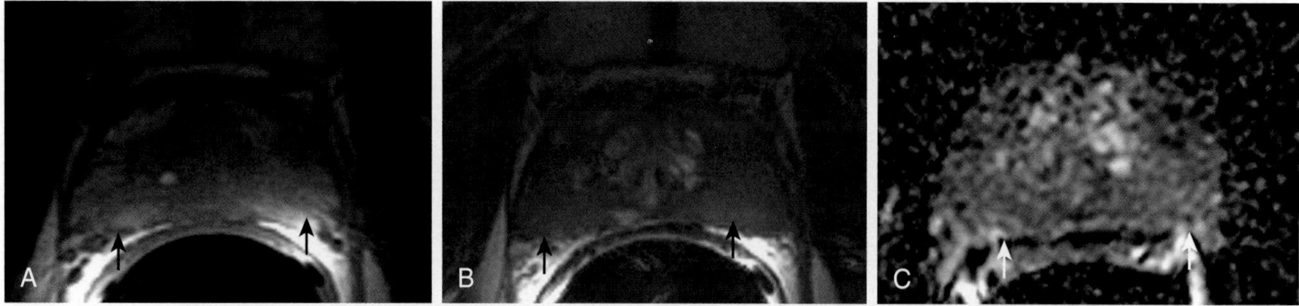

Figure 23.7. Hemorrhage (*arrows*) seen as increased signal on T1-weighted images (**A**), decreased signal on T2-weighted images (**B**), and apparent diffusion coefficient reconstruction (**C**), confounding interpretation.

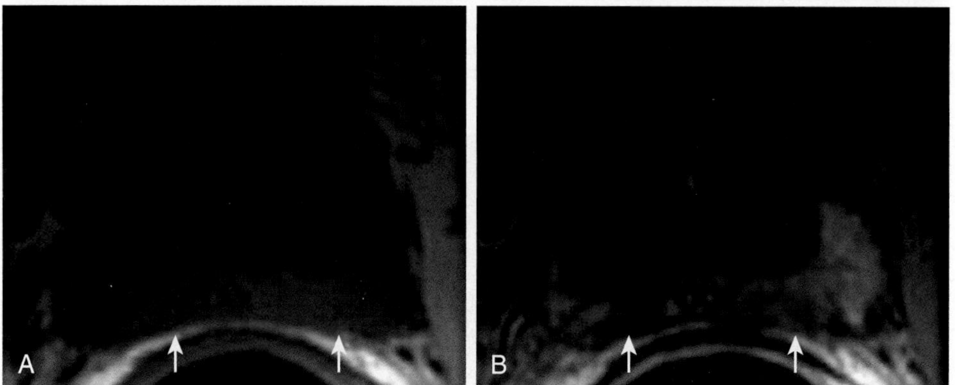

Figure 23.8. Focal prostate cancer (*arrows*) presenting as intermediate signal on T1-weighted axial magnetic resonance imaging (MRI) (**A**) and low signal on T2-weighted axial MRI (**B**). Notice that prostate cancer is often multifocal.

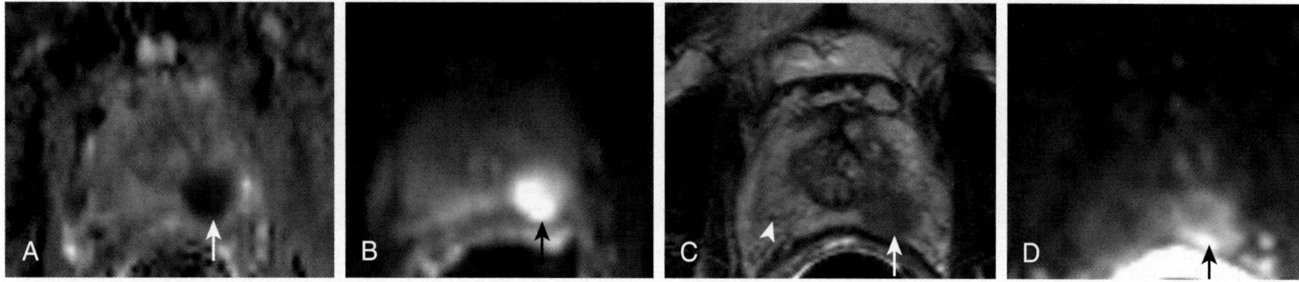

Figure 23.9. Peripheral zone prostate tumor (*arrow*) seen as low signal on apparent diffusion coefficient (**A**), increased signal on diffusion0weighted imaging (**B**), low signal on T2-weighted imaging (**C**), and enhancement on dynamic contrast-enhanced (**D**). Linear or band-like areas (*arrow*) can be seen in normal prostate peripheral zone but tend to be more marked and diffuse with current or prior prostatitis.

difference was found in the ROC curves, suggesting that visual evaluation of the enhancement is similar to more computer-intensive semiquantitative methods.[28] The likelihood of prostate cancer within the prostate using T2W DWI with ADC reconstruction and DCE can be categorized using the Likert scale (from 0 [unlikely] to 5 [highly likely]).

A standardized report, Prostate Imaging Reporting and Data System (PIRADS), has been proposed for detecting prostate cancer; version v2.1 was published in 2019. The report suggests minimal acceptable acquisition parameters and a reading method. It recommends waiting 6 weeks postbiopsy for imaging if possible, states that 1.5 T or 3 T scanners are acceptable, and advises that there is no consensus on endorectal coils for detection, but that endorectal coils are recommended for older 1.5 T systems.[43] Endorectal coils may be advantageous for increased signal-to-noise ratio, particularly for DWI and for staging, particularly with balloon distension to better separate the neurovascular bundles from the prostate gland. For interpretation, PIRADS is divided into five categories, with 1 being very low, 3 intermediate, and 5 very high clinical suspicion of prostate cancer. A dominant sequence strategy is used for interpretation. For the PZ (Fig. 23.9) it is DWI. Interpretation is usually of the ADC, where tumor appears to have low signal, and, if available, of a late B_0 DWI ($\geq$1400 sec/mm^2), where the tumor appears to have high signal. The latter is commonly calculated (synthetic) instead of directly measured because of signal loss. PIRADS 1 is normal, 2 is linear or wedge-shaped, 3 is focal, 4 is focal with marked signal change and less than 1.5 cm, and 5 is great than 1.5 cm. If the lesion is equivalent (PIRADS 3), enhancement on DCE increase score to 4; otherwise there is no change. DCE is considered positive if there is focal enhancement earlier than or contemporaneous with adjacent tissue and corresponds to suspicious DWI or T2 lesion. T2 is not used in the PZ unless DWI is not available, and DCE is used as above if available. If T2 is used, 1 is normal, 2 is linear or wedge-shaped, 3 is heterogeneous rounded, 4 is a rounded homogeneous mass less than 1.5 cm, and 5 is greater than 1.5 cm. For TZ (Fig. 23.10) T2 is dominant, and DCE is not used. Differentiating from BPH is the main difficulty. For TZ, T2 1 is normal, 2 is mostly encapsulated and homogeneous, 3 is heterogeneous with obscured margins, 4 is lenticular or noncircumscribed less than 1.5 cm, and 5 is greater than or equal to 1.5cm or definite EPE. PIRADS 1 is normal, T2 of 2 and DWI less than or equal to 3 is 2, T2 of 2 and DWI greater than or equal to 4 or T2 of 3 and DWI less than or equal to 4 is 3, T2 of 3 and DWI of 5 or T2 of 4 and any DWI is 4, and T2 of 5 and any DWI is 5.

PIRADS uses imaging alone and does not incorporate clinical data such as PSA or a radiologist's experience, which can both be a positive and a negative. It was created to make more consistent reads, but prior versions of PIRADS were found to have interreader agreement scores (kappa) equal to or lower than Likert,[44] and evaluations of version 2 found kappa values of 0.46 to 0.81 at single institutions[45–50] and 0.52 (moderate) in a multiinstitutional study.[51] Version 2 was noted to have greater sensitivity in the CZ but less specificity in the PZ compared with version 1. From version 1 to 2, spectroscopy was removed, and dominant sequence was introduced: DWI for PZ and T2 for CZ.[52] PIRADS v2.1 primarily clarified benign PIRADS 2 findings. New studies have suggested that biparametric MRI without DCE but with T2 and DWI may be sufficient.[53–57] Diagnostic ability improves with reader experience.[58]

Among benign mimics, BPH presents as homogeneous or heterogeneous well-defined nodules in the central zone (see Fig. 23.10). Occasionally, these will herniate into the PZ. These can have low ADC signal and can enhance confounding distinction from a central zone tumor. Unlike prostate cancer, prostatitis, if seen, commonly presents on T2W imaging as diffuse or band-like low signal instead of an oval or lenticular signal (see Fig. 23.9). Wedge or band-like abnormalities may also be seen with atrophy and fibrosis.

MRI/ultrasound fusion and in-bore MRI are being used to guide biopsy. The former is more widely used. Image-guided biopsy can improve detection of "significant," higher Gleason grade lesions that are more likely to affect the patient, although a fraction of such lesions are only detected by random biopsy. Siddiqui reported detection sensitivities of 77%, 53%, and 85% for intermediate to high-risk prostate cancer by MRI/ultrasound fusion, random extended sextant, and combined, respectively, whereas the negative predictive values (NPVs) were 70%, 53%, and 73%, suggesting that more, but not all, "significant" lesions are detected by the fusion method, and that negative biopsy has strong NPV, but does not exclude prostate cancer; and also suggesting that less clinically insignificant lesions are detected.[59] Other studies have noted the utility of combined systemic and targeted therapy.[60] The PRECISION trial compared mpMRI- guided MRI/ultrasound fusion biopsy with 12-core systematic biopsy. Initial images were acquired at 1.5T or 3T, and PIRADS 3 to 5 was considered positive and biopsied, with ultrasound fusion leading to 38% detection rate of Gleason greater than or equal to 3 + 4, whereas the detection rate for systemic TRUS was 26%; moreover, percent positive increased with increasing PIRADS score from 12% to 60% to 83% for PIRADS 3 to 4 to 5, respectively.[61] MRI-guided biopsy is being explored as the primary biopsy method, as it may lead to the identification of more clinically significant lesions than systematic biopsy.[62] The negative predictive value of biparametric MRI for clinically significant prostate cancer has been reported as 95% to 97%, suggesting that such imaging may aid in avoiding unnecessary biopsies.[63,64] Techniques in the future that may aid prostate cancer detection and characterization may include metabolic functional imaging, for example, with hyperpolarization of pyruvate to boost detection of it and its metabolic products by MRI spectroscopy.

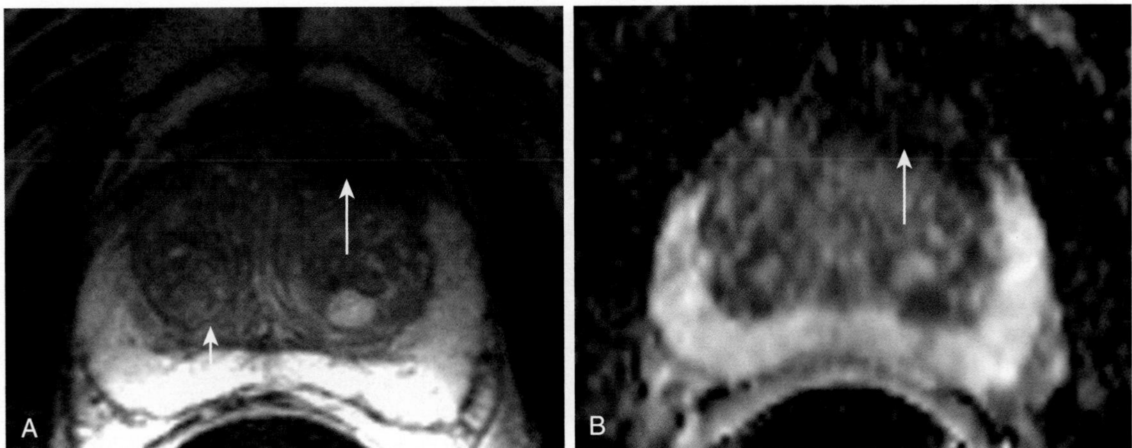

FIGURE 23.10. Central-zone prostate tumor (*long arrows*) seen as low signal on T2-weighted imaging (**A**) and on apparent diffusion coefficient (**B**). Benign prostatic hyperplasia nodules (*short arrow*) are better defined on T2-weighted imaging.

Key Points Imaging

- Ultrasound is used primarily to visualize the prostate and guide biopsy. It is limited in detecting prostate cancer. New techniques include magnetic resonance imaging (MRI)-guided biopsy and MRI/ultrasound fusion biopsy.
- MRI offers anatomic and functional evaluation.
- Detection of prostate cancer is an emerging field for MRI or MRI/ultrasound fusion biopsy.
- Diffusion-weighted imaging is the primary sequence for detecting prostate cancer in the peripheral zone.
- T2-weighted imaging is the primary sequence for detecting prostate cancer in the transition zone.
- Increased signal on T1 implies hemorrhage and confounds interpretation.

Local Staging

For staging, T1 axial of the prostate, three-plane T2, T1 of the pelvis, and DWI of the pelvis often supplement mpMRI of the prostate. Traditionally, MRI has been used to locally stage prostate cancer. This includes evaluation of EPE, neurovascular bundle invasion, and seminal vesicle invasion and, more rarely, detection of bladder neck, external sphincter, or rectal invasion. EPE is more accurately diagnosed by TRUS or endorectal MRI than by DRE.[65] Most studies have shown that high-resolution endorectal MRI provides higher accuracy in staging local disease than does TRUS.[66–68] Moreover, adding data from endorectal MRI to Partin nomograms improves prediction of organ-confined prostate cancer versus extraprostatic disease at radical prostatectomy (area under ROC curve [AUC] 0.81 vs. 0.90, nomogram vs. nomogram plus MRI) in all risk groups, with greatest impact on intermediate- and high-risk groups.[69] An endorectal coil significantly improves signal quality and allows thinner slices for improved spatial resolution. These are directional, and greatest signal is seen near the coil highlighting the areas of the neurovascular bundles, where EPE and neurovascular bundle invasion tends to occur. Inflation of the balloon with the coil tends to displace the neurovascular bundles outward, better exposing the critical fat plane between the prostate and the neurovascular bundles.

Jager and colleagues[70] suggested that MRI is cost-effective when used for the patients with a prior probability of EPE of at least 30% (PSA >10 ng/mL or Gleason score >7). In practice, patients with PSA less than10 ng/mL are routinely imaged for staging. EPE or seminal vesicle invasion is associated with a higher risk of recurrence after resection.[71] The accuracy of endorectal MRI in detecting EPE can vary between 58% and 90%, depending on the criteria and techniques used.[72] For patients at intermediate risk, it has shown approximately 80% accuracy in predicting the pathologic stage.[67,68] Specificity can be more important than sensitivity for determining EPE to prevent patients from being excluded from potentially curative treatment.[73] The most specific findings for EPE include asymmetry of the neurovascular bundle, blunting of the rectoprostatic angle, and direct tumor extension outside of the capsule (Fig. 23.11); these provide a specificity of greater than 90%.[72] Focal bulging (Fig. 23.12) is often used but is less specific.[72] Because microscopic extracapsular tumor extension does not affect patient survival, subtle findings suggesting capsular penetration, such as irregular bulge, irregular gland contour, focal capsular thickening, or retraction, may not influence management.[74] Capsule contact length greater than 1cm, morphology, and tumor dimension all had similar sensitivity of approximately 75% and specificity of approximately 65% for detecting EPE.[75] The first is easy to assess. Metaanalysis found that MRI has a sensitivity and specificity of 80% and 69%, respectively, for EPE.[76] Although there is some controversy, pathologic EPE has been associated with earlier biochemical relapse, but did not affect prostate cancer specific survival or overall survival.[77]

Located at 5 and 7 o'clock, the neurovascular bundles appear as oval in axial and linear in long axis hypointense structures surrounded by hyperintense fat on T1W imaging. Because overall survival is high with localized disease, morbidity is a significant issue, and compromise of the neurovascular bundle at surgery can lead to decreased erection or impotence. Neurovascular bundle–sparing surgery can

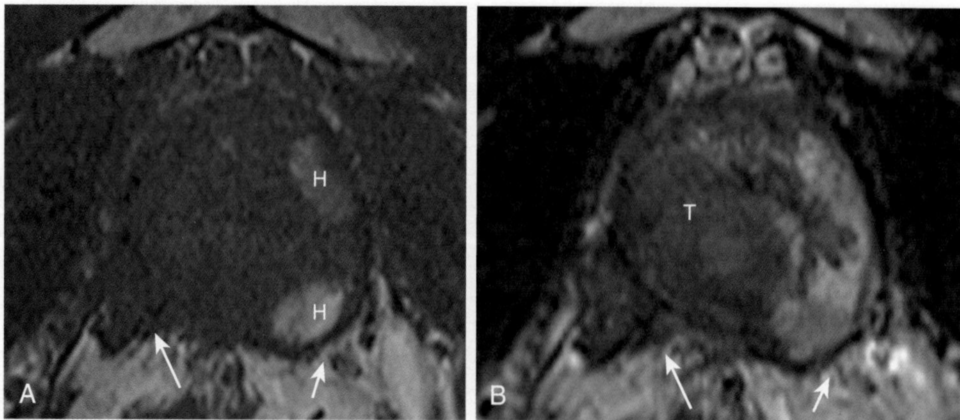

Figure 23.11. Locally advanced prostate cancer with neurovascular bundle invasion on the left (*long arrows*) seen as direct tumor extension on T1 (**A**) and T2-weighted (**B**) images. The fat plane (*short arrows*) between the prostate and the neurovascular bundle on the left is lost on the right, and this fat plane and neurovascular bundle itself is most often better appreciated on T1-weighted images. *T*, Tumor; *H*, hemorrhage.

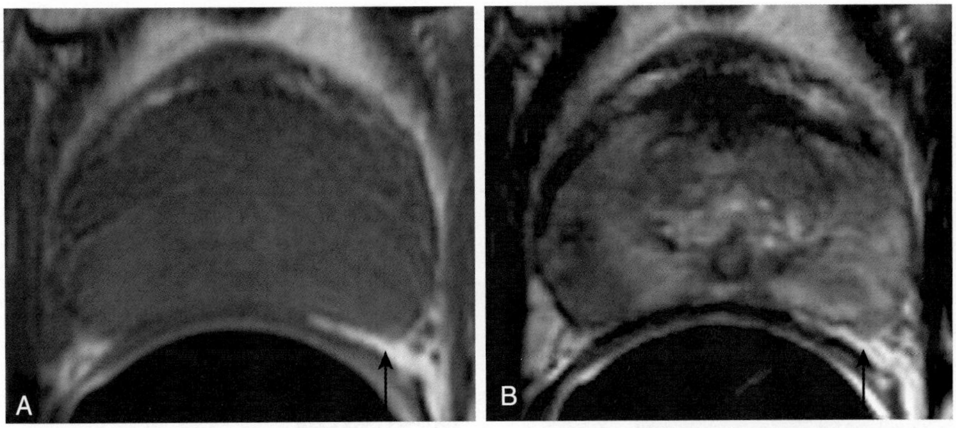

FIGURE 23.12. Focal bulge (*arrows*) is not a specific sign for extraprostatic extension. Axial magnetic resonance imaging. **A**, T1-weighted. **B**, T2-weighted.

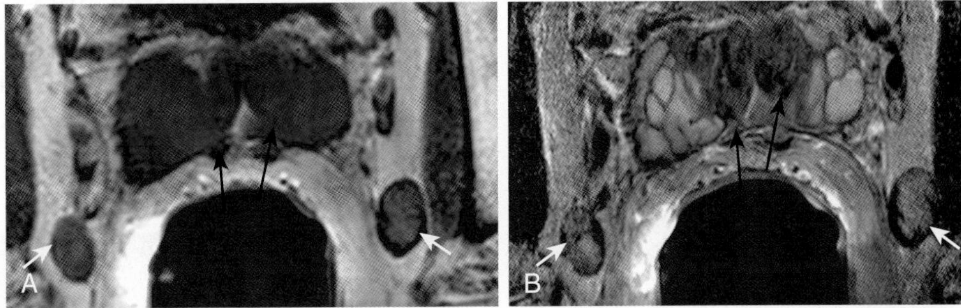

FIGURE 23.13. Seminal vesicle invasion (*black arrows*) and lymph node metastases (*white arrows*) seen as intermediate T1 signal (**A**) and low T2 signal (**B**) in the seminal vesicles.

be performed, including of one of the two bundles; thus, describing involvement and laterality (i.e., right or left side) is important. Neurovascular bundle invasion is often better assessed on T1W than T2W imaging, owing to better delineation of the prostate margin and fat between it and the neurovascular bundle (see Fig. 23.5). Neurovascular bundle invasion may appear as asymmetric enlargement with loss of the intervening periprostatic fat plane or as gross tumor extension (see Fig. 23.11).[78] Sensitivity has been reported to be 60% and negative predictive value 92%,[79] which may give confidence when making decisions regarding nerve-sparing surgery.

In the seminal vesicles, tumor appears as a low-signal area within the high-signal fluid on T2W imaging and as low signal on T1W imaging (Fig. 23.13). It may appear as increased signal on DWI. In contrast, postbiopsy hemorrhage usually has high T1 signal and either low or high T2 signal. Seminal vesicle involvement is also suggested by asymmetry or loss of the fat plane between the base of the bladder and the inferior aspect of the seminal vesicle, focal or diffuse seminal wall thickening, or nonvisualization of the ejaculatory ducts or seminal vesicle wall,[80] and is commonly better seen on sagittal images. An AUC of 0.76 has been reported, and MRI findings aid Kattan nomograms.[81] MRI evaluation can improve nomogram performance for detection of EPE and seminal vesicle invasion.[82]

Periprostatic vessels appear as serpiginous or honeycomb iso- to hyperintense structures on T2W imaging (Fig. 23.14), usually adjacent to the apex of the prostate, and should be identified, owing to the possibility of hemorrhage at the time of surgery.

T4 disease involves invasion into structures other than the seminal vesicles and is indicated by the loss of the fat plane between the tumor and the adjacent structure or by direct tumor visualization of tumor in the adjacent structure (Fig. 23.15).

To screen the pelvis, T1W imaging is typically used to evaluate for lymph nodes and bone metastases. DWI imaging, typically with b-value of 500 to 800, can be helpful for visualizing lymph nodes and bone metastases. Commonly, lymph nodes greater than 1 cm on the short axis are considered potentially metastatic. Because of Bateson's plexus, lymph node metastases may skip the pelvis, and if the patient is not scheduled to have an abdominal CT, MRI covering retroperitoneal lymph nodes may be considered. Bone marrow can appear heterogeneous on T1W imaging. Bone metastases tend to be focal and have decreased T1 signal and increased DWI signal, and such lesions, particularly if focal and in the setting of PSA greater than 10 ng/mL, can signify metastatic disease and warrant confirmatory imaging such as bone scan, which would show increased uptake or CT or radiographs that usually show sclerotic lesions.

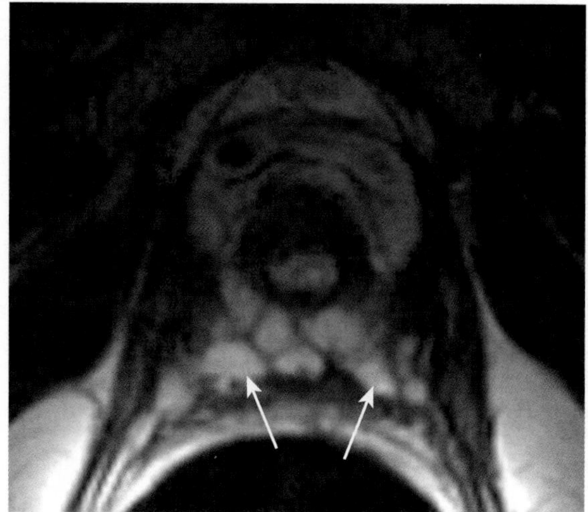

FIGURE 23.14. Axial magnetic resonance imaging demonstrates periprostatic blood vessels (*arrows*) adjacent to the prostate apex.

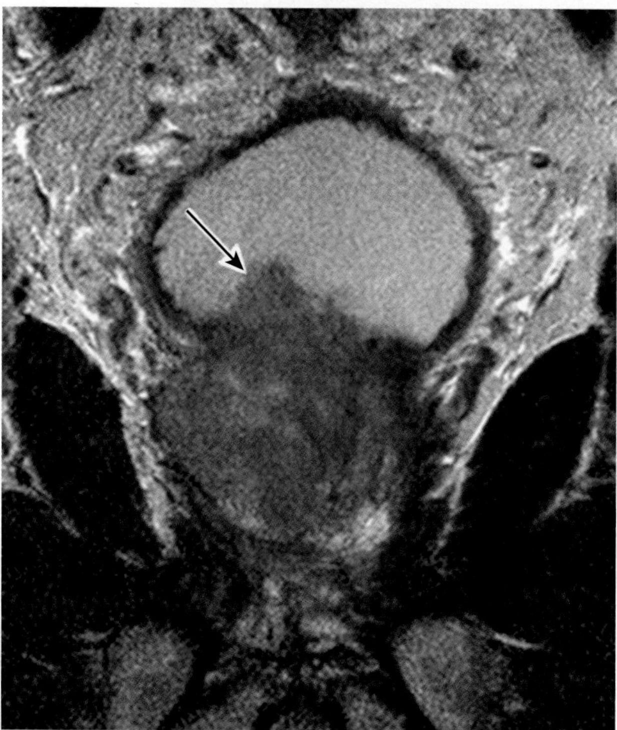

FIGURE 23.15. Coronal magnetic resonance imaging demonstrates prostate cancer (*arrow*) invading the bladder.

KEY POINTS Prostate Magnetic Resonance Imaging Radiology Report

- Location of disease
- Extraprostatic tumor extension
- Neurovascular bundle invasion (key for potential morbidity)
- Seminal vesicle invasion, other organ invasion
- Lymph node metastases and location
- Bone metastases and location
- Prostate size

Imaging Advanced Disease and Lymphatic and Hematogenous Metastases

Computed Tomography

CT scans of the abdomen and pelvis are obtained primarily in patients with suspected metastatic disease to lymph node (Fig. 23.16) and/or bone. As on MRI (see Figs. 23.13 and 23.16), lymph nodes greater than 1 cm on the short axis are considered suspicious for metastasis by CT. Rare metastases to other solid organs, such as lung, liver, pleura, and adrenal glands, may also be detected by CT (Fig. 23.17)

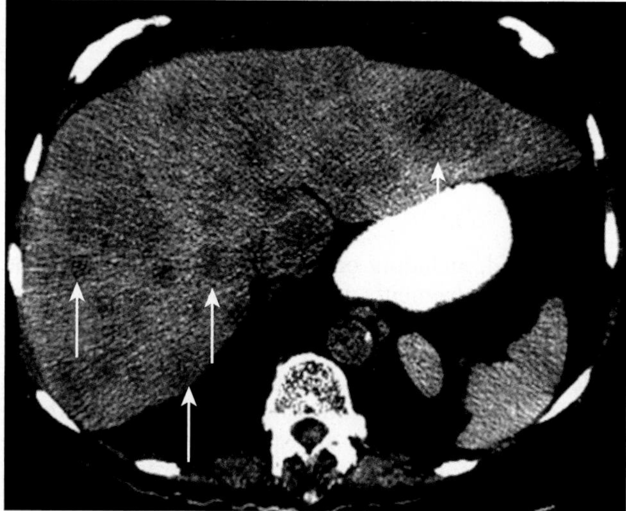

FIGURE 23.17. Axial computed tomography demonstrates multiple liver metastases (*arrows*) from a Gleason 9 prostate cancer.

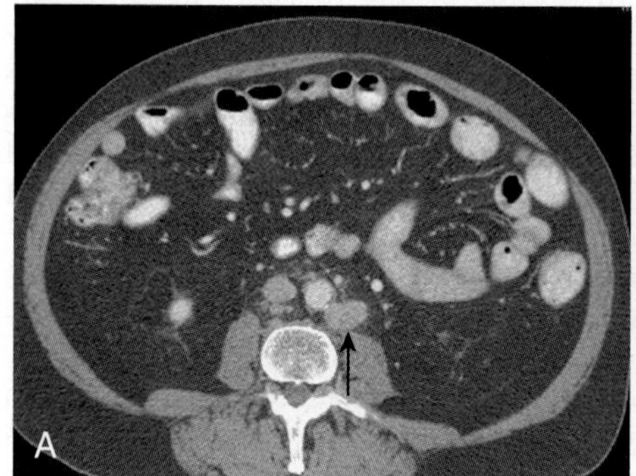

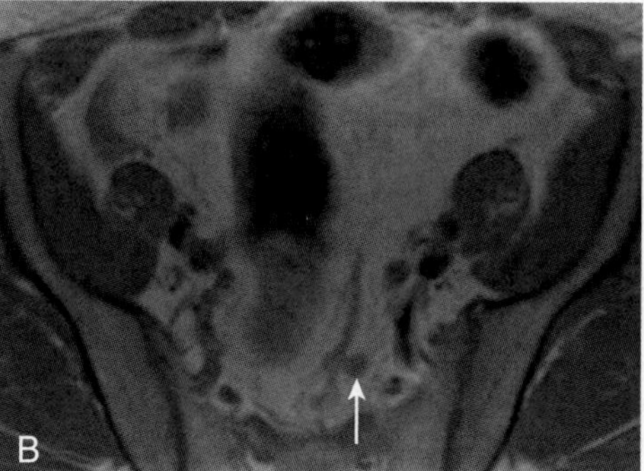

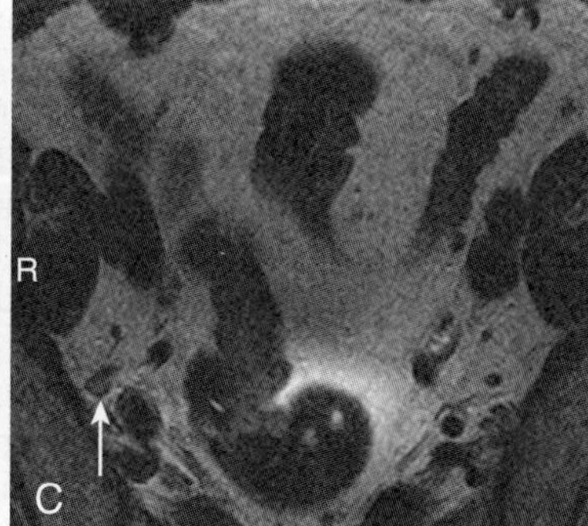

FIGURE 23.16. Lymph nodes (*arrows*). **A**, Computed tomography. **B**, T1-weighted magnetic resonance imaging (MRI). **C**, T2-weighted MRI.

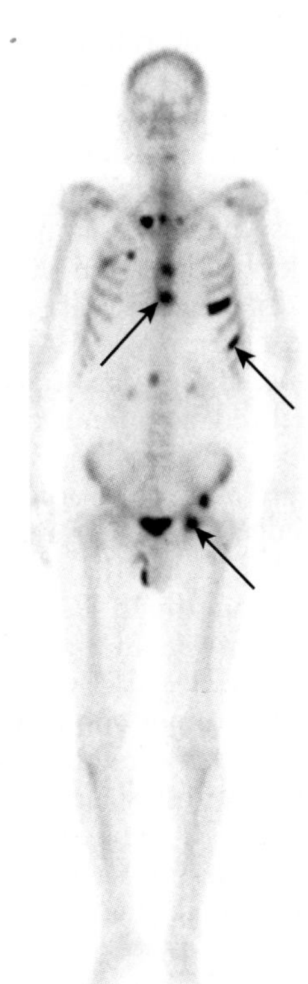

FIGURE 23.18. Multiple bone metastases seen as areas of increased uptake (*arrows*) on bone scan.

or MRI.[28,29] The thorax is commonly evaluated by radiography and/or chest CT.

Bone Scan, Magnetic Resonance Imaging, Computed Tomography, and Radiographs

Bone scan, MRI, CT, and radiographs are used for detecting visceral and bone metastases. Bone scan most commonly employs technitium-99m methyl diphosphonate (MDP) and is performed on patients with elevated PSA or clinically suspected bone metastasis, for example, because of pain. Because of the low likelihood of skeletal metastasis, a bone scan has been considered unnecessary in patients with newly diagnosed, untreated prostate cancer with PSA less than 10 ng/mL and no clinical signs of bone pathology.[83] Patients with PSA greater than 20 ng/mL have a relatively higher risk of bone metastasis. Metastases from prostate cancer usually present as focal areas of increased uptake on bone scan (Figs. 23.18 and 23.19). When there are diffuse bone metastases, the radiopharmaceutical may become incorporated into multiple metastases without apparent focal uptake or apparent excretion of the radiopharmaceutical. Nonvisualization of the kidneys is the classic finding of such a "superscan." Late in disease, very rarely, an aggressive prostate cancer bone metastasis may appear as normal bone or as a cold spot on bone scan. A flare reaction of increased uptake can be seen when therapy decreases the size of a metastasis and healing results. MDP mimics calcium phosphate and is incorporated into newly formed bone matrix; thus, it assesses mineralized bone

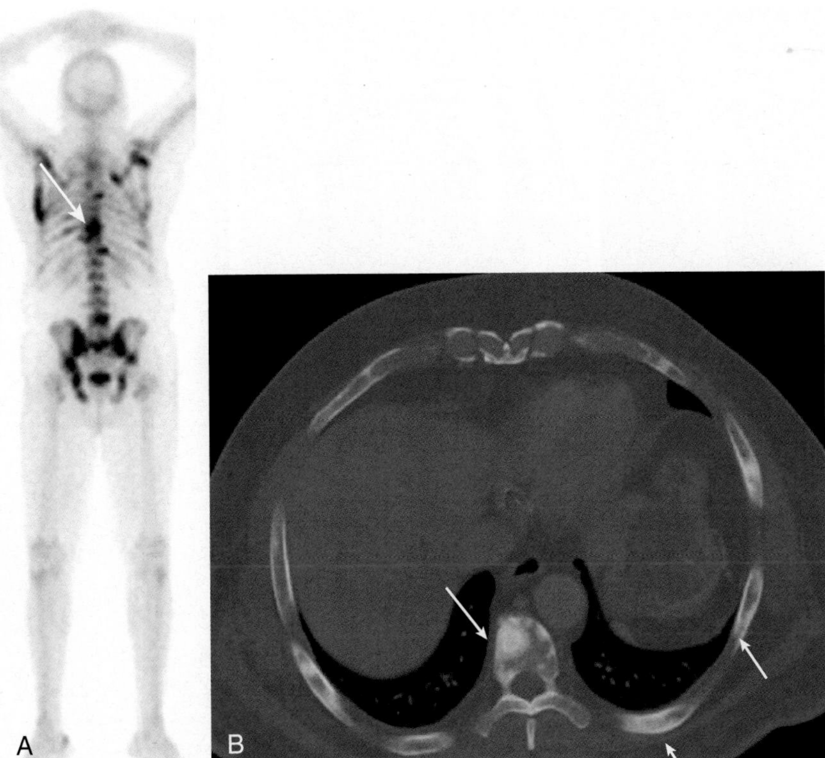

FIGURE 23.19. Multiple bone metastases (*white arrow*) seen as increased uptake on bone scan (**A**) and sclerotic lesions on axial computed tomography (**B**). Nonvisualization of the kidneys on bone scan can be seen in a "superscan" where the ratiopharmaceutical is taken up by the bone metastases with little to no excretion, suggesting widespread bone metastases; with widespread disease, individual bone metastases may not be seen.

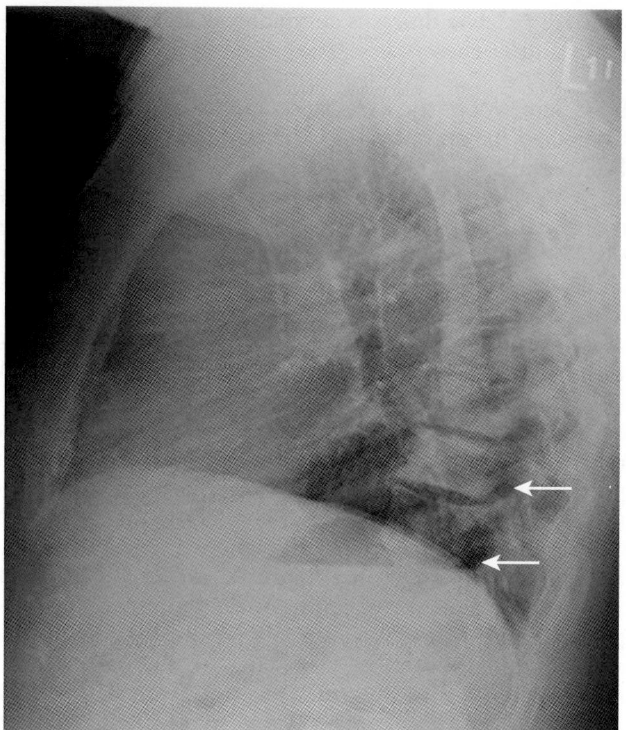

FIGURE 23.20. Sclerotic bone metastases (*arrows*) seen on the lateral chest radiograph.

turnover, not the soft-tissue tumor itself. Bone scan is a functional technique that is more sensitive for bone metastasis than anatomic CT or plain radiographs. However, the latter two can aid in distinguishing increased uptake on bone scan because of metastasis from other etiologies, such as degenerative disease, healing fractures, or metabolic disorders and their complications. On the x-ray–based techniques, prostate cancer metastases are most often sclerotic (Fig. 23.20). Unlike radiographs, CT can separate bone from overlying tissue. Bone scan, radiographs, and CT visualize the mineralized component of bone primarily. Whereas CT is more sensitive than conventional radiographs for detecting cortical invasion, it is less sensitive than MRI for medullary bone or marrow involvement, where metastasis begins.[84] On MRI, bone metastases demonstrate low T1 signal and high T2 signal, and enhance, but highly sclerotic metastases may appear dark on each of these sequences (Fig. 23.21). MRI can delineate the soft-tissue component of the tumor and is more sensitive than bone scan for detecting bone metastasis.[85] An advantage of bone scan is its ability to visualize the entire skeleton. However, whole-body MRI techniques[86,87] have become available. Major indications for MRI include evaluation for epidural disease and resolving ambiguity or discrepancy between other modalities, as well as metastasis detection and response evaluation. PET using $Na^{18}F$ can be used for detecting bone metastases but has not been widely adopted

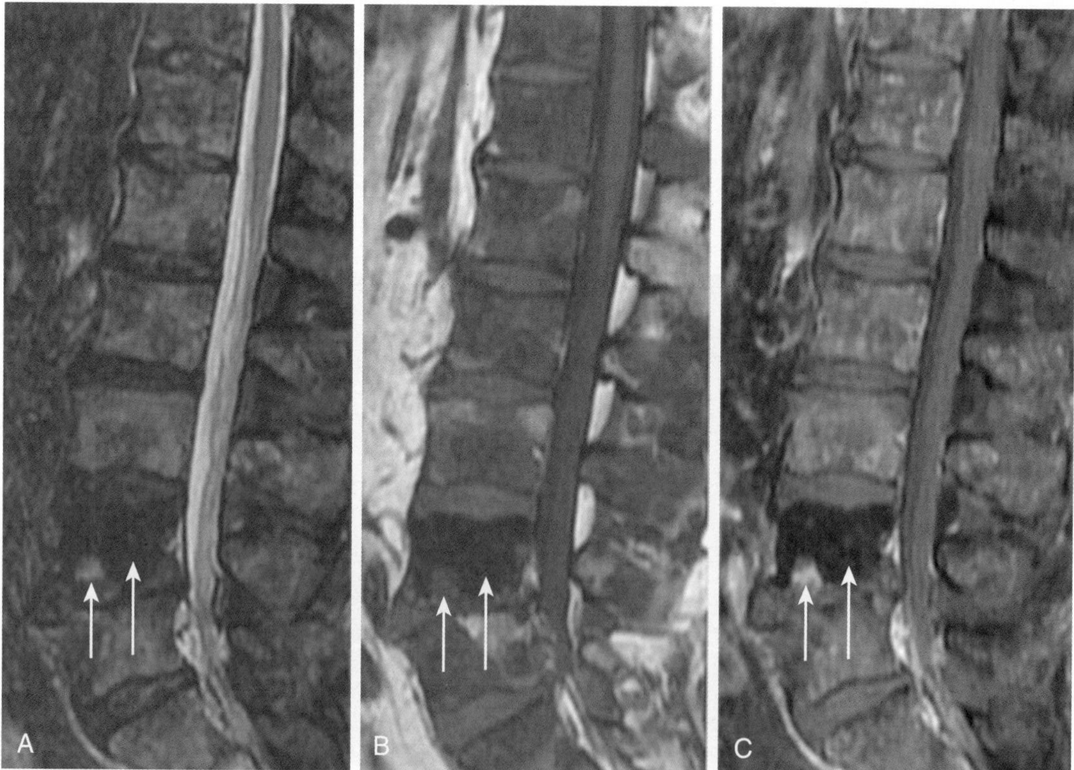

FIGURE 23.21. Diffuse bone metastases appear as areas of increased signal on T2-weighted fat-suppressed images (**A**), decreased signal on T1-weighted images (**B**), and increased signal on T1 post–intravenous contrast–enhanced fat-suppressed images (**C**). Note the vertebrae with generally very low signal on all sequences (*long arrows*), with an area of enhancement anteroposteriorly (*short arrows*) consistent with essentially an ivory (very sclerotic) vertebra because of metastatic disease.

as providing greater utility over other methods such as bone scan. Other PET methods such as ^{11}C-choline and ^{18}F-fluciclovine available in the United States and ^{68}Ga- or ^{18}F-labeled prostate-specific membrane antigen (PSMA) analogs, which are available under investigational new drug application (IND) in the United States but more commonly used in Europe, can aid in metastasis detection[88] but currently are more commonly used in evaluation of recurrence. These have generally replaced ProstaScint.[89]

Key Points

- Magnetic resonance imaging (MRI) is used for local and metastatic disease.
- Computed tomography is better used for metastatic disease.
- Bone scan is used for detecting bone metastases and is of little value if prostate-specific antigen (PSA) is under 10 ng/mL, unless there is bone pain or other symptoms, and one can suggest not obtaining a bone scan unless PSA is greater than 20 ng/mL.
- Whole-body techniques for MRI and for positron emission tomography to stage metastatic disease are emerging.

TREATMENT

Prostate cancer treatment options depend on the stage and severity of the tumor. There are several treatment options for localized tumors. Active surveillance (AS), cryotherapy, high-intensity focused ultrasound (HIFU), brachytherapy, and external beam radiation are options for this disease state. Cancer-specific survival is similar among all curative therapies. Additionally, each treatment option has different side effects.[90–93] Therefore, there is no best treatment option for localized disease, and treatment selection is dependent on patient preference after having an in-depth discussion about the benefits and potential side effects of treatment options, which can require a patient visiting multiple specialists. For patients who have metastatic disease, systemic therapy consists of hormonal therapy to inhibit androgen production. Development of castration-resistant disease can occur at a median of 18 to 24 months. This disease state requires the use of second-generation antiandrogen therapy or chemotherapy.

Active Surveillance

Prostate cancer can be stratified (Table 23.2).[94] Men diagnosed with low-risk and favorable intermediate-risk prostate cancer have AS as an option. The goal of AS is to monitor the cancer with the intent of curative treatment upon progression. The rationale behind AS is that small-volume, low-grade prostate cancers detected on screening have a low chance of becoming lethal. Studies have shown that the rate of death from prostate cancer while under AS is less than 2%[95,96]; thus, intervention has little effect on survival. AS inclusion criteria and monitoring protocols differ among institutions, but all protocols involve serial PSA values, DREs, and intermittent prostate biopsies.[95–100] Approximately one-third of patients on AS will receive treatment within 10 years, meaning the majority of men who start AS are able to continue AS.[95,101] There has not been any evidence that men who progress to treatment fare any worse than those who had initial treatment.

The use of prostate MRI for patients under AS is evolving. Similar to its use in initial staging, prostate MRI can detect disease, evaluate for change in size, and help guide subsequent fusion biopsies. Repeated MRIs while on AS are increasingly used. More research and follow-up are required to determine how to optimally use MRI for patients under AS.[102–104]

Surgery

The goal of surgery is to remove the prostate gland while attaining negative margins. Radical prostatectomy via an open approach was refined by Walsh et al.[105] The principles of the open technique were applied to laparoscopic, and eventually robotic, techniques. Robotic-assisted radical prostatectomy (RARP) is the most common type of prostatectomy performed in the United States today. When compared with open prostatectomy, RARP allows for a shorter hospital stay, less blood loss, and quicker recovery from surgery.[106,107] No studies have shown a difference in disease-control or quality-of-life metrics between the two approaches. The steps of surgery involve disconnecting the bladder from the prostate, truncating the vas deferens and performing *en bloc* resection of the seminal vesicles, separating the prostate from the rectum, disconnecting the prostate from the urethra, and anastomosing the bladder to the urethral stump. Potential complications include erectile dysfunction, urinary incontinence, urethral stricture, and rectourethral fistula. Classically, the decision to preserve the cavernosal nerves depends on preoperative erectile function, PSA level, Gleason score, and clinical stage. The use of MRI in decision-making on nerve sparring is becoming more prevalent.[108,109] A pelvic lymph node dissection can be performed if there is a high chance of nodal metastasis based on established nomograms.[110–112]

Cryotherapy

Cryotherapy is a technique in which probes are passed into the prostate to induce freezing to −40° C, which destroys cancer cells via protein denaturation and cell membrane rupture.[113] Transrectal ultrasound is used to monitor the extent of the ice ball to minimal damage to adjacent structure. A urethral warming catheter is used to minimize the risk of urethral sloughing. Complications include erectile dysfunction, urethral sloughing, urinary retention, urinary incontinence, and rectourethral fistula.[114] Short and intermediate follow-up have shown disease control similar to that following surgery or radiation; however, longer follow-up is needed to determine true efficacy.

High-Intensity Focused Ultrasound

HIFU uses a transrectal probe to deliver focused ultrasound waves to the prostate that result in a temperature elevation to 65° C. This produces both thermal and mechanical damage to tissue.[115,116] Potential complications include erectile dysfunction, urinary retention, urethral stricture, and rectourethral fistula. Similar to cryotherapy, short and intermediate follow-up has shown similar disease control to radiation and surgery; however, long-term follow-up is required to determine true equivalence.

Radiation Therapy

External Beam Therapy

Methods for accurate tumor imaging and computer-based planning and treatment systems have been key to the necessary dose escalation and tumor targeting for prostate cancer radiation therapy. CT-based three-dimensional treatment planning is now standard, as are sophisticated delivery techniques such as intensity-modulated radiation therapy (IMRT; Fig. 23.22). For the latter, multiple beams of high-energy x-rays (photons) generated in linear accelerators are consecutively applied at different angles, and a portion of the radiation field is blocked at a specified time during each angled application. This enables intensity modulation and convergence to maximize dose to the target but limits the dose to nearby critical structures such as the bladder, rectum, and bowel. Volumetric arc therapy is a type of IMRT that delivers radiation while the machine rotates in an arc, thereby shortening the treatment time and using a lower overall dose of radiation. Proton beam radiation therapy is increasingly used for the treatment of prostate cancer and uses accelerated protons generated in a cyclotron or synchrotron. Protons interact with tissue and deposit dose differently than the photons used in IMRT. The appeal of proton radiation therapy is that it delivers a lower radiation dose to nontarget organs than does IMRT. The safety and efficacy of proton beam radiation therapy is supported by multiple publications; however, to date there is no level 1 evidence directly comparing proton radiation therapy to IMRT.[117–119]

CT and MRI in the preplanning stage can help identify structures to target or avoid, including tumor, prostate, neurovascular bundles, seminal vesicles, bladder, lymph nodes, rectum, and bowel, as well as postsurgical (such as postprostatectomy) changes. Computer-based planning allows calculation of radiation dose to each structure.

Because treatment fields conform tightly to the treatment targets, it is usually necessary to image the prostate or prostate resection bed location daily. Several techniques are used to aid daily treatment planning, including transabdominal ultrasound, implanted radiopaque (fiducial) markers imaged by daily x-ray, and CT units attached to the linear accelerator. Recently, MRI imaging has been integrated into radiation treatment systems.

Outcome Studies for Primary Radiation Therapy

Randomized trials demonstrate improved biochemical disease–free survival when dose-escalated external beam radiation therapy is delivered compared with lower dose radiation,[120–127] and the former is currently standard treatment for localized prostate cancer.[128,129] Addition of brachytherapy to external beam radiation can escalate dose to the prostate and improves biochemical progression-free survival, but at the cost of increased physician-reported and patient-reported toxicity.[130–133]

It can take 8 to 10 weeks to complete dose-escalated external beam radiation therapy when treatment is delivered using conventional daily doses of 1.8 or 2.0 Gy per fraction. Shorter 4- to 6-week treatment regimens, called moderate hypofractionation, have been developed that deliver larger daily doses of radiation. Over 6000 men have been treated in randomized trials comparing moderate hypofractionation to standard fractionation.[134,135]

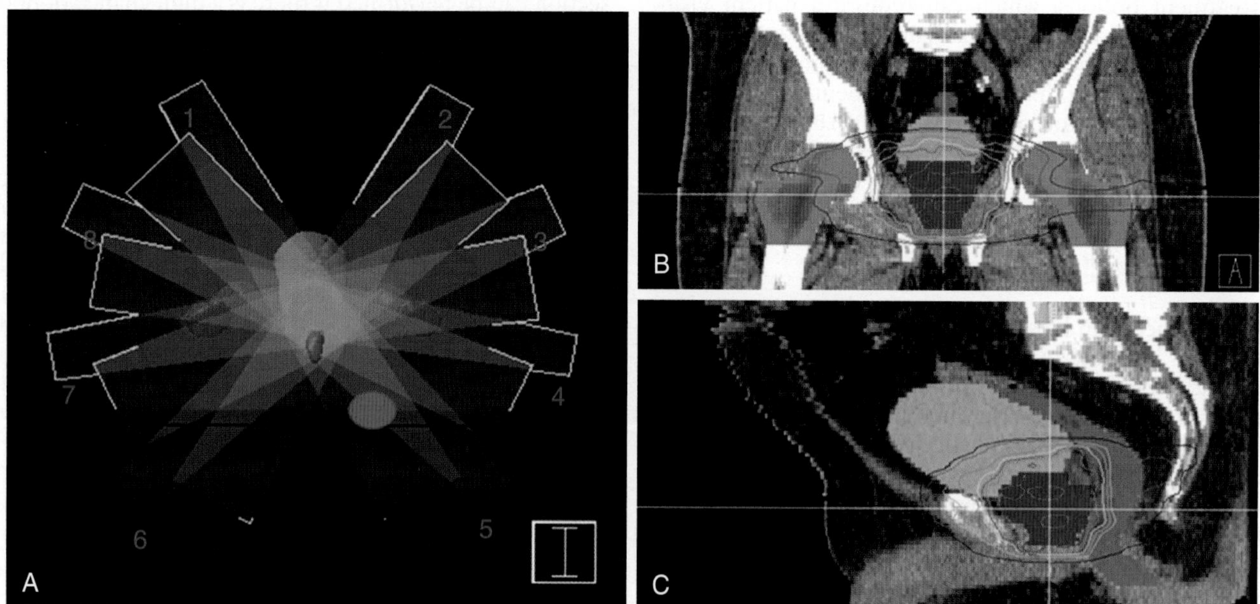

FIGURE 23.22. Intensity-modulated radiation therapy. **A**, Radiation is delivered from multiple angles, resulting in more focused delivery at the center, where the beams intersect. Thus, the dose is directed more specifically to the object of interest and is limited to the surrounding normal tissue. Coronal (**B**) and sagittal (**C**) images of dose plan.

Moderate hypofractionation provides similar cancer control, similar rates of late toxicity, and only a slight excess of acute gastrointestinal toxicity. By shortening treatment duration, moderate hypofractionation regimens are more convenient for patients and decrease treatment cost. The 2018 evidence-based American Society of Radiation Oncology, American Society of Clinical Oncology, and American Urologic Association (ASTRO/ASCO/AUA) guideline on Hypofractionated Radiation Therapy for Localized Prostate Cancer recommends offering moderate hypofractionation to men choosing external beam radiation therapy for prostate cancer.[136]

Ultrahypofractionated external beam therapy regimens further shortens treatment duration to just 1 to 2.5 weeks by delivering even larger daily doses of 5.0 Gy or higher. Studies generally show excellent biochemical control and low toxicity[137]; however, published evidence largely consists of prospective single-arm trials in men with low-risk and, to a lesser extent, intermediate-risk disease. Several large-scale randomized trials comparing ultrahypofractionation to moderate hypofractionation and standard fractionation are in progress. The 2018 ASTRO/ASCO/AUA guideline on Hypofractionated Radiation Therapy for Localized Prostate Cancer conditionally recommends ultrahypofractionation as a treatment option for low- and intermediate-risk prostate cancer.[138]

Adding androgen deprivation therapy (ADT) to external beam radiation therapy improves prostate cancer control, prostate cancer–specific survival, and overall survival for men with intermediate-risk and high-risk prostate cancer.[139] However, ADT has multiple adverse effects, including hot flashes, sexual dysfunction, bone loss, gynecomastia, metabolic syndrome, and increased risk of cardiovascular disease.[140] Several studies have evaluated the optimal duration of ADT in this setting.[141–143] Among patients with intermediate-risk disease, benefit appears greatest for those men with 4 + 3 = 7 disease, large-volume disease, and no or mild comorbidities.[144,145] The National Comprehensive Cancer Network Prostate Cancer Guidelines recommend adding 18 to 36 months of ADT to external beam radiation therapy alone for high-risk disease, 12 to 36 months of ADT to external beam radiation therapy with brachytherapy boost for high-risk disease, and 4 months of ADT to radiation for men receiving external beam radiation therapy alone for unfavorable intermediate-risk disease.[128] There is no cancer control benefit to adding ADT to external beam radiation therapy for men with low-risk disease. In contemplating adding ADT, considerations include duration of ADT, cancer characteristics, patient age, comorbidities, and preference.

Brachytherapy

Although not as widely applicable as external beam radiation, brachytherapy[146] can be low–dose-rate with permanently implanted radioactive seeds[147] or high–dose-rate with temporary radiation sources that are inserted and removed.[148] It is more commonly performed in patients with low-risk prostate cancer. It may be used alone in patients with favorable intermediate-risk cancer, but if unfavorable, it is often combined with ADT. Combinations of brachytherapy and ERBT + ADT are also under evaluation.[146] Permanent brachytherapy can be seen on MRI, such as on T2W imaging, and tends to be better appreciated with intravenous contrast-enhanced imaging.

Hormone Therapy/Chemotherapy

If medical therapy is needed, it commonly begins with hormone therapy. This entails either reducing production of testosterone to castrated levels (e.g., by surgical orchiectomy or medical castration by administration of a gonadotropin-releasing hormone analog) or blocking the effect of testosterone by inhibiting the testosterone receptor. Hormone therapy remains the primary treatment for metastatic prostate cancer. It also serves a role for treatment of intermediate- and high-risk disease treated with radiation, and, based on data showing synergy and improved survival with multimodality therapy, hormone therapy may be given before, during, and after radiation therapy.[149] Both hormone and radiation therapy result in shrinkage of the prostate gland and low signal on T2W imaging in the PZ that can limit identification of prostate cancer (Fig. 23.23). Functional techniques have the potential to allow evaluation of such a posttherapy prostate gland. The use of hormone therapy before surgery has been investigated, and although it has been shown to improve surgical outcomes, such as lower positive margin rates, it does not appear to affect survival.[150] Thus, efforts continue on finding the ideal neoadjuvant drug or combination drugs to use in such cases.[151] More recently, there has been the recognition that hormone therapy, even for short courses of 1 to 2 years, can have deleterious systemic effects, and these are briefly reviewed in the section later on "Complications of Therapy." Inevitably and unpredictably, metastatic disease treated with hormone therapy becomes androgen-independent (or, conversely, hormone-resistant) prostate cancer, defined by either clinical or PSA progression in the face of a castrated level of testosterone. Newer therapies include those with increased testosterone suppression activity (enzalutamide, apalutamide, and abiraterone) and are now in some cases being used/tested before metastatic disease or castration resistance develops. Taxane-based therapies have been shown to improve survival in this population and are now considered first-line therapy for androgen-independent prostate cancer, and can be combined with the advanced ADT agents.[146] Skeletal-related events are a major source of morbidity in this population, but the introduction of bisphosphonates has lowered this risk.[152] For bone metastases, systemic radiotherapy with ^{223}radium can be used, including with hormonal or taxane-based therapy.[153] Efforts continue, with newer agents including tyrosine kinase inhibitors and immunotherapies, as well as combination regimens, to improve the outcomes of patients with androgen-independent prostate cancer.

KEY POINTS Therapy

- Localized disease: surgery or radiation therapy
- Systemic disease: hormone therapy
- Systemic disease after hormone therapy failure: taxane-based chemotherapy

Recurrence

Following radical prostatectomy, recurrence risk correlates with preoperative serum PSA, pathologic tumor stage, Gleason score, and positive surgical margins.[154,155] MRI findings can contribute to nomograms. Approximately 50% of patients with preoperative serum PSA greater than 10 ng/mL and 70% of patients with a Gleason score of 8 to 10 experience recurrence within 7 years after radical prostatectomy. Approximately 25% of patients with positive tumor margins experience recurrence within 5 years.[146,147] After radical prostatectomy, PSA should drop to 0 ng/mL, and two PSA assessments greater than 0.2 ng/mL suggests recurrence. In comparison, after radiation therapy, PSA remains detectable at a low level; and in general, biochemical failure or recurrent disease is suspected when PSA rises to 2 ng/mL above the postradiotherapy nadir.[156]

When suspected, PSA kinetics can suggest the site of recurrence but cannot definitively differentiate between local recurrence and distant metastases. In general, local recurrence is suggested by biochemical failure after a long duration posttreatment (>24 months after local treatment), low PSA velocity (change in serum PSA over time), and long PSA doubling time (>6 months). In contrast, recurrence at a distant site is suggested by rapid biochemical failure, high PSA velocity, and short PSA doubling time.[157,158]

Thus, recurrent tumor after therapy may present as a distant metastasis, lymph node metastasis, or a new mass in the prostatectomy bed. For the latter, MRI is superior to CT. TRUS, CT, 2-[^{18}F] fluoro-2-deoxy-D-glucose–PET, and DRE are limited in detecting local recurrence. On MRI, the key sequence to detect recurrence either post-prostatectomy or post–radiation therapy is DCE,[159] where the lesion enhances. Because T2 low signal occurs post–radiation therapy and post–hormone therapy, utility of T2 is limited (see Fig. 23.23). This can also limit DWI evaluation. Postprostatectomy, on MRI, the recurrent lesion may be hyperintense on T2 (instead of hypointense on T2 when the tumor is in the context of the prostate) and isointense on T1 (Fig. 23.24).[160,161] Clips or brachytherapy seeds can lead to artifacts on all imaging, but in particular on DWI and then DCE. In the postprostatectomy setting, DWI may be more valuable than ADC for recurrence detection. mpMRI of the pelvis, including the prostatectomy bed, has

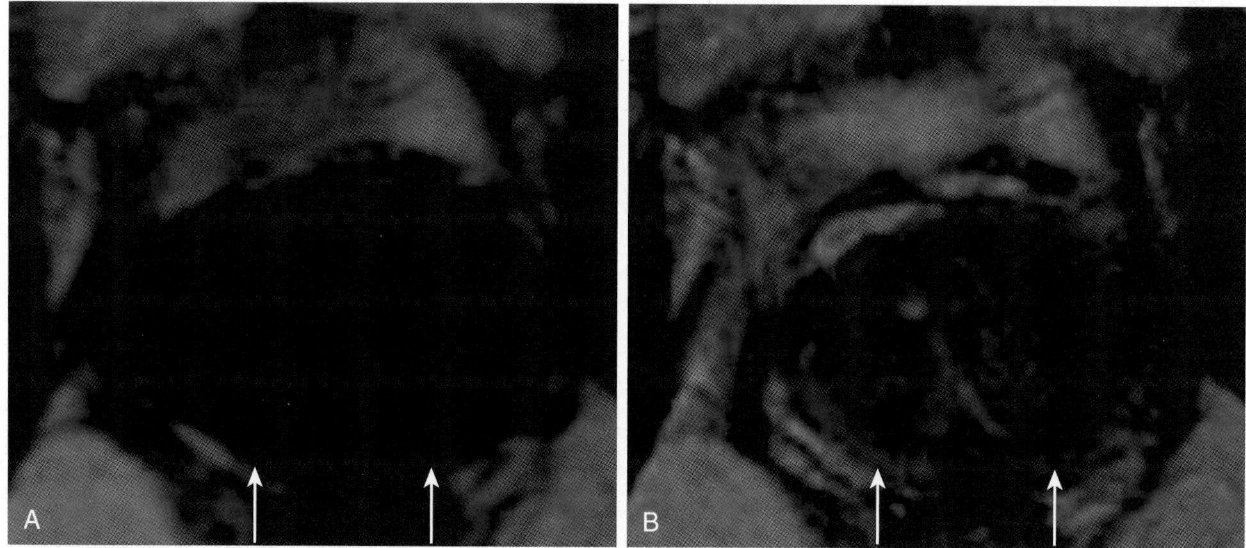

FIGURE 23.23. Low signal in the peripheral zone (*arrows*) on T1-weighted (**A**) and T2-weighted (T2W) (**B**) imaging because of treatment with hormonal therapy. The low signal can confound interpretation of prostate cancer on T2W images. Hormonal or radiation therapy can also result in a small gland because of shrinkage of the gland, as noted in this example.

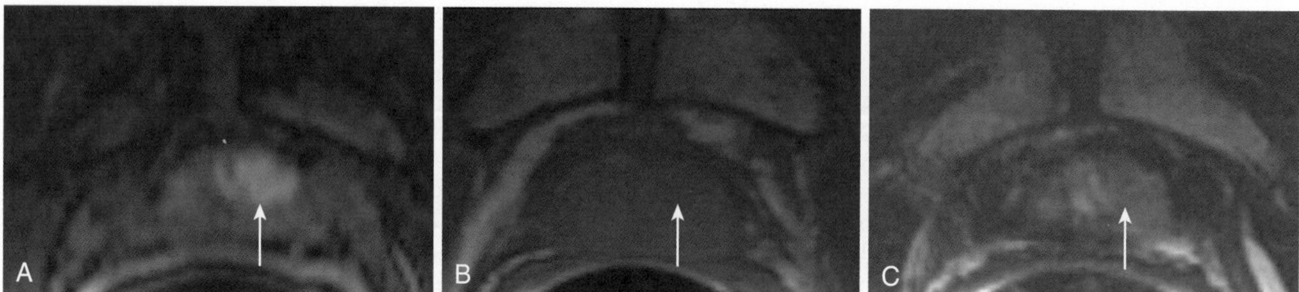

FIGURE 23.24. History of prior prostatectomy with slowly rising prostate-specific antigen. An intermediate signal area (*arrows*) is seen at the expected location of the prostatic apex on T2-weighted imaging (**A**), and low signal is seen in this same location on T1-weighted imaging (**B**). **C**, Early enhancement is seen just to the right of center anteriorly. Overall, the findings suggest incomplete prostatectomy with residual prostate cancer.

emerged as the most accurate imaging modality to identify local recurrence in patients with biochemical recurrence postprostatectomy, especially at low PSA levels (<1.0 ng/mL).[162–164] Endorectal coil is preferred for high-resolution imaging. Although infrequently used, MRI spectroscopy has shown promise in evaluating for metabolic atrophy posttreatment and for distinguishing recurrence post–radiation therapy.[165] When combined with endorectal MRI, MRI spectroscopy improved detection of recurrence within 4 months of hormone therapy compared with endorectal MRI alone for a less experienced reader.[166] Improved spatial, temporal, and spectral resolution, and potentially new markers, should improve spectroscopy. Local recurrence postprostatectomy is most commonly at the vesicourethral anastomosis, followed by the anterior or posterior bladder neck.[167] Differential considerations include residual glandular tissue or seminal vesicles, granulation tissue, hemorrhage, and fibrosis.[168]

If local recurrence is suspected, a biopsy is usually required for confirmation. However, an ultrasound-guided biopsy is unlikely to be of value unless the PSA is greater than 0.5 ng/mL, there is a palpable abnormality on DRE, or a target lesion is seen near the site of anastomosis after prostatectomy.[169] MRI-guided or MRI/ultrasound fusion biopsy is preferred. Posttreatment changes can make histologic confirmation of recurrence difficult after radiation therapy. mpMRI of the prostate with endorectal coil has been found to be superior to C-11 choline PET/CT for detection of local recurrence[170] postprostatectomy.

After systemic therapy, lymph node metastasis may be pelvic, retroperitoneal, retrocrural, or rarely, mediastinal; but after pelvic radiation or lymph node dissection, metastasis to pelvic lymph nodes is less common, and evaluation of nodes outside the treatment field is advisable.[171] For the uncommon patient with a poor PSA-producing tumor, radiographic surveillance plays an even more important role.

For identifying lymph node and distant metastatic disease, bone scan, CT, or MRI are commonly employed. Bone scan tends to have more value if PSA is greater than 10 ng/mL.[172] In addition to whole-body MRI, various PET tracers can be used when there is suspicion of lymph node or distant metastasis. Two PET tracers, C-11 choline and F-18 fluciclovine, are FDA-approved, whereas PSMA-based agents are not, but are used at some institutions under an IND application. Uptake of C-11 choline on PET/CT is as a result of increased synthesis of phosphatidylcholine, a component of the cell membrane[173,174] in prostate cancer. F-18 fluciclovine, or anti-1-amino-3-F-18-fluorocyclobutane1-1carboxylic acid, is a radiolabeled synthetic amino acid analog that is transported inside the cells via the ASCT2 and LAT1 transmembrane amino acid transporters, which are overexpressed by prostate cancer cells.[173,175] PSMA is a type II transmembrane glycoprotein that is overexpressed to 100 to 1000 times the normal level in prostate cancer[173,176] and other tumor cell types. PSMA expression increases with dedifferentiated, metastatic, and hormone refractory prostate cancer and also serves as a prognostic factor in disease outcome.[177,178] Of note, approximately 5% to 10% of prostate cancers do not show PSMA overexpression[179,180]; thus, false negatives can occur. There are several PSMA analogs and labels that can be administered under an IND application. All three radiotracers can be used to detect distant recurrence (Fig. 23.25), and some have been advocated for use in detecting local recurrence. All three appear to have similar detection at PSA levels greater than 2 ng/mL, F-18 fluciclovine and Ga-68 PSMA-11 appear superior to C-11 choline at PSA levels of 1 to less than 2 ng/mL, and PSMA-11 appears superior to F-18 fluciclovine and C-11 choline at PSA levels of less than 1 ng/mL,[181] although more formal analyses with direct comparisons are needed. Because local salvage therapies such as radiation therapy are more successful for long-term control if metastases are not present, imaging with the above PET agents has been suggested to evaluate for metastatic disease first. Although PSMA-based agents are being evaluated for local recurrence, currently mpMRI is preferred for local recurrence, whereas prostate cancer–targeted radiopharmaceuticals are preferred for lymph node and distant metastases. PET-MRI is being evaluated as a one-stop shop for assessing the local posttreatment bed and for distant metastases. DWI can aid detection of both lymph nodes and bone/visceral metastases, but MRI is limited compared with CT for lung metastases. PSMA ligands can also be labeled with beta and alpha emitters, such as lutetium-177 and actinium-225, respectively, for targeted radiotherapy[182] that is being evaluated in clinical trials.

KEY POINTS Recurrence

- Slowly rising prostate-specific antigen (PSA): local recurrence is more likely; multiparametric magnetic resonance imaging (MRI) is most commonly used.
- Rapidly rising PSA: metastatic disease is more likely, and bone scan or cross-sectional imaging such as computed tomography or MRI is employed. Recently, targeted radiopharmaceuticals evaluating choline turnover, amino acid transporter activity, or prostate-specific membrane antigen expression are also being employed.

Complications of Therapy

Immediately after prostatectomy, cystography may be used to evaluate for an anastomotic leak. Most leaks heal on their own. Initial urinary incontinence, if present, tends to resolve. Rates of complete incontinence in mature series and experienced hands are generally in the 1% to 2% range.[183] However, it is not unusual for 10% to 30% of patients to experience stress urinary incontinence, with loss of minor urine volumes during periods of abdominal straining. Total incontinence is addressed by placement of an artificial urinary sphincter, and stress incontinence may be treated with various less extensive measures. Recuperation of erectile function depends primarily on three factors: the quality of preoperative erectile function, patient age (men <60 years old have better recovery), and the quality and extent of nerve sparing.[183] Complete erectile function recovery can take up to 2 years. A variety of treatments are available for treatment

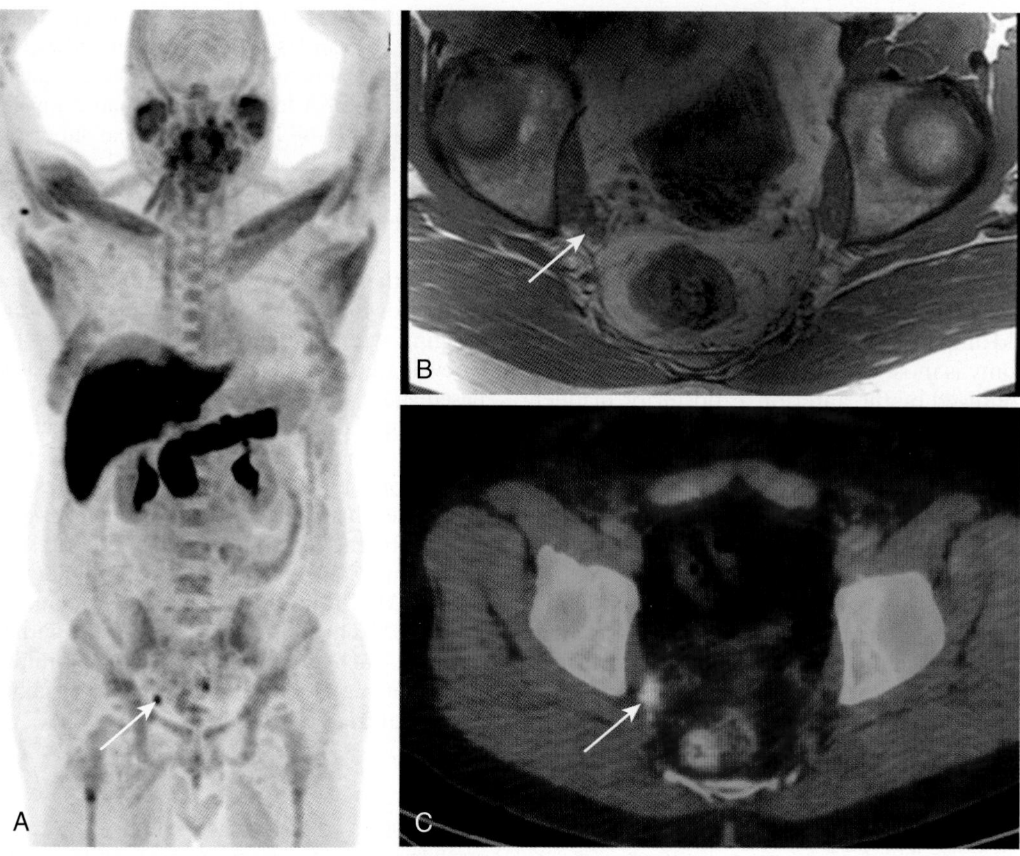

FIGURE 23.25. Rising prostate-specific antigen postprostatectomy. Whole-body fluciclovine (**A**), T1-weighted pelvis magnetic resonance imaging (**B**), and fluciclovine positron emission tomography–computed tomography fusion (**C**) demonstrate lymph node recurrence.

of postoperative erectile function, including use of oral phosphodiesterase inhibitors, vacuum erectile device, pharmacologic injection therapy, and placement of a prosthesis. The latter can be seen upon imaging. Urethral stricture disease is not uncommon after open radical prostatectomy, ranging from 10% to 20%, but is rare after RARP.[184] Retrograde urethrogram may be performed to evaluate for such strictures.

Hormone therapy, particularly when sustained for over a year, is associated with several important systemic adverse outcomes. Common side effects include hot flashes and lethargy; others may include anemia, muscle wasting, central obesity, increased rates of heart disease, decreased cognitive function, and osteoporosis with ensuing higher risk of fractures.[185] In some patients, the complications may negatively affect overall survival to the point of potentially negating any benefit from treatment of the cancer; this has prompted the concept of reserving therapy or considering other treatments that might prolong the time to initiation of hormones.[186] Patients treated with hormone therapy commonly have active intervention for some of the known adverse sequelae, such as bisphosphonates for osteoporosis.

Complications of radiation therapy similar to prostatectomy include impotence, urinary incontinence, and urethral strictures. Additional complications may include strictures of bowel and blood vessels, with the latter potentially resulting in ischemia. Radiation enteritis and osteonecrosis may also be noted. These are more commonly evaluated by cross-sectional imaging such as CT or MRI.

KEY POINTS Complications

- Surgery: cystograms employed to look for leaks and retrograde urethrograms employed for strictures.
- Radiation therapy: computed tomography/magnetic resonance imaging and retrograde urethrograms commonly employed to evaluate for strictures, ischemia, or osteonecrosis.
- Hormone therapy complications are not commonly evaluated by imaging.

CONCLUSION

Radiology plays an essential role in an integrative approach to prostate cancer. The armamentarium of imaging studies, when performed in the appropriate laboratory and clinical context, contributes crucial information for diagnosing, staging, individualizing risk stratification, formulating a suitable treatment strategy, and monitoring prostate cancer.

REFERENCES

1. American Cancer Society. Cancer Facts & Figures 2019.
2. Howlader N NA, Krapcho M, Miller D, et al. SEER Cancer Statistics Review. Bethesda: National Cancer Institute; 1975–2016.
3. Albright F, Stephenson RA, Agarwal N, et al. Prostate cancer risk prediction based on complete prostate cancer family history. *Prostate*. 2015;75:390–398.
4. Bratt O, Drevin L, Akre O, et al. Family history and probability of prostate cancer, differentiated by risk category: a nationwide population-based study. *J Nat Cancer Instit*. 2016:108.
5. Haraldsdottir S, Hampel H, Wei L, et al. Prostate cancer incidence in males with Lynch syndrome. *Genetic in Med*. 2014;16:553–557.
6. Mersch J, Jackson MA, Park M, et al. Cancers associated with BRCA1 and BRCA2 mutations other than breast and ovarian. *Cancer*. 2015;121:269–275.
7. McNeal JE, Redwine EA, Freiha FS, et al. Zonal distribution of prostatic adenocarcinoma. Correlation with histologic pattern and direction of spread. *Am J Surg Pathol*. 1988;12:897–906.
8. Cannon Jr GM, Pound CR, Landsittel DP, et al. Perineural invasion in prostate cancer biopsies is not associated with higher rates of positive surgical margins. *Prostate*. 2005;63:336–340.
9. O'Malley KJ, Pound CR, Walsh PC, et al. Influence of biopsy perineural invasion on long-term biochemical disease-free survival after radical prostatectomy. *Urology*. 2002;59:85–90.
10. Wheeler TM. Anatomy of the prostate and the pathology of prostate cancer. In: Vogelzang NJ, Shipley WU, Scardino PT, eds. *Comprehensive Textbook of Genitourinary Oncology*. Philadelphia: Lippincott Williams & Wilkins; 2000:587–604.
11. Presti Jr. JC. Prostate cancer: assessment of risk using digital rectal examination, tumor grade, prostate-specific antigen, and systematic biopsy. *Radiol Clin North Am*. 2000;38:49–58.
12. Makarov DV, Sanderson H, Partin AW, et al. Gleason score 7 prostate cancer on needle biopsy: is the prognostic difference in Gleason scores 4 + 3 and 3 + 4 independent of the number of involved cores? *J Urol*. 2002;167:2440–2442.
13. Epstein JI, Egevad L, Amin MB, et al. The 2014 International Society of Urological Pathology (ISUP) consensus conference on Gleason grading of prostatic carcinoma: definition of grading patterns and proposal for a new grading system. *Am J Surg Pathol*. 2016;40:244–252.
14. Epstein JI, Zelefsky MJ, Sjoberg DD, et al. A contemporary prostate cancer grading system: a validated alternative to the Gleason score. *Eur Urology*. 2016;69:428–435.
15. Thompson IM, Ankerst DP, Chi C, et al. Operating characteristics of prostate-specific antigen in men with an initial PSA level of 3.0 ng/ml or lower. *JAMA*. 2005;294:66–70.
16. Thompson IM, Pauler DK, Goodman PJ, et al. Prevalence of prostate cancer among men with a prostate-specific antigen level < or = 4.0 ng per milliliter. *N Engl J Med*. 2004;350:2239–2246.
17. Vickers A, Cronin A, Roobol M, et al. Reducing unnecessary biopsy during prostate cancer screening using a four-kallikrein panel: an independent replication. *J Clin Oncol*. 2010;28:2493–2498.
18. Catalona WJ, Partin AW, Sanda MG, et al. A multicenter study of [-2]pro-prostate specific antigen combined with prostate specific antigen and free prostate specific antigen for prostate cancer detection in the 2.0 to 10.0 ng/ml prostate specific antigen range. *J Urol*. 2011;185:1650–1655.
18a. McKiernan J, Donovan MJ, O'Neill V, et al. A novel urine exosome gene expression assay to predict high-grade prostate cancer at initial biopsy. *JAMA Oncol*. 2016;2:882–889.
20. Van Neste L, Hendriks RJ, Dijkstra S, et al. Detection of high-grade prostate cancer using a urinary molecular biomarker-based risk score. *Eur Urol*. 2016;70:740–748.
21. Smith RA, Andrews KS, Brooks D, et al. Cancer screening in the United States, 2019: A review of current American Cancer Society guidelines and current issues in cancer screening *CA: Cancer J Clin*. 692019184–210.
22. Carter HB, Albertsen PC, Barry MJ, et al. Early detection of prostate cancer: AUA Guideline. *J Urol*. 2013;190:419–426.
23. Grossman DC, Curry SJ, Owens DK, et al. Screening for prostate cancer: US Preventive Services Task Force Recommendation Statement. *JAMA*. 2018;319:1901–1913.
24. Jackson AS, Sohaib SA, Staffurth JN, et al. Distribution of lymph nodes in men with prostatic adenocarcinoma and lymphadenopathy at presentation: a retrospective radiological review and implications for prostate and pelvis radiotherapy. *Clin Oncol (R Coll Radiol)*. 2006;18:109–116.
25. Prostate AJCC. American Joint Committee on Cancer, American Cancer Society. In: Greene FL, ed. *AJCC Cancer Staging Manual*. New York: Springer-Verlag; 2002:337–345.
26. Yu KK, Hawkins RA. The prostate: diagnostic evaluation of metastatic disease. *Radiol Clin North Am*. 2000;38:139–157. ix.
27. Spencer J, Golding S. CT evaluation of lymph node status at presentation of prostatic carcinoma. *Br J Radiol*. 1992;65:199–201.
28. Saitoh H, Yoshida K, Uchijima Y, et al. Two different lymph node metastatic patterns of a prostatic cancer. *Cancer*. 1990;65:1843–1846.
29. Bubendorf L, Schopfer A, Wagner U, et al. Metastatic patterns of prostate cancer: an autopsy study of 1,589 patients. *Hum Pathol*. 2000;31:578–583.
30. Littrup PJ, Bailey SE. Prostate cancer: the role of transrectal ultrasound and its impact on cancer detection and management. *Radiol Clin North Am*. 2000;38:87–113.
31. Lee F, Torp-Pedersen S, Littrup PJ, et al. Hypoechoic lesions of the prostate: clinical relevance of tumor size, digital rectal examination, and prostate-specific antigen. *Radiology*. 1989;170:29–32.
32. Keetch DW, Catalona WJ, Smith DS. Serial prostatic biopsies in men with persistently elevated serum prostate specific antigen values. *J Urol*. 1994;151:1571–1574.
33. Roehrborn CG, Pickens GJ, Sanders JS. Diagnostic yield of repeated transrectal ultrasound-guided biopsies stratified by specific histopathologic diagnoses and prostate specific antigen levels. *Urology*. 1996;47:347–352.
34. Ellis WJ, Brawer MK. Repeat prostate needle biopsy: who needs it? *J Urol*. 1995;153:1496–1498.
35. Presti Jr JC, Chang JJ, Bhargava V, et al. The optimal systematic prostate biopsy scheme should include 8 rather than 6 biopsies: results of a prospective clinical trial. *J Urol*. 2000;163:163–166. discussion 166–167.
36. Singh H, Canto EI, Shariat SF, et al. Improved detection of clinically significant, curable prostate cancer with systematic 12-core biopsy. *J Urol*. 2004;171:1089–1092.
37. Kuligowska E, Barish MA, Fenlon HM, et al. Predictors of prostate carcinoma: accuracy of gray-scale and color Doppler US and serum markers. *Radiology*. 2001;220:757–764.
38. Halpern EJ, Rosenberg M, Gomella LG. Prostate cancer: contrast-enhanced us for detection. *Radiology*. 2001;219:219–225.
39. Sanchez-Chapado M, Angulo JC, Ibarburen C, et al. Comparison of digital rectal examination, transrectal ultrasonography, and multicoil magnetic resonance imaging for preoperative evaluation of prostate cancer. *Eur Urol*. 1997;32:140–149.
40. Tan CH, Wang J, Kundra V. Diffusion weighted imaging in prostate cancer. *Eur Radiol*. 2011;21(3):593–603.
41. Tan CH, Wei W, Johnson V, et al. Diffusion-weighted MRI in the detection of prostate cancer: meta-analysis. *AJR Am J Roentgenol*. 2012;199(4):822–829.
42. Tan CH, Hobbs BP, Wei W, et al. Dynamic contrast-enhanced MRI for the detection of prostate cancer: meta-analysis. *AJR Am J Roentgenol*. 2015;204(4):W439–W448.
43. P-RADS Prostate Imaging-Reporting and Data System 2019 version 2.1. ACR American College of Radiology. 2019.
44. Vaché T, Bratan F, Mège-Lechevallier F, et al. Characterization of prostate lesions as benign or malignant at multiparametric MR imaging: comparison of three scoring systems in patients treated with radical prostatectomy. *Radiology*. 2014;272(2):446–455.
45. Polanec S, Helbich TH, Bickel H, et al. Head-to-head comparison of PI-RADS v2 and PI-RADS v1. *Eur J Radiol*. 2016;85(6):1125–1131.
46. Muller BG, Shih JH, Sankineni S, et al. Prostate cancer: interobserver agreement and accuracy with the revised Prostate Imaging Reporting and Data System at multiparametric MR imaging. *Radiology*. 2015;277(3):741–750.
47. Kasel-Seibert M, Lehmann T, Aschenbach R, et al. Assessment of PI-RADS v2 for the detection of prostate cancer. *Eur J Radiol*. 2016;85(4):726–731.
48. Park SY, Shin SJ, Jung DC, et al. PI-RADS version 2: quantitative analysis aids reliable interpretation of diffusion-weighted imaging for prostate cancer. *Eur Radiol*. 2017;27(7):2776–2783.

49. Baldisserotto M, Neto EJ, Carvalhal G, et al. Validation of PI-RADS v.2 for prostate cancer diagnosis with MRI at 3T using an external phased-array coil. *J Magn Reson Imaging*. 2016;44(5):1354–1359.
50. Mussi TC, Yamauchi FI, Tridente CF, et al. Interobserver agreement and positivity of PI-RADS version 2 among radiologists with different levels of experience. *Acad Radiol*. 2019;26(8):1017–1022.
51. Rosenkrantz AB, Ginocchio LA, Cornfeld D, et al. Interobserver reproducibility of the PI-RADS version 2 lexicon: a multicenter study of six experienced prostate radiologists. *Radiology*. 2016;280(3):793–804.
52. Weinreb JC, Barentsz JO, Choyke PL, et al. PI-RADS prostate imaging - reporting and data system: 2015, version 2. *Eur Urol*. 2016;69(1):16–40.
53. Barth BK, De Visschere PJL, Cornelius A, et al. Detection of clinically significant prostate cancer: short dual-pulse sequence versus standard multiparametric MR imaging—a multireader study. *Radiology*. 2017;284:725–736.
54. Cuocolo R, Stanzione A, Rusconi G, et al. PSA-density does not improve bi-parametric prostate MR detection of prostate cancer in a biopsy naïve patient population. *Eur J Radiol*. 2018;104:64–70.
55. Kuhl CK, Bruhn R, Kramer N, et al. Abbreviated biparametric prostate MR imaging in men with elevated prostate-specific antigen. *Radiology*. 2017;285:493–505.
56. Stanzione A, Imbriaco M, Cocozza S, et al. Biparametric 3T magnetic resonance imaging for prostate cancer detection in a biopsy-na€ıve patient population: a further improvement of PI-RADS v2? *Eur J Radiol*. 2016;85:2269–2274.
57. Alabousi M, Salameh JP, Gusenbauer K, et al. Biparametric vs multiparametric prostate magnetic resonance imaging for the detection of prostate cancer in treatment-naïve patients: a diagnostic test accuracy systematic review and meta-analysis. *BJU Int*. 2019;124(2):209–220.
58. Gatti M, Faletti R, Calleris G, et al. Prostate cancer detection with biparametric magnetic resonance imaging (bpMRI) by readers with different experience: performance and comparison with multiparametric (mpMRI). *Abdom Radiol (NY)*. 2019;44(5):1883–1893.
59. Siddiqui MM, Rais-Bahrami S, Turkbey B, et al. Comparison of MR/ultrasound fusion-guided biopsy with ultrasound-guided biopsy for the diagnosis of prostate cancer. *JAMA*. 2015;313(4):390–397.
60. Borkowetz A, Hadaschik B, Platzek I, et al. Prospective comparison of transperineal magnetic resonance imaging/ultrasonography fusion biopsy and transrectal systematic biopsy in biopsy-naïve patients. *BJU Int*. 2018;121(1):53–60.
61. Kasivisvanathan V, Rannikko AS, Borghi M, et al. MRI-targeted or standard biopsy for prostate-cancer diagnosis. *N Engl J Med*. 2018;378(19):1767–1777.
62. Porpiglia F, Manfredi M, Mele F, et al. Diagnostic pathway with multiparametric magnetic resonance imaging versus standard pathway: results from a randomized prospective study in biopsy-naïve patients with suspected prostate cancer. *Eur Urol*. 2017;72(2):282–288.
63. Boesen L, Nørgaard N, Løgager V, et al. Assessment of the diagnostic accuracy of biparametric magnetic resonance imaging for prostate cancer in biopsy-naive men. *JAMA Netw Open*. 2018;1:e180219.
64. Jambor I, Verho J, Ettala O, et al. Validation of IMPROD biparametric MRI in men with clinically suspected prostate cancer: A prospective multi-institutional trial. *PLoS Med*. 2019;16(6):e1002813.
65. Sanchez-Chapado M, Angulo JC, Ibarburen C, et al. Comparison of digital rectal examination, transrectal ultrasonography, and multicoil magnetic resonance imaging for preoperative evaluation of prostate cancer. *Eur Urol*. 1997;32:140–149.
66. Ekici S, Ozen H, Agildere M, et al. A comparison of transrectal ultrasonography and endorectal magnetic resonance imaging in the local staging of prostatic carcinoma. *BJU Int*. 1999;83:796–800.
67. D'Amico AV, Whittington R, Malkowicz SB, et al. Role of percent positive biopsies and endorectal coil MRI in predicting prognosis in intermediate-risk prostate cancer patients. *Cancer J Sci Am*. 1996;2:343.
68. Perrotti M, Kaufman Jr RP, Jennings TA, et al. Endo-rectal coil magnetic resonance imaging in clinically localized prostate cancer: is it accurate? *J Urol*. 1996;156:106–109.
69. Wang L, Hricak H, Kattan MW, et al. Prediction of organ-confined prostate cancer: incremental value of MR imaging and MR spectroscopic imaging to staging nomograms. *Radiology*. 2006;238:597–603.
70. Jager GJ, Severens JL, Thornbury JR, et al. Prostate cancer staging: should MR imaging be used?—A decision analytic approach. *Radiology*. 2000;215:445–451.
71. D'Amico AV, Whittington R, Malkowicz SB, et al. Combined modality staging of prostate carcinoma and its utility in predicting pathologic stage and postoperative prostate specific antigen failure. *Urology*. 1997;49:23–30.
72. Barentsz JO, Jager GJ, Engelbrecht MR. MR imaging of prostate cancer. *Cancer Imaging*. 2000;1:44–51.
73. Langlotz C, Schnall M, Pollack H. Staging of prostatic cancer: accuracy of MR imaging. *Radiology*. 1995;194:645–646. discussion 647–648.
74. Jager GJ, Ruijter ET, van de Kaa CA, et al. Local staging of prostate cancer with endorectal MR imaging: correlation with histopathology. *AJR Am J Roentgenol*. 1996;166:845–852.
75. Ahn H, Hwang SI, Lee HJ, et al. Prediction of extraprostatic extension on multi-parametric magnetic resonance imaging in patients with anterior prostate cancer. *Eur Radiol*. 2020;30(1):26–37.
76. Bai K, Sun Y, Li W, Zhang L. Apparent diffusion coefficient in extraprostatic extension of prostate cancer: a systematic review and diagnostic meta-analysis. *Cancer Manag Res*. 2019;11:3125–3137.
77. Ball MW, Partin AW, Epstein JI. Extent of extraprostatic extension independently influences biochemical recurrence-free survival: evidence for further pT3 subclassification. *Urology*. 2015;85(1):161–164.
78. Cheng D, Tempany CM. MR imaging of the prostate and bladder. *Semin Ultrasound CT MR*. 1998;19:67–89.
79. Tanaka K, Shigemura K, Muramaki M, et al. Efficacy of using three-tesla magnetic resonance imaging diagnosis of capsule invasion for decision-making about neurovascular bundle preservation in robotic-assisted radical prostatectomy. *Korean J Urol*. 2013;54(7):437–441.
80. Cheng L, Darson MF, Bergstralh EJ, et al. Correlation of margin status and extraprostatic extension with progression of prostate carcinoma. *Cancer*. 1999;86:1775–1782.
81. Wang L, Hricak H, Kattan MW, et al. Prediction of seminal vesicle invasion in prostate cancer: incremental value of adding endorectal MR imaging to the Kattan nomogram. *Radiology*. 2007;242:182–188.
82. Morlacco A, Sharma V, Viers BR, et al. The incremental role of magnetic resonance imaging for prostate cancer staging before radical prostatectomy. *Eur Urol*. 2017;71:701–704.
83. Haukaas S, Roervik J, Halvorsen OJ, et al. When is bone scintigraphy necessary in the assessment of newly diagnosed, untreated prostate cancer? *Br J Urol*. 1997;79:770–776.
84. Gold RI, Seeger LL, Bassett LW, et al. An integrated approach to the evaluation of metastatic bone disease. *Radiol Clin North Am*. 1990;28:471–483.
85. Algra PR, Bloem JL, Tissing H, et al. Detection of vertebral metastases: comparison between MR imaging and bone scintigraphy. *Radiographics*. 1991;11:219–232.
86. Ma J, Costelloe CM, Madewell JE, et al. Fast dixon-based multisequence and multiplanar MRI for whole-body detection of cancer metastases. *J Magn Reson Imaging*. 2009;29(5):1154–1162.
87. Padhani AR, Lecouvet FE, Tunariu N, et al. METastasis reporting and data system for prostate cancer: practical guidelines for acquisition, interpretation, and reporting of whole-body magnetic resonance imaging-based evaluations of multiorgan involvement in advanced prostate cancer. *Eur Urol*. 2017;71(1):81–92.
88. Fanti S, Minozzi S, Antoch G, et al. Consensus on molecular imaging and theranostics in prostate cancer. *Lancet Oncol*. 2018;19(12):e696–e708.
89. Yao D, Trabulsi EJ, Kostakoglu L, et al. The utility of monoclonal antibodies in the imaging of prostate cancer. *Semin Urol Oncol*. 2002;20:211–218.
90. Barocas DA, Alvarez J, Resnick MJ, et al. Association between radiation therapy, surgery, or observation for localized prostate cancer and patient-reported outcomes after 3 years. *JAMA*. 2017;317(11):1126–1140.
91. Chen RC, Basak R, Meyer AM, et al. Association between choice of radical prostatectomy, external beam radiotherapy, brachytherapy, or active surveillance and patient-reported quality of life among men with localized prostate cancer. *JAMA*. 2017;317(11):1141–1150. Donovan JL, Hamdy FC, Lane JA, et al. Patient-Reported Outcomes after Monitoring, Surgery, or Radiotherapy for Prostate Cancer. *N Engl J Med*. 2016;375(15):1425–1437.
92. Hoffman KE, Penson DF, Zhao Z, et al. Patient-reported outcomes through 5 years for active surveillance, surgery, brachytherapy, or external beam radiation with or without androgen deprivation therapy for localized prostate cancer. *JAMA*. 2020;323(2):149–163.

93. Donovan JL, Hamdy FC, Lane JA, et al. Patient-reported outcomes after monitoring, surgery, or radiotherapy for prostate cancer. *N Engl J Med*. 2016;375(15):1425–1437.
94. D'Amico AV, Whittington R, Malkowicz SB, et al. Pretreatment nomogram for prostate-specific antigen recurrence after radical prostatectomy or external-beam radiation therapy for clinically localized prostate cancer. *J Clini Onco*. 1999;17:168–172.
95. Klotz L, Vesprini D, Sethukavalan P, et al. Long-term follow-up of a large active surveillance cohort of patients with prostate cancer. *J Clin Oncol*. 2015;33:272–277.
96. Tosoian JJ, Mamawala M, Epstein JI, et al. Intermediate and longer-term outcomes from a prospective active-surveillance program for favorable-risk prostate cancer. *J Clin Oncol*. 2015;33:3379–3385.
97. Tosoian JJ, Trock BJ, Landis P, et al. Active surveillance program for prostate cancer: an update of the Johns Hopkins experience. *J Clin Oncol*. 2011;29:2185–2190.
98. Adamy A, Yee DS, Matsushita K, et al. Role of prostate specific antigen and immediate confirmatory biopsy in predicting progression during active surveillance for low risk prostate cancer. *J Urol*. 2011;185:477–482.
99. Davis JW, Ward 3rd JF, Pettaway CA, et al. Disease reclassification risk with stringent criteria and frequent monitoring in men with favourable-risk prostate cancer undergoing active surveillance. *BJU international*. 2016;118:68–76.
100. Newcomb LF, Brooks JD, Carroll PR, et al. Canary Prostate Active Surveillance Study: design of a multi-institutional active surveillance cohort and biorepository. *Urology*. 2010;75:407–413.
101. Loeb S, Folkvaljon Y, Makarov DV, et al. Five-year nationwide follow-up study of active surveillance for prostate cancer. *Eur Urol*. 2015;67:233–238.
102. Schoots IG, Petrides N, Giganti F, et al. Magnetic resonance imaging in active surveillance of prostate cancer: a systematic review. *Eur Urol*. 2015;67:627–636.
103. Eineluoto JT, Jarvinen P, Kenttamies A, et al. Repeat multiparametric MRI in prostate cancer patients on active surveillance. *PloS One*. 2017;12:e0189272.
104. Moore CM, Giganti F, Albertsen P, et al. Reporting magnetic resonance imaging in men on active surveillance for prostate cancer: The PRECISE Recommendations-A report of a European School of Oncology Task Force. *European Urology*. 2017;71:648–655.
105. Walsh PC, Partin AW, Epstein JI. Cancer control and quality of life following anatomical radical retropubic prostatectomy: results at 10 years. *J Urol*. 1994;152:1831–1836.
106. Gandaglia G, Sammon JD, Chang SL, et al. Comparative effectiveness of robot-assisted and open radical prostatectomy in the postdissemination era. *J Clin Oncol*. 2014;32:1419–1426.
107. Yaxley JW, Coughlin GD, Chambers SK, et al. Robot-assisted laparoscopic prostatectomy versus open radical retropubic prostatectomy: early outcomes from a randomised controlled phase 3 study. *Lancet*. 2016;388:1057–1066.
108. Lebacle C, Roudot-Thoraval F, Moktefi A, et al. Integration of MRI to clinical nomogram for predicting pathological stage before radical prostatectomy. *World J Urol*. 2017;35:1409–1415.
109. Schiavina R, Bianchi L, Borghesi M, et al. MRI displays the prostatic cancer anatomy and improves the bundles management before robot-assisted radical prostatectomy. *J Endourol*. 2018;32:315–321.
110. Briganti A, Chun FK, Salonia A, et al. A nomogram for staging of exclusive nonobturator lymph node metastases in men with localized prostate cancer. *Eur Urol*. 2007;51:112–119. discussion 119–120.
111. Cagiannos I, Karakiewicz P, Eastham JA, et al. A preoperative nomogram identifying decreased risk of positive pelvic lymph nodes in patients with prostate cancer. *J Urol*. 2003;170:1798–1803.
112. Gandaglia G, Fossati N, Zaffuto E, et al. Development and internal validation of a novel model to identify the candidates for extended pelvic lymph node dissection in prostate cancer. *Eur Urol*. 2017;72:632–640.
113. Han KR, Belldegrun AS. Third-generation cryosurgery for primary and recurrent prostate cancer. *BJU International*. 2004;93:14–18.
114. Rees J, Patel B, MacDonagh R, et al. Cryosurgery for prostate cancer. *BJU International*. 2004;93:710–714.
115. Van Leenders GJ, Beerlage HP, Ruijter ET, et al. Histopathological changes associated with high intensity focused ultrasound (HIFU) treatment for localised adenocarcinoma of the prostate. *J Clin Pathol*. 2000;53:391–394.
116. Madersbacher S, Marberger M. High-energy shockwaves and extracorporeal high-intensity focused ultrasound. *J Endourol*. 2003;17:667–672.
117. Royce TJ, Efstathiou JA. Proton therapy for prostate cancer: A review of the rationale, evidence, and current state. *Urol Oncol*. 2019;37(9):628–636.
118. Pugh TJ, Choi S, Nogueras-Gonzalaez GM, et al. Proton beam therapy for localized prostate cancer: results from a prospective quality-of-life trial. *Int J Part Ther*. 2016;3(1):27–36.
119. Bryant C, Smith TL, Henderson RH, et al. Five-year biochemical results, toxicity, and patient-reported quality of life after delivery of dose-escalated image guided proton therapy for prostate cancer. *Int J Radiat Oncol Biol Phys*. 2016;95(1):422–434.
120. Kuban DA, Tucker SL, Dong L, et al. Long-term results of the M. D. Anderson randomized dose-escalation trial for prostate cancer. *Int J Radiat Oncol Biol Phys*. 2008;70:67–74.
121. Zietman AL, DeSilvio ML, Slater JD, et al. Comparison of conventional-dose vs high-dose conformal radiation therapy in clinically localized adenocarcinoma of the prostate: a randomized controlled trial. *JAMA*. 2005;294:1233–1239.
122. Zietman AL. Correction: inaccurate analysis and results in a study of radiation therapy in adenocarcinoma of the prostate *JAMA*. 2992008898–899.
123. Al-Mamgani A, van Putten WL, Heemsbergen WD, et al. Update of Dutch multicenter dose-escalation trial of radiotherapy for localized prostate cancer. *Int J Radiat Oncol Biol Phys*. 2008;72:980–988.
124. Dearnaley DP, Sydes MR, Graham JD, et al. Escalated-dose versus standard-dose conformal radiotherapy in prostate cancer: first results from the MRC RT01 randomised controlled trial. *Lancet Oncol*. 2007;8:475–487.
125. Kuban DA, Levy LB, Tucker S, et al. Long-term failure patterns and survival in a randomized dose-escalation trial for prostate cancer. *Who dies of disease? Int J Radiat Oncol Biol Phys*. 2008;72:S93.
126. Zelefsky MJ, Yamada Y, Fuks Z, et al. Long-term results of conformal radiotherapy for prostate cancer: impact of dose escalation on biochemical tumor control and distant metastases-free survival outcomes. *Int J Radiat Oncol Biol Phys*. 2008;71:1028–1033.
127. Cahlon O, Zelefsky MJ, Shippy A, et al. Ultra-high dose (86.4 Gy) IMRT for localized prostate cancer: toxicity and biochemical outcomes. *Int J Radiat Oncol Biol Phys*. 2008;71:330–337.
128. NCCN Guidelines Version 4.2019. Prostate Cancer.
129. Sanda MG, Cadeddu JA, Kirkby E, et al. Clinically Localized Prostate Cancer: AUA/ASTRO/SUO Guideline. Part II: recommended approaches and details of specific care options. *J Urol*. 2018;199(4):990–997.
130. Morris WJ, Tyldesley S, Rodda S, et al. Androgen Suppression Combined with Elective Nodal and Dose Escalated Radiation Therapy (the ASCENDE-RT Trial): an analysis of survival endpoints for a randomized trial comparing a low-dose-rate brachytherapy boost to a dose-escalated external beam boost for high- and intermediate-risk prostate cancer. *Int J Radiat Oncol Biol Phys*. 2017;98:275–285.
131. Hoskin PJ, Rojas AM, Bownes PJ, et al. Randomised trial of external beam radiotherapy alone or combined with high-dose-rate brachytherapy boost for localised prostate cancer. *Radiother Oncol*. 2012;103:217–222.
132. Sathya JR, Davis IR, Julian JA, et al. Randomized trial comparing iridium implant plus external-beam radiation therapy with external-beam radiation therapy alone in node-negative locally advanced cancer of the prostate. *J Clin Oncol*. 2005;23:1192–1199.
133. Lee DJ, Barocas DA, Zhao Z, et al. Comparison of patient-reported outcomes after external beam radiation therapy and combined external beam with low-dose-rate brachytherapy boost in men with localized prostate cancer. *Int J Radiat Oncol Biol Phys*. 2018;102(1):116–126.
134. Hoffman KE, Voong KR, Levy LB, et al. Randomized trial of hypofractionated, dose-escalated, intensity-modulated radiation therapy (IMRT) versus conventionally fractionated IMRT for localized prostate cancer. *J Clin Oncol*. 2018;36(29):2943–2949.
135. Pollack A, Walker G, Horwitz EM, et al. Randomized trial of hypofractionated external-beam radiotherapy for prostate cancer. *J Clin Oncol*. 2013;31(31):3860–3868.
136. Morgan SC, Hoffman K, Loblaw DA, et al. Hypofractionated radiation therapy for localized prostate cancer: executive summary

of an ASTRO, ASCO and AUA evidence-based guideline. *J Urol.* 2019;201(3):528–534.

137. King CR, Freeman D, Kaplan I, et al. Stereotactic body radiotherapy for localized prostate cancer: pooled analysis from a multi-institutional consortium of prospective phase II trials. *Radiother Oncol.* 2013;109(2):217–221.
138. Morgan SC, Hoffman K, Loblaw DA, et al. Hypofractionated radiation therapy for localized prostate cancer: executive summary of an ASTRO, ASCO, and AUA evidence-based guideline. *Pract Radiat Oncol.* 2018;8(6):354–360.
139. Bolla M, Van Tienhoven G, Warde P, et al. External irradiation with or without long-term androgen suppression for prostate cancer with high metastatic risk: 10-year results of an EORTC randomised study. *Lancet Oncol.* 2010;11(11):1066–1073.
140. Gupta D, Lee Chuy K, Yang JC, et al. Cardiovascular and metabolic effects of androgen-deprivation therapy for prostate cancer. *J Oncol Pract.* 2018;14(10):580–587.
141. Lawton CAF, Lin X, Hanks GE, et al. Duration of androgen deprivation in locally advanced prostate cancer: long-term update of NRG Oncology RTOG 9202. *Int J Radiat Oncol Biol Phys.* 2017;98(2):296.
142. Bolla M, de Reijke TM, Van Tienhoven G, et al. Duration of androgen suppression in the treatment of prostate cancer. *N Engl J Med.* 2009;360(24):2516.
143. Nabid A, Carrier N, Martin AG, et al. Duration of Androgen Deprivation Therapy in High-risk Prostate Cancer: A Randomized Phase III Trial. *Eur Urol.* 2018;74(4):432.
144. Bian SX, Kuban DA, Levy LB, et al. Addition of short-term androgen deprivation therapy to dose-escalated radiation therapy improves failure-free survival for select men with intermediate-risk prostate cancer. *Ann Oncol.* 2012;23(9):2346–2352.
145. Nguyen PL, Chen MH, Beard CJ, et al. Radiation with or without 6 months of androgen suppression therapy in intermediate- and high-risk clinically localized prostate cancer: a post-randomization analysis by risk group. *Int J Radiat Oncol Biol Phys.* 2010;77(4):1046–1052.
146. Kamran SC, D'Amico AV. Radiation therapy for prostate cancer. *Hematol Oncol Clin North Am.* 2020;34(1):45–69.
147. Potters L, Morgenstern C, Calugaru E, et al. 12-year outcomes following permanent prostate brachytherapy in patients with clinically localized prostate cancer. *J Urol.* 2005;173:1562–1566.
148. Grills IS, Martinez AA, Hollander M, et al. High dose rate brachytherapy as prostate cancer monotherapy reduces toxicity compared to low dose rate palladium seeds. *J Urol.* 2004;171:1098–1104.
149. Lee AK. Radiation therapy combined with hormone therapy for prostate cancer. *Semin Radiat Oncol.* 2006;16:20–28.
150. Soloway MS, Pareek K, Sharifi R, et al. Neoadjuvant androgen ablation before radical prostatectomy in cT2bNxMo prostate cancer: 5-year results. *J Urol.* 2002;167:112–116.
151. Pettaway CA, Pisters LL, Troncoso P, et al. Neoadjuvant chemotherapy and hormonal therapy followed by radical prostatectomy: feasibility and preliminary results. *J Clin Oncol.* 2000;18:1050–1057.
152. Pinski J, Dorff TB. Prostate cancer metastases to bone: pathophysiology, pain management, and the promise of targeted therapy. *Eur J Cancer.* 2005;41:932–940.
153. Cursano MC, Iuliani M, Casadei C, et al. Combination radium-223 therapies in patients with bone metastases from castration-resistant prostate cancer: A review. *Crit Rev Oncol Hematol.* 2020;146:102864.
154. Pound CR, Partin AW, Eisenberger MA, et al. Natural history of progression after PSA elevation following radical prostatectomy. *JAMA.* 1999;281:1591–1597.
155. Han M, Partin AW, Pound CR, et al. Long-term biochemical disease-free and cancer-specific survival following anatomic radical retropubic prostatectomy. The 15-year Johns Hopkins experience. *Urol Clin North Am.* 2001;28:555–565.
156. Roach 3rd M, Hanks G. Thames H Jr. et al. Defining biochemical failure following radiotherapy with or without hormonal therapy in men with clinically localized prostate cancer: recommendations of the RTOG-ASTRO Phoenix Consensus Conference. *Int J Radiat Oncol Biol Phys.* 2006;65:965–974.
157. Partin AW, Pearson JD, Landis PK, et al. Evaluation of serum prostate-specific antigen velocity after radical prostatectomy to distinguish local recurrence from distant metastases. *Urology.* 1994;43:649–659.
158. Lee AK, D'Amico AV. Utility of prostate-specific antigen kinetics in addition to clinical factors in the selection of patients for salvage local therapy. *J Clin Oncol.* 2005;23:8192–8197.
159. Panebianco V, Barchetti F, Sciarra A, et al. Prostate cancer recurrence after radical prostatectomy: the role of 3-T diffusion imaging in multi-parametric magnetic resonance imaging. *Eur Radiol.* 2013;23:1745–1752.
160. Manzone TA, Malkowicz SB, Tomaszewski JE, et al. Use of endorectal MR imaging to predict prostate carcinoma recurrence after radical prostatectomy. *Radiology.* 1998;209:537–542.
161. Silverman JM, Krebs TL. MR imaging evaluation with a transrectal surface coil of local recurrence of prostatic cancer in men who have undergone radical prostatectomy. *AJR Am J Roentgenol.* 1997;168:379–385.
162. Cirillo S, Petracchini M, Scotti L, et al. Endorectal magnetic resonance imaging at 1.5 Tesla to assess local recurrence following radical prostatectomy using T2-weighted and contrast-enhanced imaging. *Eur Radiol.* 2009;19:761–769.
163. Casciani E, Polettini E, Carmenini E, et al. Endorectal and dynamic contrast-enhanced MRI for detection of local recurrence after radical prostatectomy. *AJR Am J Roentgenol.* 2008;190:1187–1192.
164. Sella T, Schwartz LH, Swindle PW, et al. Suspected local recurrence after radical prostatectomy: endorectal coil MR imaging. *Radiology.* 2004;231:379–385.
165. Pickett B, Kurhanewicz J, Coakley F, et al. Use of MRI and spectroscopy in evaluation of external beam radiotherapy for prostate cancer. *Int J Radiat Oncol Biol Phys.* 2004;60:1047–1055.
166. Mueller-Lisse UG, Vigneron DB, Hricak H, et al. Localized prostate cancer: effect of hormone deprivation therapy measured by using combined three-dimensional 1H MR spectroscopy and MR imaging: clinicopathologic case-controlled study. *Radiology.* 2001;221:380–390.
167. Leventis AK, Shariat SF, Slawin KM. Local recurrence after radical prostatectomy: correlation of US features with prostatic fossa biopsy findings. *Radiology.* 2001;219:432–439.
168. Gaur S, Turkbey B, Prostate MR. imaging for posttreatment evaluation and recurrence. *Urol Clin North Am.* 2018;45:467–479.
169. Naya Y, Okihara K, Evans RB, et al. Efficacy of prostatic fossa biopsy in detecting local recurrence after radical prostatectomy. *Urology.* 2005;66:350–355.
170. Kitajima K, Murphy RC, Nathan MA, et al. Detection of recurrent prostate cancer after radical prostatectomy: comparison of 11C-choline PET/CT with pelvic multiparametric MR imaging with endorectal coil. *J Nucl Med.* 2014;55:223–232.
171. Spencer JA, Golding SJ. Patterns of lymphatic metastases at recurrence of prostate cancer: CT findings. *Clin Radiol.* 1994;49:404–407.
172. Okotie OT, Aronson WJ, Wieder JA, et al. Predictors of metastatic disease in men with biochemical failure following radical prostatectomy. *J Urol.* 2004;171:2260–2264.
173. Jadvar H. Molecular imaging of prostate cancer with PET. *J Nucl Med.* 2013;54 1685–1658.
174. Apolo AB, Pandit-Taskar N, Morris MJ. Novel tracers and their development for the imaging of metastatic prostate cancer. *J Nucl Med.* 2008;49:2031–2041.
175. Savir-Baruch B, Zanoni L, Schuster DM. Imaging of prostate cancer using fluciclovine. *Urol Clin North Am.* 2018;45:489–502.
176. Hofman MS, Iravani A, Nzenza T, et al. Advances in urologic imaging: prostate-specific membrane antigen ligand PET imaging. *Urol Clin North Am.* 2018;45:503–524.
177. Fendler WP, Eiber M, Beheshti M, et al. (68)Ga-PSMA PET/CT: Joint EANM and SNMMI procedure guideline for prostate cancer imaging: version 1.0. *Eur J Nucl Med Mol Imaging.* 2017;44:1014–1024.
178. Giovacchini G, Giovannini E, Riondato M, et al. PET/CT with (68)Ga-PSMA in prostate cancer: radiopharmaceutical background and clinical implications. *Curr Radiopharm.* 2018;11:4–13.
179. Silver DA, Pellicer I, Fair WR, et al. Prostate-specific membrane antigen expression in normal and malignant human tissues. *Clin Cancer Res.* 1997;3:81–85.
180. Maurer T, Gschwend JE, Rauscher I, et al. Diagnostic efficacy of (68)Gallium-PSMA positron emission tomography compared to conventional imaging for lymph node staging of 130 consecutive patients with intermediate to high risk prostate cancer. *J Urol.* 2016;195:1436–1443.

181. Evans JD, Jethwa KR, Ost P, et al. Prostate cancer-specific PET radiotracers: A review on the clinical utility in recurrent disease. *Pract Radiat Oncol*. 2018;8:28–39.
182. Afshar-Oromieh A, Babich JW, Kratochwil C, et al. The rise of PSMA ligands for diagnosis and therapy of prostate cancer. *J Nucl Med*. 2016;57:79S–89S.
183. Kundu SD, Roehl KA, Eggener SE, et al. Potency, continence and complications in 3,477 consecutive radical retropubic prostatectomies. *J Urol*. 2004;172:2227–2231.
184. Webb DR, Sethi K, Gee K. An analysis of the causes of bladder neck contracture after open and robot-assisted laparoscopic radical prostatectomy. *BJU Int*. 2009;103:957–963.
185. Kumar RJ, Barqawi A, Crawford ED. Preventing and treating the complications of hormone therapy. *Curr Urol Rep*. 2005;6:217–223.
186. Gomella LG. Contemporary use of hormonal therapy in prostate cancer: managing complications and addressing quality-of-life issues. *BJU Int*. 2007;99(suppl 1):25–29. discussion 30.

CHAPTER

24 Primary Retroperitoneal Tumors

Corey T. Jensen, M.D.; Bharat Raval, M.D.; Christina L. Roland, M.D., M.S.; Andrew J. Bishop, M.D.; and Shreyaskumar Patel, M.D.

INTRODUCTION

Primary retroperitoneal tumors are exceedingly rare. Primary masses in the retroperitoneum can be categorized as one of three entities: lymphomas, extragonadal germ cell tumors, and sarcomas. Although gastrointestinal stromal tumors (GISTs) arise in the intraperitoneal compartment, they can also mimic these retroperitoneal masses because of their large size. This chapter reviews primary retroperitoneal sarcomas (RPSs), which form about one third of all primary retroperitoneal tumors. RPSs lack specific clinical symptoms beyond the effect manifested from their impact on adjacent structures. As a result, they often progress to a large size before initial presentation. Successful management of RPSs requires the collaborative efforts of the radiologist, pathologist, radiation oncologist, medical oncologist, surgical oncologist, and other specialists. Imaging plays a key role in the initial detection, therapeutic planning, and follow-up of these patients.

EPIDEMIOLOGY AND RISK FACTORS

Soft tissue sarcomas (STSs) form 1% of all newly diagnosed malignancies in the United States, and 15% of these arise in the retroperitoneum.[1] STSs in children account for up to 15% of all pediatric malignancies. The mean annual incidence of RPS is 2.7 per million persons, and no significant change has been observed over time.[2]

RPSs arise from the embryonic mesoderm. The vast majority do not have any identifiable predisposing cause. A small proportion of STSs may arise as a result of prior radiation exposure or in association with a genetic syndrome.

Exposure to ionizing radiation increases the incidence of STSs, with a median interval of 10 years (range 2–50 years) after exposure. These occur in the irradiated field, commonly in patients who receive radiation therapy for breast cancer, cervical cancer, lymphoma, or testicular tumors or for benign conditions.[3–5] Patients treated with prior radiation exposure can develop either STSs or bone sarcomas.

Several genetic syndromes are associated with the development of STS.[6] Neurofibromatosis type 1, also known as von Recklinghausen disease, is an autosomal dominant condition that arises because of a mutation in the *NF1* gene. These patients have a high incidence of neurofibromas, as well as approximately a 10% increased risk of developing malignant peripheral nerve sheath tumors during their lifetime. Gardner syndrome, another autosomal dominant disease, is caused by mutation of the *APC* gene and is associated with multiple colonic polyps, colon cancer, and desmoid tumors. STS has also been reported in patients with Li–Fraumeni syndrome, which is caused by a germline mutation in the *P53* tumor suppressor gene. Children with hereditary retinoblastoma owing to a germline mutation in the *RB1* tumor suppressor gene face a higher risk of STS and osteosarcoma. The risk is further increased because these patients receive radiotherapy for the initial treatment of retinoblastoma.

ANATOMY AND PATHOLOGY

Anatomy

Macroscopically, parts of the genitourinary tract, gastrointestinal (GI) tract, aorta and its branches, inferior vena cava and its tributaries, retroperitoneal fat, and lymphatic and nervous systems form important components of the retroperitoneum (Fig. 24.1). The pancreas, ascending colon, descending colon, and duodenum are located anteriorly within the anterior pararenal space, and the aorta, inferior vena cava, and lymph nodes are in the midline. Laterally, the kidneys and adrenals are surrounded by renal fascia within the perirenal space. The psoas, quadratus lumborum, paraverterbral muscles, and bony skeleton form the posterior boundary of the retroperitoneum. Retroperitoneal fat, vessels, lymphatics, and nerves continue from the retroperitoneum into the small bowel mesentery, providing anatomic continuity between these compartments (Fig. 24.2). The displacement or contiguous involvement of these major organs, and in particular of the major vascular branches, is of critical importance when planning surgical resection.

KEY POINTS Anatomy

- Duodenum, ascending and descending colon, and pancreas lie anteriorly in the anterior pararenal space.
- Kidneys with perinephric fat and adrenals surrounded by renal fascia laterally lie within the perirenal space.
- Muscles and bones form the posterior boundary of the retroperitoneum.
- Arterial encasement, venous involvement, and the displacement or invasion of adjacent organs are important considerations in surgical planning.

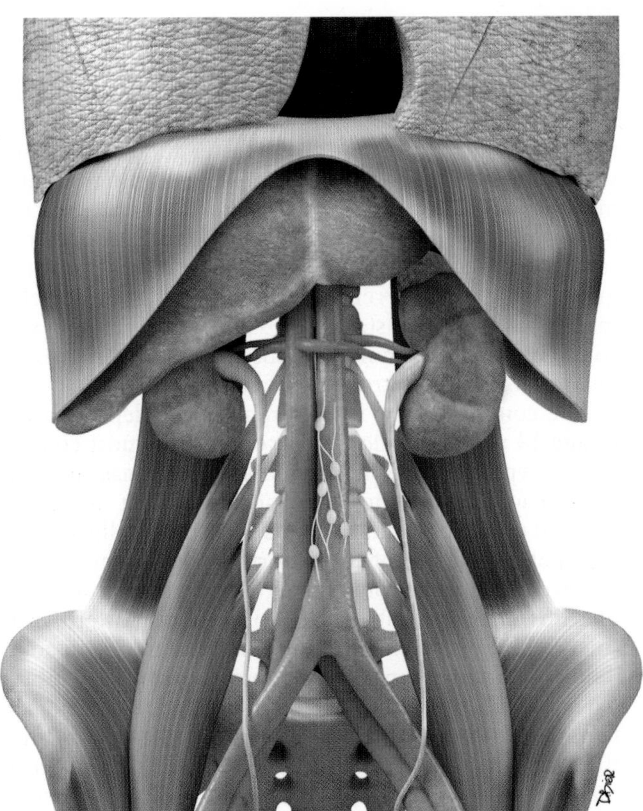

FIGURE 24.1. The major organs in the retroperitoneum are shown without the gastrointestinal tract. The aorta, inferior vena cava, renal vessels, and lymphatics lie close to the midline, and the kidneys and ureters are located more laterally. The psoas and quadratus lumborum muscles are visible posteriorly.

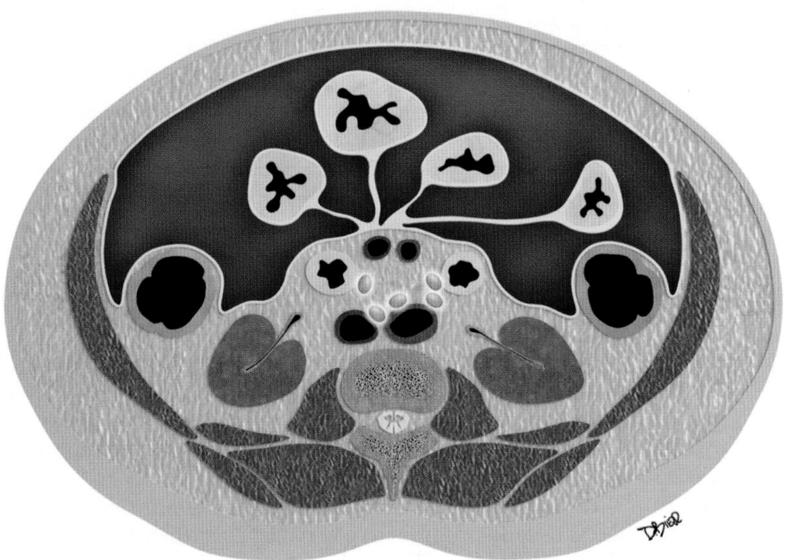

FIGURE 24.2. The position of all components of the retroperitoneum, including the gastrointestinal tract, tract are well depicted in the cross-sectional format. The duodenum, ascending colon, descending colon, their vascular supply, and lymphatic drainage lie within the retroperitoneum.

Pathology

Microscopically, primary sarcomas can arise from fat, smooth or skeletal muscle, fibrous connective tissue, peripheral nerve cells, vascular tissue, or other mesenchymal cells (Table 24.1). STSs are classified according to the adult cell type that the tumor cells most closely resemble. However, this does not mean that the tumor arose from that cell type. The use of immune markers provides important additional information in the classification of STS. Liposarcomas are the most common type of retroperitoneal STS in adults, followed by leiomyosarcoma.[7] Undifferentiated pleomorphic sarcomas (UPSs), solitary fibrous tumors, and malignant peripheral nerve sheath tumors are much less common but can arise in the retroperitoneum. In reviews from single institutions, the most

TABLE 24.1 World Health Organization Classification of Soft Tissue Sarcomas

ADIPOCYTIC TUMORS
Atypical lipomatous tumor/well-differentiated liposarcoma
Dedifferentiated liposarcoma
Myxoid/round cell liposarcoma
Pleomorphic liposarcoma
SMOOTH MUSCLE TUMORS
Leiomyosarcoma
SKELETAL MUSCLE TUMORS
Rhabdomyosarcoma (embryonal, alveolar, and pleomorphic)
FIBROBLASTIC/MYOFIBROBLASTIC TUMORS
Fibrosarcoma
Low-grade myxofibrosarcoma
Low-grade fibromyxoid sarcoma
Sclerosing epithelioid fibrosarcoma
SO-CALLED FIBROHISTIOCYTIC TUMORS
Undifferentiated pleomorphic sarcoma/malignant fibrous histiocytoma (including pleomorphic, giant-cell, myxoid high-grade myxofibrosarcoma, and inflammatory forms)
TUMORS OF PERIPHERAL NERVES
Malignant peripheral nerve sheath tumor
VASCULAR TUMORS
Epithelioid hemangioendothelioma
Deep angiosarcoma
CHONDROOSSEOUS TUMORS
Extraskeletal chondrosarcoma or osteosarcoma
TUMORS OF UNCERTAIN DIFFERENTIATION
Synovial sarcoma
Epithelioid sarcoma
Alveolar soft part sarcoma
Clear-cell sarcoma of soft tissue
Extraskeletal myxoid chondrosarcoma
Primitive neuroectodermal tumor/extraskeletal Ewing tumor
Desmoplastic round cell tumor
Extrarenal rhabdoid tumor
Undifferentiated sarcoma

(From Fletcher C, Unni KK, Mertens F. *Pathology and Genetics of Soft Tissue and Bone: World Health Organization Classification of Tumors.* Lyon: IARC Press; 2002.)

common RPS in the pediatric age is rhabdomyosarcoma, followed by fibrosarcoma and liposarcoma.[8,9]

Liposarcomas are tumors composed of fat cells. The most common form that arises in the retroperitoneum is well-differentiated liposarcoma (WDLPS). Morphologically, it can appear similar to a lipoma; histologically, the presence of lipoblasts allows its recognition, along with associated *MDM2* gene amplification, which is diagnostic for liposarcoma. WDLPSs typically demonstrate slow but progressive growth over many years without development of any metastasis, but there is a high risk of local recurrence after resection. In approximately 25% of cases, there is transformation into a higher grade of tumor. When dedifferentiation occurs, there is loss of mature fat, and the tumor grows faster and has the capacity to metastasize. These areas that show dedifferentiation may display features of leiomyosarcoma or other sarcoma on histology and by immune markers. Dedifferentiation is characterized by more aggressive local growth, a greater risk of recurrence after resection, and development of distant metastases in 15% to 30%. The myxoid/round cell and pleomorphic subtypes of liposarcomas are uncommon in the retroperitoneum.[10]

The common STSs in children are age dependent. Up to age 14 years, rhabdomyosarcoma is the most common tumor type, whereas nonrhabdomyosarcomas are common in adolescents and young adults.[9,11] In a single institutional report covering 30 years that specifically looked at retroperitoneal site of tumor origin, rhabdomyosarcoma followed by fibrosarcoma were reported as common types of RPSs in the pediatric age group.[8] This pattern is distinctly different from common tumor histology in adults. The common subtype of rhabdomyosarcoma is embryonal arising in the genitourinary system. These tumors are large, infiltrative, and liable to involve adjacent organs at the time of initial presentation; thus, negative margins may be difficult to obtain in certain cases. Microscopically, these tumor cells resemble but do not arise from skeletal myoblasts.[10]

KEY POINTS Pathology

- The most common retroperitoneal sarcoma (RPS) in adults is liposarcoma. In children, the most common RPSs are rhabdomyosarcoma (<14 years) and nonrhabdomyosarcoma (>14 years).
- Microscopic appearance is the traditional basis for determining tumor type, assisted by specific markers.[12]

CLINICAL PRESENTATION

Primary retroperitoneal tumors are rare. In essence, primary masses in the retroperitoneum can be categorized as one of three entities: extragonadal germ cell tumors, lymphoma (particularly non-Hodgkin lymphoma), and RPSs.

RPSs lack specific symptoms or laboratory findings. RPSs usually progress to a very large size before prompting clinical suspicion. Examples of potential presenting signs and symptoms include painless abdominal mass, abdominal distention, back pain or pain referred to the hip, urine retention, hematuria, early satiety, or weight loss, occurring singly or in combination. Neurologic deficits may be a presenting symptom when there is spinal cord, nerve root, or sciatic plexus involvement. Venous compromise can result in lower extremity edema. Although there is a broad age range, the sixth decade is a common time for presentation in adults. There is slight male predominance. Imaging, typically computed tomography (CT), leads to discovery of the tumor. Some 11% of patients with RPS have metastases to the liver or lungs at presentation.[13,14] Two-thirds of the tumors are high-grade at the time of diagnosis.[13,14] Therefore, at initial presentation, RPSs are at a higher stage and, consequently, their prognosis is worse than for extremity sarcomas.

The differential diagnosis of retroperitoneal tumors can frequently be narrowed based on initial history, physical examination, and laboratory testing. For example, testicular examination and ultrasonography coupled with standard germ cell serum markers will strongly suggest the possibility of germ cell tumor, whereas elucidating a history of B symptomatology such as night sweats, fever, and weight loss suggests the possibility of a lymphoma. However, image-guided tissue biopsy provides the definitive diagnosis of RPS from these entities and is crucial for treatment planning before surgical resection.

STAGING EVALUATION

The eighth edition American Joint Committee on Cancer (AJCC) staging system changed significantly for STS and now has a separate staging system for RPS and is based on a combination of anatomic as well as pathologic data (Fig. 24.3).[15] Previous versions of the AJCC staging system included tumor depth, but this is not included in the current edition. The tumor-node-metastasis (TNM) characteristics of the tumor are provided by imaging and may be modified after surgery. The histologic subtype and grade of the primary tumor are determined after biopsy or surgical excision to yield tumor stage as defined by AJCC criteria.

T Definition: Tumor Size

T1 = Maximum tumor size 5 cm or less.
T2 = Tumor size greater than 5 cm but less than or equal to 10 cm.
T3 = Tumor size greater than 10 cm but less than or equal to 15 cm.
T4 = Tumor size greater than 15 cm.

N Definition

N0 = No nodal involvement.
N1 = Nodal involvement.

Clinical, imaging, or pathologic criteria are accepted for N designation. Note that involvement of nodes is uncommon for most STSs but can occur in selected subtypes such as angiosarcoma, epithelioid sarcoma, clear-cell sarcoma, and small-cell sarcoma.[15a]

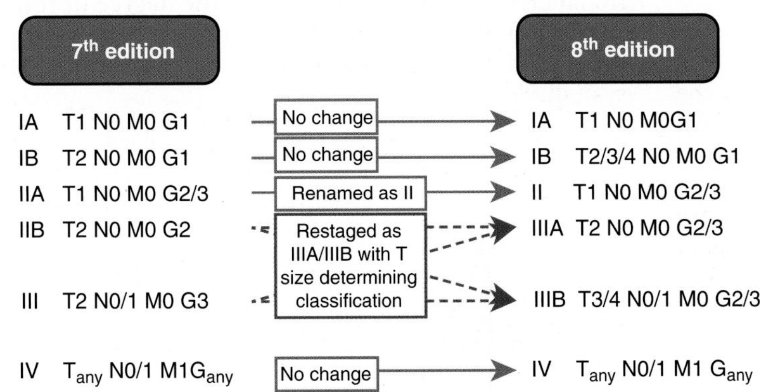

T category	T criteria
TX	Primary cannot be assessed
T0	No evidence of primary
T1	≤ 5 cm
T2	> 5 cm and ≤ 10 cm
T3	> 10 cm and ≤ 15 cm
T4	> 15

(8th edition; 7th edition)

B

AJCC 7th edition	IA	IB	II	IIIA	IIIB	IV	Total
	AJCC 8th edition						
IA	240	0	0	0	0	0	240
IB	0	2,143	0	0	0	0	2,143
IIA	0	0	256	0	0	0	256
IIB	0	0	0	186	450	0	636
III	0	0	0	422	1,707	0	2,129
IV	0	0	0	0	0	1,023	1,023
Total	240	2,143	256	608	2,157	1,023	6,427

Changes in stage between the AJCC 7th and 8th editions (n=6,427)

C

FIGURE 24.3. **A**, Schema of the changes between the seventh and eighth editions of the American Joint Committee on Cancer (*AJCC*) staging systems for soft tissue sarcoma of the retroperitoneum, with the updated T definitions (in red) (**B**) and the resulting changes in stages IIB/III (*outlined*) within the National Cancer Database study population (**C**). (From Fisher SB, Chiang YJ, Feig BW, et al. An evaluation of the eighth edition of the American Joint Committee on Cancer (AJCC) Staging System for retroperitoneal sarcomas using the National Cancer Data Base (NCDB): does size matter? *Am J Clin Oncol.* 2019;42(2):160–165.)

M Definition

M0 = No distant metastasis.
M1 = Distant metastasis.

Pathologic Criteria: Grading

A three-point grade from G1 to G3 using the French system (the French Federation of Cancer Centers Sarcoma Group) is used. It is based on scores obtained from:

- Histology-specific differentiation: high-, intermediate-, or low-grade. Also, certain histologic types (synovial sarcoma, undifferentiated sarcoma, and sarcomas of unknown type) are always assigned a high score.
- Mitotic count.
- Tumor necrosis.

Limitations of American Joint Committee on Cancer Classification

Site of Origin

The previous (seventh) edition of the AJCC classification system did not differentiate retroperitoneal origin from extremity origin or other sites of origin. The eighth edition of the AJCC staging manual includes a system that is specific to RPSs; for example, the superficial/deep category that was previously used for nonretroperitoneal tumors has been removed.

Size of Primary Tumor

The prior T staging that used a single 5-cm size as the cutoff has been shown to be limited for retroperitoneal tumors, which are very often large at presentation. It is recognized that tumor size represents a continuous variable: the greater the size at initial presentation, the worse the outcome.[16] The eighth edition of the AJCC staging manual now accounts for larger tumors, such that previous stage IIB/III groups in the seventh edition are now considered stage IIIA/IIIB. Initial evaluation suggests that the expanded T stage classification has only had a minimal impact on overall survival prognosis.15[a] (Figure 24.4)

Margin Status of Resected Tumor

R definition
R0 = Resection with negative microscopic margin.
R1 = Resection with positive microscopic margin.
R2 = Macroscopic disease remaining after surgery.

The status of the resected margin after surgery is an important prognostic factor but not a part of the AJCC staging[17–19] (Fig. 24.5).

Tumor Recurrence

AJCC staging does not differentiate between primary tumor and locally recurrent tumor. However, studies reveal that previous recurrence is a major factor for subsequent local recurrence and decreased survival.[19]

Other Staging Systems

The most important common variables in the AJCC system for RPSs are the presence of distant metastasis M1 and the tumor grade G1 to G3. Therefore, alternate staging systems based only on tumor grade or with additional criteria of multifocality and the degree of residual tumor left after surgery (R0, R1, or R2) have been proposed and are as good as or even better than the AJCC system.[20,21]

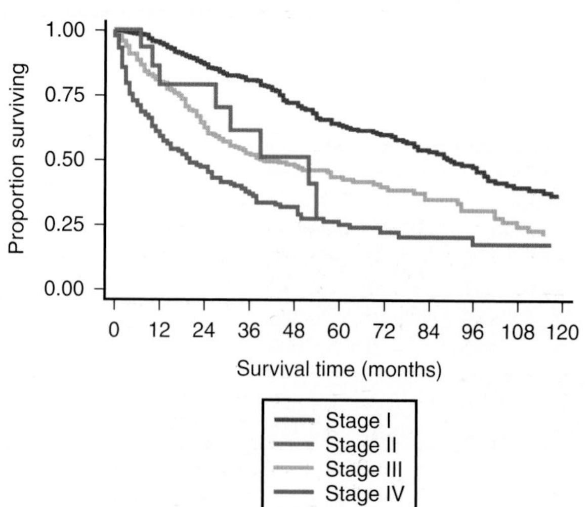

FIGURE 24.4. Overall survival by stage according to the American Joint Committee on Cancer (AJCC) seventh edition (**A**) and eighth edition (**B**); stratified by T stage in the AJCC seventh edition (**C**) and eighth edition (**D**).

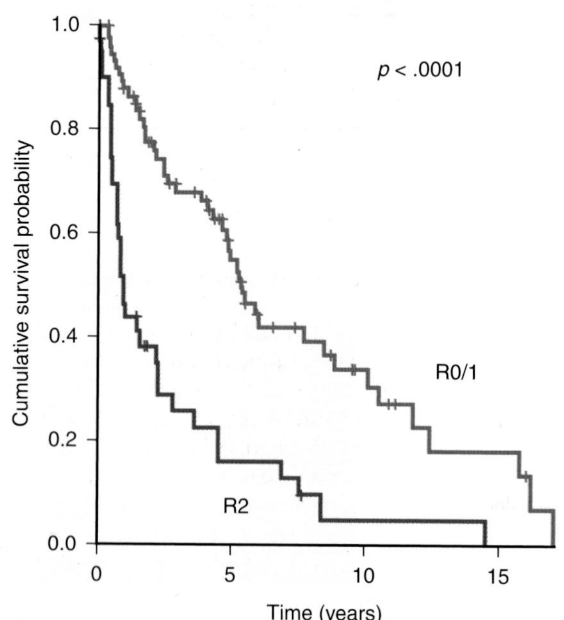

FIGURE 24.5. Resection with residual disease, particularly R2, carries a poorer prognosis. (Modified from Alldinger I, Yang Q, Pilarsky C, et al. Retroperitoneal soft tissue sarcomas: prognosis and treatment of primary and recurrent disease in 117 patients. *Anticancer Res.* 2006;26:1577–1581.)

We are poised at the brink of important change, with the availability of high-throughput technology of genomic, proteomic, and tissue microarray analysis in sarcoma. As data about relevant genes and molecular markers are integrated with disease progression, tumor response, and survival, future modifications can be made to AJCC staging.

PATTERNS OF TUMOR SPREAD

Local Spread

Local involvement of an adjacent organ is common because these tumors are large at presentation. This will manifest as displacement or invasion, particularly with high-grade tumors. When tumors arise from the upper retroperitoneum, displacement of liver, spleen, kidney, aorta, inferior vena cava, small bowel, or colon is commonly seen. Bladder displacement occurs when the tumor involves the pelvis. When the tumor invades an adjacent organ such as the ureters, bladder, or GI tract, urinary or bowel obstruction can occur. Bone involvement of the lumbar spine, sacrum, or pelvis can occur through contiguous spread. Malignant peripheral nerve sheath tumors, in particular, exhibit spread along the nerve sheath. This is an important consideration when surgical excision is undertaken. A negative frozen section is used intraoperatively to determine the extent of surgery.

Hematogenous, Lymphatic, and Peritoneal Spread

RPSs primarily spread to the liver via the hematogenous route. Such a pattern is seen in 44% of patients.[13] Liver metastases, particularly from leiomyosarcoma and angiosarcoma, can have marked enhancement. As the disease spreads further through the bloodstream, metastases can involve the lungs in 38% of cases, with additional sites of involvement including the adrenals, muscles, subcutaneous tissue, bones, and brain.

Lymph node metastases are distinctly uncommon, occurring in only 3.5% of patients with STS.[15a,22] Lymph node involvement is more likely in patients with rhabdomyosarcoma, clear-cell sarcoma, angiosarcoma, and epithelioid sarcoma.

Peritoneal spread can occur in the abdomen with seeding to produce disseminated implants in omentum, mesentery, and peritoneum.

All possible sites for tumor spread must be evaluated thoroughly on CT of the chest, abdomen, pelvis, and other appropriate imaging modalities to inform therapeutic decisions.

KEY POINTS Patterns of Tumor Spread

- Local spread occurs to organs in anatomic contiguity; thus, extensive resection may still be undertaken.
- Distant spread occurs hematogenously or by lymphatics or peritoneal dissemination and will preclude curative surgery.

IMAGING

Primary Tumor Detection and Characterization

The initial imaging workup of a patient with suspected RPS consists of a contrast-enhanced CT scan of the abdomen and pelvis performed with oral contrast. CT permits the determination of size and location of primary tumor and its relationship to adjacent organs. Coronal and sagittal reconstructions are especially useful in demonstrating proximity to or invasion of small bowel, colon, kidneys, ureters, and the major vasculature. When there is a question of major arterial or venous involvement, a dedicated CT arteriogram or venogram can be useful for further assessment. Magnetic resonance imaging (MRI) of the abdomen and pelvis can serve as an alternate modality when the patient is unable to receive intravenous contrast for CT related to either renal dysfunction or a past history of severe reaction to intravenous contrast. Although an ultrasound can detect large RPSs, its shortcomings are in the characterization of fat and calcification from bowel and delineation of the relationship of the tumor with adjacent organs. If an ultrasound examination is initially obtained in a patient in whom RPS is being considered, follow-up cross-sectional imaging should be performed.

Radiologic considerations are critical in the successful management of RPS. The important imaging features to report are size, internal attenuation characteristics (fat, soft tissue, or calcification), enhancement or necrosis, relationship to adjacent organs (displacement or invasion), the spread of disease to distant organs, and the degree of any treatment response at follow-up. These are important considerations as the surgeon considers anatomic constraints to complete resection. The key imaging characteristics of the common RPSs are presented next.

Liposarcoma

Liposarcoma is the most common RPS. Its typical appearance on CT is a bulky tumor with fat attenuation. It is recognized from generalized excess fat deposition seen with obesity by the mass effect it may exert, such as in displacement of bowel loops or adjacent viscera. Liposarcomas may contain a few septations (Fig. 24.6). These tumors are regarded as atypical lipomatous tumor or WDLPS. When the attenuation of any area of tumor is greater than that of normal fat or has the attenuation of soft tissue, or particularly if contrast enhancement is seen, there is concern for dedifferentiation (Figs. 24.7 and 24.8). Such areas may be targeted for subsequent biopsy or surgery, because dedifferentiated liposarcoma (DDLPS) can be seen in as many as 15% of WDLPSs.[21] Whereas WDLPSs lack metastatic capacity, DDLPS can disseminate and, consequently, have a worse prognosis.[23]

Leiomyosarcoma

Leiomyosarcoma is the second most common histologic type of RPS, often with a CT appearance of a large mass with a central necrotic core because of the rapidity with which it can proliferate and outgrow its blood supply. The most common location for vascular leiomyosarcoma to arise is in the inferior vena cava, which commonly

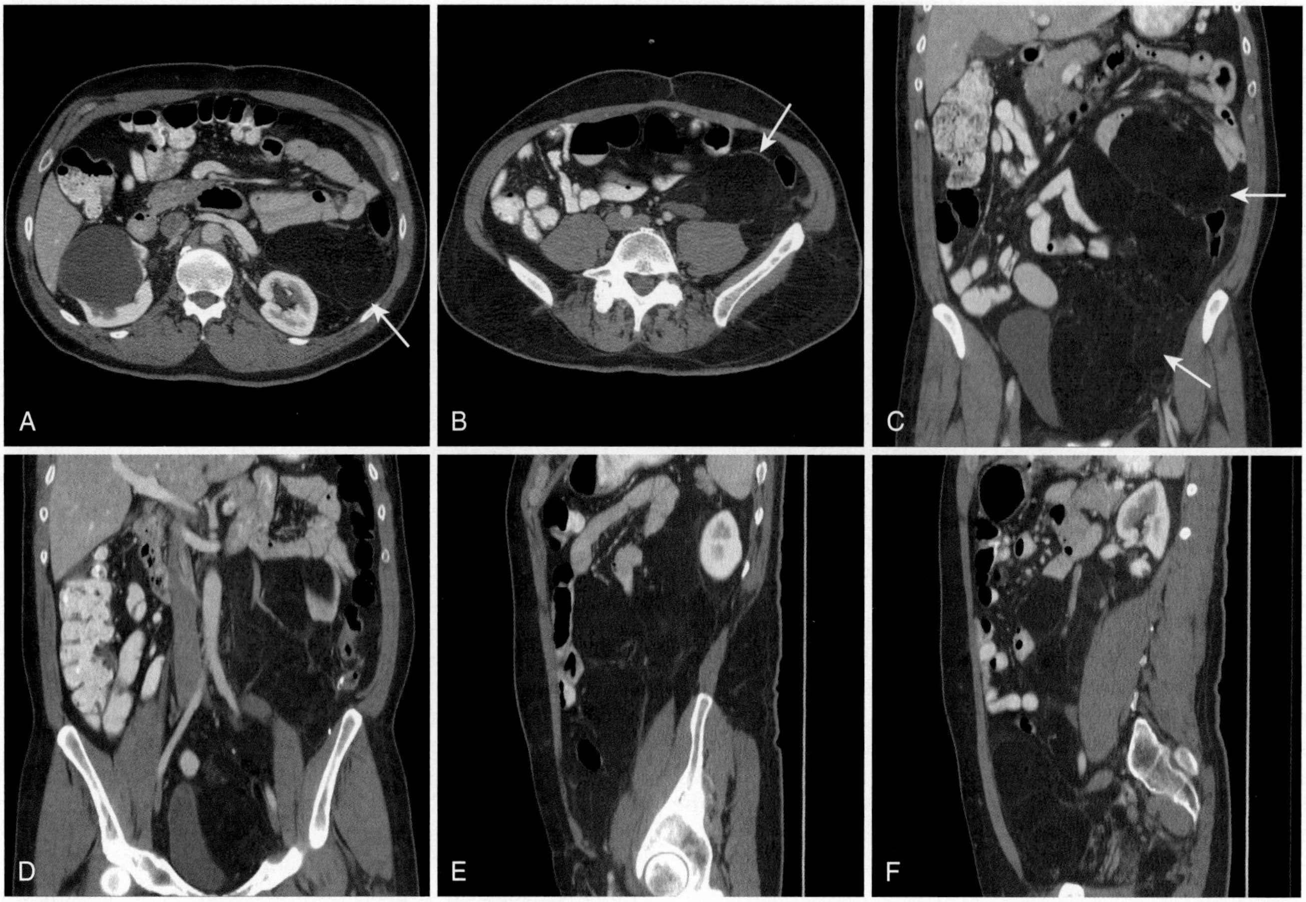

Figure 24.6. **A** and **B**, An atypical lipomatous tumor/well-differentiated liposarcoma demonstrates fat density with a few septations (*arrows*) extending from the left midabdomen into the upper pelvis. The craniocaudal extent is easier to appreciate on the reformatted coronal (**C** and **D**) and sagittal (**E** and **F**) images. The arrows in (C) denote the location of the septations.

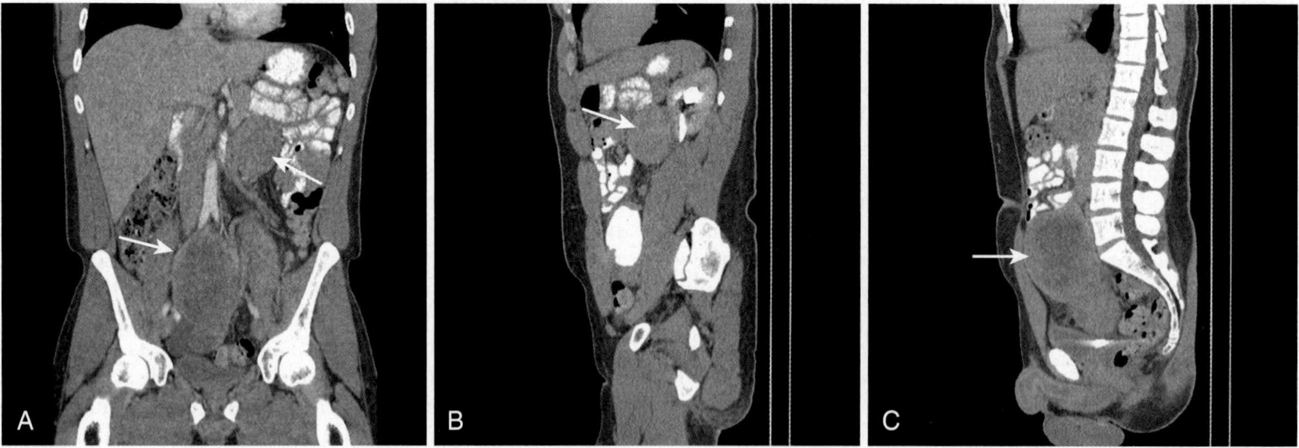

Figure 24.7. Coronal (**A**) and midline sagittal (**B** and **C**) reformatted computed tomography scans show two tumors: one in the left retroperitoneum and the second one in the pelvis (*arrows*), representing multifocal liposarcoma.

produces venous narrowing or occlusion (Figs. 24.9 and 24.10). Leiomyosarcoma, high-grade UPS (formerly called "malignant fibrous histiocytoma"), and synovial sarcoma are infiltrative tumors (Fig. 24.11). Thus, invasion of adjacent organs and the development of distant metastases are seen much more frequently with these tumors than with liposarcomas (Figs. 24.12 and 24.13).

Sarcomas Related to Genetic Syndromes

The manifestations of certain underlying genetic syndromes should induce a search for related sarcomas. For example, desmoid tumors, typically in the root of the mesentery, can be multiple and are seen as a component of Gardner syndrome. In a patient with neurofibromatosis-1,

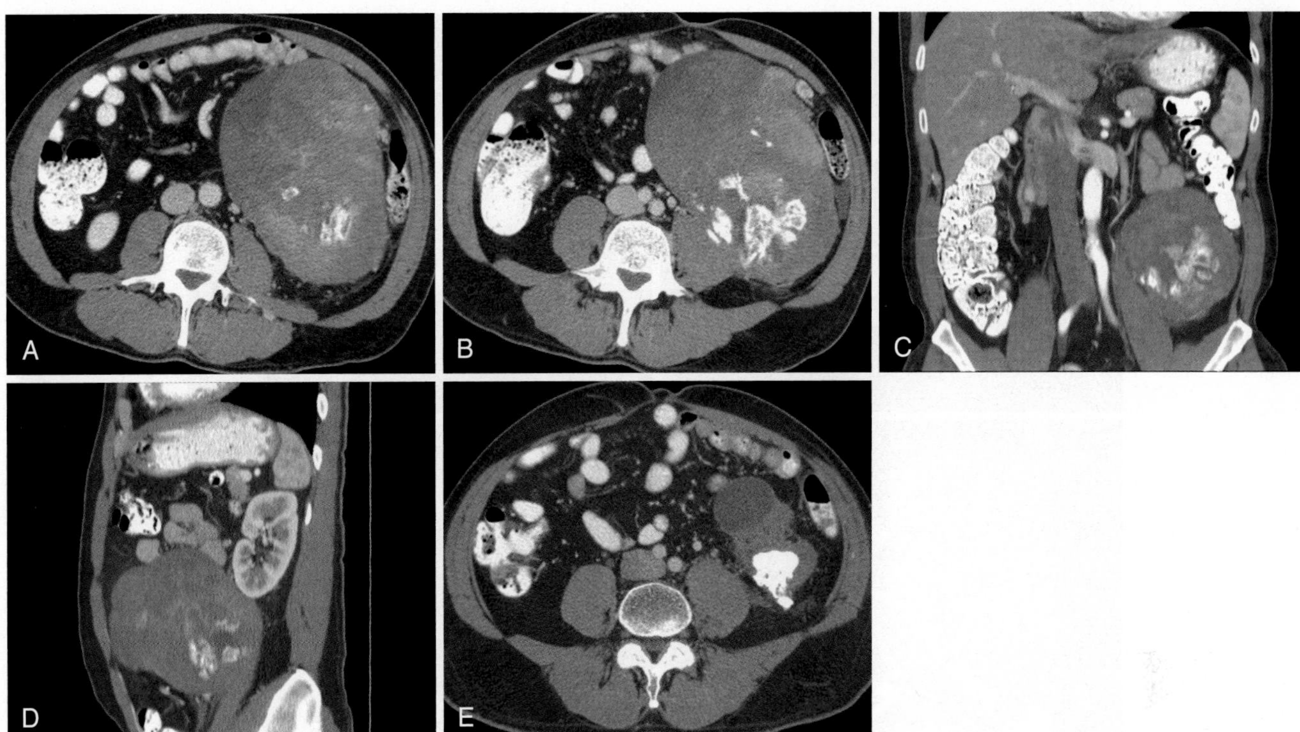

FIGURE 24.8. **A–D**, A dedifferentiated liposarcoma shows areas of calcification and soft tissue density without any recognizable fat. It is in close contact with the left kidney, ureter, psoas muscle, jejunum, and descending colon. **E**, After chemotherapy, a follow-up computed tomography scan shows response with reduction in tumor size. At surgery, the tumor was resected with R0 (microscopic negative) margin and preservation of the left kidney.

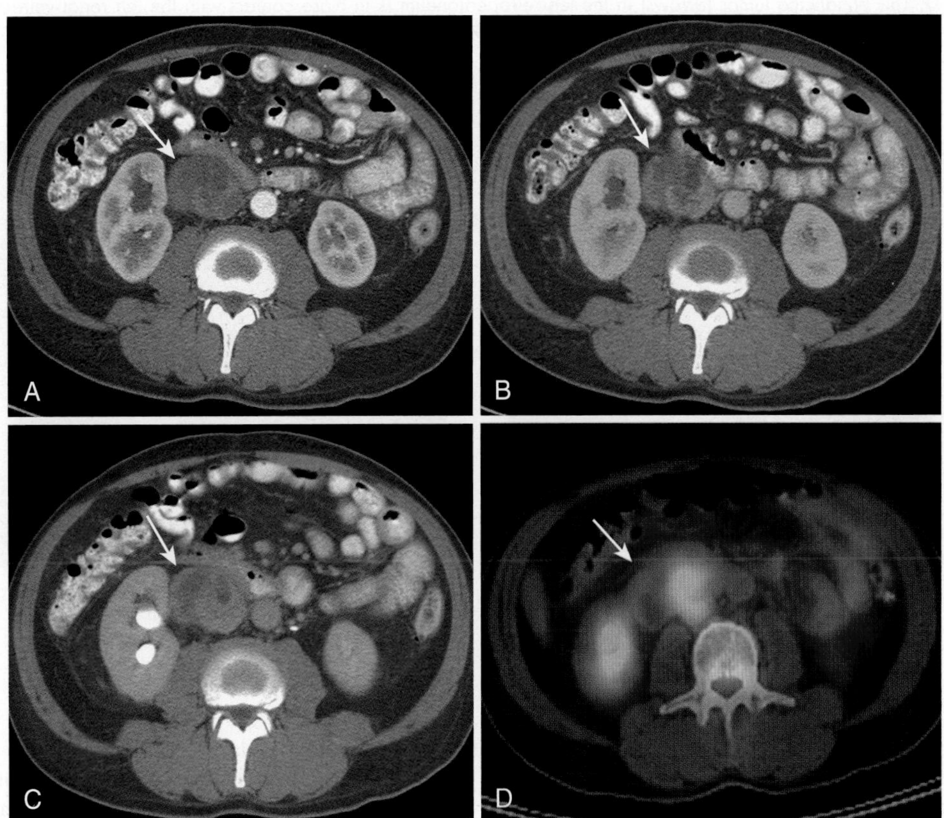

FIGURE 24.9. **A–C**, A leiomyosarcoma arises from the inferior vena cava and produces right hydronephrosis. Its intra- and extraluminal extent is depicted on arterial, venous, and delayed phases of computed tomography (CT) (*arrows*). **D**, On the fused positron emission tomography/CT scan, the tumor (*arrow*) is 2-[^{18}F] fluoro-2-deoxy-D-glucose–avid.

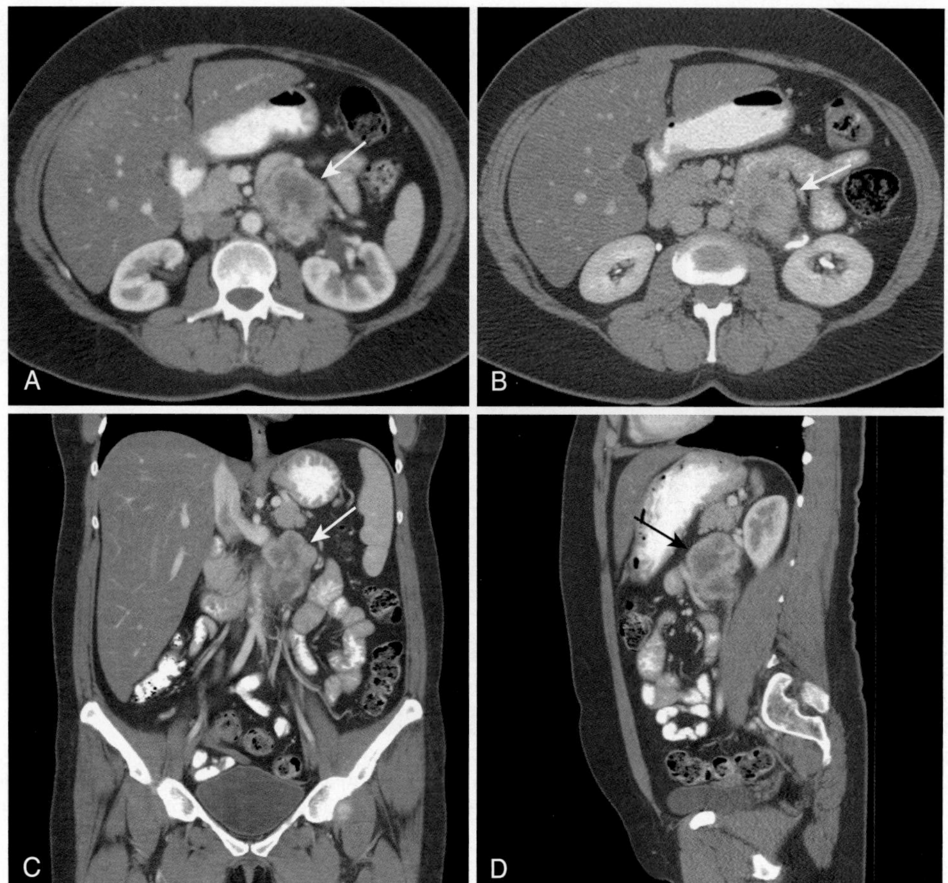

FIGURE 24.10. A–D, This enhancing tumor (*arrows*) in the left retroperitoneum is in close contact with the left renal vein and left ureter. It was removed at surgery with preservation of the left kidney and resection with reanastomosis of the left ureter. At pathology, it was a leiomyosarcoma with R1 margin.

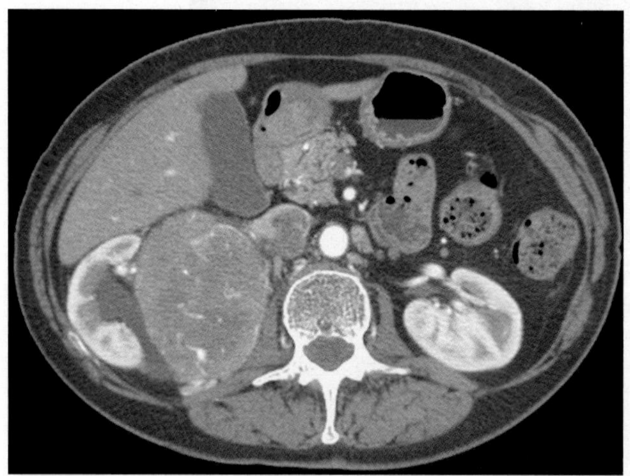

FIGURE 24.11. This tumor involves the right renal hilum and renal pelvis. It was resected with the right kidney and, at pathology, was found to be a well-capsulated epithelioid leiomyosarcoma.

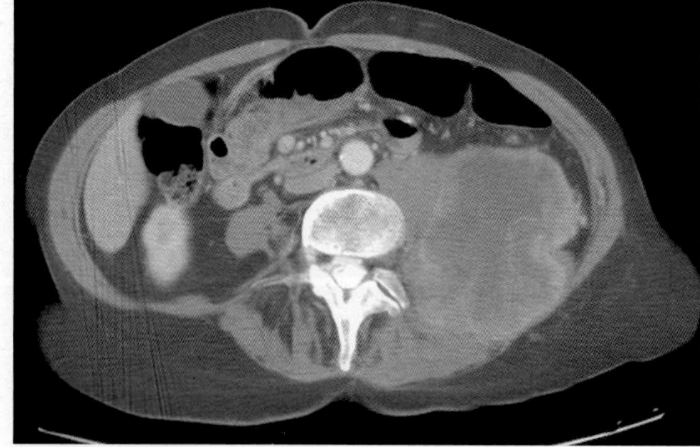

FIGURE 24.12. High-grade pleomorphic sarcoma of the retroperitoneum shows local invasion of the psoas and left paraspinal muscles.

any tumor associated with pain or enlargement of a plexiform neurofibroma should be assumed to represent malignant transformation and confirmed with a biopsy (Figs. 24.14 and 24.15).

The most common RPS in children is rhabdomyosarcoma.[8] It frequently arises from the genitourinary tract. These tumors are large, infiltrative, and liable to involve adjacent organs at the time of initial presentation (Fig. 24.16). Nonrhabdomyosarcomas in pediatric patients can be desmoplastic small round cell tumors (Figs. 24.17 and 24.18), Ewing sarcomas (Fig. 24.19), fibrosarcomas, and liposarcomas, among others.

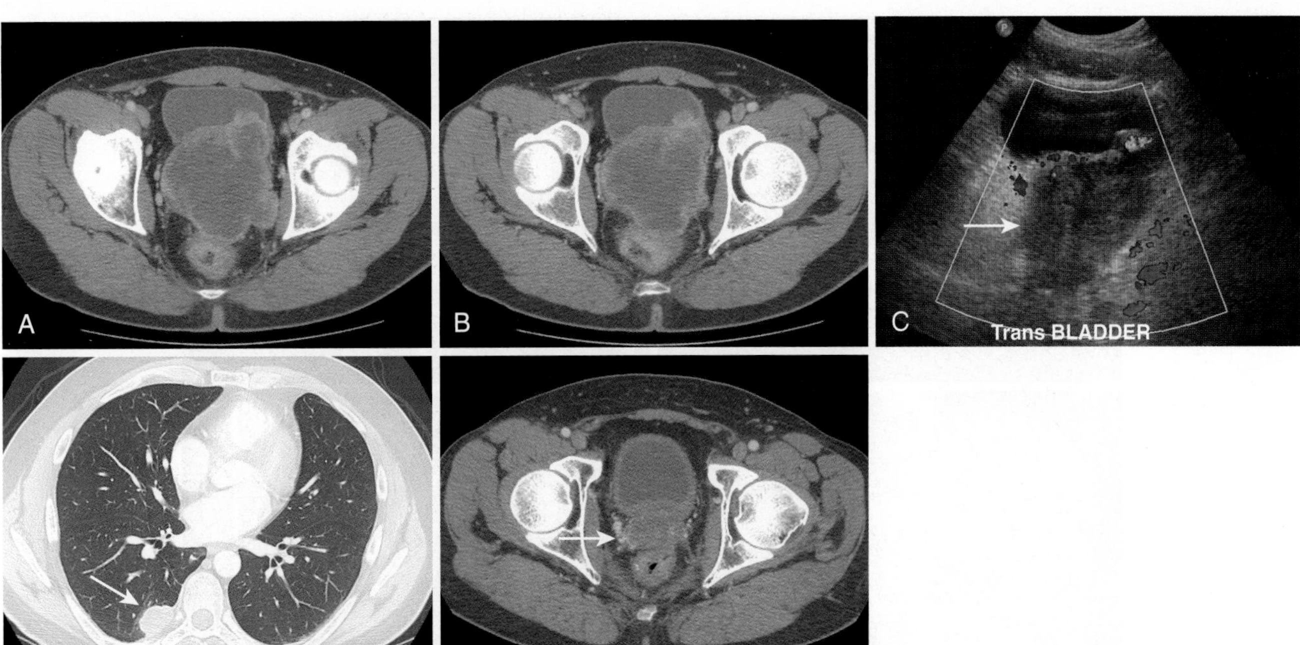

FIGURE 24.13. High-grade sarcoma arising in the pelvis shows direct invasion of the bladder on computed tomography (CT) (**A** and **B**) and pelvic ultrasound (**C**). Note the vascularity of the tumor component in the bladder with color Doppler (*arrow*). **D**, A CT scan of the chest reveals one of multiple lung metastases (*arrow*). **E**, After receiving systemic chemotherapy and radiation therapy to the pelvis, there is a decrease in tumor size (*arrow*) and relief of urinary symptoms from bladder involvement.

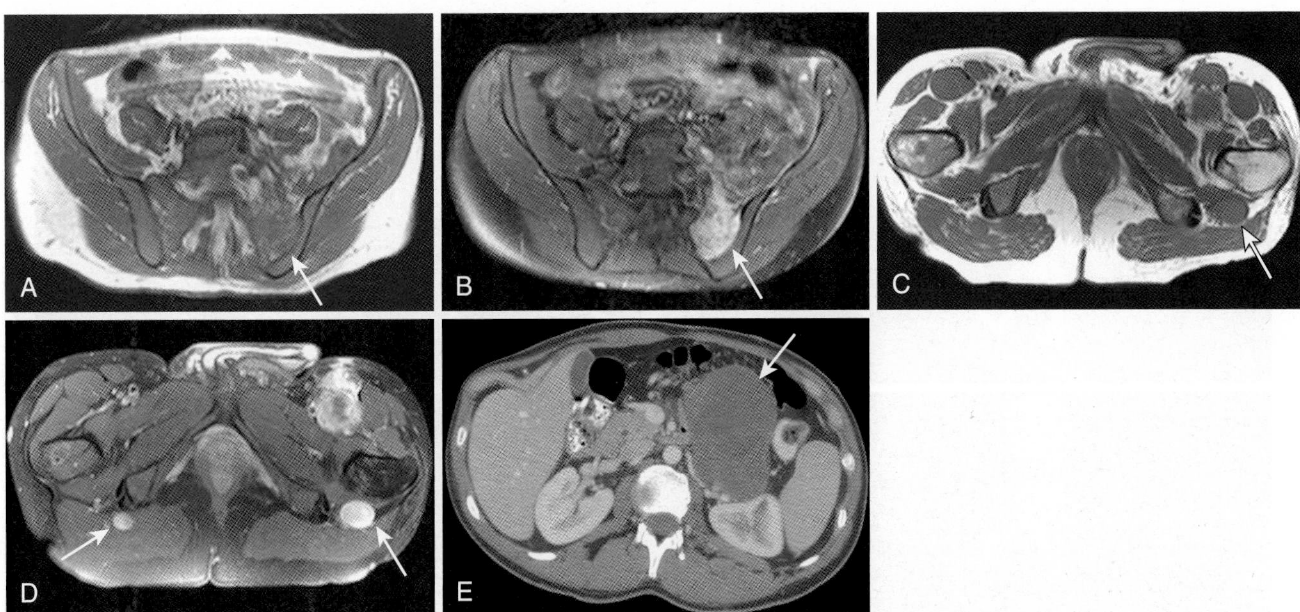

FIGURE 24.14. **A–E**, In this patient with neurofibromatosis-1, numerous plexiform neurofibromas (*arrows*) are seen on T1- and T2-weighted magnetic resonance imaging studies. There is transformation into a malignant peripheral nerve sheath tumor in the left retroperitoneum (*arrow* in **E**).

Lymph Node Metastases (N)

Although metastatic involvement of lymph nodes is defined as stage III or IV disease in the AJCC scheme, it is a distinctly uncommon occurrence.[15] Nodal metastasis is estimated to occur in 3.5% of all STSs in adults and is slightly more common in children. When CT detects and characterizes RPS, attention should be directed to the regional lymph node drainage. Enlargement or any abnormal nodal enhancement pattern must be included in the imaging findings. MRI can detect adenopathy using size, abnormal signal characteristics, and enhancement as criteria for involvement. Metastatic adenopathy is characterized on positron emission tomography (PET)/CT studies

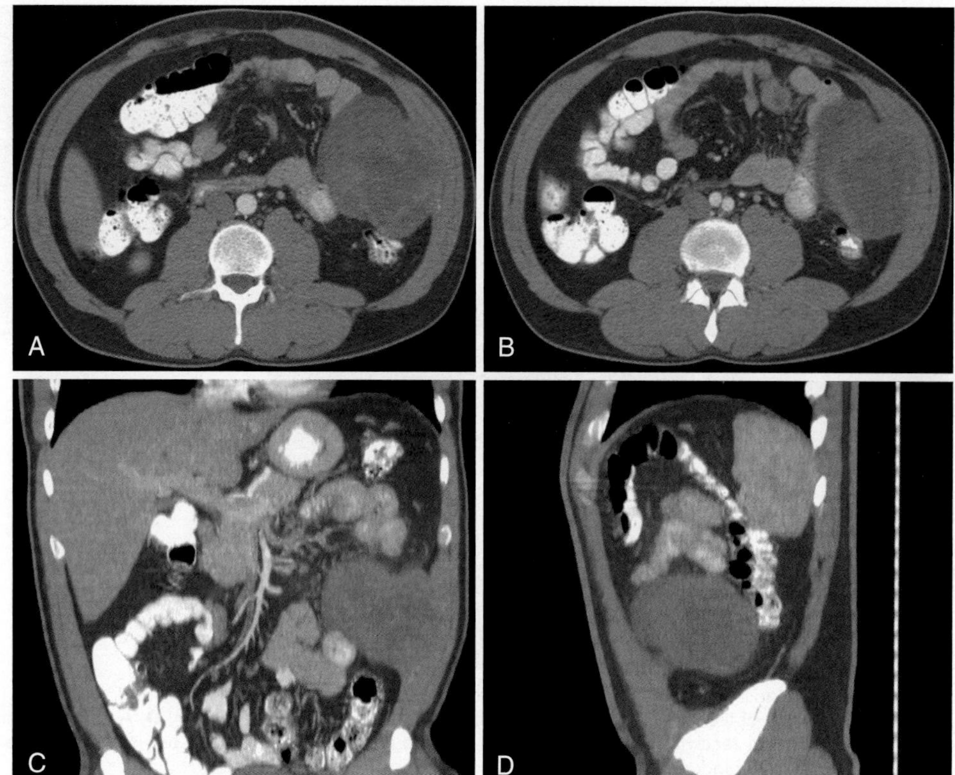

FIGURE 24.15. A–D, A malignant nerve sheath tumor arises in the left retroperitoneum laterally. Its overall extent and relationship to small bowel and descending colon are clearly seen on the coronal and sagittal reformatted computed tomography scans.

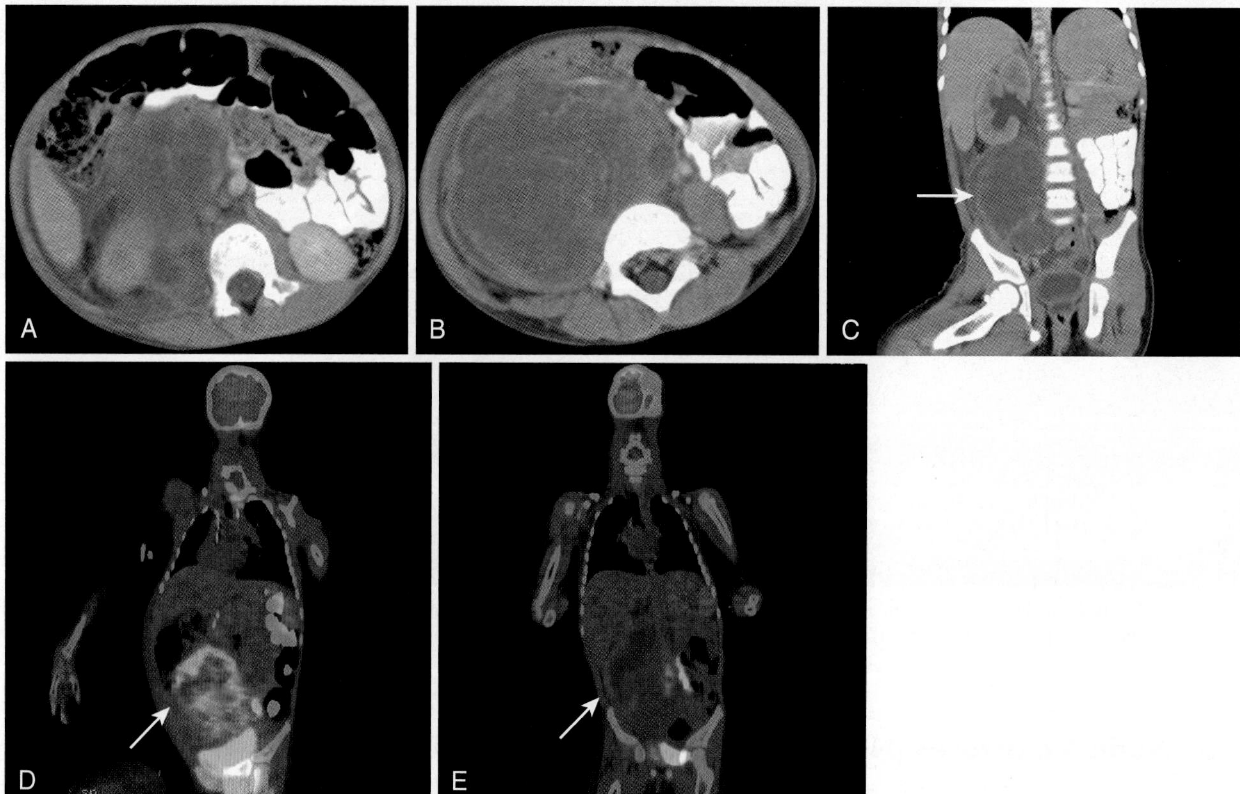

FIGURE 24.16. A 3-year-old presented with an inability to bear weight on the right side. **A–C**, Axial and coronal computed tomography (CT) scans reveal a retroperitoneal tumor with right hydronephrosis. Note local invasion of the psoas muscle and low-attenuation center, representing necrosis (*arrow* in **C**). A biopsy revealed this to be an embryonal rhabdomyosarcoma. **D**, 2-[^{18}F] fluoro-2-deoxy-D-glucose (FDG) fusion positron emission tomography (PET)/CT reveals metabolic activity at the periphery with diminished activity in the center in areas of necrosis (*arrow*). **E**, After 8 weeks of chemotherapy, follow-up FDG-PET/CT shows no change in size but a decrease in FDG uptake by the tumor (*arrow*), providing an early indication of response to chemotherapy.

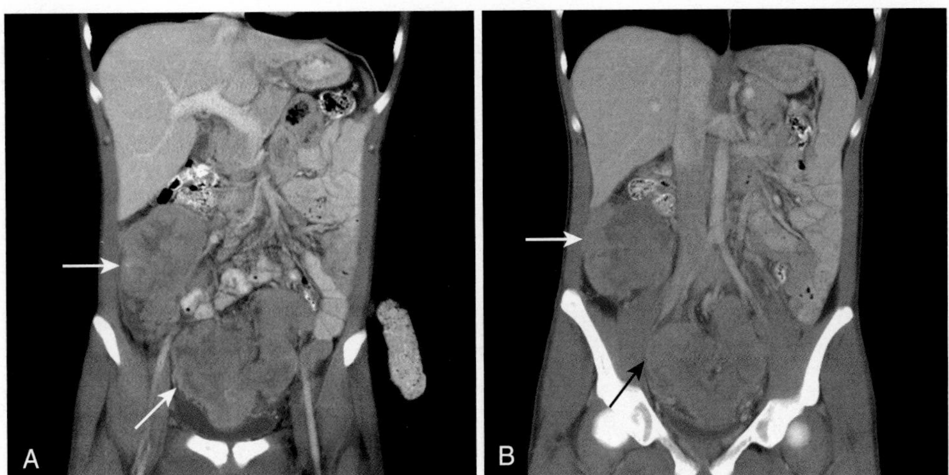

FIGURE 24.17. A 19-year-old presented with tumors (*arrows*) in the right lower quadrant and pelvis that, at pathology, were multifocal desmoplastic small round cell tumors.

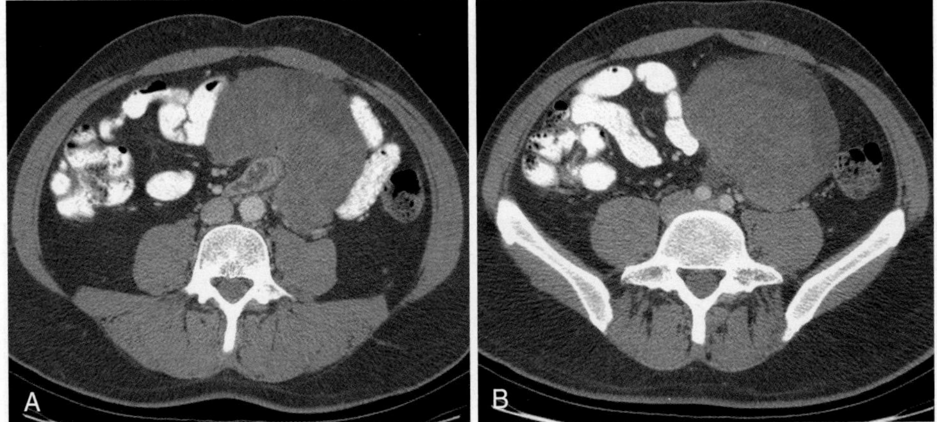

FIGURE 24.18. **A** and **B**, This desmoplastic small round cell tumor involves the retroperitoneum and contiguous mesentery. The third portion of duodenum had to be resected *en bloc* with the tumor at surgery.

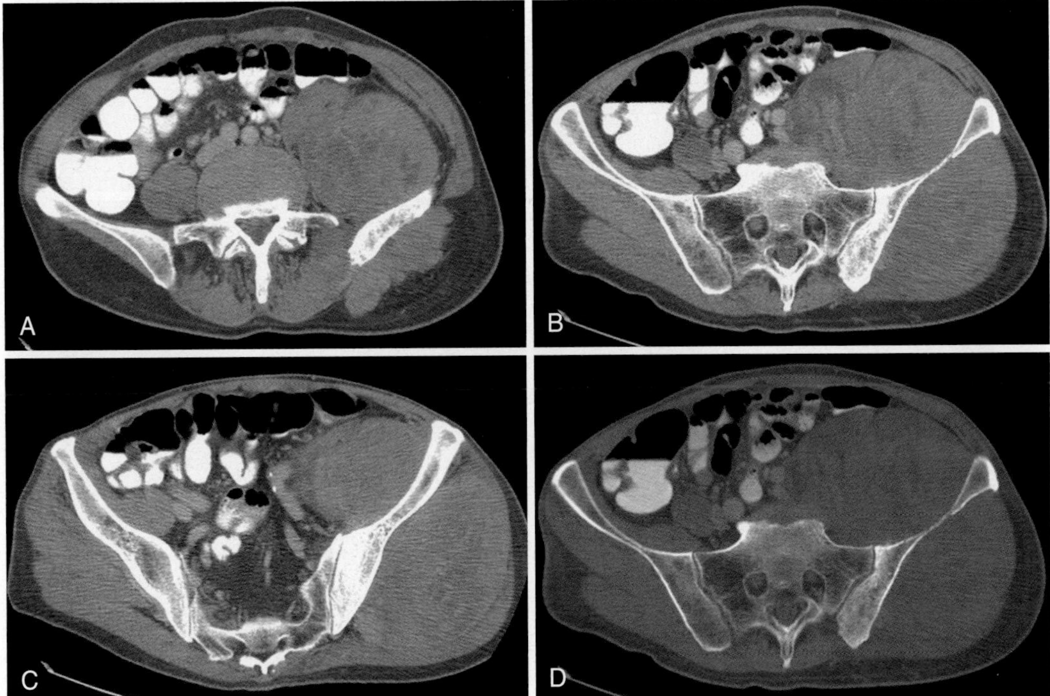

FIGURE 24.19. **A–D**, Retroperitoneal and gluteal disease is seen in multicompartment involvement by Ewing sarcoma. There is permeative metastatic involvement of the left iliac wing appreciated on the bone windows.

as 2-[^{18}F] fluoro-2-deoxy-D-glucose (FDG)-avid areas that correspond to lymph nodes anatomically.

Distant Metastases (M)

When CT is initially employed for the detection and characterization of RPSs, simultaneously an evaluation is made of the liver, which is a common site for hematogenous metastases (Fig. 24.20). Other sites of metastases (i.e., adrenals, peritoneum, bones, and intramuscular or subcutaneous sites) are also assessed at the same time (Figs. 24.21 and 24.22). This is especially important when CT demonstrates tumors other than WDLPS. A CT of the chest is very helpful for the detection of any metastasis to the lungs. MRI is necessary in the assessment of the brain and spine, especially when the patient has neurologic symptoms

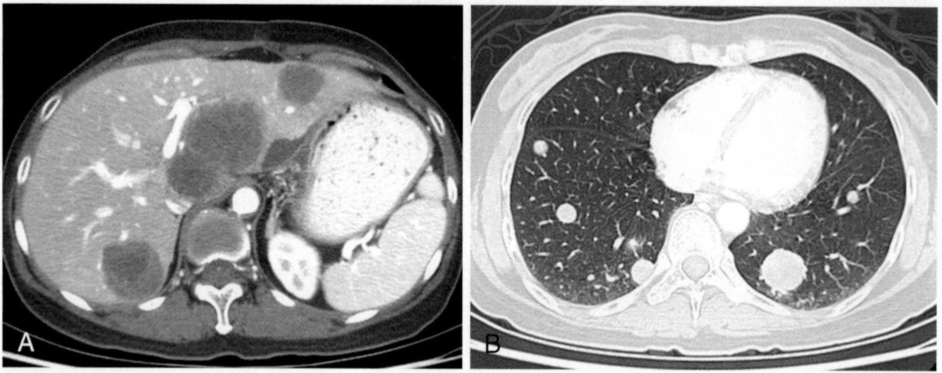

FIGURE 24.20. **A** and **B**, Metastatic sarcoma has spread to the liver and lungs (M1) by the hematogenous route, making this stage IV disease.

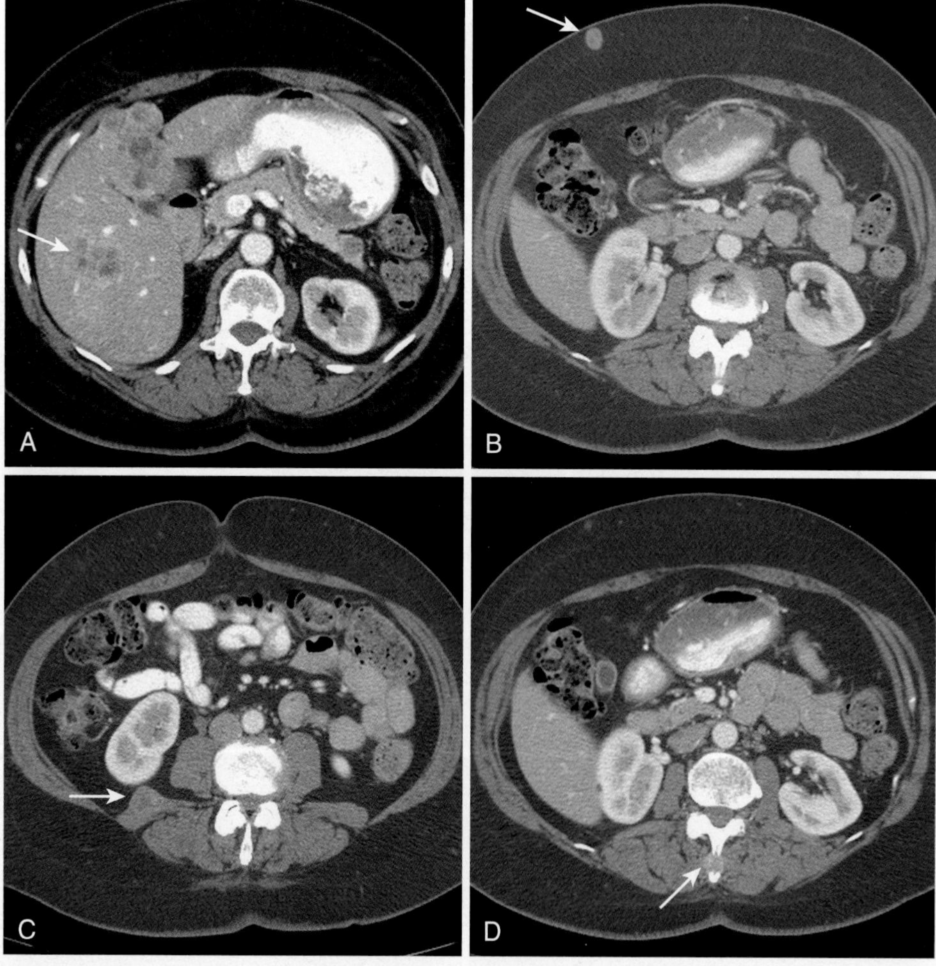

FIGURE 24.21. **A–D**, Computed tomography scans reveal leiomyosarcoma (*arrows*) spread by the hematogenous route to involve the liver, tail of pancreas, abdominal wall, right quadratus lumborum muscle, and spinous process of the L2 vertebra.

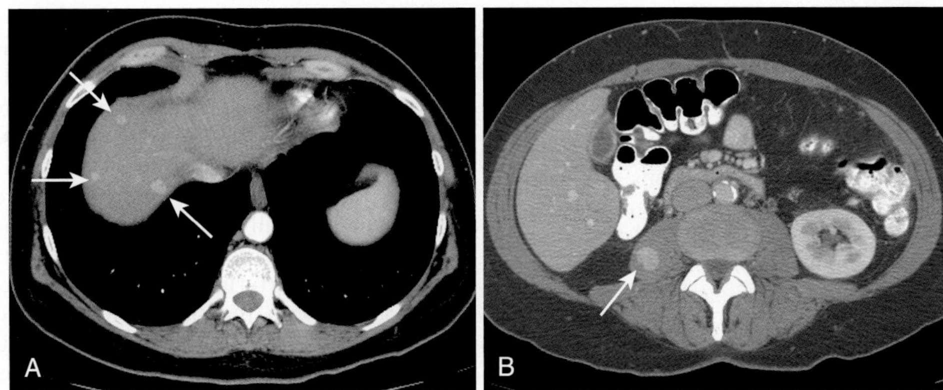

FIGURE 24.22. **A** and **B**, Enhancing sarcoma metastases (*arrows*) involve the liver and right psoas muscle.

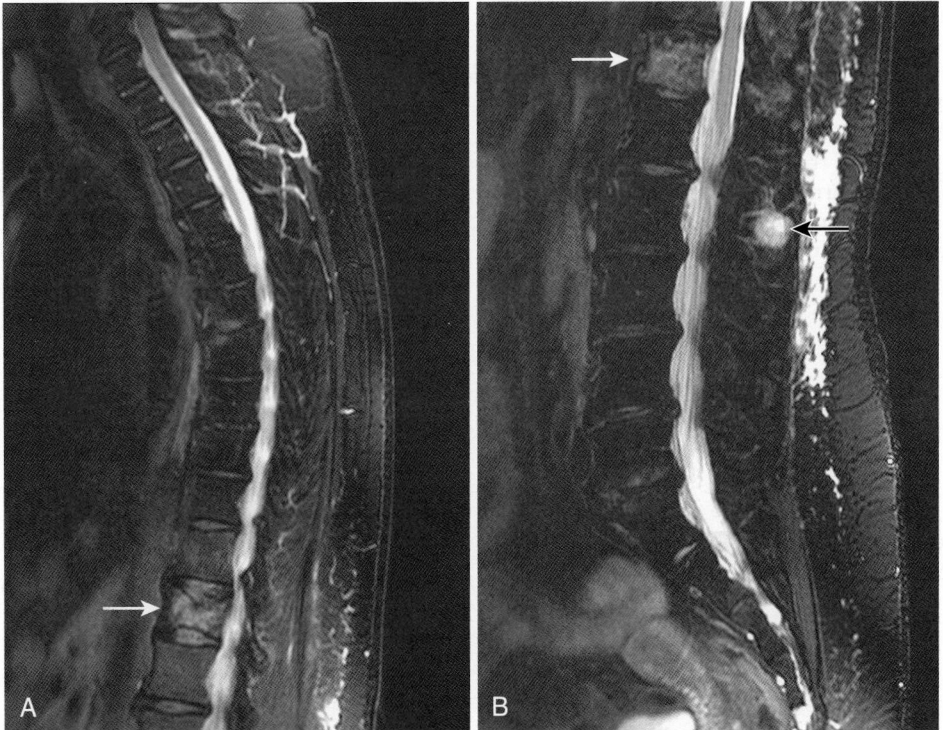

FIGURE 24.23. **A** and **B**, The extent of vertebral involvement is well-depicted on magnetic resonance imaging of the thoracic and lumbar spine (*arrows*). There is no cord compression in this patient.

(Fig. 24.23). FDG-PET/CT will accumulate in distant sites of high-grade tumors, but these should be differentiated from areas of physiologic uptake or sites of infection. A nuclear medicine bone scan is useful in the detection of bony metastases.

After the initial CT, it is possible to provide a clinical (TNM) stage of disease. Then, for the pathologic aspects to complete staging, tissue diagnosis is necessary. The differential diagnosis of retroperitoneal masses is broad, including STS as well as germ-cell tumors, lymphomas, and benign entities such as schwannoma. Therefore, preoperative biopsy is recommended before surgical resection for treatment planning.[23a] CT can guide the targeting of solid, nonnecrotic portions of the tumor for biopsy. Although fine-needle biopsy can yield material for the diagnosis of malignancy, a core biopsy is preferred for a more definitive diagnosis. This allows determination of tumor grade based on the criteria of cellular differentiation and necrosis to be made for a comprehensive AJCC staging. With the imaging detection of metastases, a biopsy can be obtained from either the primary tumor or the metastatic site, as appropriate.

KEY POINTS The Radiology Report: What to Include

- Size, location, and internal characteristics of tumor.
- Arterial encasement, venous displacement or involvement.
- Displacement or invasion of adjacent organs and ureters.
- Evaluation for metastases to liver, lungs, and bones.

THERAPY

RPSs, like all STSs, are a heterogeneous group of tumors. The general principles guiding therapy include evaluating the stage of tumor, the expected biologic behavior of the given histology, and the pros and cons of available therapeutic options. It is important that a multidisciplinary team at a specialized center review all the clinical information before implementation of treatment. The definitive treatment that can lead to cure in RPSs is *en bloc* surgical resection.

Surgical Therapy

From the surgical perspective, the radiologist can help in patient management by providing initial insight into possible histologic subtype and confirmation of the diagnosis by image-directed biopsy necessary for access to neoadjuvant treatment protocols, and by helping the surgeon reach decisions regarding resectability. Before surgical intervention, it is important to be aware of the involvement of stomach, small intestine, colon, rectum, pancreas, liver, spleen, kidney, ureter, bladder, vertebral bodies (including possible intramedullary extension of tumor), aorta, vena cava, celiac axis vasculature, and superior mesenteric artery and vein. Tumor involvement with many, if not most, of these anatomic structures can be successfully managed intraoperatively but is greatly aided by advanced presurgical planning. Hence, the role of diagnostic imaging is central in the formulation of specific surgical strategies.

Complete resection is much more difficult to achieve with infiltrating lesions versus the more indolent sarcomas, which usually abut and displace but do not invade critical structures that are in immediate proximity to the tumor. Major arterial and venous reconstruction can be undertaken with the simultaneous resection of GI tract and multiple organs during *en bloc* surgery for RPSs (Fig. 24.24).[24,25] Although complete resection improves overall survival, local recurrence continues to be a significant problem.[26]

Contraindications to resection must be individualized; however, long-segment superior mesenteric vein encasement is particularly worrisome because of the high likelihood of venous compromise after resection. Although R0 resection is the goal, it may not be possible owing to tumor size or location. R1 resection for primary and recurrent lesions, particularly in well-differentiated, low-grade liposarcomas, may create a meaningful span of disease-free survival. It may, therefore, be quite favorable for the individual patient.[27,28] Unfortunately, recurrence occurs eventually in the vast majority of cases (Fig. 24.25).

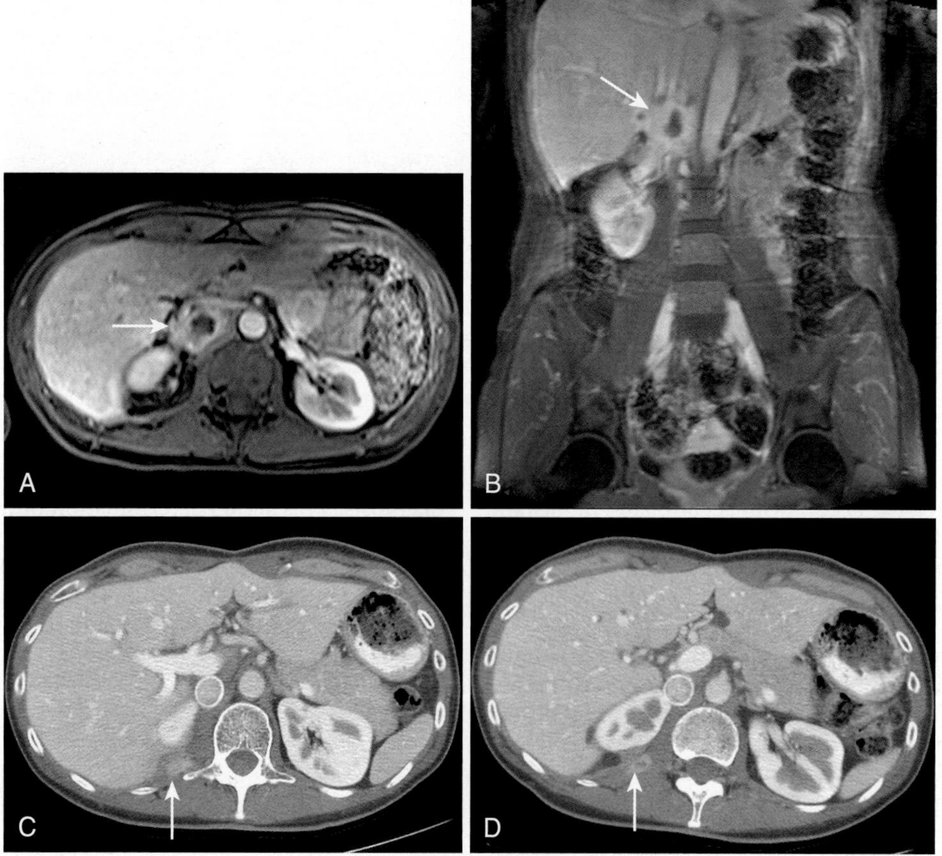

FIGURE 24.24. **A** and **B**, Magnetic resonance imaging obtained after gadolinium contrast reveals a high-grade pleomorphic sarcoma (formerly regarded as malignant fibrous histiocytoma) (*arrows*). Radical surgical excision of tumor with adjacent inferior vena cava required a venous graft. **C** and **D**, Follow-up computed tomography scans 20 months later show a patent venous graft. There is tumor recurrence (*arrows*) adjacent to the right psoas muscle.

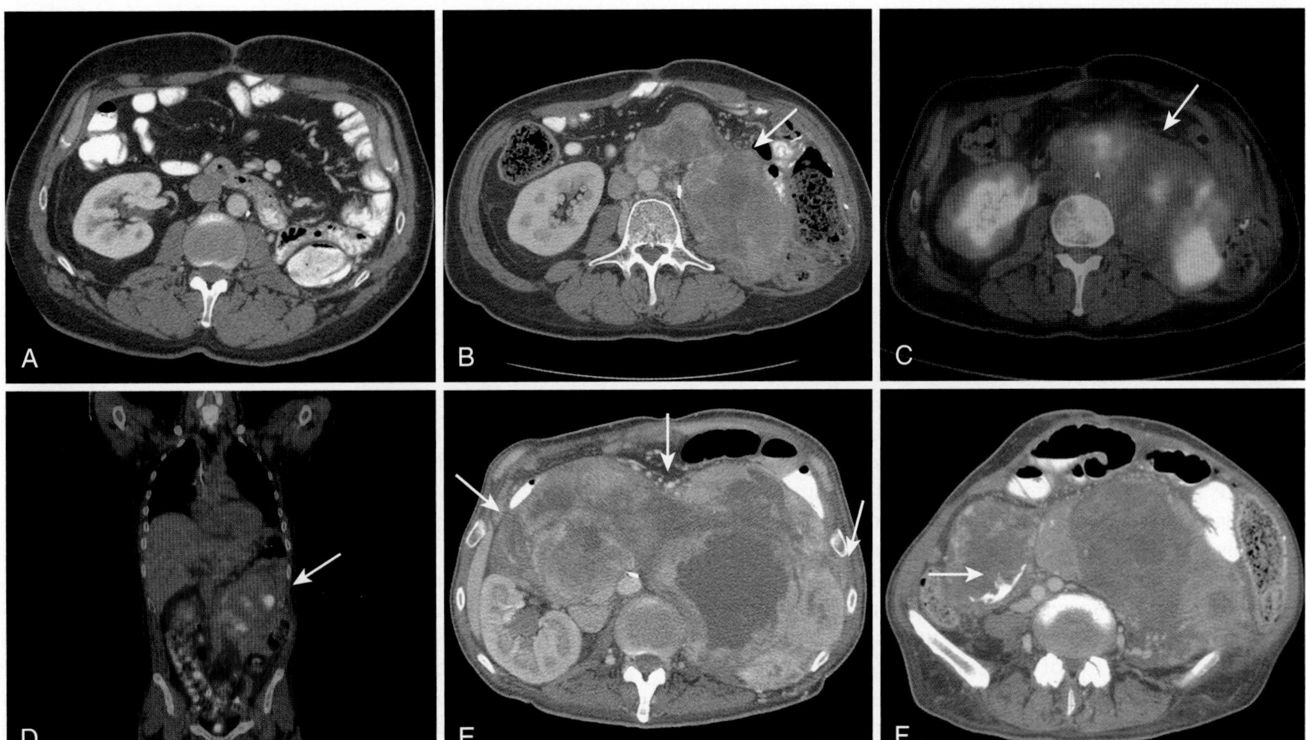

FIGURE 24.25. **A** and **B**, There is tumor recurrence of a high-grade sarcoma (*arrow*) 18 months after a baseline postoperative study. **C** and **D**, Fusion images from 2-[^{18}F] fluoro-2-deoxy-D-glucose positron emission tomography/computed tomography in the axial and coronal planes show that the tumor is metabolically active (*arrows*). **E** and **F**, Three months later there is interval enlargement of the tumor with areas of enhancement and necrosis (*arrows*). There is now obstruction of a solitary right kidney and invasion of a loop of ileum in the lower right quadrant (*arrow* in **F**), presenting clinically with bowel obstruction.

Radiation Therapy

Whereas surgical resection is the mainstay of management for RPSs, radiation therapy is sometimes employed for primary local management in an effort to improve local control of these tumors.[29] The decision to use radiation therapy as an adjuvant to surgical management can hinge on many factors, and it should be undertaken in a multidisciplinary team setting. The diagnostic imaging and its interpretation are critical to the decision-making process and in planning delivery of radiation treatment. When radiation therapy is recommended, it should be delivered preoperatively, as postoperative radiation requires increased dose that exceeds the tolerance of nearby critical structures.[7] Preoperative doses range between 45 to 50.4 Gy and must be delivered with attention to nearby critical structures because even these doses exceed the tolerance of several truncal organs (i.e., kidney, spinal cord, etc.). CT is the preferred imaging modality for radiotherapy management decisions, as well as treatment planning.

An appreciation on imaging studies of the size and extent of RPS is important to decide the feasibility of and technique for radiation therapy. Particularly for well-differentiated liposarcomas, radiology input on the extent of disease based on the appearance of "abnormal fat" is essential. Also, it is important to assess multifocality of tumor deposits because such patients are generally not suitable candidates to receive radiation therapy. The amount of small bowel approximating the tumor is important to assess, because a radiation therapy field that would include a large volume of small bowel is considered in determining feasibility and toxicity of treatment. For right-sided retroperitoneal tumors, the proximity to liver is of importance, because significant volumes (>30%) of the liver tissue cannot be irradiated to the prescribed dose without risk of unacceptable toxicity.[30] If a large volume of liver must be irradiated to cover the area at risk, radiotherapy may not be advisable. Proximity of the tumor to the kidneys is important to assess. Radiation impacts kidney function, so clearly delineating the extent of disease to guide dose volumes is important. In cases that a nephrectomy is required, dose to the ipsilateral kidney is less of a factor, but particular attention should be spent on sparing the contralateral kidney. If nephrectomy is not required, and radiation may impact kidney function, a renal scan is advisable to ascertain the function of the contralateral kidney to ensure that adequate renal function will remain after radiation therapy. In children, consideration should be given to the proximity to any growth plates that could result in subsequent bone deformity.

Prospective data supporting the use of preoperative radiation therapy for the treatment of RPSs is lacking. Recommendations have been based on retrospective series and on extrapolation from the literature supporting its use in extremity and superficial trunk STS.[30a,30b,30c] Because of the low incidence of these tumors and low enthusiasm for study enrollment, accrual to prospective studies has been difficult.[31] However, the STRASS trial, a multicenter randomized trial evaluating the role of preoperative radiation therapy in RPSs, has completed accrual; evaluation of these data will be important for shaping the conversation regarding the role of preoperative radiation therapy.

Chemotherapy

It is imperative that a multidisciplinary review of the clinical information at a specialized center precede implementation of chemotherapy. Tumors that are small or low-grade are unlikely to metastasize and are therefore, well managed with surgery with or without radiation therapy. Large or high-grade tumors have a greater propensity for metastases and need to be discussed in a multidisciplinary conference to determine the appropriateness of systemic therapy and the most beneficial sequence (preoperative vs. postoperative), acknowledging that the standard of care is complete surgical resection.[32] Systemic therapy remains the palliative standard of care for patients who have metastatic disease. Surgical consolidation may be appropriate for a select minority of these patients who can be resected completely and rendered free of all gross disease.

Conventional chemotherapy remains the standard of care for the majority of patients with RPSs. The three most common histologies encountered in the retroperitoneum include liposarcomas (predominantly WDLPS and DDLPS), leiomyosarcomas, UPS, and unclassified sarcomas. Other less common subsets include desmoid tumors, proximal/central variant of epithelioid sarcomas, solitary fibrous tumors, inflammatory myofibroblastic tumors, desmoplastic small round cell tumors, malignant peripheral nerve sheath tumors, and angiosarcomas. Low-grade liposarcomas are chemoresistant and managed with local therapies. All other subsets have variable sensitivity of standard systemic therapies. Commonly used drugs with known activity include doxorubicin, ifosfamide, dacarbazine, gemcitabine, and docetaxel. Our usual front-line regimen includes the combination of doxorubicin and ifosfamide. Special caution needs to be exercised with the use of ifosfamide in patients older than 65 years and those who have had a nephrectomy. Gemcitabine with or without docetaxel is generally used as a second-line regimen, although it may be used up front in patients with leiomyosarcomas, especially of gynecologic origin. Pazopanib is a broad-spectrum inhibitor of vascular endothelial growth factor receptors and is approved for use in soft-tissue sarcomas except liposarcomas. Trabectedin was approved in October 2015 for use in liposarcomas and leiomyosarcomas based on improved progression-free survival compared with dacarbazine.[32a] Eribulin was approved in February 2016 for use in liposarcomas based on improved survival compared with dacarbazine.[32b]

KEY POINTS Therapy Considerations

- Surgery can often provide definitive treatment for retroperitoneal sarcomas.
- Radiation therapy is used at specialized centers selectively in a preoperative setting to reduce local recurrence.
- Chemotherapy may be used in large or high-grade tumors in either the preoperative or postoperative setting and as palliation for metastatic disease.

KEY POINTS What the Surgeon, the Radiation Oncologist, and the Medical Oncologist Want to Know

- Surgeon: Tumor size, presence of fat, displacement or invasion of organs, multifocality, and vascular involvement to plan resection.
- Radiation oncologist: Tumor borders, tumor size, and the relationship of tumor to radiosensitive organs to guide radiation field design.
- Medical oncologist: Tumor size, metastases, and measurement of response to chemotherapy on follow-up imaging.

SURVEILLANCE

Monitoring Tumor Response

Radiation or chemotherapy may be directed at preoperative tumor reduction so that subsequent surgery will provide tumor-free (R0) resection margins. Alternatively, in some instances, adjuvant therapy may be considered after surgery when there is microscopic (R1) or gross residual disease (R2) for local control. In addition, conventional chemotherapy is used for palliation in the patient with distant metastatic disease (M1). It is important to be able to evaluate tumor response in all these settings. Reduction in the size of tumor and target lesions using Response Evaluation Criteria In Solid Tumors score has been used as a sign of response historically. However, such response does not necessarily lead to increased survival. Recent experience in the treatment of GISTs has shown the utility of tumor metabolism as an indicator of tumor response when evaluated with PET. A change in tumor attenuation but not tumor size by CT is a consequence of such targeted therapy.[33] PET is valuable in assessment of early tumor response in high-grade RPSs.[34] Whereas different parameters of glucose kinetics have been suggested, the standard uptake value (SUV) is used most commonly in everyday practice.[35] FDG-PET may also prove very useful when novel targeted therapy is being investigated, because reduction in SUV can provide an early separation of responders from nonresponders. Newer radiotracers such as thymidine analogue 3'-deoxy-3' ^{18}F fluorothymidine hold promise as even better means of evaluating tumor metabolism.[36]

Detection of Recurrence

The risk of local recurrence is the highest early after surgery, with two thirds occurring within 2 years.[6] The overall local recurrence rate in RPS ranges from 40% to 90%. Recurrence in the abdomen is common, with metastases to lung and liver being most common, depending on histology. It is therefore recommended that, in patients with high-grade tumors, CT of the chest, abdomen, and pelvis be performed at 3- to 4-month intervals for 3 years, subsequently at 6-month intervals for 2 years, and then annually. For low-grade tumors, the recommendation is to undergo CT of the abdomen and pelvis at 3- to 6-month intervals for 2 to 3 years and then annually. Such surveillance frequency is widely used in clinical practice, but its benefit has not been proved in a prospective trial.[37] The 5-year overall survival rate in RPS is from 40% to 52%, and it drops to 28% if there is local recurrence.[38,39] The duration of surveillance should continue beyond the conventional timeframe, because recurrence and metastases in RPS do occur beyond 5 years.

Although local recurrence occurs in 40% to 90% of RPS cases, the recurrence rate in extremity sarcoma is only approximately 10%. The resection of recurrent tumor in the retroperitoneum has been shown to provide prolonged local control, and it can be undertaken multiple times, especially in patients with low-grade, well-differentiated liposarcoma. However, whereas primary resection results in complete resection in 80% of patients, with recurrence, complete resection is only achieved in 57%, and it decreases with each subsequent recurrence.[13,14]

There remain many unanswered questions in the management of the patient with metastatic sarcoma. What is the place of metastatectomy of liver or lung lesions? What is the optimal combination and sequence for chemotherapy, radiation therapy, and surgery? Such topics can best be addressed definitively in large, multiple-institution clinical trials. Until then, multiinstitutional cooperative groups can work to provide the best possible data for the care of the patient with RPS to improve quality of life and prolong survival.

Key Points Detecting Recurrence

- Surveillance with computed tomography of chest, abdomen, and pelvis is performed more frequently with high-grade tumor and continued annually beyond 5 years.
- Recurrence commonly occurs within the abdomen at the resection site, followed by metastases to liver and lung.
- Complete resection of recurrent tumor is less successful with each subsequent surgery.

COMPLICATIONS OF THERAPY

The majority of complications are minor and treatable. Occasionally, severe complications can be life-threatening.

Surgical Therapy

The overall complication rate is 5% to 10%.[40] Complications are usually in the early postoperative period and, when severe, can include bleeding, myocardial infarction, or sepsis. Wound dehiscence, abscess, anastomotic leak, or bowel obstruction may also occur.[41]

Radiation Therapy

Acute GI toxicity may occur, depending on the size and location of the tumor. Patients with upper abdominal tumors are more likely to experience nausea or decreased appetite, whereas patients with lower abdominal or pelvic tumors more likely will notice increased bowel movements and bowel irritation. Symptom management may include antiemetics, antidiarrheals, and dietary modifications. Late toxicities are dependent on the dose and volume each organ receives. Bowel stricture and obstruction can occur.[41,42] Bowel ulceration or perforation is very uncommon with preoperative radiation, as the doses delivered do not generally cause these toxicities. Radiation therapy does impact kidney function, so field design needs to aim to spare as much ipsilateral kidney as possible; renal scans should be obtained when indicated to ensure adequate reserve renal function following radiation therapy and/or surgery when nephrectomy is required. In the pediatric population, radiation can impact bone growth and bony formation, depending on the age of the patient. Finally, secondary malignancies are a low but potential risk. These are all factors that must be weighed when recommending preoperative radiation; in many instances, the potential benefits outweigh the risks, but not in every case.

Chemotherapy

Nausea and vomiting are seen frequently and will respond to antiemetic therapy. Neutropenia, anemia, and thrombocytopenia may be seen from myelosuppression. These may manifest as neutropenic fever, infection, fatigue, or a tendency to bleed. Mucositis is usually of short duration. Cardiac toxicity can occur with doxorubicin. Ifosfamide may lead to impaired renal function or neurotoxicity.

Key Points Complications of Therapy

- Surgical complications may be early (hemorrhage, infection, or anastomotic leak) or late (bowel obstruction).
- Potential complications related to radiation therapy impact organs in the treatment field and may include enteritis, bowel stricture, organ function, and a low risk of secondary malignancy.
- Chemotherapy commonly results in nausea and vomiting; myelosuppression may predispose to infection; and cardiac, renal, and neurotoxicity can occur, as well as secondary malignancy.

NEW THERAPIES

Several ongoing and recently completed trials have investigated immunotherapy with checkpoint inhibitors with some signal of activity in UPS, alveolar soft-part sarcomas, DDLPSs, and vascular sarcomas. The development of optimal treatment strategies for sarcoma has been complicated by the large number of subtypes, the heterogeneity in their biologic behavior, and the small number of patients with particular subtypes enrolled in trials. Lessons learned from the experience of targeted therapy with imatinib in GISTs have encouraged basic and translational research in different subsets, with limited success.[43] Potential new targets relevant to sarcomas originating in the retroperitoneum are CDK4 and MDM2 in WDLPSs/DDLPSs; mammalian target of rapamycin (mTOR) in malignant peripheral nerve sheath tumors, PEComas, and lymphangioleiomyomatosis; and ALK1 in inflammatory myofibroblastic tumors. These will need to be studied extensively and validated in the clinic with appropriate inhibitors. It is essential that clinical trials archive pretreatment biopsy material to allow molecular analysis for later studies. Continued attempts at finding a relevant target and its well-tolerated inhibitor are likely to improve outcomes in patients with this rare group of diseases. Given the limitations of available systemic therapy agents, participation in any available phase 1 or 2 clinical trial of new agents in an investigational setting is always encouraged.

CONCLUSION

RPSs present a challenge in management because of their heterogeneity, location, local invasion, and propensity for local recurrence. Surgical therapy offers the best hope for cure; however, even with aggressive resection, local recurrence occurs frequently. For patients with high-grade RPSs, distant metastases also contribute to mortality. Optimal disease control with surgery and adjuvant therapy with minimal morbidity is the desired goal of therapy. Large randomized controlled trials designed to identify the most effective adjuvant therapy are essential to provide evidence-based treatment for the patient with RPS.[44,45]

REFERENCES

1. Jemal A, Siegel R, Ward E, et al. Cancer statistics, 2009. *CA Cancer J Clin*. 2009;59:225–249.
2. Porter GA, Baxter NN, Pisters PW. Retroperitoneal sarcoma: a population-based analysis of epidemiology, surgery, and radiotherapy. *Cancer*. 2006;106:1610–1616.
3. Patel SR. Radiation-induced sarcoma. *Curr Treat Options Oncol*. 2000;1:258–261.
4. Brady MS, Gaynor JJ, Brennan MF. Radiation-associated sarcoma of bone and soft tissue. *Arch Surg*. 1992;127:1379–1385.
5. Amendola BE, Amendola MA, McClatchey KD, et al. CH. Radiation-associated sarcoma: a review of 23 patients with postradiation sarcoma over a 50-year period. *Am J Clin Oncol*. 1989;12:411–415.
6. Clark MA, Fisher C, Judson I, Thomas JM. Soft-tissue sarcomas in adults. *N Engl J Med*. 2005;353:701–711.
7. Thomas DM, O'Sullivan B, Gronchi A. Current concepts and future perspectives in retroperitoneal soft-tissue sarcoma management. *Expert Rev Anticancer Ther*. 2009;9:1145–1157.
8. Pham TH, Iqbal CW, Zarroug AE, et al. Retroperitoneal sarcomas in children: outcomes from an institution. *J Pediatr Surg*. 2007;42:829–833.
9. Herzog CE. Overview of sarcomas in the adolescent and young adult population. *J Pediatr Hematol Oncol*. 2005;27:215–218.
10. Wu JM, Montgomery E. Classification and pathology. *Surg Clin North Am*. 2008;88:483–520. v-vi.
11. Loeb DM, Thornton K, Shokek O. Pediatric soft tissue sarcomas. *Surg Clin North Am*. 2008;88:615–627. vii.
12. Fletcher C, Unni KK, Mertens F. Pathology and Genetics of Soft Tissue and Bone: World Health Organization Classification of Tumors. Lyon: IARC Press; 2002.
13. Lewis JJ, Leung D, Woodruff JM, et al. Retroperitoneal soft-tissue sarcoma: analysis of 500 patients treated and followed at a single institution. *Ann Surg*. 1998;228:355–365.
14. Hueman MT, Herman JM, Ahuja N. Management of retroperitoneal sarcomas. *Surg Clin North Am*. 2008;88:583–597. vii.
15. Fisher SB, Chiang YJ, Feig BW, et al. An evaluation of the eighth edition of the American Joint Committee on Cancer (AJCC) Staging System for retroperitoneal sarcomas using the National Cancer Data Base (NCDB): does size matter? *Am J Clin Oncol*. 2019;42(2):160–165.
15a. Keung EZ, Chiang YJ, Voss RK, et al. Defining the incidence and clinical significance of lymph node metastasis in soft tissue sarcoma. *Eur J Surg Oncol*. 2018;44(1):170–177.
16. Kotilingam D, Lev DC, Lazar AJ, et al. Staging soft tissue sarcoma: evolution and change. *CA Cancer J Clin*. 2006;56:282–291. quiz 314–315.
17. Stojadinovic A, Leung DH, Hoos A, et al. Analysis of the prognostic significance of microscopic margins in 2,084 localized primary adult soft tissue sarcomas. *Ann Surg*. 2002;235:424–434.
18. Zagars GK, Ballo MT, Pisters PW, et al. Prognostic factors for patients with localized soft-tissue sarcoma treated with conservation surgery and radiation therapy: an analysis of 1225 patients. *Cancer*. 2003;97:2530–2543.
19. Alldinger I, Yang Q, Pilarsky C, et al. Retroperitoneal soft tissue sarcomas: prognosis and treatment of primary and recurrent disease in 117 patients. *Anticancer Res*. 2006;26:1577–1581.
20. Nathan H, Raut CP, Thornton K, et al. Predictors of survival after resection of retroperitoneal sarcoma: a population-based analysis and critical appraisal of the AJCC staging system. *Ann Surg*. 2009;250:970–976.
21. Anaya DA, Lahat G, Wang X, et al. Establishing prognosis in retroperitoneal sarcoma: a new histology-based paradigm. *Ann Surg Oncol*. 2009;16:667–675.
22. Fong Y, Coit DG, Woodruff JM, et al. Lymph node metastasis from soft tissue sarcoma in adults. *Analysis of data from a prospective database of 1772 sarcoma patients. Ann Surg*. 1993;217:72–77.
23. Anaya DA, Lahat G, Liu J, et al. Multifocality in retroperitoneal sarcoma: a prognostic factor critical to surgical decision-making. *Ann Surg*. 2009;249:137–142.
23a. Wilkinson MJ, Martin JL, Khan AA, Hayes AJ, Thomas JM, Strauss DC. Percutaneous core needle biopsy in retroperitoneal sarcomas does not influence local recurrence or overall survival. *Ann Surg Oncol*. 2015;22(3):853–858.
24. Schwarzbach MH, Hormann Y, Hinz U, et al. Clinical results of surgery for retroperitoneal sarcoma with major blood vessel involvement. *J Vasc Surg*. 2006;44:46–55.
25. Song TK, Harris Jr EJ, Raghavan S, et al. Major blood vessel reconstruction during sarcoma surgery. *Arch Surg*. 2009;144:817–822.
26. Hassan I, Park SZ, Donohue JH, et al. Operative management of primary retroperitoneal sarcomas: a reappraisal of an institutional experience. *Ann Surg*. 2004;239:244–250.
27. Anaya DA, Lev DC, Pollock RE. The role of surgical margin status in retroperitoneal sarcoma. *J Surg Oncol*. 2008;98:607–610.
28. Anaya DA, Lahat G, Wang X, et al. Postoperative nomogram for survival of patients with retroperitoneal sarcoma treated with curative intent. *Ann Oncol*. 2010;21:397–402.
29. Pawlik TM, Pisters PW, Mikula L, et al. Long-term results of two prospective trials of preoperative external beam radiotherapy for localized intermediate- or high-grade retroperitoneal soft tissue sarcoma. *Ann Surg Oncol*. 2006;13:508–517.
30. Emami B, Lyman J, Brown A, et al. Tolerance of normal tissue to therapeutic irradiation. *Int J Radiat Oncol Biol Phys*. 1991;21:109–122.
30a. Bishop AJ, Zagars GK, Torres KE, et al. Combined modality management of retroperitoneal sarcomas: a single-institution series of 121 patients. *Int J Radiat Oncol Biol Phys*. 2015;93(1):158–165.
30b. Yang JC, Chang AE, Baker AR, et al. Randomized prospective study of the benefit of adjuvant radiation therapy in the treatment of soft tissue sarcomas of the extremity. *J Clin Oncol*. 1998;16(1):197–203.
30c. Pisters PW, Harrison LB, Leung DH, Woodruff JM, Casper ES, Brennan MF. Long-term results of a prospective randomized trial of adjuvant brachytherapy in soft tissue sarcoma. *J Clin Oncol*. 1996;14(3):859–868.
31. Kane 3rd JM. At the crossroads for retroperitoneal sarcomas: the future of clinical trials for this "orphan disease. *Ann Surg Oncol*. 2006;13:442–443.
32. Schuetze SM, Patel S. Should patients with high-risk soft tissue sarcoma receive adjuvant chemotherapy? *Oncologist*. 2009;14:1003–1012.

32. Demetri GD, von Mehren M, Jones RL, et al. Efficacy and safety of Trabectedin or DTIC in patients with metastatic liposarcoma and leiomyosarcoma following failure of conventional chemotherapy: Results of a phase III randomized multicenter clinical trial. *J Clin Oncol*. 2016;34(8):786–793.
32b. Schoffski P, Chawla S, Maki R, et al. Eribulin vs. *Dacarbazine in advanced adipocytic sarcoma or leiomyosarcoma. Lancet*. 2016;387:1629–1637.
33. Choi H. Response evaluation of gastrointestinal stromal tumors. *Oncologist*. 2008;13:4–7.
34. Schwarzbach MH, Dimitrakopoulou-Strauss A, Willeke F, et al. Clinical value of [18-F] fluorodeoxyglucose positron emission tomography imaging in soft tissue sarcomas. *Ann Surg*. 2000;231:380–386.
35. Dimitrakopoulou-Strauss A, Strauss LG, Egerer G, et al. Impact of dynamic 18F-FDG PET on the early prediction of therapy outcome in patients with high-risk soft-tissue sarcomas after neoadjuvant chemotherapy: a feasibility study. *J Nucl Med*. 2010;51:551–558.
36. Schmitt T, Kasper B. New medical treatment options and strategies to assess clinical outcome in soft-tissue sarcoma. *Expert Rev Anticancer Ther*. 2009;9:1159–1167.
37. Windham TC, Pisters PW. Retroperitoneal sarcomas. *Cancer Control*. 2005;12:36–43.
38. Billingsley KG, Burt ME, Jara E, et al. Pulmonary metastases from soft tissue sarcoma: analysis of patterns of diseases and postmetastasis survival. *Ann Surg*. 1999;229:602–610. discussion 610–612.
39. Eilber FC, Eilber KS, Eilber FR. Retroperitoneal sarcomas. *Curr Treat Options Oncol*. 2000;1:274–278.
40. Singer S, Eberlein TJ. Surgical management of soft-tissue sarcoma. *Adv Surg*. 1997;31:395–420.
41. Mendenhall WM, Zlotecki RA, Hochwald SN, et al. Retroperitoneal soft tissue sarcoma. *Cancer*. 2005;104:669–675.
42. Caudle AS, Tepper JE, Calvo BF, et al. Complications associated with neoadjuvant radiotherapy in the multidisciplinary treatment of retroperitoneal sarcomas. *Ann Surg Oncol*. 2007;14:577–582.
43. Patel S, Zalcberg JR. Optimizing the dose of imatinib for treatment of gastrointestinal stromal tumours: lessons from the phase 3 trials. *Eur J Cancer*. 2008;44:501–509.
44. Katz MH, Choi EA, Pollock RE. Current concepts in multimodality therapy for retroperitoneal sarcoma. *Expert Rev Anticancer Ther*. 2007;7:159–168.
44a. Matushansky I, Charytonowicz E, Mills J, et al. MFH classification: differentiating undifferentiated pleomorphic sarcoma in the 21st century. *Expert Rev Anticancer Ther*. 2009;9:1135–1144.

PART VII GYNECOLOGIC AND WOMEN'S IMAGING

CHAPTER 25 Tumors of the Uterine Corpus

Chunxiao Guo, M.D., Ph.D.; Priya R. Bhosale, M.D.; Gaiane M. Rauch, M.D., Ph.D.; Aurelio Matamoros Jr., M.D.; Christine Menias, M.D.; Kathleen M. Schmeler, M.D.; Revathy B. Iyer, M.D.; and Aradhana M. Venkatesan, M.D.

Malignant tumors of the uterine corpus can be divided into epithelial and mesenchymal types (sarcomas). In 2019, there were an estimated 61,880 cases of cancer involving the uterine corpus in the United States, of which 3% were uterine sarcomas, with an estimated 12,160 deaths.[1,2]

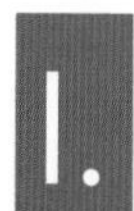

I. ENDOMETRIAL CANCER

INTRODUCTION

The most common epithelial tumor of the uterine corpus is endometrial cancer, representing more than 95% of uterine corpus cancers. It is the fourth most common cancer in women in the United States, where its incidence is increasing. Globally, it is the sixth most common malignancy in women, following breast, colorectal, lung, cervical, and thyroid cancer.[1]

Because the disease is commonly detected in the setting of abnormal uterine bleeding, 70% of patients present with early stage I disease, for which the mean 5-year survival is 85%.

> **KEY POINTS**
>
> **Introduction**
>
> - Endometrial cancer is the most common epithelial tumor of the uterine corpus.
> - Abnormal uterine bleeding is the most common symptom.
> - Endometrial cancer is confined to the uterus in the majority of patients.

EPIDEMIOLOGY AND RISK FACTORS

Age is the most important risk factor for endometrial cancer. This is a disease predominantly seen in the postmenopausal female, with a median age at diagnosis of 60 years.[3] Risk factors associated with the development of endometrial cancer include long-term exposure to unopposed estrogens, metabolic syndrome (obesity, diabetes), increased number of years of menstruation, nulliparity, history of breast cancer, long-term use of tamoxifen, Lynch syndrome, and a first-degree relative with endometrial cancer.[4]

African American women tend to be diagnosed with higher-stage, -grade, and -risk histologies than non-Hispanic White women. They also have higher rates of aggressive endometrial cancers (clear-cell, serous, high-grade endometrioid and carcinosarcomas) and lower 5-year relative survival rates for each stage and subtype compared with non-Hispanic White and Asian women.[5–7] These disparities underscore the importance of research evaluating the epidemiologic, social, and genetic factors influencing clinical outcomes across ethnic groups. Moreover, they highlight the importance of prospective clinical trials with adequate representation of patients at risk for aggressive disease. To date, the vast majority of endometrial cancers are thought to be sporadic, with a subset having a known hereditary basis (the majority of which are attributed to Lynch syndrom). Also known as hereditary nonpolyposis colorectal cancer syndrome, Lynch syndrome is an autosomal-dominant inherited cancer susceptibility syndrome caused by a germline mutation in a DNA mismatch repair gene.[8] Patients with Lynch syndrome present with early-onset colon, rectal, ovary, small bowel, renal pelvis/ureteric, and endometrial cancers.[6] Gynecologic cancer (either endometrial or ovarian) presents earlier than colon cancer in about half of all patients with Lynch syndrome.[4,9,10]

Key Points

Epidemiology and Risk Factors

- Age is the most important risk factor in the development of endometrial cancer.
- Different racial profiles have different clinical outcomes.
- Lynch syndrome/hereditary nonpolyposis colorectal cancer syndrome is associated with 5% of endometrial cancers.

ANATOMY AND PATHOLOGY

The uterus is a pear-shaped, hollow, thick-walled organ located between the bladder and the rectum, and can be divided anatomically into four regions: fundus, body, isthmus, and cervix. The fallopian tubes enter each superolateral angle of the uterus and are known as the cornu. The uterine body narrows to a waist (the isthmus), which contains the cervix. The cavity of the uterus is triangular in coronal section and slit-like in sagittal section, communicating with the cervical canal via the internal os. The cervical canal opens into the vagina via the external os.[11] The endometrium lines the uterine cavity. Uterine arterial blood supply is primarily from the uterine arteries, which are branches of the internal iliac arteries that supply the uterus, medial fallopian tubes, and vagina. The uterine artery gives off a descending branch to the cervix, as well as branches to the upper vagina that anastomose with ascending branches of the vaginal artery. The uterine vein accompanies the artery and drains into the internal iliac vein. It also communicates with the ovarian vein and with the veins of the vagina and bladder through the pelvic venous plexus.[11]

Three main routes constitute the uterine lymphatic drainage. The lymphatic vessels of the uterine fundus and superior uterine body, as well as the fallopian tubes and ovaries, drain to the preaortic and paraaortic lymph nodes. The lymphatic vessels of the cornu drain to the superficial inguinal nodes via the round ligament. The uterine body drains via the broad ligament to the external iliac lymph nodes. The cervix drains laterally via the broad ligament to the external iliac nodes, posterolaterally via the uterine vessels to the internal iliac nodes, and posteriorly along the rectouterine space to the sacral lymph nodes.[11]

Endometrial cancers are classified as type 1 and type 2. Type 1 (low-grade) endometrial adenocarcinomas are the most common (~80%–85%), are associated with long-standing estrogen exposure, and develop in a background of endometrial hyperplasia. The endometrioid type of endometrial carcinoma accounts for approximately 80% of all endometrial carcinomas. These neoplasms tend to have minimal myometrial invasion and a favorable prognosis. Based upon their degree of differentiation, endometrial adenocarcinomas are subdivided into well differentiated (grade I), moderately differentiated (grade 2), and poorly differentiated (grade 3) subtypes. Type 2 tumors (~10%) are often high grade and have a high risk of relapse and metastases, poor prognosis, and no clear association with estrogen stimulation. Their histologic pattern is that of a poorly differentiated or nonendometrioid carcinoma, with deep myometrial and vascular invasion frequently present. Type 2 tumors include grade 3 endometrioid tumors as well as tumors of nonendometrioid histology, that is, serous, clear-cell, and carcinosarcomas as well as rare nonendometrioid histologies, including mucinous, squamous, transitional cell, mesonephric, and undifferentiated subtypes.

Among the most common type 2 tumors are uterine serous and clear-cell carcinomas. Uterine serous carcinomas are associated with a papillary histologic architecture, similar to serous carcinoma of the ovary. These are in contrast to conventional endometrioid adenocarcinomas, which are characterized by proliferation of endometrial glands lacking intervening stroma.[12] Clear-cell carcinomas may demonstrate solid, papillary, or tubulocystic histologic patterns, with clear cells observed at histologic assessment because of the presence of intracellular glycogen. Myometrial invasion occurs in approximately 80% of these cases.[12]

Uterine carcinosarcomas (previously known as malignant mixed Müllerian tumors), are a rare, biphasic, aggressive neoplasm containing both malignant epithelial and malignant mesenchymal elements. Previously classified as a uterine sarcoma, carcinosarcomas are now classified as poorly differentiated metaplastic endometrial adenocarcinoma and type 2 endometrial carcinoma.[13] Patients typically present with advanced disease, often with diffuse uterine involvement by tumor, that is associated with extensive areas of necrosis and cystic and hemorrhagic change.[2,13–18]

Molecular analyses reveal distinct alterations for type 1 versus type 2 tumors. Type 1 tumors are commonly associated with microsatellite instability and mutations in the *PTEN*, *PIK3R1*, *KRAS*, and *ARID1A* genes. In contrast, type 2 tumors are associated with *P53* mutations, as well as *PPP2R1A* mutations, *P16* gene inactivation, and, in a minority of cases, *HER2* amplification. *PIK3CA* mutations can be found in either type of endometrial cancer.[19] Women taking tamoxifen for the treatment of breast cancer are at an increased risk of developing endometrial cancer; however, the risk-benefit ratio favors the use of tamoxifen, with the absolute increase in endometrial cancer rates being small. Aromatase inhibitors are an alternative to tamoxifen in patients with breast cancer and are associated with a lower incidence of endometrial cancer.[20]

Key Points

Anatomy and Pathology

- The anatomic components of the uterus are the fundus, body, isthmus, and cervix.
- The endometrium lines the uterine cavity.
- Two types of endometrial cancer have been described.
- Type 1 endometrial cancers are the most common, occur in younger women, develop in a background of endometrial hyperplasia, and have a favorable prognosis.
- Type 2 endometrial cancers are generally associated with more aggressive clinical behavior than type I tumors. These tumors are often high-grade, have a high rate of relapse and metastatic spread, and have no clear association with estrogen stimulation.

CLINICAL PRESENTATION

Abnormal uterine bleeding is the classic symptom for endometrial carcinoma. This is more common in postmenopausal women and those with risk factors. Occasionally, a thickened endometrium may be detected incidentally in female patients undergoing a pelvic sonogram, or abnormal Papanicolaou (Pap) smear results may suggest the presence of tumor. Abdominal distention, pain, and pressure may be presenting symptoms indicating intraperitoneal spread, and may mimic those of ovarian cancer.

An office endometrial biopsy is commonly used to sample the endometrium. Other diagnostic procedures include dilatation and curettage or hysteroscopy.

> **KEY POINTS**
>
> **Clinical Presentation**
> - The classic clinical presentation for endometrial carcinoma is abnormal uterine bleeding in a postmenopausal woman.
> - Worrisome symptoms include abdominal distention, pain, and pressure. Symptoms can mimic those of ovarian cancer.

PATTERNS OF TUMOR SPREAD

Endometrial cancer can spread in many different patterns. Initial tumor spread is to the myometrium, with the depth of invasion integral to the International Federation of Gynecology and Obstetrics (FIGO) staging system for this tumor (Table 25.1). The adnexa and cervix can also be invaded. Lymphatic and vascular invasion leads to spread of tumor to regional and distant lymph nodes, and is typified by the presence of positive pelvic and paraaortic lymph nodes. Transtubal peritoneal seeding and hematogenous spread are also possible, particularly with type II tumors, which have a higher incidence of both lymphatic involvement and extrauterine spread.[4] The location of tumor within the uterus is associated with the distribution of metastatic adenopathy. When cancer affects the middle and lower third of the uterus, the external iliac lymph nodes are involved; parametrial and paracervical adenopathy may also be observed.[3] For tumors located in the upper corpus or fundus of uterus, common iliac and paraaortic nodes are more commonly involved.[21] Imaging features of lymph node metastases include those greater than 0.8 to 1 cm on the short axis and those demonstrating a rounded or irregular contour, central necrosis, diffusion restriction on magnetic resonance imaging (MRI), and hypermetabolic activity on 2-[^{18}F] fluoro-2-deoxy-D-glucose (FDG)–positron emission tomography (PET)/computed tomography (CT) or PET/MRI, although metastatic disease can be present in morphologically normal–appearing, nonenlarged lymph nodes.[22] Those less than 0.6 cm on the short axis, in particular, may harbor metastatic involvement, but will also typically be below the resolution for visible metabolic activity with FDG-PET/CT and PET/MRI. The dictated radiology report should include a description of any suspicious pelvic and retroperitoneal lymph nodes to the level of the renal vascular pedicles. These data are informative in the preoperative setting before lymph node dissection, and in radiotherapy candidates will facilitate radiotherapy treatment planning.

> **KEY POINTS**
>
> **Patterns of Tumor Spread**
> - Initial spread of endometrial carcinoma is into the myometrium.
> - Lymphatic and vascular spread is typified by the presence of positive pelvic and paraaortic lymphadenopathy.
> - Type II tumors have a higher incidence of lymphatic involvement and extrauterine spread.

STAGING EVALUATION

Endometrial cancer is staged surgically. The FIGO staging system incorporates the depth of myometrial invasion and the presence or absence of extrauterine spread in determining the overall tumor stage.

Stage I endometrial carcinoma is confined to the corpus uteri, whereas stage II disease involves the corpus uteri and the cervix but has not extended outside of the uterus. Stage III endometrial carcinoma extends outside of the uterus but is confined to the true pelvis. In stage IV, endometrial cancer involves the bladder or bowel mucosa or has metastasized to distant sites (Fig. 25.1). Survival for stage I disease is 85%, for stage II is 70%, for stage III is 50%, and for stage IV is 15% to 17%.[3,21] Prognostic factors include the clinical stage, histologic grade, depth of tumor myometrial invasion, presence or absence of lymphovascular invasion, and lymph node status.[23] Using a combination of stage and histology, endometrial cancer can be subclassified as high-risk (stage >1B and high grade) or low-risk (stage IA and low grade). Depth of myometrial invasion is the factor most responsible for variation in the 5-year survival rate in patients with stage I disease: 40% to 60% in stage I patients with deep invasion versus 90% to 100% in stage I patients with minimal or no myometrial invasion.[21,22,24–26] Specifically, women with tumors confined to the corpus (stage I) and with only superficial myometrial invasion have a 3% prevalence of paraaortic lymphadenopathy, whereas women with stage I disease and deep myometrial invasion have a 46% prevalence of lymph node involvement.[27] Patients with grade 3 histologic subtype and myometrial invasion depth greater than 50% depth have an increased likelihood of pelvic and paraaortic nodal metastases and reduced survival.[23,28]

IMAGING EVALUATION

Primary Tumor

Various imaging modalities are used to evaluate the patient with endometrial cancer preoperatively, postoperatively, and during surveillance (Figs. 25.2 to 25.12). These include ultrasound, MRI, CT, PET/CT, and PET/MRI.[29]

TABLE 25.1 International Federation of Gynecology and Obstetrics Surgical Staging Systems for Endometrial Cancer

INTERNATIONAL FEDERATION OF GYNECOLOGY AND OBSTETRICS[a] STAGES	SURGICAL-PATHOLOGIC FINDINGS
I	Tumor is confined to the corpus uteri
IA	Tumor is limited to endometrium or invades less than one-half of the myometrium
IB	Tumor invades one-half or more of the myometrium
II	Tumor invades stromal connective tissue of the cervix but does not extend beyond uterus[b]
III	Tumor involves serosa, adnexa, or parametrium
IIIA	Tumor involves serosa and/or adnexa (direct extension or metastasis)[c]
IIIB	Vaginal involvement (direct extension or metastasis) or parametrial involvement[c]
IIIC	Metastases to pelvic and/or paraaortic lymph nodes[c]
IIIC1	Regional lymph node metastasis to pelvic lymph nodes (positive pelvic nodes)
IIIC2	Regional lymph node metastasis to paraaortic lymph nodes, with or without positive pelvic lymph nodes
IV	Tumor invades bladder and/or bowel mucosa, and/or there are distant metastases
IVa	Tumor invades bladder, bowel mucosa, or both
IVB	Distant metastasis (includes metastasis to inguinal lymph nodes, intraperitoneal disease, or metastasis to lung, liver, or bone; excludes metastasis to paraaortic lymph nodes, vagina, pelvic serosa, or adnexa)

[a]Grade 1, 2, or 3.
[b]Endocervical glandular involvement only should be considered as stage I, and no longer as stage II.
[c]Positive cytology has to be reported separately, without changing the stage.
(From Pecorelli S, Denny L, Ngan H, et al. Revised FIGO staging for carcinoma of the vulva, cervix and endometrium. FIGO Committee on Gynecologic Oncology. *Int J Gynaecol Obstet.* 2009;105:103-104. Copyright 2009, with permission from International Federation of Gynecology and Obstetrics.)

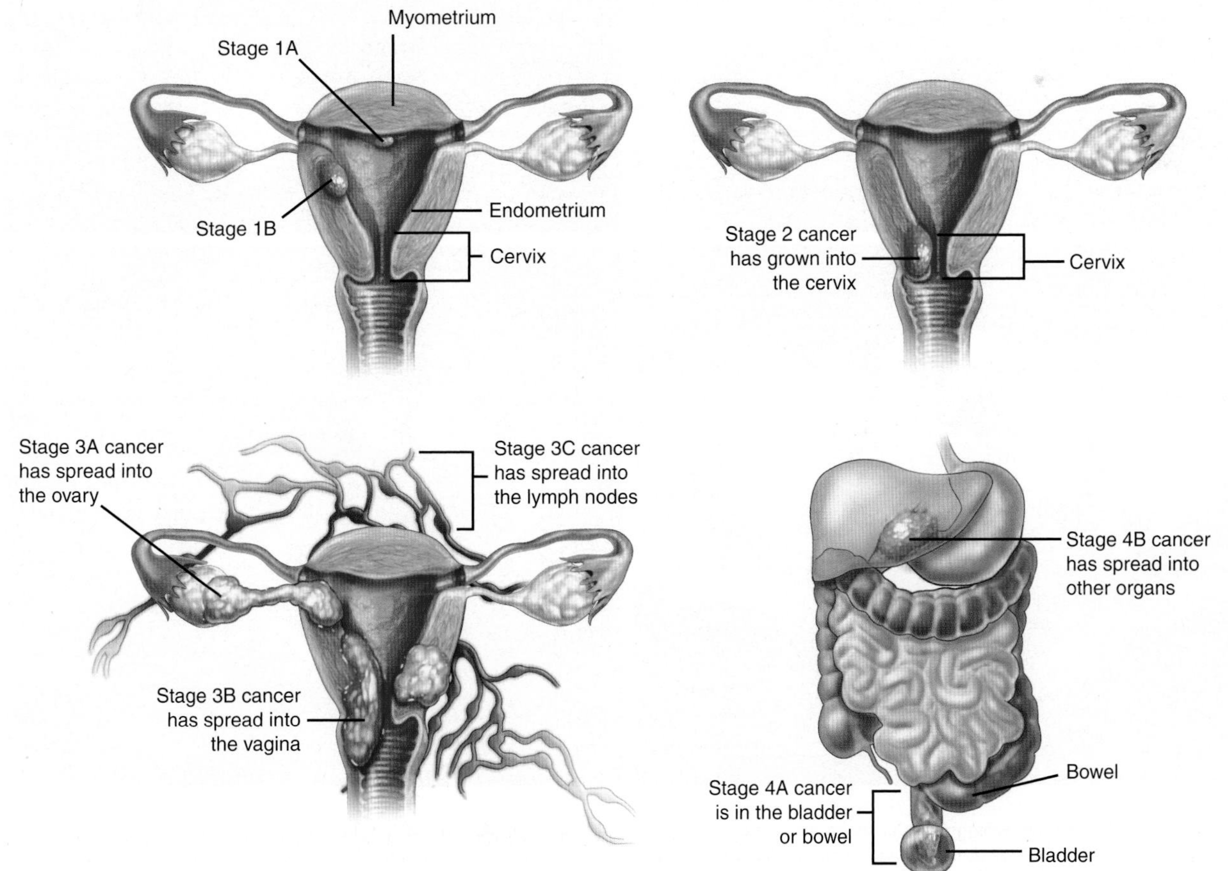

FIGURE 25.1. Staging of uterine cancer.

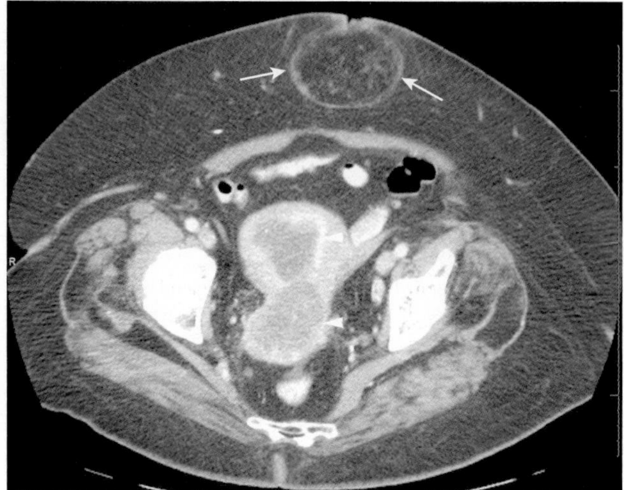

FIGURE 25.2. An 80-year-old woman with postmenopausal bleeding. Contrast-enhanced axial computed tomography scan shows an intrauterine mass with invasion of the lower uterine segment and cervix (*white arrowheads*), histologically confirmed as endometrial carcinoma.

Ultrasound

Pelvic and transvaginal ultrasound are routinely used as the first-line imaging modality to assess postmenopausal patients with abnormal vaginal bleeding. A dual-layer endometrial thickness measurement on ultrasound of less than 5 mm in a postmenopausal woman has been previously noted to have a sensitivity of 96% and specificity of 61% for the detection of endometrial cancer.[30] Ultrasound can, to an extent, evaluate the depth of myometrial invasion, with a prior metaanalysis of 184 publications indicating a pooled sensitivity of 82% and specificity of 82% for the presence of deep myometrial invasion.[31] However, ultrasound cannot assess for tumor spread to adjacent organs.[32,33] Sonohysterography can help to differentiate endoluminal mural masses from a more diffuse and uniformly thickened endometrium.

Magnetic Resonance Imaging

MRI is the imaging modality of choice to preoperatively evaluate the distribution of disease in the pelvis, including the depth of myometrial invasion, the presence or absence

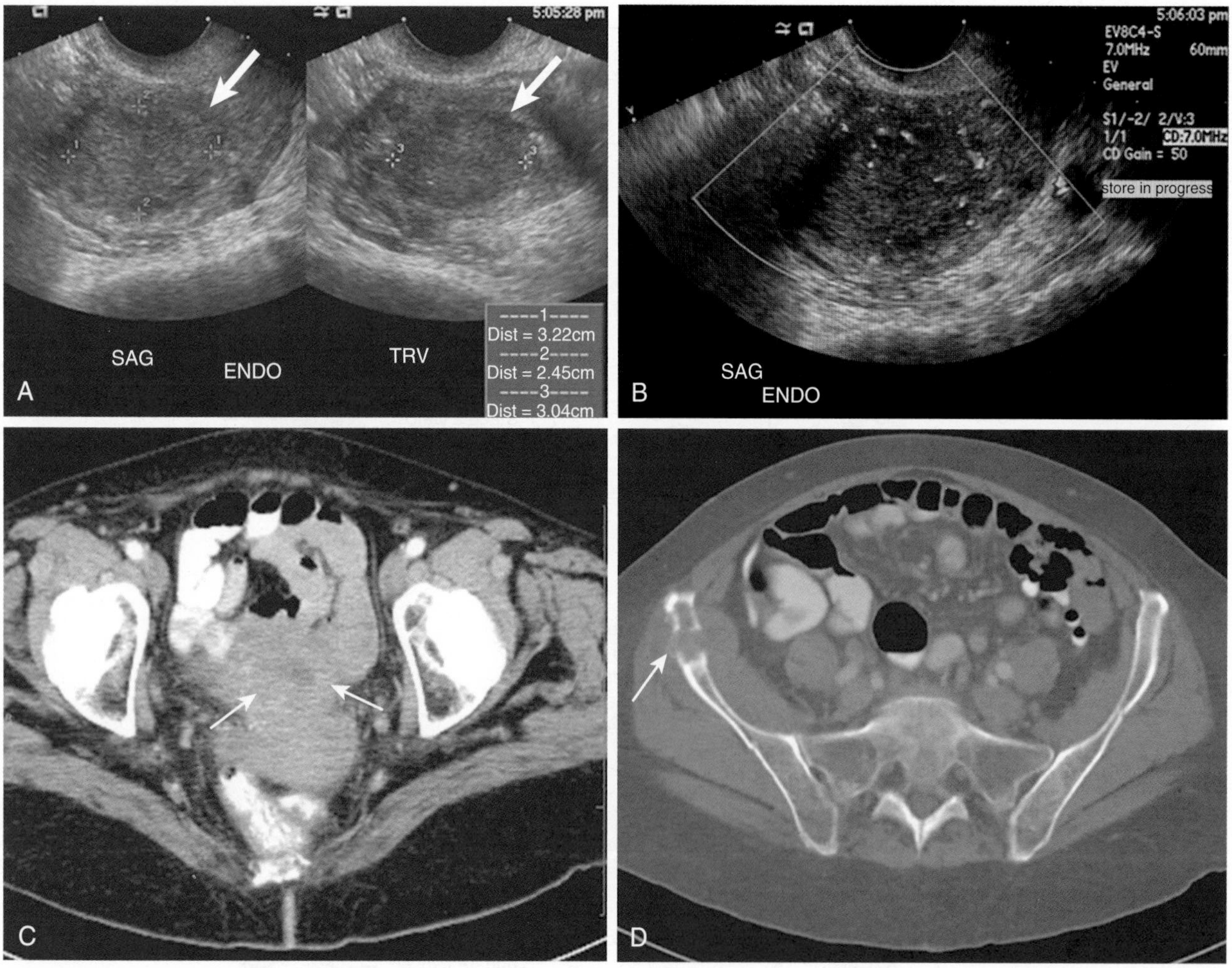

FIGURE 25.3. A 69-year-old woman with postmenopausal bleeding and right hip pain. **A**, Transvaginal ultrasound (sagittal and transverse images) demonstrate a heterogeneous solid, mildly hypoechoic, intrauterine mass (*white arrows*). **B**, Transvaginal ultrasound sagittal view with color Doppler demonstrates intralesional blood flow. **C**, Contrast-enhanced axial computed tomography (CT) scan demonstrates a poorly defined solid intrauterine mass (*white arrows*). **D**, Axial CT scan demonstrates an osteolytic metastatic lesion (*white arrow*) of the anterior right iliac bone, histologically confirmed as metastatic endometrial carcinoma. *ENDO, SAG, TRV*.

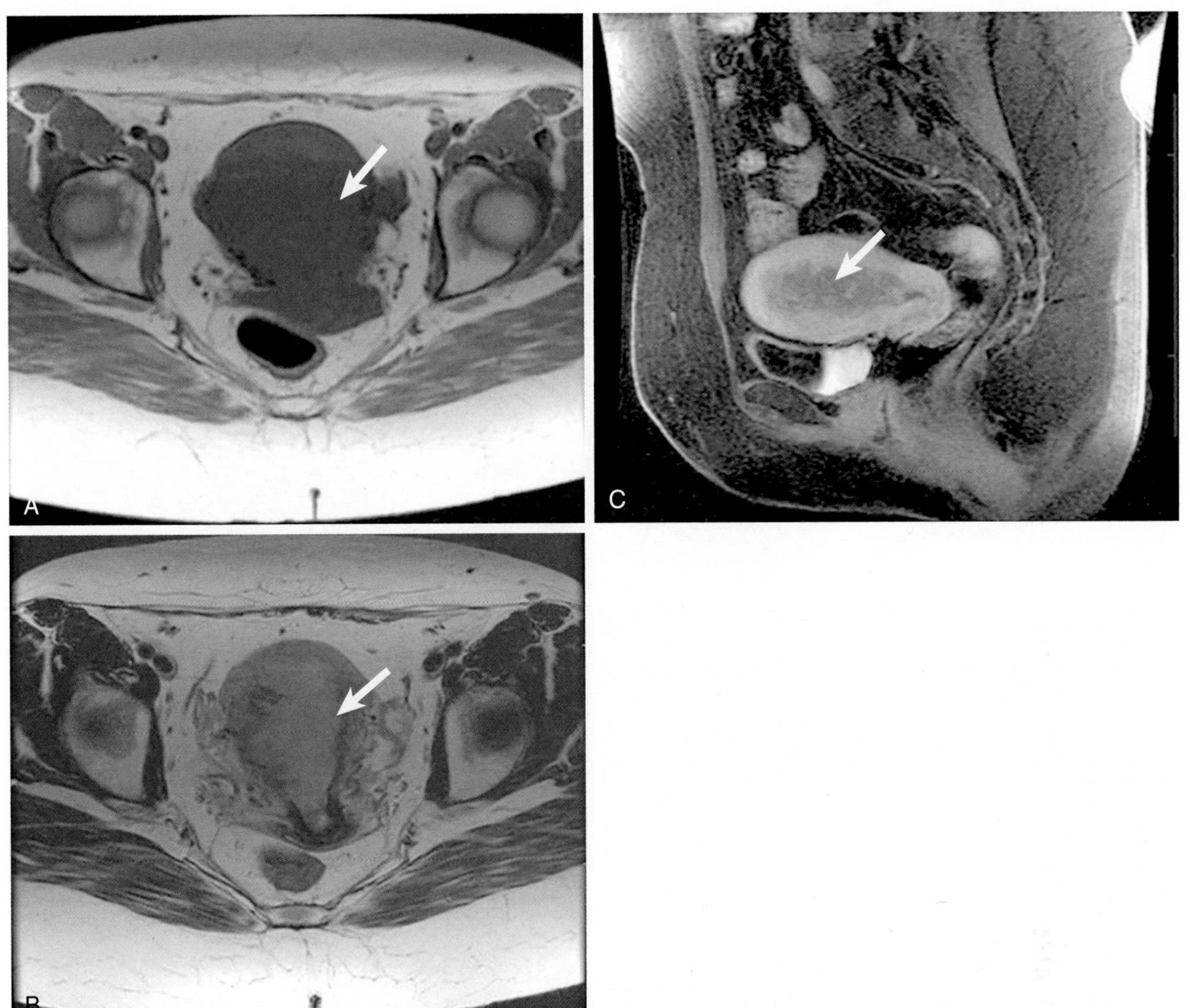

FIGURE 25.4. A 51-year-old woman with postmenopausal bleeding. **A**, Axial T1-weighted magnetic resonance imaging (MRI) study with an isointense uterus without a definable mass. **B**, Axial T2-weighted MRI study demonstrates a mass that is hyperintense relative to the normal uterine myometrium, junction zone, and cervical stroma (*white arrows*) **C**, Sagittal T1 fat-suppressed MRI following contrast administration redemonstrates the intrauterine mass (*white arrow*) that enhances less avidly than the subjacent myometrium.

of adenopathy, and invasion of adjacent soft tissue. A dedicated pelvic MRI protocol tailored to the evaluation of gynecologic anatomy is essential to maximize diagnostic accuracy. MRI images may be acquired using an eight-channel torso-pelvis coil after instructing the patient to void and instilling endovaginal gel to aid in the delineation of tumor involvement in relation to the vagina or cervix. Endovaginal gel also helps minimize susceptibility artifact, which reduces the quality of diffusion-weighted (DW) images. At our institutions (C.G., P.R.B., G.M., A.M., K.S., A.M.V., C.M.), patients are provided with a plastic tube filled with 60 mL of ultrasound gel at body temperature (Aquasonic 100; Parker Laboratories, Fairfield, NJ). They are instructed to instill the gel in the vagina per their individual tolerance, typically while lying on their left side on the MRI table. In general, instillation of 30 to 60 mL of gel into the vagina is adequate.[34–36]

On MRI, the normal uterus has three distinct layers, best seen on T2-weighted (T2W) images: (1) a high–signal intensity inner layer constituting the endometrium, (2) a low–signal intensity middle layer depicting the junctional zone or inner myometrium, and (3) the outer myometrium demonstrating intermediate signal intensity. Foci of hemorrhage will be of high signal intensity on T1-weighted (T1W) images, whereas foci of necrosis will be of high signal intensity on T2W images.

Critical elements of any gynecologic MRI protocol are small field of view ([FOV], e.g., 24 cm) imaging of the uterus, cervix, vagina, and pelvic sidewalls. These facilitate visualization of the primary tumor and assessment of parametrial involvement, specifically multiplanar or three-dimensional isotropic T2W acquisitions without fat saturation. Obtaining oblique axial T2W images can be useful for interpretation when the uterus is tilted to the left or

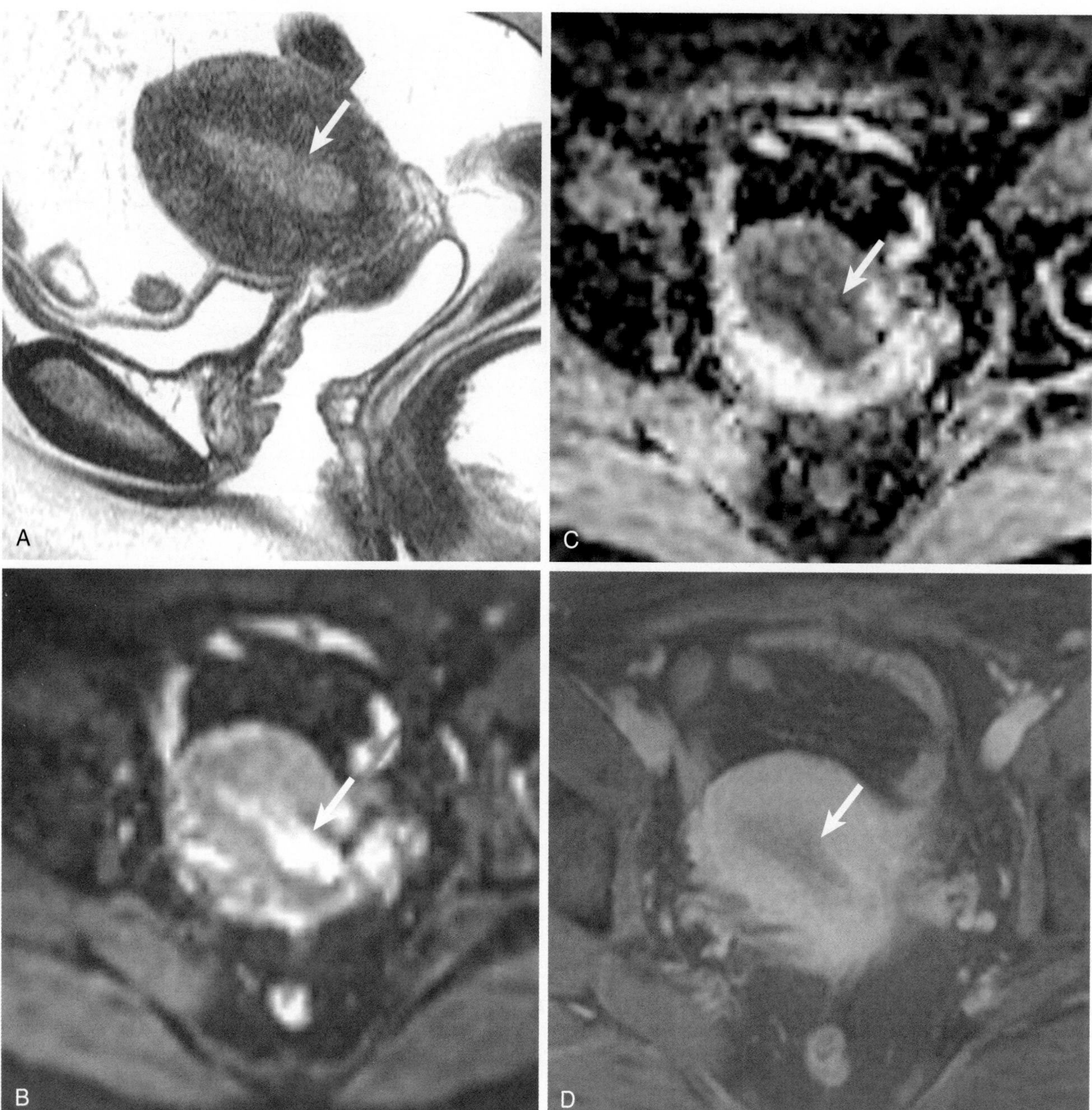

FIGURE 25.5. A 34-year-old woman with intermenstrual bleeding. **A**, Sagittal T2-weighted magnetic resonance imaging of the pelvis demonstrates a nonspecific mildly prominent endometrial stripe (*white arrow*). **B**, Axial diffusion-weighted (DW) images and **C**, axial ADC images demonstrate the restricted diffusion associated with the endometrium, with increased signal on the DW images and corresponding reduced signal on the apparent diffusion coefficient map (*white arrows* in **B** and **C**). **D**, Axial T1-weighted images with fat suppression demonstrate hypoenhancement of the endometrium (white arrow) compared with the myometrium. This was a clinical and histologically confirmed International Federation of Gynecology and Obstetrics stage I endometrioid adenocarcinoma, and the patient underwent fertility-sparing therapy (progestin-containing intrauterine device).

right of the midline, as the images are accurately obtained along the short axis of the uterus, ensuring accurate delineation of parametrial invasion in these instances.[37] Axial and/or sagittal DW imaging with apparent diffusion coefficient (ADC) mapping is used to identify tumor in relation to normal cervix, uterus, or vagina and, in the posttreatment setting, to distinguish viable tumor from posttherapy fibrosis. Images of the pelvis obtained after the administration of contrast material are useful for defining the extent of enhancing tumors, adjacent organ invasion, or, in the posttherapy setting, fistulous tracts. Axial unenhanced T1W images of the pelvis are useful for detecting regional nodal metastatic disease.

Endometrial cancer is typically apparent as a hypointense mass on T1W imaging and as an intermediate-signal mass on T2W imaging. It is typically lower in signal on T2W imaging than the endometrium and higher in signal on T2W imaging than the junctional zone. Both myometrial invasion and cervical stromal invasion are delineated on MRI. Myometrial invasion is best demonstrated on

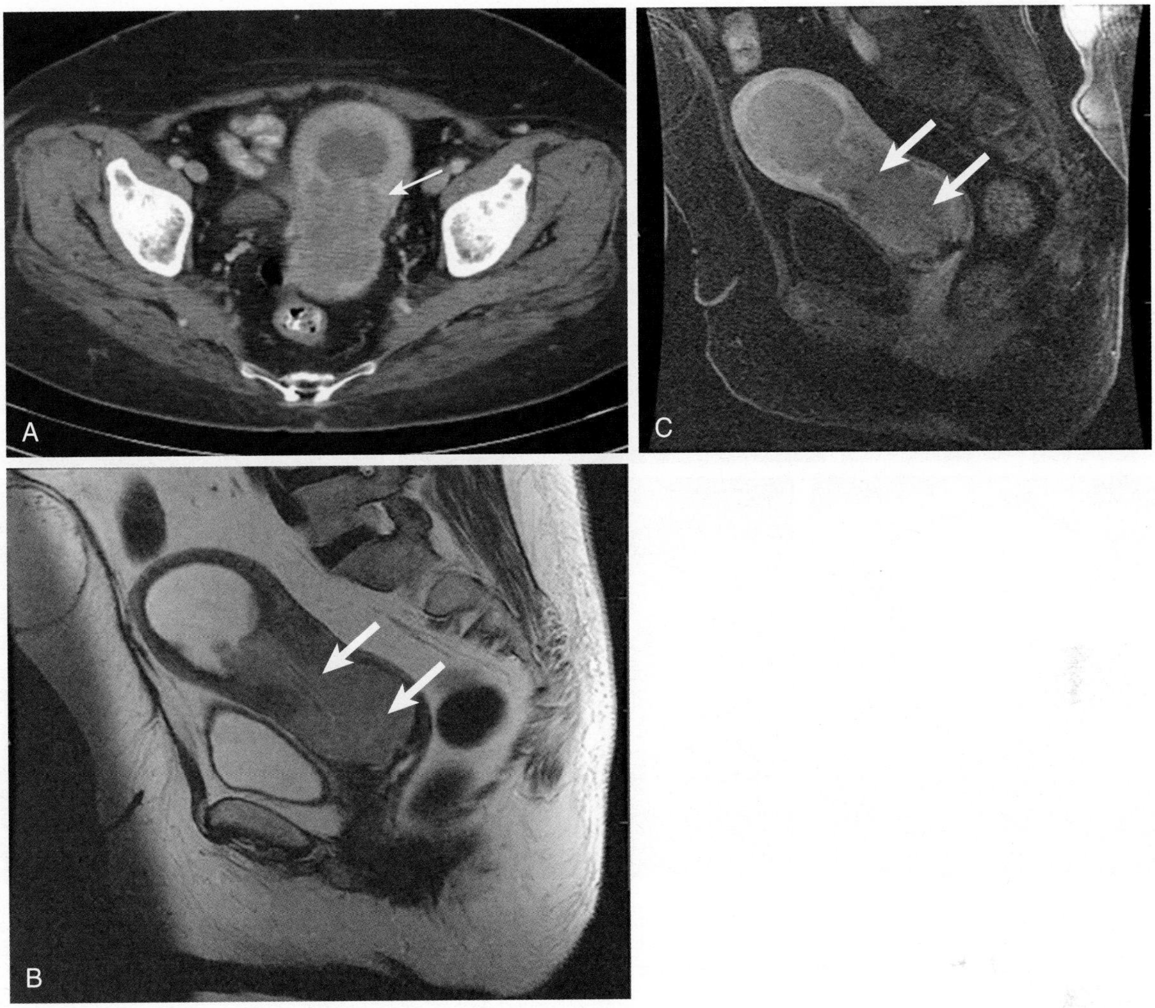

FIGURE 25.6. A 62-year-old woman with postmenopausal bleeding. **A**, Contrast-enhanced computed tomography scan demonstrates an intrauterine mass (*white arrow*) extending from the uterine body segment to involve the cervix. **B**, Sagittal T2-weighted magnetic resonance imaging (MRI) study demonstrates the intrauterine mass extending from the mid uterine body to the cervix (*white arrows*). **C**, Sagittal fat-suppressed postcontrast MRI of the pelvis demonstrates the relative hypoenhancement of the tumor (*white arrows*) as compared with the adjacent myometrium.

T2W images and is associated with disruption of the low–signal intensity junctional zone images by tumor that is intermediate in T2 signal. Tumors, particularly in the untreated setting, are associated with areas of restricted diffusion, with increased signal on DWI and reduced signal on the corresponding ADC maps. Contrast administration enhances assessment of the depth of myometrial invasion, with endometrial cancers enhancing less avidly than the normal endometrium, particularly on delayed sequences. Together, T2W images and contrast-enhanced images have an accuracy of 98% for assessing myometrial invasion.[37] Type 2 tumors tend to exhibit heterogeneous morphology, areas of hemorrhage and necrosis, and deep myometrial invasion.[38] Tumor involvement of the cervical stroma distinguishes patients as stage II, compared with stage I patients who do not exhibit cervical stromal involvement. Cervical stromal invasion is denoted by the presence of tumor that is intermediate- to high-signal on T2W images relative to the normal cervical stroma, which is low-signal on T2W images. The sensitivity and specificity of MRI for cervical stromal involvement approach 95% and 80%, respectively, with the overall reported accuracy of MRI for endometrial cancer staging reported to be between 85% and 93%.[39–48] Depth of myometrial invasion and cervical tumor involvement have important clinical implications. The prevalence of lymph node metastases increases from 3% with superficial myometrial invasion to 46% with deep myometrial invasion.[27,49,50] For stage I and II tumors, if there is greater than 50% myometrial invasion, positive cervical or extrauterine spread. The increased risk of lymph node metastasis warrants lymphadenectomy at some institutions.[21] For more advanced (stage III) disease, MRI provides the surgeon information about the extent of tumor spread, uterine size, the presence or absence of ascites, and adnexal disease, which can help with selecting the surgical approach (i.e., open laparotomy vs. transvaginal vs. laparoscopic approaches, and the need for lymphadenectomy).[51,52]

Computed Tomography

CT of the chest and abdomen is useful to evaluate for nodal and distant metastatic disease, given the feasibility of fast

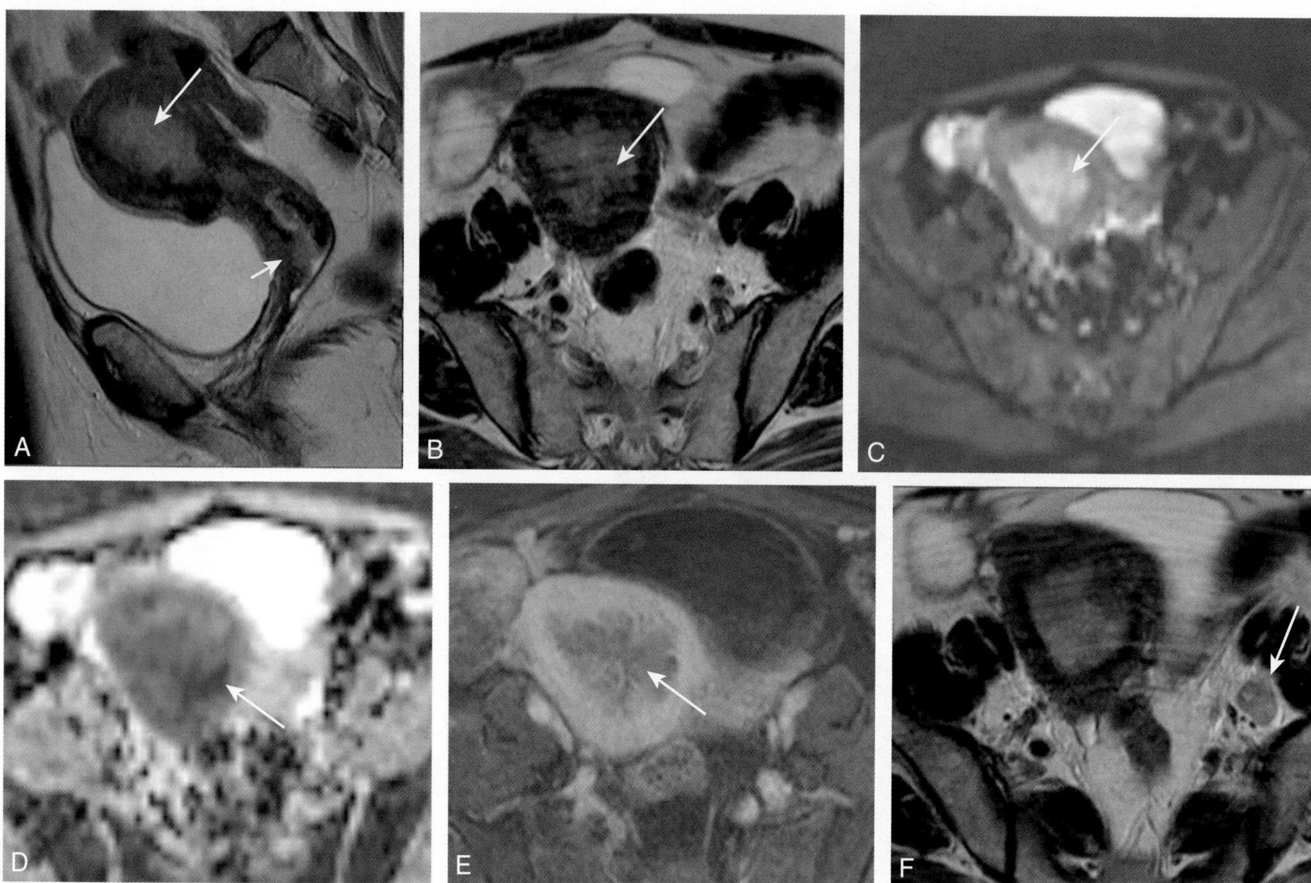

FIGURE 25.7. A 61-year-old woman with postmenopausal bleeding and International Federation of Gynecology and Obstetrics IIIc endometrioid carcinoma with clear-cell features involving the upper vagina and left external iliac lymph nodes. **A**, Sagittal T2-weighted (T2W) magnetic resonance imaging (MRI) of the pelvis demonstrates abnormal thickening of the endometrial stripe (*long white arrow*), with concomitant tumor involvement detected at the level of the cervical canal, protruding through the external cervical os and into the upper vagina (*short white arrow*). **B**, Axial T2W MRI redemonstrates a T2-hyperintense mass at the level of the endometrium (white arrow) associated with myometrial tumor involvement. Axial diffusion-weighted (DW) imaging (**C**) and axial apparent diffusion coefficient (ADC) (**D**) images demonstrate the restricted diffusion associated with the endometrial tumor, with increased signal on the DW images and corresponding reduced signal on the ADC map (*white arrows* in **C** and **D**). **E**, Axial T1W images with fat suppression demonstrate hypoenhancement of irregularly marginated endometrial tumor (*white arrow*) compared with the myometrium. **F**, Axial T2W image of the pelvis demonstrates metastatic left external iliac adenopathy (*white arrow*). The patient was dispositioned to chemoradiotherapy.

acquisition and larger FOV imaging with CT compared with MRI.[53,54] Primary endometrial cancers will typically appear as a hypoattenuating mass in the endometrial cavity, although this appearance is not pathognomonic and can be seen with endometrial polyps or submucosal leiomyomas. The suboptimal soft tissue resolution afforded by CT as compared with MRI limits its utility for primary staging, with its sensitivity and specificity for detecting myometrial invasion ranging from 40% to 83% and from 42% to 75%, respectively.[55]

Positron-Emission Tomography/Computer Tomography

FDG-PET/CT is an integral tool for whole-body oncologic staging and functional assessment. Intrinsic hypermetabolic activity, typically assessed using the FDG maximal standardized uptake value (SUVmax), is observed in many malignancies. Changes in FDG uptake are not only useful for detection of early tumor recurrence, but are also indicative of tumor response to therapy and a predictor of relapse. There has been interest in the prognostic value of PET/CT with respect to "T" staging.[56] A prospective study demonstrated that patients with high initial SUVmax had significantly lower disease-free survival (DFS) and overall survival (OS) compared with patients with low FDG uptake values. Multivariate analysis revealed that SUVmax is an independent prognostic factor of both DFS and OS that is superior to CA-125 serum levels and minimum apparent diffusion coefficient (ADCmin) on MRI.[57,58] Ongoing practical limitations of PET/CT for primary staging in this setting relate to the low soft-tissue resolution of CT as compared with MRI. Recent data suggest that PET/CT may not accurately detect extrauterine disease in patients with newly diagnosed high-risk endometrial cancer.[59] PET/CT does have value in the detection of nodal metastases, with prior publications demonstrating a high specificity (99.6%) and accuracy (97.8%) for the detection of pelvic and paraaortic nodal metastases, albeit with a sensitivity that decreases with lymph node diameter (from 93.3% to 16.7% for lesions of 10 mm and 4 mm, respectively).[60]

Positron-Emission Tomography/Magnetic Resonance Imaging

Integrated PET/MRI is a recently developed imaging modality enabling simultaneous acquisition of PET and

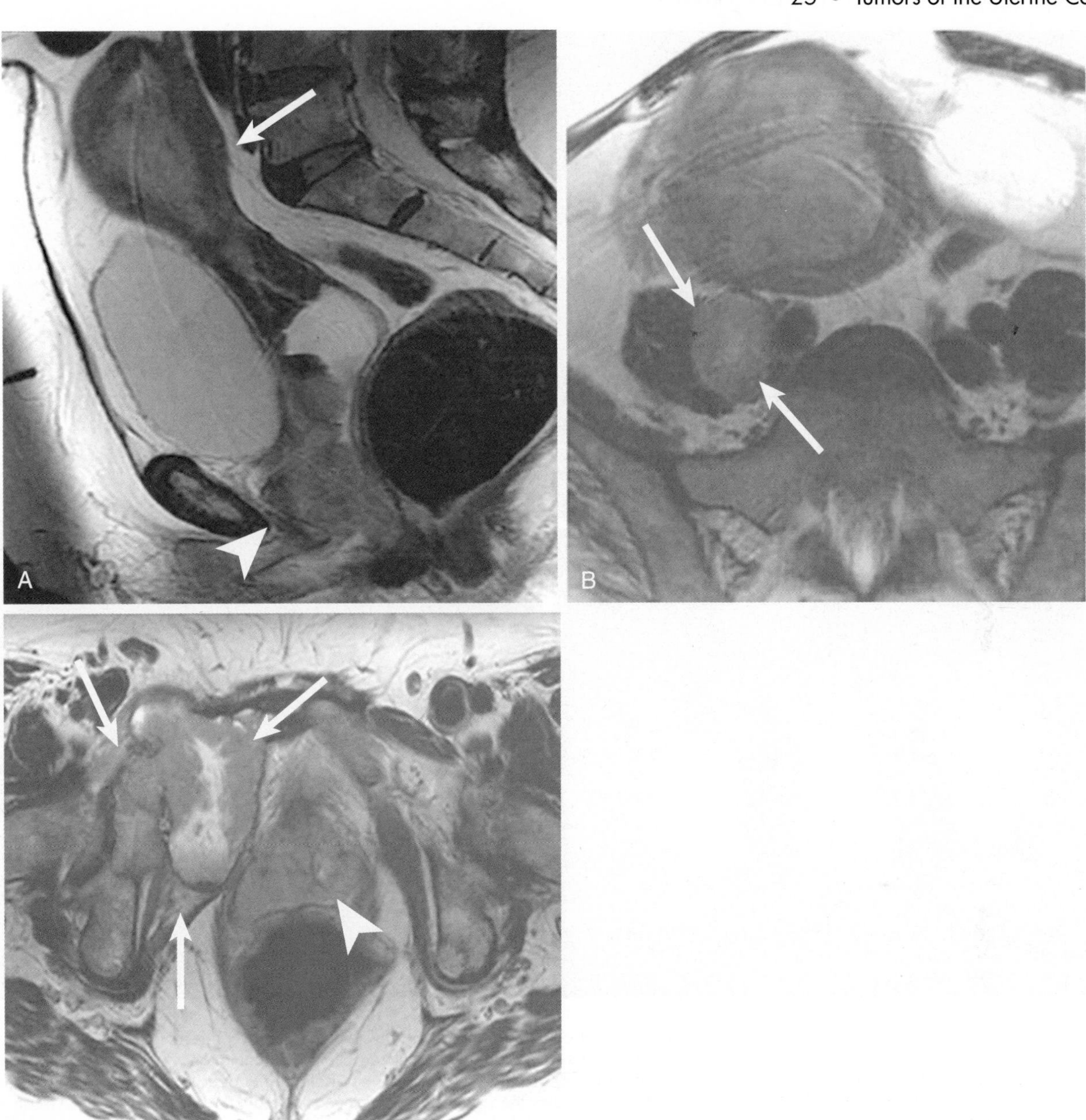

FIGURE 25.8. A 73-year-old woman with postmenopausal bleeding and International Federation of Gynecology and Obstetrics stage IVb endometrial carcinoma with right common iliac lymph nodes and pelvic osseous metastases. **A**, Sagittal T2-weighted magnetic resonance imaging (MRI) of the pelvis demonstrates a T2-hyperintense mass replacing the normal endometrial cavity (*white arrow*), with concomitant tumor involvement detected at the level of the lower vagina (*white arrowhead*) involving the posterior wall of urinary bladder. **B**, Axial T2-weighted (T2W) MRI demonstrates concomitant right common iliac metastatic adenopathy (*paired white arrows*). **C**, Axial T2W image inferiorly in the pelvis redemonstrates tumor at the level of the lower vagina (*white arrowhead*) and a right acetabular and right parasymphyseal pubis metastasis (white arrows).

MRI data in a single examination. Compared with PET/CT, it imparts less radiation to the patient and combines the strengths of PET imaging with respect to detecting extrauterine spread with those of MRI with respect to high soft tissue resolution. It enables assessment of quantitative functional imaging biomarkers derived from both PET and MRI (e.g., DWI and dynamic contrast-enhanced imaging), which can inform therapeutic response.[61] Prior work to date has investigated the diagnostic accuracy of integrated PET/MRI to detect primary or recurrent tumors in heterogeneous groups of patients with gynecologic malignancy, a subset of whom had endometrial cancer.[62–64] The diagnostic accuracy of PET/MRI has been reported to be superior to that of MRI alone and comparable to that of PET/CT. Research is underway to explore the diagnostic accuracy of integrated PET/MRI for primary staging of endometrial cancer. Prior work employed PET/MRI in 47 patients with newly diagnosed

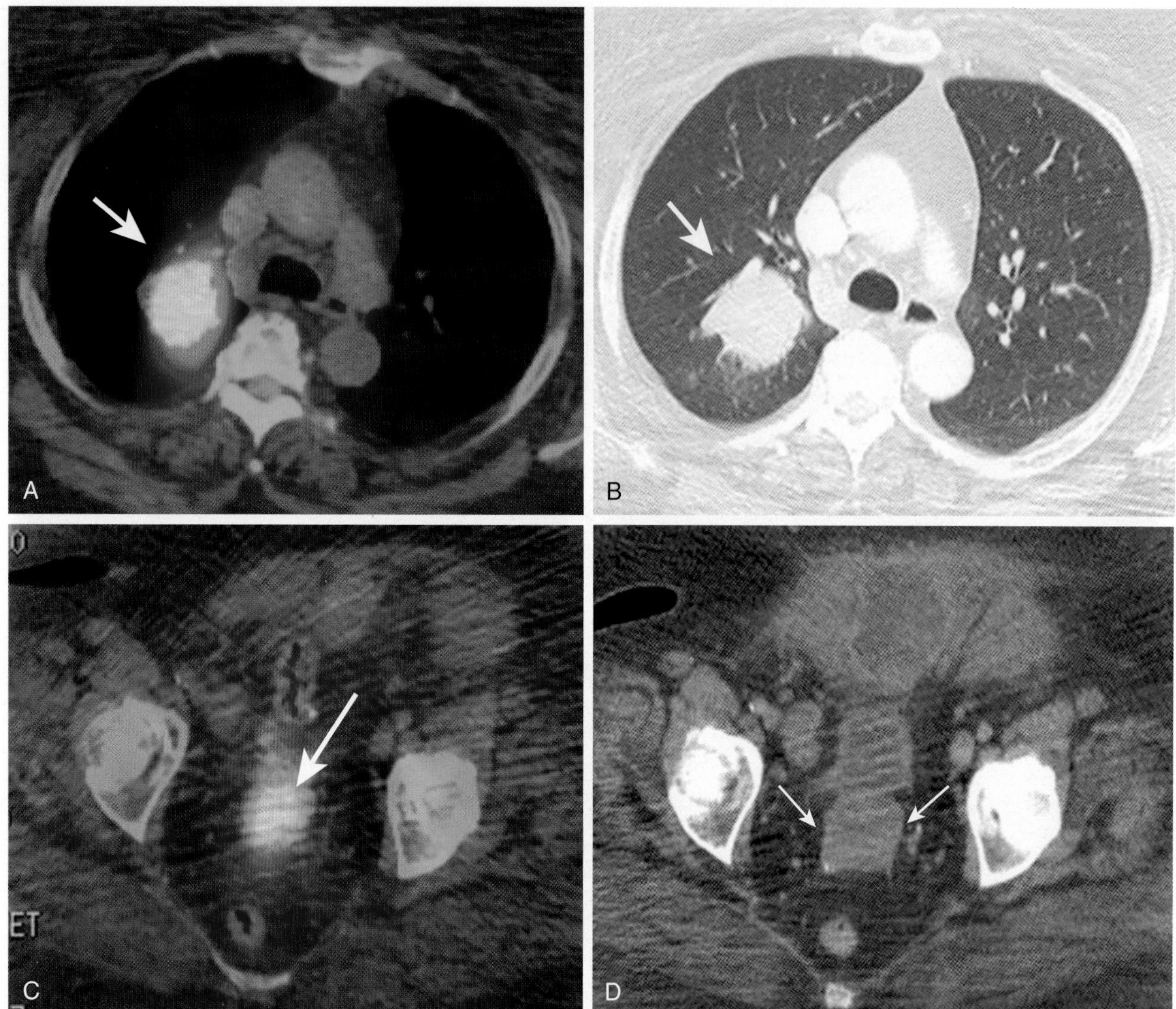

Fig. 25.9 A 61-year-old woman with prior history of endometrial carcinoma, status posthysterectomy, now presenting with abnormal vaginal bleeding, suspicious for recurrence. A solid mass at the apex of the vaginal cuff was found on clinical examination. **A**, 2-[^{18}F] fluoro-2-deoxy-D-glucose positron emission tomography (PET)/computed tomography (CT) demonstrates a hypermetabolic right upper lobe lung mass (*white arrow*), consistent with metastatic disease. **B**, CT with lung windows demonstrates the right upper lobe metastasis (*white arrow*). **C**, PET/CT scan shows a focal area of increased metabolic activity in the vaginal cuff, consistent with recurrent disease (*white arrow*). **D**, Contrast-enhanced CT scan delineates the solid mass (*white arrows*) at the apex of the vaginal cuff.

endometrial cancer, evaluating correlations between imaging biomarkers and pathologic prognostic factors, demonstrating a significant inverse correlation between SUVmax and ADCmin ($r = -0.53$; $P = .001$).[65] In addition, SUVmax was significantly higher in tumors with advanced stage, deep myometrial invasion, cervical invasion, lymphovascular space involvement, and lymph node metastasis. ADCmin was found to be lower in tumors with higher grade, advanced stage, and cervical invasion.[66] These and other data suggest the value of FDG-PET metabolic activity and DWI to provide prognostic information when evaluating patients with endometrial cancer, underscoring potential benefits of simultaneous acquisition with PET/MRI as a one-stop comprehensive imaging modality.

Key Points

Imaging Evaluation

- Preoperative imaging should identify the tumor location and extent, including the depth of myometrial invasion and cervical stromal involvement, suspected locations of adenopathy, extent of invasion into adjacent soft tissues, and presence of metastatic disease.
- Magnetic resonance imaging (MRI) is the imaging modality of choice to preoperatively evaluate the origin of the disease, the depth of myometrial invasion, the presence or absence of adenopathy, and the extent of adjacent soft tissue invasion.
- Computed tomography (CT), positron emission tomography (PET)/CT, and, more recently, PET/MRI are useful for the assessment of distal metastatic disease.

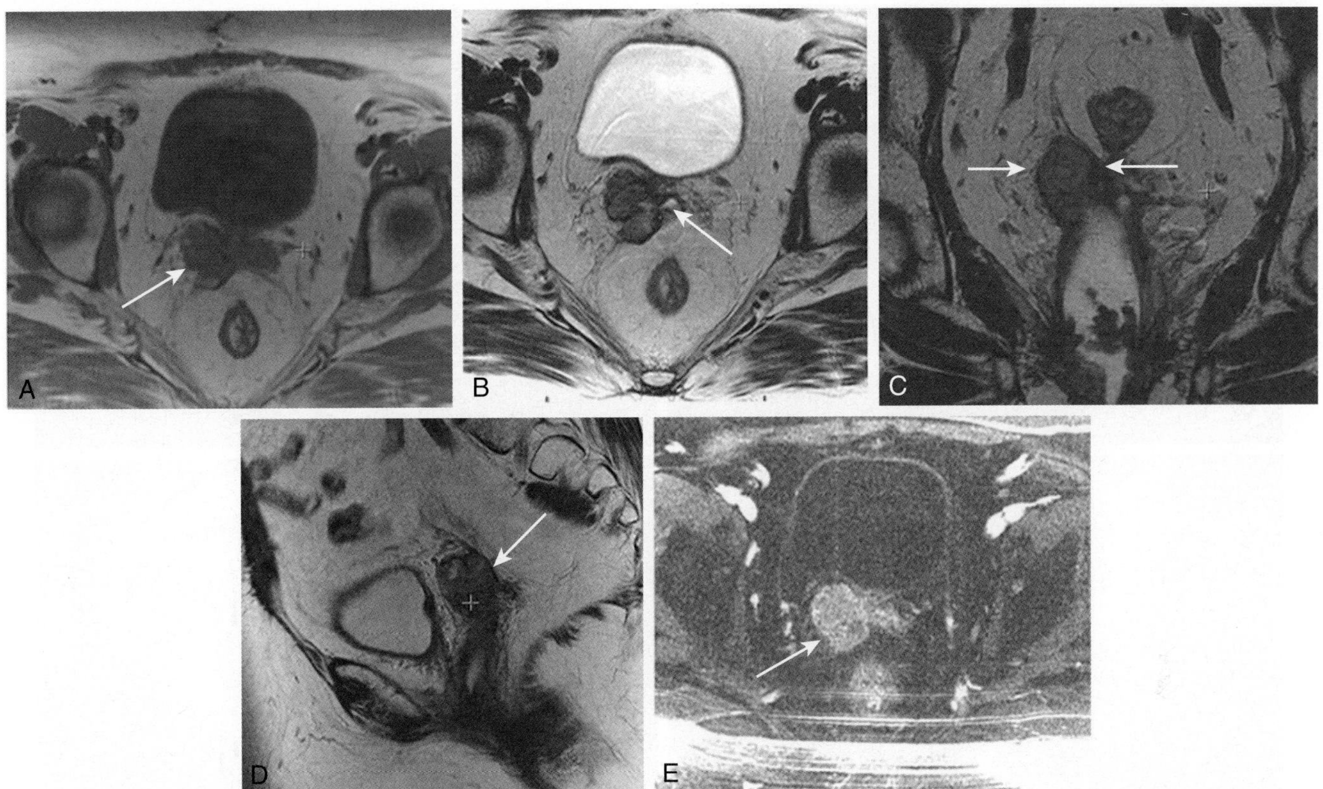

Figure 25.10. A 61-year-old woman with prior history of endometrial carcinoma, status post total abdominal hysterectomy and bilateral salpingo-oophorectomy in 2011, now presenting with vaginal bleeding. Axial T1-weighted (T1W) magnetic resonance imaging (MRI) (**A**), axial T2-weighted (T2W) MRI (**B**), coronal T2W MRI (**C**), and sagittal T2W MRI (**D**) demonstrate a lobulated mass that is heterogenous in T2 signal intensity at the level of the right lateral aspect of the vaginal cuff (*white arrows* in **A–D**). **E**, Axial T1W fat-suppressed image demonstrates avid enhancement of this mass (*white arrow*), which was histologically confirmed to be an endometrial carcinoma recurrence, for which the patient was dispositioned to pelvic exenteration.

TREATMENT

Standard-of-care first-line therapy for endometrial cancer is surgery, including hysterectomy and bilateral salpingo-oophorectomy (BSO). Peritoneal cytologic evaluation, although excluded from the FIGO staging system, can still be performed via peritoneal fluid present at the time of surgery or peritoneal washings. At times, the omentum is sampled if suspicious areas are detected intraoperatively. Carcinosarcoma is treated as high-grade endometrial carcinoma because of similar biology and clinical behavior.

The decision for lymph node dissection of the pelvic and paraaortic nodal groups superior and inferior to the inferior mesenteric artery is made at the time of surgery and is a controversial issue among different centers and geographic regions.[66] In the United States, when endometrial carcinoma is confined to the uterus, a limited staging procedure is performed, with pelvic and paraaortic lymphadenectomy.[66] Arguments for and against pelvic and paraaortic lymphadenectomy are described in the literature, with thorough lymph node dissection in patients with type II and selected patients with type I endometrial cancers.[4,67–70]

Chemotherapy for locally advanced or metastatic endometrial carcinoma usually consists of a protocol based on taxanes, platinum compounds, and anthracyclines used in combination (e.g., carboplatin/paclitaxel) rather than as single agents. In some instances, these are used in combination with radiation therapy. Hormonal therapy can be used if there are appropriate steroid hormone receptors in the tumor.

Radiation therapy is used to treat endometrial cancer in nonoperative candidates. Definitive radiation therapy with external beam radiation and/or brachytherapy is a reasonable primary treatment for endometrial cancer in patients who cannot undergo surgery. There is controversy in the literature with respect to the optimal modality, particularly in intermediate- to high-risk endometrial carcinomas, with respect to the radiotherapy regimen employed, which in part relates to patient selection, experience in grading, and depth of myometrial invasion of these neoplasms by various pathologists.[4,24–27,71–73]

Several trials and various treatment options that use cytotoxic and novel targeted agents are summarized in the literature.[4,67,74–76]

Key Points

Therapy

- Surgery represents first-line therapy for patients with endometrial cancer.
- Definitive radiotherapy with external beam radiation and/or brachytherapy is a primary treatment for endometrial cancer in patients who cannot undergo surgery.
- Chemotherapy and radiotherapy may be used for palliation; with newer targeted agents, a longer period of survival with less toxicity may be possible.

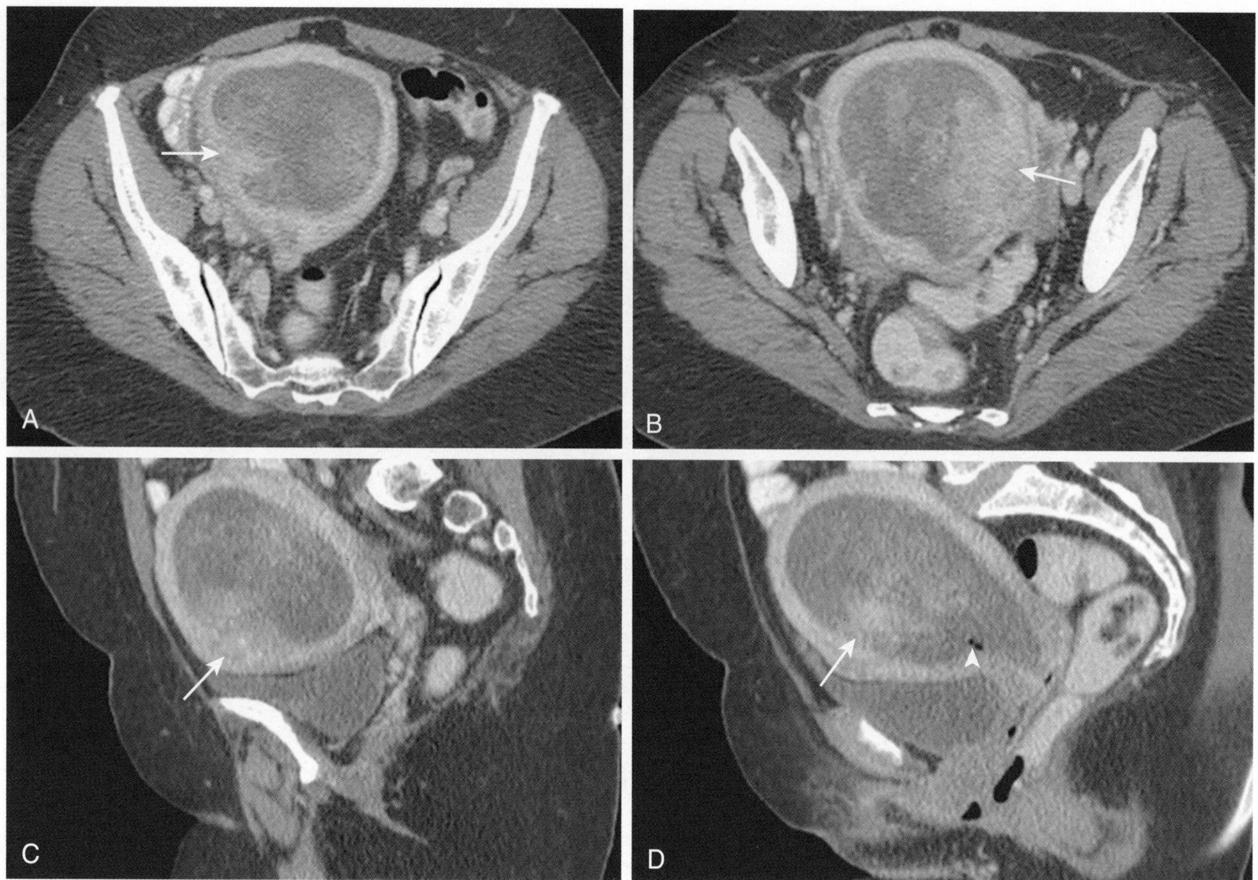

FIGURE 25.11. A 62-year-old woman with postmenopausal bleeding caused by carcinosarcoma. **A**, Contrast-enhanced computed tomography (CT) scan demonstrates extensive infiltrative enhancement (*white arrow*) along the right side of the endometrial cavity with surrounding hypoattenuation within a dilated endometrial cavity, suspicious for necrosis. **B**. Contrast-enhanced CT scan demonstrates an eccentric left-sided polypoid enhancing mass (*white arrow*) with surrounding hypoattenuation within the endometrial cavity, suspicious for necrosis. **C**, Sagittal CT reformat demonstrates anterior nodular enhancement along the myometrium (*white arrow*) with surrounding hypoattenuation within a dilated endometrial cavity. **D**, Sagittal CT reformat demonstrates a dilated uterine cavity and intraluminal mass (*white arrow*) associated with stippled foci of gas (*arrowhead*) from prior biopsy.

SURVEILLANCE, POSTTHERAPY COMPLICATIONS, AND RECURRENT DISEASE

Following surgery and appropriate staging, patients are followed closely for the first 2 to 3 years, evaluating for pain, weight loss, and vaginal bleeding, which are the most common symptoms alerting the attending physician to recurrence and/or metastatic disease. Imaging plays a role in determining the extent of recurrent or metastatic disease, usually by using CT, MRI, and PET/CT. Depending on the treatment given (fertility sparing vs. nonfertility sparing), CT or MRI can be performed every 6 months according to National Comprehensive Cancer Network guidelines.[77] Risks of recurrence are typically low, but are higher in patients with type II tumors, those with negative prognostic factors at the time of initial therapy, and those with advanced disease. CA-125 is a useful biomarker during the surveillance period to assess for recurrent disease. At one of our institutions (C.G., P.R.B., G.R., A.M., K.S., A.M.V.), CA-125 levels are assessed every 3 to 6 months for the first 2 years and annually thereafter in high-risk patients.

Potential complications may arise from the surgical procedure and postoperative recovery, such as ileus, fistulas, and wound infection. Toxicity from chemotherapy includes various grades of nausea, vomiting, and infection, as well as gastrointestinal, renal, hematologic, and neurotoxicity.

Complications from radiation therapy depend on the technique that is used: vaginal versus pelvic brachytherapy, extended field or whole abdominal radiation. Organs in the radiation fields will sustain damage based on the radiation dose, with the typical organs at risk including the sigmoid colon, rectum, and urinary bladder.

Postoperatively, patients are seen every 3 months for the first year, every 4 months for the second year, every 6 months for years 3 to 5, and then annually. A pelvic examination is performed at every visit. Also, a Pap test is done every 6 months for the first year and then annually. A chest x-ray is performed annually. Additional imaging is ordered as clinically indicated.

CT, MRI, and PET/CT are all commonly used to evaluate for recurrence. Prior published reports have described the median time to recurrence as 13 months. The most frequently observed sites of relapse are the pelvic lymph nodes, vagina, peritoneum, and lung.[78]

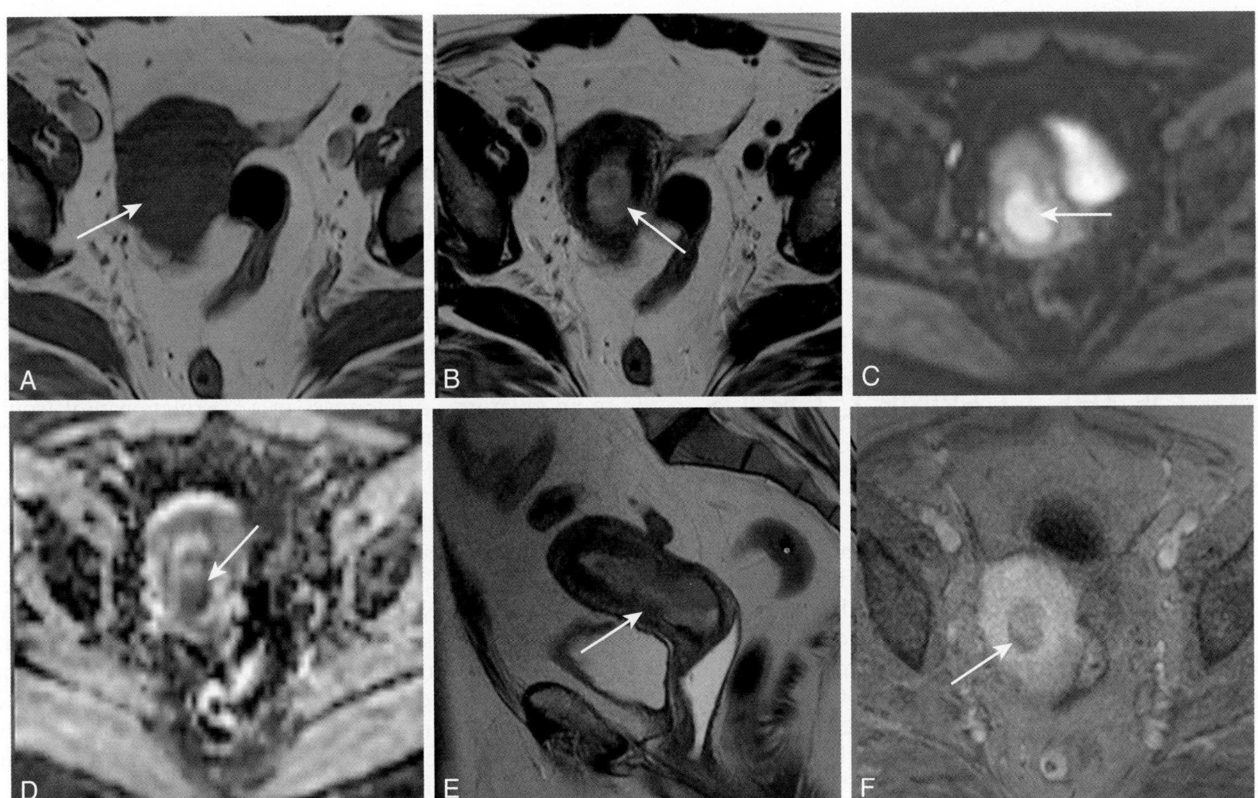

FIGURE 25.12. A 55-year-old woman with postmenopausal bleeding caused by carcinosarcoma. Axial T1-weighted (**A**) and axial T2-weighted (T2W) (**B**) magnetic resonance imaging (MRI) demonstrate a T1-isointense, T2-hyperintense mass (*white arrows*). Axial diffusion-weighted (DW) (**C**) and axial apparent diffusion coefficient (ADC) (**D**) images demonstrate the restricted diffusion of this mass (*white arrows*), associated with increased signal on DW images and reduced signal on the corresponding ADC images. **E**, Sagittal T2W images demonstrate the extent of tumor (*white arrow*) occupying the endometrial cavity and extending inferiorly to distend the cervical canal. **F**, Axial postcontrast fat-suppressed MRI demonstrates the relative hypoenhancement of this mass (*white arrow*), a nonspecific finding that can also be seen with conventional endometrial carcinomas.

KEY POINT

Surveillance, Posttherapy Complications, and Recurrent Disease

- Imaging plays a role in determining the extent of recurrent or metastatic disease, usually by using computed tomography (CT), magnetic resonance imaging, and positron emission tomography/CT.
- CA-125 is a useful biomarker during the surveillance period to assess for recurrent disease.

NEW THERAPIES

Advances have been made in our understanding of the molecular biology of endometrial cancer.[74–76,79] The molecular changes described for endometrial cancer include alteration of the tumor suppressor protein PTEN and associated pathways, microsatellite instability, *KRAS* mutations, *P53* mutations, and altered HER-2/neu expression. Subsets of these findings have been translated to clinical practice. For example, the addition of trastuzumab, a HER-2 inhibitor, to combined chemotherapy outperformed chemotherapy alone in HER-2–positive uterine serous carcinomas.[80] Lenvatinib, a kinase inhibitor targeting vascular endothelial growth factor (VEGF) receptor signaling, combined with the anti–PD-1 antibody pembrolizumab, has also been approved by the United States Food and Drug Administration for advanced recurrent endometrial cancer.[81] Other targeted therapies have been directed to mammalian target of rapamycin, human epithelial growth factor receptor, and VEGF. A comprehensive discussion of all available targeted therapies for malignancies of the uterine corpus is beyond the scope of this chapter.

CONCLUSION

Endometrial cancer is the most common malignancy of the uterine corpus. The most important risk factor for this cancer is age. Primary therapy for endometrial cancer is surgery. Definitive radiation is employed for nonsurgical candidates, and chemotherapy is used accordingly. Multidisciplinary team management for the evaluation and triage of these patients is recommended. There are ongoing controversies with respect to the use of upfront lymphadenectomy, radiation therapy technique, and chemotherapeutic regimens in selected populations. With improvements in the understanding of the biology of endometrial cancer, the development of targeted agents is expected to advance the field.

Imaging plays an integral role in diagnosis, staging, and surveillance of endometrial cancer patients, with MRI primarily being used for local staging and CT and PET/CT being used to detect distant metastatic disease. PET/MRI is a newer imaging modality that enables concomitant PET and whole-body MRI imaging, offering a one-stop comprehensive imaging modality for endometrial cancer.

II. Malignant Mesenchymal Tumors of the Uterine Corpus

INTRODUCTION

Uterine sarcomas are aggressive, and can be subdivided into pure homologous or mixed types. The pure homologous types include leiomyosarcoma (LMS) and endometrial stromal sarcoma (ESS). Adenosarcoma is the most common mixed-type tumor. Carcinosarcoma (malignant mixed Müllerian tumor) has, more recently, been reclassified as a carcinoma because it bears greater resemblance to high-grade endometrial carcinoma in pathology and clinical behavior. It is well known that uterine sarcomas have different biological underpinnings compared with conventional endometrial carcinoma, resulting in distinct, typically more aggressive, clinical profiles. However, the low incidence of these tumors (3% of all uterine cancers) can pose a challenge for patient management, as few randomized studies evaluating treatment options have been published.[2] In general, pathologic diagnosis dictates both therapeutic and prognostic implications for the patient and her attending physician. Prior studies in patients with uterine adenosarcoma, for example, have demonstrated that sarcomatous overgrowth of tumor and lymphovascular space invasion confer a higher risk of recurrence and worse PFS and OS. Although surgical management of these tumors does not require routine lymphadenectomy, as lymph node metastases are rare, recurrence can occur many years after initial diagnosis, warranting prolonged surveillance.[82]

EPIDEMIOLOGY AND RISK FACTORS

Certain risk factors, such as obesity, age, African American race, and parity, are associated with these uterine sarcomas.[2,83,84] Prior pelvic radiation is a weak risk factor for LMS.[85–87] An increased risk of uterine sarcoma has been identified with the use of tamoxifen.[88–90]

CLINICAL PRESENTATION

The most common presentation for women with uterine sarcomas is abnormal vaginal bleeding and a palpable pelvic mass. Other signs and symptoms include abdominal and/or pelvic pain or pressure and vaginal discharge, with some patients on examination having a mass protruding through the cervical os (Figs. 25.13 to 25.15). Rarely, these tumors are detected on a Pap smear. If the uterine sarcoma does not involve the endometrium, the endometrial biopsy may be unrevealing.

Although the clinical presentation of uterine sarcomas is somewhat similar, the pathology and pattern of spread vary with these neoplasms and are described separately.

The most common pure mesenchymal uterine sarcoma is LMS, which accounts for 30% of all uterine sarcomas and 1% to 2% of all uterine malignancies. It tends to present in women older than 40 years. Preoperatively, LMS is not usually suspected, because the surgeon presumes that the clinical pattern is that of benign leiomyoma discovered during the surgical exploration or at the time of pathologic review. However, malignancy should be suspected in an enlarging pelvic mass in a postmenopausal woman who is not on hormonal replacement therapy. Typically, LMS is a solitary intramural necrotic mass that is poorly circumscribed, has an infiltrating margin, and often does not project outside of the myometrium. These tumors classically have severe nuclear atypia, hypercellularity, and a high mitotic rate exceeding 15 mitotic figures per 10 high-power fields.[2] Nodal metastases are uncommon unless the LMS extends outside of the uterus, in which case the regional nodal basins and the paraaortic nodes may become involved. At times, LMS can have positive lymph nodes despite palpably normal lymph node tissue and lack of evidence of extrauterine spread.[2,91,92] LMS spreads hematogenously to the lungs, liver, brain, kidney, and bone.

The second most common type of pure malignant mesenchymal uterine tumors is ESS. These neoplasms have cells that resemble endometrial stromal cells of the proliferative endometrium. Currently, they are classified as endometrial stromal nodules, low-grade ESSs, and undifferentiated endometrial sarcomas. The latter used to be classified as high-grade ESS.[2] The term ESS is now restricted to low-grade ESS. The endometrial stromal nodule, the least common of the pure endometrial stromal tumors, is usually a solitary, well-circumscribed, expansile but not infiltrating tumor that has a smooth margin.[2] These tumors are cured by hysterectomy and have a good prognosis.

The ESSs constitute 10% to 15% of uterine malignancies with a mesenchymal component. These neoplasms are more common in the 40- to 55-year-old age group, with both high- and low-grade subtypes; 25% of these patients may be asymptomatic. These tumors have mild nuclear atypia, are usually not necrotic, have a low mitotic index (<5 mitotic figures per 10 high-power fields), have variable degrees of myometrial penetration and irregular margins, and tend to involve the parametrial veins and lymphatics.[2] Some of these neoplasms fill the uterine cavity and may extend into the cervical canal. Recurrences tend to develop in the abdomen and pelvis, and also in the lungs.[2,91,93,94] The undifferentiated endometrial sarcoma is very aggressive and has severe nuclear pleomorphism, a high degree of destructive myometrial invasion, necrosis, and high mitotic activity (>10 mitotic figures per high-power field). It typically lacks smooth muscle or endometrial differentiation.[2] This biologic behavior is associated with a propensity for local recurrence and distant metastasis.

The rarer adenosarcoma is a mixed tumor that tends to occur in postmenopausal women but has been reported in adolescents and young adults. These neoplasms are of a low malignant potential and arise from the endometrium.

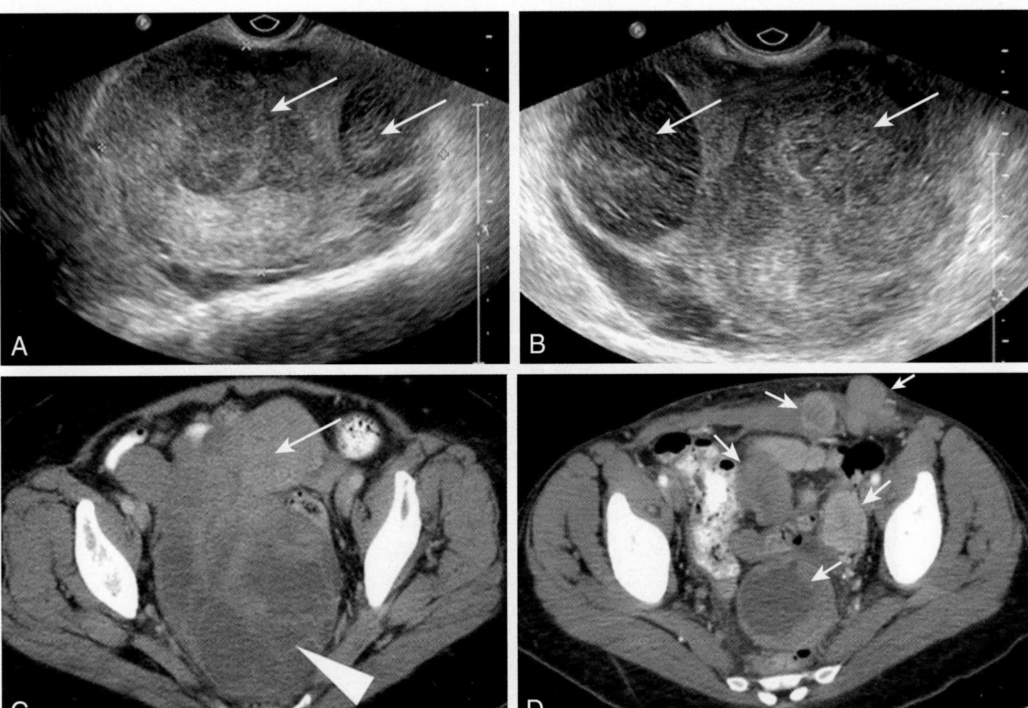

FIGURE 25.13. A 60-year-old woman presents with abdominal pain. Diagnosis: Uterine leiomyosarcoma. **A** and **B**, Sagittal images from a transabdominal pelvic ultrasound demonstrate a large lobulated uterus containing rounded hypoechoic and heterogenous masses (*white arrows*). The whole uterus cannot be seen in a single view. **C**, Axial view, contrast-enhanced computed tomography (CT) demonstrates multilobulated and heterogeneously enhancing tumor replacing the normal uterus, with areas of hyperenhancement (*white arrow*) and hypoenhancement (*white arrowhead*). **D**, Axial view, contrast-enhanced CT scan of pelvic nodal metastases, peritoneal implants, and intramuscular and subcutaneous anterior abdominal wall implants (*white arrows*).

This tumor can fill the uterine cavity and project through the cervical os. Adenosarcomas can have focal hemorrhage, necrosis, and cystic changes. They are a mixture of benign epithelium and low-grade sarcoma, usually of the endometrial stromal type.[2] Depending on the percentage of the sarcomatous component, the spread of disease is mainly to the pelvic lymph nodes, and recurrences tend to occur in the pelvis and vagina.[2,67,68]

KEY POINTS

Clinical Presentation

- Uterine sarcomas are aggressive, and can be subdivided into pure homologous or mixed types.
- The most common presentation is that of abnormal vaginal bleeding and a pelvic mass in a peri- or postmenopausal patient. These are typically large masses with foci of necrosis and hemorrhage.
- Spread of tumor depends on the tumor type.

STAGING EVALUATION

Compared with endometrial carcinomas, uterine sarcomas behave more aggressively and are associated with a poorer prognosis. The FIGO staging system for endometrial cancer was used for uterine sarcomas before 2009 (Table 25.2).[95,96] In 2009, FIGO released a staging system specific for uterine sarcomas. This system actually comprises two distinct staging systems: one for LMS and ESS (see Table 25.2), and another for adenosarcoma. Carcinosarcomas should be staged using the endometrial cancer staging system.

KEY POINT

Staging

- Staging of uterine sarcomas follows the 2010 International Federation of Gynecology and Obstetrics staging criteria (see Table 25.2).[8]

IMAGING

At the present time, there are no pathognomonic imaging features to distinguish uterine sarcomas. Clinical suspicion for a uterine sarcoma is raised in the setting of a rapidly enlarging mass in a peri- or postmenopausal woman who is not undergoing hormonal replacement therapy. Multiple imaging modalities are used initially and in follow-up to evaluate the status of these patients (see Figs. 25.8 to 25.11). Analogous to the imaging regimens for endometrial cancer, transvaginal ultrasound and pelvic MRI are used for primary tumor staging, with CT or PET/CT to evaluate mainly for metastatic disease.[97] Radionuclide bone scans may be used to evaluate for osseous metastatic disease.

On pelvic and transvaginal ultrasound, uterine sarcomas tend to be heterogeneous with mixed echogenicity and

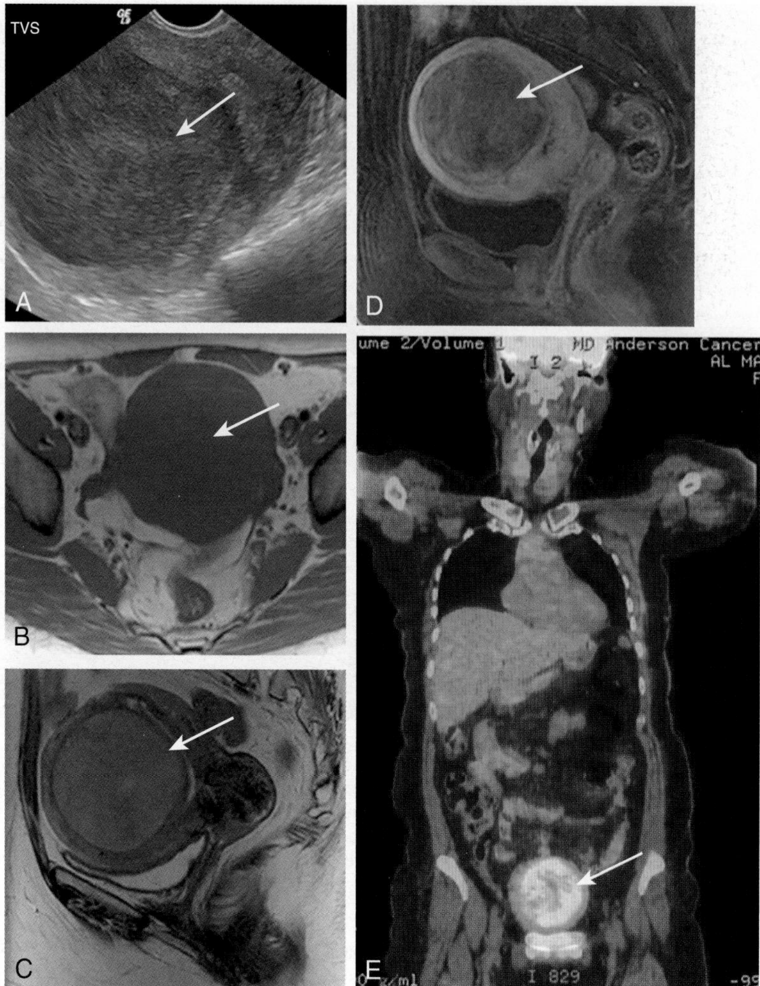

FIGURE 25.14. A 54-year-old woman presents with vaginal bleeding. Diagnosis: Endometrial stromal sarcoma. **A**, Transvaginal ultrasound demonstrates a solid, slightly hypoechoic, heterogeneous uterine mass (*white arrow*). **B**, Axial T1-weighted (T1W) magnetic resonance imaging (MRI) demonstrates an enlarged uterus of uniform hypointense signal. The location of the mass (*white arrow*) is indistinguishable from the adjacent junctional zone and myometrium. **C**, Sagittal T2-weighted MRI demonstrates a hyperintense mass within the endometrial cavity (*white arrow*). **D**, Sagittal postcontrast T1W fat-suppressed image demonstrates hypoenhancement of this mass (*white arrow*) relative to the myometrium. **E**, Coronal multiplanar reformation fused positron emission tomography/computed tomography image demonstrates hypermetabolic activity corresponding to the intrauterine mass (*white arrow*).

poorly defined margins, and can occupy the entire uterine cavity. The endometrial and myometrial junctions may not be well seen. If the uterine mass is very large, the sonographic FOV may not completely image the uterine mass, and penetration of the mass may be limited by the ultrasound frequency. The yield from vascular evaluation of these masses by color Doppler and power Doppler is mixed and nonspecific; for example, low impedance of tumoral vessels can be observed, but this may or may not aid in suggesting a malignant process.[91,98–101] Ultrasound imaging of LMS typically reveals a large heterogeneous mass of mixed echogenicity. The LMS may be large enough to exceed the FOV for the ultrasound transducers.

CT of uterine sarcomas cannot reliably differentiate between subtypes. Typical findings on CT include an enlarged uterus, heterogeneous enhancement, low-density areas of hemorrhage, and necrosis. CT is a useful imaging modality to evaluate for ascites, adenopathy, and distant metastatic disease, which are more commonly observed at presentation in these patients as compared with those with endometrial cancer.[102,103] Certain individual features have been described on CT for uterine sarcomas. LMS will present as a mass in an enlarged uterus that, on noncontrast imaging, may show areas of necrosis and/or hemorrhage. Following the administration of intravenous contrast, LMS has heterogeneous enhancement and is of lower attenuation than the normal uterine tissue. The absence of calcifications in a rapidly growing uterine mass can indicate the presence of an underlying LMS and distinguish this entity from typical leiomyomas.[104]

As is the case for endometrial cancer, MRI plays a central role in the primary staging of uterine sarcomas owing to its higher soft tissue contrast between endometrium and muscular layers of the uterine corpus and cervix. The use of intravenous contrast further enhances the delineation of disease. Pelvic MRI is used preoperatively to assess the uterine mass and to stage and evaluate for local tumor extent, deep myometrial and cervical stromal invasion, metastatic adenopathy, and pelvic metastatic disease to the regional nodes, soft tissues, and osseous structures. Following

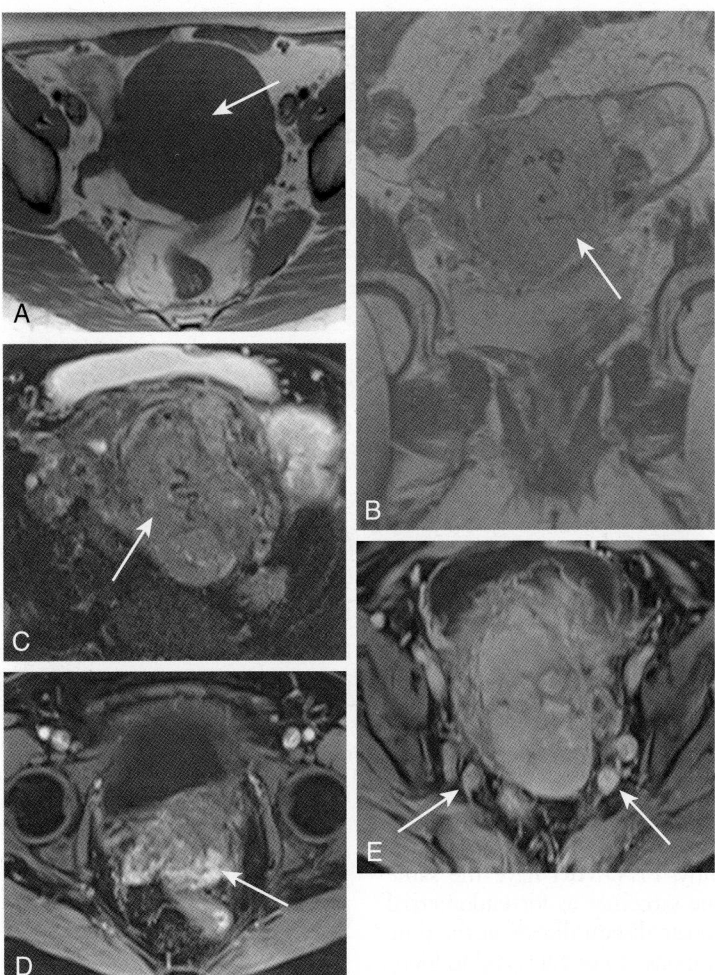

FIGURE 25.15. A 54-year-old female presents with left hip pain. Diagnosis: Undifferentiated endometrial sarcoma. Sagittal T2-weighted (T2W) magnetic resonance imaging (MRI) (**A**) and coronal T2W MRI (**B**) demonstrate a large, lobulated, T2-hyperintense mass (*white arrows* in **A** and **B**). **C**, Axial T2-weighted image redemonstrates the T2-hyperintense mass. Prominent intratumoral vessels appearing as punctate and serpiginous signal voids are seen throughout the mass. **D**, Postcontrast arterial phase images demonstrate areas of hyperenhancing tumor in the lower pelvis (*white arrow*). **E**, Axial postcontrast delayed phase images demonstrate confluent enhancing tumor in the midline pelvis, as well as metastatic bilateral internal iliac adenopathy (*paired white arrows*).

therapy, MRI can also be used in follow-up to assess disease recurrence and response to therapy. On T1W imaging, LMS tends to be of low or intermediate signal. The signal from the hemorrhagic foci depends on the age of the hemorrhage. In comparison with the signal from the normal myometrium, LMS tends to be of intermediate signal. Following the administration of intravenous contrast, there is heterogeneous enhancement, which can demonstrate both increased and reduced signal relative to the normal myometrium. Early hematogenous spread is common. MRI can be limited in distinguishing LMS from a degenerating fibroid, although marked growth in the setting of irregular margins and necrosis can be helpful. Features that have been described as distinguishing LMS from leiomyoma including nodular borders, hemorrhage, and central unenhanced area(s), which can also be helpful in assessment.[105] ESS can also appear as heterogeneous mass of variable signal intensity on both T1W and T2W pulse sequences. Of note, the endometrial stromal nodule can appear similar to normal endometrial stromal cells and mimic adenomyosis at MRI, appearing as an area of expanded low signal at the level of the junctional zone on MRI. Undifferentiated endometrial sarcoma is more likely to present with a polypoid mass that is increased in signal on T2W images, associated with hemorrhage and necrosis. Following contrast administration, these masses will demonstrate heterogeneous signal that is isointense to hyperintense relative to normal myometrium, with poor delineation between the tumor and myometrium, and with intratumoral bands of tissue typically present in the myometrium. Prominent neovessels are typically observed with undifferentiated endometrial sarcoma, as is contiguous tumor extension along vessels, ligaments, and the fallopian tubes, early lymphovascular invasion, and separate myometrial tumor deposits.[36,91,102,106,107] On MRI, adenosarcomas are heterogeneous enhancing masses associated with restricted diffusion and rapid contrast washin and washout on dynamic contrast-enhanced MRI, reflecting the low-resistance network of blood vessels supplying tumor. Polypoid components can be seen, along with potential myometrial invasion and cystic changes. The mass can protrude through the cervical os, a finding best delineated on sagittal T2W images.[108]

TABLE 25.2 International Federation of Gynecology and Obstetrics Surgical Staging Systems for Uterine Sarcomas (includes Leiomyosarcoma and Endometrial Stromal Sarcoma)

INTERNATIONAL FEDERATION OF GYNECOLOGY AND OBSTETRICS STAGES	DEFINITION
I	Tumor limited to the uterus
IA	Tumor ≤5 cm in greatest dimension
IB	Tumor >5 cm
II	Tumor extends beyond the uterus, within the pelvis
IIA	Tumor involves adnexa
IIB	Tumor involves other pelvic tissues
III[a]	Tumor infiltrates abdominal tissues
IIIA	One site
IIIB	More than one site
IVA	Tumor invades bladder or rectum
	Regional lymph nodes cannot be assessed
	No regional lymph node metastasis
IIIC	Regional lymph node metastasis
	No distant metastasis
IVB	Distant metastasis (excluding adnexa, pelvic, and abdominal tissues)

Carcinosarcomas should be staged as carcinomas of the endometrium (see Table 25.1).
[a]For stage III disease, lesions must infiltrate abdominal tissues and not just protrude into the abdominal cavity.
From D'Angelo E, Prat J. Uterine sarcomas: a review. *Int J Gynaecol Obstet.* 2010;116:131–139. Copyright 2010, with permission from International Federation of Gynecology and Obstetrics.

PET/CT and, more recently, PET/MRI have the same clinical applicability for uterine sarcomas as for endometrial cancers in their ability to delineate distant disease at the time of primary staging, to assess response to therapy, and to identify areas of recurrence. However, very few PET or PET/CT studies have been published involving uterine sarcomas.[53,54,109]

METASTATIC DISEASE

Metastatic disease to the uterus is rare, but has been reported from various extragenital cancers, including primary tumors of the breast, stomach, colon, and lung.[110,111] Metastases will alter the shape and size of the organ, with heterogeneity of the involved myometrium. MRI is the primary modality to delineate suspected metastases to the uterus. CT and PET/CT can also be considered when concomitant extrauterine metastatic disease is suspected.

KEY POINTS

Imaging

- No pathognomonic imaging features can distinguish uterine sarcomas, although many imaging findings, including diffuse uterine tumor involvement, hemorrhage, and necrosis, can raise suspicion for these aggressive entities.
- Similar to endometrial cancer, the best imaging modality for primary tumor staging is magnetic resonance imaging (MRI).
- Computed tomography (CT), positron emission tomography (PET)/CT, and, more recently, PET/MRI can be used for the evaluation of distant disease, recurrent disease, and, in appropriate cases, response to therapy.

TREATMENT

Leiomyosarcoma

LMSs are very aggressive tumors with recurrence rates of 53% to 71% even if diagnosed at an early stage.[112,113] Standard treatment includes hysterectomy and tumor debulking if disease is present outside of the uterus. In women with LMS, the rate of lymph node involvement in the absence of visible extrauterine disease has been shown to be low, and lymphadenectomy is therefore not recommended.[15–17] Removal of the ovaries is controversial. In a large retrospective study of 1396 women with LMS, a subset analysis was performed on 341 women younger than 50 years with stage I and II disease, and no differences in survival were found between the women who underwent BSO and those who did not.[95] Ovarian preservation is, therefore, acceptable in premenopausal women with early-stage LMS.

Observation after surgical resection is believed to be reasonable in patients with LMS confined to the uterus.[114] However, adjuvant therapy is often considered. Although postoperative radiation therapy may reduce the rate of local recurrence, improvement in survival has not been demonstrated.[91,115–118] Given these findings, as well as the propensity of LMS to relapse distantly, adjuvant radiation therapy is generally not recommended. However, adjuvant chemotherapy is commonly used for women with LMS, with docetaxel and gemcitabine being the preferred combination.[91]

In patients with locally recurrent LMS, reresection or radiation therapy is sometimes used. If metastatic disease or multiple sites of recurrence are noted, systemic therapy with chemotherapy or hormonal therapy is used.

Metastasectomy or local radiation for metastasis can be beneficial for certain patients.[119–121] Response rates of 15% to 42% have been reported using the combination of docetaxel and gemcitabine for metastatic LMS in both the first-line and the second-line setting.[122,123] In addition, hormonal therapy may be beneficial in women with recurrent or metastatic LMS. Approximately 50% to 60% of patients have tumors that express hormone receptors.[124,125] Responses have been described in these patients using agents such as aromatase inhibitors and mifepristone.[126,127]

Endometrial Stromal Sarcomas

ESSs are less aggressive tumors with a more favorable prognosis than LMS.[93] Standard treatment is primarily surgical and includes hysterectomy with BSO, because these tumors are often hormonally sensitive. Whether or not to perform lymphadenectomy in patients with ESS is controversial. The incidence of nodal involvement in ESSs has been reported to range from 0% to 33%.[128–131] However, these studies have not shown a survival benefit associated with lymphadenectomy, and it therefore remains unclear whether it should be performed in women with ESS.

Given the favorable prognosis and long remissions associated with ESS, observation is generally recommended for early-stage disease after surgery. Adjuvant radiation therapy and cytotoxic chemotherapy are not usually used. However, most ESS tumors express estrogen receptor (ER) and progesterone receptor (PR), so hormonal therapy may be considered.[132–134] Agents used include progestins, gonadotropin-releasing hormone (GnRH) analogs, and aromatase inhibitors.[131,134–137] There is no consensus regarding which patients with ESS should be treated with hormonal therapy and/or which agents should be used. In general, it is recommended that aromatase inhibitors or progestins should be used in patients who are postmenopausal or who have undergone BSO and whose tumors express ER and PR. In premenopausal women with retained ovaries, adjuvant treatment with GnRH analogs is recommended.[138] Treatment should be continued for 5 years. Given the high level of hormone sensitivity of ESS tumors, estrogen therapy and tamoxifen should be avoided in these patients, because they may increase the risk of recurrence.[139–141]

In patients with recurrent or metastatic ESSs, surgical resection is considered for isolated areas of disease. Disseminated or residual disease is typically treated with hormonal therapy, with chemotherapy reserved for patients who progress on hormonal therapy or those with undifferentiated endometrial sarcoma. [142]

Undifferentiated Endometrial Sarcoma

Because undifferentiated endometrial sarcomas were previously classified as high-grade ESSs and combined with low-grade ESSs, there is limited literature specifically addressing the treatment of these tumors. They are highly aggressive malignancies with a very poor prognosis. The treatment is primarily surgical, but, because of the high risk of recurrence, adjuvant treatment with radiation and/or chemotherapy is usually given. There is no consensus on chemotherapy regimens for adjuvant or palliative treatment, but carboplatinum and paclitaxel are frequently used.

Adenosarcoma

Adenosarcomas generally have a favorable prognosis, except when associated with myometrial invasion or sarcomatous overgrowth. Standard treatment consists of surgery with hysterectomy and BSO, because the tumors are usually localized. Adjuvant treatment with radiation therapy and/or chemotherapy is considered in patients with myometrial invasion or sarcomatous overgrowth.

> **Key Points**
>
> **Treatment**
> - Treatment recommendations vary by histologic type.
> - These tumors are aggressive and associated with a poor prognosis.
> - The staging of these tumors is based on the International Federation of Gynecology and Obstetrics staging system.

PROGNOSIS

In general, uterine sarcomas have a much poorer prognosis compared with other gynecologic malignancies. The most important prognostic factor for each type of uterine sarcoma is stage. Additional factors associated with poor prognosis include high histologic grade, suboptimal tumor reduction, lymphatic and/or vascular space invasion, and high mitotic count.[95,143] Although survival differences have been difficult to demonstrate between histologic types, owing to the low incidence of these cancers, ESSs and adenosarcomas have been observed to have a better prognosis and LMS tumors a worse prognosis compared with other uterine sarcomas.

> **Key Points**
>
> **Prognosis**
> - When compared with the other gynecologic malignancies, uterine sarcomas have a much poorer prognosis.
> - Stage is the most important prognostic factor.

SURVEILLANCE

Patients with uterine sarcomas are followed with physical examination and CT every 3 to 6 months for 3 years, and every 6 to 12 months thereafter.[144] Subsequent and/or additional with CT, MRI, or PET/CT is performed as clinically indicated. Patients are educated regarding symptoms associated with recurrence. In women with ESS and adenosarcoma, prolonged follow-up is warranted owing to the propensity for long disease-free intervals and late recurrences.

KEY POINTS

Surveillance

- Physical examination and computed tomography (CT), initially every 3 to 6 months for 3 years and every 6 to 12 months thereafter or as indicated.
- Other imaging modalities as clinically indicated.
- Complications of therapy are evaluated clinically, typically with CT.

NEW THERAPIES

A subset of targeted agents have been approved to treat uterine sarcoma in the past decade. Pazopanib, a multitargeted tyrosine kinase inhibitor, is used to treat uterine sarcoma patients who have failed first-line chemotherapy.[145] Trabectedin combined with doxorubicin has shown promise as first-line treatment for advanced uterine LMS in a phase 2 trial.[146] Eribulin has also demonstrated superior efficacy compared with dacarbazine in advanced or metastatic uterine sarcomas.[147] Immune checkpoint blockade has revolutionized cancer treatment in the last decade, and the era of using immune checkpoint blockade to treat gynecological cancer has recently started. Unfortunately, initial attempts employing anti–PD-1 antibodies in uterine sarcoma patients have not demonstrated promising results.[148,149] Nevertheless, ongoing trials are testing the efficacy and safety of combination therapy with anti–PD-1, radiation, and immunomodulatory agents for uterine sarcoma.[150]

CONCLUSION

Uterine sarcomas are rare and aggressive and carry a poor prognosis. These tumors are of the pure homologous or mixed type. Peri- or postmenopausal women generally present with abnormal uterine bleeding and a pelvic mass. Because of the rarity of these tumors, few randomized trials are available to aid in the standardization of their management. Treatment is based on the histologic type, and the most important clinical factor is the stage at presentation. No pathognomonic imaging features are available to definitively distinguish these entities. MRI is the imaging modality of choice for local staging of these tumors, with CT and PET/CT used for the assessment of distant disease.

REFERENCES

1. American Cancer Society *Cancer Facts & Figures 2019*. Atlanta: American Cancer Society; 2019.
2. D'Angelo E, Prat J. Uterine sarcomas: a review. *Gynecol Oncol*. 2010;116:131–139.
3. Creaseman W, Odicino F, Maisonneuve P, et al. Carcinoma of the corpus uteri. *Int J Gynecol Oncol*. 2006;95(Suppl 1):S105–S143.
4. Amant F, Moerman P, Neven P, et al. Endometrial cancer. *Lancet*. 2005;366:491–505.
5. Trimble EL, Harlan LC, Clegg LX, et al. Pre-operative imaging, surgery and adjuvant therapy for women diagnosed with cancer of the corpus uteri in community practice in the United States. *Gynecol Oncol*. 2005;96:741–748.
6. Hill HA, Coates RJ, Austin H, et al. Racial differences in tumor grade among women with endometrial cancer. *Gynecol Oncol*. 1995;56:154–163.
7. Cote ML, Ruterbusch JJ, Olson SH, et al. The Growing Burden of Endometrial Cancer: A Major Racial Disparity Affecting Black Women. *Cancer Epidemiol Biomarkers Prev*. 2015;24:1407–1415.
8. Mayer LA, Broaddus RR, Lu KH. Endometrial cancer and Lynch syndrome: clinical and pathologic considerations. *Cancer Control*. 2009;16:14–22.
9. Watson P, Lynch H. Extracolonic cancer in hereditary nonpolyposis colorectal cancer. *Cancer*. 1993;71:677–685.
10. Aarnio M, Mecklin JP, Aaltonen LA, et al. Life-time risk of different cancers in hereditary non-polyposis CRC (LS) syndrome. *Int J Cancer*. 1995;64:430–433.
11. Ellis H. Anatomy of the uterus. *Anaesthesia and Intensive Care Medicine*. 2005;6(3):74–75.
12. Suh GK, Hennessy BT, Markman M. Chapter 29. Tumors of the Uterine Corpus. In: Kantarjian HM, Wolff RA, Koller CA, eds. *The MD Anderson Manual of Medical Oncology*. 2nd ed. New York: McGraw-Hill; 2011.
13. McCluggage WG. Uterine sarcomas (malignant mixed müllerian tumors) are metaplastic carcinomas. *J Gynecol Cancer*. 2002;10:687–690.
14. Kernochan LE, Garcia RL. Carcinosarcomas (malignant mixed müllerian tumor) of the uterus: advances in elucidation of biologic and clinical characteristics. *J Natl Cancer Compr Netw*. 2009;7:550–557.
15. Brooks SE, Zhan M, Cote T, et al. Survival epidemiology and end results analysis of 267 cases of uterine sarcomas, 1989-1999. *Gynecol Oncol*. 2004;93:204–208.
16. Silverberg SG, Major FJ, Blessing JA, et al. Carcinosarcoma (malignant mixed mesodermal tumor) of the uterus. A Gynecologic Oncology Group pathologic study of 203 cases. *Int J Gynecol Pathol*. 1990;9:1–19.
17. Doss LL, Llorenas AS, Henriquez EM. Carcinosarcoma of the uterus: a 40-year experience from the state of Missouri. *Gynecol Oncol*. 1984;18:43–53.
18. Yamada DS, Burger RA, Brewster WR, et al. Pathologic variables and survival for patients with surgically evaluated carcinosarcoma of the uterus. *Cancer*. 2000;88:2782–2786.
19. Murali R, Soslow RA, Weigelt B. Classification of endometrial carcinoma: More than two types. *Lancet Oncol*. 2014;15:e268–e278.
20. Chlebowski RT, Schottinger JE, Shi J, et al. Aromatase inhibitors, tamoxifen, and endometrial cancer in breast cancer survivors. *Cancer*. 2015;121:2147–2155.
21. Ascher SM, Reinhold C. Imaging of cancer of the endometrium. *Radiol Clin N Am*. 2002;40:563–576.
22. Patel S, Liyanage SH, Sahdev A, et al. Imaging of endometrial and cervical cancer. *Insights Imaging*. 2010;1(5-6):309–328.
23. Sorosky JI. Endometrial cancer. *Obstet Gynecol*. 2012;120:383–397.
24. Chen SS, Lee L. Retroperitoneal lymph node metastases in Stage I carcinoma of the endometrium: correlation with risk factors. *Gynecol Oncol*. 1985;16:319–325.
25. DiSaia PF, Creasmean WT, Boronow RC, et al. Risk factors and recurrent patterns in stage I endometrial cancer. *Am J Obstet Gynecol*. 1985;151:1009–1115.
26. Figge DC, Otto PM, Tamini HK, et al. Treatment variables in the management of endometrial cancer. *Am J Obstet Gynecol*. 1983;146:495–500.
27. Piver MS, Lele SB, Barlow JJ, et al. Paraaortic lymph node evaluation in stage I endometrial carcinoma. *Obstet Gynecol*. 1982;59:97–100.
28. Amin MB, Edge S, Greene F, et al. *AJCC Cancer Staging Manual*. 8th ed. New York: Springer; 2017.
29. Pandharipande PV, Choy G, del Carmen MG, et al. MRI and PET/CT for triaging stage ib clinically operable cervical cancer to appropriate therapy: Decision analysis to assess patient outcomes. *Am J Roentgenol*. 2009;192:802–814.
30. Smith-Bindman R, Kerlikowske K, Feldstein VA, et al. Endovaginal ultrasound to exclude endometrial cancer and other endometrial abnormalities. *JAMA*. 1998;280:1510–1517.
31. Alcazar JL, Orozco R, Martinez-Astorquiza CT, et al. Transvaginal ultrasound for preoperative assessment of myometrial invasion in patients with endometrial cancer: a systematic review and meta-analysis. *Ultrasound Obstet Gynecol*. 2015;46:405–413.
32. Fotopoulou C, Sehouli J, Schefold JC, et al. Preoperative transvaginal ultrasound (TVS) in the description of pelvic tumor spread in endometrial cancer: Results of a prospective study. *Anticancer Res*. 2008;28:2453–2458.

33. Lane BF, Wong YC, Jade J. Imaging of endometrial pathology. *Clin Obstet Gynecol*. 2009;52:57–72.
34. Frei KA, Kinkel K, Bonél HM, et al. Prediction of deep myometrial invasion in patients with endometrial cancer: clinical utility of contrast-enhanced MR imaging-a meta-analysis and Bayesian analysis. *Radiology*. 2000;216(2):444–449.
35. Kinkel K, Forstner R, Danza FM, et al. Staging of endometrial cancer with MRI: guidelines of the European Society of Urogenital Imaging. *Eur Radiol*. 2009;19(7):1565–1574.
36. Whitten CR, DeSouza NM. Magnetic resonance imaging of uterine malignancies. *Top Magn Reson Imaging*. 2006;17:365–377.
37. Peungjesada S, Bhosale PR, Balachandran A, et al. Magnetic resonance imaging of endometrial carcinoma. *J Comput Assist Tomogr*. 2009;33:601–608.
38. Meissnitzer M, Forstner R. MRI of endometrium cancer-how we do it. *Cancer Imaging*. 2016;16:1–9.
39. Barwick TD, Rockall AG, Barton DP, et al. Imaging of endometrial carcinoma. *Clin Radiol*. 2006;61:545–555.
40. Larson DM, Connor GP, Broste SK, et al. Prognostic significance of gross myometrial invasion with endometrial cancer. *Obstet Gynecol*. 1996;88(3):394–398.
41. Yamashita Y, Harada M, Sawada T, et al. Normal uterus and FIGO stage I endometrial carcinoma: dynamic gadolinium-enhanced MR imaging. *Radiology*. 1993;186:495–501.
42. Manfredi R, Mirk P, Maresca G, et al. Local-regional staging of endometrial carcinoma: role of MR imaging in surgical planning. *Radiology*. 2004;231:372–378.
43. Ito K, Matsumoto T, Nakada T, et al. Assessing myometrial invasion by endometrial carcinoma with dynamic MRI. *J Comput Assist Tomogr*. 1994;18:77–86.
44. Joja I, Asakawa M, Asakawa T, et al. Endometrial carcinoma: dynamic MRI with turbo-FLASH technique. *J Comput Assist Tomogr*. 1996;20:878–887.
45. Seki H, Kimura M, Sakai K. Myometrial invasion of endometrial carcinoma: assessment with dynamic MR and contrast-enhanced T1-weighted images. *Clin Radiol*. 1997;52:18–23.
46. Kim SH, Kim HD, Song YS, et al. Detection of deep myometrial invasion in endometrial carcinoma: comparison of transvaginal ultrasound, CT, and MRI. *J Comput Assist Tomogr*. 1995;19:766–772.
47. Hricak H, Stern JL, Fisher MR, et al. Endometrial carcinoma staging by MR imaging. *Radiology*. 1987;162:297–305.
48. Hricak H, Rubinstein LV, Gherman GM, et al. MR imaging evaluation of endometrial carcinoma: results of an NCI cooperative study. *Radiology*. 1991;179:829–832.
49. Boronow RC, Morrow CP, Creasman WT, et al. Surgical staging in endometrial cancer: clinical-pathologic findings of a prospective study. *Obstet Gynecol*. 1984;63:825–832.
50. Sironi S, De Cobelli F, Scarfone G, et al. Carcinoma of the cervix: value of plain and gadolinium-enhanced MR imaging in assessing degree of invasiveness. *Radiology*. 1993;188:797–801.
51. Jujii S, Matsusue E, Kigawa J, et al. Diagnostic accuracy of the apparent diffusion coefficient in differentiating benign from malignant uterine endometrial cavity lesions. *Eur Radiol*. 2008;18:18–23.
52. Whittaker CS, Coady A, Culver L, et al. Diffusion-weighted MR imaging of female pelvic tumors: a pictorial review. *Radiographics*. 2009;29:759–774.
53. Lai CH, Yen TC, Chang TC. Positron emission tomography imaging for gynecologic malignancy. *Curr Opin Obstet Gynecol*. 2007;19:37–41.
54. De Gaetano AM, Calcagni ML, Rufini V, et al. Imaging of gynecologic malignancies with FDG PET-CT: case examples, physiologic activity, and pitfalls. *Abdom Imaging*. 2009;34:696–711.
55. Hardesty LA, Sumkin JH, Hakim C, et al. The ability of helical CT to preoperatively stage endometrial carcinoma. *Am J Roentgenol*. 2001;176:603–606.
56. Musto A, Grassetto G, Marzola MC, et al. Role of 18F-FDG PET/CT in the carcinoma of the uterus: a review of literature. *Yonsei Med J*. 2014;55:1467–1472.
57. Nakamura K, Hongo A, Kodama J, et al. The measurement of SUVmax of the primary tumor is predictive of prognosis for patients with endometrial cancer. *Gynecol Oncol*. 2011;123:82–87.
58. Nakamura K, Joja I, Fukushima C, et al. The preoperative SUVmax is superior to ADCmin of the primary tumour as a predictor of disease recurrence and survival in patients with endometrial cancer. *Eur J Nucl Med Mol Imaging*. 2013;40:52–60.
59. Stewart KI, Chasen B, Erwin W, et al. Preoperative PET/CT does not accurately detect extrauterine disease in patients with newly diagnosed high-risk endometrial cancer: A prospective study. *Cancer*. 2015;125:3347–3353.
60. Kitajima K, Murakami K, Yamasaki E, et al. Accuracy of 18F-FDG PET/CT in detecting pelvic and paraaortic lymph node metastasis in patients with endometrial cancer. *Am J Roentgenol*. 2008;190:1652–1658.
61. Shih IL, Shih TTF. PET/MRI hybrid imaging of cervical and endometrial cancer. *J Cancer Res Pract*. 2018;5:91–98.
62. Grueneisen J, Schaarschmidt BM, Beiderwellen K, et al. Diagnostic value of diffusion-weighted imaging in simultaneous 18F-FDG PET/MR imaging for whole-body staging of women with pelvic malignancies. *J Nucl Med*. 2014;55:1930–1935.
63. Grueneisen J, Schaarschmidt BM, Heubner M, et al. Implementation of FAST-PET/MRI for whole-body staging of female patients with recurrent pelvic malignancies: a comparison to PET/CT. *Eur J Radiol*. 2015;84:2097–2102.
64. Sawicki LM, Kirchner J, Grueneisen J, et al. Comparison of 18F-FDG PET/MRI and MRI alone for whole-body staging and potential impact on therapeutic management of women with suspected recurrent pelvic cancer: a follow-up study. *Eur J Nucl Med Mol Imag*. 2018;45:622–629.
65. Shih IL, Yen RF, Chen CA, et al. Standardized uptake value and apparent diffusion coefficient of endometrial cancer evaluated with integrated whole-body PET/MR: correlation with pathological prognostic factors. *J Magn Reson Imaging*. 2015;42:1723–1732.
66. Frost JA, Webster KE, Bryant A, et al. Lymphadenectomy for the management of endometrial cancer. *Cochrane Database Syst Rev*. 2017;10:CD007585.
67. Masciullo V, Amadio G, Lo Russo D, et al. Controversies in the management of endometrial cancer. *Obstet Gynceol Int.*. 2010:638165.
68. Pacini PB, Basile S, Maneschi F, et al. Systematic pelvic lymphadenectomy in early-stage endometrial carcinoma: randomized clinical trial. *J Natl Cancer Inst*. 2008;100:1707–1716.
69. Lu KH. Management of early-stage endometrial cancer. *Semin Oncol*. 2009;36:137–144.
70. Bassarak N, Blankestein T, Bruning A, et al. Is lymphadenectomy a prognostic marker in endometrioid adenocarcinoma of the human endometrium? *BMC Cancer*. 2010;10:224–236.
71. Nout RA, van de Poll-Franse LV, Lybeert MLM, et al. Long-term outcome and quality of life of patients with endometrial carcinoma treated with or without pelvic radiotherapy in the post operative radiation therapy in endometrial carcinoma 1 (PORTEC-1) trial. *J Clin Oncol*. 2011;29:1692–1700.
72. Wortman BG, Creutzberg CL, Putter H, et al. Ten-year results of the PORTEC-2 trial for high-intermediate risk endometrial carcinoma: improving patient selection for adjuvant therapy. *Br J Cancer*. 2018;119:1067–1074.
73. de Boer SM, Powell ME, Mileshkin L, et al. Adjuvant chemoradiotherapy versus radiotherapy alone for women with high-risk endometrial cancer (PORTEC-3):final results of an international, open-label, multicentre, randomised, phase 3 trial. *Lancet Oncol*. 2018;19:295–309.
74. Dellinger TH, Monk BJ. Systematic therapy for recurrent endometrial cancer: a review of North American trials. *Expert Rev Anticancer Ther*. 2009;9:905–916.
75. Dizon DS. Treatment options for advanced endometrial carcinoma. *Gynecol Oncol*. 2010;117:373–381.
76. Makker V, Green AK, Wenham RM, et al. New therapies for advanced, recurrent and metastatic endometrial cancers. *Gynecol Oncol Res Pract*. 2017;4:19.
77. National Comprehensive Cancer Network. Bone Cancer (Version 4.2021). http://www.nccn.org/professionals/physician_gls/pdf/uterine.pdf. Accessed Oct 15, 2021.
78. Sohaib SA, Houghton SL, Meroni R, et al. Recurrent endometrial cancer: patterns of recurrent disease and assessment of prognosis. *Clin Radiol*. 2007;62:28–34.
79. Bansal N, Yendluri V, Wenham RM. The molecular biology of endometrial cancers and the implications for pathogenesis, classification, and targeted therapies. *Cancer Control*. 2009;16:8–13.
80. Fader AN, Roque DM, Siegel E, et al. Randomized phase II trial of carboplatin-paclitaxel versus carboplatin-paclitaxel-trastuzumab in uterine serous carcinomas that overexpress human epidermal growth factor receptor 2/neu. *J Clin Oncol*. 2018;36:2044–2051.

81. Makker V, Rasco D, Vogelzang NJ, et al. Lenvatinib plus pembrolizumab in patients with advanced endometrial cancer: an interim analysis of a multicentre, open-label, single-arm, phase 2 trial. *Lancet Oncol*. 2019;20:711–718.
82. Carroll A, Ramirez PT, Westin SN, et al. Uterine adenosarcoma: An analysis on management, outcomes, and risk factors for recurrence. *Gynecol Oncol*. 2014;135:455–461.
83. Albrektsen G, Heuch I, Wik E, et al. Prognostic impact of parity in 493 uterine sarcoma patients. *Int J Gynecol Cancer*. 2009;19:1062–1067.
84. Sherman ME, Devesa SS. Analysis of racial differences in incidence, survival, and mortality for malignant tumors of the uterine corpus. *Cancer*. 2003;98:176–186.
85. Varela-Duran J, Nochomovitz LE, Prem KA, et al. Post irradiation mixed Müllerian tumors of the uterus. *Cancer.*. 1980;45:1625–1631.
86. Meredith RJ, Eisert DR, Kaka Z, et al. An excess of uterine sarcomas after pelvic irradiation. *Cancer.*. 1986;58:2003–2007.
87. Giuntoli RL, Metzinger DS, DiMarco CS, et al. Retrospective review of 208 patients with leiomyosarcoma of the uterus: prognostic indicators, surgical management, and adjuvant therapy. *Gynecol Oncol*. 2003;89:460–469.
88. Treilleux T, Mignotte H, Clement-Chassagne C, et al. Tamoxifen and malignant epithelial-nonepithelial tumors of the endometrium: report of six cases and review of the literature. *Eur Surg Oncol*. 1999;25:477–482.
89. McCluggage WG, Abdulkader M, Price JH, et al. Uterine carcinosarcomas in patients receiving tamoxifen: a report of 19 cases. *Int J Gynecol Cancer*. 2000;10:280–284.
90. Wickerham DL, Fisher B, Wolmark N, et al. Association of tamoxifen and uterine sarcoma. *J Clin Oncol*. 2002;20:2758–2760.
91. Amant F, Coosemans A, Debiec-Rychter M, et al. Clinical management of uterine sarcomas. *Lancet Oncol*. 2009;10:1188–1198.
92. Leitao M, Sonoda Y, Brennan M, et al. Incidence of lymph node and ovarian metastases in leiomyosarcoma of the uterus. *Gynecol Oncol*. 2003;91:209–212.
93. Dionigi A, Oliva E, Clement PB, et al. Endometrial stromal nodules and endometrial stromal tumors with limited infiltration: a clinicopathologic study of 50 cases. *Am J Surg Pathol*. 2002;26:567–581.
94. Chang KL, Crabtree GS, Kim Lim-Tan S, et al. Primary uterine endometrial stromal neoplasms: a clinicopathologic study of 117 cases. *Am J Surg Pathol*. 1990;14:415–438.
95. Kapp DS, Shin JY, Chan JK. Prognostic factors and survival in 1396 patients with uterine leiomyosarcomas: emphasis on impact of lymphadenectomy and oophorectomy. *Cancer.*. 2008;112:820–830.
96. Brooks SE, Zhan M, Cote T, et al. Surveillance, epidemiology, and end results analysis of 2677 cases of uterine sarcoma 1989-1999. *Gynecol Oncol*. 2004;93:204–208.
97. Haldorsen IS, Salvesen HB. What is the best preoperative imaging for endometrial cancer? *Curr Oncol Rep*. 2016;18:25.
98. Clement PB, Scully RE. Mullerian adenosarcoma of the uterus: a clinicopathologic analysis of 100 cases with a review of the literature. *Hum Path.*. 1990;21:363–381.
99. Kim JA, Lee MS, Choi JS. Sonographic findings of uterine endometrial stromal sarcoma. *Korean J Radiol*. 2006;7:281–286.
100. Chen CD, Huang CC, Wu CC, et al. Sonographic characteristics in low-grade endometrial stromal sarcoma: report of two cases. *J Ultrasound Med*. 1995;14:165–168.
101. Gandolfo N, Gandolfo NG, Serafini G, et al. Endometrial stromal sarcoma of the uterus: MR and US findings. *Eur Radiol*. 2000;10:776–779.
102. Rha SE, Byun JY, Jung SE, et al. CT and MRI of uterine sarcomas and their mimickers. *Am J Roentgenol.*. 2003;181:1369–1374.
103. Smith T, Moy L, Runowicz C. Müllerian mixed tumors: CT characteristics with clinical and pathologic observations. *Am J Roentgenol.*. 1997;169:531–535.
104. Van den Bosch T, Coosemans A, Morina M, et al. Screening for uterine tumours. *Best Pract Res Clin Obstet Gynaecol*. 2012;26:257–266.
105. Lakhman Y, Veeraraghavan H, Chaim J, et al. Differentiation of uterine leiomyosarcoma from atypical leiomyoma: diagnostic accuracy of qualitative MR imaging features and feasibility of texture analysis. *Eur Radiol.*. 2017;27(7):2903–2915.
106. Sala E, Wakely S, Senior E, et al. MRI of malignant neoplasms of the uterine corpus and cervix. *Am J Roentgenol.*. 2007;188:1577–1587.
107. Ueda M, Otsuka M, Hatakenaka S, et al. MR imaging findings of uterine endometrial stromal sarcoma: differentiation from endometrial carcinoma. *Eur Radiol.*. 2001;11:28–33.
108. Lee HK, Kim SH, Cho JY, et al. Uterine adenofibroma and adenosarcoma: CT and MR findings. *J Comput Assist Tomogr*. 1998;22:314–316.
109. Iyer RB, Balachandran A, Devine CE, et al. PET/CT and cross sectional imaging of gynecologic malignancy. *Cancer Imaging*. 2007;7(Spec No A):S130–S138.
110. Kumar NB, Hart WR. Metastases to the uterine corpus from extragenital cancers. A clinicopathologic study of 63 cases. *Cancer.*. 2006;50:2163–2169.
111. Parini CL, Mathis D, Leath CA. Occult metastatic lung carcinoma presenting as locally advanced uterine carcinoma on positron emission tomography/computed tomography imaging. *Int J Gynecol Oncol*. 2007;17:731–734.
112. Major FJ, Blessing JA, Silverberg SG, et al. Prognostic factors in early-stage uterine sarcoma. A Gynecologic Oncology Group study. *Cancer*. 1993;71(Suppl 4):1702–1709.
113. Abeler VM, Royne O, Thoresen S, et al. Uterine sarcomas in Norway. A histopathological and prognostic survey of a total population from 1970 to 2000 including 419 patients. *Histopathology*. 2009;54:355–564.
114. Chern JY, Boyd LR, Blank SV. Uterine sarcomas: the latest approaches for these rare but potentially deadly tumors. *Onology (Williston Park)*. 2017;31:229–236.
115. Giuntoli 2nd RL, Metzinger DS, DiMarco CS, et al. Retrospective review of 208 patients with leiomyosarcoma of the uterus: prognostic indicators, surgical management, and adjuvant therapy. *Gynecol Oncol*. 2003;89:460–469.
116. Sorbe B. Radiotherapy and/or chemotherapy as adjuvant treatment of uterine sarcomas. *Gynecol Oncol.*. 1985;20:281–289.
117. Ferrer F, Sabater S, Farrus B, et al. Impact of radiotherapy on local control and survival in uterine sarcomas: a retrospective study from the Grup Oncologic Catala-Occita. *Int J Radiat Oncol Biol Phys*. 1999;44:47–52.
118. Hensley ML, Ishill N, Soslow R, et al. Adjuvant gemcitabine plus docetaxel for completely resected stages I-IV high grade uterine leiomyosarcoma: Results of a prospective study. *Gynecol Oncol*. 2009;112:563–567.
119. Dhakal S, Corbin KS, Milano MT, et al. Stereotactic body radiotherapy for pulmonary metastases from soft-tissue sarcomas: excellent local lesion control and improved patient survival. *Int J Radiat Oncol Biol Phys*. 2012;82(2):940–945.
120. Mehta N, Selch M, Wang PC, et al. Safety and efficacy of stereotactic body radiation therapy in the treatment of pulmonary metastases from high grade sarcoma. *Sarcoma.*. 2013;2013:360214.
121. Leitao MM, Brennan MF, Hensley M, et al. Surgical resection of pulmonary and extrapulmonary recurrences of uterine leiomyosarcoma. *Gynecologic Oncology*. 2002;87(3):287–294.
122. Hensley ML, Blessing JA, Mannel R, et al. Fixed-dose rate gemcitabine plus docetaxel as first-line therapy for metastatic uterine leiomyosarcoma: a Gynecologic Oncology Group phase II trial. *Gynecol Oncol*. 2008;109:329–334.
123. Hensley ML, Blessing JA, Degeest K, et al. Fixed-dose rate gemcitabine plus docetaxel as second-line therapy for metastatic uterine leiomyosarcoma: a Gynecologic Oncology Group phase II study. *Gynecol Oncol*. 2008;109:323–328.
124. Bodner K, Bodner-Adler B, Kimberger O, et al. Estrogen and progesterone receptor expression in patients with uterine leiomyosarcoma and correlation with different clinicopathological parameters. *Anticancer Res*. 2003;23:729–732.
125. Zhai YL, Nikaido T, Orii A, et al. Frequent occurrence of loss of heterozygosity among tumor suppressor genes in uterine leiomyosarcoma. *Gynecol Oncol*. 1999;75:453–459.
126. Hardman MP, Roman JJ, Burnett AF, et al. Metastatic uterine leiomyosarcoma regression using an aromatase inhibitor. *Obstet Gynecol*. 2007;110:518–520.
127. Koivisto-Korander R, Leminen A, Heikinheimo O. Mifepristone as treatment of recurrent progesterone receptor-positive uterine leiomyosarcoma. *Obstet Gynecol*. 2007;109:512–514.
128. Shah JP, Bryant CS, Kumar S, et al. Lymphadenectomy and ovarian preservation in low-grade endometrial stromal sarcoma. *Obstet Gynecol*. 2008;112:1102–1108.
129. Leath 3rd CA, Huh WK, Hyde Jr J, et al. A multi-institutional review of outcomes of endometrial stromal sarcoma. *Gynecol Oncol*. 2007;105:630–634.

130. Goff BA, Rice LW, Fleischhacker D, et al. Uterine leiomyosarcoma and endometrial stromal sarcoma: lymph node metastases and sites of recurrence. *Gynecol Oncol*. 1993;50:105–109.
131. Amant F, De Knijf A, Van Calster B, et al. Clinical study investigating the role of lymphadenectomy, surgical castration and adjuvant hormonal treatment in endometrial stromal sarcoma. *Br J Cancer*. 2007;97:1194–1199.
132. Reich O, Regauer S, Urdl W, et al. Expression of oestrogen and progesterone receptors in low-grade endometrial stromal sarcomas. *Br J Cancer*. 2000;82:1030–1034.
133. Chu MC, Mor G, Lim C, et al. Low-grade endometrial stromal sarcoma: hormonal aspects. *Gynecol Oncol*. 2003;90:170–176.
134. Ioffe YJ, Li AJ, Walsh CS, et al. Hormone receptor expression in uterine sarcomas: prognostic and therapeutic roles. *Gynecol Oncol*. 2009;115:466–471.
135. Reich O, Regauer S. Is tamoxifen an option for patients with endometrial stromal sarcoma? [author reply]. *Gynecol Oncol*. 2005;96:561.
136. Burke C, Hickey K. Treatment of endometrial stromal sarcoma with a gonadotropin-releasing hormone analogue. *Obstet Gynecol*. 2004;104:1182–1184.
137. Gadducci A, Cosio S, Genazzani AR. Use of estrogen antagonists and aromatase inhibitors in breast cancer and hormonally sensitive tumors of the uterine body. *Curr Opin Investig Drugs*. 2004;5:1031–1044.
138. Thanopoulou E, Judson I. Hormonal therapy in gynecological sarcomas. *Expert Rev Anticancer Ther*. 2012;12(7):885–894.
139. Reich O, Regauer S. Hormonal therapy of endometrial stromal sarcoma. *Curr Opin Oncol*. 2007;19:347–352.
140. Pink D, Lindner T, Mrozek A, et al. Harm or benefit of hormonal treatment in metastatic low-grade endometrial stromal sarcoma: single center experience with 10 cases and review of the literature. *Gynecol Oncol*. 2006;101:464–469.
141. Beer TW, Buchanan R, Buckley CH. Uterine stromal sarcoma following tamoxifen treatment. *J Clin Pathol*. 1995;48:596.
142. Pang LC. Endometrial stromal sarcoma with sex cord-like differentiation associated with tamoxifen therapy. *South Med J*. 1998;91:592–594.
143. García-Del-Muro X, López-Pousa A, Maurel J, et al. Randomized phase II study comparing gemcitabine plus dacarbazine versus dacarbazine alone in patients with previously treated soft tissue sarcoma: a Spanish Group for Research on Sarcomas study. *J Clin Oncol*. 2011;29(18):2528–2533.
144. Rovirosa A, Ordi J, Ascaso C, et al. Prognostic factors in uterine sarcomas: a 21-year retrospective study at the Clinic and Provincial Hospital of Barcelona in Spanish. *Med Clin (Barc)*. 1998;111:172–176.
145. Benson C, Ray-Coquard I, Sleijfer S, et al. Outcome of uterine sarcoma patients treated with pazopanib: A retrospective analysis based on two European Organisation for Research and Treatment of Cancer (EORTC) Soft Tissue and Bone Sarcoma Group (STBSG) clinical trials 62043 and 62072. *Gynecol Oncol*. 2016;142:89–94.
146. Pautier P, Floquet A, Chevreau C, et al. Trabectedin in combination with doxorubicin for first-line treatment of advanced uterine or soft-tissue leiomyosarcoma (LMS-02):a non-randomised, multicentre, phase 2 trial. *Lancet Oncol*. 2015;16:457–464.
147. Schöffski P, Chawla S, Maki RG, et al. Eribulin versus dacarbazine in previously treated patients with advanced liposarcoma or leiomyosarcoma: a randomised, open-label, multicentre, phase 3 trial. *Lancet.*. 2016;387:1629–1637.
148. Paoluzzi L, Cacavio A, Ghesani M, et al. Response to anti-PD1 therapy with nivolumab in metastatic sarcomas. *Clin Sarcoma Res.*. 2016;6:24.
149. Ben-Ami E, Barysauskas CM, Solomon S, et al. Immunotherapy with single agent nivolumab for advanced leiomyosarcoma of the uterus: Results of a phase 2 study. *Cancer.*. 2017;123(17):3285–3290.
150. Tuyaerts S, Van Nuffel AMT, Naert E, et al. PRIMMO study protocol: a phase II study combining PD-1 blockade, radiation and immunomodulation to tackle cervical and uterine cancer. *BMC Cancer*. 2019;19:506.

CHAPTER

26 Cervical Cancer

Amritjot Kaur, M.B.B.S., M.D.; Claire F. Verschraegen, M.D.; and Harmeet Kaur, M.B.B.S., M.D.

INTRODUCTION

Cervical cancer is the third most common gynecologic malignancy in the United States. In 2019, 13,170 new cases and 4250 deaths are expected in the United States.[1] Across the world cervical cancer is the fourth most common cancer in women, with 575,000 cases and 311,000 deaths in 2018. However, the incidence varies widely across developed and underdeveloped countries, ranging from 2 to 75 per 100,000 women, with 85% of all cases occurring in the less developed world. In many African countries cervical cancer is the leading cause of cancer death, while countries like China and India contribute over a third of cases worldwide.[2]

The introduction of screening in the early decades of the twentieth century using exfoliative cytology obtained with the Papanicolaou (Pap) smear resulted in a steep decline in mortality from cervical cancer. However, recent data from countries with established screening programs suggest that the method may have reached its limits, with several countries reporting either stable or a slight rise in the incidence of cervical cancer.[3] Recent randomized trials suggest that screening with human papillomavirus (HPV) assays protects better against invasive cancers then screening with cytology.[4]

EPIDEMIOLOGY AND RISK FACTORS

In the early half of the twentieth century, cervical cancer was the leading cause of cancer-related mortality in women. In the developed world, the incidence has declined significantly. This success has partly been as a result of the development and implementation of an effective screening test but also to the nature of cervical cancer, in which the development of invasive cervical cancer is preceded by a long precancerous phase, and the fact that these lesions, once detected, are then accessible and amenable to treatment.

There are numerous predisposing factors in the development of cervical cancer; however, epidemiologic studies have implicated an infectious agent as the most important factor. In 1983, this was identified as HPV.[5] Although HPV infection is widespread, the majority of infections are cleared by cell-mediated immunity within 2 years, and less than 10% of individuals will develop persistent infection. Persistent infection with HPV plays a central role in the development of cervical cancer and can be identified in almost all cases. There are numerous HPV genotypes, and HPV-16 and HPV-18 have been determined to be the most potently carcinogenic. HPV-16 alone accounts for almost 60% of cervical cancers.[3] In addition to its causative role in the development of squamous cell carcinoma of the cervix, HPV has also been implicated in the development of cervical adenocarcinoma, neuroendocrine carcinoma, and other noncervical cancers.

HPV targets the immature basal cells of the cervical epithelium; mature squamous cells, in contrast, are resistant to infection. In the cervix, there is a significant area of immature squamous metaplastic cells at the squamocolumnar junction. This is also called the transformation zone and anatomically is located where the squamous lining of the ectocervix meets the columnar cells of the endocervix at the level of the external os. This ring of metaplastic tissue is most susceptible to the carcinogenic effects of HPV infection.

In addition, numerous factors function in concert with exposure to high–oncogenic risk HPV infection and an inefficient immune response to increase the risk of developing cervical cancer, including:

1. Multiple sexual partners and high-risk sexual partners.
2. History of sexually transmitted diseases (e.g., chlamydia or herpes simplex).
3. Prolonged use of oral contraceptives.
4. Smoking.
5. High parity.
6. Young age at first intercourse.
7. Low socioeconomic status.
8. Immunosuppression.
9. Exposure to diethylstilbestrol.

Smoking has been shown to be an independent risk factor. Smoking, even passive smoking, is associated with an increased risk of squamous carcinoma but not adenocarcinoma. The presence of cigarette carcinogens in the cervical mucus may be the explanation for this observation.

Approximately 80% of people will get an HPV infection in their lifetime, and vaccination provides a reliable defense against persistent infection. The first HPV vaccine was approved in 2014. Two doses of HPV vaccine administered at least 5 months apart are recommended for all 11- to 12-year-olds.[3]

A three-dose schedule is recommended for people older than 14 years, as well as for people with certain immunocompromising conditions. Each vaccine was found to be safe and effective in clinical trials. From 2008 to 2014, the proportion of grade II cervical intraepithelial dysplasias positive for HPV16/18 has declined.[6]

ANATOMY AND PATHOLOGY

Cervix

The female genital tract arises from the Müllerian ducts, which are formed by an invagination of the coelomic epithelium. The Müllerian ducts give rise to the fallopian tubes, the corpus or body of the uterus, the cervix, and the vagina. This common embryologic origin accounts for the similarities among tumors arising in different parts of the genital system and the peritoneum.

The uterus has three distinct anatomic parts: the corpus or body, the lower uterine segment, and the cervix. The cervix is divided into the supravaginal cervix (also called the cervical isthmus) and the vaginal portions. The vaginal portion of the cervix, or portio vaginalis, is covered by stratified nonkeratinized squamous epithelium, which also lines the vagina. This meets the columnar epithelium of the endocervix at the external os. This is the squamocolumnar junction, or transformation zone, described. In this area, a gradual transformation of columnar to squamous epithelium proceeds through life, leading to a gradual migration of this zone from the level of the external os in young women to a position within the endocervical canal in older women. This has consequences for the location of squamous tumors, which may present as endocervical masses in older women.

Squamous cell carcinoma is by far the most common malignancy of the cervix and accounts for 85% of all tumors in this region. This is followed by adenocarcinoma, which arises from the columnar epithelium of the endocervical canal and accounts for 10% of cervical tumors. The remaining 5% is composed of uncommon pathologies such as neuroendocrine and adenosquamous tumors.

The gross morphologic appearance of invasive squamous tumors is as either infiltrative or fungating masses that generally arise at the level of the external os. Adenocarcinomas, in contrast, arise within the lumen of the cervical canal; consequently, they are difficult to evaluate on physical examination. This makes magnetic resonance imaging (MRI) particularly important in the assessment of these tumors.

As previously mentioned, squamous carcinoma is preceded by a long premalignant phase of epithelial dysplasia originating in the squamocolumnar junction. Cervical dysplasia is classified depending upon severity as cervical intraepithelial dysplasia I to III (CIN I–III). This classification has been recently simplified into a two-tiered system that reflects clinical management. CIN I is now called low-grade squamous intraepithelial lesion (LSIL), and CIN II and III are high-grade squamous intraepithelial lesion (HSIL). The majority of LSILs will regress, with only 10% progressing to HSIL. Similarly, the majority of HSILs, which most frequently arise from LSILs, will also disappear, and only 10% will develop into invasive squamous carcinoma. In the United States, approximately 1 million of these precancerous lesions are detected every year, but only approximately 11,000 cases of invasive cancer are diagnosed. This implies that, with screening, early cancers are diagnosed and eradicated, many of which would have progressed to invasive disease.

It is important to note that, in spite of its effectiveness, Pap smear has a false-negative rate of 15% to 20%, hence the need for repeat screening, particularly in high-risk patients. A number of techniques such as computerized screening, liquid-based sampling technique, and HPV typing are being used to improve accuracy. HPV assays have proven particularly effective in screening for invasive carcinomas.[4]

An additional limitation of the Pap smear is that it is ineffective in the detection of adenocarcinoma, adenosquamous, and neuroendocrine tumors. Consequently, these tumors generally present with more advanced disease.

Pelvic Anatomy

A basic overview of pelvic anatomy is important for staging cervical cancer, because an understanding of pelvic ligaments, vessels, peritoneal reflections, and pelvic lymph node stations is vital in evaluating cross-sectional computed tomography (CT) and MRI.[7]

The important ligaments from the imaging perspective that are found in relation to the uterus, cervix, and ovaries include the broad ligament, round ligaments, uterosacral ligaments, cardinal ligaments, and suspensory ligament of the ovary (Fig. 26.1).

The broad ligament is a peritoneal reflection that extends from the uterus to the pelvic sidewall. It contains the fallopian tubes along the upper margin; the cardinal ligament runs in the base of the broad ligament. It contains fat, connective tissue, the uterine and ovarian vessels, lymphatics, and the ovarian and round ligament. It is difficult to see except in the presence of ascites. The round ligament runs from the anterior wall of the uterus through the inguinal canal to the labia and is easy to see on CT. The cardinal ligament is an important structure that runs from the supravaginal cervix/isthmus and upper vagina to the obturator internus muscle. The uterine arteries run along the superior aspect of this ligament and help define this structure. As these arteries course from their origin from the internal iliac arteries to the edge of the uterus, they arch over the ureters, creating the "arc sign," which can frequently be seen on CT. The uterosacral ligament arises from the cervix and upper vagina to arc on either side of the rectum to the S2 to S3 segments of the sacrum. This structure is thickened after radiation therapy. The suspensory ligament of the ovary carries the gonadal vessels to the ovary and is defined by the course of these vessels on cross-sectional imaging.

The main vascular supply to the uterus is the uterine arteries that arise from the internal iliac vessels, run along the superior aspect of the cardinal ligament, and then ascend on either side of the uterus to trifurcate and supply the fallopian tubes, fundus of the uterus, and ovaries (Fig. 26.2). The ovarian arteries arise from the aorta below the renal arteries; the vaginal arteries arise from the internal iliac arteries.

The parametrium refers to tissue surrounding the uterine artery cranial to the ureter extending between the uterus and pelvic sidewall, whereas the paracervix, lateral parametrium, or cardinal ligament is caudal to the ureter. The paracervix surrounds the isthmus of the cervix and upper third of the vagina and is divided into medial and lateral parts by the ureter. The medial paracervix is composed

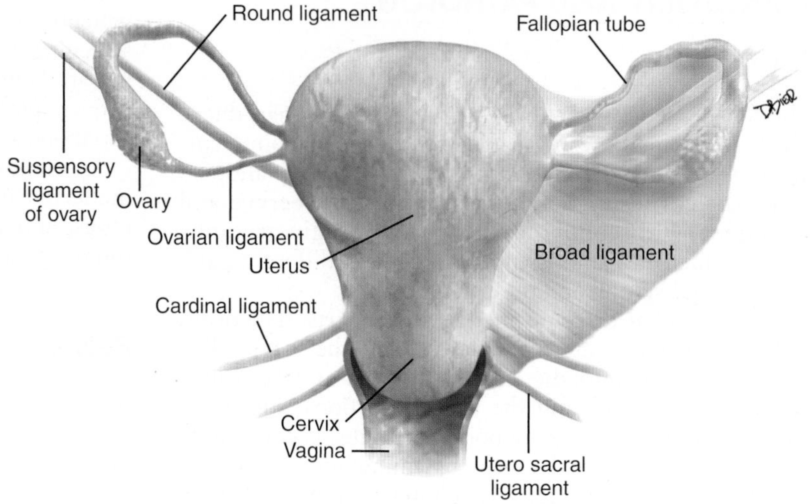

Round ligament
Fallopian tube
Suspensory ligament of ovary
Ovary
Ovarian ligament
Uterus
Broad ligament
Cardinal ligament
Cervix
Vagina
Utero sacral ligament

FIGURE 26.1. Uterine anatomy.

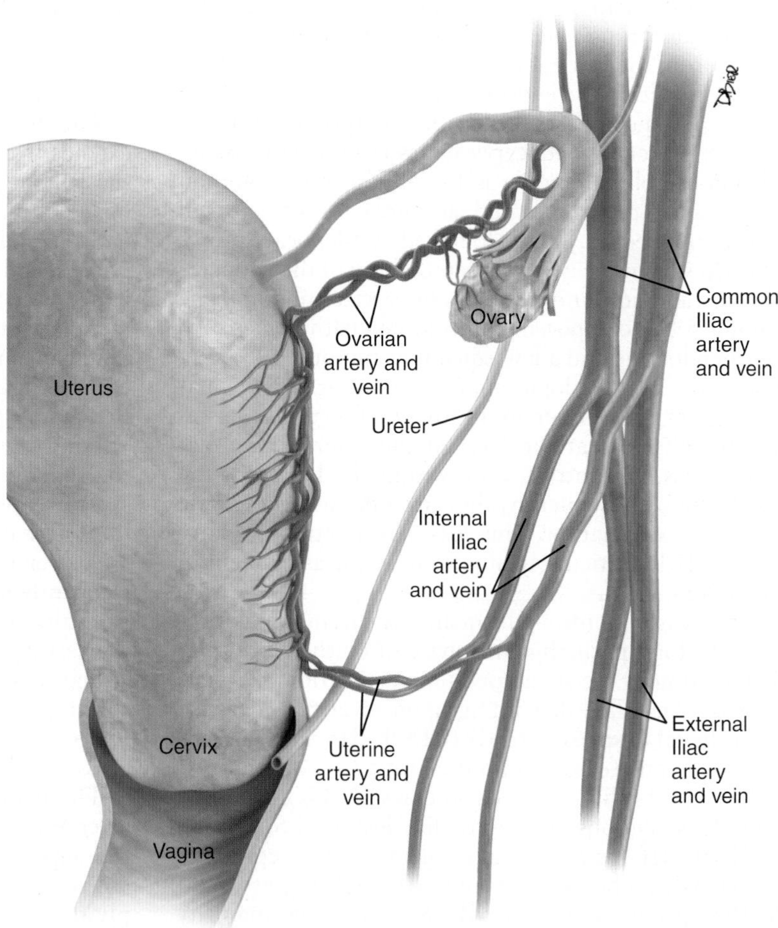

FIGURE 26.2. Vascular supply to the uterus.

of dense fibrous tissue and the lateral paracervix of lymph nodes that surround nerves and branches of the internal iliac vessels and uterine arteries.

The anterior parametrium or bladder pillar is composed medially of the vesicouterine ligament and lateral to the ureters of the lateral ligament of the bladder. The posterior parametrium or rectal pillar refers to the rectouterine ligament medially and the ureterosacral ligaments laterally.[8]

Pelvic Nodal Anatomy

Disease spread to pelvic nodes is the most common pathway of tumor dissemination from the cervix. An understanding of the pathways of spread is essential for image analysis because these are the nodes that should be most closely scrutinized when evaluating cross-sectional imaging studies (Fig. 26.3).

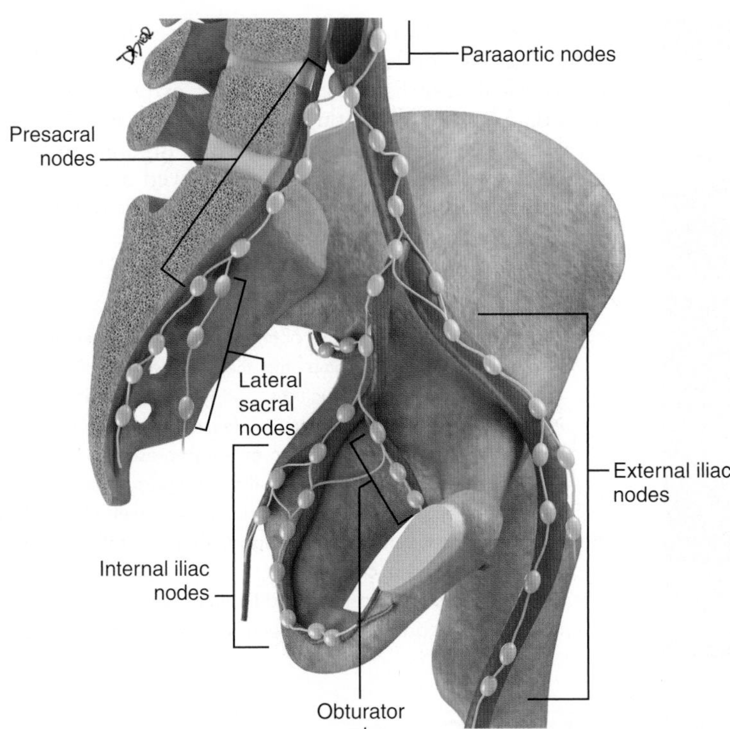

FIGURE 26.3. Pelvic nodes.

The nodal group most commonly first involved by tumor spread from pelvic tumors is the perivisceral nodes, which in the instance of cervical cancer are nodes in the lateral paracervical region. This is followed by spread to pelvic sidewall nodes. Lymphatic spread from cervical tumors can spread to the pelvic nodes by three routes: (1) the lateral pathway of spread toward external iliac nodes, (2) the hypogastric route toward nodes along the internal iliac vessels, and (3) the posterior route, where lymphatics course along the uterosacral ligament to nodes along lateral sacral vessels and nodes anterior to the sacral promontory.[9] The nodes along the external iliac vessels are subclassified into middle, medial, and lateral groups. The lateral chain nodes are located, as the name implies, lateral to the vessels; the middle chain nodes are between the external iliac artery and vein; and the medial chain nodes are located posterior and medial to the artery and vein. The nodes medial to the external iliac arteries are the group most commonly involved by metastatic spread from cervical cancer. These nodes are located in close proximity to nodes along the obturator vessels and are frequently grouped together with obturator nodes, although there is some controversy in this regard (Fig. 26.4). All the pelvic nodal chains drain to the common iliac nodes. The common iliac nodes are also classified similar to external iliac nodes into middle, lateral, and medial subgroups. The middle subgroup is located posterior to the common iliac vein in the lumbosacral fossa, which is bordered posteriorly by the sacral vertebral body.[10] This node is in close proximity to the L5 nerve root and can impinge on this root when enlarged, causing back pain (Fig. 26.5). Spread from common iliac nodes is most commonly to the para-aortic nodes.

KEY POINTS Anatomy, Pathology, and Epidemiology

- Persistent infection with human papillomavirus-16 and -18 is the most important risk factor in the development of cervical cancer.
- Cervical cancer has a long premalignant phase and, therefore, can be managed by screening and early intervention.
- Squamous carcinoma accounts for 85% of cervical tumors, arises from the zone located at the level of the external os, and may present as exophytic or infiltrative masses.
- The uterine arteries and ureters as they course in the paracervix/cardinal ligament define the level of the supravaginal cervix and site of lateral parametrial invasion.

CLINICAL PRESENTATION

In early cervical cancer, there may be no clinical symptoms as the disease progresses. Common clinical complaints are vaginal discharge, postcoital bleeding, irregular vaginal bleeding, or postmenopausal bleeding. In more advanced disease, lower abdominal or back pain or weight loss may also develop.

PATTERNS OF TUMOR SPREAD

The most common pathways of tumor spread in cervical cancer are direct invasion of contiguous pelvic structures and through lymphatics to lymph nodes; hematogenous spread is an uncommon pathway.

Direct spread occurs from penetration through the cervical stroma of the supracervical cervix or isthmus into the lateral paracervix, where the ureters and uterine arteries are located, and into the anterior or posterior parametrium.

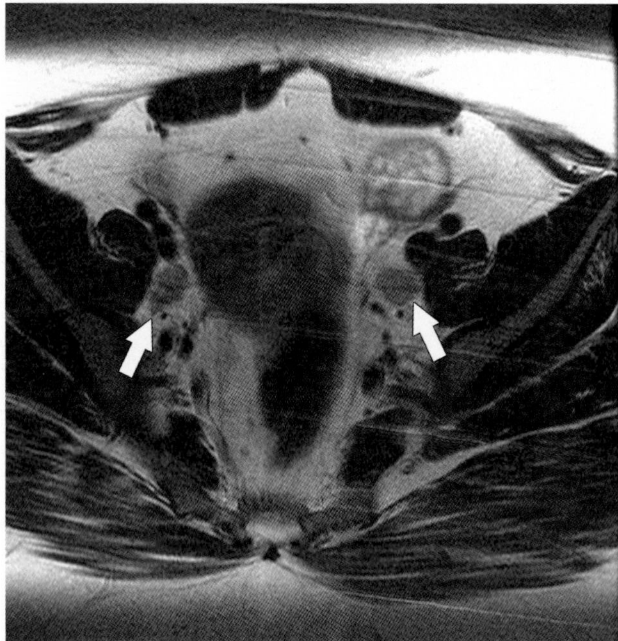

FIGURE 26.4. Bilateral obturator adenopathy (*arrows*) is identified on the axial T2-weighted fast spin echo magnetic resonance imaging study. These nodes are seen to be 2-[^{18}F] fluoro-2-deoxy-D-glucose–avid on the fused positron emission tomography/computed tomography images.

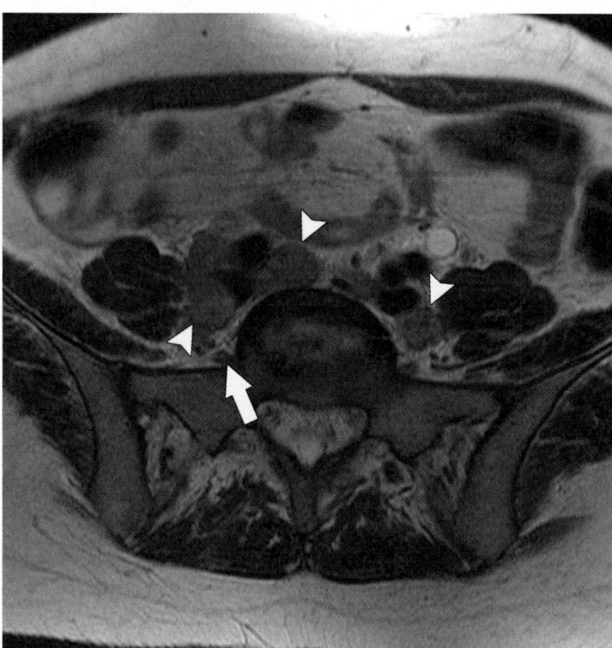

FIGURE 26.5. Common iliac adenopathy shows enlarged nodes involving the medial, middle, and lateral radial groups on the right (*arrowheads*). The right L5 nerve (*arrow*) root is in close proximity to the lateral chain nodes.

Lymph node spread in cervical cancer generally occurs in a sequential fashion, with paracervical nodal involvement followed by external or internal iliac adenopathy, common iliac adenopathy, and then paraaortic adenopathy. It is very uncommon for paraaortic nodes to be involved in the absence of pelvic nodal disease.

As with all tumors, it is important to define regional and nonregional nodal groups; involvement of the latter upstages the tumor to stage IV, because these nodes are viewed as M1 nodes. In the case of cervical cancer, the paracervical, internal iliac, obturator, external iliac, common iliac, presacral, lateral sacral, and paraaortic nodes are viewed as regional nodes, whereas the inguinal, mediastinal, and supraclavicular nodes are viewed as nonregional nodes, and consequently qualify as metastatic disease.[11]

KEY POINTS Patterns of Tumor Spread

- The most common pathways of tumor spread are direct invasion through the cervical stroma into the paracervix, extending to involve adjacent pelvic structures, and lymphatic spread.
- Nodal spread in cervical cancer occurs in a stepwise progressive manner from the paracervical to external, presacral, or internal iliac nodes, followed by common iliac and paraaortic nodes.
- The recent, eighth edition of the tumor-node-metastasis (TNM) classification system has recategorized paraaortic nodes as regional for cervical cancer.
- Supraclavicular, mediastinal, and inguinal adenopathy constitute nonregional nodes and, consequently, metastatic disease.

STAGING

Unlike most other tumors, the initial staging of cervical cancer, recommended by the International Federation of Gynecology and Obstetrics (FIGO) committee, has been primarily clinical, to maintain uniformity between clinical trials across nations. This is because, in most countries where this disease is prevalent, elaborate cross-sectional staging techniques such as MRI, CT, and positron emission tomography (PET)/CT historically have not been available. However, clinical staging is inaccurate, with understaging of 20% to 40% of stage IB-IIIB cancers and overstaging of 64% of IIIB cancers.[12] The decade since the publication of the prior FIGO guidelines in 2009 has seen the rapid dissemination of imaging technology and minimally invasive surgical procedures across the world, including into low- and middle-income countries. Because of the clear benefits of the additional information provided by these techniques, the current iteration of the FIGO guidelines published in 2019 offer the optional incorporation of imaging and pathological findings into the allocation of stage.[13] This position is now at odds with the American Joint Committee on Cancer (AJCC) eighth edition (2017) guidelines, which still require the baseline stage to be obtained on the basis of clinical examination, colposcopy, endocervical curettage, hysteroscopy, cystoscopy, proctoscopy, and basic imaging studies such as intravenous pyelogram and x-ray of the lungs and bones. The results from more advanced imaging test such as CT, MRI and PET/CT cannot be used to determine the clinical stage but can be used to formulate a treatment plan and assess prognosis (Fig. 26.6).

In contrast to the significant changes in FIGO 2018, the current TNM staging for cervical cancer published in 2017 has only one change, which was the removal of paraaortic nodes from M1 disease and their redefinition as regional nodes for cervical cancer.[11]

In the assessment of stage, FIGO 2018 mandates that the final stage should clearly document the method used

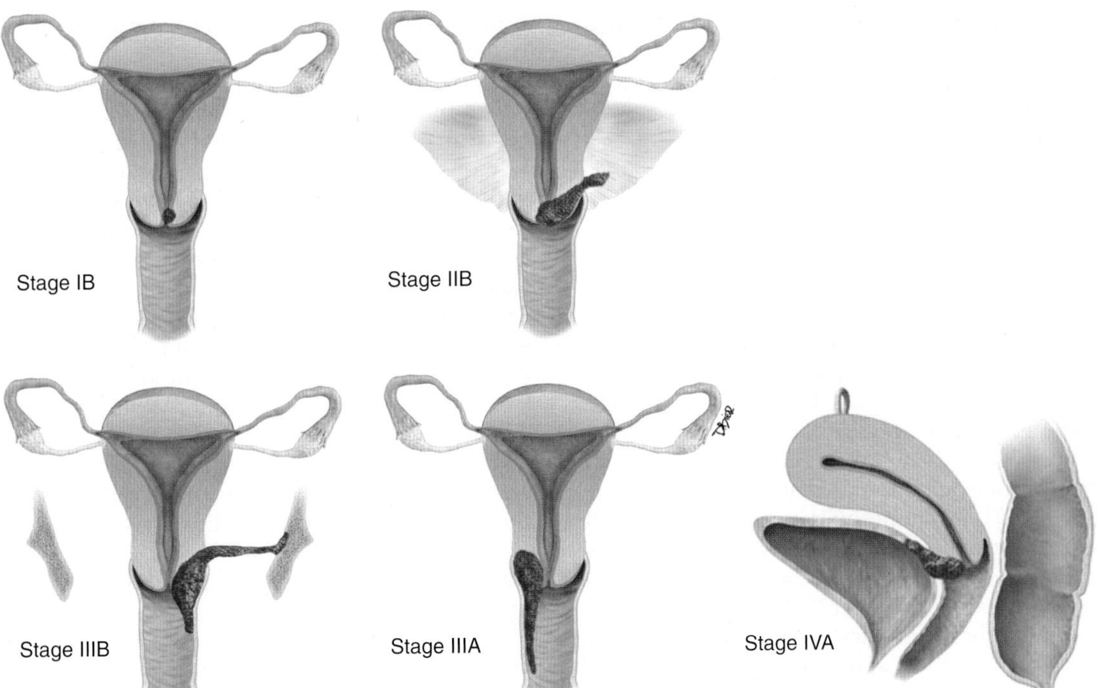

Figure 26.6. Stages I–IV of cervical cancer.

for staging, whether radiological (annotated with an "r"), pathological (annotated with a "p"), or purely clinical. This information should be included in the staging summary.

FIGO 2018 has also introduced staging modifications in stages IA, IB, and III. The definitions of FIGO stages II and IV remain unchanged.

FIGO stage 1A, which is tumors diagnosed only by microscopy, has been modified to exclude lateral extension of the lesion. However, this remains a component of the AJCC staging guidelines at the current time.

The modifications in stage 1B are related to an improved understanding of the prognostic implications of tumor size. It is now recognized that tumors less than 2 cm in size have significantly lower recurrence rates compared with tumors 2 to 4 cm in size.[14,15] Stage IB is now classified into three subgroups instead of two; and IB1 now includes tumors smaller than 2 cm, IB2 tumors between 2 and 4 cm, and IB3 tumor larger than 4 cm. The AJCC eighth edition staging for IA and IB tumors remains unchanged, and consequently there is now a discrepancy between T staging and FIGO staging for stages IA and B.

Because the previous FIGO staging system was entirely clinical, nodal involvement has not been part of the staging system. The incorporation of imaging and/or pathology in FIGO 2019 into assessment of initial stage has permitted the inclusion of nodal involvement as a separate stage IIIC, whereas stage IIIA and IIIB remain unchanged. Any patient with nodal involvement is now upstaged to IIIC, irrespective of the extent of the primary tumor. Stage IIIC further subclassifies pelvic adenopathy as stage IIIC1 and paraaortic adenopathy as stage IIIC2.

Nodal status has always been a part of the TNM staging of cervical cancer. The patterns of nodal spread have been described in a previous section; regional nodes for cervical cancer previously included obturator, internal iliac, sacral, presacral, external iliac, and common iliac nodes,[10] with spread to paraaortic nodes constituting metastatic spread. However, the AJCC eighth edition has moved paraaortic nodes into the category of regional nodes for cervical cancer, with supraclavicular, mediastinal, and other distant lymph nodes included in the category of M1 or metastatic disease. This is based on data that suggest that patients with paraaortic nodal disease have better outcomes then patients with more distant sites of metastatic disease.[16] FIGO 2018, however, separates pelvic nodal involvement from paraaortic nodal involvement, which is upstaged to IIIC2 based on data indicating poorer survival outcomes in nodal spread above the level of the common iliac nodal station.[17]

The definition of metastatic spread in the TNM classification, or IVB in the FIGO classification, includes distant spread, which most frequently presents as supraclavicular or mediastinal nodes, peritoneal spread, or involvement of lung, liver, or bones.

The National Comprehensive Cancer Network 2019 guidelines for use of imaging in cervical cancer suggest MRI with contrast for local staging in FIGO stage IB2 and optional use of MRI for stage 1B1 and below, with a very limited role for PET/CT or CT for metastatic spread. In stages II to IV PET/CT is the preferred diagnostic modality and may be supplemented by MRI for local disease if required.[18]

Key Points Staging

- International Federation of Gynecology and Obstetrics (FIGO) staging of cervical cancer now incorporates imaging and pathological information in assessment of clinical stage and has added nodal status as a separate stage, stage IIIC.

- Modified FIGO stage IA and IB no longer correspond to T stages in the tumor-node-metastasis (TNM) classification.
- TNM eighth edition and National Comprehensive Cancer Network 2019 guidelines continue to suggest the use of cross-sectional imaging to facilitate treatment planning, but not for clinical staging.

IMAGING

The staging of cervical cancer up until now has been primarily clinical, but this has changed with the current FIGO staging update. The imaging modalities most commonly deployed in the assessment of cervical cancer include MRI, CT, PET/CT, PET/MRI, and ultrasound.

A multiinstitutional trial found that the overall accuracy of MRI and CT in the preoperative staging of early cervical cancer were comparable; however, in single-institution studies, MRI is the most accurate technique for local staging of cervical cancer.[19] The primary objective is to define tumors with parametrial invasion, which precludes surgical resection and directs patients toward radiation and chemotherapy. MRI has proved to be the most effective technique in this regard, with a high negative predictive value.

Primary Tumor

Magnetic Resonance Imaging

MRI is more useful than CT because of its superior soft-tissue resolution. Its primary role is in determining tumor size, evaluating parametrial invasion, evaluating extent of uterine and vaginal involvement, and determining the involvement of adjacent pelvic structures. The patients who most benefit from an MRI are those with endocervical tumors, tumors larger than 2 cm at clinical examination, possible parametrial invasion, and pregnant patients.[20]

The goal of MRI is to guide clinical decision making. In this regard, parametrial invasion and pelvic nodal involvement are the most important aspects to be evaluated. The presence or absence of parametrial involvement determines whether surgical resection can be performed. Nodal involvement has significant prognostic value; however, also it determines whether nodal dissection should be performed and the extent of radiation coverage if chemoradiation is the chosen treatment modality. In these different goals, MRI performs with variable accuracy. These are discussed because the limitations of a modality are important in its appropriate deployment.

Technique. A phased array coil is used to improve resolution and signal-to-noise ratio of the acquired images and is preferred over use of the body coil. Patient preparation can include fasting for 4 to 6 hours to decrease bowel peristalsis, which frequently degrades image quality on the sagittal T2-weighted (T2W) images. Alternatively, frequency can be swapped to the anterior to posterior direction by adding no phase wrap for new images within a small field. In addition, vaginal gel may be used, because it improves delineation of vaginal wall involvement, particularly the fornices.

The basic principles of high-quality MRI for staging of pelvic tumors are fundamentally similar, whether staging cervical, endometrial, or rectal cancer (Table 26.1). These rely on small–field-of-view, high-resolution T2W images without fat suppression obtained perpendicular to the long axis of the cervix, preferably in two orthogonal planes (most commonly sagittal and oblique axial in the case of cervical cancer). This entails using thin sections, preferably 3 to 4 mm (with a 0.25-mm gap), with a small field of view of 16 to 20 mm and the matrix tailored to obtain an in-plane resolution of 0.04 to 0.06 cm. These basic sequences can be supplemented with a coronal T2W image with thin slices. The most important sequence for evaluation of parametrial invasion is the oblique thin-section T2W image obtained at right angles to the axis of the cervix, most importantly the supravaginal portion of the cervix.[21]

Intravenous contrast has limited value in the staging of cervical tumors. It has no role in evaluation of parametrial invasion; however, it can be used to assess involvement of adjacent structures such as the bladder. The dynamic images show small tumors as hypervascular lesions and are reported to have a high accuracy in determining depth of stromal invasion in small tumors.[22] However, larger tumors appear as centrally hypovascular with only marginal enhancement.

Diffusion-weighted imaging (DWI) (b-value 500–100 sec/mm^2) is being increasingly used in detection, characterization, staging, and response assessment for cervical tumors. Diffusion-weighted images should be interpreted in conjunction with anatomic T2W images matched by slice and apparent diffusion coefficient (ADC) maps to avoid pitfalls[23] (Figs. 26.7 and 26.8). Because diffusion-weighted images assist in delineation of the primary tumor, when superimposed on T2W images there is marginal improvement in assessment of parametrial invasion and vaginal involvement (see Fig. 26.8) related largely to a decline in false positives.[24]

TABLE 26.1 Magnetic Resonance Protocol for Cervical Center

Protocol
Axial T1-weighted images (large field of view [FOV]): 5 mm/0.5 mm
Sagittal T2-weighted images without fat suppression: FOV 20–24, 3–4 mm/0.2–0.04 mm
Oblique axial T2-weighted images without fat suppression perpendicular to cervix: FOV 18–24, 3–4 mm/0.2–0.4 mm
Diffusion-weighted imaging: b-value 0–1000 sec/mm^2 sagittal and or oblique axial matched to T2-weighted images
Optional
Sagittal dynamic three-dimensional LAVA images.
Coronal T2 without fat suppression
Postcontrast axial T1-weighted images.
It is recommended that the large FOV axial images be obtained from the level of the kidneys down through the pelvis to evaluate for retroperitoneal adenopathy and hydronephrosis.

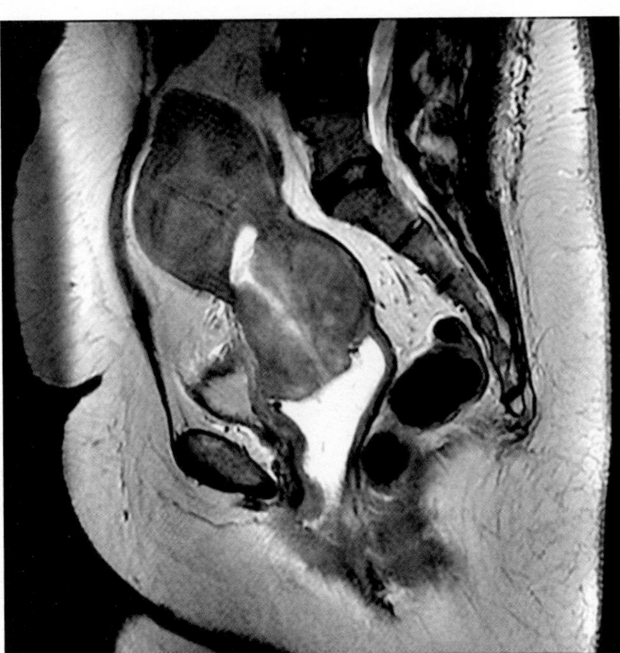

FIGURE 26.7. Sagittal T2-weighted image shows the cervical tumor expanding the cervix with possible invasion of the anterior parametrium and of the vaginal fornix.

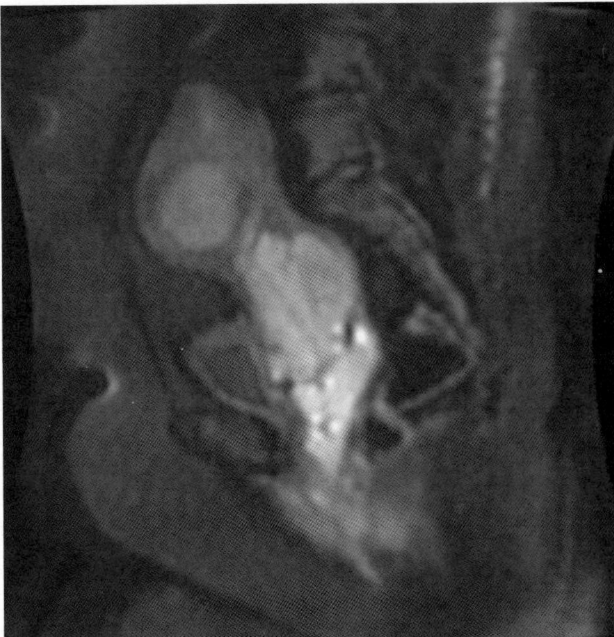

FIGURE 26.8. Sagittal diffusion-weighted image (800 m/sec^2) shows a large cervical tumor expanding the cervix extending from the external os to the lower uterine segment. There is restricted diffusion confirming involvement of the anterior vaginal fornix and into the anterior parametrium.

Evaluation of Images.

Stage I. For tumors confined to the cervix, the smaller microinvasive tumors fall into category IA. In this subgroup, the role of imaging is limited, as disease is by definition microscopic and not visible on imaging. There has been some work with dynamic contrast-enhanced MRI that identified tumors with greater than 4 mm depth of penetration into the stroma as hypervascular lesions.[22] The larger tumors that fall into the IB2 and IB3 category (FIGO 2018) are seen on T2W images as hyperintense masses that invade the hypointense stroma. However, in younger women, the stroma is occasionally hyperintense, and the tumors may be harder to delineate. The size of tumors is an important prognostic indicator; this is reflected by the decline in 5-year survival rate from 84% to 66% in patients with tumors larger than 3 cm.[25] The larger tumors are also associated with an increased likelihood of nodal spread. The assessment of tumor size by MRI has an excellent correlation with size assessed by pathology and should be assessed on two orthogonal views.

Stage II. Stage II is defined by tumor spread outside the cervix into the upper third of the vagina or parametrium.

The most important information from the perspective of treatment planning is evaluation of parametrial invasion, the presence of which categorizes the tumor as locally advanced and excludes surgical resection. In the assessment of parametrial invasion, MRI has a high negative predictive value (94%–100%) with an intact dark stromal ring (>3 mm) virtually excluding parametrial invasion (Fig. 26.9).[25,26] Disruption of the circumscribed cervical ring on oblique T2W images generally indicates parametrial invasion, with additional signs such as spiculated tumor–parametrium interface and abutment of uterine vessels improving diagnostic confidence (Figs. 26.10 and 26.11). The presence of associated hydronephrosis confirms parametrial invasion. An important limitation to keep in mind is that large tumors may be associated with peritumoral edema, which can be mistaken for parametrial invasion. This leads to a decline in staging accuracy from 90% for small lesions to 70% for larger tumors.[26,27] This important fact should be kept in mind at the time of image evaluation. Diffusion-weighted images can improve accuracy in this subgroup of patients.[24]

In terms of evaluation of the vaginal vault, disruption of the normal low signal of the vaginal wall by tumor is best identified on the sagittal T2W images and reflects invasion. However, occasionally with large tumors the vaginal fornices may be stretched over the mass, and it becomes difficult to assess for invasion. This can be overcome, to some extent, by the use of vaginal gel. However, in this circumstance, the information provided on MRI is not critical because it can also be obtained by visualization of the vaginal wall by clinical examination.

The assessment of invasion of the lower uterine segment can be obtained with MRI. Although it does not fall into information required for staging, it is important in young women who wish to retain fertility and are considering trachelectomy. In this subgroup of patients, information such as length of the cervical canal and relationship of the tumor to the internal os can be assessed on MRI with high accuracy.[27]

Stage III. In stage III, a vaginal involvement extends into the lower third of the vagina, and in IIIB, the extension is lateral until the pelvic sidewall. The MRI findings that suggest pelvic sidewall involvement include tumor within 3 mm of or abutment of the pelvic sidewall musculature.[28,29] MRI findings in vaginal involvement have been mentioned previously.

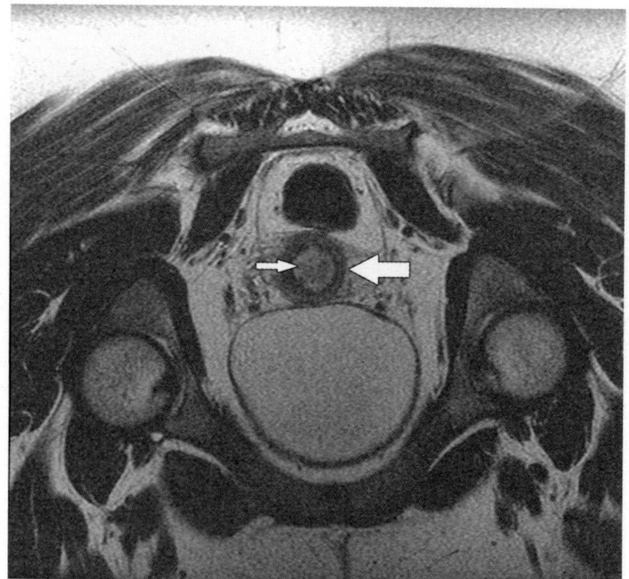

FIGURE 26.9. A 31-year-old with poorly differentiated adenocarcinoma. The oblique axial T2-weighted magnetic resonance imaging study shows a hyperintense mass in the endocervical canal (*small arrow*) with an intact stromal ring (*large arrow*) excluding parametrial invasion.

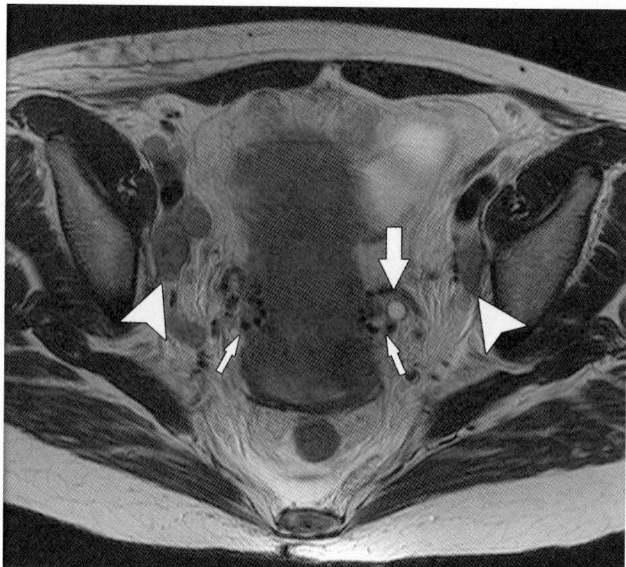

FIGURE 26.10. A 44-year-old with poorly differentiated squamous carcinoma of the cervix presenting as an infiltrative mass involving the full thickness of the cervical stroma with bilateral parametrial invasion. Tumor encases both uterine vessels (*thin arrows*) and is occluding the left ureter (*thick white arrow*). There are enlarged bilateral obturator nodes (*arrowheads*).

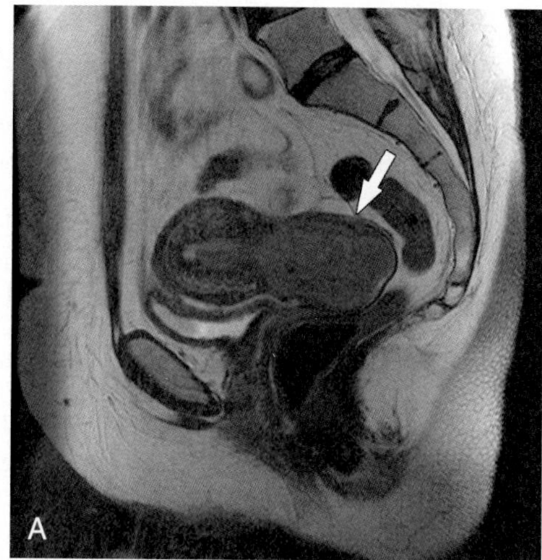

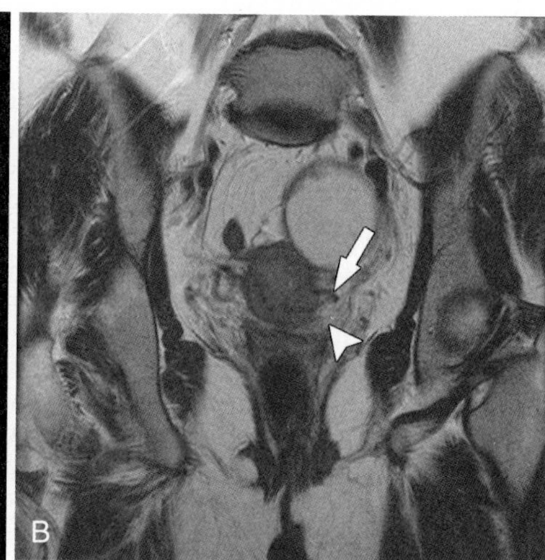

FIGURE 26.11. **A** and **B**, A 53-year-old with cervical adenocarcinoma. Sagittal T2-weighted images show a hyperintense mass expanding the endocervical canal (*arrow* in **A**). The T2-weighted images orthogonal to the plane of the tumor show parametrial invasion on the left with a spiculated tumor-parametrium interface (*arrowhead in B*) and abutment of the left uterine artery (*arrow in B*).

Stage IV. Invasion of adjacent pelvic structures such as the bladder or rectum or development of distant spread qualifies as stage IV disease. MRI has a high negative predictive value in excluding bladder or rectal involvement. However, the positive predictive value is lower. This is because abutment of the bladder or focal loss of the normal low signal of the bladder wall and development of hyperintense T2 foci along the anterior aspect of the posterior bladder wall do not always reflect tumor invasion. The sensitivity of bladder invasion is in the range of 71% to 100%, and the specificity is in the range of 88% to 91%.[30,31] This limitation has led to an evaluation of dynamic MRI, and some studies have suggested that this leads to improved accuracy over evaluation of only T2W images.[32] The more advanced cases of bladder invasion are relatively easier to diagnose as defined by nodular masses projecting into the bladder or development of a vesicovaginal fistula.

It is noted that recent multiinstitutional studies have found both CT and MRI suboptimal in evaluating depth of stromal invasion, parametrial extension, and pelvic nodal metastasis. These studies also report lower accuracies for MRI staging than those seen in single-institution studies. However, the accuracy for assessment of tumor size and lower uterine invasion remains high. It is to be noted that the technique used in these studies did not incorporate high-resolution T2 scans or imaging in the orthogonal plane, which are important in the assessment of parametrial invasion.[19,33,34]

Computed Tomography

CT has limited value in the assessment of local disease, because 50% of the tumors are isodense to the cervical stroma on contrast-enhanced CT. CT is also suboptimal in its ability to distinguish tumor from normal parametrial structures, leading to overestimation of parametrial involvement.[35]

Key Points Imaging of Primary Tumor

- Tumor size, parametrial invasion, and nodal spread are the most important factors to be evaluated on imaging and determine whether treatment will be surgical vs. nonsurgical, as well as the extent of treatment.
- T2-weighted images obtained perpendicular to the cervical canal are key to the evaluation of parametrial invasion.

Lymph Node Involvement

The presence and extent of nodal involvement are the most important prognostic factors in cervical cancer. In surgically treated cervical cancer, survival rates decline from 85% to 90% to 50% to 55% in the presence of nodes that are positive for tumor. In addition, the presence of metastatic adenopathy is important in treatment planning, defining radiation ports, and assessing need for and extent of surgical resection. It has been established in a multiinstitutional study that the incidence of metastatic adenopathy in early cervical cancer stage IIA and below is in the range of 32%.34 The breakup of the likelihood of nodal metastasis on the basis of stage is less than 1% with stromal invasion less than 3 mm. However, in the presence of stromal invasion between 3 and 5 mm, this increases to 7%. In the larger stage IB2 tumors, this increases to 20% to 25%.

Computed Tomography and Magnetic Resonance Imaging in Evaluation of Nodal Involvement

CT and MRI have comparable accuracies, in the range of 83% to 85%, in the assessment of nodal involvement. This is because both techniques rely on nodal enlargement (current definition of metastatic nodes: >1 cm on the short axis) as the criterion for malignant involvement.[11] The limitation of both techniques is a low sensitivity, in the range of 24% to 70%, which is owing to the inability to detect metastasis in normal-sized nodes. However, although neither technique can distinguish inflammatory from malignant nodes, the specificity is reportedly high, in the range of 89% to 93%. It has also been observed that there is an up to 27% incidence of necrotic adenopathy in cervical cancer, which has a positive predictive value of 100%[36] (Fig. 26.12). In an effort to improve accuracy in the assessment of nodal involvement, a variety of new MRI techniques are being evaluated, including the use of ultrasmall supraparamagnetic iron oxide (USPIO) particles and DWI. The use of USPIO particles has been reported to improve sensitivity on MRI from 29% to 93%; however, this agent is currently not available in the United States.[37] Although initial work suggested the calculation of ADC values on DWI improved sensitivity of nodal involvement, the value of DWI remains controversial and unproven at the current time.[23,38,39]

At our institution, we believe that, in the assessment of nodal disease, it is important to incorporate the location of nodes into the evaluation of involvement. In other words, nodes along the anticipated pathways of spread such as the obturator, internal iliac, and common iliac should be scrutinized with a higher sensitivity than areas in which it is less common for spread to occur, such as the lateral chain external iliac nodes. In addition, location of the tumor should also be incorporated into the assessment—for instance, if extension into the lower third of the vagina has occurred, the superficial inguinal nodes should be carefully assessed. Nodal morphology is also important in improving specificity and can be best assessed with the use of high-resolution (small–field-of-view/thin-section) images. The morphologic features most useful for assessing metastatic adenopathy are irregular or spiculated margins and, as mentioned previously, necrotic or heterogeneous nodes.[40]

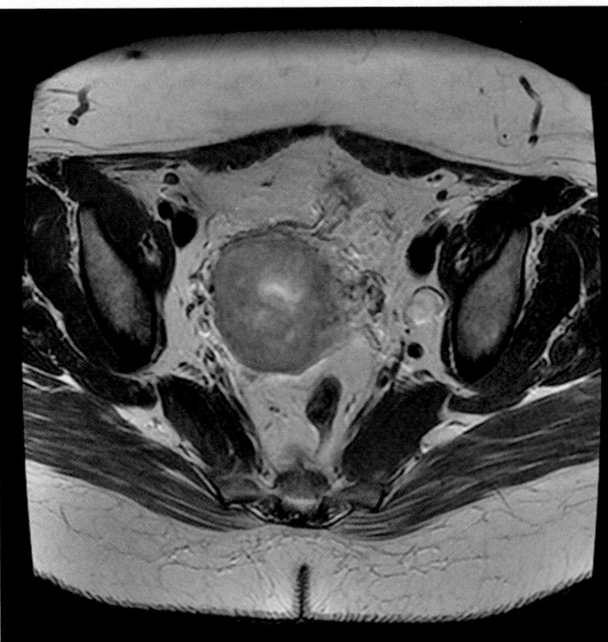

Figure 26.12. Necrotic left obturator adenopathy is identified as hyperintense nodes on T2-weighted images.

Positron Emission Tomography/Computed Tomography

In view of the low sensitivity of cross-sectional imaging in the evaluation of nodal involvement, efforts have been made to improve accuracy with the use of functional imaging modalities such as PET/CT.

The use of PET/CT has improved the accuracy of staging in that it has a high specificity in the detection of nodal metastasis. In addition, it improves sensitivity from the low sensitivities reported with MRI and CT to 83% to 91%; however, the problem with micrometastasis remains an issue. Metastatic nodes smaller than 5 mm are generally negative on PET.[41]

The role of PET/CT in advanced cervical tumors (1B2–IV) is supported in a number of studies.[42,43] It establishes the presence of paraaortic adenopathy with high accuracy (Fig. 26.13). It adds to the information available on CT, either by identifying nodes that were not enlarged on CT or by defining unexpected sites of disease. However, the value of PET in primary lymph staging is related to a high pretest probability of distant spread and is primarily

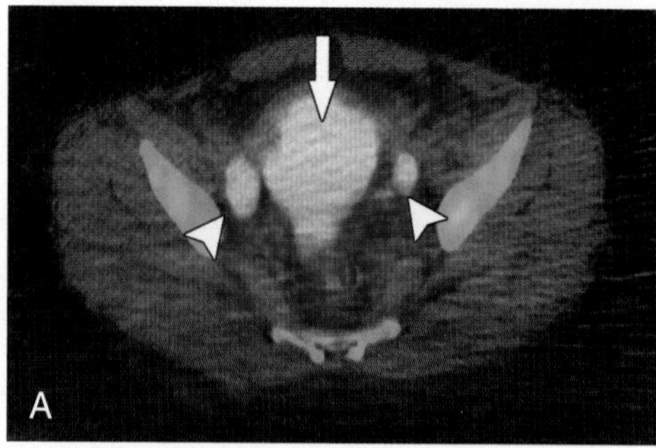

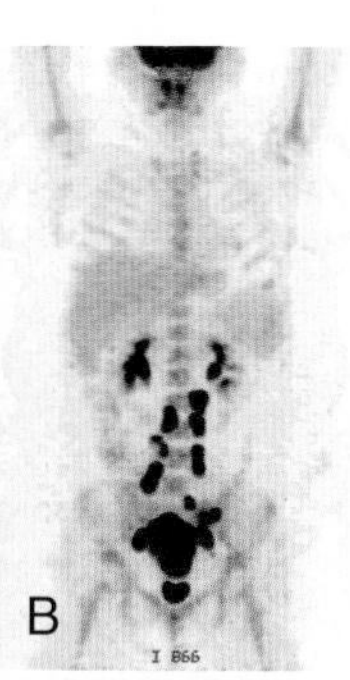

FIGURE 26.13. A 31-year-old with poorly differentiated adenocarcinoma. **A**, Axial fused positron emission tomography/computed tomography scan shows 2-[18F] fluoro-2-deoxy-D-glucose (FDG) uptake in enlarged bilateral obturator nodes (*arrowheads*). There is significant FDG uptake seen in the primary cervical tumor (*arrow*). **B**, A coronal maximum intensity projection image shows extensive FDG-avid adenopathy in the retroperitoneum along the common iliac and external iliac vessels.

in patients with locally advanced disease. Its role in early resectable cancer stages IA to IIA is questionable, because the sensitivity has been found to be low, in the range of 10% to 53%.[44,45]

This has been confirmed in more recent and larger studies of 1B1- to IIA-stage cervical tumors and is related to the high incidence of micrometastases that fall below the resolution of PET-CT. In spite of the high negative predictive value of PET/CT in early-stage cervical cancer, the impact on clinical management is minimal, and lymphadenectomy along with sentinel node involvement should be performed for staging purposes in these patients.[23,46]

KEY POINTS Lymph Node Staging

- Computed tomography and magnetic resonance imaging have comparable accuracies in the evaluation of nodal involvement because both rely on nodal size as the criterion for assessment.
- Positron emission tomography/computed tomography improves the assessment of nodal involvement in patients with advanced disease but has no value in early-stage cervical cancer.

TREATMENT

The treatment of cervical cancer is surgery in early stages (stage IA and B and IIA) and chemoradiation in more advanced stages.

The treatment of advanced cervical cancer is multidisciplinary. Women with malignant adenopathies, bulky stage IB2 tumors (primary tumor >4 cm), and higher stages are at higher risk for local and/or distant recurrences. However, the significant decline in mortality associated with cervical cancer is related primarily to early diagnosis. In advanced disease, there has been no significant improvement in survival statistics.

Concurrent Chemoradiation

In 1999, the National Cancer Institute (NCI) consensus established the standard of care in the United States, which is still valid today (available online at http://www.nih.gov/news/pr/feb99/nci-22.htm). The addition of platinum-based chemotherapy with radiation improved survival by approximately 10%.[47–49] For the last 10 years, there has been very little outcome improvement for women with cervical cancer.

A metaanalysis that included 4580 patients from [19] randomized trials confirmed the NCI consensus. If modern radiation facilities are available, concurrent chemoradiation is superior to radiotherapy alone in terms of higher local control and decreased incidence of distant relapses with both platinum and nonplatinum chemotherapy.[50]

Chemotherapy Considerations

Most chemotherapy regimens for cervical cancer are based on the use of cisplatin. Two regimens are recommended by the NCI 1999 consensus: either weekly cisplatin at 40 mg/m2 for six doses or two cycles of cisplatin and 5-fluorouracil during days 1 through 5 and days 22 through 26 of radiation.2,20 The most commonly used regimen is cisplatin at a dose of 40 mg/m2 for 6 weeks during radiation treatment. The number of cisplatin chemotherapy cycles is independently predictive of progression-free survival (PFS) and overall survival (OS). Patients who received fewer than six cycles of cisplatin have a worse PFS and OS. In addition, advanced stage, longer time to radiotherapy completion, and absence of brachytherapy are associated with decreased PFS and OS ($P < 0.05$).

Neoadjuvant Chemotherapy Followed by Surgery

The administration of chemotherapy, in a neoadjuvant setting, reduces tumor volume, potentially kills micrometastases, and renders radical surgery feasible in initially inoperable cases. The rationale for neoadjuvant chemotherapy is that a viable tumor will be more sensitive to the cytocidal effects of the anticancer drugs because of the uncompromised blood supply. A metaanalysis of individual patient data reviewed the efficacy of neoadjuvant chemotherapy followed by surgery compared with radiotherapy alone.[50] The combined results from five trials indicated a highly significant reduction in the risk of death with neoadjuvant chemotherapy, despite some differences in design and results between trials, in a population of 872 women. The timing and dose intensity of the cisplatin-based neoadjuvant chemotherapy are essential, with a dose-dense strategy being the most beneficial. Dose-dense neoadjuvant chemotherapy was investigated in a randomized study of 142 patients. The regimen was well-tolerated, with an overall clinical response rate of 69.4%. Benefits included reduction in tumor size, elimination of pathologic risk factors, and improvement of prognosis in responding patients. Dose-dense also avoids delays of other primary treatments for nonresponders.

Two phase II studies compared neoadjuvant chemotherapy followed by surgery to chemoradiation.[51,52] No difference in outcome was observed. Randomized phase III studies are ongoing to definitely answer whether this strategy is also optimal. When modern radiation facilities are not available, or if the patient prefers, neoadjuvant chemotherapy before radical surgery is an acceptable treatment approach.

Neoadjuvant Chemotherapy Followed by Radiotherapy

This sequential therapy has been studied for 30 years. A metaanalysis showed a trend for inferior survival when this treatment strategy was used.[53] Altered growth kinetics after chemotherapy probably decreases the effectiveness of radiotherapy.

A recent metaanalysis of 2946 patients reviewed data from 23 trials. Chemotherapy cycle lengths of 14 days or shorter ($P = 0.046$) or cisplatin dose intensities greater than or equal to 25 mg/m2 per week ($P = 0.20$) provided a survival advantage in favor of neoadjuvant chemotherapy. Longer cycle lengths or low cisplatin dose were detrimental. The metaanalysis reported an increase of 7% in the 5-year survival rate with chemotherapy cycles shorter than 14 days versus an 8% decrease in 5-year survival for those treated with longer cycles. The absolute reduction in the 5-year survival for the group with low intensity was 11%, whereas in the second group with high-dose intensity an increase of 3% in 5-year survival was noted. Adjuvant neoadjuvant chemotherapy followed by radiation, even with a dose-dense strategy, is not recommended until further clinical data are available from a randomized study comparing dose-dense neoadjuvant before radiation with concurrent chemoradiation.[54]

Role of Adjuvant Chemotherapy After Completion of Primary Treatment

There are scant data to support adjuvant chemotherapy after completion of concurrent chemoradiation or neoadjuvant chemotherapy followed by surgery. This topic is currently under active clinical investigation. The Radiation Therapy Oncology Group is sponsoring a trial of four courses of chemotherapy with paclitaxel and carboplatin every 21 days versus observation after concurrent chemoradiation in patients with positive pelvic or paraaortic nodes or invasion of the parametrium who have undergone radical hysterectomy with complete resection for clinical stage IA2, IB, or IIA disease. Another phase III study evaluated the role of gemcitabine in addition to cisplatin during chemoradiation followed by two courses of adjuvant gemcitabine and cisplatin in patients with stage IB2 and greater.[54] This study showed a significantly improved survival for the gemcitabine addition arm compared with concurrent radiation with single-agent cisplatin. Survival outcome results in the control arm are consistent with those reported in other studies of concomitant chemotherapy and radiation therapy for cervical cancer, suggesting that the superiority of the gemcitabine-containing arm is not as a result of underperformance of the control arm. The main survival improvement was related to improved distant control with the gemcitabine-containing regimen. However, the rate of adverse events was increased with the addition of gemcitabine, but grade 3 to 4 events were clinically manageable in the context of a survival benefit. This study does not dissociate the adjuvant chemotherapy with the addition of gemcitabine during chemoradiation. Patients with a poor response to initial multidisciplinary treatment may benefit from adjuvant chemotherapy, but results from randomized studies are necessary before this strategy is used as a standard of care.

Treatment of Stage IV Disease

The most common site of distant disease is the lungs, via the lymph vessels. Peritoneal seeding occurs in 20% to 30% of patients and may be associated with ascites, abdominal pain, and bowel obstruction. The adenocarcinomas histologic subtype spreads often to the liver. These patients should be treated primarily with chemotherapy, but palliative radiation may be indicated in some circumstances.

KEY POINTS Management Strategies for Patients With Primary Cervical Cancer

Early Stages
- Surgery.
- Radiotherapy.

Advanced Disease
- Primary chemoradiation, which is the standard of care in the United States.
- Neoadjuvant chemotherapy, followed by radical hysterectomy and subsequent chemoradiation as indicated.
- In very selected cases, primary radical hysterectomy and lymphadenectomy followed by tailored radiotherapy with concomitant chemotherapy.

Treatment of Recurrence

An isolated metastasis should be treated with curative intent. If the recurrence is small (<3 cm), chemoradiation is used. For larger areas, the lesion should be resected first and followed by chemoradiation. If the lesion is unresectable because of location or size, neoadjuvant chemotherapy with the combination of drugs that offers the best chances of response should be used, followed by surgery if the patient has a response.

Patients with multiple sites of metastases should be enrolled in a clinical trial. Patients who are ineligible for clinical trials should be offered simple palliative chemotherapy focusing on minimizing morbidity. For recurrent cervical cancer, the current treatment remains carboplatin and paclitaxel.[55] Non–platinum-based regimens are being explored in patients with recurrent disease who had prior platinum exposure.[56]

KEY POINTS Treatment of Recurrence

- Central recurrence: Exenteration.
- Isolated recurrence anywhere: Curative treatment intent with multimodalities.
- Widespread recurrence: Clinical trial; if clinical trial not available, palliative treatment with single-agent chemotherapy to minimize adverse events or palliative radiotherapy.

NEW THERAPIES

Bevacizumab, a monoclonal antivascular endothelial growth factor antibody, and pazopanib, a vascular endothelial growth factor receptor inhibitor, have been evaluated in clinical trials and have increased the progression-free interval in patients with recurrent disease.[57,58] Epidermal growth factor receptor (EGFR) tyrosine kinase inhibitors are ineffective in patients with refractory cervical cancer.[59] Cetuximab, a monoclonal inhibitor of the extracellular domain of EGFR, may have modest efficacy in patients with refractory recurrence.[60,61]

KEY POINTS New Therapies

- Antiangiogenic agents.
- Possibly monoclonal antibodies against epidermal growth factor receptor.
- Clinical trials.

SURVEILLANCE

The majority of patients who develop recurrent disease do so within 2 years of treatment of the primary malignancy. Consequently, for this period, there should be close follow-up every 3 months. Subsequently, a 6-month evaluation can be obtained for the next 3 years, and after 5 years, an annual follow-up is standard of care.

In cervical cancer, half of the recurrences are within the pelvis; the most common sites are the vaginal cuff, cervix, parametrium, and pelvic sidewalls. Patients at high risk for recurrence or those who develop symptoms such as pain or vaginal bleeding should immediately be evaluated with imaging, particularly in the initial 2-year period. This can be with MRI, CT, or PET/CT. The goal remains the early detection of local disease and accurate characterization of local and distant spread to identify patients who may be eligible for a pelvic exenteration.

Traditionally, CT is the most widely used modality in the follow-up of patients. However, it is limited in distinguishing posttreatment change from tumor.[62] The presence of baseline posttreatment scans can somewhat obviate this problem by providing a comparison for follow-up CT scans. Any interval change identified on subsequent scans raises the possibility of recurrent disease.

MRI with superior soft-tissue resolution has some advantages over CT, particularly when combined with dynamic scanning. The combination of T2W images and early enhancement on dynamic scanning (<90 sec) has a high sensitivity (91%) but the specificity, although improved over evaluation with only T2W images, remains low (67%).[63]

Recent reports suggest that PET/CT detects recurrence earlier than CT or MRI.[64] Studies using PET for surveillance of patients with no evidence of disease after primary treatment found a high sensitivity (90.3%) but a lower specificity (76.1%) for detection of recurrent disease. The recurrences were also detected earlier (at 9 to 12 months) than the historical average of 2 years, suggesting that this technique is more sensitive than previously used modalities and clinical examination. The additional value of PET/CT is the documentation of distant sites of disease, the presence of which could influence treatment decisions. The disadvantage of PET remains its low specificity and poor anatomic detail. Consequently, a reasonable strategy in the follow-up of patients with a high probability for recurrence would be to leverage the sensitivity of PET or MRI, supplemented by biopsy. If PET is used and identifies recurrence, an MRI of the pelvis should then be added in patients who are potential surgical candidates for pelvic exenteration or other radical surgeries. Alternatively, if MRI is the primary follow-up modality and if equivocal, a PET may be obtained to clarify the issue.

KEY POINTS Surveillance

- Tumor recurrence is most common in the 2 years after primary treatment, and close follow-up should be obtained every 2 to 3 months during this time period.
- Three fourths of recurrences are within the pelvis; the most common sites are the vaginal cuff, cervix, parametrium, and pelvic sidewalls.
- Follow-up should preferably be with positron emission tomography/computed tomography or magnetic resonance imaging.

REFERENCES

1. Siegel RL, Miller KD, Jemal A. Cancer statistics, 2019. *CA Cancer J Clin*. 2019;69:7–34.
2. Arbyn M, Weiderpass E, et al. *Lancet Glob Health*. 2020;8:e191–e203.
3. de Kok IM, van der Aa MA, van Ballegooijen M, et al. Trends in cervical cancer in the Netherlands until 2007: has the bottom been reached? *Int J Cancer*. 2011;128:2174–2181.
4. Ronco G. *Lancet*. 2014;383:524–532.
5. Gissmann L, Wolnik L, Ikenberg H, et al. Human papillomavirus types 6 and 11 DNA sequences in genital and laryngeal papillomas and in some cervical cancers. *Proc Natl Acad Sci U S A*. 1983;80(2):560–563.
6. McClung NM, Gargano JW, Bennett NM, et al. Trends in human papillomavirus vaccine types 16 and 18 in cervical precancers, 2008-2014. *Cancer Epidemiol Biomarkers Prev*. 2019;28(3):602–609.
7. Folgasher M, Walsh J. CT anatomy of the female pelvis: a second look. *Radiographics*. 1994;14:51–66.
8. Querleu D. *Lancet Oncol*. 2008;9:297–303.
9. Kaur H, Silverman P, Iyer R, et al. Diagnosis, staging and surveillance of cervical carcinoma. *AJR Am J Roentgenol*. 2003;180:1621–1631.
10. McMohan C, Rofsky NM, Pedrosa I. Lymphatic metastasis for pelvic tumors: anatomic classification, characterization and staging. *Radiology*. 2010;254:31–46.
11. Cervix uteri . In: Amin MB, ed. *AJCC Cancer Staging Manual*. 8th ed. New York: Springer; 2017:649–659.
12. Amendola MA, Hricak H, Mitchell DG, et al. Utilization of diagnostic studies in the pretreatment evaluation of invasive cervical cancer in the United States: results of intergroup protocol ACRIN 6651/GOG 183. *J Clin Oncol*. 2005;23:7454–7459.

13. Bhatla N, et al. *Int J Gynecol Obstet*. 2019;145:129–135.
14. Poka R, et al. *Int Journal of Gynecological Cancer*. 2017;27:1438–1445.
15. Ramirez P, et al. *Gynecologic Oncology*. 132(1):254–259.
16. Petereit D, et al. *Int J of Gynecolog Canc*. 1998:353–364.
17. Martimbeau PW, et al. *Obstet Gynecol*. 1982;60:215–218.
18. Koh W, et al. *J Natl Comp Canc Netw*. 2019;17(1):64–84.
19. Hricak H, Gatsonis C, Chi D, et al. Role of imaging in pretreatment evaluation of early cervical cancer: results of the Intergroup Study American College of Radiology Imaging Network 6651—Gynecologic Oncology Group 183. *J Clin Oncol*. 2005;23:9329–9337.
20. Sala E, Wakely S, Senior E, et al. MRI of malignant neoplasms of the uterine corpus and cervix. *AJR Am J Roentgenol*. 2007;188:1577–1587.
21. Balleyguier C, et al. *European Radiology*. 2011;21:1102–1110. Rauch, et al. *Radiographics*. 2014;34:1082–1098.
22. Kojima Y, Yoichi A, Hiroaki K, et al. Carcinoma of the cervix: value of dynamic magnetic resonance imaging in assessing early stromal invasion. *Int J Clin Oncol*. 1998;3:143–146.
23. Sala E, et al. *Radiology*. 2013;266:717–740.
24. Park JJ. *Radiology*. 2014;274:734–741.
25. Hricak H, Lacey CG, Sandles LG, et al. Invasive cervical carcinoma comparison of MR imaging and surgical findings. *Radiology*. 1998;166:623–631.
26. Kim SH, Choi BI, Lee HP, et al. Uterine cervical carcinoma: comparison of CT and MR findings. *Radiology*. 1990;175:45–51.
27. Peppercorn PD, Jeyarajah AR, Woolas R, et al. Role of MR imaging in the selection of patients with early cervical cancer for fertility preserving surgery: initial experience. *Radiology*. 1999;212:395–399.
28. Togashi K, Morikawa K, Kataoka LM, et al. Cervical cancer. *J Magn Reson Imaging*. 1998;8:391–397.
29. Hricak H, Yu KK. Radiology in invasive cervical cancer. *AJR Am J Roentgenol*. 1996;167:1101–1108.
30. Bipat S, Glas AS, van der Velden J, et al. Computed tomography and magnetic resonance imaging in staging of uterine cervical carcinoma: a systemic review. *Gynecol Oncol*. 2003;91:59–66.
31. Rockall AG, Ghosh S, Alexander-Sefre F, et al. Can MRI rule out bladder and rectal invasion in cervical cancer to help select patients for limited EUA? *Gynecol Oncol*. 2006;101:244–249.
32. Hawighort H, Knapstein PG, Weikel W, et al. Cervical carcinoma: comparison of standard and pharmokinetic MR imaging. *Radiology*. 1996;201:531–539.
33. Mitchell DG, Snyder B, Coakley F, et al. Early invasive cervical cancer: tumor delineation by magnetic resonance imaging, computed tomography and clinical examination, verified by pathologic results in the ACRIN 6651/GOG 183 intergroup study. *J Clin Oncol*. 2006;24:5687–5694.
34. Hricak H, Gatsonis C, Coakley F, et al. Early invasive cervical cancer: CT and MR imaging in preoperative evaluation—ACRIN/GOG comparative study of diagnostic performance and interobserver variability. *Radiology*. 2007;245:495–498.
35. Kim SH, Choi BI, Kim JK, et al. Preoperative staging of uterine cervical carcinoma: comparison of CT and MRI in 99 patients. *J Comput Assist Tomogr*. 1993;17:633–640.
36. Yang WT, Lam WW, Yu MY, et al. Comparison of dynamic helical CT and dynamic MRI in the evaluation of pelvic nodes in cervical carcinoma. *AJR Am J Roentgenol*. 2000;175:759–766.
37. Rockall AG, Sohaib SA, Harisinghani MG, et al. Diagnostic performance of nanoparticle-enhanced magnetic resonance imaging in the diagnosis of lymph node metastasis in patients with endometrial and cervical cancer. *J Clin Oncol*. 2005;23:2813–2821.
38. Dappa E, et al. *Insights Imaging*. 2017;8:471–481.
39. Lin G, Ho KC, Wang JJ, et al. Detection of lymph node metastasis in gynecologic cancer by diffusion weighted magnetic resonance imaging at 3 Tesla. *J Magn Reson Imaging*. 2008;28:128–135.
40. Choi HJ, Seung HK, San-Soo S, et al. MRI for pretreatment lymph node staging in uterine cervical cancer. *AJR Am J Roentgenol*. 2006;187:W538–W543.
41. Sironi S, Picchio M, Perego P, et al. Lymph node metastasis in patients with clinical early stage cervical cancer: detection with integrated FDG PET/CT. *Radiology*. 2006;238:272–279.
42. Rose PG, Adler LP, Rodriguez M, et al. Positron emission tomography for evaluating para-aortic nodal metastasis in locally advanced cervical cancer before surgical staging: a surgicopathologic study. *J Clin Oncol*. 1999;17:41–45.
43. Chao A, Ho KC, Wang CC, et al. Positron emission tomography in evaluating the feasibility of curative intent in cervical cancer patients with limited distant lymph node metastases. *Gynecol Oncol*. 2008;110:172–178.
44. Wright JD, Dehdashti F, Herzog TJ, et al. Preoperative lymph node staging of early stage cervical carcinoma by FDG PET. *Cancer*. 2005;104:2484–2491.
45. Chou HH, Chang TC, Yen TC, et al. Low value of FDG-PET in primary staging of early-stage cervical cancer prior to radical hysterectomy. *J Clin Oncol*. 2006;24:123–128.
46. Signorelli M, et al. *Gynecologic Oncology*. 2011;123:236–240.
47. Keys HM, Bundy BN, Stehman FB, et al. Cisplatin, radiation, and adjuvant hysterectomy compared with radiation and adjuvant hysterectomy for bulky stage IB cervical carcinoma. *N Engl J Med*. 1999;340:1154–1161. Erratum in: *N Engl J Med*. 1999;341:708.
48. Morris M, Eifel PJ, Lu J, et al. Pelvic radiation with concurrent chemotherapy compared with pelvic and para-aortic radiation for high-risk cervical cancer. *N Engl J Med*. 1999;340:1137–1143.
49. Rose PG, Bundy BN, Watkins EB, et al. Concurrent cisplatin-based radiotherapy and chemotherapy for locally advanced cervical cancer. *N Engl J Med*. 1999;340:1144–1153. Erratum in: *N Engl J Med*. 1999;341:708.
50. Neoadjuvant chemotherapy for locally advanced cervical cancer. A systematic review and meta-analysis of individual patient data from 21 randomised trials. *Eur J Cancer*. 2003;39:2470-2486.
51. Whitney CW, Sause W, Bundy BN, et al. Randomized comparison of fluorouracil plus cisplatin versus hydroxyurea as an adjunct to radiation therapy in stage IIB-IVA carcinoma of the cervix with negative para-aortic lymph nodes: a Gynecologic Oncology Group and Southwest Oncology Group study. *J Clin Oncol*. 1999;17:1339–1348.
52. Dueñas-González A, Lopez-Graniel C, Gonzalez-Enciso A, et al. Concomitant chemoradiation versus neoadjuvant chemotherapy in locally advanced cervical carcinoma: results from two consecutive phase II studies. *Ann Oncol*. 2002;13:1212–1219.
53. Shueng PW, Hsu WL, Jen YM, et al. Neoadjuvant chemotherapy followed by radiotherapy should not be a standard approach for locally advanced cervical cancer. *Int J Radiat Oncol Biol Phys*. 1998;40:889–896.
54. Dueñas-González A, Zarba JJ, Alcedo JC, et al. A phase III study comparing concurrent gemcitabine (Gem) plus cisplatin (Cis) and radiation followed by adjuvant Gem plus Cis versus concurrent Cis and radiation in patients with stage IIB to IVA carcinoma of the cervix. *J Clin Oncol*. 2009:27 CRA5507.
55. Monk BJ, Sill MW, McMeekin DS, et al. Phase III trial of four cisplatin-containing doublet combinations in stage IVB, recurrent, or persistent cervical carcinoma: a Gynecologic Oncology Group study. *J Clin Oncol*. 2009;27:4649–4655.
56. Tewari KS, Monk BJ. The rationale for the use of non-platinum chemotherapy doublets for metastatic and recurrent cervical carcinoma. *Clin Adv Hematol Oncol*. 2010;8:108–115.
57. Monk B, Mas L, Zarba JJ, et al. A randomized phase II study: Pazopanib (P) versus lapatinib (L) versus combination of pazopanib/lapatinib (L+P) in advanced and recurrent cervical cancer (CC). *J Clin Oncol*. 2009;27:A5520.
58. Monk BJ, Sill MW, Burger RA, et al. Phase II trial of bevacizumab in the treatment of persistent or recurrent squamous cell carcinoma of the cervix: a gynecologic oncology group study. *J Clin Oncol*. 2009;27:1069–1074.
59. Goncalves A, Fabbro M, Lhomme C, et al. A phase II trial to evaluate gefitinib as second- or third-line treatment in patients with recurring locoregionally advanced or metastatic cervical cancer. *Gynecol Oncol*. 2008;108:42–46.
60. Kurtz JE, Hardy-Bessard AC, Deslandres M, et al. Cetuximab, topotecan and cisplatin for the treatment of advanced cervical cancer: A phase II GINECO trial. *Gynecol Oncol*. 2009;113:16–20.
61. Farley JH, Sill M, Walker JL, et al. Phase II evaluation of cisplatin plus cetuximab in the treatment of recurrent and persistent cancers of the cervix: A limited access phase II study of the Gynecologic Oncology Group. *J Clin Oncol*. 2009;27:A5521.
62. Walsh JW, Goplerud DR. Prospective comparison between clinical and CT staging in primary cervical carcinoma. *AJR Am J Roentgenol*. 1981;137:997–1003.
63. Kinkel K, Ariche M, Tardivon AA, et al. Differentiation between recurrent tumor and benign conditions after treatment of gynecologic pelvic carcinoma: value of dynamic contrast-enhanced subtraction MR imaging. *Radiology*. 1997;204:55–63.
64. Ryu SY, Kim MH, Choi SC, et al. Detection of early recurrence with 18F-FDG PET in patients with cervical cancer. *J Nucl Med*. 2003;44:347–352.

CHAPTER

27 Ovarian Cancer

Abdelrahman K. Hanafy, M.D.; Ajaykumar C. Morani, M.D.; Corey T. Jensen, M.D.; Aparna Kamat, M.D.; Patricia J. Eifel, M.D.; and Priya R. Bhosale, M.D.

INTRODUCTION

In general, the role of imaging in ovarian cancer screening is limited, because gynecologic oncologists depend more on the clinical examination and tumor markers cancer antigen 125 (CA125) to make the diagnosis. Ovarian cancers are usually detected when patients become symptomatic and are often quite large and disseminated throughout the abdomen and pelvis at the time of diagnosis. Ovarian cancers comprise a wide variety of neoplasms that differ variably in histology, grade of malignancy, and prognosis.

EPIDEMIOLOGY

Ovarian carcinoma is an aggressive disease that usually presents at an advanced stage, and remains the deadliest of all gynecologic malignancies, being the most common cause of gynecologic cancer deaths. Ovarian cancer accounts for 5% of overall cancer deaths in women.[1] In the United States, approximately 22,240 new cases and 14,070 deaths because of ovarian cancer were recorded in 2018.[1]

Ovarian cancer occurs sporadically in 90% of patients but it is part of an inherited cancer-predisposition syndrome in 10% of cases.[2] Various etiologies are associated with ovarian cancer, but the most important risk factor is a family history of the disease.[3] The familial cases are usually middle-aged, and most of them are premenopausal at presentation, in contrast to patients with sporadic disease, who are predominantly postmenopausal. Three main hereditary syndromes have been linked to these tumors. The most common of these is the breast-ovarian cancer syndrome, which has been linked to mutations in *BRCA1* and *BRCA2* tumor suppressor genes.[3,4] The lifetime risk for developing ovarian cancer ranges from 15% to 30%, although some have reported a risk as high as 60% in women with *BRCA1/2* mutations.[4] The other two syndromes are the site-specific ovarian cancer syndrome and the nonpolyposis colorectal cancer, or Lynch syndrome II. Lynch syndrome is characterized by early-onset upper gastrointestinal tract cancer, colorectal carcinoma, upper urothelial tract cancer, endometrial cancer, and ovarian cancer.[5]

BRCA1 mutations have also been found in 8% to 10% of sporadic ovarian cancers.[6] One of the theories suggested for ovarian cancer development is "incessant ovulation," although this is still controversial.[7–9] This hypothesis suggests that repeated minor trauma related to ovulation and repair predisposes the ovary to neoplasia. Several observations support this theory, such as the higher risk associated with nulliparity, early menarche, and late menopause. Conversely, multiparity, late menarche, early menopause, and use of oral contraceptives (i.e., fewer ovulation cycles) are associated with lower risk.[10] This theory can also describe the geographic differences in prevalence of ovarian cancer rates, as ovarian cancer prevalence is higher in industrialized countries where women tend to have fewer children, while the risk is lower in countries where birth rates are higher.[11]

Key Points Epidemiology

- Ovarian cancer is the deadliest gynecologic cancer.
- It usually occurs in older, postmenopausal females and is sporadic in 90% of cases.
- However, 10% of cases are associated with hereditary syndromes such as breast-ovarian cancer syndrome, site-specific ovarian cancer syndrome, and Lynch syndrome II. These tend to occur at a younger age and in premenopausal patients.

ANATOMY

The ovaries are oval intraperitoneal structures located within the pelvis that measure between 3 and 5 cm. Each ovary is attached to the broad ligament by the mesovarium, to the uterine body by the uteroovarian ligament, to the fallopian tubes by the tuboovarian ligament, and to the lateral pelvic wall by the suspensory ligaments. Tumor can spread via these ligaments to the adjacent pelvic organs. The ovarian surface epithelial cells (Fig. 27.1), which are derived from the coelomic epithelium, form the outer lining of the ovaries. The internal structure of the ovary is made of dense fibrous tissue, also called the stroma, and is derived from the mesenchymal cells. The oocytes, which are also known as the germ cells, are located along the periphery of the stroma. These germ cells form the follicles, which are surrounded by specialized cells of the mesonephric origin called granulosa cells. Stromal cells immediately surrounding the follicle are called theca cells. The hilus cells of the ovary are similar

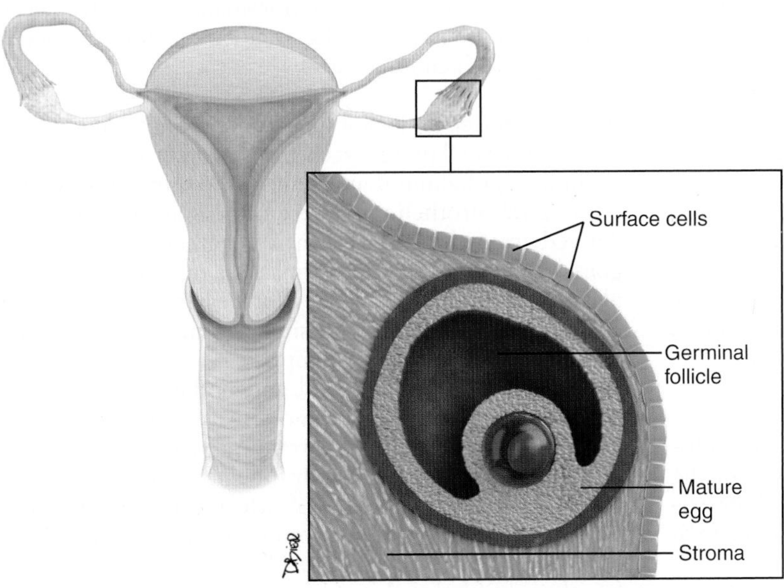

FIGURE 27.1. Anatomy of the ovary.

to the testicular cells, known as Leydig cells, and produce hormones. The rete ovary is a network of cellular cords and tubes that is similar to the rete testes of the testicles.[12]

KEY POINTS Ovarian Anatomy

- The ovary is attached via various ligaments, through which tumor dissemination can occur.
- The ovarian surface is covered by epithelial cells.
- The internal structure of the ovary is derived from the mesenchymal cells.
- Oocytes form the germinal follicles, which are surrounded by granulosa and theca cells.

CLASSIFICATION

Histopathologic classification of ovarian tumors was developed by the World Health Organization, while staging is most commonly performed following the International Federation of Gynecology and Obstetrics (FIGO) system, which was revised and republished in 2014.[13,14]

Ovarian tumors can be divided according to their cell of origin into three major categories—surface epithelial tumors, sex cord–stromal tumors, and germ cell tumors (GCTs). Approximately 90% of primary ovarian malignancies arise from the surface epithelium, which is similar to peritoneal mesothelium, the lining of peritoneal cavities, and both are derived from the coelomic epithelium.[12] Ovarian GCTs arise from germ cells. Sex cord–stromal tumors include tumors of mesonephric and mesenchymal origin. Combinations of different tumor histologies can also exist within a single lesion. When two or more tumor subtypes coexist, they are designated as *mixed* tumor and are named after the dominant contributing subtypes, provided that they constitute greater than 10% of the entire tumor.

KEY POINT Histopathologic Classification

- Ovarian tumors are divided, according to their cell of origin, into three major categories—epithelial tumors, sex cord–stromal tumors, and germ cell tumors.

Epithelial Tumors

Epithelial tumors account for 90% of malignant ovarian tumors and approximately 60% of all ovarian tumors. The prevalence of these tumors usually increases with age and has a peak incidence between 60 and 70 years old. They are further divided into benign, borderline (atypical proliferation/low malignant potential), and malignant depending on their cellular proliferation.[12,15] Based on the degree of differentiation, malignant tumors can be categorized as well differentiated (10%), moderately differentiated (25%), and poorly differentiated (65%); poorly differentiated tumors are associated with worse prognosis. The most common subtype of epithelial neoplasms is are the serous tumors, followed by mucinous neoplasms and then endometrioid carcinomas. Clear-cell carcinoma and Brenner tumor are the rare entities.[16] Although sometimes difficult, the goal of radiologic assessment is to differentiate malignant tumors from benign tumors, rather than determining their histologic subtype. Sometimes it may be possible to suggest the histologic subtype based on imaging features.[17]

Serous Tumors

Most serous tumors are benign (60%), whereas 15% are borderline, and approximately 25% are malignant, which are further subdivided into high-grade and low-grade serous carcinomas. Benign serous tumors are usually unilocular and filled with watery straw-colored fluid, but can also be multilocular with thin walls.[12] They usually do not have papillary projections, but, if present, they are small compared with those in the borderline tumors. In up to

57% of patients, benign serous tumors are bilateral, occurring simultaneously in both ovaries.[16]

The malignant form of these tumors tends to have a larger soft tissue component than the benign form and may also show focal areas of hemorrhage and necrosis.[18] Microcalcifications (psammoma bodies) are seen in 30% of the malignant serous tumors at histologic analysis.[19]

Serous carcinomas are also commonly bilateral in more than 50% of cases.[16] The primary neoplasm in these cases is small but may be associated with large-volume ascites. These tumors show large polypoid excrescences and may contain punctuate calcifications. Peritoneal carcinomatosis and omental caking are invariably seen in this setting.

Mucinous Tumors

Mucinous tumors cells can resemble the cells of the endocervical epithelium (endocervical or müllerian type) or the epithelium of the intestine (intestinal type).[12] Approximately 80% of mucinous tumors are benign, 10% to 15% are borderline, and 5% to 10% are malignant.[17]

Benign mucinous tumors are usually multilocular with thin-walled locules filled with mucin, but they can also be complicated with hemorrhage. One fourth of all benign ovarian neoplasms are mucinous tumors, and 75% to 85% of all mucinous ovarian tumors are benign.[12] Benign mucinous tumors most frequently occur between the third and the fifth decades of life[20] and are bilateral 21% of the time.[16] Borderline mucinous tumors are similar to benign mucinous tumors, but they may have solid soft tissue nodules or papillary projections. The malignant counterpart has more solid components than borderline tumors. Following rupture of these tumors, the endocervical mucinous type may be associated with mucinous implants whereas the intestinal type may cause pseudomyxoma peritonei. However, it should be noted that most cases of pseudomyxoma peritonei arise from mucinous tumors of the appendix with secondary involvement of ovaries.[12]

Endometrioid Tumors

Endometrioid tumors arise from transformed cells of the coelomic epithelium that resemble the endometrium. They are thought to be due to aberrant endometrial cells present outside the uterus in situations such as endometriosis, and are associated with hyperplasia or cancer of the endometrium that is deposited on the ovary.

These tumors are often malignant and may be cystic or predominantly solid.[21] These are the second most common malignant ovarian surface epithelial tumors, after malignant mucinous tumors, and occur in the sixth decade of life.[20,21] Approximately 26% of these tumors are bilateral.[16] Most malignant endometrioid tumors are confined to the ovaries and adjacent pelvic structures; 20% to 25% are associated with endometrial carcinoma.[12] Malignant ovarian endometrioid carcinomas are considered to have a better prognosis than either mucinous or serous carcinomas.

Clear-Cell Tumors

Clear-cell tumors are the epithelial ovarian tumors that are formed by clear, peglike or hobnail-like cells.[12,22] These tumors are usually cystic and unilocular, containing solid rounded intramural nodules. Most clear cell tumors are malignant, and represent 4% to 5% of all malignant ovarian epithelial tumors.[12] They predominate in the fifth decade of life.[20] Approximately 50% to 70% of these tumors are associated with endometriosis.[12]

Transitional Cell Epithelial Tumors or "Brenner Tumors"

Transitional cell tumors arise from transformed cells of the coelomic epithelium that resemble the transitional epithelium or the urothelium. These tumors are thought to be derived from the surface ovarian epithelium that undergoes urothelium-like transformation (e.g., urothelial metaplasia, Walthard nests).[23] They can be benign or malignant, and may be associated with similar tumors in the urinary bladder. Brenner tumors comprise 1% to 3% of all ovarian tumors.[24] They are solid and nodular, and most are unilateral, but malignant tumors may contain intermixed solid and cystic areas with intramural nodules.[25] They can be found in conjunction with mucinous cystadenomas or other epithelial tumors.[17,21,26] Most transitional ovarian tumors are very small, asymptomatic, incidentally discovered, and clinically irrelevant. They are usually seen in the fourth and fifth decades of life.[24]

Borderline tumors (tumors with atypical proliferation and low malignant potential) are intermediate in their histologic and prognostic features between benign tumors and the clearly malignant carcinomas. Although they could be of any histologic subtype, they lack the stromal invasion. Approximately 15% to 20% of all ovarian epithelial neoplasms are of borderline subtypes. Serous tumors are the most common borderline tumors, followed by mucinous tumors.[27] Patients with borderline tumors are commonly younger by 10 to 15 years than those with malignant tumors. Malignant tumors are seen at approximately 45 years of age[17,28] and account for one fourth of all ovarian neoplasms and two thirds of all ovarian serous tumors,[12] whereas the borderline tumors occur most commonly in childbearing age, show an indolent course, and usually have a better prognosis. Serous tumors are frequently bilateral, unlike mucinous tumors. Borderline tumors are usually diagnosed at surgery, and more than 90% are stage I at presentation.[29] These tumors are usually associated with elevated CA125, similar to other epithelial tumors.[29]

KEY POINTS Epithelial Tumors

- Serous cystadenomas are cystic tumors that are usually unilocular, may be bilateral, and contain punctuate calcifications.
- Mucinous cystadenomas are cystic multilocular tumors with different fluid consistencies and no solid component.
- Endometrioid tumors have solid and cystic components and are often associated with endometrial hyperplasia or carcinoma.
- Most clear-cell cancers are malignant, and many are associated with endometriosis.
- Most transitional or Brenner ovarian tumors are very small, asymptomatic, incidentally discovered, and clinically irrelevant.

Germ Cell Tumors

GCTs arise from cells that are believed to be derived from primordial germ cells.[12] GCTs usually occur in girls and adolescent females (the peak incidence is at 15 to 19 years) and comprise 20% to 25% of all ovarian neoplasms.[21,30] Only one-third of these tumors are malignant.[31,32] Conversely, most GCTs occurring in adults are benign. Most tumors are large at presentation, and 85% of patients present with abdominal pain, which sometimes mimics appendicitis due to rupture, torsion, or hemorrhage; other symptoms include vaginal bleeding.[33]

Of all the GCTs, mature teratomas are benign, while the rest are malignant. Malignant GCTs may be divided into dysgerminomatous (the most common type) and nondysgerminomatous GCT. The most common nondysgerminomatous tumors are immature teratomas, yolk sac tumors, and mixed GCTs. Less common variants of nondysgerminomatous GCT are embryonal carcinoma, polyembryoma, and nongestational choriocarcinoma.[34]

Benign Tumors

Mature teratomas are the most common GCTs and are seen in the reproductive-age years.[12] They are made of two or more mature embryonic germ cell layers. They are almost always cystic, in which case they are called mature cystic teratomas (MCTs). MCTs are unilocular in more than 80% of cases, and are filled with sebaceous material and lined by squamous epithelium.[35] MCTs have variable appearance depending on their contents, such as hair follicles, skin glands, muscle, teeth, and other tissues. In rare cases, MCTs may undergo malignant transformation, which may occur in postmenopausal patients, and most commonly results in squamous cell carcinoma.[12]

Monodermal Teratomas. Monodermal teratomas are rare benign ovarian tumors composed predominantly of one tissue type. The most commonly described subtype is struma ovarii, which is mostly a benign tumor composed mainly of thyroid tissue, and may cause thyrotoxicosis in rare cases. Ovarian carcinoids which are usually seen in postmenopausal women and can occur as part of MCT in majority of the cases or as part of mucinous tumors. These are considered benign, but with malignant potential. Subtypes with neuroectodermal differentiation are also encountered, and these can form benign ependymoma-like tumors or more aggressive and poorly prognostic primitive neuroectodermal tumors. No imaging findings can predict or differentiate different types of monodermal teratomas; instead, type is suspected mainly based on clinical picture and Lab findings.

Malignant Tumors

Dysgerminoma. Dysgerminomas are rare and occur predominantly in young women. This tumor has a striking similarity to seminoma of the testis.[36] Dysgerminomas account for 2% or less of all ovarian tumors and only 3% to 5% of all malignant ovarian tumors; nevertheless, they represent the most common malignant ovarian germ cell neoplasm.[12,21] Unilateral tumors are more common, but 10% to 20% of dysgerminomas can be bilateral. They can be associated with congenital malformations of the genital tract and Turner syndrome. These tumors are usually solid and may contain cystic areas with hemorrhage and necrosis. Most of the dysgerminomas occur in the second and third decades of life.

Nondysgerminomas.

Immature Teratomas. Immature teratomas are rare neoplasms that represent less than 1% of all teratomas and contain primitive, immature, or embryonal structures in addition to well-developed or mature tissues.[36,37] These tumors are usually unilateral, large, and predominantly solid, grow rapidly, and occur in the first two decades of life.[12] They have a solid soft tissue component, are invariably malignant, and grow rapidly. They disseminate via the lymphatic system but may rupture and spread throughout the peritoneal cavity.

Yolk Sac Tumor (Endodermal Sinus Tumor). Endodermal sinus tumor is a rare malignant tumor, also known as yolk sac tumor, and displays cellular structures that resemble those of the primitive yolk sac.[36] The tumor usually occurs in second and third decades of life, manifests as a large unilateral, complex pelvic mass that extends into the abdomen, contains both solid and cystic components, and tends to secrete alpha-fetoprotein, which serves as the serum tumor marker for diagnosis and assessing therapy response.[12] Imaging features are noncharacteristic compared with other ovarian neoplasms.

Choriocarcinoma. Choriocarcinomas are malignant GCTs that arise from trophoblastic cellular elements.[12] They typically are solid and have a hemorrhagic appearance. The majority of the primary ovarian choriocarcinomas are not related to pregnancy (nongestational). These occur in children and young adults. They secrete beta–human chorionic gonadotropin (β-hCG), which may lead to precocious puberty and abnormal uterine bleeding. Choriocarcinomas are highly malignant and locally invasive and spread mainly via lymphatics, but seeding of the peritoneal cavity can also occur.[12]

Key Points Germ Cell Tumors

- Germ cell tumors account for 15% to 20% of all ovarian tumors.
- Mature teratomas are benign and show calcifications within mural nodules; immature teratomas are malignant and show scattered calcifications.
- Yolk sac tumors are the second most common germ cell tumors and secrete alpha-fetoprotein.
- Choriocarcinomas are rare aggressive tumors known for beta–human chorionic gonadotropin secretion and are usually widely metastatic at the time of presentation.

Sex Cord–Stromal Tumors

Sex cord–stromal tumors are thought to originate from sex cords or mesenchymal cells of the embryonic gonads. They account for approximately 8% of all ovarian tumors and affect all age groups. These tumors can be divided into two groups: the first group arises from the sex cords, such as granulosa cell tumors and Sertoli-Leydig tumors, whereas the second group arises from the gonadal stroma, such as fibromas, thecomas, and sclerosing stromal tumors.[38]

Granulosa Cell Tumor

Granulosa cell tumors are rare sex cord ovarian tumors that arise from the cells surrounding the germinal cells in the ovarian follicles. There are two major forms of granulosa cell tumors: the *adult* form, which predominantly occurs in middle-aged and older women, and the *juvenile* form, which typically occurs in children and younger women.

Adult granulosa cell tumors represent 95% of the sex cord tumors of the ovary. These tumors occur commonly in peri- and postmenopausal women. This tumor is known to secrete estrogen, which may cause endometrial hyperplasia, polyps, or even carcinoma in 5% to 25% of cases.[12,38] Juvenile granulosa cell tumors account for 5% of this category and are also associated with secretion of estrogen, which may lead to precocious puberty.

These tumors generally have nonspecific imaging findings; they usually appear as solid masses with cystic changes, but may be completely cystic, and intratumoral hemorrhage may be seen. Compared with epithelial tumors, sex cord–stromal tumors do not usually show intracystic papillary projections and are often confined to the ovary. Associated endometrial thickening may be visualized as well.

Sertoli–Leydig Cell Tumors

Sertoli–Leydig cell tumors are mostly benign tumors that arise from cells that resemble epithelial and stromal testicular cells[12] and usually occur in nulliparous women younger than 25 years.[39] These tumors are rare, produce androgens, and may cause a virilization syndrome in 30% of cases.[38]

Fibromas

Fibromas are benign tumors arising from the spindle stromal cells that form collagen.[12] They are usually seen in postmenopausal women and do not produce estrogen. Fibromas may be associated with nevoid basal cell carcinoma syndrome, also known as Gorlin syndrome.[40]

Thecomas

Thecomas arise from stromal cells, which normally surround the ovarian follicles. They are usually seen in postmenopausal women and are uncommon before the third decade of life. Unlike fibromas, thecomas are hormonally active, produce estrogen, and may cause postmenopausal uterine bleeding, endometrial hyperplasia, and endometrial cancer.

Fibrothecomas are linked to Meigs syndrome, which is associated with bilateral pleural effusions and ascites. On ultrasound (US) they are homogeneous and hypoechoic and demonstrate posterior acoustic shadowing similar to that of fibroids.

Key Points Sex Cord–Stromal Tumors

- Sex cord–stromal tumors account for 5% to 10% of all ovarian tumors.
- Granulosa cell tumors are the most common tumors in this class. They are usually seen in postmenopausal women, and secrete estrogen, which may cause postmenopausal bleeding, while estrogen secretion from juvenile granulosa cell tumors may cause precocious puberty.
- Sertoli–Leydig cell tumors are seen in females of reproductive age. They may secrete testosterone/androgens, resulting in virilization.
- Fibromas and fibrothecomas may mimic fibroids and can be associated with Meigs syndrome or Gorlin syndrome.

Metastatic Ovarian Tumors

Metastatic ovarian tumors account for approximately 15% of ovarian malignancies. Most metastatic ovarian tumors seen are of gastrointestinal origin (39%), particularly the colon and stomach, followed by breast cancer (28%).[41] These tumors are usually bilateral, large (5–10 cm), have solid and cystic components, and may mimic primary ovarian neoplasms in 25% of cases.[41]

It is important to differentiate between primary and metastatic ovarian carcinoma, because this affects both treatment and prognosis. However, there are no definite characteristic imaging findings of metastatic ovarian malignancies that can differentiate them from primary ovarian cancers.

PATTERNS OF OVARIAN TUMOR SPREAD

To recognize the radiologic findings for ovarian cancer staging, it is important to thoroughly understand the mechanism of tumor spread. Ovarian carcinoma may spread directly to the surrounding pelvic tissues, such as the fallopian tubes, uterus, and contralateral adnexa, which are commonly involved, but direct extension of the tumor to the rectum, bladder, and pelvic sidewall can also be seen.[42] Tumor dissemination beyond the pelvis can occur via three mechanisms: intraperitoneal seeding, lymphatic invasion, and hematogenous dissemination.

The most common mode of tumor spread in ovarian cancer is intraperitoneal dissemination (Fig. 27.2), and approximately 70% of patients have peritoneal metastases at staging laparotomy. Greater omentum, right subphrenic region, and pouch of Douglas are the three most commonly involved sites found at laparotomy.[43] Tumor deposits are uncommonly seen in the left subdiaphragmatic space, because the inframesocolonic space is separated by the phrenicocolic ligament on the left. Malignant cells are shed from the tumor surface into the peritoneal cavity, and they follow the normal routes of peritoneal circulation. In the upright position, they will first fall into the cul-de-sac and other dependent portions of the pelvis; in the supine position, the fluid then flows into the paracolic gutters and eventually to the diaphragm.[44] The fluid then flows more commonly to the right paracolic gutter, along the liver capsule and the diaphragm.[44] Peritoneal fluid normally drains via the lymphatics of the diaphragm to the mediastinum and via the internal mammary chain of lymph nodes.[45,46] When these diaphragmatic lymphatics become occluded by tumor cells, absorption of the peritoneal fluid is impaired, resulting in accumulation of malignant ascites.

Dissemination of the ovarian cancer tumor cells can also occur through the lymphatic system. Lymphatic metastases may result from direct absorption by the lymphatic channels of the ovary versus absorption of tumor cells by the diaphragm.[47] Ovaries have three pathways of lymphatic drainage. The main lymphatic drainage follows the ovarian veins to the left paraaortic and the right paracaval lymph nodes at the level of the renal hilum, which are the most common sites for metastatic adenopathy. Lymphatics of the broad ligament drain into pelvic lymph nodes, external iliac, hypogastric, and obturator chain.[19,45] Metastatic

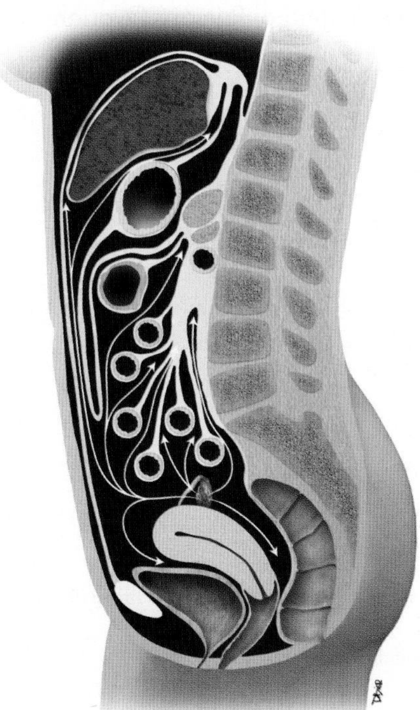

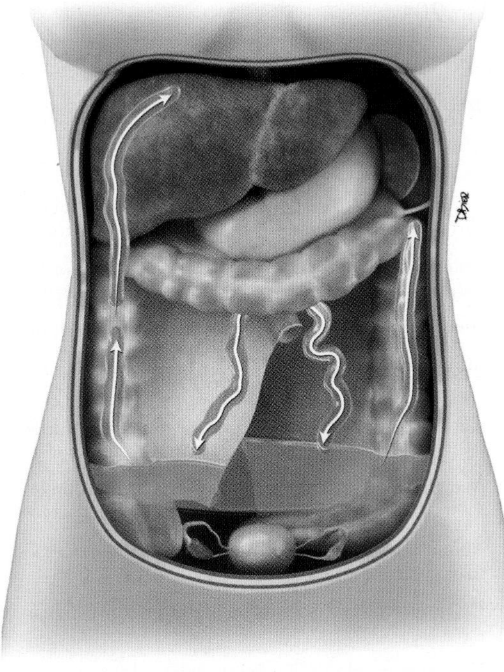

Figure 27.2. *Left,* Sagittal view. The flow of fluid in the peritoneal cavity. *Right,* Coronal view. The flow toward the left hemidiaphragm is limited by the phrenicocolic ligament.

spread to the superficial and deep inguinal nodes can be seen when tumor spreads via the round ligaments.

Hematogenous spread of disease is rare at presentation, although it has been reported in up to 50% of patients at autopsy.[19,48] The most common site of hematogenous metastasis is the liver, followed by lungs, but other locations including the brain, bone, adrenal gland, kidney, and spleen have all been reported.[19,48,49] Although most tumors may spread in this fashion, serous and clear-cell cancers predominantly spread via the lymphatics.[50,51] Some aggressive tumors such as choriocarcinoma and embryonal carcinomas commonly spread hematogenously.

STAGING

The overall prognosis for ovarian cancer is poor and decreases further when these tumors become metastatic. However, tumors of low malignant potential, formerly called "borderline ovarian tumors," have a better prognosis.[15,52] Epithelial malignancies (carcinomas) constitute the vast majority of the malignant ovarian tumors, and others include dysgerminoma, immature teratoma, yolk sac tumor, granulosa cell tumor, and metastases.[21,51] Approximately two-thirds of patients have advanced disease at the time of diagnosis.[53] Surgical exploration is typically performed to assign a disease stage based on the FIGO criteria, debulk the tumor, and confirm tumor histology.

There are two staging systems: the tumor-node-metastasis (TNM) system and the surgically-based FIGO staging system that is used worldwide and was updated in 2014.[54] The FIGO staging system is shown in Table 27.1 and Figs. 27.3 and 27.4. Accurate staging is performed with a staging laparotomy, which includes hysterectomy with bilateral salpingooophorectomy, pelvic and paraaortic lymph node biopsies, omentectomy, peritoneal biopsies, and washings.[52,55] Tumor stage is a major prognostic factor.[52] The overall 5-year survival rate depends on the tumor stage at presentation.[53] The 5-year survival rate in descending order is 80% for stage I disease, 50% for stage II, 30% for stage III, and 8% for stage IV. Almost 60% to 65% of ovarian cancer patients present with stage III disease at the time of diagnosis, making ovarian cancer one of the most lethal malignancies.[15] Several other factors can affect prognosis, such as histologic type, tumor grade, amount of residual disease after the initial cytoreductive surgery (debulking), and patient characteristics (age and performance status).[52]

Patients can be understaged if a complete staging laparotomy is not performed. In fact, ovarian cancer is understaged at initial laparotomy in more than 30% of the patients. The tumor is presumed to be localized to the pelvis in 77% of these cases, but it is subsequently found to be stage III when a full staging procedure is performed.[56] Incorrect staging may result in erroneous counselling about treatment options and prognosis. Sites of unsuspected disease most often include the pelvic peritoneum and tissues, ascitic fluid, paraaortic nodes, and diaphragm.[57]

Stage I

In stage I disease, the tumor is confined to the ovary, and the ovarian capsule is intact; or the tumor is confined to the fallopian tube, with no extension to the ovarian or fallopian tube surface, and no malignant cells are present in the ascites or peritoneal washings. Involvement of one side suggests stage IA disease, and stage IB is when both sides are involved. Surgical spill, capsular rupture before surgery, or the presence of malignant cells in the ascites or peritoneal washings upgrades the tumor to stage IC.

TABLE 27.1 The Current International Federation of Gynecology and Obstetrics Staging of Primary Ovarian Cancer, Published in 2014

CURRENT INTERNATIONAL FEDERATION OF GYNECOLOGY AND OBSTETRICS STAGING	DESCRIPTION
Stage I (T1-N0-M0)	Tumor confined to ovaries or fallopian tube(s)
IA (T1a-N0-M0)	Tumor limited to one ovary (capsule intact) or fallopian tube; no tumor on ovarian or fallopian tube surface; no malignant cells in the ascites or peritoneal washings
IB (T1b-N0-M0)	Tumor limited to both ovaries (capsules intact) or fallopian tubes; no tumor on ovarian or fallopian tube surface; no malignant cells in the ascites or peritoneal washings
IC	Tumor limited to one or both ovaries or fallopian tubes, with any of the following:
IC1 (T1c1-N0-M0)	Surgical spill
IC2 (T1c2-N0-M0)	Capsule ruptured before surgery or tumor on ovarian or fallopian tube surface
IC3 (T1c3-N0-M0)	Malignant cells in the ascites or peritoneal washings
Stage II (T2-N0-M0)	Tumor involves one or both ovaries or fallopian tubes with pelvic extension (below pelvic brim) or primary peritoneal cancer
IIA (T2a-N0-M0)	Extension and/or implants on uterus and/or fallopian tubes and/or ovaries
IIB (T2b-N0-M0)	Extension to other pelvic intraperitoneal tissues
Stage III (T1/T2-N1-M0)	Tumor involves one or both ovaries or fallopian tubes, or primary peritoneal cancer, with cytologically or histologically confirmed spread to the peritoneum outside the pelvis and/or metastasis to the retroperitoneal lymph nodes
IIIA1	Positive retroperitoneal lymph nodes only (cytologically or histologically proven): IIIA1(i) Metastasis up to 10 mm in greatest dimension IIIA1(ii) Metastasis more than 10 mm in greatest dimension
IIIA2 (T3a2-N0/N1-M0)	Microscopic extrapelvic (above the pelvic brim) peritoneal involvement with or without positive retroperitoneal lymph nodes
IIIB (T3b-N0/N1-M0)	Macroscopic peritoneal metastasis beyond the pelvis up to 2 cm in greatest dimension, with or without metastasis to the retroperitoneal lymph nodes
IIIc (T3c-N0/N1-M0)	Macroscopic peritoneal metastasis beyond the pelvis more than 2 cm in greatest dimension, with or without metastasis to the retroperitoneal lymph nodes (includes extension of tumor to capsule of liver and spleen without parenchymal involvement of either organ)
Stage IV (Any T, any N, M1)	Distant metastasis excluding peritoneal metastases
IVA	Pleural effusion with positive cytology
IVB	Parenchymal metastases and metastases to extraabdominal organs (including inguinal lymph nodes and lymph nodes outside of the abdominal cavity)

(From Prat J, FIGO Committee on Gynecologic Oncology. Staging classification for cancer of the ovary, fallopian tube, and peritoneum. *Int J Gynaecol Obstet.* 2014;124(1):1–5.)

Stage II

In stage II disease, there is local extension of the tumor into the pelvis to involve surrounding organs. Primary peritoneal cancer also falls into this stage. In this stage, tumor is confined to the pelvis without upper abdominal involvement. Stage IIA disease is characterized by either direct extension or presence of implants on the uterus and/or fallopian tubes and/or ovaries. In stage IIB disease, tumor extends to involve the surrounding pelvic tissues, rectum, bladder, and/or peritoneum. Imaging findings that suggest local extension of tumor are loss of the tissue planes between the tumor and the bladder or colon, less than 3 mm of space between the tumor and pelvic sidewall, and

FIGURE 27.3. **A**, *Top left*, Tumor in the left ovary consistent with stage IA disease. *Middle*, Tumor in both ovaries consistent with stage IB disease. *Right*, Bilateral ovarian masses and presence of malignant ascites consistent with stage IC disease. *Bottom left*, Tumor in the ovary along with tumor involving extraovarian site, however, confined to the uterus, consistent with stage IIA disease. *Bottom right*, Tumor involving the ovary and extending into other pelvic tissue, such as the rectum, consistent with stage IIB disease. **B**, The spread of tumor outside the pelvis to the abdominal area, including involvement of the right hemidiaphragm, is considered stage III. Tumor involves one or both ovaries or fallopian tubes, or primary peritoneal cancer, with cytologically or histologically confirmed spread to the peritoneum outside the pelvis and/or metastasis to the retroperitoneal lymph nodes. **C**, Parenchymal metastases and metastases to extraabdominal organs (including inguinal lymph nodes and lymph nodes outside of the abdominal cavity) are considered stage IV cancer. Tumor spread to the lungs, which may present as a pleural effusion, consistent with stage IV disease.

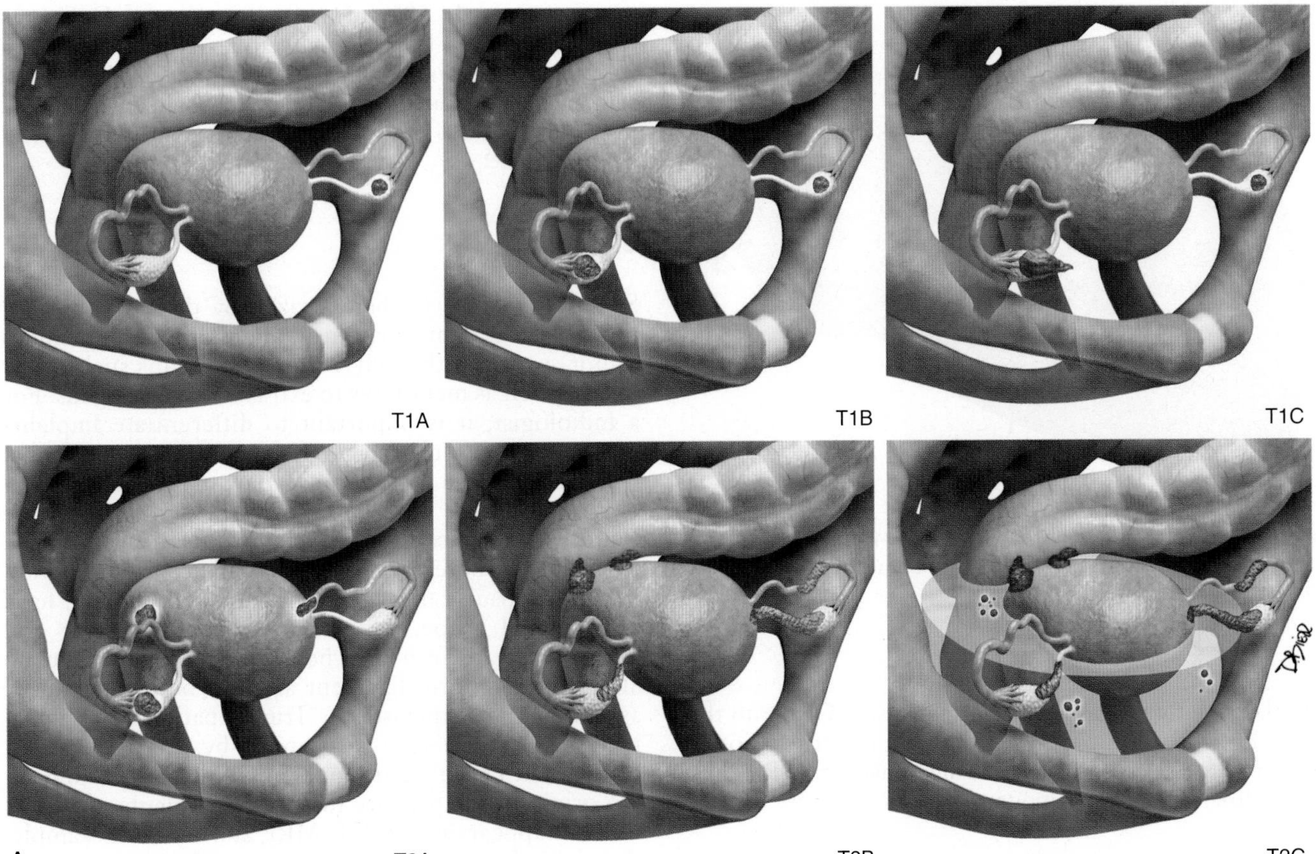

T1A T1B T1C

A T2A T2B T2C

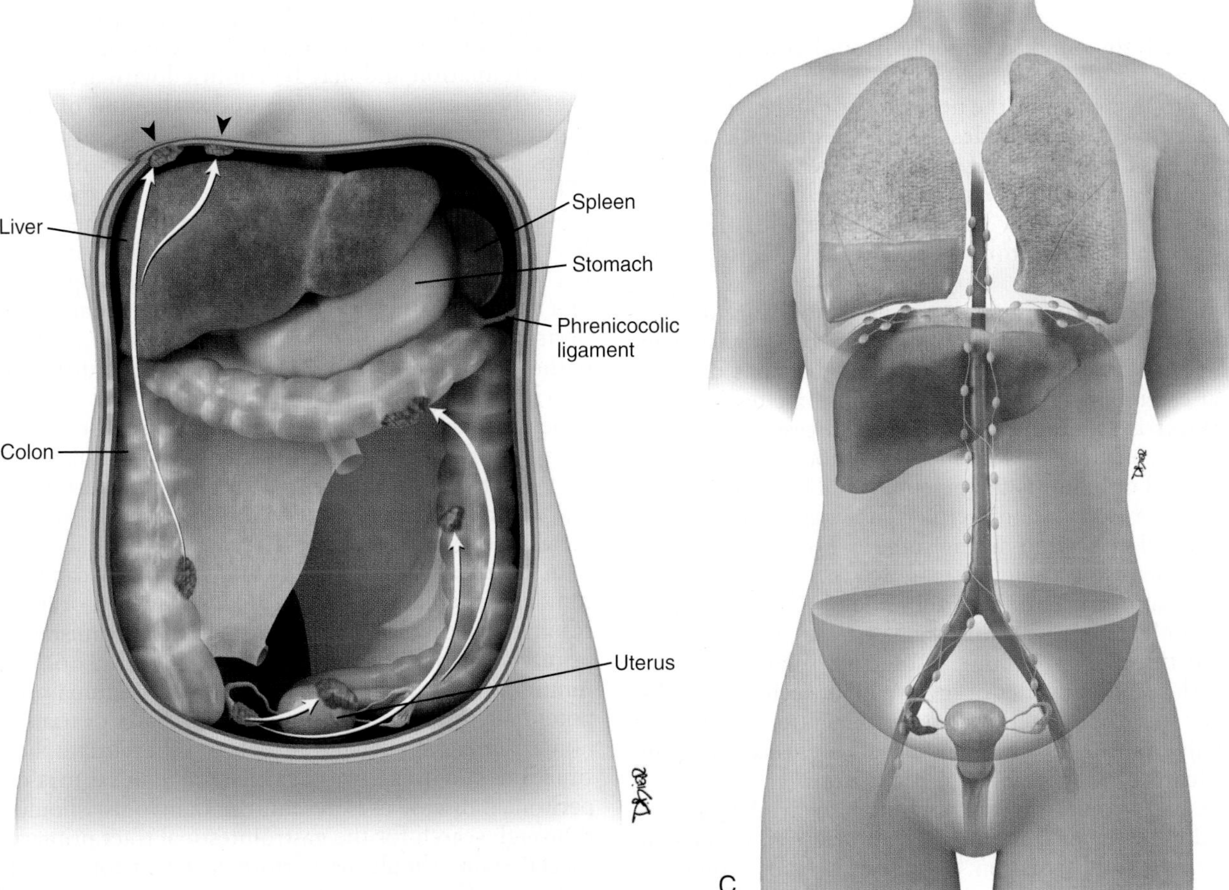

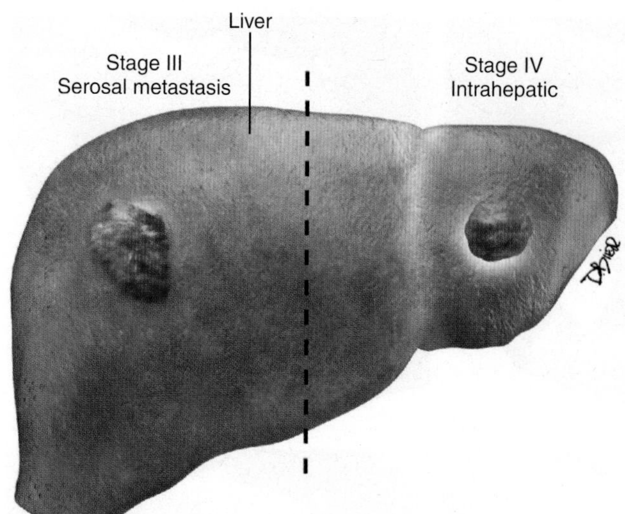

Figure 27.4. Implants on the serosal surface of the liver are consistent with stage III disease. However, liver metastases indicate stage IV disease.

displacement or encasement of iliac vessels. Owing to the superior soft tissue contrast resolution, direct invasion is better seen with magnetic resonance imaging (MRI) than with either computed tomography (CT) or US.[58]

Stage III

In stage III, the tumor is either unilateral or bilateral, but with cytologically or histologically confirmed spread to the peritoneum outside the pelvis and/or metastasis to the retroperitoneal lymph nodes. Extension of tumor outside the pelvis is considered stage III disease with the presence of peritoneal, omental, and mesenteric implants. Tiny peritoneal nodules may be undetectable with imaging, and a complete laparotomy is always indicated to detect such disease.

While interpreting images, one should look carefully for subtle peritoneal thickening, nodularity, or enhancement of the peritoneal surfaces, which are indications of peritoneal carcinomatosis.[59] The presence of ascites in ovarian cancer is suggestive of peritoneal disease and aids in lesion conspicuity.[60,61] The most common site of peritoneal spread of tumor is the omentum.[62] This involvement may be microscopic, and therefore not visible on imaging or on visual inspection during surgery; however, it can be detected on histopathology (stage IIIA2).[63] A fine reticulonodular pattern may be seen on radiology initially, but is often subtle. Later, as the disease progresses, there is often marked thickening resulting in omental caking. In addition, other common sites of involvement, such as the subphrenic space, mesentery, and paracolic gutters, should be carefully evaluated. Coronal reformats are usually helpful in evaluating the subdiaphragmatic regions.[62]

The small bowel is most commonly involved, by either serosal implants or frank bowel wall invasion, which can lead to bowel obstruction.[48] This is the most common cause of morbidity in patients and has been reported in approximately 50% of cases at autopsy.[48] On imaging, the involved bowel usually appears thickened, with resultant narrowing of the lumen. In stage III disease, retroperitoneal adenopathy has also been reported in 27% to 44% of patients, along with peritoneal disease.[62,64,65]

Stage IV

Stage IV disease is characterized by distant spread of tumor other than peritoneal metastasis, and includes tumor spread to the pelvis and solid organs such as the liver, as well as metastases to extraabdominal organs. For a radiologist, it is important to differentiate implants on the liver capsule (stage III) from true parenchymal metastases (stage IV), because they are treated differently and have a different prognostic significance (see Fig. 27.4). Surgically, capsular implants are considered resectable, whereas parenchymal metastases are not. Hepatic capsular masses are usually well defined, have an elliptical shape, and may compress the liver and rarely infiltrate into it. These implants can insinuate along the falciform ligament and can be misdiagnosed as parenchymal metastases. True hepatic parenchymal metastases are usually surrounded by the liver parenchyma and can have irregular margins. Depending on the origin of the primary tumor, the implants may have variable appearance on CT, MRI, and US. For example, the mucinous peritoneal implants exhibit low attenuation on CT scans and do not calcify. They are diffuse and insinuate between the leaves of the mesentery, bowel loops, and solid organs.[15] These implants exhibit low attenuation and may be confused with ascites; however, these cause mass effect and scalloping of the liver capsule and solid organs. Mesenteric sides of the bowel loops get matted, and subtle septations may be noted on CT. Because these implants are gelatinous, their insinuating nature makes complete resection rather difficult. It is important to know that the pseudomyxoma peritonei is now believed to originate from the appendix and metastasize to the ovary.[66] Thus, when pseudomyxoma peritonei is suspected, thorough evaluation and special pathologic staining should be performed to differentiate ovarian from gastrointestinal origin.

Serous cystadenocarcinoma implants are associated with microcalcifications, which are known as psammoma bodies.[15,45] These implants can calcify along the peritoneal lining, and this finding has been reported in 33% of cases of metastatic serous tumors.

In cases of gastric cancers and colorectal cancers, the tumor's malignant cells may deposit on the ovaries and result in large ovarian masses that can be mistaken for primary ovarian tumors (Figs. 27.5 and 27.6). These tumors may present with peritoneal carcinomatosis and potentially can be confused with metastatic ovarian carcinoma.[59] Imaging may not be able to differentiate these. In situations like this, in which bilateral adnexal masses and peritoneal disease are present, the radiologist should do a thorough search for the gastrointestinal tract primary, and special stains should be performed on histopathology in order to differentiate these entities. Other tumors such as

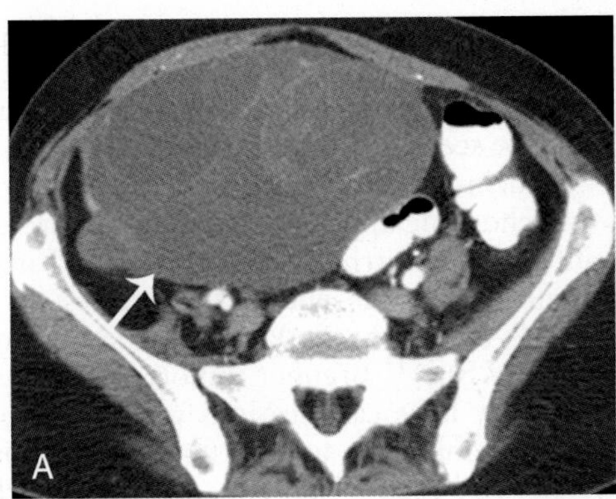

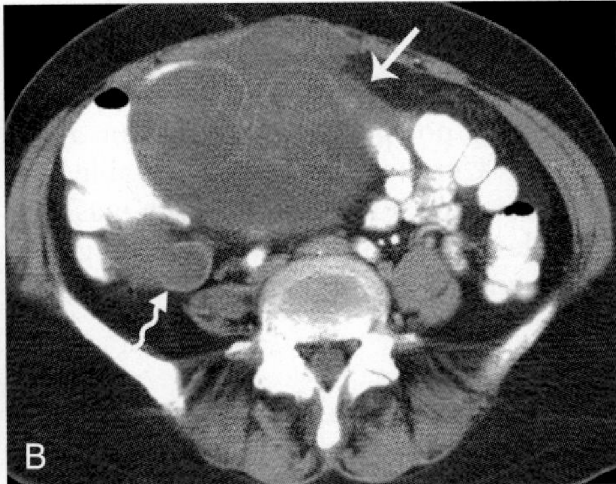

FIGURE 27.5. A 55-year-old woman with an abdominal mass. **A**, Axial contrast-enhanced computed tomography (CT) scan of the pelvis shows a large complex adnexal mass (*arrow*) with internal septations. **B**, Axial contrast-enhanced CT scan of the pelvis shows a mass in the left adnexa (*straight arrow*) and an enlarged tubular structure arising from the appendix (*wavy arrow*), representing an appendiceal mucocele with metastases to the ovary. When an adnexal mass is present, one should carefully evaluate the entire abdomen and pelvis to make sure that no other primary neoplasm is evident.

mesothelioma and papillary serous carcinoma of the peritoneum may also present in a similar manner.[51] Although rare, in the right clinical settings, infectious or inflammatory processes such a tuberculous peritonitis should also be considered as differential in these cases.[51]

KEY POINTS Federation of Gynecology and Obstetrics Staging of Ovarian Tumors

- Stage I tumor is limited to the ovaries or fallopian tubes. It has a 5-year survival rate of 73%. Treatment is surgery with or without postoperative chemotherapy.
- Stage II tumor involves pelvic extension or includes primary peritoneal cancer. It has a 5-year survival rate of 45%. Treatment is surgery with postoperative chemotherapy.
- Stage III designation is based on metastasis to the retroperitoneal lymph nodes and/or spread to the peritoneum outside the pelvis. It has a 5-year survival rate of 30%. Treatment is surgery with postoperative chemotherapy.
- Stage IV has distant metastases. It has a 5-year survival rate of 5%. Treatment is neoadjuvant chemotherapy and/or surgery.

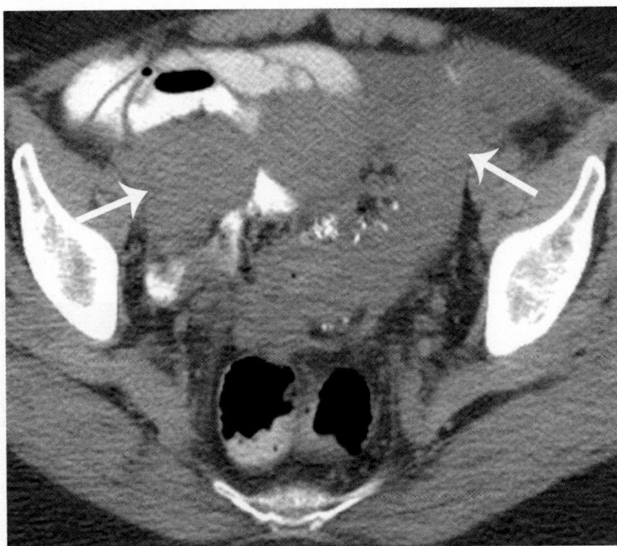

FIGURE 27.6. A 62-year-old woman, with a newly diagnosed metastatic signet-ring adenocarcinoma of unknown primary. Axial contrast-enhanced computed tomography scan of the pelvis shows enlarged enhancing ovaries (*arrows*) and a small amount of free fluid within the pelvis, suggestive of malignancy and representing Krukenberg neoplasm.

IMAGING

Role of Imaging in Diagnosing Primary Ovarian Neoplasms

Primary Tumor

Imaging helps confirm the presence of a pelvic mass, determine its site of origin, and characterize the mass. The primary role of imaging is to differentiate benign from malignant tumors. Most common modalities for clinical use are US, MRI, CT, and positron emission tomography (PET)/CT. Endovaginal US can be used to screen patients with a high risk for the development of ovarian malignancies, and is often the first modality used to determine the origin and character of a clinically-suspected pelvic mass. US is relatively inexpensive and widely available. Because tumors of the ovary arise from a variety of cells, they have different imaging appearances, which makes it difficult to definitely characterize them. Their imaging features may overlap many times, and making a subtype diagnosis is deferred until pathologic examination. However, some imaging features may point towards a specific diagnosis.

US plays an important role in the initial evaluation of a suspected adnexal mass.[67,68] When the patient's menopausal status is taken into account, CA125 levels and imaging findings facilitate the distinction between a benign from a malignant mass. This is referred to as the risk malignancy index (Table 27.2).[69] A score of 1 is given to a premenopausal female, and a score of 3 is given to a postmenopausal woman. A total score greater than 200 has high specificity for diagnosing the ovarian malignancy.[70]

Epithelial tumors usually present as large cystic masses on imaging.[51,71] The following features are suggestive of malignancy: septations greater than 3 mm; mural nodules or nonfatty solid components; homogeneous, solid masses or complex masses with cystic/solid areas; or cystic masses greater than 10 cm in diameter.[51,68] Although these features are useful, absolute characterization of the mass and prediction of histology are not possible with US or any other imaging technique. Certain features may be able to predict histology of the tumor; for example, large masses containing mural nodules and thick septations are suggestive of cystic adenocarcinomas. Serous cystic tumors are usually unilocular and may mimic physiologic cysts. However, malignancy is suspected when these unilocular cysts display papillary projections along the cystic wall, which may be seen on US, CT, or MRI (Fig. 27.7).

Mucinous tumors are typically multilocular, may have an echogenic appearance due to the presence of mucin or internal hemorrhage on the US, and may show variable signal intensities within the locules on MRI ("stained-glass" appearance). Most of these tumors are benign (Fig. 27.8).[15,17] Brenner tumors appear hypoechoic on US and may have calcifications within them. They are indistinguishable from uterine fibroids. Teratomas are typically cystic and usually contain an eccentric echogenic fat nodule, or may be completely cystic with fluid-fluid levels. The morphologic information provided by gray-scale imaging is complemented by color flow Doppler techniques. The introduction of harmonics and unique pulse sequences have improved signal-to-noise ratios and structural conspicuity, and the use of sonographic intravenous contrast agents improves the accuracy of detection and quantification of vascularity and blood flow. Contrast agents may significantly improve the diagnostic ability of US and identify early microvascular changes that are known to be associated with early-stage ovarian cancer.[72] Some of the features that predict malignancy on color Doppler include detection of central blood flow within the solid components, waveforms

TABLE 27.2 Risk Malignancy Index Based on the Product of Ultrasound Findings, Cancer Antigen 125, and Menopausal Status

	SCORE			
VARIABLE	**0**	**1**	**2**	**3**
Wall structure	Smooth <3 mm		Solid	Papillary >3 mm
Shadowing	Yes	No		
Septa	None/thin	Thick		
Echogenicity	Sonolucent, low-level echoes			Mixed or high

(From Jeong YY, Outwater EK, Kang HK. Imaging evaluation of ovarian masses. *Radiographics.* 2000;20:1445–1470.)

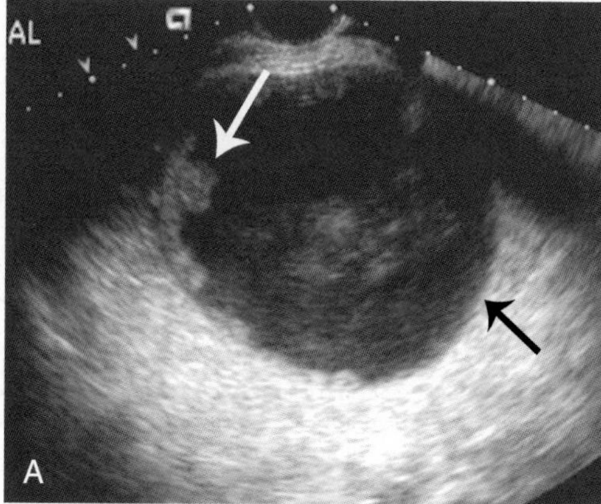

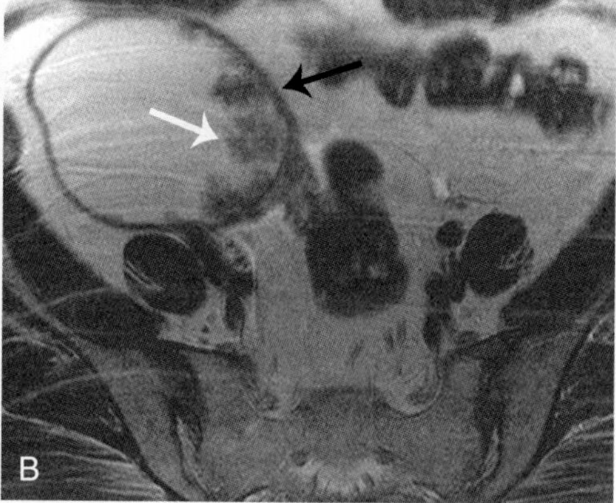

FIGURE 27.7. A 50-year-old woman with pelvic fullness on physical examination and elevated cancer antigen 125 (3800 U/mL). **A**, An endovaginal ultrasound of the pelvis shows a hypoechoic mass in the left ovary (*black arrow*) with mural nodularity (*white arrow*). **B**, Axial T2-weighted magnetic resonance imaging of the pelvis shows a unilocular cystic mass (*white arrow*) in the left ovary (*black arrow*), with mural nodularity suggesting a serous cystadenoma or a carcinoma.

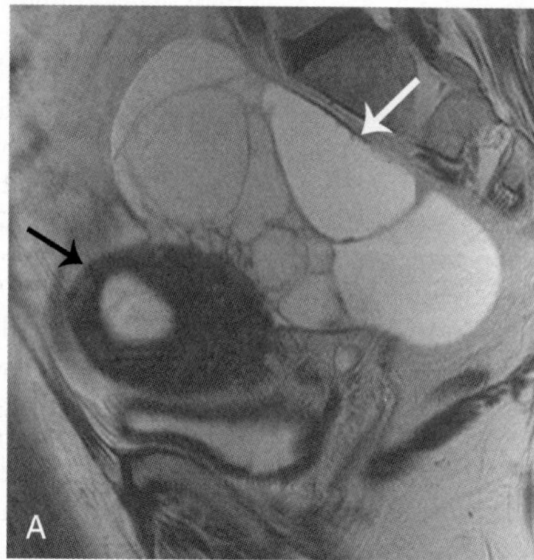

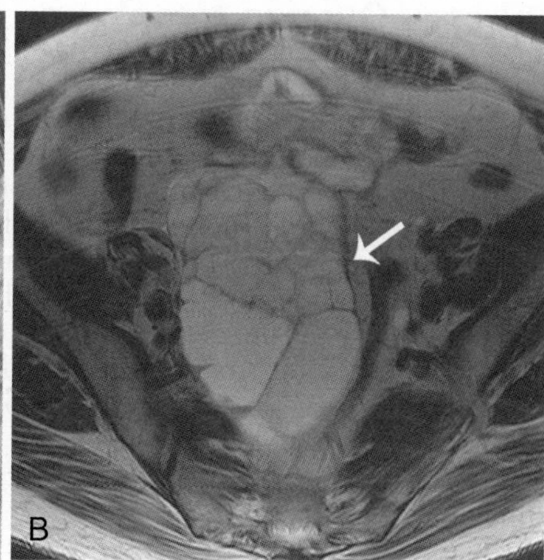

FIGURE 27.8. A 55-year-old woman with cervical cancer and pelvic mass. **A**, Sagittal T2-weighted (T2W) sequence of the pelvis shows a mass in the left ovary, which is multilocular (*white arrow*) and has varied signal intensity within the locules, representing the classic "stained-glass" appearance pathognomonic of a mucinous cystadenoma. The uterus is also seen (*black arrow*). **B**, Axial T2W image showing the multilocular mass (*arrow*).

with low resistive index (< 0.4), and a pulsatility index of 1 because ovarian cancers tend to have low-resistance flow from tumor neovascularity and arteriovenous shunting.[43] However, there is some overlap between the flow characteristics of benign and malignant lesions.[68,73] The literature suggests that adding color Doppler to morphologic information from gray-scale imagining increases the specificity of US for detection of ovarian malignancy from 82% to 97% and, the positive predictive value (PPV) from 63% to 97%.[74] Even though US is helpful in characterizing pelvic masses, its accuracy to stage cancer is low, at 60% or less.[75] The CT appearance of ovarian tumors may also vary by tumor histology. Its overall accuracy in the detection of ovarian masses approaches 95%, but its specificity in distinguishing between benign and malignant lesions ranges from 66% to 94%.[43,76] Morphologic findings such as cystic masses with septations, nodules, vegetations, or papillary projections and necrosis within solid masses suggest malignancy, as with US. However, the imaging features of ovarian masses on CT are also not entirely specific.[77] One study concluded that thin-section CT may be able to distinguish a benign from a malignant ovarian neoplasm with an accuracy of 89%.[78] Several early studies have addressed the value of CT in preoperative staging of ovarian cancer, with reported accuracies of 70% to 90%.[58,79–82]

Many adnexal lesions, particularly endometriomas and cystic teratomas, are still classified as indeterminate on US despite advances in US technology. In these situations, MRI can be used as a problem-solving tool. MRI is superior to CT in characterizing adnexal masses because it provides excellent soft tissue characterization owing to its ability to detect fat and blood products.[83,84] MRI has an overall accuracy in distinguishing benign from malignant ovarian masses of 83% to 91%.[83,85] MRI features of malignancy—such as cyst wall irregularity, intramural nodules, papillary projections, septations, complex masses containing solid and cystic components, large lesions, and early enhancement on dynamic contrast-enhanced MRI studies—are similar to those seen on CT and US. Ancillary findings such as ascites, peritoneal disease, or adenopathy help clinch the diagnosis of malignancy.[85]

On CT imaging, MCTs display fat attenuation within the cyst and often show calcifications within the cyst wall or within the cyst itself. On MRI, the sebaceous component of MCTs shows high signal intensity on T1-weighted (T1W) imaging similar to that of the subcutaneous fat. On T2-weighted (T2W) imaging, the signal intensity of the sebaceous component is variable and may be similar to that of fat (Fig. 27.9).

Dysgerminomas

On imaging, dysgerminomas are multilobulated solid masses with prominent fibrovascular septa. They may show high signal on T1W imaging owing to internal hemorrhage.

Immature Teratomas

On imaging, immature teratomas are large, complex masses with cystic and solid components, and may have scattered calcifications and small foci of fat.

Monodermal Teratomas

Monodermal teratomas, such as struma ovarii, show nonspecific imaging findings that vary by tissue type. They may have solid and cystic components. The cystic components may have a high signal on T1W imaging and T2W imaging owing to the presence of serous or mucinous fluid. Nonetheless, they may still show low signal on T1W imaging and T2W imaging owing to the thick, gelatinous colloid of the struma. Similarly, the imaging appearance of ovarian carcinoid is not well described, but high signal on T2W imaging may be noted in mucinous carcinoid tumors.

Choriocarcinomas

Choriocarcinomas contain hemorrhagic components and may show a high signal on T1W imaging. Fibromas and fibrothecomas have fibrous components that have a low signal on T1W imaging and T2W imaging and can mimic uterine fibroids (Fig. 27.10).

PET/CT is not widely used for ovarian staging, and its ability to characterize ovarian masses as benign or malignant based on metabolic activity is controversial. Hypermetabolism in an ovarian lesion in a premenopausal female may represent a benign or physiologic lesion, such as corpus luteum cysts, rather than a malignancy; however, ovarian uptake in postmenopausal women needs further evaluation with either US or MRI. Whole-body 2-[^{18}F] fluoro-2-deoxy-D-glucose (FDG)-PET scanning is not routinely used in the diagnosis and staging of primary ovarian cancer. Early studies showed sensitivities and specificities of 83% to 86% and 54% to 86%, respectively.[86–88]

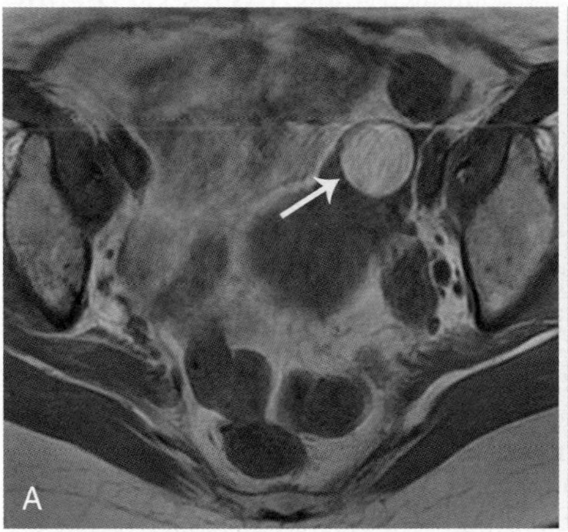

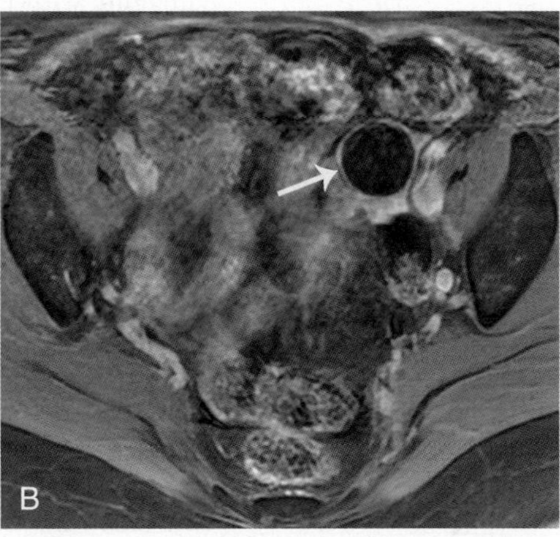

Figure 27.9. A 57-year-old woman with pelvic fullness and pain. **A**, Axial T1-weighted (T1W) magnetic resonance imaging (MRI) study of the pelvis shows a well-circumscribed high–signal intensity mass (*arrow*) in the left adnexa, comparable with fat. **B**, Axial T1W fat-suppressed contrast-enhanced MRI study of the pelvis shows that the mass (*arrow*) loses signal on the fat-suppressed image, suggesting a dermoid.

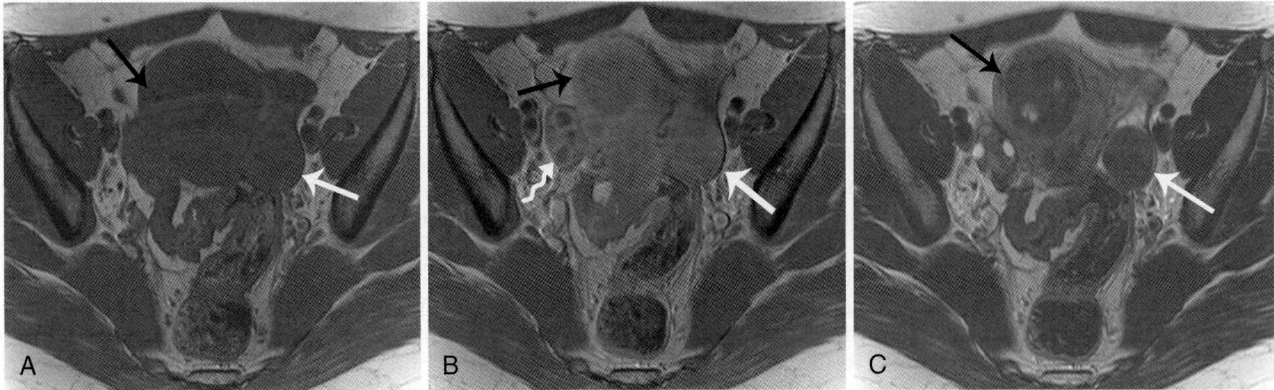

FIGURE 27.10. A 37-year-old woman with newly diagnosed right-sided colon adenocarcinoma and left adnexal mass. The images mark the uterus (*black arrows*), fibroma (*white arrows*), and right ovary (*wavy arrow*). **A**, Axial T1-weighted (T1W) sequence through the pelvis shows a low–signal intensity mass in the left adnexa similar to the fibroid seen on the uterus. **B**, Axial T2-weighted image of the pelvis shows a low-signal mass in the left adnexa, similar to the fibroid seen in the uterus. **C**, Axial T1W contrast-enhanced sequence of the pelvis shows an enhancing mass in the left adnexa suggestive of a fibroma.

In a study by Rieber and coworkers,[84] FDG-PET had a lower sensitivity and specificity than MRI and endovaginal US for the diagnosis of ovarian cancers. The author speculated that this was owing to the presence of a high percentage of low–malignant potential tumors and early-stage ovarian cancers, whereas earlier studies showed higher sensitivities owing to a greater proportion of advanced-stage tumors.[86–88] Borderline tumors (low malignant potential) and early-stage carcinomas may not demonstrate hypermetabolism because only a small amount of transformed/malignant tissue is present for glucose uptake.

KEY POINTS Imaging

- Pelvic ultrasound (US) can help determine the origin of pelvic masses.
- US provides hints for distinguishing malignant from benign lesions, but there is a considerable overlap between the two categories, as well as with borderline tumors.
- Color Doppler US is a valuable tool for determination of malignancy in the proper clinical settings.
- Magnetic resonance imaging (MRI) can be beneficial for further characterization and as a problem-solving modality.
- Serous cystadenoma is usually unilocular and can mimic physiologic cysts. However, papillary projections or mural nodules within the lesion are suggestive of malignancy.
- Mucinous cystadenoma appears as a large multilocular mass that shows varied signal intensity on MRI owing to differences in degree of hemorrhage or protein content.
- Granulosa cell tumor, endometrioid carcinoma, and occasionally thecoma or fibrothecoma are associated with endometrial hyperplasia or carcinoma.
- Fibromas and Brenner tumors have low signal intensity on T2-weighted MRI and may resemble fibroids.
- Endometrioid carcinoma or clear-cell carcinoma may rarely arise from endometriosis; hence, endometriomas should be followed.
- Teratomas, both mature and immature, can contain fat. The presence of solid soft tissue components and scattered calcifications points towards a diagnosis of immature teratoma. Serum tumor markers may help to differentiate further.
- Serous epithelial tumors and metastatic ovarian tumors may present as bilateral complex ovarian masses.

Imaging of Lymphadenopathy and Peritoneal Disease

Lymphadenopathy

The presence of lymph node metastases in ovarian cancer is an important prognostic feature. The frequency of nodal metastases in patients with stage I or II disease is close to 17% and increases to 37% in advanced stages.[89] Superior diaphragmatic adenopathy is detected in approximately 15% of patients with advanced ovarian cancer and is usually associated with a grave prognosis.[90] However, nodal spread of the disease remains a challenge to detect. A major limitation of cross-sectional imaging techniques such as CT and MRI is that they rely on nodal size as the primary criterion for determining the presence of metastatic disease within the lymph nodes. Large nodal metastases can easily be detected with CT or MRI (Fig. 27.11). The overall reported accuracy for detection of metastatic disease in lymph nodes is approximately 85%. Although an enlarged lymph node is likely to be involved, it is not possible to exclude metastatic disease in a normal-sized lymph node. Using a size threshold of greater than 1 cm on the short axis to define abnormal lymph nodes, the sensitivity and specificity of preoperative CT for nodal staging are 50% and 92%, and for MRI are 83% and 95%, respectively.[58]

Metabolic imaging with FDG-PET or hybrid molecular imaging with PET combined with CT (PET-CT) or MRI (PET-MRI) is an alternative for detecting metastatic lymph nodes, as well as recurrence, in patients with pelvic malignancies.[91] PET relies on the increased metabolic activity in lymph nodes and may be able to detect metastases in normal-sized lymph nodes. At the same time, PET resolution and detection capacity may be limited for smaller nodes/lesions. Overall, it has a reported sensitivity of 50% to 82% and a specificity of 92% to 95% for the detection of nodal metastases.[92]

Peritoneal Disease

Imaging can identify disease that can complicate primary surgical debulking or is unresectable. Usually, the disease is considered inoperable when there is invasion of the pelvic sidewall, rectum, sigmoid colon, or bladder; when the tumor deposits are greater than 1 to 2 cm; or when implants are present at the porta hepatis, along the intersegmental fissure of the liver, lesser sac, gastrosplenic ligament or in the subphrenic space, root of the mesentery, or presacral space. Suprarenal adenopathy and/or hepatic (parenchymal), pleural, or pulmonary metastases also make disease inoperable.[58,93,94]

Computed Tomography. Currently, CT is the modality of choice for staging of ovarian cancer, particularly given its wide availability. CT examination is used to evaluate the primary tumor site and the extent of disease, as well as potential sites of peritoneal implants, lymphadenopathy, and solid organ metastases. CT can depict tumor implants larger than 1 cm (see Fig. 27.11) throughout the abdomen and pelvis, with a sensitivity of 85% to 93% and a specificity of 91% to 96%.[62,95–97] However, it has a negative predictive value of only 20%, and its sensitivity decreases to 25$ to 50% for detecting implants measuring 1 cm or smaller.[62] Opacifying the gastrointestinal tract with contrast during CT helps distinguish peritoneal implants from bowel and is useful for determining the presence of bowel invasion. It is, however, important to know that calcified metastases may be obscured by positive bowel contrast, and hence, some believe in using negative contrast such as water as a contrast agent.[60,98]

Intravenous contrast is useful to define the solid organs in the abdomen and pelvis and more clearly delineate peritoneal deposits. Detection of peritoneal tumor deposits is largely dependent on their location as well as their size. Ascites and lymphadenopathy in the pelvis and retroperitoneum are well-demonstrated by CT, and the presence of ascites or calcification may increase conspicuity of the metastases.[71] Hemidiaphragms are difficult to evaluate, and axial imaging can miss small plaquelike deposits. Thin-section imaging allows the data to be manipulated; the images can be reconstructed in the coronal and sagittal planes, where these subdiaphragmatic lesions can be better seen.[60] These reconstructed images also aid in delineation of peritoneal tumor deposits from the unopacified bowel loops. The presence of isolated splenic recurrence is an important finding and can be detected by CT; splenectomy should be performed in these cases for improved long-term survival.[99,100]

Historically, CT scans were performed with intraperitoneal instillation of iodinated contrast, which was theorized to improve the sensitivity for detecting peritoneal disease compared with standard CT.[101] However, this technique fails to detect flat peritoneal metastases and has low sensitivity in patients with prior abdominal surgery; such studies are not performed currently.[102]

Dual-energy CT (DECT) is a recent CT technical development that can be utilized in a dose-neutral approach. It enables CT images to be viewed at multiple energy levels and allows generation of iodine images and virtual noncontrast (water only) CT images from the acquired source CT data. Iodine images with a high contrast-to-noise ratio may enhance lesion conspicuity and detection. Subtle subdiaphragmatic implants may be better seen on lower keV monoenergetic images and may improve the detection and staging of ovarian malignancy, with potential impact on tumor debulking efficacy. DECT may also help differentiate simple ovarian cystic lesions from ovarian malignancy, in addition to improving the detection of hepatic and musculoskeletal metastases.[103]

Ultrasound. US is operator dependent.[104,105] Bowel gas can obscure pathology and make complete evaluation of all possible areas of peritoneal involvement difficult, even in the hands of an experienced sonologist. MRI and CT are superior to US, especially in evaluation of the subdiaphragmatic and hepatic surfaces. A study performed by Tempany and colleagues[62] found that the sensitivity of Doppler US in the detection of peritoneal metastases is lower, at 69%, compared with 95% for MRI, and 92% for spiral CT in patients with advanced cancer (stages III and IV).

Magnetic Resonance Imaging. MRI has staging accuracy similar to that of both conventional and spiral CT.[58,83] MRI also helps identify invasion of pelvic organs, owing to its superior soft tissue contrast resolution.[58] Technique optimization includes the use of oral and intravenous contrast agents to define bowel and the use of fat suppression. Fast sequences performed with breathholding, fasting, and

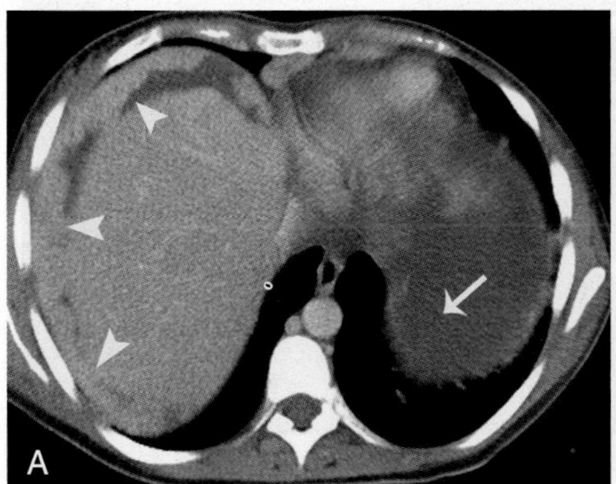

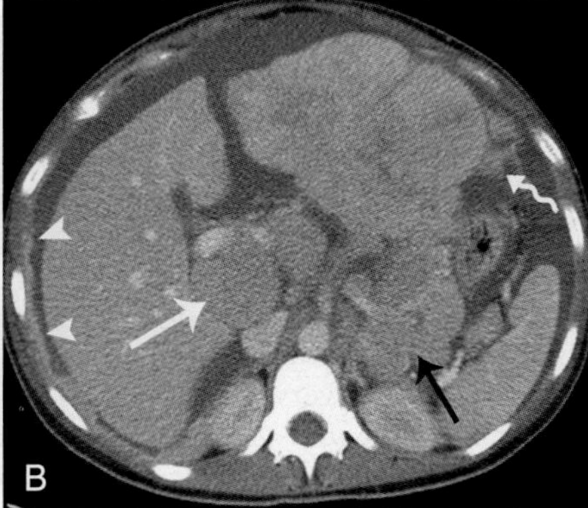

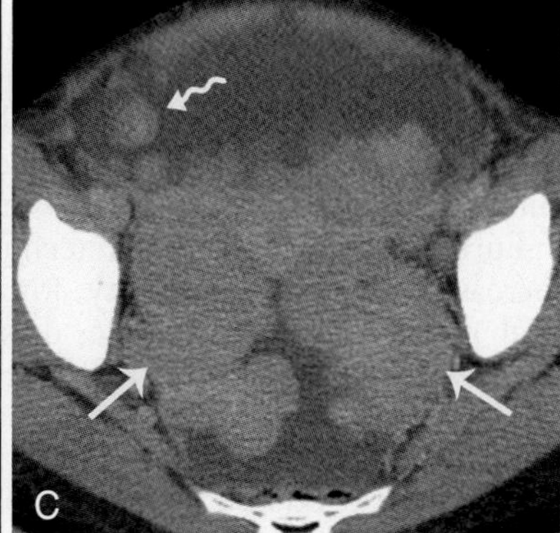

FIGURE 27.11. A 27-year-old woman with clear-cell cancer of the ovary with abdominal pain and discomfort. **A**, Axial contrast-enhanced computed tomography (CT) scan of the abdomen shows subdiaphragmatic nodules (*arrowheads*) and ascites (*arrow*). **B**, Axial contrast-enhanced CT scan of the abdomen shows portocaval adenopathy (*white arrow*) and adenopathy (*black arrow*) along the splenic vein and peritoneal nodules (*wavy arrow*) and subdiaphragmatic nodules (*arrowheads*). **C**, Axial contrast-enhanced CT scan of the pelvis shows bilateral adnexal masses (*straight arrows*) and peritoneal nodules (*wavy arrow*) and ascites.

pharmacologic agents may be useful to decrease the bowel motion.[62,83] All patients undergoing MRI for ovarian cancer assessment should have imaging of both the abdomen and pelvis. A phased array coil is recommended whenever possible to maximize signal-to-noise and in-plane image resolution for imaging of the pelvis; a body coil can be used for obese patients.

MRI can detect extraovarian spread of tumor within the pelvis. However, MRI is used less frequently than CT for evaluation of distant spread of disease in the abdomen, owing to lack of availability and high cost. Currently, improvements in technology with the advent of parallel imaging have dramatically improved the efficiency of MRI and have resulted in decreased scan time owing to the ability to acquire volumetric data and reconstruct them into multiple planes. Peritoneal deposits larger than 1 cm can be detected when the MRI technique is optimal.

There is no statistical difference in the accuracy between CT and MRI in determining the location, distribution, and size of implants in stages III and IV disease.[62] Compared with spiral CT, MRI is able to detect small or equivocal peritoneal implants.[106] However, mesenteric and bowel wall implants are still probably better detected with CT, because bowel motion is still a problem on MRI, and also because calcified deposits are more clearly seen with CT. Performance of MRI deteriorates compared with CT when there ascites is present. Given the greater availability and ease of performance, CT is considered the modality of choice for staging ovarian cancer.[71]

Oral barium can act as a negative contrast in the bowel on T1W imaging, and studies have shown that use of dilute barium in conjunction with intravenous contrast-enhanced MRI improves detection of serosal and omental implants compared with contrast-enhanced CT.[107]

Respiratory-gated fast spin echo T2W imaging helps in delineation of pelvic anatomy. Pre- and postcontrast three-dimensional dynamic imaging is performed through the abdomen, and pre- and postcontrast T1W fat-suppressed imaging through the pelvis is recommended in all cases. Contrast-enhanced studies not only helps characterize the tumor but also improves detection of peritoneal and omental implants. Although peritoneal enhancement and nodularity are sensitive findings for detection of peritoneal malignancy, they are not specific.[108–110] Compared with unenhanced T1W imaging and T2W imaging sequences, gadolinium-enhanced T1W imaging helps to identify small peritoneal implants on free peritoneal surface and bowel serosa.[59,111] Coronal and axial fast imaging employing steady state acquisition sequence can freeze the bowel and may help identify implants easier.[59]

Further advances in MRI technology are helping to increase the MRI sensitivity for detection of peritoneal metastases. For example, diffusion-weighted imaging (DWI) is a functional MRI technique with potential to detect small peritoneal metastases and may be very important in cases with potentially early malignant ovarian masses.[112] DWI can also be clinically useful in distinguishing tumor recurrence from early posttreatment or inflammatory change.[113] DWI/MRI may outperform CT in characterizing the primary tumor, detecting surgically critical metastases, detecting serosal and distant metastases, overall staging, predicting for complete or incomplete resection, and assessing for operability (Fig. 27.12). Whole-body DWI/MRI can aid in surgical planning and may also help minimize unnecessary exploratory laparotomies.[114–116] Other MRI techniques like dynamic contrast-enhanced (DCE) MRI, intrinsic susceptibility-weighted or blood oxygen level-dependent (BOLD) MRI, and magnetic resonance spectroscopy (MRS) can be useful to assess tumor vascularity, hypoxic status, and metabolism, respectively. DCE-MRI is of clinical value in detecting peritoneal carcinomatosis and differentiating malignant from benign ovarian/adnexal disease.[113] DCE-MRI may be the appropriate biomarker to assess treatment response in case of antiangiogenic drug therapy, whereas DWI may be more appropriate to assess tumor necrosis

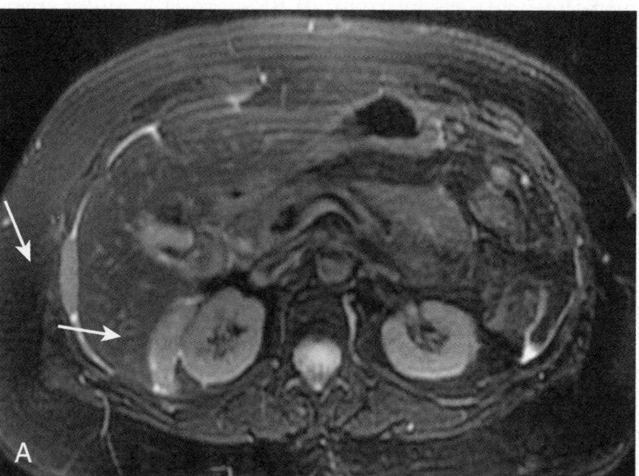

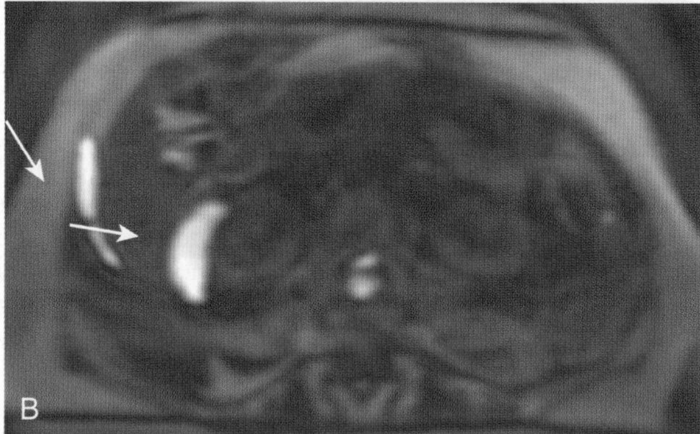

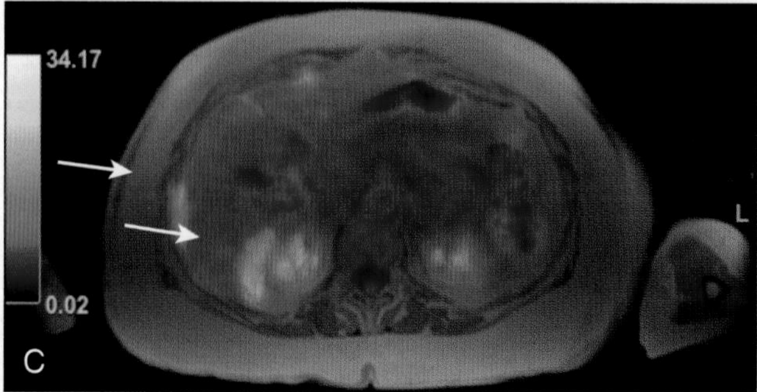

FIGURE 27.12. Whole body positron emission tomography–magnetic resonance imaging (PET-MRI) in a 71-year-old woman with high-grade serous ovarian cancer. **A**, Axial T2-weighted image shows intermediate–signal intensity implants in the perihepatic and hepatorenal regions (arrows). These were bright and more conspicuous on diffusion-weighted imaging (**B**) owing to restricted diffusion, and were hypermetabolic as shown on color-fused PET-MRI (**C**).

in response to traditional chemotherapy drugs.[113] Proton MRS can quantitatively evaluate tumor metabolite concentration, and a high choline-to-creatine ratio is helpful for differentiating malignant from benign adnexal tumors.[117] However, MRS and intrinsic susceptibility-weighted-BOLD MRI need robust magnetic resonance techniques and scanners, and remain investigational tools.[113]

Positron Emission Tomography/Computed Tomography. Although PET/CT has a limited role in characterizing ovarian masses, it is helpful in staging ovarian cancer.[118,119] FDG-PET has limited ability to visualize small (<1 cm) tumor deposits, due to limited spatial resolution. False-positive findings may be seen with inflammatory processes, corpus luteum cysts, and physiologic gastrointestinal activity.[84] FDG-PET and PET/CT can be used in the setting of recurrent disease, when CT and MRI are negative or inconclusive but tumor markers are increasing.[120–125] PET/CT scanning allows better restaging than CT alone and can alter staging and clinical management in patients with suspected ovarian carcinoma recurrence.[126] PET/CT can help in optimizing site-specific treatment, including radiotherapy, and aids in selection of optimal surgical candidates.[127,128]

PET/CT metabolic parameters including maximum standard uptake value, metabolic tumor volume, and total lesion glycolysis can help in determining prognosis and assessing treatment response. Recently, PET/MRI is gaining popularity because it combines the advantages of superior anatomic assessment on MRI and metabolic assessment on PET while avoiding the ionizing radiation associated with CT. DWI, MRS, and functional MRI can also be incorporated with molecular imaging, with added valuable information and less radiation exposure. However, added accuracy or value and added cost of these modalities needs to be justified by improved survival in these patients.[91]

Overall, although MRI has the highest sensitivity and FDG-PET/CT has the highest specificity, there are no significant differences among multidetector computed tomography (MDCT), MRI, and FDG-PET/CT for detection of peritoneal carcinomatosis. Hence, MDCT is the examination of choice if a standalone technique is needed because CT is the fastest, most economical, and most widely available of the three modalities. If inconclusive, PET/CT or MRI may be used to aid in problem-solving and offer additional help. Whole-body FDG-PET/CT may be more accurate for assessment of the supradiaphragmatic metastatic spread.[129] Recent studies suggest that pretreatment FDG-PET/CT may help select surgical approaches or alternative treatment options in ovarian cancer patients due to its low false-positive rate.[130]

Key Points Utility of Imaging

- Imaging has its limitations for distinguishing benign from malignant disease, as well as for detecting small metastases. Newer imaging techniques show more promise in such situations but are still investigational. As detection of clinically important microscopic disease remains a challenge so far, negative imaging findings do not obviate the necessity for complete surgical staging.
- Computed tomography (CT) can reliably detect peritoneal nodules >1 cm and is the study of choice to stage ovarian cancer.
- CT can be used to assess the extent of disease, identify sites of inoperable disease, and determine cases that may benefit from preoperative chemotherapy rather than primary cytoreduction.
- Radiologic staging guides subspecialty referral. For example, for stage III disease the patient should be referred directly to a gynecologic oncologist for optimal cytoreduction.
- 2-[^{18}F] fluoro-2-deoxy-D-glucose (FDG) uptake in the ovary in postmenopausal women needs further evaluation to exclude malignancy.
- FDG uptake in the ovaries in a premenopausal female is usually physiologic.

Recurrent Disease

Computed Tomography

CT has a low sensitivity for detection of recurrent peritoneal carcinomatosis and lymphatic metastasis. However, it may still play a role in the preoperative evaluation of recurrent ovarian cancer patients because it can detect nonresectable recurrent disease.[131] Significant indicators of tumor nonresectability are presence of hydronephrosis and pelvic sidewall invasion, whereas the presence of small bowel obstruction, nodal or perihepatic metastases, ascites, and the level of CA125 are not the strong indicators of tumor nonresectability.

Magnetic Resonance Imaging

MRI has 90% sensitivity, 88% specificity, and 89% accuracy for detecting ovarian cancer recurrence.[132–134] Studies suggest that there is no statistically significant difference between CT and MRI for the detection of recurrent ovarian cancer.[135] However, MRI may be better for assessing the resectability of recurrent disease, owing to its better contrast resolution (Fig. 27.13). When a localized implant is seen, it is crucial for a radiologist to report its proximity to the bowel, ureter, major vessels, and other structures so that surgery can be planned accordingly. MRI may be superior in these cases as well.

Positron Emission Tomography Alone and Positron Emission Tomography Computed Tomography

The use of combined PET/CT for detecting recurrent ovarian cancer was first described by Makhija and associates in 2002.[136] PET has a sensitivity, specificity, and accuracy of 84.6%, 100%, and 86.2%, respectively, for the diagnosis of recurrent ovarian cancer. These parameters can be even higher in patients in whom the suspicion of recurrence is based on rising serum CA125 levels. PET/CT may help in assessing metabolic activity in suspected recurrence, in the setting of small volume metastases, or in patients with serous tumors developing calcified metastases to the peritoneum or lymph nodes (Fig. 27.14).

A metaanalysis suggested that the difference between PET alone and PET/CT in detecting recurrence was slight.[137] Combined PET/CT is used to assess morphologic as well as functional information, and to assess

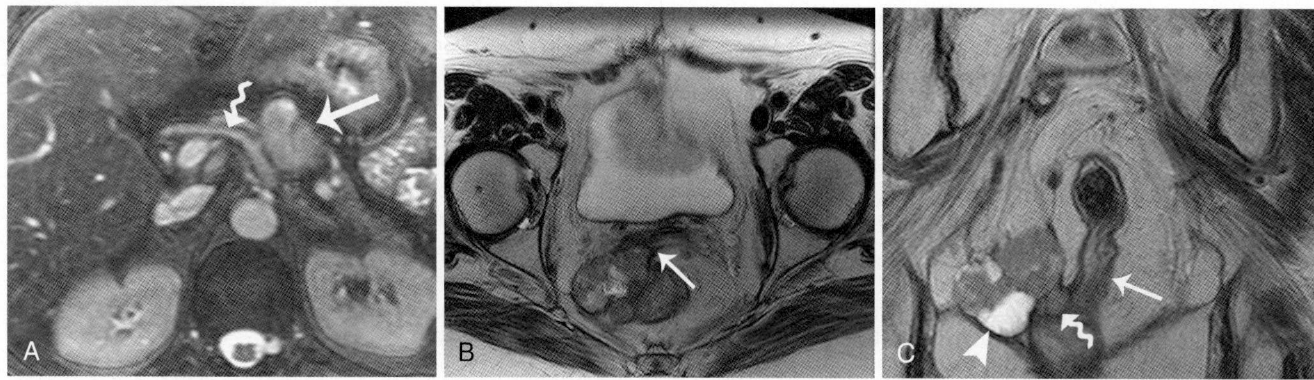

FIGURE 27.13. A 68-year-old woman with low-grade papillary serous ovarian cancer after optimal debulking surgery followed by carboplatin/taxol chemotherapy, now with recurrent disease. **A**, Axial T2-weighted (T2W) magnetic resonance imaging (MRI) sequence shows the inferior extent of the implant (*straight arrow*) adjacent to the celiac axis (*wavy arrow*). **B**, Axial T2W MRI study of the pelvis shows a mass (*arrow*) in the left hemipelvis infiltrating into the left vaginal cuff and the left rectal wall. **C**, Coronal T2W MRI of the pelvis shows that the heterogeneous signal intensity implant (*arrowhead*) infiltrates (*wavy arrow*) into the rectal wall (*straight arrow*) and abuts the levator ani muscle. This suggests that, if the patient is going to be reoperated, negative margins may not be achieved in the abdomen; in the pelvis, the patient may require pelvic exenteration, which can increase morbidity.

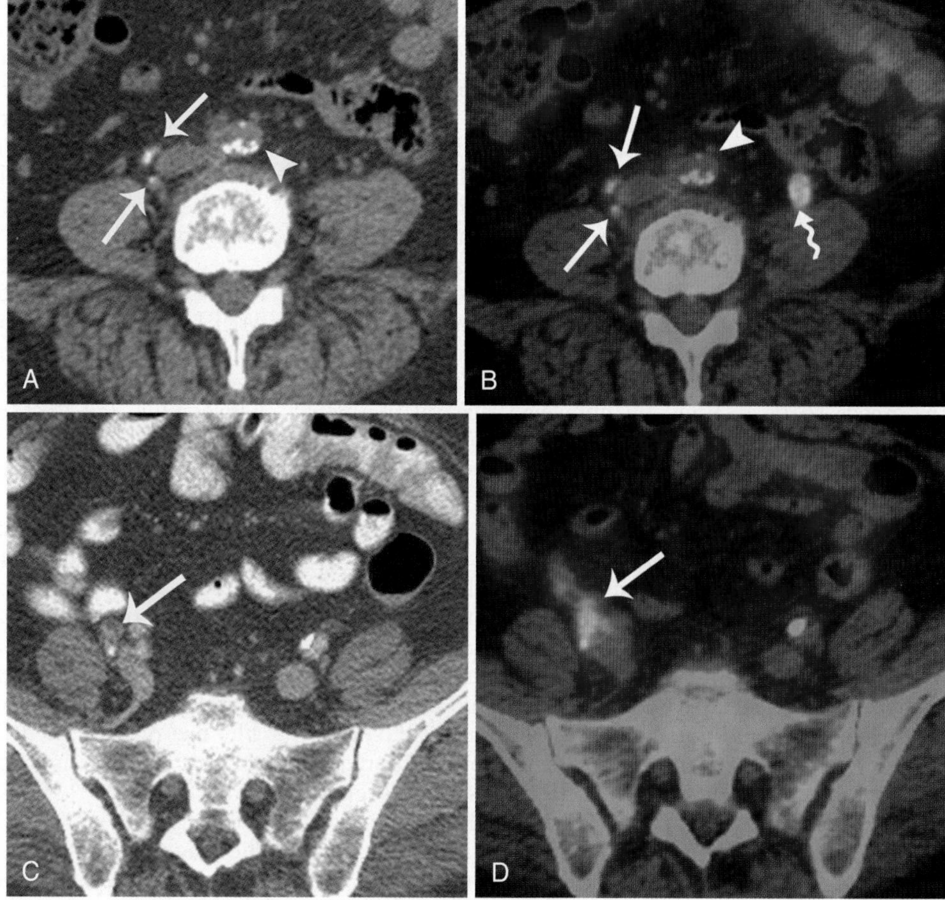

FIGURE 27.14. A 72-year-old woman with a history of stage IIIC papillary serous ovarian cancer status postoptimal debulking and postoperative chemotherapy with carboplatin and taxol with rising cancer antigen 125 (from 12.2 to 22.1 U/mL). **A**, Axial noncontrast computed tomography (CT) scan of the abdomen shows 7-mm right retroperitoneal lymph nodes (*arrows*) with punctuate calcifications and a left enlarged retroperitoneal lymph node (*arrowhead*). **B**, Axial fused positron emission tomography (PET)/CT image shows low-grade 2-[^{18}F] fluoro-2-deoxy-D-glucose (FDG) uptake in the right retroperitoneal lymph node with a maximum standard uptake value (SUVmax) of 2.5 (*arrowhead*), activity in the ureter (*wavy arrow*), and no activity in the left retroperitoneal node (*straight arrows*). **C**, Axial-contrast enhanced CT scan of the pelvis shows a right 1.2-cm lateral common iliac lymph node containing calcifications (*arrow*). **D**, Axial fused PET/CT image shows mild FDG-avid right lateral common iliac lymph node (*arrow*) with an SUVmax of 2.5. Given the patient's history of papillary serous cancer and calcified lymph nodes, these are metastatic.

response to therapy. At the authors' institution, PET/CT is performed at the time of recurrence, followed by CT scans during the therapy. If the disease is stable over time during chemotherapy, PET/CT may be performed to assess its functional status; and eventually, the chemotherapy is stopped if the disease is not metabolically active (Figs. 27.15 and 27.16).[138]

KEY POINT Imaging Recurrent Disease

- Computed tomography, magnetic resonance imaging, and positron emission tomography/computed tomography are helpful in detecting suspected recurrence and response to therapy and can help in appropriate surgical planning.

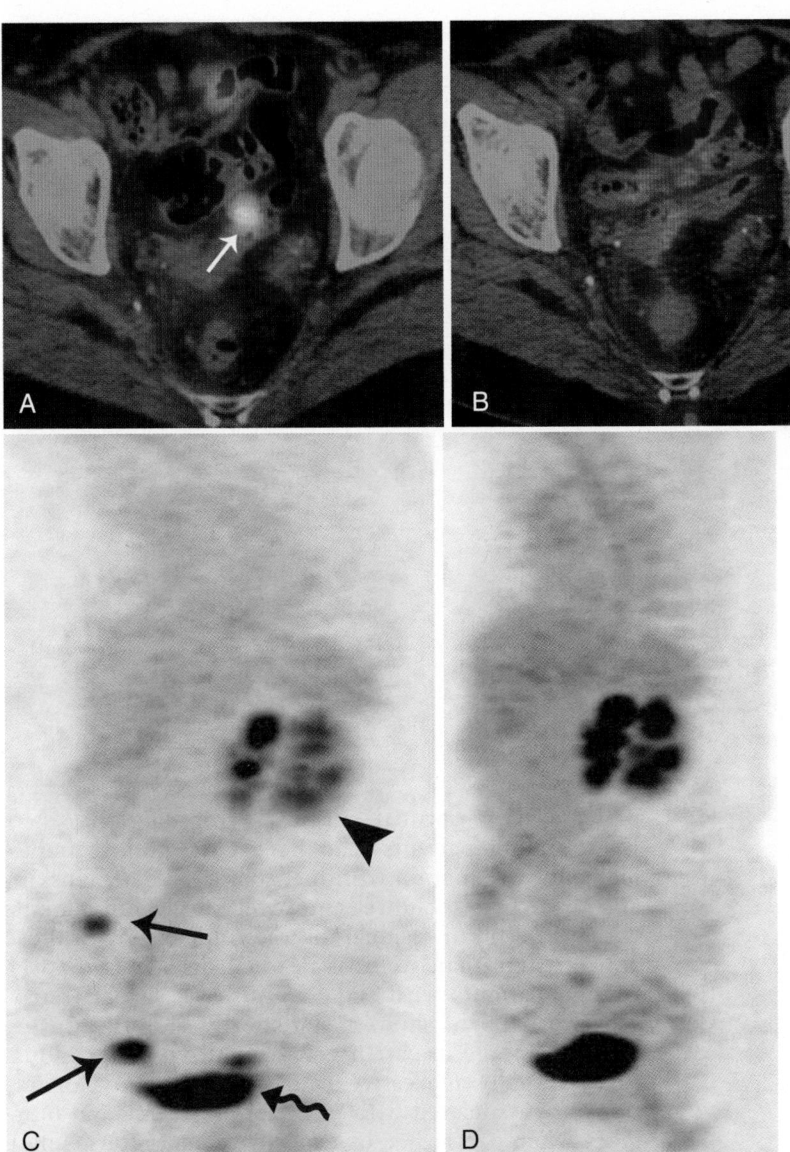

FIGURE 27.15. A 70-year-old woman with a history of recurrent high-grade ovarian cancer with recurrent disease. She received optimal debulking with neoadjuvant chemotherapy and had relapse. **A**, Fused positron emission tomography/computed tomography (PET/CT) images show recurrent tumor (implant) intimately associated with the sigmoid colon (*arrow*). **B**, Fused PET/CT scan shows complete metabolic response to therapy. **C**, Sagittal maximum intensity projection (MIP) images show recurrent disease in the abdomen (*straight arrows*), kidneys (*arrowhead*), and bladder (*wavy arrow*). **D**, MIP images show complete metabolic response to therapy.

SURVEILLANCE

CA125 is expressed on the surface of epithelial cells, which are found in approximately 80% of epithelial ovarian carcinomas, and can be used for screening for ovarian cancer. Serum CA125 is widely used to detect recurrence and monitor response to treatment in ovarian cancer cases, and is a sensitive tumor marker.[139–142] A rise in CA125 level above the upper limit of normal (35 U/mL) in patients with previous normalization suggests recurrent disease, although elevated CA125 does not justify initiation of treatment in asymptomatic patients.[143] Rising serum CA125 levels may precede clinical detection of relapse in 56% to 94% of cases, with a median lead time of 3 to 5 months.[144] However, it should be kept in mind that elevated CA125 is nonspecific and can be occur in patients with or without recurrent disease. In 3% of patients previously treated for ovarian malignancy, CA125 may be elevated, with no evidence of recurrent cancer.[145] Patients with cirrhosis, pancreatic cancer, endometriosis, pelvic inflammatory disease, and other malignancies can also have elevated levels of CA125, and the PPV of screening with serum marker is low, at 1%.[139,140] The absolute value of CA125 has not been linked to a particular pattern of recurrence,[146] although in the absence of clinically or radiographically demonstrable recurrence the significance of a rising serum CA125 level has not yet been determined. CT, MRI, and PET/CT can be used in such situations. Even when the patient does not have elevated tumor markers or is symptomatic, these imaging modalities may be useful to find the recurrent tumor.

Many Sex Cord-Stromal Tumors also produce serum markers. For example, granulosa and theca cell tumors release estrogen, Sertoli–Leydig cell tumors release testosterone, yolk sac tumors release alpha-fetoprotein, and choriocarcinomas release β-hCG.

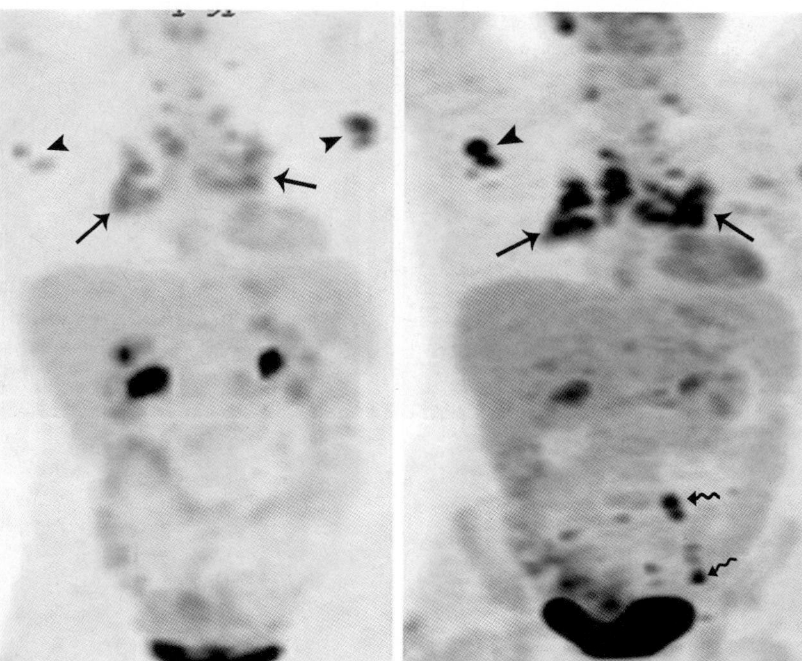

FIGURE 27.16. A 57-year-old woman with a history of stage IIIC high-grade serous carcinoma treated with abraxane and avastin. **A**, Coronal maximum intensity projection (MIP) images show recurrent disease in the mediastinum (*arrows*) and bilateral axilla (*arrowheads*). **B**, Coronal positron emission tomography MIP scan of the body shows progression of the mediastinal adenopathy (*straight arrows*), the right axillary adenopathy (*arrowhead*), and interval appearance of left pelvic adenopathy (*wavy arrows*).

KEY POINTS Surveillance

- Cancer antigen 125 is the tumor marker used for surveillance of epithelial ovarian tumors.
- Treatment of disease cannot be based on elevation of tumor marker alone without radiologic evidence of disease in an asymptomatic patient.
- Cross-sectional imaging should be used to assess for recurrent disease in patients with elevated tumor markers.

TREATMENT

Surgery

Owing to a lack of effective tools for screening and early detection, the majority of patients with ovarian cancer present with advanced disease. It is now well established that the cornerstone of treatment for advanced epithelial ovarian cancer (stages III and IV) is a combination of surgical cytoreductive and systemic or intraperitoneal chemotherapy.

For most patients with advanced disease, the goal of surgery is to provide optimal tumor reduction with removal of all visible tumor. This generally includes removal of ovarian masses, a total abdominal hysterectomy, omentectomy, and excision of any other tumor implants. Removal of bulky tumors provides symptomatic relief for patients. Munnel et al.[147] were the first to show that "maximal surgical effort" significantly improves survival (28% vs. 9%) compared with "partial removal" or "biopsy alone." Over the years, several groups have shown significant survival advantage for patients with optimal surgical cytoreduction.[42,56,148] Even among patients who have undergone suboptimal tumor reduction (residual tumor >1 cm), Hoskins and coworkers[148] showed improved survival in patients with 1 to 2 cm of residual disease compared with those with greater than 2 cm of residual disease ($P < .01$). Among patients with stage IV disease, several retrospective reports show a statistically significant survival advantage in patients with small-volume residual tumor. Finally, aggressive primary cytoreductive operations are associated with minimal morbidity and mortality when performed by experienced surgeons. These data led the National Institutes of Health Consensus Development Conference on Ovarian Cancer to conclude in 1994 that "aggressive" attempts at cytoreductive surgery as the primary management of ovarian cancer will improve the patient's opportunity for long-term survival.[5]

Chemotherapy

Surgery alone, however, is rarely curative for patients with advanced ovarian cancer. Currently, the standard of care consists of a combination of paclitaxel and carboplatin. This regimen can be administered in an outpatient setting. The combination is well tolerated, with fewer than 2% of cycles associated with grade 4 thrombocytopenia or febrile neutropenia, and is associated with an overall response rate of approximately 75%.[149] Some groups have also advocated the use of intraperitoneal chemotherapy as the preferred adjuvant treatment following optimal tumor reductive surgery, due to improved progression-free survival and overall survival.[150]

Key Points Surgery and Chemotherapy

- Primary cytoreductive surgery is the mainstay of treatment for ovarian cancer, and consists of total abdominal hysterectomy, bilateral salpingo-oophorectomy, omentectomy, and lymphadenectomy to the level of the renal hilum.
- Presence of subdiaphragmatic implants results in suboptimal cytoreduction.
- Features suggesting unresectability include implants invading pelvic sidewall, rectum, sigmoid colon, or bladder; tumor deposits greater than 1 to 2 cm in the porta hepatis, intersegmental fissure of the liver, lesser sac, gastrosplenic ligament, subphrenic space, root of mesentery, or presacral space; suprarenal adenopathy; and/or hepatic (parenchymal), pleural, or pulmonary metastases.
- Intraperitoneal chemotherapy with cisplatin and paclitaxel is the preferred adjuvant treatment for patients after optimal tumor reductive surgery.

Radiation Therapy

The role of radiation therapy in the management of ovarian cancer has evolved dramatically since the early 1960s and continues to be refined. Before the development of modern chemotherapy agents, radiation therapy played an important role in the treatment of patients with early or completely resected disease.[151] Some patient were also treated with intraperitoneal administration of radioactive phosphorus based on early results; but this may cause bowel complications.[151] In the 1980s and 1990s, the advent of more effective chemotherapy agents such as cisplatin and the taxanes led many clinicians to abandon the use of radiation therapy in the curative management of ovarian cancer. During this time, some investigators used whole abdominal radiation (WAR) as a treatment for incomplete responders to platinum-based chemotherapy. However, acute side effects (particularly hematologic) were substantial, and most investigators reported poor overall disease control rates.[152–155] Although there were isolated reports of long-term survival of patients treated with postchemotherapy WAR, this approach is not commonly used today.

Although the role of radiation therapy in the curative treatment of ovarian cancer is relatively minor today, local treatment of persistent or recurrent pelvic or nodal disease can result in long disease-free intervals in carefully selected patients.[155,156] Modern, highly conformal radiation therapy techniques facilitate administration of tumoricidal doses with minimized risk to adjacent critical structures.

Radiation therapy is also a highly effective tool in the management of tumor-related symptoms from uncontrolled local disease, painful bone metastases, or other symptomatic lesions.[157,158] A variety of radiation schedules may be used according to the nature of the lesion and life expectancy of the patient. In some cases, one or two treatments of 8 to 10 Gy can provide very effective palliation. If two treatments are given, they are generally spaced 1 month apart. Other common fractionation schedules include 20 Gy in five fractions or 30 Gy in 10 fractions. With these fractionated regimens, the risk of serious radiation-related complications is low.

Investigational Therapy

Several investigational agents are being studied in the setting of relapsed ovarian cancers. Bevacizumab is a humanized antibody that recognizes and deactivates vascular endothelial growth factor, an angiogenic factor that is often secreted by ovarian cancer cells. As a single agent, bevacizumab was shown to induce responses in 18% of patients with relapsed ovarian cancer who were either platinum-sensitive or platinum-resistant, and 39% of patients had progression-free survival at 6 months.[159] Bevacizumab can cause proteinuria, hypertension, and bleeding, and may also result in other uncommon, but potentially life-threatening, side effects such as arterial thromboembolism, wound healing complications, and gastrointestinal perforation or fistulae.[160] The risk of bowel perforation with bevacizumab in the recurrent ovarian cancer setting may be related to prior multiple treatment regimens, radiographic evidence of bowel wall involvement by the tumor, or the presence of bowel obstruction.[161] Other investigational agents with reported activity in platinum-sensitive (and, to a lesser degree, platinum-resistant) disease include ET743 (trabectedin), halichondrin B, pertuzumab, and epothilones. Her-2/neu is usually not overexpressed in ovarian cancer, and this limits the use of humanized monoclonal antibodies such as trastuzumab.[162] At present, none of these agents is approved by the U.S. Food and Drug Administration for treating patients with relapsed ovarian cancer, and their significance needs to be better defined.

Key Points Radiation and Investigational Therapy

- Radiation therapy can be used to treat localized recurrent disease.
- Radiotherapy can also be used to manage tumor-related symptoms from uncontrolled local disease, painful bone metastases, or other symptomatic lesions.
- Bevacizumab can cause bowel perforation, thromboembolism, and fistulae.
- Platinum-based chemotherapy can cause nausea, vomiting, and fatigue.

THE RADIOLOGY REPORT

Imaging does not preclude the necessity for surgical debulking; however, it can predict optimal and suboptimal surgical resections, which may lead to preoperative chemotherapy. Thus, the radiology report should include as much relevant information as possible to allow the surgeon to decide upon the treatment options. The report should include a detailed description of the location of implants and whether they involve the diaphragm and are present in locations that may preclude optimal debulking. Describing the relationship of the tumor to vessels and the bowel is important to determine whether the bowel resection is needed. Complete radiologic staging with evaluation of hepatic or distant metastases should also be included in the report. After therapy, the radiology report should include not only evidence of residual disease but also any evidence of complications from therapy such as bowel perforation if the patient received bevacizumab.

Key Points The Radiology Report

- Location of implants and whether they involve the diaphragm and are present in locations that may preclude optimal debulking.
- Adenopathy extending above or below the level of renal hilum.
- Presence of a retroaortic renal vein.

CONCLUSION

Ovarian cancer is often a fatal disease and is usually detected at late stages; survival decreases as the stage of the disease increases. In this chapter we have reviewed the clinical, pathologic, radiologic, and therapeutic features of this malignancy. Management of this malignancy requires a team approach. At MD Anderson, the clinical management of ovarian cancer necessitates opinions from the radiologist, gynecologic oncologist, surgeon, radiation oncologist, and pathologist. This team approach helps in formulating optimal treatment plans and providing better patient management. Continued newer imaging techniques and improvements in imaging will enhance appropriate patient management. Newer therapies are being developed to help treat recurrent disease in platinum-resistant patients and may improve progression-free and overall survival.

Key Points Overall Review of Ovarian Cancer

- Ovarian cancer is the most common cause of death from cancer in women with gynecologic malignancy, and accounts for 5% of overall deaths due to cancer.
- Risk factors are hormonal, genetic, and environmental.
- Ovarian cancers can be of different histologic varieties, with different ages of presentation, pathways of dissemination, tumor markers, and prognosis.
- Epithelial tumors comprise the majority of ovarian cancers and usually present at an advanced stage.
- Sex cord–stromal tumors occur in the reproductive or postmenopausal age group, and can produce estrogen or testosterone depending on their origin.
- Usually, ovarian cancers produce cancer antigen 125, whereas germ cell neoplasms produce alpha-fetoprotein and beta–human chorionic gonadotropin.
- The most common method of epithelial ovarian tumor spread is via peritoneal dissemination.
- Staging of ovarian tumors is based on International Federation of Gynecology and Obstetrics staging, which includes a staging laparotomy, in which the patient undergoes total abdominal hysterectomy, bilateral salpingo-oophorectomy, pelvic lymphadenectomy, and omentectomy.
- Surgical cytoreduction for stages II and IV disease can be quite complex, and macroscopic disease may be left behind in some cases. More importantly, miliary or microscopic implants cannot be surgically removed, and the role of adjuvant chemotherapy is therefore critical.
- Ultrasound, computed tomography (CT), and magnetic resonance imaging (MRI) can help characterize adnexal masses, although there is considerable overlap between benign and malignant lesions.
- MRI and CT are equally accurate in the staging of abdominal and pelvic disease.
- CT is the modality of choice to stage intraabdominal and pelvic disease, as well as to detect recurrence.
- Positron emission tomography/CT can detect disease above the diaphragm and can help in assessing response to therapy.
- Imaging can help assess residual disease after primary cytoreductive surgery and detect recurrent disease.

REFERENCES

1. Siegel RL, Miller KD, Jemal A. Cancer statistics, 2018. *CA Cancer J Clin*. 2018;68(1):7–30.
2. Bristow RE, et al. A model for predicting surgical outcome in patients with advanced ovarian carcinoma using computed tomography. *Cancer*. 2000;89(7):1532–1540.
3. Holschneider CH, Berek JS. Ovarian cancer: epidemiology, biology, and prognostic factors. *Semin Surg Oncol*. 2000;19(1):3–10.
4. Berchuck A, et al. Managing hereditary ovarian cancer risk. *Cancer*. 1999;86(11 Suppl):2517–2524.
5. NIH consensus conference Ovarian cancer. Screening, treatment, and follow-up. NIH Consensus Development Panel on Ovarian Cancer. *JAMA*. 1995;273(6):491–497.
6. Godwin AK, Hamilton TC, Knudson Jr. AG. Oncogenes and tumor suppressor genes. In: Hoskins WJ, Young RC, eds. *Principles and practice of gynecologic oncology*. 2nd ed. Philadelphia: Lippincott-Raven; 1997:107–148.
7. Chen X, et al. Early alterations in ovarian surface epithelial cells and induction of ovarian epithelial tumors triggered by loss of FSH receptor. *Neoplasia*. 2007;9(6):521–531.
8. Fathalla MF. Incessant ovulation-a factor in ovarian neoplasia? *Lancet*. 1971;2(7716):163.
9. Chene G, et al. Ovarian epithelial dysplasia after ovulation induction: time and dose effects. *Hum Reprod*. 2009;24(1):132–138.
10. Daly MB. The epidemiology of ovarian cancer. *Hematol Oncol Clin North Am*. 1992;6(4):729–738.
11. Hall HI, et al. Regional variations in ovarian cancer incidence in the United States, 1992–1997. *Cancer*. 2003;97(10 Suppl):2701–2706.
12. Chen VW, et al. Pathology and classification of ovarian tumors. *Cancer*. 2003;97(10 Suppl):2631–2642.
13. Przybora LA. [International classification of ovarian neoplasms elaborated by the WHO Commission in 1971]. *Patol Pol*. 1974;25(2):203–211.
14. Prat J. Staging classification for cancer of the ovary, fallopian tube, and peritoneum. *Int J Gynaecol Obstet*. 2014;124(1):1–5.
15. Wagner BJ, et al. From the archives of the AFIP. Ovarian epithelial neoplasms: radiologic-pathologic correlation. *Radiographics*. 1994;14(6):1351–1374. quiz 1375–1376.
16. Boger-Megiddo I, Weiss NS. Histologic subtypes and laterality of primary epithelial ovarian tumors. *Gynecol Oncol*. 2005;97(1):80–83.
17. Jung SE, et al. CT and MR imaging of ovarian tumors with emphasis on differential diagnosis. *Radiographics*. 2002;22(6):1305–1325.
18. Outwater EK, et al. Papillary projections in ovarian neoplasms: appearance on MRI. *J Magn Reson Imaging*. 1997;7(4):689–695.
19. Kawamoto S, Urban BA, Fishman EK. CT of epithelial ovarian tumors. *Radiographics*. 1999;19(Spec No):S85–S102. quiz S263–S264.
20. Scully RE. *Histological typing of ovarian tumours*. New York: Springer Berlin; 1999.
21. Scully RE, Young RH, Clement PB. Tumors of the ovary, maldeveloped gonads, fallopian tube, and broad ligament. In: *Atlas of Tumor Pathology*. Washington DC: Armed Forces Institute of Pathology; 1999.
22. Scully RE. World Health Organization classification and nomenclature of ovarian cancer. *Natl Cancer Inst Monogr*. 1975;42:5–7.
23. Seldenrijk CA, et al. Malignant Brenner tumor. A histologic, morphometrical, immunohistochemical, and ultrastructural study. *Cancer*. 1986;58(3):754–760.

24. Silverberg SG. Brenner tumor of the ovary. A clinicopathologic study of 60 tumors in 54 women. *Cancer*. 1971;28(3):588–596.
25. Oh SN, et al. Transitional cell tumor of the ovary: computed tomographic and magnetic resonance imaging features with pathological correlation. *J Comput Assist Tomogr*. 2009;33(1):106–112.
26. Imaoka I, et al. Developing an MR imaging strategy for diagnosis of ovarian masses. *Radiographics*. 2006;26(5):1431–1448.
27. Vereczkey I, Toth E, Orosz Z. [Diagnostic problems of ovarian mucinous borderline tumors]. *Magy Onkol*. 2009;53(2):127–133.
28. deSouza NM, et al. Borderline tumors of the ovary: CT and MRI features and tumor markers in differentiation from stage I disease. *AJR Am J Roentgenol*. 2005;184(3):999–s1003.
29. Wong HF, et al. Ovarian tumors of borderline malignancy: a review of 247 patients from 1991 to 2004. *Int J Gynecol Cancer*. 2007;17(2):342–349.
30. Smith HO, et al. Incidence and survival rates for female malignant germ cell tumors. *Obstet Gynecol*. 2006;107(5):1075–1085.
31. Tewari K, et al. Malignant germ cell tumors of the ovary. *Obstet Gynecol*. 2000;95(1):128–133.
32. Talerman A. Germ cell tumors of the ovary. *Curr Opin Obstet Gynecol*. 1997;9(1):44–47.
33. Gershenson DM, et al. Mixed germ cell tumors of the ovary. *Obstet Gynecol*. 1984;64(2):200–206.
34. Gershenson DM. Management of ovarian germ cell tumors. *J Clin Oncol*. 2007;25(20):2938–2943.
35. Comerci Jr JT, et al. Mature cystic teratoma: a clinicopathologic evaluation of 517 cases and review of the literature. *Obstet Gynecol*. 1994;84(1):22–28.
36. Brammer 3rd HM, et al. From the archives of the AFIP. Malignant germ cell tumors of the ovary: radiologic-pathologic correlation. *Radiographics*. 1990;10(4):715–724.
37. Outwater EK, Siegelman ES, Hunt JL. Ovarian teratomas: tumor types and imaging characteristics. *Radiographics*. 2001;21(2):475–490.
38. Outwater EK, et al. Sex cord-stromal and steroid cell tumors of the ovary. *Radiographics*. 1998;18(6):1523–1546.
39. Roth LM, et al. Sertoli-Leydig cell tumors: a clinicopathologic study of 34 cases. *Cancer*. 1981;48(1):187–197.
40. Tsuji T, Catasus L, Prat J. Is loss of heterozygosity at 9q22.3 (PTCH gene) and 19p13.3 (STK11 gene) involved in the pathogenesis of ovarian stromal tumors? *Hum Pathol*. 2005;36(7):792–796.
41. de Waal YR, et al. Secondary ovarian malignancies: frequency, origin, and characteristics. *Int J Gynecol Cancer*. 2009;19(7):1160–1165.
42. Hoskins WJ, et al. The influence of cytoreductive surgery on recurrence-free interval and survival in small-volume stage III epithelial ovarian cancer: a Gynecologic Oncology Group study. *Gynecol Oncol*. 1992;47(2):159–166.
43. Buy JN, et al. Epithelial tumors of the ovary: CT findings and correlation with US. *Radiology*. 1991;178(3):811–818.
44. Meyers MA, et al. The peritoneal ligaments and mesenteries: pathways of intraabdominal spread of disease. *Radiology*. 1987;163(3):593–604.
45. Feldman GB, Knapp RC. Lymphatic drainage of the peritoneal cavity and its significance in ovarian cancer. *Am J Obstet Gynecol*. 1974;119(7):991–994.
46. Coakley FV, Hricak H. Imaging of peritoneal and mesenteric disease: key concepts for the clinical radiologist. *Clin Radiol*. 1999;54(9):563–574.
47. Meyers MA. *Dynamic radiology of the abdomen: normal and pathologic anatomy in distribution of intra-abdominal malignant seeding: dependency on dynamics of flow of ascitic fluid*: Springer; 2000:198–206.
48. Dvoretsky PM, et al. Distribution of disease at autopsy in 100 women with ovarian cancer. *Hum Pathol*. 1988;19(1):57–63.
49. Dauplat J, et al. Distant metastases in epithelial ovarian carcinoma. *Cancer*. 1987;60(7):1561–1566.
50. Di Re F, et al. Pelvic and para-aortic lymphadenectomy in cancer of the ovary. *Baillieres Clin Obstet Gynaecol*. 1989;3(1):131–142.
51. Coakley FV. Staging ovarian cancer: role of imaging. *Radiol Clin North Am*. 2002;40(3):609–636.
52. Friedlander ML. Prognostic factors in ovarian cancer. *Semin Oncol*. 1998;25(3):305–314.
53. Jemal A, et al. Cancer statistics, 2007. *CA Cancer J Clin*. 2007;57(1):43–66.
54. Prat J, Oncology FCOG. Staging classification for cancer of the ovary, fallopian tube, and peritoneum. *Int J Gynaecol Obstet*. 2014;124(1):1–5.
55. Marsden DE, Friedlander M, Hacker NF. Current management of epithelial ovarian carcinoma: a review. *Semin Surg Oncol*. 2000;19(1):11–19.
56. Young RC, et al. Staging laparotomy in early ovarian cancer. *JAMA*. 1983;250(22):3072–3076.
57. Leblanc E, et al. Surgical staging of early invasive epithelial ovarian tumors. *Semin Surg Oncol*. 2000;19(1):36–41.
58. Forstner R, et al. Ovarian cancer: staging with CT and MR imaging. *Radiology*. 1995;197(3):619–626.
59. Coakley FV, et al. Peritoneal metastases: detection with spiral CT in patients with ovarian cancer. *Radiology*. 2002;223(2):495–499.
60. Pannu HK, et al. Multidetector CT of peritoneal carcinomatosis from ovarian cancer. *Radiographics*. 2003;23(3):687–701.
61. Walkey MM, et al. CT manifestations of peritoneal carcinomatosis. *AJR Am J Roentgenol*. 1988;150(5):1035–1041.
62. Tempany CM, et al. Staging of advanced ovarian cancer: comparison of imaging modalities-report from the Radiological Diagnostic Oncology Group. *Radiology*. 2000;215(3):761–767.
63. Steinberg JJ, Demopoulos RI, Bigelow B. The evaluation of the omentum in ovarian cancer. *Gynecol Oncol*. 1986;24(3):327–330.
64. Carnino F, et al. Significance of lymph node sampling in epithelial carcinoma of the ovary. *Gynecol Oncol*. 1997;65(3):467–472.
65. Sakai K, et al. Relationship between pelvic lymph node involvement and other disease sites in patients with ovarian cancer. *Gynecol Oncol*. 1997;65(1):164–168.
66. Ronnett BM, et al. Disseminated peritoneal adenomucinosis and peritoneal mucinous carcinomatosis. A clinicopathologic analysis of 109 cases with emphasis on distinguishing pathologic features, site of origin, prognosis, and relationship to "pseudomyxoma peritonei". *Am J Surg Pathol*. 1995;19(12):1390–1408.
67. Brown DL. A practical approach to the ultrasound characterization of adnexal masses. *Ultrasound Q*. 2007;23(2):87–105.
68. Brown DL, et al. Benign and malignant ovarian masses: selection of the most discriminating gray-scale and Doppler sonographic features. *Radiology*. 1998;208(1):103–110.
69. Jeong YY, Outwater EK, Kang HK. Imaging evaluation of ovarian masses. *Radiographics*. 2000;20(5):1445–1470.
70. Mansour GM, et al. Adnexal mass vascularity assessed by 3-dimensional power Doppler: does it add to the risk of malignancy index in prediction of ovarian malignancy?: four hundred-case study. *Int J Gynecol Cancer*. 2009;19(5):867–872.
71. Mironov S, et al. Ovarian cancer. *Radiol Clin North Am*. 2007;45(1):149–166.
72. Leen E. Ultrasound contrast harmonic imaging of abdominal organs. *Semin Ultrasound CT MR*. 2001;22(1):11–24.
73. Jokubkiene L, Sladkevicius P, Valentin L. Does three-dimensional power Doppler ultrasound help in discrimination between benign and malignant ovarian masses? *Ultrasound Obstet Gynecol*. 2007;29(2):215–225.
74. Buy JN, et al. Characterization of adnexal masses: combination of color Doppler and conventional sonography compared with spectral Doppler analysis alone and conventional sonography alone. *AJR Am J Roentgenol*. 1996;166(2):385–393.
75. Khan O, et al. Ovarian carcinoma follow-up: US versus laparotomy. *Radiology*. 1986;159(1):111–113.
76. Johnson RJ. Radiology in the management of ovarian cancer. *Clin Radiol*. 1993;48(2):75–82.
77. Sohaid S, Husband JRR. *Ovarian cancer*. *Imaging in Oncology*. 1st ed. Oxford: Isis Medical Media Ltd; 1998:277–308.
78. Tsili AC, et al. Adnexal masses: accuracy of detection and differentiation with multidetector computed tomography. *Gynecol Oncol*. 2008;110(1):22–s31.
79. Amendola MA. The role of CT in the evaluation of ovarian malignancy. *Crit Rev Diagn Imaging*. 1985;24(4):329–368.
80. Ferrandina G, et al. Role of CT scan-based and clinical evaluation in the preoperative prediction of optimal cytoreduction in advanced ovarian cancer: a prospective trial. *Br J Cancer*. 2009;101(7):1066–1073.
81. Sanders RC, et al. A prospective study of computed tomography and ultrasound in the detection and staging of pelvic masses. *Radiology*. 1983;146(2):439–442.
82. Shiels RA, et al. A prospective trial of computed tomography in the staging of ovarian malignancy. *Br J Obstet Gynaecol*. 1985;92(4):407–412.
83. Kurtz AB, et al. Diagnosis and staging of ovarian cancer: comparative values of Doppler and conventional US, CT, and MR

imaging correlated with surgery and histopathologic analysis-report of the Radiology Diagnostic Oncology Group. *Radiology*. 1999;212(1):19–s27.
84. Rieber A, et al. Preoperative diagnosis of ovarian tumors with MR imaging: comparison with transvaginal sonography, positron emission tomography, and histologic findings. *AJR Am J Roentgenol*. 2001;177(1):123–129.
85. Hricak H, et al. Complex adnexal masses: detection and characterization with MR imaging-multivariate analysis. *Radiology*. 2000;214(1):39–46.
86. Romer W, et al. [Metabolic characterization of ovarian tumors with positron-emission tomography and F-18 fluorodeoxyglucose]. *ROFO*. 1997;166(1):62–68.
87. Hubner KF, et al. Assessment of primary and metastatic ovarian cancer by positron emission tomography (PET) using 2-[18F]deoxyglucose (2-[18F]FDG). *Gynecol Oncol*. 1993;51(2):197–s204.
88. Zimny M, et al. [18F-fluorodeoxyglucose PET in ovarian carcinoma: methodology and preliminary results]. *Nuklearmedizin*. 1997;36(7):228–233.
89. Bidzinski M, et al. [Risk of lymph node metastases in patients with ovarian cancer]. *Ginekol Pol*. 2003;74(9):671–676.
90. Holloway BJ, et al. The significance of paracardiac lymph node enlargement in ovarian cancer. *Clin Radiol*. 1997;52(9):692–697.
91. Suppiah S, et al. Systematic review on the accuracy of positron emission tomography/computed tomography and positron emission tomography/magnetic resonance imaging in the management of ovarian cancer: is functional information really needed? *World J Nucl Med*. 2017;16(3):176–185.
92. Nam EJ, Yun MI, Oh YK, et al. Diagnosis and staging of primary ovarian cancer: Correlation between PET/CT, Doppler US, and CT or MRI. *Gynecol Oncol*. 2010;116(3):389–394.
93. Nelson BE, Rosenfield AT, Schwartz PE. Preoperative abdominopelvic computed tomographic prediction of optimal cytoreduction in epithelial ovarian carcinoma. *J Clin Oncol*. 1993;11(1):166–172.
94. Heintz AP, et al. Cytoreductive surgery in ovarian carcinoma: feasibility and morbidity. *Obstet Gynecol*. 1986;67(6):783–788.
95. Pannu HK, Horton KM, Fishman EK. Thin section dual-phase multidetector-row computed tomography detection of peritoneal metastases in gynecologic cancers. *J Comput Assist Tomogr*. 2003;27(3):333–340.
96. Buy JN, et al. Peritoneal implants from ovarian tumors: CT findings. *Radiology*. 1988;169(3):691–694.
97. Jacquet P, et al. Evaluation of computed tomography in patients with peritoneal carcinomatosis. *Cancer*. 1993;72(5):1631–s1636.
98. Jensen CT, et al. Utility of CT oral contrast administration in the emergency department of a quaternary oncology hospital: diagnostic implications, turnaround times, and assessment of ED physician ordering. *Abdom Radiol (NY)*. 2017;42(11):2760–2768.
99. Gemignani ML, et al. Splenectomy in recurrent epithelial ovarian cancer. *Gynecol Oncol*. 1999;72(3):407–s410.
100. Lee SS, et al. Splenectomy for splenic metastases: a changing clinical spectrum. *Am Surg*. 2000;66(9):837–s840.
101. Halvorsen Jr RA, et al. Intraperitoneal contrast material improves the CT detection of peritoneal metastases. *AJR Am J Roentgenol*. 1991;157(1):37–40.
102. Gryspeerdt S, et al. Intraperitoneal contrast material combined with CT for detection of peritoneal metastases of ovarian cancer. *Eur J Gynaecol Oncol*. 1998;19(5):434–437.
103. Benveniste AP, et al. Potential application of dual-energy CT in gynecologic cancer: initial experience. *AJR Am J Roentgenol*. 2017;208(3):695–705.
104. Goerg C, Schwerk WB. Peritoneal carcinomatosis with ascites. *AJR Am J Roentgenol*. 1991;156(6):1185–1187.
105. Hanbidge AE, Lynch D, Wilson SR. US of the peritoneum. *Radiographics*. 2003;23(3):663–684. discussion 684-685.
106. Low RN, et al. Extrahepatic abdominal imaging in patients with malignancy: comparison of MR imaging and helical CT, with subsequent surgical correlation. *Radiology*. 1999;210(3):625–632.
107. Low RN, Francis IR. MR imaging of the gastrointestinal tract with I.V., gadolinium and diluted barium oral contrast media compared with unenhanced MR imaging and CT. *AJR Am J Roentgenol*. 1997;169(4):1051–1059.
108. Low RN, et al. Peritoneal tumor: MR imaging with dilute oral barium and intravenous gadolinium-containing contrast agents compared with unenhanced MR imaging and CT. *Radiology*. 1997;204(2):513–520.
109. Outwater EK, et al. Benign and malignant gynecologic disease: clinical importance of fluid and peritoneal enhancement in the pelvis at MR imaging. *Radiology*. 1996;200(2):483–488.
110. Semelka RC, et al. Primary ovarian cancer: prospective comparison of contrast-enhanced CT and pre-and postcontrast, fat-suppressed MR imaging, with histologic correlation. *J Magn Reson Imaging*. 1993;3(1):99–106.
111. Arai K, et al. Enhancement of ascites on MRI following intravenous administration of Gd-DTPA. *J Comput Assist Tomogr*. 1993;17(4):617–622.
112. Grabowska-Derlatka L, et al. Diffusion-weighted imaging of small peritoneal implants in "potentially" early-stage ovarian cancer. *Biomed Res Int*. 2016:9254742.
113. Wakefield JC, et al. New MR techniques in gynecologic cancer. *AJR Am J Roentgenol*. 2013;200(2):249–260.
114. Dresen RC, et al. Whole-body diffusion-weighted MRI for operability assessment in patients with colorectal cancer and peritoneal metastases. *Cancer Imaging*. 2019;19(1):1.
115. Michielsen K, et al. Diagnostic value of whole body diffusion-weighted MRI compared to computed tomography for preoperative assessment of patients suspected for ovarian cancer. *Eur J Cancer*. 2017;83:88–98.
116. Garcia Prado J, et al. Diffusion-weighted magnetic resonance imaging in peritoneal carcinomatosis from suspected ovarian cancer: Diagnostic performance in correlation with surgical findings. *Eur J Radiol*. 2019;121:108696.
117. Ma FH, et al. MR Spectroscopy for Differentiating Benign From Malignant Solid Adnexal Tumors. *AJR Am J Roentgenol*. 2015;204(6):W724–730.
118. Yoshida Y, et al. Incremental benefits of FDG positron emission tomography over CT alone for the preoperative staging of ovarian cancer. *AJR Am J Roentgenol*. 2004;182(1):227–233.
119. Sheng XG, et al. [Value of positron emission tomography-CT imaging combined with continual detection of CA125 in serum for diagnosis of early asymptomatic recurrence of epithelial ovarian carcinoma]. *Zhonghua Fu Chan Ke Za Zhi*. 2007;42(7):460–463.
120. Cho SM, et al. Usefulness of FDG PET for assessment of early recurrent epithelial ovarian cancer. *AJR Am J Roentgenol*. 2002;179(2):391–395.
121. Cuenca JI, et al. [Clinical impact of FDG-PET in patients with suspected recurrent ovarian cancer]. *Rev Esp Med Nucl*. 2008;27(6):411–417.
122. Iagaru AH, et al. 18F-FDG PET/CT evaluation of patients with ovarian carcinoma. *Nucl Med Commun*. 2008;29(12):1046–1051.
123. Garcia-Velloso MJ, et al. Diagnostic accuracy of FDG PET in the follow-up of platinum-sensitive epithelial ovarian carcinoma. *Eur J Nucl Med Mol Imaging*. 2007;34(9):1396–1405.
124. Chung HH, et al. Role of [18F]FDG PET/CT in the assessment of suspected recurrent ovarian cancer: correlation with clinical or histological findings. *Eur J Nucl Med Mol Imaging*. 2007;34(4):480–486.
125. Funicelli L, Travaini LL, Landoni F, et al. Peritoneal carcinomatosis from ovarian cancer: the role of CT and [(18)F]FDG-PET/CT. *Abdom Imaging*. 2010;35(6):701–707.
126. Risum S, et al. Does the use of diagnostic PET/CT cause stage migration in patients with primary advanced ovarian cancer? *Gynecol Oncol*. 2010;116(3):395–398.
127. Soussan M, et al. Impact of FDG PET-CT imaging on the decision making in the biologic suspicion of ovarian carcinoma recurrence. *Gynecol Oncol*. 2008;108(1):160–165.
128. Thrall MM, et al. Clinical use of combined positron emission tomography and computed tomography (FDG-PET/CT) in recurrent ovarian cancer. *Gynecol Oncol*. 2007;105(1):17–22.
129. Schmidt S, et al. Peritoneal carcinomatosis in primary ovarian cancer staging: comparison between MDCT, MRI, and 18F-FDG PET/CT. *Clin Nucl Med*. 2015;40(5):371–377.
130. Han S, et al. Performance of pre-treatment (1)(8)F-fluorodeoxyglucose positron emission tomography/computed tomography for detecting metastasis in ovarian cancer: a systematic review and meta-analysis. *J Gynecol Oncol*. 2018;29(6):e98.
131. Funt SA, et al. Role of CT in the management of recurrent ovarian cancer. *AJR Am J Roentgenol*. 2004;182(2):393–398.
132. Low RN, et al. Treated ovarian cancer: MR imaging, laparotomy reassessment, and serum CA-125 values compared with clinical outcome at 1 year. *Radiology*. 2005;235(3):918–926.

133. Balestreri L, et al. Abdominal recurrence of ovarian cancer: value of abdominal MR in patients with positive CA125 and negative CT. *Radiol Med*. 2002;104(5–6):426–436.
134. Ricke J, et al. Prospective evaluation of contrast-enhanced MRI in the depiction of peritoneal spread in primary or recurrent ovarian cancer. *Eur Radiol*. 2003;13(5):943–949.
135. Kubik-Huch RA, et al. Value of (18F)-FDG positron emission tomography, computed tomography, and magnetic resonance imaging in diagnosing primary and recurrent ovarian carcinoma. *Eur Radiol*. 2000;10(5):761–767.
136. Makhija S, et al. Positron emission tomography/computed tomography imaging for the detection of recurrent ovarian and fallopian tube carcinoma: a retrospective review. *Gynecol Oncol*. 2002;85(1):53–58.
137. Gu P, et al. CA 125, PET alone, PET-CT, CT and MRI in diagnosing recurrent ovarian carcinoma: a systematic review and meta-analysis. *Eur J Radiol*. 2009;71(1):164–174.
138. Gadducci A, et al. Are surveillance procedures of clinical benefit for patients treated for ovarian cancer?: A retrospective Italian multicentric study. *Int J Gynecol Cancer*. 2009;19(3):367–374.
139. Hartge P. Designing early detection programs for ovarian cancer. *J Natl Cancer Inst*. 102(1):3-4.
140. Partridge E, et al. Results from four rounds of ovarian cancer screening in a randomized trial. *Obstet Gynecol*. 2009;113(4):775–782.
141. Skates SJ, et al. Toward an optimal algorithm for ovarian cancer screening with longitudinal tumor markers. *Cancer*. 1995;76(10 Suppl):2004–2010.
142. Hogberg T, Kagedal B. Long-term follow-up of ovarian cancer with monthly determinations of serum CA 125. *Gynecol Oncol*. 1992;46(2):191–198.
143. Goonewardene TI, Hall MR, Rustin GJ. Management of asymptomatic patients on follow-up for ovarian cancer with rising CA-125 concentrations. *Lancet Oncol*. 2007;8(9):813–821.
144. Gadducci A, Cosio S. Surveillance of patients after initial treatment of ovarian cancer. *Crit Rev Oncol Hematol*. 2009;71(1):43–52.
145. Crombach G, Zippel HH, Wurz H. [Experiences with CA 125, a tumor marker for malignant epithelial ovarian tumors]. *Geburtshilfe Frauenheilkd*. 1985;45(4):205–212.
146. Gadducci A, et al. Serum CA125 assay at the time of relapse has no prognostic relevance in patients undergoing chemotherapy for recurrent ovarian cancer: a multicenter Italian study. *Int J Gynecol Cancer*. 1997;7(1):78–83.
147. Munnell EW. The changing prognosis and treatment in cancer of the ovary. A report of 235 patients with primary ovarian carcinoma 1952–1961. *Am J Obstet Gynecol*. 1968;100(6):790–805.
148. Hoskins WJ, et al. The effect of diameter of largest residual disease on survival after primary cytoreductive surgery in patients with suboptimal residual epithelial ovarian carcinoma. *Am J Obstet Gynecol*. 1994;170(4):974–979. discussion 979–980.
149. Ozols RF. Paclitaxel (Taxol)/carboplatin combination chemotherapy in the treatment of advanced ovarian cancer. *Semin Oncol*. 2000;27(3 Suppl 7):3–s7.
150. Armstrong DK, et al. Intraperitoneal cisplatin and paclitaxel in ovarian cancer. *N Engl J Med*. 2006;354(1):34–43.
151. Thomas GM. Radiotherapy in early ovarian cancer. *Gynecol Oncol*. 1994;55(3 Pt 2):S73–79.
152. Klaassen D, et al. External beam pelvic radiotherapy plus intraperitoneal radioactive chronic phosphate in early stage ovarian cancer: a toxic combination. A National Cancer Institute of Canada Clinical Trials Group Report. *Int J Radiat Oncol Biol Phys*. 1985;11(10):1801–1804.
153. Cmelak AJ, Kapp DS. Long-term survival with whole abdominopelvic irradiation in platinum-refractory persistent or recurrent ovarian cancer. *Gynecol Oncol*. 1997;65(3):453–460.
154. Dowdy SC, et al. Salvage whole-abdominal radiation therapy after second-look laparotomy or secondary debulking surgery in patients with ovarian cancer. *Gynecol Oncol*. 2005;96(2):389–394.
155. Hoskins WJ, et al. Whole abdominal and pelvic irradiation in patients with minimal disease at second-look surgical reassessment for ovarian carcinoma. *Gynecol Oncol*. 1985;20(3):271–280.
156. Albuquerque KV, et al. Impact of tumor volume-directed involved field radiation therapy integrated in the management of recurrent ovarian cancer. *Gynecol Oncol*. 2005;96(3):701–704.
157. Davidson SA, et al. Limited-field radiotherapy as salvage treatment of localized persistent or recurrent epithelial ovarian cancer. *Gynecol Oncol*. 1993;51(3):349–354.
158. Adelson MD, et al. Palliative radiotherapy for ovarian cancer. *Int J Radiat Oncol Biol Phys*. 1987;13(1):17–21.
159. Burger RA, et al. Phase II trial of bevacizumab in persistent or recurrent epithelial ovarian cancer or primary peritoneal cancer: a Gynecologic Oncology Group Study. *J Clin Oncol*. 2007;25(33):5165–5171.
160. Sanchez-Munoz A, et al. Current status of anti-angiogenic agents in the treatment of ovarian carcinoma. *Clin Transl Oncol*. 2009;11(9):589–595.
161. Cannistra SA, et al. Phase II study of bevacizumab in patients with platinum-resistant ovarian cancer or peritoneal serous cancer. *J Clin Oncol*. 2007;25(33):5180–5186.
162. Cannistra SA, et al. Expression and function of beta 1 and alpha v beta 3 integrins in ovarian cancer. *Gynecol Oncol*. 1995; 58(2):216–225.

CHAPTER

28 Breast Cancer

Huong Le-Petross M.D.; R. Jason Stafford Ph.D.; Isabelle Bedrosian M.D.; Patrick B. Garvey M.D.; Wendy A. Woodward M.D., Ph.D.; and Stacy L. Moulder-Thompson M.D.

INTRODUCTION

The management of breast cancer has evolved into a highly multidisciplinary endeavor that includes specialists from medical and radiation oncology, surgery, radiology, and cancer prevention services. Despite advances in the knowledge and technology associated with diagnosis and treatment, breast cancer continues to be a substantial source of morbidity in women, and efforts to improve proper staging and effective treatment of advanced disease are ongoing. However, early detection of breast cancer is associated with a more favorable prognosis. For example, ductal carcinoma *in situ* (DCIS), an early stage of breast cancer, is associated with an excellent prognosis fairly independent of treatment approach. Therefore, considerable effort in breast cancer research has also been focused on the development of methods for early detection and management of patients with early-stage disease. Whereas clinical breast examinations have long been at the forefront of the screening movement, breast imaging that uses digital mammography and sonography in conjunction with magnetic resonance imaging (MRI), when indicated, currently provides the most effective screening for early detection of breast cancer. In addition, the efficacy of imaging is enhanced substantially when a patient-specific risk assessment is integrated with image-based screening. Thus, breast imaging has come to play a pivotal role in the management of patients with breast cancer. Highly specialized protocols, with an accompanying lexicon for highly nuanced interpretation, facilitate the use of advanced imaging for highly sensitive longitudinal screening, biopsy guidance, presurgical staging, assessment of treatment efficacy, and risk of disease spread or local recurrence. In this chapter, we discuss this evolving role of imaging in the management of breast cancer patients.

EPIDEMIOLOGY

Breast cancer remains the most common cancer diagnosis and the number two cause of cancer-related death in women in the United States.[1] Worldwide, breast cancer remains the most frequently diagnosed cancer in women in the majority of countries.[2] Breast cancer survival rates vary greatly around the world, ranging from less than 40% in impoverished or developing nations to 80% and higher in North America.[3] This disparity in breast cancer–related mortality is most likely related to the lack of or variability in screening programs, education on awareness of symptoms, treatment facilities, and healthcare resources between countries.[3] Screening mammography has been demonstrated to reduce breast cancer–specific mortality by 20% to 30% in randomized clinical trials. The overall death rate from breast cancer decreased by 40% from 1989 to 2016 in the United States.[1] This decrease was most likely related to progress such as expanded treatment options and the implementation of the Mammography Quality Standard Act of 1992, which established a national screening program. A national and government-funded mammography screening program is too costly for many countries because it requires a substantial financial investment to build the healthcare infrastructure required to maintain this program long term. However, the financial investment in preventive healthcare would be worthwhile, because mammography screening in the community setting has been shown to reduce breast cancer mortality not only in the United States but also in other developed countries.[4,5]

The incidence of breast cancer increases with age. In the United States, the segment of the population 65 years and older is expected to exhibit an increase in breast cancer incidence.[1–6] In addition to age and country of residence, other factors affecting the incidence of and mortality from breast cancer include race and ethnicity. The breast cancer incidence is higher in African American and White women living in the United States than in women of any ethnicity living in Asia, South America, or Eastern Europe. Asian American women born in the West have a higher risk of breast cancer than those who were born in Asia; this finding suggests that environmental and behavioral factors, rather than genetic predisposition alone, contribute to the risk of breast cancer.[7] Studies identifying potentially modifiable risk factors for breast cancer provide better opportunities for breast cancer prevention among women who have an average-to-high risk of developing breast cancer.

SCREENING

Mammography

Mammography is used for two major purposes: (1) to screen asymptomatic women for breast cancer and (2) to evaluate breast problems or abnormalities. Although the United States does not have a government-funded screening program, the screening guidelines recommended by the National Cancer Institute advise that women 40 years and older who are at average risk of breast cancer undergo screening mammography every 1 to 2 years.[8] Since the introduction of screening mammography, the number of deaths from breast cancer has declined in every age and racial group of women in the United States.[9] Some investigators attribute this decline to mammography screening, whereas others believe it is related to advances in therapy. The 2002 Swedish screening trial reported that screening mammography reduced breast cancer mortality by 30%, supporting the concept that the decline in breast cancer mortality rates is related to the utilization of screening mammography.[10] Today, the benefits of screening mammography for women between the ages of 50 and 69 years are universally accepted, whereas screening for women between the ages of 40 and 49 years remains controversial, despite the statistically significant reduction in breast cancer mortality[11] and significant increase in survival rates[12] reported.

Screening mammography consists of mediolateral oblique and craniocaudal views of each breast. In the United States, a standardized terminology for interpreting mammograms, the Breast Imaging Reporting and Data System (BI-RADS), has been developed by the American College of Radiology to help facilitate uniformity in mammography reporting across facilities.[13]

Historically, mammography studies were performed using either film screen or full-field digital mammography (FFDM) technologies. FFDM technology slowly replaced film screen mammography, because FFDM provides a lower radiation dose in large breasts; increased image quality associated with a higher contrast resolution; shorter examination times, and hence higher patient throughput; elimination of costs associated with film such as film storage, film, and processing; and facilitation of teleradiology for mammography.[14] Digital breast tomosynthesis (DBT) has become the standard of care in the last several years, in a hybrid setting with FFDM or totally replacing mammography. DBT has been demonstrated in clinical trials to result in decreased recall rate and increased detection rate.[15] Additional advanced techniques such as computer-assisted diagnosis algorithms and/or contrast-enhanced mammography are current areas of research that may improve the detection of small early-stage cancers and decrease the false-positive recall rate (Fig. 28.1).

The potential role of physician-performed screening ultrasound (US) as an adjunct to mammography screening has been evaluated in a multiinstitutional trial that demonstrated many barriers to widespread implementation, such as high false-positive rates and low reimbursement rates.[16] In high-risk populations, such as women with a genetic predisposition for breast cancer, MRI has been reported to have a higher sensitivity than either US or mammography for the detection of breast cancer; therefore, MRI is a more appropriate adjunct to screening mammography in these cases.

Magnetic Resonance Imaging

Use of screening mammography in the general population has been shown to reduce the mortality associated with breast cancer by at least 24%.[17] Women at high risk of breast cancer owing to a known genetic predisposition should be engaged in aggressive surveillance and screening, which should begin at a younger age than screening for women in the general population because of the potential for early onset associated with familial breast cancer. Current surveillance protocols for screening women with a *BRCA1* or *BRCA2* mutation include a clinical breast examination every 6 months and annual mammography and MRI.[18]

Multiple studies have demonstrated higher cancer detection rates with MRI than with mammography, although the differences were not statistically significant.[19–21] Despite variations in breast cancer screening techniques between facilities, MRI is consistently reported to have a higher sensitivity (77%–100%) than mammography (25%–40%).[22–24] MRI detects more breast cancers than either mammography or sonography.[22–24] However, MRI also consistently demonstrates a higher false-positive rate and, thus is associated with a higher biopsy rate (8.2%) than mammography (2.3%) or sonography (2.3%).[24] The majority of breast cancers detected on MRI screening demonstrate the typical conspicuous morphologic and dynamic enhancing patterns expected for malignant lesions (Fig. 28.2). However, in a trial studying patients at high risk of breast cancer, 20% of the breast cancers detected on MRI screening presented with nonmasslike enhancement, and 33% presented with an enhancing pattern typical for benign lesions.[25] This lack of specificity associated with current morphologic and kinetic MRI features makes MRI detection of breast cancers in high-risk patients challenging. A study by Kuhl and coworkers[26] compared clinical breast examination, mammography, sonography, and MRI in 529 study participants. The combination of mammography and MRI yielded the highest sensitivity (93%), which agrees with the findings from other published trials. In this trial, MRI and mammography had the same specificity (97%), as opposed to a higher specificity for mammography than MRI reported in prior studies. This improved specificity of MRI may be as a result of improved imaging techniques.[26]

Although the role of MRI in breast screening programs continues to evolve, the full impact of modern MRI screening technology on mortality from breast cancer is still unknown. Patients for whom MRI is being considered should be informed of the current status of MRI in the detection of breast cancer, and appropriate management strategies are best determined on an individual basis. At the present time, no consensus exists as to the appropriateness of MRI as an adjunct to screening mammography in the general population.

Key Points Screening

Clinical Breast Examination

- Every 3 years, starting at age 20 to 39 years.
- Annually after age 40 years.

Mammography

- Annual, starting at age 40 years, with no specific upper age.[1]

Magnetic Resonance Imaging

- Annual magnetic resonance imaging with mammography in at with high risk for breast cancer, such as those with the following risk factors:

[1]Annual screening interval is recommended by American College of Radiology, American Cancer Society, and National Comprehensive Cancer Network. Biennial screening interval is recommended by American College of Physicians and US Preventive Services Task Force.

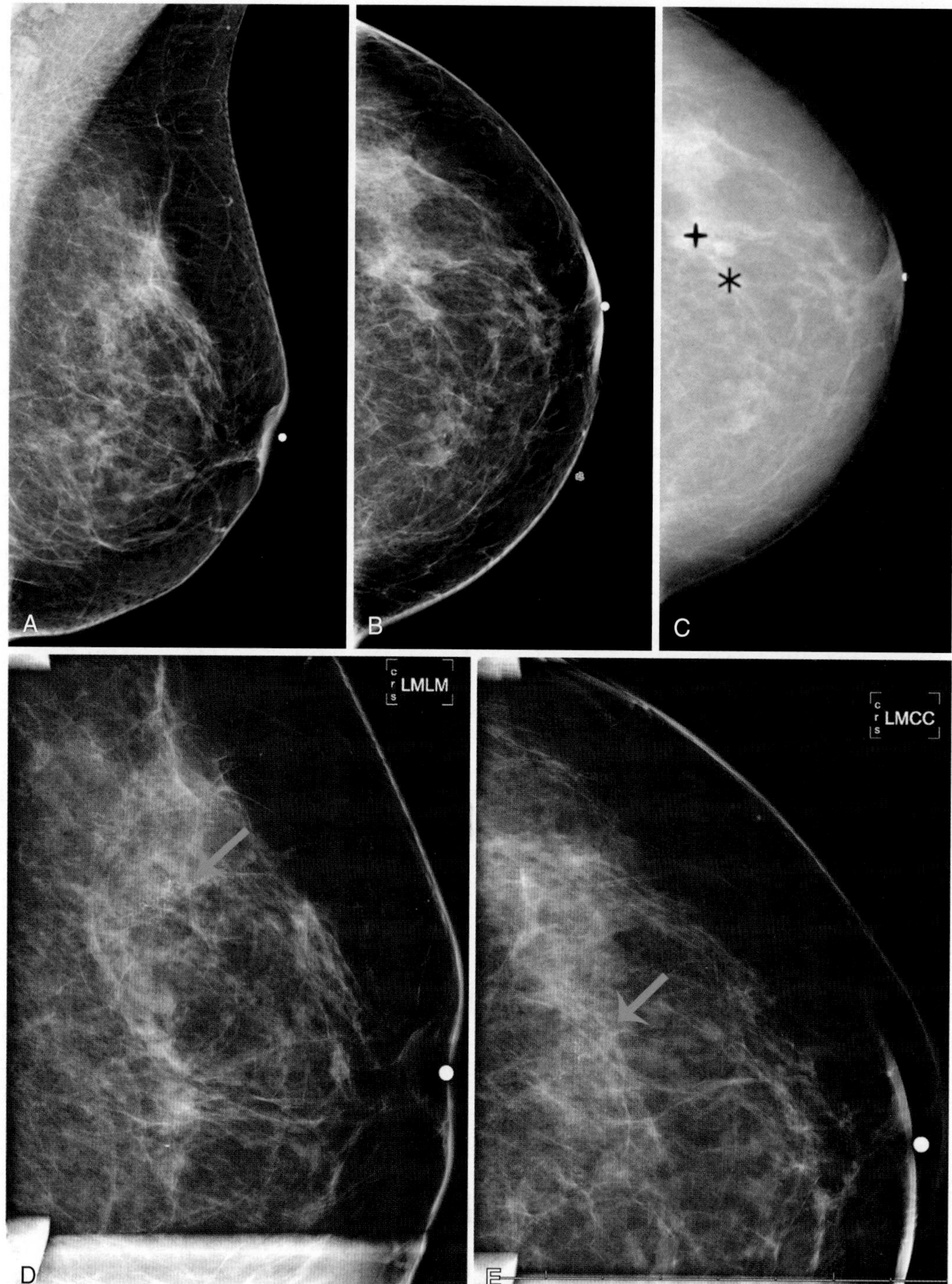

FIGURE 28.1. A 53-year-old woman had a screening mammogram (**A**, craniocaudal [CC] view and **B**, mediolateral [ML] view) that demonstrated a cluster of suspicious microcalcifications at the 12 to 1 o'clock position of the left breast, measuring 10 mm. **C**, Computer-assisted diagnosis software digitally annotated the suspicious calcifications (*asterisk*). **D** and **E**, Magnification ML and CC views confirm that the calcifications (*arrows*) have suspicious characteristics. Stereotactic-guided biopsy confirms that the calcifications represent intraductal carcinoma, grades 1 to 2.

- *BRCA1/2* mutation carrier.
- First-degree relative of *BRCA1/2* mutation carrier, but untested.
- Lifetime risk approximately 20% to 25% or greater.
- Radiation to chest between ages 10 and 30 years.
- Li–Fraumeni syndrome and first-degree relatives with breast cancer.
- Cowden or Bannayan-Riley-Ruvalcaba syndrome and first-degree relatives with breast cancer.

ANATOMY AND PATHOLOGY

Anatomy

The breast is composed of 15 to 20 lactiferous ducts that open in the subareolar tissue. The areolar tissue and nipple contain smooth muscle fibers, sensory nerve cell endings, sebaceous glands, sweat glands, and accessory areolar

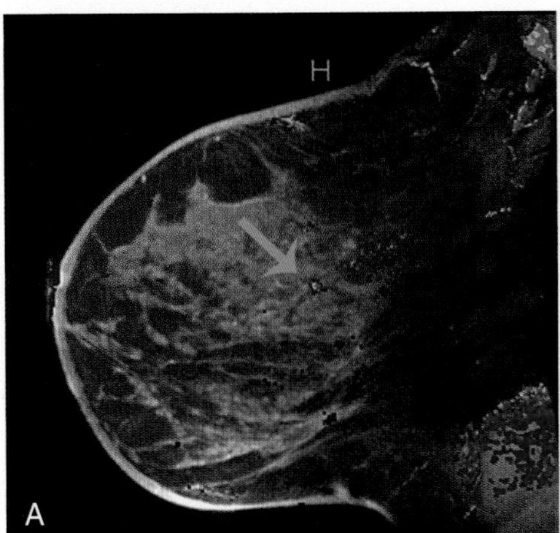

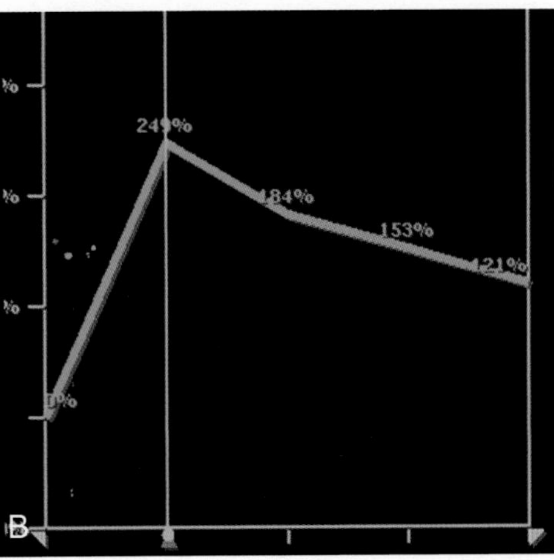

FIGURE 28.2. A 49-year-old woman with a history of right segmentectomy for breast cancer 3 years before this screening magnetic resonance imaging study. The recent screening mammography examination was negative for cancer. Sagittal T1-weighed contrast-enhanced image (**A**) and kinetic curve analysis image (**B**) of the right breast revealed a 6-mm invasive ductal carcinoma (*arrow* in **A**) with initial rapid enhancement and delayed washout pattern.

glands (also called Montgomery glands). The breast is attached to the skin by fibrous connective tissue and suspensory structures called Cooper's ligaments. Posterior to the breast tissue is the retromammary bursa, located between the deep layer of the superficial fascia and the deep layer of the pectoralis major muscle.[27] The breast extends from the second or third rib to the sixth or seventh rib. The breast rests on the pectoralis major, serratus anterior, and external abdominal oblique muscles and the upper extent of the rectus sheath. The mammary gland growth is influenced by the levels of estrogen, progesterone, and adrenal corticoids; during pregnancy or lactation, growth of the mammary gland is also influenced by prolactin (from the adenohypophysis) and somatomammotropin (from the placenta).

The axilla contains important structures, such as vessels, nerves, connective tissue, and lymph nodes. The boundaries of the axilla are the four walls, the apex, and the base. The four walls are the anterior wall (pectoralis major and minor muscles and associated fasciae), posterior wall (subscapularis muscle, teres major, and latissimus dorsi muscles and associated tendons), lateral wall (humerus and bicipital groove), and medial wall (serratus anterior muscle). The apex is the aperture into the cervicoaxillary canal, whose borders consist of the clavicle, scapula, and the first rib. The base consists of the axillary fascia and skin.

Pathology

Breast cancer is a heterogeneous disease and has been traditionally categorized as *in situ* lesions (DCIS and lobular carcinoma *in situ*) or invasive cancers. The *in situ* or noninvasive disease encompasses a spectrum of lesions and is not as simple as the original definition implies[28]; *in situ* lesions develop in a linear progression from normal breast tissue to atypical ductal hyperplasia, DCIS, and invasive cancers. DCIS predominantly arises from the terminal ductal-lobular unit and may extend into the extralobular ducts.

The conventional pathologic classifications of invasive breast cancers include invasive ductal carcinoma, invasive lobular carcinoma, tubular carcinoma, mucinous carcinoma, medullary carcinoma, papillary carcinoma, metaplastic carcinoma, and other less common types. Tubular carcinoma accounts for 3% to 5% of all invasive breast carcinomas, is low-grade with excellent prognosis, and usually occurs in older women.[29] Mucinous or colloid carcinoma is characterized on histologic examination as having extracellular pools of mucin and low-grade tumor aggregates. Pure mucinous carcinoma also has a very favorable prognosis, with a 10-year survival rate of 90%.[29] Medullary carcinoma is commonly seen on imaging as a circumscribed mass consistent with the distinctive smooth pushing border seen on pathology.[30] Medullary carcinoma also has a favorable prognosis, but is less common than tubular and mucinous carcinomas. This type of carcinoma comprises a higher proportion of *BRCA1/2*-related breast cancers than sporadic cases but still represents a minority of the breast cancers in women with *BRCA1/2* mutations. Metaplastic carcinomas include tumors that show both epithelial and mesenchymal features and exhibit an aggressive clinical course with sarcoma-like behavior.[31] Inflammatory breast cancer is a rare but aggressive disease with a poor prognosis; it is usually diagnosed clinically owing to the inflammatory symptoms. In addition to the type of breast cancer, the receptor or tumor marker status of the cancer (estrogen receptor [ER], progesterone receptor [PR], and human epidermal growth factor receptor 2 [HER2]) is very important for determining the treatment options in patients with invasive breast carcinoma and for considering hormonal therapy in patients with *in situ* disease.

Molecular classification, based on genetic profiling, divides breast cancer into five subtypes: luminal A, luminal B, normal breast–like, HER2+, and basal-like carcinomas.[32] Luminal A breast cancer is characterized by the high expression of ERs and PRs, tends to be of a lower grade, and has a better prognosis than the other subtypes. Luminal B breast cancers not only express ERs and/or PRs but also overexpress HER2. They are more aggressive, with high tumor grade. The normal breast–like type or unclassified subtype is a triple-negative tumor with a molecular profile similar to that of basal-like carcinoma; however, normal breast–like carcinoma has a better prognosis than basal-like carcinoma. The HER2+ subtype includes ER-negative and ER-positive types and is often associated with DCIS. The basal-like breast carcinomas lack ER, PR, and HER2 expression and, therefore, are often called triple-negative tumors. These tumors show a high rate of *P53* mutations and are common in *BRCA1/2* mutation carriers. Triple-negative cancers tend to be more sensitive

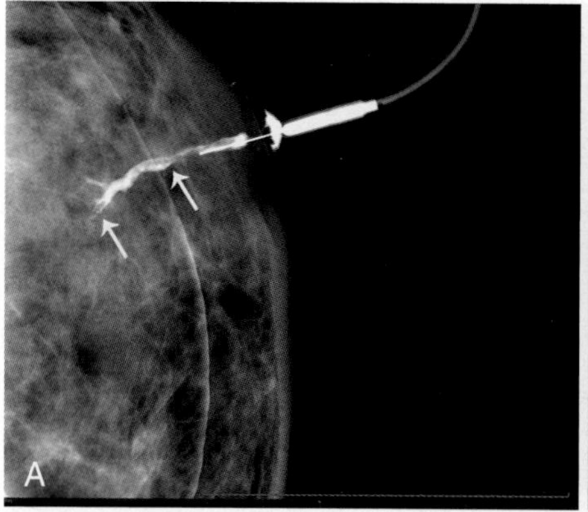

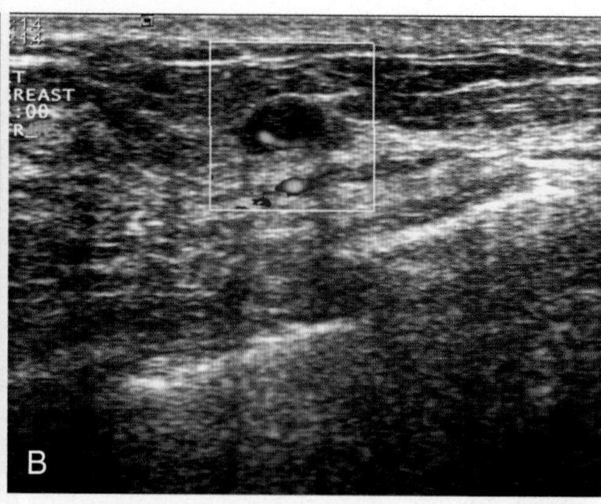

FIGURE 28.3. A 53-year-old woman with a history of bloody nipple discharge from the left breast. **A**, She underwent ductography, which demonstrated filling defects (*arrows*) within a duct. **B**, An ultrasound of the same duct revealed a circumscribed solid nodule with internal vascularity. At surgery, this central duct was excised, and final pathology demonstrated intraductal papillomas.

to chemotherapy but have a worse prognosis than other subtypes.[2,33] However, not all triple-negative breast cancers are basal-like tumors. Some data suggest that 76% of triple-negative breast cancers are basal-like, and 77% of the basal-like tumors are triple negative.[29] This molecular classification will likely be further modified as additional molecular features are discovered. Future classifications should help predict the sensitivity of particular tumors to targeted therapies, thereby improving the selection of patients for specific therapeutic approaches.

KEY POINTS Pathology

- Breast cancer is a heterogeneous disease and can be *in situ*, invasive, or both.
- Invasive breast cancers are classified by morphology: ductal, lobular, tubular, mucinous, medullary, papillary, metaplastic, and others.
- Breast cancer subtypes are determined by gene profiling: luminal A, luminal B, normal, receptor 2 (HER2)+, and basal-like.
- Estrogen receptor, progesterone receptor, HER2, and lymphovascular invasion status are important risk factors for relapse.

CLINICAL PRESENTATION

The detection of cancer at an early stage, when the cancer is small, may reduce cancer-related mortality and improve survival. Cancers can be detected on palpation or present with symptoms rather than with imaging screening, such as mammography or US. In a national survey of 41,000 breast cancer patients, approximately 70% presented with a palpable breast mass.[34] A more recent study of 592 breast cancer cases reported that the cancer was detected as a palpable mass and not at screening in 43% of patients.[35] The investigators evaluated the role of breast self-examination as a screening tool and reported that women who performed breast self-examinations did not have lower breast cancer mortality rates than women who did not practice breast self-examinations.[35]

Common clinical presentations of breast cancer on clinical breast examination include a breast mass, asymmetrical thickening or nodularity, nipple retraction, bloody nipple discharge, skin dimpling, and erythema. For a palpable breast mass, further evaluation on imaging, and possibly a core needle or fine-needle aspiration biopsy, would be needed. For asymmetrical thickening or nodularity, further evaluation with US is needed, and possibly mammography for women 30 years or older. For nonspontaneous nipple discharge and discharge from multiple ducts, the suspicion of breast cancer is low, and patients are advised to stop compression of the breast and elicitation of the nipple discharge. For spontaneous unilateral or single-duct nipple discharge, or serous, sanguineous, or serosanguineous nipple discharge, investigation with mammography, US, MRI, or ductography is recommended to determine the etiology and rule out a malignancy (Fig. 28.3). Skin changes in women older than 40 years would raise a concern of either infection or inflammatory breast cancer. Skin changes may include peau d'orange or skin thickening, Paget disease with scaling, eczema, or nipple excoriation. Other associated clinical symptoms of concern include lymphadenopathy and weight loss.

In addition to performing a clinical or physical examination, many medical clinics offer risk assessment analysis for women who request this service. A risk assessment includes a detailed analysis of relevant personal and family history (such as family members with breast or ovarian cancers), counseling on risk factors, genetic testing, and surveillance and chemoprevention options.

STAGING CLASSIFICATION

Staging at the time of initial diagnosis is essential to determine the extent and severity of the breast cancer, to determine the best choice of therapy, to estimate the prognosis, and to identify those patients eligible for clinical trials. The most popular staging system is the anatomic stage or tumor-node-metastasis (TNM) system (Table 28.1, p. 481), which includes the primary breast tumor size, the regional lymph nodes involvement, and the spread of cancer to distant sites.[36] The latest (eighth) edition of the American Joint Committee on Cancer staging system made significant changes to prior versions, with two stage group options: the anatomic stage for use when biomarkers (grade, ER, PR, HER2) are not available, and prognostic stage for patients for whom T, N, M, tumor grade, ER, PR, and HER2 status information are available.[36] The pathologic staging is based on the tumor size of the

TABLE 28.1 Tumor-Node-Metastasis Classification of Breast Cancer

STAGE	CHARACTERISTICS
T	Primary tumor
Tx	Primary tumor not assessed
To	Primary tumor not detected
Tis	DCIS, LCIS, Paget disease of nipple with no tumor
T1	Tumor ≤2 cm in greatest dimension
T1mic	Microinvasion ≤0.1 cm or smaller in greatest dimension
T1a	Tumor >0.1 cm but ≤0.5 cm in greatest dimension
T1b	Tumor >0.5 cm but ≤1 cm in greatest dimension
T1c	Tumor >1 cm but ≤2 cm in greatest dimension
T2	Tumor >2 cm but ≤5 cm in greatest dimension
T3	Tumor >5 cm in greatest dimension
T4	Tumor of any size with direct extension to chest wall or skin
T4a	Extension to chest wall, but not pectoralis muscle
T4b	Edema
T4c	T4a and 4b
T4d	Inflammatory carcinoma
N	Regional lymph nodes
pNx	Regional lymph nodes cannot be assessed
pN0	No regional lymph node metastasis identified histologically
pN1	Micrometastasis, or metastases in one to three axillary lymph nodes with or without internal mammary nodes
pN2	Metastases in ≥10 axillary lymph nodes, or infraclavicular lymph nodes (level III), or clinically detected internal mammary lymph nodes, or >3 axillary lymph nodes and internal mammary nodes, or ipsilateral supraclavicular lymph nodes
pN3	Metastases in ≥10 axillary lymph nodes, or metastases to infraclavicular lymph nodes (level III)
M	Distant metastases
M0	No distant metastases
cM0 (i+)	Circulating tumor cells or microscopic tumor cells in bone marrow; no clinical or radiologic distant metastasis
M1	Distant metastases

final pathology specimen and is to be used when surgical resection is the initial treatment, before systemic or radiation therapy. For multiple synchronous ipsilateral primary carcinomas, the largest tumor is used. Once the tumor size, node status, and presence of metastatic disease have been determined, one of the five breast cancer stages is assigned. Stage 0 is assigned to precancerous lesions or carcinoma *in situ* with no local or distant metastasis; this stage is associated with a nearly 100% cure rate. Stage I is assigned to small cancers confined to the breast, and these patients have an excellent prognosis. Stage II cancers have regional lymph node metastases, and stage III breast cancers involve large tumors or locally advanced disease at the time of initial diagnosis. Stages II and III are associated with a poor prognosis. Stage IV cancers have a distant metastasis and are associated with a poor survival (Fig. 28.4).

PATTERNS OF TUMOR SPREAD

Recurrent disease and distant metastases occur when cancer cells remain after treatment or spread beyond the breast and axillary lymph nodes, representing a major source of morbidity in breast cancer patients. Breast cancer cells can spread via the lymphatic system to the regional lymph nodes, involving the level I axillary lymph nodes first, followed by levels II and III. Level I lymph nodes are lateral to the lateral border of the pectoralis minor muscle. Level II lymph nodes are between the medial and the lateral borders of the pectoralis minor muscle, as well as the interpectoral lymph nodes (Rotter's nodes). Level III lymph nodes are medial to the medial margin of the pectoralis minor muscle and inferior to the clavicle. Standard axillary nodal dissection often involves removal of level I and II axillary lymph nodes. Involvement of the internal mammary chain is observed in approximately 20% of patients, often with large and deep medially located breast cancer, and tends to be associated with extensive metastasis.

Tumor cells may spread to distant sites via the lymphatic or circulatory system. Four major sites of distant metastasis are bone, lung, brain, and liver. Bone is the most common site of metastasis from most subtypes of breast cancer,[37] and the presence of tumor cells in the bone marrow is a strong predictor for distant metastases. Cutaneous metastasis is not common, but breast carcinoma is the most common primary malignancy to spread to the skin and accounts for 24% of all cutaneous metastases.[38] The pattern of spread is not a random process, and a better understanding of this process and a rational approach to preventing this sequence of selective events are essential to improving the survival of patients with metastatic breast cancer.

KEY POINTS Metastases

- May be local, regional, or distant disease.
- May be lymphatic or hematogenous spread.
- Most commonly occurs in bone and visceral organs.
- Nonrandomized process with distinct pattern associated with cancer subtypes and survival.

IMAGING

Several modalities available to image the breasts include mammography, US, ductography, and MRI. Once a woman has been diagnosed with breast cancer, cross-sectional imaging with computed tomography (CT), positron emission tomography (PET), MRI, or bone scintigraphy are often indicated to image the rest of the body. Most often, using a combination of imaging modalities is crucial for the accurate staging of breast cancer. Here, an overview of the role of imaging in the diagnosis and staging of this common disease is presented.

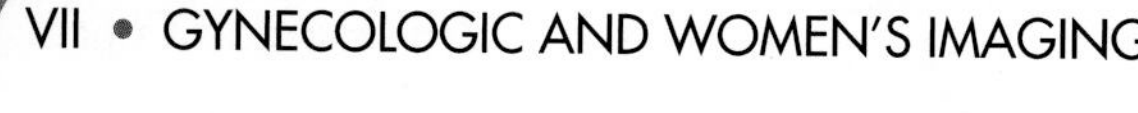

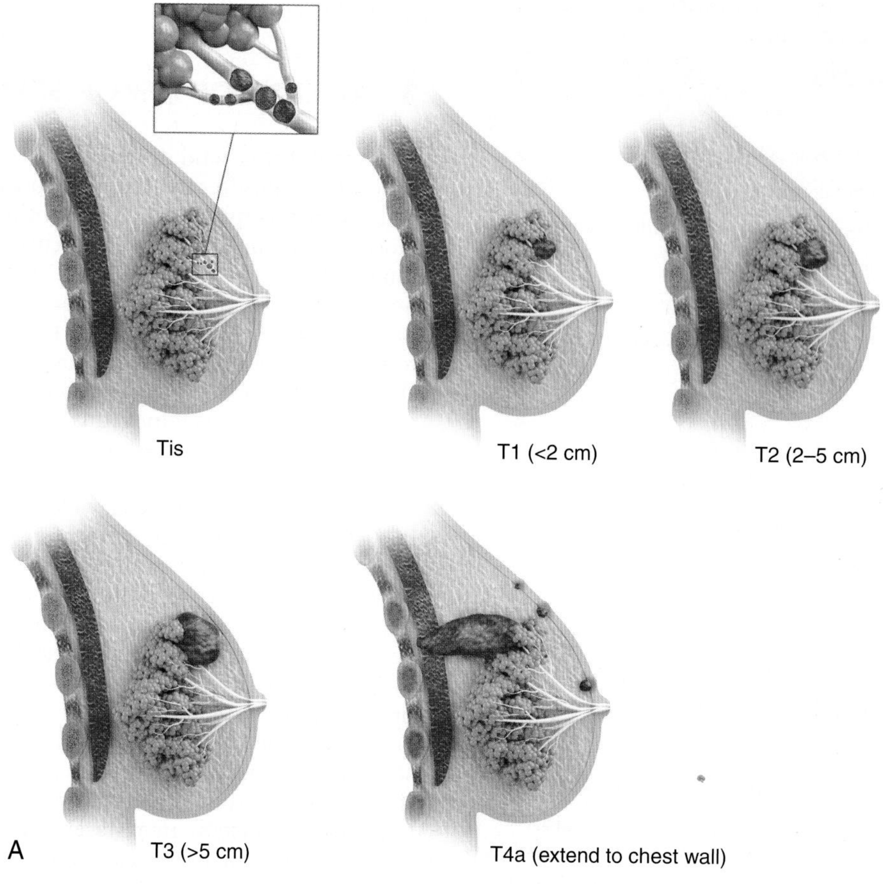

FIGURE 28.4. cont'd

Primary Tumor

Breast imaging is used to detect primary or recurrent breast cancer, to determine the extent of disease, to evaluate lymph nodes involvement, and to identify distant metastatic disease. Cancer within the affected breast may be described as unifocal (Fig. 28.5), multifocal (two or more lesions in the same quadrant [Fig. 28.6]), or multicentric (lesions in two or more quadrants [Fig. 28.7]). Currently, mammography, US, and MRI are the primary modalities indicated in the detection and staging of breast cancer.

Mammography

Diagnostic mammography or problem-solving mammography is performed when a patient presents with a palpable finding or when a suspicious finding is detected with screening mammography. A radiopaque BB or skin marker is placed directly over the suspicious region before the mammogram is obtained. In addition to the mediolateral oblique and craniocaudal (CC) views, additional views may be indicated to properly evaluate the abnormality. A 90-degree lateral view can assist in triangulating the abnormality. Spot compression views in CC and lateral projections are incorporated to evaluate a possible mass, asymmetrical density, or superimposition of normal breast parenchyma. Magnification views (in CC or lateral projections) facilitate characterization of microcalcifications. With digital tomosynthesis (DBT) becoming commonly used with or in place of mammography, spot compression views with DBT may increase the sensitivity and specificity of mammography for cancer detection and diagnosis.[39] Studies to date have demonstrated DBT to be equivalent to mammography in a diagnostic setting and to increase cancer detection in a screening setting.[40]

Mammography or DBT is also used to guide biopsy (stereotactic-guided core biopsy with vacuum-assisted devices) and guide preoperative localization of a lesion. Immediately after resection of the targeted lesion, the biopsy or resected specimen can be imaged while the patient is still under anesthesia to verify the margins. This "specimen radiography" provides additional information in patients who had a complete response to preoperative chemotherapy, because the only image-detectable finding is often the biopsy clip placed at the time of the initial biopsy, or residual calcifications (Fig. 28.8).

Ultrasound

Breast US is widely used as a screening tool or a diagnostic tool for characterization of lesions detected via mammography or clinical examination and for staging of newly diagnosed breast cancer. The BI-RADS risk assessment

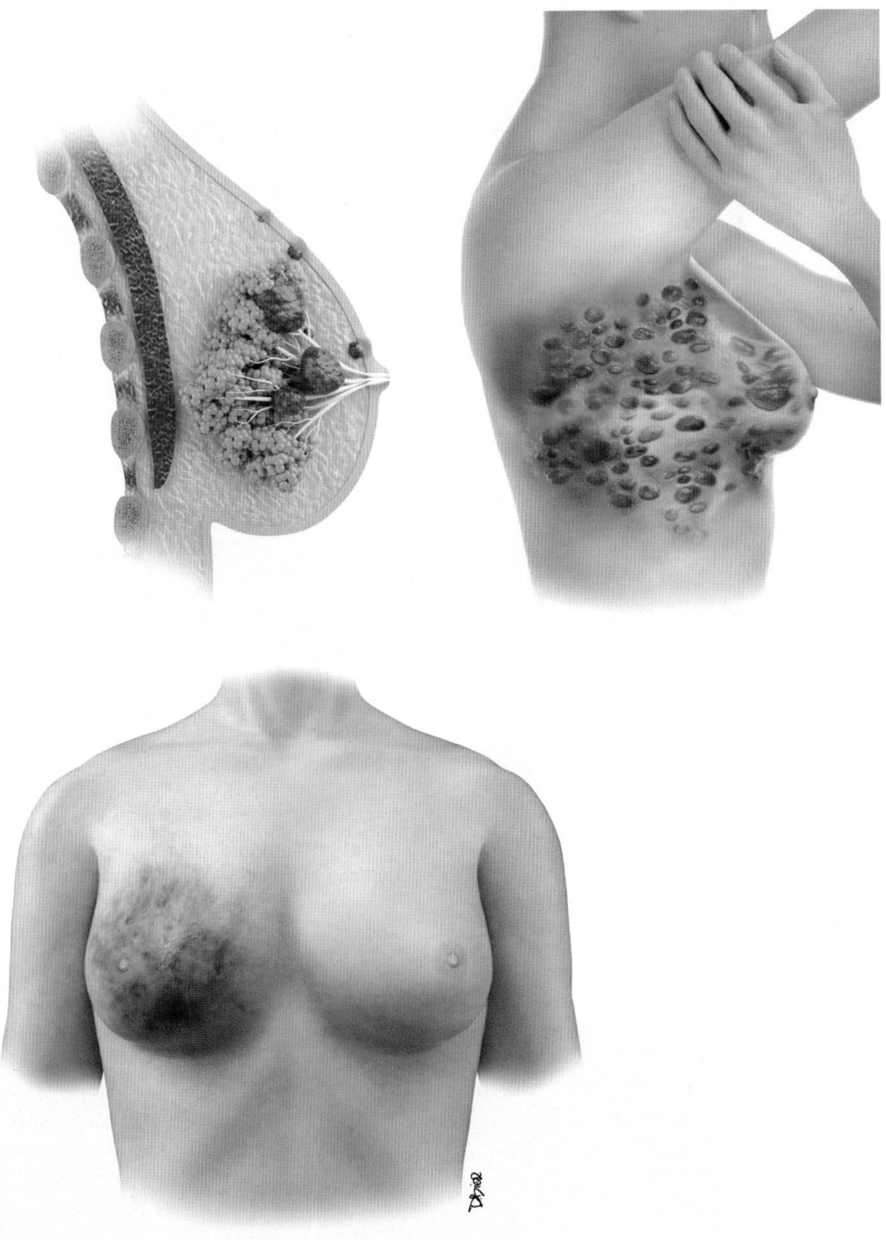

FIGURE 28.4. cont'd

categories should be adhered to in the reporting of breast US findings.[13] A linear array transducer should be used to perform the examination, using the highest center frequency (7.5–15 MHz) possible that still penetrates to the chest wall. Both longitudinal and transverse planes are commonly used to characterize findings.[41] However, a radial and orthogonal antiradial pattern has been demonstrated to be superior and is preferred.[41] Breast tumors are usually hypoechoic solid masses with irregular margins, posterior acoustic shadowing, and internal vascularity on color Doppler imaging (Fig. 28.9). US of the ipsilateral axilla should be conducted for all newly diagnosed breast cancer cases to assess for morphologically abnormal nodes and guide biopsy via US-guided core biopsy or fine-needle aspiration. Radiologic marker placement at the time of the US-guided breast or nodal biopsy can aid in facilitating subsequent confirmation of proper node recovery or ensuring the complete removal of the breast cancer that has disappeared after the completion of neoadjuvant chemotherapy. At our institution, the infraclavicular (level II) and internal mammary regions are also evaluated during the staging US examination of all new breast cancer cases (Fig. 28.10, p. 488).

Magnetic Resonance Imaging

A breast MRI is performed with the patient lying in a prone position within a 1.5-Tesla or higher magnetic field strength scanner. Only breast-dedicated multiphase array coils should be used, to ensure adequate spatial resolution. The examination usually uses bilateral imaging techniques for several reasons, including the ability to assess

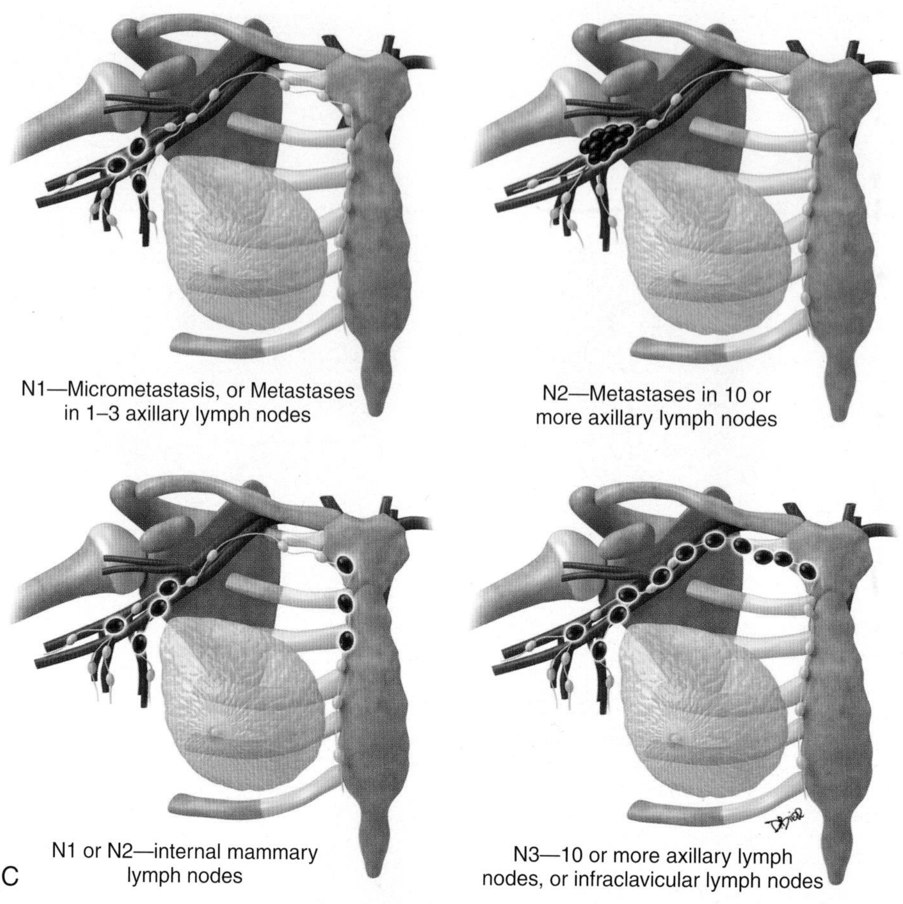

FIGURE 28.4. Staging breast cancer. **A** and **B**, Primary tumor (T). **C**, Lymph nodes (N).

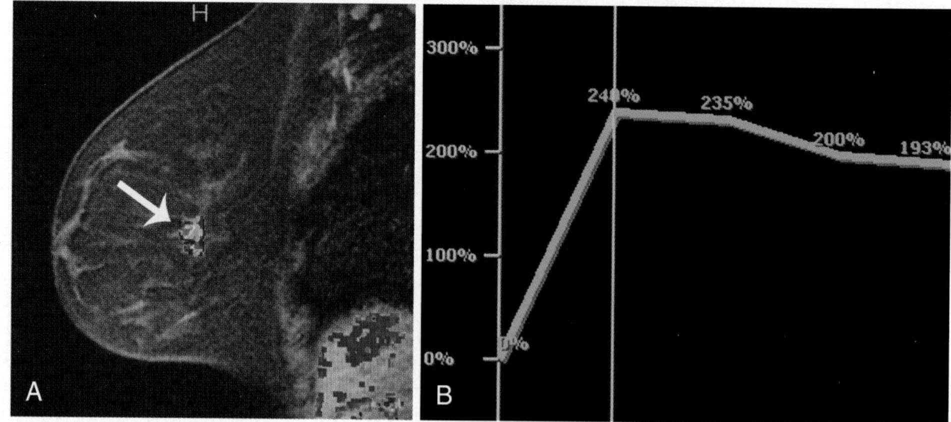

FIGURE 28.5. **A**, A 52-year-old woman with a newly diagnosed unifocal invasive ductal carcinoma in the right breast (*arrow*) measuring 1.8 cm. **B**, The kinetic analysis demonstrates the rapid initial enhancement with delayed washout pattern, typical for malignancy.

asymmetrical enhancement between the breasts as well as evaluation for contralateral carcinoma in patients with newly diagnosed breast cancer. Common sequences of a standard examination include a precontrast T1-weighted (T1W) pulse sequence to delineate fat from a lesion or lymph node, a precontrast T2-weighted (T2W) pulse sequence with or without fat suppression to separate cysts from most solid masses, a time series of contrast-enhanced T1W sequences to detect enhancing breast masses, or a dynamic contrast-enhanced series. This series usually consists of a minimum of three time points after the intravenous administration of the contrast medium over a 6- to 8-minute period. The minimal imaging parameter requirements for the dynamic acquisition recommended by the American College of Radiology include a slice thickness of mm or less and in-plane resolution of 1 mm or less to facilitate the evaluation of essential morphologic details such as lesion margins, spiculations, and internal enhancement. Interpretation is based on the descriptors from the BI-RADS MRI lexicon.

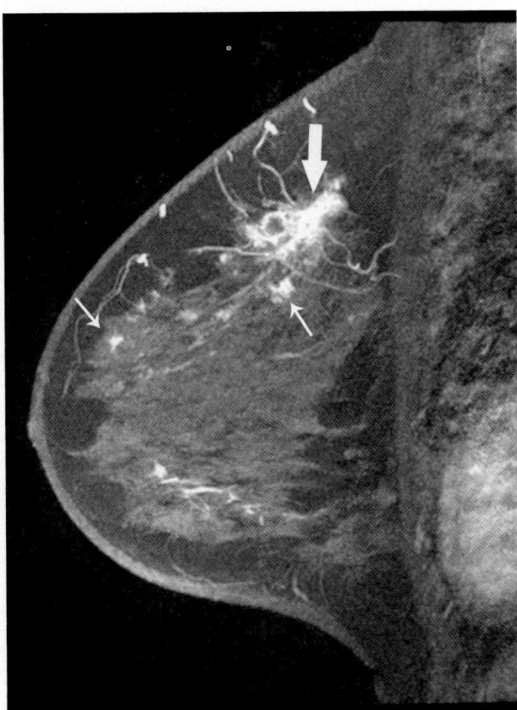

Figure 28.6. A 46-year-old woman with a newly diagnosed 3.2-cm invasive ductal carcinoma in the left breast seen on mammography and ultrasound. Sagittal postcontrast fat-suppressed T1-weighted (T1W) gradient echo magnetic resonance imaging study of the left breast revealed multifocal disease with the known carcinoma (*thick arrow*) and additional enhancing foci extending toward the nipple in a ductal distribution (*thin arrows*). The high T1W signals within the ducts in the inferior breast are related to fibrocystic changes; no malignancy was seen on pathology after mastectomy.

The use of preoperative breast MRI in staging newly diagnosed breast cancers remains a source of considerable discussion and research.[42] MRI used in conjunction with a computer-aided detection software can be helpful in defining the extent and size of the primary breast carcinoma and has been used to detect additional foci of malignancy within the ipsilateral breast in up to 16% of patients and malignancies that were occult on mammography within the contralateral breast in up to 4% of patients.[43,44] A metaanalysis of 19 studies and a prospective randomized Comparative Effectiveness of MRI in Breast Cancer trial reported that MRI demonstrated no benefit on the reoperation rate but did result in more extensive breast surgery.[43,45] Another metaanalysis of 50 studies reported that 67% of additional MRI findings in two-thirds of studies were malignant but only impacted treatment in 20% of patients.[46] Unfortunately, the additional disease detected on MRI has not translated into improved outcomes. The impact of preoperative MRI-based decisions on reduction in recurrent disease was not significant.[47] Preoperative MRI is not necessarily indicated in every patient; the ability of MRI to detect additional tumor foci and contralateral cancers that are not detected via physical examination or mammography should not be discounted.

For less common and more aggressive invasive breast cancers, such as invasive lobular carcinoma or inflammatory breast cancer, MRI can provide useful information regarding tumor extension, as well as involvement of skin, nipple, or chest wall.[48,49] Because of the diffuse infiltrative growth pattern of invasive lobular carcinoma, a prebiopsy MRI may be helpful in accurately localizing the disease and facilitating a more effective biopsy and surgical plan (Fig. 28.11, p. 489). In patients who present with adenocarcinoma in the axilla without a diagnosis of a primary carcinoma, MRI has been demonstrated to be beneficial in identifying the primary tumor.[50] When a primary breast lesion can be detected (Fig. 28.12, p. 490), proper staging can be performed, facilitating targeted therapy or consideration for breast-conservation therapy in conjunction with radiotherapy, depending on the stage of the carcinoma.

DCIS is a noninvasive malignancy, and the patient is often asymptomatic. However, DCIS is associated with increased risk of developing invasive carcinoma that can involve multiple sites. The prevalence of DCIS diagnoses in the United States has increased with the introduction of screening mammography and currently accounts for 25% to 30% of all reported breast cancers. Mammography tends to underestimate both the size and the extent of DCIS.[51] MRI, conversely, has a reported sensitivity of 67% to 100% for the detection DCIS, whereas mammography has a sensitivity of 70% to 80%.[52,53] Common MRI features indicative of DCIS include clumped or heterogeneous enhancement in a linear, ductal, or segmental distribution (Fig. 28.13, p. 490). MRI may be useful in cases where mammography, US, and clinical findings are inconclusive and no focal finding is apparent; currently, approximately 95% of DCIS cases are diagnosed via calcifications identified on mammography.

Unconventional Breast Imaging

In contrast to conventional breast imaging tools (mammography, US, and MRI) that focus primarily on anatomic and morphologic detail, many molecular imaging techniques focus on the functional differences between normal and cancerous tissues. For example, positron emission mammography (PEM) shows glucose analog 2-[^{18}F] fluoro-2-deoxy-D-glucose uptake by metabolically active cells such as tumor cells. PEM is approved by the US Food and Drug Administration for imaging the breast (Fig. 28.14, p. 491) and is reported to have comparable sensitivity to but greater specificity than MRI.[54] Breast magnetic resonance spectroscopy (MRS) detects metabolic byproducts such as choline within a suspicious lesion, as an elevated choline concentration tends to be indicative of a malignant process. As an adjuvant tool to breast MRI, MRS may improve the specificity of MRI.[55] The limited resolution and imaging of only one lesion at a time limit the practical use of MRS (Fig. 28.15, p. 491) Other promising technologies, such as dedicated breast CT and optical coherence tomography, are still being researched and are not widely used at this time (Fig. 28.16, p. 492)[56]

Nodal Disease

Evaluation of the local regional nodal basin is among the key prognostic factors in the newly diagnosed breast cancer patient. Increasingly, this evaluation is initially performed noninvasively with US. In a metaanalysis of 16 selected studies, axillary US combined with needle biopsy had a

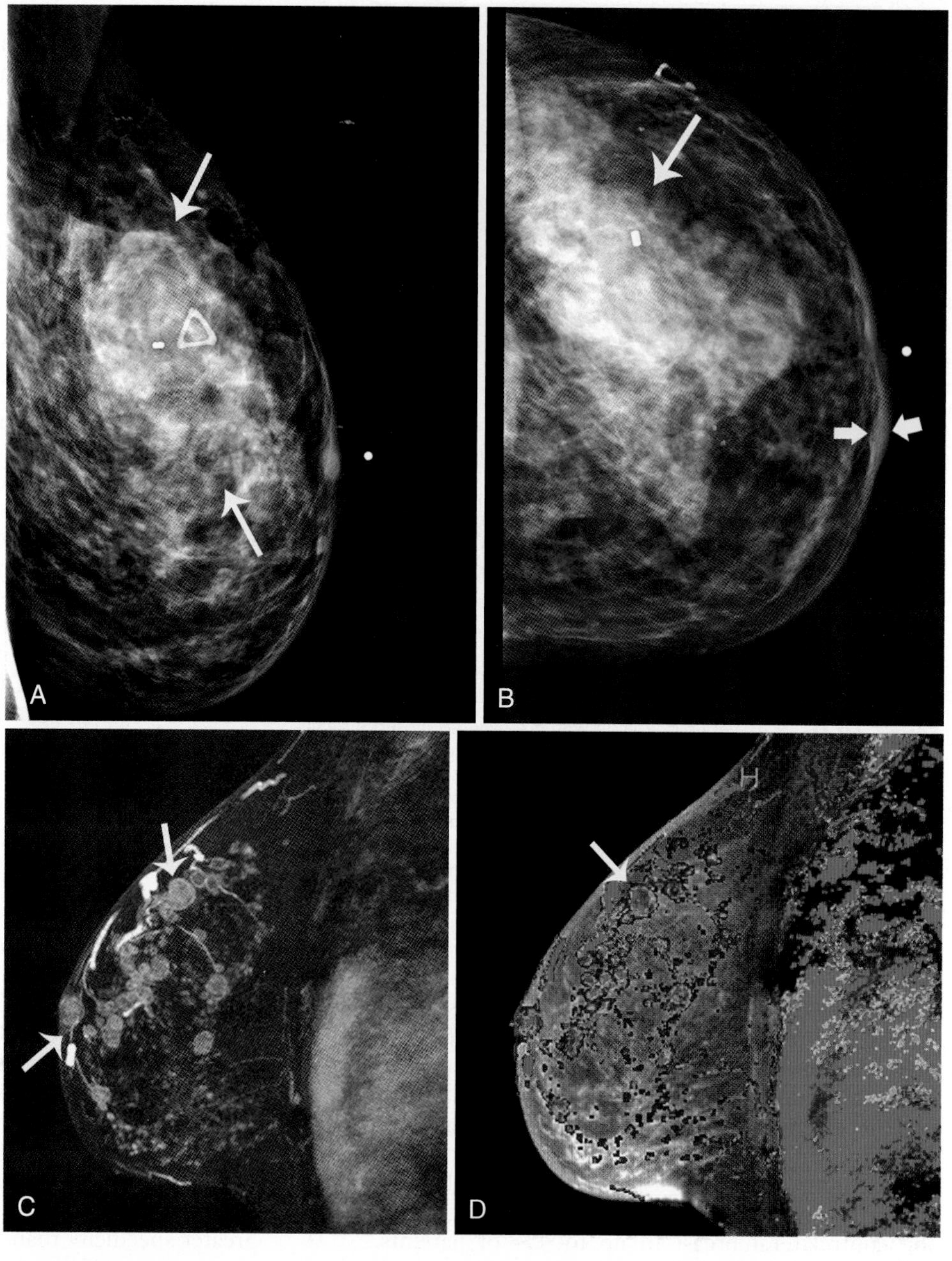

FIGURE 28.7. A 45-year-old woman with newly diagnosed multicentric invasive ductal carcinoma in the left breast. The mediolateral (**A**) and craniocaudal (**B**) mammography views showed multiple obscured masses in the left breast, measuring at least 7.7 cm (*thin arrows*), with global skin thickening (*thick arrows* in **B**). **C** and **D**, The postcontrast maximum intensity projection and colorized magnetic resonance imaging studies revealed multiple rim-enhancing masses (*arrows*) in all four quadrants of the left breast, compatible with locally advanced multicentric carcinoma.

specificity of 88.5% to 98.3% in diagnosing axillary metastasis.[57] The reported sensitivity is more heterogeneous, ranging from 43.5% to 94.9%.[57]

It is important that this noninvasive evaluation of the regional nodal basins be inclusive of both the axilla as well as the internal mammary nodes, particularly for cancers located in the inner quadrants of the breast, given the propensity of the disease to involve both lymphatic chains.[58] Further, identification of internal mammary nodal involvement substantially affects staging and impacts decisions regarding the scope of adjuvant radiation therapy. For women with negative US evaluation, sentinel node biopsy has replaced the traditional approach of axillary node dissection, with multicenter trials confirming the high overall accuracy of this more limited surgical technique.[59] This shift towards more minimal axillary surgery has recently been extended to select women with limited nodal metastasis identified with sentinel node biopsy. With the publication of the results from the American College of Surgeons Oncology Group Z0011 trial, many such women are now able to avoid the need for completion axillary node dissection, with no impact on long-term recurrence and survival.[60]

Management of the axilla in women who are found by US to harbor nodal metastasis has been more challenging. Many of these women will undergo neoadjuvant chemotherapy, and 25% to 50% will experience a complete response in the axilla. Efforts at developing minimal invasive surgical techniques, such as sentinel node biopsy, to identify women who have had a complete pathologic response and who can thus forgo the need for axillary node dissection have had limited success. Several trials have shown that sentinel node biopsy in this population has unacceptably high false-negative rates, in excess of

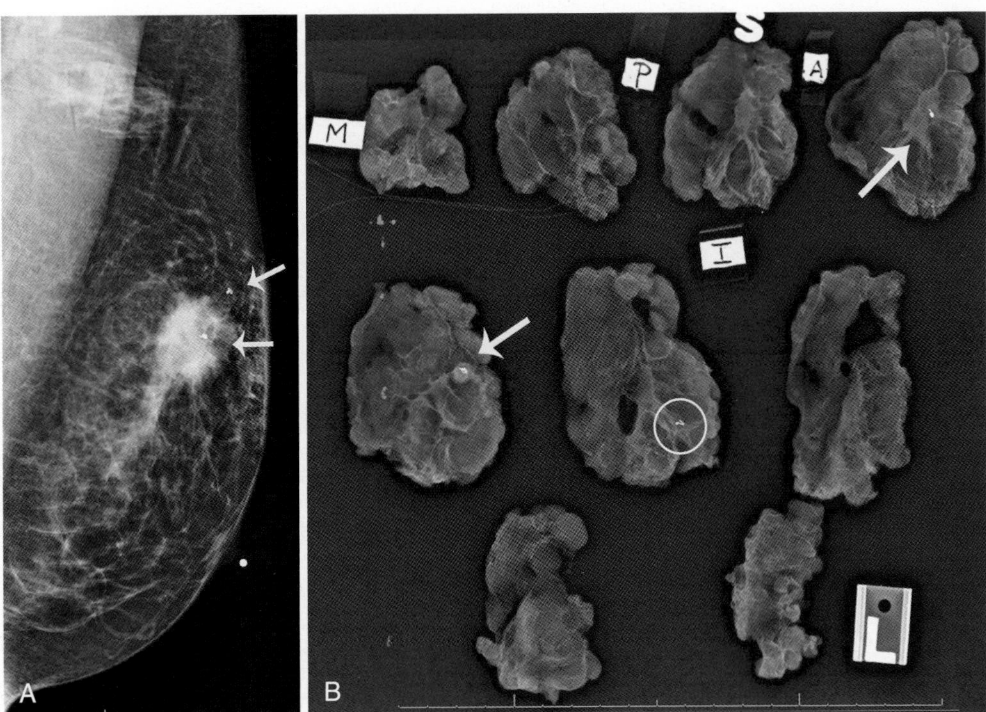

FIGURE 28.8. A 37-year-old female with multifocal invasive ductal carcinoma in the left breast. **A**, On the mediolateral view of the pretreatment mammogram, two biopsy clips are associated with the spiculated 2.5-cm mass and satellite lesion (*arrows*). After neoadjuvant chemotherapy, the masses have decreased in size. **B**, The left segmentectomy specimen radiograph confirmed resection of the targeted biopsy clips with associated residual subcentimeter nodules (*arrows*). A third biopsy clip (*circle*) is seen, related to location of an ultrasound-guided biopsy denoting a satellite lesion.

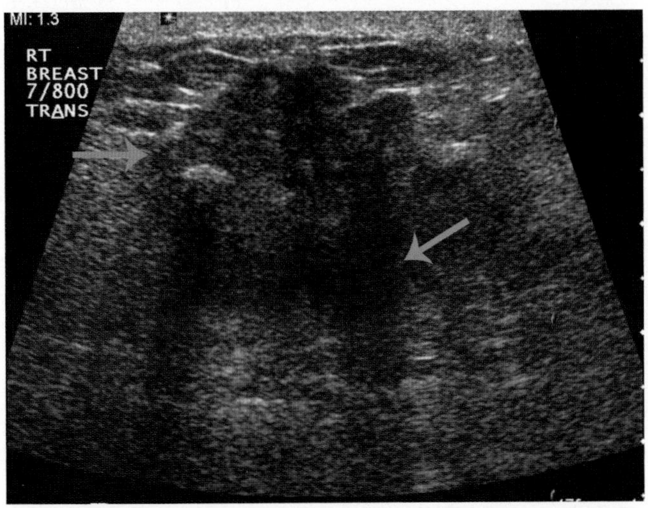

FIGURE 28.9. Ultrasound of the right breast in a 41-year-old woman with newly diagnosed invasive ductal carcinoma demonstrates an ill-defined hypoechoic mass with irregular margins (*blue arrow*) and posterior acoustic shadowing (*green arrow*).

10%.[61,62] Efforts at refining the surgical technique have been focused on combining sentinel node biopsy with removal of the known metastatic node identified by US and needle biopsy (and generally marked by placement of biopsy clip). These early studies have been promising, showing a significant improvement in the accuracy of restaging the axilla after neoadjuvant chemotherapy.[63] Larger studies and longer-term data on recurrence outcomes are needed to verify these early results. Nonetheless, these early data underscore the importance of thorough evaluation of the regional nodal basin needle biopsy to assess the histologic status of any abnormal nodes and the placement of a clip to denote a positive node.

The nodal US evaluation at our institution include the axillary level I, II, and III and internal mammary regions. Lymph nodes are assessed for both size and morphology. A short-axis, or minimum, diameter larger than 1 cm has been suggested as the threshold criterion for an abnormal lymph node diagnosis.[41] However, many nodes that are normal can measure over 1 cm, whereas a malignant node can be less than 1 cm. For this reason, the morphologic findings of the lymph node are crucial for an accurate diagnosis. Morphology suggestive of a malignant node includes a diffuse or focal hypoechoic and thickened cortex of 3 mm or more, partial or complete hilar compression or displacement, and perinodal invasion (Fig. 28.17, p. 492) If a suspicious lymph node is detected, a biopsy can be performed using a hypodermic needle (21- to 23-gauge attached to a 10-mL syringe). The management of internal mammary nodes remains controversial, and many medical centers do not perform US-guided or surgical percutaneous biopsies owing to concerns about morbidity and the lack of a demonstrated impact on survival.

Metastatic Disease

Metastatic disease of the breast is a heterogeneous disease and ranges from a solitary metastasis to diffuse disease within multiple organs. Approximately 30% of patients with early-stage breast cancer will develop a distant

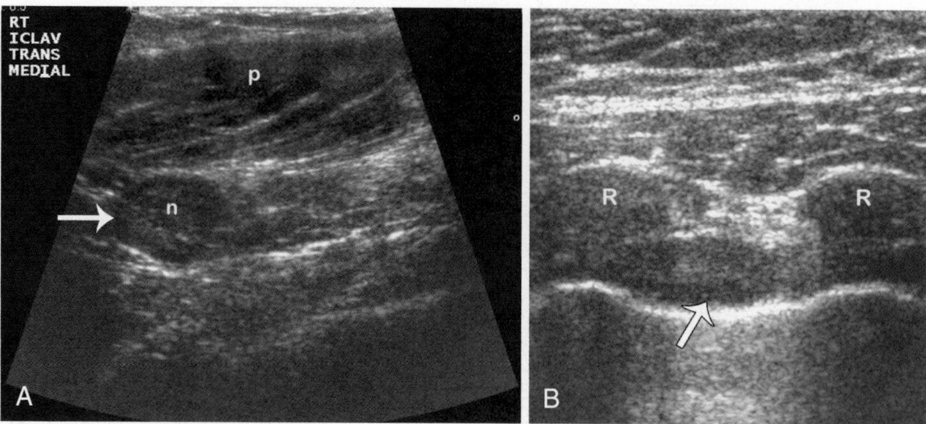

FIGURE 28.10. **A**, Gray-scale ultrasonographic image of a biopsy-proven malignant infraclavicular lymph node (*n; arrow*) diagnosed at the staging ultrasound examination of a 44-year-old woman with newly diagnosed right breast invasive mucinous carcinoma. The node is deep to the pectoralis muscle (*p*). **B**, Gray-scale ultrasonographic image of an enlarged metastatic internal mammary lymph node (*arrow*) in a 41-year-old woman with locally advanced invasive ductal carcinoma and ductal carcinoma *in situ* of the right breast. *R*, Ribs.

metastasis.[64] A subset of oligometastatic disease refers to a few metastatic lesions within one organ and has a more optimistic prognosis than the cases with diffuse disease when treated with an intensified multidisciplinary therapeutic approach.[65] Currently, we do not have a clear understanding of the patterns of spread or specific sites of recurrence. Advances in whole-body imaging may aid in the early detection of metastases and in facilitating a better understanding of how and why breast cancer spreads in spite of therapy.

Bone Metastases

Metastases develop in approximately 69% of patients, and bone is the most common site of distant metastases from breast cancer.[64] Imaging modalities commonly indicated for the detection and management of osseous metastases include plain-film radiography, skeletal scintigraphy, CT, MRI, PET, and single-proton emission radiography, as well as combination techniques such as PET/CT, dual-modality single-photon emission CT, and whole-body MRI.[66] For a newly diagnosed breast cancer patient with no bone symptoms, skeletal scintigraphy is the modality of choice for screening for osseous metastases (Fig. 28.18, p. 492) If focal bony symptoms are present, plain-film radiography of the symptomatic area(s) would be helpful to visualize the bony anatomy. If the radiography fails to identify osteolysis, CT can be performed to evaluate the cortex and associated soft tissue calcifications. CT is also preferred over MRI for rib lesions. When evaluation of bone marrow or soft tissue is indicated, high-contrast MRI is the preferred imaging modality. MRI carries the added advantage of being able to differentiate metastatic breast cancer from osteoporotic compression fractures (Fig. 28.19, p. 493) If radiography, CT, or MRI studies remain discordant in the presence of highly suspicious clinical symptoms, PET/CT is indicated.

Liver Metastasis

Liver metastasis from breast cancer is less common than bone metastasis, yet is observed in 55% to 75% of autopsies in patients with breast cancer.[67] Common clinical presentation includes hepatomegaly and abnormally elevated liver function tests. Imaging tests commonly incorporated to investigate these clinical symptoms include abdominal US and contrast-enhanced CT, MRI, and PET studies.

US is the least expensive and most widely available modality, with a reported sensitivity of 94% in the detection of liver lesions larger than 2 cm and 56% for smaller lesions.[68] Hepatic metastasis is usually presented as a hypoechoic focal lesion compared with normal liver parenchyma, or it may have a "target" appearance, displaying as an echogenic center surrounded by a hypoechoic halo (Fig. 28.20, p. 493) Diffuse hepatic metastases may present as a diffusely inhomogeneous liver parenchyma. US is primarily used for further characterization of liver lesions and for guiding biopsies, but not as a surveillance tool. US is a strong alternative choice for patients with allergies or contraindications to CT or MRI contrast agents.

Unlike US, CT is not operator-dependent, is easily reproducible, and can detect subcentimeter liver lesions. Hepatic metastases from breast cancer typically present as irregular, ill-defined, hypodense masses on the precontrast image and during the portal venous phase. The periphery of the mass may demonstrate mild enhancement. Against the background of hepatic steatosis, hepatic metastasis can be difficult to detect on CT, and MRI is a superior modality for this clinical scenario. The liver may be shrunken or have the appearance of cirrhosis as a result of diffuse disease related to periportal fibrosis. Hepatic steatosis can also be a posttreatment appearance from tamoxifen or cytotoxic drugs.[69] Because of its usefulness in lesion detection and prevalence in interventional clinics, CT is also used to guide biopsies of suspicious lesions. For nonspecific liver CT findings, MRI may be useful in both confirming the presence of liver lesions and further characterizing the lesions.

Breast carcinoma has variable appearances on MRI, ranging from a military pattern with ring-enhancing masses to confluent segmental abnormalities. Metastases are typically hypervascular tumors that do not contain Kupffer cells. Therefore, the contrast agent does not accumulate in these lesions, and metastases tend to appear as hypointense lesions compared with liver parenchyma on delayed-phase

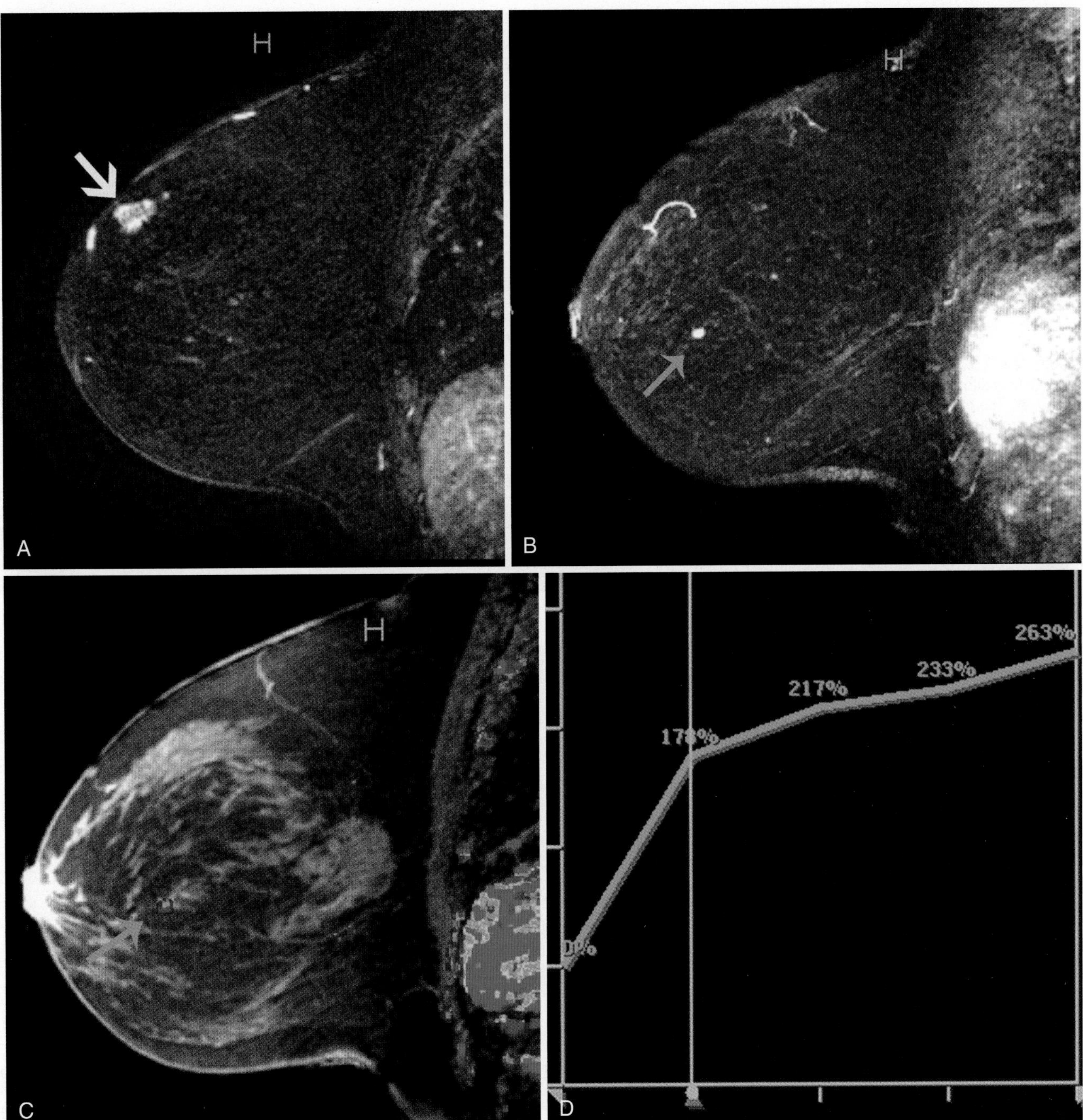

FIGURE 28.11. A 60-year-old woman with a newly diagnosed right breast invasive ductal carcinoma who had a preoperative staging magnetic resonance imaging (MRI) study. **A**, A sagittal maximum intensity projection (MIP) MRI study of the right breast revealed an irregular 2.1-cm carcinoma (*arrow*). **B**, A sagittal MIP MRI study of the left breast revealed a 6-mm enhancing focus (*arrow*). **C** and **D**, The kinetic analysis (**D**) demonstrated that the left breast lesion has rapid initial and delayed progressive enhancing patterns. MRI-guided biopsy confirmed the left breast lesion (*arrow* in **C**) to be a contralateral invasive ductal carcinoma.

imaging. Regardless of the imaging modality performed, information acquired from imaging of metastatic liver lesions includes the number and size of each liver lesion, the characteristics of the lesion, and the resectability or relationship to vital vessels.

Intrathoracic Metastasis

The thorax is a common site of metastasis and involves the lung, pleura or mediastinum, and airway. Pulmonary metastasis may be a single pulmonary mass, multiple pulmonary nodules, an airspace-pattern metastasis, a lymphangitic metastasis, or an endobronchial metastasis (Fig. 28.21, p. 494). The metastatic pulmonary nodules or masses can be irregular or circumscribed lesions and tend to be in the periphery of the lung. Centrally located metastases or mediastinal metastases can extend into the bronchial walls, resulting in endobronchial metastasis. The pulmonary metastases rarely cavitate or present as a consolidation or airspace pattern, mimicking pneumonia. Breast cancer cells can spread to the pulmonary lymphatic

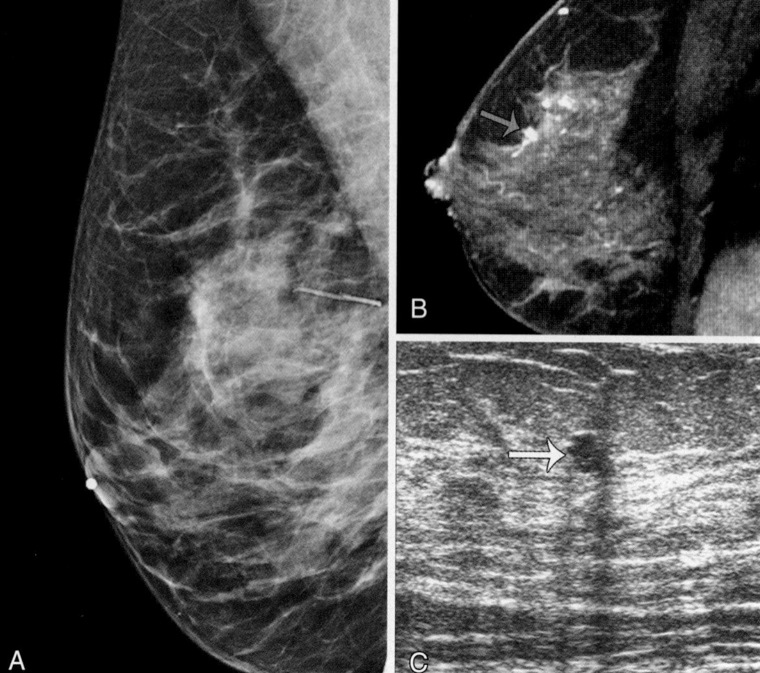

FIGURE 28.12. A 40-year-old woman with diagnosis of metastatic axillary lymphadenopathy from an excisional biopsy. **A**, The mammogram (mediolateral view) and initial breast ultrasound did not reveal a suspicious finding for malignancy. **B**, A magnetic resonance imaging (MRI) study of the right breast (sagittal T1-weighted after intravenous contrast) demonstrated a 4-mm irregular enhancing focus with a linear enhancement toward the nipple (*arrow*). **C**, A targeted breast ultrasound, performed after the MRI examination, revealed a 4-mm hypoechoic mass (*arrow*). A core biopsy was performed and confirmed an invasive ductal carcinoma.

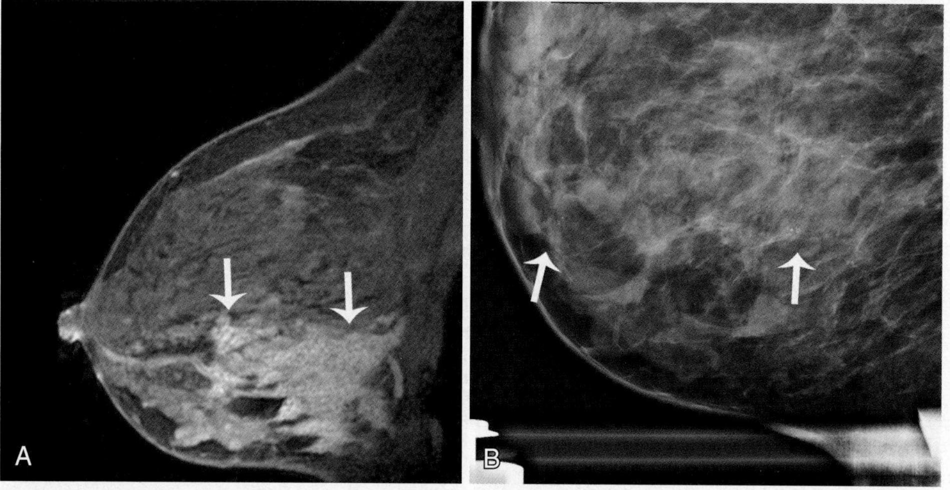

FIGURE 28.13. A 42-year-old woman with a new diagnosis of advanced left breast carcinoma who received a magnetic resonance imaging (MRI) examination for staging assessment. **A**, Sagittal postcontrast T1-weighted MRI study demonstrated nonmasslike and ductal enhancement in a segmental distribution (*arrows*) concerning for ductal carcinoma *in situ* (DCIS) within the contralateral or right breast. **B**, The corresponding magnification mammographic views revealed a few small clusters of microcalcifications (*arrows*) in the area of abnormal enhancement seen on MRI. The entire area of abnormal enhancement corresponds to high-grade DCIS at surgery.

system, resulting in lymphangitic metastasis. This pattern of spread presents as a thickening and nodularity of the interlobular septa or Kerley B lines. Unilateral involvement is more common than bilateral involvement. Other intrathoracic metastases include pleural effusions, pleural thickening, or pleural-based masses. The effusion tends to be unilateral and ipsilateral to the primary breast cancer. Pleural metastasis is thought to be caused by lymphatic dissemination of breast cancer.[38] Most patients receive a chest radiograph at the initial staging evaluation, even though CT better delineates the metastatic pulmonary lesions, the endobronchial lesions, and the pleural nodules.

Brain Metastasis

The most common intracranial malignancy is metastases, with lung and breast cancers as the most common primary cancers.[70] Breast cancer cells spread to the brain via the bloodstream, and the location of the metastases parallels the intracranial blood flow, with the cerebral hemispheres being the most common location. Metastases can also involve the meninges, skull, and dura. Brain metastases may present as a solitary lesion or oligometastases. On MRI, the metastases tend to be hypointense to isointense to brain parenchyma on T1W images and hyperintense with peritumoral edema on T2W images. On contrast-enhanced T1W images, the metastatic lesions are typically moderate

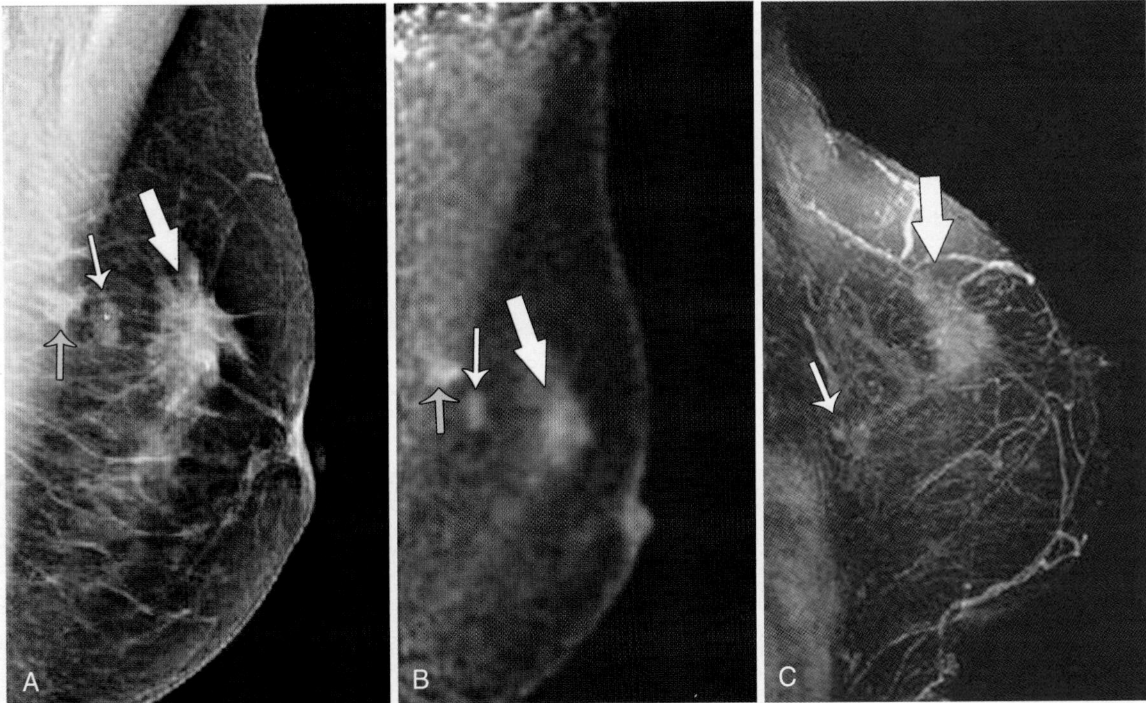

Figure 28.14. Positron emission mammography. **A–C**, A 58-year-old female who presented with two biopsy-proven invasive ductal carcinomas of the left breast, as denoted by the biopsy clips at both sides (*white arrows*). The positron emission mammography confirms the presence of another lesion that was suspected on mammography but subtle on the magnetic resonance imaging sagittal image (*yellow arrows*).

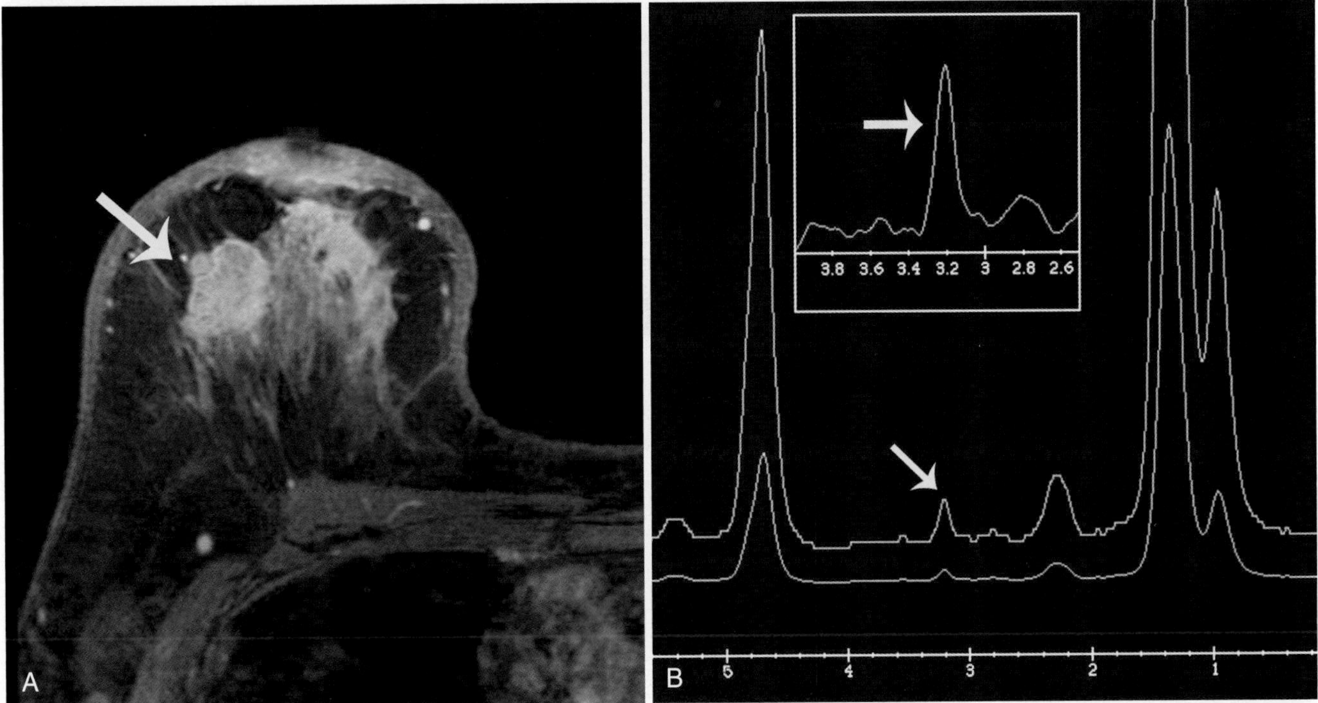

Figure 28.15. **A** and **B**, A 44-year-old woman with locally advanced right breast invasive ductal carcinoma and ductal carcinoma *in situ*, with global skin thickening and global breast enlargement. Magnetic resonance spectroscopy was performed on the index largest breast mass in the lateral right breast (*arrow* in **A**), and demonstrated the presence of a choline peak (*arrows* in **B**).

to marked nodular-enhancing lesions or ringlike enhancing lesions with central nonenhancement. Single intracranial metastatic lesions treated with surgery followed by whole-brain radiation therapy have been reported to improve survival.[71]

Abdominal Metastasis

Besides the liver, other organs that breast cancer cells can spread to include the spleen, adrenal glands, lymph nodes, and peritoneum (Fig. 28.22, p. 494). Splenic metastases tend to be microscopic rather than macroscopic disease, and appear

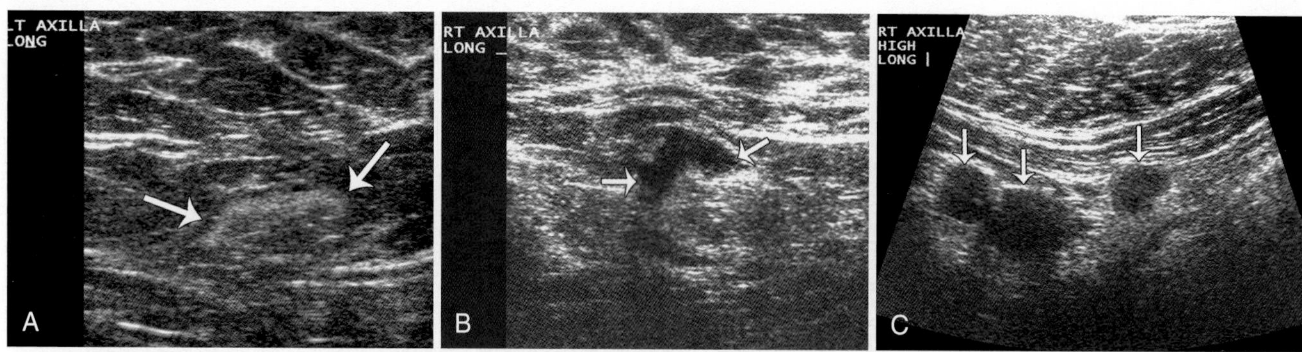

Fig. 28.16 **A**, The spectrum of normal lymph node appearance includes a thin cortex (*arrows*) with echogenic hilum. Abnormal lymph node secondary to tumor infiltration or replacement of the lymph node by metastatic disease can have variable ultrasonographic appearances such as cortical thickening (**B**) and irregularity (*arrows* in **B**) or complete mediastinal obliteration and rounding of the lymph node (*arrows* in **C**).

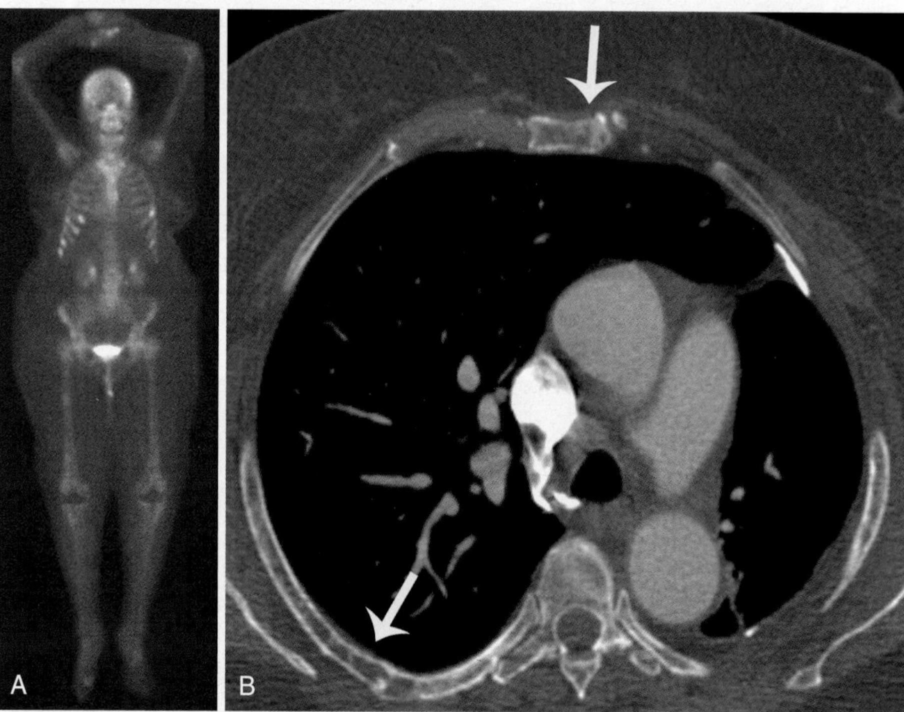

Figure 28.17. Abnormal bone scan in an 83-year-old woman with newly diagnosed breast cancer. **A**, A bone scan demonstrated multiple foci of increased radiotracer technitium-99m methyl diphosphonate uptake in the bilateral ribs, sternum, vertebral bodies, and iliac bones. **B**, Computed tomography scan of the chest demonstrates corresponding osteolytic lesions throughout the ribs and sternum (*arrows*).

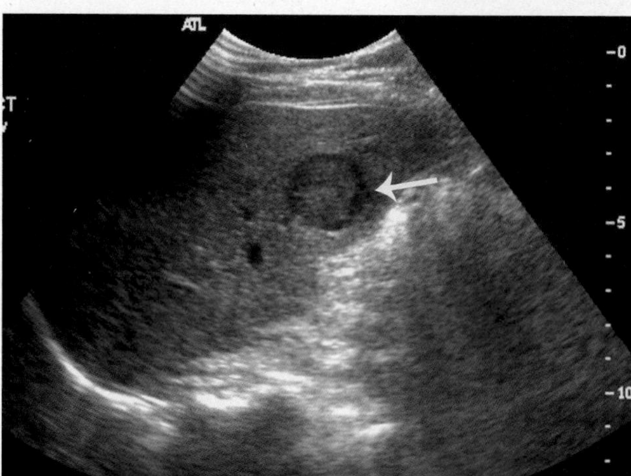

Figure 28.18. Ultrasound of liver metastases in a 61-year-old woman with a history of invasive ductal carcinoma of the right breast who subsequently developed liver metastasis. Ultrasonographic image demonstrates a 2.5-cm isoechoic liver mass with a hypoechoic halo (*arrow*), compatible with metastatic disease.

as irregular, ill-defined hypodense lesions on CT. If there is diffuse disease, splenomegaly may also be present. Metastases to the adrenal glands are more common than to other endocrine organs, such as the thyroid or pituitary glands. Adrenal metastases demonstrate as hypodense lesions with irregular, ill-defined margins and can be unilateral or bilateral; however, a new lesion is suspicious for metastases. Nodal metastases in the abdomen can involve the retrocrural, paraaortic, retroperitoneal, and intrapelvic nodes. Ascites and peritoneal spread to the bowel wall, mesentery, and omentum are not uncommon, especially with invasive lobular carcinoma.[70] Other distant sites include the kidneys, ovaries, and uterus, although metastasis to the uterus is uncommon.

Key Points The Radiology Report

What the Surgeon Needs to Know

- Tumor size, number, and total volume to be taken out *en bloc*.
- Tumor location.

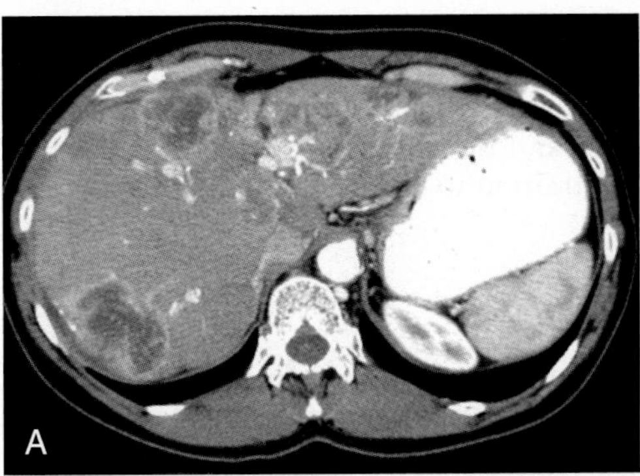

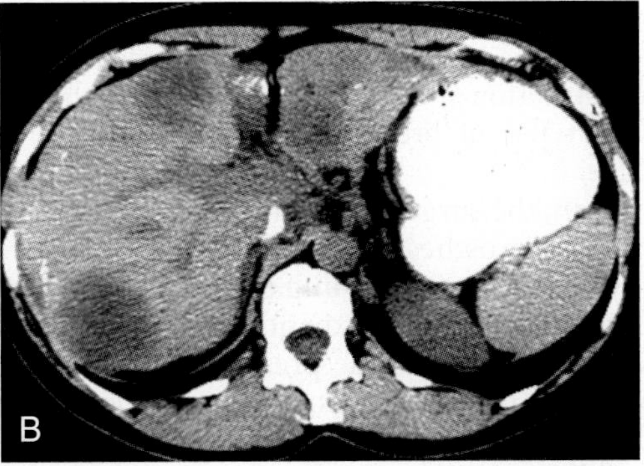

FIGURE 28.19. A 57-year-old woman with a history of left breast carcinoma who subsequently developed liver metastasis 3 years later. Computed tomography images of the abdomen revealed multiple irregular hypodense hepatic masses on the precontrast image (**A**), typical of hepatic metastasis from breast cancer. **B**, On the postcontrast image, the lesions mildly enhance along the periphery.

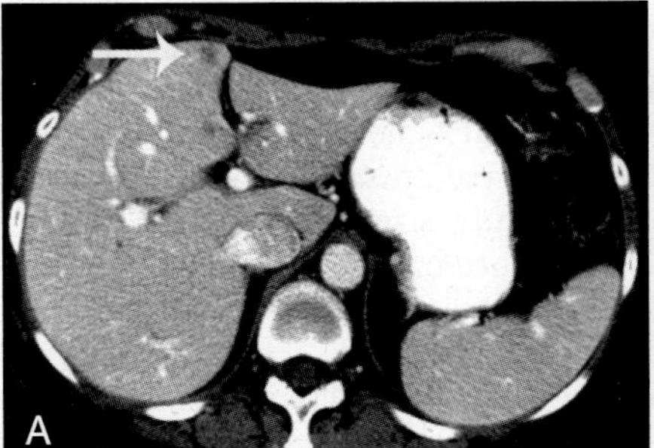

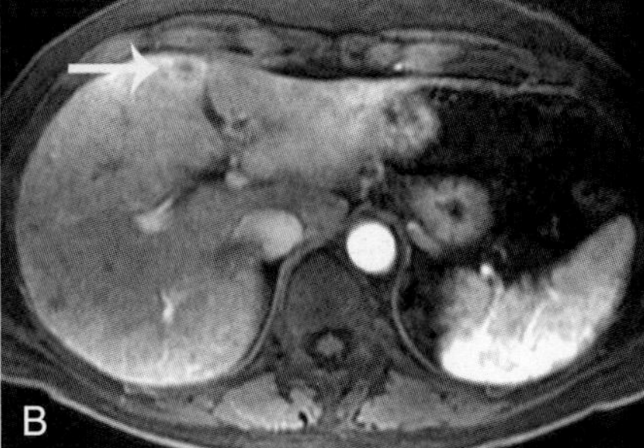

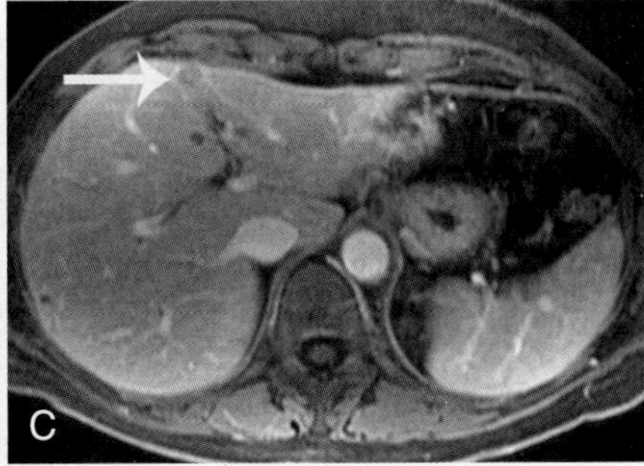

FIGURE 28.20. A 58-year-old woman with a history of invasive ductal carcinoma of the left breast. **A**, Staging computed tomography of the abdomen demonstrated one indetermined hypodense liver lesion (*arrow*) and a few hepatic cysts. **B** and **C**, Magnetic resonance imaging studies performed for further tissue characterization demonstrate a hypointense liver lesion (*arrows*) with peripheral enhancement and washout on delayed-phase imaging.

What the Medical Oncologist Needs to Know

- Tumor size, skin or chest wall involvement, and absence or presence of regional lymph node involvement.
- Metastatic disease: location of metastasis, extent of disease, and related complications from the metastasis.

What the Radiation Oncologist Needs to Know

- Location of existing and resected gross disease.
- Location of adjacent vital structures, such as carotid vessels or the thyroid gland.
- Location of malignant lymph nodes.

TREATMENT

Surgical Treatment

Surgical management of breast cancer involves the appropriate extirpation of the primary tumor, as well as assessment of the regional lymph nodes. The National Surgical Adjuvant Breast and Bowel Project B-4 and B-6 trials clearly established that less extensive surgery is as effective in curing patients of their disease as more extensive surgery and opened the door to breast-conserving therapy.[31,72] Thus, most breast cancer patients have the option of undergoing breast-conserving surgery as an alternative to mastectomy for treatment of their primary tumor. Currently, oncologic exclusions to breast-conserving surgery include inflammatory breast cancer, multicentric breast cancer, and T4 tumors involving the skin. Breast-conserving surgery requires the complete removal of all macroscopic and microscopic disease, as determined by achieving negative margins; after surgery, the patient must undergo radiation therapy to the breast. Margin-positive excisions are clearly recognized as increasing the risk of local failure,[73] which in turn may compromise long-term survival.[74]

The second component in the surgical management of breast cancer is the evaluation of regional lymph nodes to provide accurate regional staging and prognostic data. Traditionally, this was accomplished by axillary dissection with its attendant morbidities, in particular lymphedema and paresthesia. In 1994, however, sentinel node biopsy was introduced as an accurate and less morbid means of staging the axilla[75] and has now become the standard practice for this purpose. Considerable debate remains about whether women with sentinel node metastasis require complete dissection, because many will have no metastasis beyond the sentinel node.[76] Among the underlying issues in this debate is whether axillary dissection has therapeutic value in addition to providing prognostic information. At a minimum, it is becoming clear that, even if a survival benefit owing to complete node dissection cannot be proved, in-basin recurrences are higher if completion node dissection is omitted.[77,78] It is also theoretically possible that failure to remove additional foci of nonsentinel nodal disease may result in understaging of the patient and, potentially, undertreatment as well. Despite this ongoing debate, it should be noted that, although in individual cases a decision may be made to forego complete node dissection, the American Society of Clinical Oncology recommends node dissection for all women with micro- or macrometastasis in the sentinel lymph node.[79]

For women who require a mastectomy, breast reconstructive surgery is offered to improve the physical and psychosocial effects of the physical deformity caused by mastectomy. The two broad categories of breast reconstruction are implant-based reconstruction and autologous tissue–based reconstruction. The types of breast reconstruction are listed in Table 28.2.

For implant-based reconstruction, the surgeon initially creates a breast mound by placing a prosthesis or tissue expander within the mastectomy skin pocket extending to the pectoralis major muscle. Patients with tissue expanders should avoid undergoing an MRI owing to the presence of metal in the infusion port. The decision to use either a silicone- or a saline-filled implant is largely based upon the patient's preference. Silicone implants offer a more natural appearance and feel, whereas saline implants are perceived as a safer choice, even though studies have not shown a difference in the safety profiles of the two types of implants.

Autologous tissue–based reconstructions, also described as flap reconstruction, are the second major classification of breast reconstruction.[80] Flaps are classified by both the source of their arterial perfusion and the method of their transfer (see Table 28.2). Pedicled flaps entail the transfer of skin and subcutaneous fat based on a vascular leash that remains attached to its source vessels. Free flaps are created when the vascular supply to the tissue is detached from the source vessels, and the vessels are anastomosed under microscopic visualization to distant recipient vessels.[81]

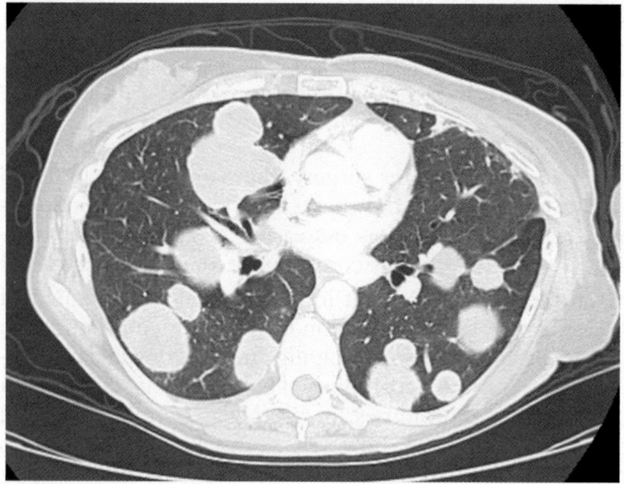

FIGURE 28.21. A 51-year-old woman with triple negative (estrogen receptor–negative, progesterone receptor–negative, human epidermal growth factor receptor 2–negative) invasive ductal carcinoma of the left breast who developed pulmonary metastasis 1 year later. Computed tomography of the lungs revealed multiple masses bilaterally, compatible with pulmonary metastasis.

Chemotherapy

Chemotherapy treatment for breast cancer depends on disease stage, patient symptoms, and tumor features such as receptor status and grade. Chemotherapy may be administered after surgical resection (adjuvant therapy) to reduce the risk of developing metastatic disease in high-risk patients. Adjuvant therapy reduces the risk of breast cancer recurrence by 30% to 50%.[82,83] The administration of chemotherapy before surgical resection (neoadjuvant therapy) offers the same survival benefit as adjuvant therapy and is often considered in patients with locally advanced breast cancer to reduce tumor size, which results in a less extensive operative procedure in certain patients. Chemotherapy is also used to palliate symptoms in patients with metastatic breast cancer.

Many chemotherapy drugs have activity against breast cancer (Table 28.3). Anthracyclines, such as doxorubicin and epirubicin, are commonly used to treat breast cancer and exert their action by inhibiting topoisomerase II, an enzyme that relieves torsional stress during DNA replication and transcription.[84] To increase cytotoxicity, anthracycline-based regimens usually include cyclophosphamide with or without fluoropyrimidines, such as 5-deoxyfluorouridine (5-FU).[85] Taxanes, such as paclitaxel, docetaxel, and nab-paclitaxel (an albumin-bound formulation of paclitaxel that reduces hypersensitivity reactions), exert their cytotoxic effects by binding to alpha-tubulin, stabilizing microtubule formation, and blocking the progression of mitosis.[86] Epothilones, such as ixabepilone, also bind to alpha-tubulin but have demonstrated activity in taxane-resistant cell lines.[87] Vinca alkaloids, such as vinorelbine, interfere with mitosis by exerting their effects on microtubule assembly.[88] Nucleoside analogs, such as 5-FU, capecitabine, and gemcitabine, induce apoptosis through their effects on DNA replication.[89,90] Alkylating agents, such as cyclophosphamide, or platinum salts, such as cisplatin and carboplatin, induce apoptosis by cross-linking DNA strands.

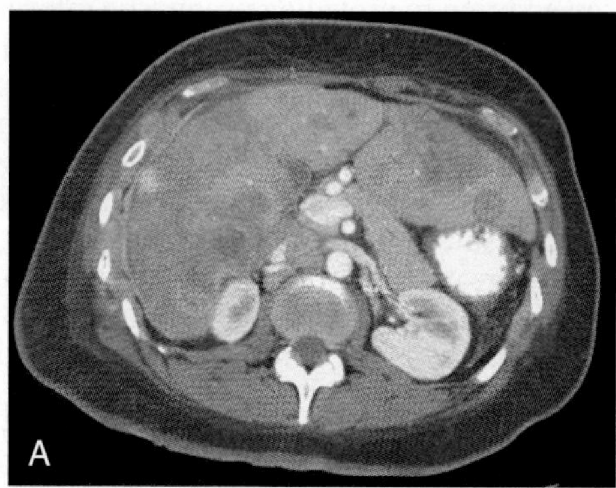

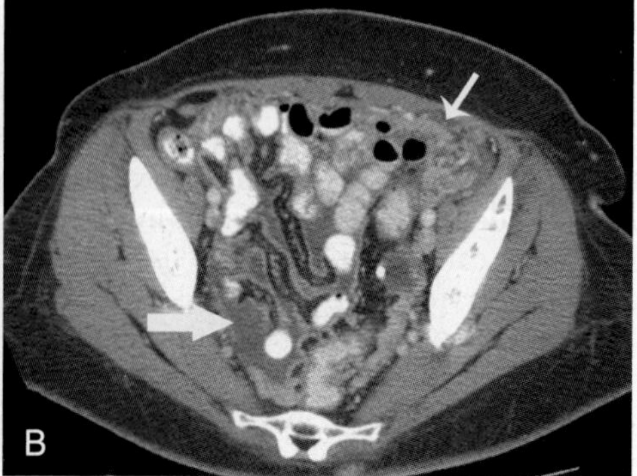

FIGURE 28.22. A 48-year-old woman with a history of right breast invasive ductal carcinoma and ductal carcinoma *in situ* who developed lung metastasis, liver metastasis (**A**), malignant ascites (*thick arrow* in **B**), and peritoneal carcinomatosis (*thin arrow* in **B**) 3 years later.

TABLE 28.2 Types of Breast Reconstruction

TYPES	DESCRIPTIONS	COMPLICATIONS	IMAGING
Implants			MRI, US
Single-lumen saline	Saline in silicone shell	• Rupture • Capsular contracture malposition • Extrusion • Periprosthetic seroma/hematoma • Infection	
Single-lumen silicone	Silicone gel in silicone shell		
Double-lumen	Outer: saline Inner: silicone		
Autologous	(Based on arterial source)	• Partial or total flap necrosis • Fat necrosis • Hematoma/seroma • Infection • Abdominal hernia • Weakness/bulging	
Pedicled			
pTRAM	Superior epigastric artery		
Latissimus	Thoracodorsal artery		
Free			
TRAM	(Based on arterial source)		
DIEA	Inferior epigastric arteries		CT, MRI, US
SGAP	Superior gluteal artery	• Partial or total flap necrosis • Fat necrosis • Hematoma/seroma • Infection • Leg weakness or numbness	
IGAP	Inferior gluteal artery		
TUG	Ascending branch of medial circumflex femoral artery		

CT, Computed tomography; *MRI*, magnetic resonance imaging; *US*, ultrasound; *PTRAM*, pedicled traverse rectus abdominal muscle; *TRAM*, traverse rectus abdominal muscle; *DIEA*, deep inferior epigastric artery; *SGAP*, superior gluteal artery perforator; *IGAP*, superior gluteal artery perforator; *TUG*, transverse upper gracilis.

Common toxicities associated with chemotherapy drugs used to treat breast cancer are listed in Table 28.3. Anthracyclines and/or taxanes are the most frequently used neoadjuvant and adjuvant chemotherapy regimens and may also be used to treat patients with metastatic disease. Taxanes, nucleoside analogs, vinca alkaloids, and platinum salts are commonly combined with targeted agents, such as trastuzumab, bevacizumab, or lapatinib, to enhance their cytotoxic effects.

Radiation Therapy

Adjuvant radiation therapy is indicated after a lumpectomy for virtually all patients; this recommendation is based on data from a phase III randomized trial.[91–93] Women older than 70 years with small, low-grade, ER-negative invasive tumors who take tamoxifen have been reported to have sufficiently low risk of recurrence without radiation therapy, indicating that observation may be considered.[94] Women with early-stage breast cancer who undergo segmental mastectomy now have several adjuvant radiation therapy options, including a shorter course of radiation therapy to the whole breast (higher dose per day than the standard 5- to 6-week regimens)[95,96] and accelerated partial breast irradiation (treats only the tissue adjacent to the lumpectomy cavity with high dose per fraction twice a day for 1 week). Selection of patients and techniques for the latter approach are still under investigation and should be carefully considered.[97] Adjuvant radiation therapy in the postmastectomy setting reduces the risk of locoregional recurrence by two thirds and should be offered to all patients with stage III breast cancer and to high-risk node-positive patients with stage II breast cancer.[91] Common toxicities are summarized in Table 28.4. Adjuvant radiation therapy for patients who receive neoadjuvant systemic therapy has not been studied extensively but is routinely given to patients who presented with stage III disease, regardless of response, and to stage II patients with residual disease, particularly in the lymph nodes.[98,99] Adjuvant radiation therapy has been shown to improve survival by preventing locoregional recurrences.[91] A 21-gene expression signature has recently been shown to predict for locoregional recurrence, and in the future it may be possible to better select patients who are at the highest risk of locoregional recurrence.[36]

KEY POINTS Treatment

Therapies

- Neoadjuvant chemotherapy: to reduce tumor size and possibly enable breast conservation.
- Surgery: to remove the primary breast tumor and nodes; breast reconstruction.
- Postoperative chemotherapy: to decrease risk of metastases; to treat palliative symptoms.
- Radiation therapy: to improve overall survival after breast-conservation surgery.

Complications

- Surgery: infection, lymphedema, paresthesia.
- Chemotherapy: myelosuppression (most common).
- Radiation therapy: postradiation dermatitis, contracture.

SURVEILLANCE

Monitoring Tumor Response

Increasingly, neoadjuvant chemotherapy is used in the management of locally advanced and inflammatory breast cancer, T2 tumors (2–5 cm), and triple-negative or HER2+ breast cancers. Early initiation of systemic therapy can

TABLE 28.3 Chemotherapy Agents Commonly Used to Treat Breast Cancer, and Their Associated Toxicities

DRUGS	SINGLE-AGENT RESPONSE RATE	TOXICITIES
Anthracyclines		
Doxorubicin[104,105]	10%–50%	Myelosuppression, nausea/vomiting, alopecia, fatigue, damage to myocardium/congestive heart failure, diarrhea, mucositis
Epirubicin[106]	13%–48%	Myelosuppression, nausea/vomiting, alopecia, fatigue, damage to myocardium/congestive heart failure, diarrhea, mucositis
Liposomal doxorubicin[107,108]	10%–50%	Myelosuppression, nausea/vomiting, fatigue, damage to myocardium/congestive heart failure (less than is seen with other anthracyclines), diarrhea, mucositis
Agents affecting microtubules		
Docetaxel[109,110]	18%–68%	Myelosuppression, neuropathy, hypersensitivity reactions, alopecia, fatigue, nausea, diarrhea
Paclitaxel[111]	16%–62%	Myelosuppression, neuropathy, hypersensitivity reactions, alopecia, fatigue, nausea, diarrhea
Nab-paclitaxel[112]	33%–48%	Myelosuppression, neuropathy, alopecia, fatigue, nausea
Ixabepilone[112,113]	12%–57%	Myelosuppression, neuropathy, alopecia, fatigue, nausea, diarrhea
Vinorelbine[114]	25%–50%	Myelosuppression, neuropathy, fatigue, nausea
Nucleoside analogs		
Capecitabine[115]	20%–35%	Myelosuppression, fatigue, diarrhea, hand foot syndrome
Gemcitabine[116]	12%–37%	Myelosuppression, fatigue, nausea
Platinum salts		
Cisplatin/carboplatin[117]	9%–51%	Myelosuppression, neuropathy, fatigue, nausea/vomiting, hypersensitivity reactions, renal insufficiency/failure

TABLE 28.4 Radiation Therapy and Toxicities

RADIATION THERAPY	TOXICITIES
Short-term	
During treatment	Fatigue
1–2 months after treatment	Radiation dermatitis
Long-term	Soft tissue fibrosis Soft tissue contracture Telangiectasia Pneumonitis Cardiovascular disease

improve overall and disease-free survival for patients. By downstaging the primary tumor, neoadjuvant chemotherapy can make surgery or breast-conservation therapy an option for patients whose cancer was initially considered inoperable. Nodal disease can be eradicated in 40% of patients who have node-positive disease at initial presentation,[100] and the eradication of nodal disease is likely to increase with the improvement in targeted therapies, such as trastuzumab in combination with chemotherapy.[101] Therefore, it is important to determine early in the course of the disease which patients are most likely to respond to neoadjuvant chemotherapy.

Physical examination, digital mammography, digital breast tomosynthesis, US, and MRI have all been used to assess the response to neoadjuvant chemotherapy. The principal value of these techniques is in measuring the size of the residual lesion based on morphologic changes in the tumor. Treatment-induced fibrosis or inflammation can result in an overestimation or underestimation of the residual disease, meaning the true response to therapy is not reflected in these imaging tests. MRI with intravenous contrast and advanced MRI techniques provide new opportunities for assessing tumor morphologic changes, tumor vascularity, tumor cellularity, and tumor metabolic features. MRI and molecular breast imaging provide additional functional information about factors such as tumor vascularity and metabolism and are promising imaging modalities for tumor response assessment over conventional methods of physical examination, mammography, and US.[102,103]

Detection of Recurrence

After mastectomy or breast-conserving surgery for breast cancer, disease can reappear locally, regionally, or at distant sites. Locoregional recurrent disease refers to the reappearance of the original breast cancer in the treated breast within the skin flaps, mastectomy scars, or ipsilateral chest wall. Regional recurrent disease refers to the breast cancer recurring in the regional lymphatic system of the treated breast, such as the ipsilateral axillary level I/II/III, supraclavicular, or internal mammary lymph nodes. The recurrent disease may present as a small solitary tumor or a palpable lesion or as diffuse disease involving the entire chest wall or regional lymph nodes. The majority of recurrences occur in the first decade after the diagnosis of the primary breast cancer, with peak incidence at 2 years and a second peak incidence at 5 years after initial diagnosis.[118] Therefore, the goal of an intensive surveillance program after treatment is to detect potential curable recurrences or secondary primary tumors.

The modes of surveillance recommended by the American Society for Clinical Oncology 2016 clinical guidelines[119] include clinical history, breast self-examination, and mammography. However, routine laboratory tests and imaging studies (such as breast MRI, radionuclide scans, CT, or PET scans) are not routinely recommended. Locoregional recurrent disease, with or without simultaneous distant metastasis, occurs in up to 49% of cases during 18 years of follow-up.[120] At least half of the patients with locoregional recurrent disease develop distant metastases.[121,122] Some prognostic factors associated with an increased likelihood of locoregional recurrence include a tumor greater than 5 cm in diameter, disease-positive lymph nodes, and initial disease involving the skin or fascia. More than half of patients with locoregional recurrent disease will develop distant metastases within 5 years, and approximately two thirds of these patients will develop distant metastases within 10 years.[123]

CONCLUSION

Early detection and treatment of breast cancer has substantially decreased the morbidity associated with this disease, and breast imaging, particularly via uniform imaging standards and interpretation, has played an integral role in decreasing morbidity. New imaging tests with improved specificity may reduce unnecessary interventions. Advanced imaging techniques, in addition to the multidisciplinary team approach in both clinical practice and research settings, are critical for establishing current and emerging imaging techniques to improve the detection of breast cancer and the survival of patients with breast cancer.

REFERENCES

1. American Cancer Society. *Cancer Facts & Figures 2019*. Atlanta: American Cancer Society; 2019:10-71. Available at: https://www.cancer.org/content/dam/cancer-org/research/cancer-facts-and-statistics/annual-cancer-facts-and-figures/2019/cancer-facts-and-figures-2019.pdf. Accessed November 14, 2019.
2. Bray F, Ferlay J, Soerjomataram I, et al. Global cancer statistics 2018: GLOBOCAN estimates of incidence and mortality worldwide for 36 cancers in 185 countries. *CA Cancer J Clin*. 2018;68(6):394–424.
3. Coleman MP, Quaresma M, Berrino F, et al. Cancer survival in five continents: a worldwide population-based study (CONCORD). *Lancet Oncol*. 2008;9:730–756.
4. Shapiro S. Evidence on screening for breast cancer from a randomized trial. *Cancer*. 1977;39:2772–2782.
5. Nystrîm L, Rutqvist LE, Wall S, et al. Breast cancer screening with mammography: overview of Swedish randomized trials. *Lancet*. 1993;341:973–978.
6. Hetzel L, Smith AA. *The 65 Years and Over Population*. Washington, DC: United States Census Bureau; 2000. Available at: www.census.gov/prod/2001pubs/c2kbr01-10.pdf. Accessed March 25, 2010.
7. Ziegler RG, Hoover RN, Pike MC, et al. Migration patterns and breast cancer risk in Asian-American women. *J Natl Cancer Inst*. 1993;85:1819–1827.
8. von Eschenbach AC. NCI remains committed to current mammography guidelines. *Oncologist*. 2002;7:170–171.
9. Howe HL, Wingo PA, Thun MJ, et al. Annual report to the nation on the status of cancer (1973 through 1998), featuring cancers with recent increasing trends. *J Natl Cancer Inst*. 2001;93:824–842.
10. Tabár L, Fagerberg CJ, Gad A, et al. Reduction in mortality from breast cancer after mass screening with mammography: randomised trial from the Breast Cancer Screening Working Group of the Swedish National Board of Health and Welfare. *Lancet*. 1985;1:829–832.
11. Smart CR, Hendrick RE, Rutledge 3rd JH, Smith RA. Benefit of mammography screening in women ages 40–49 years. *Current evidence from randomized controlled trials. Cancer*. 1995;75:1619–1626.
12. Thurfjell EL, Lindgren JA. Breast cancer survival rates with mammographic screening: similar favorable survival rates for women younger and those older than 50 years. *Radiology*. 1996;201:421–426.
13. American College of Radiology (ACR) *ACR-RADS®—Mammography. ACR Breast Imaging Reporting and Data System, Breast Imaging Atlas*. 4th ed. Reston: American College of Radiology;; 2003.
14. Schulz-Wendtland R, Fuchsjäger M, Wacker T, et al. Digital mammography: an update. *Eur J Radiol*. 2009;72:258–265.
15. Destounis S. Role of digital breast tomosynthesis in screening and diagnostic breast imaging. *Semin Ultrasound CT MR*. 2018; 31(1):35–44.
16. Berg WA, Blume JD, Cormack JB, et al. Combined screening with ultrasound and mammography versus mammography alone in women at elevated risk of breast cancer. *JAMA*. 2008;299:2151–2163.
17. Kuhl CK, Kuhn W, Schild H. Management of women at high risk for breast cancer: new imaging beyond mammography. *Breast*. 2005;14:480–486.
18. Saslow D, Boetes C, Burke W, et al. American Cancer Society guidelines for breast screening with MRI as an adjunct to mammography. *CA Cancer J Clin*. 2007;57:75–89.
19. Lehman CD, Blume JD, Weatherall P, et al. Screening women at high risk for breast cancer with mammography and magnetic resonance imaging. *Cancer*. 2005;103:1898–1905.
20. Morris EA, Liberman L, Ballon DJ, et al. MRI of occult breast carcinoma in a high-risk population. *AJR Am J Roentgenol*. 2003; 181:519–525.
21. Lehman CD, Blume JD, Thickman D, et al. Added cancer yield of MRI in screening the contralateral breast of women recently diagnosed with breast cancer: results from the International Breast Magnetic Resonance Consortium (IBMC) trial. *J Surg Oncol*. 2005;92:9–15.
22. Warner E, Plewes DB, Shumak RS, et al. Comparison of breast magnetic resonance imaging, mammography, and ultrasound for surveillance of women at high risk for hereditary breast cancer. *J Clin Oncol*. 2001;19:3524–3531.
23. Stoutjesdijk MJ, Boetes C, Jager GJ, et al. Magnetic resonance imaging and mammography in women with a hereditary risk of breast cancer. *J Natl Cancer Inst*. 2001;18(93):1095–1102.
24. Lehman CD, Isaacs C, Schnall MD, et al. Cancer yield of mammography, MR, and US in high-risk women: prospective multi-institution breast cancer screening study. *Radiology*. 2007;244:381–388.
25. Schrading S, Kuhl CK. Mammographic, US, and MR imaging phenotypes of familial breast cancer. *Radiology*. 2008;246:58–70.
26. Kuhl CK, Schrading S, Leutner CC, et al. Mammography, breast ultrasound, and magnetic resonance imaging for surveillance of women at high familial risk for breast cancer. *J Clin Oncol*. 2005;20 (23):8469–8476.
27. Cowie AT. Overview of mammary gland. *J Invest Dermatol*. 1974;63:2–9.
28. Wellings SR, Jensen HM. On the origin and progression of ductal carcinoma in the human breast. *J Natl Cancer Inst*. 1973;50:1111–1118.
29. Diab SG, Clark G, Osborne CK, et al. Tumor characteristics and clinical outcome of tubular and mucinous carcinomas. *J Clin Oncol*. 1999;17:1442–1449.
30. Rubens JR, Lewandrowski KB, Kopans DB, et al. Medullary carcinoma of the breast: Overdiagnosis of a prognostically favorable neoplasm. *Arch Surg*. 1990;125:601–604.
31. Fisher B, Wolmark N, Redmond C, et al. Findings from NSABP Protocol No. B-04: comparison of radical mastectomy with alternative treatments. II. The clinical and biologic significance of medial-central breast cancers. *Cancer*. 1981;48:1863–1872.
32. Haupt B, Ro JY, Schwartz MR. Basal-like breast carcinoma: a phenotypically distinct entity. *Arch Pathol Lab Med*. 2010;134:130–133.
33. Anders CK, Carey LA. Biology, metastatic patterns, and treatment of patients with triple-negative breast cancer. *Clin Breast Cancer*. 2009;9(suppl 2):S73–S81.
34. Osteen RT, Cady B, Chmiel JS, et al. survey of carcinoma of the breast by the Commission on Cancer. *J Am Coll Surg*. 1991;1994 (178):213–219.
35. Mathis KL, Hoskin TL, Boughey JC, et al. *Palpable presentation of breast cancer persists in the era of screening mammography*. 2010;210:314–331.

36. Hortobabyi GN, Connolly JL, D'Orsi CJ, et al. *AJCC Cancer Staging Manual. Updates and Corrections. AJCC Breast Cancer Staging System, 2017*. 8th ed. New York: Springer; 2017:1–96. https://cancerstaging.org/About/news/Pages/Updated-Breast-Chapter-for-8th-Edition.aspx.
37. Kennecke H, Yerushalmi R, Woods R, et al. Metastatic behavior of breast cancer subtypes. *J Clin Oncol*. 2010;28:3271–3277.
38. Thomas JM, Redding WH, Sloane JP. The spread of breast cancer: importance of the intrathoracic lymphatic route and its relevance to treatment. *Br J Cancer*. 1979;40:540–547.
39. Tingberg A. X-ray tomosynthesis: a review of its use for breast and chest imaging. *Radiat Prot Dosimetry*. 2010;139:100–107.
40. Destounis S. Role of digital breast tomosynthesis in screening and diagnostic breast imaging. *Semin Ultrasound CT MR*. 2018;39: 35–44.
41. Stavros AT. *Breast ultrasound technique. Breast Ultrasound*. Philadelphia: Lippincott Williams & Wilkins; 2004:42–55.
42. Le-Petross H, Stafford R. The need for MRI before breast conserving surgery. *Curr Breast Cancer Rep*. 2009;1:98–103.
43. Houssami N, Ciatto S, Macaskill P, et al. Accuracy and surgical impact of magnetic resonance imaging in breast cancer staging: systematic review and meta-analysis in detection of multifocal and multicentric cancer. *J Clin Oncol*. 2008;26:3248–3258.
44. Brennan ME, Houssami N, Lord S, et al. Accuracy and surgical impact of magnetic resonance imaging in breast cancer staging: systematic review and meta-analysis in detection of multifocal and multicentric cancer. *J Clin Oncol*. 2009;27:5640–5649.
45. Turnbull L, Brown S, Harvey I, et al. Comparative effectiveness of MRI in breast cancer (COMICE) trial: a randomised controlled trial. *Lancet*. 2010;375:563–571.
46. Plana MN, Carreira C, Muriel A, et al. Magnetic resonance imaging in the preoperative assessment of patients with primary breast cancer: systematic review of diagnostic accuracy and meta-analysis. *Eur Radiol*. 2012;22(1):26–38.
47. Hill MV, Beeman JL, Jhala K, et al. Relationship of breast MRI to recurrence rates in patients undergoing breast-conservation treatment. *Breast Cancer Res Treat*. 2017;163(3):615–622.
48. Mann RM. The effectiveness of MR imaging in the assessment of invasive lobular carcinoma of the breast. *Magn Reson Imaging Clin North Am*. 2010;18:259–276.
49. Le-Petross CH, Bidaut L, Yang WT. Evolving role of imaging modalities in inflammatory breast cancer [review]. *Semin Oncol*. 2008;35:51–63.
50. Kuhl C. The current status of breast MR imaging. Part I. Choice of technique, image interpretation, diagnostic accuracy, and transfer to clinical practice. *Radiology*. 2007;244:356–378.
51. Kuerer H, Albarracin C, Yang W, et al. Ductal carcinoma in situ: state of the science and roadmap to advance the field. *J Clin Oncol*. 2009;27:279–288.
52. Kuhl CK, Schrading S, Bieling HB, et al. MRI for diagnosis of pure ductal carcinoma in situ: a prospective observational study. *Lancet*. 2007;370:485–492.
53. Ernster V, Ballard-Barbash R, Barlow W, et al. Detection of ductal carcinoma in situ in women undergoing screening mammography. *J Natl Cancer Inst*. 2002;94:1546–1554.
54. Berg WA, Madsen KS, Schilling K, et al. Breast cancer: comparative effectiveness of positron emission mammography and MR imaging in presurgical planning for the ipsilateral breast. *Radiology*. 2011;258:59–72.
55. Bartella L, Morris EA, Dershaw DD, et al. Proton MR spectroscopy with choline peak as malignancy marker improves positive predictive value for breast cancer diagnosis: preliminary study. *Radiology*. 2006;239:686–692.
56. Boone JM, Kwan AL, Yang K, et al. Computed tomography for imaging the breast. *J Mammary Gland Biol Neoplasia*. 2006;11: 103–111.
57. Alvarez SA, Añorbe E, Alcorta P. Role of sonography in the diagnosis of axillary lymph node metastases in breast cancer: a systematic review. *Am J Roentgenol*. 2006;186:1342–1348.
58. Estourgie SH, Tanis PJ, Nieweg OE, et al. Should the hunt for internal mammary chain sentinel nodes begin? An evaluation of 150 breast cancer patients. *Ann Surg Oncol*. 2003;10:935–941.
59. Garcia-Etienne CA, Ferrari A, Della Valle A, et al. Management of the axilla in patients with breast cancer and positive sentinel lymph node biopsy: An evidence-based update in a European breast center. *Eur J Surg Oncol*. 2020 Jan;46(1): 15-23.
60. Giuliano AE, Ballman KV, McCall L, et al. Effect of axillary dissection versus no axillary dissection on 10-year overall survival among women with invasive breast cancer and sentinel node metastasis. The ACOSOG Z0011 (Alliance) randomized clinical trial. *JAMA*. 2017;318(10):918–926.
61. Boughey JC, Suman VJ, Mittendorf EA, et al. Sentinel lymph node surgery after neoadjuvant chemotherapy in patients with node-positive breast cancer: the ACOSOG Z1071 (Alliance) clinical trial. *JAMA*. 2013;310(14):1455–1461.
62. Kuehn T, Bauerfeind I, Fehm T, et al. Sentinel-lymph-node biopsy in patients with breast cancer before and after neoadjuvant chemotherapy (SENTINA): a prospective, multicentre cohort study. *Lancet Oncol*. 2013;14(7):609–618.
63. Caudle AS, Yang WT, Krishnamurthy S, et al. Improved axillary evaluation following neoadjuvant therapy for patients with node-positive breast cancer using selective evaluation of clipped nodes: implementation of targeted axillary dissection. *J Clin Oncol*. 2016;34(10):1072–1078.
64. Early Breast Cancer Trialists' Collaborative Group . Effects of chemotherapy and hormonal therapy for early breast cancer on recurrence and 15-year survival: an overview of the randomized trials. *Lancet*. 2005;365:1687–1717.
65. Hanrahan EO, Broglio KR, Buzdar AU, et al. Combined-modality treatment for isolated recurrences of breast carcinoma: update on 30 years of experience at the University of Texas M.D. Anderson Cancer Center and assessment of prognostic factors. *Cancer*. 2005;104:1158–1171.
66. Mueller GC, Hussein HK, Carlos RC, et al. Effectiveness of MR imaging in characterizing small hepatic lesions: routine versus expert interpretation. *AJR Am J Roentgenol*. 2003;180:673–680.
67. Hoe AL, Royle GT, Taylor I. Breast liver metastases—incidence, diagnosis and outcome. *J R Soc Med*. 1991;84:714–716.
68. Sheu JC, Sung SL, Chen DS, et al. Ultrasonography of small hepatic tumors using high-resolution linear-array real time instruments. *Radiology*. 1984;150:797–802.
69. Saphner T, Triest-Robertson S, Li H, et al. The association of nonalcoholic steatohepatitis and tamoxifen in patients with breast cancer. *Cancer*. 2009;115:3189–3195.
70. Brookes M, MacVicar D, Husband J. Metastatic carcinoma of the breast: the appearances of metastatic spread to the abdomen and pelvis as demonstrated by CT. *Br J Radiol*. 2007;80:284–292.
71. Eichler AF, Loeffler JS. Multidisciplinary management of brain metastases. *Oncologist*. 2007;12:884–898.
72. Fisher ER, Anderson S, Redmond C, et al. Pathologic findings from the National Surgical Adjuvant Breast Project protocol B-06. 10-year pathologic and clinical prognostic discriminants. *Cancer*. 1993;71:2507–2514.
73. Park C, Mitsumori M, Nixon A, et al. Outcome at 8 years after breast conserving surgery and radiation therapy for invasive breast cancer: influence of margin status and systemic therapy on local recurrence. *J Clin Oncol*. 2000;18:1668–1675.
74. Clarke M, Collins R, Darby S, et al. Effects of radiotherapy and of differences in the extent of surgery for early breast cancer on local recurrence and 15-year survival: an overview of the randomised trials. *Lancet*. 2005;366:2087–2106.
75. Giulano AE, Kirgan DM, Guenther JM, et al. Lymphatic mapping and sentinel lymphadenectomy for breast cancer. *Ann Surg*. 1994;220:391–401.
76. Chu K, Turner R, Hansen N, et al. Do all patients with sentinel node metastasis from breast carcinoma need complete axillary node dissection? *Ann Surg*. 1999;229:536–541.
77. Naik AM, Fey J, Gemignani M, et al. The risk of axillary relapse after sentinel lymph node biopsy for breast cancer is comparable with that of axillary lymph node dissection: a follow-up study of 4008 procedures. *Ann Surg*. 2004;240:462–468. discussion 468-471.
78. Bilimoria KY, Bentrem DJ, Hansen NM, et al. Comparison of sentinel lymph node biopsy alone and completion axillary lymph node dissection for node-positive breast cancer. *J Clin Oncol*. 2009;27:2946–2953.
79. Wasif N, Ye X, Giuliano AE. Survey of ASCO members on management of sentinel node micrometastases in breast cancer: variation in treatment recommendations according to specialty. *Ann Surg Oncol*. 2009;16:2442.
80. Elliott LF. Breast reconstruction. In: Thorne CH, Beasley RW, Aston SJ, eds. *Grabb & Smith's Plastic Surgery*. Philadelphia: Lippincott Williams & Wilkins; 2007:648–656.

81. Blondeel PN, Morrison CM. Deep inferior epigastric artery perforator flap. In: Blondeel PN, Morris SF, Hallock GG, eds. *Perforator Flaps: Anatomy, Technique, & Clinical Applications*. St. Louis: Quality Medical Publishing; 2006:385–403.
82. Early Breast Cancer Trialists' Collaborative Group Polychemotherapy for early breast cancer: an overview of the randomised trials. *Lancet*. 1998;352:930–942.
83. Early Breast Cancer Trialists' Collaborative Group Tamoxifen for early breast cancer: an overview of the randomised trials. *Lancet*. 1998;351:1451–1467.
84. Walker JV, Nitiss JL. DNA topoisomerase II as a target for cancer chemotherapy. *Cancer Invest*. 2002;20:570–589.
85. Bull JM, Tormey DC, Li SH, et al. A randomized comparative trial of adriamycin versus methotrexate in combination drug therapy. *Cancer*. 1978;41:1649–1657.
86. Schiff PB, Fant J, Horwitz SB. Promotion of microtubule assembly in vitro by taxol. *Nature*. 1979;277:665–667.
87. Bollag DM, McQueney PA, Zhu J, et al. Epothilones, a new class of microtubule-stabilizing agents with a taxol-like mechanism of action. *Cancer Res*. 1995;55:2325–2333.
88. Abeloff MD. Vinorelbine (Navelbine) in the treatment of breast cancer: a summary. *Semin Oncol*. 1995;22:1–4. discussion 41-44.
89. Galmarini CM, Jordheim L, Dumontet C. Pyrimidine nucleoside analogs in cancer treatment. *Expert Rev Anticancer Ther*. 2003;3:717–728.
90. Adema AD. Bijnsdorp IV, Sandvold ML, et al. Innovations and opportunities to improve conventional (deoxy)nucleoside and fluoropyrimidine analogs in cancer. *Curr Med Chem*. 2009;16:4632–4643.
91. Early Breast Cancer Trialists' Collaborative Group Radiotherapy for early breast cancer. *Cochrane Database Syst Rev*. 2002;2:CD003647.
92. Bijker N, Meijnen P, Peterse JL, et al. Breast-conserving treatment with or without radiotherapy in ductal carcinoma-in-situ: ten-year results of European Organisation for Research and Treatment of Cancer randomized phase III trial 10853—a study by the EORTC Breast Cancer Cooperative Group and EORTC Radiotherapy Group. *J Clin Oncol*. 2006;24:3381–3387.
93. Hughes KS, Schnaper LA, Berry D, et al. Lumpectomy plus tamoxifen with or without irradiation in women 70 years of age or older with early breast cancer. *N Engl J Med*. 2004;351:971–977.
94. Bentzen SM, Agrawal RK, Aird EG, et al. The UK Standardisation of Breast Radiotherapy (START) Trial A of radiotherapy hypofractionation for treatment of early breast cancer: a randomised trial. *Lancet Oncol*. 2008;9:331–341.
95. Whelan TJ, Pignol JP, Levine MN, et al. Long-term results of hypofractionated radiation therapy for breast cancer. *N Engl J Med*. 2010;362:513–520.
96. Smith BD, Arthur DW, Buchholz TA, et al. Accelerated partial breast irradiation consensus statement from the American Society for Radiation Oncology (ASTRO). *J Am Coll Surg*. 2009;209:269–277.
97. Buchholz TA, Lehman CD, Harris JR, et al. Statement of the science concerning locoregional treatments after preoperative chemotherapy for breast cancer: a National Cancer Institute conference. *J Clin Oncol*. 2008;26:791–797.
98. Buchholz TA, Tucker SL, Masullo L, et al. Predictors of local-regional recurrence after neoadjuvant chemotherapy and mastectomy without radiation. *J Clin Oncol*. 2002;20:17–23.
99. Mamounas EP, Tang G. Fisher B, et al. Association between the 21-gene recurrence score assay and risk of locoregional recurrence in node-negative, estrogen receptor–positive breast cancer: results from NSABP B-14 and NSABP B-20. *J Clin Oncol*. 2010;28:1677–1683.
100. Kuerer HM, Sahin AA, Hunt KK, et al. Incidence and impact of documented eradication of breast cancer axillary lymph node metastases before surgery in patients treated with preoperative chemotherapy. *Ann Surg*. 1999;230:72–78.
101. Buzdar AU, Ibrahim NK, Francis D, et al. Significantly higher pathologic complete remission rate after preoperative therapy with trastuzumab, paclitaxel, and epirubicin chemotherapy: results of a randomized trial in human epidermal growth factor receptor 2-positive operable breast cancer. *J Clin Oncol*. 2005;23:3676–3685.
102. Le-Petross H, Hylton N. Role of breast MR imaging in neoadjuvant chemotherapy. *Magn Reson Imaging Clin North Am*. 2010;18:249–258. viii-ix.
103. Slanetz PJ, Moy L, Baron P, et al. ACR appropriateness criteria monitoring response to neoadjuvant systemic therapy for breast cancer. *J Am Coll Radiol*. 2017;14(11S):S462–S475.
104. Sledge GW, Neuberg D, Bernardo P, et al. Phase III trial of doxorubicin, paclitaxel, and the combination of doxorubicin and paclitaxel as front-line chemotherapy for metastatic breast cancer: an intergroup trial (E1193). *J Clin Oncol*. 2003;21:588–592.
105. Norris B, Pritchard KI, James K, et al. Phase III comparative study of vinorelbine combined with doxorubicin versus doxorubicin alone in disseminated metastatic/recurrent breast cancer: National Cancer Institute of Canada Clinical Trials Group Study. *J Clin Oncol*. 2000;18:2385–2394.
106. Hortobagyi GN, Yap HY, Kau SW, et al. A comparative study of doxorubicin and epirubicin in patients with metastatic breast cancer. *Am J Clin Oncol*. 1989;12:57–62.
107. Keller AM, Mennel RG, Georgoulias VA, et al. Randomized phase III trial of pegylated liposomal doxorubicin versus vinorelbine or mitomycin C plus vinblastine in women with taxane-refractory advanced breast cancer. *J Clin Oncol*. 2004;22:3893–3901.
108. O'Brien ME, Wigler N, Inbar M, et al. Reduced cardiotoxicity and comparable efficacy in a phase III trial of pegylated liposomal doxorubicin HCl (CAELYX/Doxil) versus conventional doxorubicin for first-line treatment of metastatic breast cancer. *Ann Oncol*. 2004;15:440–449.
109. Nabholtz JM, Senn HJ, Bezwoda WR, et al. Prospective randomized trial of docetaxel versus mitomycin plus vinblastine in patients with metastatic breast cancer progressing despite previous anthracycline-containing chemotherapy. *J Clin Oncol*. 1999;17:1413–1424.
110. Jones SE, Erban J, Overmoyer B, et al. Randomized phase III study of docetaxel compared with paclitaxel in metastatic breast cancer. *J Clin Oncol*. 2005;23:5542–5551.
111. Gradishar WJ, Tjulandin S, Davidson N, et al. Superior efficacy of albumin-bound paclitaxel, ABI-007, compared with polyethylated castor oil-based paclitaxel in women with metastatic breast cancer: results of a phase III trial. *J Clin Oncol*. 2005;23:7794–7803.
112. Moulder S, Li H, Wang M, et al. A phase II trial of trastuzumab plus weekly ixabepilone and carboplatin in patients with HER2-positive metastatic breast cancer: an Eastern Cooperative Oncology Group Trial. *Breast Cancer Res Treat*. 2010;119:663–671.
113. Perez EA, Lerzo G, Pivot X, et al. Efficacy and safety of ixabepilone (BMS-247550) in a phase II study of patients with advanced breast cancer resistant to an anthracycline, a taxane, and capecitabine. *J Clin Oncol*. 2007;25:3407–3414.
114. Seidman AD, O'Shaughnessy J, Misset JL. Single-agent capecitabine: a reference treatment for taxane-pretreated metastatic breast cancer? *Oncologist*. 2002;7(suppl 6):20–28.
115. Silvestris N, D'Aprile M, Andreola G, et al. Rationale for the use of gemcitabine in breast cancer [review]. *Int J Oncol*. 2004;24:389–398.
116. Decatris MP, Sundar S, O'Byrne KJ. Platinum-based chemotherapy in metastatic breast cancer: current status. *Cancer Treat Rev*. 2004;30:53–81.
117. Clarke M, Collins R, Darby S, et al. Effects of radiotherapy and of differences in the extent of surgery for early breast cancer on local recurrence and 15-year survival: an overview of the randomised trials. *Lancet*. 2005;366:2087–2106.
118. Jatoi I, Tsimelzon A, Weiss H, et al. Hazard rates of recurrence following diagnosis of primary breast cancer. *Breast Cancer Res Treat*. 2005;89:173–178.
119. Runowics CD, Leach CR, Henry NL, et al. American Cancer Society/American Society of Clinical Oncology Breast Cancer Survivorship Care Guideline. *CA Cancer J Clin*. 2016;66:43–73.
120. Nielsen HM, Overgaard M, Grau C, et al. Loco-regional recurrence after mastectomy in high-risk breast cancer—risk and prognosis. An analysis of patients from the DBCG 82 b&c randomization trials. *Radiother Oncol*. 2006;79:147–155.
121. Ragaz J, Olivotto IA, Spinelli JJ, et al. Locoregional radiation therapy in patients with high-risk breast cancer receiving adjuvant chemotherapy: 20-year results of the British Columbia randomized trial. *J Natl Cancer Inst*. 2005;97:116–126.
122. Tennvall-Nittby L, Tenegrup I, Landberg T. The total incidence of loco-regional recurrence in a randomized trial of breast cancer TNM stage II: the South Sweden Breast Cancer Trial. *Acta Oncol*. 1993;32:641–646.
123. Willner J, Kiricuta IC, Kolbl O. Locoregional recurrence of breast cancer following mastectomy: always a fatal event? Results of univariate and multivariate analysis. *Int J Radiat Oncol Biol Phys*. 1997;37:853–863.

Visit ExpertConsult.com for algorithms

BREAST CANCER SCREENING

Note: This algorithm is intended for women who have not undergone prophylactic mastectomy. Breast cancer screening may continue as long as a woman has a 10-year life expectancy and no co-morbidities that would limit the diagnostic evaluation or treatment of any identified problem. Women should be counseled about the benefits, risks and limitations of mammography.

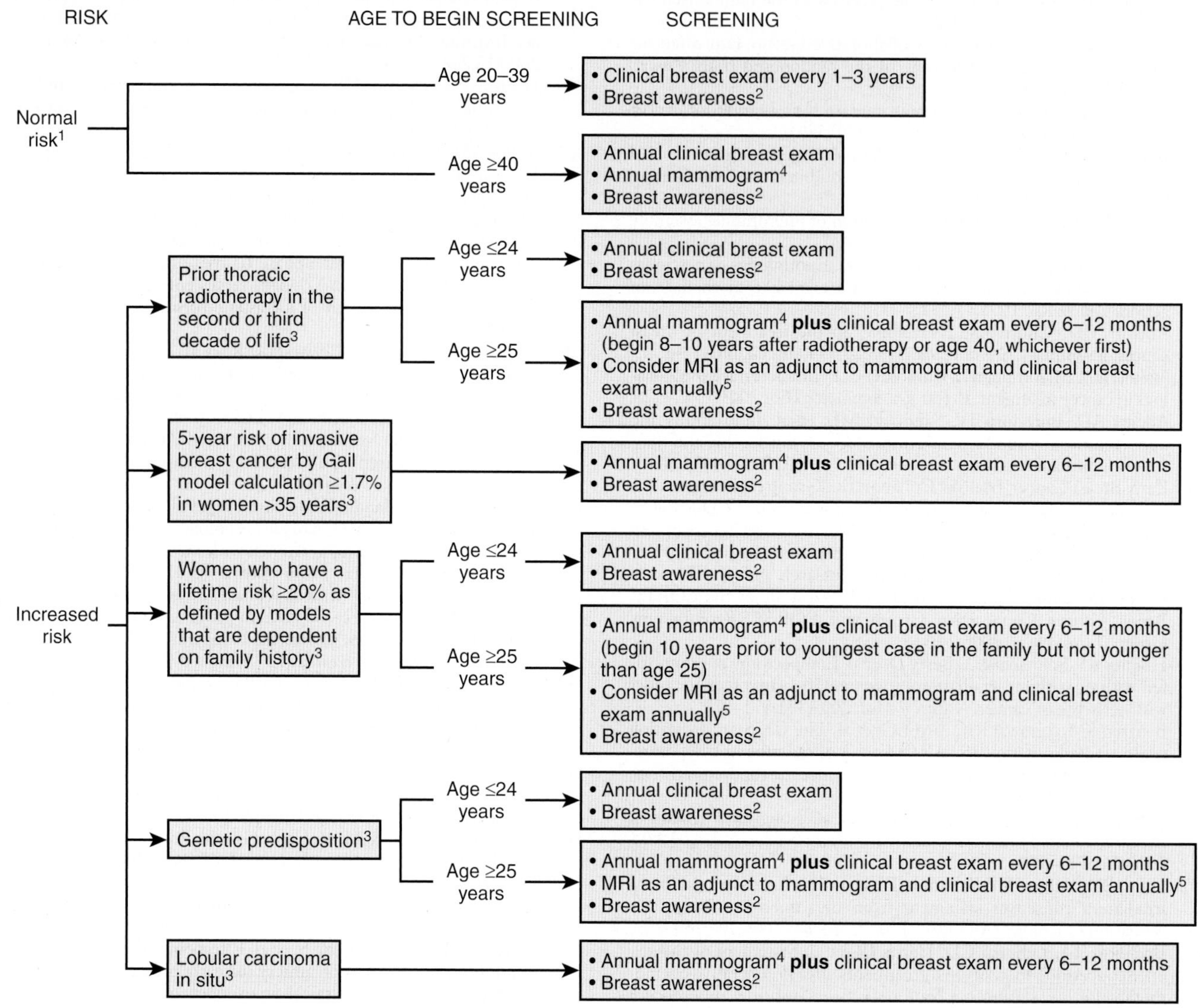

RISK		AGE TO BEGIN SCREENING	SCREENING
Normal risk[1]		Age 20–39 years	• Clinical breast exam every 1–3 years • Breast awareness[2]
Normal risk[1]		Age ≥40 years	• Annual clinical breast exam • Annual mammogram[4] • Breast awareness[2]
Increased risk	Prior thoracic radiotherapy in the second or third decade of life[3]	Age ≤24 years	• Annual clinical breast exam • Breast awareness[2]
Increased risk	Prior thoracic radiotherapy in the second or third decade of life[3]	Age ≥25 years	• Annual mammogram[4] **plus** clinical breast exam every 6–12 months (begin 8–10 years after radiotherapy or age 40, whichever first) • Consider MRI as an adjunct to mammogram and clinical breast exam annually[5] • Breast awareness[2]
Increased risk	5-year risk of invasive breast cancer by Gail model calculation ≥1.7% in women >35 years[3]		• Annual mammogram[4] **plus** clinical breast exam every 6–12 months • Breast awareness[2]
Increased risk	Women who have a lifetime risk ≥20% as defined by models that are dependent on family history[3]	Age ≤24 years	• Annual clinical breast exam • Breast awareness[2]
Increased risk	Women who have a lifetime risk ≥20% as defined by models that are dependent on family history[3]	Age ≥25 years	• Annual mammogram[4] **plus** clinical breast exam every 6–12 months (begin 10 years prior to youngest case in the family but not younger than age 25) • Consider MRI as an adjunct to mammogram and clinical breast exam annually[5] • Breast awareness[2]
Increased risk	Genetic predisposition[3]	Age ≤24 years	• Annual clinical breast exam • Breast awareness[2]
Increased risk	Genetic predisposition[3]	Age ≥25 years	• Annual mammogram[4] **plus** clinical breast exam every 6–12 months • MRI as an adjunct to mammogram and clinical breast exam annually[5] • Breast awareness[2]
Increased risk	Lobular carcinoma in situ[3]		• Annual mammogram[4] **plus** clinical breast exam every 6–12 months • Breast awareness[2]

[1]Women who do not meet one of the increased risk categories.
[2]Women should be familiar with their breasts and promptly report changes to their healthcare provider.
[3]For women at increased risk, see Risk Reduction Algorithm (currently in development).
[4]Augmented breasts need additional views for complete assessment.
[5]Current practice at M.D. Anderson is to alternate the mammogram and breast MRI every 6 months. While there is no data to suggest that this is the optimal approach, it is done with the expectation that interval cancers may be identified earlier. Other screening regimens, such as breast MRI done at the time of the annual mammogram, are also acceptable.

This practice algorithm has been specifically developed for M.D. Anderson using a multidisciplinary approach and taking into consideration circumstances particular to M.D. Anderson, including the following: M.D. Anderson's specific patient population; M.D. Anderson's services and structure; and M.D. Anderson's clinical information. Moreover, this algorithm is not intended to replace the independent medical or professional judgment of physicians or other health care providers. This algorithm should not be used to treat pregnant women.

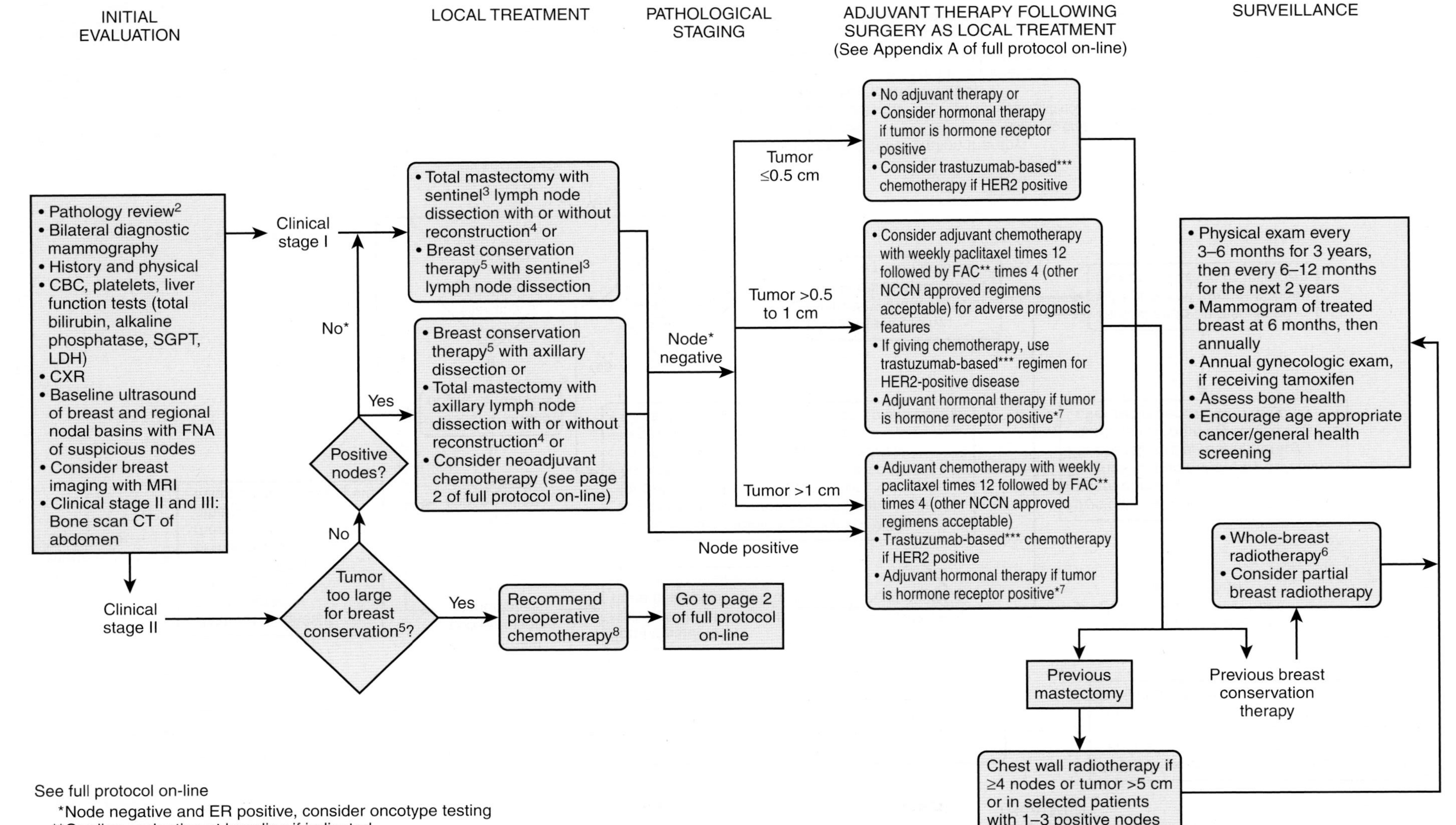

See full protocol on-line

*Node negative and ER positive, consider oncotype testing

**Cardiac evaluation at baseline if indicated

***Cardiac evaluation at baseline, during and after treatment and as clinically indicated

This practice algorithm has been specifically developed for M.D. Anderson using a multidisciplinary approach and taking into consideration circumstances particular to M.D. Anderson, including the following: M.D. Anderson's specific patient population; M.D. Anderson's services and structure; and M.D. Anderson's clinical information. Moreover, this algorithm is not intended to replace the independent medical or professional judgment of physicians or other health care providers. This algorithm should not be used to treat pregnant women.

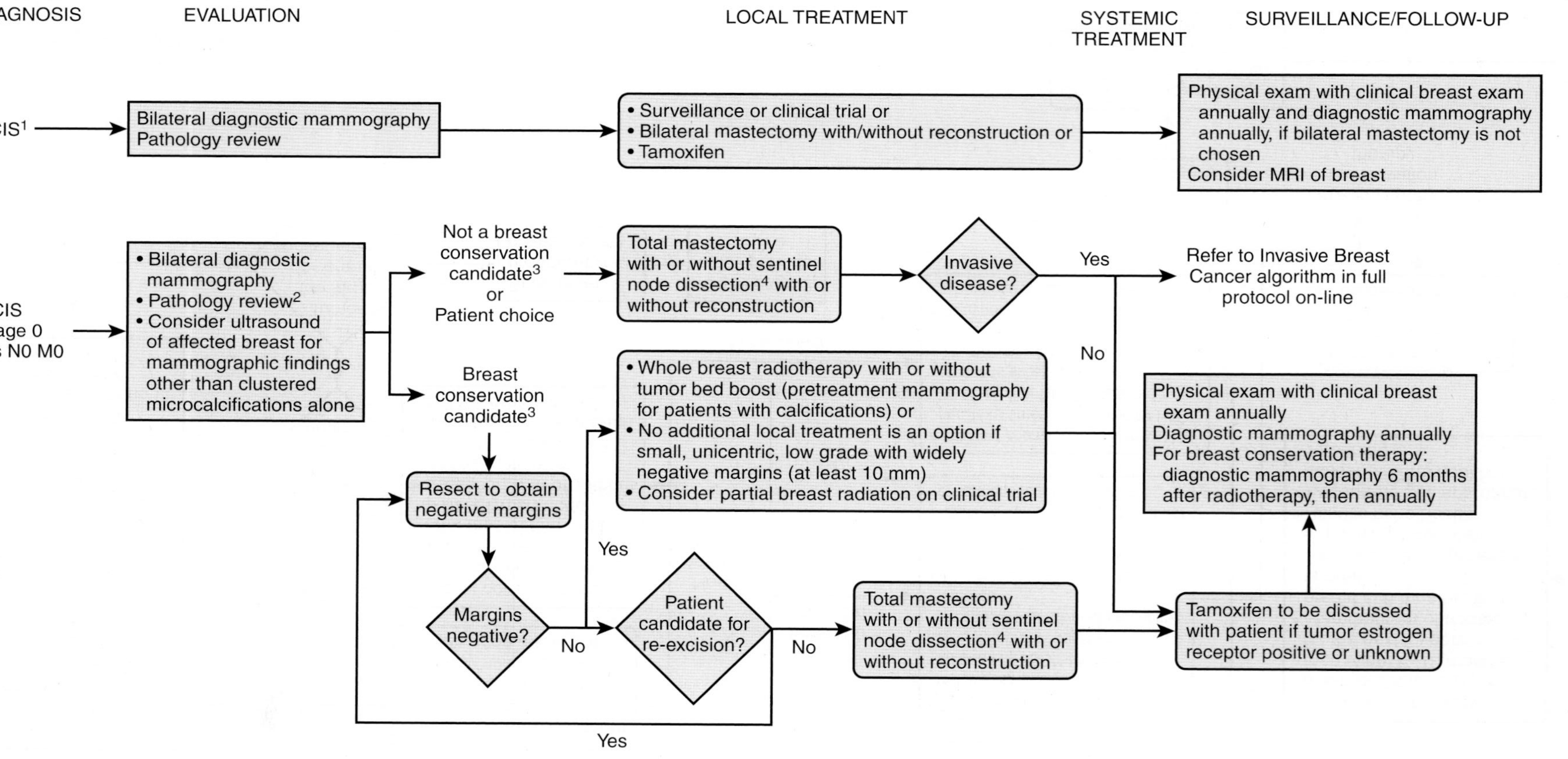

[1]Consider a marker for a future risk of breast cancer.

[2]Pathology review to include:
- Tumor size
- Rule out invasive component
- Lymph node status, if lymph node surgery performed
- Margin status
- Nuclear grade
- Histologic type/necrosis
- Estrogen receptor and progesterone receptor

[3]Candidates for breast conservation therapy:
- unicentric disease
- attempt margins ≥2 mm
- no contraindication to radiotherapy
- tumor to breast size ratio allows for acceptable cosmetic result
- no evidence of diffuse microcalcifications on mammography

[4]DCIS lymph node evaluation not recommended unless patient having total mastectomy which would preclude mapping at a later date if invasive disease noted on final pathology.

This practice algorithm has been specifically developed for M.D. Anderson using a multidisciplinary approach and taking into consideration circumstances particular to M.D. Anderson, including the following: M.D. Anderson's specific patient population; M.D. Anderson's services and structure; and M.D. Anderson's clinical information. Moreover, this algorithm is not intended to replace the independent medical or professional judgment of physicians or other health care providers. This algorithm should not be used to treat pregnant women.

PART

VIII LYMPHOMAS AND HEMATOLOGIC IMAGING

CHAPTER

29 Myeloma and Leukemia

Sameh Nassar, M.D.; Gregory P. Kaufman, M.D.; Ahmed Taher, M.D.; John E. Madewell, M.D.; and Bilal Mujtaba, M.D.

INTRODUCTION

Myeloma and leukemia share a common origin as hematologic malignancies. Both are usually systemic at the time of the diagnosis, although occasionally a plasmacytoma may exist as an isolated collection of plasma cells without systemic involvement. Both also have unclear boundaries from each other and from other related malignancies. For example, plasma cell leukemia is usually considered to be in the myeloma family rather than the leukemia family, despite its name, and pathologists may argue over whether a patient has lymphoma with a plasmacytic component or myeloma. Many of the chemotherapeutic agents that work for one of these diseases will have some efficacy for others as well.

Despite the similarities between myeloma and leukemia, each of them is a spectrum of diseases having distinct presentations, treatments, and prognoses. The use of imaging differs significantly between these two broad categories of malignancy. In myeloma, imaging is mainly used as a part of the staging process, to monitor response to treatment, and to look for evidence of disease progression. However, in leukemia there is little role for imaging in diagnosis and staging, and imaging is usually reserved for the diagnosis of treatment-related complications.

MYELOMA

Epidemiology and Risk Factors

Multiple myeloma is a malignant disorder that results from a clonal proliferation of marrow plasma cells that usually results in the production of monoclonal immunoglobulin in the serum or urine. Its the second most common hematologic malignancy in the United States, with approximately 32,110 patients diagnosed and 12,960 dying annually in the United States. The disease is more frequent in males than in females (1.3:1).[1] Multiple myeloma incidence in the African American population is twofold to threefold higher than the incidence in the White population. The exact reason for this disparity is still unknown, but may be attributed to the higher prevalence of monoclonal gammopathy of undetermined significance (MGUS) in Blacks.[2,3] The disease most commonly occurs during the seventh and eighth decades of life; only 2% of patients are younger than 40 years at the time of diagnosis.[4]

There is no undisputable risk factor for myeloma, but ionizing radiation or work in the paper, pulp, and leather tanning industries, as well as other chemical exposures, have been implicated.[5] There are numerous reports of myeloma in people with chronic exposure to low-dose ionizing radiation, including radiology technicians/physicians before routine shielding and radium watch dial painters; perhaps the best evidence was among atomic bomb survivors at Hiroshima in an initial report, but the follow-up of this report failed to confirm those initial findings.[6] Similarly, benzene has been implicated, but a thorough retrospective analysis of available reports eliminated this factor as well.[7] Hereditary factors have not previously been thought to play a prominent role as risk factors for multiple myeloma, but recent reports suggest that, at least among certain populations, the incidence of MGUS/myeloma may have a familial/genetic association.[8]

PATHOLOGY

Myeloma begins with the clonal expansion of a malignant plasma cell that is usually positive for CD38, CD138, and monoclonal cytoplasmic immunoglobulin, with a clonal light chain of either kappa or lambda type. These cells typically have an eccentric nucleus within a large cytoplasm and often have an area of central clearing that corresponds to intracytoplasmic immunoglobulin. Cells of plasmacytic origin are usually negative for other markers of the B-cell lineage such as CD19 and CD20. Recent studies suggest the existence of different categories of myeloma that may separate the disease into different levels of outcome.[9] A heterogeneous array of cytogenetic abnormalities has been described in patients. Deletions of chromosomes 13 or 17p, certain translocations involving chromosome 14, on which the immunoglobulin heavy chain locus resides (t(4;14) is present in approximately 11% of patients, and t(14;16) is present in approximately 3% of patients), and chromosome 1 abnormalities have predicted shortened survival. In contrast, t(11;14), which is found in approximately 14% of patients, has usually been associated with either an average or an improved prognosis, and is rarely noted to have a subgroup with poor prognosis. The median time to progression from smoldering multiple myeloma (SMM) to multiple myeloma was found to be shorter in patients with t(4;14) than in patients with t(11;14), with a median time of 28 months and 55 months, respectively.[9,10]

Abnormal clonal proliferation usually results in the production of monoclonal immunoglobulin in the serum and/or urine: immunoglobin (Ig)G is secreted in approximately 60%, IgA in 20%, IgD in 2%, and IgE in less than 1%, whereas biclonal secretion is rare. Secretion of light chain as the sole monoclonal protein is noted in 18%.[11] Previously, 3% of patients were noted to have the nonsecretory disease; this number has declined with the advent of serum free light chain detection (detection of free kappa, free lambda, and the free kappa:free lambda ratio in the serum).

Key Points

Monoclonal Plasma Cell Proliferation

- Cells are usually:
  - CD38- and CD138-positive
  - CD19- and CD20-negative
  - Either kappa or lambda light chain–positive

Numerous Chromosomal Aberrations Possible

- Shortened survival with:
  - Chromosome 13 deletion by karyotype
  - Chromosome 17p deletion by karyotype
  - Chromosome 14 translocations t(4;14), t(14;16), or t(14;20)
  - Chromosome 1 abnormalities
- Average or improved prognosis with:
  - Chromosome 14 translocation t(11;14)

Cells Usually Produce a Monoclonal Immunoglobulin

- Immunoglobin (Ig)G in 60%
- IgA in 20%
- IgD in 2%
- IgE in less than 1%
- Light chain only in 18%

CLINICAL PRESENTATION

Multiple myeloma may present with a number of characteristic clinical features and complications such as those that result from bone marrow infiltration (anemia), subsequent bone destruction (lytic bone lesions, fractures, bone pain, and hypercalcemia), complications of circulating monoclonal proteins, or reduced uninvolved immunoglobulins and/or light chains (hyperviscosity, increased infections, and renal failure). Patients with multiple myeloma most commonly present with fatigue and bone pain, with anemia, which contributes to fatigue, occurring in approximately 75% of patients.[4]

Bone disease occurs in nearly 70% of newly diagnosed patients with multiple myeloma and results, in part, from RANKL overexpression and OPG inhibition resulting in unbridled activation of osteoclasts. Other cytokines such as interleukin (IL)-1β, IL-6, and tumor necrosis factor-α also have a role in lytic bone disease.[12,13] Progressive bone destruction results in hypercalcemia in approximately 20% of patients with newly diagnosed myeloma.

Marrow infiltration with plasma cells results in normocytic, normochromic anemia in the majority of patients with previously untreated myeloma. Recently, upregulation of hepcidin mRNA in myeloma patients has been noted and may play a causative role in this complication.[14] In patients with high levels of circulating monoclonal serum protein, stacking of red blood cells on the peripheral blood smear, known as rouleaux formation, may occur.

Nearly half of the patients will develop renal failure at some time during the course of their disease. Cast nephropathy, resulting from accumulation of light chains in the distal tubule where they can combine with Tamm–Horsfall urinary glycoprotein to form obstructing casts, is the most common cause of this complication. However, hypercalcemia, dehydration, hyperuricemia, and concomitant conditions such as amyloidosis and light or heavy chain deposition diseases may also be contributing factors.[15,16]

Frequent bacterial infections may also be noted in patients with myeloma because of suppression of uninvolved immunoglobulins, decreased antibody response, and impaired opsonization, among other abnormalities reflective of the impaired immune response in patients with multiple myeloma.[17,18]

Although the diagnosis of myeloma by a fixed criteria may be difficult, the International Myeloma Working Group (IMWG) proposed has revised diagnostic criteria for MGUS, SMM, and multiple myeloma. The term multiple myeloma refers to multiple myeloma requiring therapy, based on measurement of serum monoclonal protein levels, assessment of the bone marrow, and presence or absence of myeloma-defining events (MDEs). MDEs include "CRAB" (hypercalcemia, renal failure, anemia, bone lesions) features and the presence of one or more of the following malignancy biomarkers: a clonal bone marrow plasma cell (BMPC) percentage of greater than or equal to 60%, an involved:uninvolved serum free light chain ratio of greater than or equal to 100, or the presence of two or more focal lesions on magnetic resonance imaging (MRI).

CRAB features are used to determine whether there has been end-organ damage, which would classify a patient as having a symptomatic disease that would require initiation of treatment. These features include serum calcium levels of greater than 1 mg/dL higher than the upper limit of normal levels (or serum calcium levels of >11 mg/dL), Renal insufficiency (creatinine clearance of <40 mL/min or serum creatinine levels of >2 mg/dL), Anemia (hemoglobin levels of >2 g/dL below the lower limit of normal levels or <10 g/dL), Bone lesions (presence of one or more bone lytic lesions detected by conventional radiology, computed tomography (CT) imaging or positron-emission tomography (PET)/CT, or osteoporosis with compression fractures), or other complications (hyperviscosity, amyloidosis, and light chain deposition diseases).[19]

It is important to distinguish multiple myeloma from other related plasma cell dyscrasias such as MGUS, SMM, and solitary bone plasmacytoma (SBP) or extramedullary plasmacytoma (EMP). The diagnosis of MGUS relies on the presence of less than 10% clonal BMPC infiltration and serum monoclonal protein levels of less than 3 g/dL in a patient who has no evidence of end-organ/tissue damage, including anemia, hypercalcemia, renal failure, or lytic bone lesions attributable to myeloma and no evidence of a B-cell proliferative disorder.[19] The diagnosis of SMM requires the presence of 10% to 60% clonal bone marrow plasma cell infiltration and/or serum monoclonal protein levels of greater than or equal to 3 g/dL, plus the absence of MDEs or amyloidosis.[19] SBP or EMP is diagnosed when a single lesion of biopsy-proven clonal plasma cells is detected without evidence of another disease, including negative MRI of the spine and pelvis (except for the primary solitary lesion), and absence of end-organ damage that can be attributed to myeloma with no or minimal (<10% clonal plasma cells in the bone marrow) bone marrow plasmacytosis; it is particularly important to identify these patients, because they have about a 10% progression rate to multiple myeloma within 3 years, and around 35% to 65% of these patients may be curable when given radiation therapy with a curative intent.[20–22]

Key Points

Monoclonal Gammopathy of Unknown Significance

- <10% clonal marrow plasma cells
- And serum monoclonal protein level of less than 3.0 g/dL
- Without hypercalcemia, renal failure, anemia, bone lesions (CRAB) features or any of the complications (attributable to myeloma) listed below

Solitary Plasmacytoma

- Single lesion of biopsy-proven clonal plasma cells without other evidence of myeloma, including negative magnetic resonance imaging (MRI) of the spine and pelvis, and negative or minimal bone marrow plasmacytosis (clonal plasma cells <10%)

Smoldering Multiple Myeloma

- Between 10% and 60% clonal bone marrow plasma cell infiltration
- And/or serum monoclonal protein level of 3 g/dL or greater
- Absence of myeloma-defining events (MDEs) or amyloidosis

Multiple Myeloma

- Clonal bone marrow plasma cell percentage of 10% (or more) or biopsy-proven bony or extramedullary plasmacytoma
- And the presence of one or more of the MDEs listed

Myeloma-Defining Events

- CRAB features
- A clonal bone marrow plasma cell percentage of 60% or more
- An involved:uninvolved serum free light chain ratio of 100 or more
- Two or more focal lesions on MRI

Myeloma Complications

- Elevated serum calcium
- Renal insufficiency
- Bone lesions
- Serum hyperviscosity
- Amyloidosis
- More than two bacterial infections in 12 months

STAGING

Numerous factors have been suggested to determine the prognosis of patients with myeloma. In the 1970s, Durie and Salmon proposed a staging system based on the degree of anemia, level of paraprotein, presence or absence of hypercalcemia, bone lytic lesions, and renal insufficiency that subsequently became the standard staging system for myeloma for several decades (Table 29.1). Although this system was predictive of the degree of myeloma tumor mass, several components were imprecise, such as the extent of bone lesions and the inclusion of factors such as anemia, hypercalcemia, and renal function, which may be affected by factors other than myeloma infiltration. Subsequently, multiple new prognostic factors emerged, including plasma cell hypodiploidy, C-reactive protein, lactate dehydrogenase, labeling index, cytogenetic abnormalities, and β-2 microglobulin (β2M).[23]

In 2005, Greipp and coworkers proposed the International Staging System (ISS) that separated patients into three stages based on the level of serum albumin and β_2M.[24] The data from 10,750 patients were analyzed by univariate and multivariate analysis; the system was designed using half of the data set and validated in the other half of the population (Table 29.2). This system effectively identified a group of patients with a relatively short median survival of 29 months (β_2M ≥5.5 mg/L, stage III), another with longer median survival of 62 months (β_2M <3.5 mg/L and albumin >3.5 g/dL, stage I), and a group with intermediate survival (stage II). Although some patients in the data set may have received thalidomide, the impact on survival of novel agents including bortezomib, lenalidomide, and multiple combinations utilizing both of these drugs will likely lead to improved median survivals for one or more stages defined by the ISS. The Greek Myeloma Study Group also confirmed the validity of the ISS in the era of novel agents.[25] The ISS has subsequently become a standard staging system for patients with myeloma.

Although the Durie–Salmon staging system and ISS effectively separate patients into different survival categories, the impact of chromosomal abnormalities (CAs) on prognosis is significant, and some have even suggested a

TABLE 29.1 Durie–Salmon Staging System for Multiple Myeloma

STAGE	CRITERIA	MYELOMA CELL MASS (× $10^{12}/M^2$)
I	Hemoglobin >10 g/dL Serum calcium levels: normal or ≤12 mg/dL Normal bone or solitary plasmacytoma on x-ray Low production rates of M-component IgG <5 g/dL IgA <3 g/dL Urine light chains <4 g/24 hours	<0.6 (low)
II	Not fitting stage I or III	0.6–1.2 (intermediate)
III	Hemoglobin <8.5 g/dL Serum calcium >12 mg/dL Multiple (>3) lytic bone lesions on x-ray High production rates of M-component IgG >7 g/dL IgA >5 g/dL Urine light chains >12 g/24 hours	>1.2 (high)
SUBCLASSIFICATION	**CRITERION**	
A	Normal renal function (serum creatinine level <2.0 mg/dL)	
B	Abnormal renal function (serum creatinine level ≥2.0 mg/dL)	

(From Durie BG, Salmon SE. A clinical staging system for multiple myeloma: correlation of measured myeloma cell mass with presenting clinical features, response to treatment, and survival. Cancer. 1975;36:842–854.)

molecular classification of myeloma.[9] Certain translocations involving chromosome 14 (t(4;14), t(14;16)) and deletion of chromosome 13 have previously predicted a poor prognosis, but treatment with novel agents such as bortezomib appears to partially ameliorate the prognostic impact of these abnormalities; the same data with lenalidomide are premature and need to be validated over time.[9,26,27] Deletion of chromosome 17p remains prognostic even in the era of novel agents; other considerations include the poor prognosis of chromosome 1 abnormalities and the possibility of an improved prognosis with t(11;14).[9]

In 2015, Palumbo et al. developed the Revised International Staging System by incorporating CAs and serum lactate dehydrogenase (LDH) levels into the ISS to predict the prognosis and overall survival (OS) in patients with newly diagnosed multiple myeloma. They pooled data from 11 international trials involving 4,445 patients.[28] CAs, detected by interphase fluorescence *in situ* hybridization after CD138 plasma cell purification, classified patients into two groups: a high-risk group characterized by the presence of high-risk CAs, including deletion of chromosome 17 (17p), translocation t(4;14), and translocation t(14;16), and a standard-risk group characterized by the absence of high-risk CAs. Serum LDH levels were classified as high or normal: high LDH was defined as serum LDH levels above the upper limit of the normal range, whereas normal LDH was defined as serum LDH levels lower than the upper limit of the normal range. Later, they assessed the prognosis and 5-year OS rates in each group (Table 29.3).

TABLE 29.2 International Staging System for Multiple Myeloma

STAGE	CRITERIA	SURVIVAL (MONTHS)
I	β_2M <3.5 mg/L And albumin ≥3.5 g/dL	62
II	β_2M 3.5–5.5 mg/L irrespective of serum albumin level *Or* β_2M <3.5 mg/L and albumin <3.5 g/dL	44
III	β_2M ≥5.5 mg/L	29

β2M, β-2 microglobulin.
(From Greipp PR, San Miguel J, Durie BG, et al. International staging system for multiple myeloma. J Clin Oncol. 2005;23:3412–3420.)

TABLE 29.3 Revised International Staging System for Multiple Myeloma

STAGE	CRITERIA	FREQUENCY (% OF PATIENTS)	5-YEAR SURVIVAL RATE (%)
I	International Staging System (ISS) stage I and Standard risk (no high-risk) CA and Normal LDH	28	82
II	Not R-ISS stage I or III	62	62
III	ISS stage III and Either high-risk CA or high LDH	10	40

CA, Chromosomal abnormality; *LDH*, lactate dehydrogenase.
(From Palumbo A, Avet-Loiseau H, Oliva S, et al. Revised international staging system for multiple myeloma: a report from International Myeloma Working Group. *J Clin Oncol.* 2015;33:2863.)

IMAGING

Goals

Imaging strategies are somewhat different for MGUS, plasmacytoma, and multiple myeloma. MGUS is a benign condition with a small (1%/year) chance of progression to multiple myeloma or occasionally to other malignancies. Imaging in this condition is limited to evaluation of any specific patient complaint that could be attributed to myeloma and to staging to exclude myeloma.

When a patient is suspected of having an isolated plasmacytoma, imaging initially serves two roles. The first is similar to its role in any focal solid tumor—to define the anatomy of the tumor and its relationship to other structures to assist with local treatment planning, which will usually be radiation therapy with a curative intent. The second is to determine whether the seemingly isolated plasmacytoma is the only site of disease, or whether it is merely the tip of the iceberg in a patient who should properly be classified as having multiple myeloma. To that end, one may weigh and choose between the various forms of systemic imaging, to be discussed later. If no other tumor is found elsewhere, and the patient remains classified as having solitary plasmacytoma, then follow-up imaging also serves two purposes. The first is again similar to its role in other solid tumors—to evaluate the site of the primary disease for evidence of healing or, alternatively, recurrence or progression (Fig. 29.1). The second is surveillance for the development of multiple myeloma, again by the use of systemic imaging along with other criteria.

For patients with multiple myeloma, imaging helps at the initial evaluation to distinguish those with smoldering or asymptomatic myeloma, who have no visible bone disease, from those with symptomatic myeloma. Once the patient has been categorized into the symptomatic or smoldering group, imaging is used to assess stability versus progression of the disease.

KEY POINTS

Radiology Report

- Identify and characterize focal bone lesions: number, location, and size when practical. (For multiple lesions, it is often impractical to discuss each separately.)
- Clearly indicate when a bone lesion is thought to be attributed to disease other than myeloma, such as a geode because of degenerative joint disease.
- Discuss specific lesions with a significantly elevated risk of pathological fracture.
- Assess subjective bone mineralization—normal, decreased absolutely, decreased allowing for age and gender.
- Look for and discuss compression fractures in the spine.
- Follow-up examinations: indicate whether the disease is stable, progressive, or shows signs of healing; include resolution of 2-[^{18}F] fluoro-2-deoxy-D-glucose avidity at positron-emission tomography/computed tomography scans or decrease in contrast enhancement at magnetic resonance imaging.

Techniques

Conventional Radiography

Skeletal surveys have for decades been a mainstay of imaging in multiple myeloma and related diseases and are included in the original Durie and Salmon staging system.[23] They consist of a series of images intended to include all the bones that have a reasonable likelihood of

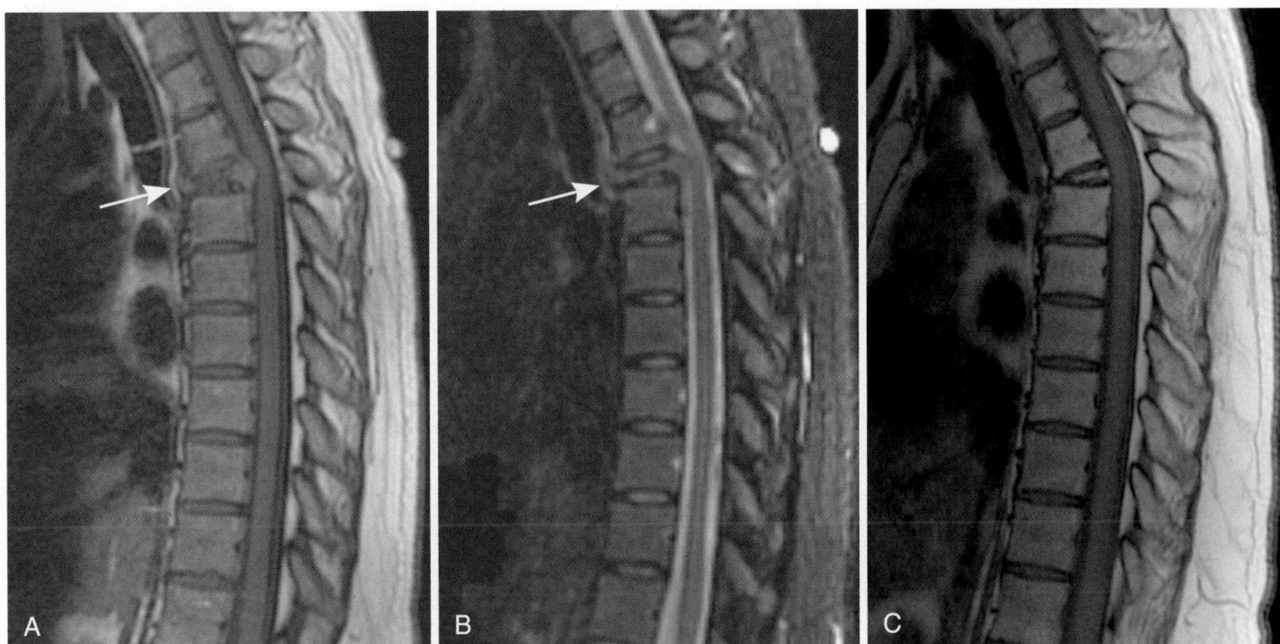

FIGURE 29.1. Plasmacytoma in a 46-year-old woman with a compression fracture of T4. Thoracic vertebrae are the most common site of solitary plasmacytoma of bone. T1-weighted sagittal magnetic resonance imaging (MRI) **(A)** and short tau inversion recovery (STIR) sagittal MRI **(B)** demonstrate loss of height of the vertebral body (*arrows*) with a convex contour to the central part of the posterior cortical margin, a shape that is more common in pathologic than in traumatic or osteoporotic compression fractures. The STIR image is atypical in that the signal in the collapsed vertebral body approximates that in other nearby vertebrae instead of being of higher intensity. Biopsy revealed a plasma cell neoplasm. No evidence was found of additional focal lesions, and so a plasmacytoma was diagnosed and treated by radiation with curative intent. **C**, T1-weighted sagittal MRI obtained 4.5 years later shows that the bulging of the posterior cortex has resolved, and the marrow signal in the collapsed T4 vertebral body matches that of other vertebrae.

developing visible signs of multiple myeloma. There is no generally agreed-upon grouping of images to be included in a skeletal survey, and so there will be variation from one institution to another as to exactly what is included. Based on observation not only of our own practice pattern but also of the assortment of images obtained at outside institutions and then reviewed within our institution, the minimum number and type of views might reasonably be lateral skull, lateral cervical spine, frontal and lateral thoracic and lumbar spine, frontal chest or ribs, frontal pelvis, and frontal views of each humerus and femur. That would be 12 views. The assortment of images suggested by the IMWG[29] is listed in a key point text box later. Whole-body radiography has been suggested as an alternative to the individual views obtained with skeletal surveys.[30]

Skeletal surveys have the advantage of being relatively cheap and easy to perform using widely available equipment. They are adequate for finding lytic bone lesions, appearing as punched out lesions that have reached a sufficient size. Generally, that means loss of 30% to 50% of bone mineralization.[31,32] For an individual lesion, the size needed for it to be visible will depend greatly on which bone is involved and where the lesion is in the bone. For example, if a femoral lesion is located along the lateral or medial margin of the bone, it will erode the endosteal surface of the cortex and create a scalloped border that will be noticeable earlier than a similarly sized lesion located either anteriorly or posteriorly, assuming that the bone is being imaged in the frontal projection. Lesions in the pelvis and sacrum often have to attain a size of several centimeters before they are noticed because overlying bowel gas may mask them. In the skull, the presence of normal lucencies owing to venous lakes can make it difficult to decide whether a particular lucent area is normal or abnormal.

Skeletal surveys are obtained as part of the initial diagnostic workup of patients with MGUS or suspected SBP because the presence of unexpected lytic bone lesions would necessitate recategorization, probably to multiple myeloma. Skeletal surveys are also obtained in patients with myeloma to help determine the stage of disease when diagnosed. If the skeletal survey shows lytic lesions, more advanced imaging may be unnecessary. The skeletal survey is also useful for searching for progression after treatment.[33]

Skeletal surveys and other conventional radiographs can reveal disease progression but are of limited utility in assessing response to therapy, because lytic bone lesions heal very slowly, if at all. Thus, even if there is treatment response, they rarely show radiologically distinct changes (Figs. 29.2 and 29.3).[32]

Another use of conventional radiography is in assessing the risk of pathological fracture once a lytic lesion has been identified by any means. For this, one usually needs both frontal and lateral views of the area in question (Fig. 29.4).

Limitations of conventional radiography include low sensitivity, limited specificity, restricted visualization of the spine and pelvis, limited ability to diagnose myeloma-related osteoporosis, failure to detect extraosseous lesions, and limited assessment of therapy response.

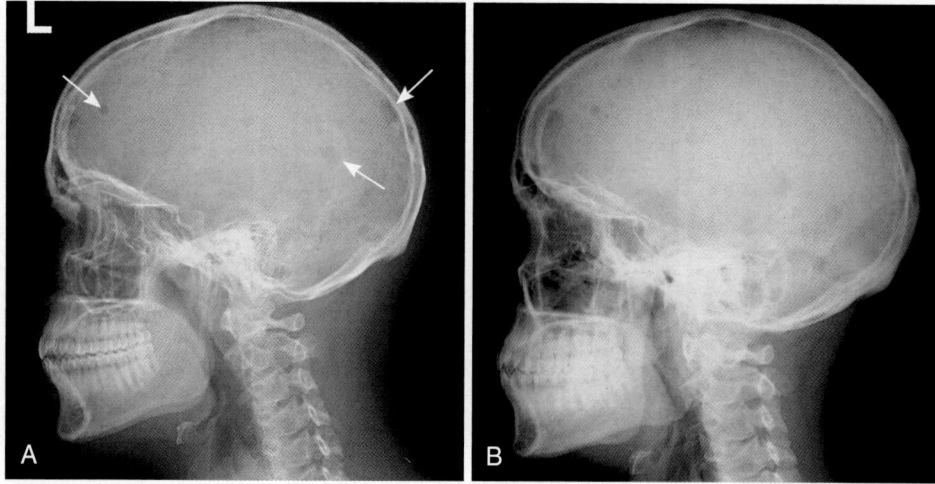

FIGURE 29.2. Stable lytic lesions. **A**, Conventional lateral radiograph of the skull in a 23-year-old man with multiple myeloma. There are multiple typical, sharply defined lytic lesions of myeloma (*arrows*). **B**, Conventional lateral radiograph of the skull 8 months later shows the same well-circumscribed lytic lesions of myeloma that, allowing for slight differences in technique and positioning, have not changed despite a good response to chemotherapy and bone marrow transplantation.

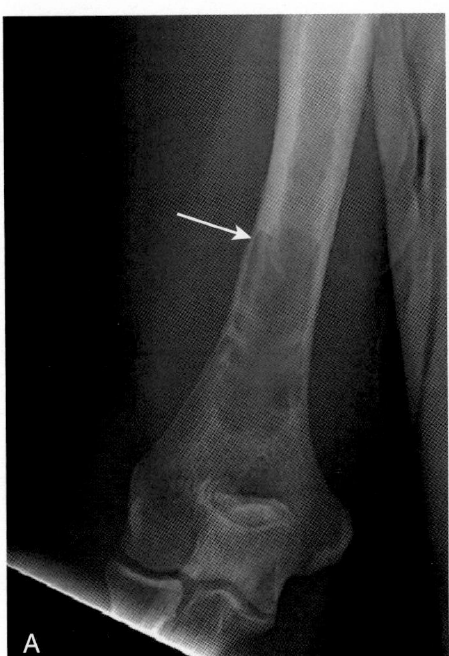

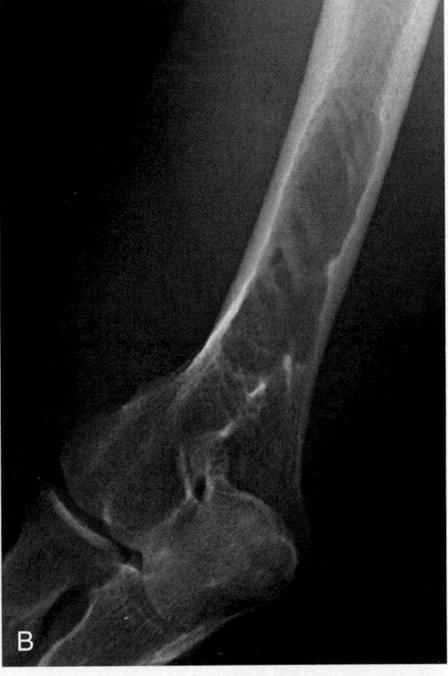

FIGURE 29.3. Healing lytic lesion. **A**, Anteroposterior (AP) radiograph of the right humerus in a 48-year-old man with a newly diagnosed myeloma. A well-defined lytic lesion in the distal humerus narrows the cortex medially and laterally by approximately 80% (*arrow* shows the lateral junction between normal and eroded cortex). Because the lesion is lucent, it is clearly narrowing the anterior and posterior cortex as well. **B**, AP radiograph of the distal right humerus obtained 5 years, 4 months after the preceding one again demonstrates a sharply defined lytic lesion, but now both the lateral and the medial cortex have thickened. The lateral cortex now approaches a normal thickness, and the medial cortex is now narrowed by approximately 30%.

KEY POINTS

Skeletal Survey

Views suggested for inclusion in the skeletal survey by the International Myeloma Working Group

- Skull anteroposterior (AP) and lateral
- Cervical spine AP, open-mouth odontoid, and lateral
- Thoracic spine AP and lateral
- Lumbar spine AP and lateral
- Pelvis AP
- Chest AP
- Femurs AP and lateral
- Humeri AP and lateral

This would total 15 images, but the femurs often have to be covered in two views each, proximal and distal, so this may require 17 images.

Computed Tomography

CT provides cross-sectional radiographic images of the body and can serve many purposes. Myeloma's most common anatomic manifestation is in the bones. CT can demonstrate smaller lytic lesions than would be apparent by conventional radiography and can, like conventional radiography, help estimate the risk of pathologic fracture (Fig. 29.5).[29–31] With attention to the difference in attenuation between tumor (water density) and marrow (fat density), CT can also demonstrate marrow involvement. Despite these capabilities, CT is not commonly used for evaluation of osseous myeloma, although low-dose whole-body CT has been suggested as an alternative to the skeletal survey.[34] The sensitivity of whole-body CT is superior to that of whole-body x-ray, especially for lesions located in the ribs, spine, or pelvis.[34,35] CT is also quite useful for detecting and characterizing the uncommon soft tissue manifestations of myeloma or complications of its treatment.

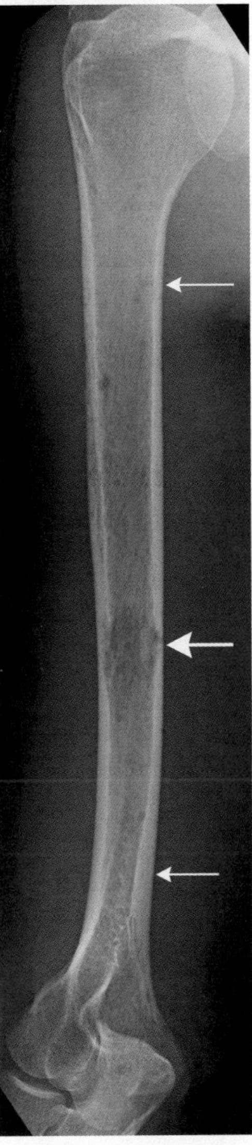

FIGURE 29.4. Increased fracture risk. Conventional radiograph of the right humerus in external rotation demonstrates numerous tiny lucencies in the bone extending at least as far up and down the diaphysis as between the two *small arrows*, with a central area of more focal destruction (*large arrow*). The amount of destruction in this bone confers an excessive risk of pathologic fracture.

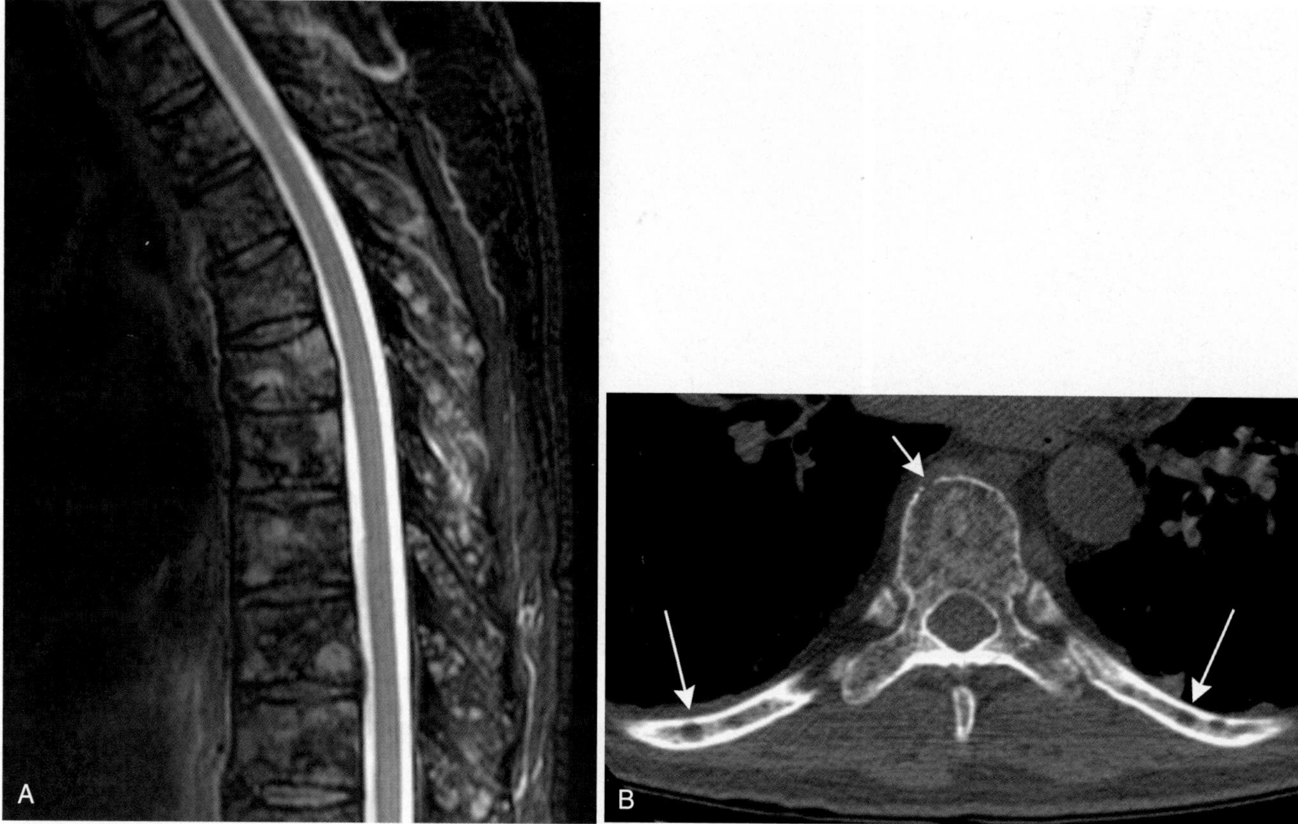

FIGURE 29.5. Computed tomography (CT) in myeloma. **A**, T2-weighted sagittal magnetic resonance imaging (MRI) of the thoracic spine in a 47-year-old man with innumerable rounded areas of abnormally bright signal ranging in size from a few millimeters to a little over a centimeter. No vertebral level is spared. These are consistent with myeloma. **B**, Axial CT image of the same patient obtained through the T9 vertebral body clearly shows multiple small lytic lesions in the vertebra and both ribs (*long arrows*). Similar findings were present in every imaged bone. In one place at the anterior vertebral body, the cortex has been breached (*short arrow*). These areas of cortical damage are more obvious on CT than on MRI. In the cancellous bone of the vertebral body, however, the abnormality is evident primarily as a greater variegation in opacity than would be normally expected, but individual lesions are not as easily distinguished as on the MRI.

Magnetic Resonance Imaging

MRI is also a cross-sectional imaging technique that differs from CT in having an inherently lower spatial resolution but greater contrast resolution, an advantage in imaging the bone marrow that makes MRI highly sensitive for early detection of marrow infiltration by myeloma cells, compared with other imaging modalities, before the incidence of myeloma-related bone destruction. Because of this, MRI is typically used in myeloma for staging assessment of bone marrow involvement. Myeloma can involve any bone, but spine MRI has been used traditionally for assessing a large amount of bone marrow in one MRI examination. With the advancement of new techniques using coils adapted to image large areas, imaging from the skull base to the proximal thighs can be done, including assessment of the entire body in one scan. This whole-body MRI examination gives a very broad view of the marrow at the cost of spatial resolution. Whole-body MRI has recently been tested as a staging method for plasma cell neoplasms. Ghanem and colleagues compared whole-body MRI and skeletal surveys in patients with either myeloma or MGUS. Among 54 patients, whole-body MRI found bone marrow involvement in 10 who had negative skeletal surveys.[36] Walker and associates also found MRI to be more sensitive than skeletal survey in detecting focal bone lesions.[37] Evaluating 100 patients with MGUS or myeloma, Bäuerle and coworkers compared spinal MRI with whole-body MRI and found nine patients with isolated extraaxial disease that was identified only with whole-body MRI.[38]

Myeloma lesions usually demonstrate decreased signal intensity on T1-weighted (T1W) images, increased signal intensity on T2-weighted (T2W) and short time inversion recovery images, and increased enhancement on gadolinium-enhanced images.[39,40]

Five patterns of myeloma involvement have been seen on MRI: normal marrow (which does not exclude low-level infiltration of myeloma cells), focal involvement (lesion with a diameter ≥5 mm) (Fig. 29.6), diffuse homogeneous involvement (Fig. 29.7), combined diffuse and focal involvement, and heterogeneous involvement with combinations of fatty marrow and tiny areas of myeloma creating a salt-and-pepper appearance.[41,42] Low tumor burden is typically associated with normal MRI appearance, whereas high tumor burden is typically associated with diffuse hypointensity on T1W sequences and diffuse hyperintensity on T2W sequences.[42] Shorter time to progression and worse response to therapy have been found with diffuse and focal disease as opposed to normal marrow or heterogeneous involvement.[41,43,44] With successful treatment, the marrow pattern should become more normal.[32]

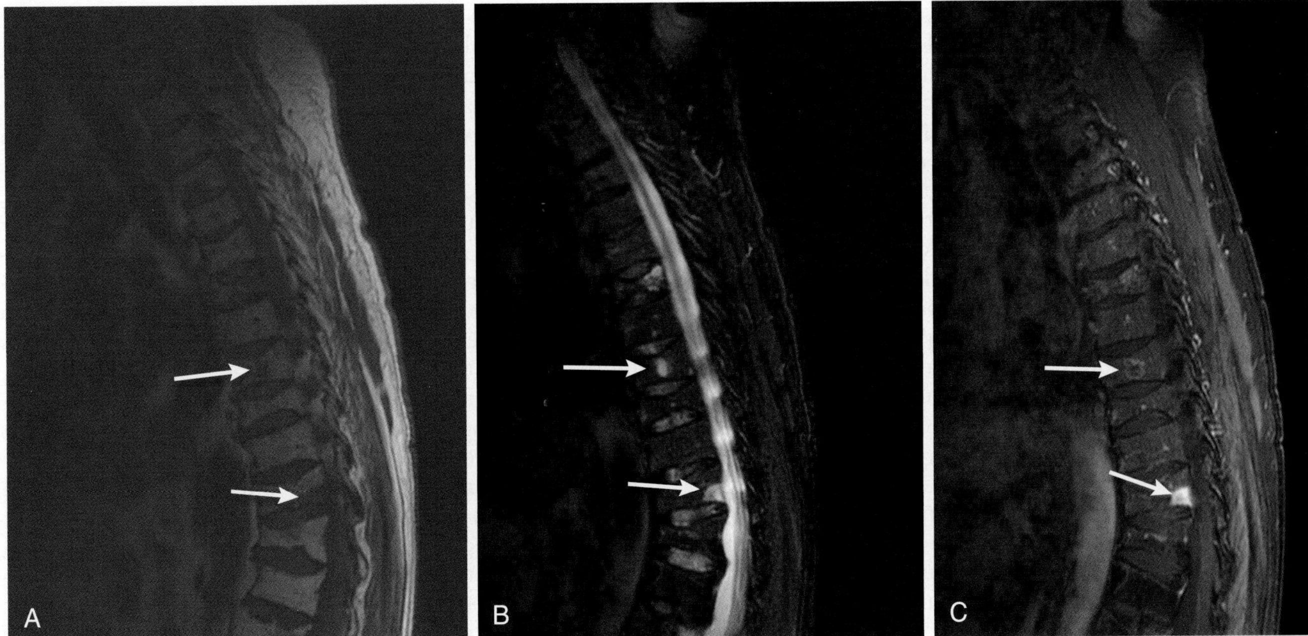

FIGURE 29.6. Focal myeloma. A 55-year-old man with relapsed refractory multiple myeloma. **A**, T1-weighted sagittal magnetic resonance imaging (MRI) of the thoracic spine shows focal lesions with decreased signal intensity (*arrows*). **B**, T2-weighted sagittal MRI through the same area causes the lesions (*arrows*) to appear bright. **C**, Following intravenous gadolinium administration, the lesions (*arrows*) show contrast enhancement.

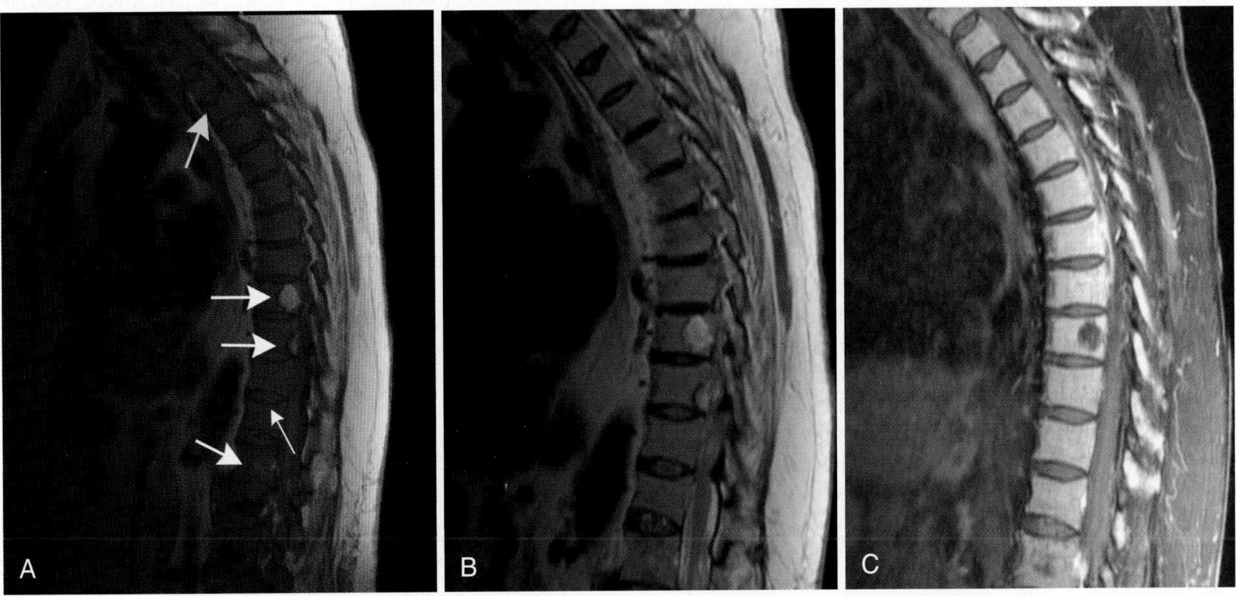

FIGURE 29.7. Diffuse myeloma in a 66-year-old woman. **A**, T1-weighted sagittal magnetic resonance imaging (MRI) of the thoracic spine looks deceptively normal. In particular, there are no focal areas of low signal as one expects with myeloma; however, the marrow is diffusely too dark, as dark as or darker than the signal in the intervertebral discs. The subcutaneous fat and fat in three hemangiomas (*large white arrows*) is bright, and the fat in the marrow of the remainder of the spine should approach fatty signal as well. Other subtle clues to abnormality are slightly excessive concavity to the superior endplate of a lower thoracic vertebra (*thin white arrow*), a Schmorl node (*yellow arrow*), and mildly accentuated kyphosis. These subtle findings, however, are nonspecific and may be seen in many people without myeloma. **B**, T2-weighted sagittal MRI of the thoracic spine also looks relatively normal, but this image has been obtained with fat saturation. Notice that the subcutaneous fat is now darker, yet the bone marrow is not noticeably darker. In fact, it may be just a little brighter compared with its appearance on the T1-weighted (T1W) image. **C**, On T1W fat-saturated sagittal MRI of the thoracic spine following gadolinium administration, the bone marrow is now diffusely bright. The fat in the hemangiomas appears dark because of fat saturation, and this is approximately how all the marrow should normally appear. The middle of the three hemangiomas is not apparent because it is slightly out of plane in this image.

All patients with smoldering or asymptomatic myeloma should undergo whole-body MRI or spine and pelvic MRI if whole-body MRI is not available. If MRI detects the presence of more than one focal lesion greater than 5 mm in diameter, the patient should be considered to have symptomatic myeloma that requires treatment. In case of equivocal small lesions, MRI should be repeated 3 to 6 months later to detect any progression. If present, the patient should be treated as having symptomatic disease.[45]

Other advantages of MRI include its ability to distinguish between benign (e.g., osteoporosis) and malignant (e.g., myeloma) causes of a vertebral fracture, as well as diagnose any concomitant spinal cord and/or nerve root compression.[29,46] Limitations include high cost, unsuitability for patients with metallic devices in their bodies, and a relatively long scanning time, making it difficult for ill and claustrophobic patients.

A weakness of MRI is that normal marrow may vary considerably in its appearance from person to person, and it may be difficult to decide in individual cases whether the pattern is within the range of normal variation or indicates the presence of myeloma. In our experience, administering gadolinium contrast can help with this discrimination, because islands of red marrow will not enhance as noticeably as pockets of myeloma.

Positron Emission Tomography

PET can be performed with different radiopharmaceuticals, but the one most commonly used is 2-[18F] fluoro-2-deoxy-D-glucose (FDG), which functions as a sugar analog. Because myeloma cells are metabolically hyperactive, FDG is taken up by them in greater amounts than by normal tissue and then enters the glycolytic pathway, where it becomes phosphorylated, generating FDG-6 phosphate. However, because of an abnormal hexose-phosphate bond, FDG-6 phosphate cannot be further metabolized; thus, it becomes trapped within the malignant cell, where it can be detected by PET/CT. To overcome the low resolution inherent in nuclear medicine studies, nowadays PET scans are performed in conjunction with CT. The CT serves for attenuation correction, and then the CT images are fused with the PET images, providing both excellent localization and the important anatomic information inherent in the CT study.

The purpose of PET/CT varies depending on the stage of the disease. In newly diagnosed patients, it helps find locations of the disease, both osseous and in the soft tissues, which may be occult by conventional radiography. In this way, it can help distinguish a solitary plasmacytoma from multiple myeloma.[47] Kim and colleagues found PET to be positive in 13 of 14 known plasmacytomas, and in one of 21 patients with suspected SBP, PET imaging resulted in upstaging of the disease to multiple myeloma by disclosing previously unsuspected additional disease.[48] In contrast with multiple myeloma, PET is usually negative in patients with MGUS.[29,49] Depending on the equipment available, PET/CT will usually cover at least the head, trunk, and proximal humeri and femurs, and it may be able to include literally the entire body, so, like large field of view MRI, it is a way to obtain more sensitive screening of most or all of the body than is available with a bone survey. In patients who have been treated, PET/CT is used to identify sites of disease progression and to distinguish the osseous lesions that are still apparent anatomically but are no longer metabolically active from those that are resistant to treatment and remain active (Fig. 29.8).[50,51] Complete suppression of abnormal PET activity after treatment may be linked to longer progression-free survival (PFS) than for patients without complete suppression.[52] PET allows quantitative assessment of FDG uptake by a given lesion, known as the standardized uptake value (SUV). A number of studies have demonstrated that higher SUV values correlate with more progressive disease with a worse prognosis.[29,53,54] When compared with MRI, PET/CT tends to be less sensitive to diffuse marrow infiltration and perhaps more sensitive to the presence of focal lesions.[55]

Both MRI and PET/CT are more sensitive than conventional radiography, yet each has limitations.[51,56] Shortt and associates compared whole-body MRI and PET/CT with bone marrow aspiration. Bone marrow aspiration was taken as the gold standard, although it can also suffer from sampling error if the myeloma cells are patchy in distribution rather than fairly widespread through the marrow. For the 34 sets of paired MRI and PET/CT studies they obtained in 24 patients, MRI had an overall accuracy rate of 65%, and PET/CT had an overall accuracy rate of 74%. When both MRI and PET/CT were either positive or negative, the combined accuracy rate rose to 81%. The routine use of both examinations is probably not justified owing to their financial impact.[57]

One promising technique is combining PET with MRI, where PET detects the presence of active focal lesions, while MRI provides data about the site of the lesions and marrow myeloma cell infiltration. This technique will be useful, especially in patients in complete remission, to determine the location of residual disease activity and therefore guide therapy.[58]

Both the presence and the number of focal lytic bone lesions, particularly those that are FDG-avid and remain so after induction therapy, may be of a prognostic significance. Bartel and coworkers found that the presence of more than three lytic lesions correlated with an inferior survival, whereas complete suppression of FDG avidity during induction therapy correlated with an improved outcome.[52] Additionally, FDG-PET/CT is considered the gold standard technique for evaluating and monitoring the response to therapy by comparing the metabolic activity of the lesions in posttreatment images with pretreatment images.[59]

Key Points

Imaging Algorithm for Multiple Myeloma

- Start with the skeletal survey. (Whole-body radiography or low-dose whole-body computed tomography [CT] are possible alternatives.)
- If positive, perform focal imaging of any areas that may be at risk of pathologic fracture. Consider either positron emission tomography (PET)/CT or magnetic resonance imaging (MRI) of the spine or whole-body MRI as a baseline to allow an anatomic method of monitoring the response to therapy.
- If negative, obtain MRI of the spine (consider whole-body MRI or PET/CT if available) to look for radiographically occult marrow infiltration or focal lesions.

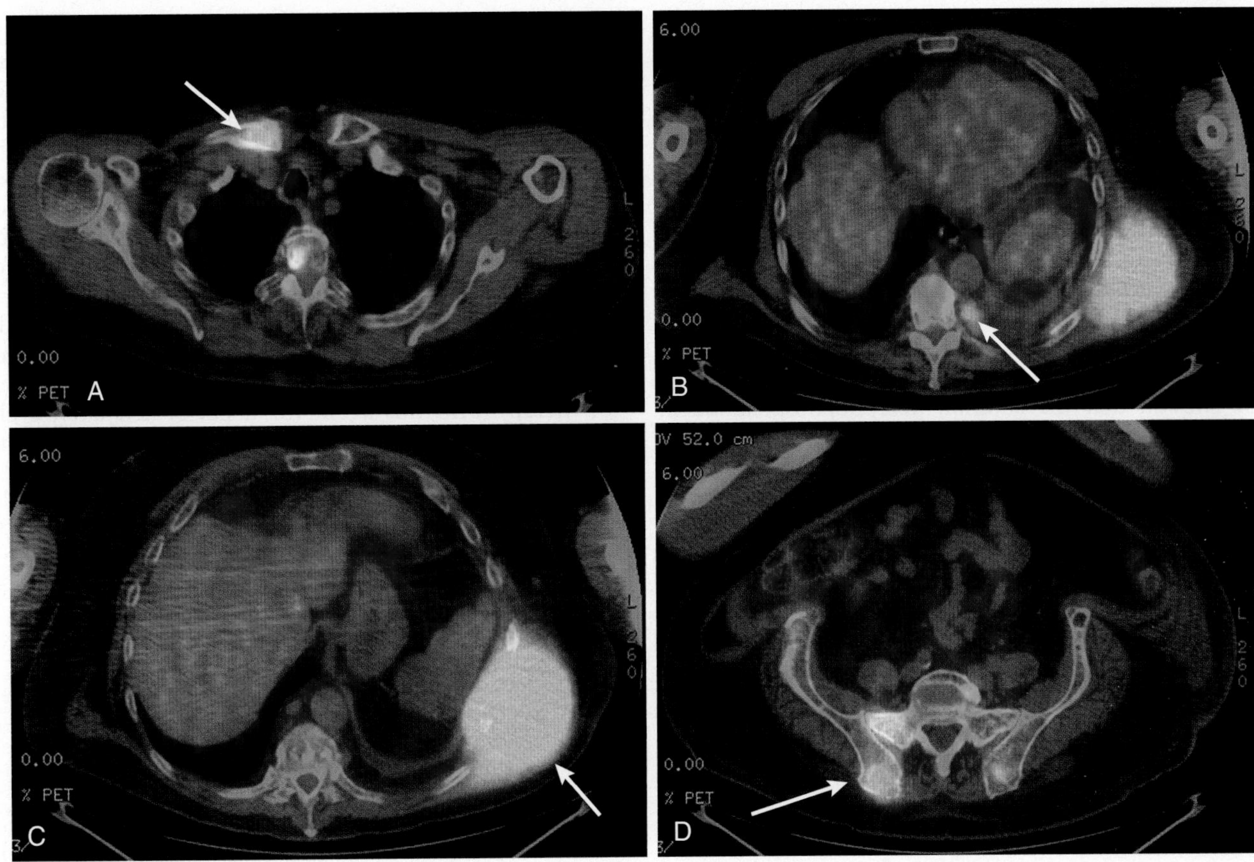

FIGURE 29.8. Positron-emission tomography (PET) in myeloma. Fused PET/computed tomography (CT) images of a 61-year-old man with multiple myeloma show numerous sites of 2-[^{18}F] fluoro-2-deoxy-D-glucose (FDG)-avid lesions within the skeleton. **A**, PET/CT shows FDG-avidity at the right clavicular head with a standardized uptake value (SUV) of 8.7 (*arrow*). **B**, A gadolinium-avid soft tissue nodule measuring 1.6 × 2.8 cm at the level of tenth costovertebral junction with an SUV of 6.4 (*arrow*). **C**, Very large soft tissue mass associated with the left posterolateral ninth rib lesion, measuring 11.2 × 8.4 cm with an SUV of 16.1 (*arrow*). **D**, FDG-avidity at the right posterior iliac bone with an SUV of 8.1 (*arrow*).

TREATMENT

Approximately 20% of patients are diagnosed with multiple myeloma by chance while in an asymptomatic phase. For these patients without CRAB criteria defining symptomatic disease, the standard of care is observation with frequent follow-up, without treatment. However, in patients with high-risk SMM, early treatment might prolong the time of progression to multiple myeloma. In a randomized clinical trial, early treatment of high-risk SMM with lenalidomide and dexamethasone showed a significantly longer median time to progression to multiple myeloma compared with patients who underwent observation only, after a median follow-up of 40 months.[60] This study included some patients who today would be classified as having active multiple myeloma per updated criteria, although without active classic end organ damage. However, a subsequent randomized study, E3A06, also showed improvement in time to progression in patients with high-risk SMM.[61] However, questions remain, given limited follow-up and uncertainty regarding long-term outcomes.

The first treatment strategy in multiple myeloma has classically been to determine whether the patient is eligible for autologous stem cell transplantation (ASCT) or not, as some drugs, like melphalan, can disrupt the ability to collect stem cells.[62] For decades, melphalan and prednisone induction therapy and vincristine-doxorubicin-dexamethasone (VAD) for relapsing multiple myeloma remained the standard of care for patients with symptomatic disease.[63,64] In the 1990s, myeloablative therapy with ASCT provided the first major improvement in survival for myeloma patients and subsequently became the standard of care for eligible patients.[65]

The introduction of thalidomide in 1999 to therapy for myeloma provided not only a new therapeutic avenue for patients with myeloma but also enthusiasm for investigation of novel pathways and mechanisms of action of the disorder.[66] Soon after, novel agents including bortezomib and lenalidomide changed the landscape of therapy and ushered in the "novel agent" era of myeloma therapy. Treatment with either the proteasome inhibitor bortezomib or the immunomodulatory derivative (ImiD) lenalidomide in combination with dexamethasone for induction results in overall response rates of approximately 80%, with complete response (CR) rates of 10% to 20%.[67–69] However, treatment with bortezomib and lenalidomide in combination with dexamethasone (the VRD regimen) has demonstrated improved response rates, depth of response, PFS, and OS for patients with multiple myeloma, compared with patients who received either bortezomib or lenalidomide in combination with dexamethasone.[70–73] Thus, it is not unexpected that this combination (VRD) is now the backbone of induction therapy for this disorder.[74] Other induction combinations including bortezomib-cyclophosphamide-dexamethasone (VCD), and in some countries bortezomib-thalidomide-dexamethasone, remain standard considerations for newly diagnosed symptomatic disease. Overall, these three drug regimens have improved overall response rates for induction therapy to 85% to 100%, and CR rates to approximately 25% to 45%.[75–78] The addition of a fourth agent with the goal of deepening response to induction therapy while balancing toxicity and considering long-term patient outcomes has proven challenging. The EVOLUTION study showed that the addition of cyclophosphamide in multiple dosing strategies to the VRD backbone did not significantly improve outcomes, and increased toxicity.[79] Similarly, the CYCLONE trial showed no substantial advantage of four-drug combination therapy including carfilzomib, thalidomide, cyclophosphamide, and dexamethasone over three-drug combinations.[80] Likewise, Ludwig and associates' phase 2 randomized trial showed similar efficacy of the three-drug VTD combination (bortezomib, thalidomide, and dexamethasone) when compared with VTD plus cyclophosphamide, but with an increased incidence of serious adverse events with the four-drug combination.[81] However, the development of well-tolerated monoclonal antibodies has reopened the door for the consideration of four-drug induction combinations. Several trials are currently ongoing to assess the efficacy of triplet regimens (VRD, VTD, VCD) in combination with either of the CD38 monoclonal antibodies daratumumab or elotuzumab, particularly in patients with high-risk features, and the preliminary results are promising.

For patients eligible for consolidation with myeloablative therapy with ASCT, randomized trials have demonstrated an improvement in OS compared with chemotherapy alone; similar results have been noted at first relapse and for primary refractory disease.[65,82,83] However, in the current era of novel agents, there has been increasing debate regarding the role of ASCT and whether the same results will be obtained with randomized trials using these novel agents. Regimens using novel agent induction therapy followed by ASCT have resulted in some of the highest CR rates noted to date. Notably, the IFM/DFCI DETERMINATION study has shown improvement in PFS with an early ASCT strategy as upfront consolidation in the context of VRD induction, although long-term follow up and OS endpoints remain pending. ASCT is still considered an essential part of a multistep treatment strategy. Metaanalysis of several trials has showed improved OS in patients who received lenolidomide maintenance therapy following ASCT, compared with the use of ASCT alone.[84–86] For patients ineligible for myeloablative therapy, treatment approaches should be modified depending on patient characteristics, like age, physical capacity, and comorbidities. In the VISTA trial, bortezomib-melphalan-prednisone combination therapy demonstrated excellent response rates and PFS/OS benefits even among patients with high-risk CAs.[27] In the FIRST trial, treatment with lenalidomide and dexamethasone until progression demonstrated improved PFS and OS compared with patients who received melphalan, prednisone, and thalidomide; therefore, it is considered an excellent treatment strategy for older and more fragile patients.[87] Based on the Southwest Oncology Group S0777 trial results, the triplet VRD or modified versions referred to as VRD "lite" are often considered for patients who are not eligible for ASCT, given the OS advantage of the triplet regimen VRD compared with RD only without upfront ASCT.[73]

Prolonged therapy with melphalan may impair stem cell collection and should be avoided in transplant candidates. Radiation to large areas of marrow should also be avoided for similar reasons.[88] Stem cell harvest may also be impaired after prolonged therapy with lenalidomide; thus, stem cell harvest should proceed early in the course of therapy with this agent (or if performed later, cyclophosphamide mobilization or plerixafor may be used) for transplant-eligible patients.[88]

Key Points

Treatment

Monoclonal Gammopathy of Undetermined Significance

- No specific treatment.
- Monitor for progression to myeloma.

Solitary Bone Plasmacytoma

- Radiation therapy with a curative intent.

Asymptomatic Smoldering Multiple Myeloma

- Observation with regular follow-up is still the standard of care.
- However, selected high-risk smoldering multiple myeloma patients could be considered for therapy.

Symptomatic Myeloma

- Combination chemotherapy (bortezomib-lenalidomide-dexamethasone, bortezomib-cyclophosphamide-dexamethasone, and carfilzomib-lenalidomide-dexamethasone are the most commonly used combinations in the United States, whereas bortezomib-thalidomide-dexamethasone is still commonly used in Europe and Australia) induce remission followed, when possible, by myeloablative therapy and autologous stem cell transplantation.
- Radiation therapy for palliation of selective symptomatic focal lesions. (Avoid large fields whenever possible in stem cell–transplant candidates.)
- Bisphosphonate therapy for 2 years for patients with lytic bone disease, to be resumed if there is a progression of bone disease.

SURVEILLANCE

Response criteria for myeloma have often varied between institutions and investigators, prompting the European Bone Marrow Transplant (group to propose uniform response criteria that were later revised by the IMWG.[89,90] In the revised criteria, partial response (PR) is determined by at least a 50% reduction in serum myeloma protein and at least a 90% reduction in Bence–Jones proteinuria, along with additional criteria for special circumstances.[89] CR is determined by the complete absence of serum and urine monoclonal protein by immunofixation and less than 5% marrow plasma cells, among other criteria for less common circumstances. Other categories include stringent CR (sCR), which includes additional normalization of free light chains and absence of clonal marrow plasma cells as detected by immunohistochemistry or immunofluorescence, and very good PR (VGPR), in which M-protein can be detected in serum and urine by immunofixation but not on electrophoresis or there is at least a 90% reduction in the serum M-protein plus a urine M-protein level of less than100 mg/24 hours. After achieving a PR or better, the question of maintenance therapy arises.

The use of maintenance or continuous therapy has become common among both transplant-eligible and transplant-ineligible patients. A metaanalysis of several phase III trials showed improved PFS and OS with lenalidomide maintenance therapy following ASCT.[86,91] Therefore, post-ASCT maintenance therapy is currently considered the standard care with consideration to bortezomib use in intermediate-risk and high-risk patients.[92] However, the pros and the cons of lenalidomide maintenance therapy should be considered carefully because there has been evidence of increased risk of secondary primary malignancies with continuous lenalidomide therapy. Thus, lenalidomide maintenance therapy is recommended in standard-risk patients who tolerated lenalidomide-based induction therapy and did not achieve VGPR following ASCT.[93] In nontransplant patients, analysis of several phase III studies showed improved PFS and OS with continuous lenalidomide therapy compared with fixed-duration therapy.[94] Some investigators, however, have noted worse survival after thalidomide maintenance therapy in patients with deletion of 17p.[95] The question of maintenance therapy remains unresolved, although for patients achieving less than VGPR, maintenance therapy appears warranted based on survival benefits and may be considered in all patients based on benefits in depth of response and PFS. The benefits of maintenance therapy for patients not receiving ASCT are less clear, although recent reports demonstrate similar benefits.[96]

Patients should be monitored every 2 to 3 months (although, if continued on maintenance therapy, this may be more frequent) until relapse, with continued monitoring of serum and urine protein electrophoretic studies, serum free light chain analyses, routine chemistries, and blood counts, particularly focusing on hemoglobin and creatinine, and bone x-rays annually or for persistent pain. Criteria for relapse have also been proposed by the IMWG and include recurrence of paraprotein, marrow plasmacytosis of 5% or greater, or progression and/or new lytic lesions for relapse from CR and for VGPR or less; a 25% increase in monoclonal protein; marrow plasmacytosis of 10% or greater with similar bone parameters; an absolute rise in monoclonal serum protein of 0.5 g/dL or greater; and an absolute rise of at least 200 mg/day of Bence–Jones protein.[89] Parameters for clinical relapse have also been proposed by this group.

Patients with bone disease should receive therapy with bisphosphonates after performance of a careful dental examination to evaluate for predisposing factors for osteonecrosis of the jaw (ONJ).[97] Careful monitoring for ONJ and renal function (with dose reduction as appropriate) is also necessary, and bisphosphonates should be held if complications occur. Denosumab is also a United States Food and Drug Administration (FDA)-approved option widely adopted in patients with renal dysfunction as an alternative to bisphosphonates. The ideal duration of bisphosphonate therapy is not clear, but a consensus panel has recommended 2 years of therapy, followed by a resumption of bisphosphonates in case of progression of the bony disease.[97–99] Vertebroplasty or kyphoplasty may be performed for eligible patients with vertebral compression factors; it is important to note that compression fractures may occur after response, without progression of the disease.[100] Radiotherapy can also be useful for pain associated with vertebral fractures.[101]

Patients with neuropathy secondary to thalidomide or bortezomib, and, much less frequently, lenalidomide, may find symptoms alleviated with dose reduction or, if severe, cessation of the offending agent and initiation of drugs for symptom control, such as gabapentin, pregabalin, duloxetine, or acetyl-l-carnitine. Prophylactic acyclovir/valacyclovir is recommended for patients receiving treatment with proteasome inhibitor–based therapies and patients receiving ASCT, owing to an increased incidence of herpes zoster, and the antiviral drugs should be continued for 6 weeks after discontinuation of the proteasome inhibitor.[98,102] Prophylactic anticoagulation with aspirin, warfarin, or low-molecular-weight heparin is recommended per IMWG guidelines for patients on thalidomide or lenalidomide, particularly in combination with steroids and/or anthracyclines.[98,103,104]

KEY POINTS

Detecting Progression

- Established indicators of relapse or progression include:
  - Rising urine or serum paraprotein levels
  - Increase in marrow plasmacytosis
  - Development of new lytic bone lesions
  - Enlargement of previous lytic bone lesions
- Consider relapse or progression for:
  - New or increasing skeletal foci of 2-[^{18}F] fluoro-2-deoxy-D-glucose avidity on positron emission tomography/computed tomography
  - New or increasing marrow infiltration on magnetic resonance imaging
  - Worsening anemia
  - Rising creatinine

PROMISING THERAPIES

Eventually, the disease relapses in nearly all myeloma patients; depending on the duration of remission, the same initial regimen may be repeated. However, if the remission duration is relatively short, a new regimen or combination of the previously discussed agents should be initiated. In addition, several new novel agents hold promise for the future.

The success of the reversible proteasome inhibitor bortezomib has led to further investigation of more specific and/or other targets within the ubiquitin-proteasome system. Carfilzomib is a second-generation, irreversible proteasome inhibitor that has a higher degree of chymotrypsin-like activity and a lower affinity for caspase- and trypsin-like binding sites within the proteasome. Because of these differences in affinity for proteasome-binding sites, differences in the toxicity and efficacy profile compared with bortezomib appeared feasible. Carfilzomib carries a lower risk of neurotoxicity compared with bortezomib, but around 5% of patients may develop serious cardiac adverse events.[105] Carfilzomib-based combinations are currently an important strategy for the treatment of relapsed multiple myeloma. In a phase 3 trial, the carfilzomib-lenalidomide-dexamethasone (KRD) combination was associated with better response rates, PFS, and OS.[106] The use of upfront KRD in newly diagnosed patients is actively being compared with VRD in ongoing clinical trials as well. Because proteasome inhibition has provided such a successful new avenue of treatment for patients with myeloma, it is natural to consider a more convenient, oral route of administration for these agents. Ixazomib is an oral proteasome inhibitor that has been approved in the United States for the treatment of relapsed, refractory, and newly diagnosed multiple myeoloma.[107]

After the introduction of thalidomide and lenalidomide as active agents in myeloma, it became clear that side effects such as neuropathy and thromboembolic events were frequent. The ImiD pomalidomide has demonstrated significant activity in combination with dexamethasone and has been approved for the treatment of relapsed and refractory multiple myeloma, even in patients in whom lenalidomide or lenalidomide plus bortezomib has been ineffective.[108–111] Toxicity included myelosuppression, one thrombotic event (on aspirin), and mild neuropathy in 30%, but only one patient developed grade 3 or higher neuropathy.

Panobinostat is another drug that was approved in 2015 for the treatment of relapsed and refractory multiple myeloma.[112] Panobinostat is a pan–histone deacetylase inhibitor that acts by blocking the aggresome pathway, an alternative way for cells to bypass proteasome inhibition. Therefore, combining panobinostat with bortezomib leads to simultaneous blockade of both the proteasome and aggresome pathways.[113,114] Caution should be taken with the use of Panobinostat because it was associated with grade 3 diarrhea in around 25% of patients.

Monoclonal antibodies have shown promising results for the treatment of relapsed and refractory multiple myeloma. Daratumumab is a monoclonal antibody targeting CD38 that has been approved for the treatment of relapsed and refractory multiple myeloma and is being investigated in earlier lines of therapy.[115] Elotuzumab is another monoclonal antibody targeting the signaling lymphocytic activation molecule F7 and has been approved for the treatment of relapsed multiple myeloma. Elotuzumab has a synergistic effect when used in combination with RD or lenalidomide/pomalidomide-dexamethasone in terms of PFS.[116,117] Additional therapies including bispecific antibodies and CAR-T cells, and others are in development currently.

LEUKEMIA

Although additional diseases are included in the family of hematologic malignancies known as leukemia, this discussion is restricted to the four major types: acute lymphoblastic leukemia (ALL), chronic lymphocytic leukemia (CLL), acute myeloid leukemia (AML), and chronic myeloid (or myelogenous) leukemia (CML).

Epidemiology and Risk Factors

Acute Lymphoblastic Leukemia

ALL is the most frequent cancer, and the most common form of leukemia among children, accounting for approximately 30% of all cancers in children and around 80% of all childhood leukemia.[118–120] The incidence decreases with age, even among children. Around 6000 cases are diagnosed annually in the United States, and approximately 80% of these cases occur in children.[1,121] The incidence of ALL is characterized by a bimodal distribution, with the first peak occurring during childhood (3–5 years) followed by another peak around the age of 50 years.[122] The etiology is unknown, although many different factors including genetics (such as Down syndrome), exposure to ionizing radiation, some viruses (such as Epstein–Barr virus and human immunodeficiency virus [HIV]), pesticides, and toxins are under investigation.[123–127] However, in the majority of patients, ALL develops as a result of *de novo* malignant proliferation in a previously healthy individual. Clinical presentation is usually acute, and the most common symptoms include fever, fatigue, bone pain, arthralgia, infections, and abnormal bleeding.[128]

Acute Myeloid Leukemia

AML is the most common type of acute leukemia among adults, with an estimated incidence of approximately 21,450 cases in the United States in 2019.[1] The peak age at diagnosis is approximately 67 years, so this is primarily a disease of older adults.[129] When AML occurs in children, it is usually in infants.[126] People with Down syndrome are at a distinctly increased risk, with approximately 1% of children with Down syndrome developing leukemia. This is usually a form of AML that is sufficiently distinct from other variants of AML that it may be referred to as myeloid leukemia of Down syndrome.[130] Children with Down syndrome are also at increased risk for ALL.[124,126]

Chronic Lymphocytic Leukemia

In the United States, CLL is the second most common form of leukemia after AML, with an estimated incidence of approximately 20,720 new cases in 2019.[1] To diagnose CLL, the patient must have an absolute B-lymphocyte count of 5000/mL or greater for a duration of at least 3 months.[131] This leukocytosis may be found on routine laboratory tests run on asymptomatic individuals. Patients who present with symptoms may complain of painless lymphadenopathy, or occasionally of typical B symptoms, as seen in lymphoma—weakness, night sweats, weight loss, or fever. Some patients will present with symptoms of immune dysfunction, particularly infection or an autoimmune syndrome.[132]

Chronic Myeloid (or Myelogenous) Leukemia

The incidence of CML varies from one population to another, with an estimated incidence of 8990 in the United States in 2019, with a slight male predominance.[1] The median age at the time of diagnosis is 57 to 60 years.[133] CML is brought on by a single oncogene, *BCR-ABL1*, formed owing to stem cell acquisition of the Philadelphia (Ph) chromosome that, in turn, is the product of a characteristic translocation between the long arms of chromosomes 9 and 22 causing fusion between the breakpoint cluster regions gene (*BCR*) and the Abelson murine leukemia (*ABL1*) tyrosine kinase protooncogene. The resulting oncogene, *BCR-ABL1*, produces a protein that acts as a tyrosine kinase. Diagnosis requires, in the setting of persistent unexplained leukocytosis, evidence via cytogenetics, polymerase chain reaction, or western blot test of this characteristic translocation.[134–137]

Staging

Acute Lymphoblastic Leukemia

In 1997, ALL was divided into three types: precursor B-cell ALL, mature B-cell ALL (Burkitt ALL), and T-cell ALL.[138] However, in 2008 in the revised World Health Organization (WHO) classification, Burkitt cell leukemia was removed, and ALL was classified, based on the cell type, into T-lymphoblastic leukemia and B lymphoblastic leukemia (B-ALL). B-ALL was further classified into two subgroups: B-ALL with recurrent genetic abnormalities and B-ALL not otherwise specified.[139] Beyond the categorization based on cell type, patients may also be divided into prognostic categories based on the presence or absence of risk factors. Older age is the single most important risk factor. Long-term cure rates are over 80% for children but only 40% to 50% for adults. Not only is prognosis much better among children than among adults, but younger adults do better than older ones; the prognosis is especially dismal for patients older than 60 years. The unfavorable prognosis of older patients may relate not directly to their age but rather to the greater tendency of older individuals to manifest unfavorable chromosomal states. For example, the Ph chromosome, found in 20% to 30% of adults with ALL, is associated with a worse prognosis than in patients without this mutation.[120,128,140,141] Other factors that worsen prognosis include high leukocyte count, CD20 expression by the tumor cells, and longer time to achieve initial CR.[120] The International Childhood Acute Lymphoblastic Leukemia Workshop has recommended the division of pediatric patients into four prognostic groups (low risk, standard risk, high risk, and very high risk),[142] whereas adult patients are usually divided into just two categories: low or standard risk and high risk.[143] These categories pertain to newly diagnosed patients and patients who have completed front-line therapy and have hopefully gone into remission. Once a patient relapses, the prognosis depends on the length of prior remission(s) and the availability of a suitable donor for allogeneic stem cell transplantation.[141]

Chronic Lymphocytic Leukemia

Two staging systems are used in CLL: the Rai staging system and the Binet staging system, both of which were named after the first authors of the original publications.[144,145] The Rai system divides the disease into five stages (0 through IV), whereas the Binet system uses only three stages (stages A, B, and C). Later, in 1987, the Rai staging system was modified to decrease the number of prognostic categories from five to three (low, intermediate, and high risk).[131] There are, however, factors that affect prognosis that are not included in either of these staging systems. About half of CLL cases will have undergone a mutation in the immunoglobulin heavy chain variable region gene. Patients with this mutation have a favorable prognosis compared with patients lacking this mutation.[146,147] Two proteins, ZAP-70 and CD38, may be associated with more aggressive disease and a worse prognosis.[132] Therefore, a more relevant prognostic score has been developed using clinical, biological, and genetic data from 3472 treatment-naïve patients to develop an international scoring system called the CLL International Prognostic Index (CLL-IPI). The CLL-IPI categorizes patients with CLL into four groups: low, intermediate, high, and very high risk.[148]

Acute Myeloid Leukemia

Genetic abnormalities associated with the population of leukemic cells constitute the single most important prognostic factor in AML, and the cytogenetic risk groups can be stratified into favorable, intermediate, and unfavorable strata. The division into these risk groups not only helps predict outcome, but also allows tailoring of therapy to individual patients.[149] In 2008, the WHO classified AML into four major categories: AML with recurrent genetic abnormalities, AML with myelodysplasia-related changes, therapy-related AML, and AML not otherwise specified.[150]

Chronic Myeloid (or Myelogenous) Leukemia

Patients with CML may be divided into prognosis-related categories using the Sokal formulation. This method uses risk factors including age, spleen size, platelet count, and the percentage of blast cells in the peripheral blood to obtain a Sokal score. On the basis of this score, the patients are divided into low-, intermediate-, and high-risk groups that correlate with a stratified tendency to develop longer-term PFS remission.[151,152] In 1998, with the introduction of interferon-α (IFN-α), a new prognostic scoring system (the EURO risk score) was developed to estimate survival of patients with CML treated with IFN-α using the following variants: age, spleen size, blast count, platelet count, eosinophil count, and basophil count.[153] Later on, with the introduction of tyrosine kinase inhibitors, a new prognostic score (the EUTOS prognostic score) was developed to predict complete cytogenetic response, PFS, and OS in patients with CML treated with imatinib using only two variables: spleen size and basophil count.[154]

Imaging of the Disease and its Relapse after Treatment

When imaging plays a role in the diagnosis of leukemia, it is often because the leukemia is an unexpected finding discovered when evaluating a symptom. For example, leukemia may present with joint pain. If the joint pain is confined to one or a few joints, an MRI may be ordered to evaluate for causes of joint pain such as mechanical derangement. Acute leukemia may replace normal fatty marrow with a monotonous sea of disease that will appear abnormally dark on T1W images and bright on T2W images and enhance with contrast administration (Fig. 29.9). The appearance is not specific, however,

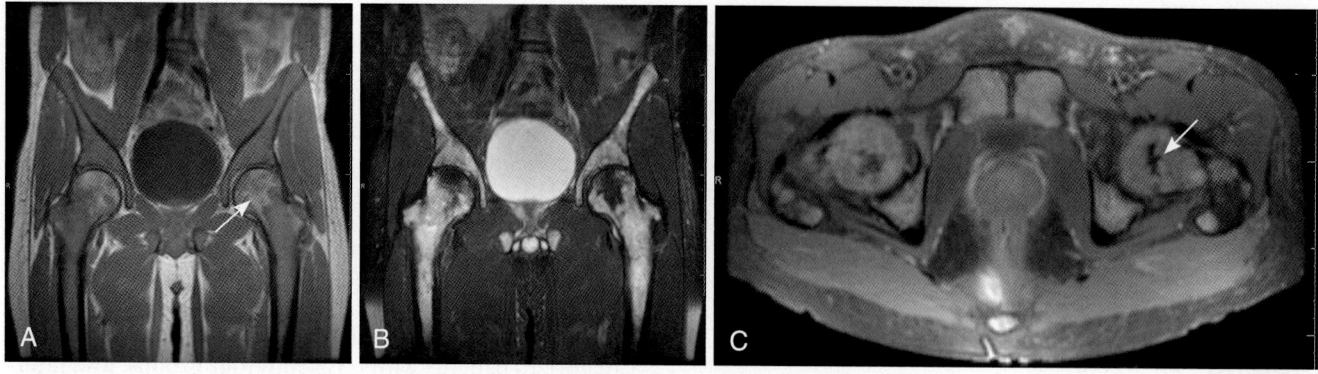

FIGURE 29.9. Marrow replacement in leukemia in a 23-year-old man with chronic myelogenous leukemia in an accelerated phase. **A**, T1-weighted coronal magnetic resonance imaging (MRI) demonstrates near-complete replacement of expected fatty signal with abnormally low signal consistent with infiltration of bone marrow by leukemic cells. The higher-signal marrow remaining in parts of the femoral head, neck, and greater trochanters is normal. The *arrow* shows one example of marrow with normal signal. **B**, T2-weighted, fat-saturated coronal MRI shows the small islands of normal marrow to be dark, and the leukemic infiltration to be bright. **C**, T1-weighted, fat-saturated, postcontrast axial MRI through the femoral heads demonstrates abnormally bright signal throughout most of the bone marrow with a few islands of more normal, low-signal marrow remaining in the femoral heads. The *arrow* shows one example of marrow with normal signal.

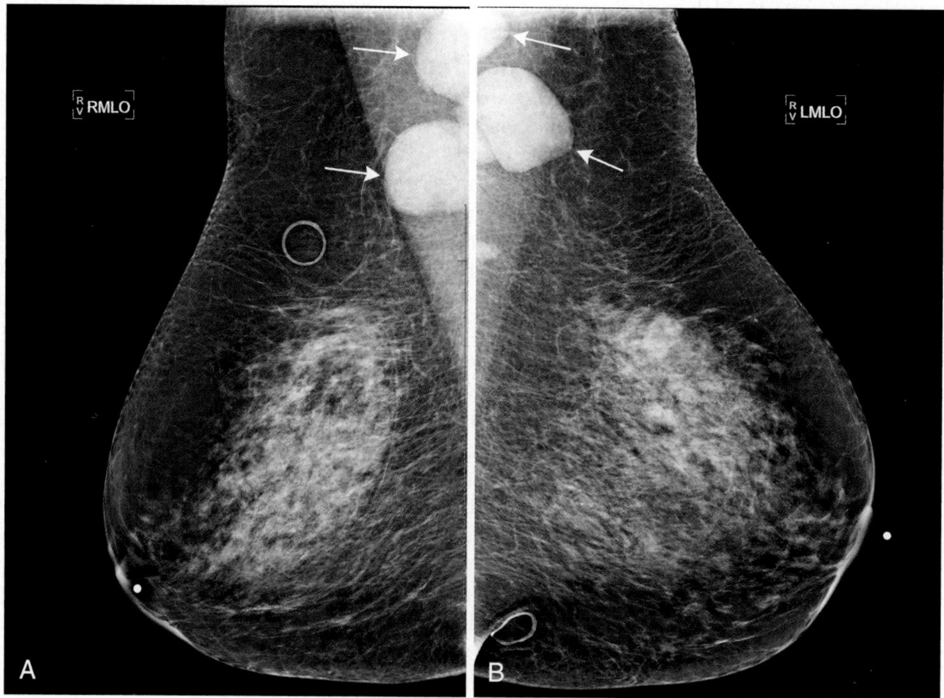

FIGURE 29.10. Axillary adenopathy at mammography. Right **(A)** and left **(B)** mediolateral oblique views from a screening mammogram of a 71-year-old woman with chronic lymphocytic leukemia (CLL). Large, dense, bilateral axillary lymph nodes (*arrows*) are consistent with the patient's leukemia and disappeared over the following 2 years as the patient responded to therapy. If the adenopathy were unilateral rather than bilateral, occult breast cancer would be a more pressing concern. In our experience, axillary lymphadenopathy attributed to leukemia is more likely because of chronic myelogenous leukemia than to CLL.

because other marrow-replacing disorders, including diffuse myeloma, may have the same appearance. Another common incidental imaging finding of leukemia is axillary lymphadenopathy noted in patients with leukemia who undergo screening mammography (Fig. 29.10).

Marrow involvement with leukemia is usually assessed clinically rather than with imaging. Zha and coworkers, however, have suggested that dynamic contrast-enhanced MRI of spinal bone marrow may prove useful for assessing leukemic marrow involvement.[155] In a mixed group of 26 patients with a variety of hematologic malignancies, 18 of whom had leukemia, these authors found that, even at low levels of marrow infiltration (5%–25%), time to peak enhancement was significantly shorter, and the slope of the time-enhancement curve was significantly greater in patients than in normal controls. There were also statistically significant differences among different grades of infiltration, but this may not be of practical use in individual patients owing to large amounts of overlap between categories.

Chloromas (granulocytic sarcoma), extramedullary masses of leukemia cells, are uncommon on initial evaluation but may occur in up to 21% of patients relapsing after allogeneic stem cell transplantation, especially for myelogenous leukemias. Such a local recurrence may potentially be cured with radiation. PET/CT plays an important role in identifying clinically undetectable extramedullary sites of disease, which subsequently influence future management.[156] The morphologic imaging appearance of these masses is nonspecific, and biopsy is often needed to distinguish them from secondary primary cancers or focal areas of opportunistic infection.[157,158] Extramedullary relapse of AML has been identified using PET/CT. Following successful treatment, the abnormal FDG-avidity resolved.[159,160] In the same way, focal areas of disease within bone marrow have a nonspecific appearance and also commonly require biopsy for diagnosis (Fig. 29.11).

The central nervous system is a sanctuary area for leukemia. Relapse in this region may manifest either as focal masses that may be visible on CT or MRI or as a leptomeningeal disease (leukemic meningitis). Leptomeningeal involvement is caused by sheets of tumor cells spreading over the surface of the brain and/or spinal cord. Intracranially, the tumor cells infiltrate into the sulci and can mimic leptomeningeal hemorrhage or infectious meningitis.[161] In the spinal canal, they create an enhancing lumpy coating on the surface of the spinal cord. The main task is to distinguish them from vessels that normally run on the surface of the cord. Ulu and colleagues reported leptomeningeal disease in five of 15 patients with childhood leukemia.[162] All five of these had ALL.

CLL is the most common form of leukemia in adults and, at times, may present with extensive adenopathy (Fig. 29.12). Although imaging may have a greater role in CLL than in other leukemias in terms of staging and disease surveillance, it rarely changes management of this disease. In CLL, imaging is mainly reserved for the complications of the disease, either identifying infections these patients are prone to develop owing to their abnormal immune system because of the disease itself and/or therapy or the dreaded complication of Richter's transformation (RT), in which CLL progresses to other, more aggressive neoplasms, most often large B-cell lymphoma. Differentiating the adenopathy associated with CLL from RT can be difficult with morphologic imaging. However, because the FDG activity in CLL-involved lymph nodes is low-grade, and with large B-cell lymphoma it is high, imaging with FDG-PET would seem ideal. Indeed, PET/CT was found to have a sensitivity of 91% and a specificity of 80% for RT in a study of 37 patients with CLL. If not only RT but also transformation into an accelerated phase of CLL or development of a new malignancy of any sort were considered positive results, then the sensitivity and specificity improved to 94% and 90%, respectively.[163] Although PET/CT can be very valuable in detecting RT, it cannot replace tissue biopsy. Instead, PET/CT can guide the need for and the site of biopsy to confirm the diagnosis in clinically suspected patients.[164]

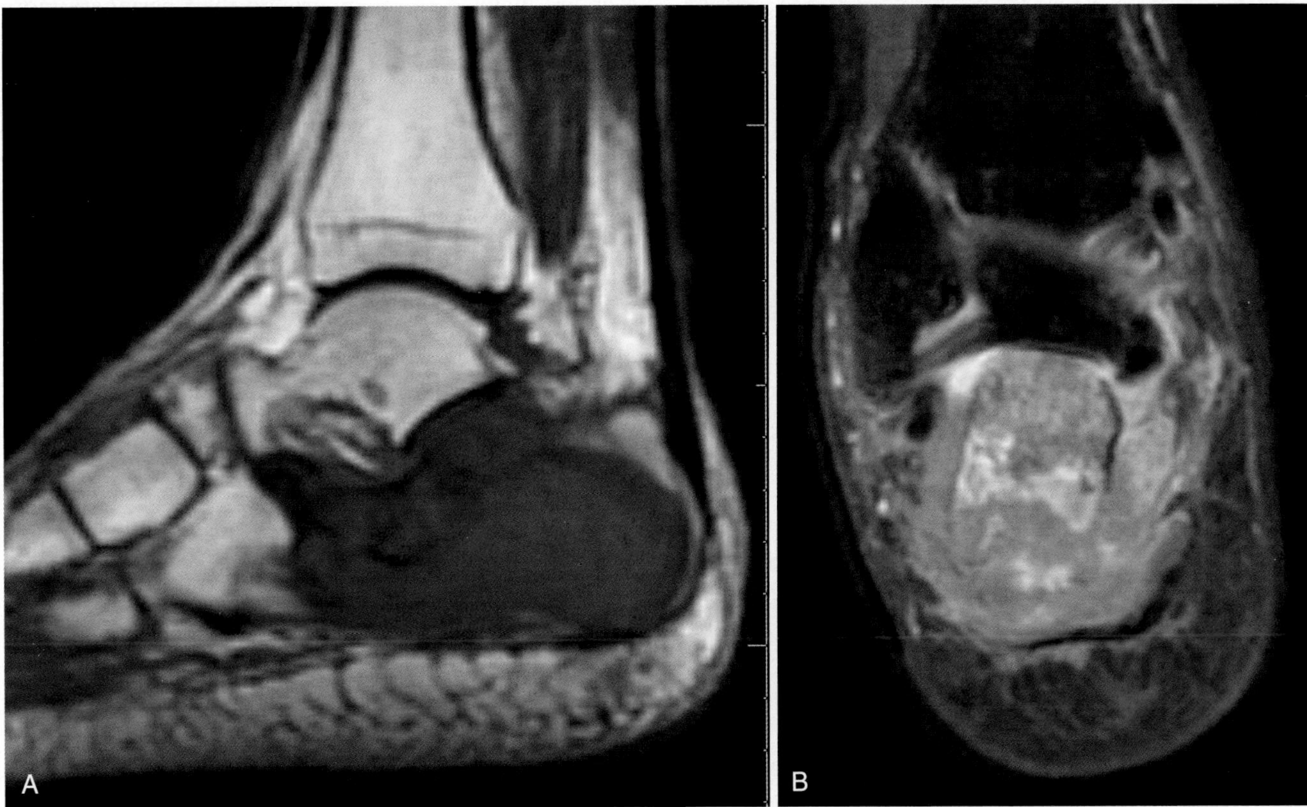

Figure 29.11. Focal recurrence of chronic myelogenous leukemia (CML) in a 46-year-old man with CML in complete remission who presented with pain in the right foot of 1 year's duration but increasing in intensity over the preceding 2 months. **A**, T1-weighted (T1W) sagittal magnetic resonance imaging (MRI) demonstrates abnormally decreased signal in the calcaneus with ill-defined cortical borders and infiltration into the adjacent soft tissues, most obvious at the plantar surface of the bone. **B**, T1W, fat-saturated, postcontrast coronal MRI of the foot shows enhancement of the calcaneus and of the infiltrated soft tissues for approximately 15 mm on either side of the bone. Bone marrow aspirate was negative, but a biopsy of the calcaneus demonstrated CML in a myeloid blast phase. The patient was treated with local radiation and dasatinib.

IMAGING OF COMPLICATIONS

Leukemia patients are immune suppressed both from the disease itself, which affects the function of the immune system, and from the chemotherapy used to treat the disease. The lungs are a common source of infection in these patients, and thus, when a leukemic patient presents with fever, imaging usually starts with a chest radiograph to assess for pneumonia, as well as imaging studies that may be directed toward specific symptomatic sites. In addition to ordinary community-acquired bacterial infections, leukemic patients are susceptible to invasive fungal infections that may involve any area of the body, commonly the lungs and sinuses. Of the fungal infections, invasive pulmonary aspergillosis is by far the most common. Invasive pulmonary fungal infections, whether because of aspergillosis, mucormycosis, candidiasis, or fusariosis, produce local infarcts in the lungs. Imaging wise, these differ from other bacterial and viral infection in that they produce large (>1 cm) pulmonary nodules.[165] Thus, in a leukemic febrile patient, the finding of pulmonary nodules or masses is consistent with invasive fungal pneumonia until proven otherwise. These nodular lesions can be solid or consolidative or have a rim of ground glass surrounding them that is caused by surrounding hemorrhage, the so-called halo sign. Mortality from these invasive fungal pneumonias is higher than 50%, and early identification by CT with early initiation of antifungal agents improves survival.[166] Management of invasive pulmonary aspergillosis in neutropenic patients has improved through the use of early thoracic CT scan and surgery (Fig. 29.13). In the liver, fungal infections, especially caused by *Candida*, often appear as multiple, small, uniform, low-attenuation regions that may be surrounded by a rim of enhancement (Fig. 29.14).

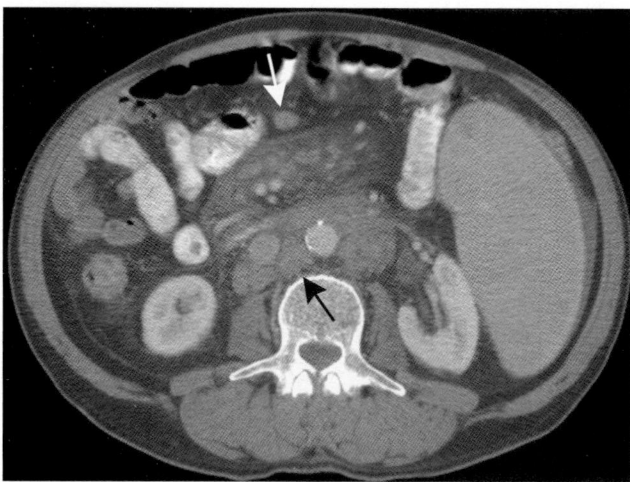

FIGURE 29.12. Chronic lymphocytic leukemia (CLL) with adenopathy. Axial computed tomography image through the midabdomen of a 71-year-old man with CLL. There is extensive retroperitoneal and mesenteric adenopathy (*white arrow* shows a mesenteric node; *black arrow* shows an interaortocaval node). The spleen is also enlarged.

Another common complication in leukemia patients is osteonecrosis. Steroids, which are a part of some chemotherapy regimens for leukemia, and which may also play a role in suppressing graft-versus-host disease after stem cell transplantation, predispose to osteonecrosis, as does leukemia itself. Osteonecrosis most often occurs in the femoral heads, followed by the humeral heads, but can be seen in numerous bones. On radiographs, it may be occult. Later, it may be visible, usually as a vague area of sclerosis in the femoral or humeral head. In long bones, where it is often referred to as an area of bone infarction, it may appear as a jagged area of sclerosis that may be difficult to distinguish from an enchondroma. Bone infarcts, however, are inclined to calcify around their periphery more than centrally, whereas an enchondroma tends to do the opposite. Eventually, osteonecrosis may weaken the bone sufficiently to cause fracture of the adjacent cortex. This typically occurs at the femoral head and is manifested first by a thin radiolucent rim running just under the articular surface and then by the collapse of the articular surface (Fig. 29.15). On MRI, osteonecrosis usually appears centrally to be the same as nearby fatty bone marrow. At the periphery, areas of osteonecrosis are surrounded by a narrow, sharply defined band of contrasting signal, generally dark on T1W and bright on T2W images, resembling the guiding outlines in a child's coloring book (Fig. 29.16).

Patients with leukemia can also experience hemorrhage secondary to abnormal clotting mechanisms. If intracranial hemorrhage is suspected, CT is the appropriate means to detect it (Fig. 29.17).

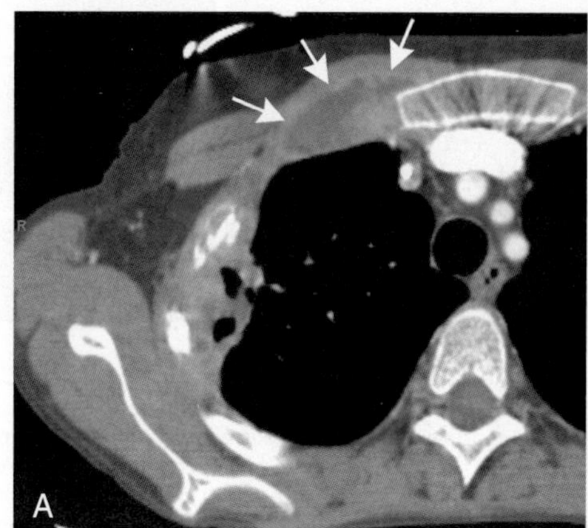

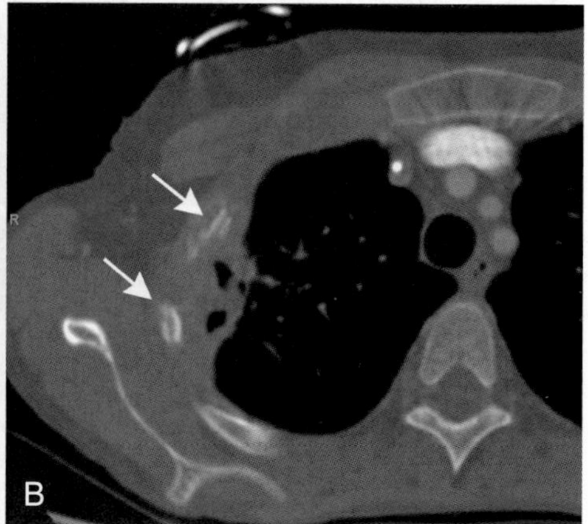

FIGURE 29.13. Mucormycosis of the chest wall. Axial computed tomography images through the upper chest of a 25-year-old woman with relapsed/refractory acute myelogenous leukemia are displayed in soft tissue **(A)** and bone windows **(B)**. They demonstrate a pleural-based right chest wall mass eroding ribs (*arrows* in **B**) and creating a fluid density abscess anteriorly (*arrows* in **A**). Zygomycetes were cultured from a similar fluid collection in the neck. The patient was treated with triple antifungal drugs and underwent bone marrow transplantation.

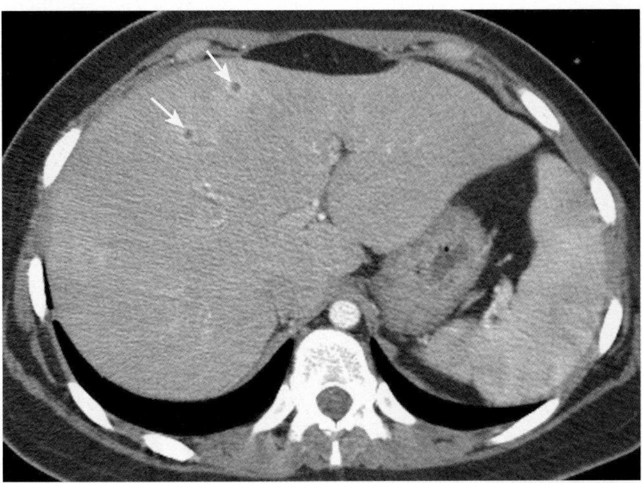

FIGURE 29.14. Hepatic *Candida* infection in an 18-year-old woman with relapsed acute myelogenous leukemia who presented with fever of 102° F. Multiple small lucencies in the liver with enhancing rims (*arrows*) were typical of *Candida* infection, and the patient was placed on antifungal medication.

KEY POINTS

Predominant Role of Imaging in Leukemia

- Identify Richter's transformation: positron emission tomography imaging is useful
- Identify fungal infection with computer-generated imaging
  - Highly suspected when the following are present:
    - Nodules larger than 1 cm
    - Masses
    - Halo sign
    - Reversed halo sign
- Identify other complications
  - Bacterial infection
  - Chloroma
  - Hematoma

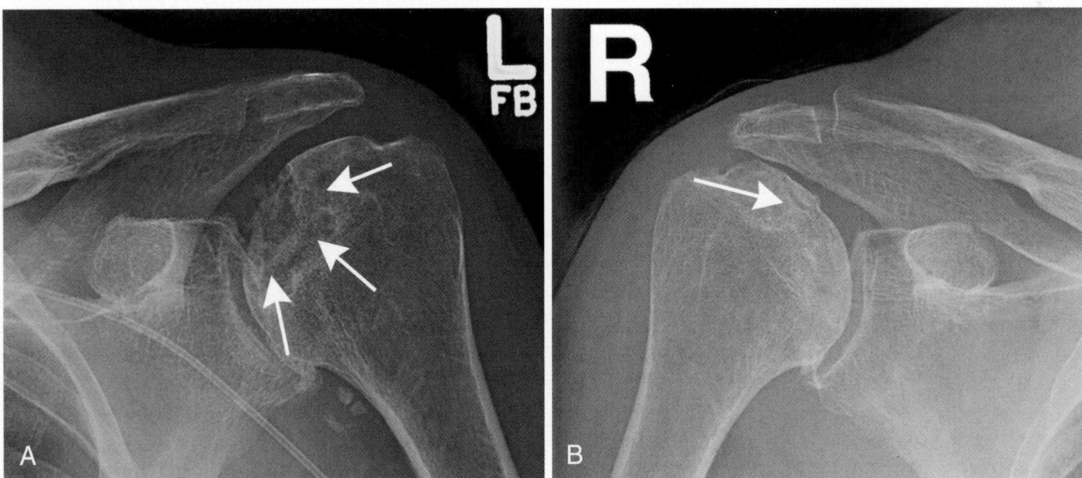

FIGURE 29.15. Osteonecrosis of the proximal humeri in a 59-year-old man with chronic lymphocytic leukemia. **A**, Radiograph of the left shoulder demonstrates a crescentic area of increased opacity in the epiphysis (*arrows*). **B**, Radiograph of the right shoulder demonstrates a slender lucency (*arrow*) running beneath the articular cortex represents a subcortical fracture; the articular cortex has lost its usual smooth, round contour, and spurs at the caudal edge of the glenohumeral joint indicate secondary osteoarthritis. There is more advanced articular collapse in the left shoulder.

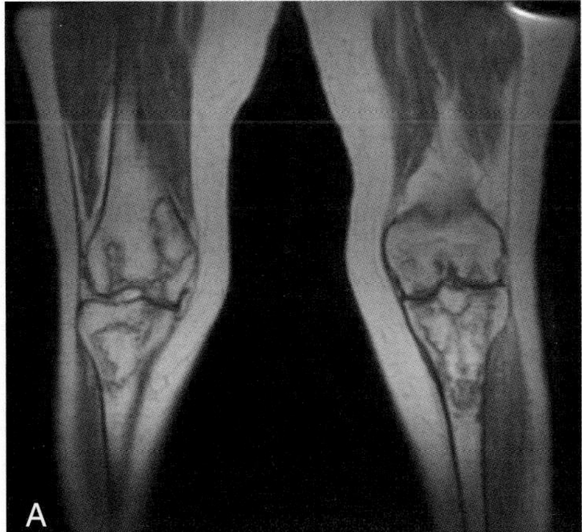

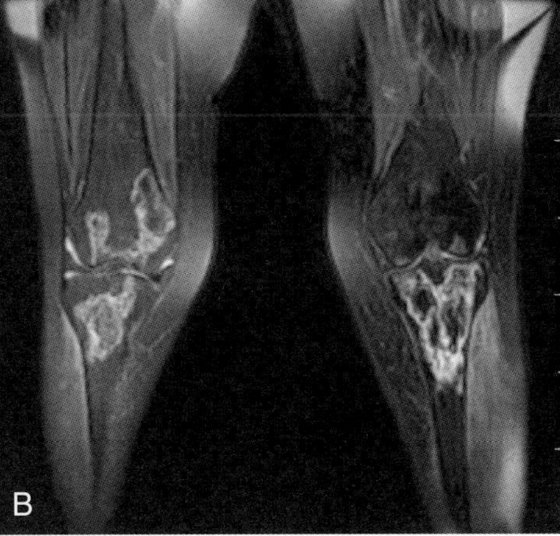

FIGURE 29.16. Bone infarcts. T1-weighted (T1W) (**A**) and T2-weighted (**B**) coronal magnetic resonance imaging of both knees in an 18-year-old woman with acute lymphocytic leukemia demonstrate the typical appearance of multiple bilateral bone infarctions. Centrally, the lesions are similar in signal to other, normal areas of fatty bone marrow. Peripherally, they are surrounded by a crisply defined, serpiginous line of abnormal signal, dark on the T1W images and bright on the T2-weighted images.

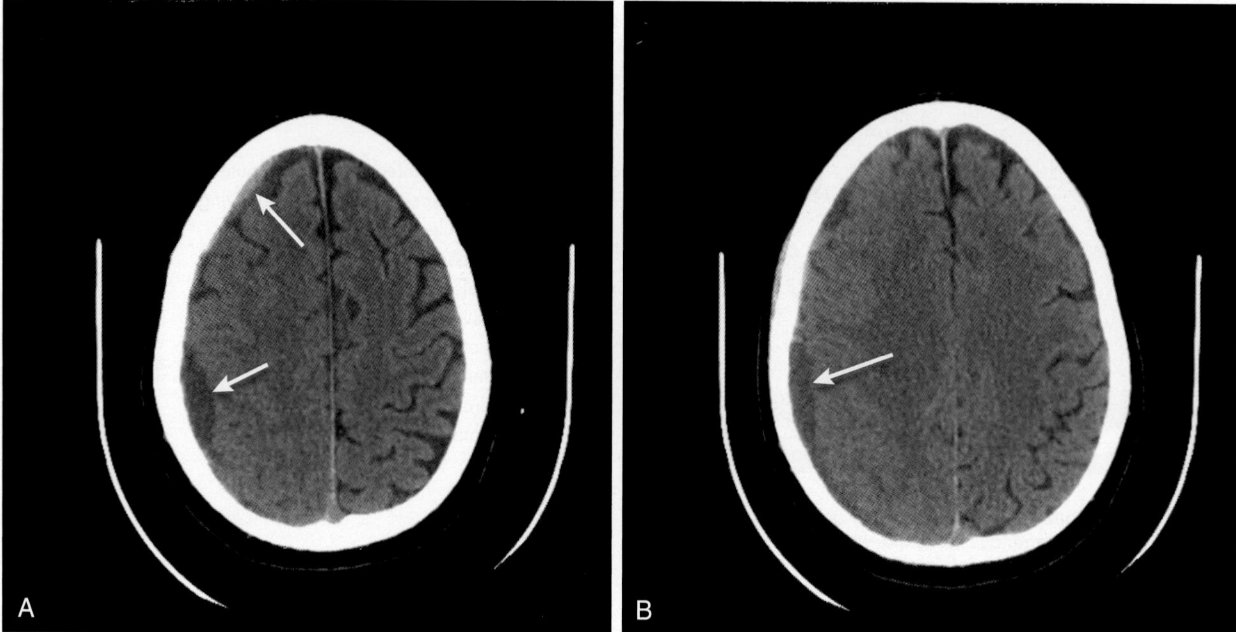

Figure 29.17. Intracranial hemorrhage in a 26-year-old man with acute lymphocytic leukemia who complained of persistent headache. Computed tomography of the head without contrast reveals the presence of a subacute subdural hemorrhage along the right hemisphere and acute subdural hemorrhage along the falx and right tentorium (*arrows*).There is mild mass effect on the right hemisphere, but there is no significant midline shift (only 1–2 mm).

TREATMENT

Leukemia is treated chemically, although the particular type of medication differs from one type of leukemia to another. Radiation therapy can play a role; for example, central nervous system radiation has been used to decrease the likelihood of relapse in that location in childhood ALL, but side effects of this radiation have caused its use to be minimized in favor of other treatments such as intrathecal chemotherapy.[167,168] Stem cell transplantation is usually reserved for specific situations and is not standard therapy for most patients.

Acute Lymphoblastic Leukemia

Treatment of ALL can be divided into three stages: induction, consolidation, and maintenance. The goal of initial chemotherapy is to induce a CR as quickly as possible. A combination of vincristine, corticosteroid (dexamethasone or prednisone), and an anthracycline will achieve remission in 72% to 92% of patients. Hyperfractionated cyclophosphamide, vincristine, doxorubicin, and dexamethasone (HCVAD) alternating with methotrexate and high-dose cytarabine has also been used recently. In children, L-asparaginase also plays an important role in initial therapy. Because the central nervous system can be the site of relapse in 10% to 16% of patients, intrathecal chemotherapy for central nervous system (CNS) prophylaxis maybe indicated, depending on the predetermined risk of CNS disease.[120,121] The HCVAD regimen has demonstrated a 92% CR rate and a 32% 5-year disease-free survival.[169] After induction, eligible patients may proceed with allogenic stem cell transplantation, while the rest proceed with consolidation and maintenance therapy.[170]

Consolidation regimens vary. For patients with the Ph chromosome, allogeneic stem cell transplantation is recommended for consolidation, as it improves the rate of long-term survival to 35% to 55%. However, because of limited availability of matched donors, the emergence of tyrosine kinase inhibitors (TKIs) represented a turning point in the treatment of Ph-positive ALL. In one study, imatinib combined with traditional HCVAD led to an increase in the 3-year OS rate from 15% to 54%.[171,172] However, despite these promising results, some patients, especially those with CNS diseases where imatinib has limited penetration, developed resistance or relapse.[173] For patients with CNS disease, resistance, or relapse, dasatinib, a second-generation ABL kinase inhibitor with better penetration of the blood-brain barrier, is used instead of imatinib. In a multicenter trial, dasatinib combined with HCVAD achieved a 3-year OS rate of 71% in adult patients younger than 60 years.[174,175] For Ph-negative patients, consolidation treatment is often a modified continuation of the same drugs used for induction and, occasionally, cranial radiation for CNS prophylaxis.[120,121]

Maintenance therapy is usually given over 2 to 3 years and includes daily 6-mercaptopurine, weekly methotrexate, and vincristine and a 5-day prednisone pulse every 3 months.[121] Stem cell transplantation may be used for refractory or relapsed ALL.[176]

Chronic Lymphocytic Leukemia

Patients with asymptomatic, early-stage CLL are monitored for disease progression but are not treated unless there is evidence of rapid disease progression. Early treatment has not been associated with improved outcomes, and because some patients will never require treatment, it is good to avoid the side effects of treatment.[132]

For symptomatic and physically fit patients, a standard front-line chemoimmunotherapy should be offered: a combination of a purine analog, typically fludarabine, with rituximab, a murine anti-CD20 monoclonal antibody, and cyclophosphamide. However, patients over the age of 65 years may benefit from an alternative regimen: a combination of bendamustine and rituximab.[177] Patients with impaired physical activity should be treated with either a combination of chlorambucil and an anti-CD20 antibody (particularly obinutuzumab) or with ibrutinib monotherapy. Currently, there is no strong evidence to support the use of one regimen over the other.[131]

Acute Myeloid Leukemia

Patients with AML are treated with standard chemotherapy to achieve remission. This includes cytarabine combined with anthracyclines or anthacenediones to achieve remission, followed by additional cytarabine, either alone or in combination, for consolidation. CR is achieved in 60% to 85% of patients 60 years old or younger, compared with 40% to 60% in patients older than 60 years.[150] In children and younger adults, intensive cytarabine therapy may be pursued with the goal of cure.[129,130] Allogeneic stem cell transplantation is commonly used in remission, primarily for patients with intermediate or unfavorable cytogenetics, to lengthen the time to relapse and possibly achieve cure. Indeed, AML is the most common indication for stem cell transplantation.[149]

In the older adults who make up most of the AML patient population, the relapse rate is high, and the outcome is poor, with survival often measured in weeks.[129] Treatment decisions in these individuals involve both an estimation of the added life span that may result from aggressive therapy and consideration of the patient's quality of life, which may be better with less aggressive therapy.[178]

Cytogenetic testing and stratification allow some tailoring of chemotherapeutic regimens. For example, one subtype of AML with favorable cytogenetics is acute promyelocytic leukemia. This subtype has an excellent prognosis if all-*trans*-retinoic acid and arsenic are added to induction chemotherapy.[149,179–182] Chen and associates have also suggested that dynamic contrast-enhanced MRI of the spinal bone marrow may also help stratify treatment by identifying patients at greater and lesser risk of relapse after the achievement of remission.[183]

Chronic Myeloid (or Myelogenous) Leukemia

Because CML is triggered by a single oncogene that, with its resulting protein, has been well-studied, it has lent itself very well to specific, targeted therapies that are distinctly more efficacious than ordinary chemotherapy. The abnormal protein is a tyrosine kinase, and therefore TKIs are active against CML. Three TKIs are available for frontline therapy: imatinib, dasatinib, and nilotinib. Almost all patients will go into remission with frontline therapy and continued therapy may result in a long period of PFS. In one trial, 61% of patients were still progression free at 6 years.[134,136,152,184,185]

If relapse occurs, options include continued treatment with higher doses of imatinib or a trial of another TKI, either dasatinib or nilotinib.[134,136,152] If these are ineffective, or if control is lost, then allogeneic stem cell transplantation may be helpful.[134]

In case of development of drug resistance and failure of frontline therapy, salvage therapy with second- or third-generation TKIs is indicated. The choice of second- or third-generation TKIs drug depends on disease phase, cytogenetics, and the patient's comorbidities.[137]

When CML progresses, it may go into blast crisis, and at that stage the TKIs are of little use. Allogeneic stem cell transplantation should be attempted.[134]

PROMISING THERAPIES

Most types of leukemia initially respond to therapy, and patients will achieve PR or CR. This is followed by a period of minimal residual disease, then eventually refractory relapse or relapses will occur, and the patient may eventually die owing to these relapses. Refractory relapses are likely caused by the persistence of a small colony of leukemic stem cells.[186] These cells are resistant to therapy because they have a relatively low level of metabolic activity and an impressive group of protective mechanisms. They also tend to migrate to and immobilize themselves in sanctuary areas that protect them from therapy. Although first found in AML, leukemic stem cells have now been found in all major forms of leukemia.[187–190]

Ultimate cure of leukemia will probably require elimination of leukemic stem cells, and current research is therefore directed at devising methods of attacking the leukemic stem cells, preferably while sparing the patient's normal stem cells. One approach has been to target cell surface antigens. No antigen has been identified that is unique to leukemic stem cells, but some antigens have been found that are more active in leukemic stem cells than in normal cells. One of these is CD33, which is mainly expressed in cells of the myeloid lineage. Several experimental therapies are being tested that target CD33. One, for example, is gemtuzamab ozogamicin, an anti-CD33 monoclonal antibody conjugated with calicheamicin (a cytotoxic antineoplastic antibiotic). The antibody adheres to the cell membrane, enters the cell, and releases the cytotoxic antibiotic. The antibiotic subsequently enters the nucleus, where it causes double-stranded DNA breaks resulting in apoptosis. This therapy has been FDA-approved in the United States for patients older than 60 years with AML who are not considered candidates for routine chemotherapy, and in a trial produced a 26% remission rate.[186,191,192] Another approach, which is still under investigation, focuses on targeting CD123, the transmembrane alpha chain of the IL-3 receptor that is preferentially expressed on leukemic stem cells.[193] In CML, there is also intense interest in investigating methods of attacking the leukemic stem cells.[135]

Because drugs that are effective against one hematologic malignancy often are effective against others as well, research is also ongoing regarding the application of drugs already known to be useful in other diseases in new settings. In CLL, for example, thalidomide and lenalidomide, both known to be useful against myeloma, have been tested as potential salvage therapy for relapsed or refractory disease. Because one of their effects is to support the immune system, it is hoped that they can stimulate the immune system to battle the disease, while also avoiding the infection-promoting effects of immune compromise encountered with many chemotherapies.[194]

CONCLUSION

In conclusion, the role of imaging is different in myeloma and leukemia. In myeloma, imaging assists in staging evaluation and in searching for signs of progression. It helps to find evidence of myeloma in patients thought to have MGUS or SBP. In leukemia, imaging plays only a minor role in diagnosis or staging. It may be useful to evaluate focal masses called chloromas but plays a critical role in the evaluation of complications and can be useful in identifying and guiding biopsy for RT in patients with CLL.

REFERENCES

1. Siegel RL, Miller KD, Jemal A. Cancer statistics. *2019. Cancer J Clin*. 2019;69(1):7–34.
2. VanValkenburg M, Pruitt G, Brill I, et al. Family history of hematologic malignancies and risk of multiple myeloma: differences by race and clinical features. *Cancer Causes & Control*. 2016;27:81–91.
3. Landgren O, Gridley G, Turesson I, et al. Risk of monoclonal gammopathy of undetermined significance (MGUS) and subsequent multiple myeloma among African American and white veterans in the United States. *Blood*. 2006;107:904.
4. Kyle RA. Review of 1027 patients with newly diagnosed multiple myeloma. (Mayo Clinic Proceedings) (Author Abstract). *JAMA*. 2003;289:2047.
5. Riedel DA, Pottern LM. The epidemiology of multiple myeloma. *Hematology/Oncology Clinics of North America*. 1992;6:225–247.
6. Preston DL, Kusumi S, Tomonaga M, et al. Cancer incidence in atomic bomb survivors. Part III. Leukemia, lymphoma and multiple myeloma, 1950-1987. *Radiation research*. 1994;137:S68.
7. Berenson JR, Bergsagel PL, Munshi N. Initiation and maintenance of multiple myeloma. *Seminars in hematology*. 1999;36:9–13.
8. Kristinsson SY, Björkholm M, Goldin LR, et al. Patterns of hematologic malignancies and solid tumors among 37,838 first-degree relatives of 13,896 patients with multiple myeloma in Sweden. *International Journal of Cancer*. 2009;125:2147–2150.
9. Fonseca R, Bergsagel PL, Drach J, et al. International Myeloma Working Group molecular classification of multiple myeloma: spotlight review. *Leukemia*. 2009;23:2210–2221.
10. Rajkumar SV, Gupta V, Fonseca R, et al. Impact of primary molecular cytogenetic abnormalities and risk of progression in smoldering multiple myeloma. *Leukemia*. 2013;27:1738.
11. Kyle R, Child J, Anderson K, et al. Criteria for the classification of monoclonal gammopathies, multiple myeloma and related disorders: a report of the International Myeloma Working Group. *British Journal of Haematology*. 2003;121:749–757.
12. Sezer O, Heider U, Zavrski I, et al. RANK ligand and osteoprotegerin in myeloma bone disease. *Blood*. 2003;101:2094–2098.
13. Roodman GD, Dougall WC. *RANK ligand as a therapeutic target for bone metastases and multiple myeloma*: *Elsevier Ltd*; 2008:92–101.
14. Sharma S, Nemeth E, Chen Y-H, et al. Involvement of hepcidin in the anemia of multiple myeloma. *Clinl Canr Res Offl Jourl Ameri Associ Can Res*. 2008;14:3262–3267.
15. Dimopoulos MA, Kastritis E, Rosinol L, et al. Pathogenesis and treatment of renal failure in multiple myeloma. *Leukemia*. 2008;22:1485.
16. Batuman V. The pathogenesis of acute kidney impairment in patients with multiple myeloma. *Advances in Chronic Kidney Disease*. 2012;19:282–286.
17. Cheson BD, Plass RR, Rothstein G. Defective opsonization in multiple myeloma. *Blood*. 1980;55:602–606.
18. Fahey JL, Scoggins R, Utz JP, et al. Infection, antibody response and gamma globulin components in mutiple myeloma and macroglobulinemia. *The American Journal of Medicine*. 1963;35:698–707.
19. Rajkumar SV, Dimopoulos MA, Palumbo A, et al. International Myeloma Working Group updated criteria for the diagnosis of multiple myeloma. *The Lancet Oncology*. 2014;15:e538–e548.
20. Weber DM. Solitary bone and extramedullary plasmacytoma. *ASH Education Program Book*. 2005;2005:373–376.
21. Paiva B, Chandia M, Vidriales M-B, et al. Multiparameter flow cytometry for staging of solitary bone plasmacytoma: new criteria for risk of progression to myeloma. *Blood*. 2014;124:1300–1303.
22. Dimopoulos MA, Kiamouris C, Moulopoulos LA. Solitary plasmacytoma of bone and extramedullary plasmacytoma. *Hematology/Oncology Clinics*. 1999;13:1249–1257.
23. Durie BG, Salmon SE. A clinical staging system for multiple myeloma correlation of measured myeloma cell mass with presenting clinical features, response to treatment, and survival. 1975.
24. Greipp PR, San Miguel J, Durie BGM, et al. International staging system for multiple myeloma. *Jourl Clin Oncol: Offl Jourl Ameri Soci Clin Oncol*. 2005;23:3412–3420.
25. Kastritis E, Zervas K, Symeonidis A, et al. Improved survival of patients with multiple myeloma after the introduction of novel agents and the applicability of the International Staging System (ISS): an analysis of the Greek Myeloma Study Group (GMSG). *Leukemia*. 2009;23:1152.
26. Jagannath S, Richardson PG, Sonneveld P, et al. Bortezomib appears to overcome the poor prognosis conferred by chromosome 13 deletion in phase 2 and 3 trials. *Leukemia*. 2006;21:151.
27. San Miguel JF, Schlag R, Khuageva NK, et al. Bortezomib plus melphalan and prednisone for initial treatment of multiple myeloma. *The New England Journal of Medicine*. 2008;359:906–917.
28. Palumbo A, Avet-Loiseau H, Oliva S, et al. Revised international staging system for multiple myeloma: A report from International Myeloma Working Group. *Journal of Clinical Oncology: Official Journal of the American Society of Clinical Oncology*. 2015;33:2863–2869.
29. Dimopoulos M, Terpos E, Comenzo RL, et al. *International myeloma working group consensus statement and guidelines regarding the current role of imaging techniques in the diagnosis and monitoring of multiple myeloma*: *Nature Publishing Group*; 2009:1545.
30. Mulligan M, Smith S, Talmi D. Whole body radiography for bone survey screening of cancer and myeloma patients. *Cancer Investigation*. 2008;26:916–922.
31. Schmidt GP, Reiser MF, Baur-Melnyk A. Whole-body imaging of bone marrow. *Semin Musculoskelet Radiol*. 2009;13:120–133.
32. Hanrahan CJ, Christensen CR, Crim JR. Current concepts in the evaluation of multiple myeloma with MR imaging and FDG PET/CT. *Radiographics: a Review Publication of the Radiological Society of North America, Inc*. 2010;30:127–142.
33. Mulligan ME. *Imaging techniques used in the diagnosis, staging, and follow-up of patients with myeloma*. London, England: *SAGE Publications*; 2005:716–724.
34. Horger M, Claussen CD, Bross-Bach U, et al. Whole-body low-dose multidetector row-CT in the diagnosis of multiple myeloma: an alternative to conventional radiography. *European Journal of Radiology*. 2005;54:289–297.
35. Gleeson T, Moriarty J, Shortt C, et al. Accuracy of whole-body low-dose multidetector CT (WBLDCT) versus skeletal survey in the detection of myelomatous lesions, and correlation of disease distribution with whole-body MRI (WBMRI). *Skeletal Radiology*. 2009;38:225–236.
36. Ghanem N, Lohrmann C, Engelhardt M, et al. Whole-body MRI in the detection of bone marrow infiltration in patients with plasma cell neoplasms in comparison to the radiological skeletal survey. *Clinical Imaging*. 2006;30:440–441.
37. Walker R, Barlogie B, Haessler J, et al. Magnetic resonance imaging in multiple myeloma: diagnostic and clinical implications. *Journal of Clinical Oncology: Official Journal of the American Society of Clinical Oncology*. 2007;25:1121.
38. Bäuerle T, Hillengass J, Fechtner K, et al. Multiple myeloma and monoclonal gammopathy of undetermined significance: importance of whole-body versus spinal MR imaging. *Radiology*. 2009;252:477.
39. Weininger M, Lauterbach B, Knop S, et al. Whole-body MRI of multiple myeloma: Comparison of different MRI sequences in assessment of different growth patterns. *European Journal of Radiology*. 2009;69:339–345.
40. Libshitz HI, Malthouse SR, Cunningham D, et al. Multiple myeloma: appearance at MR imaging. *Radiology*. 1992;182:833–837.

41. Moulopoulos LA, Dimopoulos MA, Smith TL, et al. Prognostic significance of magnetic resonance imaging in patients with asymptomatic multiple myeloma. *Journal of Clinical Oncology: Official Journal of the American Society of Clinical Oncology*. 1995;13:251–256.
42. Moulopoulos LA, Gika D, Anagnostopoulos A, et al. Prognostic significance of magnetic resonance imaging of bone marrow in previously untreated patients with multiple myeloma. *Annals of Oncology*. 2005;16:1824–1828.
43. Dimopoulos MA, Moulopoulos LA, Datseris I, et al. Imaging of myeloma bone disease - implications for staging, prognosis and follow-up. *Acta Oncologica*. 2000;39:823–827.
44. Lecouvet FE, Vande Berg BC, Michaux L, et al. Stage III multiple myeloma: clinical and prognostic value of spinal bone marrow MR imaging. *Radiology*. 1998:209653.
45. Dimopoulos MA, Hillengass J, Usmani S, et al. Role of magnetic resonance imaging in the management of patients with multiple myeloma: a consensus statement. *J Clin Oncol*. 2015;33:657–664.
46. Moulopoulos LA, Dimopoulos MA. Magnetic resonance imaging of the bone marrow in hematologic malignancies. *Blood*. 1997;90:2127–2147.
47. Nanni C, Rubello D, Zamagni E, et al. 18F-FDG PET/CT in myeloma with presumed solitary plasmocytoma of bone. *In vivo (Athens, Greece)*. 2008;22:513.
48. Kim PJ, Hicks RJ, Wirth A, et al. Impact of 18F-fluorodeoxyglucose positron emission tomography before and after definitive radiation therapy in patients with apparently solitary plasmacytoma. *International Journal of Radiation Oncology, Biology, Physics*. 2009;74:740–746.
49. Nosàs-Garcia S, Moehler T, Wasser K, et al. Dynamic contrast-enhanced MRI for assessing the disease activity of multiple myeloma: A comparative study with histology and clinical markers. *Journal of Magnetic Resonance Imaging*. 2005;22:154–162.
50. Cholewinski IW, Castellon II, Raphael IB, et al. Value of precise localization of recurrent multiple myeloma with F-18 FDG PET/CT. *Clinical Nuclear Medicine*. 2009;34:1–3.
51. Durie BGM, Waxman AD, D'Agnolo A, et al. Whole-body (18)F-FDG PET identifies high-risk myeloma. *Journal of Nuclear Medicine: Official Publication, Society of Nuclear Medicine*. 2002;43:1457–1463.
52. Bartel TB, Haessler J, Brown TLY, et al. F18-fluorodeoxyglucose positron emission tomography in the context of other imaging techniques and prognostic factors in multiple myeloma. *Blood*. 2009;114:2068.
53. Zamagni E, Patriarca F, Nanni C, et al. Prognostic relevance of 18-F FDG PET/CT in newly diagnosed multiple myeloma patients treated with up-front autologous transplantation. *Blood*. 2011;118:5989–5995.
54. Haznedar R, Akı SZ, Akdemir ÖU, et al. Value of 18F-fluorodeoxyglucose uptake in positron emission tomography/computed tomography in predicting survival in multiple myeloma. *European Journal of Nuclear Medicine and Molecular Imaging*. 2011;38:1046–1053.
55. Delorme S, Baur-Melnyk A. Imaging in multiple myeloma. *European Journal of Radiology*. 2009;70:401–408.
56. Fonti R, Salvatore B, Quarantelli M, et al. 18F-FDG PET/CT, 99mTc-MIBI, and MRI in evaluation of patients with multiple myeloma. *Journal of Nuclear Medicine: Official Publication, Society of Nuclear Medicine*. 2008;49:195.
57. Shortt CP, Gleeson TG, Breen KA, et al. Whole-body MRI versus PET in assessment of multiple myeloma disease activity. *AJR*. 2009;192:980.
58. Fraioli F, Punwani S. Clinical and research applications of simultaneous positron emission tomography and MRI. *The British Journal Of Radiology*. 2014;87 20130464-20130464.
59. Cavo M, Terpos E, Nanni C, et al. Role of 18F-FDG PET/CT in the diagnosis and management of multiple myeloma and other plasma cell disorders: a consensus statement by the International Myeloma Working Group. *The Lancet Oncology*. 2017;18:e206–e217.
60. Mateos M-V, Hernández M-T, Giraldo P, et al. Lenalidomide plus dexamethasone for high-risk smoldering multiple myeloma. *The New England Journal Of Medicine*. 2013;369:438.
61. Lonial S, Jacobus SJ, Weiss M, et al. E3A06: Randomized phase III trial of lenalidomide versus observation alone in patients with asymptomatic high-risk smoldering multiple myeloma. *Journal of Clinical Oncology*. 2019;37 8001–8001.
62. Meldgaard Knudsen L, Rasmussen T, Jensen L, Johnsen HE. Reduced bone marrow stem cell pool and progenitor mobilisation in multiple myeloma after melphalan treatment. *Medical Oncology*. 1999;16:245–254.
63. Barlogie B, Smith L, Alexanian R. Effective treatment of advanced multiple myeloma refractory to alkylating agents. *The New England Journal Of Medicine*. 1984;310:1353–1356.
64. Alexanian R, Haut A, Khan AU, et al. Treatment for multiple myeloma: combination chemotherapy with different melphalan dose regimens. *JAMA*. 1969;208:1680–1685.
65. Attal M, Harousseau J-L, Stoppa A-M, et al. A prospective, randomized trial of autologous bone marrow transplantation and chemotherapy in multiple myeloma. *The New England Journal of Medicine*. 1996;335:91–97.
66. Singhal S, Mehta J, Desikan R, et al. Antitumor activity of thalidomide in refractory multiple myeloma. *The New England Journal of Medicine*. 1999;341:1565–1571.
67. Jagannath S, Durie BGM, Wolf JL, et al. Extended follow-up of a phase 2 trial of bortezomib alone and in combination with dexamethasone for the frontline treatment of multiple myeloma. *British Journal of Haematology*. 2009;146:619–626.
68. Kropff MH, Bisping G, Wenning D, et al. Bortezomib in combination with dexamethasone for relapsed multiple myeloma. *Leukemia Research*. 2005;29:587–590.
69. Rajkumar S, Jacobus S, Callander N, et al. Lenalidomide plus high-dose dexamethasone versus lenalidomide plus low-dose dexamethasone as initial therapy for newly diagnosed multiple myeloma: an open-label randomised controlled trial. *Lancet Oncology*. 2010;11:29–37.
70. Richardson PG, Barlogie B, Berenson J, et al. A phase 2 study of bortezomib in relapsed, refractory myeloma. *The New England Journal of Medicine*. 2003;348:2609–2617.
71. Dimopoulos M, Spencer A, Attal M, et al. Lenalidomide plus dexamethasone for relapsed or refractory multiple myeloma. *The New England Journal of Medicine*. 2007;357:2123–2132.
72. Weber DM, Chen C, Niesvizky R, et al. Lenalidomide plus dexamethasone for relapsed multiple myeloma in North America. *The New England Journal of Medicine*. 2007;357:2133–2142.
73. Durie BGM, Hoering A, Abidi MH, et al. Bortezomib with lenalidomide and dexamethasone versus lenalidomide and dexamethasone alone in patients with newly diagnosed myeloma without intent for immediate autologous stem-cell transplant (SWOG S0777): a randomised, open-label, phase 3 trial. *The Lancet*. 2017;389:519–527.
74. Shaji KK, Vincent R, Robert AK, et al. Multiple myeloma. *Nature Reviews Disease Primers*. 2017:3.
75. Anderson KC, Weller E, Lonial S, et al. Lenalidomide, bortezomib, and dexamethasone in patients with newly diagnosed multiple myeloma (MM): Final results of a multicenter phase I/II study. *Journal of Clinical Oncology*. 2010;28 8016-8016.
76. Reeder CB, Reece DE, Kukreti V, et al. Once- versus twice-weekly bortezomib induction therapy with CyBorD in newly diagnosed multiple myeloma. *Blood*. 2010;115:3416–3417.
77. Oakervee HE, Popat R, Curry N, et al. PAD combination therapy (PS-341/bortezomib, doxorubicin and dexamethasone) for previously untreated patients with multiple myeloma. *British Journal of Haematology*. 2005;129:755–762.
78. Wang M, Giralt S, Delasalle K, et al. Bortezomib in combination with thalidomide-dexamethasone for previously untreated multiple myeloma. *Hematology*. 2007;12:235–239.
79. Kumar SK, Flinn I, Noga SJ, et al. Bortezomib, dexamethasone, cyclophosphamide and lenalidomide combination for newly diagnosed multiple myeloma: phase 1 results from the multicenter EVOLUTION study. *Leukemia*. 2010;24:1350.
80. Reeder CB, Libby EN, Costa LJ, et al. A Phase I/II trial of cyclophosphamide, carfilzomib, thalidomide and dexamethasone (CYCLONE) in patients with newly diagnosed multiple myeloma: final results of MTD expansion cohort. *Blood*. 2013;122:3179.
81. Ludwig H, Viterbo L, Greil R, et al. Randomized phase II study of bortezomib, thalidomide, and dexamethasone with or without cyclophosphamide as induction therapy in previously untreated multiple myeloma. *Journal of Clinical Oncology: Official Journal of the American Society of Clinical Oncology*. 2013;31:247.
82. Fermand JP, Ravaud P, Chevret S, et al. High-dose therapy and autologous peripheral blood stem cell transplantation in multiple myeloma: up-front or rescue treatment? Results of a multicenter sequential randomized clinical trial. *Blood*. 1998;92:3131.
83. Alexanian R, Dimopoulos MA, Delasalle KB, et al. Myeloablative therapy for primary resistant multiple myeloma. *Stem Cells*. 1995;13:118–121.

84. Attal M, Lauwers-Cances V, Marit G, et al. Lenalidomide maintenance after stem-cell transplantation for multiple myeloma. *The New England Journal of Medicine*. 2012;366:1782–1791.
85. McCarthy P, Owzar K, Hofmeister C, et al. Lenalidomide after stem-cell transplantation for multiple myeloma. *New England Journal Of Medicine*. 2012;366:1770–1781.
86. McCarthy P, Palumbo A, Holstein SA, et al. A meta-analysis of overall survival in patients with multiple myeloma treated with lenalidomide maintenance after high-dose melphalan and autologous stem cell transplant. *Haematologica*. 2016;101:2-+.
87. Benboubker L, Dimopoulos MA, Dispenzieri A, et al. Lenalidomide and dexamethasone in transplant-ineligible patients with myeloma. *The New England Journal of Medicine*. 2014;371:906–917.
88. Giralt S, Stadtmauer EA, Harousseau JL, et al. International myeloma working group (IMWG) consensus statement and guidelines regarding the current status of stem cell collection and high-dose therapy for multiple myeloma and the role of plerixafor (AMD 3100). *Leukemia*. 2009;23:1904.
89. Durie BGM, Harousseau JL, Miguel JS, et al. International uniform response criteria for multiple myeloma. *Leukemia*. 2006;20:2220.
90. Bladé J, Samson D, Reece D, et al. Criteria for evaluating disease response and progression in patients with multiple myeloma treated by high-dose therapy and hemopoietic stem cell transplantation. *British Journal of Haematology*. 1998;102:1115–1123.
91. McCarthy P, Holstein S, Petrucci MT, et al. Lenalidomide (LEN) maintenance following high-dose melphalan and autologous stem cell transplant (ASCT) in patients (Pts) with newly diagnosed multiple myeloma (MM): A meta-analysis of overall survival (OS). *Clinical Lymphoma Myeloma and Leukemia*. 2017;17 e6-e6.
92. Sonneveld P, Schmidt-Wolf IGH, Holt B, et al. Bortezomib induction and maintenance treatment in patients with newly diagnosed multiple myeloma: Results of the randomized phase III HOVON-65/GMMG-HD4 trial. *Journal of Clinical Oncology*. 2012;30:2946–2955.
93. Mikhael J, Dingli D, Roy V, et al. Management of newly diagnosed symptomatic multiple myeloma: updated mayo stratification of myeloma and risk-adapted therapy (mSMART) consensus guidelines 2013. *Mayo Clinic Proceedings*. 2013;88:360–376.
94. Palumbo A, Gay F, Cavallo F, et al. Continuous therapy versus fixed duration of therapy in patients with newly diagnosed multiple myeloma. *Journal of clinical oncology: official journal of the American Society of Clinical Oncology*. 2015;33:3459.
95. Morgan GJ, Jackson GH, Davies FE, et al. Maintenance thalidomide may improve progression free but not overall survival; results from the myeloma IX maintenance randomisation. *Blood*. 2008;112 656–656.
96. Mateos M-V, Oriol A, Martínez-López J, et al. Bortezomib, melphalan, and prednisone versus bortezomib, thalidomide, and prednisone as induction therapy followed by maintenance treatment with bortezomib and thalidomide versus bortezomib and prednisone in elderly patients with untreated multiple myeloma: a randomised trial. *Lancet Oncology*. 2010;11:934–941.
97. Kyle RA, Yee GC, Somerfield MR, et al. American Society of Clinical Oncology 2007 clinical practice guideline update on the role of bisphosphonates in multiple myeloma. *Journal of Clinical Oncology: Official Journal Of the American Society of Clinical Oncology*. 2007;25:2464–2472.
98. Terpos E, Kleber M, Engelhardt M, et al. European Myeloma Network guidelines for the management of multiple myeloma-related complications. *Haematologica*. 2015;100:1254–1266.
99. Tu KN, Lie JD, Wan CKV, et al. Osteoporosis: a review of treatment options. *P & T: a Peer-Reviewed Journal for Formulary Management*. 2018;43:92–104.
100. Berenson J, Pflugmacher R, Jarzem P, et al. Balloon kyphoplasty versus non-surgical fracture management for treatment of painful vertebral body compression fractures in patients with cancer: a multicentre, randomised controlled trial. *Lancet Oncology*. 2011;12:225–235.
101. Leigh BR, Kurtts TA, Mack CF, et al. Radiation therapy for the palliation of multiple myeloma. *International Journal of Radiation Oncology. Biology and Physics*. 1993:25.
102. Chanan-Khan A, Sonneveld P, Schuster MW, et al. Analysis of herpes zoster events among bortezomib-treated patients in the phase III APEX study. *Journal of Clinical Oncology: Official Journal of the American Society of Clinical Oncology*. 2008;26:4784.
103. Palumbo A, Rajkumar SV, Dimopoulos MA, et al. Prevention of thalidomide- and lenalidomide-associated thrombosis in myeloma. *Leukemia*. 2007;22:414.
104. Larocca A, Cavallo F, Bringhen S, et al. Aspirin or enoxaparin thromboprophylaxis for patients with newly diagnosed multiple myeloma treated with lenalidomide. *Blood*. 2012;119:933.
105. Rajkumar SV, Kumar S. Multiple myeloma: diagnosis and treatment. *Mayo Clinic Proceedings*. 2016;91:101–119.
106. Stewart AK, Rajkumar SV, Dimopoulos MA, et al. Carfilzomib, lenalidomide, and dexamethasone for relapsed multiple myeloma. *New England Journal of Medicine*. 2015;372:142–152.
107. Moreau P, Masszi T, Grzasko N, et al. Oral ixazomib, lenalidomide, and dexamethasone for multiple myeloma. *New England Journal of Medicine*. 2016;374:1621–1634.
108. Lacy MQ, Hayman SR, Gertz MA, et al. Pomalidomide (CC4047) plus low dose dexamethasone (Pom/dex) is active and well tolerated in lenalidomide refractory multiple myeloma (MM). *Leukemia*. 2010;24:1934.
109. Lacy MQ, Hayman SR, Gertz MA, et al. Pomalidomide (CC4047) plus low-dose dexamethasone as therapy for relapsed multiple myeloma. *Journal of Clinical Oncology: Official Journal of the American Society of Clinical Oncology*. 2009;27:5008.
110. Richardson PG, Siegel DS, Vij R, et al. Pomalidomide alone or in combination with low-dose dexamethasone in relapsed and refractory multiple myeloma: a randomized phase 2 study. *Blood*. 2014;123:1826.
111. Lacy MQ, Allred JB, Gertz MA, et al. Pomalidomide plus low-dose dexamethasone in myeloma refractory to both bortezomib and lenalidomide: comparison of 2 dosing strategies in dual-refractory disease. *Blood*. 2011;118:2970.
112. San-Miguel JF, Hungria VTM, Yoon S-S, et al. Panobinostat plus bortezomib and dexamethasone versus placebo plus bortezomib and dexamethasone in patients with relapsed or relapsed and refractory multiple myeloma: a multicentre, randomised, double-blind phase 3 trial. *Lancet Oncology*. 2014;15:1195–1206.
113. San-Miguel JF, Richardson PGG, Sezer O, et al. A phase lb study of oral panobinostat and IV bortezomib in relapsed or relapsed and refractory multiple myeloma. *Journal of Clinical Oncology*. 2011;29 8075–8075.
114. Hideshima T, Bradner JE, Wong J, et al. Small-molecule inhibition of proteasome and aggresome function induces synergistic antitumor activity in multiple myeloma. *Proceedings of the National Academy of Sciences of the United States of America*. 2005;102:8567.
115. Lonial S, Weiss BM, Usmani SZ, et al. Phase II study of daratumumab (DARA) monotherapy in patients with ≥ 3 lines of prior therapy or double refractory multiple myeloma (MM): 54767414MMY2002 (Sirius). *Journal of Clinical Oncology*. 2015;33 LBA8512-LBA8512.
116. Lonial S, Vij R, Harousseau J-L, et al. Elotuzumab in combination with lenalidomide and low-dose dexamethasone in relapsed or refractory multiple myeloma. *Journal of Clinical Oncology*. 2012;30:1953–1959.
117. Lonial S, Dimopoulos M, Palumbo A, et al. Elotuzumab therapy for relapsed or refractory multiple myeloma. *The New England Journal of Medicine*. 2015;373:621–631.
118. Smith MA, Seibel NL, Altekruse SF, et al. Outcomes for children and adolescents with cancer: challenges for the twenty-first century. *Journal of Clinical Oncology: Official Journal of the American Society of Clinical Oncology*. 2010;28:2625.
119. Linabery AM, Ross JA. Trends in childhood cancer incidence in the U.S. (1992–2004. *Cancer*. 2008;112:416–432.
120. Fullmer A, O'Brien S, Kantarjian H, et al. Novel therapies for relapsed acute lymphoblastic leukemia. *Current Hematologic Malignancy Reports*. 2009;4:148–156.
121. Terwilliger T, Abdul-Hay M. *Acute lymphoblastic leukemia: a comprehensive review and 2017 update: Nature Publishing Group*; 2017:e577.
122. Paul S, Kantarjian H, Jabbour EJ. Adult acute lymphoblastic leukemia. *Mayo Clinic Proceedings*. 2016;91:1645–1666.
123. Jabbour E, O'Brien S, Konopleva M, et al. New insights into the pathophysiology and therapy of adult acute lymphoblastic leukemia. *In*. 2015;2517–2528.
124. Chessells JM, Harrison G, Richards SM, et al. Down's syndrome and acute lymphoblastic leukaemia: clinical features and response to treatment. *Archives of Disease in Childhood*. 2001;85:321–325.
125. Sehgal S, Mujtaba S, Gupta D, et al. High incidence of Epstein Barr virus infection in childhood acute lymphocytic leukemia: a preliminary study. *Indian Journal of Pathology & Microbiology*. 2010;53:63.
126. Eden T. Aetiology of childhood leukaemia. *Cancer Treatment Reviews*. 2010:286–297.

127. Gérinière L, Bastion Y, Dumontet C, et al. Heterogeneity of acute lymphoblastic leukemia in HIV-seropositive patients. *Annals of Oncology: Official Journal of the European Society for Medical Oncology*. 1994;5:437–440.
128. Onciu M. Acute lymphoblastic leukemia. *Hematol Oncol Clin North Am*. 2009;23:655–674.
129. Duong H, Sekeres M. Targeted treatment of acute myeloid leukemia in older adults: role of gemtuzumab ozogamicin. *Clinical Interventions in Aging*. 2009;4:197–205.
130. Kaspers GJL, Zwaan CM. Pediatric acute myeloid leukemia: towards high-quality cure of all patients. *Haematologica*. 2007;92:1519–1532.
131. Hallek M. Chronic lymphocytic leukemia: 2017 update on diagnosis, risk stratification, and treatment. *American Journal Of Hematology*. 2017;92:946–965.
132. Kaufman M, Rubin J, Rai K. Diagnosing and treating chronic lymphocytic leukemia in 2009. *Oncology*. 2009;23:1030–1037.
133. Höglund M, Sandin F, Simonsson B. Epidemiology of chronic myeloid leukaemia: an update. *Annals of Hematology*. 2015;94:241–247.
134. Von Bubnoff N, Duyster J. Chronic myelogenous leukemia: treatment and monitoring. *Deutsches Arzteblatt International*. 2010;107:114–121.
135. Copland M. Chronic myelogenous leukemia stem cells: What's new? *Current Hematologic Malignancy Reports*. 2009;4:66–73.
136. Sullivan C, Peng C, Chen Y, et al. Targeted therapy of chronic myeloid leukemia. *Biochemical Pharmacology*. 2010;80:584–591.
137. Jabbour E, Kantarjian H. Chronic myeloid leukemia: 2018 update on diagnosis, therapy and monitoring. *American Journal of Hematology*. 2018;93:442–459.
138. Harris NL, Jaffe ES, Diebold J, et al. World Health Organization classification of neoplastic diseases of the hematopoietic and lymphoid tissues: report of the Clinical Advisory Committee meeting-Airlie House, Virginia, November 1997. *Journal of Clinical Oncology: Official Journal of the American Society of Clinical Oncology*. 1999;17:3835–3849.
139. Vardiman JW, Thiele J, Arber DA, et al. The 2008 revision of the World Health Organization (WHO) classification of myeloid neoplasms and acute leukemia: rationale and important changes. 2009;114:937-951.
140. Ribera J-M, Oriol A. Acute lymphoblastic leukemia in adolescents and young adults. *Hematology/Oncology Clinics of North America*. 2009;23:1033–1042.
141. Rowe JM. *Prognostic factors in adult acute lymphoblastic leukaemia*. Oxford, UK: Blackwell Publishing Ltd; 2010:389–405.
142. Pui CH, Sallan S, Relling MV, et al. International childhood Acute Lymphoblastic Leukemia workshop: Sausalito, CA, 30 November–1 December 2000. *Leukemia*. 2001;15:707–715.
143. Hoelzer D, Thiel E, Löffler H, et al. Prognostic factors in a multicenter study for treatment of acute lymphoblastic leukemia in adults. *Blood*. 1988;71:123.
144. Rai KR, Sawitsky A, Cronkite EP, et al. Clinical staging of chronic lymphocytic leukemia. *Blood*. 1975;46:219.
145. Binet JL, Auquier A, Dighiero G, et al. A new prognostic classification of chronic lymphocytic leukemia derived from a multivariate survival analysis. *Cancer*. 1981;48:198.
146. Damle RN, Wasil T, Fais F, et al. Ig V gene mutation status and CD38 expression as novel prognostic indicators in chronic lymphocytic leukemia. *Blood*. 1999;94:1840.
147. Hamblin TJ, Davis Z, Gardiner A, et al. Unmutated Ig V(H) genes are associated with a more aggressive form of chronic lymphocytic leukemia. *Blood*. 1999;94:1848–1854.
148. An international prognostic index for patients with chronic lymphocytic leukaemia (CLL-IPI): a meta-analysis of individual patient data. *The Lancet Oncology*. 2016;17:779-790.
149. Hill BT, Copelan EA. Acute myeloid leukemia: when to transplant in first complete remission. *Current Hematologic Malignancy Reports*. 2010;5:101–108.
150. Döhner H, Weisdorf DJ, Bloomfield CD. Acute myeloid leukemia. *The New England Journal of Medicine*. 2015;373:1136–1152.
151. Sokal JE, Cox EB, Baccarani M, et al. Prognostic discrimination in "good-risk" chronic granulocytic leukemia. *Blood*. 1984;63:789–799.
152. Saglio G, Baccarani M. First-line therapy for chronic myeloid leukemia: new horizons and an update. *Clinical Lymphoma, Myeloma & Leukemia*. 2010;10:169–176.
153. Hasford J, Pfirrmann M, Hehlmann R, et al. A new prognostic score for survival of patients with chronic myeloid leukemia treated with interferon alfa. *Journal of the National Cancer Institute*. 1998;90:850–859.
154. Hoffmann V, Baccarani M, Lindörfer D, et al. The EUTOS prognostic score: review and validation in 1288 patients with CML treated frontline with imatinib. *Leukemia*. 2013;27:2016.
155. Zha Y, Li M, Yang J. Dynamic contrast enhanced magnetic resonance imaging of diffuse spinal bone marrow infiltration in patients with hematological malignancies. *Korean Journal of Radiology*. 2010;11:187–194.
156. Elojeimy S, Luana AS, Parisi MT. Use of 18F-FDG PET-CT for detection of active disease in acute myeloid leukemia. *Clinical Nuclear Medicine*. 2016;41:e137–e140.
157. Fritz J, Vogel W, Bares R, et al. Radiologic spectrum of extramedullary relapse of myelogenous leukemia in adults. *AJR. American Journal of Roentgenology*. 2007;189:209–218.
158. Zhou WL, Wu HB, Wang LJ, et al. Usefulness and pitfalls of F-18-FDG PET/CT for diagnosing extramedullary acute leukemia. *European Journal of Radiology*. 2016;85:205–210.
159. Rao RS, Langston KA, Galt KJ, et al. Extramedullary acute myeloid leukemia and the use of FDG-PET/CT. *Clinical Nuclear Medicine*. 2009;34:365–366.
160. Cunningham I, Kohno B. 18FDG-PET/CT: 21st century approach to leukemic tumors in 124 cases. *American Journal of Hematology*. 2016;91:379–384.
161. Konuma T, Ooi J, Takahashi S, et al. Central nervous system leukemia on magnetic resonance imaging. *Internal Medicine (Tokyo, Japan)*. 2008;47 477–477.
162. Ulu EMK, Töre HG, Bayrak A, et al. MRI of central nervous system abnormalities in childhood leukemia. *Diagnostic and Interventional Radiology*. 2009;15:86–92.
163. Bruzzi JF, Macapinlac H, Tsimberidou AM, et al. Detection of Richter's transformation of chronic lymphocytic leukemia by PET/CT. *Journal of Nuclear Medicine: Official Publication, Society of Nuclear Medicine*. 2006;47:1267–1273.
164. Rhodes JM, Mato AR. PET/computed tomography in chronic lymphocytic leukemia and Richter transformation. *PET Clinics*. 2019;14:405–410.
165. Escuissato DL, Gasparetto EL, Marchiori E, et al. Pulmonary infections after bone marrow transplantation: high-resolution CT findings in 111 patients. *AJR*. 2005;185:608–615.
166. Caillot D, Casasnovas O, Bernard A, et al. Improved management of invasive pulmonary aspergillosis in neutropenic patients using early thoracic computed tomographic scan and surgery. *Journal of Clinical Oncology: Official Journal of the American Society of Clinical Oncology*. 1997;15:139.
167. Hochberg J, Cairo MS. Childhood and adolescent lymphoblastic lymphoma: End of the beginning and future directions. *Pediatric Blood & Cancer*. 2009;53:917–919.
168. Nathan PC, Wasilewski-Masker K, Janzen LA. Long-term outcomes in survivors of childhood acute lymphoblastic leukemia. In Nathan PC (*ed*). 2009;1065–1082.
169. Kantarjian HM, O'Brien S, Smith TL, et al. Results of treatment with hyper-CVAD, a dose-intensive regimen, in adult acute lymphocytic leukemia. *Journal of Clinical Oncology: Official Journal of the American Society of Clinical Oncology*. 2000;18:547.
170. Narayanan S, Shami PJ. Treatment of acute lymphoblastic leukemia in adults. *Critical Reviews in Oncology/Hematology*. 2012;81:94–102.
171. Thomas D, O'Brien SM, Faderl S, et al. Long-term outcome after hyper-CVAD and imatinib (IM) for de novo or minimally treated Philadelphia chromosome-positive acute lymphoblastic leukemia (Ph-ALL). *Journal Of Clinical Oncology*. 2010:28.
172. Thomas DA, Faderl S, Cortes J, et al. Treatment of Philadelphia chromosome-positive acute lymphocytic leukemia with hyper-CVAD and imatinib mesylate. *Blood*. 2004;103:4396–4407.
173. Jones D, Thomas D, Yin CC, et al. Kinase domain point mutations in Philadelphia chromosome-positive acute lymphoblastic leukemia emerge after therapy with BCR-ABL kinase inhibitors. *Cancer*. 2008;113:985–994.
174. Porkka K, Koskenvesa P, Lundán T, et al. Dasatinib crosses the blood-brain barrier and is an efficient therapy for central nervous system Philadelphia chromosome-positive leukemia. *Blood*. 2008;112:1005.
175. Ravandi F, Othus M, O'Brien S, et al. Multi-center US intergroup study of intensive chemotherapy plus dasatinib followed by allogeneic stem cell transplant in patients with Philadelphia chromosome

positive acute lymphoblastic leukemia younger than 60. *Blood.* 2015:126.

176. Jude V, Chan K. Recent advances in hematopoietic stem cell transplantation for childhood acute lymphoblastic leukemia. *Current Hematologic Malignancy Reports*. 2010;5:129–134.
177. Eichhorst B, Fink A-M, Bahlo J, et al. First-line chemoimmunotherapy with bendamustine and rituximab versus fludarabine, cyclophosphamide, and rituximab in patients with advanced chronic lymphocytic leukaemia (CLL10): an international, open-label, randomised, phase 3, non-inferiority trial. *The Lancet Oncology*. 2016;17:928–942.
178. Deschler B, de Witte T, Mertelsmann R, et al. Treatment decision-making for older patients with high-risk myelodysplastic syndrome or acute myeloid leukemia: problems and approaches. *Haematologica.* 2006;91:1513–1522.
179. Sanz MA, Lo-Coco F. Modern approaches to treating acute promyelocytic leukemia. *Journal of Clinical Oncology: Official Journal of the American Society of Clinical Oncology*. 2011;29:495–503.
180. Estey E, Koller C, Tsimberidou AM, et al. Potential curability of newly diagnosed acute promyelocytic leukemia without use of chemotherapy: the example of liposomal all-trans retinoic acid. *Blood.* 2005;105:1366.
181. Mathews V, George B, Chendamarai E, et al. Single-agent arsenic trioxide in the treatment of newly diagnosed acute promyelocytic leukemia: long-term follow-up data. *Journal of Clinical Oncology: Official Journal of the American Society of Clinical Oncology*. 2010;28:3866.
182. Hu J, Liu Y-F, Wu C-F, et al. Long-term efficacy and safety of all-trans retinoic acid/arsenic trioxide-based therapy in newly diagnosed acute promyelocytic leukemia. *Proceedings of the National Academy of Sciences of the United States of America*. 2009;106:3342–3347.
183. Chen B-B, Hsu C-Y, Yu C-W, et al. Dynamic contrast-enhanced MR imaging measurement of vertebral bone marrow perfusion may be indicator of outcome of acute myeloid leukemia patients in remission. *Radiology.* 2011;258:821.
184. O'Brien SG, Guilhot F, Larson RA, et al. Imatinib compared with interferon and low-dose cytarabine for newly diagnosed chronic-phase chronic myeloid leukemia. *New England Journal of Medicine*. 2003;348:994–1004.
185. Hochhaus A, Larson RA, Guilhot F, et al. Long-Term Outcomes of Imatinib Treatment for Chronic Myeloid Leukemia. *The New England Journal of Medicine*. 2017;376:917–927.
186. Ten Cate B, de Bruyn M, Wei Y, et al. Targeted elimination of leukemia stem cells; a new therapeutic approach in hemato-oncology. *Current Drug Targets*. 2010;11:95–110.
187. Misaghian N, Ligresti G, Steelman LS, et al. Targeting the leukemic stem cell: the Holy Grail of leukemia therapy. *Leukemia*. 2008;23:25.
188. Anders C, Lars N, Ingbritt Å-G, et al. Distinct patterns of hematopoietic stem cell involvement in acute lymphoblastic leukemia. *Nature Medicine*. 2005;11:630.
189. Tsvee L, Christian S, Josef V, et al. A cell initiating human acute myeloid leukaemia after transplantation into SCID mice. *Nature.* 1994;367:645.
190. Dominique B, John ED. Human acute myeloid leukemia is organized as a hierarchy that originates from a primitive hematopoietic cell. *Nature Medicine*. 1997;3:730.
191. Larson RA, Sievers EL, Stadtmauer EA, et al. Final report of the efficacy and safety of gemtuzumab ozogamicin (Mylotarg) in patients with CD33-positive acute myeloid leukemia in first recurrence. *Cancer.* 2005;104:1442–1452.
192. Castaigne S, Pautas C, Terré C, et al. Effect of gemtuzumab ozogamicin on survival of adult patients with de-novo acute myeloid leukaemia (ALFA-0701): a randomised, open-label, phase 3 study. *The Lancet.* 2012;379:1508–1516.
193. Gill S, Tasian SK, Ruella M, et al. Preclinical targeting of human acute myeloid leukemia and myeloablation using chimeric antigen receptor-modified T cells. *Blood.* 2014;123:2343.
194. Awan FT, Johnson AJ, Lapalombella R, et al. *Thalidomide and lenalidomide as new therapeutics for the treatment of chronic lymphocytic leukemia*: *Taylor & Francis*; 2010:27–38.

CHAPTER 30

Hematologic Malignancy: The Lymphomas

Sarah J. Vinnicombe, M.R.C.P., F.R.C.R.; and Naveen Garg, M.D.

INTRODUCTION

The lymphomas are a diverse group of hematologic neoplasms arising primarily from lymph nodes. They vary widely in affected age group, clinical course, and prognosis. Hodgkin lymphoma (HL) was first described by Thomas Hodgkin in 1832, and since the early 1990s advances in therapy have been so great that HL is now curable in most patients. The non-Hodgkin lymphomas (NHLs) are far more variable in their clinical course and may be rapidly fatal. As in HL, improvements in survival are largely attributable to advances in therapy, but modern cross-sectional and functional imaging studies have also had significant impact. The accurate delineation of disease extent and identification of risk factors facilitate optimal, individualized, risk-adapted treatment with resultant survival benefits. Accurate imaging is crucial in choosing the most appropriate treatment at the time of diagnosis and staging, in monitoring response to therapy, and in detecting recurrence.

The objectives of initial staging are twofold: to define the local extent of clinically overt disease and to seek for occult disease elsewhere, in the knowledge of the likely pattern of tumor spread. Initial imaging should identify adverse prognostic features and factors that may influence delivery of therapy (e.g., central venous occlusion). Choice of the most appropriate imaging method requires an appreciation of the likelihood of particular sites being affected, the accuracy of specific tests chosen to investigate those sites, and the likely impact of a positive result on management.

EPIDEMIOLOGY

Incidence

Lymphoma is the fifth commonest malignancy in the Western world and in the United States. Within the United States, NHL annually accounts for 5% of new cancers in men and 4% of new cancers in women. It is estimated that there will be 81,560 new cases of NHL and 20,720 deaths in 2021.[1] HL accounts for approximately 15% of all lymphomas. It is estimated that there will be 8,830 new cases in 2021 and 1000 deaths.[1] Men are affected somewhat more than women: for HL, the male-to-female ratio is 1.4:1; for NHL, it is 1.1:1.

The incidence of HL has been stable for years, but that of NHL rose by approximately 60% in the United States after 1960, although it now appears to be stabilizing. This is evident for all age groups, but particularly for older persons. NHL occurs more often in men and in White ethnic groups.[2] The incidence of NHL varies geographically, being more common in the Northeast and Midwest, but the increased incidence has been observed in all geographic areas of the United States. The overall mortality for NHL has also risen over the last few decades, especially in older patients, reflecting the increased incidence, despite the fact that survival rates for each subtype of NHL have improved secondary to advances in treatment.

The reasons for the increasing incidence are only partly understood. Some may be artifactual, in that new lymphoma classifications have led to a diagnosis of NHL in patients who would previously have received other diagnoses,[3] including HL, in up to 15% of cases. Much of the increase from the late 1980s resulted from the increased incidence of lymphomas associated with immune deficiency, notably secondary to human immunodeficiency virus (HIV) infection. However, the occurrence of some HIV-associated NHL has started to fall since the introduction of highly active combined antiretroviral therapy (cART).[4]

HL has a bimodal peak distribution, with one peak in the third decade of life and a second, smaller peak in patients older than 50 years. NHLs are diseases mainly of older persons, with a median age at diagnosis of 65 years.

Lymphomas account for around 11% of pediatric malignancies, and HL accounts for nearly 50% of all pediatric lymphomas.

KEY POINTS Incidence and Etiology

- The incidence of non-Hodgkin lymphoma (NHL) has increased by 60% since the 1960s in the United States and the United Kingdom.
- Hodgkin lymphoma (HL) has a peak incidence between the ages of 20 and 40 years, with a second peak in individuals older than 50 years.
- NHLs are seen in children and in those older than 50 years.
- There is a link between Epstein–Barr virus and lymphoma, and especially between Burkitt lymphoma and HL.
- Infective agents are also associated with NHLs.

Etiology

There is an association between Epstein–Barr virus (EBV) and HL, but the exact etiologic role of the virus is uncertain. Patients with HL have a higher titer of antibody to EBV viral capsular antigen, and the risk of HL among patients who have had infectious mononucleosis is trebled. EBV can also be found in malignant HL cells. Thus, it is classified by the International Agency for Research on Cancer as a cause of HL. Other infective agents such as HIV-1, associated with the mixed cellularity subtype of classic HL, are also implicated in the development of this disease. Infective agents are also associated with the development of certain subtypes of NHL. EBV is found in virtually 100% of cases of endemic African Burkitt lymphoma (BL); in the sporadic form, the incidence is 15% to 30%. The rare primary effusion lymphomas are associated with human herpesvirus–8 (HHV-8), as are some rare diffuse large B-cell lymphomas (DLBCLs). *Helicobacter pylori* infection is necessary for the development of gastric lymphoma of the mucosa-associated lymphoid tissue (MALT) type. Human T-cell lymphotrophic virus (HTLV-1) has a causal relationship with adult T-cell leukemia/lymphoma, as seen in South Japan and the Caribbean. The disease is believed to represent clonal expansion of HTLV-1–infected T lymphocytes. Additionally, *Borrelia burgdorferi* infection is associated with cutaneous MALT lymphoma.

Genetic factors have limited importance in the etiology of HL, with only approximately 5% of cases being familial, whereas familial aggregation of NHL is well recognized.

In NHL, immunosuppression is a very important etiologic factor. The incidence is greatly increased in patients with acquired immunodeficiency syndrome (AIDS) and in patients on long-term immunosuppressant therapy (e.g., following renal transplantation). Up to 25% of patients with congenital immunodeficiency syndromes including ataxia-telangiectasia, Wiskott–Aldrich syndrome, and X-linked immunodeficiencies will develop malignancies, of which lymphoproliferative disorders account for over 50%. Non–organ-specific autoimmune diseases (e.g., rheumatoid arthritis, systemic lupus erythematosus) are associated with HL and DLBCL, whereas organ-specific autoimmune diseases predispose to the development of MALT-type lymphomas within the affected organs (e.g., the thyroid and salivary glands). Finally, occupational exposure to certain chemicals such as pesticides and organic solvents may be a risk factor for the development of NHL.

PATHOLOGY

There have been several pathologic classifications of lymphoma in the past; however, the functional anatomy of the lymph node is key to understanding the pathologic classification of lymphomas (Fig. 30.1).

Non-Hodgkin Lymphoma

Over 90% of NHLs in the Western world are of B-cell origin. In general, those arising at stages of development within the germinal center of the node have a follicular or nodular architecture, whereas those arising outside the germinal center have a diffuse pattern. New insights into the pathogenesis of NHL, in terms of cellular and immunologic origins, resulted in the introduction of the Revised European American Classification of Lymphoid

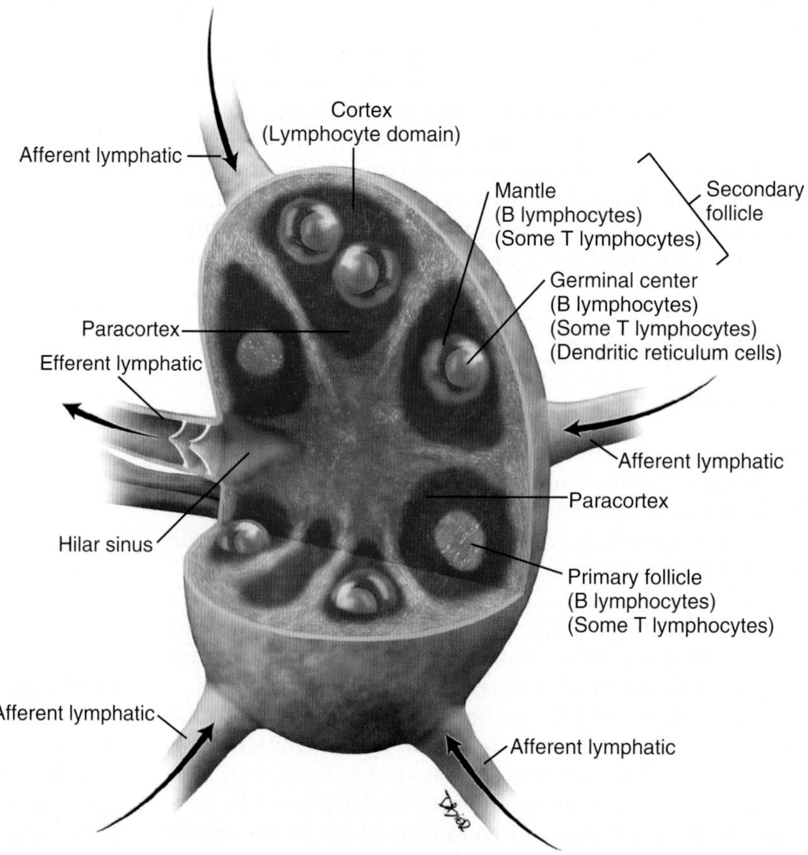

FIGURE 30.1. The functional anatomy of the lymph node.

Neoplasms classification in 1994. This, in turn, led to the adoption of the definitive World Health Organization (WHO) Classification of Tumors of Hematopoietic and Lymphoid Tissues in 1995, which was most recently revised in 2016 (Table 30.1).[5,6]

The WHO classification is a list of distinct disease entities defined by a combination of morphology, immunophenotype, and genetic and clinical features. It stratifies neoplasms according to myeloid, lymphoid, and histiocytic/dendritic cell lineages and recognizes three major categories of lymphoid neoplasms: B-cell, T-cell/natural killer cell, and HL. *Precursor* neoplasms, corresponding to the early stages of differentiation and including lymphoblastic leukemias and lymphomas, are separated from the more mature or peripheral neoplasms. For example, chronic lymphocytic leukemia (CLL) is the circulating form of small lymphocytic lymphoma, a mature B-cell neoplasm, and is classified as such.

TABLE 30.1 Summary of the World Health Organization Classification of Tumors of Lymphoid Tissue. Major Subdivisions are Shown With the Most Common Entities Listed.

Precursor Lymphoid Neoplasms	
B lymphoblastic leukemia/lymphomas not otherwise specified	
B-lymphoblastic leukemia/lymphoma with genetic abnormalities, e.g., *BCR-ABL*	
T lymphoblastic leukemia/lymphoma	
Mature B-Cell Neoplasms	**Mature T-Cell and NK-cell Neoplasms**
Chronic lymphatic leukemia/small lymphocytic lymphoma	T-cell prolymphocytic leukemia
Splenic marginal zone lymphoma	T-cell large granular lymphocytic leukemia
Hairy cell leukemia	Aggressive NK-cell leukemia
Lymphoplasmacytic lymphoma, Waldenström macroglobulinemia	Systemic EBV-positive T-cell lymphoma of childhood
Heavy chain diseases (Mu, Gamma, Alpha)	Adult T-cell leukemia/lymphoma
Plasma cell neoplasms: non-IgM monoclonal gammopathy, myeloma, solitary plasmactyoma of bone, extraosseous plasmactyoma, monoclonal immunoglobulin deposition diseases	Extranodal NK/T-cell lymphoma, nasal type
Extranodal marginal zone lymphoma of mucosa-associated lymphoid tissue (MALT)	Enteropathy-associated T-cell lymphoma
Nodal marginal zone lymphoma	Intestinal T-cell lymphoma, NOS
Follicular lymphoma (FL)	Hepatosplenic T-cell lymphoma
Pediatric type follicular lymphoma	Subcutaneous panniculitis-like T-cell lymphoma
Primary cutaneous follicle centre lymphoma	Mycosis fungoides
Mantle cell lymphoma	Sézary syndrome
Diffuse large B-cell lymphoma (DLBCL), NOS: germinal center B-cell & activated B-cell subtypes	Primary cutaneous CD30-positive T-cell lymphoproliferative disorders
T-cell–/histiocyte-rich DLBCL	Primary cutaneous gamma delta T-cell lymphoma
Primary DLBCL of the CNS	Peripheral T-cell lymphoma, NOS
Primary cutaneous DLBCL, leg type	Angioimmunoblastic T-cell lymphoma
EBV-positive DLBCL, NOS	Follicular T-cell lymphoma
DLBCL associated with chronic inflammation	Anaplastic large cell lymphoma: ALK-positive and ALK-negative
Lymphoid granulomatosis	Breast implant–associated anaplastic large-cell lymphoma
Primary mediastinal large B-cell lymphoma	
Intravascular large B-cell lymphoma	
ALK-positive large B-cell lymphoma	
Plasmablastic lymphoma	
Primary effusion lymphoma	
Multicentric Castleman disease	
HHV8-positive DLBCL	
Burkitt lymphoma	
High grade B cell lymphoma	
B-cell lymphoma, unclassifiable, with features intermediate between DLBCL and HL	
Histiocytic and Dendritic Cell Neoplasms	**Hodgkin Lymphoma (HL)**
Histiocytic sarcoma	Nodular lymphocyte predominant HL
Langerhans cell histiocytosis	Classical HL
Langerhans cell sarcoma	• Nodular sclerosis Classical HL
Erdheim–Chester disease	• Lymphocyte-rich Classical HL
	• Mixed cellularity Classical HL
	• Lymphocyte-depleted Classical HL
Immunodeficiency-Associated Disorders	
Posttransplant lymphoproliferative disorders	
– Polymorphic	
– Monomorphic	
– Classical HL	
Other iatrogenic immunodeficiency associated lymphoproliferative disorders	

NK, Natural killer; *Ig*, immunoglobulin; *EBV*, Epstein–Barr virus; *NOS*, not otherwise specified; *CNS*, central nervous system.

(Modified from Swerdlow SH, Campo E, Pileri SA, et al. The 2016 revision of the World Health Organization classification of lymphoid neoplasms, 2016. Blood. 2016;127(20):2375-2390.)

This comprehensive approach has significantly improved the consistency of classification of lymphoma, such that, if given sufficient material, expert hematopathologists agree on classification of entities in over 95% of cases.[7] Further refinements have drawn on findings from gene expression profiling and facilitate appropriate patient management.[8] For example, gene expression profiling for DLBCL enables recognition of discrete subsets (germinal center B-cell type and activated B-cell type) with independent prognostic significance.[6,9] Other changes include separation of monoclonal B-cell lymphocytosis into low-count and high-count variants, a new provisional entity of large B-cell lymphoma with *IRF4* rearrangement, renaming of *in situ* follicular lymphoma (FL) to *in situ* follicular neoplasia, and reclassification of EBV-positive DLBCL in the elderly to "not otherwise specified (EBV+ DLBCL, NOS)."[5] Histologic grade can also influence therapeutic decision-making. For example, FL is graded according to the number of centroblasts per high-power field, and grade III FL may require more intensive chemotherapy.

Hodgkin Lymphoma

Investigators have demonstrated that HL is a true lymphoma; hence, the term Hodgkin lymphoma is preferred to "Hodgkin disease." Indeed, the distinction between HL and NHL is not always straightforward, and composite cases occur. Diagnosis depends upon the demonstration of malignant Reed–Sternberg and Hodgkin cells against a background of nonneoplastic inflammatory cells. The WHO classification recognizes two distinct entities that differ in clinical features, behavior, morphology, and immunophenotype: classical HL (CHL, 95%) and nodular lymphocyte-predominant HL (NLPHL, 5%). CHL is, in turn, divided into four subgroups, based on the proportion of lymphocytes in relation to the number of malignant cells and on the connective tissue background (Table 30.2).[10] All share the same immunophenotype, with expression of CD30 by the malignant cells.

In nodular sclerosing HL, nodules of lymphoid tissue are separated by dense bands of collagen. This form of HL accounts for approximately 70% of CHLs and is the only form of HL without a male preponderance. Anterior mediastinal disease occurs in 80% of cases, and bulky disease in approximately 50%. Mixed cellularity HL accounts for 20% to 25% of CHLs and is more common in patients with HIV infection and in developing countries. Advanced-stage disease is common. EBV positivity is frequent. Lymphocyte-rich classic HL accounts for 5% of all HLs; 70% of cases are male, with a higher median age. Stage I or II peripheral nodal disease is typical. Lymphocyte-depleted CHL is the rarest subtype, accounting for less than 5% of cases; the median age at presentation is 35 to 40 years. It is associated with HIV infection and occurs more often in developing countries. Advanced-stage disease at presentation is common (70%), with frequent involvement of abdominal organs, retroperitoneal nodes, and bone marrow. Most cases of NLPHL were probably misclassified as lymphocyte-rich HL in the past. The malignant cells (called *popcorn* cells because of their striking nuclear convolutions) express CD20, not CD30. Affected patients are mostly male, aged 30 to 50 years, presenting with peripheral adenopathy affecting one or two nodal groups (axillary, cervical, or inguinal).

TABLE 30.2 Classification of Hodgkin Lymphoma and Approximate Frequency

HISTOLOGY	FREQUENCY (%)
Nodular lymphocyte-predominant Hodgkin lymphoma (HL)	5
Classical HL	95
Lymphocyte-rich	5
Nodular sclerosis	70
Mixed cellularity	20
Lymphocyte-depleted	5

KEY POINTS Classification of Lymphomas

- The WHO classification stratifies lymphoma according to myeloid, lymphoid, or histiocytic/dendritic lineage and provides distinction between disease entities.
- HL comprises two distinct entities: CHL (95%) and NLPHL (5%).
- CHL consists of four subtypes with differing presentations: nodular sclerosing (70%), mixed cellularity (20%–25%), lymphocyte-rich (5%), and lymphocyte-depleted (<5%).

CLINICAL FEATURES

Both HL and NHL are predominantly diseases of lymph nodes, which may present as a localized process involving a single nodal group or organ or as widely disseminated disease. However, there are recognizable differences in the clinical presentation of the two diseases (Table 30.3).

TABLE 30.3 Key Differences Between the Clinical Features of Hodgkin Lymphoma and Non-Hodgkin Lymphoma

	HODGKIN LYMPHOMA		NON-HODGKIN LYMPHOMA
Age	Young adults		More common ages 40–70 years
B symptoms	40%		20%
Spread	Generally contiguous nodal groups		Multiple remote nodal groups often involved
Stage at presentation	>80% early stage I and II		>85% late stage III and IV
Nodal groups	Thoracic	65%–85%	25%–40%
	Paraaortic	25%–35%	45%–55%
	Mesenteric	5%	50%–60%
Extranodal disease	Central nervous system	<1%	2%
	Gastrointestinal tract	<1%	5%–15%
	Genitourinary tract	<1%	1%–5%
	Bone marrow	5%	20%–40%
	Lung parenchyma	8%–12%	3%–6%
	Bone	<1%	1%–2%

Hodgkin Lymphoma

Most patients with HL present with painless asymmetrical lymph node enlargement, which may be accompanied by sweats, fever, weight loss ("B" symptoms), and pruritus in approximately 40% of patients. B symptoms are more common in advanced-stage disease, and thus in the mixed cellularity and lymphocyte-depleted subtypes of CHL. Alcohol-induced pain is rare.

The cervical lymph nodes are affected in 60% to 80% of patients, the axillary nodes in 6% to 20%, and the inguinal/femoral nodes in 6% to 15%. Exclusive infradiaphragmatic lymphadenopathy occurs in less than 10% of patients at diagnosis. Splenomegaly is found on clinical examination in approximately 30% of patients. Some 80% of patients present with early-stage disease, and the incidence of splenic or bone marrow involvement is low, although it varies with the histologic subtype.

Non-Hodgkin Lymphomas

Although most patients with NHL present with nodal enlargement, extranodal disease is far more frequent than in HL, as is bone marrow involvement, with over 80% of patients having advanced-stage disease at diagnosis, depending on the subtype. Despite this, B symptoms are less frequent at diagnosis compared with HL, occurring in approximately 20% of patients.

So-called indolent lymphomas account for up to 35% of NHL, and lymphadenopathy may be intermittent. FL is typically indolent, accounting for 25% to 30% of all newly diagnosed NHL. It is usually diagnosed in the sixth decade. Conversely, DLBCL is termed aggressive, but generally responds well to therapy. DLBCL accounts for 35% of all NHL and is the most common B-cell NHL, usually presenting with rapidly enlarging lymph nodes.

The most aggressive subtypes include BL and lymphoblastic lymphoma; these are histologically characterized by very high proliferation fractions, and patients often exhibit rapidly progressive systemic disease that requires urgent treatment.

Key Points Clinical

- Most patients with Hodgkin lymphoma (HL) and non-Hodgkin lymphoma (NHL) present with painless enlargement of a group of lymph nodes.
- In HL, most patients present with stage I or II disease; in NHL most patients have stage III or IV disease at diagnosis.
- Systemic symptoms are twice as common in HL as in NHL.

STAGING SYSTEMS AND PROGNOSTICATION

Because lymphomas are primarily neoplasms of lymphoid tissues (whether nodal or extranodal), the tumor-node-metastasis (TNM) staging system is not appropriate. The Ann Arbor staging system for HL was introduced in 1970 and took into account the extent of nodal disease and the presence of extranodal extension. Increasing recognition of the influence of tumor bulk as an independent prognostic indicator within each stage and the routine application of computed tomography (CT) in the 1980s led to a modification of the classification in 1989, the Cotswolds classification.[11] This system was routinely used until a few years ago. It was similar to the original Ann Arbor classification, but stage III was subdivided, and an additional qualifier "X" denoted bulky disease (Table 30.4).

The prognosis of HL depends upon a number of factors, including:

- Age. Older patients have a worse prognosis (for early-stage disease, 5-year survival is 45% in patients older than age 65 years, as opposed to over 90% in younger patients).
- Tumor subtype. Mixed cellularity and lymphocyte-depleted HL have a poorer prognosis.
- Raised erythrocyte sedimentation rate (ESR).
- Multiple sites of involvement (more than three or four involved regions).
- Bulky mediastinal disease.
- Systemic B symptoms.

In 2014, the Cotswolds modification of the Ann Arbor system was replaced by the Lugano classification. Here the key distinction is between limited or early-stage disease and advanced-stage disease (Table 30.5).[12]

The modified Ann Arbor classification, although applied, was never as useful as for NHL, as the prognosis in NHL is more dependent on histologic subtype, tumor bulk, and specific organ involvement, rather than stage. In NHL, the critical questions are whether or not disease is limited, the effect of the disease on end organs such as bone marrow,

Table 30.4 Staging of Lymphoma (Cotswolds Classification)

STAGE	AREA OF INVOLVEMENT	
I	One lymph node region or extralymphatic site	
II	Two or more lymph node regions on the same side of the diaphragm	
III	Involvement of lymph node regions or structures on both sides of the diaphragm, subdivided: 1. With involvement of spleen and/or splenic hilar, celiac, and portal nodes 2. With pararaortic, iliac, or mesenteric nodes	
IV	Extranodal sites beyond those designated "E"	
Additional qualifiers	A	No symptoms
	B	Fever, sweats, weight loss (to 10% body weight)
	E	Involvement of a single extranodal site, contiguous in proximity to a known nodal site
	X	Bulky disease; mass >10 cm maximum dimension
	CS	Clinical stage
	PS	Pathologic stage; denoted by a subscript at a given site (M, marrow; H, liver; L, lung; O, bone; P, pleural; D, skin; S, spleen)

(Modified from Lister TA, Crowther D, Sutcliffe SB, et al. Report of a committee convened to discuss the evaluation and staging of patients with Hodgkin's disease: Cotswolds meeting. *J Clin Oncol.* 1989;7:1630-1636.)

TABLE 30.5 The Lugano Staging Classification[a]

STAGE	DESCRIPTION
Limited stage	
I	Involvement of a single lymphatic site (e.g., nodal region, spleen, Waldeyer's ring)[b]
IE	Single extralymphatic site, no nodal disease
II	Two or more nodal regions on the same side of the diaphragm
IIE	Contiguous extralymphatic extension from a nodal site ± involvement of other nodal regions on the same side of the diaphragm
II bulky[c]	Can be limited or advanced stage depending on histology and prognostic factors
	The maximum diameter of the largest mass should be measured
	HL: mass >10 cm or >1/3 thoracic diameter on CT
	FL: mass >6 cm
	DLBCL: mass >10 cm
A PA CXR is no longer required	
Advanced stage	
III	Nodal regions on both sides of the diaphragm or nodes above the diaphragm and splenic involvement. IIIE and IIIS are no longer recognized
IV	Diffuse/disseminated involvement of ≥1 extralymphatic organ ± nodal involvement or noncontiguous extranodal involvement with stage II nodal disease or any extralymphatic organ involvement in stage III disease
NB: includes any involvement of CSF, bone marrow, liver, or lungs except by direct extension in stage IIE disease[d]	

[a]The main differences between the Cotswolds and Lugano classification systems are described.
[b]Waldeyer's ring, the thymus, and the spleen are considered nodal or lymphatic sites.
[c]The "X" subscript is no longer used.
[d]Any liver involvement by contiguous or noncontiguous spread should be regarded as stage IV disease.
"B" symptoms are used for HL only.
HL, Hodgkin lymphoma; *CT*, computed tomography; *FL*, follicular lymphoma; *DLBCL*, diffuse large B-cell lymphoma; *PA CXR*, posteroanterior chest radiograph; *CSF*, cerebrospinal fluid.
(Modified from Cheson BD, Fisher RI, Barrington SF et al. Recommendations for the initial evaluation, staging and response assessment of Hodgkin and non-Hodgkin lymphoma: the Lugano classification. *J Clin Oncol*. 2014; 32:3059-3068.)

and symptomatology. As NHL spreads more randomly than HL, the Cotswolds staging system is less helpful in defining prognostic subgroups. The Lugano classification is also applied to NHL, and the definition of bulky disease is subtype-dependent (Table 30.5).

Considerable effort has been applied to the development of robust prognostic indices in NHL that are simple and discriminant. Such indices not only aid in the management of the individual patient but also facilitate meaningful comparison of results from clinical trials. The International Prognostic Index (IPI) was developed by an international collaborative group.[13] For DLBCL, five factors have prognostic significance: age greater than 60 years, elevated serum lactate dehydrogenase (LDH), Eastern Cooperative Oncology Group performance status greater than 1 (i.e., nonambulatory), advanced-stage (III or IV) disease, and more than one extranodal site of disease.

Four risk groups are recognized depending on the number of adverse prognostic features that are present. Before the monoclonal antibody era, patients in the low-risk group (no or one prognostic factor present) had a 5-year survival rate greater than 70%, whereas patients in the high-risk group (four or five factors present) had only a 25% 5-year survival rate. More recently, the prognostic importance of gene expression profiling within individual subtypes of NHL has become evident, as described previously for DLBCL,[9] where the better prognosis of the germinal center–like subtype compared with the activated B-cell subtype is independent of the IPI. A similar prognostic index has been developed for FL, the FLIPI.[14] In the initial index, prognostic factors were age over 60 years, elevated serum LDH, hemoglobin less than 12 g/dL, stage III or IV disease, and more than four nodal sites of disease. The more recent modification (FLIPI 2) includes elevated serum beta-2 microglobulin and the presence of a lymph node over 6 cm in longest diameter.

For the purposes of the index, nine nodal sites are recognized (right and left cervical; right and left axillary; mediastinal; paraaortic; mesenteric; and right and left inguinal). Histologic factors are also important; grades I, II, and IIIa FL are treated similarly, whereas grade IIIb FL is now treated as DLBCL. Recent work also suggests that gene expression profiling yields significant prognostic information in FL. In other NHL subtypes, other prognostic factors are important. In mantle cell lymphoma (MCL), which has until recently had a dismal prognosis, the Ki-67 proliferation index has greater predictive value than any other histologic or clinical criterion.

The clinical spectrum of childhood lymphoma differs from adult lymphoma, with more frequent extranodal involvement, especially of the gastrointestinal (GI) tract, solid viscera including the kidneys and pancreas, and extranodal sites in the head and neck.[15] In these situations, the St. Jude, or Murphy's, staging classification is applied, because it takes into account the increased frequency of extranodal disease (Table 30.6).

For primary extranodal lymphoma (see later), a modified Ann Arbor staging classification may be used. Other staging systems in use include the Rai or Binet systems for SLL/CLL.

PATTERNS OF TUMOR SPREAD

HL tends to spread predictably in contiguous fashion from one lymph node group or region to the next adjacent group via lymphatic pathways. Thus, clinical involvement of the cervical lymph nodes should prompt careful scrutiny of the anterior and middle mediastinal nodal groups at staging CT. Similarly, in the presence of bulky mediastinal disease, attention should be paid to the upper retroperitoneal, celiac, portal, and splenic hilar nodal stations. Lymph node involvement is usually the only manifestation of disease. Primary extranodal HL is exceptionally rare and is a diagnosis of exclusion, although it is not uncommon for nodal HL to affect contiguous organs. For example, bulky anterior mediastinal disease can involve the adjacent lung

TABLE 30.6 Murphy's Staging System for Childhood Non-Hodgkin Lymphoma

STAGE	CRITERIA FOR EXTENT OF DISEASE
I	A single tumor (extranodal) or single nodal region, except in the mediastinum or abdomen
II	A single tumor (extranodal) with regional nodal involvement Two or more nodal areas on the same side of the diaphragm Two single (extranodal) tumors with or without regional node involvement on the same side of the diaphragm A primary gastrointestinal tract tumor, usually ileocecal, with or without involvement of associated mesenteric nodes only, grossly completely resected
III	Two single tumors (extranodal) on opposite sides of the diaphragm Two or more nodal areas above and below the diaphragm All primary intrathoracic tumors (mediastinal, pleural, thymic) All extensive primary intraabdominal disease, unresected All paraspinal or epidural tumors, regardless of other tumor site(s)
IV	Any of the above with initial central nervous system and/or bone marrow involvement

parenchyma or the chest wall, but this does not affect the disease stage or prognosis and would be designated "E" at staging. By contrast, the presence of peripheral subpleural pulmonary nodules discontiguous with the mediastinal mass indicates hematogenous spread and disseminated disease, which would be designated stage IV. With disease progression or relapse, visceral involvement occurs, and tumoral deposits may be seen in the liver, spleen, lungs, and bones.

NHL is generally a disseminated disease at presentation, involving lymph node groups through hematogenous spread, and multiple organs may be involved as well as the bone marrow. Thus, nodal enlargement might be seen at CT in the neck and pelvis, with no nodal abnormality in the chest or abdomen, whereas this distribution would be most unusual for HL. This unpredictability makes a whole-body staging technique imperative. However, individual subtypes of NHL are associated with certain patterns of disease. Marked splenomegaly is a feature of splenic marginal zone lymphoma and MCL, the latter often in association with bowel involvement. The constellation of a large anterior mediastinal mass with central venous obstruction and disease in the liver, kidneys, or adrenal glands but little or no nodal disease makes primary mediastinal large B-cell lymphoma (PMBL) the most likely diagnosis, whereas widespread peritoneal disease at presentation, with involvement of the viscera and female genital tract, suggests BL. Certain types of NHL are strongly associated with central nervous system (CNS) or meningeal disease, especially testicular and head and neck lymphoma, and this association may warrant screening of the craniospinal axis or prophylactic intrathecal therapy. With disease progression, nodal lymphoma may spread to involve adjacent structures. In the retroperitoneum, this can affect the paravertebral and paraspinal structures, with resultant neural compression. In the mesentery, spread into adjacent bowel loops is common, causing displacement, encasement, or compression. As disease advances, peritoneal involvement can occur that is radiologically indistinguishable from peritoneal carcinomatosis.

Often, the pattern of disease at CT may suggest the diagnosis. Thus, involvement of cervical lymph nodes and the tissues of Waldeyer's ring suggests NHL rather than HL. Nodal enlargement in the anterior and middle mediastinum suggests HL, whereas disease in the mesentery, with or without concomitant bowel involvement, strongly favors NHL (see Table 30.3).

IMAGING TECHNIQUES

Nodal Disease

Cross-sectional Imaging

For some time, contrast-enhanced CT (CE-CT) has been the modality of choice for the staging and follow-up of lymphoma. It enables localization of the most appropriate lesion for percutaneous image-guided biopsy. Ultrasound has limited value in staging. Involved lymph nodes have nonspecific appearances, although the pattern of nodal vascular perfusion on power Doppler sonography may suggest the diagnosis. The main value of ultrasound is in providing image guidance for biopsy. Although magnetic resonance imaging (MRI) is as accurate as CT in detecting lymph node enlargement, its role has been essentially adjunctive. As with CT and ultrasound, involved lymph nodes cannot be diagnosed other than by size criteria (Fig. 30.2). Advances in scanner technology including high–field strength magnets enable whole-body MRI studies, and in the last decade there has been much research into the use these techniques as a staging tool, particularly in pediatric patients, where radiation dose is an important consideration. Whole-body diffusion-weighted imaging (DWI) of lymphoma may have a role in the differentiation of lymphoma from other causes of malignant nodal enlargement.[16]

Functional Imaging With Positron Emission Tomography and Positron Emission Tomography/Computed Tomography

Detection of disease in normal-sized nodes is not possible with cross-sectional imaging, nor is it possible to differentiate between nodal enlargement secondary to lymphoma or reactive hyperplasia. Functional radioisotope studies permit this distinction. Gallium-67 citrate scintigraphy has been superseded by 2-[^{18}F] fluoro-2-deoxy-D-glucose–positron emission tomography (FDG-PET). In most lymphomas, increased glucose metabolism results in increased cellular uptake of FDG with an accuracy comparable with or better than CT for the detection of nodal and extranodal disease.[17,18] Upstaging with PET/CT occurs in up to 40% of patients, although changes of therapy as a consequence are more common in HL than in NHL. In NHL, staging FDG-PET gives important information by indicating tumor burden as well as the presence of extranodal disease (Fig. 30.3). Most NHLs show increased uptake, the exceptions being some MALT, cutaneous, and small lymphocytic lymphomas. In FL, the presence of relatively high FDG uptake in a given nodal group may suggest histologic transformation, which can then be confirmed by

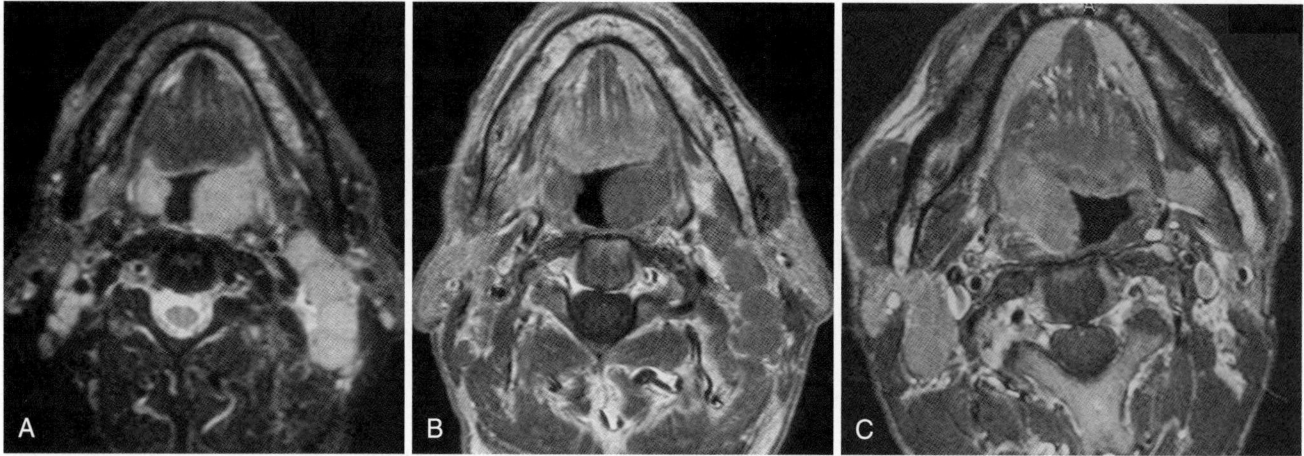

FIGURE 30.2. **A**, Axial T2-weighted magnetic resonance imaging scan demonstrates lymphomatous involvement of both tonsillar fossae with enlarged high–T2 signal lymph nodes on the left. Notice high T2 signal in multiple normal-sized right level 2 lymph nodes. **B**, Corresponding T1-weighted scan demonstrates uniform intermediate signal in the involved lymph nodes. **C**, Same patient at a higher level. After intravenous contrast, there is uniform moderate enhancement of a right level 2 node and a right tonsillar fossa mass.

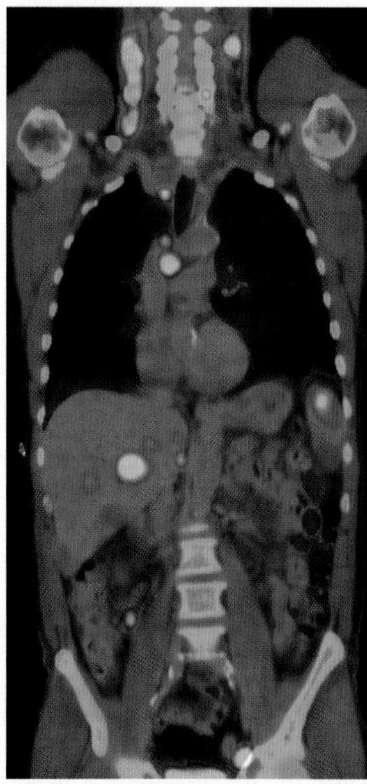

FIGURE 30.3. Coronal fused positron emission tomography computed tomography (PET/CT) image in a patient with stage II Hodgkin lymphoma on conventional CT. There are regions of increased tracer uptake in the liver, spleen, and bone, indicating stage IV disease.

targeted percutaneous biopsy. PET/CT allows accurate co-localization of morphologic abnormalities and their associated functional changes. Debate continues as to whether it is always necessary to carry out a full diagnostic CE-CT as part of the PET/CT study or whether a low-dose CT for the purposes of attenuation correction and anatomic correlation is sufficient.[19] Current guidelines recommend performing a diagnostic CE-CT at presentation, after which it can be omitted if noncontributory.[20]

For nonavid and variably FDG-avid histologies, CE-CT remains the staging technique of choice.[12] CE-CT is also recommended for enumerating nodes for clinical trials and for radiotherapy planning.[12,20] In these guidelines, a lymph node with longest diameter (LDi) greater than 1.5 cm is considered enlarged, and it is recommended that up to six nodes measurable in two orthogonal diameters are used as target lesions.[12,20]

KEY POINTS Nodal Imaging: General

- Recognition of nodal disease with computed tomography (CT) and magnetic resonance imaging (MRI) depends on size criteria alone.
- CT and MRI have equal sensitivity below the diaphragm.
- Ultrasound has a role in problem-solving and biopsy guidance.
- FDG PET/CT may enable identification of disease in normal-sized lymph nodes.
- Nodal disease in the lymphomas may involve any anatomic lymph node site.

Neck

Cervical lymph node enlargement is seen in 60% to 80% of patients with HL at presentation. It typically involves the internal jugular chain of nodes initially, with further spread to the spinal accessory and transverse cervical chains. In NHL, the pattern of involvement is more haphazard than in HL (Fig. 30.2). Enhancement after administration of contrast medium is usually mild to moderate, and central necrosis within a lymph node is rare. MRI may be particularly useful for defining the extent of lymphomatous masses in the lower neck and supraclavicular fossa.

Thorax

Intrathoracic nodes are involved at presentation in 60% to 85% of patients with HL and 25% to 40% of patients with NHL. Almost all patients with nodular sclerosing HL have disease in the anterior mediastinum. Nodal involvement in mediastinal presentations includes prevascular and paratracheal (84%; Fig. 30.4A), hilar (28%), subcarinal (22%), and other sites (~5%), including aortoplumonary, internal mammary, and anterior diaphragmatic (Fig. 30.4B and C).[21] In NHL, the incidence varies, but may include superior mediastinal (34%), hilar (9%), subcarinal (13%), and other sites (≤10%).[22]

The majority of cases of HL show enlargement of two or more nodal groups, whereas only one nodal group is involved in up to half of NHL cases. Hilar nodal enlargement is rare without associated mediastinal involvement, particularly in HL. Although nodes in the internal mammary chains and paracardiac regions are rarely involved at presentation, they become important as sites of recurrence because they may not be included in conventional radiation fields. It is important to review these sites because minimally enlarged nodes are easily overlooked.

Nodal calcification before therapy is extremely rare. Cystic degeneration may be seen in both HL and NHL, especially with large anterior mediastinal masses, and is a particular feature of PMBL[23] (Fig. 30.5). Thymic infiltration occurs in both HL and NHL and is often indistinguishable from anterior mediastinal nodal disease. A large anterior mediastinal mass is an adverse prognostic factor in HL. Axillary nodes are also frequently detected on CT in HL and NHL (Fig. 30.4B). Preservation of the normal fatty hilum may be helpful in distinguishing benign reactive hyperplasia from lymphomatous involvement.

Key Points Supradiaphragmatic Nodal Disease

- Some 60% to 80% of patients with (HL) present with enlarged neck nodes. This is also a common presentation in (NHL).
- Some 60% to 80% of patients with HL and 25% to 40% of patients with NHL have prevascular and paratracheal lymphadenopathy at diagnosis.
- A large anterior mediastinal mass may represent lymphomatous infiltration of the thymus.

Abdomen and Pelvis

At presentation, retroperitoneal nodes are involved in 25% to 35% of patients with HL and in 45% to 55% of patients with NHL. Mesenteric lymph nodes are involved in more than 50% of patients with NHL but less than 5% of patients with HL. Other intraabdominal sites are also less frequently involved in HL than in NHL. Given the mode of spread of HL, involvement of retrocrural nodes should prompt close scrutiny of the celiac axis nodes. The celiac axis, splenic hilar, and porta hepatis nodes are involved in approximately 33% of patients, and splenic hilar nodal involvement is almost always associated with diffuse splenic infiltration. The node of the foramen of Winslow (portacaval node) between the portal vein and the inferior vena cava should be carefully evaluated, as enlargement is easily overlooked (Fig. 30.6).

In NHL, nodal involvement is frequently noncontiguous and bulky, and is often associated with extranodal disease (Fig. 30.7A). Discrete mesenteric nodal enlargement or masses may be seen with or without retroperitoneal nodal enlargement. Regional nodal involvement is frequently observed in primary extranodal lymphoma involving an abdominal viscus. In a patient with lymphoma, the presence of multiple normal-sized mesenteric nodes is suspicious for involvement (Fig. 30.7B). Nodularity and streakiness within the mesentery is also suspicious, lymphoma being one cause of a misty mesentery. Any pelvic nodal group may be involved in HL and NHL. Presentation with enlarged inguinal/femoral lymphadenopathy is seen in fewer than 20% of cases of HL.

Key Points Abdominal Nodal Disease

- Retroperitoneal lymphadenopathy is more commonly seen in (NHL) than in (HL).
- Mesenteric lymphadenopathy is seen in over 50% of cases of NHL.
- The celiac, splenic hilar, and porta hepatis nodes are involved in approximately 30% of patients with HL.

Extranodal Disease

Approximately 30% of cases of NHL arise primarily in extranodal sites other than the spleen or bone marrow. The most common pathologic subtypes with extranodal involvement are DLBCL, MALT, and FL, and the most common locations affected in decreasing order of frequency are Waldeyer's ring, the stomach and small intestine, the soft tissues, and the orbit. Secondary extranodal

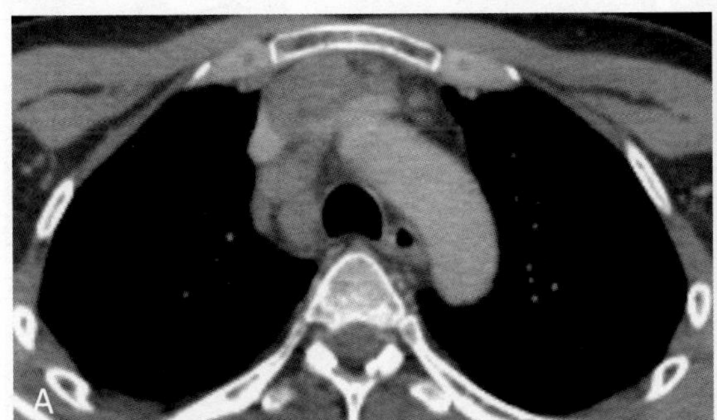

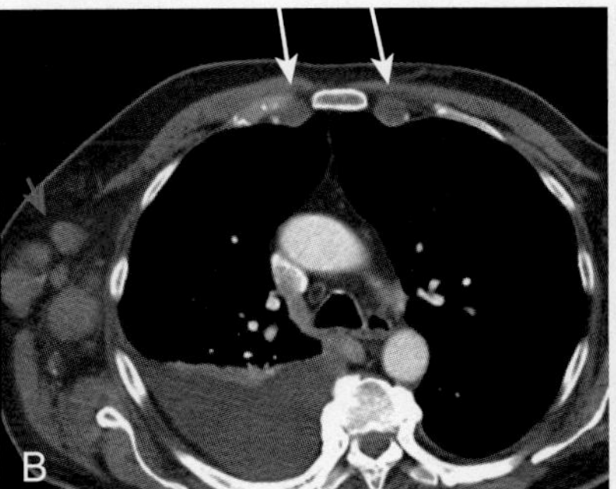

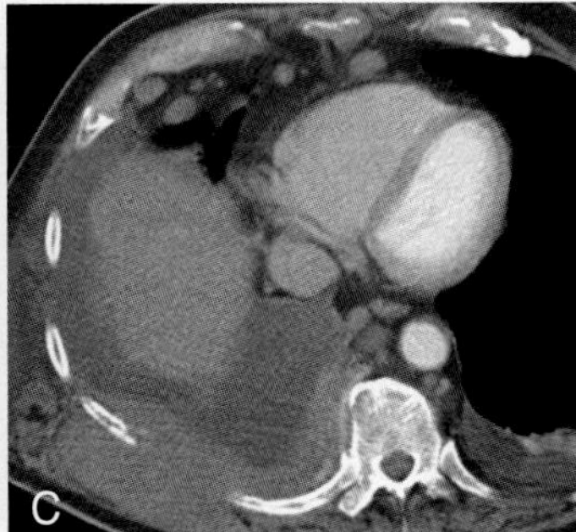

Figure 30.4. **A**, Anterior and middle mediastinal nodal enlargement in a patient with Hodgkin lymphoma. **B**, Bilateral internal mammary (*white arrows*) and right axillary lymph node (*red arrow*) enlargement in association with a right pleural effusion. **C**, Multiple peridiaphragmatic and paracardiac lymph nodes. There is also an abnormal right retrocrural lymph node and a large posterior chest wall mass involving the pleura anteriorly and the chest wall musculature posteriorly.

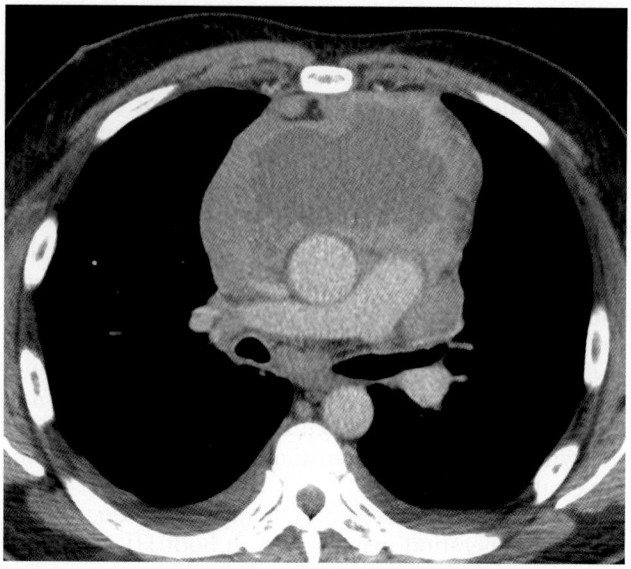

FIGURE 30.5. Primary mediastinal large B-cell lymphoma. Axial contrast-enhanced computed tomography scan demonstrates a large anterior mediastinal mass replacing the normal thymus. Notice low attenuation within the mass, indicating cystic necrosis.

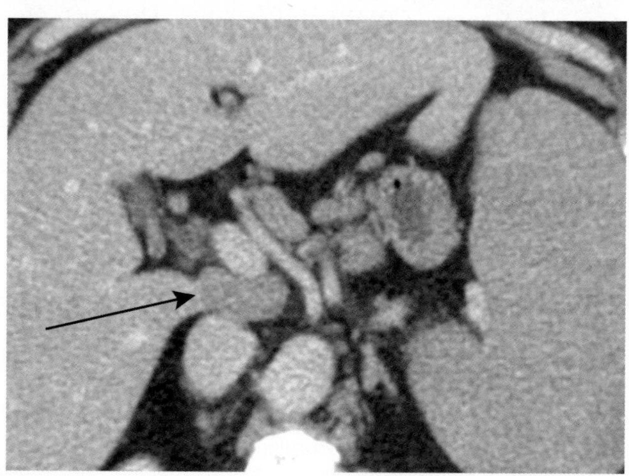

FIGURE 30.6. Axial contrast-enhanced computed tomography. An enlarged portacaval lymph node (*black arrow*) in a patient with Hodgkin lymphoma.

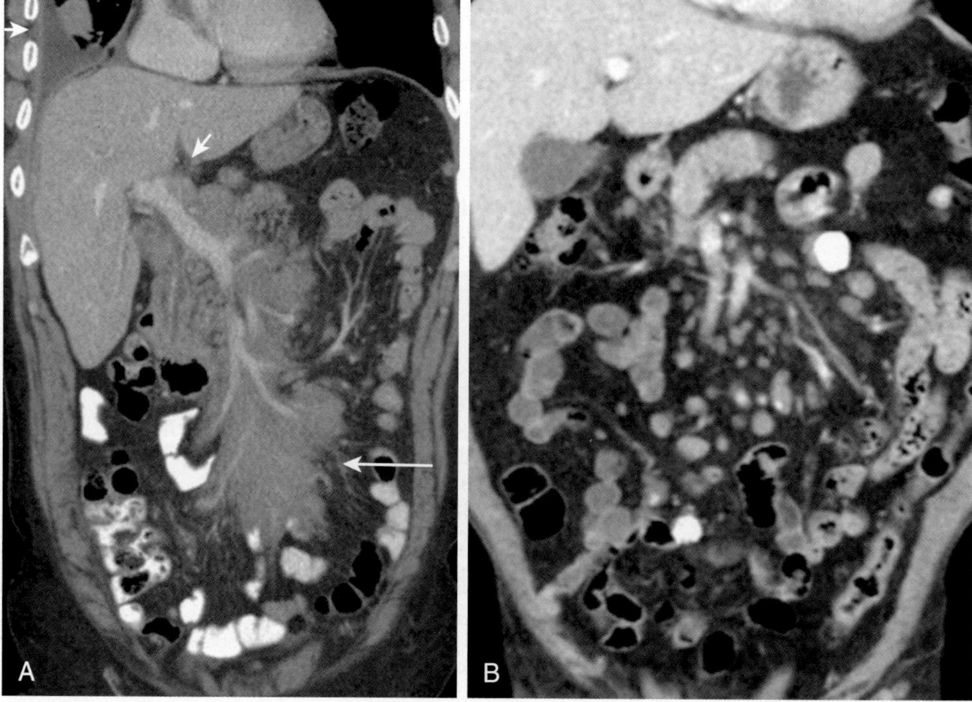

FIGURE 30.7. **A**, Coronal reformatted computed tomography scan demonstrates massive lymphomatous involvement of the mesentery (*long arrow*) with accompanying nodal enlargement in the porta hepatis (*short arrow*). **B**, Multiple discrete minimally enlarged mesenteric lymph nodes and a misty mesentery in a different patient with non-Hodgkin lymphoma.

lymphoma occurs owing to spread of lymph node disease into adjacent structures and organs or as part of widespread disease. Although the latter is an adverse prognostic factor in the IPI,[13] stage IE or IIE DLBCL does not have as poor a prognosis as stage IV disease unless it arises in the testis. There has been a marked increase in incidence of extranodal NHL, especially in the GI tract and CNS. Visceral lymphoma can mimic many other disease entities, and it is important to recognize its protean radiologic appearances.

FDG-PET is generally more sensitive than CT in the staging of extranodal disease, largely because of its ability to demonstrate bone marrow involvement.[17] FDG-PET/CT is also more sensitive than CT in identifying organ involvement, reaching sensitivities of up to 85%, with only 37% sensitivity for CT (Fig. 30.3). Use of PET or PET/CT can result in upstaging in up to 40% of cases. However, in some instances of low-grade NHL, CT is more sensitive.

Thorax

Secondary involvement of the pulmonary parenchyma in HL is most commonly by direct invasion from involved hilar or mediastinal nodes. On chest radiography, lung parenchymal involvement is seen three times more frequently in HL (12%) than in NHL. Parenchymal involvement in HL is almost invariably accompanied by intrathoracic adenopathy unless there has been prior mediastinal irradiation, whereas in NHL pulmonary or pleural lesions occur in isolation in up to 50% of cases. The radiographic changes in both HL and NHL are extremely varied. The most common pattern is one or more discrete nodules resembling primary or metastatic carcinoma, which may cavitate (Fig. 30.8). Primary (or isolated) pulmonary lymphoma is uncommon (1% of all extranodal presentations) and is usually attributed to NHL, particularly low-grade B-cell lymphomas such as MALT-type lymphomas, with DLBCL accounting for the remaining 15% to 20%. MALT type lymphomas are often indolent with large nodules, or with consolidation that is often stable over time. DLBCL is more aggressive, with well-recognized rapid growth and cavitation. The diverse appearances of pulmonary lymphoma provide a particular diagnostic challenge because many of these patients have other reasons for developing lung disease.

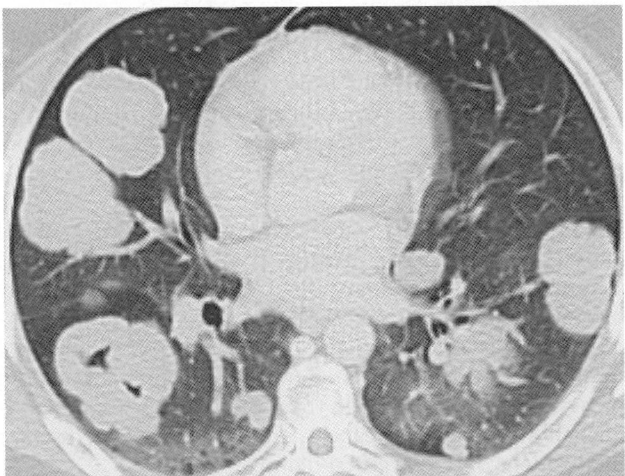

FIGURE 30.8. Axial computed tomography of the chest in a patient with posttransplant lymphoproliferative disorder demonstrates multiple nodules of varying sizes.

Pleural effusions are nearly always accompanied by mediastinal lymph node enlargement and, by CT, are present in over 50% of cases with mediastinal nodal disease (Fig. 30.4B). Most effusions are unilateral exudates from venous or lymphatic obstruction rather than direct neoplastic involvement.[24] Chest wall involvement in HL is usually as a result of direct extension from an anterior mediastinal mass. Less commonly, NHL may arise in the thoracic wall. Bony destruction is relatively uncommon. Pericardial effusions are seen on CT in 6% of patients with HL at presentation and are associated with coexistent bulky mediastinal adenopathy abutting the pericardium. Intracardiac masses can occur with T-cell lymphomas and aggressive lymphomas, especially in the setting of AIDS-related lymphomas (ARLs).

Thymic involvement occurs in 30% of patients with newly diagnosed HL[25] and is a particular feature of PMBL (Fig. 30.5). As the thymus is regarded as lymphoid tissue, thymic involvement does not impact staging. Cysts and calcification may be seen within the thymus at presentation or during follow-up on both CT and MRI.[26] Benign thymic rebound hyperplasia after completion of chemotherapy can be difficult to differentiate from recurrent disease.

KEY POINTS

- Secondary involvement of the lung parenchyma is seen three times more frequently in Hodgkin lymphoma (HL) than in non-Hodgkin lymphoma.
- Lung involvement in HL is almost invariably associated with mediastinal lymphadenopathy.
- Most primary low-grade lymphomas of the lung are MALT or bronchus-associated lymphoid tissue (BALT) tumors.

Primary breast lymphoma is rare, accounting for less than 1% of all breast tumors and approximately 2% of all lymphomas. Masses are usually solitary, but synchronous bilateral disease and metachronous contralateral disease have been described. In secondary lymphoma, there may be multiple masses with associated large-volume axillary adenopathy. Breast implant–associated anaplastic large cell lymphoma is a new provisional entity that presents as recurrent seroma accumulation within the capsule surrounding both saline and silicone implants.[6]

Abdomen

Spleen and Liver. The spleen is involved in approximately 30% of patients with HL, usually with nodal disease above and below the diaphragm. The spleen is regarded as a lymph node for the purposes of staging, but an enlarged spleen is not a reliable indicator of disease in HL. Cross-sectional imaging is unreliable in the detection of splenic involvement because infiltration is usually microscopic. Occasionally, focal splenic nodules larger than 1 cm are seen on cross-sectional imaging (Fig. 30.9). However, the failure of imaging to detect splenic infiltration in HL is now of less

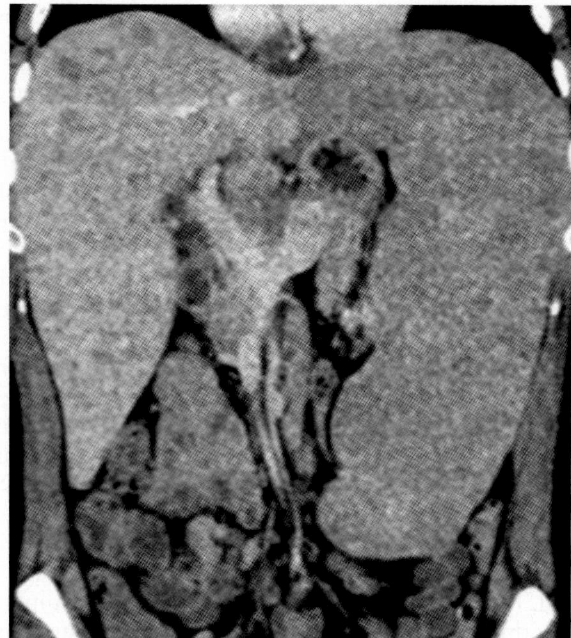

FIGURE 30.9. Coronal contrast-enhanced computed tomography in a patient with non-Hodgkin lymphoma demonstrates massive splenomegaly and focal hepatic and splenic nodules.

clinical importance, because patients with early-stage disease and occult splenic infiltration will receive multiagent chemotherapy, and because involvement is well shown with FDG-PET/CT.[18,27]

Up to 40% of patients with NHL have splenic involvement at some stage. It is a particular feature of MCL and splenic marginal zone lymphoma, where massive splenomegaly can occur. Primary splenic lymphoma usually presents as a mass or masses rather than splenomegaly alone, and miliary nodules may be seen. The presence of splenomegaly generally indicates diffuse infiltration, and infarction is a frequent complication. Splenomegaly is present if the craniocaudal length of the spleen at CT is 13 cm or more.

In HL, approximately 5% of patients have hepatic involvement at presentation, nearly always with accompanying splenic involvement. In NHL, approximately 15% of patients have hepatic infiltration, although the incidence is higher in the pediatric population. Primary lymphoma of the liver, indistinguishable radiologically from other forms of hepatic malignancy, is extremely rare.

As with splenic disease, hepatic lymphoma usually takes the form of microscopic infiltration around the portal triads, and detection by cross-sectional imaging is usually difficult, although periportal low attenuation may be seen at CT.[15] The presence of hepatomegaly suggests infiltration. Larger foci of involvement are seen in only 5% to 10% of patients and resemble metastatic disease from other sources (Fig. 30.9).

KEY POINTS Spleen and Liver Involvement

- In 10% of Hodgkin lymphomas (HLs), the spleen is the only site of subdiaphragmatic disease.
- An enlarged spleen is not a reliable indicator of disease in HL.
- Liver involvement is almost invariably associated with splenic infiltration.
- Only 5% to 10% of patients with liver disease have focal lesions detectable on cross-sectional imaging, resembling metastases.
- Enlargement of the liver is a strong indicator of lymphomatous infiltration.

The GI tract is the most common site of primary extranodal lymphoma, constituting approximately 1% of GI tumors and being the initial site of involvement in 5% to 10% of adult patients. Primary GI lymphoma is usually unifocal. Secondary involvement is common because of the frequent origin of lymphoma in the mesenteric or retroperitoneal nodes. Typically, multiple sites are involved. In both the primary and the secondary forms, the stomach is the most commonly involved organ (50%), followed by the small bowel (35%), large bowel (15%), and esophagus (<1%). In children, the disease is almost exclusively ileocecal.

Primary lymphoma of the stomach accounts for approximately 2% to 5% of gastric tumors, commonly appearing radiologically as multiple nodules, some with central ulceration; a large fungating lesion; diffuse infiltration with marked mural thickening, sometimes with extension into the duodenum; and localized polypoid forms.[28] A rare pattern is gastric rugal hypertrophy, similar to the pattern seen in hypertrophic gastritis. CT often shows extensive gastric wall thickening, as well as associated nodal disease (Fig. 30.10A). Spread into adjacent organs is variable. Gastric MALT lymphomas are usually localized at diagnosis and often result in minimal gastric mural thickening, which may not be recognizable even with dedicated CT studies, but which can be recognized with endoscopic ultrasound.[29] The European Society of Medical Oncology recommends a staging system that considers the depth of mural invasion, as this better correlates with prognosis.[30] Multiorgan involvement occurs in up to 25% of patients, so extensive imaging for staging may be necessary.[31]

Lymphoma accounts for up to 50% of all primary tumors of the small bowel, occurring most frequently in the terminal ileum and becoming less frequent proximally. Mural thickening results in constriction of segments of bowel with obstructive symptoms, which are common at presentation (Fig. 30.10B). Alternating areas of dilatation and constriction are the most common manifestations. Occasionally, multiple submucosal nodules or polyps of varying size are seen, predominantly in the terminal ileum. This form is prone to intussusception (usually ileocecal or ileoileal).

Primary lymphoma accounts for only 0.05% of all colonic neoplasms and usually involves the cecum and rectum, whereas secondary involvement is usually widely distributed and multicentric. The most common manifestation is a diffuse or segmental distribution of submucosal nodules 0.2 to 2 cm in diameter. Focal exophytic polypoid masses can be seen, often in the cecum, which are indistinguishable from colonic cancer, unless there is concomitant involvement of the terminal ileum.

Primary pancreatic lymphoma usually results in a solitary mass lesion or diffuse infiltration and is extremely rare, accounting for only 1.3% of all cases of pancreatic

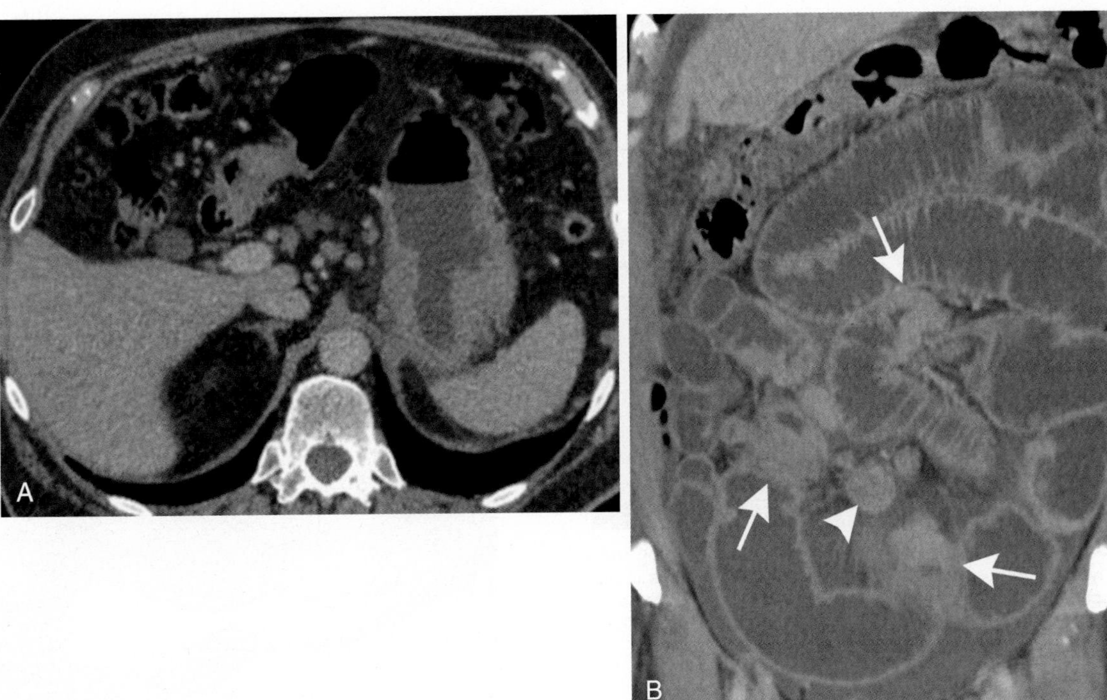

Figure 30.10. **A**, Diffuse large B-cell lymphoma of the stomach. There is marked circumferential gastric mural thickening of the fundus of the stomach extending into the proximal greater and lesser curves with multiple pathologic gastrohepatic lymph nodes. **B**, Coronal reformatted computed tomography scan demonstrates widespread small bowel lymphoma with multiple areas of mural thickening causing partial obstruction (*arrows*) and accompanying mesenteric lymph node enlargement (*arrowhead*).

malignancy and 2% of patients with NHL. Secondary pancreatic involvement is most commonly attributed to direct infiltration from adjacent nodal masses and may be focal or massive (Fig. 30.11).

Key Points Gastrointestinal Tract

- The stomach is the most frequent site of gastrointestinal lymphoma, which may be primary or secondary.
- Lymphoma accounts for up to 50% of all primary tumors of the small bowel and is multifocal in 50% of cases.
- Involvement of the colon and rectum accounts for only 0.5% of colonic neoplasms.

Genitourinary Tract

Although the genitourinary tract is infrequently involved at the time of presentation, in end-stage disease more than 50% of cases will have involvement of some part of it. The testicle is the most commonly involved organ, followed by the kidney and perirenal space. Involvement of the bladder, prostate, uterus, vagina, and ovaries is rare.

Close to 90% of renal cases are attributed to high-grade NHL (DLBCL, BL). In more than 40% of patients, the disease occurs at the time of recurrence only, and renal involvement is seen at staging CT in under 5% of cases.[32] The most frequent pattern of disease is multiple masses (60%),[33] followed by solitary masses (10%–20%) and direct infiltration from the retroperitoneum into the renal hilum and sinus (25%). In over 50% of cases, there is no accompanying retroperitoneal lymph node enlargement on CT.[33]

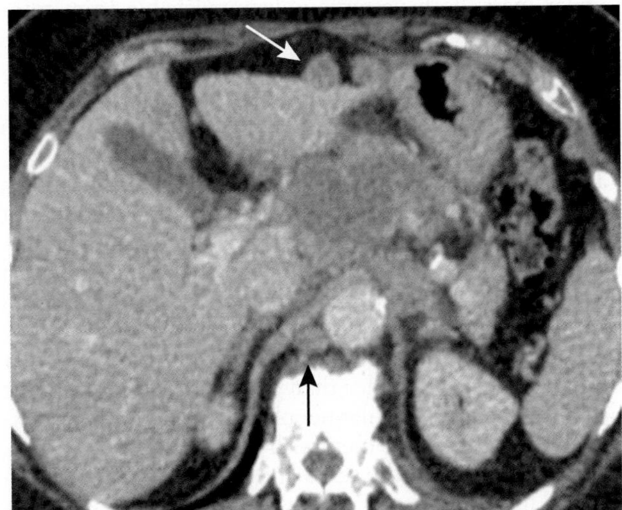

Figure 30.11. Contrast-enhanced axial computed tomography in a patient with diffuse large B cell lymphoma of the pancreas. An irregular, poorly defined relatively hypodense mass infiltrates the head and body of the pancreas. Notice peritoneal deposits (*white arrow*) and a pathologic retrocrural lymph node (*black arrow*).

Frequently, a soft tissue mass is seen in the perirenal space, occasionally encasing the kidney, without evidence on CT of invasion of the parenchyma. Diffuse infiltration of the kidneys with global renal enlargement is a rare manifestation. The appearance after intravenous contrast medium injection is variable, but usually homogeneous hypoenhancing tissue replaces the normal enhancing parenchyma (Fig. 30.12). A particularly rare form of disease is isolated periureteric lymphoma, described in both NHL and HL.

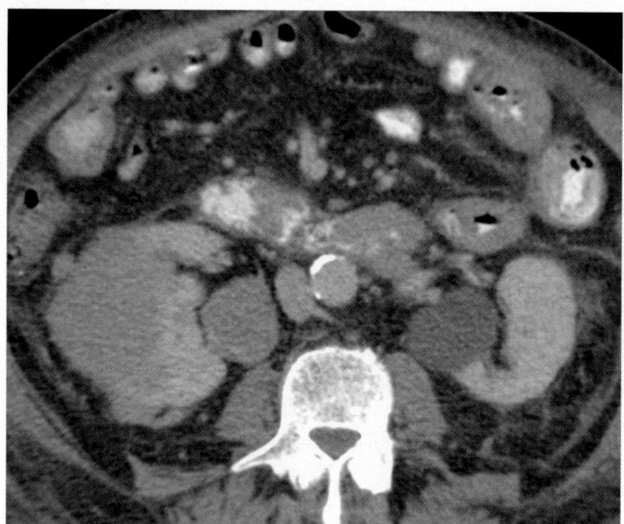

FIGURE 30.12. Axial contrast-enhanced computed tomography scan shows lymphomatous infiltration of the right kidney. There is also a discrete nodule in the perinephric space laterally and plaque-like infiltration of the space posteriorly. Notice also multifocal small bowel involvement in this patient with non-Hodgkin lymphoma.

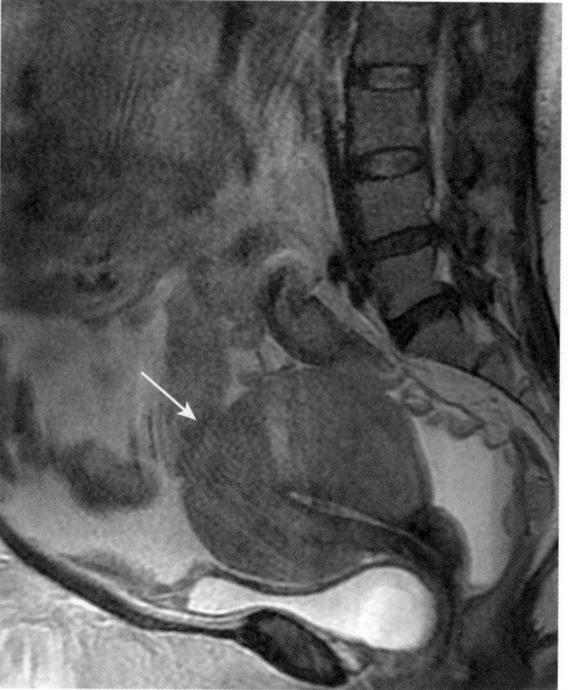

FIGURE 30.13. Lymphoma of the uterine corpus. Sagittal T2-weighted magnetic resonance imaging scan shows global enlargement of the corpus (*arrow*) with uniform intermediate T2 signal replacing the normal low–signal intensity myometrium.

Primary lymphoma of the bladder is extremely rare, although secondary lymphoma of the bladder is found in 10% to 15% of patients with lymphoma at autopsy. The appearances on CT and MRI are nonspecific, with either diffuse widespread thickening of the bladder wall or a large nodular mass, both patterns indistinguishable from transitional cell carcinoma. Indolent MALT type lymphomas are recognized in elderly women, often with a history of frequent cystitis.

Renal excretion of FGD limits the utility of PET/CT in the diagnosis of renal tract lymphoma.

Primary prostatic lymphoma carries a poor prognosis. In the majority of cases, there is diffuse infiltration throughout the prostate and periprostatic tissue. Secondary involvement of the gland is far more common; direct extension into the prostate from pelvic lymph nodes is often seen in very advanced disease.

Testicular lymphoma is the most common testicular tumor in individuals older than age 60 years but accounts for only 5% of all testicular neoplasms. It is seen in approximately 1% to 2% of men with NHL. At presentation, 80% are localized to the testis and abdominopelvic lymph nodes. There is an association with lymphoma of Waldeyer's ring, the CNS, and skin. On ultrasound, the lesions usually have a nonspecific appearance, with focal areas of decreased echogenicity. A well-recognized pattern is a diffuse decrease in reflectivity of the entire testicle. Involvement is bilateral in 10% to 25% of cases.

In advanced, widespread lymphomatous disease, the female genital organs are frequently involved secondarily. Isolated lymphomatous involvement is rare. Tumors originate predominantly in the uterine cervix, and CT and MRI may demonstrate a large mass (Fig. 30.13). Involvement of the uterine body usually produces diffuse enlargement, often with a lobular contour similar to that of a fibroid, with relatively homogeneous signal intensity at MRI on all sequences despite the large tumor size, with preservation of the epithelium (Fig. 30.13).[34] Similarly, primary lymphoma of the cervix and/or vagina is characterized by a large, exophytic mass. Ovarian lymphoma is less common and carries a poorer prognosis because tumors are usually more advanced at the time of discovery. As with primary epithelial ovarian carcinoma, involvement is often bilateral and the appearances on cross-sectional imaging are identical. DLBCL and BL are the commonest subtypes to affect the ovary.

KEY POINTS Genitourinary Tract

- Testis is the most frequent site of involvement of the genitourinary tract with lymphoma, although it accounts for only 5% of all testicular tumors.
- Lymphomatous involvement of the kidneys is not usually associated with renal impairment.
- Primary lymphoma of the prostate carries a poor prognosis, whereas primary lymphoma of the bladder has a good prognosis.
- Primary lymphoma of the female genital tract is rare and best demonstrated on magnetic resonance imaging.

Primary adrenal lymphoma is rare, usually occurring in men older than age 60 years. Secondary involvement of the adrenal glands is usually demonstrated on routine abdominal CT for staging (where it is seen in ≤6% of cases of NHL), although adrenal insufficiency is extremely rare. Involvement is usually bilateral and indistinguishable from metastases, although it is readily distinguishable from adenomas.

Central Nervous System

Primary CNS lymphoma (PCNSL) is initially localized to the CNS. It occurs almost exclusively within the brain rather than the spinal cord and presents most frequently between the fourth and the sixth decades, with a separate peak in the first decade of life. Nearly all PCNSLs are DLBCL. The marked increase in incidence seen in the 1990s as a consequence of AIDS has now started to reverse with the advent of cART.[35] On CT or MRI, more than 50% of lesions occur within the cerebral white matter, close to or within the corpus callosum (Fig. 30.14). Most occur about the ependymal surface of the ventricles. A butterfly distribution with spread across the corpus callosum is characteristic.[36] In approximately 15% of cases, the deep cortical gray matter of the basal ganglia and thalamus are involved. In 10%, lymphoma develops in the posterior fossa and is multifocal in 20%. In AIDS-related PCNSL, multifocality is much more common, being seen in up to 50% of cases. At CT, increased density is typical on unenhanced CT with homogeneous enhancement after intravenous injection of contrast medium; only approximately 10% of lesions do not enhance.[36] Calcification is very rare, and surrounding vasogenic edema relatively mild.[36] On MRI, the typical appearance is of a hyper- or isointense tumor mass, relative to the surrounding normal tissue on T2-weighted (T2W) sequences.[37] Restricted diffusion is seen with DWI, and there is usually uniform enhancement after injection of gadolinium-based contrast (Fig. 30.14). Ring enhancement can be a feature of AIDS-related PCNSL. PCNSL is usually markedly FDG-avid, which can aid in the differential diagnosis from infective entities such as toxoplasmosis.

Secondary cerebral involvement occurs in 10% to 15% of patients with NHL at some time during the course of their disease. Patients with testicular, orbital, or paranasal sinus disease are at increased risk, as are those with multiple sites of extranodal disease. Secondary cerebral involvement is so rare in HL that a space-occupying lesion in the brain of a patient with known HL should prompt a second diagnosis. Secondary lymphoma is distinguishable from the primary form to some extent by its propensity to involve the extracerebral spaces (epidural, subdural, and subarachnoid; Fig. 30.15A) and the spinal epidural and subarachnoid spaces. MRI typically shows extracerebral plaquelike tumor deposits in the subdural or epidural spaces, made more obvious on 'gadolinium-based contrast-enhanced T1-weighted (T1W) images. CT is less sensitive, not only in the detection of these extracerebral lesions but also in demonstrating leptomeningeal deposits around the cranial nerves,[38] particularly when resulting in cranial nerve palsies.

Gadolinium-enhanced MRI is relatively sensitive in demonstrating spinal leptomeningeal cord and nerve root involvement. Epidural extension of tumor into the spinal canal from a paravertebral nodal mass may also be elegantly demonstrated on MRI (Fig. 30.15B). Compression of the spinal cord or cauda equina attributed to lymphoma is a late manifestation of HL, but it is often an earlier manifestation of NHL. In both conditions, the usual cause is extension of nodal disease through the intervertebral foramina. Tumor compresses the dura, but the latter usually acts as an effective barrier to the intrathecal spread of tumor.

NHL is the most common primary orbital malignancy in adults, accounting for 10% to 15% of orbital masses and approximately 5% of all primary extranodal NHLs. *Primary orbital* lymphomas occur most commonly in patients aged 40 to 70 years. They can arise from the conjunctiva, eyelids, lacrimal glands, or retrobulbar tissues. Up to 50% will be found to have an extra-CNS primary site of origin. *Secondary* orbital involvement occurs in approximately 3% to 5% of NHL. Involvement of the lacrimal glands is bilateral in over 20% of cases. Involvement of the eyelids

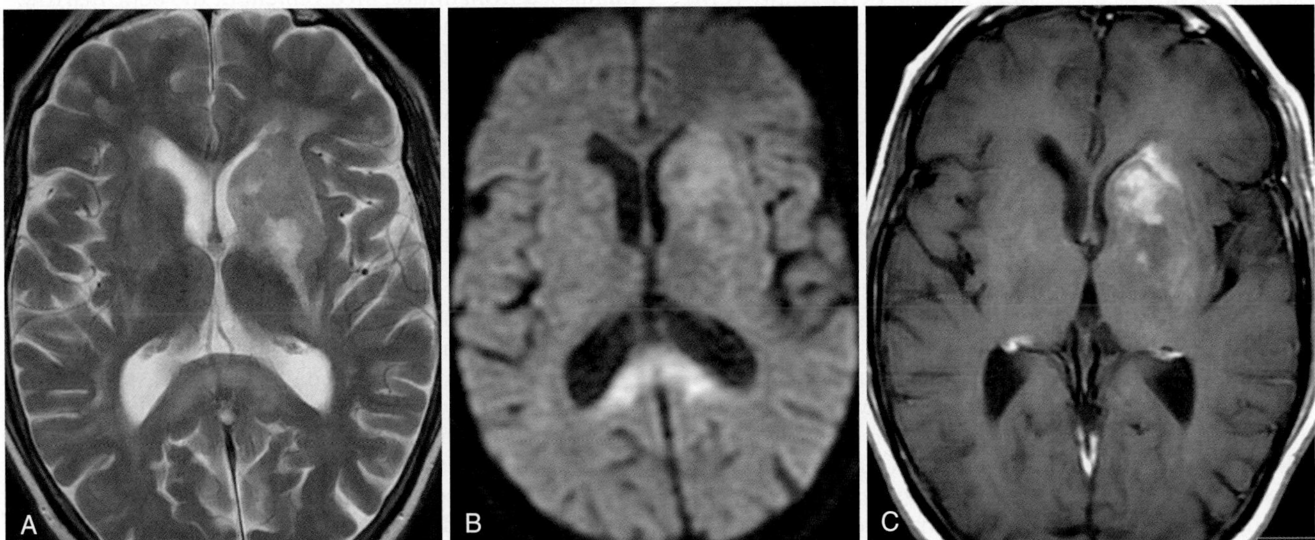

FIGURE 30.14. Primary central nervous system lymphoma. **A**, Axial T2-weighted magnetic resonance imaging scan. **B**, Axial high b-value diffusion-weighted image. **C**, Axial T1-weighted scan after intravenous contrast at a slightly lower level. There is an intermediate–signal intensity mass in the caudate nucleus extending into the internal capsule and abutting the left lateral ventricle with minimal vasogenic edema. Notice restricted diffusion in the mass and also in the splenium of the corpus callosum. After intravenous contrast, there is marked heterogeneous enhancement of the mass.

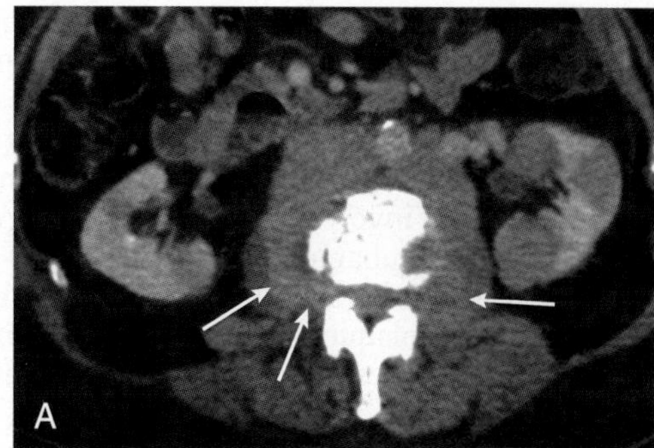

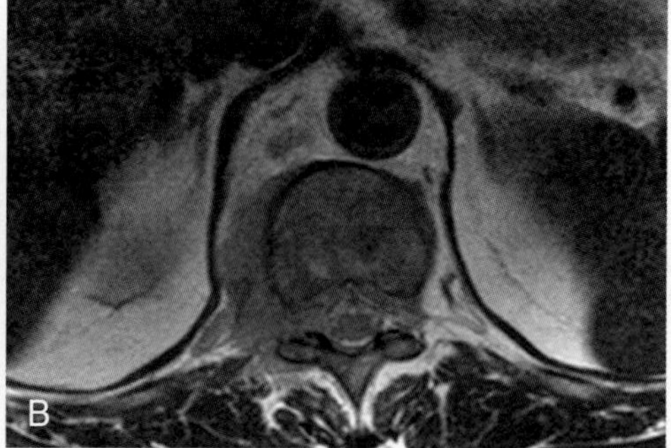

FIGURE 30.15. **A**, Axial contrast-enhanced CT scan demonstrates a large enhancing retroperitoneal paraspinal mass extending posteriorly into the spinal canal through both intervertebral foramina (*arrows*). **B**, Axial T2-weighted magnetic resonance imaging scan in a different patient clearly demonstrates lymphomatous infiltration from the right retrocrural region into the spinal canal.

and subconjunctival spaces is readily assessed on clinical examination, whereas MRI best depicts the presence and extent of any intracranial extension.

KEY POINTS Central Nervous System

- Primary central nervous system lymphoma almost exclusively involves the cerebral white matter.
- Secondary lymphoma preferentially involves the extracerebral spaces and the spinal epidural and subarachnoid spaces.
- Non-Hodgkin lymphoma is the most common primary orbital malignancy in adults.

True extranodal involvement of sites in the *head and neck* in HL is very rare. In NHL, 10% of patients present with extranodal head and neck involvement, and NHL accounts for approximately 5% of head and neck malignancies. Waldeyer's ring is the most common site of disease, and there is a pronounced link with involvement of the gut, which may be synchronous or metachronous. A diagnosis of NHL is suggested by circumferential involvement or multifocality (see Fig. 30.2). Intense FGD avidity is the norm. Middle-aged women are most often affected.

NHL accounts for 8% of tumors of the paranasal sinuses. In the West, the disease affects middle-aged men, and the maxillary sinus is most commonly involved, nearly always with DLBCL, whereas the aggressive T-cell type affects younger Asian patients and is linked to EBV. These tumors are aggressive and can transgress normal anatomic barriers, as a consequence of which intracranial spread through the base of the skull is seen in up to 40% of cases. MRI is the preferred imaging technique. Fat-suppressed T1W sequences pre- and postintravenous gadolinium-based contrast medium are most helpful.

NHL accounts for 2% to 5% of malignant tumors of the thyroid.[39] There is an association with Hashimoto disease, so the disease tends to occur in women in their 60s with MALT types. However, DLBCL also occurs, and these patients present with a rapidly growing mass involving adjacent structures causing obstructive symptoms. On CT, these masses usually have a lower attenuation than the normal gland, and peripheral enhancement can be seen after administration of intravenous contrast. PET/CT can exclude the presence of synchronous disease elsewhere.

KEY POINTS Head and Neck

- Extranodal non-Hodgkin lymphoma (NHL) accounts for approximately 5% of all head and neck cancers.
- Waldeyer's ring is the most common site of head and neck lymphoma.
- NHL accounts for up to 5% of all malignant thyroid tumors.

Bone and Bone Marrow

Skeletal involvement may occur in both HL and NHL. Because the bone marrow is an integral part of the reticuloendothelial system, lymphomas may arise within the marrow as a true primary disease. More often, however, the marrow is involved as part of a disseminated process (stage IV disease). Bone and bone marrow are important sites of disease relapse. Involvement of osseous bone does not necessarily imply bone marrow involvement, and skeletal radiography has no predictive value in determining marrow involvement. Infiltration of bone may also occur by direct invasion from adjacent soft tissue masses. This is designated with the suffix "E" added to the appropriate stage. For the purposes of clarity, involvement of the bone is distinguished from diffuse involvement of the bone marrow.

Primary lymphoma of bone is almost exclusively due to NHL. The criteria for the diagnosis of primary lymphoma require that only a single bone is involved, there is unequivocal histologic evidence of lymphoma, other disease is limited to regional areas at the time of diagnosis, and the primary tumor precedes metastasis by at least 6 months. Most patients present in their 50s and 60s. Males are affected more often than females. Secondary involvement of bones is present in 5% to 6% of patients with NHL but is more common in children with NHL.[15] Systemic (secondary) NHL involves the axial skeleton more frequently than the appendicular skeleton.

Primary NHL of bone is radiologically indistinguishable from secondary lymphoma or other bone tumors. However, whereas bone lesions in NHL (primary or secondary) are usually permeative osteolytic (77%) or mixed lytic/sclerotic (16%), bony involvement in HL typically gives a sclerotic or mixed picture (86%) and is infrequently lytic. In HL, soft tissue disease typically may involve adjacent bones. A classic finding is the sclerotic ivory vertebra. MRI is the imaging modality of choice for staging and follow-up[40] (Fig. 30.16). Bone scintigraphy is of limited usefulness

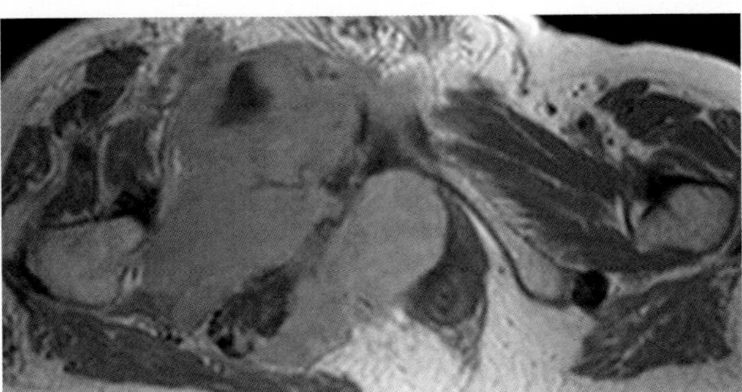

FIGURE 30.16. Axial T1-weighted magnetic resonance imaging scan after intravenous contrast shows an enormous lymphomatous mass arising from the right inferior pubic ramus infiltrating the adjacent musculature, the sciatic notch and the pelvic floor with distortion and displacement of the urethra and introitus.

compared with FDG-PET or PET/CT, and there is also some evidence that FDG-PET can demonstrate response to treatment earlier and more accurately than conventional modalities including MRI.[41]

Involvement of the bone marrow indicates stage IV disease. It is rare at presentation in HL but is found in 20% to 40% of patients with NHL and is associated with a worse prognosis than involvement of the liver, lung, or osseous bone. During the course of HL, marrow involvement occurs in 5% to 15% of patients. Bone marrow biopsies may not be indicated as part of the initial staging of early-stage HL, but the high incidence in NHL justifies its use as a staging procedure in many cases. Marrow involvement in FL is typically paratrabecular, whereas in other subtypes it is more likely to be diffuse.

MRI is extremely sensitive in the demonstration of bone marrow involvement (Fig. 30.17). Tumor infiltration is of low signal on T1W sequences and high signal intensity on short tau inversion recovery. T1W spin echo sequences are the most sensitive.[42] MRI can upstage as many as 33% of patients with negative iliac crest biopsies (Fig. 30.17).

The accuracy of PET/CT is subtype-dependent.[43] Thus, in HL, bone marrow biopsy is not indicated if staging PET/CT is negative.[44] Similarly in DLBCL, it is not required if there is obvious PET/CT positivity.[45] False-negative PET findings occur with indolent lymphoma, often PET-negative elsewhere, or with microscopic infiltration, whereas reactive marrow hyperplasia can lower specificity.[43]

KEY POINTS Bone and Bone Marrow

- Primary lymphoma of bone accounts for only 1% of all cases of non-Hodgkin lymphoma (NHL); secondary involvement is seen in 5%–6% of cases.
- Secondary bone involvement is seen in 20% of patients with Hodgkin lymphoma (HL). Primary HL of bone is extremely rare.
- In HL, soft tissue disease may invade adjacent bone, but this is rare in NHL.
- Bone marrow involvement indicates stage IV disease and is present in 20%–40% of patients with NHL at presentation.
- Bone marrow biopsy in NHL increases the stage of disease in up to 30% of cases (usually from stage III to stage IV).
- In HL, bone marrow involvement occurs in 5%–15% of patients during the course of disease.

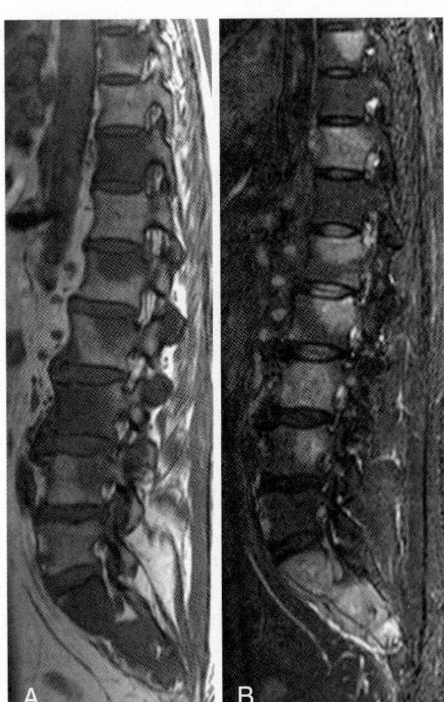

FIGURE 30.17. Bone marrow involvement of the spine. Sagittal T1-weighted (**A**) and sagittal short tau inversion recovery (**B**) magnetic resonance imaging sequences show multiple foci of infiltration with low T1 and high T2 signal with excellent contrast between tumor and surrounding fatty marrow.

- Although positron emission tomography/computed tomography is more sensitive than contrast-enhanced computed tomography or bone scintigraphy, false-negative examinations occur with microscopic infiltration and indolent lymphomas.

LYMPHOMA IN THE IMMUNOCOMPROMISED

The WHO classification recognizes four broad groupings associated with an increased incidence of lymphoma and lymphoproliferative disorders: primary immunodeficiency syndromes, lymphomas associated with HIV infection, posttransplant lymphoproliferative disorders (PTLDs), and other iatrogenic immunodeficiency-associated lymphoproliferative disorders. The development of lymphoma in these settings appears to be largely related to defective immune surveillance, with or without chronic antigenic stimulation.

Acquired Immunodeficiency Syndrome–Related Lymphomas

The incidence of all subtypes of NHL is increased 60- to 200-fold in patients with HIV. Although the risk of ARL has decreased in the cART era, it is now more often the first AIDS-defining illness, in up to 10% of patients. The incidence of HL is increased up to eightfold and is increasing further in the cART era. Various histologic subtypes of

NHL are seen: those occurring in the normal population (BL, DLBCL, and PCNSL), and others occurring much more frequently in the HIV population (e.g., primary effusion lymphoma and plasmablastic lymphoma of the oral cavity). EBV positivity occurs in up to 70%, depending on the precise morphologic variant; PCNSL is associated with EBV in over 90% of cases, as is HIV-related HL.

Most ARL are aggressive, presenting with advanced stage, bulky disease, and a marked propensity to involve extranodal sites, especially the GI tract, CNS (less frequent with the advent of HAART), liver, and bone marrow. Multiple sites of extranodal involvement are seen in over 75% of cases. Peripheral lymph node enlargement was seen in only 30% before the introduction of cART but is now seen at presentation in up to 50% of patients. In the chest, NHL is usually extranodal; pleural effusion and lung disease are common, often with nodules, and acinar and interstitial opacities. There is a wide differential diagnosis, especially mycobacterial infection.[46] Within the abdomen, the GI tract, lower genitourinary tract, and major viscera are commonly involved. Regarding PCNSL, features such as rim enhancement and multifocality are seen more often than in the immunocompetent population. The differential diagnosis includes cerebral toxoplasmosis, although the location of PCNSL in the deep white matter is suggestive. Quantitative FDG-PET/CT uptake may help in the differentiation of PCNSL, toxoplasmosis, and progressive multifocal leucoencephalopathy, being higher in the former.[47] Magnetic resonance spectroscopy and ^{201}thallium single-photon emission CT may also be useful.[48]

Posttransplant Lymphoproliferative Disorders

PTLD occurs in 2% to 4% of solid organ transplant recipients, depending on the type of transplant, with the lowest frequency being seen in renal transplant recipients (1%). Marrow allograft recipients have a low risk (<1%). Most appear to represent EBV-induced monoclonal or, more rarely, polyclonal B-cell or T-cell proliferation in a setting of reduced immune surveillance. The clinical features are variable, correlating with the type of allograft and type of immunosuppression. In all cases, extranodal disease is common. In patients receiving azathioprine, the allograft itself and the CNS are often involved, whereas in patients receiving cyclosporin A the GI tract is affected more often. The bone marrow, liver, and lung are frequently involved. In the lung, pulmonary nodules or airspace opacity and pleural effusions are common, with or without mediastinal adenopathy (Fig. 30.8). Abdominal PTLD is characterized by frequent extranodal disease. Multiple segments of bowel may be affected along with the allograft itself.[49]

KEY POINTS Lymphoma in the Immunocompromised

- Lymphomas associated with human immunodeficiency virus have a propensity to involve extranodal sites (especially the gastrointestinal tract, central nervous system, liver, and bone marrow).
- Most tumors are aggressive, with advanced-stage bulky disease.
- Posttransplant lymphoproliferative disorder occurs in 2% to 4% of solid organ and 1% of marrow allograft recipients and typically causes solitary or multiple lung nodules. In the abdomen, this disorder is characterized by involvement of the gastrointestinal tract and liver.

THE RADIOLOGIST'S REPORT

Lymph Nodes

- Enumerate the number of nodal regions involved.
- Bidimensional measurement of a marker lymph node at each involved site.
- Presence or absence of bulky disease (>10 cm).
- In cases of follicular lymphoma, presence of any single nodes with long-axis measurement >6 cm.
- Presence or absence of "E" lesions.

Extranodal Disease

- Major viscera: splenomegaly, focal lesions; hepatomegaly, focal lesions.
- Other viscera if involved.
- Lungs.
- Careful review areas: the bones and epidural spaces.

Local Complications of Disease

- Central venous occlusion.
- Hydronephrosis.

Conclusion

- Computed tomography stage.
- Presence or absence of adverse prognostic features (bulk disease, number of sites of extranodal disease).
- Suitable biopsy site.

TREATMENT

Hodgkin Lymphoma

There has been a dramatic improvement in survival from HL in the past 40 years, with mortality rates falling by over 50% since 1975. Current mortality rates are approximately 0.3/100,000 for both men and women. Early-stage disease has a 5-year survival rate of over 90%. The histologic subtype does not usually affect treatment decisions, except for NLPHL.

Patients with HL have traditionally been divided into two or three prognostic groups, each associated with a standard treatment strategy; but treatment has changed markedly in recent years with the development of more efficacious chemotherapy and with recognition of the late effects of radiotherapy. For many years, mantle radiotherapy for cervical disease was the treatment of choice. It included irradiation to the cervical, supraclavicular, axillary, and mediastinal nodes, down to the lower border of the T10 vertebral body. However, with the prolonged survival of most patients with HL, the long-term consequences of this treatment have become apparent, including a huge excess of breast cancer in women and thyroid cancer in men and women treated with mantle radiotherapy.[50] In patients with early-stage disease treated when they were younger than 50 years, the absolute excess mortality actually increases with time because of the increased incidence of cardiac disease and second tumors consequent upon treatment.[51] New chemotherapeutic regimens have, therefore, been developed with the aim of reducing toxicity while maintaining efficacy. Only in NLPHL, which commonly presents with stage I disease, would involved field radiotherapy or surgical excision alone be considered now. Both yield excellent results, with a long-term progression-free survival (PFS) rate of over 80%.

HL is chemosensitive, and chemotherapy with or without radiotherapy is used depending on whether disease is early-stage (with or without unfavorable factors) or late-stage. Precise definitions of prognostic groups vary in different centers, but, as a rule, early stages designated favorable (CS I, IIA, no bulk) can receive short-course combination chemotherapy with or without involved field radiotherapy. For early-stage HL, patients with masses over 7 cm have better outcomes if radiotherapy is given. Early stages designated unfavorable (CS IIB, bulk disease) usually require more intensive chemotherapy plus radiotherapy, and advanced-stage disease is managed with intensive chemotherapy with or without consolidation radiation to sites of bulk disease or a residual mass.

Duration and intensity of chemotherapy is increasingly response-adapted as assessed by PET/CT. The most common chemotherapy regimen is doxorubicin, bleomycin, vinblastine, and dacarbazine (ABVD). It is well tolerated, through bleomycin lung toxicity is an issue. Thus, if interim PET/CT demonstrates a good response, bleomycin may be omitted from subsequent cycles.[52] For patients with more advanced disease, 30% to 50% of patients treated with ABVD will relapse within 5 years. Therefore, intensified chemotherapy regimens are justified for poor-risk patients (CS IIB, III and IV) despite the increased toxicity, including the bleomycin, etoposide, adriamycin, cyclophosphamide, oncovin, procarbazine, and prednisolone (BEACOPP) regimen. The Stanford V protocol uses polypharmacy with low-dose small-field irradiation of all sites originally larger than 5 cm or to the spleen if it is clinically involved. However, regimens such as BEACOPP are highly toxic, and therefore trials such as the Risk-Adapted Therapy in Hodgkin Lymphoma (RATHL) trial have evaluated the use of interim PET/CT to escalate or deescalate treatment according to response.[52] Patients failing initial chemotherapy for advanced HL have a poor prognosis, but for relapsed or refractory HL salvage chemotherapy with high-dose treatment and autologous hemopoietic stem cell rescue (ASCT) is increasingly employed.[53]

In the last decade many novel biologic therapies have been developed that have activity against HL, for example, brentuximab vedotin, an anti-CD30 antibody conjugated with the antimicrotubule agent vedotin. This is efficacious in patients who relapse after ASCT and is recommended by the National Institute of Clinical Excellence (NICE) agency in the United Kingdom.[54,55]

Second Malignancies After Treatment for Hodgkin Lymphoma

Aside from the risk of cardiovascular disease, breast cancer, and thyroid cancer in survivors of HL treated with mantle radiotherapy, the most important long-term complication of treatment is the development of a second malignancy. The most common are acute myeloid leukemia (AML) and NHL (DLBCL or BL-like). AML usually develops 2 to 5 years after successful treatment. The risk of NHL is relatively low (2% for CHL) but increases after combined modality treatment. DLBCL can occur after NLPHL, and this may represent clonal expansion of the original malignancy because composite forms occur.

Non-Hodgkin Lymphoma

As indicated previously, the prognosis and, therefore, treatment of NHL varies markedly according to histologic subtype. FL is regarded as an indolent lymphoma. The 10-year overall survival rate for patients with FL is now over 70%. With time, FL may undergo histologic transformation, with increasing numbers of blast cells in the affected lymph node. Such transformation has a grave prognosis and may be a terminal event in up to 70% of cases.[56]

Before the monoclonal antibody era, 40% of patients with DLBCL were cured with anthracycline-based combination chemotherapy, and patients in the low-risk group (IPI 0 or 1) had an 87% CR rate with a 5-year survival rate greater than 70%, whereas patients in the high-risk group (IPI 4 or 5) had only a 25% 5-year survival.

Histologic subtype also determines when that treatment should start. For asymptomatic patients with FL, surveillance alone may be appropriate until symptoms develop or transformation supervenes. In contrast, patients presenting with DLBCL generally require treatment with multiagent anthracycline-containing chemotherapy immediately. Standard treatment for DLBCL now comprises cyclophosphamide, doxorubicin, vincristine, and prednisone (CHOP) chemotherapy combined with rituximab, a chimeric monoclonal antibody against CD20, which is expressed by over 95% of B-cell NHLs; this combination is referred to as CHOP-R. Most relapses occur within the first 2 years after treatment. Once relapse occurs, particularly if remission is short, further response to salvage chemotherapy, with or without immunotherapy, is difficult to sustain, and high-dose therapy, supported by ASCT because consolidation of second remission offers the best chance of cure. However, the development of novel targeted therapies has increased the number of options available to the patient with relapsed disease.

B-cell lymphomas express several surface antigens, against which antibodies have been raised. A number now have U.S. Food and Drug Administration and NICE approval. Rituximab, the best known, can be used as a single agent in indolent NHL, but is mostly used with chemotherapy, as in CHOP-R. For FL requiring chemotherapy, rituximab combined with bendamustine appears efficacious.[57]

Monoclonal antibodies can also be conjugated to radioactive isotopes to form radioimmunoconjugates, the antibody delivering the isotope to the tumor cells. The anti-CD20 antibody tositumomab combined with iodine-131 (Bexxar) has been used successfully to treat FL. It is a gamma emitter and can be used for imaging as well as treatment. Ibritumomab, combined with yttrium-90 (ibritumomab tiuxetan [Zevalin]) has also been used for FL. This beta emitter has higher energies and is better for larger tumors, as well as being safe to administer on an outpatient basis. Both drugs induce high response rates and improve PFS. However, recurrence remains a problem, and, increasingly, rituximab is being used to maintain remission, although development of rituximab-refractory disease is well-recognized.

Like HL, NHL are extremely radiosensitive. Radiotherapy still has a role in some MALT lymphomas and in rare instances of stage I or II FL, where regional or involved field radiotherapy may be curative. However, 80% of NHL are widespread at diagnosis, making primary radiotherapy impractical, although it is frequently used as consolidation, for palliative intent.

Experimental Therapies

Today, research is directed at the development of novel classes of therapeutic agents that target specific molecular and cellular pathways, such as the proteosome inhibitor bortezomib. Bortezomib is approved for use in MCL, and is also active in FL, with and without rituximab. Thalidomide and lenalidomide have antiangiogenic and immunomodulatory properties and have some activity in a number of indolent and aggressive lymphomas. Novel BCL2 inhibitors such as antisense oligonucleotides, which prevent BCL2-induced inhibition of apoptosis, are also generating considerable interest. One such inhibitor, venetoclax, has recently been shown to be an effective regimen for CLL when combined with ibrutinib, a Bruton's tyrosine kinase inhibitor.[58] Other classes of agents under development include histone deacetylase, protein kinase C, and other inhibitors, which can modulate cell proliferation, differentiation, and apoptosis.

KEY POINTS Treatment

- In Hodgkin lymphoma (HL), disease stage is the most important prognostic factor and determines the intensity and nature of treatment.
- HL is curable in the vast majority of cases.
- In non-Hodgkin lymphoma, the histologic subtype is the major determinant of treatment.
- Paradoxically, cure is most often achieved in the more aggressive large cell lymphomas.

SURVEILLANCE

The advent of FDG-PET/CT has resulted in a paradigm shift in response assessment in lymphoma, although cross-sectional imaging still plays a vital role, especially in non FDG-avid lymphomas, and most clinical trials still use CT.

Monitoring Response to Therapy

Achievement of a CR after treatment is the most important factor for prolonged survival in lymphoma, and final evaluation of response after completion of therapy is critical. Most centers assess patients approximately 1 month after completion of therapy, but a longer interval (6–8 weeks) is required if FDG-PET/CT is used.

An imaging CR is documented only when no abnormality is seen at the site of previously demonstrated disease. Assessment of response necessitates measurement of a number of marker lesions before and after therapy, especially for clinical trials. CT permits accurate reproducible measurements of well-defined masses, but there is significant interobserver variation for poorly defined masses.

Radiographic Predictors of Outcome

Many centers favor an interim CT scan after a few cycles of chemotherapy to confirm some response to treatment, but recently, numerous studies have shown that an interim FDG-PET/CT scan yields much more prognostic information, especially in HL. Early PET/CT in aggressive NHL is a more accurate predictor of PFS and overall survival than other prognostic indicators.[59,60] A similar association has been shown in patients with HL,[61,62] even after just one cycle of treatment[63] (Fig. 30.18). Thus, for HL, interim PET/CT is an integral part of response-adapted therapy. The RAPID trial demonstrated that patients with early-stage HL and a negative interim PET after three cycles of ABVD can avoid radiotherapy (though the impact on long-term survival is as yet unknown, and longer follow-up is needed).[64] Conversely, in advanced HL, interim PET can be used for deescalation if negative (through omission of bleomycin) or intensification if positive (through escalation to BEACOPP or similar).[52,65] However, for aggressive NHL, the existing data are heterogeneous, and therefore interim scans should be done only in large clinical trials, especially because there is evidence that the positive predictive value (PPV) of interim scans for NHL has diminished in the rituximab era.

Residual Masses and Functional Imaging

Though treated lymphomatous masses may resolve completely, residual sterile masses of fibrous tissue may persist in up to 40% to 50% of patients in clinical complete remission (CR) after treatment for HL and NHL. Before the advent of PET/CT, determination of the nature of the residual mass was a major challenge for the oncologic radiologist. Strategies included serial CT scans, MRI, and gallium scintigraphy. In recognition of this issue, an international workshop was convened to standardize response criteria for NHL.[66] The National Cancer Institute–sponsored International Working Group criteria (IWC), published in 1999, included the category CR_u (complete response, unconfirmed) to encompass those patients in whom there was clinical and

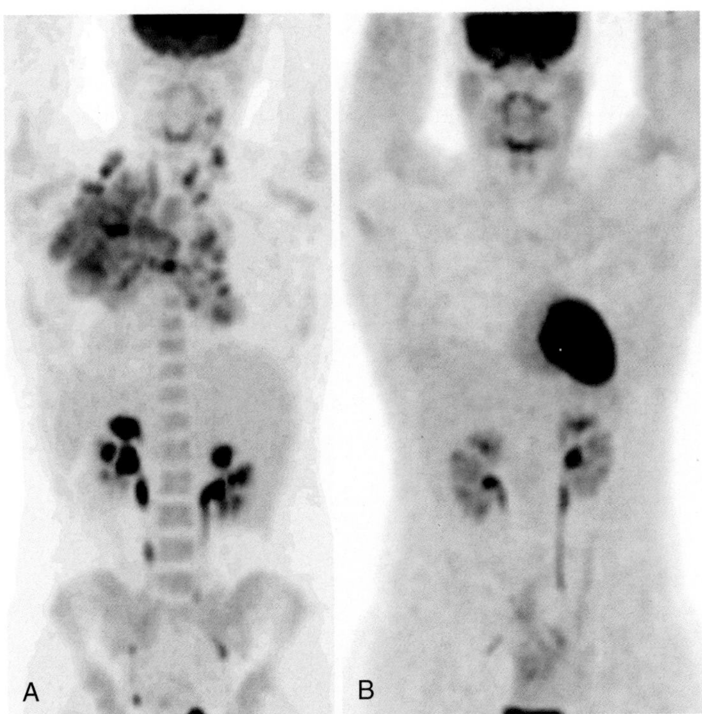

Figure 30.18. Coronal maximum intensity projection images from a 2-[^{18}F] fluoro-2-deoxy-D-glucose positron emission tomography scan before (**A**) and after (**B**) one cycle of doxorubicin, bleomycin, vinblastine, and dacarbazine chemotherapy in a patient with Hodgkin lymphoma. Multiple foci of abnormal tracer uptake in the neck, supraclavicular fossa, and mediastinum have resolved completely.

biological complete response with a persistent residual mass, greater than 1.5 cm maximum transverse diameter, but regressed by more than 75% of the sum of the products of greatest diameter.

However, numerous studies have subsequently shown that FDG-PET/CT has a very high PPV in the differentiation between active tumor and fibrosis (Fig. 30.19). Indeed, a positive PET/CT at the end of treatment has a high PPV for early relapse, even without a residual mass at CT.[67–69] There is evidence that the PPV of PET/CT may be lower in patients treated with rituximab.[70] Therefore, clinical correlation is essential when interpreting FDG-PET results.

Functional Imaging and Response Criteria

In the 2000s it became apparent that incorporation of end-of-treatment PET/CT results had a profound effect on response categorization. In one study, patients with a partial response by standard IWC who were PET-negative did as well as those who were in CR by IWC and IWC plus PET.[71] Thus, in 2007, an International Harmonization Project (IHP) was convened to revise the IWC to include PET/CT, bone marrow evaluation, and flow cytometry.[72] The IHP guidelines supported the use of PET/CT for end-of-therapy response assessment in DLBCL and HL, but not for other NHL. In the revised criteria, patients with residual PET-negative masses were assigned to the CR category, provided the mass was, or could have expected to have been, PET-positive before treatment. A partial response was assigned when there was residual FDG-PET positivity in at least one previously involved site.[73]

The Lugano Classification

The initial guidelines described earlier did not address a few key issues. There was no defined cutoff for measurable disease, nor a defined minimal size of a qualifying lesion. No set number of lesions was determined for follow-up. Finally, a 25% size increase in one lesion was used to denote progression, which, importantly, may be within measurement error.

In June 2011, the 11th International Conference on Malignant Lymphoma in Lugano, Switzerland held a workshop to improve staging and response criteria for HL and NHL. Subsequent workshops at the 12th International Conference on Malignant Lymphoma in 2013 culminated with the development of The Lugano Classification.[12] Under the Lugano Classification, PET/CT is the preferred imaging modality in determining nodal and extranodal target lesions for FDG-avid lymphomas such as HL, DLBCL, FL, and MCL. PET/CT is also the preferred method to assess bone marrow involvement over biopsy.

CT is the imaging modality of choice for non–FDG-avid lymphomas. In this setting, measurable disease is defined as lymph nodes with longest diameter greater than 1.5 cm or extranodal lesions greater than 1 cm in length. Up to six of the largest lesions are selected as target lesions for follow-up. The remaining lesions, as well as unmeasurable disease such as pleural effusions, are deemed nontarget lesions.[20]

PET/CT-based response evaluation uses the Five Point Scale or Deauville Criteria. The Five Point Scale was initially developed as an easily reproducible method of scoring treatment response based on FDG uptake of a lesion compared with reference organs.[20] This scale was devised by the First International Workshop on PET in

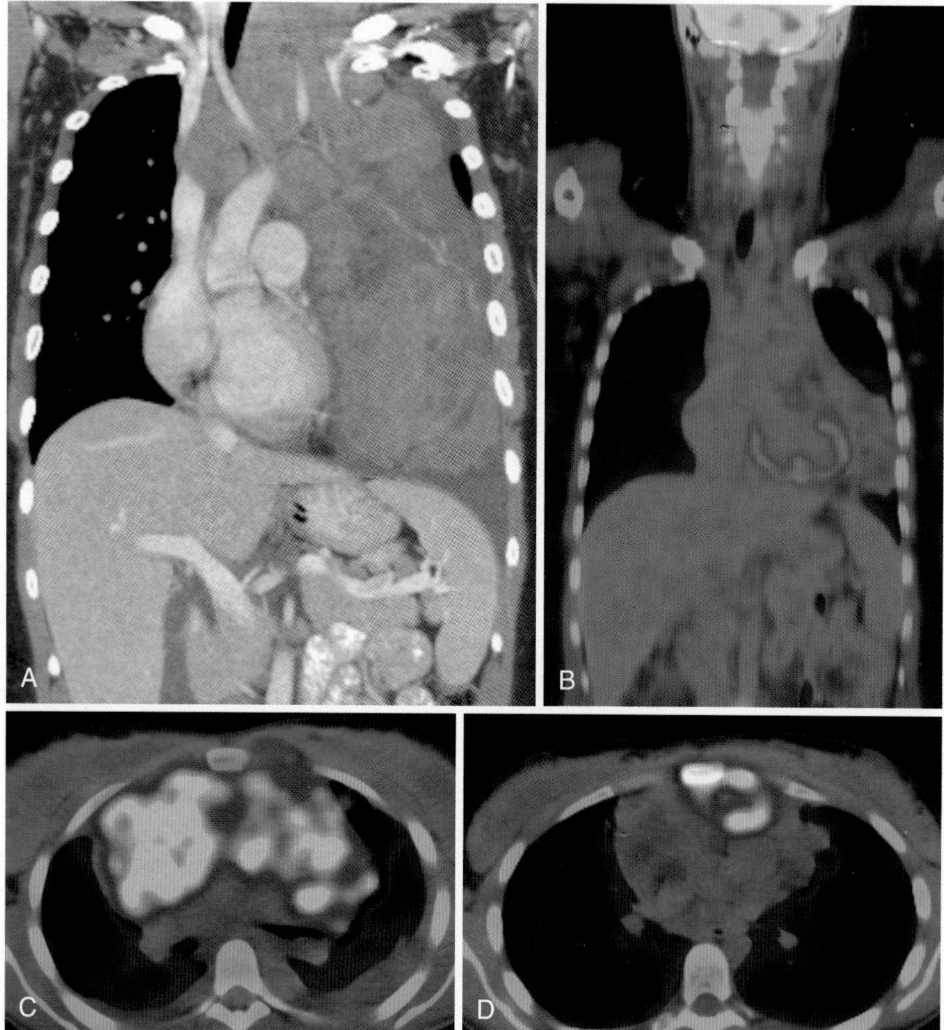

FIGURE 30.19. Evaluation of the residual mass. **A** and **B**, Coronal reformatted computed tomography (CT) scan in a patient with Hodgkin lymphoma. There is an enormous mediastinal mass filling most of the left hemithorax, encasing the great vessels and extending up into the root of the neck. **B**, Coronal fused positron emission tomography (PET)/CT image. Posttreatment, there is a residual mass draped over the left ventricle, which shows no metabolic activity, indicating a complete response. **C** and **D**, A different patient with Hodgkin lymphoma. **C**, Pretreatment, the axial fused PET/CT image demonstrates a very large anterior mediastinal mass involving the chest wall with intense metabolic activity. **D**, Posttreatment, the mass has reduced significantly in size, but there is a focus of persistent metabolic activity indicating residual disease and placing the patient in the partial response category.

Lymphoma in Deauville, France as the preferred method in assessing interim and post therapy response (Deauville Criteria). The Deauville Criteria are most reproducible when applied to HL, DLBCL, and FL and have now been adopted internationally. The scale enables use of a different threshold to define scan positivity according to the clinical question.

The most intense uptake in a site of initial disease is scored as follows:

1. No uptake
2. Uptake less than or equal to mediastinum
3. Uptake greater than mediastinum but less than or equal to liver
4. Uptake moderately higher than liver
5. Uptake markedly higher than liver (>2–3 times higher) and/or new lesions

X. New areas of uptake unlikely to be related to lymphoma

The Lugano Classification PET/CT-based response evaluation and CT-based response evaluation are summarized in Table 30.7. Of note, in this classification the term CR_u is no longer used, and a partial response should be assigned if there is a residual mass.

FDG-PET can also be used to predict outcome before high-dose treatment.[74] Patients commencing high-dose therapy with a positive pretreatment PET scan have a much poorer prognosis.

Percutaneous core biopsy is of proven value in determining the nature of soft tissue masses in lymphoma and can direct appropriate management in up to 90% of cases. It can be used for definition of the nature of a residual mass after treatment, detection of transformation of NHL to a higher grade, and establishing the primary diagnosis in patients who present with unusual manifestations of disease. In general, if a PET/CT study is available, the most metabolically active lesion should be targeted for biopsy.

International Workshop on Chronic Lymphocytic Leukemia

Specific criteria have been developed for the management of CLL, particularly when performing clinical trials. These were first created by a National Cancer Institute–sponsored Working Group in 1988. The most recent update of the International Workshop on Chronic Lymphocytic Leukemia (iwCLL) guidelines from 2018 incorporates recent discoveries in genomics and updated assessment methods.[75] These guidelines not only govern the design and conduct of clinical trials, but also provide a standard for management in general practice. Overall, the iwCLL guidelines rely largely on physical examination and laboratory data. Initial staging of disease is performed with the Rai and Binet staging systems, neither of which include imaging.

The iwCLL uses seven parameters in assessment of treatment response: lymph node size, liver/spleen size, constitutional symptoms, circulating lymphocyte count, platelet count, hemoglobin, and marrow evaluation. Imaging is nonetheless valuable in evaluating lymphadenopathy and organomegaly, particularly for clinical trials where objective measurements are needed. As CLL is the leukemic counterpart of SLL, the Lugano CT response criteria can be used (Table 30.7). There is no consensus on objective measurement of hepatomegaly; therefore, hepatic involvement is determined by the presence or absence of hepatic nodules.

To qualify as progressive disease (PD) in lymph nodes, there must be either a new enlarged lymph node (>1.5 cm in longest diameter) or a greater than 50% increase in longest diameter of a previously chosen lymph node. PD in the spleen is defined as a greater than 50% increase in splenomegaly beyond baseline, or an increase in size of the spleen of 2 cm or more if there is no splenomegaly at baseline.

Detection of Recurrence

Relapse following satisfactory response to initial treatment occurs in 10% to 20% of patients with HL and up to 50% of patients with NHL. In HL, relapse usually occurs within the first 2 years after treatment, and patients are followed up closely during this period, but extended surveillance is not indicated. For patients with HL or aggressive NHL in whom CR is achieved, there is very little evidence for routine surveillance with imaging.[76] Routine follow-up tests, including CT, only rarely detect relapse before patients become symptomatic.[76,77]

TABLE 30.7 The Lugano Response Criteria

A. PET/CT–BASED RESPONSE EVALUATION

RESPONSE	5-POINT SCALE SCORE	BONE MARROW
CR	Score of 1, 2, or 3 with or without residual mass Any lesion with increased uptake previously has the same activity of the background	No evidence of FDG-avid disease
PR	Score of 4 or 5 with uptake < baseline and residual mass of any size during treatment[a]	Residual focal uptake < baseline[b]
SD	Score of 4 or 5 with no uptake change from baseline	No change from baseline
PD	Score of 4 or 5 with uptake > baseline and/or new FDG-avid lesions consistent with lymphoma	New or recurrent FDG-avid foci

[a]If these findings are present at the end of treatment, this indicates residual disease.
[b]Diffuse uptake is compatible with reactive changes to chemotherapy and is a normal finding. If there is focal uptake in the context of nodal response, further magnetic resonance imaging evaluation or interval scan should be considered.

B. CT–BASED RESPONSE EVALUATION

RESPONSE	TARGET LESIONS	NONTARGET LESIONS	SPLENOMEGALY (>13 CM IN VERTICAL LENGTH)
CR (all criteria)	Nodal disease ≤1.5 cm in LD No extranodal disease	Absent	No splenomegaly
PR (all criteria)	≥50% decrease in SPD[a]	Absent or decreased	>50% decrease in splenomegaly[b]
SD (all criteria)	<50% decrease in SPD from baseline, no criteria for progressive disease	No progression	No progression
PD (any one of these criteria)	Individual lesion: ≥50% increase from nadir PPD and increased LD or SD from nadir by: 0.5 cm for lesions ≤2 cm 1 cm for lesions >2 cm New lesion or regrowth of previously involved lesions	Clear progression New or recurrent bone marrow involvement	Prior splenomegaly: >50% decrease in enlargement ≥2 cm increase in size if no splenomegaly at baseline

CR, Complete response; *PR*, partial response; *SD*, stable disease; *PD*, progressive disease; *FDG*, 2-[^{18}F] fluoro-2-deoxy-D-glucose.*PPD*, Product of perpendicular diameter; *SPD*, sum product perpendicular diameter; *LD*, longest diameter; *SD*, shortest axis perpendicular to longest diameter; *CR*, complete response; *PR*, partial response; *SD*, stable disease; *PD*, progressive disease.
[a]If a lesion is too small to measure, it is assigned 5 × 5 mm. If a lesion is not visible, it is assigned 0 × 0 mm.
[b]That is if the spleen is 15 cm at baseline, this is 2 cm larger than normal size of 13 cm. There must be at least a 1-cm decrease in size (50% of 2 cm) to be considered a partial response.

FDG-PET/CT can detect relapse before there is any clinical evidence, but the false-positive rate is high, with an even lower PPV than CE-CT, and it appears to offer little clinical benefit.[78,79] Thus, most oncological societies do not advise routine surveillance imaging. On the other hand, in cases of clinically suspected relapse, the development of a positive PET scan is highly suggestive and facilitates image-guided percutaneous biopsy of FDG-avid suspicious lesions.

COMPLICATIONS OF THERAPY

KEY POINTS Complications of Therapy

Short-Term

- Drug-induced pulmonary toxicity (diffuse alveolar damage, organizing pneumonia, pulmonary hemorrhage, nonspecific interstitial pneumonia).
- Opportunistic pulmonary infection (*Pneumocystis* spp., viral pneumonia, invasive fungal infection, tuberculosis).
- Neutropenic sepsis.
- Enterocolitis, pseudomembranous colitis, neutropenic typhlitis.
- Posterior reversible leucoencephalopathy syndrome.
- Tumor lysis syndrome.
- Immunotherapy-related adverse events.

Long-Term

- Pulmonary fibrosis (radiation- and drug-induced).
- Secondary malignancies (hematologic, radiation-induced—sarcomas, breast cancer, thyroid cancer).
- Graft-versus-host disease.

These can be divided into short-term and long-term consequences. Short-term complications are usually related to the side effects of combination chemotherapy or to the immunosuppression that results from it. The lungs are particularly vulnerable. Long-term consequences relate mostly to the side effects of chemoradiation and high-dose treatments. With the development of intensity-modulated radiotherapy, florid radiation pneumonitis is rarely seen, but the role of FDG-PET/CT in defining tumor volumes requires further investigation so as to minimize toxicity to normal structures and the development of radiation-induced malignancies. The main complications are shown in the text box.

CONCLUSION

The lymphomas are a diverse group of hematologic malignancies primarily involving lymph nodes. Patients with HL typically present with early-stage malignancy involving the supradiaphragmatic nodal groups. Treatment is dictated by stage, and the majority of patients are cured. The incidence of NHL is increasing, and most patients present with advanced disease, often involving extranodal sites. The prognosis depends mostly on tumor subtype. In both conditions, imaging is crucial at every stage of patient management, and PET/CT has added a new dimension to the assessment of the patient with lymphoma.

REFERENCES

1. American Cancer Society *Cancer Facts and Figures 2019*. Atlanta: American Cancer Society; 2019:4.
2. Ries LA, Kosary CL, Hankey BP, eds. *SEER Cancer Statistics Review, 1973-1996*. Bethesda, MD: National Cancer Institute; 1999.
3. Rabkin CS, Devesa SS, Zahm SH, Gail MH. Increasing incidence of non-Hodgkin's lymphoma. *Semin Hematol*. 1993;30:286–296.
4. International collaboration on HIV and cancer Highly active antiretroviral therapy and the incidence of cancer in HIV-infected adults. *J Natl Cancer Inst*. 2000;92:1823–1830.
5. Harris NL, Jaffe ES, Diebold J, et al. World Health Organization classification of neoplastic diseases of the hematopoietic and lymphoid tissues: report of the Clinical Advisory Committee meeting—Airlie House, Virginia, November 1997. *J Clin Oncol*. 1999;17:3835–3849.
6. Swerdlow SH, Campo E, Pileri SA, et al. The 2016 revision of the World Health Organization classification of lymphoid neoplasms, 2016. *Blood*. 2016;127(20):2375–2390.
7. A clinical evaluation of the International Lymphoma Study Group classification of non-Hodgkin's lymphoma The Non-Hodgkin's Lymphoma Classification Project. *Blood*. 1997;89:3909–3918.
8. Jaffe ES. The 2008 WHO Classification of lymphomas: implications for clinical practice and translational research. *Hematology Am Soc Hematol Educ Program*. 2009:523–531.
9. Alizadeh AA, Eisen MB, Davis RE, et al. Distinct types of diffuse large B-cell lymphoma identified by gene expression profiling. *Nature*. 2000;403:503–511.
10. Lukes RJ, Butler JJ. The pathology and nomenclature of Hodgkin's disease. *Cancer Res*. 1966;26:1063–1083.
11. Lister TA, Crowther D, Sutcliffe SB, et al. Report of a committee convened to discuss the evaluation and staging of patients with Hodgkin's disease: Cotswolds meeting. *J Clin Oncol*. 1989;7:1630–1636.
12. Cheson BD, Fisher RI, Barrington SF, et al. Recommendations for the initial evaluation, staging and response assessment of Hodgkin and non-Hodgkin lymphoma: the Lugano classification. *J Clin Oncol*. 2014;32:3059–3068.
13. Shipp MA, Harrington DP, Anderson JR, et al. A predictive model for aggressive non-Hodgkin's lymphoma. The International Non-Hodgkin's Lymphoma Prognostic Factors Project. *N Engl J Med*. 1993;329:987–994.
14. Solal-Celigny P. Follicular Lymphoma International Prognostic Index. *Curr Treat Option Oncol*. 2006;7:270–275.
15. Ng YY, Healy JC, Vincent JM, et al. The radiology of non-Hodgkin lymphoma in childhood: a review of 80 cases. *Clin Radiol*. 1994;49:594–600.
16. King AD, Ahuja AT, Yeung DK, et al. Malignant cervical lymphadenopathy: diagnostic accuracy of diffusion-weighted MR imaging. *Radiology*. 2007;245:806–813.
17. Moog F, Bangerter M, Diederichs CG, et al. Lymphoma: role of whole-body 2-deoxy-2-[F-18]fluoro-D-glucose (FDG) PET in nodal staging. *Radiology*. 1997;203:795–800.
18. Moog F, Bangerter M, Diederichs CG, et al. Extranodal malignant lymphoma: detection with FDG PET versus CT. *Radiology*. 1998;206:475–481.
19. Rodríguez-Vigil B, Gómez-León N, Pinílla I, et al. PET/CT in lymphoma: prospective study of enhanced full-dose PET/CT versus unenhanced low-dose PET/CT. *J Nucl Med*. 2006;47:1643–1648.
20. Barrington S, Mikhaeel N, Kostakoglu L, et al. Role of Imaging in the Staging and Response Assessment of Lymphoma: Consensus of the International Conference on Malignant Lymphomas Imaging Working Group. *J Clin Oncol*. 2014;32:3048–3058.
21. Castellino RA, Blank N, Hoppe RT, Cho C. Hodgkin disease: contributions of chest CT in the initial staging evaluation. *Radiology*. 1986;160:603–605.
22. Castellino RA, Hilton S, O'Brien JP, Portlock CS. Non-Hodgkin's lymphoma: contribution of chest CT in the initial staging evaluation. *Radiology*. 1996;199:129–132.
23. Shaffer K, Smith D, Kirn D, et al. Primary mediastinal large-B-cell lymphoma: radiologic findings at presentation. *AJR Am J Roentgenol*. 1996;167:425–430.
24. Lewis ER, Caskey CI, Fishman EK. Lymphoma of the lung: CT findings in 31 patients. *AJR Am J Roentgenol*. 1991;156:711–714.
25. Wernecke K, Vassallo P, Rutsch F, et al. Thymic involvement in Hodgkin disease: CT and sonographic findings. *Radiology*. 1991;181:375–383.

26. Spiers AS, Husband JE, MacVicar AD. Treated thymic lymphoma: comparison of MR imaging with CT. *Radiology*. 1997;203:369–376.
27. Rini JN, Manalili EY, Hoffman MA, et al. F-18 FDG versus Ga-67 for detecting splenic involvement in Hodgkin's disease. *Clin Nucl Med*. 2002;27:572–577.
28. Fishman EK, Urban BA, Hruban RH. CT of the stomach: spectrum of disease. *Radiographics*. 1996;16:1035–1054.
29. Fujishima H, Chijiiwa Y. Endoscopic ultrasonographic staging of primary gastric lymphoma. *Abdom Imaging*. 1996;21:192–194.
30. Zucca E, Copie-Bergman C, Ricardi U, et al. Gastric marginal zone lymphoma of MALT type: ESMO clinical practice guidelines for Diagnosis, Treatment and Follow-up. *Ann Oncol*. 2013;24:144–148.
31. Raderer M, Vorbeck F, Formanek M, et al. Importance of extensive staging in patients with mucosa-associated lymphoid tissue (MALT)-type lymphoma. *Br J Cancer*. 2000;83:454–457.
32. Bach AG, Behrmann C, Holzhausen HJ, et al. Prevalence and patterns of renal involvement in imaging of malignant lymphoproliferative diseases. *Acta Radiol*. 2012;53:343–348.
33. Reznek RH, Mootoosamy I, Webb JA, Richards MA. CT in renal and perirenal lymphoma: a further look. *Clin Radiol*. 1990;42:233–238.
34. Kim YS, Koh BH, Cho OK, Rhim HC. MR imaging of primary uterine lymphoma. *Abdom Imaging*. 1997;22:441–444.
35. Crum-Cianflone N, Hullsiek KH, Marconi V, et al. Trends in the incidence of cancers among HIV-infected persons and the impact of antiretroviral therapy: a 20-year cohort study. *AIDS*. 2009 Jan 2;23(1):41–50.
36. Jenkins CN, Colquhoun IR. Characterization of primary intracranial lymphoma by computed tomography: an analysis of 36 cases and a review of the literature with particular reference to calcification haemorrhage and cyst formation. *Clin Radiol*. 1998;53:428–434.
37. Küker W1, Nägele T, Korfel A, et al. Primary central nervous system lymphomas (PCNSL): MRI features at presentation in 100 patients. *J Neurooncol*. 2005;72:169–177.
38. Chamberlain MC, Sandy AD, Press GA. Leptomeningeal metastasis: a comparison of gadolinium-enhanced MR and contrast-enhanced CT of the brain. *Neurology*. 1990;40:435–438.
39. Takashima S, Ikezoe J, Morimoto S, et al. Primary thyroid lymphoma: evaluation with CT. *Radiology*. 1988;168:765–768.
40. Mengiardi B, Honegger H, Hodler J, et al. Primary lymphoma of bone: MRI and CT characteristics before and after successful treatment. *AJR Am J Roentgenol*. 2005;184:185–192.
41. Park YH, Kim S, Choi SJ, et al. Clinical impact of whole-body FDG-PET for evaluation of response and therapeutic decision-making of primary lymphoma of bone. *Ann Oncol*. 2005;16:1401–1402.
42. Yasumoto M, Nonomura Y, Yoshimura R, et al. MR detection of iliac bone marrow involvement by malignant lymphoma with various MR sequences including diffusion-weighted echo-planar imaging. *Skeletal Radiol*. 2002;31:263–269.
43. Elstrom R, Guan L, Baker G, et al. Utility of FDG-PET scanning in lymphoma by WHO classification. *Blood*. 2003;101:3875–3876.
44. El-Galaly TC, d'Amore F, Mylam KJ, et al. Routine bone marrow biopsy has little or no therapeutic consequence for positron emission tomography/computed tomography-staged treatment-naive patients with Hodgkin lymphoma. *J Clin Oncol*. 2012; 30:4508–4514.
45. Khan AB, Barrington SF, Mikhaeel NG, et al. PET-CT staging of DLBCL accurately identifies and provides new insight into the clinical significance of bone marrow involvement. *Blood*. 2013;122:61–67.
46. Jasmer RM, Gotway MB, Creasman JM, et al. Clinical and radiographic predictors of the etiology of computed tomography-diagnosed intrathoracic lymphadenopathy in HIV-infected patients. *J Acquir Immune Defic Syndr*. 2002;31:291–298.
47. O'Doherty MJ, Barrington SF, Campbell M, et al. PET scanning and the human immunodeficiency virus-positive patient. *J Nucl Med*. 1997;38:1575–1583.
48. Yang M, Sun J, Bai HX, et al. Diagnostic accuracy of SPECT, PET, and MRS for primary central nervous system lymphoma in HIV patients. A systematic review and meta-analysis. *Medicine*. 2017;96:e6676.
49. Pickhardt PJ, Siegel MJ. Abdominal manifestations of posttransplantation lymphoproliferative disorder. *AJR Am J Roentgenol*. 1998;171:1007–1013.
50. Henry-Amar M. Second cancer after the treatment for Hodgkin's disease: a report from the International Database on Hodgkin's Disease. *Ann Oncol*. 1992;3(Suppl 4):117–128.
51. Ng AK, Bernardo MP, Weller E, et al. Long term survival and competing causes of death in patients with early stage Hodgkin's disease treated at age 50 or younger. *J Clin Oncol*. 2002;20:2101–2108.
52. Johnson P, Federico M, Kirkwood A, et al. Adapted Treatment Guided by Interim PET-CT Scan. *New Engl J Med*. 2016;374:2419–2429.
53. von Treskow B, Moskowitz C. Treatment of relapsed and refractory Hodgkin Lymphoma. *Semin Hematol*. 2016;53:180–185.
54. Younes A, Ansell S. Novel agents in the treatment of Hodgkin lymphoma: Biological basis and clinical results. *Semin Hematol*. 2016;53:186–189.
55. NICE Technology Appraisal Guidance 524 https://www.nice.org.uk/guidance/ta524 June 2018
56. Montoto S, Davies AJ, Matthews J, et al. Risk and clinical implications of transformation of follicular lymphoma to diffuse large B cell lymphoma. *J Clin Oncol*. 2007;25:2426–2433.
57. Rummel MJ, Niederle N, Maschmeyer G, et al. Bendamustine plus rituximab versus CHOP plus rituximab as first-line treatment for patients with indolent and mantle cell lymphomas: an open label, multicenter randomized, phase 3 non-inferiority trial Study Group Indolent Lymphomas (StiL). *Lancet*. 2013;381:1203–1210.
58. Jain N, Keating M, Thompson P, et al. Ibrutinib and Venetoclax for First-Line Treatment of CLL. *N Engl J Med*. 2019;380(22):2095–2103.
59. Spaepen K, Stroobants S, Dupont P, et al. Early restaging positron emission tomography with (18)F-fluorodeoxyglucose predicts outcome in patients with aggressive non-Hodgkin's lymphoma. *Ann Oncol*. 2002;13:1356–1363.
60. Haioun C, Itti E, Rahmouni A, et al. [18F]fluoro-2-deoxy-d-glucose positron emission tomography (FDG-PET) in aggressive lymphoma: an early prognostic tool for predicting patient outcome. *Blood*. 2005;106:1376–1381.
61. Hutchings M, Loft A, Hansen M, et al. FDG-PET after two cycles of chemotherapy predicts treatment failure and progression-free survival in Hodgkin lymphoma. *Blood*. 2006;107:52–59.
62. Gallamini A, Hutchings M, Rigacci L, et al. Early interim 2-[18F] fluoro-2-deoxy-d-glucose positron emission tomography is prognostically superior to international prognostic score in advanced-stage Hodgkin's lymphoma: a report from a joint Italian-Danish study. *J Clin Oncol*. 2007;25:3746–3752.
63. Kostakoglu L, Goldsmith SJ, Leonard JP, et al. FDG-PET after 1 cycle of therapy predicts outcome in diffuse large cell lymphoma and classic Hodgkin disease. *Cancer*. 2006;107:2678–2687.
64. Radford J, Illidge T, Counsell N, Hancock B, Pettengell R, Johnson P, et al. Results of a trial of PET-directed therapy for early-stage Hodgkin's lymphoma. *N Engl J Med*. 2015 Apr 23;372(17):1598–1607.
65. Gallamini A, Tarella C, Viviani S, et al. Early Chemotherapy Intensification with escalated BEACOPP in Patients with Advanced-Stage Hodgkin Lymphoma with a positive Interim Positron Emission Tomography/Computed Tomography Scan after two ABVD Cycles: Long-Term Results of the GITIL/FIL HD 0607 Trial. *J Clin Oncol*. 2018;36:454–462.
66. Cheson BD, Horning SJ, Coiffier B, et al. Report of an international workshop to standardize response criteria for Non-Hodgkin's lymphomas. NCI Sponsored International Working Group. *J Clin Oncol*. 1999;17:1244.
67. Naumann R, Vaic A, Beuthien-Baumann B, et al. Prognostic value of positron emission tomography in the evaluation of post-treatment residual mass in patients with Hodgkin's disease and non-Hodgkin's lymphoma. *Br J Haematol*. 2001;115:793–800.
68. Weihrauch MR, Re D, Scheidhauer K, et al. Thoracic positron emission tomography using 18F-fluorodeoxyglucose for the evaluation of residual mediastinal Hodgkin disease. *Blood*. 2001;98:2930–2934.
69. Zinzani PL, Chierichetti F, Zompatori M, et al. Advantages of positron emission tomography (PET) with respect to computed tomography in the follow-up of lymphoma patients with abdominal presentation. *Leuk Lymphoma*. 2002;43:1239–1243.
70. Han HS, Escalon MP, Hsiao B, et al. High incidence of false positive PET scans in patients with aggressive non-Hodgkin's lymphoma treated with rituximab-containing regimens. *Ann Oncol*. 2009;20:309–318.
71. Juweid M, Wiseman GA, Vose J, et al. Response assessment of aggressive non-Hodgkin's lymphoma by Integrated International Workshop criteria and fluorine-18-fluordeoxyglucose positron emission tomography. *J Clin Oncol*. 2005;23:4652–4661.
72. Cheson BD, Pfistner B, Juweid ME, et al. Revised response criteria for malignant lymphoma. *J Clin Oncol*. 2007;25:579–586.

73. Juweid ME, Stroobants S, Hoekstra OS, et al. Use of positron emission tomography for response assessment of lymphoma: consensus of the Imaging Subcommittee of International Harmonization Project in Lymphoma. *J Clin Oncol*. 2007;25:571–578.
74. Becherer A, Mitterbauer M, Jaeger U, et al. Positron emission tomography with [18F]2-fluoro-D-2-deoxyglucose (FDG-PET) predicts relapse of malignant lymphoma after high-dose therapy with stem cell transplantation. *Leukemia*. 2002;16:260–267.
75. Hallek M, Cheson BD, Catovsky D, et al. iwCLL guidelines for diagnosis, indications for treatment, response assessment, and supportive management of CLL. *Blood*. 2018;131(25):2745–2760.
76. Guadagnolo BA, Punglia RS, Kuntz KM, et al. Cost-effectiveness analysis of computerized tomography in the routine follow-up of patients after primary treatment for Hodgkin's disease. *J Clin Oncol*. 2006;24:4116–4122.
77. Elis A, Blickstein D, Klein O, et al. Detection of relapse in non-Hodgkin's lymphoma: role of routine follow-up studies. *Am J Hematol*. 2002;69:41–44.
78. Jerusalem G, Beguin Y, Fassotte MF, et al. Early detection of relapse by whole-body positron emission tomography in the follow-up of patients with Hodgkin's disease. *Ann Oncol*. 2003;14:123–130.
79. Zinzani PL, Stefoni V, Ambrosini V, et al. FDG-PET in the serial assessment of patients with lymphoma in complete remission. *Blood*. 2007;110:71 (abstract 216).

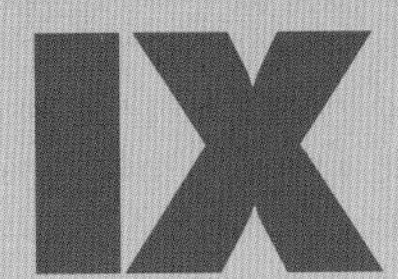

PART IX METASTATIC DISEASE

CHAPTER 31 Thoracic Metastatic Disease

Girish S. Shroff M.D.; Chad D. Strange M.D.; Jitesh Ahuja M.D.; and Bradley S. Sabloff M.D.

INTRODUCTION

Metastatic disease is the most common chest malignancy, and the chest acquires more metastases than any system.[1] In autopsy series, pulmonary metastases are present in 20% to 54% of patients with a primary malignancy.[2,3] The most common extrathoracic malignancies to metastasize to the chest include breast cancer, gastrointestinal (GI) malignancies (colon, pancreatic, and gastric cancer), melanoma, head and neck tumors, and renal cell cancer.[1] Rarely, metastatic disease to the thorax can be the initial presentation of a malignancy. Tumor spread to the chest can occur via hematogenous, lymphatic, or endobronchial routes. Chest radiographs and computed tomography (CT) are the main modalities used to assess thoracic metastatic disease. Other modalities currently serve complementary roles and include magnetic resonance imaging (MRI), ultrasound (US), and positron emission tomography (PET)/CT. Technique and typical and atypical CT imaging manifestations of pulmonary, pleural, and cardiac metastases are addressed.

TECHNIQUE

In the evaluation of patients with a primary tumor, imaging serves to stage patients and to detect or exclude metastatic disease. Achieving this goal with the appropriate technique is essential. Chest radiographs (posteroanterior and lateral views) generally serve as the initial evaluation tool in patients with possible metastatic disease. In patients whose radiographs demonstrate obvious metastatic disease, additional imaging modalities may not be necessary, and radiographic follow-up may be sufficient.[4] However, chest radiographs lack sensitivity, and CT has been shown to be superior to radiography in the detection of pulmonary nodules. CT is now the state-of-the-art modality for both the detection and characterization of intrathoracic metastatic disease.[5,6] The evolution of CT as the standard began with several improvements in CT technology: the ability to obtain thinner collimation and the development of spiral, and subsequently multidetector row CT (MDCT), scanners. Thinner collimation enabled the development of high-resolution CT to assess diffuse lung disease and improved anatomic assessment and characterization of small lesions. Current MDCT scanners acquire a continuous volume and thus decrease misregistration artifacts and improve nodule detection by eliminating interslice gaps. This aids assessment of diffuse lung diseases, increases sensitivity for small lung nodules, and improves multiplanar reconstructions. Other benefits of CT include its ability to quantify disease in the case of possible metastectomy, assess response to therapy, and provide a detailed roadmap to guide biopsy.

Our present CT chest protocol for assessing patients with possible metastatic disease includes MDCT scan parameters that allow image review in both standard and lung algorithms at 2.5- and 1.25-mm image thickness. Images are also reconstructed in both coronal and sagittal planes and reviewed at workstations with cine mode capabilities.

Intravenous contrast (100 mL) is used in patients in whom there is no contraindication, at a rate of 3 mL/sec after a 30-second delay. The rationale for intravenous contrast is multiple:

1. Contrast enhancement permits better delineation of the mediastinum and hilar regions and is also useful for detecting subtle pleural metastatic disease.
2. Patients with primary malignancy are at increased risk for developing pulmonary emboli. In retrospective reviews of CT scans of oncologic patients, between 3.3% and 4.0% of patients had incidentally discovered pulmonary emboli, with higher risks associated with inpatients, advanced disease, gynecologic malignancy, and melanoma.[7,8]
3. Patients undergoing chemotherapy often have indwelling catheters that may lead to thrombotic occlusion of vessels and collateral vessel formation.

Although sensitive, CT is not specific in the assessment of metastatic disease. False-positive nodules are often caused by intraparenchymal lymph nodes and noncalcified granulomas. Image processing can improve image interpretation. Maximum intensity projection images increase sensitivity to small lung nodules by demonstrating vascular structures as tubular branching structures.[9]

Other modalities such as US, MRI, and PET serve complementary roles in evaluating thoracic metastatic disease. Electrocardiogram (ECG)-gated cardiac MRI (CMRI) is useful in evaluating the heart and surrounding structures for findings on either CT or echocardiography that may suggest metastatic disease. CMRI is a cardiac-gated study that eliminates cardiac motion and has excellent temporal resolution and excellent soft tissue contrast. ECG-gated CT is an alternative to CMRI in the evaluation of cardiac tumors in patients who are unable to undergo CMRI, for example, those patients who have an implanted ferromagnetic device or who experience discomfort lying on the MRI table for prolonged periods of time.[10]

Key Points Technique

- Computed tomography (CT) is the gold standard in the evaluation of metastatic disease.
- Cine mode review, thin image thickness, and image processing improve sensitivity.
- Electrocardiogram-gated cardiac magnetic resonance imaging and CT are useful for characterizing cardiac tumors.

PATTERNS OF METASTATIC DISEASE

Simple Nodules

Most metastases to the chest are spread hematogenously. The characteristic appearance of these metastatic lesions includes multiple bilateral spherical or ovoid sharply marginated nodules of variable sizes predominantly affecting the periphery of the lungs and the lower lobes (where the majority of the blood flow is directed)[1,3,11] (Fig. 31.1A). The typical sharply marginated edges of metastatic lesions help differentiate these tumors from primary lung cancers, as well as their characteristic ill-defined, spiculated margins that extend into the adjacent lung parenchyma. Growth of metastatic lesions is extremely variable, and volume doubling times (an increase in the diameter of a nodule by 26%) have been reported to range from 1 to 2 weeks for rapidly growing lesions such as sarcomas, melanomas, and germ cell tumors to months for thyroid malignancy.[12] Hematogenous metastases can also simulate a miliary pattern, typical of medullary thyroid malignancy.[1] Occasionally, imaging metastatic nodules with contrast-infused CT demonstrates areas of enhancement with dilated, tortuous, tubular enhancing vessels. This feature can be seen in sarcomas, particularly alveolar soft part sarcoma or leiomyosarcoma[6,13] (Fig. 31.1B).

Benign tumors rarely metastasize, and benign tumors that can metastasize to lung include leiomyoma of the uterus, hydatidiform mole, giant cell tumor of bone, chondroblastoma, pleomorphic adenoma of the salivary gland, and meningioma. Slow growth of these solid benign nodules is typical, but the appearance is indistinguishable from other malignant metastatic nodules.[6]

Metastatic nodules that remain stable on serial exams may represent sterilized metastatic disease. These residual nodules are indistinguishable from viable tumor on CT scans. Biopsied materials show areas of necrosis and/or areas of fibrosis. Testicular cancer, breast cancer, and choriocarcinoma are common tumors that present in this manner.[14,15] In some cases, following serum markers such as beta–human chorionic gonadotropin or alpha-fetoprotein or, alternatively, PET scanning can be helpful in following and assessing viability. In addition, growth of metastatic nonseminomatous germ cell lesions with negative serum markers frequently represents a conversion to a benign mature teratoma.[16]

Nodules With a Ground Glass "Halo"

Hemorrhage around a metastasis can produce the halo sign, a solid nodule surrounded by a ground glass rim. Metastatic tumors that can exhibit this appearance include choriocarcinoma and angiosarcoma[17,18] (Fig. 31.1C). The halo sign is not pathognomonic for metastatic disease and can be

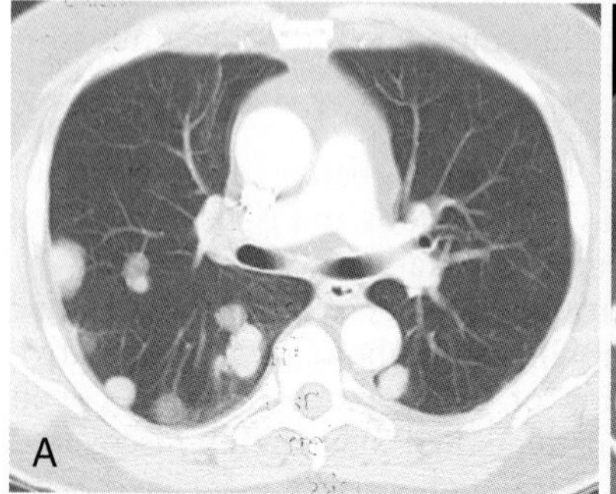

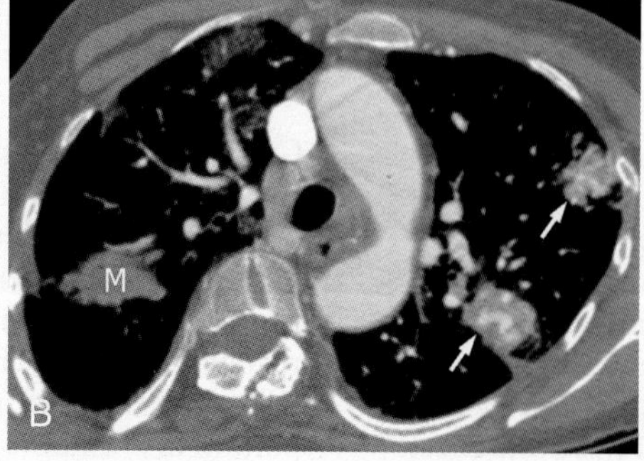

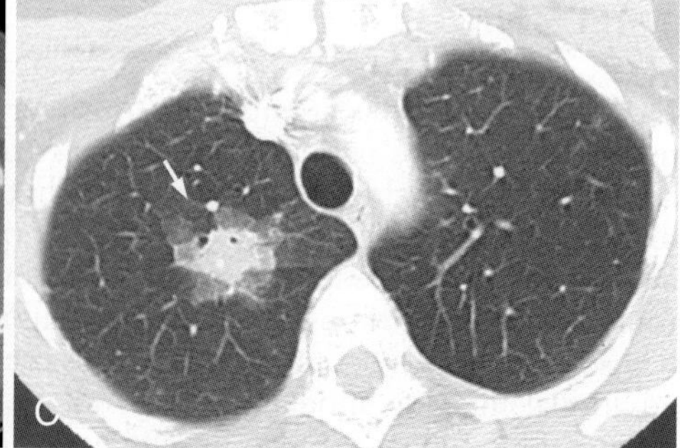

Figure 31.1. Solid nodules. **A**, Typical pattern of hematogenous metastatic disease dissemination. Computed tomography (CT) scan of a patient with metastatic nonseminomatous germ cell tumor demonstrates multiple soft tissue nodules that predominate in the periphery of the lungs and are sharply demarcated. **B**, Vascular nodule. CT scan of a patient with adrenal cancer with intravenous contrast. Image shows bilateral masses, two lesions on the left (*arrows*) show tubular branching vessels coursing through the lesion. The lesion on the right (*M*) is solid. **C**, Nodule with "halo." Right upper lobe solid nodule has a rim of ground-glass density, known as "CT halo sign." (arrow) The appearance is attributed to hemorrhage around metastatic lesions related to fragility of the neovascular bed.

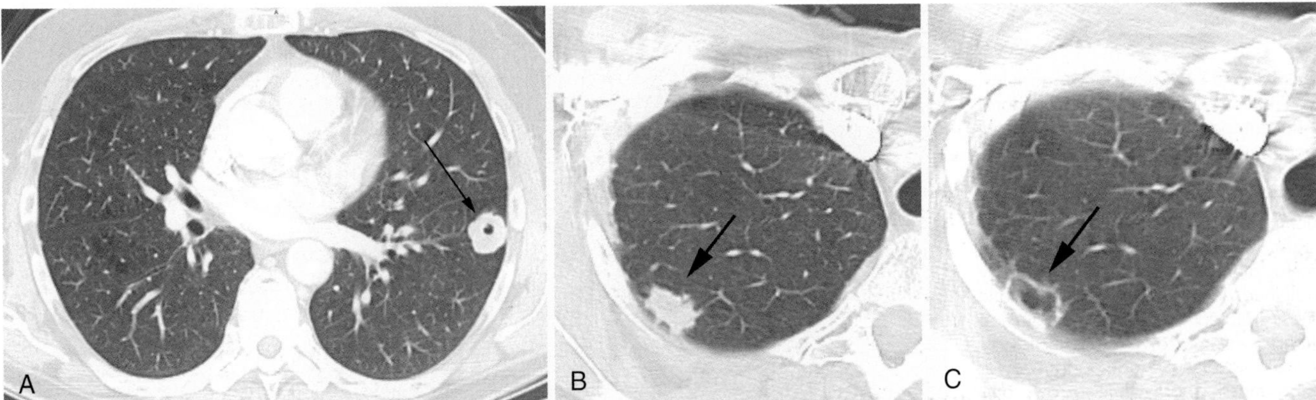

Figure 31.2. Cavitary nodules. **A**, Typical cavitary metastases. Computed tomography scan of a patient with a head and neck squamous cell cancer of the piriform sinus shows a well-defined thick-walled cavitary left lower lobe nodule (*arrow*). Cavitation with therapy in a patient with metastatic breast cancer. Solid soft tissue nodule (*arrows*) in the right upper lobe **B** cavitates and develops thin walls after 6 weeks of therapy **C**.

seen with other hemorrhagic lesions, including infections such as invasive aspergillosis (the most common condition showing the halo sign in immunocompromised patients) and inflammatory processes such as Wegener granulomatosis. In addition, primary malignancy can simulate this appearance; examples include minimally invasive adenocarcinoma (the most common condition showing the halo sign in immunocompetent patients) and lymphoma.[6,18]

Cavitary Nodules

Cavitation in metastases is less frequent than in primary lung cancers. Metastatic squamous cell lesions, from any source, were thought to have the highest rate of cavitation, at approximately 10%. However, a similar rate of cavitation was demonstrated in a series of metastatic adenocarcinoma.[6] Typical cavitary metastases have thick, irregular walls (Fig. 31.2A); less frequently, they can have thin walls, and this feature is particularly noted in patients with metastatic adenocarcinoma or sarcoma. Chemotherapy can induce cavitation, and this is more common in sarcomatous metastases than in other cancers[1,6,19] (Fig. 31.2B and C).

Calcified Nodules

Calcification is often considered a sign of benignity, representing either a granuloma or a hamartoma; however, infrequently calcification can occur in various metastases through different mechanisms. Most frequently, calcification in metastases is associated with matrix-forming primary tumors such as osteosarcoma and chondrosarcoma[11,20] (Fig. 31.3A). Mucoid-producing tumors, including tumors of the GI tract and breast cancer, can produce calcified metastases (Fig. 31.3B). Dystrophic calcification can be seen in metastatic thyroid cancer, synovial sarcoma, and giant cell tumors[20–23] and can also occur in areas of necrosis after therapy.[12] Aside from the four characteristic patterns of benign calcification (diffuse, central, popcorn, and laminar), CT cannot reliably differentiate benign and malignant lesions based on other patterns of calcifications.[6,12]

Airspace Nodules, Airspace Disease

An airspace pattern of disease, mimicking pneumonia, can be seen in metastatic disease. These lesions can be ground-glass, consolidative, or a mixture of these densities and may contain air bronchograms. Adenocarcinomas of the GI tract and the breast can spread to the lung and then grow along the lung scaffolding (lepidic growth) to create this appearance.[24–26] In one study of metastatic GI tumor, an airspace pattern of metastatic disease was identified in approximately 10% of patients.[26] The lepidic growth pattern is characteristic of well-differentiated primary lung adenocarcinoma.

Key Points Nodular Pattern

- Nodules are the most common form of metastatic disease.
- Calcification in metastatic disease is possible but overlaps with forms of calcification in benign lesions.
- Metastatic nodules can mimic nonmalignant forms of disease and include solid nodules, (granuloma), airspace nodules (pneumonia), and nodules with a halo (including invasive aspergillosis).

BRANCHING METASTATIC DISEASE

Reticular and Nodular Opacities (Lymphangitic Carcinomatosis)

Reticular and nodular opacities in the lung can be caused by lymphangitic carcinomatosis. Lymphangitic carcinomatosis is usually a result of hematogenous spread of malignancy to the lung and secondary invasion of the lymphatic system. Less frequently, lymphangitic carcinomatosis can be a result of direct spread from mediastinal and hilar lymph nodes. Only 50% of lymphangitic carcinomatosis

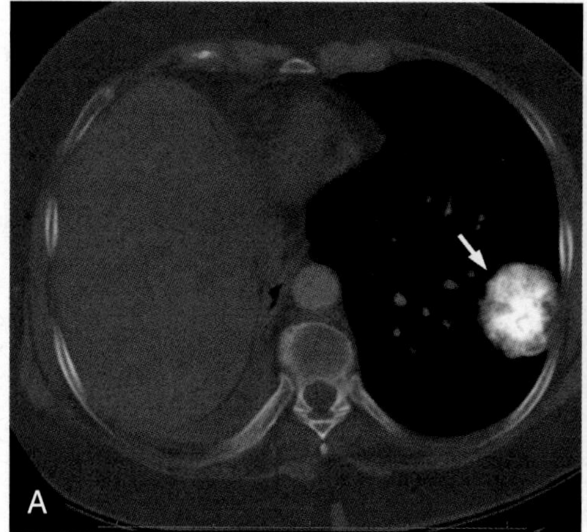

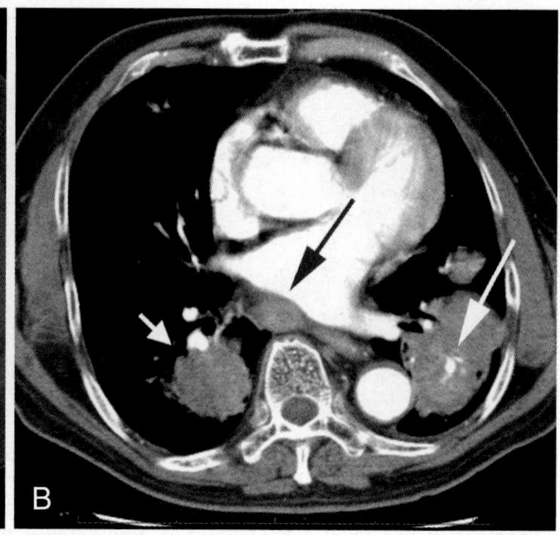

FIGURE 31.3. Calcified nodules. **A**, Patient with a distal femoral osteosarcoma with previous right pneumonectomy. Computed tomography scan, bone windows, shows a calcified mass with trabeculation compatible with an ossified metastatic lesion (*arrow*). **B**, Patient with metastatic colon cancer with a partially calcified left lower lobe metastatic mass related to mucoid production (*long white arrow*). Other sites of metastatic disease are a right lower lobe mass (*short white arrow*) and paraesophageal adenopathy (*black arrow*).

cases have hilar adenopathy supporting a hematogenous mechanism as the primary mode of lymphangitic tumor spread. Lymphangitic carcinomatosis most often results from spread of carcinomas of the lung; breast cancer; upper GI malignancies including pancreas and stomach; prostate, uterus, cervical, or thyroid cancer; and adenocarcinomas of unknown primary site.[1] The process can be a focal, unilateral, or diffuse and bilateral and is associated with pleural effusions in 60% of cases. Radiographic findings in lymphangitic carcinomatosis include reticulonodular opacities and interlobular septal thickening. Typical CT features include thickening of the bronchovascular bundles and smooth or beaded interlobular septal thickening. Smooth peripheral interlobular septal thickening needs to be differentiated from the Kerley-B lines of pulmonary edema, which are typically bilateral and symmetric. Unlike other reticular parenchymal processes such as fibrosis, the architecture of the secondary pulmonary lobule is preserved in lymphangitic carcinomatosis[27,28] (Fig. 31.4A).

Endovascular Metastases

Two other forms of branching nodular metastatic disease can occur: lesions to the pulmonary artery, known as tumor emboli, and lesions to the airway, or endobronchial metastases. Tumor emboli are similar to hematogenous metastatic lesions in mode of spread but differ in that they proliferate only in the vasculature. At autopsy, microscopic tumor emboli were seen in up to 26% of patients with solid malignancy.[29] CT findings include multifocal dilatation and areas of beading generally affecting mid to small pulmonary arteries (Fig. 31.4B). Infrequently, central vessels are involved.[30] Peripheral airspace disease can be seen secondary to infarction.[30–32] Tumors most frequently associated with tumor emboli include hepatoma, breast cancer, renal cancer, prostate cancer, gastric cancer, and choriocarcinoma.[33]

Endobronchial Metastases

Endobronchial metastases are infrequent, seen in less than 2% to 4% of patients at autopsy.[34,35] Routes of metastatic disease spread to bronchi include (1) direct deposition, either aspiration of tumor cells or lymphatic or hematogenous spread, and (2) direct invasion from tumor in the adjacent lung or lymph nodes. Endobronchial metastases are only rarely visible on radiographs, most often manifesting with postobstructive atelectasis. On CT, endobronchial metastases manifest as small soft-tissue filling defects in the airways, areas of narrowing, or obstruction[34] (Fig. 31.4C). Symptoms may include dyspnea, cough, and hemoptysis.[36] Generally, endobronchial metastases are a late manifestation of disease, with a median survival after diagnosis of 9 to 18 months[36,37]; they are most frequently associated with renal, breast, and colorectal primary malignancies.[36,37] Occasionally, it is difficult to differentiate the branching patterns of endobronchial and endovascular metastases. Differentiation is facilitated by sequential thin-cut image review, often in the cine mode, allowing separation of the normal pulmonary artery or bronchus from the involved structure.

KEY POINTS Branching Pattern

- Branching metastatic disease includes lymphangitic carcinomatosis and endobronchial and endovascular metastases.
- Lymphangitic carcinomatosis can be smooth or beaded and spares the architecture of the secondary pulmonary lobule.
- Examination of sequential thin-cut images helps establish the origin of the branching pattern.

ADENOPATHY

Metastatic Intrathoracic Adenopathy

Metastatic intrathoracic adenopathy can be seen in all nodal groups. Generally, metastatic adenopathy occurs with parenchymal lung metastases but can occasionally develop in their absence. Metastatic intrathoracic adenopathy from tumors other than lung cancer is most frequently associated with cancers of the genitourinary system, head and neck tumors, breast cancer, and melanoma.[12]

Enlarged mediastinal and hilar nodes can also be secondary to sarcoidosis or sarcoid-like reaction. In these

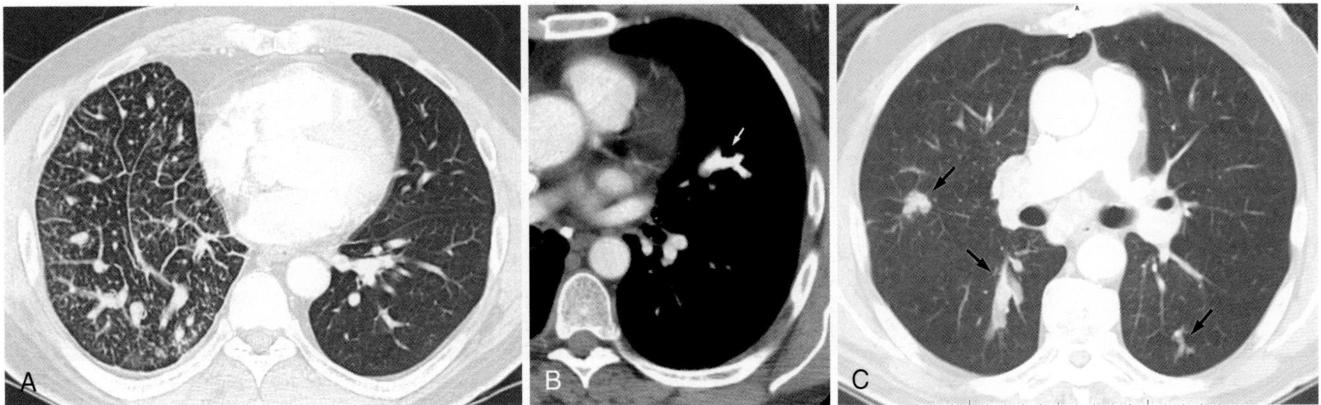

FIGURE 31.4. Branching metastases. **A**, Lymphangitic carcinomatosis, primary lung adenocarcinoma. Diffuse smooth thickening of the secondary pulmonary lobule with smooth thickened septal lines extending out to the periphery in the right lung with preservation of the secondary pulmonary lobule architecture. Within the center of the secondary pulmonary lobule is a "dot" that represents thickening of the central lymphatics. **B**, Endovascular metastases in a patient with osteosarcoma. Branching calcified metastatic lesion in the left lung shows enlargement of the involved pulmonary artery with dense calcification (*arrow*). The lesion enlarged on sequential computed tomography scans. **C**, Endobronchial metastases in a patient with renal cell cancer. Multiple branching opacities bilaterally in the lungs (*arrows*). Differentiation of the branching patterns between endobronchial and endovascular metastases is difficult and requires an examination of sequential thin-cut images to separate the normal pulmonary artery or bronchus from the involved structure.

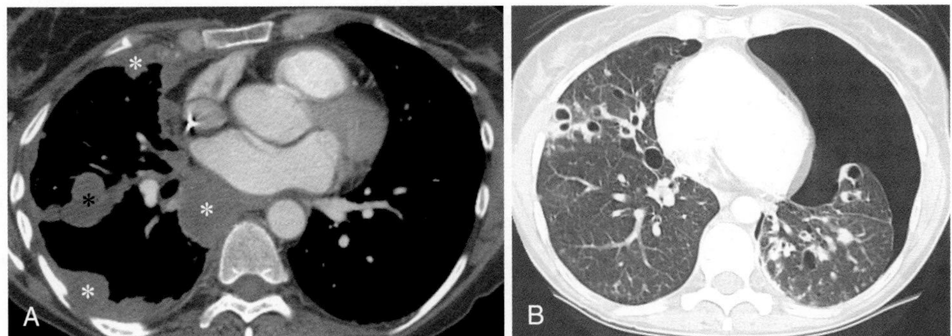

FIGURE 31.5. Pleural lesions. **A**, A patient with metastatic endometrial cancer. Typical pleural metastases with diffuse thickening of the peripheral pleura (*white asterisks*) and along the major fissure (*black asterisk*). **B**, Large left pneumothorax associated with metastatic disease in a patient with placental site trophoblastic tumor. Pneumothorax could be related to one of the multiple thin-walled cavitary metastatic lesions or to one of the subpleural nodules. Clinically, the patient experienced bilateral pneumothoraces throughout the course of the illness.

conditions, biopsy shows noncaseous necrosis, without evidence of malignancy.[38]

KEY POINTS Lymphadenopathy

- Any nodal group can be affected.
- Occasionally, enlarged nodes develop in patients with malignancy and are secondary to a sarcoid-like reaction. Biopsy shows noncaseous necrosis.

PLEURAL MANIFESTATIONS OF METASTATIC DISEASE

Pleural Metastases

Pleural metastases are generally associated with metastatic adenocarcinoma and are frequently associated with tumors of the lung, breast, pancreas, and stomach.[1] Pleural metastases most frequently are a result of hematogenous spread but can also be secondary to lymphangitic spread or related to hepatic metastases.[1] Pleural metastases can present as an effusion or as smooth or nodular pleural thickening (Fig. 31.5A). In the absence of irregular or nodular pleural thickening, it is difficult to distinguish a benign from a malignant pleural effusion. Occasionally, diffuse thickening can mimic mesothelioma, and this pattern is typically associated with metastatic lesions from renal cell carcinoma and lymphoma.[1]

Pneumothorax Associated With Metastatic Disease

A pneumothorax can result from a metastatic lesion. Proposed mechanisms include cavitation of a metastatic nodule adjacent to the pleura or an aggressive tumor that creates a bronchopleural fistula. A pneumothorax associated with metastatic disease is frequently related to osteosarcoma but

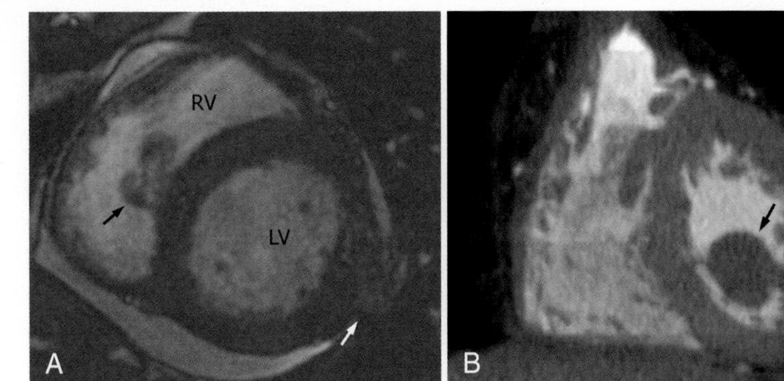

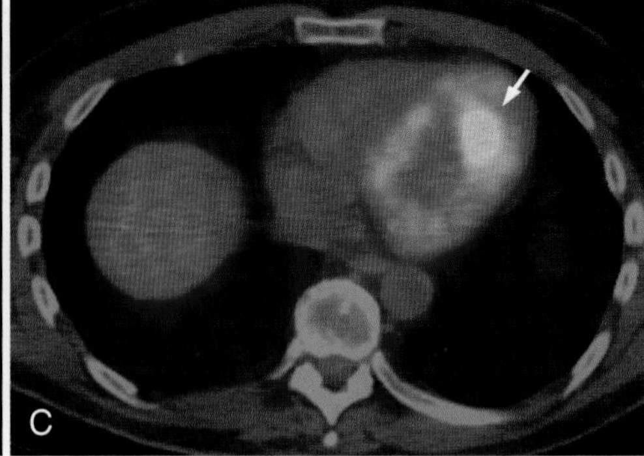

FIGURE 31.6. Cardiac metastases. **A**, Squamous cell cancer of the tongue. Short-axis cardiac magnetic resonance imaging of the heart shows two metastatic foci: one arising from the lateral wall of the left ventricle (*LV*), on the epicardial surface (*white arrow*), and the other from the endocardial surface of the right ventricle (*RV; black arrow*). **B** and **C**, Melanoma metastasis. **B**, Short-axis gated cardiac computed tomography (CT) scan shows a left ventricular mass (*arrow*) attached to the lateral wall by a stalk. **C**, Fused positron emission tomography (PET)/CT axial image shows increased 2-[^{18}F] fluoro-2-deoxy-D-glucose uptake by the mass (*arrow*).

can occur with other sarcomas or aggressive tumors[11,39] (see Fig. 31.5B). The incidence of pneumothorax in a patient with osteosarcoma is estimated to be 5% to 7%. When a pneumothorax occurs secondary to metastatic disease, patients usually have other known metastatic disease; occasionally, a pneumothorax can be the initial manifestation of a metastatic lesion.[40] In people who present with a pneumothorax, fewer than 1% will have an underlying malignancy.[41]

KEY POINTS Pleural Disease

- Manifestations of pleural metastases include effusion or smooth or nodular pleural thickening.
- Pleural metastases are most frequently associated with adenocarcinoma.
- Infrequently, a pneumothorax is a result of metastatic disease, most frequently associated with osteosarcoma.

CARDIAC METASTASES

Metastatic disease to the heart and pericardium is 22 times more frequent than primary tumors.[42] In a retrospective autopsy review of patients with a primary malignancy, 10.7% of patients were found to have cardiac metastases, with most metastases arising from lung cancer (36.4%).[43] Nonsolid primary tumors (lymphoma, leukemia, and Kaposi sarcoma) are also relatively common.[42,43] By cell type, adenocarcinoma accounted for the most cardiac metastases; however, melanoma had the highest propensity to involve the heart, occurring in approximately 50% of cases.[43] The majority of the lesions are located in the pericardium and epicardium, followed by myocardium and endocardium. Approximately one-third of epicardial lesions have an associated pericardial effusion. Most cardiac metastases are clinically silent.

The typical imaging pattern for cardiac metastases includes multiple nodules or masses, but they can be diffusely infiltrative (Fig. 31.6). In many cases, the appearance of cardiac metastases is relatively nonspecific. CMRI is the preferred method to evaluate these lesions, and most lesions show a low T1 signal and a high T2 signal. Occasionally, in patients with metastatic melanoma, CMRI characteristics are helpful in distinguishing metastases from other lesions in which the T1 signal may be high. Enhancement is generally heterogeneous. CT imaging is also nonspecific, demonstrating soft tissue lesions.[10]

KEY POINTS Cardiac

- Metastatic disease to the heart is 22 times more common than a primary tumor.
- More than one-third of cardiac metastases are from lung cancer.
- Melanoma is the tumor with the highest association of cardiac metastases.
- Epicardium is the most frequently involved layer, followed by the myocardium and endocardium.

Differential Diagnosis

Generally, when multiple nodules in the chest are detected in patients with a known primary malignancy, no further diagnostic tests are necessary, and nodules can be assumed to be metastatic. The appearance of multiple nodules in patients with more than one known primary is problematic; tissue sampling may be required to make a more specific diagnosis and institute appropriate therapy. Also problematic is the detection of a solitary pulmonary nodule in a patient with an extrathoracic primary malignancy. In these cases, differentiation between a primary and a secondary malignancy is important. In one series of breast cancer patients, the incidence of a second primary lung cancer was higher than that of a metastatic lesion.[44] The propensity for a second primary to develop is highest in cases in which the initial primary originated from a head and neck cancer, but is also common when there is a primary in the lung, breast, prostate, or stomach, especially in patients who smoke.[1] Conversely, solitary lung nodules in patients with melanoma and sarcoma are more likely to be metastases than primary lung malignancies.[1]

A difficult issue that frequently arises in the evaluation of possible metastatic disease in the workup of a patient with a primary malignancy is small nodules that are detected on CT. It should be stressed that most small (<4 mm), solid, noncalcified nodules discovered at CT scanning, even in patients with a known primary extrathoracic malignancy, are benign, and most often sequelae of granulomatous disease. Despite this fact, the current recommendation is to follow these nodules to exclude metastatic disease. In our experience, the vast majority of metastatic nodules will show changes at 3-month follow-up.

CONCLUSION

There are varied patterns of metastatic disease to the thorax. Hematogenous dissemination is the most frequent mode of spread and is the reason the thorax acquires more metastases than any other anatomic region. Some patterns of metastases mimic nonmalignant processes, necessitating differentiation. CT scanning is the gold standard in the evaluation of metastatic disease to the thorax. CT scanning is a sensitive but nonspecific modality, and additional imaging modalities serve complementary roles.

REFERENCES

1. Herold CJ, Bankier AA, Fleischmann D. Lung metastases. *Eur Radiol.* 1996;6:596–606.
2. Crow J, Slavin G, Kreel L. Pulmonary metastasis: a pathologic and radiologic study. *Cancer.* 1981;47:2595–2602.
3. Davis SD. CT evaluation for pulmonary metastases in patients with extrathoracic malignancy. *Radiology.* 1991;180:1–12.
4. Davis SD, Westcott J, Fleishon H, et al. Screening for pulmonary metastases. American College of Radiology. ACR Appropriateness Criteria. *Radiology.* 2000;215(Suppl):655–662.
5. Peuchot M, Libshitz HI. Pulmonary metastatic disease: radiologic-surgical correlation. *Radiology.* 1987;164:719–722.
6. Seo JB, Im JG, Goo JM, et al. Atypical pulmonary metastases: spectrum of radiologic findings. *Radiographics.* 2001;21:403–417.
7. Gladish GW, Choe DH, Marom EM, et al. Incidental pulmonary emboli in oncology patients: prevalence, CT evaluation, and natural history. *Radiology.* 2006;240:246–255.
8. Cronin CG, Lohan DG, Keane M, et al. Prevalence and significance of asymptomatic venous thromboembolic disease found on oncologic staging CT. *AJR Am J Roentgenol.* 2007;189:162–170.
9. Gruden JF, Ouanounou S, Tigges S, et al. Incremental benefit of maximum-intensity-projection images on observer detection of small pulmonary nodules revealed by multidetector CT. *AJR Am J Roentgenol.* 2002;179:149–157.
10. Hoey ET, Mankad K, Puppala S, et al. MRI and CT appearances of cardiac tumours in adults. *Clin Radiol.* 2009;64:1214–1230.
11. Libshitz HI, North LB. Pulmonary metastases. *Radiol Clin North Am.* 1982;20:437–451.
12. McLoud TC. *Thoracic. Radiology: The Requisites.* St. Louis: CV Mosby; 1998:336–337.
13. Choi JI, Goo JM, Seo JB, et al. Pulmonary metastases of alveolar soft-part sarcoma: CT findings in three patients. *Korean J Radiol.* 2000;1:56–59.
14. Libshitz HI, Jing BS, Wallace S, et al. Sterilized metastases: a diagnostic and therapeutic dilemma. *AJR Am J Roentgenol.* 1983;140:15–19.
15. Swett HA, Westcott JL. Residual nonmalignant pulmonary nodules in choriocarcinoma. *Chest.* 1974;65:560–562.
16. Panicek DM, Toner GC, Heelan RT, et al. Nonseminomatous germ cell tumors: enlarging masses despite chemotherapy. *Radiology.* 1990;175:499–502.
17. Tateishi U, Hasegawa T, Kusumoto M, et al. Metastatic angiosarcoma of the lung: spectrum of CT findings. *AJR Am J Roentgenol.* 2003;180:1671–1674.
18. Lee YR, Choi YW, Lee KJ, et al. CT halo sign: the spectrum of pulmonary diseases. *Br J Radiol.* 2005;78:862–865.
19. Thalinger AR, Rosenthal SN, Borg S, et al. Cavitation of pulmonary metastases as a response to chemotherapy. *Cancer.* 1980; 46:1329–1332.
20. Maile CW, Rodan BA, Godwin JD, et al. Calcification in pulmonary metastases. *Br J Radiol.* 1982;55:108–113.
21. deSantos LA, Lindell Jr MM, Goldman AM, et al. Calcification within metastatic pulmonary nodules from synovial sarcoma. *Orthopedics.* 1978;1:141–144.
22. Maxwell JR, Yao L, Eckardt JJ, et al. Case report 878: densely calcifying synovial sarcoma of the hip metastatic to the lungs. *Skeletal Radiol.* 1994;23:673–675.
23. Hall FM, Frank HA, Cohen RB, et al. Ossified pulmonary metastases from giant cell tumor of bone. *AJR Am J Roentgenol.* 1976;127:1046–1047.
24. Ohnishi H, Haruta Y, Yokoyama A, et al. Metastatic breast cancer presenting as air-space consolidation on chest computed tomography. *Intern Med.* 2009;48:727–731.
25. Jung JI, Kim HH, Park SH, et al. Thoracic manifestations of breast cancer and its therapy. *Radiographics.* 2004;24:1269–1285.
26. Gaeta M, Volta S, Scribano E, et al. Air-space pattern in lung metastasis from adenocarcinoma of the GI tract. *J Comput Assist Tomogr.* 1996;20:300–304.
27. McLoud TC. *Thoracic Radiology.* St. Louis: CV Mosby; 1998: 216–218.
28. Webb WR, Müller NL, Naidich DP. *High-resolution CT of the Lung.* Philadelphia: Lippincott-Raven; 1996:149–150.
29. Winterbauer RH, Elfenbein IB, Ball Jr WC. Incidence and clinical significance of tumor embolization to the lungs. *Am J Med.* 1968;45:271–290.
30. Shepard JA, Moore EH, Templeton PA, et al. Pulmonary intravascular tumor emboli: dilated and beaded peripheral pulmonary arteries at CT. *Radiology.* 1993;187:797–801.
31. Kang CH, Choi JA, Kim HR, et al. Lung metastases manifesting as pulmonary infarction by mucin and tumor embolization: radiographic, high-resolution CT, and pathologic findings. *J Comput Assist Tomogr.* 1999;23:644–646.
32. Kim AE, Haramati LB, Janus D, et al. Pulmonary tumor embolism presenting as infarcts on computed tomography. *J Thorac Imaging.* 1999;14:135–137.
33. Chan CK, Hutcheon MA, Hyland RH, et al. Pulmonary tumor embolism: a critical review of clinical, imaging, and hemodynamic features. *J Thorac Imaging.* 1987;2:4–14.
34. Ikezoe J, Johkoh T, Takeuchi N, et al. CT findings of endobronchial metastasis. *Acta Radiol.* 1991;32:455–460.
35. Braman SS, Whitcomb ME. Endobronchial metastasis. *Arch Intern Med.* 1975;135:543–547.
36. Akoglu S, Ucan ES, Celik G, et al. Endobronchial metastases from extrathoracic malignancies. *Clin Exp Metastasis.* 2005;22: 587–591.
37. Katsimbri PP, Bamias AT, Froudarakis ME, et al. Endobronchial metastases secondary to solid tumors: report of eight cases and review of the literature. *Lung Cancer.* 2000;28:163–170.
38. Hunsaker AR, Munden RF, Pugatch RD, et al. Sarcoidlike reaction in patients with malignancy. *Radiology.* 1996;200:255–261.
39. Dines DE. Pneumothorax and metastatic sarcomas. *Chest.* 1978;73:681–682.
40. Furrer M, Althaus U, Ris HB. Spontaneous pneumothorax from radiographically occult metastatic sarcoma. *Eur J Cardiothorac Surg.* 1997; 11:1171–1173.
41. Smevik B, Klepp O. The risk of spontaneous pneumothorax in patients with osteogenic sarcoma and testicular cancer. *Cancer.* 1982;49:1734–1737.
42. Lam KY, Dickens P, Chan AC. Tumors of the heart. A 20-year experience with a review of 12,485 consecutive autopsies. *Arch Pathol Lab Med.* 1993;117:1027–1031.
43. Klatt EC, Heitz DR. Cardiac metastases. *Cancer.* 1990;65: 1456–1459.
44. Cahan WG, Castro EB. Significance of a solitary lung shadow in patients with breast cancer. *Ann Surg.* 1975;181:137–143.

CHAPTER 32

Metastases to Abdominal-Pelvic Organs

Silvana Castro Faria, M.D., Ph.D.; Wen-Jen Hwu, M.D., Ph.D.; and Steven A. Curley M.D., F.A.C.S.

INTRODUCTION

Metastasis is a complex process in which tumor cells leave the original site of disease, called the primary tumor, to spread to other parts of the body. Cancer cells can break away from a primary tumor, enter the blood vessels, circulate through the bloodstream, and be deposited in other organs far from the primary tumor. When tumor cells metastasize to distant organs, the new tumor is called a secondary or metastatic tumor.[1]

EPIDEMIOLOGY

Most tumors can metastasize. The most common sites of metastasis from solid tumors are the lungs, liver, and bones. However, the frequency, location, and patterns of metastases will depend on the primary tumor. Certain tumors rarely metastasize, whereas some cancers tend to metastasize earlier than others.[2] The presence of metastatic disease may also be correlated with the tumoral histology. Undifferentiated, anaplastic, and high-grade tumors have a tendency to generate more metastases than well-differentiated and low-grade tumors.[3] The cells in a metastatic tumor resemble those in the primary tumor. However, when the metastatic tumor is undifferentiated, the pathologist can use several adjuvant techniques, such as immunohistochemistry, to try to identify the origin of the primary tumor. In rare cases, patients will have metastatic disease without a primary tumor found, and these patients are considered to have a cancer of an unknown primary tumor.[4]

CLINICAL PRESENTATION

Metastatic disease is usually present in late stages of the cancer. However, when metastases are present early in the course of the disease, the type and frequency of the symptoms will depend on the location and size of the metastatic lesions. For example, symptoms of liver impairment including development of jaundice and hepatomegaly can indicate that the cancer has spread to the liver, and neurological symptoms such as headaches and seizures may indicate the presence of brain metastases, whereas bone metastases usually present as bone pain.

DIAGNOSIS

The diagnosis of metastatic disease is one of the most important steps in the staging of patients with cancer. The detection of metastatic disease has an important role on the prognosis and treatment of cancer patients. Several imaging modalities can be used in the assessment of presence of metastatic disease, including ultrasound (US), computed tomography (CT), magnetic resonance imaging (MRI) and 2-[^{18}F] fluoro-2-deoxy-D-glucose positron emission tomography (FDG-PET)/CT.[5] Among them, US has advantages such as noninvasiveness, ready availability, and relatively low cost. CT scans of the chest, abdomen, and pelvis are the most common imaging methods used for the initial staging of oncologic patients, as CT is widely available and is a noninvasive diagnostic tool. MRI, a nonionizing imaging technique, is very helpful in patients who are allergic to iodinated contrast agents and has intrinsic multiplanar capabilities that offer increased sensitivity in the detection of metastatic disease due to high soft-tissue contrast resolution. PET and CT performed in a single scanning session (PET/CT) is used for staging of oncologic patients. FDG uptake is an important discriminating factor in the evaluation of potentially malignant cells. Additionally, newly developed PET radionuclides are being used to image neuroendocrine tumors and prostate cancer, among others. More recently, simultaneous PET and MRI (PET/MRI), which combines the anatomic and quantitative strengths of MRI with physiologic information obtained from PET, has been used for the detection and characterization of metastatic disease.[5]

TREATMENT

Treatment for metastatic disease usually depends on several factors, including the size and location of the metastasis, the patient's age and general health, and the types of treatments the patient has had in the past. Patients with single metastasis or single site of metastatic disease need to be evaluated for possible curative treatment, usually with surgical resection. However, when there are multiple metastases, systemic treatment such as chemotherapy, and in some cases radiation therapy and clinical trials or a combination of these, may be necessary. Recent exciting developments in cancer immunotherapy, which involves priming the host's natural immune defenses to recognize, target, and destroy cancer cells effectively, and advances in targeted therapy have provided some hope in fighting metastatic disease.[6]

PATTERNS OF TUMOR SPREAD

The three principal pathways of tumor dissemination include: hematogenic, lymphatic, and local invasion. The purpose of this chapter is to review hematogenous metastasis to intraabdominal and pelvic organs. We will divide our chapter by individual organ.

Key Points General Principles

- Metastasis is a complex process in which tumor cells leave the original site to spread to other parts of the body.
- The most common sites of metastasis from solid tumors are the lungs, liver, and bones.
- The diagnosis of metastatic disease is one of the most important steps in staging patients.
- The three principal pathways of tumor dissemination are hematogeneous, lymphatic, and local invasion.
- Several imaging modalities may be used in staging, including ultrasound, computed tomography, and magnetic resonance imaging.

Key Points What the Surgeon, Radiation Oncologist, and Medical Oncologist Want to Know

- The surgeon wants to know the presence of metastases, the number and size of the lesions, multifocality, and vascular involvement to plan resection.
- The radiation oncologist needs to know the location, size, and relationship of tumor to radiosensitive organs to plan the radiation therapy field.
- The medical oncologist wants to know the number, location, and size of the lesions in the baseline study and the response to chemotherapy on follow-up imaging.

Liver

The most common solid organ to receive metastatic disease is the liver. Approximately 50% to 60% of patients who die of cancer have hepatic metastases at autopsy.[7] The tumors that most commonly metastasize to the liver include: lung tumors, breast tumors, gastrointestinal tract tumors (such as esophageal, gastric, and colorectal tumors), pancreas tumors, and melanoma. Liver metastases usually appear as multiple solid lesions; however, in some cases they may present as a solitary lesion, confluent masses, and infiltrative lesions that may mimic cirrhosis.[8] Various imaging modalities may be used in the assessment of presence of hepatic metastases.

On US, liver metastases can have a variety of different appearances. Generally, the majority of liver metastases present as multiple solid hypoechoic lesions from hypovascular tumors such as breast and lung cancers (Fig. 32.1). They may show a peripheral hypoechoic rim, known as the halo sign, which has been shown to represent a zone of proliferating tumor, a pseudocapsule, and/or compressed liver parenchyma.[9] Other liver metastases may appear isoechoic or hyperechoic and with an anechoic cystic component. Hyperechoic lesions are frequently associated with gastrointestinal primary tumor, renal cell carcinoma (RCC), or hepatocellular carcinoma (Fig. 32.2). Cystic metastases may demonstrate mural solid nodules or thick septations. Calcified metastases present with posterior acoustic shadowing and are usually seen with mucinous adenocarcinoma of the gastrointestinal and genitourinary tracts.[10]

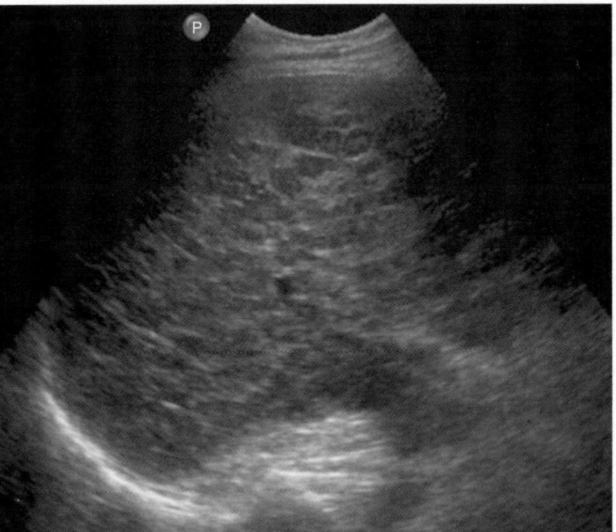

Figure 32.1. A 69-year-old woman with lung cancer. Gray-scale ultrasound image demonstrates replacement of the hepatic parenchyma by multiple small, round, hypoechoic solid lesions, consistent with metastatic disease.

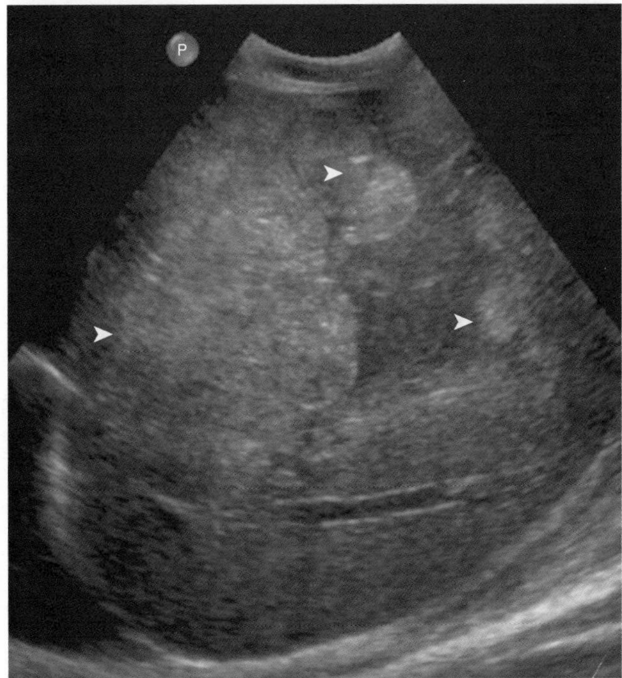

Figure 32.2. A 65-year-old man with colon cancer. Gray-scale ultrasound image demonstrates several hyperechoic solid lesions (*arrowheads*) within the liver parenchyma, consistent with metastatic disease.

Although US has been widely used to detect liver metastases, the sensitivity of US in detecting liver metastases is lower than that of CT or MRI. Wernecke et al. reported a sensitivity of 53% for US in the detection of hepatic masses.[11] The use of microbubble intravenous (IV) contrast agent improves differentiation between the metastatic lesions and liver parenchyma, increasing the sensitivity of US in detecting hepatic metastases, even though it use is still limited to only some centers.[12] Additional limitations of US include being operator-dependent, nonreproducible, and limited by abdominal gas and patient body habitus.

On unenhanced CT, the majority of liver metastases appear as low-attenuating lesions compared with the surrounding liver parenchyma (Fig. 32.3). Calcifications may be seen in metastatic lesions from a primary mucin-secreting tumor of the gastrointestinal tract or ovary, as well as after chemotherapy treatment (Fig. 32.4). The use of IV contrast medium facilitates the distinction between focal lesions and the underlying liver parenchyma, improving the detection and characterization of hepatic lesions.[13]

On enhanced CT, the imaging features of a liver metastasis will depend on the primary tumor. The most common liver metastases are hypovascular compared with the adjacent liver and appear as low-attenuation lesions on the portal venous phase of imaging when the surrounding normal liver is at its peak of enhancement (Figs. 32.5 and 32.6). Liver metastasis may also present a hypoattenuating halo and areas of hemorrhage and necrosis when the growth exceeds the tumor neovascularity (Figs. 32.7, 32.8, and 32.9). Hypovascular metastases usually originate from primary tumors from the gastrointestinal tract, including colon, rectum, esophagus, and stomach, as well as others site such as lung, pancreas, and prostate.[14]

Alternatively, hepatic metastases with increased arterial flow relative to normal liver are best seen as hypervascular lesions during the arterial-dominant phase of enhancement. Moreover, they may show washout and become hypoattenuating on delayed images (Fig. 32.10). Hypervascular metastases usually originate from RCCs and neuroendocrine tumors. Other primary tumors that may present with hypervascular liver metastases include medullary thyroid cancer, melanoma, and gastrointestinal stromal tumors.[15]

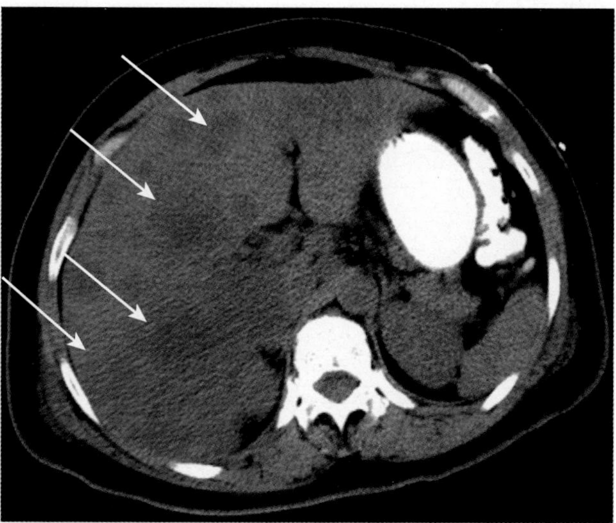

Figure 32.3. A 56-year-old woman with melanoma. Axial unenhanced computed tomography scan shows multiple solid, low-attenuation lesions (*arrows*) within the liver parenchyma, consistent with metastatic disease.

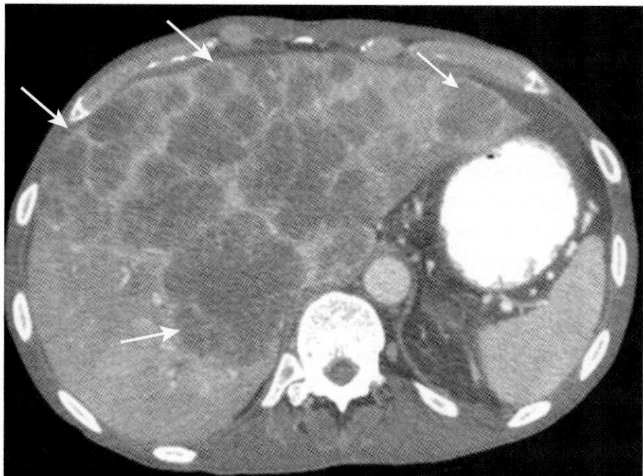

Figure 32.5. A 65-year-old man with colon cancer. Axial contrast-enhanced computed tomography scan in the portal venous phase of enhancement shows multiple solid, low-attenuation lesions (*arrows*) compared with the surrounding liver parenchyma, consistent with metastatic disease.

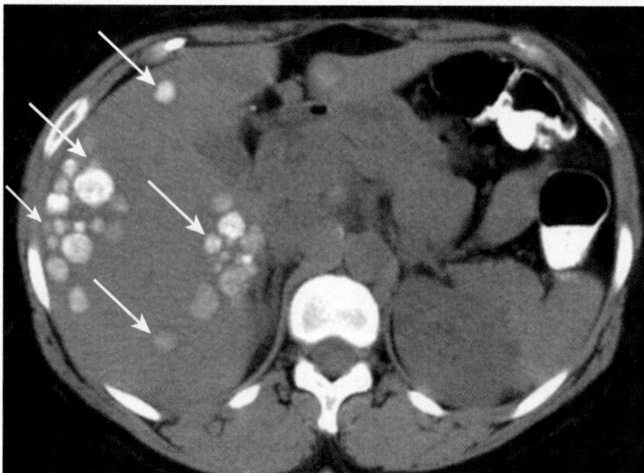

Figure 32.4. A 44-year-old woman with moderately differentiated adenocarcinoma of the gastroesophageal junction. Axial unenhanced computed tomography scan demonstrates multiple high-attenuation calcified lesions (*arrows*) within the liver, consistent with metastatic disease.

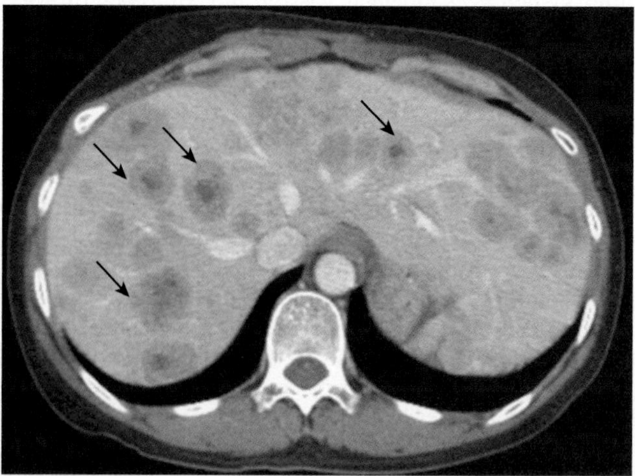

Figure 32.6. A 41-year-old woman with breast cancer. Axial contrast-enhanced computed tomography scan in the portal venous phase of enhancement shows multiple solid, low-attenuation lesions (*arrows*) within the liver, consistent with metastatic disease. Note that some lesions present a more hypodense center, probably representing areas of necrosis.

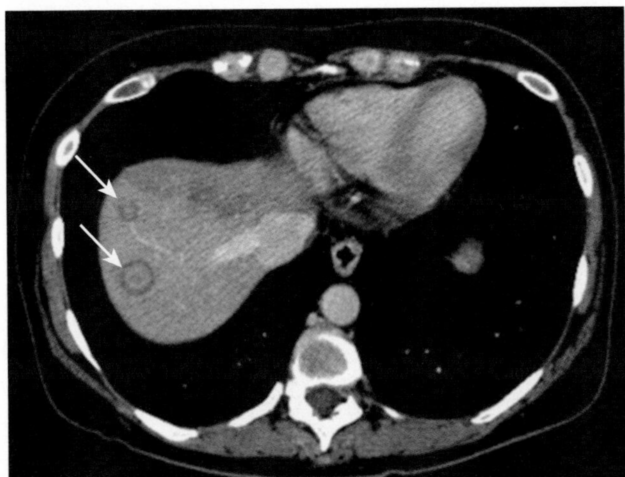

FIGURE 32.7. A 53-year-old woman with islet cell pancreatic tumor. Axial contrast-enhanced computed tomography scan in the portal venous phase of enhancement shows two solid lesions that present a thin, low-attenuating halo (*arrows*) surrounding an ovoid center of more intense enhancement, consistent with metastatic disease.

The reported accuracy of CT in detecting hepatic metastases ranges from 75% to 96%, based on studies of patients with colorectal cancer.[16,17] The limitations of CT include radiation exposure and the risk of adverse reaction with the use of IV contrast agents.

Hepatic metastases may have a variable appearance on MRI. However, the majority of liver metastases appear as low signal intensity on unenhanced T1-weighted (T1W) MRI images. Some tumors that contain melanin or fat, such as metastases from melanomas and liposarcomas, respectively, can appear hyperintense on T1W images. Hemorrhagic metastases may also appear hyperintense on T1W images. On T2-weighted (T2W) images, most liver metastases exhibit high signal intensity (Fig. 32.11). Lesions with central necrosis or cystic metastases can result in even higher signal intensity on T2W images, whereas calcified lesions may be hypointense on T2W images.[18]

After IV injection of gadolinium, most liver metastases show a peripheral ring of enhancement and are seen in the portal-venous phase of imaging as hypointense lesions in comparison with the enhancing surrounding liver parenchyma (Fig. 32.11). Larger lesions may show

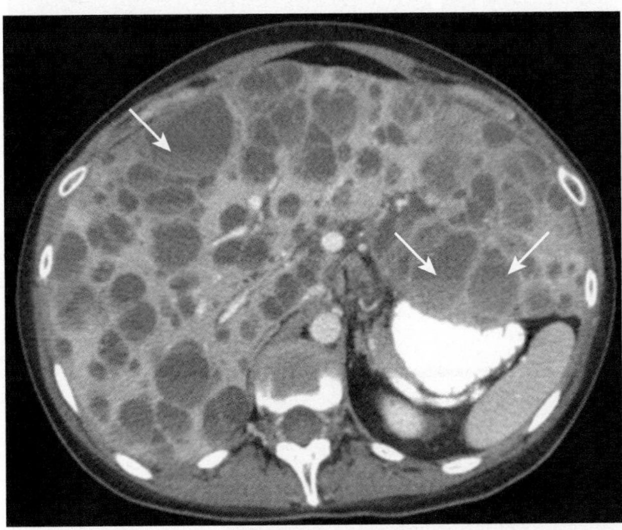

FIGURE 32.8. A 33-year-old woman with melanoma. Axial contrast-enhanced computed tomography scan in the portal venous phase of enhancement shows innumerous hypodense lesions within the liver, consistent with metastatic disease. Note fluid levels in some of the lesions that may represent hemorrhage (*arrows*).

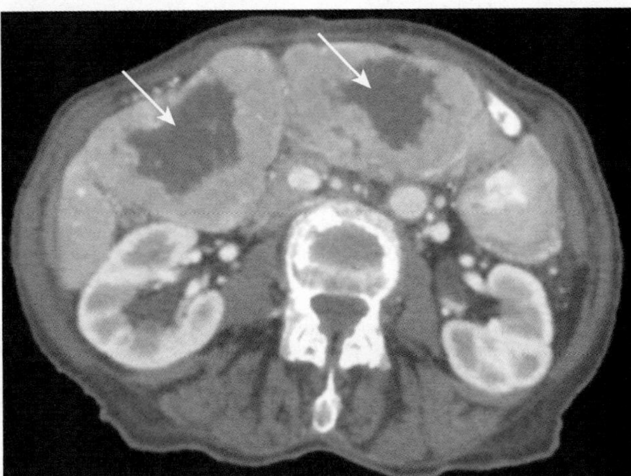

FIGURE 32.9. A 56-year-old woman with ovarian cancer. Axial contrast-enhanced computed tomography scan in the portal venous phase of enhancement shows two large metastatic liver lesions with peripheral enhancement of the solid portions and central hypodensity, representing areas of necrosis (*arrows*).

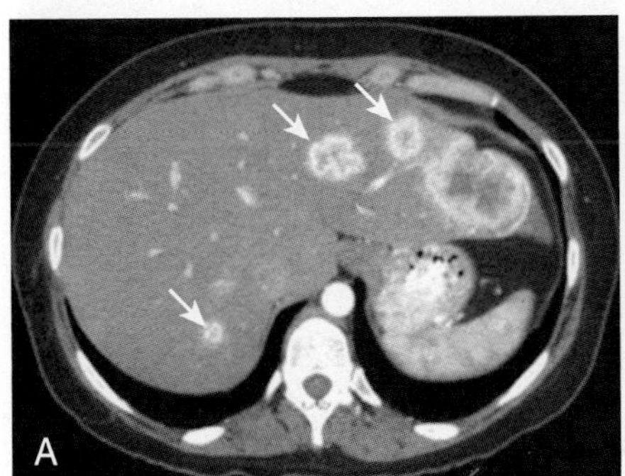

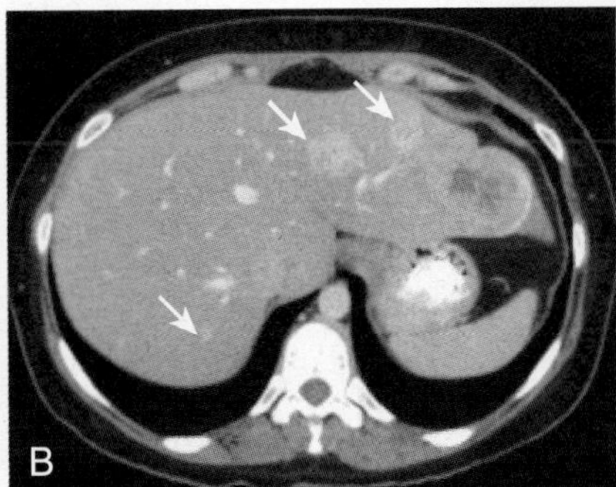

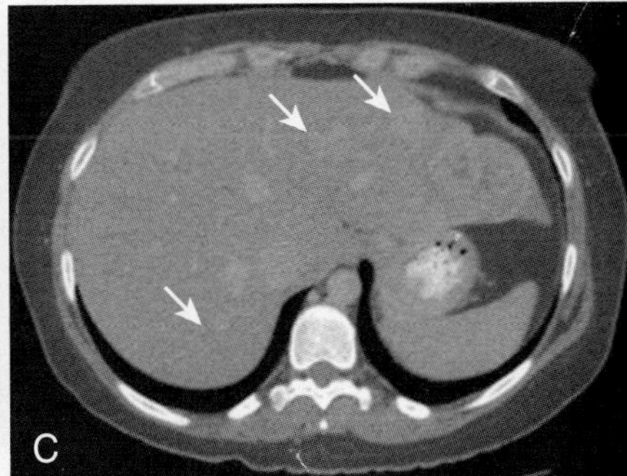

FIGURE 32.10. A 54-year-old woman with gastric carcinoid tumor. **A**, Axial contrast-enhanced computed tomography (CT) scan shows few lesions that present intense early enhancement in the arterial phase of enhancement (*arrows*) compared with the background liver parenchyma, characterizing hypervascular metastases. Axial contrast-enhanced CT scans in the portal venous (**B**) and delayed (**C**) phases of enhancement show that the lesions are progressively less conspicuous (*arrows*) than the background liver parenchyma.

cauliflower-like enhancement. Hypervascular metastases appear as foci of intense enhancement versus the background liver parenchyma during the arterial phase of enhancement (Fig. 32.12). The presence of washout of the contrast from the lesion on delayed images is highly suspicious for malignancy.[19] The reported sensitivity of MRI for

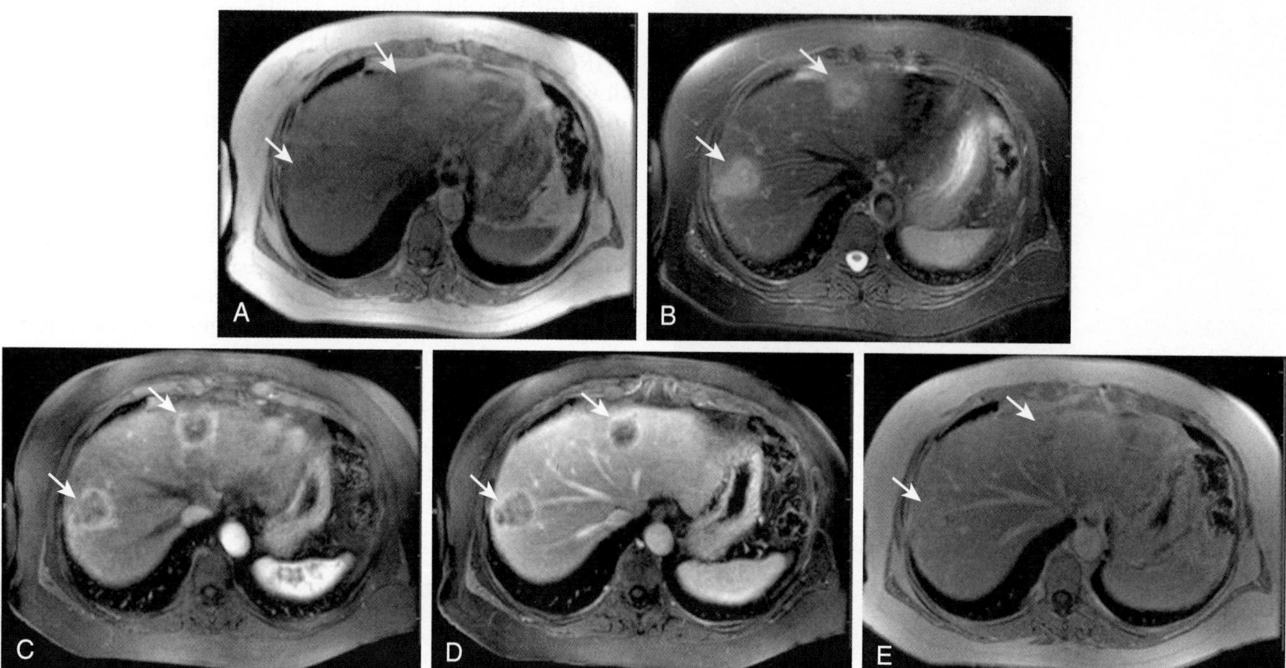

FIGURE 32.11. A 62-year-old woman with colon cancer. **A**, Axial T1-weighted (T1W) magnetic resonance imaging (MRI) demonstrates two dominant low–signal intensity lesions (*arrows*) in the liver. **B**, Axial T2-weighted MRI demonstrates two dominant metastatic foci of high signal intensity (*arrows*) in the liver. **C–E**, Axial postcontrast T1W dynamic MRI obtained after intravenous injection of contrast during the arterial (**C**), portal venous (**D**), and delayed (**E**) phases demonstrates early rim enhancement (*arrows* in **C**), hypointense lesions in the portal venous phase of enhancement (*arrows* in **D**) compared with the background liver, and subsequent washout of the rim in later images, as well as a progressive accumulation of contrast in the central portion of the lesion (*arrows* in **E**).

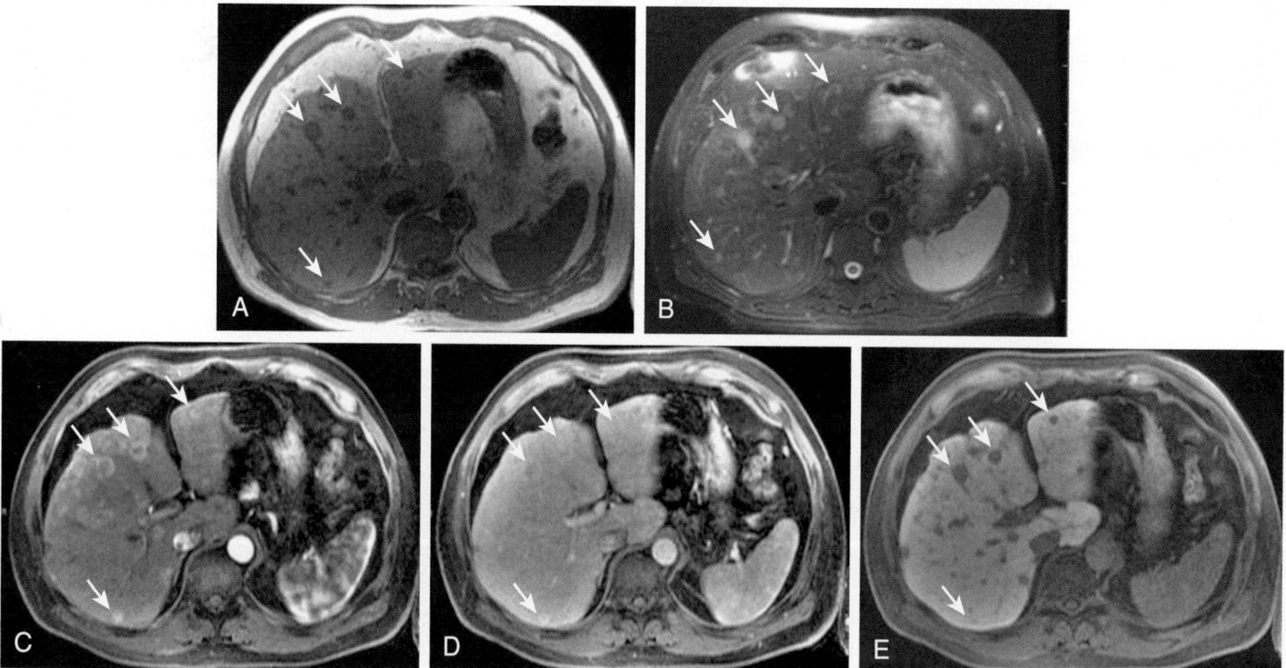

FIGURE 32.12. A 63-year-old man with islet cell pancreatic tumor. **A**, Axial T1-weighted (T1W) magnetic resonance imaging (MRI) demonstrates a few small, low–signal intensity lesions (*arrows*) in the liver. **B**, Axial T2-weighted MRI demonstrates a few small, metastatic foci with high signal intensity (*arrows*) in the liver. **C**, Axial T1W dynamic MRI obtained after intravenous injection of contrast shows intense enhancement during the arterial phase of enhancement, with some lesions presenting ring enhancement and smaller lesions presenting more homogeneous early enhancement (*arrows*). Note the progressive washout of the lesions in the portal venous phase (**D**) and delayed phase (**E**) of contrast enhancement (*arrows*).

the evaluation of suspected hepatic metastases ranges from 80% to 99%.[20,21] The limitations of MRI include restriction to large centers and contraindication for patients with pacemakers or ferromagnetic implants.

Key Points

- The liver is the most common solid organ to receive metastatic disease.
- Approximately 50% to 60% of patients who die of cancer have hepatic metastases at autopsy.
- Liver metastases may have a variable appearance, and imaging features depend on the primary tumor.
- Most common liver metastases are hypovascular and appear as low-attenuation lesions compared with the adjacent liver parenchyma in the portal venous phase.
- Some hepatic metastases are hypervascular, presenting with increased arterial flow relative to normal liver, and are best seen during the arterial phase of enhancement.

Spleen

The spleen is an infrequent site of tumor metastasis, which usually occurs in late stages of cancer as a manifestation of widely disseminated disease. The incidence of neoplastic involvement of the spleen ranges from 0.3% to 33%, depending on the type of primary tumor and the extent of disease on autopsy studies.[22] The lack of afferent lymphatic vessels, the presence of a sharp angle at the origin of the splenic artery, the contractile nature of the spleen, and the inhibitory effect of the splenic reticuloendothelial system are some of the theories that have been proposed to explain the relative paucity of splenic metastases.[23]

The most common primary sources of splenic metastases are breast cancer, lung cancer, ovarian cancer, melanoma, colorectal cancer, and gastric cancer. In cases of isolated splenic metastasis, ovarian and colorectal carcinomas are the most common causes. Most metastases to the spleen occur by hematogenous involvement resulting in parenchymal disease. The presence of surface/capsular lesions is often associated with peritoneal dissemination, usually from ovarian cancer, while direct splenic invasion is more commonly observed in gastric cancer and left RCC.[24]

Patients with splenic metastases are usually asymptomatic, and the diagnosis is generally made by routine imaging studies. Eventually, patients may present with abdominal pain, splenomegaly or a palpable mass. In rare cases, it may present as spontaneous rupture of the spleen.[25]

Parenchymal splenic metastases usually appear as multiple round solid hypoechoic lesions on US. In some cases, it may be a hypoechoic solitary lesion. Splenic surface involvement also appears hypoechoic on US.

On CT scans, splenic metastases are typically solid round areas of slightly decreased attenuation in relation to the normal splenic parenchyma (Fig. 32.13). Capsular metastases result in indentation of the splenic surface. Melanoma and ovarian cancers may also cause cystic splenic metastases, and ovarian metastatic lesions may calcify (Figs. 32.14 and 32.15).[26]

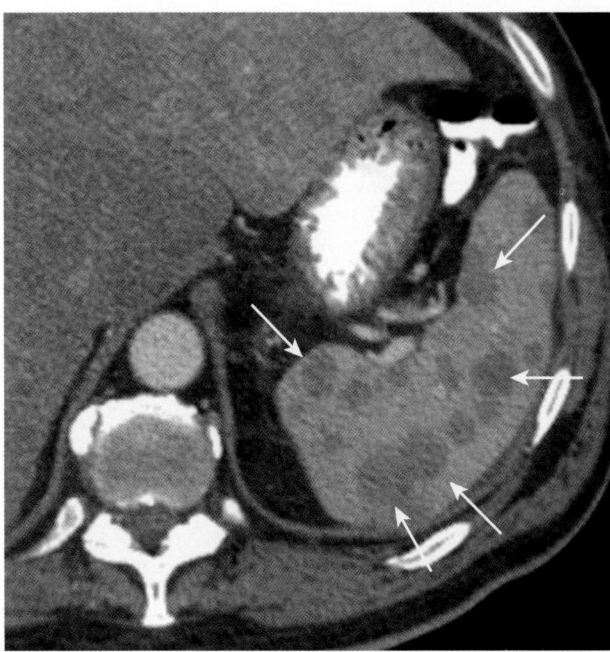

Figure 32.13. A 69-year-old man with melanoma. Axial contrast-enhanced computed tomography scan in the portal venous phase of enhancement shows multiple solid, low-attenuation lesions (*arrows*) within the spleen, consistent with metastatic disease.

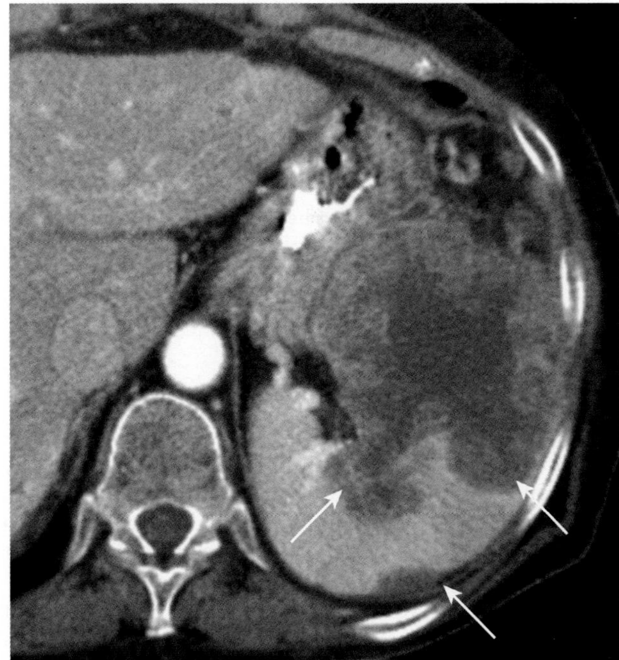

Figure 32.14. A 56-year-old woman with ovarian cancer. Axial contrast-enhanced computed tomography scan in the portal venous phase of enhancement shows peritoneal implants involving the spleen with indentation of the splenic surface (*arrows*), consistent with metastatic disease.

On MRI, splenic metastases typically appear as hypointense to isointense lesions on T1W images and as hyperintense lesions on T2W images. They usually enhance after IV injection of contrast.[27]

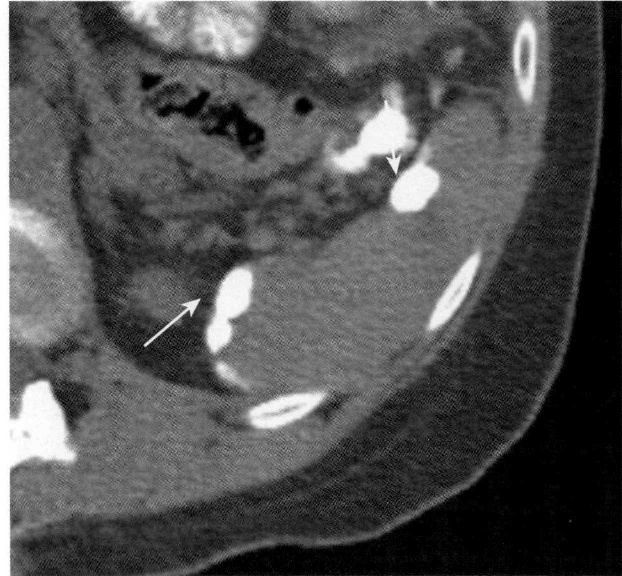

FIGURE 32.15. A 60-year-old woman with ovarian cancer. Axial unenhanced computed tomography scan shows calcified peritoneal implants (*arrows*) involving the surface of the spleen, consistent with metastatic disease.

KEY POINTS

- The incidence of neoplastic involvement of the spleen ranges from 0.3% to 16%, depending on the type of primary tumor and the extent of disease on autopsy studies.
- Most common primary sources of splenic metastases are breast cancer, lung cancer, ovarian cancer, melanoma, colorectal cancer, and gastric cancer.
- Metastases to the spleen may be due to parenchymal disease, surface/capsular lesions, or direct invasion.

Gallbladder

Metastases to the gallbladder are rare in clinical practice. Although infrequent, there are some reports in the literature of metastases to the gallbladder from some primary cancers such as melanoma, RCC, lung cancer, breast cancer, and stomach cancer.[28] Among these, malignant melanoma is reported to be the most common origin of gallbladder metastases, accounting for 50% to 60% of cases of gallbladder metastases. According to Shimkin et al., malignant melanoma can metastasize to the gallbladder in 4% to 20% of cases.[29]

Gallbladder metastases generally do not cause clinical symptoms and are usually an incidental postmortal finding. However, in symptomatic cases, the most frequent presentation is acute cholecystitis. Nassenstein reported a case of a 45-year-old man who developed symptoms of an acute cholecystitis caused by a metastasis from a nonsmall cell lung cancer to the wall of the gallbladder.[30]

The most used modality in the assessment of both primary and metastatic lesions of the gallbladder is US. US can demonstrate focal thickening of the gallbladder wall, intraluminal polipoid mass, or an exophytic echogenic mass. It is usually not associated with presence of calculi, as in cases of primary gallbladder malignancy.[31]

CT may also show focal thickening of the gallbladder wall, intraluminal polipoid mass, or an exophytic mass that usually enhances after administration of contrast. Some cases may involve the biliary tree, causing bile ductal dilation (Fig. 32.16).[32]

On MRI, metastatic lesions of the gallbladder may appear as hyperintense lesions on T2W images and hypointense to isointense on T1W images, and usually enhance after IV injection of contrast.[33]

KEY POINTS

- Gallbladder metastases are rare in clinical practice.
- Although infrequent, some primary tumors, such as melanoma, renal cell carcinoma, lung cancer, breast cancer, and stomach cancer, metastasize to the gallbladder.

Pancreas

The pancreas is rarely a site of metastatic disease, which is found at autopsy in 3% to 12% of patients with disseminated malignant disease.[34] The most common primary tumor associated with solitary pancreatic metastases is RCC. Other primary malignancies that may metastasize to the pancreas include lung, stomach, breast, colon, and esophageal cancer, melanoma, and lymphoma.[35]

According to Thompson and Heffess, RCC metastatic disease to the pancreas may occur many years after nephrectomy, with an average of 8.4 years (range, 0.5–27 years), and they are usually potentially amenable to surgery.[36] Thus, patients must be followed closely, as most patients with pancreatic metastases are asymptomatic, with the lesions usually being detected incidentally on surveillance CT scans. Alternatively, symptomatic patients may present with abdominal pain, back pain, nausea, weight loss, and jaundice. In rare cases RCC metastatic disease to the pancreas may cause acute pancreatitis.

Metastatic pancreatic involvement manifests as a solitary focal mass without a predilection for a particular part of the pancreas, as multiple nodules within the pancreas, or as diffuse enlargement of the pancreas.[37] On US, single or multiple metastatic solid lesions usually appear more hypoechoic than the rest of the pancreatic parenchyma.[38] Circumscribed lesions may appear isodense or, more often, slightly hypodense compared with the normal pancreatic parenchyma on unenhanced CT images. After IV injection of contrast, most pancreatic metastases appear as single or multiple enhancing low-attenuation lesions (Fig. 32.17). Rim enhancement with heterogeneous areas of central low attenuation may be observed in large lesions, with smaller lesions enhancing more homogeneously (Fig. 32.18). Conversely, metastases from RCC appear as intense enhancing lesions, better identified in the arterial phase of contrast enhancement (Fig. 32.19). Additionally, attention should be given to the CT protocol used in

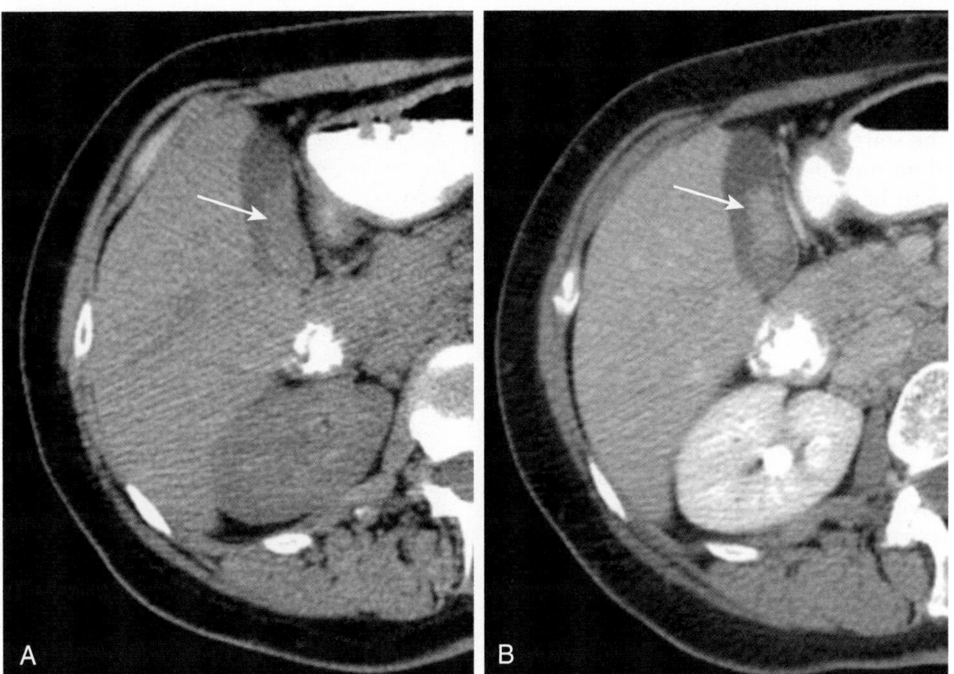

Figure 32.16. A 50-year-old man with melanoma. Axial unenhanced computed tomography scan shows soft tissue focus within the gallbladder (**A**) that enhances after the intravenous injection of contrast (**B**), consistent with metastatic disease (*arrows*).

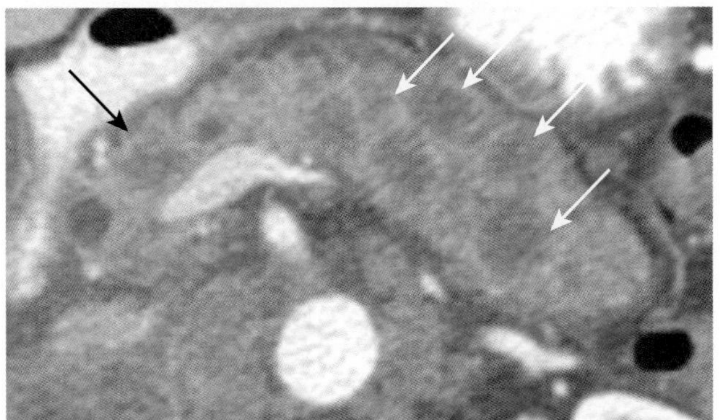

Figure 32.17. A 52-year-old woman with small-cell lung cancer. Axial enhanced computed tomography scan in the portal venous phase of enhancement shows multiple round, low-attenuation lesions (*white arrows*) within the pancreatic parenchyma (*black arrow*), consistent with metastatic disease.

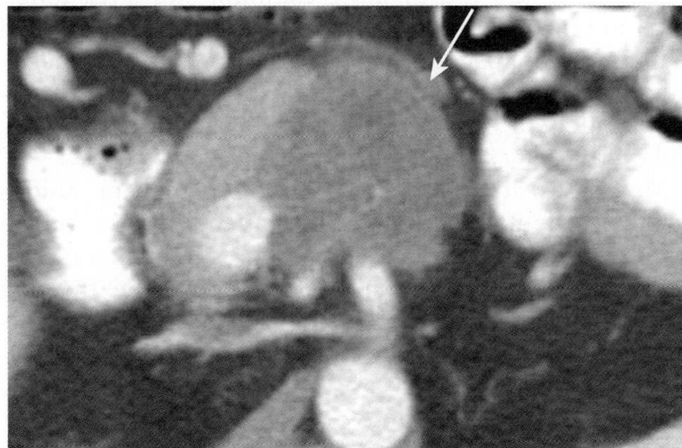

Figure 32.18. A 60-year-old man with melanoma. Axial enhanced computed tomography scan in the portal venous phase of enhancement shows a heterogeneous, predominantly low-attenuation lesion (*arrow*) in the neck/body of the pancreas, consistent with metastatic disease.

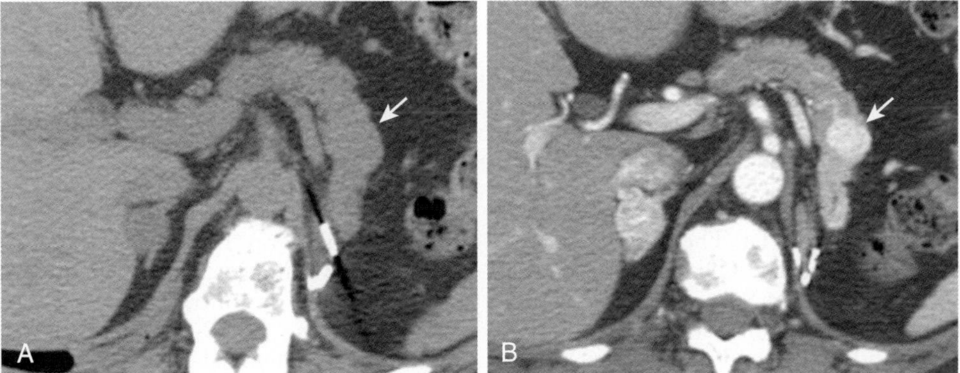

Figure 32.19. A 70-year-old woman with renal cell carcinoma. **A**, Axial unenhanced computed tomography scan shows an isodense round lesion (*arrow*) within the tail of the pancreas. **B**, After the intravenous injection of contrast, the lesion presents with intense enhancement (*arrow*) in the arterial phase of enhancement, consistent with metastatic disease.

the surveillance of RCC patients. According to Ng et al., smaller pancreatic metastases from RCC ranging from 0.6 to 11 cm in diameter enhance most conspicuously during the early arterial phase of enhancement, beginning 25 seconds from the start of injection. The enhancement is less pronounced on the 60-second portal phase images and may even fail to be appreciated on the 120-second delayed phase images.[39] On MRI, pancreatic lesions are usually hypointense on unenhanced T1W images and moderately hyperintense on T2W images and enhance after IV injection of contrast.[40]

KEY POINTS Pancreas

- Metastatic disease to the pancreas may be found in 3% to 12% of patients with disseminated malignant disease at autopsy.
- The most common primary tumors that produce pancreatic metastases include lung cancer, renal cell carcinoma, stomach cancer, breast cancer, colon cancer, esophageal cancer, melanoma, and lymphoma.

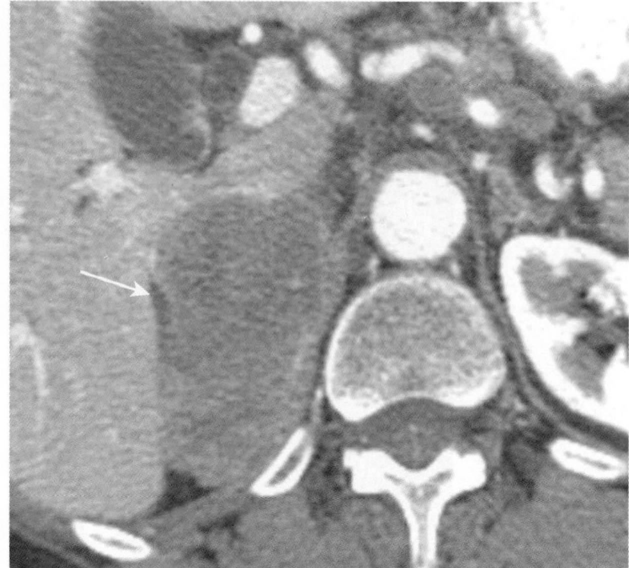

FIGURE 32.20. A 68-year-old man with small cell lung cancer. Axial contrast-enhanced computed tomography scan in the portal venous phase of enhancement shows a large heterogeneous lesion (*arrow*) in the right adrenal gland, consistent with a metastatic lesion.

Adrenal Glands

The adrenal glands are a frequent site of metastatic disease, representing the fourth most common site after lungs, liver, and bones. At autopsy, adrenal metastases are found in up to 27% of patients who did from an epithelial malignancy.[34] Common sites of origin of adrenal gland metastases include lung, breast, gastrointestinal, kidney, pancreas, and thyroid cancers and melanoma.

Metastases are the most common malignant lesions involving the adrenal glands. In patients with a known underlying malignancy, an adrenal mass may be a metastasis but also could be an unrelated benign lesion. Imaging studies may help in differentiating between them. Patients with adrenal metastases are usually clinically silent. However, in some cases metastasis to the adrenal glands may present as hypoadrenalism.[41]

The radiographic appearance of adrenal metastases is not specific. They may be unilateral or bilateral, large or small. Adrenal metastases that are smaller than 2 cm are usually difficult to diagnose by US. Additionally, US is also limited in the differentiation of benign and malignant adrenal masses.[42]

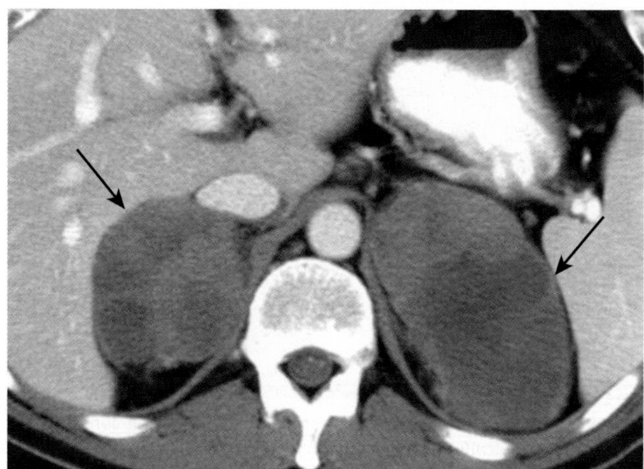

FIGURE 32.21. A 58-year-old man with melanoma. Axial contrast-enhanced computed tomography scan in portal venous phase of enhancement shows bilateral large masses within the adrenal glands, with heterogeneous enhancement due to areas of necrosis and areas of more solid enhancement (*arrows*), consistent with metastatic disease.

On CT, small adrenal metastases are usually well-defined round or ovoid lesions with a thin rim and homogeneous density. Conversely, larger adrenal metastases may be lobulated or irregular in shape, with a heterogeneous appearance owing to areas of necrosis, hemorrhage, or calcifications (Figs. 32.20 and 32.21). The demonstration of the presence of fat in an adrenal mass allows the differential diagnosis between an adrenal adenoma and adrenal metastases, which do not contain fat. The threshold of 10 Hounsfield units in an unenhanced CT scan has a sensitivity of 79% and a specificity of 96% for the diagnosis of adrenal adenomas.[43] After IV administration of contrast material, both adrenal adenomas and adrenal metastases enhance, but adenomas have a faster "washout." The use of a percentage enhancement washout with a threshold of more than 60% on delayed enhanced scans performed 15 minutes after the injection of contrast has a sensitivity of 86% and a specificity of 92% for the diagnosis of adrenal adenomas.[44]

On MRI, adrenal metastases usually demonstrate low signal intensity on T1W images and high signal intensity on T2W images. They usually enhance after the administration of contrast material. The most accurate MRI technique for distinguishing an adenoma from a metastasis is chemical-shift imaging. Because of their high fat content, adrenal adenomas demonstrate signal loss on out-of-phase images, which is not seen with adrenal metastases.[45]

Key Points

- The adrenal glands are the fourth most common site of metastatic disease after lungs, liver, and bones.
- Adrenal metastases may be found in up to 27% of patients who die from an epithelial malignancy at autopsy.
- Common origins of adrenal glands metastases include lung, breast, gastrointestinal tract, kidneys, pancreas, and thyroid cancers and melanoma.

Kidneys

Renal metastases constitute a significant percentage of kidney lesions found at autopsy. The kidney is the fifth most common site for metastatic solid tumors, following the lung, liver, bones, and adrenal glands. Renal metastases may be seen in up to 20% of patients who die of malignancy.[46]

The most common primary tumors to metastasize to the kidneys are lung cancer, breast lymphoma, melanoma, and gastrointestinal tract cancer. Most renal metastases are clinically silent, but some patients may present with microscopic or gross hematuria. Metastatic renal lesions may present as single or multiple cortical nodules and can be unilateral or bilateral. Renal metastases rarely manifest as intraluminal filling defects.[47]

On US, renal metastases usually appear as homogeneous hypoechoic masses. However, some metastases may appear heterogeneous or echogenic.[48]

On unenhanced CT, renal metastases are generally small and appear as multiple isodense or slightly hypodense lesions compared with the renal parenchyma. They are usually hypovascular and present mild enhancement after IV injection of contrast (Figs. 32.22 and 32.23). Other features include an irregular thickened wall and a blurred margin with the normal renal parenchyma. Tumor invasion of the renal vein and extension into the inferior vena cava is rare with metastatic lesions.[49] When the primary tumor is lymphoma, the renal involvement from lymphoma may have several different appearances. The most common presentation is multiple bilateral, round lesions with the same density as soft tissue that also enhance less than the normal renal parenchyma. However, a solitary mass or diffuse infiltration of the kidney by lymphoma may also be seen.[50] On MRI, renal metastases usually demonstrate low signal intensity on T1W images and high signal intensity on T2W images. They usually present mild enhancement after the administration of contrast material.[49]

Key Points

- The kidneys are the fifth most common site for metastasis of solid tumors, following the lung, liver, bones, and adrenal glands.
- Renal metastases may be seen in up to 20% of patients who die of malignancy.
- The most common primary tumors to metastasize to the kidneys are lung cancer, breast lymphoma, melanoma, and gastrointestinal tract cancer.

Urinary Bladder

The bladder is not a common site for metastasis, and bladder metastases often go undiagnosed in the clinical follow-up of cancer patients. Metastases to the bladder represent no more than 3% of all malignant bladder tumors.[51] Urinary bladder involvement by a secondary tumor occurs either as a metastasis or by direct extension. Bladder metastases originate most commonly from primary tumors in the genitourinary tract, such as those at prostate and cervical sites and from the colon and rectum. Of the malignancies arising from distant foci, melanoma is the most common tumor to generate bladder metastases, followed by breast, lung, and gastric carcinomas. Radiographically, these tumors present as one or multiple mural masses projecting into the bladder lumen. However, in some cases they may present as

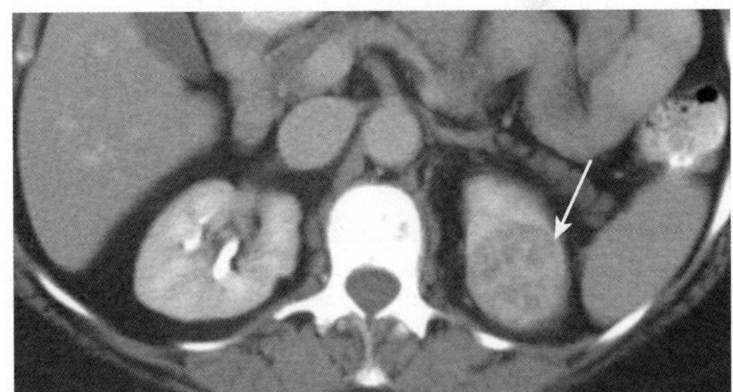

Figure 32.23. A 68-year-old woman with breast cancer. Axial contrast-enhanced computed tomography scans in the excretory phase of enhancement shows a solid heterogeneous enhancing lesion (*arrow*) in the left kidney, consistent with metastatic disease.

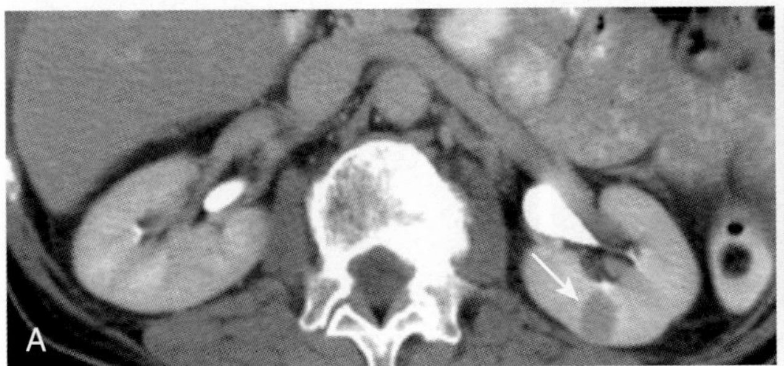

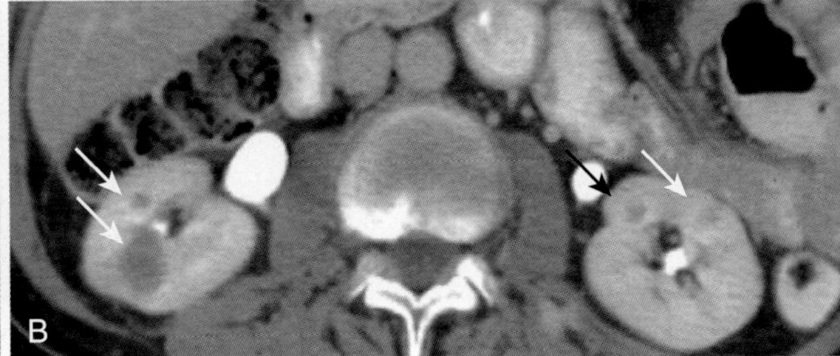

Figure 32.22. A 62-year-old man with melanoma. **A** and **B**, Axial contrast-enhanced computed tomography scans in the excretory phase of enhancement show bilateral small, solid, hypodense lesions (*arrows*) in the kidneys, consistent with metastatic disease.

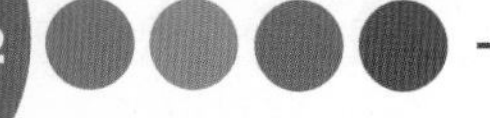

diffuse thickening of the bladder wall, which can be seen on US and CT.[52]

Female Genital Tract

Metastases to the female genital tract are uncommon. However, the most frequent metastatic sites for both extragenital and genital primaries are the ovaries and vagina. Secondary tumors of the uterus are very uncommon and account for less than 10% of all cases of metastases to the female genital tract from extragenital cancers.[53] The most common genital primary tumors to give rise to metastases to the female genital tract are uterine body and uterine cervix cancers. The most common extragenital tumors to give rise to metastases to the female genital tract include breast, colon, stomach, lung, and pancreas tumors, melanomas, and sarcomas.[53]

Metastatic tumors to the ovaries may represent 10% to 30% of malignant ovarian tumors.[54] The most common tumors that metastasize to the ovary are melanomas or tumors of the gastrointestinal tract, breast, gynecologic organs, or lungs.[54] The term "Krukenberg tumor" is usually used to describe bilateral ovarian metastases consisting of solid portions and variable amounts of fluid-filled structures and characterized by mucin-producing signet ring cells, most commonly originating from primary lesions in the gastrointestinal tract, in particular from carcinomas of the stomach (Fig. 32.24).[55]

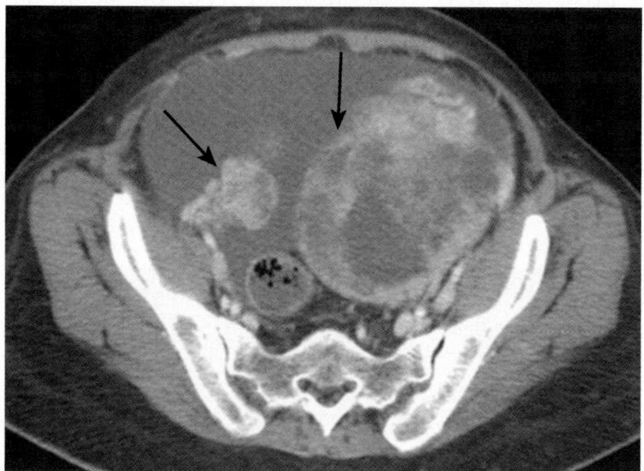

FIGURE 32.24. A 53-year-old woman with poorly differentiated adenocarcinoma of the stomach with signet-ring cells. Axial contrast-enhanced computed tomography scan in the delayed phase of enhancement shows bilateral heterogeneous lesions (*arrows*) with solid and cystic components involving the ovaries bilaterally, consistent with metastatic disease.

Colon carcinoma is one of the most frequent primary tumors that metastasizes to the ovary. Approximately 3% to 8% of female patients with colon carcinoma will develop metastases to the ovaries, and between 6% and 14% of women who die with colorectal cancer are found to have ovaries metastases at autopsy.[56]

Radiographically, ovarian metastases are difficult to differentiate from primary ovarian cancer. On US, ovarian metastastic lesions appear as complex masses with mixed echogenicity due to areas of soft tissue and cystic components.[57] On CT, ovarian metastases frequently appear as heterogeneous masses with solid and cystic areas. The solid areas enhance after IV injection of contrast (Figs. 32.25 and 32.26).[58]

On MRI, the signal intensity will vary according to the presence and extent of the solid and cystic components. The more solid areas present low signal intensity on T1W images and intermediate to low signal intensity on T2W images. Alternatively, the signal intensity of the cystic component will depend on the chemical composition of the cyst fluid. Although simple fluid cystic lesions present with low signal intensity on T1W images and high signal intensity on T2W images, some mucin-containing lesions exhibit high signal intensity on T1W images.[59]

Key Points Ovaries

- Metastatic tumors to the ovaries may represent 10% to 30% of malignant ovarian tumors.
- The most common ovarian metastases originate from melanomas or tumors of the gastrointestinal tract, breast, gynecologic organs, or lungs.
- The term "Krukenberg tumor" is usually used to describe bilateral ovarian metastases consisting of solid and cystic portions, most commonly originating from primary lesions in the gastrointestinal tract, particularly from the stomach.
- Approximately 3% to 8% of female patients with colon carcinoma will develop ovarian metastases.
- Some 6% to 14% of women who die with colorectal cancer are found to have ovarian metastases at autopsy.

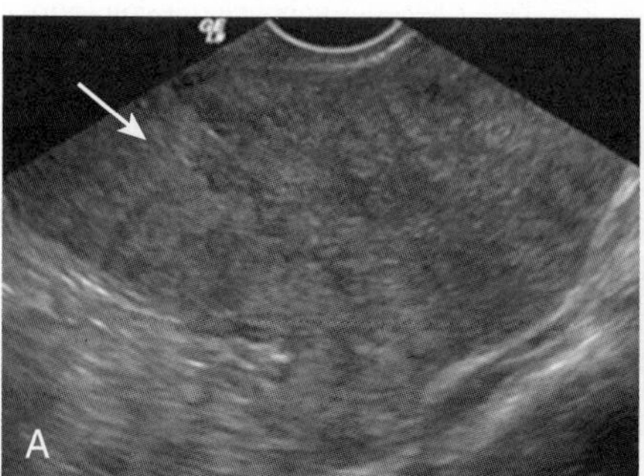

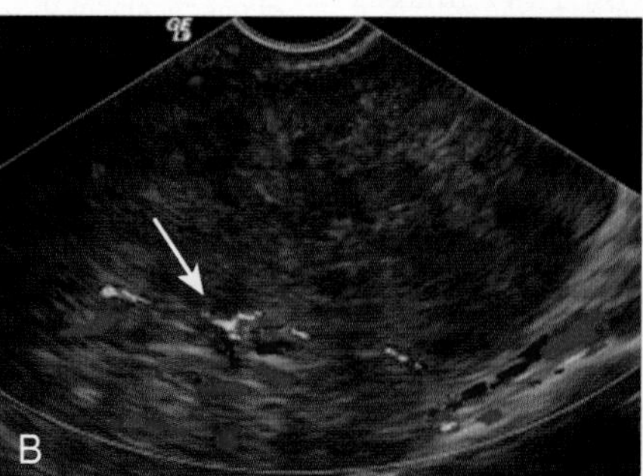

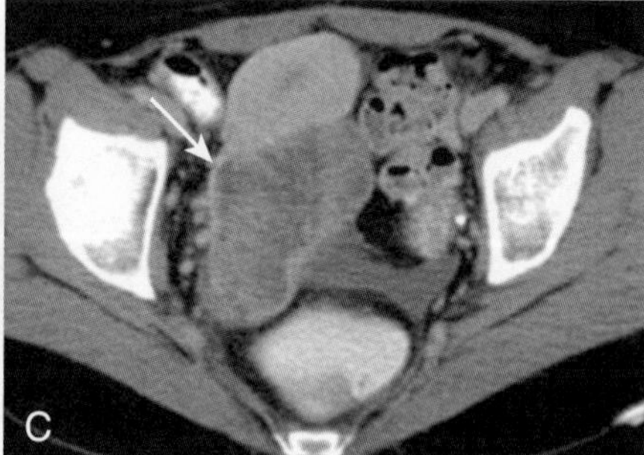

FIGURE 32.25. A 49-year-old woman with moderately differentiated appendiceal adenocarcinoma. **A**, Gray-scale endovaginal ultrasound image demonstrates a large heterogeneous mass with mixed echogenicity (*arrow*). **B**, Note some areas of increased vascularity (*arrow*) on the color Doppler image. **C**, Axial contrast-enhanced computed tomography scan in the delayed phase of enhancement shows a large heterogeneous lesion (*arrow*) involving the right ovary, consistent with metastatic disease.

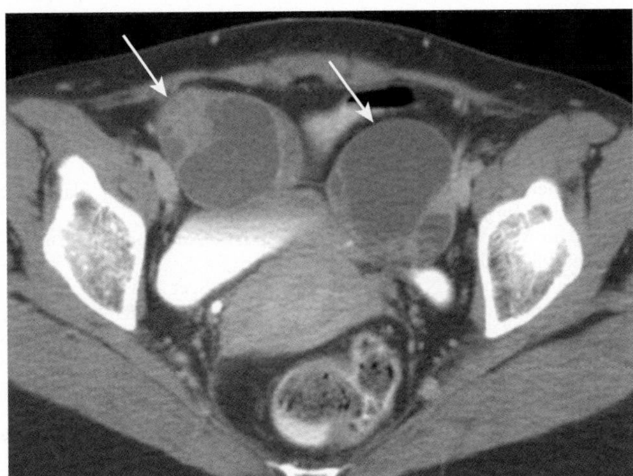

FIGURE 32.26. A 56-year-old woman with colon carcinoma. Axial contrast-enhanced computed tomography scan in the delayed phase of enhancement shows bilateral heterogeneous lesions with solid and cystic components (*arrows*) involving the ovaries bilaterally, consistent with metastatic disease.

Male Genital Tract

Metastatic tumors to the male genital tract are rare. Secondary tumors account for 1.6% to 3% of solid malignancies encountered in surgical specimens from the genitourinary tract.[60]

Prostate

Secondary neoplasms of the prostate were found in 0.5% to 5.6% of patients who died from cancer and in 2.1% of all neoplasms in surgical specimens.[60] Prostate involvement by a secondary tumor occurs either as a metastasis or by direct extension from adjacent structures. The most common primary tumors that can give rise to metastases to the prostate include melanomas and lung, gastrointestinal tract, and pancreas tumors. Tumors of the bladder and rectum usually reach the prostate by direct spread.[61]

Testicles

Secondary neoplasms of the testicles are most commonly an incidental finding at autopsy and are reported to be found in 0.5% of patients who have died of cancer. The most common primary tumors that can give rise to metastases to the testicles include melanomas and prostate, lung, colon, kidney, urinary tract, and pancreas cancers.[62]

REFERENCES

1. Poste G, Fidler IJ. The pathogenesis of cancer metastasis. *Nature*. 1980;283(5743):139–146.
2. Fidler IJ. Critical determinants of metastasis. *Semin Cancer Biol*. 2002;12(2):89–96.
3. Yokota J. Tumor progression and metastasis. *Carcinogenesis*. 2000;21(3):497–503.
4. Blaszyk A, Hartmann J. Bjornsson, Cancer of unknown primary: clinicopathologic correlations. *APMIS*. 2003;111:1089–1094.
5. Faas L. Imaging and cancer: A review. *Molecular Oncology*. 2008;2(2):115–152.
6. Dromain C, Beigelman C, Pozzessere C, et al. Imaging of tumor response to immunotheraphy. *Eur Radiol Exp*. 2020;1:2.
7. Cameron GR. The liver as a site and source of cancer. *Br Med J*. 1954;13(1):347–352.
8. Baker ME, Pelley R. Hepatic metastases: basic principles and implications for radiologists. *Radiology*. 1995;197(2):329–337.
9. Wernecke K, Henke L, Vassallo P, et al. Pathologic explanation for hypoechoic halo seen on sonograms of malignant liver tumors: an in vitro correlative study. *AJR Am J Roentgenol*. 1992;159:1011–1016.
10. Robison PJ. Imaging liver metastases: current limitations and future prospects. *Br J Radiol*. 2000;73(867):234–241.
11. Wernecke K, Rummeny E, Bongartz G, et al. Detection of hepatic masses in patients with carcinoma: comparative sensitivities of sonography, CT, and MR imaging. *AJR Am J Roentgenol*. 1991;157(4):731–739.
12. Quaia E, D'Onofrio M, Palumbo A, et al. Comparison of contrast-enhanced ultrasonography versus baseline ultrasound and contrast-enhanced computed tomography in metastatic disease of the liver: diagnostic performance and confidence. *Eur Radiol*. 2006;16:1599–1609.
13. Sica GT, Ji H, Ros PR CT. and MRI imaging of hepatic metastases. *AJR Am J Roentgenol*. 2000;174(3):691–698.
14. Kanematsu M, Kondo H, Goshima S, et al. Imaging liver metastases: review and update. *Eur J Radiol*. 2006;58(2):217–228.
15. Liu PS, Francis IR. Hepatic imaging for metastatic disease. *Cancer J*. 2010;16(2):93–102.
16. Mainenti PP, Mancini M, Mainolfi C, et al. Detection of colo-rectal liver metastases: prospective comparison of contrast enhanced US, multidetector CT, PET/CT, and 1.5 Tesla MR with extracellular and reticulo-endothelial cell specific contrast agents. *Abdom Imaging*. 2010;35:511–521.
17. Valls C, Lopez E, Gumà A, et al. Helical CT versus CT arterial portography in the detection of hepatic metastasis of colorectal carcinoma. *AJR Am J Roentgenol*. 1998;170:1341–1347.
18. Imam K, Bluemke DA. MR imaging in the evaluation of hepatic metastases. *Magn Reson Imaging Clin N Am*. 2000;8:741–756.
19. Namasivayam S, Martin DR, Saini S. *Imaging of liver metastases: MRI. Cancer Imaging*. 2007;7:2–9.
20. Hussain SM, Semelka RC. Hepatic imaging: comparison of modalities. *Radiol Clin North Am*. 2005;43:929–947.
21. Semelka RC, Schlund JF, Molina PL, et al. Malignant liver lesions: comparison of spiral CT arterial portography and MR imaging for diagnostic accuracy, cost, and effect on patient management. *J Magn Reson Imaging*. 1996;6:39–43.
22. Berge T. Splenic metastases. *Frequencies and patterns. Acta Pathol Microbiol Scand*. 1974;82:499–506.
23. Lam KY, Tang V. Metastatic tumors to the spleen. A 25-year clinicopathologic study. *Arch Pathol Lab Med*. 2000;124(4):526–530.
24. Compérat E, Bardier-Dupas A, Camparo P, et al. Splenic metastases: clinicopathologic presentation, differential diagnosis, and pathogenesis. *Arch Pathol Lab Med*. 2007;131(6):965–969.
25. Sauer J, Soblewski K, Dommish K. Splenic metastases--not a frequent problem, but an underestimate location of metastases: epidemiology and course. *J Cancer Res Clin Oncol*. 2009;135(5):667–671.
26. Federle M, Moss AA. Computed tomography of the spleen. *Crit Rev Diagn imaging*. 1983;19:1–16.
27. Elsayes KM, Narra VR, Mukundan G, et al. MR imaging of the spleen: spectrum of abnormalities. *Radiographics*. 2005;25(4):967–982.
28. Yoon WJ, Yoon YB, Kim YJ, et al. Metastasis to the gallbladder: a single-center experience of 20 cases in South Korea. *World J Gastroenterol*. 2009;15(38):4806–4809.
29. Shimkim PM, Soloway MS, Jaffe E. Metastatic melanoma of the gallbladder. *AJR Am J Roentgenol*. 1972;116:393–395.
30. Nassenstein K, Kissler M. Gallbladder metastasis of non-small cell lung cancer. *Onkologie*. 2004;27(4):398–400.
31. Dong XD, DeMatos P, Prieto VG, et al. Melanoma of the gallbladder: a review of cases seen at Duke University Medical Center. *Cancer*. 1999;85(1):32–39.
32. Takayama Y, Asayama Y, Yoshimitsu K, et al. Metastatic melanoma of the gallbladder. *Comput Med Imaging Graph*. 2007;31(6):469–471.
33. Yoshimitsu K, Honda H, Kaneko K, et al. Dynamic MRI of the gallbladder lesions: differentiation of benign from malignant. *J Magn Reson Imaging*. 1997;7(4):696–701.

34. Abrams HL, Spiro R, Goldestein N. Metastases in carcinoma. analysis of 1000 autopsied cases. *Cancer*. 1950;3:73–85.
35. Adsay NV, Andea A, Basturk O, et al. Secondary tumors of the pancreas: an analysis of a surgical and autopsy database and review of the literature. *Virchows Arch*. 2004;444(6):527–535.
36. Thompson LD, Heffess CS. Renal cell carcinoma to the pancreas in surgical pathology material. *Cancer*. 2000;89(5):1076–1088.
37. Klein KA, Stephens DH, Welch TJ. CT characteristics of metastatic disease of the pancreas. *Radiographics*. 1998;18(2):369–378.
38. Wernecke K, Peters PE, Galanski M. Pancreatic metastases: US evaluation. *Radiology*. 1986;160(2):399–402.
39. Ng CS, Loyer EM, Iyer RB, et al. Metastases to the pancreas from renal cell carcinoma: findings on three- phase contrast-enhanced helical CT. *AJR Am J Roentgenol*. 1999;172:1555–1559.
40. Merkle EM, Boaz T, Kolokythas O, et al. Metastases to the pancreas. *Br J Radiol*. 1998;71(851):1208–1214.
41. Sahagian-Edwards A, Holland JF. Metastatic carcinoma to the adrenal glands with cortical hypofunction. *Cancer*. 1954;7(6):1242–1245.
42. DeAtkine AB, Dunnick NR. The adrenal glands. *Semin Oncol*. 1991;18(2):131–139.
43. Lee MJ, Hahn PF, Papanicolaou N, et al. Benign and malignant adrenal masses: CT distinction with attenuation coefficients, size, and observer analysis. *Radiology*. 1991;179(2):415–418.
44. Caoili EM, Korobkin M, Francis IR, et al. Adrenal masses: characterization with combined unenhanced and delayed enhanced CT. *Radiology*. 2002;222(3):629–633.
45. Bilbey JH, McLoughlin RF, Kurkjian PS, et al. MR imaging of adrenal masses: value of chemical-shift imaging for distinguishing adenomas from other tumors. *AJR Am J Roentgenol*. 1995;164(3):637–642.
46. Hietala SO, Wahlqvist L. Metastatic tumors to the kidney. A postmortem, radiologic and clinical investigation. *Acta Radiol Diagn (Stockh)*. 1982;23(6):585–591.
47. Wagle DG, Moore RH, Murphy GP. Secondary carcinomas of the kidney. *J Urol*. 1975;114(1):30–32.
48. Choyke PL, White EM, Zeman RK, et al. Renal metastases: clinicopathologic and radiologic correlation. *Radiology*. 1987;162(2):359–363.
49. Bailey JE, Roubidoux MA, Dunnick NR. Secondary renal neoplasms. *Abdom Imaging*. 1998;23(3):266–274.
50. Cohan RH, Dunnick NR, Leder RA, et al. Computed tomography of renal lymphoma. *J Comput Assist Tomogr*. 1990;14(6):933–938.
51. Morichetti D, Mazzucchelli R, Lopez-Beltran A, et al. Secondary neoplasms of the urinary system and male genital organs. *BJU Int*. 2009;104(6):770–776.
52. Velcheti V, Govindan R. Metastatic cancer involving bladder: a review. *Can J Urol*. 2007;14(1):3443–3448.
53. Mazur MT. Metastases to the female tract. *Analysis of 325 cases. Cancer*. 1984;53:1978–1984.
54. Yada-Hashimoto N, Yamamoto T, Kamiura S, et al. Metastatic ovarian tumors: a review of 64 cases. *Gynecol Oncol*. 2003;89(2):314–317.
55. Young RH. From Krukenberg to today: the ever present problems posed by metastatic tumors in the ovary: part I. Historical perspective, general principles, mucinous tumors including the Krukenberg tumor. *Adv Anat Pathol*. 2006;13(5):205–227.
56. Omranipour R, Abasahl A. Ovarian metastases in colorectal cancer. *Int J Gynecol Cancer*. 2009;19(9):1524–1528.
57. Moyle JW, Rochester D, Sider L, et al. Sonography of ovarian tumors: predictability of tumor type. *AJR Am J Roentgenol*. 1983; 141(5):985–991.
58. Megibow AJ, Hulnick DH, Bosniak MA, et al. Ovarian metastases: computed tomographic appearances. *Radiology*. 1985;156(1):161–164.
59. Iyer VR, Lee SI. MRI, CT, and PET/CT for ovarian cancer detection and adnexal lesion characterization. *AJR Am J Roentgenol*. 2010;194(2):311–321.
60. Bates AW, Baithun SI. The significance of secondary neoplasms of the urinary and male genital tract. *Virchows Arch*. 2002;440(6): 640–647.
61. Bates AW, Baithun SI. Secondary solid neoplasms of the prostate: a clinico-pathological series of 51 cases. *Virchows Arch*. 2002; 440(4):392–396.
62. Ulbright TM, Young RH. Metastatic carcinoma to the testis: a clinicopathologic analysis of 26 nonincidental cases with emphasis on deceptive features. *Am J Surg Pathol*. 2008;32(11):1683–1693.

CHAPTER 33

Peritoneal Cavity and Gastrointestinal Tract

Ott Le, M.D.

INTRODUCTION

To understand metastatic disease in the abdomen and pelvis, one must appreciate the remarkable complexity of the peritoneum. By definition, the serosal peritoneum is a membrane that covers the lining of the abdominal and pelvic cavity and reflects over the viscera to form ligaments, mesenteries, and omenta. These reflections structurally support the organs and are conduits for the blood vessels, lymphatics, and nerves.

The network of connections formed by the peritoneal reflections serves to provide continuity between the abdominal walls and the organs therein and bridges the retroperitoneum with the peritoneum. These connections serve a physiologic role, but also can act as a pathway for the spread of disease.[1] These processes include inflammation, infection, trauma, and, importantly, tumor.

Primary tumors of the peritoneum are rare.[2] Metastasis is more common. Patients present with vague and nonspecific symptoms. Therefore, imaging plays a key role in the diagnosis of peritoneal disease. Because of the spaces and compartments formed by the peritoneal reflections, there are predictable patterns of disease spread. Common tumors that spread and metastasize to the peritoneum include stomach, colon, ovarian, and pancreatic cancer and lymphoma.

Peritoneal disease could not be assessed in a direct manner radiographically before the advent of cross-sectional imaging.[3] With improving technologies such as multidetector row computed tomography (CT), positron emission tomography/computed tomography (PET/CT), magnetic resonance imaging (MRI), and ultrasound, peritoneal metastasis can now be readily evaluated.

ANATOMY

Embryology

To fully understand the peritoneum, a basic understanding of its embryologic development is necessary.[4–7] The embryologic development of the peritoneum is complex. Briefly, the primitive gut is suspended within the peritoneal cavity by a dorsal and ventral primitive mesentery, which divides the peritoneum into a right and a left cavity. Unlike the ventral mesentery, the dorsal mesentery does not stop its attachment at the stomach, but continues to connect the primitive gut to the posterior abdominal wall inferiorly.

The liver develops within the ventral mesentery. The pancreas and spleen develop within the dorsal mesentery. The ventral mesentery anterior to the liver and attaching it to the anterior abdominal wall later becomes the falciform ligament, containing the umbilical vessels. The ventral mesentery between the liver and the stomach will develop into the gastrohepatic and hepatoduodenal ligaments.

Further growth, organ development, elongation, cavitation, and rotation form the adult peritoneum (Figs. 33.1 and 33.2). This includes the formation of the lesser sac, which is isolated from the remainder of the peritoneum or greater sac except at a small opening called the foramen of Winslow.

A single layer of mesothelial cells forms the peritoneum. It is separated from the submesothelial layer of connective tissue by a basal lamina. The submesothelial layer of connective tissue consists of collagen, elastic fibers, fibroblast-like cells, arteries, veins, and lymphatics.[6] The submesothelial layer or subperitoneal space is a virtual space that allows continuity between the mesenteries, the ligaments, the abdominal wall, and the retroperitoneum.

The peritoneum normally also contains a small amount of sterile fluid for lubrication, bacterial defense, and fluid transport.

Visceral and Parietal Peritoneum

The peritoneum is classified as either visceral or parietal.[8] The abdominal and pelvic walls are lined by the parietal peritoneum. Conversely, the visceral peritoneum covers the intraperitoneal organs or viscera and forms the omenta and mesenteries.

In males, the greater peritoneal cavity is a closed continuous cavity. Conversely, in females, it is discontinuous at the ostia of the oviducts, providing a communication between the peritoneal cavity and the lower pelvis, which is extraperitoneal.[6]

Double folds of the peritoneum result in formation of ligaments and mesenteries. They suspend and form the supporting structure for the peritoneal organs. For example, the mesentery suspends the small bowel within the peritoneal cavity and also serves to carry the arteries, lymphatics, and nerves. The omenta are formed from a double fold of the visceral peritoneum that extends from the stomach (Figs. 33.3 and 33.4). The peritoneal cavity is divided into various interconnecting compartments by the ligaments and mesenteries.

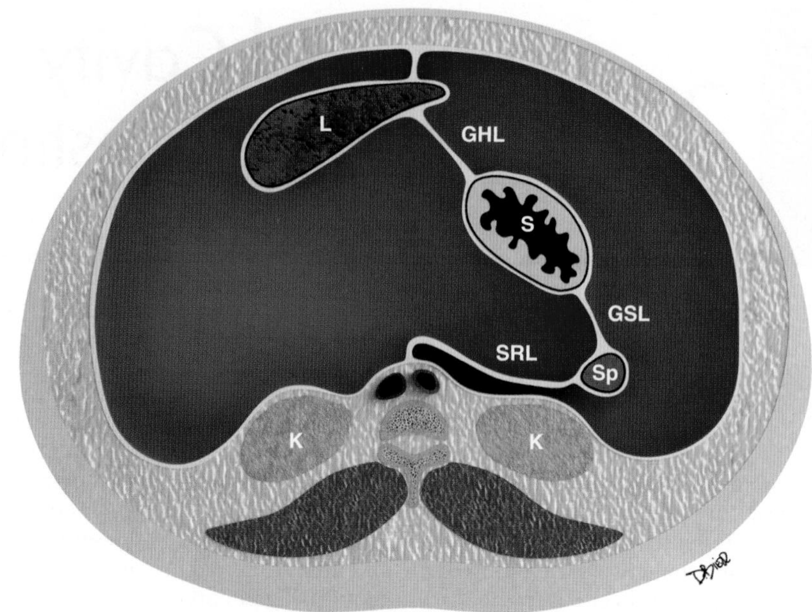

FIGURE 33.1. Embryologic rotation of the peritoneal structures to the eventual adult position. The liver (L) will grow and fill the right side of the peritoneal cavity. The spleen (Sp) moves similarly to the left. *GHL*, Gastrohepatic ligament; *GSL*, gastrosplenic ligament; *K*, kidney; *S*, stomach; *SRL*, splenorenal ligament. Illustration courtesy of David Bier.

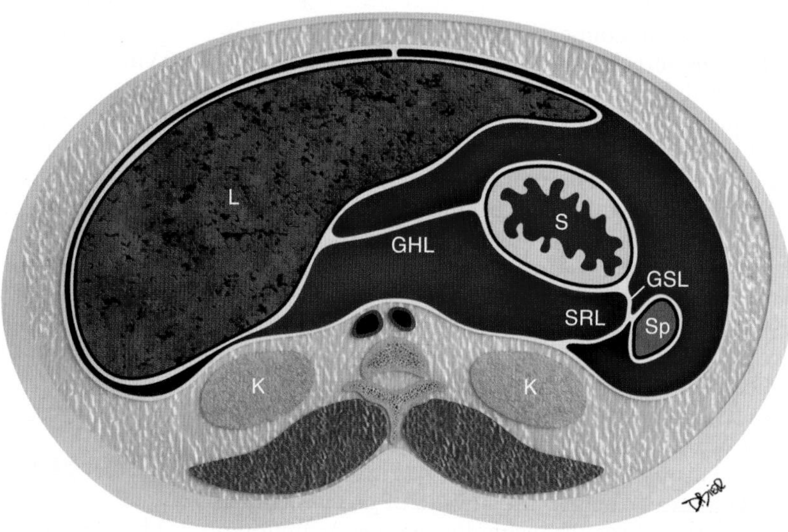

FIGURE 33.2. The adult position of the peritoneal structures and organs after embryologic rotation. *GHL*, Gastrohepatic ligament; *GSL*, gastrosplenic ligament; *L*, Liver; *Sp*, spleen; *K*, kidney; *S*, stomach; *SRL*, splenorenal ligament. Courtesy of David Bier.)

Supramesocolic and Inframesocolic Space

The peritoneal cavity is divided into a supramesocolic and an inframesocolic space by the transverse mesocolon[9] (Fig. 33.5). The supramesocolic space is further divided into the right and left supramesocolic space by the falciform ligament. The right supramesocolic space also is subdivided into the anterior perihepatic space and a posterior compartment known as the lesser sac. The right and left supramesocolic space communicates via the foramen of Winslow, allowing communication between the lesser sac and the remainder of the peritoneal cavity or greater sac.

Important supporting ligaments in the supramesocolic space include the gastrohepatic ligament, hepatoduodenal ligament, gastrocolic ligament, gastrosplenic ligament, and splenorenal ligament (Figs. 33.6 to 33.8). The ligaments are anatomically connected and continuous, and their location and relationship can be identified by certain landmarks, mostly vasculature (Table 33.1).

The inframesocolic compartment is divided into a right and a left inframesocolic space by the obliquely oriented small bowel mesentery. The ascending colon provides the lateral border of the right inframesocolic space. The inframesocolic compartment consists of the root of the mesentery, the jejunal mesentery, the ileal mesentery, the ascending mesocolon, the descending mesocolon, the sigmoid mesentery, and the pelvic floor and peritoneal folds (Table 33.2).

Paravesicular Spaces

Peritoneal folds or reflections in the pelvis also result in potential spaces and compartments[10–12] (Figs. 33.9 and 33.10). The urinary bladder, obliterated umbilical arteries,

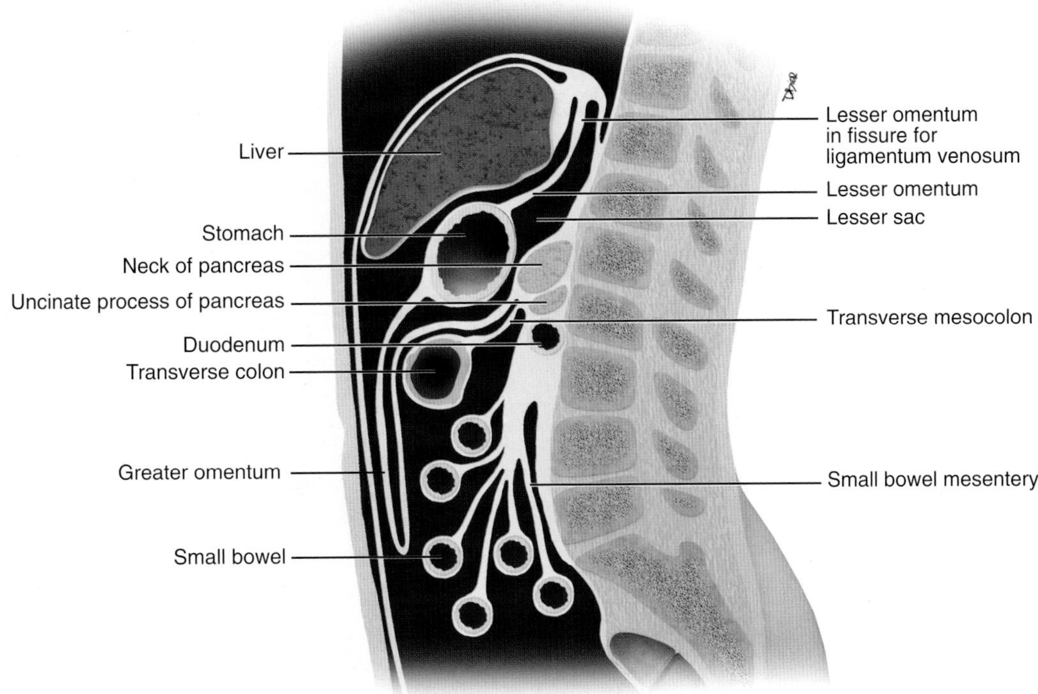

FIGURE 33.3. The peritoneal structures in midsagittal view, diagrammatic representation. (Courtesy of David Bier.)

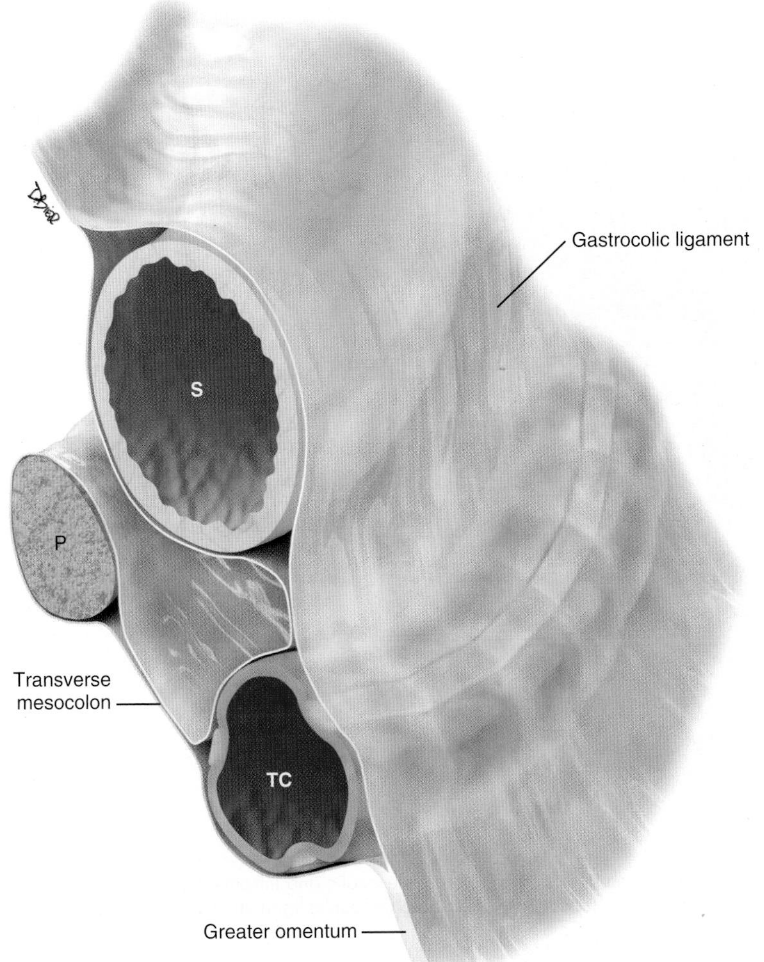

FIGURE 33.4. The peritoneal structures in oblique view. Diagrammatic representation and relationship of the stomach (*S*), pancreas (*P*), and transverse colon (*TC*) and their attachments. (Courtesy of David Bier.)

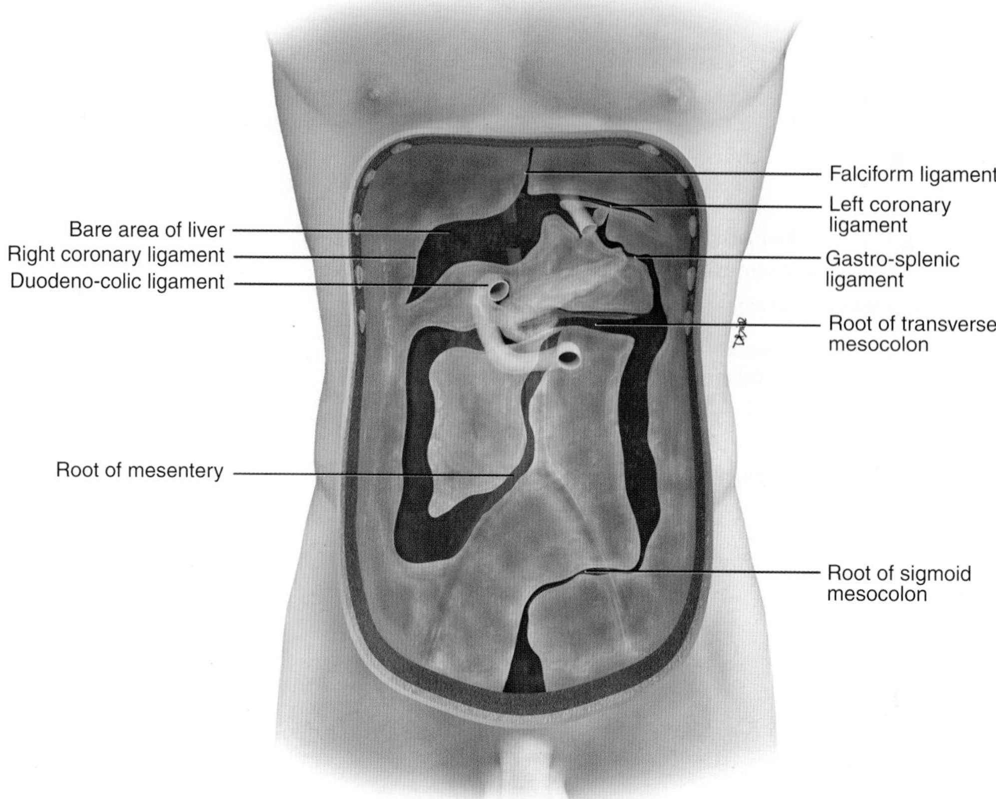

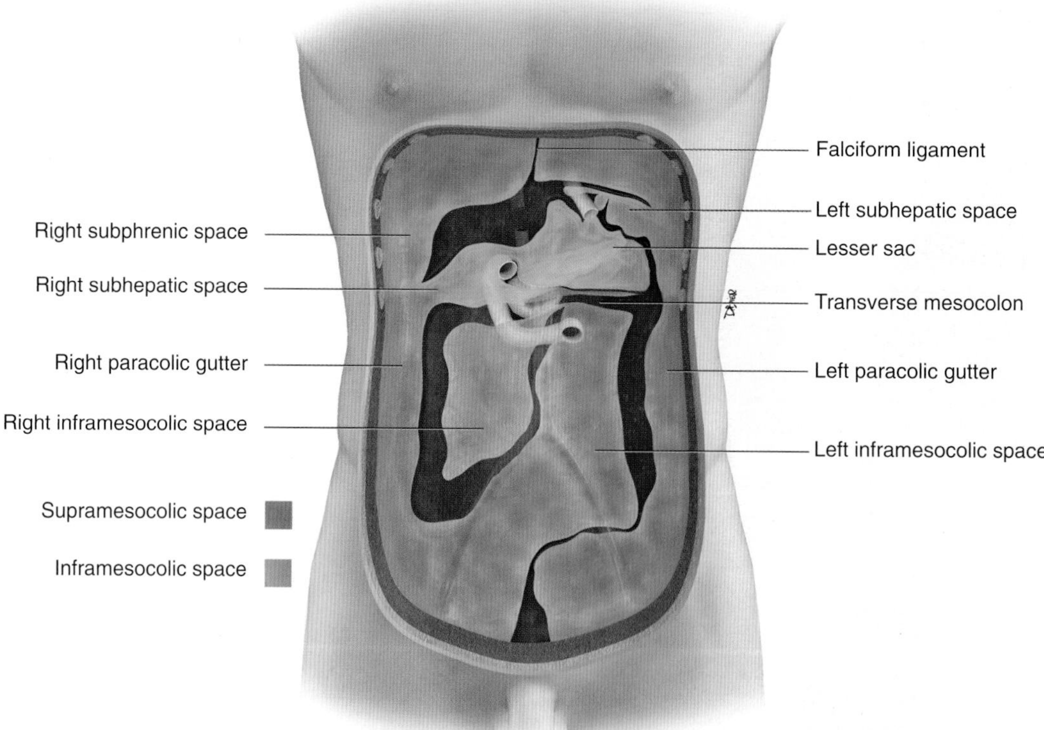

FIGURE 33.5. **A** and **B**, Coronal view of the peritoneal spaces and attachments, including the supramesocolic and inframesocolic spaces. Note that there is no communication between the left supramesocolic and the left paracolic spaces, owing to the phrenocolic ligament. (Courtesy of David Bier.)

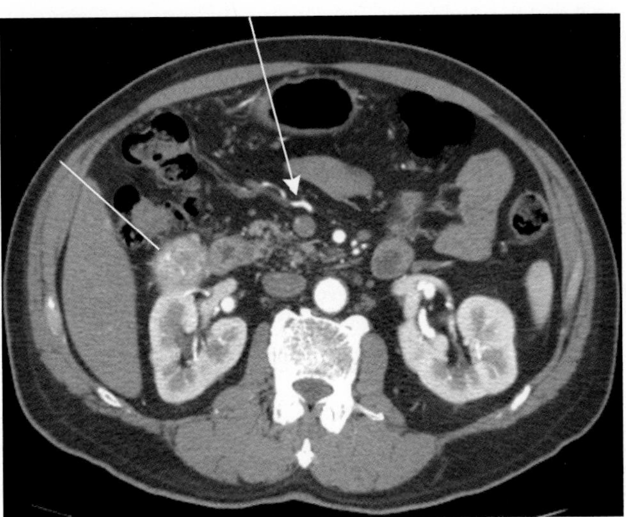

FIGURE 33.6. Computed tomography with intravenous contrast. The transverse mesocolon is delineated by the middle colic artery and its branches (*arrow*). Note the solid enhancing mass in the right kidney from renal cell carcinoma (*line*).

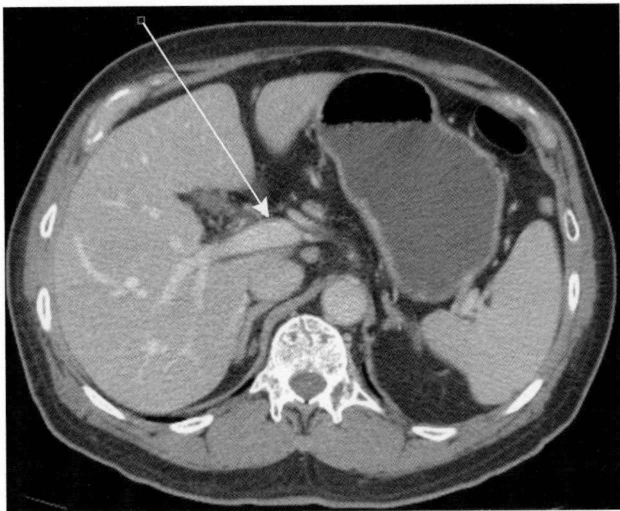

FIGURE 33.8. Computed tomography with intravenous contrast. The hepatoduodenal ligament contains the portal vein (*arrow*), hepatic artery, extrahepatic bile duct, and nodal stations. It connects the lesser curvature of the stomach to the hepatic hilum.

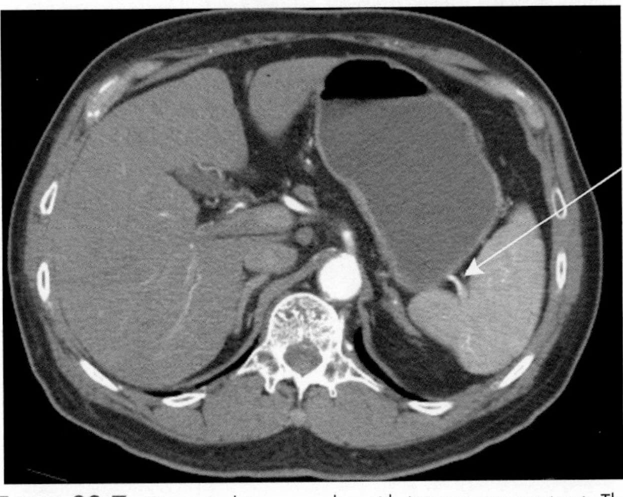

FIGURE 33.7. Computed tomography with intravenous contrast. The gastrosplenic ligament is delineated by the short gastric artery (*arrow*) and left gastroepiploic vessels (not shown). The gastrosplenic ligament extends from the greater curvature of the fundus and upper body of the stomach to the splenic hilum.

TABLE 33.1 Supramesocolic Ligaments: Their Organ Relationship and Landmarks

LIGAMENT	ORGAN RELATIONSHIP	LANDMARKS
Gastrohepatic ligament	Lesser curvature of the stomach to left hepatic lobe	Left gastric vessels and left gastric nodal station
Hepatoduodenal ligament	Lesser curvature of the stomach to the hepatic hilum	Portal vein, hepatic artery, extrahepatic bile duct, and nodal stations
Gastrocolic ligament/ supracolic omentum	Greater curvature of the stomach to the body of the transverse colon	Perigastric branches of the left gastroepiploic vessels with anastomosis to the right gastroepiploic vessels
Greater omentum	Transverse colon extending as an apron anterior to the small bowel	Epiploic vessels and branches of the gastroepiploic vessels
Gastrosplenic ligament	Continuous and to the left of the gastrocolic ligament, from the greater curvature of the fundus and upper body of the stomach to the splenic hilum	Short gastric vessels and left gastroepiploic vessels
Splenorenal ligament	Continuity between the spleen and the tail of the pancreas	Distal splenic artery or proximal splenic vein

and inferior epigastric vessels indent upon the parietal peritoneum to form the anterior and posterior paravesicular spaces.

The anterior paravesicular space is further divided into the supravesicular space and medial and lateral inguinal fossae. These compartments are demarcated by the median, medial, and lateral umbilical folds, each of which can be identified by the urachus, obliterated umbilical arteries, and inferior epigastric vessels, respectively.

The lateral inguinal fossa is the site for the internal inguinal ring and can contain portions of the cecum or sigmoid colon. The medial inguinal fossa can also contain portions of the cecum or sigmoid colon and is the site for the femoral canal.

The posterior paravesicular space is demarcated by peritoneal coverings of the rectum and bladder to form the rectovesicular and pararectal space. In the female, the rectovesicular space is further divided into the vesicouterine recess and rectouterine space (cul-de-sac).

These large potential spaces can be easily delineated when there is accumulation of ascites, abscesses, metastasis, and other disease processes (Figs. 33.11 and 33.12).

TABLE 33.2 Inframesocolic Compartment, Organ Relationship, and Landmarks

LIGAMENT	ORGAN RELATIONSHIP	VASCULAR LANDMARKS
Root of mesentery	From the horizontal portion of the duodenum to the right iliac fossa	Superior mesenteric artery, superior mesenteric vein, and ileocolic artery and vein
Ileal mesentery	From the root of the mesentery to the ileum	Ileal artery and veins
Ascending mesocolon	Root of the mesentery to the ascending colon	Right colic artery and vein, cecal artery and vein
Jejunal mesentery	From the base of the mesentery to the jejunum	Jejunal artery and vein
Descending mesocolon	Base of the transverse mesocolon along the tail of the pancreas to the descending colon	Left colic artery and vein
Sigmoid mesocolon	Root of the sigmoid mesocolon	Sigmoid arteries, superior hemorrhoidal artery and vein

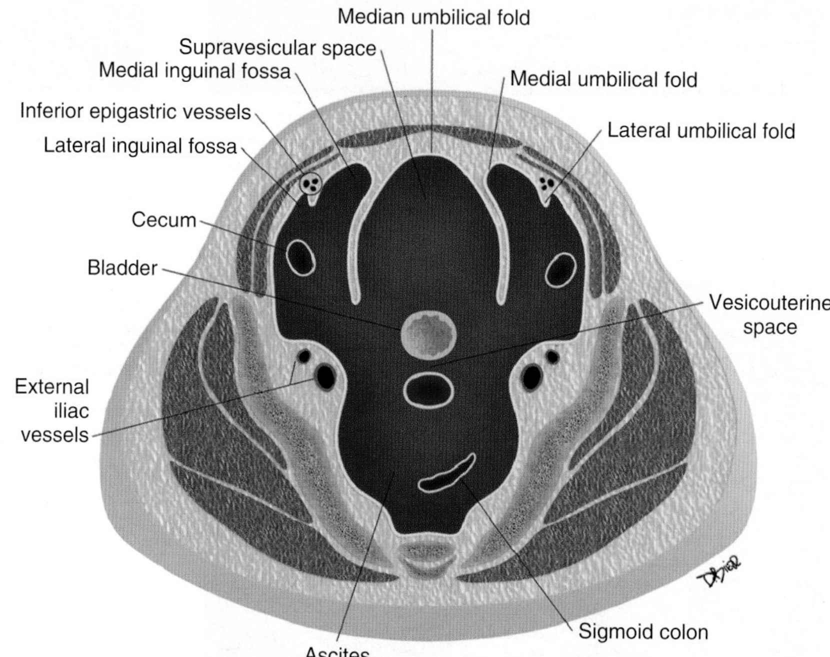

FIGURE 33.9. The paravesicular spaces in cross-sectional view. Ascites distend the pelvic cavity and help delineate the folds and spaces. The anterior paravesicular spaces are divided into the supravesicular space, medial inguinal fossae, and lateral inguinal fossae. The supravesicular space covers the dome of the urinary bladder and in between the medial umbilical folds, which is formed by indentation of the obliterated umbilical vessels. The medial and lateral inguinal folds are separated by the lateral umbilical fold, which is formed by the inferior epigastric vessels. (Courtesy of David Bier.)

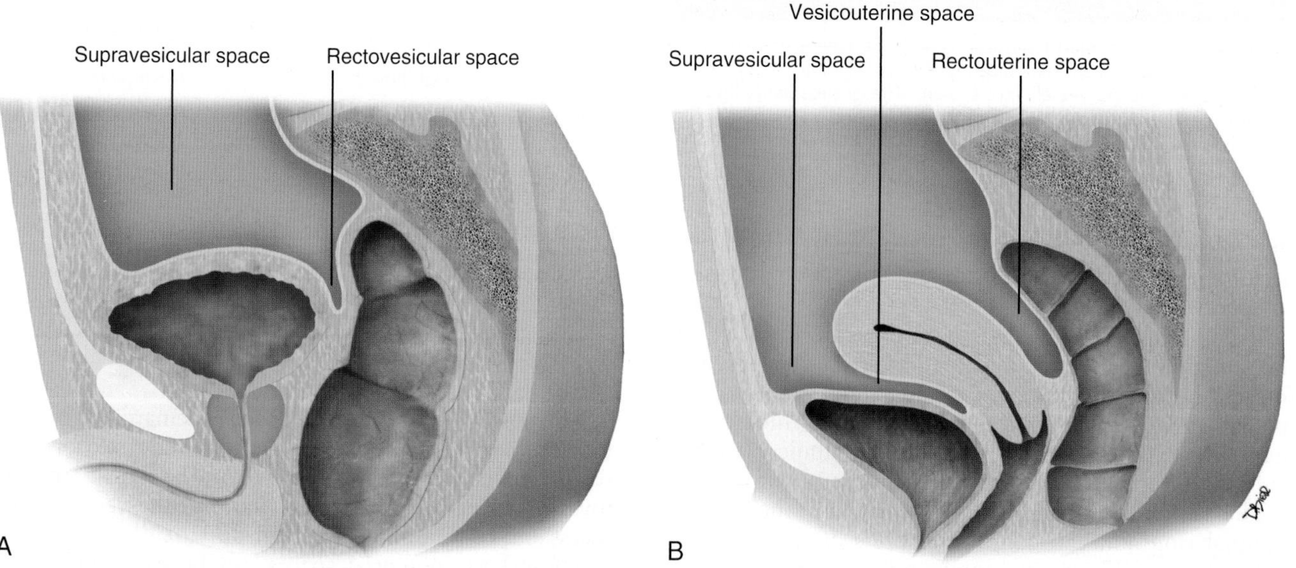

FIGURE 33.10. Posterior paravesicular spaces. Sagittal views of the male (**A**) and female (**B**) pelvis demonstrate the peritoneal covering of the superior bladder, uterus, and upper one third of the rectum. (Courtesy of David Bier.)

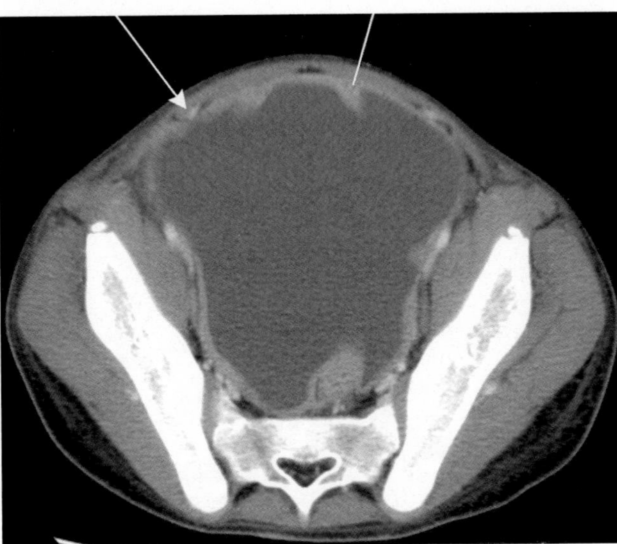

Figure 33.11. Computed tomography with intravenous contrast. Ascites in a 13-year-old with rhabdomyosarcoma. Ascites fill the pelvis, optimizing visualization of the anterior paravesicular spaces. The lateral and medial inguinal fossae are separated by the lateral umbilical fold (landmarked by the inferior epigastric vessels [*arrow*]). The supravesicular space lies in between the medial umbilical fold, which is the site of the obliterated umbilical vein (*line*).

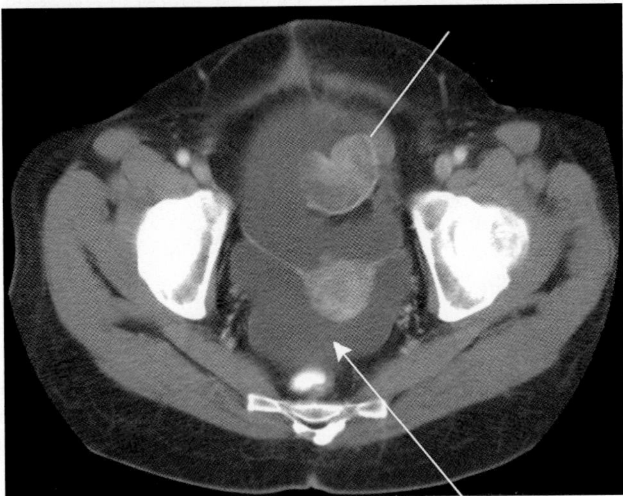

Figure 33.12. Computed tomography with intravenous contrast. A 52-year-old woman with spindle cell sarcoma with metastasis to the peritoneum. Ascites reveal the large potential space in the rectouterine space (*arrow*). Note the large enhancing metastatic deposit in the supravesicular space (*line*).

Key Points Anatomy

- Embryologic development of the peritoneum is complex; basic knowledge of its development aids in an understanding of disease spread.
- Peritoneum lines the abdominal and pelvic walls and organs, aiding in lubrication, organ support, movement, and host defense.
- Foldings of the peritoneum form the ligaments and mesenteries, suspending and supporting internal organs.
- Ligaments and mesenteries create the compartments and potential spaces within the abdominal and pelvic cavity.

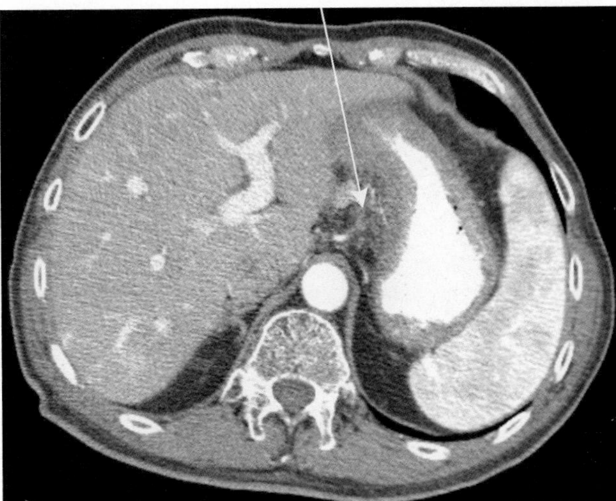

Figure 33.13. Computed tomography with intravenous contrast. A 66-year-old man with metastatic gastric cancer. Tumor spread along the gastrohepatic ligament can be identified by soft tissue infiltration and obliteration of the normal fat plane (*arrow*).

SPREAD OF DISEASE

There are four established pathways of tumor spread and metastasis in the peritoneal cavity.[1,13] First, tumor can spread directly from the tumor through the serosa, through the peritoneal lining, and to an adjacent organ. It can also spread directly within the peritoneal ligaments, mesenteries, and omenta along the "subperitoneal space" to noncontiguous organs in a perilymphatic, perineural, perivascular, or periductal manner. Second, tumor can spread by intraperitoneal seeding along the flow of ascitic fluid. Third, tumor can follow the lymphatics. Finally, tumor can also embolize hematogenously.

Direct Spread

Carcinomas of the stomach, colon, and pancreas commonly involve the subperitoneal space of the ligaments, mesenteries, and omenta.[14] For instance, gastric cancer will commonly use the lesser omentum/gastrohepatic ligament to spread metastatic disease to the left hepatic lobe. This can be identified when there is loss of a fat plane in the lesser omentum as seen on CT imaging (Fig. 33.13).

Similarly, the greater omentum and transverse mesocolon can serve as pathways for subperitoneal spread of cancer of the stomach, pancreas, and colon. When cancer has spread to the greater omentum, "omental caking" can be identified[15] (Figs. 33.14 and 33.15).

Pancreatic cancer can spread directly to the liver via the hepatoduodenal ligament. The hepatoduodenal ligament again contains the portal vein, common bile duct, and hepatic artery (Fig. 33.16). Less frequently, the lesser omentum can serve as a bidirectional bridge. That is, disease can spread in a reverse fashion from the liver back to the stomach.

The root of the mesentery extends from the horizontal portion of the duodenum to the iliac fossa. Lymphoma, carcinoid, pancreatic, and colonic cancer will commonly

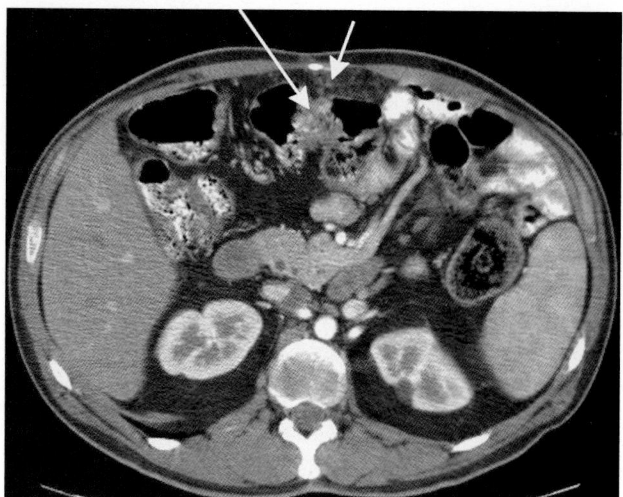

FIGURE 33.14. Computed tomography with intravenous contrast. A 45-year-old man with gastric cancer. Spread of disease along the gastrocolic ligament seen as nodular soft tissue infiltration (*short arrow*) and to the transverse colon resulting in circumferential bowel wall thickening (*long arrow*).

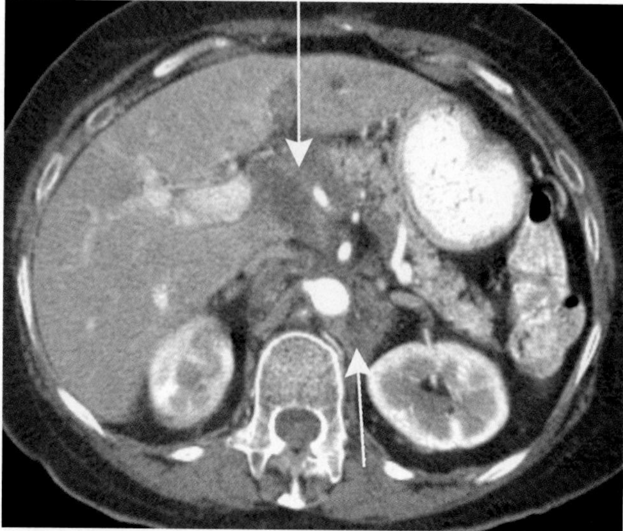

FIGURE 33.16. Computed tomography with intravenous contrast. A 63-year-old woman with intrahepatic cholangiocarcinoma. Spread of disease along the hepatoduodenal ligament (*long arrow*). Note the associated retroperitoneal lymphadenopathy (*short arrow*).

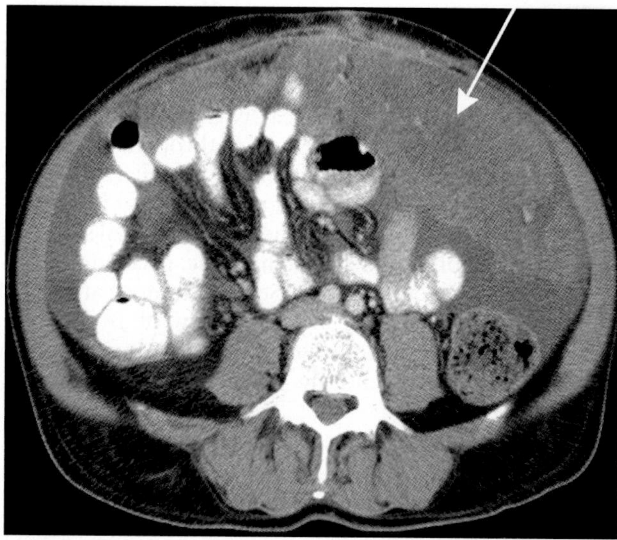

FIGURE 33.15. Computed tomography with intravenous contrast. Spread of cancer to the greater omentum, resulting in "omental caking" (*arrow*) in a patient with colon cancer. Note the associated ascites.

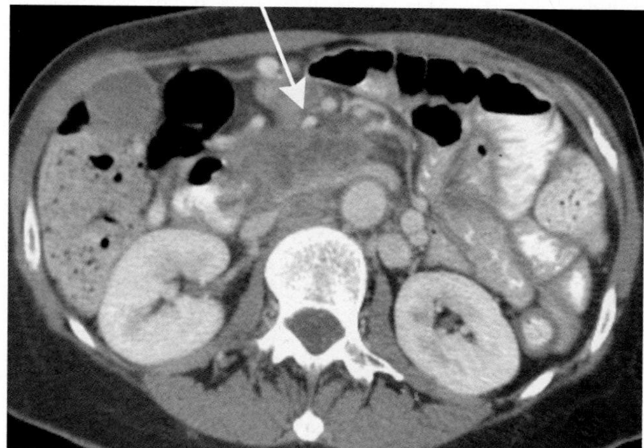

FIGURE 33.17. Computed tomography with intravenous contrast. A 62-year-old with pancreatic cancer. The disease has spread along the mesenteric root, seen as a mass with soft tissue stranding growing along the superior mesenteric artery and superior mesenteric vein (*arrow*).

involve the root of the mesentery and use it as a pathway for spread of disease. Imaging will reveal mesenteric soft tissue thickening, perivascular encasement, and tethering of bowel[1] (Fig. 33.17).

Intraperitoneal Seeding

Spread of disease such as metastasis within the peritoneal cavity is influenced by physical forces such as gravity and negative subdiaphragmatic pressure.[1] Dynamic circulation, flow, and pooling of ascites within dependent peritoneal recesses also serve to spread and deposit disease.

Common sites for intraperitoneal spread of metastatic disease are the pouch of Douglas/rectovesicular space in the pelvis, right lower quadrant at the inferior junction of the small bowel mesentery, superior aspect of the sigmoid mesocolon, and right paracolic gutter. When there are intraperitoneal metastases, they can be identified as soft tissue nodules or plaquelike soft tissue masses on imaging such as CT. There may be associated ascites. Peritoneal metastatic nodules as small as 5 mm can be identified with CT imaging. Likewise, parietal peritoneal involvement will produce smooth or nodular thickening with enhancement when visualized by CT imaging.

Serous cystadenocarcinoma may produce diffuse peritoneal calcifications, especially after treatment.[16] Carcinoid and, less commonly, gastric and colon cancer will also elicit peritoneal calcifications.[8]

Pseudomyxoma peritonei from mucinous tumor of the appendix or mucinous carcinomatosis from a gastrointestinal tract or ovarian primary can also be identified in the peritoneal cavity. Mucin secretion will be cystic in appearance by imaging and may occasionally calcify.

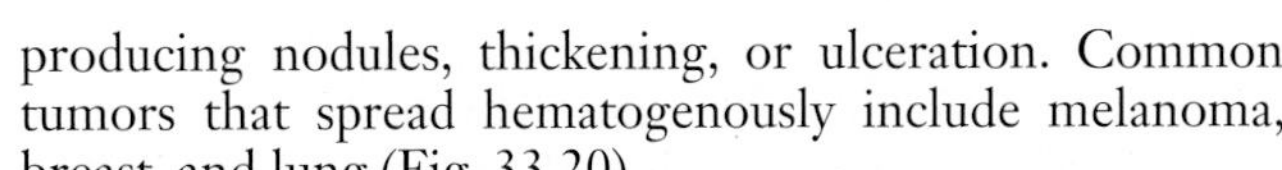

Pseudomyxoma peritonei exert pressure upon the viscera, causing scalloping along the surface of organs such as the liver, spleen, or bowel[17] (Fig. 33.18). The pressure from the mucin will occasionally prevent bowel from floating upward, unlike ascites.

Lymphatic Spread

Spread of disease can also occur via the lymphatics.[18] However, the lymphatics play a minor role, except in lymphoma, where 50% will be non-Hodgkin disease. Round or oval mesenteric masses will be manifested with displacement of bowel. A sandwich sign has also been described.[19] This is seen when mesenteric and retroperitoneal lymphadenopathy are separated by a fat plane (Fig. 33.19).

Hematogenous Spread

Finally, metastatic disease to the peritoneum can spread hematogenously. For instance, the mesenteric arteries can carry metastasis to the antimesenteric side of the bowel, producing nodules, thickening, or ulceration. Common tumors that spread hematogenously include melanoma, breast, and lung (Fig. 33.20).

Key Points Peritoneal Spread of Disease

- Directly or in the subperitoneal space along the ligaments and mesenteries, "subperitoneal space."
- Intraperitoneal seeding associated with the flow of ascites.
- Lymphatics.
- Hematogenous.

IMAGING TECHNIQUES

Computed Tomography

CT is widely used for imaging of the peritoneum. For metastatic disease, CT demonstrated sensitivities ranging from 85% to 93%, specificities of 78% to 91%, positive

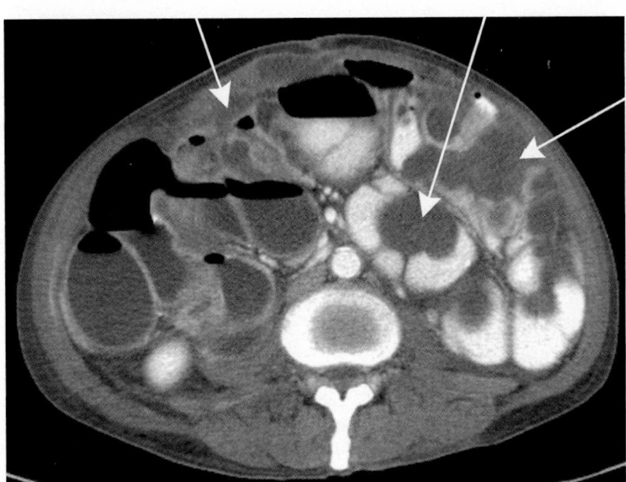

Figure 33.18. Computed tomography with intravenous contrast. A 66-year-old male with appendiceal carcinoma and pseudomyxoma peritonei. Mucin is identified as low-density collections scalloping and exerting pressure on the surface of the bowel (*arrows*).

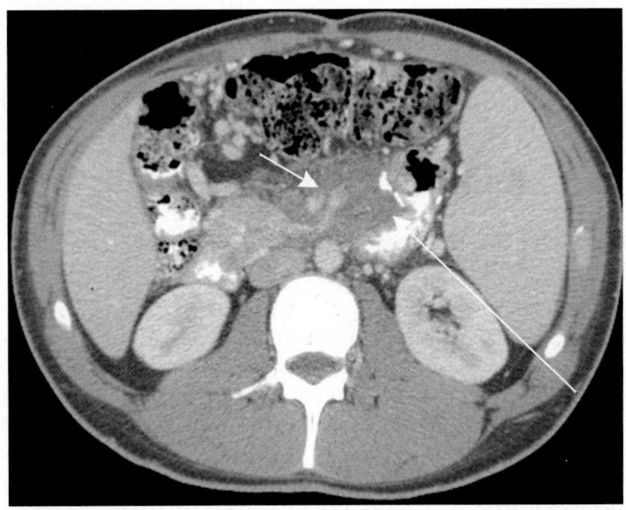

Figure 33.20. Computed tomography with intravenous contrast. A 21-year-old with melanoma of the right ear with hematogenous metastasis to the root of the mesentery (*short arrow*). Tumor infiltration to the adjacent small bowel causes wall thickening (*long arrow*).

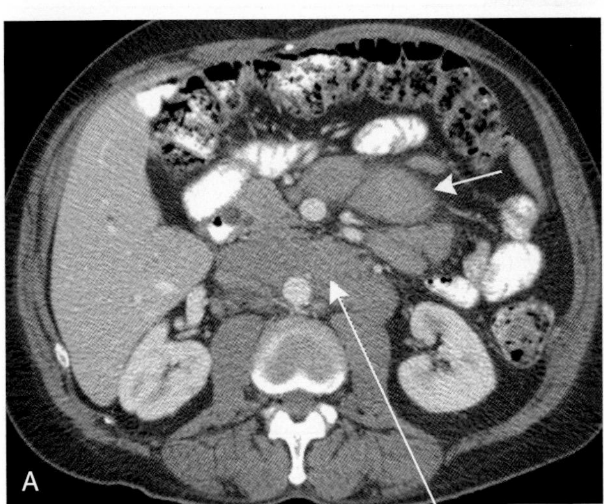

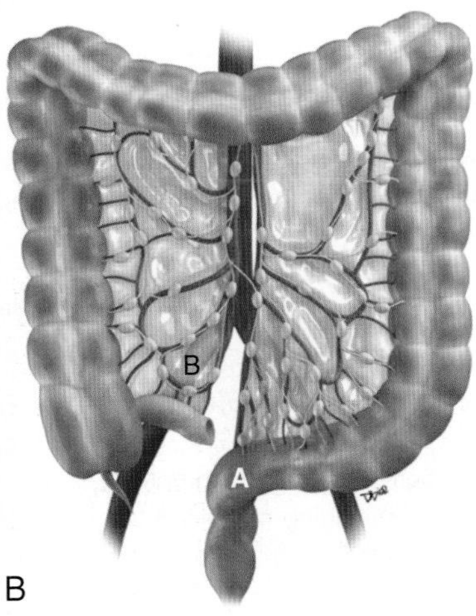

Figure 33.19. A, Computed tomography with intravenous contrast. A 66-year-old with lymphoma. Lymphatic spread of disease along the mesentery is seen as enlarged lymph nodes (*short arrow*). Note also the retroperitoneal lymphadenopathy (*long arrow*). **B**, Diagrammatic examples of additional route of lymphatic spread of disease. For example, rectal carcinoma can spread superiorly to the superior hemorrhoidal chain of lymph nodes (**A**). Cecal cancer can spread along the ileocolic chain (**B**). Illustration courtesy of David Bier.

predictive values of 88% to 98%, and negative predictive values of 78% to 88%. The sensitivity, however, is greatly reduced with nodules smaller than 1 cm (25%–50%).[3] Some studies found that sensitivities were highest for metastatic disease to the right paracolic gutter and infracolic omentum and when thin slices and multiplanar reconstruction were obtained.[20]

Magnetic Resonance Imaging

Although MRI is not as commonly used to assess for peritoneal metastasis as CT, it can be effective.[2,21] As stated, CT sensitivity for peritoneal nodules smaller than 1 cm is low (25%–50%). However, with superior contrast resolution, MRI sensitivities for peritoneal nodules smaller than 1 cm are reportedly better (85%–90%).[22]

An effective MRI sequence will include T1-weighted (T1W), fat-suppressed T2-weighted, and fat-suppressed gadolinium-enhanced T1W spoiled gradient recalled echo. Because peritoneal metastatic disease enhances slowly, delay imaging after 5 minutes has been found to be beneficial.

Although it has been reported that MRI can be better than CT in terms of sensitivity for the detection of peritoneal implants, in our experience, we generally use multidetector computed tomography as the backbone of workup, with its very excellent spatial resolution, thin sections, and minimization of motion artifact, which can compromise MRI.

Positron Emission Tomography/Computed Tomography

PET/CT has also been found to be effective in the evaluation of peritoneal metastatic disease.[23–27] Reported sensitivities for PET/CT in detection of peritoneal metastasis range from 78% to 100%.[22] However, cystic or mucinous peritoneal carcinomatosis can be non–2-[^{18}F] fluoro-2-deoxy-D-glucose (FDG)–avid and produce false-negative results on PET/CT owing to their low cellularity. In addition, like CT and MRI, PET/CT will be limited by spatial resolution. Lesions smaller than 1 cm may not have sufficient FDG uptake to be detectable.

Sonography

Sonography is sensitive for the detection of ascites and large implants. Ultrasound, however, is not sensitive in the detection of small metastatic implants.

KEY POINTS Imaging

- Computed tomography (CT) is widely available and is a robust imaging modality for the evaluation of peritoneal metastasis and tumor.
- Magnetic resonance imaging, positron emission tomography/CT, and sonography are also available imaging modalities for the evaluation of peritoneal metastasis, with the appropriate clinical indications and with radiologist expertise.

APPROACH TO AND CLASSIFYING OF PERITONEAL DISEASE

When encountering peritoneal disease, patient history, risk factors, laboratory studies, and radiographic evaluation will aid in the diagnosis. Classification of peritoneal disease can be divided into primary tumors of the peritoneum and secondary tumors and tumorlike lesions.[22] A few examples of disease classifications are outlined in Tables 33.3 and 33.4.

With a history of prior asbestos exposure, malignant mesothelioma should be suspected. Imaging findings of sheet-like thickening of the peritoneum, lack of a primary malignancy, lack of lymphadenopathy, or lack of metastasis elsewhere should aid in the differential diagnosis[6,28,29] (Fig. 33.21).

Primary peritoneal mesotheliomas are rare. These originate from mesothelial or submesothelial layers of the peritoneum, can spread along the serosal surface, and can invade hollow or solid viscera. Beginning as small nodules initially, they can coalesce to form sheetlike thickening or masses in the peritoneum and develop omental caking.

TABLE 33.3 Primary Tumors of the Peritoneum

Mesothelial Tumors
Malignant mesothelioma
Epithelial Tumors
Primary peritoneal serous carcinoma
Smooth Muscle Tumor
Leiomyomatosis peritonealis disseminate
Tumors of Uncertain Origin
Solitary fibrous tumor

(Modified from Levy AD, Shaw JC, Sobin LH. Secondary tumors and tumorlike lesions of the peritoneal cavity: imaging features with pathologic correlation. *Radiographics*. 2009;29:347–373.)

TABLE 33.4 Secondary Tumors and Other Diseases of the Peritoneal Cavity

Metastatic Neoplasms
Carcinomatosis
Pseudomyxoma peritonei
Lymphomatosis
Infection and Inflammation
Granulomatous peritonitis such as tuberculosis
Inflammatory pseudotumor
Miscellaneous
Endometriosis
Melanosis
Splenosis

(Modified from Levy AD, Shaw JC, Sobin LH. Secondary tumors and tumorlike lesions of the peritoneal cavity: imaging features with pathologic correlation. *Radiographics*. 2009;29:347–373.)

Malignant peritoneal mesothelioma usually develops in individuals exposed to high levels of asbestos. Women exposed to asbestos are noted to have a lower rate of developing malignant mesothelioma than men (23%).[6] Other risk factors suspected of contributing to the development of malignant mesothelioma can include erionite (a mineral fiber found in Turkey), therapeutic irradiation, exposure to simian virus 40, and chronic pleural or peritoneal irritation.[6] Younger patients have been found to occasionally develop the disease with no history of exposure.

When there are nodular masses with mesenteric stranding and tethering of bowel, carcinoid tumors should be suspected. Although carcinoid tumors often arise from the bowel and within Meckel's diverticulum from neuroendocrine cells, they can also originate from the mesentery and peritoneum.

Fatty and soft tissue peritoneal masses may reveal benign lipomas and neurofibromas, respectively. A history of neurofibromatosis type 1 can aid in the diagnosis. A more cystic multiloculated mass can be as a result of a rare benign condition found in women known as multicystic mesothelioma.[30,31]

Secondary disease of the peritoneum can result from inflammation and infection. Tuberculosis (TB) and histoplasmosis are examples. Patients with human immunodeficiency virus or other immunosupression, young adults between the ages of 20 and 40 years, patients with a history of illicit drug use, and patients from or with recent travel to endemic areas should be suspected of TB peritonitis in the appropriate setting. Clues to their diagnosis can be found when there is associated lymphadenopathy in the mesentery and retroperitoneum. Furthermore, the lymphadenopathy will usually contain low attenuation centrally with an enhancing rim.[22,32] This is owing to casseating necrosis (Fig. 33.22). Calcification occasionally involves the lymph nodes.

Metastatic disease is the most common manifestation of a peritoneal neoplastic process. Culprits in the order of most common will be colorectal and ovarian carcinoma, followed by gastric, pancreatic, breast, lung, and melanoma.[33]

Understanding the peritoneal anatomy and the route of disease spread aids in suggesting the most likely diagnosis. For instance, if there is isolated lymphadenopathy along the superior hemorrhoidal distribution, a rectosigmoid primary tumor can be suspected to have spread along this route (see Fig. 33.19B).

Findings of an adnexal pelvic mass with ascites, peritoneal nodules in dependent locations, and omental caking from intraperitoneal seeding will be suspicious for a primary ovarian carcinoma. Common locations for metastatic peritoneal nodules are found in the pouch of Douglas, ileocecal region, right paracolic gutter, sigmoid mesocolon, greater omentum, and right subdiaphragmatic parietal peritoneum.

The diagnosis of peritoneal disease will be apparent for most patients in certain instances because they will present with history of a known primary malignancy confirmed by clinical, pathologic, and radiologic evidence. Conversely, without a known malignancy, occasionally it will be difficult to differentiate between a primary malignant peritoneal disease (such as malignant peritoneal mesothelioma), peritoneal metastatic disease, or infection such as TB.

KEY POINTS Classifying Peritoneal Disease

- Primary tumors of the peritoneum are rare.
- Secondary disease of the peritoneum such as from metastases is most common.

CONCLUSION

In conclusion, an understanding of the embryology, anatomy, and pattern of disease spread within the peritoneum is fundamental to the detection and diagnosis of diseases affecting the peritoneal cavity.

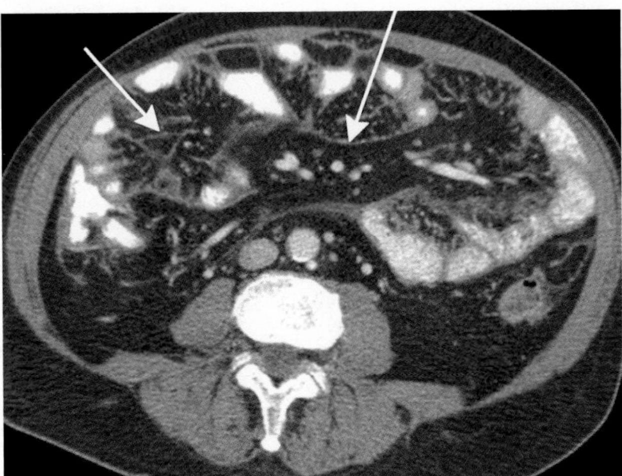

FIGURE 33.21. Computed tomography (CT) with intravenous contrast. An 80-year-old patient with malignant mesothelioma. CT with intravenous and gastrointestinal contrast reveals sheetlike thickening of the mesenteric peritoneum (*arrows*) owing to malignant mesothelioma.

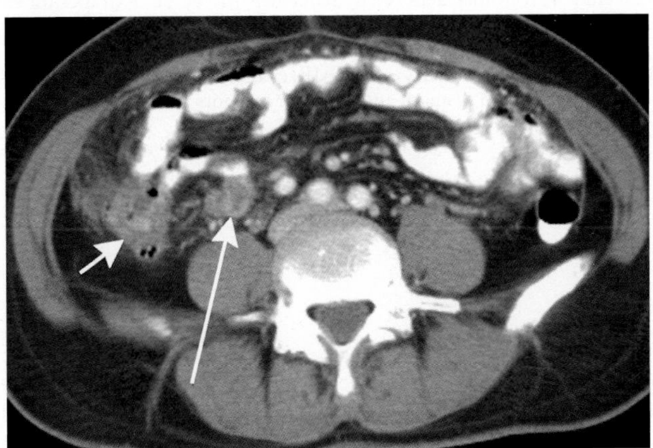

FIGURE 33.22. Computed tomography (CT) with intravenous contrast. A 58-year-old Asian female with a history of tuberculosis exposure. CT reveals mural thickening in the cecum (*short arrow*), peritoneal nodules, and central low-density ileocolic lymph nodes with rim enhancement (*long arrow*). Biopsy showed granulomatous reaction.

The peritoneal reflections and peritoneal cavities form potential spaces and pathways for the spread of many disease processes. Understanding this anatomic relationship enables better detection, staging, and evaluation of tumor recurrence or metastasis.

Besides direct, subperitoneal spread, metastasis can also involve the peritoneum by intraperitoneal seeding, the lymphatic route, or hematogenous involvement.

The clinical symptoms will often be nonspecific. Imaging will, therefore, play an important role in the diagnosis. Imaging techniques are dominated by the use of CT. MRI, PET/CT, and ultrasound can complement.

REFERENCES

1. Meyers MA, Oliphant M, Berne AS, et al. The peritoneal ligaments and mesenteries: pathways of intraabdominal spread of disease. *Radiology*. 1987;163:593–604.
2. Elsayes KM, Staveteig PT, Narra VR, et al. MRI of the peritoneum: spectrum of abnormalities. *AJR Am J Roentgenol.* 2006;186:1368–1379.
3. Healy JC, Reznek RH. Peritoneal metastasis. In: Husband JES, Reznek R, eds. *Imaging in Oncology. London: Martin Dunitz Ltd*; 1998:841–852.
4. Sompayrac SW, Mindelzun RE, Silverman PM, et al. The greater omentum. *AJR Am J Roentgenol.* 1997;168:683–687.
5. Silverman P. The subperitoneal space: mechanism of tumor spread within the peritoneal cavity, mesentery and omentum. *Cancer Imaging*. 2004;4:25–29.
6. Levy AD, Arnáiz J, Shaw JC, et al. Continuing medical education: from the archives of the AFIP: primary peritoneal tumors: imaging features with pathologic correlation. *Radiographics*. 2008;28:583–607.
7. Jeong YJ, Kim S, Kwak SW, et al. Neoplastic and nonneoplastic conditions of serosal membrane origin: CT findings. *Radiographics*. 2008;28:801–818.
8. Hamrick-Turner JE, Chiechi MV, Abbitt PL, et al. Neoplastic and inflammatory processes of the peritoneum, omentum, and mesentery: diagnosis with CT. *Radiographics*. 1992;12:1051–1068.
9. Healy JC, Reznek RH. The peritoneum, mesenteries and omenta: normal anatomy and pathological processes. *Eur Radiol.* 1998;8:886–900.
10. Auh YH, Rubenstein WA, Markisz JA, et al. Intraperitoneal paravesical spaces: CT delineation with US correlation. *Radiology*. 1986;159:311–317.
11. Gambino J, Cohen AJ, Friedenberg RM. The direction of bladder displacement by adnexal masses. *Clin Imaging*. 1983;17:8–11.
12. Auh YH, Rubenstein WA, Schneider M, et al. Extraperitoneal paravesical spaces: CT delineation with US correlation. *Radiology*. 1986;159:319–328.
13. Sheth S, Horton KM, Garland MR, et al. Mesenteric neoplasms: CT appearances of primary and secondary tumors and differential diagnosis. *Radiographics*. 2003;23:457–473.
14. Oliphant M, Berne AS. Computed tomography of the subperitoneal space: demonstration of direct spread of intraabdominal disease. *J Comput Assist Tomogr*. 1982;6:1127–1137.
15. Woodward PJ, Hosseinzadeh K, Saenger JS. from the archives of the AFIP: radiologic staging of ovarian carcinoma with pathologic correlation. *Radiographics*. 2004;24:225–246.
16. Agarwal A, Yeh BM, Breiman RS, et al. Peritoneal calcification: causes and distinguishing features on CT. *AJR Am J Roentgenol.* 2004;182:441–445.
17. Sulkin TVC, O'Neill H, Amin AI, et al. CT in pseudomyxoma peritonei: A review of 17 cases. *Clin Radiol*. 2002;57:608–613.
18. Karaosmanoglu D, Karcaaltincaba M, Oguz B, et al. CT findings of lymphoma with peritoneal, omental and mesenteric involvement: Peritoneal lymphomatosis. *Eur J Radiol*. 2009;71:313–317.
19. Hokama A, Nakamoto M, Kinjo F, et al. 'The sandwich sign' of mesenteric lymphoma. *Eur J Haematol*. 2006;77:363–364.
20. Pannu HK, Horton KM, Fishman EK. Thin section dual-phase multidetector-row computed tomography detection of peritoneal metastases in gynecologic cancers. *J Comput Assist Tomogr.* 2003;27:333–340.
21. Low RN, Barone RM, Lacey C, et al. Peritoneal tumor: MR imaging with dilute oral barium and intravenous gadolinium-containing contrast agents compared with unenhanced MR imaging and CT. *Radiology*. 1997;204:513–520.
22. Levy AD, Shaw JC, Sobin LH. Secondary tumors and tumorlike lesions of the peritoneal cavity: imaging features with pathologic correlation. *Radiographics*. 2009;29:347–373.
23. Turlakow A, Yeung HW, Salmon AS, et al. Peritoneal carcinomatosis: role of 18F-FDG PET. *J Nucl Med*. 2003;44:1407–1412.
24. Anthony M-P, Khong P-L, Zhang J. Spectrum of 18F-FDG PET/CT appearances in peritoneal disease. *AJR Am J Roentgenol.* 2009;193:W523–W529.
25. Schwarz JK, Grigsby PW, Dehdashti F, et al. The role of 18F-FDG PET in assessing therapy response in cancer of the cervix and ovaries. *J Nucl Med*. 2009;50(Suppl 1). 64S-3S.
26. Weber WA. Assessing tumor response to therapy. *J Nucl Med.* 2009;50(Suppl 1):1S–10S.
27. Funicelli L, Travaini LL, Landoni F, et al. Peritoneal carcinomatosis from ovarian cancer: the role of CT and [(18)F]FDG-PET/CT. *Abdom Imaging*. 2010;35:701–707.
28. Guest PJ, Reznek RH, Selleslag D, et al. Peritoneal mesothelioma: the role of computed tomography in diagnosis and follow up. *Clin Radiol*. 1992;45:79–84.
29. Puvaneswary M, Chen S, Proietto T. Peritoneal mesothelioma: CT and MRI findings. *Australas Radiol*. 2002;46:91–96.
30. Safioleas MC, Constantinos K, Michael S, et al. Benign multicystic peritoneal mesothelioma: a case report and review of the literature. *World J Gastroenterol*. 2006;12:5739–5742.
31. Jain KA. Imaging of peritoneal inclusion cysts. *AJR Am J Roentgenol.* 2000;174:1559–1563.
32. Ha HK, Jung JI, Lee MS, et al. CT differentiation of tuberculous peritonitis and peritoneal carcinomatosis. *AJR Am J Roentgenol.* 1996;167:743–748.
33. Gupta P. The straight line sign. *Radiology*. 2006;240:611–612.

CHAPTER

34 Bone Metastases

Colleen M. Costelloe, M.D.; Patrick P. Lin, M.D.; Hubert H. Chuang, M.D., Ph.D.; Behrang Amini, M.D., Ph.D.; Naoto T. Ueno, M.D., Ph.D.; Sudpreeda Chainitikun, M.D.; T. Kuan Yu, M.D., Ph.D.; and John E. Madewell, M.D.

INTRODUCTION

Bone metastases are common in patients with advanced malignancies. Autopsy series have shown an incidence of bone metastases of approximately 70% in breast and prostate cancer and 35% in lung cancer.[1,2] Osseous metastases can profoundly influence quality of life and prognosis. Early and accurate detection is important for therapeutic planning, and many imaging modalities can be used for this purpose. X-ray–based technologies such as radiography and computed tomography (CT) image bone calcium, skeletal scintigraphy (SS; bone scan) detects bone formation, magnetic resonance imaging (MRI) images the soft tissue of the marrow cavity, and 2-[^{18}F] fluoro-2-deoxy-D-glucose (FDG) positron emission tomography (PET) reflects the glucose metabolism of the lesions. The therapeutic response of bone metastases can be assessed through means of response criteria that are also used to determine the clinical efficacy of cancer therapy. Response criteria developed at the MD Anderson Cancer Center (MDA criteria) are useful for interpreting the behavior of bone metastases.[3,4] Successful new therapies are prolonging the lives of cancer patients, with a concomitant increase in skeletal metastasis–related complications such as pain, pathologic fractures, and spinal cord compression.[2,5] Patients with multiple painful bone metastases can be treated with systemic therapy such as bisphosphonates or radiopharmaceuticals. When symptomatic lesions are limited in number, they can be treated with radiation therapy, surgery, or percutaneous techniques such as vertebroplasty or radiofrequency ablation (RFA). This chapter discusses the role of imaging in the detection and therapeutic response of bone metastases, with a discussion of treatment, including topics such as medical therapy, radiation, surgery, and percutaneous procedures.

DISTRIBUTION AND PATHOPHYSIOLOGY

Cortical bone is compact and lamellar in structure, forming a heavily calcified, well-defined boundary for the marrow cavity and providing the structural support of the skeleton. Inside of the cortical bone resides delicate trabecular bone that supports either red hematopoietic or yellow fatty marrow. The large majority of bone metastases are hematogenous and spread primarily by invasion into and dissemination through the arterial system. Otherwise, venous backflow has been implicated. Metastatic disease can also invade directly into bone from adjacent structures.[6]

Following the distribution of highly vascular red marrow, osseous metastases occur most commonly in the medullary cavity of the bones of the axial skeleton. In a study of 4105 bone metastases in 2001 patients, Clain[7] reported the highest incidence of lesions in the vertebrae (33.5%), pelvis (19.9%), ribs (12.2%), femora (12.3%), skull (6.8%), and humeri (4.7%) (Fig. 34.1).

Bone metastases can be classified as lytic, blastic, or mixed, depending on the activity of tumor-stimulated host osteoclasts and osteoblasts.[8] Osteoclasts are large, multinucleated cells with a specialized cell membrane (the "ruffled border") that resorb bone, and osteoblasts are smaller, mononucleated cells that form new bone.[9] These cells produce lytic or blastic lesions, respectively, and a combination of the two processes results in mixed lesions.

Lesion margins can be well-defined, ill-defined, or expansile (Fig. 34.2). Unlike primary bone tumors, which typically demonstrate nonaggressive margins when benign and aggressive margins when malignant,[10] virtually all bone metastases are malignant, regardless of the appearance of the margins. Metastases from solid malignancies and myeloma are the most common bone tumors to arise in patients older than 40 years.

DETECTION

Conventional Radiography

Radiography, CT, bone scan, single-photon emission tomography with integrated CT (SPECT/CT), MRI, and PET with integrated CT (PET/CT) or with integrated MRI (PET/MRI) are methods used to detect bone metastases and evaluate their response to treatment. Radiography, like all x-ray–based technologies, primarily images bone calcium, and the majority of the calcium is found in the cortex. Radiography is specific but not sensitive for the detection of bone metastases.[11] A minimum of 30% to 50% bone loss must occur for most lytic metastases to be detectable on radiographs (XRs),[12,13] and metastases in the axial skeleton are often obscured by overlapping anatomic structures (Fig. 34.3). Nevertheless, the high specificity and low cost of radiography make it an ideal initial imaging modality for the detection of bone metastases in areas of focal pain.[3] Radiography is also optimal to assess for pathologic fracture in the appendicular skeleton.[14]

Computed Tomography

CT is an excellent modality for detailed imaging of mineralized structures.[15,16] CT is the optimal imaging modality for

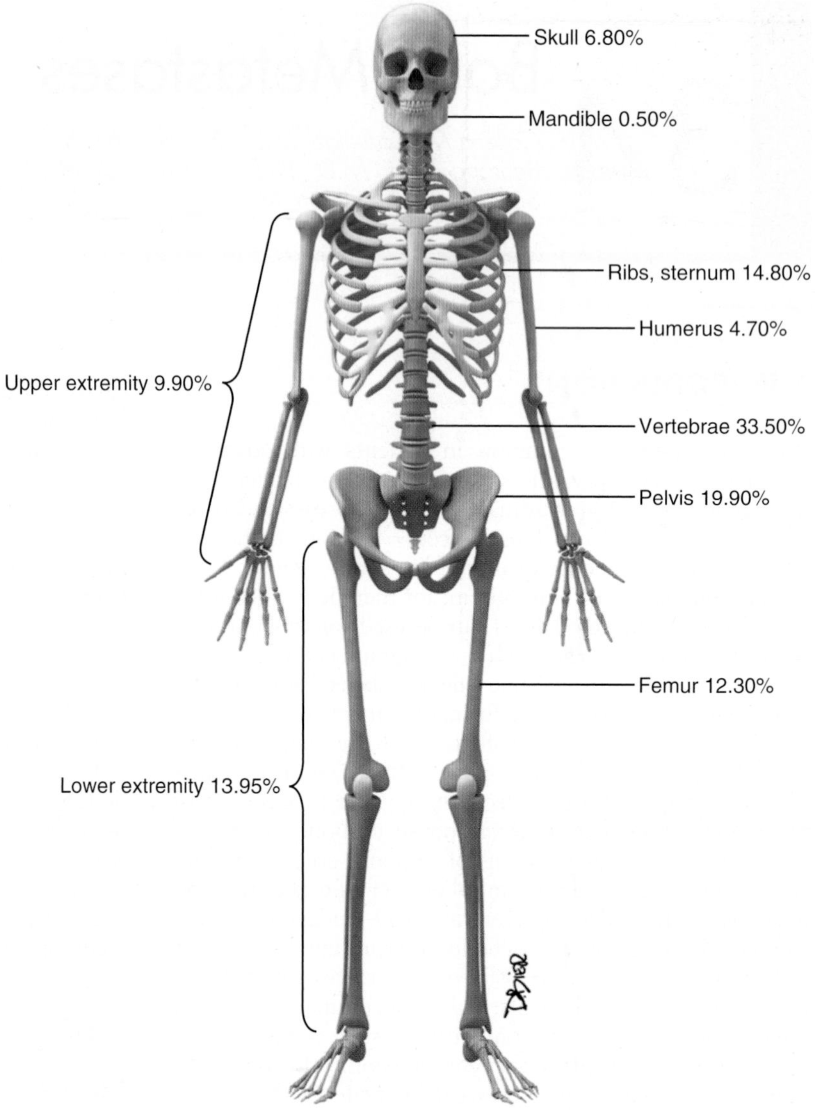

FIGURE 34.1. Distribution of bone metastases. Data are from a study of 2001 patients with 4105 bone metastases. The lesions were counted on the basis of a combination of anatomic sites and individual bones. The entire spine, all ribs, and the entire bony pelvis were each considered one anatomic site, and one or numerous metastases to these areas were counted as one lesion. Long-bone metastases were counted per bone. This is a common method of tallying bone metastases that can lead to a relative underrepresentation of axial metastases. Only 0.7% of the metastases in the study were unspecified. (Data from Clain A. Secondary malignant disease of bone. *Br J Cancer*. 1965;19:15–29.)

determining the extent of cortical bone destruction in irregular bones such as the vertebrae, and the cross-sectional nature of CT eliminates the effect of overlapping structures when assessing the axial skeleton (Fig. 34.3). For example, the cortical detail seen on CT of the spine (with sagittal and coronal reformations) can provide an estimate of spinal stability (Fig. 34.4). Owing to limited soft tissue contrast resolution, this modality is not the best choice for imaging the marrow cavity. Bone windowing displays a greater degree of fine bony detail than soft tissue windowing and is recommended for the detection and follow-up of bone lesions[17] (Fig. 34.5).

Nuclear Medicine

Bone-seeking agents, such as technitium-99m methyl diphosphonate (Tc-99m MDP), are the most commonly used tracers for SS, and uptake is related to hydroxyapatite production during bone formation.[18] Whole-body (WB) planar images allow efficient screening for asymptomatic osseous metastases in patients with malignancies that produce blastic or mixed bone metastases, such as prostate, breast, and lung cancer.[14] Lytic metastases may not allow sufficient reparative bone formation for detection on SS (Fig. 34.4), which reduces sensitivity for purely lytic metastases such as from renal cell, thyroid carcinoma, and multiple myeloma.[19–21]

Bone scans are more sensitive than specific for the detection of osseous metastases.[11] A wide range of benign findings (e.g., arthritis, healing fractures, benign bone tumors) can mimic metastatic disease.[22] Alternatively, healing sclerotic change can also result in a deceptive "flare" phenomenon.[23,24] Therefore, the sensitivity of bone scan is often combined with the specificity of radiography to provide a powerful and relatively inexpensive means of diagnosing uptake on bone scan.[3,14,22]

In addition to planar images, SPECT is used to create three dimensional (tomographic) images of a region, which improves not only sensitivity but also specificity, because the location of the activity can help in the diagnosis (e.g., degenerative uptake at a joint space) (Fig. 34.6). Hybrid SPECT/CT, when both SPECT and CT images of a region are acquired during the same session, results in even better lesion characterization.[25–27]

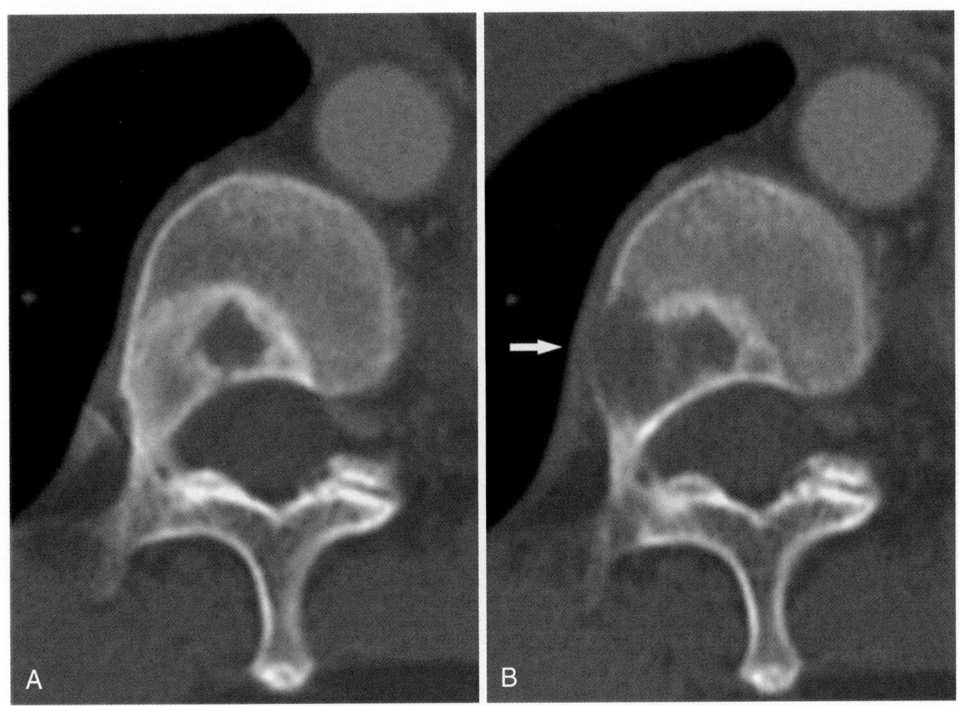

FIGURE 34.2. Appearance of bone metastases. **A**, Computed tomography of a well-defined mixed lytic/blastic bone metastases from non–small-cell lung cancer. **B**, Eight months later, lytic disease has progressed. The new area of osteolysis is ill-defined and expansile and demonstrates a permeative margin that destroys the cortex of the vertebral body (*arrow*).

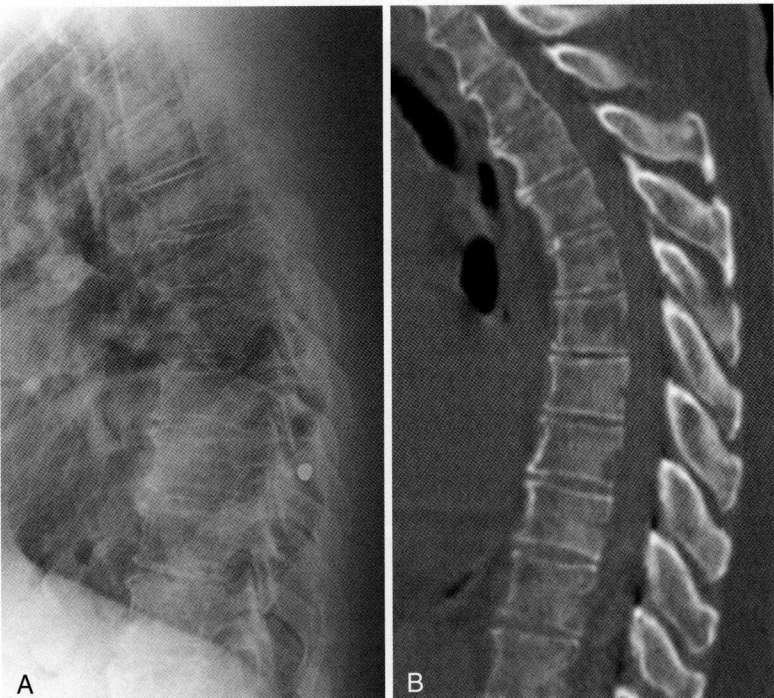

FIGURE 34.3. Effect of overlapping structures in a patient with multiple myeloma. **A**, Lateral radiograph of the thoracic spine demonstrates generalized osteopenia but no discrete lesions. **B**, Sagittal computed tomography reformation reveals numerous lytic, myelomatous lesions that were obscured by overlapping ribs and lung parenchyma on the radiograph.

However, SPECT/CT imaging requires longer imaging and generally only images a limited region with current gamma camera technology. FDG-PET/CT generates high quality WB tomographic images more rapidly. This improves lesion detection and characterization compared with SS and SPECT/CT.[28] It is also an alternative to Tc-99m MDP–based agents during regional or international shortages. However, these studies have higher complexity, and FDG-PET/CT may be better suited for select problem-solving than for routine use.

PET is commonly used to identify the high glucose metabolism of many malignancies. However, FDG uptake is not limited to tumor cells, and other processes result in FDG accumulation, such as inflammation (e.g., arthritis, infection) or normal physiology (e.g., brain and liver function). Despite these limitations, PET alone (without CT) was found to be more specific for detection of bone metastases than planar SS[29–31] owing to the higher spatial resolution of PET.[29,32,33] Evaluation of the morphology of the bone metastases has shown that PET reveals more lytic than blastic lesions,[34,35]

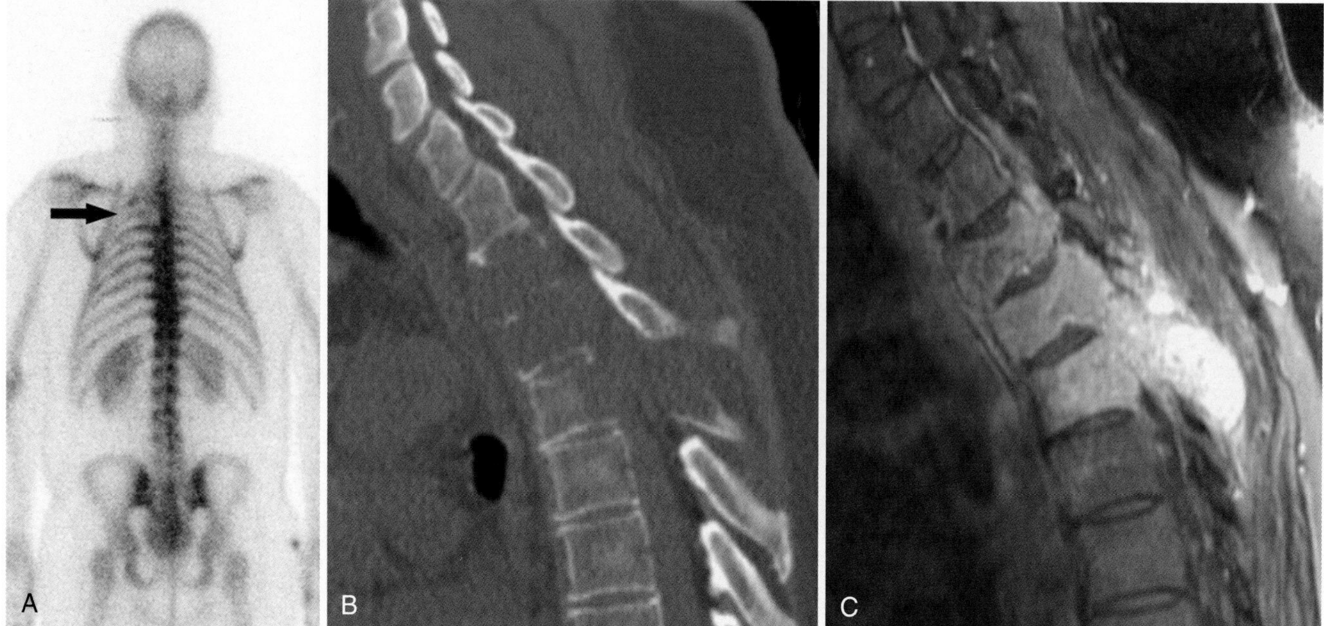

FIGURE 34.4. Metastatic renal cell carcinoma to the spine. **A**, Technitium-99m methyl diphosphonate bone scan demonstrates subtle photopenia in the upper thoracic spine (*arrow*). Lytic bone metastases such as those from renal cell and thyroid carcinoma may not induce sufficient reparative bone formation for the lesion to be detected on bone scan. **B**, Sagittal reformation of a computed tomography (CT) of the spine in bone windows demonstrates lytic metastases. CT is useful for assessment of the structural integrity of the axial skeleton. **C**, Fat-saturated T1-weighted magnetic resonance imaging (MRI) with intravenous gadolinium contrast. MRI best demonstrates the extent of disease in the marrow cavity, soft tissues, and epidural space (not shown).

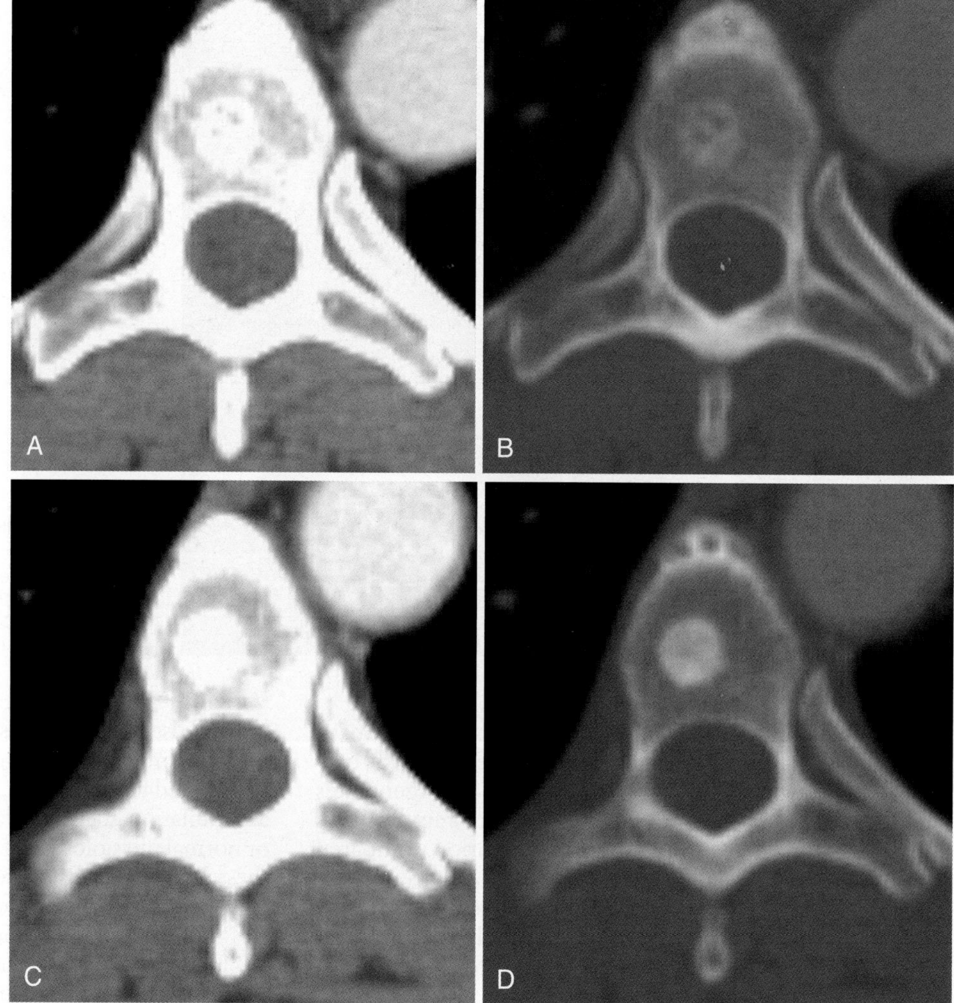

FIGURE 34.5. Computed tomography bone windows. **A**, Mixed lytic/sclerotic bone metastasis to the thoracic spine displayed with soft tissue windowing. **B**, Same study, companion bone window. Ten months later, change is difficult to perceive when the lesion is viewed with soft tissue windowing (**C**), but healing sclerosis is readily apparent on the same study using bone windows (**D**).

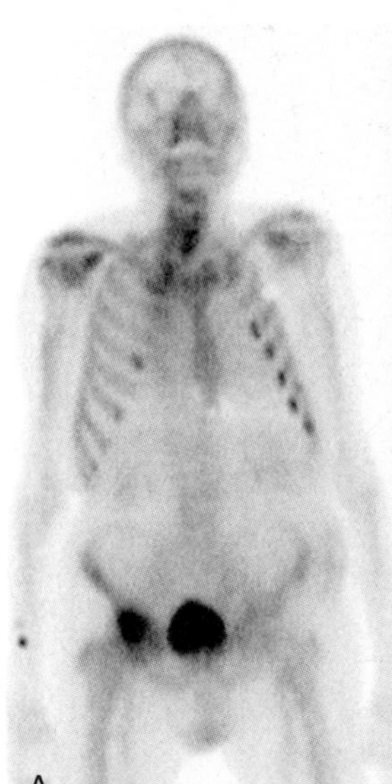

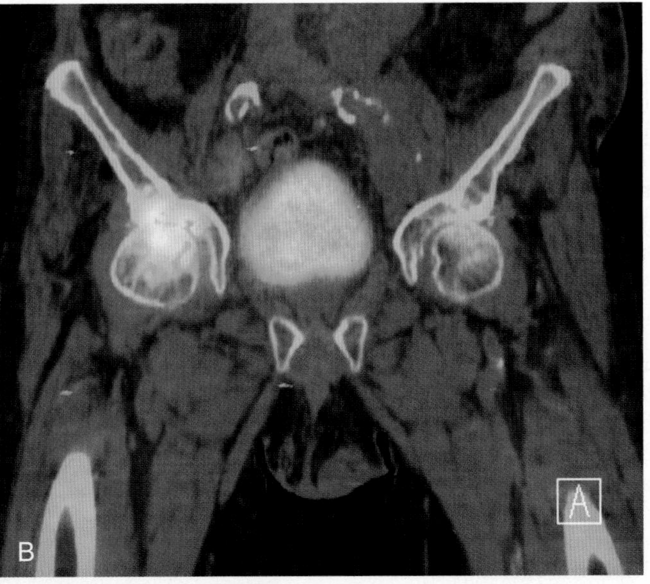

FIGURE 34.6. Planar bone scan and single-photon emission computed tomography (SPECT)/computed tomography (CT) in a patient with prostate cancer. **A**, Technitium-99m methyl diphosphonate bone scan demonstrates a large area of tracer uptake suspicious for a metastasis to the right acetabulum. Incidental note is made of benign fractures of numerous bilateral costochondral junctions and of the injection site in the right forearm. **B**, Fused coronal SPECT/CT image demonstrates tracer uptake on both sides of the narrowed right hip with subchondral sclerosis and degenerative cyst formation, indicating osteoarthritis. No bone metastases.

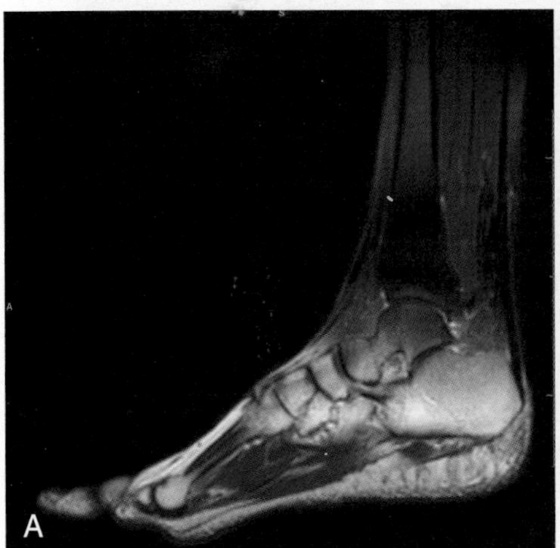

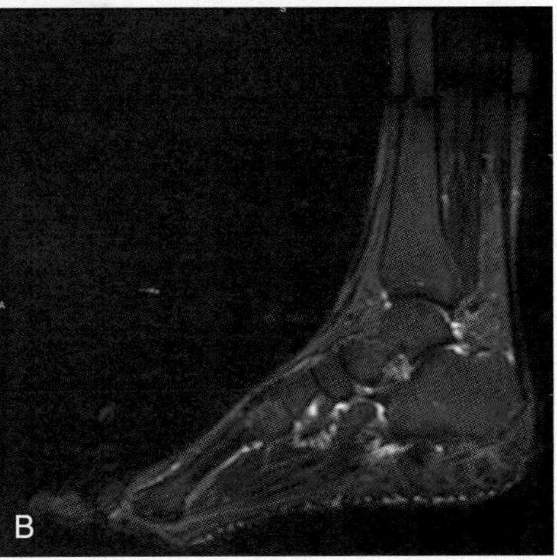

FIGURE 34.7. Reduction of magnetic resonance imaging (MRI) artifacts. **A**, Fat-saturated T2-weighted sagittal MRI of the ankle with failure of fat saturation in the lower portion of the image and uneven fat saturation in the upper part of the image. **B**, Short tau inversion recovery was performed in the same imaging session, producing more uniform fat saturation.

potentially because of the relatively lower cellularity of sclerotic, as compared with lytic, lesions.[36] Hybrid imaging with PET/CT improves sensitivity compared with PET alone (95.2% and 83.9%, respectively) while the specificity is similar (94.6% and 95.8%, respectively).[37] Whereas PET scans are expensive, and accessibility can be limited, the combination of functional and anatomic imaging makes FDG-PET/CT a powerful modality for WB tumor assessment.

Magnetic Resonance Imaging

MRI is capable of providing the greatest soft tissue resolution of all imaging modalities. The optimal MRI pulse sequences for imaging the musculoskeletal system may differ from those used to image other organs. Bone movement occurs through the conscious contraction of muscles rather than through the involuntary action of the autonomic nervous system (e.g., intestinal motion). The majority of patients are able to remain still throughout a typical examination (~45 min), allowing the routine use of several relatively lengthy pulse sequences that permit exquisite soft tissue contrast resolution. The following pulse sequences are recommended for conventional MRI of musculoskeletal oncology: fast spin echo (FSE) T1-weighted (T1W), FSE fat-saturated (FS) T2-weighted (T2W), and FSE FS T1 following intravenous gadolinium contrast. Short tau inversion recovery (STIR) can be substituted for FSE FS T2 in situations that predispose to uneven fat saturation, such as when scanning irregular anatomy (foot, ankle [Fig. 34.7]) or structures that are offset from the isocenter of the magnet (humeri). STIR is not used routinely, owing to comparatively lower signal-to-noise ratio compared with FS T2. Functional imaging sequences such as diffusion-weighted imaging (DWI) and dynamic contrast-enhanced MRI can provide additional information about the cellularity and vascularity of lesions, and are being increasingly used in musculoskeletal imaging.[38]

The interpretation of DWI in bone is different from that of DWI in soft tissue lesions, because normal yellow marrow has low apparent diffusion coefficient (ADC) values because of the low water content of densely packed adipocytes.[38] Unlike soft tissue lesions, malignant bone lesions typically have greater ADC values than normal marrow (in the range of 700–1400 μm²/sec), compared with normal marrow (<700 μm²/sec).[39]

The metal from bone reconstructions can produce significant artifacts that can be minimized through a number of techniques, including using lower field strength, excluding fat saturation from postcontrast sequences, using Dixon sequences for postcontrast imaging, replacing FS T2 with STIR, swapping the phase- and frequency-encoding directions in a direction that causes less obscuration of the area of interest, increasing the bandwidth of the receiver, increasing the bandwidth of the excitation pulse, using thinner slices, or increasing the image matrix size.[40,41] There are also new advanced techniques for reduction of metal artifact, including view angle tilting combined with isotropic three-dimensional (3D) fast spin-echo sequences (e.g., SPACE in Siemens), slice encoding for metal artifact correction (SEMAC), known as O-MAR XD (Philips, Best, Netherlands) and Advanced WARP (Siemens), multiacquisition with variable-resonance image combination (MAVRIC), as well as hybrid MAVRIC-SEMAC sequences (MAVRIC-SL, GE Milwaukee, WI).[41]

Most lytic and mixed bone metastases demonstrate low or intermediate T1 signal and high T2 signal and enhance. Sclerotic metastases may have a similar appearance or demonstrate low signal on all pulse sequences. Because the vast majority of skeletal metastases arise in the soft tissue of the marrow cavity, MRI allows early lesion detection by imaging the tumor while confined to the marrow.[42] Conversely, radiography and CT depend primarily on the interaction of the tumor with cortex, and metastases are often visible only after the tumor has grown large enough to extend from the marrow into the cortex. MRI is also the optimal imaging modality for determining the extent of tumor in the medullary cavity[16,43] and can be crucial for planning surgery or radiation therapy (Fig. 34.8). Another advantage of MRI is that excellent soft tissue resolution allows detection of impending emergencies involving adjacent structures, such as major nerves, blood vessels, or the spinal cord.[16,43–45] However, a disadvantage of MRI is that it cannot typically depict cortical bone structure, owing to a paucity of free protons, resulting in the black signal void typical of normal cortex. Ultrashort echo-time MRI allows for capture of the weak, short-lived signal from cortical bone[46] and may allow the characterization of the cortex on MRI. However, radiography and CT remain preferred for evaluating fine cortical detail in routine practice. Whereas MRI has traditionally been used for limited anatomic coverage, WB MRI is now feasible in the typical 1-hour patient scheduling allotment,[47] as is further discussed.

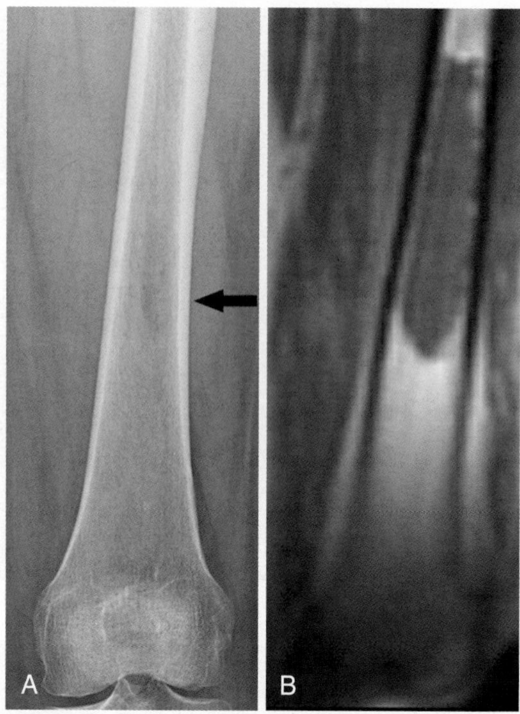

FIGURE 34.8. Magnetic resonance imaging (MRI) for evaluating the extent of marrow disease. **A**, Frontal radiograph of a patient with myeloma demonstrates subtle lucency with mild cortical permeation (*arrow*). **B**, T1-weighted coronal MRI reveals a large marrow lesion. MRI can allow accurate visualization of the extent of metastases in the medullary cavity of patients with radiographically ill-defined lesions. Depending on the histology of the primary tumor and risk of pathologic fracture, this can be helpful for planning radiation ports or surgery.

Future Imaging

WB MRI is a technology that allows MRI of the entire body to be performed in a single imaging session. Conventional MRI is limited in anatomic coverage owing to a combination of the long acquisition times of traditional pulse sequences and field inhomogeneity artifacts that increase with large coverage areas. WB MRI has been repeatedly shown to detect more bone metastases than SS.[48–56]

In many studies, completion of multiple pulse sequences of the entire body in a reasonable time frame is facilitated by use of specialized hardware, such as a rolling table platform that utilizes a combination of stationary coils embedded in the table and a fixed anterior surface coil under which the patient moves for each anatomic station.[52,57,58] Parallel imaging techniques, based on phased-array coil technology,[59] can also be used to speed up image acquisition.[60,61]

Considering the challenges of time limitation and artifact suppression, investigators of WB MRI have used a variety of rapidly acquired or robust pulse sequences. Whereas some investigators have used T2W imaging exclusively,[48,62] others have sought to increase diagnostic accuracy by performing at least two complementary sequences on each patient. T2W and STIR images have high sensitivity but lower specificity for the detection of osseous metastases. In contrast, T1W sequences have high specificity and lower sensitivity.[50–52,57,58,60,63]

Dixon techniques are increasingly used for the detection of bone marrow lesions with WB MRI (IDEAL in General Electric, DIXON in Siemens, and mDixon in Philips). Two-dimensional single-slice or 3D parallel imaging can be used with either gradient echo or spin echo (SE) Dixon sequences, increasing the versatility of the technique.[47,64] The Dixon technique can generate four sets of images: in-phase, out of phase, fat-only, and water only. The combination of T2W SE Dixon fat-only and water-only images allows for robust assessment of potential vertebral metastases.[64,65] The fat-only sequences increase lesion conspicuity compared with T1W SE images, whereas the water-only images provide fat-suppressed fluid-sensitive images.[64–66]

In addition, the fat content of bone lesions can be quantified to assist in classification of benign versus malignant lesions and in assessment of therapeutic response.[64]

WB DWI can also be used as an adjunct or replacement for T2W imaging. The low–b-value images serve as a sensitive sequence for detection of T2-hyperintense lesions, and high–b-value images serve as a more specific sequence for lesions with restricted diffusion.[38,39]

In addition to high sensitivity for the detection of bone metastases, MRI can image soft tissues (including organs such as liver and brain), making WB MRI a versatile imaging modality for total body imaging.[37,53,58,60]

WB MRI and PET/CT allow for WB evaluation for tumor, including bone metastases. The superior contrast resolution and high sensitivity of MRI combined with the functional information of various PET radiotracers makes hybrid PET/MRI an exciting option for WB imaging of cancer patients. A prospective study comparing WB MRI and FDG-PET/CT in 98 patients found that the sensitivity of WB MRI was greater than FDG-PET/CT for the detection of osseous and hepatic metastases, whereas WB MRI had lower sensitivity than FDG-PET/CT for the detection of pulmonary metastases.[58] In addition, FDG-PET/CT was found to be more accurate than WB MRI for primary tumor and nodal staging. These findings suggest that the two modalities are complementary, and that one of the major strengths of WB MRI is in the evaluation of bone metastases. Recently, commercial hybrid PET/MRI scanners have become available. One study reported similar detection of bone metastases compared with PET/CT but higher reader confidence with PET/MRI.[67] A second study reported slightly higher detection of bone metastases with PET/MRI compared with PET/CT (100% vs. 94%) but worse identification of benign osseous lesions (67% vs. 96%) that was thought to be related to the low signal of sclerotic lesions on MRI.[68] Although in theory hybrid imaging with PET and MRI should allow better lesion identification and characterization, an advantage of PET/MRI over PET/CT has yet to be clearly demonstrated, and this continues to be an active area of investigation.

Key Points Detection

- Combining the high specificity of radiography with the high sensitivity of bone scan is effective for detecting bone metastases.
- Magnetic resonance imaging (MRI) is optimal for detecting early metastases confined to the marrow, extent of disease in marrow, soft tissue extension from bone, and epidural extension.
- Positron emission tomography (PET) detects more lytic than blastic metastases, the opposite of bone scan.
- Whole-body (WB) MRI detects more bone metastases than bone scan.
- The strengths and limitations of WB MRI and PET/computed tomography may be complementary, and the hybrid PET/MRI modality is under investigation.

Response to Therapy

Cancer response criteria are used to determine the efficacy of therapeutic agents in clinical cancer trials and can be used as general guidelines for assessing therapeutic response, whether or not a patient is enrolled in a trial. The most commonly used criteria, such as the Response Evaluation Criteria In Solid Tumors, are based on the physical measurement of metastatic lesions. Bone metastases are often located in the axial skeleton, and the irregular shape of bones such as the vertebra and pelvis make physical measurement difficult. In addition, bone metastases do not always respond to therapy with a significant change in size. Therefore, these traditional methods of evaluating therapeutic response are not generally applicable to bone metastases, unless a measurable soft tissue mass extends from the cortex.[69] In response to the need for criteria that can be used to evaluate bone metastases, a bone-specific set of criteria, the MDA criteria, were developed at the MD Anderson Cancer Center.[3]

The MDA criteria include quantitative and qualitative assessments of the behavior of bone metastases. Response is divided into four categories: complete response, partial response, progressive disease, and stable disease. See Table 34.1 for the criteria and imaging examples of therapeutic response.

Table 34.1 MD Anderson Bone Response Criteria

RESPONSE CATEGORY	CRITERIA
Complete response	Complete sclerotic fill-in of lytic lesions on radiograph (XR) or computed tomography (CT). Normalization of bone density on XR or CT. Normalization of signal intensity on magnetic resonance imaging (MRI) (Fig. 34.9). Normalization of tracer uptake on skeletal scintigraphy (SS).
Partial response	Development of a sclerotic rim or partial sclerotic fill-in of lytic lesions on XR or CT. Sclerotic "flare": interval visualization of lesions with sclerotic rims or "new" sclerotic lesions in the setting of other signs of partial response and absence of progressive bone disease (Figs. 34.11 and 12). ≥50% decrease in measurable lesions on XR, CT, or MRI (Fig. 34.10). ≥50% subjective decrease in the size of ill-defined lesions on XR, CT, or MRI. ≥50% subjective decrease in tracer uptake on SS.
Progressive disease	≥25% increase in size of measurable lesions on XR, CT, or MRI. ≥25% subjective increase in the size of ill-defined lesions on XR, CT, or MRI. ≥25% subjective increase in tracer uptake on SS. New bone metastases.
Stable disease	No change. <25% increase or <50% decrease in measurable lesions. <25% subjective increase or <50% subjective decrease in ill-defined lesions. No new bone metastases.

(Modified from Hamaoka T, Madewell JE, Podoloff DA, et al. Bone imaging in metastatic breast cancer. *J Clin Oncol*. 2004;22:2942–2953.)

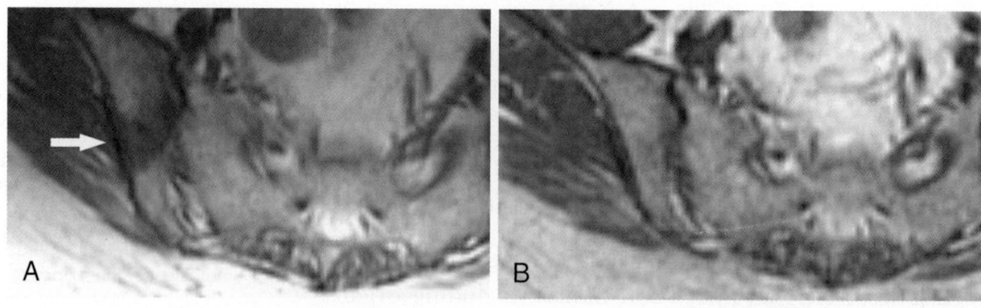

FIGURE 34.9. Complete response to therapy. **A**, Axial T1-weighted magnetic resonance imaging of the pelvis in a patient with breast cancer demonstrates a metastasis to the right iliac bone that is isointense to muscle (*arrow*). **B**, Seven months later, fat signal has returned, indicating a complete response.

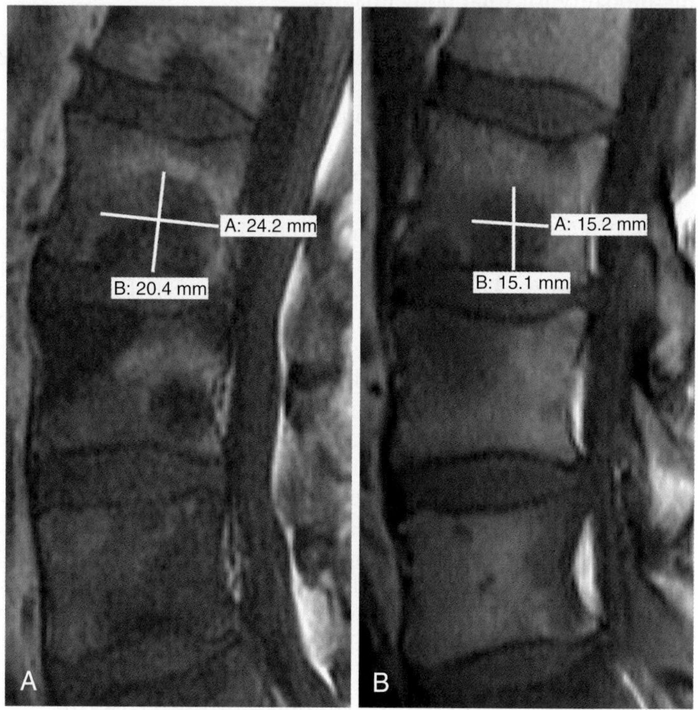

FIGURE 34.10. Partial response to therapy in a patient with prostate cancer. **A**, T1-weighted magnetic resonance imaging of the lumbar spine demonstrates numerous low–signal intensity metastases. **B**, Measurement of the perpendicular diameters of a lesion in the L2 vertebral body on a scan obtained 3 weeks later reveals a 79% decrease in the size of the lesion, meeting the MD Anderson criteria for a partial response to therapy (>50% decrease in the sum of the perpendicular diameters of a lesion). Numerous additional lesions have also decreased in size.

In comparison to the World Health Organization criteria and the International Union Against Cancer criteria, the MDA criteria were shown to be the only set of response criteria to correlate to progression-free survival in a study of 41 breast cancer patients with bone-only metastases.[4] Another study found that the MDA criteria predicted progression-free survival at 6 months in breast cancer patients with bone and measurable soft tissue metastases.[70] Clinical investigators have found the MDA criteria to be useful and have incorporated them into their study protocols.[71,72] The MDA bone response criteria reflect the behavior of bone metastases as they progress or improve and can also be used as guidelines for interpretation of imaging studies.

KEY POINTS Response to Therapy

- Lytic lesions typically heal with rim and/or central sclerosis.
- "Osteoblastic flare" can occur when lytic lesions heal, resulting in newly visualized sclerotic lesions at the site of undetected metastases, or cause lytic lesions to increase in size owing to development of rim sclerosis, mimicking disease progression.
- "Scintigraphic flare" results from increased tracer uptake in healing metastases and can mimic disease progression.
- The MD Anderson bone response criteria can be used to follow the therapeutic outcome of patients with bone metastases.

TREATMENT OF BONE METASTASES

Medical/Systemic Therapy

The systemic therapy of bone metastases can be divided into bisphosphonates and other agents such as monoclonal antibodies. Bisphosphonates, such as pamidronate (Aredia) and zoledronic acid (Zometa), have been shown to reduce serious skeletal-related events (SREs) such as fractures. Therefore, intravenous pamidronate has been established as the standard of care for breast cancer patients with bone metastasis.[73,74] Pamidronate delayed the first SREs for 3.5 to 6.1 months compared with placebo. The proportion of patients with skeletal complications decreased by approximately 11% to 13%. No overall survival benefit has been proven with the use of pamidronate.[73–75]

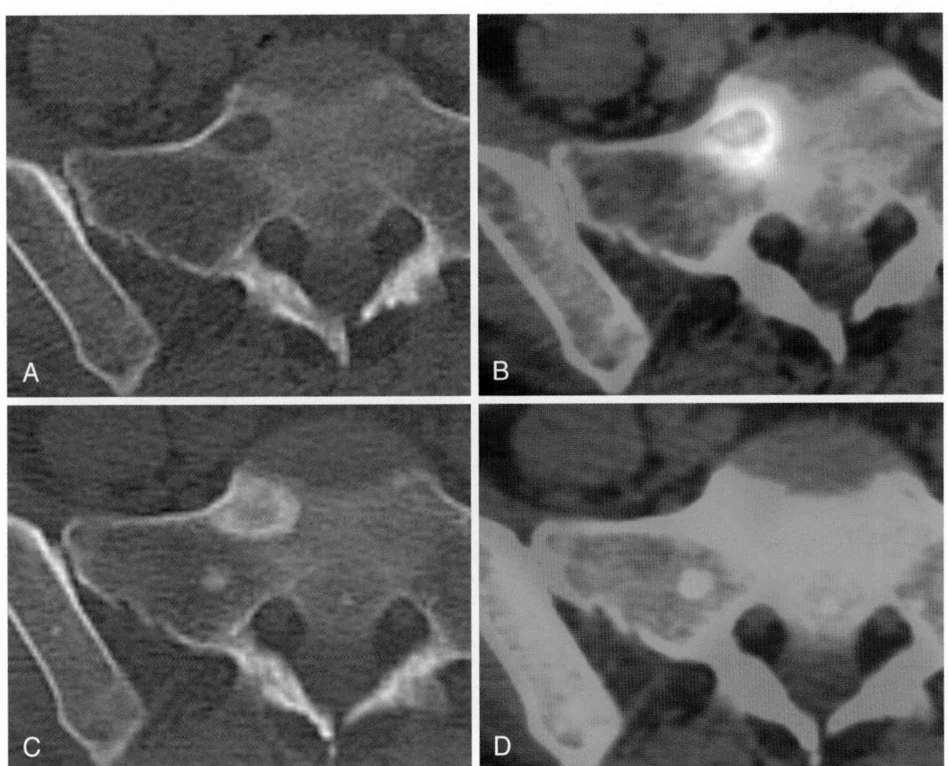

FIGURE 34.11. Osteoblastic "flare" in a patient with metastatic breast cancer. The computed tomography (CT) portion of a positron emission tomography (PET)/CT examination demonstrates a lytic metastasis in the S1 segment (**A**) that demonstrates 2-[18F] fluoro-2-deoxy-D-glucose (FDG) uptake on the fused PET/CT image (**B**). **C**, Nine months later, the lesion has undergone sclerosis and several additional sclerotic lesions are now visualized. **D**, No FDG uptake is seen on the fused PET/CT, confirmative of healing sclerosis. The "new" sclerotic lesions represent osteoblastic flare that has occurred at the site of subclinical marrow metastases, which were not visible until the development of healing sclerosis.

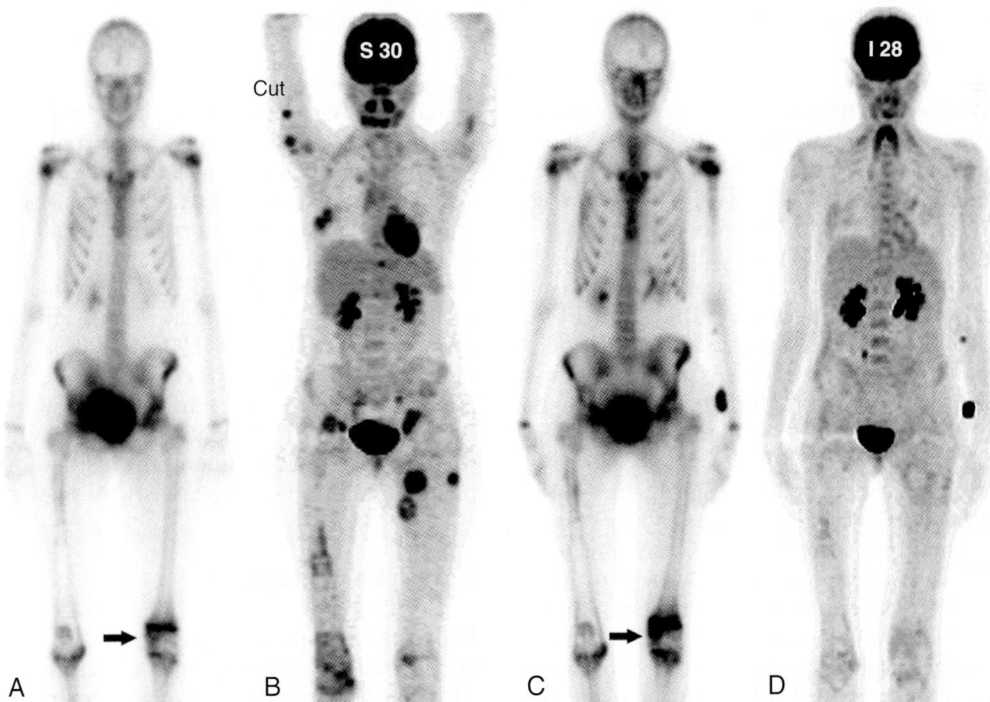

FIGURE 34.12. Scintigraphic flare in a patient with metastatic osteosarcoma. **A**, Technitium-99m methyl diphosphonate (Tc-99m MDP) bone scan demonstrates open physes and scattered bone metastases, such as in the distal left femoral metaphysis (*arrow*). The area of photopenia in the right femur corresponds to resection arthroplasty of the primary tumor. **B**, Maximum intensity projection (MIP) 2-[18F] fluoro-2-deoxy-D-glucose (FDG)–positron emission tomography (PET) image demonstrates widespread bone and soft tissue metastases. **C**, Tc-99m MDP bone scan obtained 1 month after **A** is suspicious for disease progression, with increased tracer uptake in numerous lesions such as at the left distal femoral metaphysis (*arrow*). **D**, MIP FDG-PET image obtained the same day as **C** demonstrates marked improvement in the metastases, indicating that the appearance of the left distal femoral lesion on the bone scan in **C** was a flare response to the healing lesion. Scintigraphic flares are usually seen within the first 3 months after therapy.[23,24]

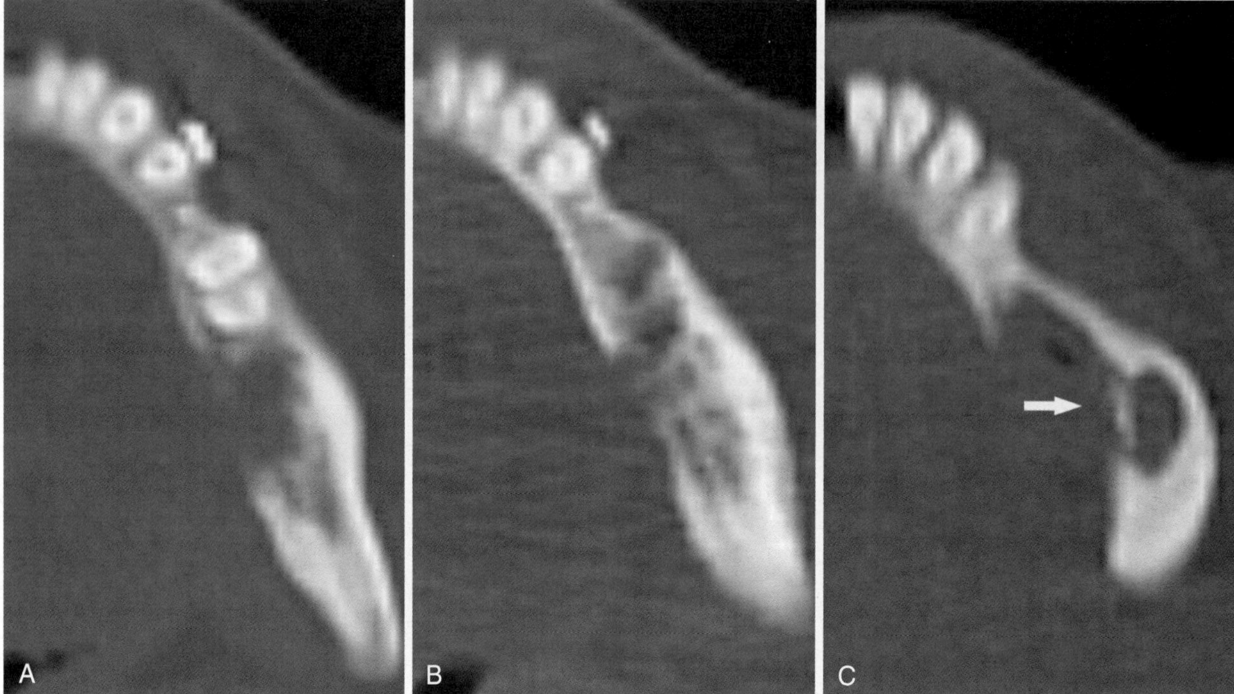

FIGURE 34.13. Osteonecrosis of the jaw (ONJ) in a breast cancer patient who had a tooth removed after intravenous bisphosphonate therapy. **A**, Osteolysis of the body of the left mandible is representative of ONJ. **B**, Seven months later, healing has occurred with increased mineralization of the lytic area. Two teeth are missing. Whereas dental extractions often perpetrate ONJ, the condition itself can destabilize the teeth. **C**, In the 4-year interval between **B** and **C**, multiple infections occurred, ultimately leading to further osteolysis and formation of a sequestrum (*arrow*). Recurrence with pain and purulent discharge is common following the discontinuation of individual courses of antibiotic therapy. Surgery is typically reserved for ONJ that is refractory to antibiotics. Because the entire skeleton is affected by the action of the bisphosphonates, surgeons are unable to resect down to normal bone. Soft-tissue flaps are not used to cover the exposed bone, owing to the likelihood that infection that may lead to fistula formation or wound dehiscence, ultimately exposing more bone. The patient was followed conservatively with intermittent removal of small portions of problematic, exposed bone. The mucosa healed to the extent that the mandible was covered.

Another bisphosphonate that is standard of care is intravenous zoledronic acid, which has been shown to be more potent than pamidronate in preclinical studies.[76,77] When zoledronic acid (4 or 8 mg intravenous [IV]) was compared with pamidronate (90 mg IV),[78,79] the annual incidence of skeletal complications decreased by 40%. In a metaanalysis comparing zoledronic acid (4 mg IV), pamidronate (90 mg IV), ibandronate (6 mg IV), ibandronate (50 mg *per os* [PO]), and clodronate (1600 mg PO), zoledronic acid was as effective as pamidronate in preventing SREs. Many oncologists choose zoledronic acid over pamidronate because of its shorter infusion time (15 minutes) as compared with that of pamidronate (2 hours).

An important complication of bisphosphate therapy is osteonecrosis of the jaw (ONJ) Fig. 34.13. ONJ may present as nonhealing oral mucosa and exposed mandibular or maxillary bone.[80] The incidence in breast cancer patients is from 1.2% to 15%.[81–88] The most important step in the prevention of ONJ is a dental evaluation[89,90] before initial administration of the bisphosphonate. If any dental work is needed, it is recommended that it be completed and the wound well healed before starting the bisphosphonate. Halting the drug and implementing observation is recommended for the treatment of ONJ, with debridement of necrotic bone reserved for refractory cases.

Denosumab is a human monoclonal antibody that specifically binds receptor activator of nuclear factor kappa-B ligand (RANKL) to inhibit osteoclast activity. This results in reduced bone resorption, tumor-induced bone destruction, and SREs. Many randomized trials with similar study design have directly compared denosumab and zoledronic acid. Patients with bone metastases from breast cancer, prostate cancer, and solid tumors were enrolled.[91–93] The results showed that denosumab was superior to zoledronic acid in delaying and preventing SREs. Denosumab reduced the risk of a first SRE by 17% (hazard ratio [HR] 0.83, 95% confidence interval [CI]: 0.76–0.90, $P < .001$). There was a similar rate of ONJ, but renal toxicity was higher with the bisphosphonate zoledronic acid. The results showed no difference in survival outcome (HR 0.99, 95%CI: 0.91–1.07, $P = .71$).[94,95] Medical therapy is an important method of simultaneously treating multiple bone metastases throughout the skeleton.

Radiation Therapy

Radiation therapy for bone metastases is mainly palliative and is used for situations such as pain that is uncontrolled with analgesics and prevention or treatment of pathologic fractures. Radiation therapy can help maintain bone integrity and prevent further progression of bone destruction. Thus, radiation is not simply used to control pain, but also can help preserve the function of bone Fig. 34.14. It is also often indicated for reducing the volume of epidural tumor that compresses or threatens to compress the spinal cord or nerve roots.

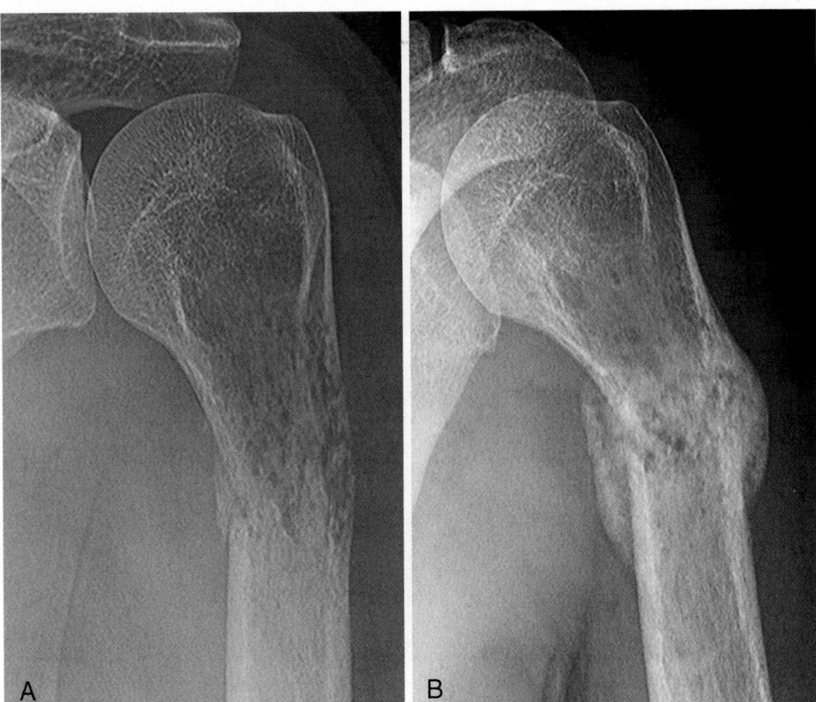

Figure 34.14. Pathologic fracture of the proximal humeral diaphysis in a patient with myeloma treated with radiation therapy. **A**, Frontal radiograph of the left humerus demonstrates innumerable tiny lytic lesions that contributed to the loss of structural integrity that resulted in a pathologic fracture. **B**, Six months after external beam radiation, healing callous and a mild degree of bony remineralization is seen at the fracture site.

External beam radiation is effective in reducing bone metastasis–associated pain in approximately 50% to 80% of patients.[96,97] For patients with poor prognosis, the most widely used regimen in the United States is to deliver 30 Gy in 10 daily treatments over 2 weeks.[96]

The overall condition of the patient is considered when choosing an appropriate treatment schedule. Shorter regimens can be chosen for patients with widespread metastases and poor prognosis and who are unable to keep multiple appointments. For example, a course of 8 Gy in one treatment rather than 20 Gy in five daily treatments can be considered. The American Society for Radiation Oncology has published guidelines that also recommend using a single treatment of 8 Gy because the pain relief was similar to that obtained with a longer treatment regimen.[98] Short regimens have been found to have no significant difference in the efficacy of pain control but lead to a higher rate of symptom relapse and need for retreatment in comparison to longer, more conventional regimens.[96,97]

For patients with better prognoses, stereotatic body radiation therapy (SBRT), which delivers high-dose radiation therapy in a small number of treatments, can achieve better and longer pain control.[99] A phase II randomized trial of patients with spine metastases that compared SBRT of 24 Gy in one treatment with 30 Gy in 10 treatments (3DRT) found that the shorter regimen achieved quicker and better pain relief. SBRT achieved significantly lower visual analog pain scale ratings at 6 months than 3DRT (13.7 vs. 35, $P = .0024$). A phase II randomized trial in patients with oligometastasis including bone reported that SBRT improved median overall survival to 41 months, compared with 28 months with standard-of-care treatment.[100] Larger phase III trials are needed to further delineate the role of SBRT in bone metastasis.

Radiation therapy is also often best combined with surgery in patients with epidural extension of tumor and subsequent compression or impending compression of the spinal cord. A prospective randomized trial[101] found that, when a single area of the spine is involved, circumferential surgical decompression of the cord before radiation therapy can result in significantly better preservation of motor function than radiation alone. Surgery is preferred in these instances, because the mass effect of the radiated tumor only resolves gradually over several days, and prolonged mass effect can cause otherwise reversible cord edema to progress into irreversible ischemia. Some 84% of the patients were ambulatory for a median duration of 122 days after combined treatment, whereas only 57% of those who received radiation alone were ambulatory for a median duration of 13 days.[101] For patients with disease at numerous spinal levels and/or a combination of poor prognosis and poor performance status, palliative radiation therapy alone can provide benefit.

For patients with extensive painful bone metastases refractory to analgesics and systemic therapy, or patients who have failed external beam radiation, radiopharmaceuticals are another option. Strontium-89 chloride (^{89}Sr) and samarium-153 ethylene diamine tetramethylene phosphonaic acid (^{153}Sm) are bone-seeking beta emitters that localize to sites of bone turnover. Pretherapeutic SS can be performed to verify osteoblastic reaction to the metastases. Unlike ^{89}Sr, ^{153}Sm emits a gamma photon that permits high-quality posttherapeutic imaging (Fig. 34.15). No significant difference has been found in the palliation of bone pain with ^{89}Sr compared with ^{153}Sm (60%–95%).[102–105] Improved pain control usually occurs within days or weeks, with a duration of several months.[106] In castrate-resistant prostate cancer patients with bone-only metastases, radium-223 dichloride (an alpha emitter that mimics calcium and binds to newly formed bone stroma, particularly sclerotic metastases) can also be used. The alpha particle delivers a much more energetic and localized dose of

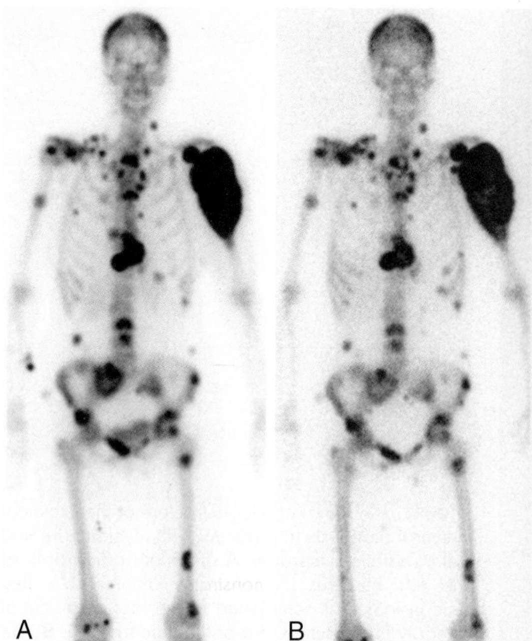

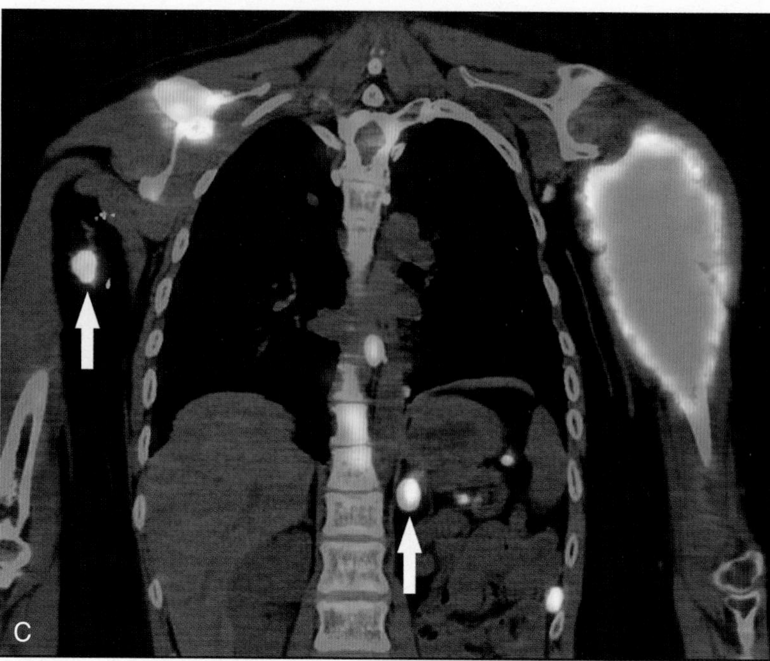

FIGURE 34.15. Samarium-153 (^{153}Sm) therapy in a patient with metastatic breast cancer. **A**, Technitium-99m methyl diphosphonate (Tc-99m MDP) bone scan demonstrates widespread bony metastases. Diphosphonate bone scans are obtained before radiopharmaceutical therapy to verify osteoblastic response to which radiopharmaceuticals can localize and thereby treat the metastases. Radiopharmaceuticals are not given to patients with negative Tc-99m MDP scans. **B**, Maximum intensity projection ^{153}Sm image with uptake paralleling the lesions on bone scan. **C**, The ^{153}Sm study was performed as a single-photon emission tomography with integrated computed tomography redundant "computed tomorgaphy" (CT) examination. The addition of CT allows localization of lesions to soft tissue (the largest are marked with *arrows*) in addition to bone on the coronal reformatted image. The soft tissue metastases were detected on the Tc-99m MDP study in **A** because they are heavily calcified. (Courtesy of Hubert H. Chuang, M.D., Ph.D., Department of Nuclear Medicine, MD Anderson Cancer Center.)

radiation than beta particles, inducing double-stranded DNA breaks that result in a potent and highly localized cytotoxic effect[107] that was found to improve both pain and median overall survival (HR 0.70; P = .002).[108] Contraindications include renal insufficiency, bone marrow suppression, spinal cord compression, and pregnancy. The side effects of these agents include mild bone marrow suppression 4 to 8 weeks after the therapy, which is reflected by leukopenia and thrombocytopenia. Bone marrow toxicity is usually transient, and the same drugs can be repeated 2 to 3 months after blood counts recover.[102]

Surgical/Interventional Therapy

Pathologic fracture or impending fracture is the main indication for surgical treatment of bone metastases. The basic goals of surgery are stabilization, preservation of mobility, and pain relief.[109] The discomfort of osseous metastases can be among the most severe that a cancer patient can experience, and the marked pain reduction after surgery typically allows patients to regain much of their lost mobility.[110]

There is controversy as to whether patients with advanced, widespread disease are reasonable candidates for surgery. Projected survival or longevity is not necessarily the primary concern, and patients with a life expectancy as short as 1 month can be appropriate surgical candidates. In fact, the improvement in pain and the reduction in opioid usage may even help increase survival. Often more important is comparison of the morbidity of the procedure to the expected benefit because patients near the end of life may not be able to tolerate the stress of lengthy procedures. Therefore, a number of minimally invasive orthopedic operations, such as closed insertion of intramedullary nails and some partial joint replacements, have been increasingly employed to address the pain of pathologic fractures. Improvements in medical treatment, with newer targeted therapies and antiresorptive treatment, have helped expand the use of such surgery.

Many factors contribute to the decision regarding whether to intervene surgically. If a pathologic fracture is present, particularly in the lower extremity, surgery is usually the best treatment option because these fractures for the most part are not expected to heal. Casts or braces are not as effective as surgical fixation with respect to pain relief and adequate stabilization for ambulation. If fracture has not yet occurred, fracture risk must be determined to decide between surgery and other options. Several methods can be used to determine fracture risk, and all involve image-based analysis of the size and character of the metastasis. It has been found that painful femoral lesions that are at least 2.5 cm in length and involve the cortex are at risk for pathologic fracture.[111] Lesions that occupy more than 50% of the circumference of the bone are also at considerable risk.[112] Mirels' scoring system can also be used to determine fracture risk[113] (Table 34.2). This system is based on four parameters: the site of the metastasis (upper extremity, lower extremity, or peritrochanteric region), pain (mild, moderate, severe/aggravated with function), tumor type (blastic, mixed, or lytic), and lesion size (involvement of less than one-third, one-third

TABLE 34.2 Mirels' Scoring System for Assessment of Fracture Risk

	SCORE		
VARIABLE	**1**	**2**	**3**
Site	Upper limb	Lower limb	Peritrochanteric
Pain	Mild	Moderate	Functional
Lesion	Blastic	Mixed	Lytic
Size	<⅓	⅓–⅔	>⅔

(From Mirels H. Metastatic disease in long bones. A proposed scoring system for diagnosing impending pathologic fractures. *Clin Orthop Relat Res.* 1989;249: 256–264. Reprinted with permission from Springer.)

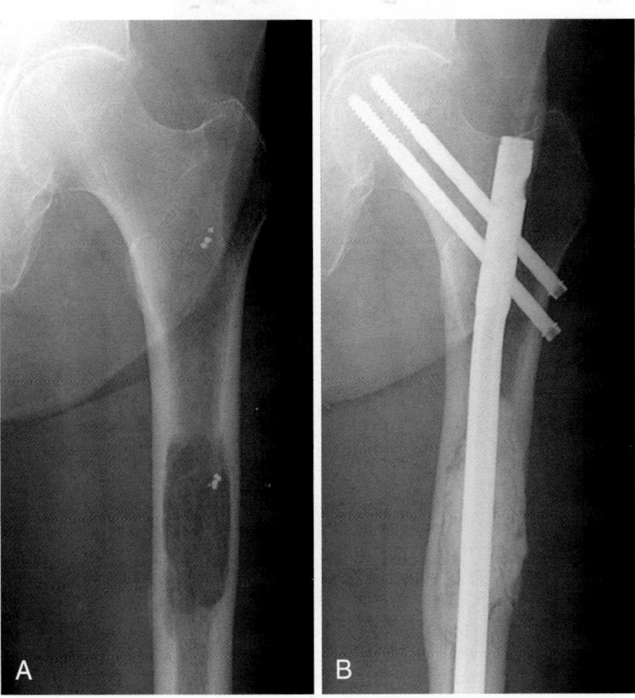

FIGURE 34.16. Impending pathologic fracture in a patient with lung cancer. **A**, A lytic metastasis is seen in the proximal diaphysis of the left femur. The lesion is greater than 2.5 cm in length and encompasses more than 50% of the diameter of the bone. The Mirels score would be 10 (lytic lesion 3 points; more than two thirds the diameter 3 points; lower extremity 2 points; moderate pain 2 points), and fracture is considered likely to occur without operative intervention. **B**, The lesion was treated with curettage and polymethylmethacrylate cementation, and the bone was stabilized with intramedullary nailing.

to two-thirds, or more than two-thirds of the diameter of the bone). Reflecting severity, 1 to 3 points are assigned per category. A total score of 8 or greater indicates significant concern for pathologic fracture, and surgery is considered the treatment of choice (Fig. 34.16). A score of less than 7 suggests less risk for fracture, and nonsurgical approaches such as functional bracing, protected weight-bearing, and radiation can be considered. Although used extensively, the Mirels score is based partially on subjective criteria. A more quantitative and accurate approach to fracture risk assessment that utilizes CT data to determine if structural rigidity has been developed, but this has not gained widespread clinical use.[114]

In addition to fracture risk, the expected response of bone metastasis to other therapies is a strong factor when determining the appropriateness and type of surgery. Response depends in part upon the histology of the primary tumor. For example, lymphoma of bone frequently resolves after chemotherapy, and the bone has the capacity to recover completely. Metastatic breast, prostate, and thyroid carcinoma and multiple myeloma also tend to demonstrate positive treatment response, whereas sarcomas, melanomas, and carcinomas from the gastrointestinal tract tend to respond poorly. In the past, it has been stated that renal cell carcinoma metastases do not respond well to medical treatment, and that the lytic lesions inexorably progress with time; however, this should no longer be considered universally true. Improvements in targeted and other therapies for renal cell cancer have resulted in better control of osseous metastases and fewer SREs.[115]

The likelihood of response to systemic or radiation therapy helps determine the most appropriate type of operation. In general, surgery may be open or closed, meaning that the tumor site or fracture may be directly exposed (open) or not exposed (closed). Closed nailings are typically performed across lesions in long bones that are expected to respond well to chemotherapy or radiation. Intramedullary nails are generally preferred over side plates, because nails can stabilize the entire length of the bone instead of just the area under the plate, and the operation can be performed percutaneously through small incisions for the entrance sites of the nail and interlocking screws. The morbidity of such operations is minimal, although blood loss through the bone may be brisk with vascular tumors such as renal cell carcinoma and thyroid carcinoma. In these cases, preoperative selective arterial embolization, typically performed by interventional radiology, can significantly reduce blood loss.

Surgical excision of the metastatic tumor, which may be done in conjunction with open nailing or more extensive reconstructive procedures, is often performed for diseases such as sarcomas, melanomas, and renal cell carcinoma that do not typically respond well to medical or radiation treatment, and is performed to prevent uncontrolled local relapse. Common excisional procedures include curettage and *en bloc* resection. Curettage is a procedure in which the tumor is intralesionally removed in a piecemeal fashion, leaving the adjacent bone intact, whereas *en bloc* resection removes the tumor as a single intact mass, often resulting in wider surgical margins. In the setting of massive local recurrence, limb amputation may be required (Fig. 34.17). Another indication for open resection of osseous metastases is for treatment of lesions that destroy the structure of the bone to such an extent that it cannot be salvaged by nailing or plating (Fig. 34.18). Advantages of wide, *en bloc* excision include reducing the likelihood of massive local recurrence (Fig. 34.19), achieving better control of bleeding vessels, and controlling refractory hypercalcemia, which can directly result from loss of large amounts of mineralized tissue.

The benefits of wide excision are not achieved without a price. In addition to the increased length of surgery, more extensive wound, and greater potential for perioperative complications, there may be limb weakness and worse function after surgery. Most large skeletal defects of long bones can now be reconstructed in a straightforward manner with modular prostheses that can be easily adapted to various sizes (Fig. 34.20). In recent years, there have been improvements in some of these prostheses to improve muscle function. For the proximal tibia, porous metal for attachment of the patellar tendon has increased quadriceps strength. For the proximal humerus, the use of reverse shoulder prostheses has compensated for the loss of the rotator cuff.

Several nonsurgical percutaneous treatment options for painful bone metastases are also available. Examples include vertebroplasty, kyphoplasty, radiofrequency ablation (RFA), and cryoablation. Vertebroplasty and kyphoplasty are performed by injecting bone cement (polymethylmethacrylate) into the collapsed vertebral body by needle, typically through the pedicles, under fluoroscopic guidance. In vertebroplasty, the cement stabilizes the segment, preventing

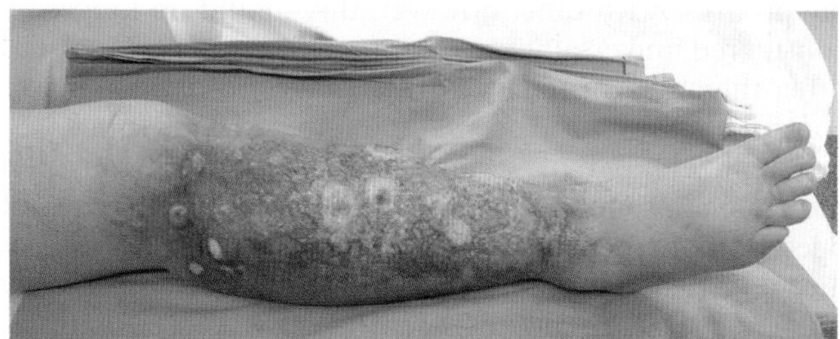

FIGURE 34.17. Massive recurrence of metastatic sarcoma of the tibia refractory to treatment resulted in an above-knee amputation of the limb. Numerous tumor deposits are seen in the skin.

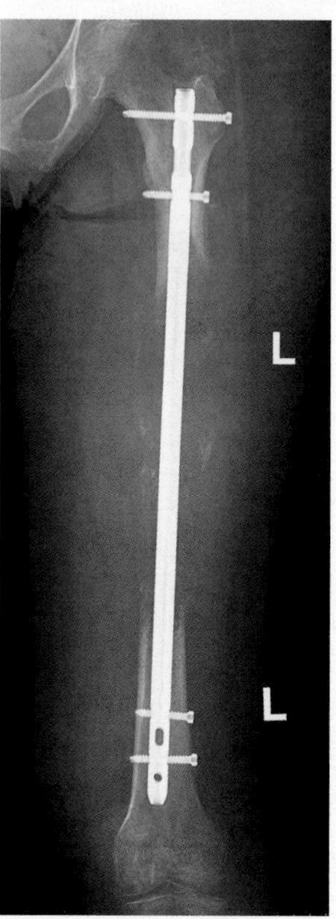

FIGURE 34.19. Metastatic uterine leiomyosarcoma to the left femur that was previously treated with a closed intramedullary nail; subsequent progression of disease led to dramatic destruction of bone.

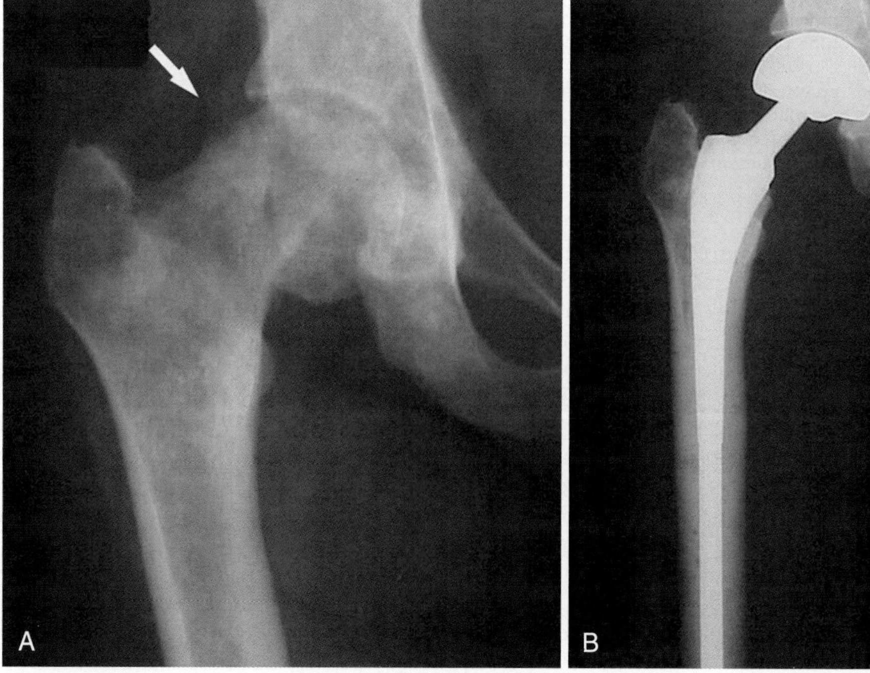

FIGURE 34.18. Displaced femoral neck fracture as a result of metastatic breast cancer. **A**, The fracture is varus displaced (*arrow*), and the femur is shortened. An attempt at reduction is likely to fail because of nonunion and avascular necrosis. **B**, The femur was reconstructed by a bipolar hemiarthroplasty with a long femoral stem to provide additional protection for the femoral shaft against future pathologic fracture.

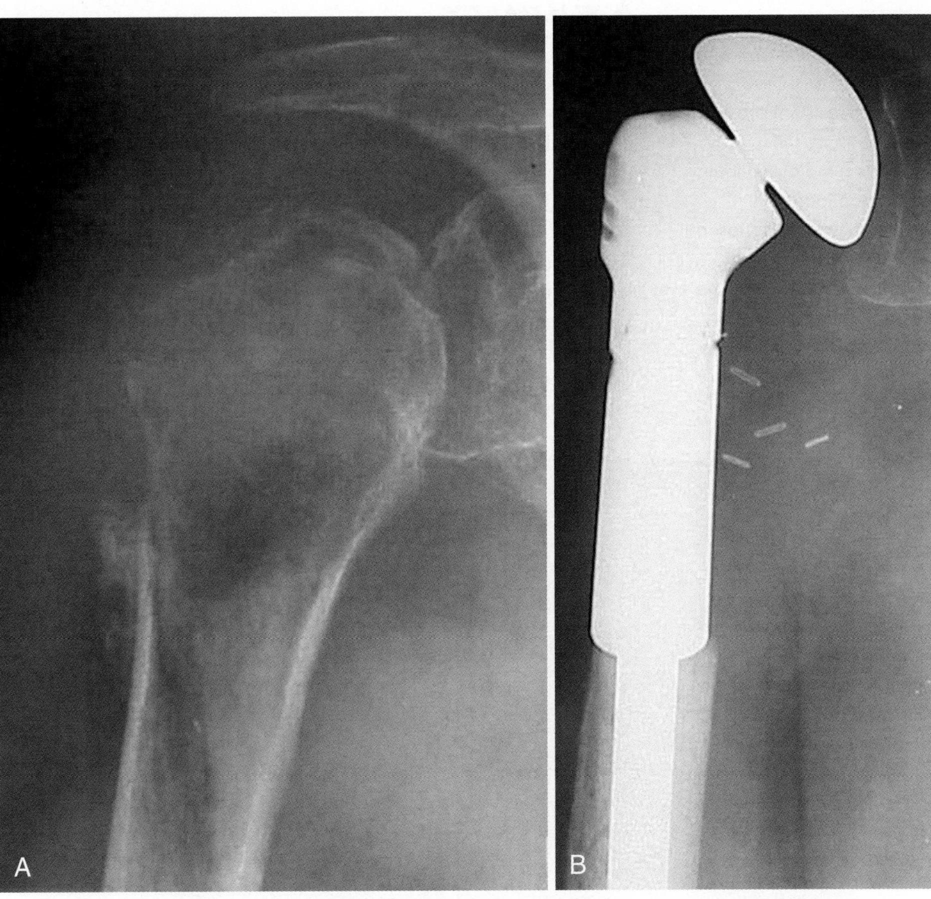

Figure 34.20. Metastatic renal cell carcinoma to the right humeral head. **A**, Preoperative radiograph shows destruction and deformity of the humeral head to the extent that preservation of the proximal humerus would not allow normal smooth articulation at the joint. **B**, Following *en bloc* resection, the proximal humerus was replaced by a modular endoprosthetic implant that can be built to varying lengths of bone resection.

further collapse. This has proved especially helpful for patients with multiple myeloma who may have extensive spinal disease and/or poor structural integrity disallowing stabilization hardware. Kyphoplasty is performed in a similar manner by injecting the cement into a balloon, with the goal of increasing the height of the segment to also help correct abnormal spinal curvature. Once the balloon is inflated, it is withdrawn, and cement is then injected into the cavity (Fig. 34.21). Pain relief has been reported in the vast majority of patients after vertebroplasty or kyphoplasty.[116–118] These procedures are contraindicated in patients with cord compression.[116] Complications have been reported at a rate of approximately 0% to 8%. Most complications are related to probe insertion (e.g., hematoma/hemothorax), cement embolism (e.g., pulmonary embolism), or radiculopathies from nerve root/spinal cord compression against extravasated cement.[117] The success with cement injection for the spine has led to its use in other areas, such as the periacetabular region, often with additional screw reinforcement. For debilitated and elderly patients who may not tolerate a complex hip reconstruction well, the percutaneous approach has intuitive appeal.

RFA is a procedure by which a thermal probe is inserted into a tumor and used to destroy the lesion by heat necrosis. RFA has been shown to provide excellent pain relief with little morbidity.[119] Goetz et al.[120] studied RFA in 43 patients with bone metastases and found that 95% experienced a clinically significant decrease in pain for up to 6 months. Lesions in this study were limited to lytic or mixed metastases, owing to inability to expand the probe into hard, blastic lesions. The procedure can sometimes be complemented by percutaneous cement injection to help support the bone. Similarly, cryoablation has emerged as a viable technique for percutaneous treatment of small, symptomatic metastatic lesions.[121,122] RFA and cryoablation may be particularly advantageous in patients who have already undergone radiotherapy and are not candidates for further radiation.

The therapy of bone metastases is a complex endeavor that encompasses the fields of diagnostic imaging, nuclear medicine, medical oncology, radiation oncology, and orthopedic surgery. A multidisciplinary effort is needed to achieve the maximum benefit for patients with bone metastasis.

Key Points Treatment

- Systemic bone-targeted therapy (e.g., bisphosphonates, receptor activator of nuclear factor kappa-B ligand (RANKL) inhibitors [denosumab], and radiopharmaceutical agents) are indicated to treat multiple bone metastases simultaneously.
- Osteonecrosis of the jaw is a serious adverse event both of bisphosphonate and RANKL inhibitors, and a dental check is required before administration.
- Denosumab is superior to bisphosphonates for preventing skeletal-related events, with less renal toxicity but with no known survival advantage.
- Radiation therapy can be used to palliate limited numbers of bone metastases and can be combined with surgery in cases of spinal cord compression or impending pathologic fracture.

- Radiopharmaceuticals can provide pain control for widespread bone metastases that are unresponsive to systemic therapy and analgesics.
- Radium-223 showed survival benefit in castrate-resistant prostate cancer with bone metastases.
- Imaging-assessed risk of pathologic fracture is a major deciding factor between surgery and other therapeutic options.
- Open surgical procedures remove the tumor, whereas closed procedures simply stabilize the bone.
- Selection of the appropriate operation often depends on the expected response of the lesion to systemic or radiation therapy.
- Percutaneous interventions (e.g., vertebroplasty, kyphoplasty, or radiofrequency ablation) should be considered for treatment of individual bone metastases.

SUMMARY

Bone metastases have a significant impact on the lives of many cancer patients. The detection of these lesions is accomplished through a variety of imaging studies. Dedicated XRs are helpful for evaluating specific abnormalities or for the initial imaging of painful areas. By imaging the marrow cavity, MRI can detect lesions early and is the optimal modality for determining the extent of bone metastases before therapy. WB MRI is more sensitive than bone scan for the detection of bone metastases. PET/CT, WB MRI, and PET/MRI are WB imaging modalities that can be used to detect bone metastases and can simultaneously image organs and soft tissues. Imaging is commonly used to evaluate the

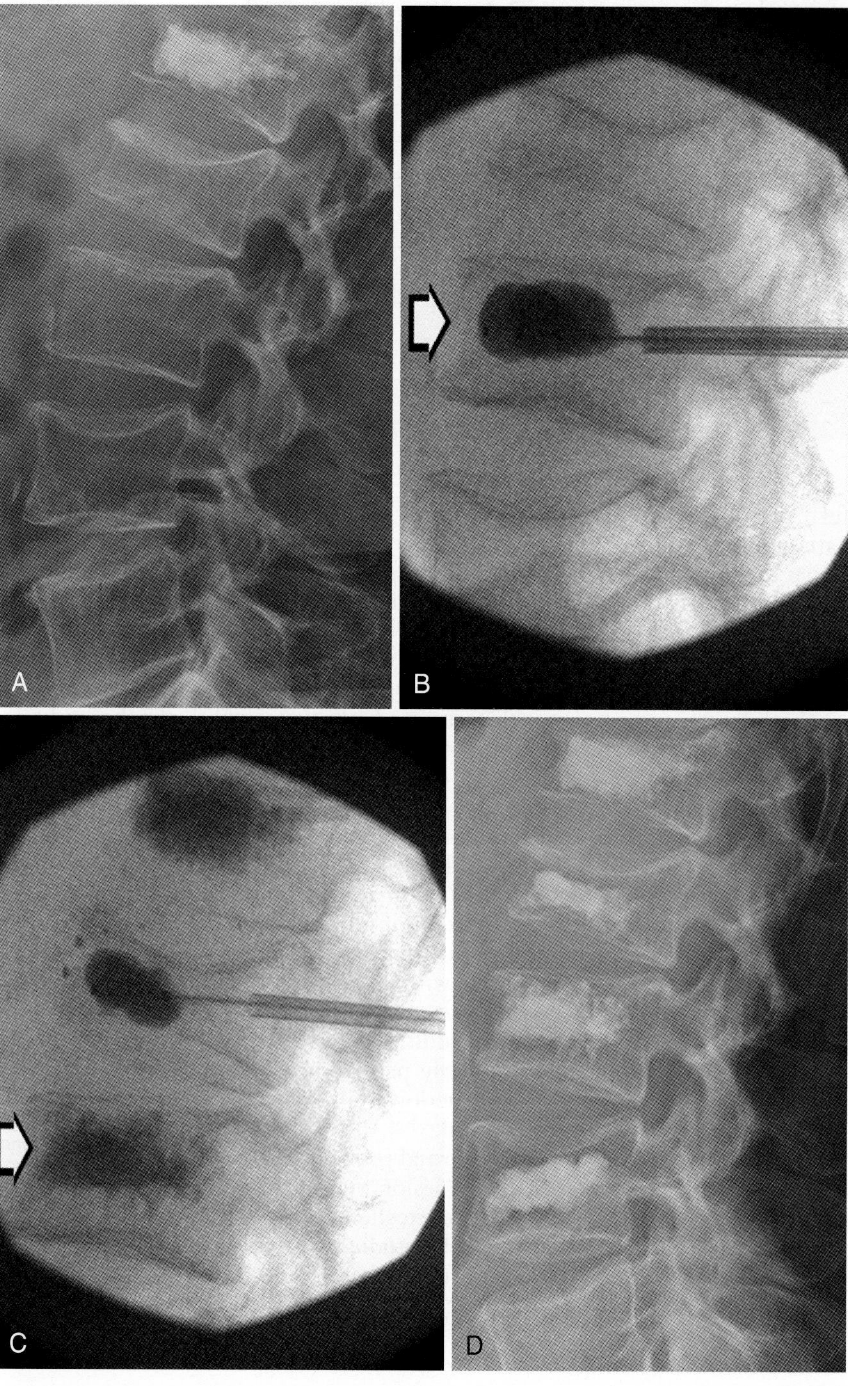

FIGURE 34.21. Kyphoplasty in a patient with myeloma. **A**, Preprocedural radiograph demonstrates compression fractures at L2, L3, and L4 and prior kyphoplasty at L1. **B**, Polymethylmethacrylate cement is injected percutaneously into balloons at L3 that are introduced into one or both pedicles under fluoroscopic guidance (*arrow*). **C**, Balloons are withdrawn and cement is injected into the cavity created in the marrow by pressure of the inflated balloons (*arrow*). This fluoroscopic image also shows kyphoplasty being performed at L2. **D**, Postprocedural radiograph demonstrates that kyphoplasty was performed at L2–4 (procedure at L4 not shown). In addition to pain relief, increased vertebral body height and correction of accentuated curvature are goals of the procedure.

response of metastases to therapy, and bone-specific response criteria can be used to guide assessment. The treatment of bone metastases is a multidisciplinary endeavor that includes imaging and the expertise of the medical oncologist, radiation oncologist, and orthopedic surgeon to properly assess and optimize therapeutic options. Practitioners from all involved specialties benefit from an understanding of the roles of the others to optimize the care of cancer patients.

KEY POINTS Summary

- Computed tomography (CT), skeletal scintigraphy (SS)/bone scan, magnetic resonance imaging (MRI), and positron emission tomography PET/CT can complement each other in detecting bone metastases.
- Response criteria provide guidelines for interpreting changes in the appearance of bone metastases after therapy.
- Widespread metastases are best treated with systemic therapy. Limited or individual metastases are addressed by external beam radiation, surgery, or percutaneous interventions.
- Treatment of bone metastases is complex and requires a knowledge of bone imaging in conjunction with a multidisciplinary approach.

REFERENCES

1. Abrams HL, Spiro R, Goldstein N. Metastases in carcinoma; analysis of 1000 autopsied cases. *Cancer.* 1950;3(1):74–85.
2. Coleman RE. Clinical features of metastatic bone disease and risk of skeletal morbidity. *Clin Cancer Res.* 2006;12(20 Pt 2):6243s–6249s.
3. Hamaoka T, Madewell JE, Podoloff DA, et al. Bone imaging in metastatic breast cancer. *J Clin Oncol.* 2004;22(14):2942–2953.
4. Hamaoka T, Costelloe CM, Madewell JE, et al. Tumour response interpretation with new tumour response criteria vs the World Health Organisation criteria in patients with bone-only metastatic breast cancer. *Br J Cancer.* 2010;102(4):651–657.
5. Langer C, Hirsh V. Skeletal morbidity in lung cancer patients with bone metastases: demonstrating the need for early diagnosis and treatment with bisphosphonates. *Lung Cancer.* 2010;67(1):4–11.
6. Schindlbeck C, Andergassen U, Jueckstock J, et al. Disseminated and circulating tumor cells in bone marrow and blood of breast cancer patients: properties, enrichment, and potential targets. *J Cancer Res Clin Oncol.* 2016;142(9):1883–1895.
7. Clain A. Secondary malignant disease of bone. *Br J Cancer.* 1965;19:15–29.
8. Roodman GD. Mechanisms of bone metastasis. *N Engl J Med.* 2004;350(16):1655–1664.
9. Dorfman HD, Czerniak B. *Bone Tumors.* St. Louis: Mosby; 1998:1–33.
10. Madewell JE, Ragsdale BD, Sweet DE. Radiologic and pathologic analysis of solitary bone lesions. *Part I: internal margins. Radiol Clin North Am.* 1981;19(4):715–748.
11. Hortobagyi GN, Libshitz HI, Seabold JE. Osseous metastases of breast cancer. *Clinical, biochemical, radiographic, and scintigraphic evaluation of response to therapy. Cancer.* 1984;53(3):577–582.
12. Ardran GM. Bone destruction not demonstrable by radiography. *Br J Radiol.* 1951;24(278):107–109.
13. Edelstyn GA, Gillespie PJ, Grebbell FS. The radiological demonstration of osseous metastases. *Experimental observations. Clin Radiol.* 1967;18(2):158–162.
14. Costelloe CM, Rohren EM, Madewell JE, et al. Imaging bone metastases in breast cancer: techniques and recommendations for diagnosis. *Lancet Oncol.* 2009;10(6):606–614.
15. Tehranzadeh J, Mnaymneh W, Ghavam C, et al. Comparison of CT and MR imaging in musculoskeletal neoplasms. *J Comput Assist Tomogr.* 1989;13(3):466–472.
16. Zimmer WD, Berquist TH, McLeod RA, et al. Bone tumors: magnetic resonance imaging versus computed tomography. *Radiology.* 1985;155(3):709–718.
17. Costelloe CM, Chuang HH, Chasen BA, et al. Bone windows for distinguishing malignant from benign primary bone tumors on FDG PET/CT. *J Cancer.* 2013;4(7):524–530.
18. Arano Y. Recent advances in 99mTc radiopharmaceuticals. *Ann Nucl Med.* 2002;16(2):79–93.
19. Roodman GD. Pathogenesis of myeloma bone disease. *Blood Cells Mol Dis.* 2004;32(2):290–292.
20. Daffner RH, Lupetin AR, Dash N, et al. MRI in the detection of malignant infiltration of bone marrow. *AJR Am J Roentgenol.* 1986;146(2):353–358.
21. Roodman GD. Skeletal imaging and management of bone disease. *Hematology Am Soc Hematol Educ Program.* 2008:313–319.
22. Corcoran RJ, Thrall JH, Kyle RW, et al. Solitary abnormalities in bone scans of patients with extraosseous malignancies. *Radiology.* 1976;121(3 Pt. 1):663–667.
23. Chao HS, Chang CP, Chiu CH, et al. Bone scan flare phenomenon in non-small-cell lung cancer patients treated with gefitinib. *Clin Nucl Med.* 2009;34(6):346–349.
24. Schneider JA, Divgi CR, Scott AM, et al. Flare on bone scintigraphy following Taxol chemotherapy for metastatic breast cancer. *J Nucl Med.* 1994;35(11):1748–1752.
25. Sedonja I, Budihna NV. The benefit of SPECT when added to planar scintigraphy in patients with bone metastases in the spine. *Clin Nucl Med.* 1999;24(6):407–413.
26. Han LJ, Au-Yong TK, Tong WC, et al. Comparison of bone single-photon emission tomography and planar imaging in the detection of vertebral metastases in patients with back pain. *Eur J Nucl Med.* 1998;25(6):635–638.
27. Romer W, Nomayr A, Uder M, et al. SPECT-guided CT for evaluating foci of increased bone metabolism classified as indeterminate on SPECT in cancer patients. *J Nucl Med.* 2006;47(7):1102–1106.
28. Even-Sapir E, Metser U, Mishani E, et al. The detection of bone metastases in patients with high-risk prostate cancer: 99mTc-MDP Planar bone scintigraphy, single- and multi-field-of-view SPECT, 18F-fluoride PET, and 18F-fluoride PET/CT. *J Nucl Med.* 2006;47(2):287–297.
29. Ohta M, Tokuda Y, Suzuki Y, et al. Whole body PET for the evaluation of bony metastases in patients with breast cancer: comparison with 99Tcm-MDP bone scintigraphy. *Nucl Med Commun.* 2001;22(8):875–879.
30. Kato H, Miyazaki T, Nakajima M, et al. Comparison between whole-body positron emission tomography and bone scintigraphy in evaluating bony metastases of esophageal carcinomas. *Anticancer Res.* 2005;25(6C):4439–4444.
31. Shie P, Cardarelli R, Brandon D, et al. Meta-analysis: comparison of F-18 Fluorodeoxyglucose-positron emission tomography and bone scintigraphy in the detection of bone metastases in patients with breast cancer. *Clin Nucl Med.* 2008;33(2):97–101.
32. Schirrmeister H, Guhlmann A, Elsner K, et al. Sensitivity in detecting osseous lesions depends on anatomic localization: planar bone scintigraphy versus 18F PET. *J Nucl Med.* 1999;40(10):1623–1629.
33. Yang SN, Liang JA, Lin FJ, et al. Comparing whole body (18) F-2-deoxyglucose positron emission tomography and technetium-99m methylene diphosphonate bone scan to detect bone metastases in patients with breast cancer. *J Cancer Res Clin Oncol.* 2002;128(6):325–328.
34. Uematsu T, Yuen S, Yukisawa S, et al. Comparison of FDG PET and SPECT for detection of bone metastases in breast cancer. *AJR Am J Roentgenol.* 2005;184(4):1266–1273.
35. Abe K, Sasaki M, Kuwabara Y, et al. Comparison of 18FDG-PET with 99mTc-HMDP scintigraphy for the detection of bone metastases in patients with breast cancer. *Ann Nucl Med.* 2005;19(7):573–579.
36. Du Y, Cullum I, Illidge TM, et al. Fusion of metabolic function and morphology: sequential [18F]fluorodeoxyglucose positron-emission tomography/computed tomography studies yield new insights into the natural history of bone metastases in breast cancer. *J Clin Oncol.* 2007;25(23):3440–3447.
37. Costelloe CM, Chuang HH, Madewell JE FDG. PET for the detection of bone metastases: sensitivity, specificity and comparison with other imaging modalities. *PET Clin.* 2010;5(3):281–295.
38. Tang H, Ahlawat S, Fayad LM, Multiparametric MR. imaging of benign and malignant bone lesions. *Magn Reson Imaging Clin N Am.* 2018;26(4):559–569.
39. Messiou C, Hillengass J, Delorme S, et al. Guidelines for acquisition, interpretation, and reporting of whole-body MRI in myeloma:

myeloma response assessment and diagnosis system (MY-RADS). *Radiology*. 2019;291(1):5–13.
40. Costelloe CM, Kumar R, Yasko AW, et al. Imaging characteristics of locally recurrent tumors of bone. *AJR Am J Roentgenol*. 2007;188(3):855–863.
41. Khodarahmi I, Isaac A, Fishman EK, et al. Metal about the hip and artifact reduction techniques: from basic concepts to advanced imaging. *Semin Musculoskelet Radiol*. 2019;23(3):e68–e81.
42. Avrahami E, Tadmor R, Dally O, et al. Early MR demonstration of spinal metastases in patients with normal radiographs and CT and radionuclide bone scans. *J Comput Assist Tomogr*. 1989;13(4):598–602.
43. Aisen AM, Martel W, Braunstein EM, et al. MRI and CT evaluation of primary bone and soft-tissue tumors. *AJR Am J Roentgenol*. 1986;146(4):749–756.
44. Sarpel S, Sarpel G, Yu E, et al. Early diagnosis of spinal-epidural metastasis by magnetic resonance imaging. *Cancer*. 1987;59(6):1112–1116.
45. Godersky JC, Smoker WR, Knutzon R. Use of magnetic resonance imaging in the evaluation of metastatic spinal disease. *Neurosurgery*. 1987;21(5):676–680.
46. Robson MD, Gatehouse PD, Bydder M, et al. Magnetic resonance: an introduction to ultrashort TE (UTE) imaging. *J Comput Assist Tomogr*. 2003;27(6):825–846.
47. Ma J, Costelloe CM, Madewell JE, et al. Fast dixon-based multisequence and multiplanar MRI for whole-body detection of cancer metastases. *J Magn Reson Imaging*. 2009;29(5):1154–1162.
48. Eustace S, Tello R, DeCarvalho V, et al. A comparison of whole-body turboSTIR MR imaging and planar 99mTc-methylene diphosphonate scintigraphy in the examination of patients with suspected skeletal metastases. *AJR Am J Roentgenol*. 1997;169(6):1655–1661.
49. Horvath LJ, Burtness BA, McCarthy S, et al. Total-body echo-planar MR imaging in the staging of breast cancer: comparison with conventional methods--early experience. *Radiology*. 1999;211(1):119–128.
50. Steinborn MM, Heuck AF, Tiling R, et al. Whole-body bone marrow MRI in patients with metastatic disease to the skeletal system. *J Comput Assist Tomogr*. 1999;23(1):123–129.
51. Engelhard K, Hollenbach HP, Wohlfart K, et al. Comparison of whole-body MRI with automatic moving table technique and bone scintigraphy for screening for bone metastases in patients with breast cancer. *Eur Radiol*. 2004;14(1):99–105.
52. Lauenstein TC, Goehde SC, Herborn CU, et al. Whole-body MR imaging: evaluation of patients for metastases. *Radiology*. 2004;233(1):139–148.
53. Costelloe CM, Kundra V, Ma J, et al. Fast Dixon whole-body MRI for detecting distant cancer metastasis: a preliminary clinical study. *J Magn Reson Imaging*. 2012;35(2):399–408.
54. Balliu E, Boada M, Pelaez I, et al. Comparative study of whole-body MRI and bone scintigraphy for the detection of bone metastases. *Clin Radiol*. 2010;65(12):989–996.
55. Kalus S, Saifuddin A, Whole-body MRI. vs bone scintigraphy in the staging of Ewing sarcoma of bone: a 12-year single-institution review. *Eur Radiol*. 2019;29(10):5700–5708.
56. Kim JR, Yoon HM, Jung AY, et al. Comparison of whole-body MRI, bone scan, and radiographic skeletal survey for lesion detection and risk stratification of Langerhans Cell Histiocytosis. *Sci Rep*. 2019;9(1):317.
57. Lauenstein TC, Freudenberg LS, Goehde SC, et al. Whole-body MRI using a rolling table platform for the detection of bone metastases. *Eur Radiol*. 2002;12(8):2091–2099.
58. Antoch G, Vogt FM, Freudenberg LS, et al. Whole-body dual-modality PET/CT and whole-body MRI for tumor staging in oncology. *JAMA*. 2003;290(24):3199–3206.
59. Larkman DJ, Nunes RG. Parallel magnetic resonance imaging. *Phys Med Biol*. 2007;52(7):R15–R55.
60. Schmidt GP, Schoenberg SO, Schmid R, et al. Screening for bone metastases: whole-body MRI using a 32-channel system versus dual-modality PET-CT. *Eur Radiol*. 2007;17(4):939–949.
61. Schlemmer HP, Schafer J, Pfannenberg C, et al. Fast whole-body assessment of metastatic disease using a novel magnetic resonance imaging system: initial experiences. *Invest Radiol*. 2005;40(2):64–71.
62. Walker R, Kessar P, Blanchard R, et al. Turbo STIR magnetic resonance imaging as a whole-body screening tool for metastases in patients with breast carcinoma: preliminary clinical experience. *J Magn Reson Imaging*. 2000;11(4):343–350.
63. Ohno Y, Koyama H, Nogami M, et al. Whole-body MR imaging vs. FDG-PET: comparison of accuracy of M-stage diagnosis for lung cancer patients. *J Magn Reson Imaging*. 2007;26(3):498–509.
64. van Vucht N, Santiago R, Lottmann B, et al. The Dixon technique for MRI of the bone marrow. *Skeletal Radiol*. 2019;48(12):1861–1874.
65. Hahn S, Lee YH, Suh JS. Detection of vertebral metastases: a comparison between the modified Dixon turbo spin echo T2 weighted MRI and conventional T1 weighted MRI: a preliminary study in a tertiary centre. *Br J Radiol*. 2018;91(1085):20170782.
66. Costelloe CM, Madewell JE, Kundra V, et al. Conspicuity of bone metastases on fast Dixon-based multisequence whole-body MRI: clinical utility per sequence. *Magn Reson Imaging*. 2013;31(5):669–675.
67. Samarin A, Hullner M, Queiroz MA, et al. 18F-FDG-PET/MR increases diagnostic confidence in detection of bone metastases compared with 18F-FDG-PET/CT. *Nucl Med Commun*. 2015;36(12):1165–1173.
68. Beiderwellen K, Huebner M, Heusch P, et al. Whole-body [(1)(8)F]FDG PET/MRI vs. PET/CT in the assessment of bone lesions in oncological patients: initial results. *Eur Radiol*. 2014;24(8):2023–2030.
69. Eisenhauer EA, Therasse P, Bogaerts J, et al. New response evaluation criteria in solid tumours: revised RECIST guideline (version 1.1). *Eur J Cancer*. 2009;45(2):228–247.
70. Hayashi N, Costelloe CM, Hamaoka T, et al. A prospective study of bone tumor response assessment in metastatic breast cancer. *Clin Breast Cancer*. 2013;13(1):24–30.
71. Tsai YC, Lee HL, Kuo CC, et al. Prognostic and predictive factors for clinical and radiographic responses in patients with painful bone metastasis treated with magnetic resonance-guided focused ultrasound surgery. *Int J Hyperthermia*. 2019;36(1):932–937.
72. Yu T, Choi CW, Kim KS. Treatment outcomes of stereotactic ablative radiation therapy for non-spinal bone metastases: focus on response assessment and treatment indication. *Br J Radiol*. 2019;92(1099):20181048.
73. Hortobagyi GN, Theriault RL, Porter L, et al. Efficacy of pamidronate in reducing skeletal complications in patients with breast cancer and lytic bone metastases. Protocol 19 Aredia Breast Cancer Study Group. *N Engl J Med*. 1996;335(24):1785–1791.
74. Hortobagyi GN, Theriault RL, Lipton A, et al. Long-term prevention of skeletal complications of metastatic breast cancer with pamidronate. Protocol 19 Aredia Breast Cancer Study Group. *J Clin Oncol*. 1998;16(6):2038–2044.
75. Theriault RL, Lipton A, Hortobagyi GN, et al. Pamidronate reduces skeletal morbidity in women with advanced breast cancer and lytic bone lesions: a randomized, placebo-controlled trial. Protocol 18 Aredia Breast Cancer Study Group. *J Clin Oncol*. 1999;17(3):846–854.
76. Green JR, Muller K, Jaeggi KA. Preclinical pharmacology of CGP 42'446, a new, potent, heterocyclic bisphosphonate compound. *J Bone Miner Res*. 1994;9(5):745–751.
77. Maxwell C, Swift R, Goode M, et al. Advances in supportive care of patients with cancer and bone metastases: nursing implications of zoledronic acid. *Clin J Oncol Nurs*. 2003;7(4):403–408.
78. Rosen LS, Gordon D, Kaminski M, et al. Zoledronic acid versus pamidronate in the treatment of skeletal metastases in patients with breast cancer or osteolytic lesions of multiple myeloma: a phase III, double-blind, comparative trial. *Cancer J*. 2001;7(5):377–387.
79. Rosen LS, Gordon D, Kaminski M, et al. Long-term efficacy and safety of zoledronic acid compared with pamidronate disodium in the treatment of skeletal complications in patients with advanced multiple myeloma or breast carcinoma: a randomized, double-blind, multicenter, comparative trial. *Cancer*. 2003;98(8):1735–1744.
80. Marx RE. Pamidronate (Aredia) and zoledronate (Zometa) induced avascular necrosis of the jaws: a growing epidemic. *J Oral Maxillofac Surg*. 2003;61(9):1115–1117.
81. Aguiar Bujanda D, Bohn Sarmiento U, Cabrera Suarez MA, et al. Assessment of renal toxicity and osteonecrosis of the jaws in patients receiving zoledronic acid for bone metastasis. *Ann Oncol*. 2007;18(3):556–560.
82. Bamias A, Kastritis E, Bamia C, et al. Osteonecrosis of the jaw in cancer after treatment with bisphosphonates: incidence and risk factors. *J Clin Oncol*. 2005;23(34):8580–8587.
83. Dimopoulos MA, Kastritis E, Anagnostopoulos A, et al. Osteonecrosis of the jaw in patients with multiple myeloma treated with bisphosphonates: evidence of increased risk after treatment with zoledronic acid. *Haematologica*. 2006;91(7):968–971.
84. Durie BG, Katz M, Crowley J. Osteonecrosis of the jaw and bisphosphonates. *N Engl J Med*. 2005;353(1):99–102. discussion 99-.
85. Ibrahim T, Barbanti F, Giorgio-Marrano G, et al. Osteonecrosis of the jaw in patients with bone metastases treated with bisphosphonates: a retrospective study. *Oncologist*. 2008;13(3):330–336.

86. Maerevoet M, Martin C, Duck L. Osteonecrosis of the jaw and bisphosphonates. *N Engl J Med*. 2005;353(1):99–102. discussion 99-.
87. Wang EP, Kaban LB, Strewler GJ, et al. Incidence of osteonecrosis of the jaw in patients with multiple myeloma and breast or prostate cancer on intravenous bisphosphonate therapy. *J Oral Maxillofac Surg*. 2007;65(7):1328–1331.
88. Zervas K, Verrou E, Teleioudis Z, et al. Incidence, risk factors and management of osteonecrosis of the jaw in patients with multiple myeloma: a single-centre experience in 303 patients. *Br J Haematol*. 2006;134(6):620–623.
89. Dimopoulos MA, Kastritis E, Bamia C, et al. Reduction of osteonecrosis of the jaw (ONJ) after implementation of preventive measures in patients with multiple myeloma treated with zoledronic acid. *Ann Oncol*. 2009;20(1):117–120.
90. Ripamonti CI, Maniezzo M, Campa T, et al. Decreased occurrence of osteonecrosis of the jaw after implementation of dental preventive measures in solid tumour patients with bone metastases treated with bisphosphonates. The experience of the National Cancer Institute of Milan. *Ann Oncol*. 2009;20(1):137–145.
91. Fizazi K, Carducci M, Smith M, et al. Denosumab versus zoledronic acid for treatment of bone metastases in men with castration-resistant prostate cancer: a randomised, double-blind study. *Lancet*. 2011;377(9768):813–822.
92. Stopeck AT, Lipton A, Body JJ, et al. Denosumab compared with zoledronic acid for the treatment of bone metastases in patients with advanced breast cancer: a randomized, double-blind study. *J Clin Oncol*. 2010;28(35):5132–5139.
93. Zunk K, Mummenhoff K, Koch M, et al. Phylogenetic relationships of Thlaspi s.l. (subtribe Thlaspidinae, Lepidieae) and allied genera based on chloroplast DNA restriction-site variation. *Theor Appl Genet*. 1996;92(3-4):375–381.
94. Lipton A, Fizazi K, Stopeck AT, et al. Superiority of denosumab to zoledronic acid for prevention of skeletal-related events: a combined analysis of 3 pivotal, randomised, phase 3 trials. *Eur J Cancer*. 2012;48(16):3082–3092.
95. Zheng GZ, Chang B, Lin FX, et al. Meta-analysis comparing denosumab and zoledronic acid for treatment of bone metastases in patients with advanced solid tumours. *Eur J Cancer Care (Engl)*. 2017;26(6).
96. Hartsell WF, Scott CB, Bruner DW, et al. Randomized trial of short-versus long-course radiotherapy for palliation of painful bone metastases. *J Natl Cancer Inst*. 2005;97(11):798–804.
97. McQuay HJ, Collins SL, Carroll D, et al. Radiotherapy for the palliation of painful bone metastases. *Cochrane Database Syst Rev*. 2000;2:CD001793.
98. Lutz S, Balboni T, Jones J, et al. Palliative radiation therapy for bone metastases: Update of an ASTRO Evidence-Based Guideline. *Pract Radiat Oncol*. 2017;7(1):4–12.
99. Spencer KL, van der Velden JM, Wong E, et al. Systematic review of the role of stereotactic radiotherapy for bone metastases. *J Natl Cancer Inst*. 2019;111(10):1023–1032.
100. Palma DA, Olson R, Harrow S, et al. Stereotactic ablative radiotherapy for the comprehensive treatment of 4-10 oligometastatic tumors (SABR-COMET-10): study protocol for a randomized phase III trial. *BMC Cancer*. 2019;19(1):816.
101. Patchell RA, Tibbs PA, Regine WF, et al. Direct decompressive surgical resection in the treatment of spinal cord compression caused by metastatic cancer: a randomised trial. *Lancet*. 2005;366(9486):643–648.
102. Turner JH, Claringbold PG. A phase II study of treatment of painful multifocal skeletal metastases with single and repeated dose samarium-153 ethylenediaminetetramethylene phosphonate. *Eur J Cancer*. 1991;27(9):1084–1086.
103. Robinson RG, Blake GM, Preston DF, et al. Strontium-89: treatment results and kinetics in patients with painful metastatic prostate and breast cancer in bone. *Radiographics*. 1989;9(2):271–281.
104. Pons F, Herranz R, Garcia A, et al. Strontium-89 for palliation of pain from bone metastases in patients with prostate and breast cancer. *Eur J Nucl Med*. 1997;24(10):1210–1214.
105. Alberts AS, Smit BJ, Louw WK, et al. Dose response relationship and multiple dose efficacy and toxicity of samarium-153-EDTMP in metastatic cancer to bone. *Radiother Oncol*. 1997;43(2):175–179.
106. Lam MG, de Klerk JM, van Rijk PP, et al. Bone seeking radiopharmaceuticals for palliation of pain in cancer patients with osseous metastases. *Anticancer Agents Med Chem*. 2007;7(4):381–397.
107. Bruland OS, Nilsson S, Fisher DR, et al. High-linear energy transfer irradiation targeted to skeletal metastases by the alpha-emitter 223Ra: adjuvant or alternative to conventional modalities? *Clin Cancer Res*. 2006;12(20 Pt 2):6250s–6257s.
108. Hoskin P, Sartor O, O'Sullivan JM, et al. Efficacy and safety of radium-223 dichloride in patients with castration-resistant prostate cancer and symptomatic bone metastases, with or without previous docetaxel use: a prespecified subgroup analysis from the randomised, double-blind, phase 3 ALSYMPCA trial. *Lancet Oncol*. 2014;15(12):1397–1406.
109. Aboulafia AJ, Levine AM, Schmidt D, et al. Surgical therapy of bone metastases. *Semin Oncol*. 2007;34(3):206–214.
110. Parrish FF, Murray JA. Surgical treatment for secondary neoplastic fractures. A retrospective study of ninety-six patients. *J Bone Joint Surg Am*. 1970;52(4):665–686.
111. Beals RK, Lawton GD, Snell WE. Prophylactic internal fixation of the femur in metastatic breast cancer. *Cancer*. 1971;28(5):1350–1354.
112. Fidler M. Prophylactic internal fixation of secondary neoplastic deposits in long bones. *Br Med J*. 1973;1(5849):341–343.
113. Mirels H. Metastatic disease in long bones. A proposed scoring system for diagnosing impending pathologic fractures. *Clin Orthop Relat Res*. 1989;249:256–264.
114. Nazarian A, Entezari V, Zurakowski D, et al. Treatment planning and fracture prediction in patients with skeletal metastasis with CT-based rigidity analysis. *Clin Cancer Res*. 2015;21(11):2514–2519.
115. Umer M, Mohib Y, Atif M, et al. Skeletal metastasis in renal cell carcinoma: A review. *Ann Med Surg (Lond)*. 2018;27:9–16.
116. Lee B, Franklin I, Lewis JS, et al. The efficacy of percutaneous vertebroplasty for vertebral metastases associated with solid malignancies. *Eur J Cancer*. 2009;45(9):1597–1602.
117. Mendel E, Bourekas E, Gerszten P, et al. Percutaneous techniques in the treatment of spine tumors: what are the diagnostic and therapeutic indications and outcomes? *Spine (Phila Pa 1976)*. 2009;34(22 Suppl):S93–100.
118. Voggenreiter G. Balloon kyphoplasty is effective in deformity correction of osteoporotic vertebral compression fractures. *Spine (Phila Pa 1976)*. 2005;30(24):2806–2812.
119. Dupuy DE, Liu D, Hartfeil D, et al. Percutaneous radiofrequency ablation of painful osseous metastases: a multicenter American College of Radiology Imaging Network trial. *Cancer*. 2010;116(4):989–997.
120. Goetz MP, Callstrom MR, Charboneau JW, et al. Percutaneous image-guided radiofrequency ablation of painful metastases involving bone: a multicenter study. *J Clin Oncol*. 2004;22(2):300–306.
121. Prologo JD, Passalacqua M, Patel I, et al. Image-guided cryoablation for the treatment of painful musculoskeletal metastatic disease: a single-center experience. *Skeletal Radiol*. 2014;43(11):1551–1559.
122. McArthur TA, Narducci CA, Lander PH, et al. Percutane image-guided cryoablation of painful osseous metastases: a retrospective single-center review. *Curr Probl Diagn Radiol*. 2017;46(4):282–287.

CHAPTER

35 Cancer of Unknown Primary

Ajaykumar C. Morani, M.D.; Abdelrahman K. Hanafy, M.D.; Aurelio Matamoros Jr., M.D.; Gauri R. Varadhachary, M.D.; and Priya R. Bhosale, M.D.

INTRODUCTION

Cancer of unknown primary (CUP) is a designation given to discordant group of metastatic carcinomas for which the primary site of origin cannot be identified, despite a thorough diagnostic workup that includes a thorough medical history, complete physical examination to include breast, pelvic, and rectal evaluations, complete blood count and biochemical analysis, urinalysis, serum prostate-specific antigen (PSA) in males, and histopathologic review of tissue specimens with immunohistochemistry. Computed tomography (CT) of the chest, abdomen, and pelvis; chest radiography; and mammography in females are performed as indicated. Despite this workup, the treating physician will more than likely still be in a quandary as to the primary site that produced the aggressive metastatic disease. Needless to say, this scenario creates stress not only to the physician but also to the patient in trying to cope with the unknown. Unproven theories regarding the localization of the primary CUP site include: (1) the primary tumor has involuted, and only the metastatic disease is evident, and (2) metastatic disease is favored over the primary growth based on the phenotype and genotype of the tumor.[1]

EPIDEMIOLOGY AND RISK FACTORS

Worldwide, CUP is one of the 10 most frequent cancers, constituting approximately 3% to 5% of all cancer cases.[2,3] In 2018, according to the American Cancer Society, there were an estimated 31,810 cases of "other & unspecified primary cancer sites" in the United States, accounting for 2% of all cancer cases and an estimated 44,560 deaths.[2,4,5] At presentation, the median age of the patient is approximately 60 years, and it is slightly more frequent in males. No risk factors have been identified for this heterogeneous group of neoplasms, and no screening programs have yet been described to detect these neoplasms.

PATHOLOGIC CLASSIFICATION AND ASSESSMENT

Because only carcinomas are included in the diagnosis of CUP, four main histologic types of CUP have been described: well to moderately differentiated adenocarcinomas (50%), undifferentiated or poorly differentiated carcinomas (30%), squamous cell carcinomas (15%), and undifferentiated neoplasms (5%). The latter group includes lymphomas, sarcomas, germ cell tumors, poorly differentiated carcinomas, neuroendocrine tumors, and embryonal malignancies that can be characterized by immunohistochemistry.[6] In children, CUPs represent less than 1% of solid tumors, and the majority of these tumors are embryonal malignancies.[2,5]

Pathologic assessment is a must to characterize the CUP and is usually accomplished by histologic and cytopathologic evaluation. As an adjunct, electron microscopy is occasionally used to evaluate those CUPs that demonstrate indeterminate features which cannot be resolved or characterized with routine pathologic evaluation. Serum tumor markers, which are mainly overexpressed glycoproteins that are released into the bloodstream by malignant tumors, can help to identify, diagnose, classify, follow-up, and aid in the assessment of response to therapy in some cases. However, these serum tumor markers have low sensitivity and specificity, as they are not expressed specifically by one organ or in one particular tumor. The number of serum tumor markers to be assessed is determined on a case-by-case basis; these markers include but are not limited to carcinoembryonic antigen (CEA), CA125, CA19-9, CDX2, CA15-3, CK-7, CK-20, thyroid transcription factor-1, PSA, alpha-fetoprotein, beta–human chorionic gonadotropin, estrogen receptors, and gross cystic disease fluid protein-15 (GCDFP-15). Some of the tumor markers can even be elevated in benign diseases, such as CEA in inflammatory bowel disease and CA19-9 in pancreatitis.

ROLE OF MOLECULAR PROFILING TO DETERMINE THE TISSUE OF ORIGIN

Molecular profiling of CUP offers a technique to determine the tissue of origin (ToO), with a possible impact on therapy. Several studies demonstrated the feasibility of using gene expression profiling with DNA microarray to classify uncertain tumors based on their ToO by identifying gene subsets whose expression pertains to a specific cancer class. These studies achieved an accuracy of 78% to 98% in identifying tumor ToO.[7–13]

Two main strategies have been used to identify the ToO: DNA microarray platforms and quantitative reverse transcription real-time polymerase chain reaction (qRT-PCR). For both of these strategies, messenger RNA is extracted from fresh frozen or formalin-fixed paraffin-embedded tumor tissue. The multigene expression pattern of a CUP cancer is compared with known primary cancers, and a ToO assigned based on the molecular signature it most

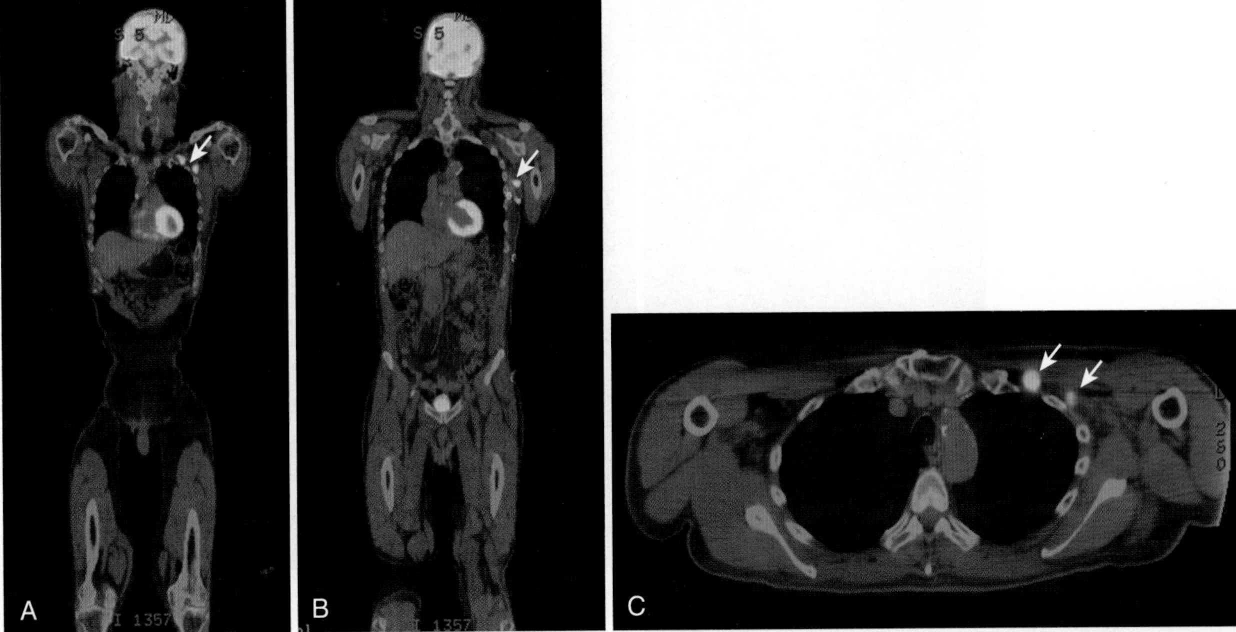

FIGURE 35.1. A 64-year-old man presented with a "lump" in the left axilla. Left axillary lymph node biopsy showed squamous cell carcinoma. Thorough workup failed to reveal site of origin. **A**, Coronal positron emission tomography/computed tomography (PET/CT) scan shows increased activity in the left subpectoral nodes (*arrow*). **B**, Coronal PET/CT scan shows increased activity in the left axillary nodes (*arrow*). **C**, Axial PET/CT scan shows increased activity in the left subpectoral nodes (*arrows*).

closely resembles. Some of the molecular assays have been commercialized and are available from several vendors.

In a large study using qRT-PCR to determine the ToO in CUP, 98% of successful assays performed for 252 patients were able to predict the ToO.[13] The most common sites predicted, in descending order, were biliary tract (11%), urothelium, and colorectal. However, the clinical utility of these assays still needs further assessment, as results-based treatment still did not change survival significantly. This testing will become even more important as specific targeted therapies emerge for known cancers, which can then be applied to CUP subsets.[14]

KEY POINTS Pathology

- Four main histologic types of cancer of unknown primary (CUP) have been described: well to moderately differentiated adenocarcinomas, poorly differentiated carcinomas, squamous cell carcinomas, and undifferentiated neoplasms.
- Metastatic disease from CUPs can appear anywhere in the body.

NATURAL HISTORY, CLINICAL PRESENTATION AND PROGNOSIS

Patients with known primary malignancy have a neoplasm with natural history and a predictable metastatic pattern that allows for staging. The opposite is true for CUPs. Given that CUPs are very aggressive and have an unpredictable metastatic pattern, no formal staging can be done in most patients. To complicate the clinical scenario, more than 50% of CUP patients present with multiple sites of metastatic disease, and approximately 30% have metastatic disease involving three or more organs. In comparison, less than 15% of patients with known primary tumors have metastatic diseas e in three or more sites.[15–17]

The clinical presentation is as a result of the symptoms created by rapid spread of metastases, rather than the primary tumor, like visual or palpable masses and constitutional symptoms. Overall, these patients face a grim prognosis. Survival rates of 6 to 10 months are reported for the patients enrolled in clinical studies.[2] On the other hand, CUP patients not enrolled in clinical trials have reported life expectancies of 2 to 3 months.[15]

Given the diverse clinical presentation of these patients, it is best to classify them into favorable and unfavorable subsets, with the former having a better prognosis.[3,18]

The favorable subsets include:

1. Squamous cell carcinoma involving cervical lymph nodes (Fig. 35.1).
2. Women with adenocarcinoma involving only axillary lymph nodes.
3. Women with peritoneal cavity papillary serous adenocarcinoma.
4. Men with elevated serum PSA and blastic osseous metastases (Fig. 35.2).
5. Poorly differentiated carcinoma with midline distribution (extragonadal germ cell tumor syndrome).
6. Isolated inguinal adenopathy with squamous cell carcinoma (Fig. 35.3).
7. Poorly differentiated neuroendocrine carcinomas.
8. Patient with a single, small, potentially resectable metastasis.

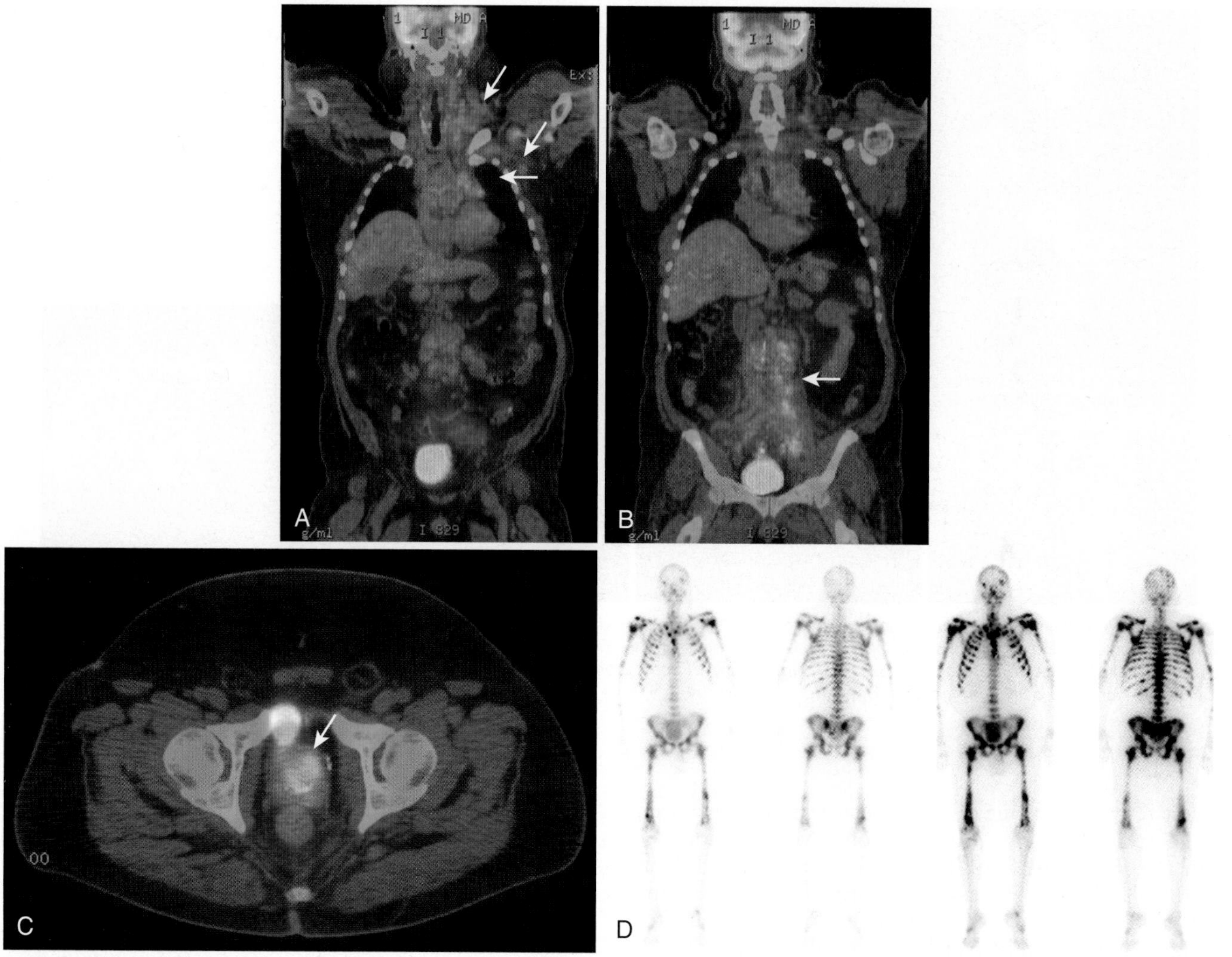

Figure 35.2. A 54-year-old man presented with a "lump" in the left lower neck. Outside initial biopsy shows poorly differentiated adenocarcinoma. Further immunohistochemistry shows prostate origin. **A**, Coronal positron emission tomography/computed tomography (PET/CT) shows increased activity in the left lower neck (*top arrow*) and left axillary (*middle arrow*), as well as left subpectoral (*bottom arrow*) adenopathy. **B**, Coronal PET/CT scan shows increased activity in the retroperitoneum and pelvis (*arrow*). **C**, Axial PET/CT scan shows increased activity in the prostate gland (*arrow*). **D**, Bone scan shows diffuse metastatic disease.

The unfavorable subsets are:

1. Adenocarcinoma primarily metastatic to the liver.
2. Adenocarcinoma with multiple metastases to the lungs (Fig. 35.4).
3. Adenocarcinoma with mainly diffuse osseous metastatic disease.
4. Multiple cerebral metastases.
5. Malignant ascites with nonpapillary adenocarcinoma histology.

Key Points Clinical Presentation and Prognosis

- Cancer of unknown primary (CUPs) are very aggressive neoplasms with an unpredictable metastatic pattern.
- Clinical presentation is owing to symptoms from the metastatic disease rather than the primary tumor.
- Prognosis is grim.
- There are favorable and unfavorable subsets of CUP.

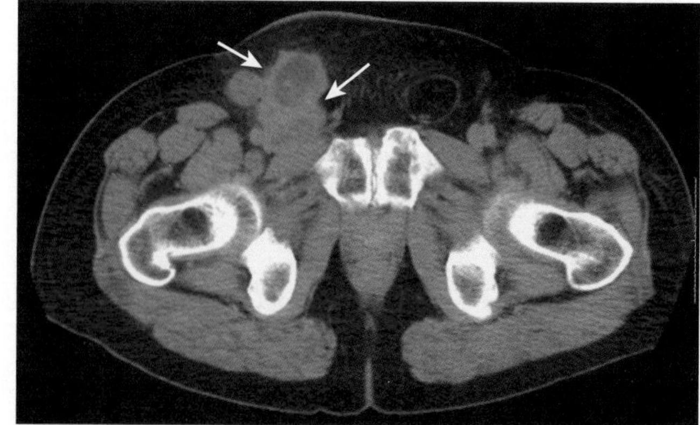

Figure 35.3. A 65-year-old man presented with a right groin mass at an outside institution. Biopsy was consistent with squamous cell carcinoma. Thorough workup failed to reveal primary site of origin. Contrast-enhanced pelvic computed tomography scan shows a large, partially necrotic inguinal nodal mass (*arrows*).

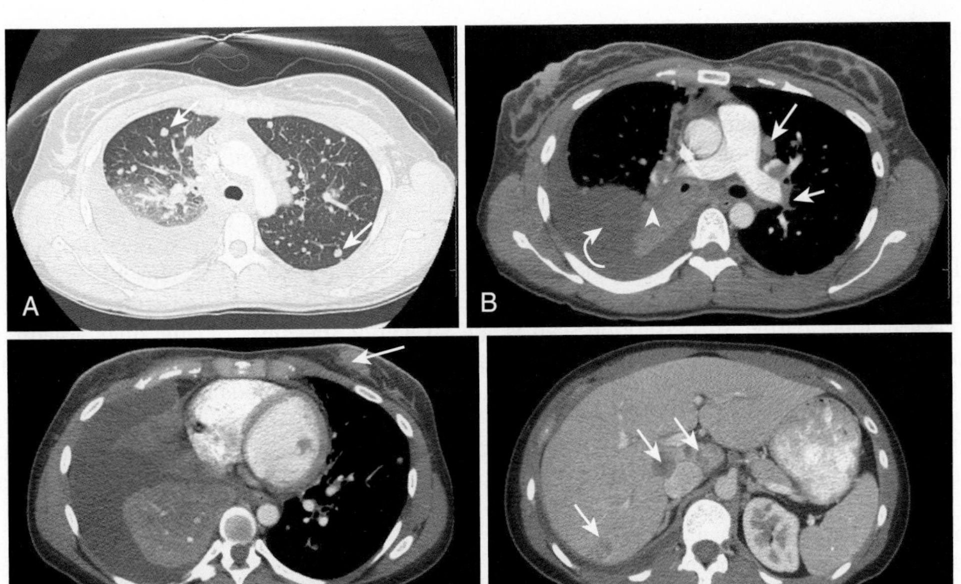

FIGURE 35.4. A 33-year-old woman presented with cough that did not resolve with conventional therapy. Computed tomography (CT) study of the chest was done to evaluate the lungs. Lung and left breast biopsies were consistent with poorly differentiated adenocarcinoma not specific for lung or breast primary. **A**, Contrast-enhanced chest CT scan shows pulmonary metastases (*arrows*) and a right pleural effusion. **B**, Contrast-enhanced chest CT scan shows mediastinal (*long straight arrow*) and hilar (*short straight arrow*) adenopathy, right pleural effusion (*curved arrow*), and collapse of the right lower lobe (*arrowhead*). **C**, Contrast-enhanced chest CT scan shows a small mass (*arrow*) in the inner lower quadrant of the left breast. **D**, Contrast-enhanced abdominal CT scan shows multiple liver metastases (*arrows*).

PATTERNS OF TUMOR SPREAD

The most common sites for CUP metastatic disease are the liver, lungs, bones, and lymph nodes. However, in contrast to tumors of known origin, CUPs typically present with unpredictable patterns of spread. For example, when pancreatic and hepatic carcinomas present as CUPs, there is a higher incidence of lung and osseous metastatic disease compared with a known primary originating in the pancreas and liver. Brain and osseous metastatic disease from a CUP originating in the gastrointestinal tract is more commonly seen than that from a known gastrointestinal primary carcinoma. Hepatic and pulmonary metastatic disease is seen more frequently in cases that present as a CUP from a prostatic carcinoma than from a known prostatic carcinoma. On the other hand, approximately 50% of lung cancers exhibit osseous metastatic disease, whereas CUPs of pulmonary origin have a lower incidence of osseous metastatic disease.[19–22]

KEY POINT Patterns of Tumor Spread

- At presentation, metastatic disease is the prevailing pattern, mainly by lymphatic or hematogenous route/spread.

STAGING EVALUATION

To stage a malignancy, the tumor needs to be identified for the tumor-node-metastasis (TNM) system. Although postmortem tumor identification yield has been reported to be higher with primary site found in approximately 51% to 79% of cases,[20,22,23] primary tumors in CUPs are identified in only approximately 11% to 20% of the patients after a thorough clinical workup in real-life scenarios so far.[24,25] Overall, CUPs do not allow for the typical staging of tumors, given their diverse clinical presentation, different subtypes, different histologies, and metastatic patterns. For optimal patient management, the best approach is to identify the subset in which that CUP patient best fits. A distinct entity according to the new 2017 cancer staging manual of The American Joint Committee on Cancer is unknown primary squamous cell cancer (UPSCC) of the head and neck.[26] Because most (90%) patients with UPSCCs that tested positive for human papilloma virus (HPV) were found to harbor the primary in the oropharynx, a newly found HPV-positive UPSCC of the head and neck is staged as an oropharyngeal cancer.[27–29] Similarly, a UPSCC that tests positive for Epstein–Bar virus (EBV) is assigned and staged as a primary nasopharyngeal cancer.

IMAGING

Plain radiographic imaging of the chest is almost always a part of the routine evaluation of CUPs, because the lungs are frequently involved with these tumors. Otherwise, the histologic diagnosis will dictate the extent of imaging that needs to be performed to hopefully identify the site of the CUP and, at the same time, limit the discomfort and distress to the patient and the overall expense. Usually CTs of the chest, abdomen, and pelvis are obtained as a baseline. A mammogram is ordered based on the clinical evaluation.

Bone scintigraphy and brain imaging by either CT or magnetic resonance imaging (MRI) is performed based on symptomatology. MRIs of body parts or cavities may yield further information regarding the site of the CUP. Positron emission tomography (PET) and PET/CT are now more frequently used to help identify not only the location of the CUP but also other metastatic sites not identified by CT or MRI. Endoscopy with or without imaging, and neck CT or MRI are done as clinically indicated, such as in those patients with a diagnosis of squamous cell carcinoma and metastatic cervical adenopathy. An octreotide scan is appropriate for patients with neuroendocrine malignancy.

The use of ultrasound is mainly for evaluation of lymph nodes and to provide biopsy guidance for the lymph nodes or suspicious soft tissues, including the superficial or moderately deep structures such as liver, testicular, breast, and renal lesions.

An example of tailored imaging in a favorable subset would be that of a female with axillary adenopathy but with a nondiagnostic mammographic study. This patient would benefit from an MRI evaluation of the breasts, in which there is a reported higher detection rate of 70% to 86%.[30–32] A testicular sonogram may help to identify a neoplasm in a male patient with midline adenopathy.

PET and PET/CT are being more frequently used to identify not only the tumor but also any unrecognized metastatic disease. These usually use the radiotracer 2-[^{18}F] fluoro-2-deoxy-D-glucose (FDG) and provide functional results; with PET/CT also providing concurrent anatomic information from its CT component compared with FDG-PET study alone. In a study reported by Kolesnikov-Gauthier and coworkers,[33] the primary tumor site was identified in six of 24 patients with CUP, and all known metastatic sites were visualized with FDG-PET/CT. Based on FDG-PET, the clinical management of metastatic cervical lymph adenopathy was altered in 25% of patients, as reported by Johansen et al.[34]

Seve and colleagues[35] performed a metaanalysis of 10 studies (published from 1998–2006) involving a combined total of 221 CUP patients. Although this metaanalysis included studies with different patient populations, study designs, and diagnostic workups, approximately 94% of these patients had a single metastatic site. Each study evaluated the role of FDG-PET in identifying the unknown primary cancer site. FDG-PET detected the primary tumor sites in 41% of these patients. Previously unrecognized metastases were detected in 37% of the patients. Of the detected tumors, 59% were in the lungs. A false-positive rate of 58% was noted in tumors of the lower digestive tract, likely because of the inherent bowel activity. Clinical management was changed in approximately 35% of these patients. Specific chemotherapy was given to those patients (53%) with lung and pancreatic cancers and to those patients (12%) with breast, ovarian, and prostate cancers, and 14% of these patients underwent potential curative surgery. In an another systematic review and metaanalysis of 11 published studies with a cohort of 433 patients with CUP, Kwee and Kwee[36] reported a primary tumor detection rate of 37% and a pooled sensitivity and specificity of 84% and 84%, respectively by FDG-PET/CT. Across the studies, the sensitivity was heterogeneous, and the specificity was homogeneous. FDG-PET/CT can also play an important role in radiation therapy planning and for monitoring response or lack of response to therapy.[37]

A recent study evaluating the diagnostic value of FDG-PET/CT versus MRI with diffusion-weighted images (DWI) on 31 patients with UPSCC of the head and neck reported a slightly higher sensitivity with for detecting the primary tumor with PET/CT (93%) compared with MRI-DWI (81%).[38] Another study comparing the diagnostic potential of PET/CT versus PET/MRI found a comparable results between the two modalities.[39]

Overall, because of the dual advantage of providing anatomic as well as metabolic information, FDG-PET/CT may be the modality of choice for evaluation of CUP patients at present; it also may be less expensive than the thorough diagnostic imaging studies that are currently used. In addition, with new radiopharmaceuticals, better results could be obtained.

Key Points Staging and Imaging Evaluation

- There is no set staging or tumor-node-metastasis system available, because the primary tumor is occult.
- Unknown primary squamous cell cancer (UPSCC) of the head and neck that tests positive for human papilloma virus is staged as a primary oropharyngeal cancer.
- UPSCC of the head and neck that tests positive for Epstein–Barr virus is staged as a primary nasopharyngeal cancer.
- Computed tomography (CT) of the chest, abdomen, and pelvis is mainly used to identify the primary tumor. Mammogram, breast magnetic resonance imaging (MRI), or bone scan is ordered as indicated. CT or MRI brain is used if the patient is symptomatic.
- PET/CT may become the main modality of choice for evaluation of a patient with cancer of unknown primary, and all or some other forms of imaging may not be needed.

Key Points The Radiology Report

- Locations of the metastatic disease should be identified.
- More isolated lesions should be identified and used as index lesions.
- Describe all soft tissue and osseous sites of disease, including any lymphadenopathy.
- Suggest possible primary tumor etiology, if possible, based on the radiographic pattern of metastatic disease.
- Suggest alternative imaging modalities that may help in evaluating the possible primary tumor or in managing potential complications such as spinal cord involvement.

General Considerations for Management

The median survival of patients with disseminated CUP is approximately 6 to 10 months. Patients with favorable prognosis do slightly better because they have a cancer biology that is either more indolent or more responsive to therapies. Prognostic factors include a patient's performance status, locations and number of metastases, response to chemotherapy, and serum lactate dehydrogenase (LDH) level.[13] Culine and coworkers[17] developed and retrospectively validated a prognostic model that uses performance status and serum LDH, allowing patients to be assigned to one of two subgroups with divergent outcomes. This model was also validated in a study performed on young adults diagnosed with CUP, who were also found to show the same distribution of the predicted primary sites and prognosis as the old model.[40] CUP can be divided into two subsets based on prognosis: a prognostically favorable subset, which includes 20% of cases, and a prognostically unfavorable subset, which includes 80% of cases.[3,41] Management of some of the favorable subsets and of disseminated or unfavorable CUP is discussed later.

Prognostically Favorable Subsets of Cancer of Unknown Primary

These subgroups are important to note, because appropriate therapies can significantly affect survival in these cases.

1. Isolated axillary adenopathy with adenocarcinoma or carcinoma in women. Women with isolated axillary adenopathy and adenocarcinoma or carcinoma are often treated for stage II or III breast cancer and are candidates for breast MRI if their mammography and sonography results are negative (as discussed previously). In addition, breast markers on immunohistochemistry including mammoglobin, GCDFP-15, estrogen and progesterone receptors, and HER2 neu are warranted to determine the appropriate treatment. If the clinical and imaging presentation suggests breast cancer, then neoadjuvant or adjuvant chemotherapy, axillary lymph node dissection, and radiation therapy (and hormonal therapy if appropriate) is the standard therapy.
2. Peritoneal carcinomatosis suggestive of primary peritoneal carcinoma in women. The term "primary peritoneal papillary serous carcinoma" (PPSC) refers to CUP with carcinomatosis and the pathologic and laboratory (elevated CA125 antigen) characteristics of a Müllerian cancer without an obvious ovarian primary identified on transvaginal sonography or laparotomy. Patients with PPSC are candidates for cytoreductive surgery followed by adjuvant taxane- and platinum-based chemotherapy. Median progression-free and overall survival of 7 and 15 months or longer, respectively (median follow-up 60 months) is reported in these cases.
3. Cervical adenopathy with squamous cell carcinoma. Patients with cervical adenopathy with squamous cell carcinoma should undergo triple endoscopy with biopsies of inconspicuous sites, bilateral tonsillectomy, and CT or PET/CT of the neck and chest to search for the primary and determine the stage of the tumor. Patients with early-stage disease are candidates for node dissection and radiation therapy, which can result in long-term survival. The utility of chemotherapy in these patients is unknown, although chemoradiation therapy or induction chemotherapy is often used and beneficial in bulky N2 and N3 disease.
4. Low-grade neuroendocrine carcinoma. It is important to differentiate between low-grade and high-grade neuroendocrine CUP. High-grade neuroendocrine cancers have a high mitotic index (Ki-67), necrosis, and hemorrhage on pathologic evaluation. Patients with low-grade neuroendocrine carcinoma may present with an indolent disease course; thus, treatment decisions are based on symptoms and tumor bulk. Current therapies include treatment with somatostatin analogs alone for hormone-related symptoms and locoregional therapies, including bland embolization, chemoembolization, or SIR-Spheres microspheres. Systemic therapy, including anti–vascular endothelial growth factor therapies and mammalian target of rapamycin inhibitors, has shown promise in these tumors and is indicated in patients with symptomatic or progressive disease.
5. Solitary metastases. Patients with solitary metastatic disease most often present with nodal, liver, bone, or brain metastasis. Some of these are candidates for aggressive management, which can result in prolonged disease-free survival and even a cure. Immunohistochemical studies, pattern of spread, age, gender, and risk factors help determine the best therapy for these patients. In selected patients, neoadjuvant chemotherapy is used to treat micrometastatic disease and downstage the cancer to maximize the potential for a margin-negative resection, which may also be done to study its biology. We do not advocate that all patients with solitary metastatic CUP follow this approach, and this is not intended to define the standard of care in this setting.

Prognostically Unfavorable Subsets of Cancer of Unknown Primary

The majority of CUP patients belong to this subset (80%). Often, these patients have bulky liver metastases, non-PPSC peritoneal carcinomatosis, and bone or adrenal metastases. Non-PPSC peritoneal carcinomatosis has a large differential diagnosis, including gastric, appendiceal, colonic, and pancreatic cancer and cholangiocarcinoma. Imaging, endoscopy, and pathologic evaluation including immunohistochemistry can help suggest the best therapy options. For example, in patients with carcinomatosis and an immunohistochemical profile favoring colon cancer (CK7-negative/CK 20-positive and CDX-2-positive), using a colon cancer regimen is a reasonable treatment approach, although data comparing response rates and survival using this approach to conventional CUP regimens are lacking.

TREATMENT HIGHLIGHTS

Traditionally, cisplatin-based combination chemotherapy regimens have been used to treat CUP patients. In a phase II study by Greco and colleagues,[42] 55 CUP patients (51 of whom were chemotherapy-naïve) were treated with paclitaxel, carboplatin, and oral etoposide every 3 weeks. The overall response rate was 47%, and the median overall survival was 13.4 months. Briasoulis and associates[43] reported similar results in 77 CUP patients treated with paclitaxel and carboplatin (without etoposide). Patients with nodal or pleural disease and peritoneal carcinomatosis had a higher response rate (than did patients with visceral disseminated disease) and an overall survival of 13 and 15 months, respectively. More recent studies have incorporated newer agents, such as gemcitabine, irinotecan, and targeted agents. In a phase II randomized trial by Culine and coworkers,[44] 80 patients were randomly assigned to receive gemcitabine plus cisplatin or irinotecan plus cisplatin. Seventy-eight patients were assessable for effectiveness and toxicity. Objective responses were observed in 21 patients (55%) in the gemcitabine and cisplatin arm and 15 patients (38%) in the irinotecan and cisplatin arm. The median survival was 8 months in the gemcitabine and cisplatin arm, compared with 6 months in irinotecan and cisplatin arm (median follow-up of 22 months).

KEY POINTS Treatment

- The vast majority of these patients are managed by the medical oncologist with radiation therapy as needed. To define the burden, location, and biology of disease, a surgeon may be needed for a biopsy, cytoreduction, and sometimes metastasectomy.
- The mainstay for cancer of unknown primary therapy is combination chemotherapy with multiple drugs.
- Response is relatively better when targeted chemotherapy regimens to a suspected tumor type can be administered.
- Evaluation for recurrence is mainly achieved through clinical examination and appropriate imaging studies.

SURVEILLANCE

A standard follow-up routine for these patients is usually based on the type of therapy used, whether chemotherapy, surgery, or a combination. Usually, patients receiving chemotherapy are reevaluated every 2 to 3 months; however, this varies based on the type of chemotherapy and number of cycles. It is also common that CUP patients are seen emergently owing to complications of therapy.

CONCLUSION

An algorithm based on immunohistochemistry, clinical presentation, and imaging facilitates selection of treatment in patients with CUP. Incorporation of molecular profiling tools to help identify the ToO appears promising and is currently being evaluated. In the current era, treatment has shifted from empiricism to individualization of therapies for each patient with a CUP.

REFERENCES

1. Lenzi R, et al. Phase II study of cisplatin, 5-fluorouracil and folinic acid in patients with carcinoma of unknown primary origin. *Euro J Cancer*. 1993;29(11):1634.
2. Pavlidis N, Fizazi K. Carcinoma of unknown primary (CUP). *Crit Rev Oncol Hematol*. 2009;69(3):271–278.
3. Pavlidis N, Pentheroudakis G. Cancer of unknown primary site. *Lancet*. 2012;379(9824):1428–1435.
4. Siegel RL, Miller KD, Jemal A. Cancer statistics, 2018. *CA Cancer J Clin*. 2018;68(1):7–30.
5. Siegel R, et al. Cancer statistics, 2011: the impact of eliminating socioeconomic and racial disparities on premature cancer deaths. *CA Cancer J Clin*. 2011;61(4):212–236.
6. Greco FA. Cancer of unknown primary site. In: *DeVita, Hellman, and Rosenberg's Cancer: Principles and Practice of Oncology*. 8th ed, Philadelphia: JB Lippincott; 2008:2363–2386.
7. Tothill RW. An expression-based site of origin diagnostic method designed for clinical application to cancer of unknown origin. *Cancer Res*. 2005;65(10):4031–4040.
8. Ma XJ, et al. Molecular classification of human cancers using a 92-gene real-time quantitative polymerase chain reaction assay. *Arch Pathol Lab Med*. 2006;130(4):465–473.
9. Monzon FA, Koen TJ. Diagnosis of metastatic neoplasms: molecular approaches for identification of tissue of origin. *Arch Pathol Lab Med*. 2010;134(2):216–224.
10. Varadhachary GR, et al. Molecular profiling of carcinoma of unknown primary and correlation with clinical evaluation. *J Clin Oncol*. 2008;26(27):4442–4448.
11. Horlings HM, et al. Gene expression profiling to identify the histogenetic origin of metastatic adenocarcinomas of unknown primary. *J Clin Oncol*. 2008;26(27):4435–4441.
12. Pentheroudakis G, Greco FA, Pavlidis N. Molecular assignment of tissue of origin in cancer of unknown primary may not predict response to therapy or outcome: a systematic literature review. *Cancer Treat Rev*. 2009;35(3):221–227.
13. Hainsworth JD, et al. Molecular gene expression profiling to predict the tissue of origin and direct site-specific therapy in patients with carcinoma of unknown primary site: a prospective trial of the Sarah Cannon research institute. *J Clin Oncol*. 2013;31(2):217–223.
14. Varadhachary GR, Raber MN. Cancer of unknown primary site. *N Engl J Med*. 2014;371(8):757–765.
15. van de Wouw AJ, et al. Epidemiology of unknown primary tumours; incidence and population-based survival of 1285 patients in Southeast Netherlands, 1984-1992. *Eur J Cancer*. 2002;38(3):409–413.
16. Hess KR, et al. Classification and regression tree analysis of 1000 consecutive patients with unknown primary carcinoma. *Clin Cancer Res*. 1999;5(11):3403–3410.
17. Culine S, et al. Development and validation of a prognostic model to predict the length of survival in patients with carcinomas of an unknown primary site. *J Clin Oncol*. 2002;20(24):4679–4683.
18. Abbruzzese JL, et al. Unknown primary carcinoma: natural history and prognostic factors in 657 consecutive patients. *J Clin Oncol*. 1994;12(6):1272–1280.
19. Blaszyk H, Hartmann A, Bjornsson J. Cancer of unknown primary: clinicopathologic correlations. *Apmis*. 2003;111(12):1089–1094.
20. Mayordomo JI, et al. Neoplasms of unknown primary site: a clinicopathological study of autopsied patients. *Tumori*. 1993;79(5):321–324.
21. Jordan 3rd WE, Shildt RA. Adenocarcinoma of unknown primary site. The Brooke Army Medical Center experience. *Cancer*. 1985;55(4):857–860.
22. Le Chevalier T, et al. Early metastatic cancer of unknown primary origin at presentation. A clinical study of 302 consecutive autopsied patients. *Arch Intern Med*. 1988;148(9):2035–2039.
23. Al-Brahim N, et al. The value of postmortem examination in cases of metastasis of unknown origin-20-year retrospective data from a tertiary care center. *Ann Diagn Pathol*. 2005;9(2):77–80.
24. Kirsten F, et al. Metastatic adeno or undifferentiated carcinoma from an unknown primary site--natural history and guidelines for identification of treatable subsets. *Q J Med*. 1987;62(238):143–161.
25. Nystrom JS, et al. Metastatic and histologic presentations in unknown primary cancer. *Semin Oncol*. 1977;4(1):53–58.
26. Amin MB, Edge S, Greene F, et al. AJCC Cancer Staging Manual. 2017.
27. Piazza C, Incandela F, Giannini L. Unknown primary of the head and neck: a new entry in the TNM staging system with old dilemmas for everyday practice. *Curr Opin Otolaryngol Head Neck Surg*. 2019;27(2):73–79.
28. Keller LM, et al. p16 status, pathologic and clinical characteristics, biomolecular signature, and long-term outcomes in head and neck squamous cell carcinomas of unknown primary. *Head Neck*. 2014;36(12):1677–1684.
29. Motz K, et al. Changes in unknown primary squamous cell carcinoma of the head and neck at initial presentation in the era of human papillomavirus. *JAMA Otolaryngol Head Neck Surg*. 2016;142(3):223–228.
30. Orel SG, et al. Breast MR imaging in patients with axillary node metastases and unknown primary malignancy. *Radiology*. 1999;212(2):543–549.
31. Olson Jr JA, et al. Magnetic resonance imaging facilitates breast conservation for occult breast cancer. *Ann Surg Oncol*. 2000;7(6):411–415.
32. Obdeijn IM, et al. MR imaging-guided sonography followed by fine-needle aspiration cytology in occult carcinoma of the breast. *AJR Am J Roentgenol*. 2000;174(4):1079–1084.

33. Gauthier H, et al. FDG PET in patients with cancer of an unknown primary. *Nuclear medicine communications*. 2006;26:1059–1066.
34. Johansen J, et al. Prospective study of 18FDG-PET in the detection and management of patients with lymph node metastases to the neck from an unknown primary tumor. Results from the DAHANCA-13 study. *Head Neck*. 2008;30(4):471–478.
35. Seve P, et al. The role of 2-deoxy-2-[F-18]fluoro-D-glucose positron emission tomography in disseminated carcinoma of unknown primary site. *Cancer*. 2007;109(2):292–299.
36. Kwee TC, Kwee RM. Combined FDG-PET/CT for the detection of unknown primary tumors: systematic review and meta-analysis. *Eur Radiol*. 2009;19(3):731–744.
37. Podoloff DA. PET/CT and occult primary tumors. *J Natl Compr Canc Netw*. 2009;7(3):239–244.
38. Noij DP, et al. Diagnostic value of diffusion-weighted imaging and (18)F-FDG-PET/CT for the detection of unknown primary head and neck cancer in patients presenting with cervical metastasis. *Eur J Radiol*. 2018;107:20–25.
39. Ruhlmann V, et al. Hybrid imaging for detection of carcinoma of unknown primary: A preliminary comparison trial of whole-body PET/MRI versus PET/CT. *Eur J Radiol*. 2016;85(11):1941–1947.
40. Raghav K, et al. Cancer of unknown primary in adolescents and young adults: clinicopathological features, prognostic factors and survival outcomes. *PLoS One*. 2016;11(5):e0154985.
41. Bochtler T, Loffler H, Kramer A. Diagnosis and management of metastatic neoplasms with unknown primary. *Semin Diagn Pathol*. 2018;35(3):199–206.
42. Greco FA, Hainsworth JD. One-hour paclitaxel, carboplatin, and extended-schedule etoposide in the treatment of carcinoma of unknown primary site. *Semin Oncol*. 1997;24(6 Suppl 19):S19-101–S19-105.
43. Briasoulis E, et al. Carboplatin plus paclitaxel in unknown primary carcinoma: a phase II Hellenic Cooperative Oncology Group Study. *J Clin Oncol*. 2000;18(17):3101–3107.
44. Culine S, et al. Cisplatin in combination with either gemcitabine or irinotecan in carcinomas of unknown primary site: results of a randomized phase II study--trial for the French Study Group on Carcinomas of Unknown Primary (GEFCAPI 01). *J Clin Oncol*. 2003;21(18):3479–3482.

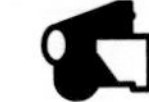

Visit ExpertConsult.com for additional algorithms.

CANCER OF UNKNOWN PRIMARY

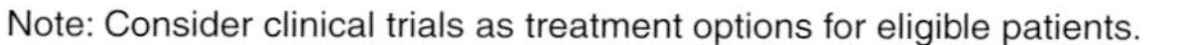

Note: Consider clinical trials as treatment options for eligible patients.

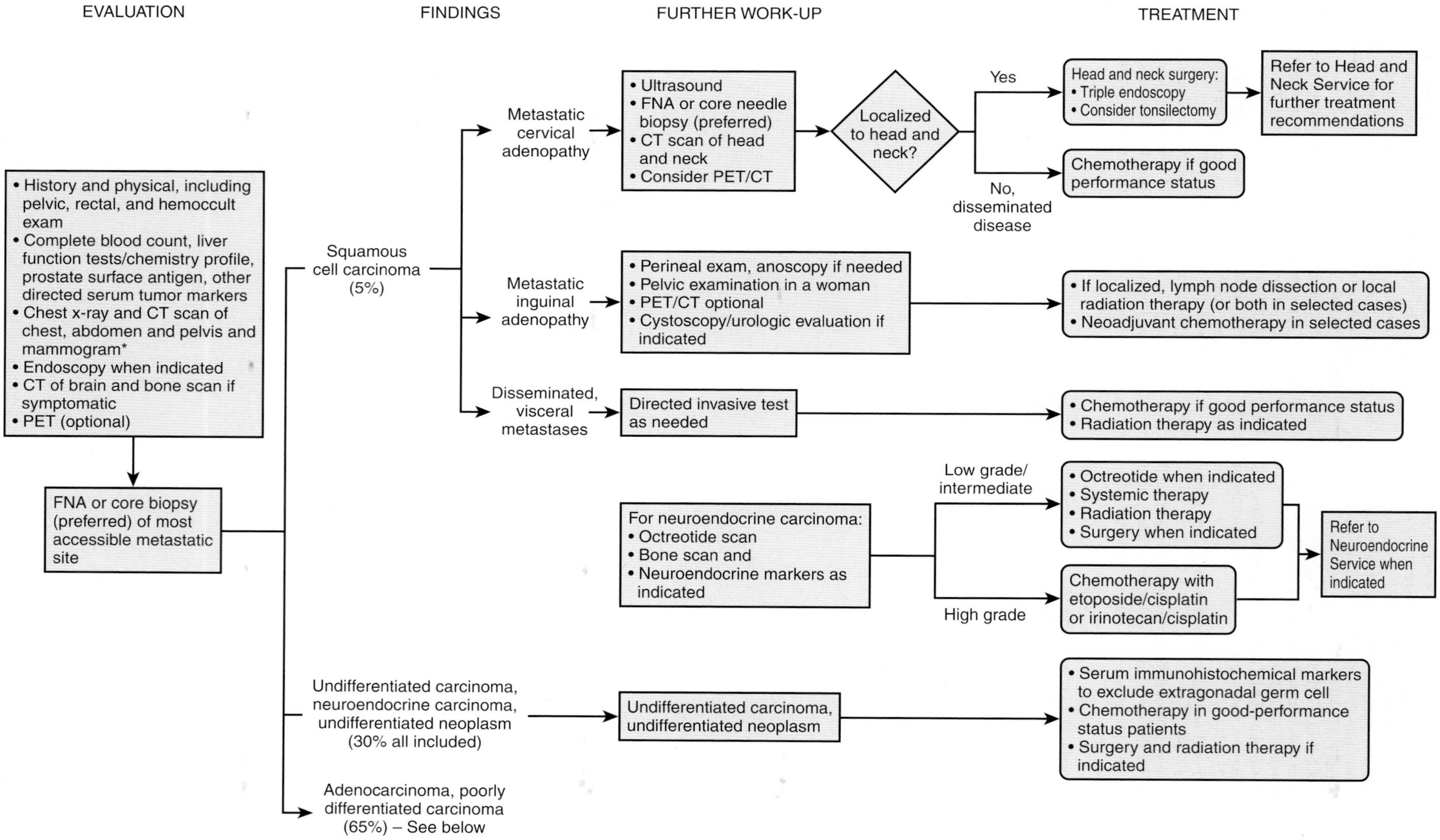

EVALUATION

- History and physical, including pelvic, rectal, and hemoccult exam
- Complete blood count, liver function tests/chemistry profile, prostate surface antigen, other directed serum tumor markers
- Chest x-ray and CT scan of chest, abdomen and pelvis and mammogram*
- Endoscopy when indicated
- CT of brain and bone scan if symptomatic
- PET (optional)

→ FNA or core biopsy (preferred) of most accessible metastatic site

FINDINGS → FURTHER WORK-UP → TREATMENT

Squamous cell carcinoma (5%)

- Metastatic cervical adenopathy → Further work-up:
  - Ultrasound
  - FNA or core needle biopsy (preferred)
  - CT scan of head and neck
  - Consider PET/CT

  → Localized to head and neck?
  - Yes → Head and neck surgery:
    - Triple endoscopy
    - Consider tonsilectomy

    → Refer to Head and Neck Service for further treatment recommendations
  - No, disseminated disease → Chemotherapy if good performance status
- Metastatic inguinal adenopathy → Further work-up:
  - Perineal exam, anoscopy if needed
  - Pelvic examination in a woman
  - PET/CT optional
  - Cystoscopy/urologic evaluation if indicated

  → Treatment:
  - If localized, lymph node dissection or local radiation therapy (or both in selected cases)
  - Neoadjuvant chemotherapy in selected cases
- Disseminated, visceral metastases → Directed invasive test as needed → Treatment:
  - Chemotherapy if good performance status
  - Radiation therapy as indicated

Undifferentiated carcinoma, neuroendocrine carcinoma, undifferentiated neoplasm (30% all included)

- For neuroendocrine carcinoma:
  - Octreotide scan
  - Bone scan and
  - Neuroendocrine markers as indicated

  - Low grade/intermediate →
    - Octreotide when indicated
    - Systemic therapy
    - Radiation therapy
    - Surgery when indicated
  - High grade → Chemotherapy with etoposide/cisplatin or irinotecan/cisplatin

  → Refer to Neuroendocrine Service when indicated
- Undifferentiated carcinoma, undifferentiated neoplasm → Treatment:
  - Serum immunohistochemical markers to exclude extragonadal germ cell
  - Chemotherapy in good-performance status patients
  - Surgery and radiation therapy if indicated

Adenocarcinoma, poorly differentiated carcinoma (65%) – See below

*In women only

This practice algorithm has been specifically developed for M.D. Anderson using a multidisciplinary approach and taking into consideration circumstances particular to M.D. Anderson, including the following: M.D. Anderson's specific patient population; M.D. Anderson's services and structure; and M.D. Anderson's clinical information. Moreover, this algorithm is not intended to replace the independent medical or professional judgment of physicians or other health care providers. This algorithm should not be used to treat pregnant women.

CANCER OF UNKNOWN PRIMARY

Note: Consider clinical trials as treatment options for eligible patients.

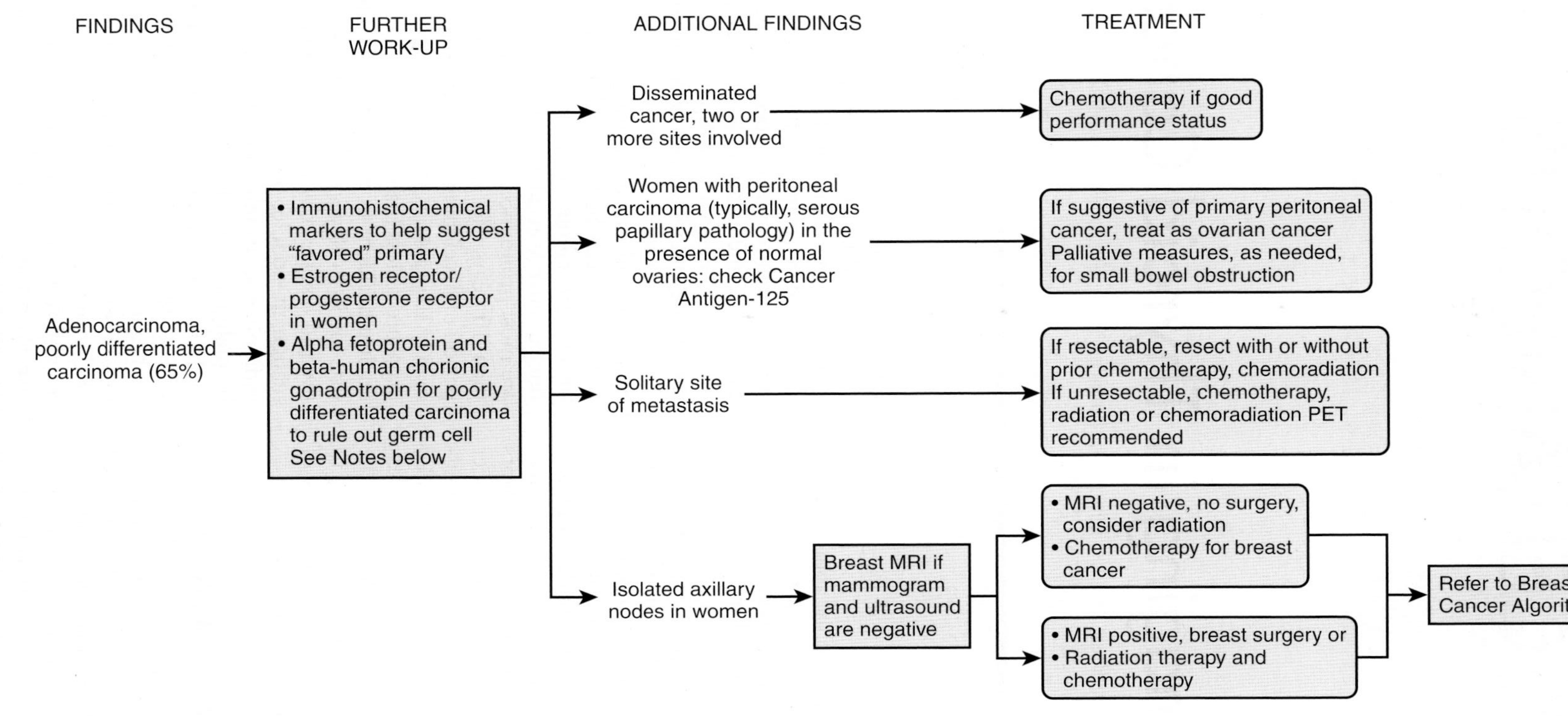

NOTES:
- Gene expression profiling to identify the putative primary cancer profile (tissue of origin) is an emerging diagnostic test; currently experimental and studies are ongoing.
- Appropriate mutation analysis studies where indicated (e.g., in a lung profile patient, EGFR mutation analysis when appropriate)

This practice algorithm has been specifically developed for M.D. Anderson using a multidisciplinary approach and taking into consideration circumstances particular to M.D. Anderson, including the following: M.D. Anderson's specific patient population; M.D. Anderson's services and structure; and M.D. Anderson's clinical information. Moreover, this algorithm is not intended to replace the independent medical or professional judgment of physicians or other health care providers. This algorithm should not be used to treat pregnant women.

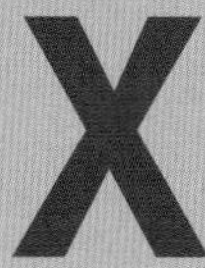

PART X MISCELLANEOUS

36 Imaging in Thyroid Cancer

Jeremy Ross, M.D.; Hemant A. Parmar, M.D.; Anca Avram, M.D.; Mohannad Ibrahim, M.D.; and Suresh K. Mukherji, M.D.

INTRODUCTION

Although thyroid cancer represents only approximately 2% of all malignancies worldwide, it is currently one of the most rapidly increasing malignancies in the Western world.[1] Thyroid nodules can be palpated in 2% to 6% of patients and can be detected on imaging in approximately 50% of the general population.[1, 2] Approximately 5% of these nodules represent cancer.[3, 4] With newly available imaging modalities, more and more asymptomatic and nonpalpable nodules are detected, making it imperative that primary care doctors and radiologists understand how to interpret these diagnostic studies, understand indications for further referral, and manage long-term survivors of thyroid cancer. Most patients who have thyroid cancer have well-differentiated cancers, with an excellent long-term prognosis. Some patients have well-differentiated cancers with a poor prognosis, and some have other less common types of thyroid cancers. The challenge for the clinician is to identify the patients who have cancers, to treat them according to the extent and aggressiveness of their disease, and to limit morbidity and mortality.

EPIDEMIOLOGY AND RISK FACTORS

Over the last few decades, the incidence of thyroid cancer has increased dramatically. It is unclear whether this increased incidence is real or whether it may be attributable to increased detection by newer diagnostic imaging techniques.[6–8] Autopsy studies have shown that up to 11% of adults have incidental cancers at the time of death.[9] The average age of diagnosis of thyroid cancer is 47 years, and the average age of death is 74 years.[7] The most common type is the papillary thyroid cancer (PTC); it accounts for approximately 80% of all thyroid cancers. Follicular thyroid carcinoma (FTC) represents approximately 12% of cancers and, in combination with PTC, composes the category of well-differentiated thyroid carcinomas. Grouped into the less common thyroid cancers are medullary (4%–6%), anaplastic (3%–4%), and others (≤5%), such as lymphoma, sarcoma, squamous cell carcinoma, and metastases to the thyroid.[7]

The most significant environmental risk factor for developing thyroid cancer is prior exposure to ionizing radiation, which can be the result of either medical treatment or nuclear fallout (e.g., atomic bomb/testing survivors, nuclear energy accidents). The effects of ionizing radiation are most pronounced in children, especially those younger than 10 years old at the time of exposure. The latency period of developing cancer from this exposure is approximately 10 years for patients having external beam radiation exposure to less than 5 years for victims of the Chernobyl nuclear accident in the Ukraine.[10] The increased risk persists for 30 to 40 years.[10, 11] Patients presenting with benign thyroid disease may also be at higher risk of harboring a malignant nodule; for example, a cold nodule found on radionuclide scanning in patients with Graves disease may be malignant 15% to 38% of the time, and complex cysts in thyroid disease may harbor a malignancy approximately 17% of the time.[10] Given that, overall, two-thirds of thyroid cancer cases occur in women, there would seem to be a link between reproductive hormones and the development of thyroid cancer. Estrogen has been linked to genomic instability, which may explain how it exerts its mutagenic effects on the thyroid.[12] There are no definite data on the role of dietary iodine and its role in the development of thyroid cancer.[13] Certain genetic syndromes increase the risk for thyroid cancer or are associated with thyroid cancer, especially medullary thyroid cancer (MTC), which has been linked to several specific genetic abnormalities. In some cases, PTC follows a familial pattern. Several rare genetic disorders, including Cowden disease, multiple endocrine neoplasia (MEN), and Gardner syndrome, are also associated with a higher incidence of thyroid cancer.[14]

ANATOMY

The thyroid is a shield-shaped gland that consists of right and left lobes connected by the isthmus in midline, although occasionally, the isthmus can be absent. The thyroid isthmus is anterior to the trachea, usually overlying the first through the third tracheal rings. The thyroid gland typically terminates above the level of the clavicle; however, substernal extension into the superior mediastinum can occur. An accessory lobe, the pyramidal lobe, may be present in 50% to 70% of people and usually arises from the isthmus and extends superiorly.[15] The visceral fascia, part of the middle layer of the deep cervical fascia, attaches the thyroid gland to the larynx and trachea. As a result, the gland or abnormalities related to it will move with the larynx during swallowing. The arterial supply to the gland is derived from two separate paired vessels. The inferior thyroid vessels come directly off of the thyrocervical trunk and supply the inferior part of the gland, as well as both the superior and the inferior parathyroids. The superior thyroid artery arises as the first branch of the external carotid artery and supplies the superior portion of the gland. Rarely, a small artery or pair of arteries may come directly from the aorta or brachiocephalic trunk, named the thyroid ima artery. There are three main paired veins that drain the thyroid. There is some variability in location and presence, but they generally drain into the internal jugular veins and innominate vein. The lymphatics of the thyroid consist of intraglandular and extraglandular components. Extraglandular lymphatics generally follow venous flow; the inferior portions of the lateral lobes drain along the tracheoesophageal groove into the central neck. The superior parts of the lobes drain toward the superior thyroid veins, and the isthmus may drain toward the delphian (prelaryngeal) lymph node or central neck nodes. More unusual, but clearly documented, are lymphatic pathways to the retropharyngeal region, accounting for metastases to the skull base. Based on clinical and anatomic review, the central lymphatics are generally considered the primary drainage pathways for thyroid cancers, with the lateral neck nodes being considered secondary levels of lymphatic spread. These facts are important from an imaging and a treatment perspective.[16] The parathyroid glands are also closely related to the thyroid anatomically. They tend to lie on the undersurface of the thyroid and receive their blood supply from the inferior thyroid artery.

PATHOLOGY

Papillary Thyroid Carcinoma

The most common type is PTC, which accounts for approximately 80% of all thyroid cancers. This cancer has a favorable prognosis: most patients who are treated are either cured of their disease or live for many years after the initial diagnosis. The cancer often retains the ability to concentrate iodine, secrete thyroglobulin, and respond to thyroid-stimulating hormone (TSH) stimulation. There are several variants of PTC. The follicular variant of PTC has a pattern of neoplastic follicles that are small with little colloid. They contain relatively fewer nuclear inclusions and psammoma bodies. The prognosis and biologic behavior are similar to that of PTC. The tall cell variant has neoplastic cells in which the height is twice the width. It is associated with more aggressive biologic characteristics and tends to metastasize earlier in its course. It is common for PTC to demonstrate multifocal disease within the thyroid gland at the time of histologic examination. The incidence has been reported to be as high as 80%.[17] When extrathyroidal extension of tumor is seen, it has prognostic significance.[18] The overlying strap muscles in the neck are the most commonly invaded structures. Cases of tracheal, laryngeal, esophageal, and other soft tissue extensions in the neck are sometimes seen.

Follicular Thyroid Carcinoma

FTC is the second most common type of thyroid cancer. It represents approximately 12% of thyroid cancers. Many authors have suggested that the prognosis is slightly poorer than that for PTC. Both benign and malignant follicular lesions demonstrate follicular cells arranged in microfollicles, rosettes, or spindles, and thus they cannot be differentiated on fine-needle aspiration. Capsular invasion is the only current method of distinguishing between the two entities, and hence, quite often, the diagnosis is made after surgery, unless extracapsular extension is seen on imaging before surgery. In patients who have minimal capsular invasion, the prognosis is excellent, and few patients develop distant metastases or die of disease.[19, 20] Unfortunately, patients with capsular invasion have a worse prognosis. Young patients and women may have a slightly better prognosis than men. Clinically, FTCs tend to present with a solitary thyroid mass. The incidence of multicentric disease within the thyroid is much lower than with PTC.

Hurthle Cell Carcinoma

Hurthle cell carcinoma is a variant of FTC, accounting for approximately 3% of all thyroid cancers.[21] It is composed of large acidophilic or oncocytic cells that do not take up radioiodine as well as classic FTC. Like FTC, the diagnosis can be made only after examination of the entire tumor capsule. The cancers generally have a slightly worse prognosis than other FTCs. They are associated with a higher rate of lymph node and distant metastasis than other FTCs.[21]

Medullary Thyroid Carcinoma

MTC arises from the parafollicular or C cells, which are a part of the amine precursor uptake and decarboxylation cell system. These cells produce calcitonin and are unrelated to the iodine-concentrating and thyroid hormone production activities of the gland. MTC is more closely related to other tumors of the neuroendocrine system, such as the carcinoid tumors and pheochromocytomas. MTC is rare, accounting for 2% to 3% of thyroid cancers.[22] The familial form, which is less common than the sporadic form of MTC, is inherited as an autosomal dominant trait. It can be inherited as a part of three distinct entities. The most common, MEN IIA, is associated with pheochromocytoma and hyperparathyroidism. The second most common, MEN IIB, is associated with pheochromocytoma, mucosal neuromas, and marfanoid body habitus. The least common, familial MTC (FMTC), consists of MTC only. The presence of MTC has been strongly linked to mutation of the *RET* oncogene, which is located on chromosome 10. This mutation has been studied extensively and has had a significant effect on diagnosis, management, and understanding of these tumors.[22] Clinically, patients tend to present with a solitary thyroid nodule. Some patients present with an enlarging neck mass or, rarely, with signs of local invasion, including hoarseness or dysphagia. Some patients can present with paraneoplastic syndromes, such as Cushing or carcinoid syndrome.

Anaplastic Thyroid Carcinoma

Anaplastic thyroid cancer is an aggressive disease, usually proving fatal within several weeks to months of diagnosis. It represents approximately 3% to 5% of thyroid cancers.[18] This cancer tends to affect elderly patients, and the peak incidence is in the seventh decade.[18] Some investigators believe that anaplastic carcinoma may represent a dedifferentiation of well-differentiated cancers.[18] Clinically, patients present with a rapidly growing neck mass, often in the context of a slow-growing mass or goiter for several decades. Patients often present with signs of local invasion such as dysphagia, dyspnea, hoarseness, sore throat, and neck pain.

Lymphoma of the Thyroid Gland

Lymphoma of the thyroid has been reported to make up 2% to 5% of thyroid cancers.[23] It tends to be non-Hodgkin B-cell type, although other types do occur. Patients with Hashimoto disease (chronic lymphocytic thyroiditis) have a 70-fold increased incidence of thyroid lymphoma compared with the general population.[23] It is suspected that chronic autoimmune stimulation is responsible for the development of this cancer.[23] Many lymphomas can be diagnosed cytologically, based on their monoclonality. Differentiating them from anaplastic carcinoma is often challenging, however, and it is not uncommon to require core or open biopsy to make an accurate diagnosis. In the clinical setting, lymphoma also mirrors anaplastic carcinoma in many ways. It tends to present with a rapidly expanding mass in the neck, often fixed to surrounding structures. Patients often have neck pain, hoarseness, dysphagia, and even facial edema. The tumor is often fixed to surrounding structures, including the trachea and larynx, the esophagus, and the skin.

Other Cancers of the Thyroid

Although rare, several other cancers can involve the thyroid, either primarily or through metastasis. Squamous cell carcinoma is a rare primary cancer of the thyroid, either as squamous metaplasia of epithelial cells or metastasis to intrathyroid lymph nodes. Once diagnosed, a thorough workup must be performed to rule out a head and neck primary that has metastasized to the thyroid. Other metastatic cancer to the thyroid are also rare, the common primary tumors include breast, lung, and renal cancers. It is suspected that the significant vascularity of the gland accounts for these metastases. In patients who have a known history of other primary cancers who have a new thyroid mass, the possibility of metastatic disease must be entertained.

GROSS AND MICROSCOPIC FEATURES

On gross pathology, PTCs are poorly encapsulated, firm, and often have calcifications (psammoma bodies) within their substance. The presence of these calcifications is of diagnostic significance, because they are rarely present in other cancers. Larger tumors may contain focal areas of hemorrhage and necrosis. PTC demonstrates papillary fronds, along with follicular components. The nuclei have a characteristic appearance, with a feature described as "Orphan Annie eyes" used to refer to the relatively empty appearance of the nucleoplasm.[16]

FTC has a thick capsule with focal necrosis and cystic changes.[21] The cells are small and monotonous and organized into follicles with sparse amount of colloid. Psammoma bodies are rare compared with PTC.

Anaplastic carcinomas consist of grossly infiltrating tumor with areas of necrosis and hemorrhage. It often has a gray-white color and may be calcified and fibrotic. Tumors generally have high mitotic rates, marked cellular pleomorphism, necrosis, vascular invasion, and tumor emboli.

MTCs are well-encapsulated tumors. Histologically, the tumor demonstrates amyloid depositions in 60% to 80% of cases.[24] The tumor often displays nuclear pleomorphism, necrosis, and multiple mitosis. Calcitonin staining is also helpful, and the level of staining may reflect the level of cellular differentiation. Serum calcitonin levels are useful as a diagnostic and measure of response to therapy. MTC have been reported to secrete multiple polypeptide hormones, adrenocorticotropic hormone, somatostatin, vasoactive intestinal peptide, chromogranin A, neuron-specific enolase, and substance P.[16] Carcinoembryonic antigen is also secreted by many MTCs and has been used as a tumor marker and a receptor for nuclear imaging with octreotide imaging. Recent studies have shown nuclear imaging with gallium-DOTATATE to be superior to octreotide in detecting recurrent MTC because of the high number of somatostatin receptors expressed by MTC cells, which are targeted by the gallium-DOTATATE.[25]

CLINICAL PRESENTATION

Most patients with thyroid cancer commonly self-diagnose after finding a lump in their neck during palpation. Other patients may present with a thyroid nodule detected incidentally on imaging ordered for other medical reasons. Other symptoms that may be seen in thyroid cancer include dysphagia, change in voice, coughing, choking, dyspnea, and pain. There may be a history of exposure to ionizing radiation and a family history of thyroid or parathyroid disease. Physical examination should assess for features of the nodule and for the presence of cervical lymphadenopathy. Suspicious features for cancer include nodules that are hard, fixed, irregular, 4 cm or larger, or with associated lymphadenopathy. A general rule to follow is that any lesion with two or more associated high-risk characteristics may have a malignancy rate greater than 80%.[26]

PATTERNS OF TUMOR SPREAD

Regional metastasis to the neck and mediastinal lymph nodes is the common pattern of spread for PTC, with incidence rates from 40% to more than 75%.[27, 28] The role of regional metastasis on overall prognosis of PTC is still being debated; however, the literature supports the idea that prognosis worsens with increasing lymph node size and number.[29] It is clear, however, that distant metastases do adversely affect prognosis. Approximately 4% of patients demonstrate metastasis to distant sites, most commonly to the lungs, brain, and bones.[30]

Although the rate of regional lymphatic metastasis is low, the presence of lymph nodes positive for follicular carcinoma is a poor prognostic indicator. Distant metastases are more common with FTC than with PTC and tend to spread primarily to bones (presenting with pathologic fracture), lung, liver, and brain (which can be hemorrhagic). The prognosis for patients with distant metastasis is poor.

Patients with anaplastic tumors may demonstrate cervical metastasis. Distant metastasis tends to be to the lungs, although other sites, including bone, brain, and mediastinum, have been demonstrated.[18]

STAGING EVALUATION

In 2017 the American Joint Committee on Cancer published the most recent tumor-node-metastasis (TNM) system for the staging of differentiated, anaplastic (undifferentiated), and medullary thyroid cancer.[18, 31]

IMAGING

Whereas clinical and biochemical assessment remains the cornerstone of the thyroid gland evaluation, imaging is considered an important adjuvant for evaluating its anatomy and functions. Imaging of the thyroid gland can be divided into anatomic and functional evaluations. Anatomic evaluation is primarily done for the assessment of thyroid nodules and thyroid cancer. Ultrasound with fine-needle aspiration is the study of choice for assessment of thyroid nodules, whereas computed tomography (CT) and magnetic resonance imaging (MRI) are reserved for evaluating the locoregional extent of thyroid cancer. Functional imaging of the thyroid gland is primarily performed with radionuclide scanning using ^{99m}Tc pertechnetate or ^{123}I.

Ultrasonography

Ultrasound is the imaging modality of choice to evaluate all palpable and nonpalpable thyroid nodules. It is extremely sensitive for the detection of thyroid nodules missed on physical examination or on other imaging modalities. In addition, ultrasound screening is recommended for all patients at high risk of thyroid malignancy (FMTC, MEN IIB, or significant radiation exposure) and for patients with multinodular goiter.[5]

Along with size determination, ultrasound helps to better characterize thyroid nodules, stratify a nodule's risk of cancer, and guide clinical management. Features of thyroid nodules including echogenicity and internal structure, shape and margin, and the presence of calcifications are important to evaluate and can help identify the presence of cancer. These features help characterize nodules and guide clinical management based on the Thyroid Imaging, Reporting and Data System lexicon and scoring (Fig. 36.12, p. 626)). A nodule's echogenicity should be described using normal thyroid tissue as a reference, with the nodule described as "hypoechoic," "isoechoic," or "hyperechoic." Hypoechoic solid nodules transmit the ultrasound wave with minimal reflection, whereas hyperechoic nodules reflect a greater proportion of the signal. Isoechoic nodules are similar to the normal thyroid tissue. A thyroid cyst is characterized as thin-walled, anechoic without internal structure, and with increased echogenicity posterior to it. Cysts are rare and benign; however, cystic degeneration of solid nodules, benign or malignant, is common. Intralesional calcifications are seen as bright echogenic densities that greatly attenuate the ultrasound beam, a phenomenon known as shadowing.

Sonographic features that increase the possibility of malignancy include hypoechogenicity, microcalcification (Fig. 36.1), irregular margins or shape, extracapsular invasion, and suspicious adjacent lymph nodes.[32] Many thyroid cancers are less echogenic than the surrounding normal thyroid tissue; however, benign nodules can also be hypoechoic on imaging. Hyperechoic lesions are generally nonmalignant and are unlikely to be of clinical significance.[33] Punctate calcifications can be seen and suggest the presence of psammoma bodies in PTCs, whereas peripheral or eggshell-like calcifications are associated with

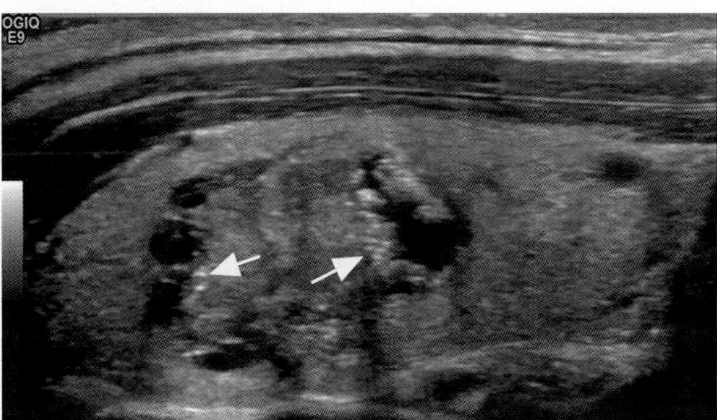

FIGURE 36.1. Papillary thyroid carcinoma in a 45-year-old woman. Thyroid ultrasonography demonstrates a predominantly solid nodule with irregular outlines and several cystic areas and presence of microcalcifications (*arrows*). (Courtesy of Dr. Amit Pandya, Ann Arbor, MI.)

benignity.[34] Coarse, scattered calcifications may be seen in benign or malignant nodules, and large areas of calcification may be seen in MTCs. Nodules with an irregular or lobulated margin are more likely to be malignant.[35] The overall positive predictive value of the sonographic evaluation of thyroid malignancy has been reported to be as high as 97%.[36]

Finally, ultrasound-guided biopsy can be used to decrease the rate of nondiagnostic fine-needle aspiration biopsy. Ultrasound-guided aspiration biopsy is valuable in patients with a palpable thyroid nodule, multinodular goiter, or high risk of malignancy, and for cervical lymphadenopathy.[5] Similarly, biopsy is appropriate in nonpalpable thyroid nodules in patients with a high risk of cancer or in those with nodules larger than 1 to 1.5 cm with ultrasound features concerning for malignancy (Fig. 36.12. p. 626).[37] Small (<1–1.5 cm) nonpalpable lesions with benign sonographic features do not require sonographic follow-up.

Isotope Scanning

Thyroid scintigraphy, using ^{99m}Tc pertechnetate or ^{123}I, is used for assessment of thyroid function, detection of autonomously functioning thyroid nodules, and evaluation of thyroid cancer extent. Thyroid follicular cells can take up iodine and ^{99m}Tc pertechnetate; however, only iodine is organified and stored (as thyroglobulin) in the lumen of thyroid follicles. ^{99m}Tc pertechnetate and ^{123}I scintigraphy is primarily recommended for functional assessment in cases in which TSH concentration is suppressed in patients with suspected hyperthyroidism (e.g., Graves disease, autonomously functioning nodule, or toxic multinodular goiter) or in which ectopic thyroid tissue is suspected.[5]

Conversely, ^{99m}Tc pertechnetate and ^{123}I scintigraphy is used to functionally classify thyroid nodules. Based on the pattern of isotope uptake, nodules are classified as cold (decreased uptake) (Fig. 36.2), hot (increased uptake), or warm (uptake similar to surrounding tissue). Thyroid scintigraphy is also recommended in a subset of patients who have indeterminate fine-needle aspiration results. Hot nodules on scintigraphy are rarely malignant.[38] A review of published reports of radionuclide scanning reveals that 84% of solitary thyroid nodules are cold, 10% are warm, and the remaining 6% are hot. A cold thyroid nodule is more likely to be malignant, but most thyroid nodules are cold (~84%), including many benign lesions.[3, 39] The sensitivity of scintigraphy for detection of cold nodule is further limited in smaller lesions (<1 cm) owing to the limited spatial resolution of the camera. Approximately 5% of thyroid nodules will concentrate ^{99m}Tc pertechnetate with no uptake on the ^{123}I scan.[40] These discordant nodules will appear as hot or warm nodules on ^{99m}Tc pertechnetate scan but as cold nodules on radioiodine scan. Although the majority of these nodules are benign, few represent thyroid cancers. As a result, patients with nodules that are functioning on ^{99m}Tc pertechnetate imaging should undergo radioiodine imaging. Radioiodine (^{131}I) can be used diagnostically to measure the uptake within the hyperfunctional gland or for localization of recurrent or metastatic thyroid cancer in patients with thyroid cancer that concentrates iodine. Conversely, ^{131}I can be delivered at a therapeutic dose for radioiodine treatment of a hyperfunctional gland or nodule. Similarly, it is considered the treatment of choice for residual, recurrent, or metastatic differentiated thyroid cancer.

2-[^{18}F] Fluoro-2-Deoxy-D-Glucose Positron Emission Tomography Scanning

The clinical role of 2-[^{18}F] fluoro-2-deoxy-D-glucose (FDG) positron emission tomography (PET) scan in preoperative evaluation of thyroid nodules is controversial, and it is not routinely used in daily clinical practice. Focal FDG uptake is incidentally seen in approximately 2% of all patients, and approximately one-third of these lesions are thyroid cancer.[41, 42] However, benign lesions also demonstrate FDG uptake. FDG-PET scan has an increasing role in the evaluation of selected patients treated for thyroid

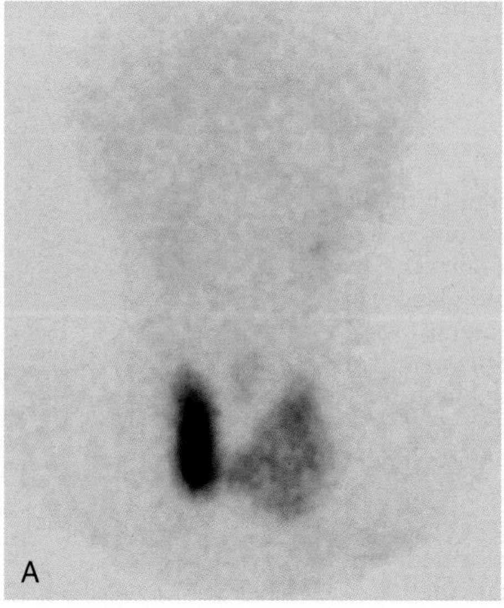

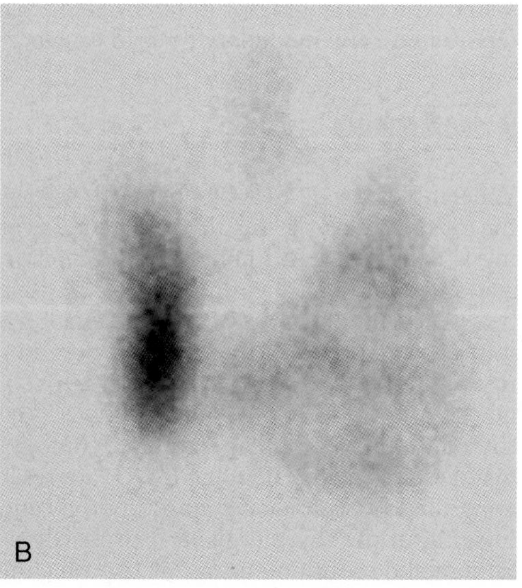

FIGURE 36.2. A 64-year-old man with hyperthyroidism attributed to Graves disease. **A**, Parallel hole image from a ^{99m}Tc pertechnetate scan demonstrates an enlarged asymmetrical heterogeneous appearance in the left thyroid lobe. The right lobe shows increased uptake associated with suppressed salivary glands and soft tissue uptake attributed to Graves disease. **B**, Pinhole image shows several photopenic nodules consistent with cold nodules. Pathology confirms the presence of a 4-cm papillary thyroid carcinoma corresponding to the left cold nodules.

cancer with clinically negative examinations and rising thyroglobulin level. The uptake of FDG in general is inversely proportional to iodine uptake/differentiation. Therefore, it may be particularly useful in metastatic thyroid tumors that do not concentrate radioiodine.[41] Potential pitfalls include indolent or well-differentiated thyroid tumors that take up FDG poorly, as well as FDG uptake that may not be related to metastatic thyroid cancer. An additional limitation of PET is that cancerous nodes may not be detected on PET owing to low cellularity or because they are predominantly cystic or necrotic.

Additional Diagnostic Imaging (Computed Tomography and Magnetic Resonance Imaging)

Cross-sectional imaging, using CT scan (Figs. 36.3 to 36.7) and MRI (Fig. 36.8), is not indicated in the evaluation of benign versus malignant thyroid nodules, as benign and malignant nodules may have a similar imaging appearance. The main role of CT and MRI is to assess for local aggressiveness, including evidence of extracapsular extension, lymph node metastasis (see Figs. 36.3 and 36.4), infiltration of the strap muscles, invasion of the airway (Fig. 36.6) and esophagus, and invasion of the prevertebral musculature. Consequently, cross-sectional imaging is usually obtained when patients present with features concerning for aggressive cancer (including a fixed, immobile thyroid mass) or are symptomatic with hoarseness, dysphagia, or respiratory symptoms. In addition, cross-sectional imaging is frequently requested for evaluation of the extent of disease in the neck and mediastinum, for surgical planning, and to identify distant metastases (Fig. 36.5). Diagnostic CT often requires iodinated contrast, which may be contraindicated if ^{131}I whole-body scanning or ablation therapy will used. MRI can be helpful, because it is highly sensitive in the evaluation of local neck disease and does not require iodinated contrast.

TREATMENT

The primary therapy for differentiated (papillary and follicular) thyroid cancer is surgery. Total thyroidectomy is usually performed in patients with nodules larger than 1 cm or if extrathryoidal extension or metastases are present. This is frequently followed by administration of ^{131}I to destroy any remaining thyroid tissue and/or microscopic tumor foci. An algorithm summarizing the management of differentiated thyroid cancer is shown in Fig. 36.11, p. 625.

Surgery

There are two potential surgical approaches to differentiated thyroid cancer: total (or near-total) thyroidectomy and unilateral lobectomy and isthmusectomy. Total thyroidectomy involves removal of all thyroid tissue. This more aggressive surgical approach is associated with lower rates of local and regional recurrence and a lower mortality in high-risk patients.[43] Near-total thyroidectomy is identical, except for preserving the posterior thyroid capsule of the lobe contralateral to the thyroid tumor. During a unilateral lobectomy and isthmusectomy, one entire lobe and the isthmus are removed, without entering the contralateral neck. Subtotal thyroidectomy is considered an inadequate procedure for

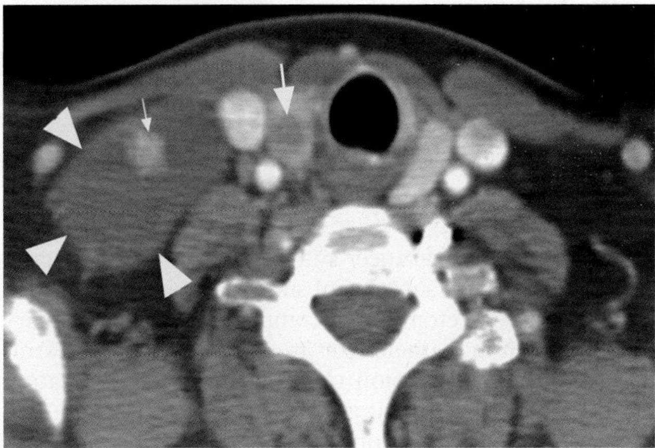

FIGURE 36.4. Papillary thyroid cancer in a 57-year-old man. Axial contrast-enhanced computed tomography scan of the neck reveals a small hypodense nodule (*large arrow*) within the right lobe of the thyroid gland. There is a large predominantly cystic metastatic lymph node (*arrowheads*) in the right lateral neck with an enhancing central component (*small arrow*). Such cystic metastatic lymph nodes from papillary thyroid cancer are a common presentation on imaging.

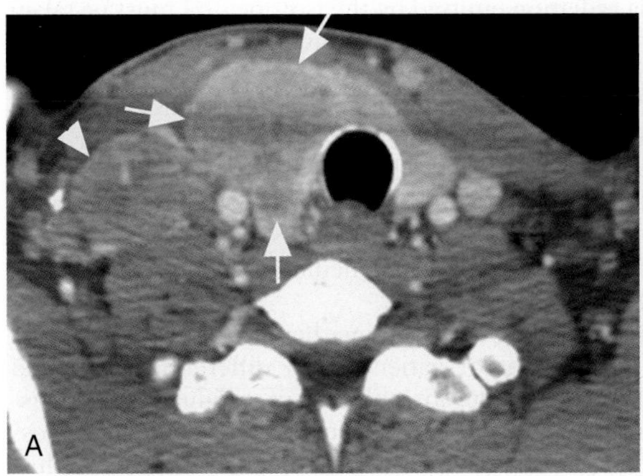

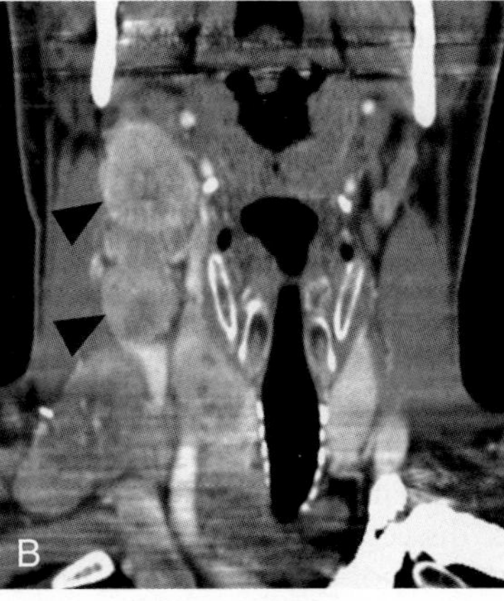

FIGURE 36.3. Papillary thyroid carcinoma in a 64-year-old man. Axial (**A**) and coronal (**B**) contrast-enhanced computed tomography scans of the neck reveal a large hypodense mass within the right lobe of the thyroid gland (*arrows* in **A**), which was found to be papillary thyroid carcinoma at surgery. Multiple metastatic lymph nodes (*arrowheads*) are seen in the right lateral neck.

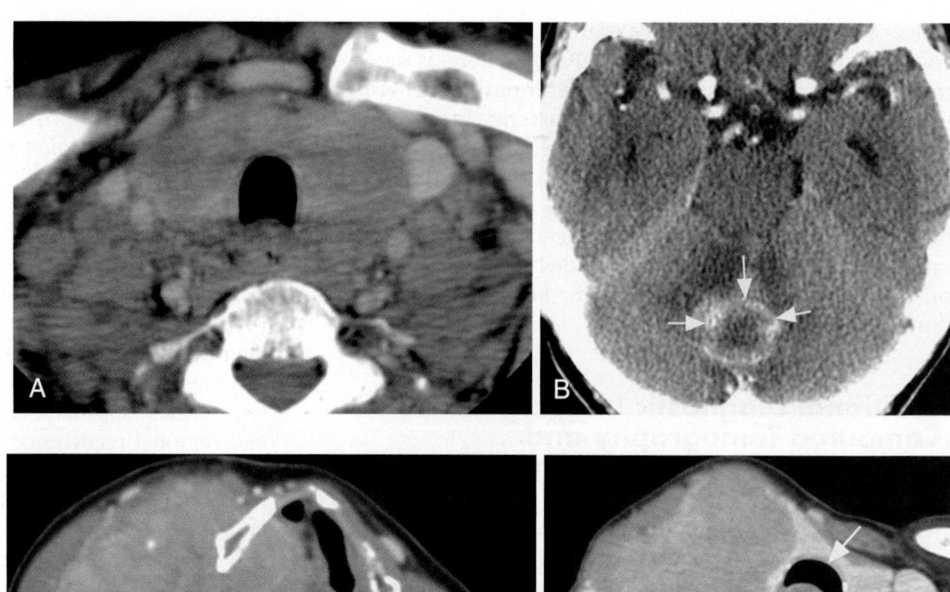

FIGURE 36.5. Follicular thyroid cancer in a 72-year-old woman. **A**, Axial contrast-enhanced computed tomography (CT) scan of the neck reveals an infiltrative, hypodense mass involving both lobes of the thyroid gland. This was found to be follicular thyroid carcinoma at biopsy. **B**, Axial contrast-enhanced CT of the brain shows a metastatic deposit (*arrows*) in the cerebellar vermis.

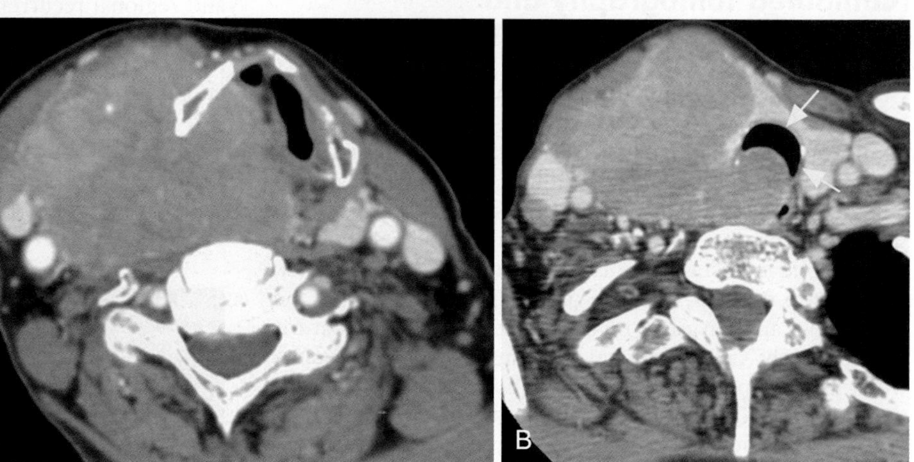

FIGURE 36.6. Anaplastic thyroid cancer in a 76-year-old man. **A** and **B**, Axial contrast-enhanced computed tomography scans of the neck reveal a large hypodense mass arising from the right lobe of the thyroid gland with extension into the adjacent neck soft tissues. There is invasion into the larynx superiorly (**A**), as well as into the trachea (*arrows* in **B**) and subsequent narrowing.

patients with thyroid cancer and is associated with a higher complication rate if subsequent surgery is required.[44]

Total thyroidectomy is recommended if the primary tumor is 1 cm in diameter (or greater) or if there is extrathyroidal tumor extension or metastases. This operation should also be performed in all patients with thyroid cancer who have a history of exposure to ionizing radiation of the head and neck, owing to the higher rate of tumor recurrence. Foci of papillary cancer have been found in both thyroid lobes in up to 36% to 85% of patients,[17, 45] with approximately 7% of thyroid cancer recurrences in the contralateral lobe.[46] In addition, radioiodine ablation of thyroid bed remnants and treatment of metastatic disease are facilitated by resection of as much thyroid tissue as possible. The specificity of measurements of serum thyroglobulin as a tumor marker is facilitated by removal of nearly all normal thyroid tissue. Unilateral lobectomy and isthmusectomy is considered if the tumor is less than 1 cm in diameter (or even $\leq$3 cm if entirely confined to the thyroid in low-risk patients) and confined to one lobe of the gland. For patients with a cytologically suspicious nodule, and without proven cancer, a unilateral lobectomy and isthmusectomy is usually performed.[47]

Lymph node dissection is typically performed if there is clinical evidence of cervical or mediastinal nodal metastases. Pathologic adenopathy of the central neck requires resection of all nodal groups in the area. The presence of pathologic adenopathy lateral to the jugular vein indicates a need for a modified radical neck dissection. The precise role of prophylactic neck dissection of microscopic lymph node metastases that are not clinically identifiable is controversial, as it is uncertain whether this improves long-term outcome. Additionally, subsequent radioiodine administration will ablate these occult foci.

Radioiodine Ablation Therapy and Chemotherapy

Well-differentiated thyroid cancers often concentrate iodine, permitting treatment with ^{131}I. Like iodine, radioiodine is taken up and concentrated in normal and malignant thyroid follicular cells. ^{131}I causes acute thyroid cell death by emission of short–path-length beta rays. The uptake of ^{131}I by thyroid tissue can be visualized by detecting the gamma radiation emitted by the isotope. ^{131}I must be taken up by thyroid tissue to be effective. As a result, it is of no value in patients with thyroid cancers that do not concentrate iodine, for example, patients with medullary cancer, anaplastic cancer, dedifferentiated thyroid cancer, or lymphoma. Radioiodine uptake is dependent upon adequate stimulation by TSH (either endogenous or recombinant) and is reduced by the presence of excess stable iodide, for example, iodine-containing medications and intravenous contrast used for CT scans.

The advantage of radioiodine therapy in the postthyroidectomy treatment of patients with differentiated thyroid cancer includes adjuvant ablation of residual thyroid tissue and/or residual microscopic cancer, imaging for possible metastatic disease, and treatment of known residual

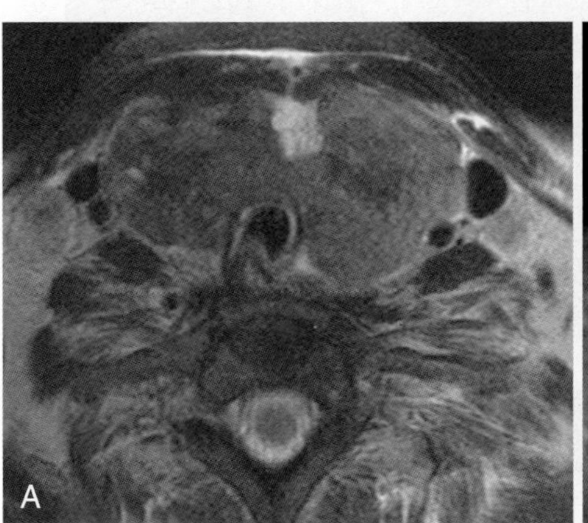

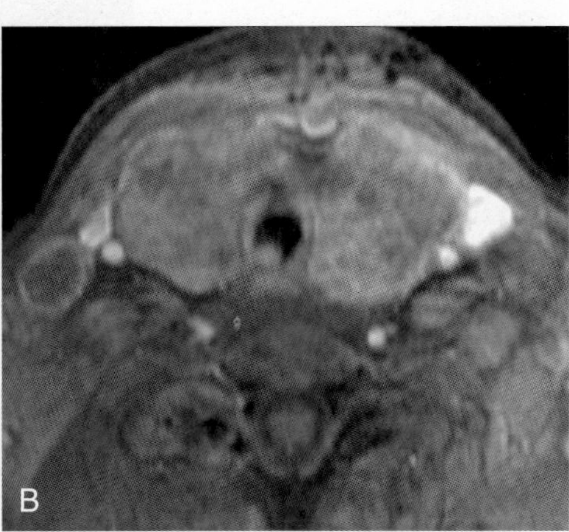

FIGURE 36.7. Medullary thyroid cancer in a 16-year-old man. **A**, Axial contrast-enhanced computed tomography scans of the neck show a small hypoenhancing nodule in the right lobe of the thyroid gland (*arrow*). **B**, Multiple heterogeneously enhancing lymph nodes were found in the right lower neck (*arrows*). Pathology revealed this to be a thyroid medullary cancer with lymph node metastasis. Genetic testing for *RET* was negative.

FIGURE 36.8. Mucoepidermoid carcinoma in 68-year-old woman. Axial T2-weighted (**A**) and post–contrast-enhanced T1-weighted (**B**) magnetic resonance imaging show a large infiltrative mass involving the thyroid gland. The mass shows heterogeneous signal on T2-weighted images and mild heterogeneous enhancement with gadolinium.

or metastatic thyroid cancer (Fig. 36.11, p. 625). In addition, the sensitivity of serum thyroglobulin measurements is improved during follow-up for recurrence. There is currently a lack of consensus regarding which specific subsets of patients benefit from ^{131}I treatment after thyroidectomy; however, it is clear that patients with high-risk features will benefit most.[48–50] Radioiodine therapy is indicated for all patients with known distant metastases, gross extrathyroidal tumor extension, or primary tumor size larger than 4 cm, even in the absence of other high-risk features.[48, 49] Radioiodine ablation is not routinely recommended for low-risk patients with cancers smaller than 4 cm that are confined to the thyroid gland (no local metastases).[38, 48] Chemotherapy may occasionally be beneficial in patients with progressive symptomatic thyroid cancer that is unresponsive or not amenable to surgery, radioiodine therapy, or external radiotherapy. Nevertheless, no chemotherapeutic regimen has been consistently successful. To date, treatment guidelines have generally been dictated by the results of case reports or small retrospective series.

Radiation

External irradiation is rarely used as adjunctive therapy in the initial management of patients with well-differentiated thyroid cancer. Radiation therapy may be beneficial, however, in patients with poorly differentiated thyroid cancers that do not concentrate radioiodine.[51] External beam radiotherapy also has been used for palliation in patients with unresectable locally advanced disease. Radiotherapy has been used in patients with all types of thyroid epithelial cancer, MTC, and thyroid lymphoma. It can be used as primary therapy to treat unresectable cancer, as adjuvant therapy after surgical resection, and as palliative therapy for recurrent cancer.[51] It can be given alone or in combination with surgery or chemotherapy.

SURVEILLANCE

Most recurrences of differentiated thyroid cancer occur within the first 5 years after initial treatment, although recurrences may occur many years later, particularly with papillary cancer.[52, 53] All patients should have periodic physical examination, biochemical testing, and anatomic or functional imaging to monitor for recurrence. Anatomic imaging using ultrasound, CT, or MRI or functional imaging using ^{131}I or PET scan is essential for evaluation of tumor recurrence. Recently there has been a shift toward using biochemical testing instead of imaging in cases where there is clinical and biochemical evidence of recurrence.

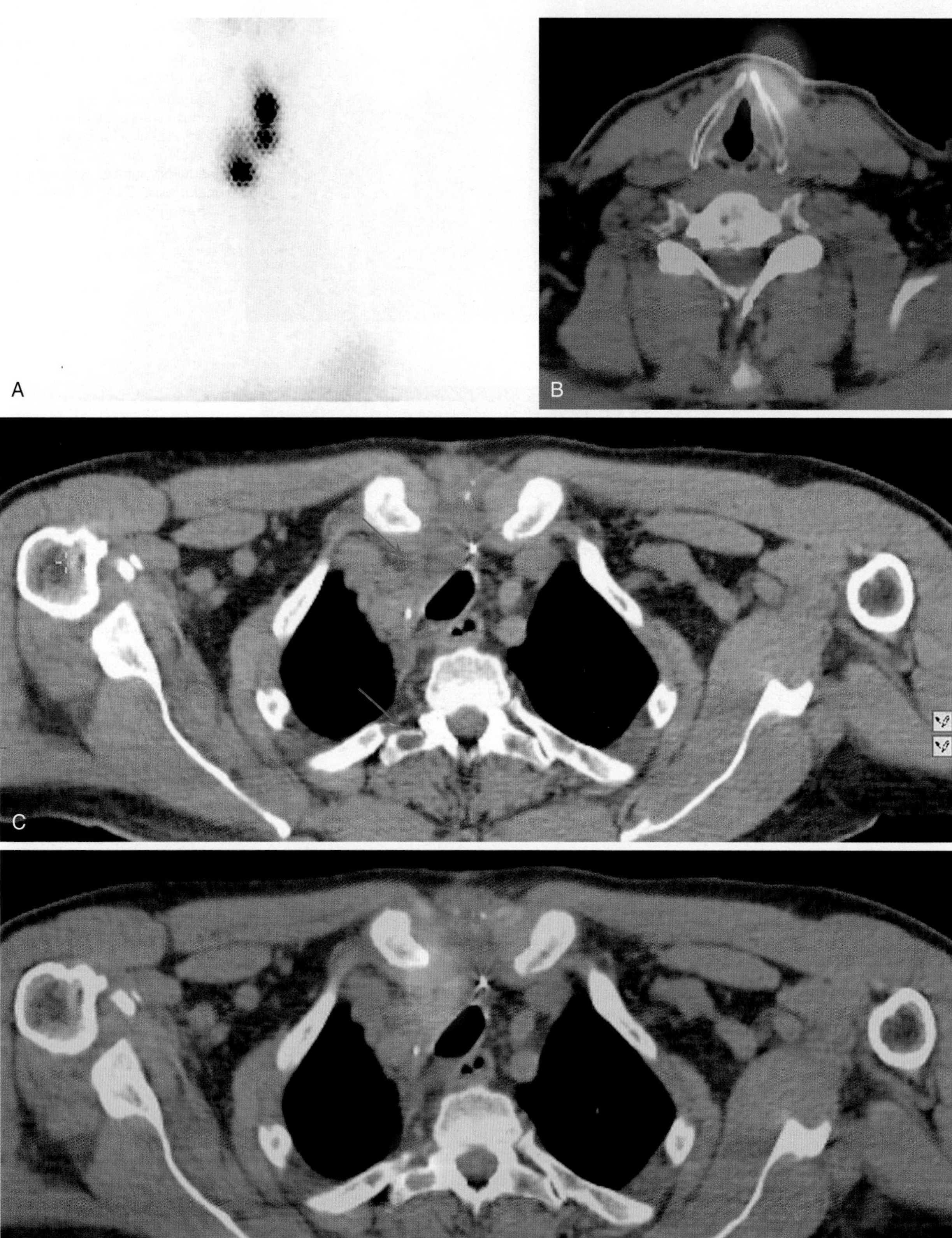

FIGURE 36.9. Diagnostic 131-I scan in a 64-year-old male with 11 cm angioinvasive follicular variant papillary thyroid carcinoma, status post resection of large substernal goiter via median sternotomy. Planar static view of the neck and chest (**A**) demonstrates intensely focal central neck activity; Transaxial fused SPECT/CT of the neck (**B**) demonstrates thyroglossal duct remnant; Transaxial chest CT (**C**) and fused SPECT/CT (**D**) demonstrate mediastinal nodal metastases (*arrow*) and lytic osseous metastasis in the right transverse process of T3 vertebra (*arrow*).

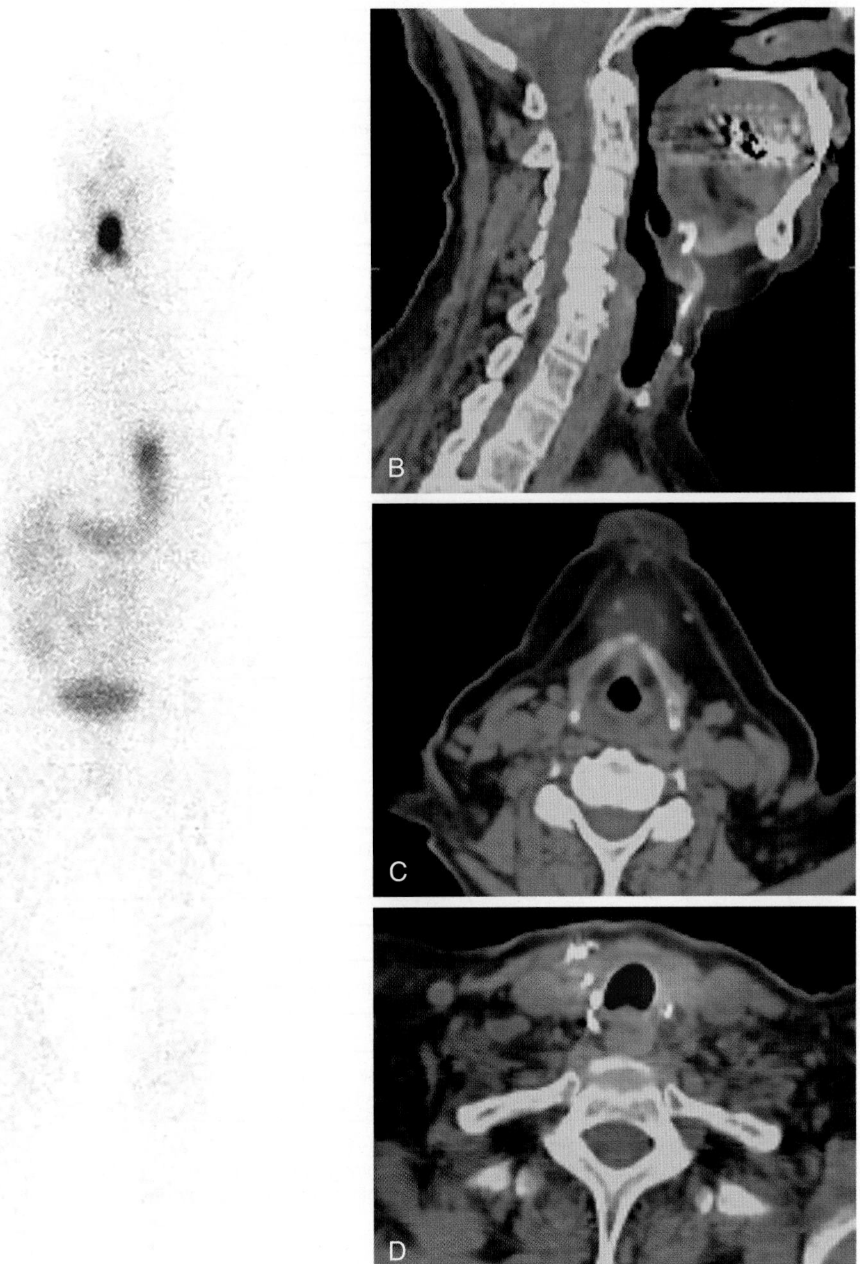

FIGURE 36.10. Diagnostic 131-I scan in a 72-year-old female with multifocal and bilateral papillary thyroid cancer (largest tumor of 1.2 cm in the left thyroid lobe), status post thyroidectomy. Planar whole body scan (**A**) demonstrates intensely focal central neck activity; Fused SPECT/CT, sagittal (**B**) and transaxial (**C**, **D**) images demonstrate thyroid remnant tissue within the thyroglossal duct (panels **B** and **C**) and the bilateral thyroidectomy bed (panel **D**), without evidence of regional or distant metastatic disease.

Serum Thyroglobulin Measurement

Thyroglobulin is a prohormone of thyroxine (T_4) and triiodothyronine (T_3). It is synthesized only by thyroid follicular cells and released into the serum along with the thyroid hormones. Given the cellular specificity of thyroglobulin, serum thyroglobulin is a very useful marker of persistent or recurrent tumor in patients after thyroidectomy and ablation of residual normal thyroid tissue. Approximately 60% of differentiated thyroid cancers take up enough iodide to be detected by radioiodine imaging, and over 90% synthesize and secrete thyroglobulin. Serum thyroglobulin has a high degree of sensitivity and specificity to detect thyroid cancer, with the highest degree of sensitivity noted after thyroid hormone withdrawal or stimulation using recombinant human TSH (rhTSH).

Following thyroidectomy and ablation of any thyroid remnant, the serum thyroglobulin concentration should be

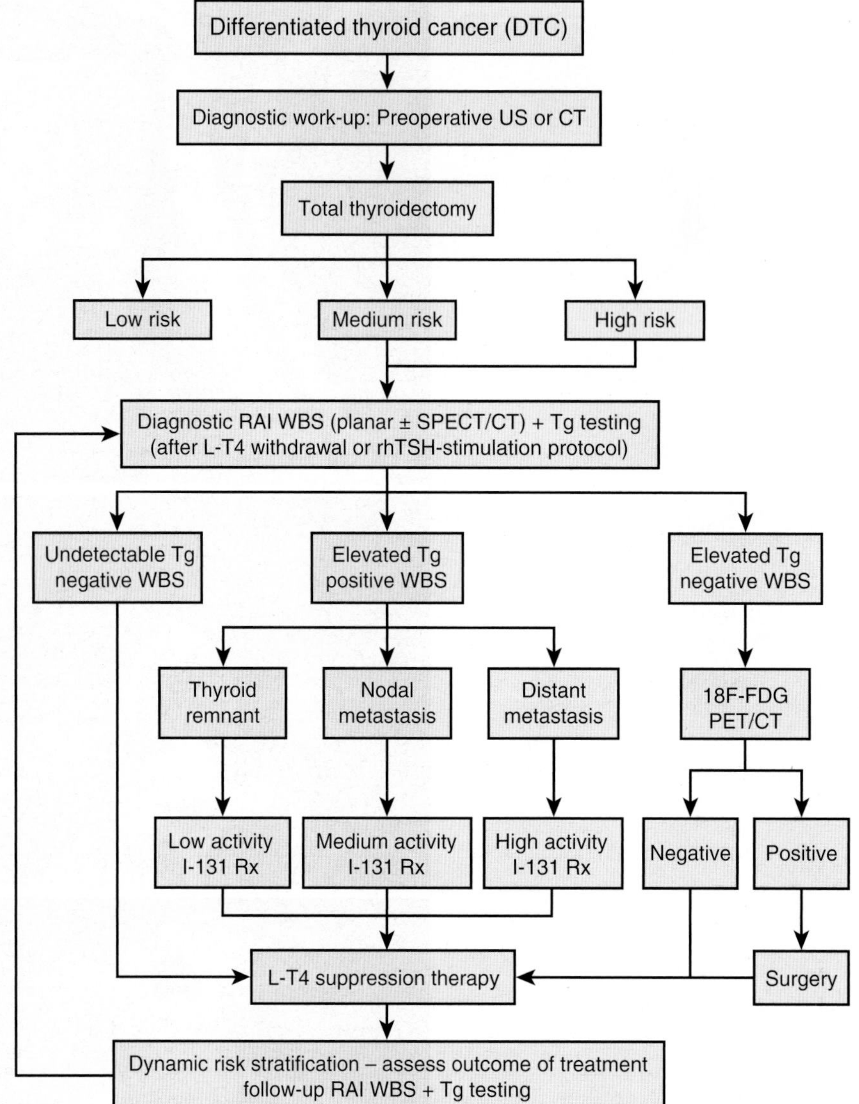

FIGURE 36.11. Algorithm for thyroid cancer management. *RAI*, Radioiodine (^{131}I or ^{123}I); *FDG*, 2-[^{18}F] fluoro-2-deoxy-D-glucose; *PET*, positron emission tomography; *CT*, computed tomography; *SPECT*, single-photon emission tomography; *WBS*, whole-body scan; *L-T4*, levothyroxine; *L-T4 withdrawal*, hypothyroid stimulation protocol; *rhTSH*, recombinant human thyroid-stimulating hormone; *Tg*, thyroglobulin; *US*, ultrasound; *Rx*, radionuclide.

very low (<1–2 ng/mL), both during T_4 therapy and after it is discontinued or stimulated by rhTSH. A stimulated thyroglobulin value of at least 2 ng/mL or higher suggests recurrence, and, consequently, more extensive evaluation is indicated.[54] Patients with lower thyroglobulin values may still present with localized recurrence during subsequent years of follow-up. The positive predictive value of an initial thyroglobulin greater than 2 ng/mL is 80%, and the negative predictive value is 98%.[55] Antithyroglobulin antibodies are present initially in approximately 25% of patients with thyroid cancer, and may interfere with assays for thyroglobulin. Therefore, the laboratory should always test for antithyroglobulin antibodies before measuring serum thyroglobulin.

In low-risk patients with a thyroglobulin level of less than 2 ng/mL, a combination of neck ultrasound and rhTSH-stimulated thyroglobulin is effective at detecting persistent/recurrent disease. A combination of rhTSH-stimulated thyroglobulin and neck ultrasound has a better predictive value than rhTSH-stimulated thyroglobulin either alone or in combination with radioiodine scanning.[56] Diagnostic whole-body radioiodine scanning is indicated for higher-risk patients (Figs. 36.9 and 36.10) but is not routinely indicated in low-risk patients with rhTSH-stimulated serum thyroglobulin concentrations of less than 2 ng/mL. A 2003 consensus statement suggests relying upon rhTSH-stimulated thyroglobulin testing instead of radioiodine scanning in all low-risk patients.[54, 57]

Surveillance Imaging

Ultrasonography is particularly useful in identifying recurrent cancer in the thyroid bed following thyroidectomy, in the contralateral lobe following hemithyroidectomy, and in neck lymph nodes. Following thyroidectomy, neck ultrasound should be performed to evaluate the thyroid bed and cervical nodal compartments at 6 and

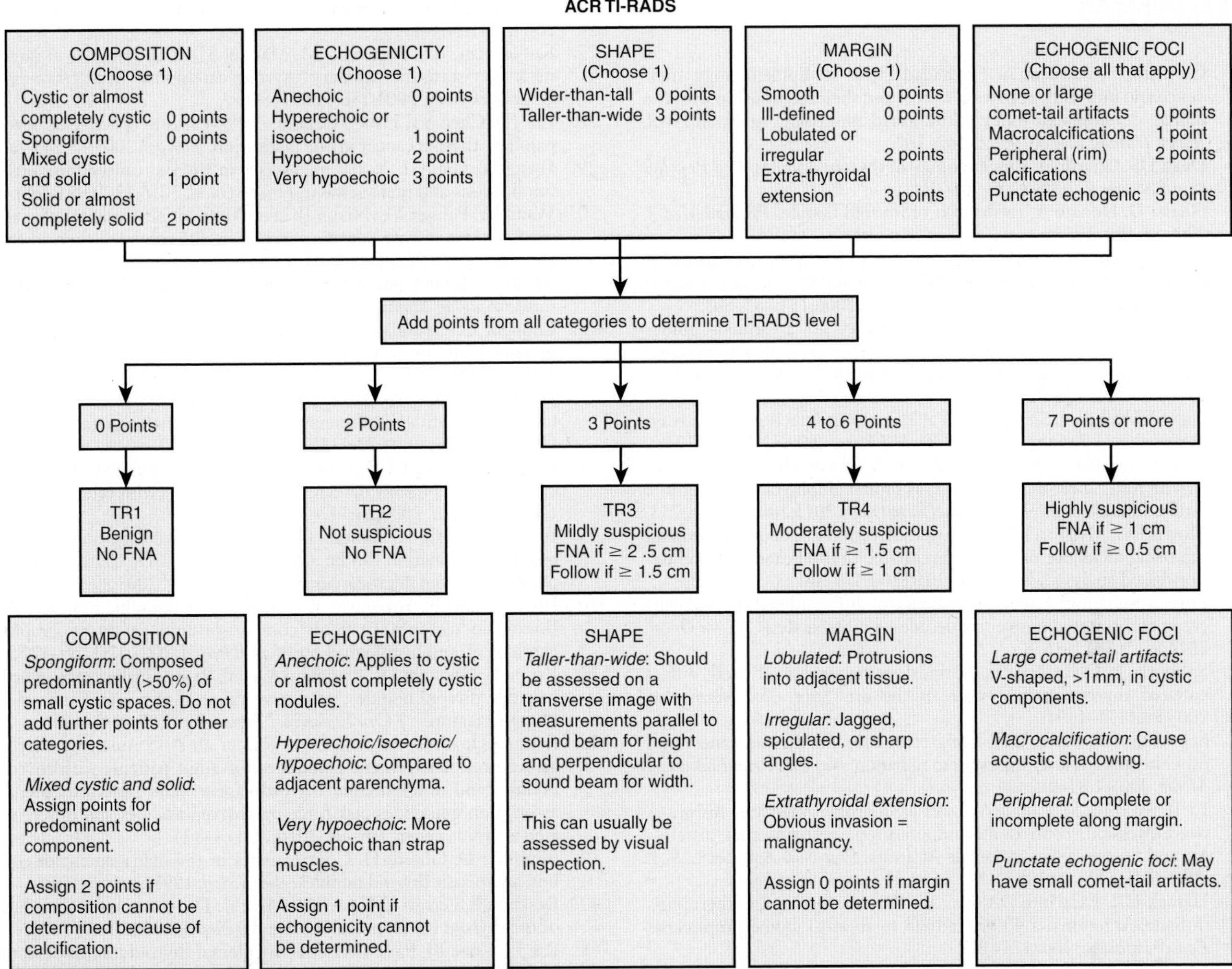

FIGURE 36.12. Chart showing five categories on the basis of the American College of Radiology Thyroid Imaging, Reporting and Data System lexicon, TI-RADS scoring, and criteria for fine-needle aspiration or follow-up ultrasound. Explanatory notes appear at the bottom. (From Tessler FN, Middleton WD, Grant EG, et al. ACR Thyroid Imaging, Reporting and Data System (TI-RADS): white paper of the ACR TI-RADS committee. *J Am Coll Radiol.* 2017;14(5):587–595.)

12 months, and then annually for at least 3 to 5 years, depending on the patient's thyroglobulin status and risk for recurrent disease. Sonographic lymph node characteristics most consistent with malignancy include cystic appearance, internal microcalcifications, loss of a fatty hilum, and peripheral vascularization.[58] In addition, ultrasound-guided fine-needle aspiration is highly effective in evaluating and detecting regional recurrence in previously treated patients. Cross-sectional imaging (CT and MRI) is essential for evaluation of the extent of recurrent disease, including evaluation of adenopathy in the neck and mediastinum.

Following radioiodine ablation, diagnostic whole-body scanning has low sensitivity and is typically unnecessary in low-risk patients who are clinically free of residual tumor (with undetectable serum thyroglobulin and a negative cervical ultrasound).

The use of rhTSH before an FDG-PET scan significantly increases the number of lesions detected on FDG-PET.[59] FDG-PET may complement ^{131}I scanning, because FDG uptake, in general, is inversely proportional to iodine uptake/differentiation. Therefore, it may be particularly useful in metastatic thyroid tumors that do not concentrate radioiodine.[41]

In patients with evidence of distant metastases, FDG-PET scanning may provide useful prognostic information.[41] A study of 125 patients with well-differentiated thyroid cancer undergoing FDG-PET scanning showed that FDG uptake in a large volume of tissue correlated with poor survival and predicted outcome better than uptake of radioiodine (Fig. 36.8).

REFERENCES

1. Goodarzi E, Moslem A, Feizhadad H, et al. Epidemiology, incidence and mortality of thyroid cancer and their relationship with the human development index in the world: an ecology study in 2018. *Advan Human Bio*. 2019;9(2):162–167.
2. Dean DS, Gharib H. Epidemiology of thyroid nodules. *Best Prac Res Clin Endocrinol*. 2008;22(6):901–911.
3. Ghassi D, Donato A. Evaluation of thyroid nodule. *Postgrad Med J*. 2009;85:190–195.
4. Pacini F, Schlumberger M, Dralle H, et al. European consensus for the management of patients with differentiated thyroid carcinoma of the follicular epithelium. *Eur J Endocrinol*. 2006;154:787–803.
5. Singer PA, Cooper DS, Daniels GH, et al. Treatment guidelines for patients with thyroid nodules and well-differentiated thyroid cancer. American Thyroid Association. *Arch Intern Med*. 1996;156:2165–2172.
6. Hall SF, Walker H, Siemens R, et al. Increasing detection and increasing incidence in thyroid cancer. *World J Surg*. 2009;33:2567–2571.
7. Aschebrook-Kilfoy B, Kaplan EL, et al. The acceleration in papillary thyroid cancer incidence rates is similar among racial and ethnic groups in the United States. *Annal Surg Oncol*. 2013;20(8):2746–2753.
8. Morris LG, Myssiorek D. Improved detection does not fully explain the rising incidence of well-differentiated thyroid cancer: A population-based analysis. *Am J Surg*. 2010;200:454–461.
9. Furuya-Kanamori L, et al. Prevalence of differentiated thyroid cancer in autopsy studies over six decades: a meta-analysis. *J Clin Oncol*. 2016;9(12):3672–3678.
10. Suliburk J, Delbridge L. Surgical management of well differentiated thyroid cancer: state of the art. *Surg Clin North Am*. 2009;89:1171–1191.
11. Schneider AB, Sarne DH. Long-term risks for thyroid cancer and other neoplasms after exposure to radiation. *Nat Clin Pract Endocrinol Metab*. 2005;1:82–91.
12. Li JJ, Weroha SJ, Lingle WL, et al. Estrogen mediates Aurora-A overexpression, centrosome amplification, chromosomal instability, and breast cancer in female ACI rats. *Proc Natl Acad Sci U S A*. 2004;101:18123–18128.
13. Harach HR, Escalante DA, Day ES. Thyroid cancer and thyroiditis in Salta, Argentina: a 40-yr study in relation to iodine prophylaxis *Endocr Pathol*. 132002175–181.
14. Cameselle-Teijeiro J, et al. Findings in Cowden syndrome: a clue for the diagnosis of the PTEN hamartoma tumor syndrome. *Am J Clin Pathol*. 2015;144(2):322–328.
15. Cady B, Sedgwick CE, Meissner WA, et al. Changing clinical, pathologic, therapeutic, and survival patterns in differentiated thyroid carcinoma. *Ann Surg*. 1976;184:541–553.
16. Newman JG, Chalian AA, Shaha AR. Surgical approaches in thyroid cancer: what the radiologist needs to know. *Neuroimag Clin North Am*. 2008;18:491–504.
17. Iacobone M, Jansson S, Barczyński M, et al. Multifocal papillary thyroid carcinoma—a consensus report of the European Society of Endocrine Surgeons (ESES). *Langenbecks Arch Surg*. 2014;399:141–154.
18. American Joint Committee on Cancer *Thyroid—Differentiated and Anaplastic*. *AJCC Cancer Staging Manual*. 8th ed. New York: Springer; 2017:873.
19. Emerick GT, Duh QY, Siperstein AE, et al. Diagnosis, treatment, and outcome of follicular thyroid carcinoma. *Cancer*. 1993;72:3287–3295.
20. Noone AM, Howlader N, Krapcho M, et al. SEER Cancer Statistics Review. Bethesda: National Cancer Institute; 1975–2015.
21. Ahmadi S, Stang M, Jiang XS, et al. Hurthle cell carcinoma: current perspectives. *Onco targets ther*. 2016;9:6873–6884.
22. Ganeshan D, Paulson E, Duran C, et al. Current update on medullary thyroid carcinoma. *Am J Radiol*. 2013;201(6):867–876.
23. Holm LE, Blomgren H, Lowhagen T. Cancer risks in patients with chronic lymphocytic thyroiditis. *N Engl J Med*. 1985;312:601–604.
24. Papaparaskeva K, Nagel H, Droese M. Cytologic diagnosis of medullary carcinoma of the thyroid gland. *Diagn Cytopathol*. 2000;22:351–358.
25. Yamaga LYI, Cunha ML, Campos Neto GC, et al. 68Ga-DOTATATE PET/CT in recurrent medullary thyroid carcinoma: a lesion-by-lesion comparison with 111In-octreotide SPECT/CT and conventional imaging. *Eur J Nucl Med Mol Imaging*. 2018;44(10):1695–1701.
26. Hegedus L. Clinical practice. The thyroid nodule. *N Engl J Med*. 2004;351:1764–1771.
27. Kupferman ME, Patterson M, Mandel SJ, et al. Patterns of lateral neck metastasis in papillary thyroid carcinoma. *Arch Otolaryngol Head Neck Surg*. 2004;130(7):857–860.
28. Lin JD, Chen ST, Hsueh C, et al. A 29-year retrospective review of papillary thyroid cancer in one institution. *Thyroid*. 2007;17:535–541.
29. Wang W, Ganly I. Nodal metastases in thyroid cancer: prognostic implications and management. *Future Oncol*. 2016;12(7):981–994.
30. Wang LY, Palmer FL, Nixon IJ, et al. Multi-organ distant metastases confer worse disease-specific survival in differentiated thyroid cancer. *Thyroid*. 2014;24(11):1594–1599.
31. American Joint Committee on Cancer *Thyroid—Medullary*. *AJCC Cancer Staging Manual*. 8th ed. New York: Springer; 2017:891.
32. Cappelli C, Castellano M, Pirola I, et al. The predictive value of ultrasound findings in the management of thyroid nodules. *QJM*. 2007;100:29–35.
33. Solivetti FM, Bacaro D, Cecconi P, et al. Small hyperechogenic nodules in thyroiditis: usefulness of cytological characterization. *J Exp Clin Cancer Res*. 2004;23:433–435.
34. Kakkos SK, Scopa CD, Chalmoukis AK, et al. Relative risk of cancer in sonographically detected thyroid nodules with calcifications. *J Clin Ultrasound*. 2000;28:347–352.
35. Ito Y, Kobayashi K, Tomoda C, et al. Ill-defined edge on ultrasonographic examination can be a marker of aggressive characteristic of papillary thyroid microcarcinoma. *World J Surg*. 2005;29:1007–1011.
36. Ito Y, Amino N, Yokozawa T, et al. Ultrasonographic evaluation of thyroid nodules in 900 patients: comparison among ultrasonographic, cytological, and histological findings. *Thyroid*. 2007;17:1269–1276.
37. Papini E, Guglielmi R, Bianchini A, et al. Risk of malignancy in nonpalpable thyroid nodules: predictive value of ultrasound and color-Doppler features. *J Clin Endocrinol Metab*. 2002;87:1941–1946.
38. Bryan RH, Alexander EK, Bible KC, et al. 2015 American thyroid association management guidelines for adult patients with thyroid nodules and differentiated thyroid cancer: The American thyroid association guidelines task force on thyroid nodules and differentiated thyroid cancer. *Thyroid*. 2016;26(1):1–131.
39. Giuffrida D, Gharib H. Controversies in the management of cold, hot, and occult thyroid nodules. *Am J Med*. 1995;99:642–650.
40. Reschini E, Ferrari C, Castellani M, et al. The trapping-only nodules of the thyroid gland: prevalence study. *Thyroid*. 2006;16:757–762.
41. Bae JS, Chae BJ, Park WC, et al. Incidental thyroid lesions detected by FDG-PET/CT: prevalence and risk of thyroid cancer. *World J Surg Oncol*. 2009;7(63):120–127.
42. Pattison DA, Bozin M, Gorelik A, et al. 18F-FDG-avid thyroid incidentalomas; the importance of contextual interpretation. *J Nucl Med*. 2018;59(5):749–755.
43. Ross DS, Litofsky D, Ain KB, et al. Recurrence after treatment of micropapillary thyroid cancer. *Thyroid*. 2009;19:1043.
44. Padur A, Kumar N, Guru A, et al. Safety and effectiveness of total thyroidectomy and its comparison with subtotal thyroidectomy and other thyroid surgeries: A systematic review. *J Thyroid Res*. 2016:1–6.
45. Pacini F, Elisei R, Capezzone M, et al. Contralateral papillary thyroid cancer is frequent at completion thyroidectomy with no difference in low- and high-risk patients. *Thyroid*. 2001;11:877–881.
46. Huang H, Liu S, Xu Z, et al. Long-term outcome of thyroid lobectomy for unilateral multifocal papillary carcinoma. *Medicine*. 2017;96(27):1–4.
47. Matsuzu K, Sugino K, Masudo K, et al. Thyroid lobectomy for papillary thyroid cancer: long-term follow-up study of 1, 088 cases. *World J Surg*. 2014;38(1):68–79.
48. Andresen NS, Buatti JM, Tewfik HH, et al. Radioiodine ablation following thyroidectomy for differentiated thyroid cancer: literature review of utility, dose, and toxicity. *Eur Thyroid J*. 2017;6:187–196.
49. Schmidt M, Gorges R, Drzezga A, et al. A matter of controversy: is radioiodine therapy favorable in differentiated thyroid carcinoma? *J Nucl Med*. 2018;59(8):1195–1201.
50. Carhill AA, Litofsky DR, Ross DS, et al. Long-term outcomes following therapy in differentiated thyroid carcinoma: NTCTCS registry analysis 1987-2012. *J Clin Endocrinol Metab*. 2015;100(9):3270.
51. Giuliani M, Brierley J. Indications for the use of external beam radiation in thyroid cancer. *Curr Opin Oncol*. 2014;26(1):45–50.
52. Shaha AR, Loree TR, Shah JP. Prognostic factors and risk group analysis in follicular carcinoma of the thyroid. *Surgery*. 1995;118:1131–1136.

53. Grant CS. Recurrence of papillary thyroid cancer after optimized surgery. *Gland Surg*. 2015;4(1):52–62.
54. Prpic M, Franceschi M, Romic M, et al. Thyroglobulin as a tumor marker in differentiated thyroid cancer—clinical considerations. *Acta Clin Croatia*. 2018;57(3):518–527.
55. Kloos RT, Mazzaferri EL. A single recombinant human thyrotropin-stimulated serum thyroglobulin measurement predicts differentiated thyroid carcinoma metastases three to five years later. *J Clin Endocrinol Metab*. 2005;90:5047–5057.
56. Pacini F, Molinaro E, Castagna MG, et al. Recombinant human thyrotropin-stimulated serum thyroglobulin combined with neck ultrasonography has the highest sensitivity in monitoring differentiated thyroid carcinoma. *J Clin Endocrinol Metab*. 2003;88:3668–3673.
57. Mazzaferri EL, Robbins RJ, Spencer CA, et al. A consensus report of the role of serum thyroglobulin as a monitoring method for low-risk patients with papillary thyroid carcinoma. *J Clin Endocrinol Metab*. 2003;88:1433–1441.
58. Leboulleux S, Girard E, Rose M, et al. Ultrasound criteria of malignancy for cervical lymph nodes in patients followed up for differentiated thyroid cancer. *J Clin Endocrinol Metab*. 2007;92:3590–3594.
59. Leboulleux S, Schroeder PR, Busaidy NL, et al. Assessment of the incremental value of recombinant thyrotropin stimulation before 2-[18F]-fluoro-2-deoxy-d-glucose positron emission tomography/computed tomography imaging to localize residual differentiated thyroid cancer. *J Clin Endocrinol Metab*. 2009;94:1310–1316.

CHAPTER

37 Melanoma

Silvana C. Faria, M.D., Ph.D; Rodabe N. Amaria, M.D.; and Madhavi Patnana, M.D.

INTRODUCTION

Cutaneous melanoma is an aggressive neoplasm that is the most common cause of death from cutaneous malignancies. Of additional concern, the incidence of melanoma has continue to rise over the past few decades.[1] Primary melanoma most commonly arises in the skin. However, melanoma can arise less commonly in other sites such as the orbit and mucosa. This chapter focuses on imaging for cutaneous melanoma.

The utility of imaging studies in patients with melanoma generally depends on the melanoma stage. There is little, if any, role for comprehensive imaging in patients with early-stage disease where surgery is often curative.[2] Preoperative lymphoscintigraphy is generally first performed to identify site(s) of regional nodal drainage and patients with multiple draining nodal basins, as well as to locate unpredictable nodal basins outside the standard nodal basins. Intraoperative lymphatic mapping and sentinel lymph node biopsy (SLNB) provide accurate staging of melanoma patients with no clinically detectable nodal disease.[2] Hematogenous dissemination is more likely in advanced regional disease and can occur in any organ system and, unfortunately, at any time. For distant metastases, computed tomography (CT), magnetic resonance imaging (MRI) and positron emission tomography (PET)/CT are the imaging modalities in general use. Ultrasound (US) is commonly performed to evaluate surgical scars, new palpable lesions, lymph nodes with equivocal findings on other examinations, and/or lymph node basins at risk for metastatic disease.[2] Imaging, therefore, plays an important role in staging, treatment planning, and posttreatment follow-up of patients with melanoma.

EPIDEMIOLOGY AND RISK FACTORS

Epidemiology

Melanoma accounts for 4% to 7% of new cancer diagnoses in the United States and is the fifth and sixth most common new cancer diagnosis in men and women, respectively.[3] In 2021, 106,110 new cases of melanoma and 7,180 deaths are projected to occur in the United States.[3] The average lifetime risk for developing melanoma is approximately 1 in 50.[4] Furthermore, its incidence continues to increase throughout much of the world.[4] Although the exact etiology for these epidemiologic trends is not entirely clear, and is certainly multifactorial, the rising incidence is thought to be at least partly related to increased sun exposure and early detection through screening programs. The incidence of melanoma also has a notable geographic variation, with the highest incidence in Australia/New Zealand, followed by Europe and then North America. Whereas the reasons for this are multiple and likely multifactorial, it is likely at least in part owing to the sun exposure and fair skin complexions of populations in these countries.[5]

Risk Factors

Cutaneous melanoma can occur in any skin location but most commonly occurs in sunlight-exposed areas, such as the head, neck, and extremities. Nonetheless, truncal melanoma is also common, particularly among males. Ultraviolet (UV) light exposure is considered to be an important environmental risk factor for cutaneous melanoma; the risk may be associated with the duration, intensity, and age of UV exposure. UV light has a damaging effect on DNA.[6]

In men, approximately one-third of melanomas are on the trunk, most commonly the back, and in women, the most common site is in the lower extremities.[6] These distributional differences may reflect sun exposure patterns between the sexes.

Melanomas are generally associated with nevi, particularly dysplastic nevi. A positive family history of melanoma is also associated with an increased risk of developing melanoma. Susceptibility for some families is due to mutation in one of the known high-penetrance melanoma predisposition genes: *CDKN2A*, *CDK4*, *BAP1*, *POT1*, *ACD*, TERF2IP, and *TERT*.[7]

KEY POINTS Epidemiology and Risk Factors

- Melanoma accounts for 4% to 7% of new cancer diagnoses in the United States.
- The lifetime risk is 1 in 50.
- The primary risk factor is ultraviolet light exposure.
- A variety of susceptibility genes has been identified.

ANATOMY AND PATHOLOGY

Anatomy

Melanomas are derived from melanocytes, the pigment-producing cells in skin, and are of neural crest origin. These cells are distributed widely throughout the skin as a result

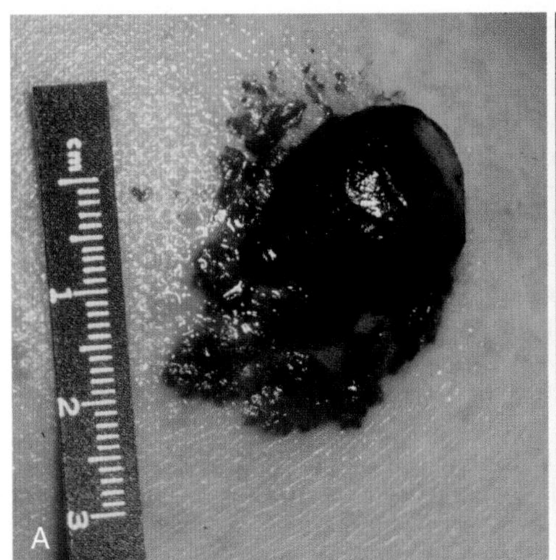

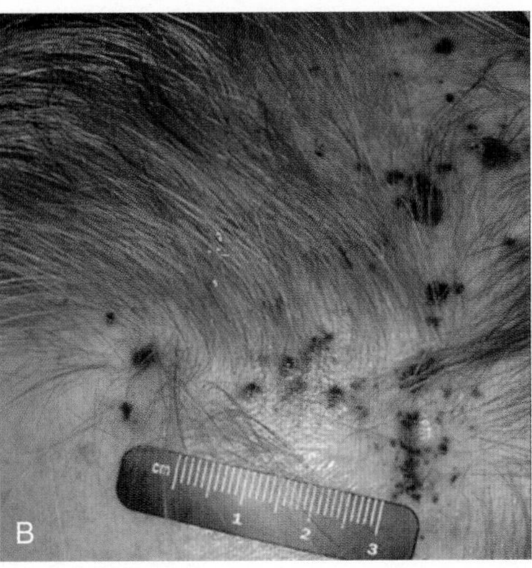

FIGURE 37.1. Cutaneous melanoma. **A**, Primary superficial spreading and polypoid ulcerated melanoma of the posterior shoulder measures 11 mm (on pathology evaluation, this lesion was found to have 5 mitoses/mm^2). **B**, Multiple pigmented metastatic melanoma lesions are seen scattered across the scalp.

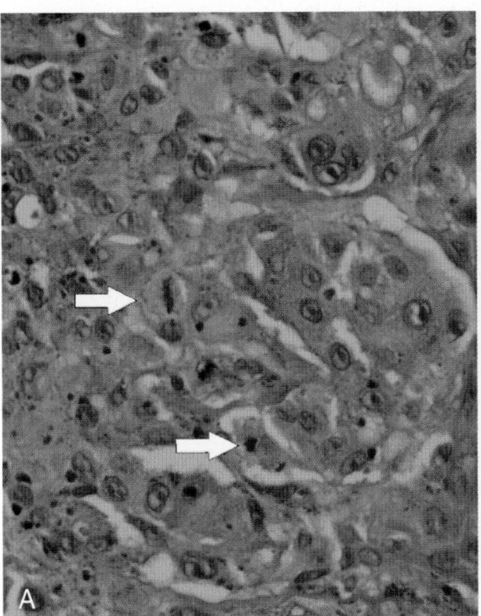

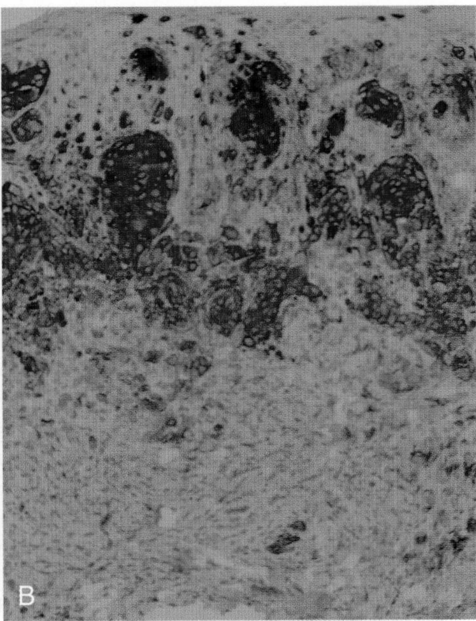

FIGURE 37.2. Cutaneous melanoma. **A**, Hematoxylin and eosin–stained histology slide of cutaneous melanoma shows large, atypical melanocytes with scattered mitotic figures (*arrows*; original magnification ×400). **B**, Tumor cells express the melanocytic marker glycoprotein 100 (with HMB45) (HMB45, aminoethylcarbazol, original magnification ×200). (**A** and **B** courtesy of Victor G. Prieto, M.D., Ph.D.)

of their embryologic origin. Melanocytes can also be found in other sites and give rise to uncommon primary melanomas. Examples of noncutaneous sites in which melanomas occur include the eye (e.g., conjunctiva, retina, and uveal tract) and mucosal surfaces (e.g., sinonasal, vulvovaginal, and anorectal).[8,9] Primary visceral melanoma is extremely rare but has also been reported.[10,11]

Melanomas typically contain melanin, which accounts for their characteristic dark appearance (Fig. 37.1). However, some melanomas do not contain obvious visible melanin and are termed amelanotic.

Although the appearance of some cutaneous lesions is highly suggestive of melanoma, definitive diagnosis is based on histologic assessment of the primary lesion. In general, the diagnosis of melanoma is based on a combination of standard hematoxylin and eosin staining, as well as confirmatory immunohistochemical studies using, for example, antibodies against melanocytic antigens such as S100 protein, melan-A, or glycoprotein 100 (as detected by the antibody HMB45) (Fig. 37.2). HMB45 can help distinguish melanoma *in situ* from sun-damaged skin/pigmented actinic keratosis. A confluent pattern of growth is observed with melanoma *in situ* compared with scattered atypical melanocytes found in sun-damaged skin or a pigmented actinic keratosis.[12]

Cutaneous melanomas typically grow from the epidermis toward the subcutaneous tissues (through papillary dermis, then reticular dermis, then subcutaneous tissues). Careful histologic evaluation of the primary melanoma is paramount, and pathologists should report important parameters such as the thickness of the primary lesion, the presence or absence of primary tumor ulceration, mitotic rate, lymphovascular invasion, neurotropism (perineural and intraneural invasion), tumor-infiltrating lymphocytes, and microsatellites.[13] Additionally, the determination of the mutational status of the melanoma tumors is of pivotal importance in the era of target therapy.[14]

> **Key Points Anatomy and Pathology**
>
> - Melanomas are derived from melanocytes, originating from the neural crest.
> - Melanomas typically contain melanin, but some do not contain significant amounts of melanin and are classified as amelanotic.
> - Melanomas most commonly arise in the skin and may arise in other areas (e.g., eye and mucosae).
> - Diagnosis must be confirmed histologically.
> - Tumor thickness is a key prognostic marker in cutaneous melanoma.
> - Other primary tumor prognostic markers include ulceration, mitotic rate, lymphovascular invasion, neurotropism (perineural and intraneural invasion), tumor-infiltrating lymphocytes, and microsatellites.

CLINICAL PRESENTATION

The vast majority of patients with cutaneous melanoma present with a new or changing skin lesion that can occur essentially anywhere on the body. These are typically, but not always, darkly pigmented; pigmentation may be heterogeneous or homogeneous. Lesions may or may not be raised and nodular (see Fig. 37.1). The diagnosis of cutaneous melanoma on clinical examination is fraught with difficulty and error; a reliable diagnosis of melanoma requires biopsy and histopathologic evaluation. Biopsies should be strongly considered for any pigmented lesions that have a change in color, size, or morphology. The ABCDEs of lesion classification as described by Rigel and coworkers[15] may be used to identify skin lesions suspicious for melanoma and deserving of biopsy. "A" describes asymmetry, "B" describes border irregularity, "C" is for color variegation, "D" denotes a diameter greater than 6 mm, and "E" is for a lesion that is evolving or enlarging. A small subset of skin lesions ultimately confirmed to be melanoma that are not hyperpigmented are classified as amelanotic. In some patients with a newly diagnosed primary melanoma, a synchronous or second primary can be found. Moreover, a small subset of newly diagnosed patients may present with metastatic melanoma to lymph nodes with an unknown primary tumor.[16] Rarely, patients my present with signs and symptoms of distant metastatic disease at initial melanoma diagnosis.

PATTERNS OF TUMOR SPREAD

Cutaneous melanoma is considered to have a high metastatic potential. Cutaneous melanoma can metastasize hematogenously or by the lymphatic system. Lymphatic dissemination is the most common first route of spread. The tumor can metastasize via lymphatics with or without hematogenous dissemination. Nodal metastases often involve regional nodal basins before distal spread. Thus, cutaneous primary melanomas in the lower extremities tend to first metastasize to ipsilateral inguinal nodes, whereas upper extremity primaries first involve axillary nodes. The lymphatic pathways for truncal lesions are not predictable and may drain to one or more of the bilateral cervical, axillary, or ilioinguinal regional basins. Melanomas arising in the head and neck also often have complex lymphatic drainage patterns.

Lymphoscintigraphy is used for localization of sentinel lymph nodes before surgery. The sentinel lymph node is the first draining lymph node on the afferent lymphatic pathway from the primary tumor. However, more than one pathway (i.e., more than one sentinel node and/or regional nodal basin) may drain a primary tumor. Thompson and associates found 13 of 4262 patients (0.31%) with primary melanomas of the distal lower extremities to develop popliteal nodal metastases.[17] Because popliteal nodal involvement from melanoma is uncommon, indications for popliteal nodal dissection include a positive histologic popliteal fossa sentinel node or clinical detection of popliteal nodal disease. Uren and coworkers observed drainage to the epitrochlear region in 36 of 218 patients (16%) with melanomas on the forearm or hand.[18]

A feature of lymphatic dissemination in cutaneous melanoma that is not commonly seen in other tumors is intralymphatic disease. Intralymphatic disease include satellite lesions and in-transit metastases. The American Joint Committee on Cancer (AJCC) defines in-transit metastases as any skin or subcutaneous metastases that are more than 2 cm from the primary lesion but are not beyond the regional nodal basin. Lesions occurring within 2 cm of the primary tumor are classified as satellite metastases.[19] Risk factors for in-transit disease include age older than 50 years, a lower extremity primary tumor, increasing Breslow depth, ulceration, and positive sentinel lymph node status.[20] Satellite metastasis, in-transit metastasis, and lymph node metastasis represent locoregional metastasis.

Hematogenous metastases from melanoma can occur essentially anywhere.[21] The more common sites of such spread include the lung (parenchyma), soft tissue, liver, and brain. However, metastases can occur in essentially any organ, such as in the gastrointestinal, genitourinary, and musculoskeletal systems. Pleural and peritoneal implants may also occur.

Primary uveal melanoma, unlike primary cutaneous melanoma, tends to preferentially metastasize hematogeneously (rather than via lymphatics), most commonly to the liver. In patients with metastatic uveal melanoma, the liver is involved in 71.4% to 87% of cases.[8] Liver metastases can appear up to 15 years after the initial diagnosis of primary uveal melanoma. Uveal melanoma cells have been shown in studies to express receptors (e.g., c-Met, insulin-like growth factor-1 receptor, and CXCR4) for ligands (e.g., hepatocyte growth factor, insulin-like growth-factor-1, and stromal-derived factor-1) produced in the liver. The binding of these receptors and ligands contributes to cell growth and motility and increased invasiveness.[22]

A disconcerting feature of metastatic melanoma is that it can affect almost any organ system. The risk of metastasis is related to the primary pathology. Metastatic disease may occur at almost any time in a patient with an advanced primary melanoma, particularly with nodal involvement. The risk, however, for a young patient with a thin T1a melanoma is rather low.

KEY POINTS Tumor Spread

- Lymphatic dissemination typically precedes hematogenous spread, most commonly to regional nodes.
- Satellite metastases are defined as lesions occurring within 2 cm of the primary tumor.
- In-transit metastases are defined as any skin or subcutaneous metastases that are more than 2 cm from the primary lesion but are not beyond the regional nodal basin.
- Risk factors for in-transit metastases include age older than 50 years, lower extremity primary tumor, increasing Breslow depth, ulceration, and positive sentinel lymph node status.
- Hematogenous metastases may occur anywhere, although "common" sites of distant metastatic melanoma include lung, soft tissue, liver, and brain.

STAGING AND PROGNOSIS

The tumor-node-metastasis (TNM) classification is used for staging melanoma. The seventh edition of the AJCC staging system for cutaneous melanoma published in 2009 has been superseded by the eighth edition of the *AJCC Cancer Staging Manual*, released in 2018.[23] The eighth edition not only includes assessment of the primary tumor and the presence or absence of regional nodal and distant metastases, which are the basis for staging (Fig. 37.3), but also consider nonanatomic factors, with the objective of improving staging and prognostic assessment.[23]

Primary Tumor Classification

The T category is based on primary tumor thickness, determined by measuring the maximal thickness from the top of the epidermal granular layer to the bottom of the tumor using an ocular micrometer.[24] Strata are primarily defined as T1 to T4. T1 lesions are melanomas that are 1 mm or less in thickness (and are also known as thin melanomas). A T2 lesion is greater than 1 mm to 2 mm, and a T3 lesion is greater than 2 mm to 4 mm (together they comprise intermediate-thickness melanomas). Melanomas greater than 4 mm in thickness are T4 lesions and are clinically classified as thick melanomas.

In the eighth edition of the AJCC staging system, there was an addition of a 0.8-mm tumor thickness criterion for subcategorizing T1 melanomas. This criterion was a more powerful prognostic factor than mitotic rate, and for this reason mitotic rate as a dichotomous variable was removed as a T1 subcategory criterion. Currently, T1a melanomas include those less than 0.8 mm without ulceration, while T1b melanomas include those that are 0.8 to 1 mm in thickness with or without ulceration and those less than 0.8 mm with ulceration.[25] In addition to these strata, in the eighth edition the definitions of Tis, T0, and TX have been clarified. Tis is used for melanoma *in situ* (i.e., no invasive component is present). T0 is designated when no evidence of a primary tumor can be found (e.g., a patient presenting with an inguinal nodal metastasis of melanoma with no evidence of a primary tumor). TX is used when the tumor thickness cannot be determined (e.g., in a curettage specimen when there is no sectioning of the tumor perpendicular to the skin surface) or there is no information about the T category for the primary tumor (e.g., a primary melanoma that was resected many years previously, and the primary melanoma report cannot be found).[19,23]

Primary tumor thickness at the time of diagnosis is the major determinant of prognosis and is used for treatment planning. For ulcerated lesions, primary tumor thickness is measured from the ulcer base to the bottom of the tumor. The level of invasion, originally defined by Clark, is no longer in use, because of its limited independent prognostic significance in contemporary multivariate modeling. Instead, tumor thickness, tumor ulceration, and tumor mitotic rate are powerful primary tumor prognostic factors in patients with primary melanoma. There is an inverse relationship between tumor thickness and prognosis, with a significant decrease in survival with increasing tumor thickness. Patients with an ulcerated melanoma have a lower survival rate than those patients with a nonulcerated primary lesion.[19,23]

Lymph Node

The most common first site of metastatic disease in patients with primary melanoma is regional lymph nodes. In patients with negative regional lymph nodes on clinical examination, intraoperative lymphatic mapping, and SLNB are often used to surgically stage otherwise clinically negative regional nodal basins in patients deemed to have sufficient risk of harboring occult stage III disease. Overall, the histologic status of the sentinel node is the most important predictor of survival in such patients.

The eighth edition of AJCC revised the N category, which reflects the number and extent of tumor-involved regional lymph nodes and the extent of nonnodal regional metastasis.[19,23] The previously used terms "microscopic" and "macroscopic" regional disease have been replaced by "clinically occult" (i.e., patients without clinical or radiographic evidence of regional lymph node metastasis but who have tumor-involved regional nodal metastasis found at SLNB) and "clinically detected" (i.e., patients with tumor-involved regional lymph nodes detected by clinical examination or radiographic imaging) to enhance clarity. These correspond to N category designations "a" and "b," respectively.[19,23]

The eighth edition of AJCC grouped nonnodal regional disease (i.e., satellites, in-transit metastases, and microsatellites) for staging purposes, due to similar survival outcomes. The presence of microsatellites, satellites, or in-transit metastases is now categorized as N1c, N2c, or N3c, based on the number of tumor-involved regional lymph nodes. The definition of a microsatellite was refined and clarified; a microsatellite is a microscopic cutaneous and/or subcutaneous metastasis adjacent or deep to, but discontinuous from, a primary melanoma detected on pathological examination of the primary tumor site. Satellite metastases are classically defined as any foci of clinically evident cutaneous and/or subcutaneous metastases occurring within 2 cm of but discontinuous from the primary melanoma. In-transit metastases are classically defined as clinically evident cutaneous and/or subcutaneous metastases occurring greater than 2 cm from the primary melanoma in the

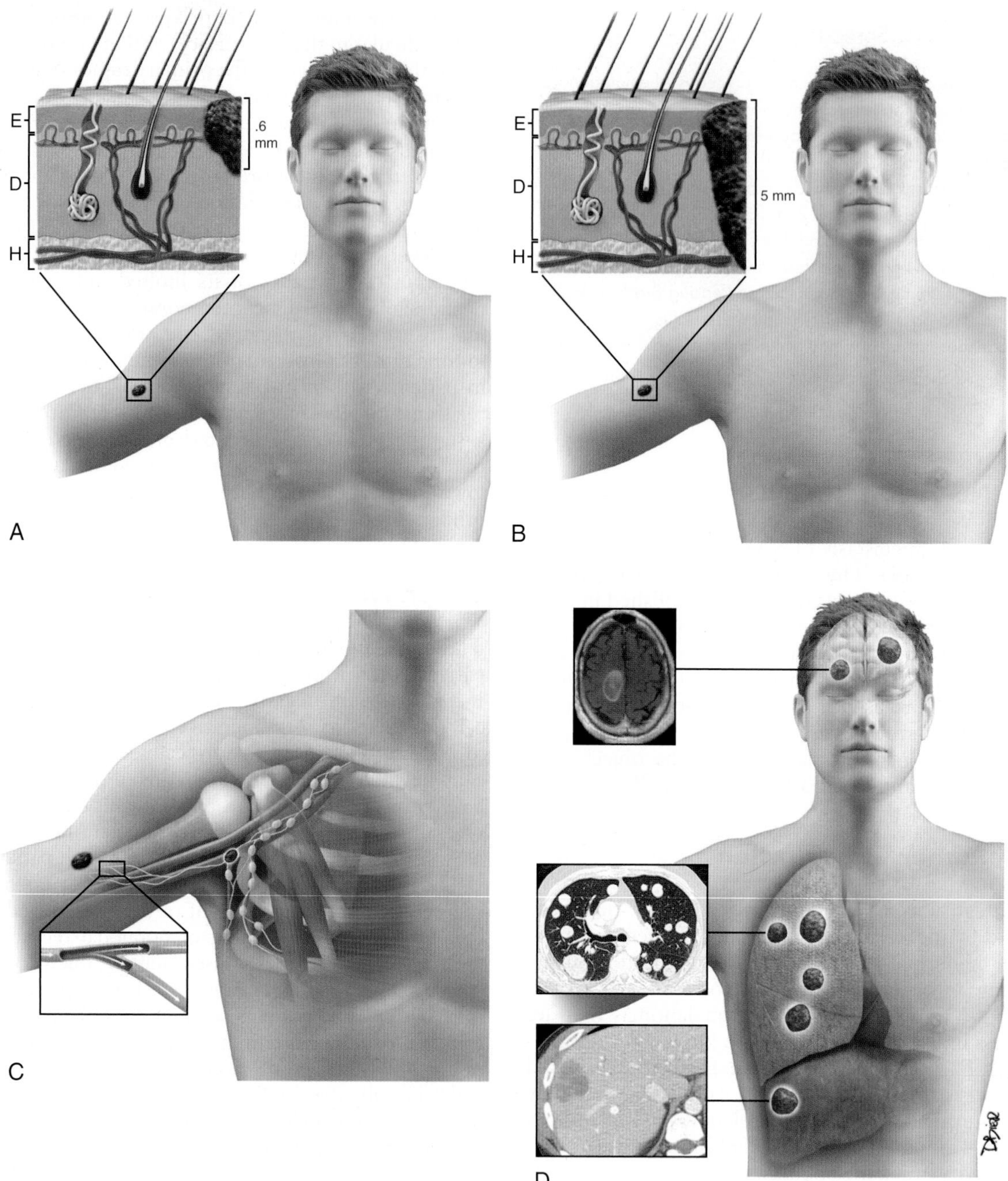

FIGURE 37.3. Tumor-node-metastatis staging schematic of primary melanoma of the right upper arm. **A**, Stage I: A magnified view demonstrates melanoma along the skin surface penetrating 0.6 mm into the dermis (D). *E*, Epidermis; *H*, hypodermis. **B**, Stage II: A magnified view demonstrates further penetration of melanoma cells to involve the subcutaneous fat. Stage I and II lesions are without evidence of nodal or metastatic disease. **C**, Stage III: Tumor has spread via lymphatics to a right axillary lymph node, located lateral and subjacent to the pectoralis musculature. Macrometastasis is demonstrated by this enlarged lymph node (as denoted in black). **D**, Stage IV disease is evidenced by distant metastases to the brain, lung, and liver.

region between the primary melanoma and the regional lymph node basin.[19,23]

Sentinel lymph node tumor burden provides important prognostic information and is a dominant independent predictor of survival in patients with nodal metastases.[19] The number of tumor-involved lymph nodes is also an important predictor of survival. The presence of nonnodal regional disease (i.e., satellites, in-transit metastases, and microsatellites) has been associated with a dverse prognosis.[26]

Metastatic Subgroups

The M category is defined as presence of distant metastatic disease and serum lactate dehydrogenase (LDH) level. M0 indicates no detectable evidence of distant metastatic disease, and the presence of distant metastatic disease is noted as M1. The M category is further subdivided based on anatomic site(s) of distant disease and LDH level. In the eighth edition of AJCC, a new M1d designation for distant metastasis to the central nervous system (CNS) has been added, and M1c no longer includes patients with CNS metastasis.[19,23] Currently, patients with nonvisceral distant metastasis (distant cutaneous, subcutaneous, nodal) are categorized as M1a, and they have a relatively better prognosis than those with distant metastases to other sites. Presence of pulmonary metastases constitutes M1b disease and is associated with an intermediate prognosis. M1c is defined as metastatic disease to non-CNS viscera. M1d is defined as metastatic disease to CNS with or without any other distant sites of disease and has a very poor prognosis. Patients with an elevated LDH level have a significant reduction in survival; therefore, the revised M category now includes a suffix (0) or (1) to signify the absence or presence of an elevated LDH, respectively, for each M1 category.[19,23]

Clinical Stage Groups

There are no changes of definitions of clinical stage groups between the seventh and eighth edition AJCC melanoma staging systems. According to the AJCC staging system, stages I and II groupings are primary melanomas without evidence of nodal or distant metastases. Stage III groupings include nodal involvement, and stage IV includes nodal and distant metastases.[23]

Pathological Stage Groups

In the eighth edition AJCC staging system, patients with pathological T1bN0M0 melanoma are included in the pathological stage IA subgroup and not in the pathological stage IB subgroup as before, due to overall better prognosis of patient with T1b melanoma with pathological negative nodes compared with patient with T1b melanoma with clinically negative nodes (some of whom will have pathologically positive nodes).[19,23] Stage II melanoma remains unchanged. Stage III melanoma is currently subdivided into four more accurate prognosis stage subgroups in the eighth edition of the AJCC staging system based on the combination of the T category (i.e., adding tumor thickness along with ulceration) and N category (number of tumor-involved lymph nodes, whether they were clinically detected or clinically occult, and the presence of microsatellite, satellite, and/or in-transit metastases) factors. There are no changes to stage IV group.[19,23]

Prognosis

Patients with stage I and II melanoma have the best prognosis, with a 5-year survival rate of over 97% in patients for stage I and between 85% and 92% for stage II.[19] However, patients with stage IIC disease (thick ulcerated tumors without involved nodes) have risk comparable to stage IIIA patients, and adjuvant treatment options for this high-risk group are under exploration. In patients with regional lymph node metastases (i.e., stage III) the prognosis is highly variable due to significant heterogeneity among the stage III population. For example, in patients with stage IIIA primary tumors (tumors <1 mm with or without ulceration and tumors >1–2 mm without ulceration, with up to three microscopically involved regional lymph nodes), the 5-year survival rate is approximately 80% to 93%%, whereas the 5-year survival for patients with stage IIID (4 mm with ulceration and four or more microscopically involved regional lymph nodes or at least one clinically positive lymph node) decreases to 32%.[19] Overall, patients with distant metastatic melanoma (stage IV) have a poor prognosis, with a 5-year overall survival between 9% and 28%. In carefully selected subsets of patients with limited metastatic disease, surgical resection may be associated with prolonged survival, even though patients with distant metastases usually have a poor 5-year survival rate.[19]

Key Points Staging

- Staging has a significant impact on prognostic and treatment decision-making.
- Tumor thickness and ulceration remain the key T category criteria and are important predictors of survival.
- Although mitotic rate was removed as a T category criteria in the eighth edition of the American Joint Committee on Cancer (AJCC) staging system, it remains a very important factor.
- The risk of metastatic disease increases with T stage.
- In patients with negative regional lymph nodes on clinical examination, intraoperative lymphatic mapping and sentinel lymph node biopsy are used to surgically stage regional nodal basins at risk.
- The N category reflects both the number and extent of tumor-involved regional nodes, as well as extent of nonnodal regional metastasis.
- Stage III groups are based on both T and N category criteria and increased from three to four subgroups in the eighth edition of the AJCC staging system.
- Patients with distant metastasis are classified by site(s) of metastases (M1a, M1b, M1c, and M1d) and lactate dehydrogenase (LDH) level. The new M1d designation was added in the eighth edition of the AJCC staging system to represent the presence of metastatic disease to the central nervous system and to reflect the poor prognosis of these patients.
- Patients with an elevated LDH level have a significant reduction in survival.

IMAGING

Imaging studies play an essential role in the multidisciplinary management of patients with melanoma. It is used for staging to evaluate the extent and presence of metastatic disease, for surgical planning, to monitor the response to treatment, and in the surveillance of high-risk patients.

Primary Tumor

The T staging of cutaneous melanoma is based on histologic evaluation of the primary tumor. In general, there is no role of imaging in T staging of cutaneous melanoma. In rare cases, high-frequency US (>20 MHz) can be used to assess large primary tumors before surgical excision to evaluate the size and depth of the tumor. Hayashi and colleagues studied melanomas with high-frequency (30-MHz) US. In 68 of 70 sonographically well-seen melanomas (excluding two melanoma *in situ* lesions), they showed good correlation between sonographic and histologic thickness ($r = 0.887$) and concluded that high-frequency sonography is quite useful in preoperative prediction of tumor thickness and may be used as a complementary method.[27]

Nodal Disease and Distant Metastatic Disease

Imaging Modalities

Lymphoscintigraphy. Regional lymph nodes are the most common first site of metastatic disease (Fig. 37.4). In patients for whom SLNB is planned, preoperative lymphoscintigraphy is generally first performed to identify site(s) of regional nodal drainage and patients with multiple draining nodal basins, as well as to locate unpredictable nodal basins outside the standard nodal basins, and thus provide a roadmap before surgery.[28] Preoperatively, technetium-99m–labeled sulfur colloid and intraoperative vital blue dye (isosulfan blue 1%) are injected intradermally around the primary melanoma to assess the regional nodal basins at risk. A handheld gamma probe is used transcutaneously in the operating room to identify the sentinel lymph nodes that need to be removed. Radiocolloid and vital blue dye mapping are complementary techniques that, when used simultaneously, increase the accuracy (>99%) of identifying the sentinel lymph nodes compared with blue dye alone (84% accuracy).[29]

Ultrasound. Sonography is often used as the preferred modality of choice for equivocal or suspicious nodal disease on clinical examination and is now used as a modality for serial monitoring of lymph node beds in patients with a positive sentinel node, in place of completion lymph node dissection. Indeterminate superficial lymph nodes as imaged on CT and MRI can also be further evaluated with US.[30] The sonographic appearance of a normal lymph node is an oval-shaped node with a thin hypoechoic cortex and echogenic hilum (Fig. 37.5). Metastatic disease is suspected when there is an increase in nodal size and loss of the normal ovoid morphology. Involved nodes are often hypoechoic and round, with loss of their fatty hila (see Fig. 37.5). Involved lymph nodes can also have preservation of the normal sonographic lymph node architecture and an enlarged cortex with a preserved hyperechoic hilum (see Fig. 37.5). On some occasions, involved lymph nodes may have a prominent focal lobulation or bulge (see Fig. 37.5). This is secondary to asymmetrical tumor involvement of the lymph node. These lymph nodes are amenable to US-guided fine needle aspiration (FNA) for pathologic confirmation. Voit and associates described US features of sentinel lymph node melanoma involvement. They evaluated 400 sentinel lymph nodes in patients with melanoma and concluded that US and FNA can identify 65% of all sentinel node metastases, thus reducing the need for surgical sentinel node procedures. US characteristics of lymph nodes as described in their study include peripheral perfusion (an early sign of involvement), loss of central echoes, and a balloon-shaped lymph node (late signs of large-volume disease).[31] Sanki and coworkers however, performed US on 871 sentinel lymph nodes in 716 patients with melanoma. They found a sensitivity of 24.3% for US

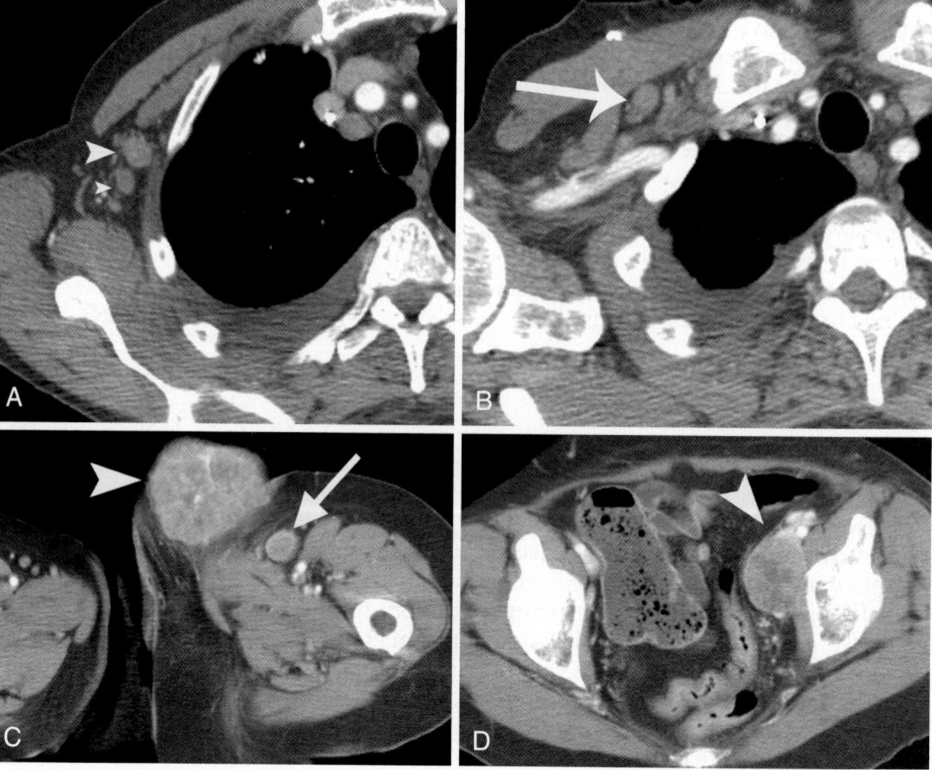

FIGURE 37.4. Nodal metastases. **A** and **B**, In this patient with a history of a primary melanoma on the back, level I right axillary adenopathy is seen lateral to the pectoralis minor muscle (*arrowheads* in **A**). Level III nodal disease is seen medial to the right pectoralis major muscle (*arrow* in **B**), an area that should be included in surgical lymph node dissection. **C**, Nodal metastasis is seen in the left inguinal nodal station (*arrow*) in this patient with primary calf melanoma who recurred after wide local excision of the primary tumor and incomplete left inguinal node dissection. Incidental bulky cutaneous disease is also present (*arrowhead*). **D**, Deep pelvic adenopathy is also in the left obturator nodal station (*arrowhead*).

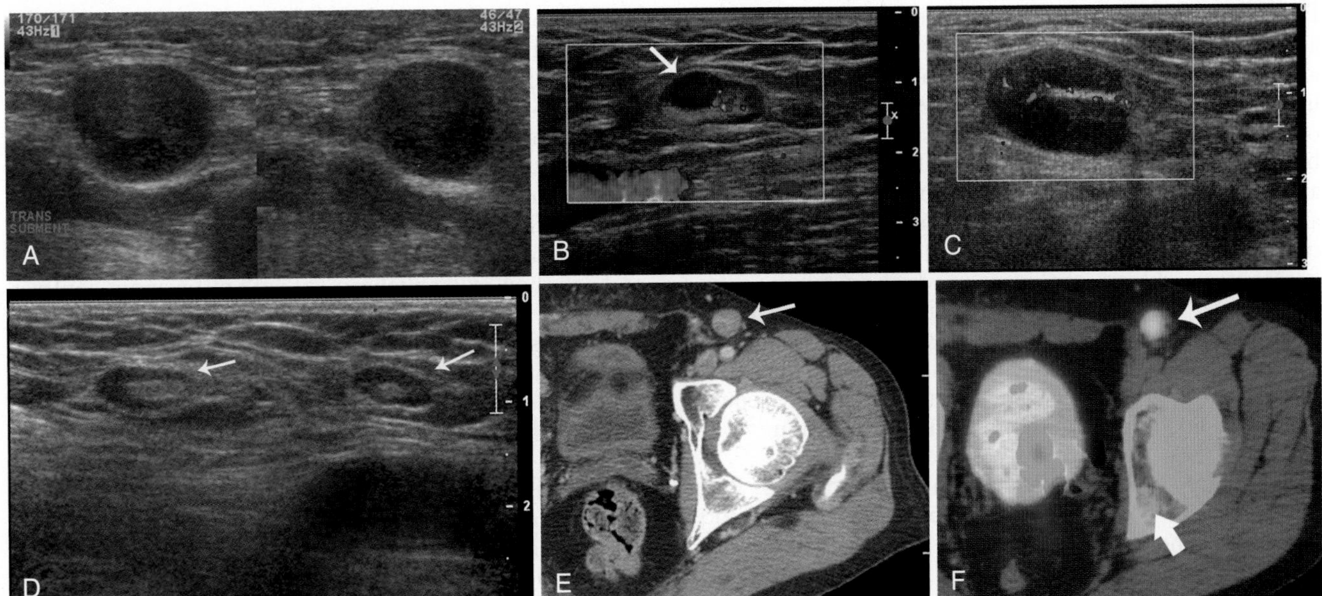

FIGURE 37.5. Ultrasound appearance of nodal metastases. **A**, Sonographic transverse and longitudinal images demonstrate a hypoechoic, round submental lymph node with absence of the fatty hilum and loss of the normal nodal architecture—an appearance suggesting melanoma involvement. **B**, Sonographic image of a right inguinal lymph node with a focal prominent hypoechoic lobulation (*arrow*) from asymmetrical tumor involvement of the lymph node in a patient with history of melanoma of the right great toe. **C**, Sonographic image of a left inguinal node demonstrates preservation of normal lymph node architecture, with normal hilar vessel color flow; however, there is enlargement of the nodal cortex. **D**, For comparison: normal appearance of inguinal lymph nodes (*arrows*) with a hyperechoic hilum and normal-sized hypoechoic cortex. **E** and **F**, Computed tomography (CT) and positron emission tomography/CT scans of the left inguinal lymph node (as shown in **C**) demonstrate diffuse enlargement and increased metabolic activity (*thin arrows*). Incidental note is made of metabolic uptake in the posterior left acetabulum (*thick arrow*) from osseous metastatic disease. The patient has other sites of osseous metastastic disease (not shown). These were not detected on the CT.

detection of positive sentinel lymph nodes and a specificity of 96.8% and concluded that US is not an adequate substitute for SLNB.[32]

Computed Tomography and Magnetic Resonance Imaging. There is no role for routine CT for *in situ*, stage I, and stage IIA, although patients with high-risk primaries (stages IIB and IIC) are often imaged before surgery to ensure absence of obvious metastatic foci. For patients with stage III disease and palpable nodal disease, CT may be useful in identifying other sites of metastatic disease that may preclude surgery in some patients.[33] CT and MRI imaging may be used in patients with stage III disease and microscopic disease in sentinel lymph nodes (asymptomatic patients), but the incidence of distant metastases is low.[33] CT may also be useful in patients with more advanced disease (stages IIIB, IIIC, and IV) to determine resectability and disease extent for surgical planning.[2]

On CT and MRI, an increase in the size of a lymph node compared with a prior examination can sometimes be an indicator of metastatic involvement. Tumor involvement may be suspected if there is a change in size, shape, or development of heterogeneity of the lymph node. However, these characteristics are not specific and may be the result of nonmalignant etiologies such as inflammation or infection, and pathological confirmation is usually necessary.

MRI is often used as a problem-solving tool, such as for the characterization of indeterminate liver lesions as imaged on CT. MRI is the modality of choice for brain metastases and for CNS surveillance in patients at high risk for developing brain metastases.

Positron Emission Tomography/Computed Tomography. PET/CT scanners provide both functional information and anatomic images in a single examination. Over the past decade, the use of PET/CT has expanded in the staging, treatment response assessment, and follow-up of patients with melanoma. The role of PET/CT in nodal disease detection is still evolving. It is important to note that PET/CT is not specific for detection of nodal disease. Enlarged lymph nodes may demonstrate increased metabolic activity on PET/CT; however, they may simply be reactive lymph nodes. Conversely, normal-sized lymph nodes may contain micrometastases below the sensitivity threshold of PET/CT, demonstrating no abnormal metabolic activity. In patients with stage I or II disease, the role of PET/CT is extremely limited, due to both the low sensitivity for occult regional lymphatic disease and the low incidence of more advanced disease in these patients.[34] The role of PET/CT in clinical stage III melanoma continues to evolve. Recently, Groen et al. reported that 18% of patients were restaged as stage IV in a retrospective study of 73 patients with stage III melanoma, which significantly affects patient management.[35]

In patients with advanced disease, PET/CT is at least as sensitive and is more specific than anatomic imaging modalities such as CT and MRI in the evaluation of disease extent and detection of distant metastases and can also identify lesions outside the field of conventional imaging.[36] Sensitivity is highest for metastases that are greater than 1 cm in diameter, but tumor deposits as small as 0.6 cm can be identified. The reported sensitivity for PET/CT in the detection of distant metastases is 80% to 91%.[36,37]

PET/CT can be used in patients with potentially resectable stage IV disease to exclude other sites of disease. It can also be used in patients with equivocal findings on other imaging such as CT or MRI. False negatives, however, can occur if there is small-volume disease in which the tumor burden is below the detection of PET/CT. False negatives are seen with bone marrow stimulation and in lymph nodes adjacent to brown fat uptake. Normal bowel concentration of tracer may obscure bowel metastases. Conversely, false-positive disease can occur in which metabolic activity may be due to inflammation, infection, postsurgical change, brown fat, exercised muscle, or normal activity in the bowel and urinary collecting systems. This can lead to misinterpretation of metastatic disease, which may require additional imaging or biopsy for further evaluation.[37]

Whole-Body Magnetic Resonance Imaging and Positron Emission Tomography/Magnetic Resonance Imaging. Whole-body MRI and PET/MRI are relatively new technologies and not yet as widely available as PET/CT, and consequently their role in the management of patients with melanoma remains to be defined.[38] Currently, when comparing PET/CT with whole-body MRI, PET/CT is usually more accurate in N-staging and detection of lung and soft tissue metastases, whereas whole-body MRI is superior in detecting liver, bone, and brain metastases.[39]

General Features

Although most patients with melanoma have localized disease at the time of diagnosis and are treated by surgical excision of the primary tumor, as many as half of patients will eventually relapse. Most of the recurrences will be local or in regional lymph nodes, and approximately one-third of patients will develop distant metastases.[40] Melanoma has the potential to metastasize to any organ. Metastatic lesions from melanoma can be round, oval, irregular, or lobulated and sometimes present as confluent masses. They can vary in size and number and can affect one organ system or several. They may be hypervascular and will show avid enhancement with intravenous contrast. However, after outgrowing their blood supply, melanoma metastases can become necrotic. Hematogenous metastases may occur essentially anywhere, although common sites of distant metastatic disease include lung, soft tissue, liver, and brain.

Metastatic Sites

Lung. The lungs are the second most common site of metastatic disease after nodal disease.[41] CT, in comparison with chest radiography, has a greater sensitivity for detection of intrathoracic metastatic disease. Pulmonary metastatic disease can present as a solitary nodule but is often multiple, rounded, and well-defined, as seen in other cancers (Fig. 37.6).[42] A single nodule in a patient with melanoma is more likely to be metastatic disease than a primary bronchogenic carcinoma.[43] Primary lung cancers may be difficult to distinguish from a melanoma metastasis, because some primary lung cancers can be round or oval and smoothly marginated. Some primary lung cancers, however, have spiculations of their margins (see Fig. 37.7).

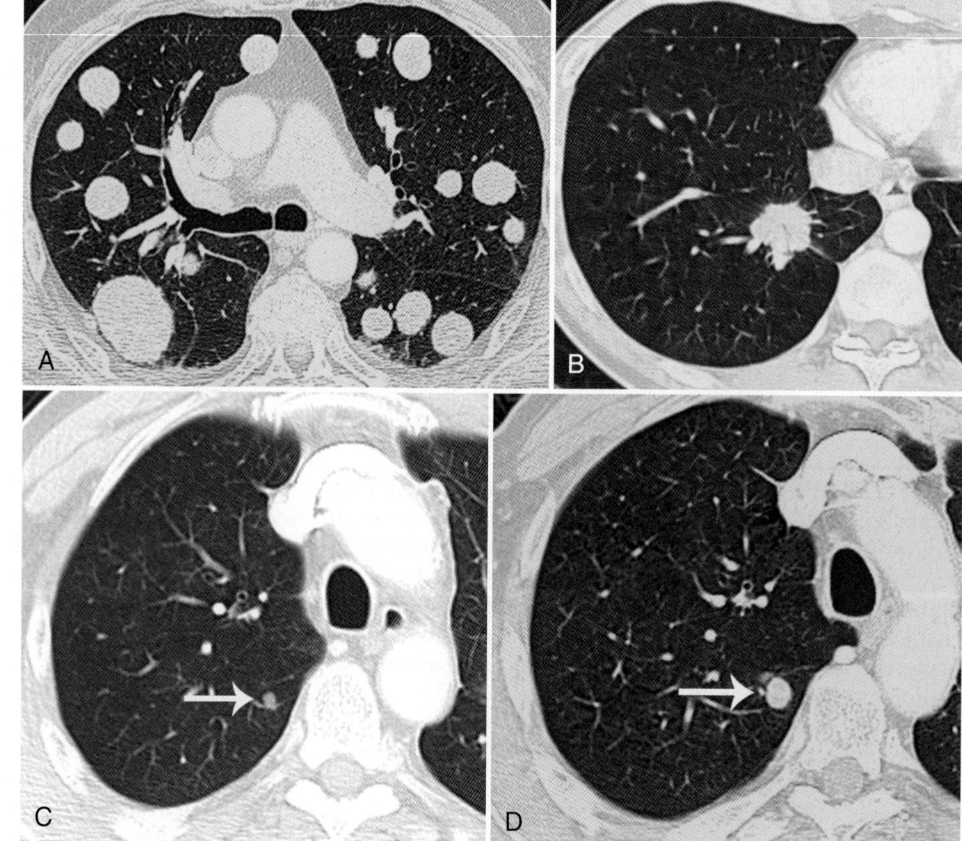

FIGURE 37.6. Computed tomography (CT) appearance of lung metastases. **A**, Axial CT scan of the chest demonstrates numerous bilateral lung metastases that are well-defined and rounded, as seen in other cancers. **B**, CT of the chest demonstrates a spiculated mass in the right lower lobe. This appearance can be seen in some primary lung cancers. **C** and **D**, Melanoma metastasis or a primary lung cancer can be round and well-defined, as seen in this growing melanoma lung metastasis (*arrow*) in the right upper lobe over a 3-month interval.

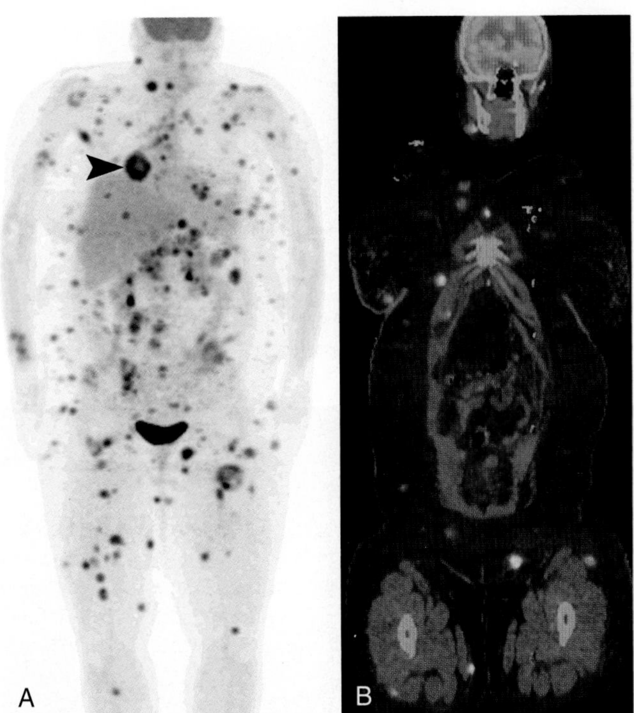

FIGURE 37.7. Widespread metastatic disease. **A** and **B**, Maximum intensity projection positron emission tomography (PET) image and fused PET/computed tomography scans demonstrate diffuse increased metabolic foci, most of which are related to subcutaneous metastatic deposits. A right lower lobe pulmonary metastasis is also seen (*arrowhead* in **A**).

Skin and Soft Tissues. Cutaneous or subcutaneous metastases are best detected by clinical examination or US. They appear as hypoechoic lesions with distal acoustic enhancement, often with increased vascularity on color Doppler.[44] On CT, these subcutaneous metastases manifest as soft-tissue–density nodules, but they may be inhomogeneous secondary to necrosis. These deposits are often detected as foci of increased metabolic activity on PET/CT (see Fig. 37.7).

Liver. As found on autopsy series, the liver is the third most common site of metastatic melanoma.[41] On US, melanoma liver metastases are typically hypoechoic relative to the surrounding liver. On CT, most melanoma metastases are low in attenuation compared with the normal liver on pre- and postintravenous contrast imaging (Fig. 37.8). Abdominal MRI is performed for indeterminate lesion characterization seen on other imaging modalities, including CT and US (Fig. 37.9). Approximately 50% of metastatic liver lesions will present with a typical melanotic appearance on MRI, with shortened T1 and T2 relaxation times indicating a high signal on T1-weighted (T1W) sequences and low signal on T2-weighted (T2W) sequences. Metastatic melanoma liver lesions that do not have a high melanin content will be hypointense on T1W MRI[45] (see Fig. 37.8). Hepatic melanoma metastases on PET/CT are 2-[^{18}F] fluoro-2-deoxy-D-glucose (FDG)-avid and appear as foci of increased metabolic activity (see Fig. 37.8).

Brain. Melanoma is the third most common cause of brain metastases, following breast and lung cancer. Until recently, melanoma brain metastases carried a very poor prognosis, with a median overall survival of approximately 4 to 5 months. However, improvements in radiation and systemic therapies are offering promise for this challenging complication, and thus more stringent CNS imaging guidelines should be considered.

Patients with melanoma can present with acute neurologic symptoms. Brain MRI is obtained based on patient symptoms; it is also performed in patients with stage IV disease to exclude asymptomatic disease. Brain MRI may also be obtained in patients with advanced regional disease to exclude brain metastasis.

If melanoma metastases are present on CT, they are hyperdense compared with the surrounding normal brain tissue on noncontrast images. Brain metastases, however, are best detected after the administration of intravenous contrast, with MRI being more sensitive than CT. Imaging characteristics of brain metastases from melanoma can vary. Melanin decreases T1 relaxation time on MRI. Therefore, if enough melanin is present, lesions will be hyperintense on T1W MRI (see Fig. 37.9). T1 hyperintensity can also be secondary to hemorrhage or fat. Melanin can shorten T2 relaxation times, so lesions will have decreased T2 signal intensity.[46] A T1 hyperintense lesion can be attributed to melanin, hemorrhage, or both.[47] Melanoma metastases have a propensity to hemorrhage, and so the paramagnetic effects of blood products (especially methemoglobin) may also result in T1 and T2 shortening in these lesions. An amelanotic pattern in which metastases contain less than 10% melanin-containing cells can also be seen and associated with a signal intensity pattern that is seen in metastases from other primary tumors. Such lesions will generally be isointense or hypointense on T1W images and isointense or hyperintense on T2W images[48] (see Fig. 37.9).

Metastatic disease to the gray-white matter junction is most common and can be solitary but is often multiple. Miliary and subependymal metastases are also seen.[46] Melanoma metastases can often present as punctuate or subtle lesions, often mistaken for normal blood vessels; owing to the rapid growth of metastatic disease, close follow-up imaging is needed (see Fig. 37.9).

Leptomeningeal disease detection can be problematic, because repeat lumbar punctures for cerebrospinal fluid testing may be inaccurate in 15% to 20% of cases.[49] MRI with intravenous contrast may be helpful in leptomeningeal disease detection, in which radiologic signs include leptomeningeal, dural, and cranial nerve enhancement; superficial cerebral metastasis; hydrocephalus; subependymal enhancement; and/or enhancement of subarachnoid nodules. False-positive leptomeningeal enhancement, however, can be seen with hemorrhage and inflammation due to infection or intrathecal chemotherapy.[50]

Head and Neck. Melanoma may metastasize not only to the brain parenchyma but also to other parts of the head and neck, including bone, muscle, skin, nasopharynx and mucosa, parotid gland, internal auditory canal, and orbit.[46] Metastatic disease to the thyroid gland is not common, but it can be seen in patients with various primary cancers, including renal, breast, lung, colon, or prostate cancer or melanoma.[51]

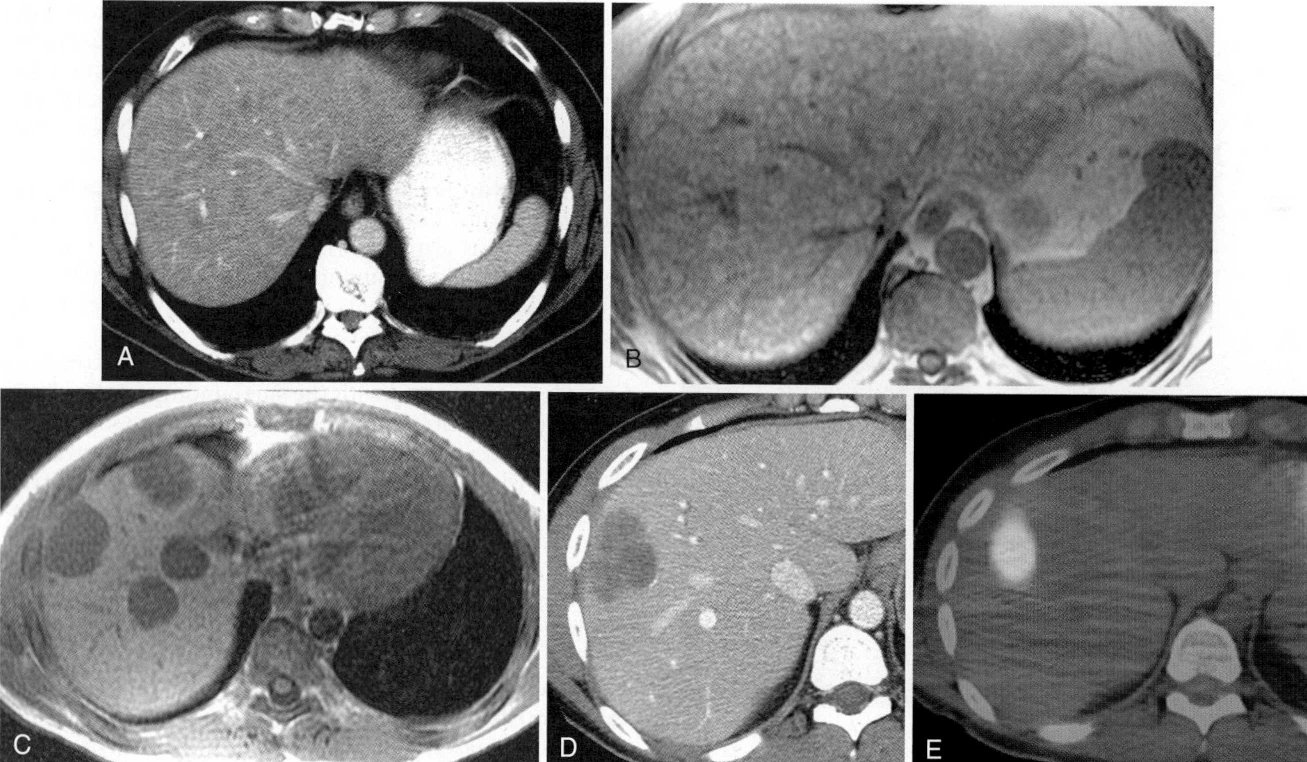

FIGURE 37.8. Hepatic metastases. **A**, Computed tomography (CT) scan of the liver after intravenous contrast in a patient with melanoma demonstrates a heterogeneous liver. Magnetic resonance imaging (MRI) was recommended, because discrete lesions could not be identified with CT. **B**, Axial T1-weighted (T1W) MRI of the liver without intravenous contrast in the same patient as in **A** demonstrates widespread hyperintense metastatic lesions throughout the liver from melanin and/or hemorrhage, a feature unique to melanoma. The MRI increased lesion conspicuity in this patient with an equivocal CT. **C**, Axial T1W MRI of the liver without intravenous contrast demonstrates multiple hypointense liver lesions from melanoma metastases, an imaging finding as seen in metastatic disease from other primary tumors and not specific to melanoma. Axial CT scan of the liver demonstrates a metastatic melanoma metastasis that is hypovascular compared with the surrounding liver parenchyma (**D**), with focal metabolic activity on fused positron emission tomography/CT scan (**E**).

Musculoskeletal System. Potepan and associates reviewed 120 melanoma bone metastases and found that most were osteolytic (87.5%). The second most common pattern was a mixed osteolytic-osteoblastic pattern, found in 10% of cases, and a pure osteoblastic pattern was seen in 2.5% of cases.[52] Heusner and coworkers studied 54 patients with nonsmall cell lung cancer and 55 patients with melanoma who underwent PET/CT as well as whole-body MRI. Of these 109 patients, 11 had bone metastases (eight patients with non–small-cell lung cancer and three with melanoma). They found that PET/CT and MRI were equal in detection of skeletal metastases in both of these patient populations[53] (Fig. 37.10). Bone scintigraphy may be negative owing to lack of bone reaction from metastases to the bone marrow. Gokaslan and colleagues studied 133 patients with melanoma metastases to the spine. Bone scan was performed in 85 of these patients, with a 15% false-negative rate compared with plain films, CT, or MRI.[54]

Muscle metastases may be the result of hematogenous spread or from extension from adjacent subcutaneous tissues or bone. On CT, these lesions may appear similar to other cancers that metastasize to muscle, manifesting as soft-tissue–density lesions that are isodense or hyperdense on preintravenous contrast images compared with the surrounding normal muscle.

Gastrointestinal Tract. The most frequently involved sites in the gastrointestinal tract are the small and large bowel (75% and 25%, respectively).[21] Disease can vary in size and present as single or multiple nodules, but can also be irregular or polypoid or have an infiltrating appearance. Complications of small bowel metastases include intussusception, small bowel obstruction, and perforation[55] (Fig. 37.11). Metastatic disease to the esophagus or stomach is uncommon. Metastatic disease can present as wall thickening with an appearance similar to adenocarcinoma.

Genitourinary Tract. Metastatic disease to the adrenal gland is nonspecific and has imaging characteristics similar to other cancers that metastasize to the adrenal gland. These metastases can present as lobulated, heterogeneously enhancing soft-tissue masses and are typically unilateral (Fig. 37.12); however, they can be bilateral in some patients.[56] Melanoma metastases to the kidney may be solid or cystic. Disease can also present as perirenal solid nodules. Urothelial metastases are less common, but, when they occur, can appear as an intraluminal filling defect on the excretory phase, as seen in transitional cell cancers. Metastases to the urinary bladder can also be similar to transitional cell carcinomas, presenting as a soft-tissue mass involving the urinary bladder wall.[21]

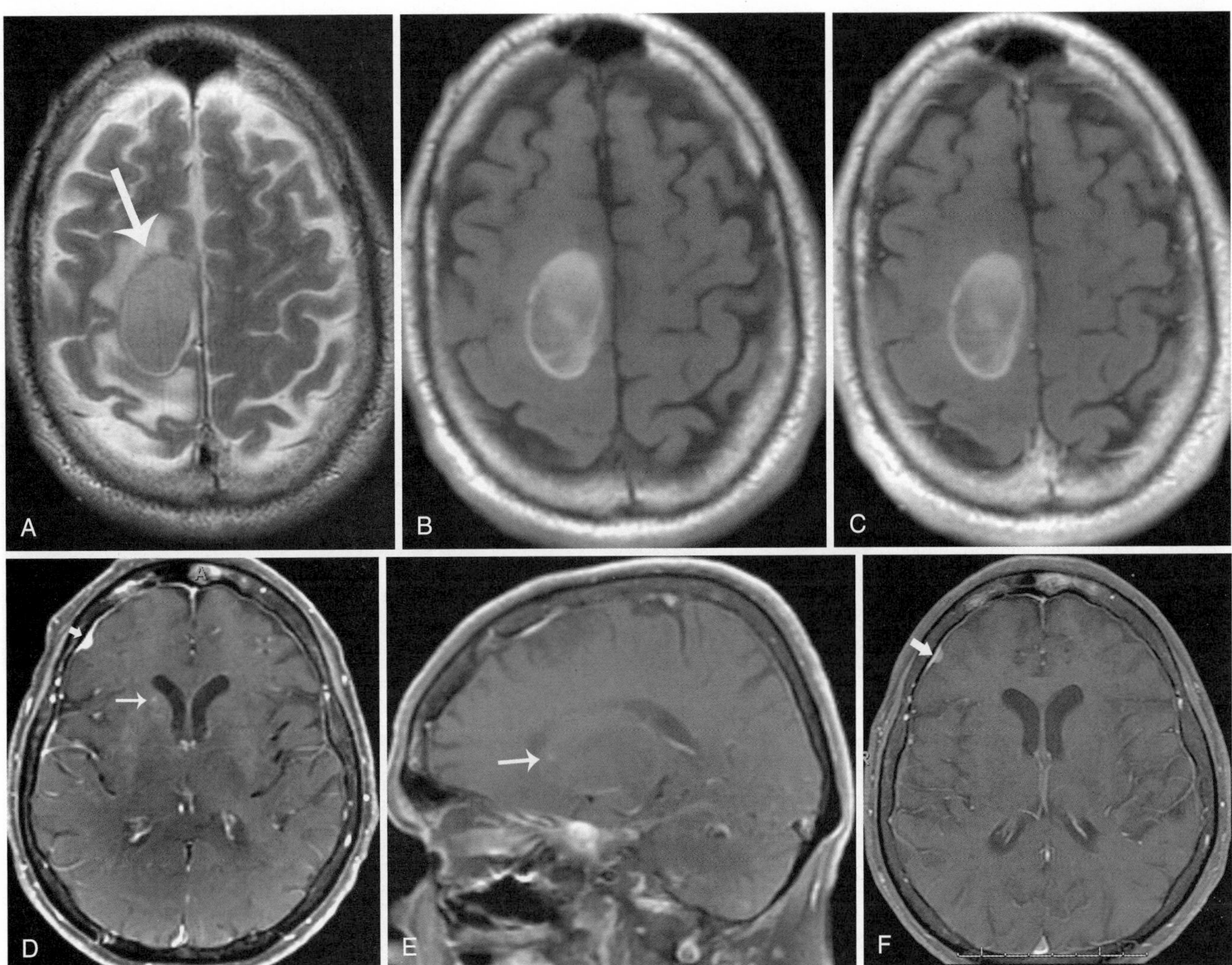

FIGURE 37.9. Brain metastasis. **A**, Axial T2-weighted magnetic resonance imaging (MRI) demonstrates a heterogeneous hyperintense mass (*arrow*) in the right parietal lobe with surrounding T2 hyperintense vasogenic edema. This lesion is hyperintense on T1-weighted MRI images before (**B**) and after (**C**) intravenous contrast. This hyperintensity on preintravenous contrast is due to hemorrhage, melanin, or a combination of the two. Sometimes metastases are punctate and can be mistaken for blood vessels. A punctate metastatic focus is seen in the right caudate lobe (*arrows* in **D** and **E**) on MRI axial (**D**) and sagittal T1 (**E**) post–intravenous contrast images not previously seen 6 months prior (**F**). Note incidental right frontal hemangioma (*short arrows* in **D** and **F**).

Metastatic disease to the ovaries can present as solid or solid/cystic masses. Metastasis from melanoma to the uterus or cervix is also rare. In an analysis of 63 cases of metastatic cancers to the uterine corpus from extragenital neoplasms, the most common extragenital neoplasm to metastasize to the uterine corpus was found to be breast cancer.[57]

Gallbladder, Pancreas, and Spleen. Primary gallbladder melanoma is very rare; however, melanoma is the most common tumor to metastasize to the gallbladder.[58] Metastatic disease to the pancreas and spleen is rare. The incidence of melanoma metastasis to the spleen is less than 5%.[59] Both splenic and pancreatic metastases can vary in size and number and may be solid or cystic (see Fig. 37.12). Metastatic disease to the pancreas may present as a hypervascular solid mass, similar to metastases from renal cell carcinoma or primary pancreatic neuroendocrine tumors.

Mesentery. Melanoma involving the small or large bowel mesenteries can manifest as single or multiple nodules or have an infiltrative appearance that is confluent, insinuating into surrounding tissues, a similar finding seen in lymphoma, carcinoid, or desmoid tumors[60] (Fig. 37.13). Jejunal small bowel adenopathy can be detected by locating the superior mesenteric vein and tracing the jejunal veins to the left side of the abdomen into the jejunal small bowel mesentery. Although uncommon, disease manifestation as seen in ovarian cancer can also occur in patients with melanoma, including peritoneal nodules or carcinomatosis (Fig. 37.14).

Thorax. Melanoma can metastasize to rare sites in the thorax, including the pleura, bronchi, breast, heart, and pericardium. Melanoma metastases have a propensity to metastasize to the myocardium[61] (Fig. 37.15).

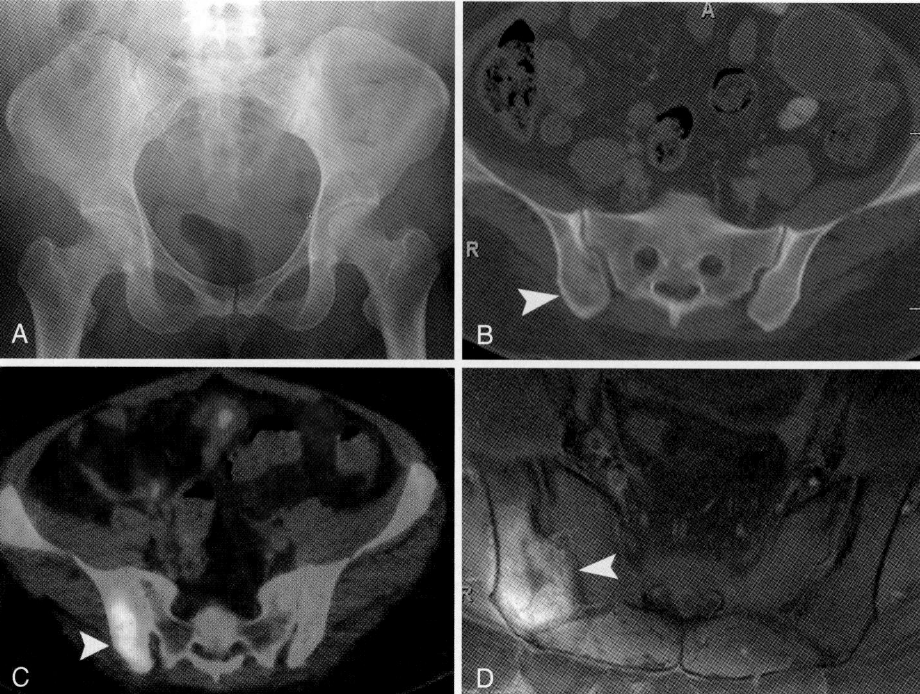

FIGURE 37.10. Bone metastasis. In this patient with widespread metastatic melanoma, osseous metastatic disease is not detected by radiography and is barely perceptible by computed tomography (CT). **A**, Plain film radiograph of the pelvis demonstrates no radiographic osseous metastatic disease or fracture. **B**, Axial CT scan of the pelvis with bone algorithm demonstrates subtle mild heterogeneity of the right posterior iliac bone (*arrowhead*). **C**, positron emission tomography/CT fused scan demonstrates increased metabolic activity in the posterior right iliac bone (*arrowhead*). **D**, Axial T1-weighted magnetic resonance imaging (MRI) after intravenous contrast demonstrates an enhancing lesion (*arrowhead*) in the posterior right iliac bone. Note the increased lesion conspicuity on MRI compared with CT.

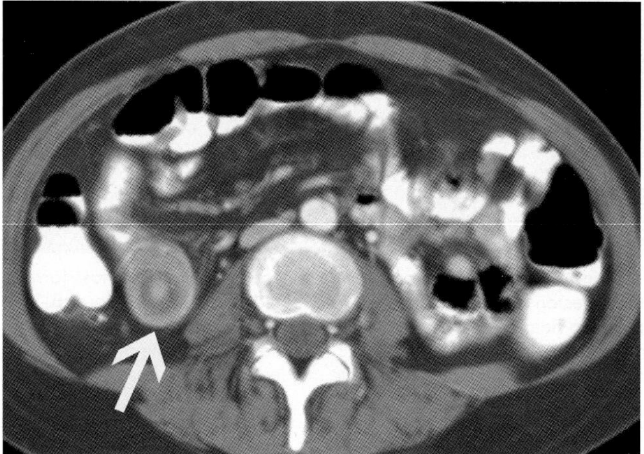

FIGURE 37.11. Small bowel metastasis with intussusception. Axial computed tomography scan of the abdomen with intravenous contrast demonstrates a nonobstructing proximal small bowel intussusception caused by metastasis to the small bowel. On cross-sectional imaging, an intussusception may appear as a "target" lesion (*arrow*).

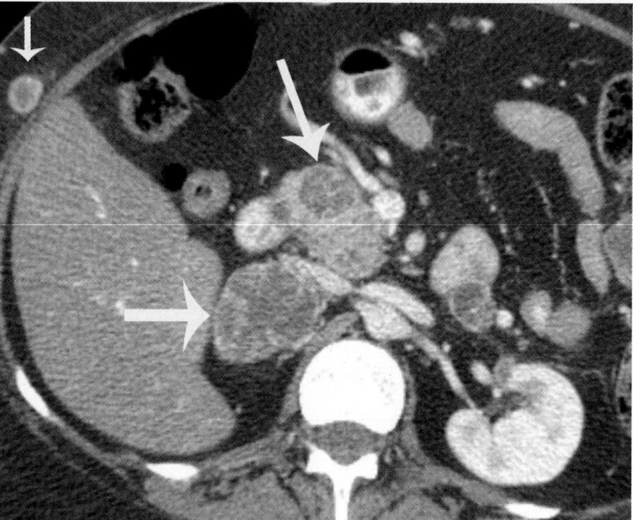

FIGURE 37.12. Adrenal and pancreas metastases. Axial computed tomography scan of the abdomen after the administration of intravenous contrast demonstrates melanoma metastases to the right adrenal gland (*short arrow*) and head of the pancreas (*long arrow*). Subcutaneous metastatic nodule is seen in the right anterior abdominal wall (*medium arrow*).

KEY POINTS Imaging

- The radiology report should include all sites of metastatic disease, with a thorough search of all organ systems including subcutaneous tissues and muscle.
- In patients undergoing sentinel lymph node biopsy, preoperative lymphoscintigraphy is generally first performed to identify site(s) of regional nodal drainage and patients with multiple draining nodal basins, as well as to locate unpredictable nodal basins outside the standard nodal basins.
- Ultrasound is now used for routine surveillance of lymph node basins with positive sentinel lymph nodes in patients who do not undergo complete lymph node dissection.
- Recognition of vertebral metastases causing spinal cord compression and neurologic compromise is important for possible radiotherapy.

TREATMENT

Treatment options include surgical and nonsurgical methods and will depend on the extent and stage of disease. The nonsurgical options include systemic chemotherapy,

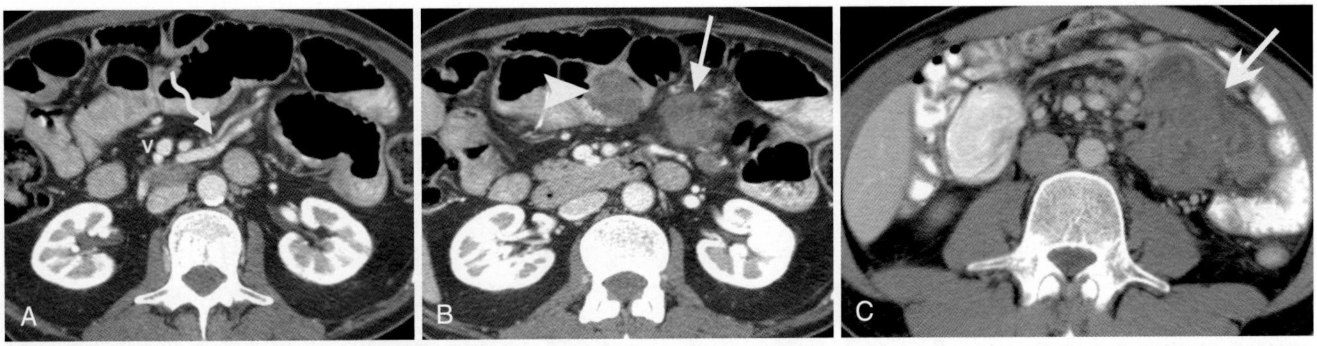

FIGURE 37.13. Confluent adenopathy. **A**, Jejunal small bowel adenopathy (as seen in **B** and **C**) can be found by locating the superior mesenteric vein (v) and tracing the jejunal veins (*squiggly arrow*) into the jejunal small bowel mesentery. **B** and **C**, Axial computed tomography scans of the abdomen with intravenous contrast demonstrate confluent adenopathy in the jejunal small bowel mesentery (*arrows*) in two different patients, a finding similarly seen in patients with lymphoma. An incidental small bowel metastasis is also seen in **B** (*arrowhead*).

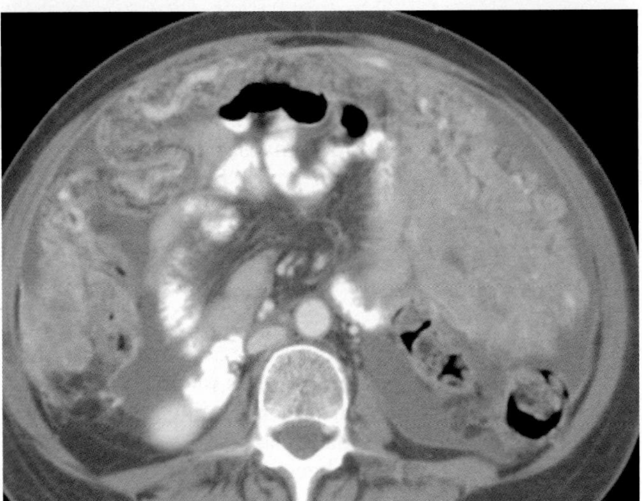

FIGURE 37.14. Axial computed tomography scan of the abdomen with intravenous contrast demonstrates diffuse peritoneal carcinomatosis and ascites in a patient with a history of a primary melanoma of her left lower back.

radiation therapy, cytokine therapy, immunotherapy, molecularly-targeted therapy, and experimental therapies.

Surgery and Lymph Node Dissection

Surgical treatment involves wide local excision that resects the primary tumor and surrounding healthy tissue, and represents the mainstay of treatment for early-stage disease. The recommended margin of excision is based on the thickness of the primary tumor, with recommendations of 1 or 2 cm based on tumor thickness.[62] Patient-specific surgical planning may vary, however, based on anatomic constraints associated with the location of the primary tumor.

The technique of intraoperative lymphatic mapping and SLNB is generally offered to patients with primary cutaneous melanoma who have intermediate to high risk of occult regional nodal disease, in an effort to identify microscopic nodal disease by accurate pathologic regional lymph node staging, and to patients who have occult disease, for regional disease control and potential cure.[63] Clinical evidence of regional lymph node metastasis is generally treated by completion lymphadenectomy; however, clinically occult metastasis (sentinel node positivity) no longer requires completion lymphadenopathy, and observation of the nodal basin by US is recommended.[64] Complete lymph node dissection is a surgery that removes all lymph nodes in a specific nodal basin. Possible complications of lymphadenectomy include lymphedema, pain, numbness, and decreased range of motion.[65]

Surgery is also often considered as a component of the treatment plan for satellite and in-transit disease, particularly when solitary or confined. Hyperthermic isolated limb perfusion or, more recently, minimally invasive isolated limb infusion—both relatively specialized techniques involving regional administration of cytotoxic agents (most commonly melphalan) to the involved extremity—is also rarely employed for the management of in-transit disease.[66] Possible complications with isolated limb infusion include myonecrosis, nerve injury, compartment syndrome, and arterial thrombosis. In rare severe cases, fasciotomy or amputation may be necessary.[66] Surgery may sometimes be performed in very highly select patients with limited distant disease for curative intent or, more commonly, for palliation of symptomatic disease (particularly for soft tissue, lung, brain, or gastrointestinal metastases).

Nonsurgical Therapy

Chemotherapy

Until 2011, the only treatment options for patients with metastatic melanoma was cytotoxic chemotherapy or high-dose interleukin-2 (IL-2). Dacarbazine, an alkylating agent, was approved by the U.S. Food and Drug Administration (FDA) for the treatment of melanoma in 1975 and until recently was the standard of care for metastatic melanoma patients, with a 1-year survival rate of only 27%.[67] With the advent of newer immunotherapies and targeted therapies, chemotherapy is used less often, mainly for patients whose disease can no longer be controlled with immunotherapy or targeted agents. Dacarbazine is generally well tolerated, with the major side effects being nausea and vomiting.

Cytokine Therapy

Melanoma antigens are recognized by cytotoxic T cells. IL-2 and interferon-alpha are two older immunotherapy

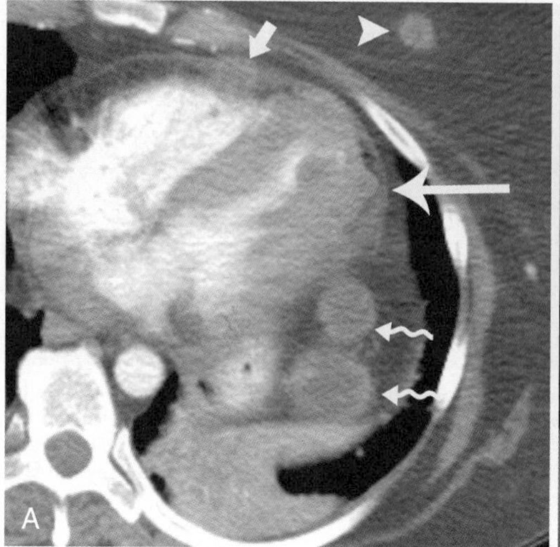

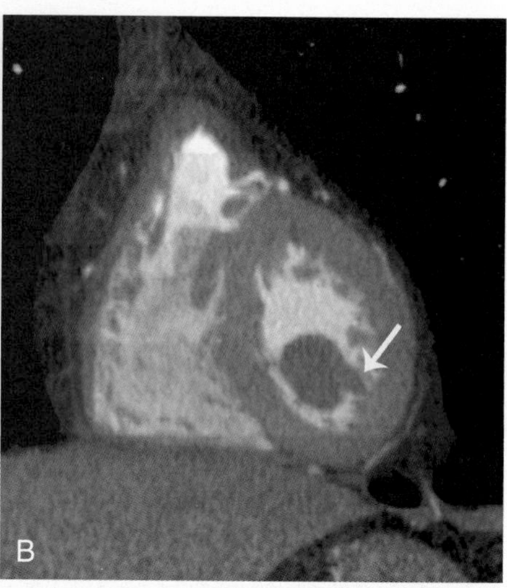

FIGURE 37.15. Cardiac metastatic disease. **A**, Axial computed tomography (CT) scan of the thorax after the administration of intravenous contrast demonstrates metastatic disease involving the myocardium of the left ventricle. Disease is also seen to involve the pericardium (*thick arrow*) and subcutaneous tissues (*arrowhead*). Peritoneal metastatic nodules are seen posterior to the left ventricle (*squiggly arrows*). **B**, A round metastatic mass is seen connected by a stalk (*arrow*) to the left ventricular free wall in a different patient on this postintravenous CT scan of the heart.

drugs used to treat melanoma. IL-2 is a cytokine that directly stimulates the immune system, promoting T-cell proliferation and antitumor activity. Infusion of IL-2 has been shown to have activity in some patients with metastatic melanoma, with an overall response rate in 16%, a complete response in 6%, and a median overall survival of 8.9 months.[68] However, its severe toxicity limited its application, and it is not used as much as in the past due to the advent of new treatments that have been shown to be less toxic and more effective. Complications of IL-2 therapy include hypotension, capillary leak syndrome, which can lead to pulmonary edema, and renal toxicity.

Radiation Therapy

Even though surgery is the mainstay of treatment for localized or regional metastatic melanoma, radiation therapy may be used for locoregional disease control in patients with high-risk features, when complete surgical resection cannot be performed, or as a palliative treatment to relieve symptoms. In some patients, radiation therapy can be used for long-term control and palliation. Sites of disease for which radiotherapy may be offered include osseous metastases or other sites not amenable to surgery, such as fungating or bleeding cutaneous metastases. Radiotherapy is often used for treatment of vertebral metastases causing spinal cord compression and neurologic compromise.[69] Stereotactic radiosurgery or whole-brain radiation may be used for brain metastasis. Radiation side effects depend on the amount of radiation given to the area being treated. Side effects can include hair loss, fatigue, or dry skin. Complications also include severe lymphedema, inflammation such as radiation-induced pneumonitis, enteritis, or cystitis, which can also lead to fistula formation.

Oncolytic Virus Therapy

The oncolytic alimogene laherparepvec (T-VEC) virus is an engineered, genetically modified herpes simplex virus type I that was designed and made in a lab to infect and kill mainly cancer cells.[70] T-VEC is used as local therapy and is given as an injection into metastatic, but not primary, melanoma tumors in the skin or lymph nodes that cannot be removed with surgery. In addition to killing the cancer cells directly, T-VEC also triggers the immune system to find and attack the cancer cells nearby, and sometimes elsewhere in the body. The most common side effects of T-VEC are fatigue, chills, fever, nausea, flu-like symptoms, and pain at the injection site.[70]

Immunotherapy for Stage III and IV Melanoma

Immunotherapy stimulates a person's own immune system to recognize and destroy cancer cells more effectively. In the last decade, advances in understanding the molecular and immune biology of melanoma led to the development of immunotherapies using checkpoint inhibitors that have resulted in improved survival for patients with locoregionally advanced and metastatic melanoma, and more recently for patients in the adjuvant and neoadjuvant settings.[71]

Immune checkpoint inhibitors are monoclonal antibodies targeting the cytotoxic T-lymphocyte–associated protein 4 (CTLA-4) and monoclonal antibodies targeting the programmed cell death protein 1 (PD-1) and its ligand (PD-L1), which are essential for self-tolerance and tumor immune escape.[71] CTLA-4 is a molecule expressed on T cells after activation that strongly binds to costimulatory molecules found on antigen-presenting cells, which results in the downregulation of any further T-cell activation and immune response expansion. The CTLA-4 molecule acts as a halting mechanism, decreasing the function of T cells. Antibodies that block CTLA-4, therefore, release this halting mechanism and increase the activation and proliferation of T cells.[71,72]

Adjuvant Immunotherapy

Ipilimumab, an anti–CTLA-4 antibody, is FDA approved for metastatic melanoma at a dose of 3 mg/kg. However, in the adjuvant therapy trial that resulted in the licensing of this drug in the adjuvant setting, a higher dose of 10 mg/kg was used. In this randomized phase III trial, ipilimumab showed a significant improvement in recurrence-free survival rate at 3 years of 46.5% compared with placebo in patients with surgically resected disease. This response is durable with longer follow-up and does improve overall survival compared with placebo.[73] Currently, ipilimumab 10 mg/kg is approved by the FDA for adjuvant treatment of stage III melanoma and has been shown to delay recurrences and lengthen life for some patients.[74]

PD-1 is a protein found on the surface of T cells. PD-1 normally helps keep T cells from attacking other cells in the body. The activation of PD-1 leads to an inhibition of T-cell activity. The anti–PD-1 antibodies nivolumab and pembrolizumab block the PD-1 receptor and boost the immune system response against melanoma cells.[75] Nivolumab demonstrated a role in the adjuvant setting. In a study comparing nivolumab with ipilimumab for patients who had undergone complete resection of locoregional or distant metastases, the recurrence-free survival rate was 62.6% for nivolumab versus 50.2 % for ipilimumab at a minimum follow-up of 24 months.[76] Currently, nivolumab is approved for use in the adjuvant treatment of patients who have undergone resection of melanoma and resection of all sites of disease. Pembrolizumab has also been approved for adjuvant treatment of patients who have melanoma with lymph node involvement who have undergone complete resection.[77]

Immunotherapy for Metastatic Melanoma

Ipilimumab was the first immune checkpoint inhibitor approved by the FDA as treatment for unresectable or metastatic melanoma, in 2011, based on a large multicenter phase III randomized study that showed a statistically significant longer overall survival of 10.1 months for ipilimumab (3 mg/kg every 3 weeks for four doses) versus 6.4 months for glycoprotein 100 peptide vaccine in a group of patients with stage III and IV melanoma whose disease had progressed in spite of previous systemic treatment.[78] This study also reported a higher 2-year-survival rate of 21.6% for patients treated with ipilimumab compared with 13.7% for those treated with glycoprotein 100.[78] An increase in the dose of ipilimumab from 3 mg/kg to 10 mg/kg resulted in a significant increase in overall survival of 15.7 months versus 11.5 months, respectively.[79] However, it also increased toxicity, with grade 3 (severe) or grade 4 (life-threatening) toxicities noted in 18% to 28% of patients at the 3 mg/kg dose versus 34% with the 10 mg/kg dose.[79]

Nivolumab was the first anti–PD-1 antibody approved for the treatment of metastatic melanoma, based on the results of a phase III trial comparing nivolumab with dacarbazine in previously untreated patients with metastatic melanoma. The overall response rates were 40% versus 13.9%, median progression-free survival rates were 5.1 months versus 2.2 months, and 1-year survival rates were 73% versus 43% for nivolumab and dacarbazine, respectively.[80] The CheckMate-067 trial showed 3-year survival rates of 52% versus 34% for previously untreated patients with unresectable stage III or IV melanoma patients receiving nivolumab or ipilimumab, respectively.[81]

Pembrolizumab, another anti–PD-1 antibody approved by the FDA in 2014, has a response rate of approximately 38% in patients with metastatic melanoma and an overall survival of 74% at 12 months.[82] Pembrolizumab showed a longer 4-year survival rate of 44% compared with 35% for ipilimumab in a phase III study of treatment-naïve patients, and the median progression-free survival was 11.2 months versus 3.7 months for pembrolizumab and ipilimumab, respectively.[83,84]

Nivolumab and pembrolizumab have overall response rates of 40% to 50% and 5-year overall survival rates of 30% to 40%, respectively, in patients with metastatic melanoma, and responses are durable.[77,85] Additionally, patients who have a good response to immunotherapy can be reassessed for possible surgical resection of residual metastases.[86]

Combination Immunotherapy

The CheckMate-067 trial evaluated the combined use of nivolumab and ipilimumab in previously untreated patients with advanced melanoma. This combination therapy achieved objective responses more frequently than either agent alone, with an overall response rate of 58% for the combination of nivolumab and ipilimumab versus 44% in the nivolumab group and 19% in the ipilimumab group and a 5-year overall survival rate of 52% with the combination versus 44% with nivolumab alone.[81,87,88] In 2015, the FDA approved the combination of ipilimumab and nivolumab for the treatment of advanced melanoma. The association of nivolumab and ipilumumab is better than either drug alone in reducing the size of tumors and improve survival. This effect was also demonstrated in patients with asymptomatic brain metastases less than 3 cm in size, where the intracranial clinical benefit rate was 57%, including 26% of patients with complete responses from drugs alone without the need for radiation.[89] Currently, it is the most efficient combination available for use in patients with metastatic or unresectable melanoma.[81,87,88] However, grade 3 and grade 4 toxicities were noted in 59% of patients for the combination versus 21% for nivolumab alone. This combination is preferentially used for select patients, particularly those with rapidly progressing disease, symptomatic disease, or active brain metastases.[89,90] Recently, survival updates for this trial were published and demonstrated 5-year overall survival rates of 52%, 44%, and 26% for combination ipilimumab with nivolumab, nivolumab alone, and ipilimumab alone, respectively.[87]

Investigators have also explored the use of flipped dosing of combination ipilimumab and nivolumab. In this regimen, low-dose ipilimumab (1 mg/kg) with nivolumab (3 mg/kg) is associated with significantly lower toxicity than traditional dosing (34% vs. 48% grade 3–5 toxicities) and showed response rates comparable to the traditional dosing, although the study was not powered to compare efficacy between regimens.[91]

Immunotherapy has also been used in the neoadjuvant setting, which allows for assessment of both imaging response and pathological response.[92,93] A phase II trial of multiple dosing combinations of ipilimumab with nivolumab demonstrated that the combination of two doses of nivolumab 3 mg/kg and ipilimumab 1 mg/kg in the neoadjuvant setting has the optimal efficacy/toxicity ratio, with radiological objective response in 57% of patients and pathological complete response (absence of any viable tumor in surgical specimen) in 77% of patients, with only 20% grade 3 and grade 4 immune-related adverse events (irAEs).[94]

Targeted Therapy

Targeted therapy is a treatment that targets specific parts of cancer cells, such as cancer-specific genes or proteins that help cancers grow and spread. A mutation within the mitogen-activated protein kinase (MAPK) pathway leads to uncontrollable growth and proliferation and is commonly found in various malignancies. The most common driver mutation in melanoma that leads to this characteristic overactivation in the MAPK pathway is the BRAF mutation.[95]

The BRAF mutation is present in approximately 40% to 50% of cutaneous melanomas.[96] BRAF mutations can be found in mucosal or acral subtypes of melanomas, but the incidence is less than 10%. BRAF mutations are not identified in uveal melanomas. Substitution of valine (V) for glutamic acid (E) at amino acid position 600 (V600E) represents 85% to 90% of BRAF mutations. A second common substitution of valine (V) for lysine (K) at amino acid position 600 (V600K) represents 10% to 15% of the BRAF mutations. Mutations at other sites in BRAF are detected in approximately 5% of cutaneous melanomas.[96] Other mutations, such as NRAS mutations, can occur in approximately 20% of cutaneous melanoma, and C-KIT mutations are more frequently present in mucosal or acral melanomas and melanoma associated with chronic sun damage.[97]

BRAF inhibitors are small-molecule inhibitors that selectively target the mutant BRAF isoform, preferentially V600E but also other isoforms such as V600K or V600D. In the majority of patients with BRAF V600 mutation–positive melanoma, BRAF inhibition produces rapid tumor regression; however, development of resistance to this therapy can occur.[98]

Targeted Therapy in the Adjuvant Setting

The regimen of dabrafenib and trametinib is FDA approved for use in patients with stage III melanoma after surgical resection. In the trial leading to its approval, 1 year of dabrafenib and trametinib demonstrated 3-year progression-free survival rates of 58% versus 39% in the placebo group.[99] Longer-term follow-up of this study confirmed improvements in relapse-free survival and distant metastasis–free survival and estimated a cure rate of 54% for dabrafenib/trametinib-treated patients versus 37% in the placebo group.[100]

Targeted Therapy in the Metastatic Setting

Vemurafenib is an oral inhibitor of the V600E BRAF mutant that produces a rapid clinical response with low toxicity. A phase III randomized clinical trial that compared vemurafenib with dacarbazine in patients with the V600E mutation showed a significant difference in progression-free survival of 6.9 months versus 2.7 months for verumafenib and dacarbazine, respectively. The overall response rates were 50% for vemurafenib and 6% for dacarbazine.[101] Verumafenib was the first FDA-approved BRAF inhibitor, approved in 2011, for the treatment of metastatic and unresectable BRAF-mutated melanoma.

Dabrafenib, another BRAF inhibitor, has a clinical efficacy similar to that of vemurafenib. A phase III randomized clinical trial that compared dabrafenib with dacarbazine in patients with BRAF V600 mutations showed an overall response rate or 50% for dabrafenib and 6% for dacarbazine, with a significantly improved progression-free survival of 5.1 months for dabrafenib versus 2.7 months for dacarbazine, respectively.[102] Dabrafenib was approved by the FDA for the treatment of metastatic and unresectable BRAF-mutated melanoma in 2013.

The most recent FDA-approved BRAF inhibitor is encorafenib, which was approved in 2018.[103] It is a BRAF inhibitor with increased affinity for BRAF, and thus a longer binding time, which allows for administration once daily compared with twice daily as with vemurafenib and dabrafenib.

An important limitation to the use of single-agent BRAF inhibitors is the eventual development of resistance. Although these drugs can be highly effective, with dramatic reduction in tumor size, the majority of patients develop secondary resistance within 6 to 8 months of therapy initiation. The median progression-free survival is approximately 6 months, and 90% of patients develop resistance within 1 year.[104] Additionally, the side-effect profile of single-agent BRAF inhibition can be challenging. The most common side effects of BRAF inhibitors include arthralgia, rash, fever, photosensitivity, fatigue, alopecia, nausea, and development of squamous cell carcinomas of the skin.[104]

BRAF V600 mutations are also associated with an increased and selective sensitivity to MEK inhibitors. MEK inhibitors are small-molecule inhibitors targeting MEK1/2 proteins in the MAPK pathway. MEK inhibitors target a molecule downstream of the BRAF protein.[105] Currently, three different MEK inhibitors are approved to be used for unresectable or metastatic melanoma with a BRAF V600E or V600K mutation.

Trametinib is a selective MEK1 and MEK2 inhibitor. In a phase III trial of patients with BRAF V600E–mutated melanoma, trametinib resulted in an improved overall response rate of 22% versus 8% for chemotherapy and a significantly prolonged progression-free survival compared with chemotherapy (4.8 months vs. 1.5 months).[106] Trametinib was the first MEK inhibitor approved by the FDA for the treatment of metastatic BRAF-mutated melanoma, in 2013. Trametinib was approved for patients who had not previously been treated with a selective BRAF inhibitor, because it fails to achieve clinical benefit in pretreated patients.[107]

Cobimetinib is a selective MEK1 inhibitor that was approved by the FDA for use in combination with vemurafenib in the treatment of metastatic BRAF V600–mutated metastatic melanoma, in 2015.[108] Binimetinib is a selective MEK1 and MEK2 inhibitor that was approved by the FDA in 2018 to be used in combination with encorafenib for the treatment of patients with unresectable or metastatic melanoma with BRAF V600E or V600K mutations.[108]

MEK inhibitors are usually well tolerated, with the most common side effects including rash, diarrhea, peripheral edema, fatigue, hypertension, ocular events, and cardiomyopathy. However, MEK inhibition does not seem to cause any cutaneous squamous-cell carcinomas or hyperproliferative skin lesions.[109] Interestingly, it is thought that the combination of BRAF and MEK inhibition together may actually lessen the side effects seen when the drugs are used as single agents.

Combination BRAF/MEK Inhibition

Patients treated with BRAF inhibitors will relapse within 6 to 8 months of treatment initiation due to acquired drug resistance, most likely as a result of reactivation of the MAPK pathway.[109] The combination of BRAF and MEK inhibitors is used in order to delay the development of resistance to BRAF inhibitor monotherapy. Both drugs block targets that act at different steps in the MAPK pathway.

Combination use of dabrafenib with trametinib resulted in a median progression-free survival of 9.4 months versus 5.8 months for dabrafenib alone and a higher response rate of 76% for complete or partial response compared with 54% for dabrafenib alone. This combined treatment with dabrafenib and trametinib was approved by the FDA in 2014 to treat BRAF V600E/K–mutated metastatic melanoma.[110]

In a more recent phase III trial, the combination of dabrafenib and trametinib was shown to improve the rate of progression-free survival and overall survival in previously untreated patients with metastatic melanoma with a BRAF V600E or V600K mutation, without increased overall toxicity.[111,112] This combination also shows some response in patients with brain metastases and BRAF mutation.[113]

The combination of cobimetinib and vemurafenib showed a progression-free survival of 12.3 months versus 7.2 months and a median overall survival of 22.3 months versus 17.4 months for vemurafenib alone.[114] The use of cobimetinib in combination with vemurafenib is approved for patients with BRAF V600E/K–mutated metastatic melanoma.

Overall, combined BRAF plus MEK inhibitor therapy is well tolerated and markedly delays the onset of resistance compared with BRAF monotherapy.[109] Therefore, the combination of BRAF and MEK inhibitors has replaced the use of single-agent BRAF inhibitors and has become the standard of care for patients with a BRAF-mutated advanced or unresectable melanoma.[105] Options include dabrafenib plus trametinib, vemurafenib plus cobimetinib, and encorafenib plus binimetinib.

The use of BRAF inhibitors has improved treatment for patients with BRAF V600–mutant metastatic melanoma. However, these therapies are not always durable, and approximately 50% of patients experience disease progression by 12 months.[109] This phenomenon highlights the need to increase our understanding of mechanisms of resistance associated with molecularly-targeted therapies. Identification of the molecular mechanisms underlying resistance and the development of drugs or drug combinations to overcome resistance are important challenges for the future treatment of this disease.

KEY POINTS Treatment

- Surgical resection of the primary tumor is performed by wide local excision and is the mainstay of treatment for early-stage melanoma.
- Sentinel lymph node biopsy is generally offered to patients with primary cutaneous melanoma who have intermediate- to high-risk primary cutaneous melanoma, in an effort to identify occult microscopic regional nodal disease.
- Microscopically involved sentinel nodes are no longer treated by lymphadenectomy, and observation with serial ultrasounds of the affected lymph node bed is recommended.
- Radiotherapy is often used for treatment of metastases causing spinal cord compression, brain metastasis, or bone metastasis.
- The development of immune checkpoint inhibitors and antibodies to the programmed cell death 1 (PD-1) receptor have revolutionized the treatment of stage III and IV melanoma.
- Ipilimumab was the first immune checkpoint inhibitor to be approved for the treatment of melanoma.
- Monotherapy with anti–PD-1 antibodies has a better efficacy and toxicity profile than ipilimumab.
- The combination of nivolumab and ipilimumab appears to be the most effective treatment available in metastatic melanoma, but the toxicity of the regimen is a limitation.
- Targeted therapies inhibit the mitogen-activated protein kinase pathway.
- Whenever possible, the tumor should be assayed for the presence of a driver mutation.
- Target therapy with BRAF inhibitors combined with MEK inhibitors is associated with rapid and high response rates in patients with metastatic melanoma in the presence of a BRAF V600 mutation.
- Treatment with targeted therapies and immunotherapies improves overall survival for patients with locoregionally advanced and metastatic melanoma and improves recurrence-free survival in the adjuvant setting.
- New therapies allows patients who have a good response to treatment to be reassessed for possible surgical resection of residual metastases

Immune-Related Adverse Events

The side effects of immune checkpoint inhibitors are usually immune-related inflammatory conditions called irAEs.[115] The frequency and severity depends on the type and dose of the drug and its use in monotherapy or in combination. IrAEs are seen in approximately 60% to 80% of patients treated with ipilimumab.[72] The most common side effects are fatigue, diarrhea, nausea, skin rashes, and itching. Severe adverse events may occur in 15% of patients treated with 3 mg/kg and in 30% of patients treated with 10 mg/kg. Common toxicities involve inflammation of the intestines, liver, nerves, lungs, skin, kidneys, and endocrine system, leading to a wide range of potential toxicities. Immune-induced colitis may appears as diffuse or a segmental colonic involvement with an inflammatory pattern characterized by wall thickening, and mucosal enhancement (Fig. 37.16). Skin-related adverse events can be expected after 2 to 3 weeks, gastrointestinal and hepatic events after 6 to 7 weeks, and endocrinologic events usually after 9 weeks.[72]

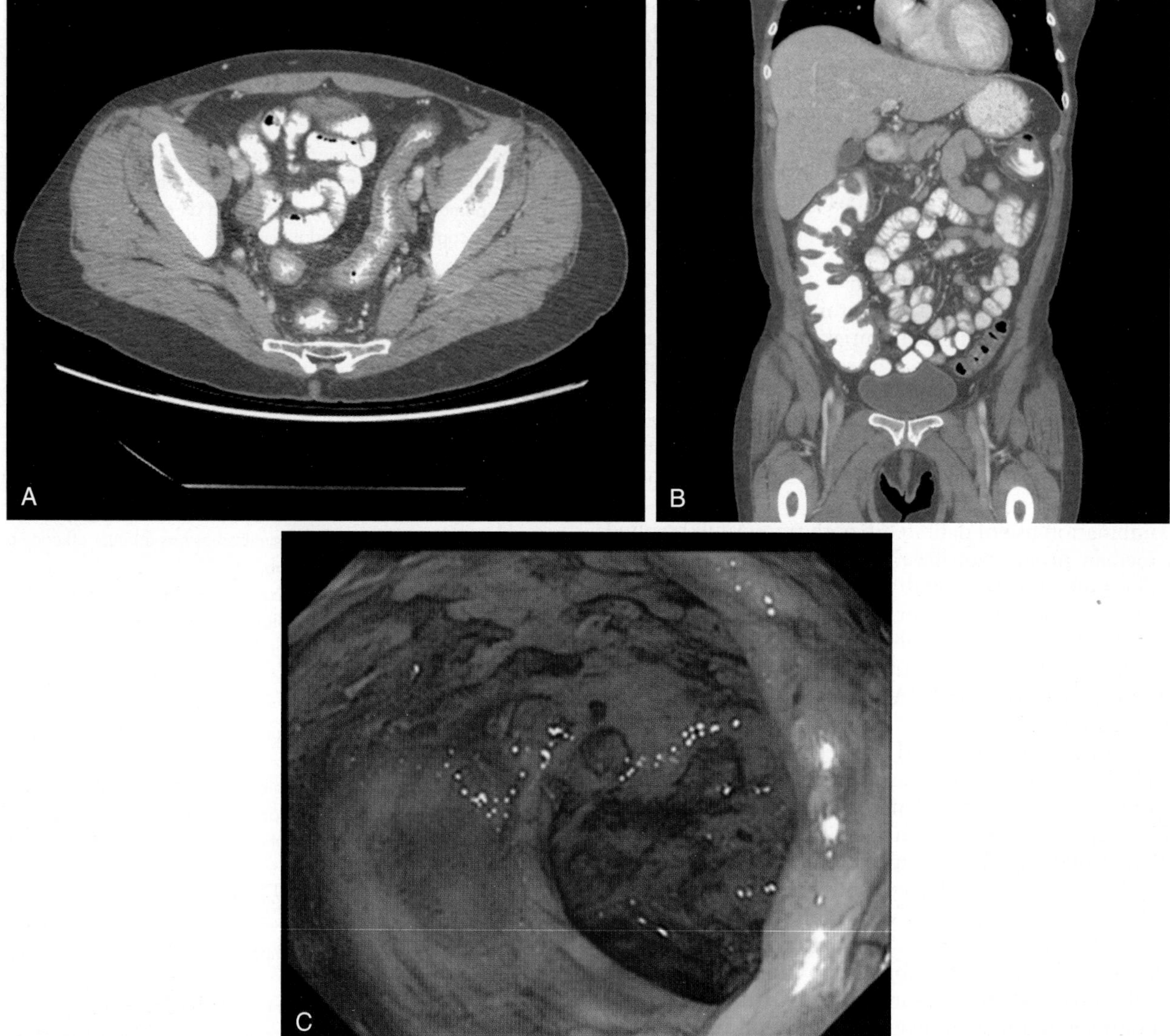

FIGURE 37.16. Immune-induced colitis. A 62-year-old male with metastatic melanoma to the left axilla and lung was treated with ipilimumab. After 1 month of treatment, he presented with diarrhea. **A** and **B**, Axial and coronal reformat postcontrast computed tomography images with intravenous and oral contrast showed diffuse thickening of the colonic walls (*arrows*). **C**, Colonoscopy revealed diffuse ulcerations suggestive of pancolitis. Patient was treated with prednisone and recovered well.

Pembrolizumab and nivolumab have similar side-effect profiles, with severe adverse events seen in approximately 15% of cases.[116] Combination immunotherapy with ipilimumab 3 mg/kg and nivolumab 1 mg/kg can cause grade 3 or higher toxicity in approximately 48% of patients, but toxicity is approximately 34% for the flipped dose regimen.[91] The most common side effects are fatigue, diarrhea, lymphopenia, cutaneous rash, pruritus, pulmonary issues, increased lipase levels, and endocrine disorders such as thyroid issues. In general, the anti–PD-1 agents have less toxicity compared with anti-CTLA-4. The most commonly affected organs include the lungs (with pneumonitis) and the kidneys.[116] Immune-induced pneumonitis may present with a wide range of clinical courses, ranging from mild dyspneia to life-threatening respiratory failure. The radiological patterns vary from minor interstitial anomalies up to acute interstitial pneumonia or acute respiratory distress syndrome patterns including organizing pneumonia, hypersensitivity pneumonitis, or nonspecific pneumonitis (Fig. 37.17).[116]

Supportive management alone is usually sufficient to manage grade 1 toxicities, and interruption of the treatment is recommended if the adverse events are grade 2 or higher. In severe cases of grade 3 toxicity or higher immunotherapy may be permanently discontinued, or in other cases it can be continued once irAEs resolve after appropriate treatment with systemic corticosteroids. Close monitoring during treatment with any immunotherapeutic agent is recommended. The most common irAEs typically resolve within 4 to 9 weeks of onset, depending on the organ system involved. The early recognition and treatment of an adverse event is important and reduces the risk of adverse sequelae.[115–118] In cases of severe toxicity, systemic corticosteroids are employed. At least 1 mg/kg of corticiosteroids should be utilized for grade 3 or higher toxicity, although more severe toxicities may require temporary use of higher

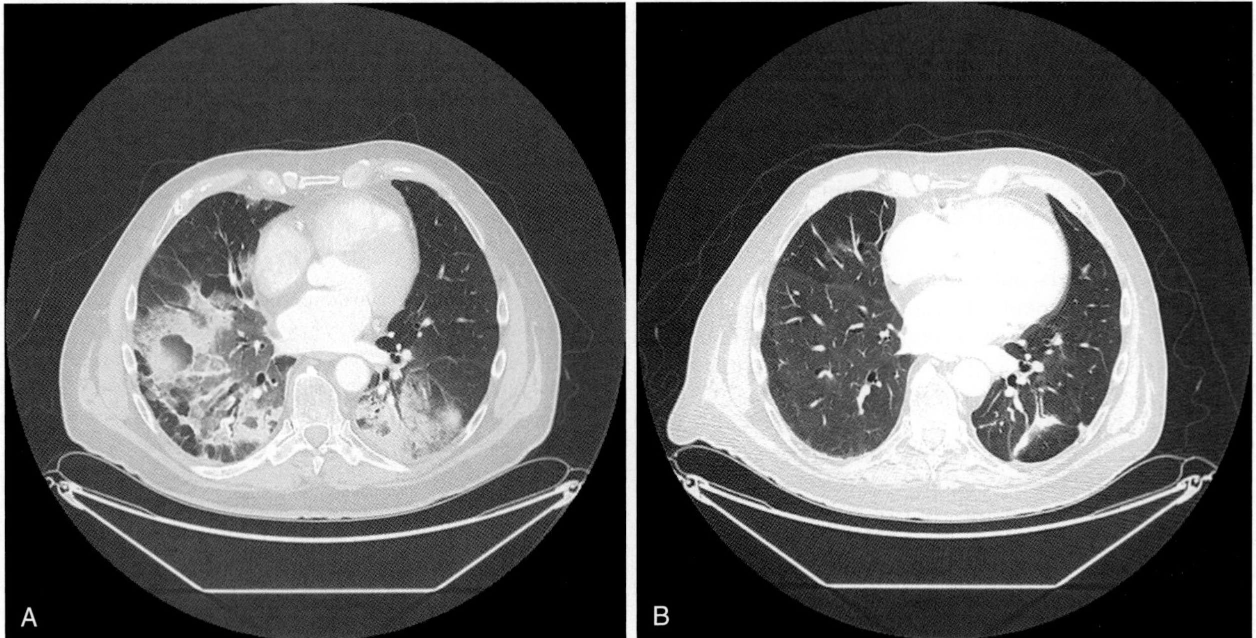

Figure 37.17. Immune-induced pneumonitis. A 75-year-old male with metastatic melanoma treated with anti–programmed cell death 1 therapy. After 2 months of therapy, he developed flu symptoms and worsening cough. **A**, Axial postcontrast chest computed tomography (CT) image with intravenous contrast showed significant ground-glass and nodular opacities, particularly in the lower lobes. Broncoscopy with bronchialveolar lavage showed inflammation. **B**, He was treated with steroids, with a follow-up axial chest CT image with intravenous contrast showing improvement.

doses. Steroid taper should begin when symptoms improve and should last for 4 to 6 weeks. In steroid-refractory colitis, alternative agents such as the tumor necrosis factor alpha inhibitor infliximab are useful and may be used as a way to taper steroids more quickly than the usual 4 to 6 weeks.[119]

Key Points

- The side effects of immune checkpoint inhibitors are usually immune-related inflammatory conditions called immune-related adverse events (irAEs).
- The frequency and severity depend on the type and dose of the drug and its use in monotherapy or in combination.
- Close monitoring during treatment with all immunotherapy is recommended.
- Treatment of irAEs includes delay/omission of drug administration and intense monitoring for moderate irAEs, and for persistent or high-grade irAEs includes discontinuation of the drug and use of systemic corticosteroids.

Monitoring Tumor Response/Treatment Response

Monitoring tumor response is traditionally based on resolution or decrease in size of solid-organ metastases and nodal metastases as detected on CT or MRI using the Response Evaluation Criteria In Solid Tumors (RECIST).[120] In RECIST 1.1, published in 2009, tumor burden for response determination is assessed by measuring the longest diameter of five lesions in the axial plane (two per organ). Lymph nodes that are 15 mm or larger in short axis are considered pathologic, and when they decrease to 10 mm or less they are considered normal. However, these measurements are not specific for tumor involvement because lymph nodes may enlarge secondary to infection or inflammation, and/or metastatic lymph nodes may be less than 10 mm.[120]

However, since the use of immunotherapies, it was observed that the patterns of treatment responses for immunotherapies may differ from those typical of cytotoxic chemotherapies. A small but measurable number of patients may experience pseudoprogression, which is characterized by clinical and radiologic worsening of disease burden in the first few weeks of treatment followed by durable tumor regression.[121] The enlargement of disease in preexisting lesions and the emergence of new lesions are related to therapy-induced inflammatory infiltration of activated T cells. Therefore, monitoring treatment response using RECIST is difficult, because tumor growth can be transient and dependent upon timing of scan. Additionally, immunotherapies are not always rapid in onset of response, and delayed response after 3 months of therapy has been appreciated.

Owing to the different patterns of response to immunotherapy, alternative criteria for monitoring treatment response called immune-related response criteria (irRC)[121] were proposed in 2009 that considers the "total tumor burden," regardless of the growth of new disease. According to irRC, the appearance of new lesions does not constitute progression of disease. The "total tumor burden" is made up by summation of the product of perpendicular diameters (bidimensional measurement) of new and preexisting measurable lesions (five lesions per organ, up to 10 visceral lesions, and five cutaneous index lesions). A complete immune response is defined as disappearance of all detectable tumor lesions. Partial response means that there has been greater than or equal to 50% reduction but less than a 100% decrease in tumor burden; immune-related stable disease is defined as less than a 50% decrease or less than a 25% increase in tumor burden. Progression of disease has to be reported if the tumor burden increases by greater than or equal to 25% relative to nadir (minimum recorded tumor burden). These new criteria require confirmation on a follow-up scan no less than 4 weeks from the date first documented.[121]

In 2013, researchers published revised irRC using unidimensional measurements instead of bidimensional measurements to assess tumor response to immunotherapy, termed immune-related Response Evaluation Criteria in Solid Tumors.[122] Partial response is defined as a 30% or more reduction in the sum of target lesions, stable disease as less than a 20% increase and less than a 30% reduction in the sum of target lesions, and progressive disease as a 20% or more increase in the sum of target lesions, plus new measurable lesions, from the nadir.[48]. These criteria have been found to provide high reproducibility compared with the irRC.[122]

In 2017 the RECIST working group published the modified RECIST 1.1 for immunotherapy, the so-called immune-related RECIST (iRECIST), to encourage consistency in immune-based radiographic data analysis.[123] The iRECIST uses unidimensional measurements and includes the measurements of new target lesions into disease assessments. The modified criteria also introduced the term "unconfirmed progressive disease," which corresponds to progressive disease that remains to be confirmed on 4- to 8-week follow-up imaging. As opposed to other criteria developed for immunotherapy, nontarget lesion progression can define progressive disease. Partial response is defined as a 30% or more reduction in the sum of target lesions, and unconfirmed progressive disease as a 20% or more increase in the sum of target lesions from the nadir or nontarget lesion progression or appearance of new lesion.[123] Progressive disease is confirmed in the case of a target lesion previously classified as unconfirmed progressive disease and an increase in the tumor burden of target lesions of 5 mm or more on the 4- to 8-week follow-up imaging; or nontarget lesion previously classified as unconfirmed progressive disease and significant increase of nontarget lesion on the 4- to 8-week follow-up imaging; or new lesions resulting from unconfirmed progressive disease and increase in tumor burden of 5 mm or more of these new lesions or increase in the number of new lesions on the 4- to 8 -week follow-up imaging.[123] The immune-modified RECIST (imRECIST) criteria were developed initially for implementation in atezolizumab studies and are modifications of the RECIST 1.1 system based on the principles of the irRC.[124]

The first PET-based response criteria including metabolic response to treatment in solid tumors were proposed by the European Organization for Research and Treatment of Cancer (EORTC) in 1999.[125] In 2009, Wahl et al. proposed the PET Response Criteria in Solid Tumors based on PET images only.[126] Subsequently, some other specific response criteria have been formulated for PET/CT to improve the diagnostic predictive value, taking into account both the combined use of metabolic (maximum standard uptake value) and the size of the lesions, including the PET/CT Criteria for Early Prediction of Response to Immune Checkpoint Inhibitor Therapy, as well as the number of newly emerging lesions at the PET study, as described in the PET Response Evaluation Criteria for Immunotherapy.[127,128]

Key Points

- The patterns of treatment responses for immunotherapies may differ from those typical of cytotoxic chemotherapy.
- Patients treated with immunotherapy may have pseudoprogression, a transient worsening of disease, manifested either by progression of known lesions or the appearance of new lesions, before the disease stabilizes or tumor regresses.
- The enlargement of preexisting lesions and new lesions is related to therapy-induced inflammatory infiltration of activated T-cells.
- New immune-related response criteria for monitoring treatment response have been created.

Biomarkers

Although immune checkpoint inhibitors have been a breakthrough for cancer therapeutic and have revolutionized the treatment of metastatic melanoma, a significant subset of patients still does not respond to these drugs, and many patient who do respond develop secondary resistance. Currently, is not possible to determine which patient will respond to treatment with immune checkpoint inhibitors. The identification of biomarkers of response is the next step to understanding the complex interactions between melanoma and the immune system. Researchers have been working to resolve these issues. Many biomarkers have been proposed and are being investigated, such as tumor expression of PD-L1, tumor T-cell infiltration, and the rate of somatic mutations in tumor (tumor mutational burden).[129]

SURVEILLANCE AND RECURRENCE

Surveillance for recurrence in patients with no evidence of disease is dependent on the melanoma stage and risk factors for recurrence. Approximately 20% to 30% of early-stage melanoma patients will develop a recurrence within 5 years.[23] Stage III and IV melanoma patients have a high risk for recurrence. The sites of relapse include local/in-transit (28%), regional nodal (21%), or systemic (51%).[130] It is important to identify these patients as soon as possible to enable earlier treatment, which will hopefully lead to better outcome.[37]

Locoregional recurrence is often found by patient self-examination or by physical examination. With the advent of more effective systemic therapies, the use of imaging in surveillance of melanoma patients is evolving. Guidelines have been provided by the National Comprehensive Cancer Network (NCCN) in approaches to the management of patients with melanoma.[2] According with the NCCN guidelines, imaging is recommend at all stages to evaluate specific signs and symptoms. In patients with an equivocal lymph node exam, short-term follow-up or additional imaging should be considered. Clinical exam and regional lymph node US in patients with a positive SLNB who did not undergo complete lymph node dissection is recommended every 3 to 4 months during the first 2 years, then every 6 months during years 3 to 5.[2]

Routine imaging to screen for asymptomatic recurrence or metastatic disease is not recommended for early-stage disease (stages 0–IIA). For these patients, an annual skin examination and patient education regarding monthly skin self-examination are recommended. For stages IIB to IV, consider cross-sectional imaging with or without brain imaging every 3 to 12 months for 2 years, then every 6 to 12 months for another 3 years to screen for recurrence or metastatic disease.[2] PET/CT also has an important role in assessing patients with suspected clinical locoregional recurrences to evaluate the presence of other sites of recurrent disease versus a single recurrent site for possible surgical resection. Additionally, PET/CT is also useful for imaging areas (arms and legs) not scanned on routine CT.[131]

Key Points Surveillance and Recurrence

- Locoregional recurrence is often found by patient self-examination or by physical examination.
- Ultrasound can be used in evaluating surgical resection scars or regional lymph node basins at risk for metastatic disease.
- The National Comprehensive Cancer Network provides guidelines for approaches to the management of patients with melanoma, and imaging is recommend at all stages to evaluate specific signs and symptoms.
- Imaging studies are not indicated for early-stage disease (stages 0–IIA).
- For stages IIB–IV, consider cross-sectional imaging with or without brain imaging every 3–12 months for 2 years, then every 6–12 months for another 3 years to screen for recurrence or metastatic disease.

CONCLUSION

Melanoma is an aggressive neoplasm that continues to rise in incidence. Primary tumor prognostic markers include tumor thickness and ulceration. Lymphatics represent the most common first route of spread and typically precede hematogenous spread. In patients with negative regional lymph nodes on clinical examination, intraoperative lymphatic mapping and SLNB are often used to surgically stage regional nodal basins at risk. In the last decade, immunotherapy and targeted therapy have revolutionized the treatment and improved the overall survival of patients with advanced melanoma. Imaging has a crucial role in staging, monitoring response to treatment, identifying irAEs, performing surveillance, and achieving early detection of metastatic disease. Knowledge of imaging features of the common and uncommon sites of metastatic spread is important for accurate follow-up of melanoma patients. As melanoma care will continue evolving over the next years, imaging is crucial in the multidisciplinary management of patients with melanoma.

REFERENCES

1. Guy Jr GP, Thomas CC, Thompson T, et al. Vital signs: melanoma incidence and mortality trends and projections - United States, 1982-2030. *MMWR Morb Mortal Wkly Rep*. 2015;64(21):591–596.
2. Coit DG, Thompson JA, Albertini MR, et al. Cutaneous Melanoma, Version 2.2019, NCCN Clinical Practice Guidelines in Oncology. *J Natl Compr Canc Netw*. 2019;17(4):367–402.
3. Siegel R, Miller K, Fuchs H, Jemal A. Cancer Statistics. *CA Cancer J Clin*. 2021;71(1):7–33.
4. Rastrelli M, Tropea S, Rossi CR, et al. Melanoma: epidemiology, risk factors, pathogenesis, diagnosis and classification. *In Vivo*. 2014;28(6):1005–1011.
5. Erdmann F, Lortet-Tieulent J, Schuz J, et al. International trends in the incidence of malignant melanoma 1953-2008-are recent generations at higher or lower risk? *Int J Cancer*. 2013;132(2):385–400.
6. Tucker MA. Melanoma epidemiology. *Hematol Oncol Clin North Am*. 2009;23(3):383–395. vii.
7. Read J, Wadt KA, Hayward NK. Melanoma genetics. *J Med Genet*. 2016;53(1):1–14.
8. Chattopadhyay C, Kim DW, Gombos DS, et al. Uveal melanoma: From diagnosis to treatment and the science in between. *Cancer*. 2016;122(15):2299–2312.
9. Yde SS, Sjoegren P, Heje M, et al. Mucosal melanoma: a literature review. *Curr Oncol Rep*. 2018;20(3):28.
10. DeMatos P, Wolfe WG, Shea CR, et al. Primary malignant melanoma of the esophagus. *J Surg Oncol*. 1997;66(3):201–206.
11. Sanchez AA, Wu TT, Prieto VG, et al. Comparison of primary and metastatic malignant melanoma of the esophagus: clinicopathologic review of 10 cases. *Arch Pathol Lab Med*. 2008;132(10):1623–1629.
12. Prieto VG, Shea CR. Use of immunohistochemistry in melanocytic lesions. *J Cutan Pathol*. 2008;35(Suppl 2):1–10.
13. Scolyer RA, Rawson RV, Gershenwald JE, et al. Melanoma pathology reporting and staging. *Mod Pathol*. 2020;33(Suppl 1):15–24.
14. Siroy AE, Boland GM, Milton DR, et al. Beyond BRAF(V600): clinical mutation panel testing by next-generation sequencing in advanced melanoma. *J Invest Dermatol*. 2015;135(2):508–515.
15. Rigel DS, Friedman RJ, Kopf AW, et al. ABCDE-an evolving concept in the early detection of melanoma. *Arch Dermatol*. 2005;141(8):1032–1034.
16. Song Y, Karakousis GC. Melanoma of unknown primary. *J Surg Oncol*. 2019;119(2):232–241.
17. Thompson JF, Hunt JA, Culjak G, et al. Popliteal lymph node metastasis from primary cutaneous melanoma. *Eur J Surg Oncol*. 2000;26(2):172–176.
18. Uren RF, Howman-Giles R, Thompson JF. Patterns of lymphatic drainage from the skin in patients with melanoma. *J Nucl Med*. 2003;44(4):570–582.
19. Gershenwald JE, Scolyer RA, Hess KR, et al. Melanoma staging: evidence-based changes in the American Joint Committee on Cancer eighth edition cancer staging manual. *CA Cancer J Clin*. 2017;67(6):472–492.
20. Pawlik TM, Ross MI, Thompson JF, et al. The risk of in-transit melanoma metastasis depends on tumor biology and not the surgical approach to regional lymph nodes. *J Clin Oncol*. 2005;23(21):4588–4590.
21. Kamel IR, Kruskal JB, Gramm HF. Imaging of abdominal manifestations of melanoma. *Crit Rev Diagn Imaging*. 1998;39(6):447–486.
22. Peruzzi B, Bottaro DP. Targeting the c-Met signaling pathway in cancer. *Clin Cancer Res*. 2006;12(12):3657–3660.
23. Gerhenwald JE, Scholyer RA, Hess KR, et al. Melanoma of the skin. In: Amin MES, Greene FL, eds. *AJCC Cancer Staging Manual*. 8th ed. Switzerland: Springer International; 2017:563–585.
24. Breslow A. Tumor thickness, level of invasion and node dissection in stage I cutaneous melanoma. *Ann Surg*. 1975;182(5):572–575.
25. Gershenwald JE, Scolyer RA. Melanoma staging: American Joint Committee on Cancer (AJCC) 8th edition and beyond. *Ann Surg Oncol*. 2018;25(8):2105–2110.
26. Read RL, Haydu L, Saw RP, et al. In-transit melanoma metastases: incidence, prognosis, and the role of lymphadenectomy. *Ann Surg Oncol*. 2015;22(2):475–481.
27. Hayashi K, Koga H, Uhara H, et al. High-frequency 30-MHz sonography in preoperative assessment of tumor thickness of primary melanoma: usefulness in determination of surgical margin and indication for sentinel lymph node biopsy. *Int J Clin Oncol*. 2009;14(5):426–430.

28. Sumner 3rd WE, Ross MI, Mansfield PF, et al. Implications of lymphatic drainage to unusual sentinel lymph node sites in patients with primary cutaneous melanoma. *Cancer*. 2002;95(2):354–360.
29. Gershenwald JE, Tseng CH, Thompson W, et al. Improved sentinel lymph node localization in patients with primary melanoma with the use of radiolabeled colloid. *Surgery*. 1998;124(2):203–210.
30. Uren RF, Sanki A, Thompson JF. The utility of ultrasound in patients with melanoma. *Expert Rev Anticancer Ther*. 2007;7(11):1633–1642.
31. Voit C, Van Akkooi AC, Schafer-Hesterberg G, et al. Ultrasound morphology criteria predict metastatic disease of the sentinel nodes in patients with melanoma. *J Clin Oncol*. 2010;28(5):847–852.
32. Sanki A, Uren RF, Moncrieff M, et al. Targeted high-resolution ultrasound is not an effective substitute for sentinel lymph node biopsy in patients with primary cutaneous melanoma. *J Clin Oncol*. 2009;27(33):5614–5619.
33. Buzaid AC, Tinoco L, Ross MI, et al. Role of computed tomography in the staging of patients with local-regional metastases of melanoma. *J Clin Oncol*. 1995;13(8):2104–2108.
34. Aviles Izquierdo JA, Molina Lopez I, Sobrini Morillo P, et al. Utility of PET/CT in patients with stage I-III melanoma. *Clin Transl Oncol*. 2019;22(8):1414–1417.
35. Groen LC, Lazarenko SV, Schreurs HW, et al. Evaluation of PET/CT in patients with stage III malignant cutaneous melanoma. *Am J Nucl Med Mol Imaging*. 2019;9(2):168–175.
36. Akcali C, Zincirkeser S, Erbagcy Z, et al. Detection of metastases in patients with cutaneous melanoma using FDG-PET/CT. *J Int Med Res*. 2007;35(4):547–553.
37. Stodell M, Thompson JF, Emmett L, et al. Melanoma patient imaging in the era of effective systemic therapies. *Eur J Surg Oncol*. 2017;43(8):1517–1527.
38. Miles K, McQueen L, Ngai S, et al. Evidence-based medicine and clinical fluorodeoxyglucose PET/MRI in oncology. *Cancer Imaging*. 2015;15:18.
39. Pfannenberg C, Schwenzer N. [Whole-body staging of malignant melanoma: advantages, limitations and current importance of PET-CT, whole-body MRI and PET-MRI]. *Radiologe*. 2015;55(2):120–126.
40. Meier F, Will S, Ellwanger U, et al. Metastatic pathways and time courses in the orderly progression of cutaneous melanoma. *Br J Dermatol*. 2002;147(1):62–70.
41. Patel JK, Didolkar MS, Pickren JW, et al. Metastatic pattern of malignant melanoma. A study of 216 autopsy cases. *Am J Surg*. 1978;135(6):807–810.
42. Fishman EK, Kuhlman JE, Schuchter LM, et al. CT of malignant melanoma in the chest, abdomen, and musculoskeletal system. *Radiographics*. 1990;10(4):603–620.
43. Quint LE, Park CH, Iannettoni MD. Solitary pulmonary nodules in patients with extrapulmonary neoplasms. *Radiology*. 2000;217(1):257–261.
44. Nazarian LN, Alexander AA, Kurtz AB, et al. Superficial melanoma metastases: appearances on gray-scale and color Doppler sonography. *AJR Am J Roentgenol*. 1998;170(2):459–463.
45. Sofue K, Tateishi U, Tsurusaki M, et al. MR imaging of hepatic metastasis in patients with malignant melanoma: evaluation of suspected lesions screened at contrast-enhanced CT. *Eur J Radiol*. 2012;81(4):714–718.
46. Escott EJ. A variety of appearances of malignant melanoma in the head: a review. *Radiographics*. 2001;21(3):625–639.
47. Marx HF, Colletti PM, Raval JK, et al. Magnetic resonance imaging features in melanoma. *Magn Reson Imaging*. 1990;8(3):223–229.
48. Isiklar I, Leeds NE, Fuller GN, et al. Intracranial metastatic melanoma: correlation between MR imaging characteristics and melanin content. *AJR Am J Roentgenol*. 1995;165(6):1503–1512.
49. Glass JP, Melamed M, Chernik NL, et al. Malignant cells in cerebrospinal fluid (CSF): the meaning of a positive CSF cytology. *Neurology*. 1979;29(10):1369–1375.
50. Freilich RJ, Krol G, DeAngelis LM. Neuroimaging and cerebrospinal fluid cytology in the diagnosis of leptomeningeal metastasis. *Ann Neurol*. 1995;38(1):51–57.
51. Yeung MJ, Serpell JW. Management of the solitary thyroid nodule. *Oncologist*. 2008;13(2):105–112.
52. Potepan P, Spagnoli I, Danesini GM, et al. [The radiodiagnosis of bone metastases from melanoma]. *Radiol Med*. 1994;87(6):741–746.
53. Heusner T, Golitz P, Hamami M, et al. "One-stop-shop" staging: should we prefer FDG-PET/CT or MRI for the detection of bone metastases? *Eur J Radiol*. 2011;78(3):430–435.
54. Gokaslan ZL, Aladag MA, Ellerhorst JA. Melanoma metastatic to the spine: a review of 133 cases. *Melanoma Res*. 2000;10(1):78–80.
55. Kawashima A, Fishman EK, Kuhlman JE, et al. CT of malignant melanoma: patterns of small bowel and mesenteric involvement. *J Comput Assist Tomogr*. 1991;15(4):570–574.
56. King DM. Imaging of metastatic melanoma. *Cancer Imaging*. 2006;6:204–208.
57. Kumar NB, Hart WR. Metastases to the uterine corpus from extragenital cancers. A clinicopathologic study of 63 cases. *Cancer*. 1982;50(10):2163–2169.
58. Giannini I, Cutrignelli DA, Resta L, et al. Metastatic melanoma of the gallbladder: report of two cases and a review of the literature. *Clin Exp Med*. 2016;16(3):295–300.
59. Silverman PM, Heaston DK, Korobkin M, et al. Computed tomography in the detection of abdominal metastases from malignant melanoma. *Invest Radiol*. 1984;19(4):309–312.
60. Sheth S, Horton KM, Garland MR, et al. Mesenteric neoplasms: CT appearances of primary and secondary tumors and differential diagnosis. *Radiographics*. 2003;23(2):457–473. quiz 535-456.
61. Gibbs P, Cebon JS, Calafiore P, et al. Cardiac metastases from malignant melanoma. *Cancer*. 1999;85(1):78–84.
62. Ross MI, Gershenwald JE. Evidence-based treatment of early-stage melanoma. *J Surg Oncol*. 2011;104(4):341–353.
63. Balch CM, Gershenwald JE. Clinical value of the sentinel-node biopsy in primary cutaneous melanoma. *N Engl J Med*. 2014;370(7):663–664.
64. Faries MB, Thompson JF, Cochran AJ, et al. Completion dissection or observation for sentinel-node metastasis in melanoma. *N Engl J Med*. 2017;376(23):2211–2222.
65. Moody JA, Botham SJ, Dahill KE, et al. Complications following completion lymphadenectomy versus therapeutic lymphadenectomy for melanoma - A systematic review of the literature. *Eur J Surg Oncol*. 2017;43(9):1760–1767.
66. Beasley GM, Caudle A, Petersen RP, et al. A multi-institutional experience of isolated limb infusion: defining response and toxicity in the US. *J Am Coll Surg*. 2009;208(5):706–715. discussion 715-707.
67. Bhatia S, Tykodi SS, Thompson JA. Treatment of metastatic melanoma: an overview. *Oncology (Williston Park)*. 2009;23(6):488–496.
68. Bedikian AY, Johnson MM, Warneke CL, et al. Systemic therapy for unresectable metastatic melanoma: impact of biochemotherapy on long-term survival. *J Immunotoxicol*. 2008;5(2):201–207.
69. Ballo MT, Ang KK. Radiation therapy for malignant melanoma. *Surg Clin North Am*. 2003;83(2):323–342.
70. Andtbacka RH, Kaufman HL, Collichio F, et al. Talimogene laherparepvec improves durable response rate in patients with advanced melanoma. *J Clin Oncol*. 2015;33(25):2780–2788.
71. Sharma P, Allison JP. Immune checkpoint targeting in cancer therapy: toward combination strategies with curative potential. *Cell*. 2015;161(2):205–214.
72. Kaehler KC, Piel S, Livingstone E, et al. Update on immunologic therapy with anti-CTLA-4 antibodies in melanoma: identification of clinical and biological response patterns, immune-related adverse events, and their management. *Semin Oncol*. 2010;37(5):485–498.
73. Eggermont AMM, Chiarion-Sileni V, Grob JJ, et al. Adjuvant ipilimumab versus placebo after complete resection of stage III melanoma: long-term follow-up results of the European Organisation for Research and Treatment of Cancer 18071 double-blind phase 3 randomised trial. *Eur J Cancer*. 2019;119:1–10.
74. Eggermont AM, Chiarion-Sileni V, Grob JJ, et al. Prolonged survival in stage iii melanoma with ipilimumab adjuvant therapy. *N Engl J Med*. 2016;375(19):1845–1855.
75. Hersey P, Kakavand H, Wilmott J, et al. How anti-PD1 treatments are changing the management of melanoma. *Melanoma Manag*. 2014;1(2):165–172.
76. Weber J, Mandala M, Del Vecchio M, et al. Adjuvant nivolumab versus ipilimumab in resected stage iii or iv melanoma. *N Engl J Med*. 2017;377(19):1824–1835.
77. Gellrich FF, Schmitz M, Beissert S, et al. Anti-PD-1 and novel combinations in the treatment of melanoma-an update. *J Clin Med*. 2020;9(1):223.
78. Hodi FS, O'Day SJ, McDermott DF, et al. Improved survival with ipilimumab in patients with metastatic melanoma. *N Engl J Med*. 2010;363(8):711–723.
79. Ascierto PA, Del Vecchio M, Robert C, et al. Ipilimumab 10 mg/kg versus ipilimumab 3 mg/kg in patients with unresectable or

metastatic melanoma: a randomised, double-blind, multicentre, phase 3 trial. *Lancet Oncol*. 2017;18(5):611–622.
80. Robert C, Long GV, Brady B, et al. Nivolumab in previously untreated melanoma without BRAF mutation. *N Engl J Med*. 2015;372(4):320–330.
81. Wolchok JD, Chiarion-Sileni V, Gonzalez R, et al. Overall survival with combined nivolumab and ipilimumab in advanced melanoma. *N Engl J Med*. 2017;377(14):1345–1356.
82. Hamid O, Robert C, Daud A, et al. Safety and tumor responses with lambrolizumab (anti-PD-1) in melanoma. *N Engl J Med*. 2013;369(2):134–144.
83. Rothermel LD, Sarnaik AA, Khushalani NI, et al. Current immunotherapy practices in melanoma. *Surg Oncol Clin N Am*. 2019;28(3):403–418.
84. Schachter J, Ribas A, Long GV, et al. Pembrolizumab versus ipilimumab for advanced melanoma: final overall survival results of a multicentre, randomised, open-label phase 3 study (KEYNOTE-006). *Lancet*. 2017;390(10105):1853–1862.
85. Moser JC, Wei G, Colonna SV, et al. Comparative effectiveness of pembrolizumab vs. nivolumab for patients with metastatic melanoma. *Acta Oncol*. 2020;59(4):434–437.
86. Deutsch GB, Kirchoff DD, Faries MB. Metastasectomy for stage IV melanoma. *Surg Oncol Clin N Am*. 2015;24(2):279–298.
87. Larkin J, Chiarion-Sileni V, Gonzalez R, et al. Five-year survival with combined nivolumab and ipilimumab in advanced melanoma. *N Engl J Med*. 2019;381(16):1535–1546.
88. Larkin J, Chiarion-Sileni V, Gonzalez R, et al. Combined nivolumab and ipilimumab or monotherapy in untreated melanoma. *N Engl J Med*. 2015;373(1):23–34.
89. Tawbi HA, Forsyth PA, Algazi A, et al. Combined nivolumab and ipilimumab in melanoma metastatic to the brain. *N Engl J Med*. 2018;379(8):722–730.
90. Carlino MS, Long GV. Ipilimumab combined with nivolumab: a standard of care for the treatment of advanced melanoma? *Clin Cancer Res*. 2016;22(16):3992–3998.
91. Lebbe C, Meyer N, Mortier L, et al. Evaluation of two dosing regimens for nivolumab in combination with ipilimumab in patients with advanced melanoma: results from the phase IIIb/IV CheckMate 511 Trial. *J Clin Oncol*. 2019;37(11):867–875.
92. Amaria RN, Menzies AM, Burton EM, et al. Neoadjuvant systemic therapy in melanoma: recommendations of the International Neoadjuvant Melanoma Consortium. *Lancet Oncol*. 2019;20(7): e378–e389.
93. Pelster MS, Amaria RN. Neoadjuvant immunotherapy for locally advanced melanoma. *Curr Treat Options Oncol*. 2020;21(2):10.
94. Rozeman EA, Menzies AM, van Akkooi ACJ, et al. Identification of the optimal combination dosing schedule of neoadjuvant ipilimumab plus nivolumab in macroscopic stage III melanoma (OpACIN-neo): a multicentre, phase 2, randomised, controlled trial. *Lancet Oncol*. 2019;20(7):948–960.
95. Patel H, Yacoub N, Mishra R, et al. Current advances in the treatment of BRAF-mutant melanoma. *Cancers (Basel)*. 2020;12(2):482.
96. Valachis A, Ullenhag GJ. Discrepancy in BRAF status among patients with metastatic malignant melanoma: A meta-analysis. *Eur J Cancer*. 2017;81:106–115.
97. Atkinson V. Recent advances in malignant melanoma. *Intern Med J*. 2017;47(10):1114–1121.
98. Cheng L, Lopez-Beltran A, Massari F, et al. Molecular testing for BRAF mutations to inform melanoma treatment decisions: a move toward precision medicine. *Mod Pathol*. 2018;31(1):24–38.
99. Long GV, Hauschild A, Santinami M, et al. Adjuvant dabrafenib plus trametinib in stage III BRAF-mutated melanoma. *N Engl J Med*. 2017;377(19):1813–1823.
100. Hauschild A, Dummer R, Schadendorf D, et al. Longer follow-up confirms relapse-free survival benefit with adjuvant dabrafenib plus trametinib in patients with resected BRAF V600-mutant stage iii melanoma. *J Clin Oncol*. 2018;36(35):3441–3449.
101. Chapman PB, Hauschild A, Robert C, et al. Improved survival with vemurafenib in melanoma with BRAF V600E mutation. *N Engl J Med*. 2011;364(26):2507–2516.
102. Hauschild A, Grob JJ, Demidov LV, et al. Dabrafenib in BRAF-mutated metastatic melanoma: a multicentre, open-label, phase 3 randomised controlled trial. *Lancet*. 2012;380(9839):358–365.
103. Shirley M. Encorafenib and binimetinib: first global approvals. *Drugs*. 2018;78(12):1277–1284.
104. Kim A, Cohen MS. The discovery of vemurafenib for the treatment of BRAF-mutated metastatic melanoma. *Expert Opin Drug Discov*. 2016;11(9):907–916.
105. Grimaldi AM, Simeone E, Festino L, et al. MEK inhibitors in the treatment of metastatic melanoma and solid tumors. *Am J Clin Dermatol*. 2017;18(6):745–754.
106. Flaherty KT, Robert C, Hersey P, et al. Improved survival with MEK inhibition in BRAF-mutated melanoma. *N Engl J Med*. 2012;367(2):107–114.
107. Kim KB, Kefford R, Pavlick AC, et al. Phase II study of the MEK1/MEK2 inhibitor Trametinib in patients with metastatic BRAF-mutant cutaneous melanoma previously treated with or without a BRAF inhibitor. *J Clin Oncol*. 2013;31(4):482–489.
108. Broman KK, Dossett LA, Sun J, et al. Update on BRAF and MEK inhibition for treatment of melanoma in metastatic, unresectable, and adjuvant settings. *Expert Opin Drug Saf*. 2019;18(5):381–392.
109. Amann VC, Ramelyte E, Thurneysen S, et al. Developments in targeted therapy in melanoma. *Eur J Surg Oncol*. 2017;43(3):581–593.
110. Flaherty KT, Infante JR, Daud A, et al. Combined BRAF and MEK inhibition in melanoma with BRAF V600 mutations. *N Engl J Med*. 2012;367(18):1694–1703.
111. Long GV, Stroyakovskiy D, Gogas H, et al. Combined BRAF and MEK inhibition versus BRAF inhibition alone in melanoma. *N Engl J Med*. 2014;371(20):1877–1888.
112. Robert C, Karaszewska B, Schachter J, et al. Improved overall survival in melanoma with combined dabrafenib and trametinib. *N Engl J Med*. 2015;372(1):30–39.
113. Glitza Oliva IC, Schvartsman G, Tawbi H. Advances in the systemic treatment of melanoma brain metastases. *Ann Oncol*. 2018;29(7):1509–1520.
114. Ascierto PA, McArthur GA, Dreno B, et al. Cobimetinib combined with vemurafenib in advanced BRAF(V600)-mutant melanoma (coBRIM): updated efficacy results from a randomised, double-blind, phase 3 trial. *Lancet Oncol*. 2016;17(9):1248–1260.
115. Weber JS. Current perspectives on immunotherapy. *Semin Oncol*. 2014;41(Suppl 5):S14–S29.
116. Dromain C, Beigelman C, Pozzessere C, et al. Imaging of tumour response to immunotherapy. *Eur Radiol Exp*. 2020;4(1):2.
117. Spain L, Diem S, Larkin J. Management of toxicities of immune checkpoint inhibitors. *Cancer Treat Rev*. 2016;44:51–60.
118. Weber JS, Kahler KC, Hauschild A. Management of immune-related adverse events and kinetics of response with ipilimumab. *J Clin Oncol*. 2012;30(21):2691–2697.
119. Shoushtari AN, Friedman CF, Navid-Azarbaijani P, et al. Measuring toxic effects and time to treatment failure for nivolumab plus ipilimumab in melanoma. *JAMA Oncol*. 2018;4(1):98–101.
120. Eisenhauer EA, Therasse P, Bogaerts J, et al. New response evaluation criteria in solid tumours: revised RECIST guideline (version 1.1). *Eur J Cancer*. 2009;45(2):228–247.
121. Wolchok JD, Hoos A, O'Day S, et al. Guidelines for the evaluation of immune therapy activity in solid tumors: immune-related response criteria. *Clin Cancer Res*. 2009;15(23):7412–7420.
122. Nishino M, Giobbie-Hurder A, Gargano M, et al. Developing a common language for tumor response to immunotherapy: immune-related response criteria using unidimensional measurements. *Clin Cancer Res*. 2013;19(14):3936–3943.
123. Seymour L, Bogaerts J, Perrone A, et al. iRECIST: guidelines for response criteria for use in trials testing immunotherapeutics. *Lancet Oncol*. 2017;18(3):e143–e152.
124. Hodi FS, Ballinger M, Lyons B, et al. Immune-Modified Response Evaluation Criteria In Solid Tumors (imRECIST): refining guidelines to assess the clinical benefit of cancer immunotherapy. *J Clin Oncol*. 2018;36(9):850–858.
125. Young H, Baum R, Cremerius U, et al. Measurement of clinical and subclinical tumour response using [18F]-fluorodeoxyglucose and positron emission tomography: review and 1999 EORTC recommendations. European Organization for Research and Treatment of Cancer (EORTC) PET Study Group. *Eur J Cancer*. 1999;35(13):1773–1782.
126. Wahl RL, Jacene H, Kasamon Y, et al. From RECIST to PERCIST: evolving considerations for PET response criteria in solid tumors. *J Nucl Med*. 2009;50(Suppl 1):122S–150S.
127. Cho SY, Lipson EJ, Im HJ, et al. Prediction of response to immune checkpoint inhibitor therapy using early-time-point (18)F-FDG

PET/CT imaging in patients with advanced melanoma. *J Nucl Med.* 2017;58(9):1421–1428.
128. Anwar H, Sachpekidis C, Winkler J, et al. Absolute number of new lesions on (18)F-FDG PET/CT is more predictive of clinical response than SUV changes in metastatic melanoma patients receiving ipilimumab. *Eur J Nucl Med Mol Imaging.* 2018;45(3):376–383.
129. Nebhan CA, Johnson DB. Predictive biomarkers of response to immune checkpoint inhibitors in melanoma. *Expert Rev Anticancer Ther.* 2020;20(2):137–145.
130. Romano E, Scordo M, Dusza SW, et al. Site and timing of first relapse in stage III melanoma patients: implications for follow-up guidelines. *J Clin Oncol.* 2010;28(18):3042–3047.
131. Lee JW, Nam SB, Kim SJ. Role of 18F-fluorodeoxyglucose positron emission tomography or positron emission tomography/computed tomography for the detection of recurrent disease after treatment of malignant melanoma. *Oncology.* 2019;97(5):286–293.

Visit ExpertConsult.com for algorithms

CUTANEOUS MELANOMA

Note: Consider clinical trials as treatment options for eligible patients.

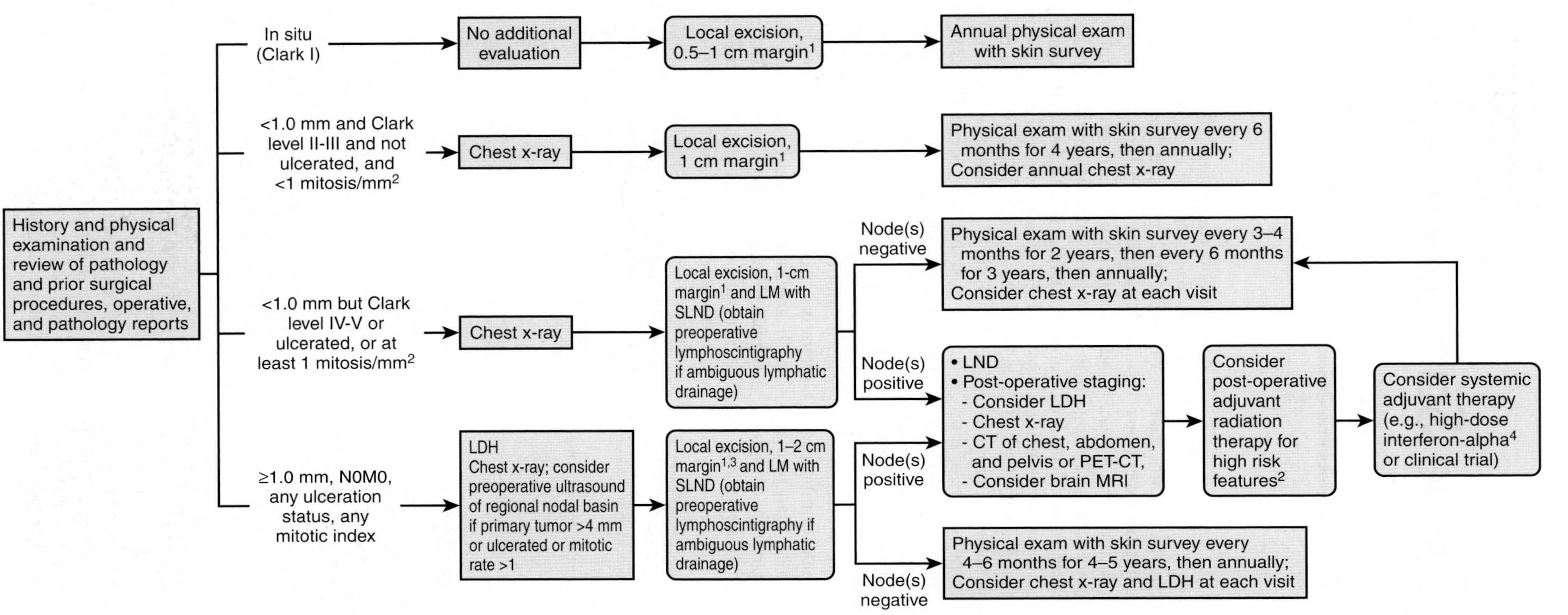

[1]Consider function and cosmesis
[2]High-risk features include: • Extracapsular extension • ≥3 cm • ≥4 nodes involved • Regional nodal or soft tissue recurrence
[3]Consider postoperative adjuvant radiation therapy for pure desmoplastic and neurotropic histology.
[4]See references in Adjuvant Interferon-Alpha section in full protocol on-line.

LM, Lymphatic mapping and sentinel lymph node biopsy LMD, Leptomeningeal disease LND, Lymph node dissection
SLND, Selective lymph node dissection based on results of sentinel lymph node evaluation

This practice consensus algorithm is not intended to replace the independent medical or professional judgment of physicians or other health care providers. Without specific instructions from an M.D. Anderson health care provider about individual patient care, this algorithm should be used for informational purposes only. This algorithm should not be used to treat pregnant women.

CHAPTER

38 Soft Tissue Sarcomas

Rajendra Kumar, M.D., F.A.C.R.; Joseph A. Ludwig, M.D.; and John E. Madewell, M.D.

INTRODUCTION

Soft tissue sarcomas are rare mesenchymal tumors that originate from the mesoderm, with the notable exceptions of those arising from primitive neuroectodermal tissue and those with unknown cell derivation, such as Ewing sarcoma or synovial sarcoma.[1, 2] Because more than 50 clinically and molecularly distinct sarcoma subtypes exist, there is tremendous clinical variation that leads to marked heterogeneity in their respective clinical behavior, prognosis, metastatic risk, and chemotherapy responsiveness.[3] For this reason, clinicians must be aware of the subtype-dependent nuances, even though many soft tissue sarcomas are treated similarly. Despite having nearly the same incidence as multiple myeloma or thyroid carcinoma, soft tissue sarcomas are responsible for more deaths than from testicular tumors, Hodgkin disease, and thyroid cancer combined.[4, 5] They are two to three times more common than primary malignant bone tumors, and, despite apparently complete surgical resection, they often metastasize to the lungs.

Key Points Introduction

- Soft tissue sarcomas are rare malignant tumors arising in mesenchymal and primitive neuroectodermal tissues.
- Soft tissue sarcomas are two to three times more common than primary malignant bone tumors.
- They often metastasize to the lungs.

EPIDEMIOLOGY AND ETIOLOGIC CONSIDERATIONS

Soft tissue sarcomas account for approximately 1% of all primary adult malignancies and 7% to 15% of pediatric neoplasms.[2, 6] The general incidence of these tumors is 1.4 per 100, 000, but rises to 8 per 100, 000 in people older than 80 years. Roughly 40% of all soft tissue sarcomas occur in people older than 50 years.[2] The American Cancer Society estimates a combined incidence of soft tissue (including heart) sarcomas in adults and children of approximately 13, 460 new cases (7720 males and 5740 females) and approximately 5270 deaths (2840 males and 2510 females) for the year 2021.[7] The overall incidence has been gradually increasing, in part because of better diagnosis.[8] A male to female ratio of approximately 1.2 to 1 has been reported, although this varies considerably depending upon the sarcoma subtype.[2] The relative frequency of each subtype of soft tissue sarcoma varies according to age. For instance, rhabdomyosarcoma mostly occurs in children, synovial sarcoma in young adults, and undifferentiated pleomorphic sarcoma (MFH) in the older population. Benign soft tissue tumors are approximately 100 times more common than malignant soft tissue tumors. Soft tissue sarcomas are most often seen in the extremities (59%), the trunk (19%), the retroperitoneum (15%), and the head and neck (9%).[2]

The vast majority of soft tissue malignancies occur sporadically without any predisposing cause. However, secondary soft tissue sarcomas may be seen 3 to 15 years following irradiation for lymphoma, cervical cancer, breast cancer, or testicular cancer.[9] Viruses have also been implicated with some soft tissue sarcomas, such as leiomyosarcoma, and with Kaposi sarcoma in patients with acquired immunodeficiency syndrome.[10] Chronic lymphedema-associated angiosarcoma (Stewart–Treves syndrome) occurs as a rare complication of breast cancer treatment.[11] An increased incidence of soft tissue sarcomas has been reported in several genetic disorders, such as neurofibromatosis, hereditary retinoblastoma, and Li–Fraumeni syndrome.[12] Chemicals, such as Agent Orange (a dioxin-containing herbicide) and immunosuppressive drugs, are an uncommon cause of soft tissue sarcoma.[13]

Key Points Epidemiology and Risk Factors

- Soft tissue sarcomas can be seen at any age; most occur after age 50 years.
- They make up for approximately 1% of all primary tumors in adults and 7% to 15% in children.
- They most commonly occur in the lower extremities.
- Most soft tissue sarcomas occur without any predisposing cause. In a few instances, genetic, infections (viral), chemicals (Agent Orange), physical agent (radiation), and immunosuppressive drugs may be contributory.

HISTOPATHOLOGIC CONSIDERATIONS

The World Health Organization (WHO) classifies various histologic subtypes of soft tissue sarcomas.[3] This classification is based on the presence of predominant constituent mesenchymal tissue of malignant soft tissue tumor, as well as whether a malignant soft tissue sarcoma is low-, intermediate-, or high-grade on histopathology. Thus, a malignant soft tissue tumor consisting of mostly malignant adipocytic cells is termed as liposarcoma. A less aggressive well-differentiated liposarcoma (atypical lipomatous tumor) may recur locally, but rarely it has distant metastases, whereas high-grade dedifferentiated liposarcoma often has distant metastases, usually to the lungs. Similarly, fibrosarcoma is named after its constituent malignant fibrous tissue. At times, a soft tissue tumor may have admixture of constituent malignant cells, as in case of myxoinflammatory fibroblastic sarcoma, which not only contains malignant fibroblasts and myxoid tissue, but also inflammatory cells. Similarly, highly malignant dedifferentiated/pleomorphic soft tissue sarcoma (malignant fibrous histiocytoma) is composed mostly of malignant fibrous and histiocytic tissues. It is therefore imperative that histopathologic diagnosis of a soft tissue mass be made before treatment to establish its tissue composition and to know whether it is benign or malignant. Also, in case of a malignant tumor, it is essential to determine whether it is low-, intermediate-, or high-grade. This histopathologic diagnosis will ultimately decide treatment, management, and patient prognosis, as different soft tissue tumors vary greatly in their clinical behavior and outcome. In general, biopsy should be performed on any symptomatic or enlarging soft tissue mass that persists longer than 4 weeks or is larger than 5 cm in diameter.[5]

Computed tomography (CT)– or ultrasound (US)-guided percutaneous fine needle aspiration (FNA) biopsy is routinely performed under local anesthesia. An FNA biopsy has low risk of complications, but a greater probability of misdiagnosis; however, it is ideal for suspected recurrent soft tissue tumors or nodal metastases.[5, 14]

A core needle biopsy is often preferred for diagnosis, as it has relatively low (~1%) rate of complications and a much higher diagnostic yield than a FNA biopsy.[14–16] Several specimens should be obtained from within a soft tissue tumor to ensure adequate tumor tissue for various pathologic stains, electron microscopic studies, cytogenetic analysis, and flow cytometric studies. US, CT, or gadolinium (Gd)-enhanced MRI is often used as a guide to determine the best area for biopsy. In addition, the biopsy site should be chosen so that it lays within the area of subsequent *en bloc* resection. Improper biopsy has been shown to be associated with greater morbidity, complications, and changes in clinical course and outcome.[17] To prevent tumor seeding, biopsy can be obtained by using a coaxial needle with its tip at the outer margin of the tumor, through which the core biopsy needle can be placed within the tumor. An adequacy rate of 93% and an accuracy rate of 95% have been reported with FNA and core needle biopsies.[16]

When a closed needle biopsy technique returns inadequate specimen, an open biopsy should be considered. For a small mass less than 3 cm in diameter, an excisional biopsy can be performed. However, for tumors larger than 5 cm in diameter, an incisional biopsy through a small longitudinal incision, preferably performed by the surgeon planning surgical resection, is recommended.

In case of a malignant retroperitoneal soft tissue tumor, needle biopsy should not be performed routinely, because of the potential danger of transperitoneal tumor spread and track seeding. Exceptions include suspected intraabdominal nodal involvement in lymphoma and germ cell tumors and for soft tissue tumors where preoperative chemotherapy or radiation is to be used.[15]

The histologic grade of soft tissue sarcoma best predicts its biologic behavior and is determined by four factors: mitotic index, degree of cellularity, intratumoral necrosis, and degree of nuclear anaplasia. A soft tissue sarcoma is graded as low-grade or high-grade malignancy on histopathology. High-grade soft tissue sarcomas can be moderately differentiated, poorly differentiated, or undifferentiated.

Key Points Histopathologic Considerations

- According to the World Health Organization, more than 50 histologic subtypes of soft tissue sarcomas exist.
- Needle aspiration or core biopsy under ultrasound, computed tomography, or magnetic resonance imaging guidance, or incisional or excisional biopsy of a soft tissue sarcoma can be performed for histologic diagnosis.
- Histopathologically, a soft tissue sarcoma may be low-grade or high-grade. A high-grade tumor may be moderately differentiated, poorly differentiated, or undifferentiated.

CLINICAL EVALUATION

Soft tissue sarcomas usually present clinically as gradually enlarging, painless masses. Diagnosis of soft tissue sarcoma relies on clinical examination, imaging, and histologic analysis. Clinical examination and imaging define tumor relationship with adjoining structures.[18–20] Because they are more superficial, soft tissue tumors in distal limbs and in the head and neck tend to be small; those in the thighs, buttocks, and retroperitoneum, being deep-seated, can be huge.

When evaluating a patient with a soft tissue mass, one must ascertain how long the mass has been present; whether the mass is slow- or fast-growing; presence of local pain and tenderness; constitutional symptoms; history of prior surgery, radiation, or trauma to the area; and recent use of anticoagulants. The growth rate of a soft tissue sarcoma can often vary with aggressiveness of the tumor. However, slow growth does not always imply benignity. It is not uncommon for epithelioid sarcoma to be mistaken for a benign tumor because of its small size, thereby leading to improper management. Presence of local pain, seen in approximately one-third of patients with rapidly growing high-grade tumors, usually indicates poor prognosis.[18] Discoloration of overlying skin or variation in size of the soft tissue mass with activity or palpation favors hemangioma. Regional lymph nodes should always be examined for metastatic spread, even though lymphangietic spread of a soft tissue sarcoma is uncommon.

Most soft tissue sarcomas expand centrifugally and tend to have a peripheral pseudocapsule of compressed normal soft tissue around them. However, this pseudocapsule is often infiltrated by tumor.[21] As a soft tissue sarcoma grows, it follows the path of least resistance and tends to remain confined to the compartment of origin. Such an intracompartmental soft tissue tumor is bounded by natural anatomical barriers, such as fascial septa, tendon, ligament, cortical bone, articular cartilage, and joint capsule. Larger tumors can cause symptoms secondary to increased pressure/stretch on adjoining neurovascular structures. This can not only cause pain, but also produce paresthesias and regional soft tissue edema. With highly aggressive soft tissue tumors, satellite soft tissue tumor foci (skip metastases) may be found frequently beyond the peritumoral reactive zone within the compartment of origin.[21]

The presence of a pseudocapsule at the periphery of a soft tissue sarcoma does not always confer benignity. A well-marginated soft tissue tumor with a pseudocapsule can be malignant, whereas an infiltrating soft tissue tumor with ill-defined borders, such as desmoid tumor, rarely metastasizes distally. The size of a soft tissue tumor does not always distinguish a benign from a malignant soft tissue tumor, as has been pointed out earlier. However, in general, a soft tissue mass smaller than 3 cm in diameter tends to be benign, with a positive predictive value of 88%, while a soft tissue mass larger than 5 cm in diameter indicates malignancy, with a sensitivity of 74%, a specificity of 59%, and an accuracy of 66%.[22]

Extracompartmental extent, involvement of adjacent bone, and encasement of neurovascular bundle are insensitive signs of malignancy, as these can also be seen with benign soft tissue tumors, such as hemangioma or desmoid tumor. A benign soft tissue lesion, such as fibromatosis, can be aggressive in behavior, while a well-differentiated liposarcoma is usually slow-growing. In some cases, both benign and malignant soft tissue tumors may be seen in the same patient. For instance, in a patient with neurofibromatosis, numerous benign soft tissue neurofibromas may coexist with a neurofibrosarcoma, and sometimes it may be difficult to distinguish between the two.

Key Points Clinical Evaluation

- Soft tissue sarcomas often present as a localized palpable mass with variable pain and tenderness.
- A soft tissue sarcoma is usually hard in consistency, and, when large, it may produce symptoms by compressing adjoining neurovascular bundle.
- When a tumor is near a joint, the patient may have limitation in range of joint motion.
- The size of a tumor does not determine whether it is benign or malignant.
- A rapidly growing soft tissue tumor usually indicates malignancy.
- A painful, rapidly growing malignant soft tissue tumor tends to have poor prognosis.
- Pseudocapsule around a soft tissue sarcoma often harbors malignancy.

CLASSIFICATION AND STAGING

Soft tissue is derived from mesenchyme and consists of skeletal muscle, fat, fibrous tissue, blood vessels, and neurovascular tissue. Soft tissue sarcomas (Greek, *sarx* means "flesh") are designated on the basis of the adult tissue they resemble microscopically, and not necessarily the tissue in which they originate.[2] For instance, the designation *lipoma* does not mean that the tumor arose from adipose tissue; instead, it means the tumor contains tissue resembling mature fat. Dedifferentiated soft tissue sarcoma contains poorly differentiated mesenchyme on microscopy, and thus lacks a specific histologic designation to the tumor. More sophisticated immunohistochemical stains and genetic markers are now available to further classify these differentiated soft tissue sarcomas. Only a few of the genetic aberrations that occur in soft tissue sarcomas are congenital; most are acquired spontaneously.[23]

Staging refers to evaluation of local and distant spread of tumor and has multiple purposes.[24–27] It provides a standardized method for determining extent of tumor, allows assessment of prognosis, and serves to guide initial treatment decisions. The French Federation of Cancer Centers Sarcoma Group (Federation Nationale des Centres de Lutte Contre le Cancer [FNCLCC]) system and the National Cancer Institution (NCI) system are most commonly used for grading soft tissue sarcomas. The FNCLCC system is based on tumor differentiation, tumor necrosis, and mitotic activity, while the NCI system uses histology, location, and tumor necrosis for grading. In comparison studies, the FNCLCC system has slightly greater ability to predict metastatic risk and mortality, as the NCI system does not directly take into consideration the histological subtype. Instead, the NCI system uses parameters such as tumor cellularity, differentiation, pleomorphism, mitotic rate, and necrosis to assign tumors to one of three possible tumor grades (low-, intermediate-, and high-grade) that indirectly predict a cancer phenotype (American Joint Committee on Cancer [AJCC] website).

The GTNM (Grade-Tumor-Node-Metastasis) system of the AJCC/Union for International Cancer Control for staging soft tissue sarcoma is based on grading, tumor, node, and metastases.[24] However, these criteria do not apply to all soft tissue sarcomas, such as visceral, retroperitoneal, and Kaposi sarcomas. The recent staging classification has undergone several critical changes. For example, several soft tissue sarcomas subtypes previously included within the general soft tissue sarcoma staging system, such as gastrointestinal stromal tumor, desmoid fibromatosis, and uterine sarcoma, now have their own respective staging classification. Conversely, dermatofibrosarcoma protuberans, angiosarcoma, extraskeletal Ewing sarcoma, and neurogenic tumor are newly included with the soft tissue sarcoma staging system.

Another change is that tumor depth, previously described as superficial or deep, is no longer used within the current AJCC staging system, and the three-tiered grading method advocated by FNCLCC for tumor grading is now preferred over the GTNM system.[24, 25]

Tumor Characteristics

Histologic grade (G): FNCLCC histologic grade

G_1 Total differentiation, mitotic count, and necrotic score 2 or 3

G_2 Total differentiation, mitotic count, and necrosis score 4 or 5

G_3 Total differentiation, mitotic count, and necrosis score 6, 7, or 8
GX Grade cannot be assessed

Primary tumor (T)
TX Primary tumor cannot be assessed
T_0 No evidence of primary tumor
T_1 Tumor 5 cm or less in greatest dimension
T_2 Tumor >5 cm and ≤10 cm in greatest dimension
T_3 Tumor >10 cm and ≤15 cm in greatest dimension
T_4 Tumor >15 cm in greatest dimension

Regional lymph nodes (N)
N_0 No regional lymph node metastases
N_1 Regional lymph node metastases

Distant metastases (M)
M_0 No distant metastasis
M_1 Distant metastasis

The most important determinants of staging of extremity soft tissue sarcoma are histologic grade and size; both have similar prognostic value.[26, 27]

The N stage refers to regional node involvement. Metastatic spread with soft tissue sarcomas is generally hematogenous; however, in less than 5% of cases, metastatic spread may occur via lymphatics. The most common tumors that metastasize to regional lymph nodes are synovial sarcoma, epithelioid sarcoma, clear cell sarcoma, rhabdomyosarcoma, and angiosarcoma.[18]

The M stage refers to local or distant metastases. Metastatic potentials for low-grade, intermediate-grade, and high-grade soft tissue sarcomas are 5% to 10%, 25% to 30%, and 50% to 60%, respectively.[18]

In general, staging of soft tissue sarcomas is as follows:

Stage I: Low-grade tumor without metastases, regardless of tumor size
Stage II: Intermediate- to high-grade sarcomas without metastases
Stage III: Large, high-grade tumors or node-positive
Stage IV: Soft tissue tumor with extranodal metastasis, regardless of lesion size or histologic grade.

Although the staging system continues to evolve, significant challenges remain to be solved.[27] Soft tissue sarcomas of the extremities, head and neck, viscera, and retroperitoneum are all staged together, regardless of different surgical approach and outcomes.[5] Also, small size alone is not always determinant of actual biological behavior of soft tissue tumors. For instance, a small epithelioid or synovial sarcoma often disseminates, whereas a much larger well-differentiated liposarcoma rarely does.

Spectrum of Soft Tissue Sarcomas

The WHO classification of soft tissue sarcomas provides uniformity of tissue diagnosis.[3] However, this classification is incomplete, as at present atypical lipoma and well-differentiated liposarcoma, having no potential for distant metastases, are considered histopathologically the same neoplasm, whereas MFH is now designated as high grade pleomorphic sarcoma.[28, 29] The most common soft tissue sarcomas in adults are dedifferentiated pleomorphic sarcoma (formerly MFH) 28%, liposarcoma 15%, leiomyosarcoma 12%, synovial sarcoma 10%, and malignant peripheral nerve sheath tumors 6%, whereas rhabdomyosarcoma is the most common soft tissue sarcoma in children.[18]

Key Points Classification and Staging

- Classification of soft tissue sarcomas is based on constituent mesenchymal tissue.
- Dedifferentiated soft tissue tumors contain poorly differentiated mesenchymal tissue on microscopy; thus, they lack a specific tissue diagnosis.
- Histologic parameters—tumor cellularity, differentiation, pleomorphism, mitotic rate, and necrosis—are used to predict tumor behavior and metastatic risk; they ultimately influence treatment and prognosis.
- The grade-tumor-node-metastasis system based upon histologic grade, size, regional lymph node involvement, and distant metastases, is used to stage soft tissue sarcomas.
- Stage I: low-grade tumor without metastases regardless of size; stage II: intermediate- to high-grade tumor without metastases; stage III: large, high-grade or node-positive tumor; and stage IV: soft tissue tumor with distant metastases, regardless of size or histologic grade.

IMAGING

Imaging of soft tissue sarcomas requires a multimodal approach, which initially includes radiography and MRI. Other imaging modalities, such as CT, positron emission tomography (PET) combined with CT, US, and magnetic resonance angiography (MRA) can be performed for further evaluation, if required. Preoperative chest radiographs and chest CT for staging are routinely done to detect lung metastases. Abdominal CT is used to detect and stage retroperitoneal tumors, such as liposarcoma, while radionuclide bone scintigraphy can detect distant bone metastases.

Radiography

Radiography has a limited role in diagnosis and staging of soft tissue tumors.[30] Small, deep-seated soft tissue tumors are often difficult to recognize on radiographs, whereas larger soft tissue tumors can be seen, as they distort fascial planes and may produce a focal surface bulge (Fig. 38.1). Other findings when present on radiographs can be useful in diagnosis. For instance, calcified phleboliths in soft tissues on radiographs indicate a soft tissue hemangioma (Fig. 38.2), while a soft tissue tumor with calcifications near a joint in a young adult is suggestive of synovial sarcoma (Fig. 38.3). A soft tissue lipoma containing radiolucent fat is often diagnosed on radiographs. Radiographs also provide useful information, such as erosion or destruction, periosteal

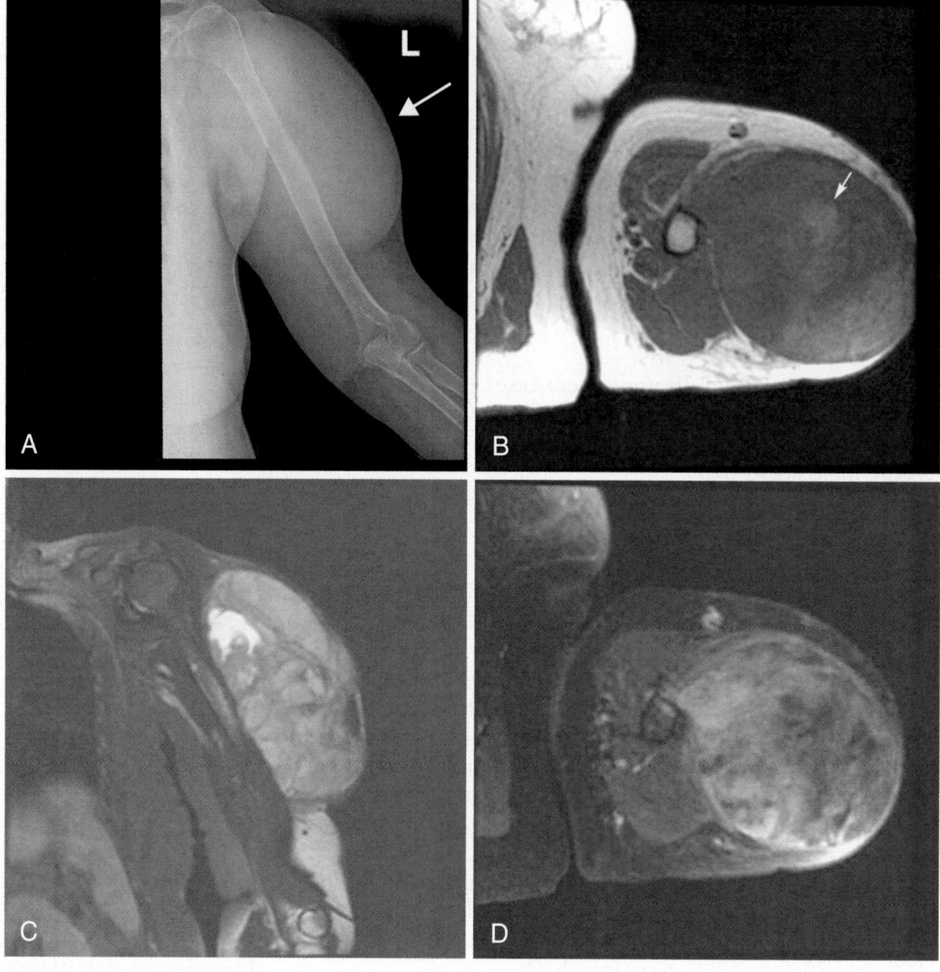

FIGURE 38.1. A 63-year-old woman with undifferentiated pleomorphic soft tissue sarcoma of left upper arm. **A**, Anteroposterior radiograph showing a large soft tissue mass in the lateral aspect of the proximal left upper arm. Note localized soft tissue bulge at left upper arm (*arrow*). **B**, Axial T1-weighted (T1W) imaging shows mostly isointense magnetic resonance (MR) signal with focal areas of hyperintense signal because of intratumoral hemorrhage (arrow). **C**, On coronal fat-suppressed T2-weighted imaging, soft tissue mass shows heterogeneous hyperintense MR signal. **D**, Axial postcontrast fat-suppressed T1W imaging demonstrates heterogeneously enhancing soft tissue tumor with well-defined pseudocapsule.

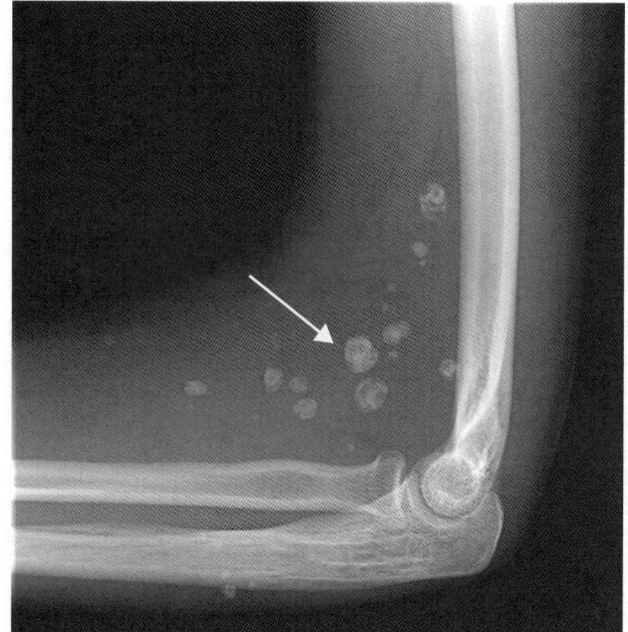

FIGURE 38.2. Hemangioma in a 22-year-old woman. Lateral radiograph of right elbow shows numerous calcified phleboliths (*arrow*) in anterior soft tissues, consistent with soft tissue hemangioma.

reaction, or pressure deformity of an adjoining bone, which may be associated with a soft tissue sarcoma (Fig. 38.4).

Magnetic Resonance Imaging

MRI is considered the imaging modality of choice for localization, characterization, and staging of a soft tissue tumor.[20, 21, 28, 30–34] Although highly sensitive, MRI has limited ability to provide specific tissue diagnosis and to distinguish benign from malignant soft tissue tumors.[30–34]

MRI provides superb contrast detail of various soft tissues, allows multiplanar imaging capability, and involves no ionizing radiation. It has the ability to assess both soft tissues and bones (Fig. 38.5). It is well-suited for postoperative evaluation in the presence of metallic hardware, with fewer susceptibility artifacts than CT. MRI is the best modality to study bone marrow and is equally as capable as CT for detecting cortical bone abnormalities.[30–35] MRI accurately demonstrates anatomic location of a soft tissue mass and its relationship to adjoining neurovascular structures and bone. Dynamic Gd-enhanced MRI can be used to guide a biopsy needle by distinguishing recurrent tumor or viable residual tumor tissue with early enhancement, as compared with poor and delayed enhancement of granulation soft tissues in the surgical bed.[36] Magnetic resonance

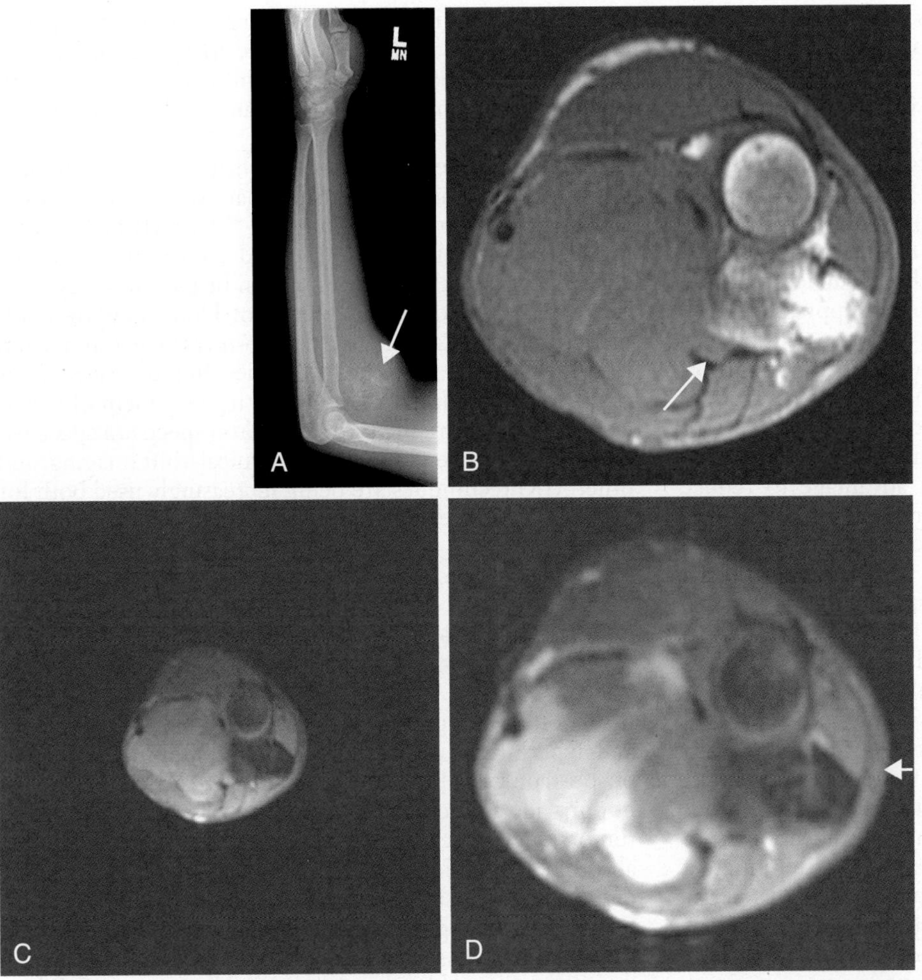

FIGURE 38.3. Synovial sarcoma in a 24-year-old man. **A**, Lateral radiograph of left elbow shows calcified soft tissue mass (*arrow*) in antecubital fossa. **B**, Axial T1-weighted (T1W) magnetic resonance imaging shows a large lobulated, mostly isointense (similar to adjoining muscle) soft tissue mass in the antecubital fossa with heterogeneous hyperintense small posterior component of tumor abutting the proximal ulna (*arrow*). **C**, Axial fat-suppressed T2-weighted (T2W) magnetic resonance imaging shows diffuse heterogeneous hyperintense soft tissue tumor with posterior area of low signal because of intratumoral calcification. Note nonsuppression of marrow fat in proximal ulna because of poor technique, often seen with T2W spin echo imaging. **D**, Axial postcontrast fat-suppressed T1W magnetic resonance imaging shows heterogeneous enhancement of calcified tumor. Note normal marrow fat suppression in ulna (*arrow*).

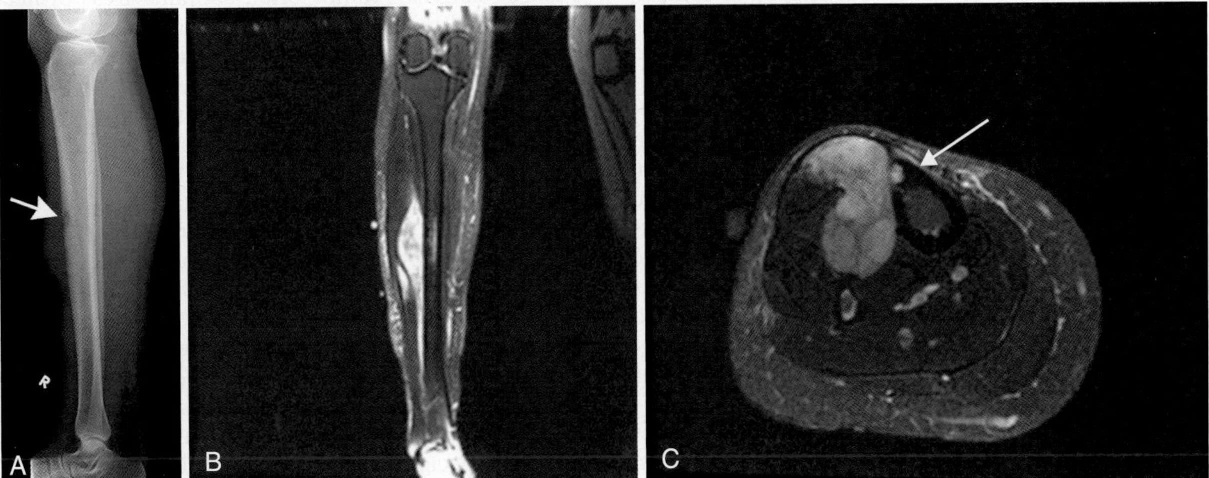

FIGURE 38.4. Undifferentiated pleomorphic soft sarcoma in a 64-year-old woman. **A**, Lateral radiograph of right lower leg shows focal pretibial soft tissue mass eroding underlying anterior cortex of left mid tibia (*arrow*). **B**, Coronal fat-suppressed T2-weighted (T2W) magnetic resonance imaging shows heterogeneous hyperintense soft tissue tumor abutting mid right lateral mid tibial shaft with hyperintense marrow signal. **C**, Axial fat-suppressed T2W image shows soft tissue tumor abutting anterolateral mid tibial cortex with small cortical erosion (*arrow*).

spectroscopy may be useful in assessing tumor response to chemotherapy where surgical resection of tumor may not be feasible.[37] However, MRI is ineffective in detection of soft tissue calcifications and air, for which plain radiography and CT are much superior.[35]

Technique

Conventional T1-weighted (T1W) imaging and T2-weighted (T2W) imaging spin echo magnetic resonance pulse sequences, preferably in the axial and coronal planes, are routinely used for imaging of a soft tissue mass.[28, 30–34] MRI in additional orthogonal (such as sagittal and oblique) planes can be done, if required. The main disadvantage of spin echo MRI is relatively long acquisition times, especially for double-echo T2W imaging. Fat-suppressed T2W imaging increases tumor-to-background signal intensity differences and demonstrates bright lesion in a suppressed fat dark background (see Fig. 38.6). Short tau inversion recovery (STIR) can be combined with the standard T1W imaging and T2W imaging spin-echo sequences because it produces tissue contrast similar to fat-suppressed T2W imaging, with a bright lesion within a suppressed fat dark background. Thus, STIR imaging enhances tumor conspicuity, but tends to have a lower signal-to-noise ratio than standard spin echo MRI, and is also more susceptible to motion artifact.[20] It is the best modality for study of bone marrow disorders and is used with advantage to reduce metallic saturation artifact in the presence of orthopedic hardware. Additional MRI sequences, such as gradient echo and turbo (fast) spin echo, can be used under special circumstances, such as in cases of suspected pigmented villonodular synovitis to assess blooming artifact related to hemosiderin.[30, 34] The routinely used MRI pulse sequences are provided in Table 38.1. Lately, subtraction MRI, which eliminates the need for fat suppression, has been found useful in surveillance for tumor recurrence in patients with metallic hardware.[30] Also, diffusion-weighted MRI of soft tissue masses has been advocated for better tumor border delineation to distinguish tumor margin infiltration from peritumoral edema and, in difficult cases, to differentiate a malignant from a benign soft tissue mass, as benign soft tissue masses usually have high apparent diffusion coefficient (ADC) value as compared with low–ADC value malignant soft tissue tumors, although some malignant soft tissue masses with cystic, cartilaginous, and myxomatous components have high ADC values.[30, 38]

Routine use of intravenous Gd for contrast-enhanced MRI of soft tissue sarcomas, except in evaluation of hemorrhagic and vascular soft tissue masses, is controversial.[30, 39, 40] Gd-enhanced MRI can differentiate between solid tumors, such as myxoma and myxoid liposarcoma, and cystic lesions, which have similar appearance on spin echo T1W imaging and T2W imaging, by demonstrating nonenhancement of cystic lesions. However, US is the best imaging modality for this purpose.[30] Gd also highlights enhanced viable tumor tissue from nonenhanced necrotic tissue within a soft tissue tumor, thereby facilitating biopsy of tumor tissue and assessment of tumor response to treatment in follow-up MRI studies. However, use of Gd adds cost and increases imaging time. It also poses a slight risk of anaphylactic adverse reactions, such as hives and bronchospasm.[41, 42] Although most of the adverse reactions to Gd are mild, at least one death has been reported.[43] Rarely, a poorly understood major adverse reaction, nephrogenic systemic fibrosis, may occur with Gd, especially in patients with impaired renal function. As a rule, patients with a glomerular filtration rate less than 30 mL/min/1.73m^2 should not be given Gd for MRI. However, use of newer group II Gd-containing contrast agents tends to have minimal risk, and they can be safely administered to patients with end-stage renal disease.[44]

The field of view should be large enough to include entire tumor, as well as the entire local area for tumor staging.[30] A marker, usually a vitamin E capsule, is routinely placed lightly on the skin surface over the area of interest.

MRA performed without or with intravenous administration of Gd is useful in multiplanar assessment of vascular anatomy of a soft tissue tumor.[45, 46] Fast MRI after bolus intravenous injection of Gd, timed with peaked contrast concentration within the tumor, can be used to study arterial, capillary, and venous phases of blood flow of a soft tissue tumor. MRA can also diagnose vascular tumors and vascular malformations in soft tissues. In most cases, it has replaced conventional angiography in assessment of vascular supply of soft tissue tumors. Proton spectrum spectroscopy, diffusion-weighted MRI, chemical-shift imaging, and other MRI techniques are being increasingly used both for qualitative, and even quantitative, analysis of soft tissue tumors.[47-49]

Magnetic Resonance Imaging Characteristics of Soft Tissue Tumors

Most soft tissue tumors are hypointense on T1W imaging and hyperintense on T2W imaging and show enhancement on postcontrast T1W imaging. In most cases, MRI cannot provide a specific diagnosis, except for a few soft tissue tumors, such as hemangioma, lipoma, or fibroma. In almost all other cases, biopsy of soft tissue tumor is required for definitive diagnosis. Also, MRI cannot reliably differentiate benign from malignant soft tissue tumors.[33, 34] In general, a malignant soft tissue tumor tends to be larger in size, and, despite increased blood supply, it quickly outgrows it. Thus, a large malignant tumor often contains areas of necrosis, which impart a nonhomogeneous appearance on T2W imaging, STIR, and postcontrast T1W imaging (see Fig. 38.5). By contrast, only approximately 5% of benign soft tissue tumors are larger than 5 cm in diameter, and most tend to be homogeneously hyperintense on T2W imaging and STIR, with homogeneous enhancement on postcontrast T1W imaging. Also, a superficial soft tissue tumor is usually benign, whereas a deep-seated tumor tends to be malignant. However, small size or superficial location of a soft tissue tumor does not always indicate that it is benign. Similarly, peritumoral soft tissue edema can be seen both with benign and malignant soft tissue tumors[5, 50].

As a rule, a malignant soft tissue tumor tends to be hypervascular with increased perfusion, and thus shows increased Gd enhancement, but many benign soft tissue tumors, especially vascular tumors, also have increased Gd enhancement. Thus, even use of intravenous Gd cannot always differentiate a benign from malignant soft tissue tumor.[30, 33, 39, 40]

For subcutaneous soft tissue tumors, except for vascular and neurogenic tumors, the presence of an obtuse angle between subcutaneous soft tissue tumor and adjoining superficial fascia is associated with a six to seven times greater probability of malignancy than a subcutaneous soft tissue tumor making an acute angle with superficial fascia.[51] In clinical practice, a soft tissue tumor that is larger than 33 mm in diameter, has intratumoral necrosis with

TABLE 38.1 Routinely Used Magnetic Resonance Imaging Sequences for Musculoskeletal Soft Tissue Tumors at the University of Texas MD Anderson Cancer Center, Houston, Texas

IMAGE TYPE	PARAMETERS	PLANE	ADVANTAGES	DISADVANTAGES
T1-weighted	Short repetition time (TR)/short echo time (TE)	Coronal	– Good anatomical detail. – Assessment of craniocaudal extent of lesion. – Bone marrow and cortex assessment. – Detects lipomatous tumors.	– Poor tumor/normal tissue contrast for nonlipomatous tumors.
T1-weighted	Short TR/Short TE	Axial	– Anatomical detail/neurovascular bundle evaluation. – Evaluation of tumor in axial plane. – Assessment of bone marrow and cortex. – Detects lipomatous tumors.	– Poor tumor/normal muscle contrast for non lipomatous tumors.
Fat-saturated T2	Long TR/Long TE	Coronal	– High tumor/normal soft tissue contrast for increased conspicuity. – Craniocaudal extent of tumor. – Bone marrow assessment. – Verification of fat seen on T1-weighted images (as fat is suppressed).	– Not good for detection of lipomatous tumors. – Poor in differentiating tumor from soft tissue edema, granulation tissue.
Fat-saturated T2	Long TR/Long TE	Axial	– High tumor/normal soft tissue contrast for increased conspicuity. – Assessment of tumor margins. – Assessment of bone marrow. – Evaluation of blood vessels and vascular tumors.	– Poor in detection of lipomatous tumors. – Poor anatomical detail.
Short tau inversion recovery (used only when metal is present)	Long TR/Short TE/ short TI	Axial	– Best for assessment of bone marrow. – High tumor/normal soft tissue conspicuity. – Reduces metal artifact. – Verification of lipomatous tumors (as fat is suppressed).	– Poor signal-to-noise ratio. – Longer scanning time. – Overestimates tumor margins.
Gadolinium-enhanced fat-saturated T1-weighted	Short TR/Short TE	Axial	– Differentiates tumor from normal soft tissue, necrotic tissue or hemorrhage. – Differentiates solid from cystic tumor. – Assessment of blood vessels/vascular lesions.	– Risk for adverse reactions. – Increased cost. – Longer scanning time.

Note: Integration of data from various magnetic resonance imaging sequences helps in diagnosis and staging of soft tissue tumors.

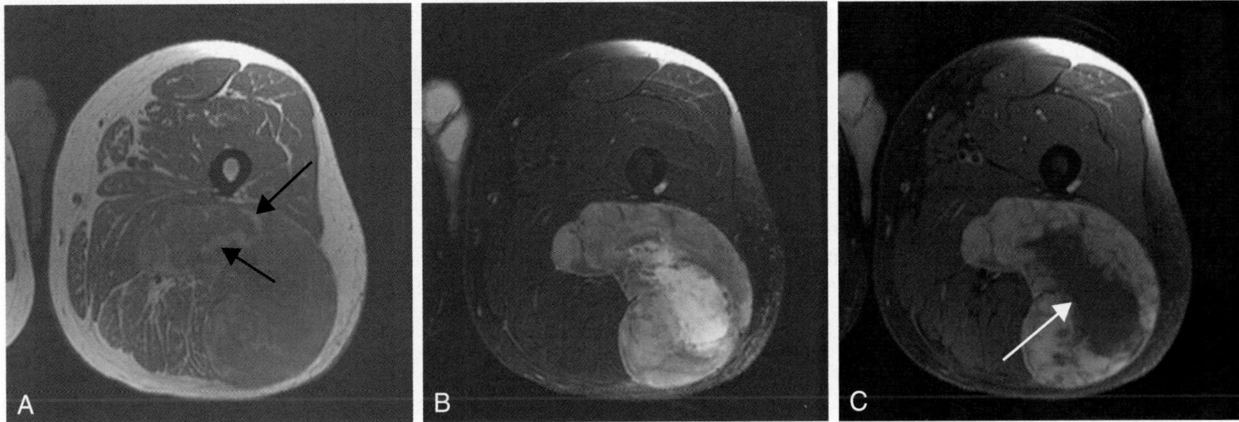

FIGURE 38.5. Myxoid liposarcoma in a 35-year-old man. **A**, Axial T1-weighted (T1W) imaging shows mildly heterogeneous isointense large soft tissue tumor (arrow) in posterior compartment of left thigh. **B**, On axial fat-suppressed T2-weighted magnetic resonance imaging, heterogeneously hyperintense soft tissue tumor has well-defined margins. **C**, Axial postcontrast fat-suppressed T1W imaging shows large nonenhancing central area of intratumoral necrosis (*arrow*), as the tumor growth has overpaced its blood supply.

heterogeneous signal on T2W imaging, STIR, and post-contrast T1W imaging, exhibits bone involvement, and entraps neurovascular bundle, has the highest probability of being malignant.[21]

Computed Tomography

CT is the preferred imaging modality for evaluation of bone and mineralized soft tissues.[30, 35, 52, 53] Although CT and MRI are considered equally good for assessment

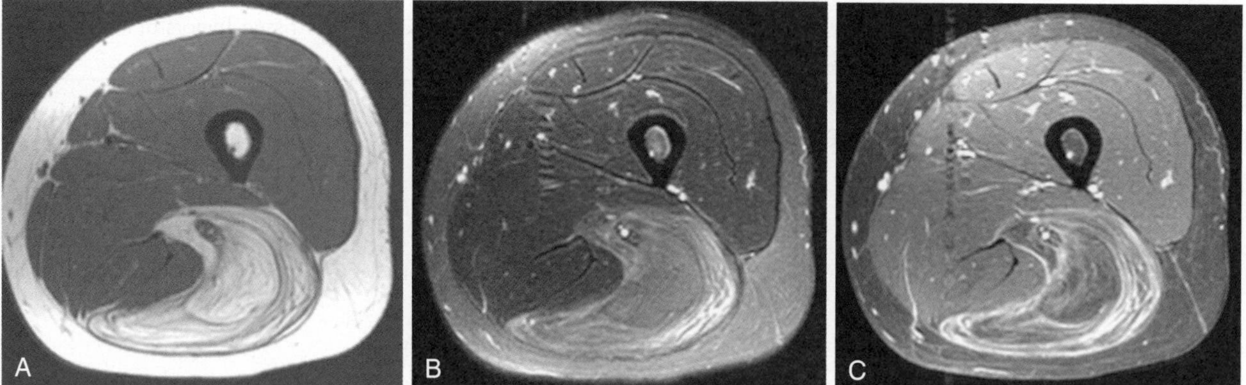

FIGURE 38.6. Well-differentiated liposarcoma (atypical lipomatous tumor) in a 46-year-old woman. **A**, Axial T1-weighted (T1W) imaging of right thigh shows a heterogeneous well-marginated fat-containing lobulated large soft tissue tumor with nonfatty dark internal septa in right thigh. **B**, Axial fat-suppressed T2-weighted imaging shows heterogeneous hyperintense lobulated tumor with suppression of fat (similar to suppressed subcutaneous fat) within the tumor. **C**, Axial postcontrast fat-suppressed T1W imaging shows heterogeneously enhancing tumor because of enhancing intratumoral septa against background of suppressed hypointense tumor fat signal.

of cortical bone, CT has an advantage over MRI in that it better demonstrates periosteal reaction, cortical erosions, tumor matrix mineralization, remodeling of bone, and gas in soft tissues. It can differentiate calcification from ossification within a tumor. It is also ideal for assessment of areas of the body with complex anatomy, such as the face, pelvis, and foot. The present-generation fast multidetector CT scanners are capable of generating high-quality reformatted multiplanar CT images, three-dimensional CT reconstructions, and even cine CT images, which can be useful to the operating surgeon. CT is especially useful in postoperative evaluation of patients with metallic orthopedic hardware, as beam-hardening artifact can be minimized with present CT imaging techniques, thereby enhancing tissue detail for diagnosis. Contrast-enhanced CT is alternative choice for imaging when a patient cannot undergo MRI. CT-guided biopsy of a soft tissue mass is routinely obtained. Lastly, CT remains the best modality for detection of pulmonary metastases in staging of soft tissue sarcomas. Contrast-enhanced CT is also routinely used in initial detection and follow-up of retroperitoneal soft tissue sarcomas (see Fig. 38.7). Dual-energy CT using 80 and 140 kVp levels to acquire CT attenuation data allows distinction of a gouty tophus containing urate crystals from other calcified soft tissue masses.[30, 54]

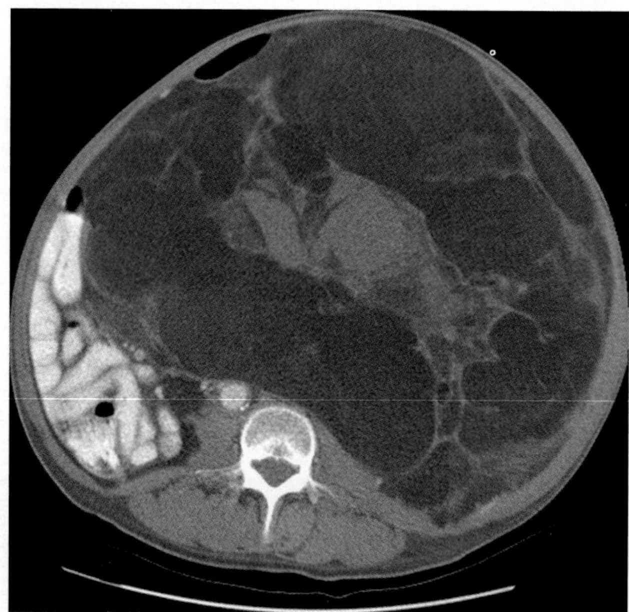

FIGURE 38.7. Retroperitoneal liposarcoma in a 78-year-old man. Axial computed tomography of abdomen following intravenous contrast administration shows a heterogeneous lobulated huge lipomatous retroperitoneal soft tissue tumor with several intratumoral areas of increased attenuation of the x-ray beam. The tumor displaces and compresses intraabdominal viscera, including contrast-filled bowel loops around it.

Positron Emission Tomography

PET provides information about metabolic activity in a soft tissue tumor.[55, 56] A PET scanner detects positron emission decay from administered radioisotope and generates an image of the entire body. The imaging agent routinely used for this purpose is 2-[^{18}F] fluoro-2-deoxy-D-glucose (FDG). Once given intravenously, FDG tagged with proton-emitting radioactive fluorine behaves like glucose and reflects glucose metabolic activity in body. However, unlike glucose, the metabolite of injected FDG is not a substrate for glycolytic enzymes, and therefore does not decay further. The proton-emitting metabolite trapped within body cells allows subsequent imaging by emitting two 512 KeV gamma energy photons perpendicular to each other. The amount of radiotracer activity within the trapping cell thus reflects its metabolic activity. As a rule, high-grade malignant soft tissue tumors have higher rates of glucose metabolic activity and show increased FDG uptake compared with benign or low-grade soft tissue malignant tumors. PET is now combined with CT for more precise anatomical correlation of tumors (Fig. 38.8). PET/CT and, more recently, PET-MRI, also have been found useful in follow-up of previously treated tumors to assess treatment response and to detect tumor recurrence (Fig. 38.9).[56, 57]

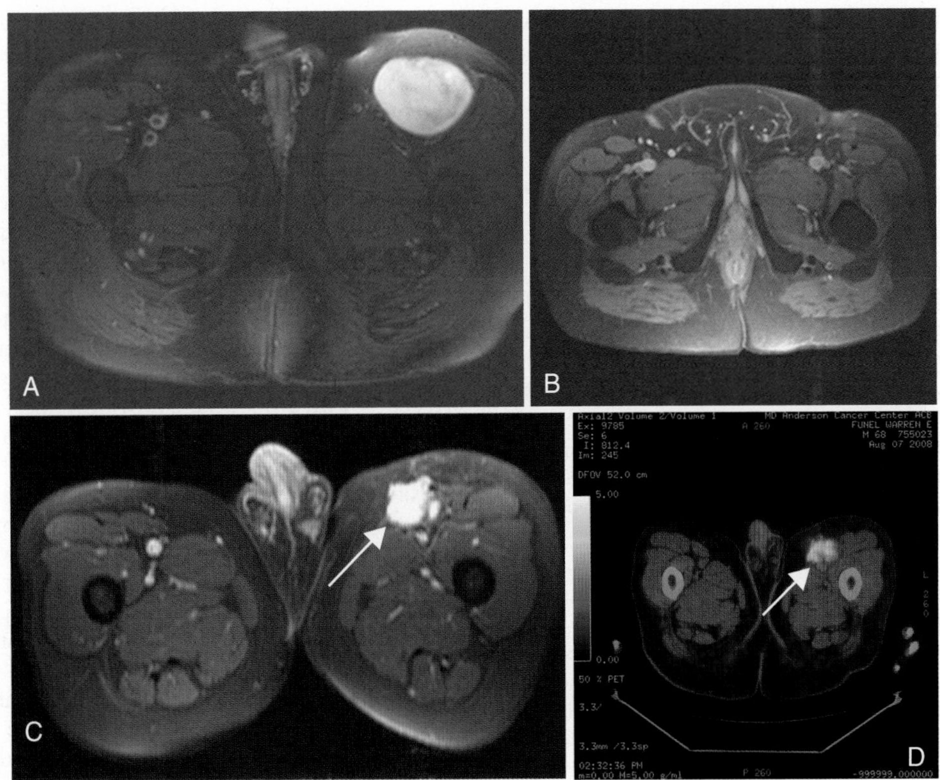

FIGURE 38.8. (arrow) Recurrent undifferentiated pleomorphic soft tissue sarcoma in left thigh of a 65-year-old man. **A**, Axial postcontrast fat-suppressed T1-weighted shows a homogeneously enhancing well-circumscribed soft tissue mass. The tumor was resected. **B**, Follow-up axial postcontrast fat-suppressed T1W imaging 6 months after surgery shows no residual or recurrent tumor in surgical bed. **C**, Further follow-up 10 months later, axial postcontrast fat-suppressed T1W MRI shows a new enhancing soft tissue mass in surgical bed, indicating recurrent tumor (*arrow*). **D**, Fused axial positron emission tomography–computed tomography with 2-[^{18}F] fluoro-2-deoxy-D-glucose shows recurrent tumor with avid radiotracer uptake (arrow).

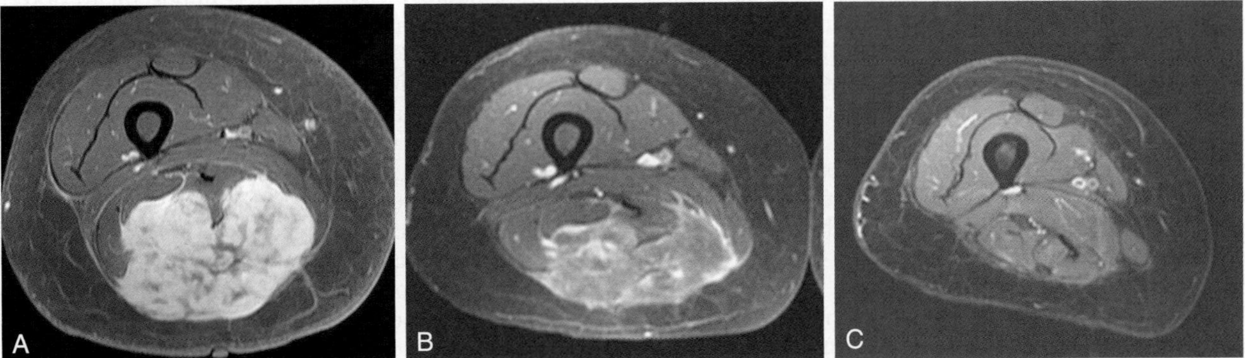

FIGURE 38.9. Excellent response to chemotherapy and radiation treatment of pleomorphic myxoid soft tissue sarcoma in left thigh of 76-year-old woman. **A**, Axial postcontrast fat-suppressed T1W1 shows heterogeneously enhancing soft tissue mass in posterior compartment of right distal thigh before treatment. **B**, Follow-up axial postcontrast fat-suppressed T1W1 obtained 6 months later shows markedly decreased enhancement of soft tissue mass, indicating excellent response to chemotherapy and radiation treatment. The patient underwent resection of the residual tumor. **C**, At 2-year postoperative follow-up, axial postcontrast fat-suppressed T1W1 shows no enhancing tissue to indicate residual or recurrent tumor in surgical bed.

Ultrasonography

The main role of US is to differentiate a solid from a cystic soft tissue tumor.[58] It is also used to guide biopsy needle for tissue diagnosis. The technique is found to be a good substitute for MRI to assess superficial soft tissue masses. Doppler US can be used for diagnosis of vascular soft tissue tumors and to distinguish malignant soft tissue tumor from benign tumor by evaluating altered intratumoral blood flow.[59]

Bone Scintigraphy

Bone scintigraphy with technitium-99m methyl diphosphonate (Tc-99m MDP), a highly sensitive, but nonspecific, imaging technique, is routinely used to detect distant bone metastases for staging.

Key Points Imaging

- Radiography provides information about tumor mineralization, bone involvement, and, in case of a lipogenic or vascular soft tissue tumor, it may even suggest a specific diagnosis. Chest radiographs are routinely used to detect lung metastases.
- Computed tomography (CT) is useful in determining size and extent of soft tissue sarcoma, tumor mineralization, and associated cortical bone involvement, if any. It is the best modality to detect lung metastases for staging and for imaging retroperitoneal soft tissue sarcomas.
- Gadolinium-enhanced MRI is the best modality for staging and characterizing a soft tissue sarcoma by determining its size, extent, associated bone involvement, and status of neurovascular bundle.
- Ultrasound is routinely used to assess superficial soft tissue masses, to differentiate cystic from noncystic soft tissue mass, and to guide biopsy needle.
- Positron emission tomography/CT can assess metabolic activity of a soft tissue tumor following treatment and for surveillance.
- Radionuclide scintigraphy with technitium-99m methyl diphosphonate is used to detect distant bone metastases for staging.

TREATMENT AND PROGNOSIS

Patients with soft tissue sarcoma should be treated at centers that specialize in treatment of soft tissue tumors, as a multidisciplinary approach is required.[5, 18, 21, 60] Surgery is the treatment of choice for resectable localized soft tissue sarcoma. The size, location, histological subtype, and grade will determine whether radiation and/or chemotherapy is used in the adjuvant or neoadjuvant setting. Approximately one-third of patients with low-grade soft tissue sarcomas will be cured by surgery alone. Limb-sparing surgery has become the norm, and amputations (forequarter, hindquarter, or joint disarticulation) are required only in approximately 5% to 10% of patients with limb soft tissue sarcomas.[19, 61]

Surgical resections can be qualified as intralesional (entering the tumor but removing all visible tumor tissue), marginal (through the surrounding pseudocapsule, often leaving microscopic tumor), wide (including a cuff of normal tissue in the resection), and radical (resection of the entire compartment). Radical resections should not be confused with amputations, because, depending on the location of the tumor, not all amputations achieve radical or even wide margins. Wide resection is recommended for all soft tissue sarcomas; however, proximity of soft tissue sarcoma to neurovascular or visceral structures, as well as patient and family preference, can play a role in the actual surgery performed.[62, 63] For soft tissue sarcomas next to bones or neurovascular structures, careful review of the CT and MRI is necessary to further investigate involvement of these structures. CT is especially useful in evaluation of bone cortex. Often, resection of periosteum is required, and resection of the underlying bone is rarely necessary. MRI is the best imaging modality for evaluation of neurovascular involvement. If neurovascular structures are encompassed by the tumor, resection and neurovascular reconstruction will be necessary, but more often these structures reside on surface of the tumor and opening of the perineurium allows their dissection free from the tumor.

Peritumoral soft tissue edema surrounding soft tissue tumor seen on T2W imaging is considered a reactive zone and should be included in the tumor resection.[64, 65] However, the amount of tissue that is needed to achieve a wide margin remains controversial. Generally, it is believed that, for definitive resection, all efforts should be made to obtain the widest margins that local anatomy and functional considerations allow; this is often quoted as 2 to 3 cm (when possible). Wide resection with limb salvage provides a local recurrence rate of less than 10%, while leaving a positive margin increases the incidence of tumor recurrence up to 90%.[66]

Radiation can be beneficial in decreasing local recurrence rate and metastases.[67, 68] Although there is a group of patients with small (<5 cm) in size, low-grade, anatomically accessible tumors in whom surgery alone should be considered as curative, radiation therapy is used as an adjuvant to surgery for the treatment of most other soft tissue sarcomas. For high-grade tumors or large, low- to intermediate- grade tumors, surgery combined with radiation therapy is the standard of care. The goal of radiation therapy is to eradicate the microscopic disease that exists beyond the surgical margin. Radiation therapy should be given before or after limb salvage surgery because there is no significant difference in tumor control, development of metastases, and progression-free survival, whether radiation is given preoperatively or postoperatively. However, preoperative radiation has been shown to be associated with an increase in early wound complications compared with postoperative radiation. It is important to note that this increase in wound complication was only seen in lower extremity tumors, and it did not affect functional outcome or long-term quality of life of these patients. Postoperative radiation does require a larger volume of tissue to be irradiated (to encompass the whole resection bed), as well as a larger radiation dose. Brachytherapy is another option in which a radioactive source is implanted into the tumor via a catheter to reduce local recurrence.[69] For those patients who are not surgical candidates, definitive treatment with radiation is an option. This requires higher doses, and the success depends on tumor size and histological subtype, treatment duration, and dose given.[69] Postoperative radiation is routinely given to the surgical bed for resected tumors with positive margins.[67, 70]

The role of chemotherapy in the treatment of soft tissue sarcomas remains controversial. The sensitivity and response to chemotherapy vary among the histological subtypes. For high-grade solitary large tumors, chemotherapy can be considered. In cases where tumors have metastasized or recurred locally, systemic chemotherapy is often employed.[71, 72] Such drug therapies, when used, are chosen by taking into consideration both host factors (such as patient age, performance score, organ function) and the factors intrinsic to the soft tissue sarcoma itself (such as tumor subtype and likelihood of chemotherapy response).

Cytotoxic drugs, such as ifosfamide, vincristine, cyclophosphamide, and doxorubicin, can be useful both for local and systemic control of tumors, and can be given either before or after surgery, depending upon the clinical scenario.[72,73] When administered as a neoadjuvant, these drugs may facilitate a margin-negative operation that might not otherwise have been possible. Chemotherapy will not, unfortunately, provide a cure to those harboring extensive metastatic disease. However, significant prolongation of life is often possible. As chemotherapeutic regimens tend to change over time, the latest treatment guidelines should be consulted in caring for soft tissue sarcoma patients. The National Comprehensive Cancer Network soft tissue sarcoma guidelines have recently been updated and provide a reasonable starting point. Fig. 38.8 illustrates the excellent treatment response of a pleomorphic dedifferentiated soft tissue sarcoma in the right thigh of a patient who received only chemotherapy and radiation treatment.

Key Points Treatment and Prognosis

- Treatment depends upon location and staging of a soft tissue sarcoma and requires a comprehensive multidisciplinary approach.
- Surgery of a soft tissue sarcoma can be intralesional, marginal, wide, or radical.
- Low-grade, small soft tissue tumors usually require only surgical resection for cure.
- High-grade tumors are treated with surgery, often combined with adjuvant radiation and chemotherapy.
- Pre- or postoperative radiation treatment may be used to reduce local tumor recurrence.
- Adjuvant chemotherapy is usually given to patients with local tumor recurrence or distant metastases.

SURVEILLANCE

Follow-up is an important part of the treatment regimen. The majority of recurrences occur in the first 2 to 3 years. Thus, follow-up is concentrated during this time interval. For the first 2 years, patients are seen every 3 months; for the next 2 years, patients are seen every 4 months; and then at 5 years, the patients are followed every 6 months. Follow-up consists of physical examination and imaging of the tumor site and chest radiograph.[5,18] Pulmonary metastases, even when multiple or bilateral, are usually resected, with a cure rate of approximately 25% to 30%.[5] Patients with unresectable pulmonary or extrapulmonary metastases should receive adjuvant chemotherapy.[5,74] Depending on location, US or MRI can provide valuable information about local tumor recurrence. MRI is still the imaging modality of choice, preferably with intravenous Gd. Presence of an enhancing soft tissue nodule or tissue in the surgical bed on postcontrast MRI is suggestive of recurrent tumor and requires biopsy. The benefit of US is that, if a postoperative nodule is seen in the surgical bed, and recurrence is suspected, immediate biopsy can be performed. For retroperitoneal soft tissue sarcomas, CT should be performed for detection of recurrent and metastatic disease, usually to liver and peritoneum, every 3 to 6 months during the first 2 years after surgery, and every 6 months for 3 years thereafter.[75,76] PET/CT and PET-MRI also can be used for surveillance.[56]

The 5-year survival rates for patients with stage I, II, III, and IV limb soft tissue sarcoma are 90%, 70%, 50%, and 10% to 20%, respectively, although these are further affected by site, histologic type, and other factors.[5,76] With the current multimodal treatment and sophisticated surgical techniques, the present overall recurrence rate for limb soft tissue sarcomas is less than 10%.[5] For retroperitoneal soft tissue tumors, because of high local recurrence rates varying from 40% to 90%, the overall prognosis is poor, regardless of the treatment modality, and the 5-year survival rate varies from 40% to 52%.[77] Large size, high histologic grade, unresectability, and gross positive margins of resected soft tissue tumor predict worse prognosis, with high mortality.[5,18]

Key Points Surveillance

- Surveillance involves periodic physical examination, obtaining magnetic resonance imaging of the surgical bed for local tumor recurrence, and chest radiographs and computed tomography (CT) for lung metastases.
- Most recurrences of resected sarcomas occur within the first 2 to 3 years after surgery.
- For the first 2 years, patients are seen every 3 months; for next 2 to 5 years, every 6 months; and thereafter, at 6-month intervals.
- For retroperitoneal soft tissue sarcomas, abdominal CT is used both for staging and surveillance.

New Therapies

Recently, biologically-targeted therapies, made possible in part through the discovery of specific oncogenic signaling cascades, have been advocated for the treatment of soft tissue tumors.[75–77] For instance, tyrosine kinase inhibitors such as imatinib and platelet-derived growth factor receptor have been effective in the treatment of gastrointestinal stromal tumors and dermatofibroma protuberance, respectively.[78,79] Similarly, RANK-B (receptor activator of nuclear factor kappa-B), its ligands and cognates, such as denosumab, are being used for treating giant cell tumors of tendon sheath and pigmented villonodular synovitis, with good results, as these tumors are susceptible to the antiosteoclastic effects of these drugs.[79] Vascular endothelial growth factor inhibitors such as bevacizumab have shown promise in treating solitary fibrous tumors, and, more recently, alveolar soft part sarcomas.[80] Also, insulin-like growth factor 1 receptor–targeted therapies have shown dramatic responses in a subset of Ewing sarcoma patients.[81] More recently, the U.S. Food and Drug Administration has approved pexidartinib (Turalio), a colony stimulating factor 1 receptor inhibitor, for adult patients with symptomatic tenosynovial giant cell tumor who are unresponsive to surgical treatment.[82] It is hoped that such biologically targeted therapies with newer therapeutic agents will become more effective for cancer treatment in future.

CONCLUSION

Soft tissue sarcomas are rare heterogeneous group of mesenchymal tumors requiring a multimodal management approach. Following clinical history and physical examination, radiographs of the affected body part should be obtained. Although it has a limited role, radiography does provide important diagnostic information about tumor mineralization and tumor effects on adjoining soft tissues and bones that may not be available from other imaging techniques. MRI is the best modality for assessment of location and size of a soft tissue tumor and for local staging; however, it cannot reliably distinguish between benign and malignant soft tissue tumors, even with use of intravenous Gd. CT, US, and PET are additional imaging modalities that provide specific information about a soft tissue tumor. CT is especially useful in detecting mineralization within a soft tissue tumor. A presumptive diagnosis of soft tissue mass is possible from clinical examination and imaging. However, in most cases, a CT- or US-guided biopsy of soft tissue mass is required for definitive diagnosis. Radionuclide scintigraphy with Tc-99m MDP is useful to detect distant bone metastases. Although surgery remains the mainstay in treatment of soft tissue sarcoma, adjunctive radiation treatment and chemotherapy, either alone or in combination, may reduce local recurrence or control distant metastases. Periodic postoperative follow-up with MRI to detect local recurrence of treated tumor, and with chest radiographs and chest CT for detection of lung metastases, should be done for at least the first 5 years after treatment.

REFERENCES

1. Kransdorf MJ. Malignant soft-tissue tumors in a large referral population: distribution of diagnoses by age, sex, and location. *AJR Am J Roentgenol*. 1995;164:129–134.
2. Enzinger FM, Weiss SW. General considerations. In: Enzinger FM, Weiss SW, eds. *Soft Tissue Tumors*. 5th ed. St. Louis: Mosby-Year Book; 1995:1–16.
3. Vilanova JC. WHO classification of soft tissue tumors. In: Vanhoenacker *Imaging of Soft Tissue Tumors*. 4th ed. Cham: Springer; 2017:187–196.
4. Hajdu SI. Soft tissue sarcomas: classification and natural history. *CA Cancer J Clin*. 1981;31:271–280.
5. Morrison BA. Soft tissue sarcomas of the extremities. *Proc (Bayl Univ Med Cent)*. 2003;16:285–290.
6. Zahm SH, Fraumeni Jr JF. The epidemiology of soft tissue sarcoma. *Semin Oncol*. 1997;24:504–514.
7. Siegel RL, Miller KD, Fuchs HE, et al. Cancer Statistics, 2019. *CA: A Cancer J Clin*. 2021;71:7–33.
8. Singer S, Nielsen T, Antonescu CR. Sarcoma of soft tissue and bone. In: DeVita Jr VT, Hellman S, Rosenberg SA, eds. *Cancer: Principle and Practice of Oncology*. 8th ed. Philadelphia: Lippincott Williams & Wilkins; 2011:1741–1793.
9. Brady MS, Gaynor JJ, Brennan MF. Radiation-associated sarcoma of bone and soft tissue. *Arch Surg*. 1992;127:1379–1385.
10. McClain KL, Leach CT, Jenson HB, et al. Association of Epstein-Barr virus with leiomyosarcomas in young people with AIDS. *N Engl J Med*. 1995;332:12–18.
11. Pincus LB, Fox LP. Images in clinical medicine. The Stewart-Treves Syndrome. *N Eng J Med*. 2008;359:950.
12. Strong LC, Williams WR, Tainsky MA. The Li-Fraumeni syndrome: from clinical epidemiology to molecular genetics. *Am J Epidemiol*. 1992;135:190–199.
13. Bertazzi PA, Consonni D, Bachetti S, et al. Health effects of dioxin exposure: A 20-year mortality study. *Am J Epidemiol*. 2001;153:1031–1044.
14. Hoeber I, Spillane AJ, Fisher C, et al. Accuracy of biopsy techniques for limb and limb girdle soft tissue tumors. *Ann Surg Oncol*. 2001;8:80–87.
15. Haslin MJ, Lewis JJ, Woodruff LM, et al. Core needle biopsy for diagnosis of extremity soft tissue sarcoma. *Ann Surg Oncol*. 1997;4:425–431.
16. Dupuy DE, Rosenberg AE, Punyaratebandhu T, et al. Accuracy of CT-guided needle biopsy of musculoskeletal neoplasm. *AJR Am J Roentngenol*. 1998;171:759–762.
17. Mankin H, Mankin CJ, Simon MA. The hazards the biopsy revisited. Minutes of the Musculoskeletal Tumor Society. *J Bone Jt Surg Am*. 1996;78:656–663.
18. Cormier JN, Pollock RE. Soft tissue sarcomas. *CA Cancer J Clin*. 2004;54:94–109.
19. Clark MA, Fisher C, Judson I, et al. Soft-tissue sarcomas in adults. *N Engl J Med*. 2005;353:701–711.
20. Kransdorf MJ, Murphey MD. Radiologic evaluation of soft-tissue masses: a current perspective. *AJR Am J Roentgenol*. 2000;175:575–587.
21. De Schepper AM, De Beuckeleer L, Vandevenne J, et al. Magnetic resonance imaging of soft tissue tumors. *Eur Radiol*. 2000;10:213–222.
22. Tung G, Davis LM. The role of magnetic imaging in the evaluation of the soft tissue mass. *Crit Rev Diagn Imaging*. 1993;24:239–308.
23. Kruzelock RP, Hansen MF. Molecular genetic and cytogenetics of sarcomas. *Hematol Oncol Clin North Am*. 1995;9:513–540.
24. Amin MB, Edge SB, Greene FL, eds. *AJCC Cancer Staging Manual*. 8th ed. New York: Springer; 2017:221–226.
25. Coindre J-M. Grading of soft tissue sarcomas: review and update. *Arch Path Lab Med*. 2006;130:1448–1453.
26. Coindre JM, Terries P, Bui NB, et al. Prognostic factors in adult patients with locally controlled soft tissue sarcoma. A study of 546 patients from French Federation of Cancer Centers Sarcoma Group. *J Clin Oncol*. 1998;14:869–877.
27. Ramanathan RC, A'Hern R, Fischer C, et al. Modified staging system for extremity soft tissue sarcomas. *Ann Surg Oncol*. 1999;6:57–69.
28. Vilanova JC, Woertler K, Narvaez JA, et al. Soft-tissue tumors update: MR imaging features according to the WHO classification. *Eur Radiol*. 2007;17:125–138.
29. Murphey MD. World Health Organization classification of bone and soft tissue tumors: modifications and implications for radiologists. *Semin Musculoskelet Radiol*. 2007;11:201–214.
30. Kransdorf M, Murphey MD. Imaging of soft-tissue masses: fundamental concepts. *RadioGraphics*. 2016;36:1931–1948.
31. Sundaram M, McGuire MH, Herbold DR. Magnetic resonance imaging of soft tissue masses: an evaluation of fifty-three histologically proven tumors. *Magn Reson Imaging*. 1988;6:237–248.
32. Totty WG, Murphy WA, Lee JKT. Soft-tissue tumors: MR imaging. *Radiology*. 1986;160:135–141.
33. Berquist TH, Ehman RL, Ding BF, et al. Value of MR imaging in differentiating benign from malignant soft-tissue masses: study of 95 lesions. *AJR Am J Roentgenol*. 1990;155:1251–1255.
34. Chhabra A, Soldatos T. Soft-tissue lesions: when can we exclude sarcoma? *AJR Am J Roentgenol*. 2012;199:1345–1357.
35. Panicek DM, Gatsonis C, Rosenthal DI, et al. CT and MR imaging in the local staging of primary malignant musculoskeletal neoplasms: report of the Radiology Diagnostic Oncology Group. *Radiology*. 1997;202:237–246.
36. Mirowitz SA, Totty WG, Lee JKT. Characterization of musculoskeletal masses using dynamic Gd-DTPA enhanced spin-echo MRI. *J Comput Assist Tomogr*. 1992;16:120–125.
37. Vaidya SJ, Payne GS, Leach MO, et al. Potential role of magnetic resonance spectroscopy in assessment of tumour response in childhood cancer. *Eur J Cancer*. 2003;39:728–735.
38. Hassanien OA, Younes RL, Dawdoud RM. Diffusion weighted MRI of soft tissue masses: can measurement of ADC value help in the differentiation between benign and malignanat lesions? *Eypt J Radiol Nuc Med*. 2018;49:681–688.
39. Beltran J, Chandnani V, McGhee RA, et al. Gadopentetate dimeglumine-enhanced MR imaging of the musculoskeletal system. *AJR Am J Roentgenol*. 1991;156:457–466.
40. Benedikt RA, Jelinek JS, Kransdorf MJ, et al. MR imaging of soft-tissue masses: role of gadopentetate dimeglumine. *J Magn Reson Imaging*. 1994;4:485–490.

41. Tisher S, Hoffman JC. Anaphylactoid reaction to IV gadopentetate dimeglumine. *Am J Neuro Rad*. 1990;174:17–23.
42. Takebayashi S, Sugiyama M, Nagase M, et al. Severe adverse reaction to IV gadopentetate dimeglumine. *AJR Am J Roentgenol*. 1993;160:659.
43. Jordan RM, Mintz RD. Fatal reaction to gadopentetate dimeglumine. *AJR Am J Roentgenol*. 1995;164:743–744.
44. Woolen SA, Shanker PR, Gagnier JJ, et al. Risk of nephrogenic systemic fibrosis in patients with stage 4 or 5 chronic kidney disease receiving a group II gadolinium-based contrast agent: a systemic review and meta-analysis. *JAMA Intern Med*. 2020;180(180):223–230.
45. Dumoulin CL, Hart HR. Magnetic resonance angiography. *Radiology*. 1986;161:717–720.
46. Glickerman DJ, Obregon RG, Schmiedl UP, et al. Cardiac-gated MR angiography of the entire lower extremity: a prospective comparison with conventional angiography. *AJR Am J Roentgenol*. 1996;167:445–451.
47. Valenzuela RF, Madewell JE, Costello CM. Advanced imaging in musculoskeletal oncology: Moving away from RECIST and embracing advanced bone and soft tissue tumor imaging (ABASTI)–Part 1–Tumor response criteria and established functional imaging techniques. *Sem Ultrasound, CT and MRI*. 2021;42:201–214.
48. Valenzuela RF, Madewell JE, Costello CM. Advanced imaging in musculoskeletal oncology: Moving away from RECIST and embracing advanced bone and soft tissue tumor imaging (ABASTI)–Part II–Novel functioning imaging techniques. *Sem Ultrasound, CT and MRI*. 2001;42:215–227.
49. de Mello R, Ma Y, Ji Y, et al. Quantitative MRI Musculoskeletal techniques: an update. *AJR Am J Roentegenol*. 2019;213:524–533.
50. Beltran J, Simon DC, Katz W, et al. Increase MR signal intensity in skeletal muscle adjacent to malignant tumors: pathologic correlation and clinical relevance. *Radiology*. 1987;162:251–255.
51. Galant J, Marti-Bonmati L, Soler R, et al. Grading of subcutaneous soft tissue tumors by means of their relationship with the superficial fascia on MR imaging. *Skelet Radiol*. 1998;27:657–663.
52. Weekes RG, McLeod RA, Reiman Pritchard DJ. CT of soft-tissue neoplasms. *AJR Am J Roentgenol*. 1985;144:355–360.
53. Demas BE, Heelan RT, Lane J, et al. Soft-tissue sarcomas of the extremities: comparison of MR and CT in determining the extent of disease. *AJR Am J Roentgenol*. 1988;150:615–620.
54. Rajiah P, Sundaram M, Subhas N. Dual-energy CT in musculoskeletal imaging. *AJR Am J Roentgenol*. 2019;213:493–505.
55. Bredella MA, Caputo GR, Steinbach LS. Value of FDG positron emission tomography in conjunction with MR imaging for evaluating therapy response in patients with musculoskeletal sarcomas. *AJR Am J Roentgenol*. 2003;179:1145–1150.
56. Bastiaannet E, Groen H, Jager PL, et al. The value of FDG-PET in the detection, grading and response to therapy of soft tissue and bone sarcomas: a systematic review and meta-analysis. *Cancer Treat Rev*. 2004;30:83–101.
57. Kubo T, Furuta T, Johan MP, et al. Prognostic significance of ^{18}F-FDG PET at diagnosis in patients with soft tissue sarcoma and bone sarcoma; systemic review and meta-analysis. *Eur J Cancer*. 2016;58:104–111.
58. Carra BJ, Bui-Mansfield LT, O'Brien Chen DC. Sonography of musculoskeletal soft-tissue masses: Techniques, pearls, and pitfalls. *AJR Am J Roentgenol*. 2014;202:1281–1290.
59. Bodner G, Schocke MF, Rachbauer F, et al. Differentiation of malignant and benign musculoskeletal tumors: combined color and power Doppler US and spectral wave analysis. *Radiology*. 2002;223:410–416.
60. Valle AA, Kraybill WG. Management of soft tissue sarcomas of the extremity in adults. *J Surg Onocol*. 1996;63:271–279.
61. Vraa S, Keller J, Nielsen OS, et al. Prognostic factors in soft tissue sarcomas: the Aarhus experience. *Euro J Cancer*. 1998;34:1876–1882.
62. Pitcher ME, Thomas JM. Functional compartmental resection for soft tissue sarcomas. *Eur J Surg Oncol*. 1994;20:441–445.
63. Clark MA, Thomas JM. Amputation for soft-tissue sarcoma. *Lancet Oncol*. 2003;4:335–342.
64. Bowden L, Booher RJ. The principles and technique of resection of soft parts for sarcoma. *Surgery*. 1958;44:963–976.
65. Watson DI, Coventry BJ, Langlois SL, et al. Soft-tissue sarcoma of the extremity: experience with limb-sparing surgery. *Med J Austral*. 1994;160:412–416.
66. Gerrand CH, Wunder JS, Kandel RA, et al. Classification of positive margins after resection of soft-tissue sarcoma of the limb predicts the risk of local recurrence. *J Bone Jt Surg (Br)*. 2001;83:1149–1155.
67. Yang JC, Chang AE, Baker AR, et al. Randomized prospective study of the benefit of adjuvant radiation therapy in the treatment of soft tissue sarcomas of the extremity. *J Clin Oncol*. 1998;6:197–203.
68. O'Sullivan B, Ward I, Catton C. Recent advances in radiotherapy for soft-tissue sarcoma. *Curr Oncol Rep*. 2003;5:274–281.
69. Pollack A, Zagars GK, Goswitz MS, et al. Preoperative vs. postoperative radiotherapy in the treatment of soft tissue sarcomas: a matter of presentation. *Int J Rad Oncol Biol Phys*. 1998;42:563–572.
70. Kepka L, Delany TL, Suit HH, et al. Results of radiation therapy for unresected soft-tissue sarcomas. *Int J Radiat Oncol Biol Phy*. 2005;63:852–859.
71. Tepper JE, Suit HD. Radiation therapy alone for sarcoma of soft tissue. *Cancer*. 1985;56:475–479.
72. Santoro A, Tursz T, Mouridsen H, et al. Doxorubicin versus CYVADIC versus doxorubicin plus ifosfamide in first-line treatment of advanced soft tissue sarcomas: a randomized study of the European Organization for Research and Treatment of Cancer Soft Tissue and Bone Sarcoma Group. *J Clin Oncol*. 1995;13:1537–1545.
73. O'Byrne K, Steward WP. The role of adjuvant chemotherapy in the treatment of adult soft tissue sarcomas. *Crit Rev Oncol/Hematol*. 1998;27:221–227.
74. Billingsley KG, Burt ME, Jara E, et al. Pulmonary metastases from soft tissue sarcoma: analysis of patterns of disease and postmetastasis survival. *Ann Surg*. 1999;229:602–612.
75. Lewis JJ, Leung D, Woodruff JM, et al. Retroperitoneal soft-tissue sarcoma: analysis of 500 patients treated and followed at a single institution. *Ann Surg*. 1998;228:355–365.
76. Catton CN, O'Sullivan BJ, Kotwall C, et al. Outcome and prognosis in retroperitoneal soft tissue sarcoma. *Int J Radiat Oncol Biol Phys*. 1994;29:1005–1010.
77. Lewis JJ, Leung D, Casper ES, et al. Multifactorial analysis of long-term follow-up (more than 5 years) of primary extremity sarcoma. *Arch Surg*. 1999;134:90–194.
78. Nakano K, Takahashi S. Current molecular targeted therapies for bone and soft tissue sarcomas. *Int J Mol Sci*. 2018;19:739.
79. Thomas D, Hinshaw R, Skubitz K, et al. Denosumab in patients with giant-cell tumour of bone: open-label, phase 2 study. *Lancet Oncol*. 2010;11:275–280.
80. Gardner K, Judson I, Leahy M, et al. Activity of cediranib, a highly potent and selective VEGF signaling inhibitor, in alveolar soft part sarcoma. *J Clin Oncol*. 2009;27:10523.
81. Sleijfer S, Ray-Coquard I, Papal Z, et al. Pazopanib, a multikinase angiogenesis inhibitor, in patients with relapsed or refractory advanced soft tissue sarcoma: a phase II study from European Organization for research and treatment of cancer-soft tissue and bone sarcoma group (EORTC study 62043). *J Clin Oncol*. 2009;27:3126–3132.
82. Tap WD, Golderblom H, Palmerini E, et al. Pexidartinib versus placebo for advanced tenosynovial giant cell tumour (ENLIVEN): a randomized phase 3 trial. *Lancet*. 2019;394(10197):478–487.

PART XI COMPLICATIONS OF THERAPY

CHAPTER 39 Interventional Imaging in the Oncologic Patient

Rony Avritscher

INTRODUCTION

The use of image-guided procedures has recently experienced tremendous growth in the setting of oncologic applications. There are several reasons for this increased use. Advances in diagnosis and therapy have led to increased survival benefit in this patient population. Earlier detection translates into more and more patients now presenting with their primary or metastatic disease still confined to a single organ. Therefore, these patients have the potential to be cured through the application of regional therapies, thus reducing systemic toxicity. A solid target lesion can now be accurately defined using novel imaging modalities, subsequently followed by the use of minimally invasive techniques to confirm the diagnosis and provide local curative or palliative therapies. In addition, recent advances in catheter technology, embolic agents, chemotherapy drugs, and delivery systems have been linked to further improvement of patient outcomes, sparking interest in combination approaches with systemic therapies. In this chapter, we discuss the most commonly performed interventional procedures in oncology and the central role of diagnostic imaging in the pre- and postprocedural care of these patients.

IMAGE-GUIDED TISSUE ABLATION

Technical Background

Image-guided tumor ablation is considered a potential first-line treatment in many patients with small tumors, and it can be accomplished using chemical agents or thermal energy.[1] Chemical ablation can be achieved by direct intratumoral percutaneous ethanol injection or, less commonly, acetic acid or chemotherapeutic agents that induce tumor cell death. Thermal ablation modalities include high-energy radiofrequency ablation (RFA), microwave ablation (MWA), cryoablation, interstitial laser photocoagulation, and high-intensity focused ultrasound (US), which causes coagulation necrosis. Irreversible electroporation constitutes a relatively novel, predominantly nonthermal, technique that is being increasingly investigated for the treatment of lesions in difficult locations, such as in the vicinity of the main bile duct in the liver.[2] These procedures can be performed under imaging guidance by interventional radiologists or by surgeons in the operating suite. A complete analysis of each image-guided tumor ablation is beyond the scope of this review; thus, the chapter focuses on RFA, MWA, and cryoablation, because these are the most commonly used ablative techniques in North America.

Radiofrequency and Microwave Ablation

Image-guided percutaneous thermal ablation is typically guided by computed tomography (CT), US, or a combination of both. RFA and MWA are performed by connecting a generator that provides an electric current to an electrode that deposits the thermal energy. The tissues surrounding the tip are destroyed within seconds as temperatures reach 55°C, and are destroyed immediately at temperatures greater than 60°C. During RFA, an alternating electrical current (frequency range 480–500 kHz) is deposited within the tissues via an electrode placed directly into the tumor. Ions in the tissue follow these high-frequency directional changes, inducing heat proportionate to the strength of applied energy in the vicinity of the electrode. RFA is subject to the heat sink effect, which limits its effectiveness for perivascular tumors (vessels >3 mm in diameter). MWA is based on dielectric heating, where thermal energy is created by electromagnetic microwaves operating at frequencies between 900 and 2450 MHz. These microwaves force the water molecules within the field to continuously realign with the oscillating electromagnetic field, producing friction and heat. This mechanism generates heat faster than radiofrequency ionic excitement and is more resistant to the heat sink effect. The primary endpoint of successful curative ablative therapy is obtaining a zone of complete necrosis of at least 5 to 10 mm around the external margin of the target lesion. The size and shape of the ablation zone will vary depending on the amount of energy, type of electrode, duration of ablation, and characteristics of the inherent tissue.[1] Image-guided RFA has been used to treat tumors in a wide variety of organs such as the liver, kidneys, lung, and bone, among many others. Initial RFA indications included the treatment of small lesions in patients who were not surgical candidates or for palliation of large lesions. However, owing to the efficacy and safety profile of the technique, its use has greatly expanded in certain diseases, to the extent that it is now used even in patients who are surgical candidates, with comparable outcomes.[3] The limitations of the techniques include incomplete ablation of large (>5 cm), complex lesions, and proximity to delicate structures, such as gastrointestinal wall, gallbladder, diaphragm, and nerves, among other effects.

Cryoablation

Cryoablation is typically guided by CT or magnetic resonance imaging (MRI). Cryoablation consists of the application of freezing temperatures to tumors to cause tissue destruction. This technique has been used to treat tumors in a variety of tissues such as the liver, kidney, prostate, lung, and cervix.[4–6] To perform cryoablation, a metallic probe is directly inserted into the target lesion. Argon gas circulates through the probe, causing a rapid drop in the local temperature. The ensuing low temperatures cause disruption of the cellular membrane and local ischemia. Ice crystals form within the cells and the adjacent interstitium, causing cell dehydration and surrounding vascular thrombosis. Subsequently, when the tissues thaw, vascular occlusion leads to further ischemic injury.[7] Consistent tumor cell death is accomplished when the tissues are exposed to temperatures of at least –20°C, corresponding to the area approximately 3 mm inside the margins of the ice ball. The temperatures along the interface between the ice ball and the adjacent tissues, as well as in the ice ball's peripheral rim, are suboptimal for tissue necrosis and represent only a reference for the interventional oncologist. As with RFA, the main limitations of cryoablation include proximity to blood vessels, gastrointestinal organs, nerves, and skin. Treatment of large tumor volumes with cryoablation can lead to the development of important systemic complications, such as cryoshock (a cytokine-mediated inflammatory response associated with coagulopathy and multiorgan failure), myoglobinuria, and severe thrombocytopenia.[8–10] Otherwise, most complications of cryotherapy—such as hemorrhage and injury to adjacent organs—are generally similar to those of RFA. Tumor antigens released after cryoablation are taken up by antigen-presenting cells and can potentially function as an *in situ* vaccination stimulating antitumor immune response.[11]

Clinical Applications

Liver Tumors

RFA and MWA are routinely performed worldwide for the curative or palliative treatment of liver tumors. There is ample literature documenting the successful use of minimally invasive thermal ablation for both resectable and nonresectable liver lesions. Hepatocellular carcinoma (HCC) and metastatic colorectal carcinoma are the most common malignancies that affect the liver. Thermal ablation is the standard of care for HCC patients with very early and early stage tumors, according to the Barcelona staging system, who are deemed not suitable for surgery, and current guidelines support the use of RFA in very early stage tumors in favorable locations, even in surgical patients. Thermal ablation in single tumors 2 to 3 cm in size is an alternative to surgical resection.[12] Recent extensive review of the literature regarding RFA in the treatment of colorectal liver metastasis by Mulier and coworkers[13] indicates a similar rate of local recurrences after open RFA versus surgical resection for colorectal liver metastasis smaller than 3 cm.

Not only is imaging essential for intraprocedural guidance, but these modalities also play a central role in preprocedural planning and postprocedural follow-up. Preprocedural scans are necessary for optimal characterization of the lesions in terms of size, number, and proximity to vital structures, namely the stomach and colon. Postprocedural imaging is critical for an accurate depiction of the zone of ablation and adequacy of the treatment, as well as for early diagnosis of any potential complications.

During the initial postprocedure follow-up imaging, the completeness of the ablation has to be carefully scrutinized. Dual-phase imaging is recommended to optimally characterize postintervention findings. The early arterial phase is essential for hypervascular lesions, such as HCC and neuroendocrine tumors. The portal venous phase is ideal for all other lesions, and the combination increases the sensitivity of the study. The zone of ablation can be readily identified as an area showing lack of contrast enhancement and overlapping the location of the original lesion. The margins of this area have to extend at least 0.5 cm beyond the original confines of the target lesion on all sides. If this safety margin is not present, the radiologist needs to have a high index of suspicion for residual disease. When CT is the modality used for guidance, a contrast-enhanced study can be performed at the end of the treatment, and any suspicious areas subjected to additional ablation. The presence of a uniform, rather than a nodular, rim of enhancement around the ablated area shortly after the procedure is usually benign and represents inflammatory reaction.[14–17] Likewise, a central area of increased attenuation on CT scans immediately after ablation is usually benign in nature.[14,15] Other expected findings commonly seen shortly after ablation that should not raise concern for complications include portal venous gas and air bubbles within the treatment cavity. Over time, the adequately ablated lesion becomes well-circumscribed and shows gradual size involution. Any areas showing enlarging nodular peripheral enhancement are concerning for residual or recurrent disease (Fig. 39.1). Comparison with prior studies is usually sufficient to establish the diagnosis. However, when an area is deemed questionable, but not definite, for recurrent or residual disease, a logical next diagnostic step is to proceed with 2-[^{18}F] fluoro-2-deoxy-D-glucose (FDG)–positron-emission tomography (PET) or PET/CT, which have been shown to be more accurate than CT in this particular scenario.[18,19]

The most common complications after hepatic RFA include: postprocedural hemorrhage, liver abscess (with

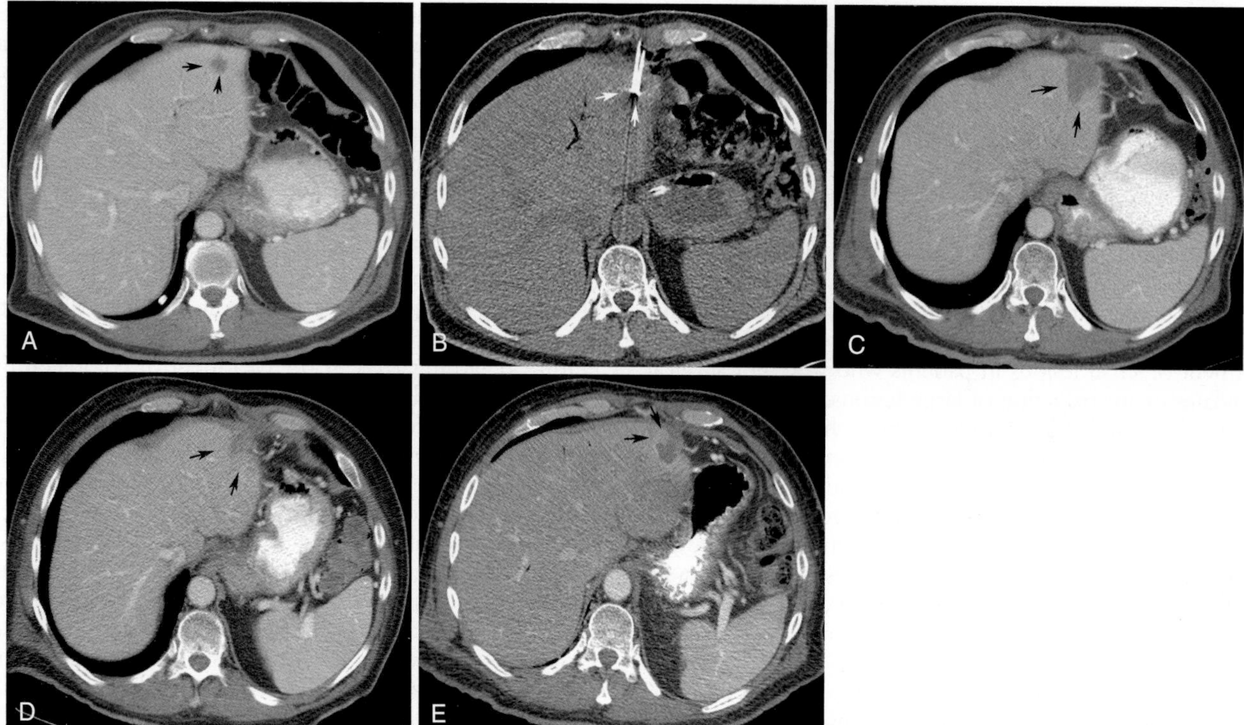

FIGURE 39.1. Computed tomography (CT)–guided percutaneous radiofrequency ablation of a left hepatic solitary metastasis in a 62-year-old man after Whipple's procedure for pancreatic adenocarcinoma. **A,** Enhanced CT scan obtained before the intervention shows a small nodular area of decreased enhancement in the left hepatic lobe consistent with a solitary metastatic focus (*arrows*). **B,** Unenhanced CT obtained during treatment shows radiofrequency ablation probes at the lesion site (*arrows*). **C,** Enhanced CT scan obtained 1 month after the intervention shows expected hypovascular defect at the ablation site (*arrows*). **D,** Enhanced CT scan obtained 6 months after the intervention shows expected size involution of the ablation defect (*arrows*). **E,** Enhanced CT scan obtained 12 months after initial treatment demonstrates new nodular enhancement at the anterolateral aspect of the ablation defect, consistent with recurrent tumor *arrows*).

an incidence of approximately 2%), bile duct injury with biloma formation, hepatic infarction, and injury to adjacent organs.[20,21] Hemorrhage is readily identified in the immediate postprocedural CT scans as a hyperattenuating fluid collection on nonenhanced images. Abscess formation should be suspected when new gas bubbles in the treatment bed are identified that were not present on the initial post-RFA scan. Focal dilatation of bile ducts peripheral to the ablation cavity is commonly observed, but usually requires no further intervention. Along the same lines, development of a low-attenuation fluid-filled cavity within the parenchyma is suggestive of biloma formation. Bilomas tend to have a benign course, rarely necessitating drainage.

Cryoablation is less commonly used than RFA in the treatment of liver tumor. This is because of the previously mentioned increased risk of severe systemic complications observed during the treatment of large lesions, such as cryoshock, myoglobinuria, and thrombocytopenia. In addition, cryotherapy of superficial lesions has been associated with potential fracture of the liver parenchyma and massive hemorrhage. However, it offers an established alternative if MRI guidance is preferred for a specific lesion.

Renal Tumors

The widespread use of US, CT, and MRI for the investigation of abdominal pathologies has led to the diagnosis of a large number of incidental renal tumors. Renal nodules displaying postcontrast enhancement of cross-sectional images are assumed to be malignant until proved otherwise. Because these lesions are increasingly being discovered when they are still small in size, therapeutic options that spare renal function are highly desirable. Minimally invasive percutaneous procedures offer a safe alternative to partial nephrectomies.[22] The thermal ablation techniques typically employed in the treatment of such tumors include RFA and cryoablation. The ideal lesion for RFA should be small in diameter (<3 cm) and peripheral in location. Central lesions are usually better treated with cryotherapy, owing to the decreased risk of ureteral stricture. A metaanalysis of 47 studies that compared cryoablation with RFA found that repeat ablation was required more frequently with RFA (8.5% of cases vs. 1.3% for cryoablation) and that local tumor progression occurred more frequently with RFA (12.9% vs. 5.2%).[23] Metastatic disease was also more common in the RFA group (2.5% of cases vs. 1%). One series comparing cryoablation with RFA found less tumor persistence or recurrence with cryoablation (11.1% of cases vs. 1.8%).[24] A more recent retrospective review from the same institution of 385 patients with 445 tumors measuring 3 cm or smaller treated with thermal ablation show that both RFA and cryoablation yield very comparable recurrence-free survival rates, with infrequent complications.[25] The radiologist has to be familiar with the different appearances of the zone of ablation in the treated kidney (Fig. 39.2). To do so, it is imperative to understand the gradual evolution of the completed area, potential complications, and signs of residual or recurrent disease. The expected natural course of a successfully treated renal mass is to slowly decrease in size over 24 months, finally reaching

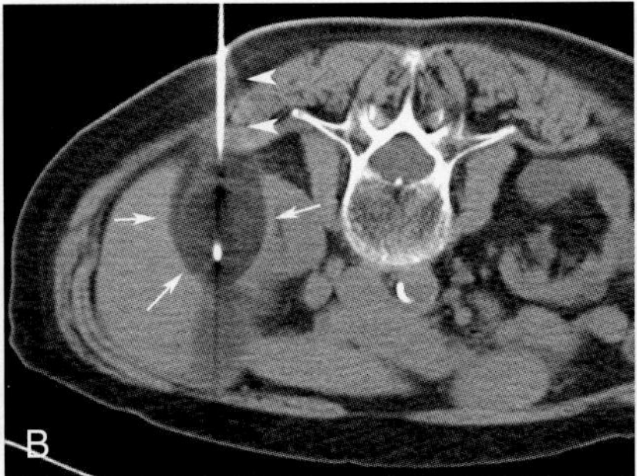

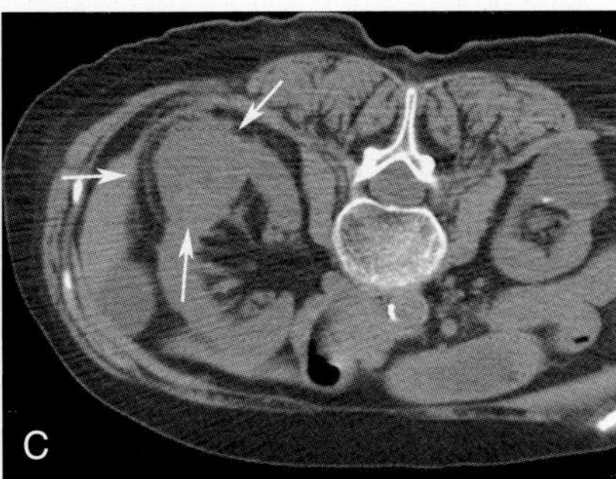

Figure. 39.2. Computed tomography (CT)–guided percutaneous cryoablation of a right renal mass in a 72-year-old woman with presumed renal cell carcinoma. **A,** Enhanced CT scan obtained before the intervention shows an enhancing heterogeneous 3.5-cm mass in the right kidney (*arrows*). **B,** Unenhanced CT scan obtained during treatment shows cryoprobe (*arrowheads*) and ice ball formation (*arrows*). Note that the ablation margin extends 0.5 to 1.0 cm beyond the mass. **C,** Unenhanced CT scan obtained immediately after the intervention shows the ablation zone as a low-attenuation area with expected small perinephric hematoma and fat stranding (*arrows*).

approximately half of its original size. A caveat is in the initial follow-up images after treatment of small lesions, when a slight increase in lesional volume is occasionally noted. This finding may be secondary to ablation of normal adjacent renal parenchyma. The typical zone of ablation does not show contrast enhancement. A focal area of enhancement should raise suspicion for residual or recurrent disease, particularly if nodular in morphology. During the precontrast phase, the ablation bed tends to be hyperattenuating compared with the adjacent renal parenchyma on CT scans. This feature indicates the presence of proteinaceous material in the treated area. Similarly, these products lead to increased signal on the nonenhanced MRI T1-weighted sequences. Particular to MRI is a thin rim of peripheral enhancement because of the presence of postablation inflammatory changes. This finding is usually not identified on CT scans, probably owing to the lower signal-to-noise ratio.

Lung Tumors

Lung cancer remains one of the most common malignancies in the world. Surgical resection is the mainstay of curative therapy. Unfortunately, only approximately 20% of all non–small cell lung cancers diagnosed are eligible for curative surgery. A substantial number of lung cancer patients do not undergo surgery on the basis of age, disease stage, underlying lung disease, and other comorbidities. Therefore, development of newer techniques that allow treatment of patients who are not surgical candidates is critical. Percutaneous RFA of lung tumors can be used for curative treatment of small local disease or palliation of large lesions that cause refractory pain, hemoptysis, and cough.

CT and PET are the imaging modalities most commonly employed to image lung lesions after ablation. Follow-up imaging is usually performed approximately 1 month after the initial treatment, and subsequently at 3- to 6-month intervals up to 24 months. Typically, the ablation zone is identified on follow-up CT scans as a nonenhancing hypoattenuating lesion, whereas areas of tumor progression tend to exhibit enhancement greater than 15 Hounsfield units. A rim of peripheral enhancement on the initial posttreatment images is usually secondary to the inflammatory reaction around the ablation cavity rather than residual or recurrent disease. In addition, ground-glass opacities may be observed around the zone of ablation in the immediate postprocedural scans.[26] Owing to these early postablative changes surrounding the target lesion, interpretation of initial posttreatment CT scans may be difficult in cases in which the target lesion appears larger in size but no obvious areas of enhancement are visualized. In this particular scenario, the use of FDG-PET/CT is useful to help distinguish areas of residual viable tumor cells. Although initial inflammatory changes around the zone of ablation may lead to early false-positive results, the presence of areas of showing increased FDG uptake after 3 months should be considered suspicious for residual disease.[27]

The most common complications of lung ablation include pleural effusion, pneumothorax, bronchopleural fistula, hemoptysis, infection, and potential worsening of the underlying lung disease. The incidence of pneumothorax is approximately 28%, with approximately 10% of patients requiring chest tube insertion.[28]

The estimated stage I lung cancer survival rates are 70%, 57%, 36%, 27%, and 27% at 1, 2, 3, 4, and 5 years, respectively, after initial lung RFA.[28] A recent combined consensus statement from both chest physicians and thoracic surgery societies evaluating the role of RFA vs. surgical resection and stereotactic body radiation therapy found that RFA was a safe treatment option that can be used as a single modality for patients with peripheral tumors 3 cm or smaller in size.[29]

Key Points Ablation

- Use curative or palliative treatment to treat these tumors.
- Cryoablation in the liver can lead to severe systemic complications.
- Radiofrequency ablation is limited by the heat sink effect and proximity to adjacent organs.

TRANSCATHETER ARTERIAL HEPATIC EMBOLIZATION AND CHEMOEMBOLIZATION

Technical Background

Hepatic arterial embolization for the treatment of liver tumors was first performed in the 1970s for local disease control. The rationale behind this approach emerges from the particularities of blood flow to liver neoplasms, which are supplied preferentially through the hepatic artery, whereas supply to the normal liver parenchyma occurs predominantly through the portal vein.[30,31]

Many different embolic agents have been used with success for bland hepatic embolization. The most common agents can be divided into proximal (large vessel), such as absorbable gelatin sponge particles and metallic coils, and distal (small vessel), including, among others, polyvinyl alcohol, fibrin glue, *N*-butyl cyanoacrylate (glue), tris-acryl gelatin microspheres, and absolute alcohol. Among the distal agents, specialized agents have been developed that function as drug-eluting beads, in which the embolic particle is loaded with a drug and delivered in a single step.[32]

Arterial chemoembolization consists of transcatheter intraarterial delivery of a combination of embolic agents and chemotherapy drugs into a liver tumor. The principles behind chemoembolization are based on the theory that tumor ischemia caused by embolization of the dominant arterial supply has a synergistic effect with the chemotherapeutic drugs. This technique was first pioneered by Yamada and colleagues in 1977.[33] The introduction of ethiodol (iodized oil), an iodinated ester derived from poppyseed oil, greatly advanced the technique. Ethiodol is well suited for chemoembolization because of its preferential tumoral uptake by certain hepatic tumors. This unique behavior is explained by the concept of enhanced permeability and retention suggested by Maeda and associates.[34] In this original study, the authors state that newly formed tumor vessels are more permeable. This increased permeability, coupled with a lack of lymphatic vessels in the neoplasm, leads to retention of molecules of higher molecular weight within the tumor interstitium for a longer period of time. This retention may explain, in part, the accumulation of iodized oil or the increase in concentration of polymer conjugates of chemotherapeutic agents in neoplasms. In addition, the iodized oil acts as both a distal embolic agent and a vehicle for the chemotherapy drugs.[35,36] It is critical to note that slow infusion of iodized oil into the hepatic artery will eventually reach the portal vein branches via the peribiliary plexus. This is important because the operator may inadvertently cause dual embolization, which may lead to parenchymal infarction.

Clinical Applications

Transarterial catheter embolization (TACE) and chemoembolization have been used to treat HCCs, cholangiocarcinomas, and a variety of hepatic metastases. The technique can be used in conjunction with liver resection or tumor ablation.

Two randomized clinical trials showed a survival advantage when chemoembolization was performed in selected HCC patients.[37–39] Owing to their better pharmacokinetic profile, drug-eluting beads are capable of delivering higher concentrations of chemotherapy agents into liver tumors with concomitant lower systemic toxicity and a prolonged intratumoral retention time. Preclinical and clinical studies have demonstrated higher and prolonged retention of doxorubicin within tumors after treatment with drug-eluting beads.[40,41] A recent randomized clinical trial by Brown et al., compared embolization with microspheres alone versus drug-eluting beads loaded with doxorubicin 150 mg in HCC patients. The results did not show significant differences in progression-free or overall between groups, but only 101 patients were enrolled, and the study was not designed to establish superiority of one approach over the other.[42] Colorectal carcinoma patients with liver-dominant disease who have not responded to systemic chemotherapy are candidates for palliative transcatheter chemotherapy. A study published by Soulen and associates evaluated the role of TACE in 121 patients with unresectable colorectal liver metastases after failure of second-line systemic therapy. The study showed partial response in 2% of the patients, stable disease in 41%, and disease progression in 57%. Survival was significantly improved when chemoembolization was performed after first- or second-line systemic therapy (11–12 months) than after third- to fifth-line therapies (6 months).[43] Several studies have evaluated the safety profile of drug-eluting bead embolic platform loaded with irinotecan (DEBIRI) for colorectal cancer patients previously treated with systemic chemotherapy. These studies have established that transarterial DEBIRI is safe and effective, and its role in their treatment algorithm is evolving.[44] In 2006, Gupta and coworkers published a study analyzing 85 patients with metastatic gastrointestinal stromal tumors.[45] Twelve patients (14%) demonstrated partial response, 63 (74%) demonstrated stable disease, and 10 (12%) demonstrated progressive disease. It is important to point out that this study was done when imatinib first became available, and a substantial number of patients in the study did not receive any treatment before the chemoembolization. Other, less frequent, metastatic tumors have also been successfully treated with TACE, including, among others, ocular melanoma and neuroendocrine, thyroid, and breast carcinoma.

Traditionally, CT scans are used to evaluate patients after hepatic embolization (Fig. 39.3). Interpretation is relatively simple, given that areas of necrosis will not show contrast enhancement, whereas viable tumors usually do. However, when iodized oil is administered concomitantly with other embolic agents and chemotherapy, assessment of residual viable tumor is complicated by the oil accumulation within the tumor because the oil is highly radiopaque. Although diffuse homogeneous accumulation of the iodized oil within the lesion portends a good general prognosis, it is important to note that the accumulation of iodized oil within the treated tumor does not always correspond to tissue death.[46]

Takayasu and associates[47] compared CT findings after chemoembolization with iodized oil for treatment of HCC with resected surgical specimens. The study found lack of correlation between tumor size reduction and the histopathologic necrosis rate in resected specimens. This finding is supported by additional studies that show complete retention of the oil within the tumors as a more specific indicator of necrosis rather than overall size reduction[46,48,49] (Fig. 39.4). The interpretation becomes difficult when the distribution of iodized oil within the lesion is nonuniform. In this scenario, studies have shown that the degree of tumor necrosis cannot be accurately predicted. Owing to this limitation, many authors advocate the use of MRI in the assessment of viability of lesions that contain iodized oil.[49] Iodized oil appears hyperintense on T1-weighted sequences during the first few months after embolization. The signal of the tumor does not change on the T2-weighted sequences, even in the presence of

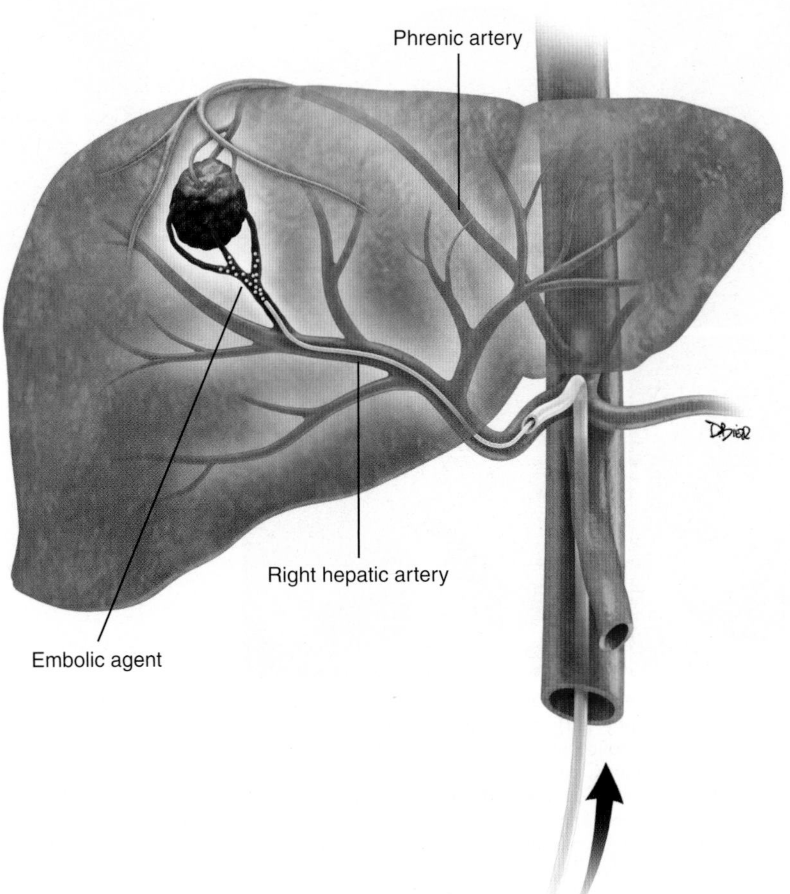

FIGURE 39.3. Partial accumulation of iodized oil within a tumor after transcatheter arterial chemoembolization may indicate the presence of extrahepatic arterial supply. Lesions near the diaphragm are commonly supplied by the inferior phrenic artery.

the oil.[50] Shortly after TACE, decrease of tumor contrast enhancement is typically seen in both the arterial and the portal venous phases. Several studies have also evaluated the role of diffusion-weighted images and apparent diffusion coefficient (ADC) maps in the assessment of tumor viability after locoregional therapy of liver tumors. The diffusion of water within viable tumors is restricted by the intact cell membranes, particularly because these lesions are typically highly cellular compared with the surrounding liver parenchyma. After treatment, the membranes are typically disrupted, which allows free water diffusion. Therefore, in the setting of tumor necrosis, ADC values are increased. However, the lesions become dehydrated after approximately 4 weeks, with subsequent decrease in apparent diffusion.[51,52] Unfortunately, these measurements are difficult to obtain in small lesions (<1 cm in diameter).

KEY POINTS Transcatheter Arterial Hepatic Embolization and Chemoembolization

- Liver neoplasms are preferentially supplied by the hepatic artery.
- Randomized clinical trials have shown a survival advantage when compare with supportive care in hepatocellular carcinoma patients.

RADIOEMBOLOTHERAPY

Technical Background

Transcatheter arterial radioembolotherapy (TARE) consists of the transarterial delivery of microspheres loaded with radioactive elements, most commonly yttrium-90 (^{90}Y). Using the same principle as other locoregional liver therapies, radioembolization relies on the preferential arterial supply to liver tumors.[30,31] Conventional radiation therapy does not have a central role in the management of patients with liver tumors, primarily because of the low tolerance of the whole liver to external beam radiation.[53] The risk of radiation-induced liver disease (RILD) after whole-liver radiation therapy delivering between 28 and 35 Gy over 3 weeks is approximately 5%,[54,55] and these doses are far less than those needed to adequately treat these lesions. Hence, delivery of the microspheres into the hepatic artery allows deposition of the particles predominantly within the tumor vascularity, leading to tissue damage while preserving the surrounding liver parenchyma. Hence, this critical feature allows delivery of substantially higher radiation doses than can be safely accomplished by external beam radiotherapy. ^{90}Y is a beta emitter with a 64.1-hour half-life. The beta radiation travels an average

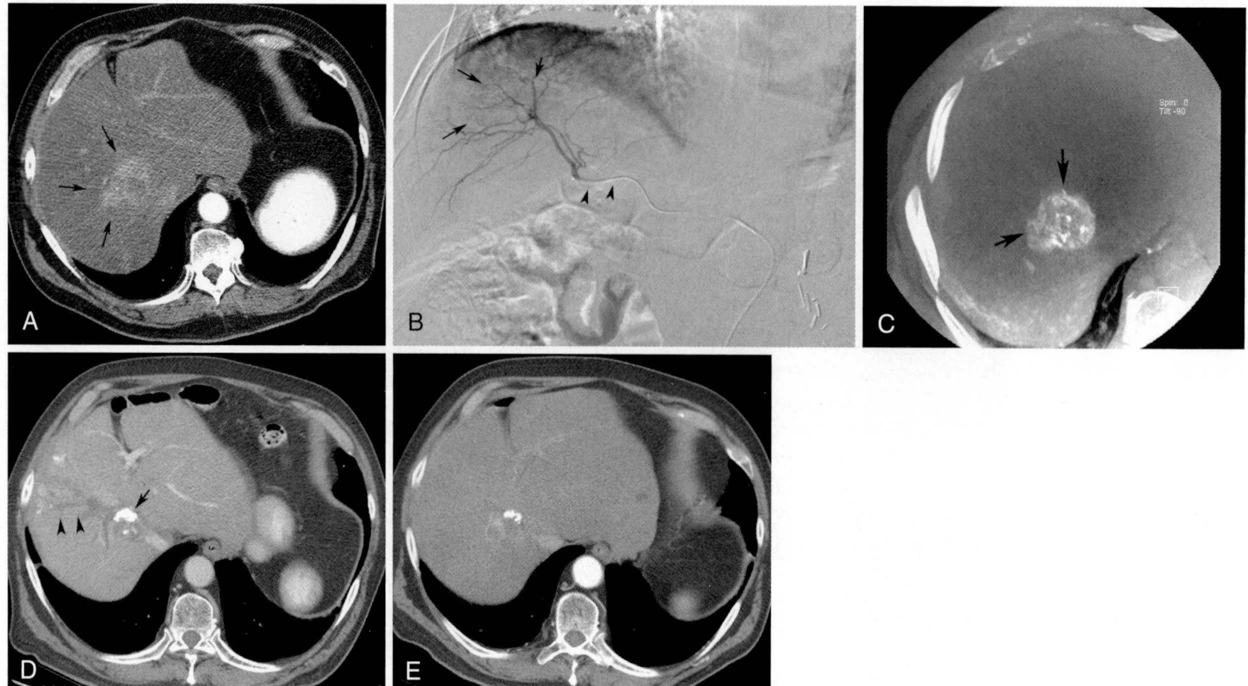

FIGURE 39.4. Transcatheter arterial chemoembolization using iodized oil performed in a 74-year-old man with diagnosis of hepatocellular carcinoma. **A,** Enhanced computed tomography (CT) scan obtained before the embolization shows a large hypervascular right hepatic mass (*arrows*). **B,** Anteroposterior selective right hepatic angiogram using a 3-Fr microcatheter (*arrowheads*) before chemoembolization demonstrates the hypervascular mass (*arrows*). **C,** Cone-beam C-arm CT scan of the right liver immediately after the chemoembolization shows homogeneous distribution of the iodized oil throughout the mass (*arrows*). **D,** Enhanced CT scan of the liver 1 month after chemoembolization shows iodized oil in the right liver mass (*arrow*) and decreased enhancement in right portal vein branches associated with distal heterogeneous parenchymal enhancement (*arrowheads*). These findings may be misinterpreted as rapid tumor progression when they actually represent portal vein thrombosis secondary to the chemoembolization procedure leading to peripheral perfusion abnormalities. **E,** Enhanced CT scan of the liver at the same level as **D** obtained 1 year later shows complete resolution of the findings, confirming their benign nature. Note that the patient did not receive any additional treatment in the interval.

of 2.5 mm (maximum 11 mm), a desirable feature because it helps minimize untoward damage.

Currently, two radioembolotherapy devices are approved for use in the United States. TheraSpheres (glass microspheres) are U.S. Food and Drug Administration–approved for neoadjuvant treatment of unresectable HCC in patients with portal vein thrombosis or as a bridge to transplantation. SIR-Spheres (resin microspheres) are approved for the treatment of metastatic colorectal cancer to the liver with concomitant use of floxuridine. Individual resin microspheres measure approximately 30 μm in diameter, with 50 Bq of activity. A whole-liver resin microsphere treatment averages an activity of 2 GBq. Glass microspheres have a diameter of 25 μm, with an activity of 2500 Bq per sphere. Single-dose whole-liver treatment using TheraSpheres has an activity of 5 GBq. Therefore, a treatment using resin microspheres requires a much greater number of particles, which leads to vessel embolization.

Clinical Applications

Multiple studies have demonstrated the safety of TARE with ^{90}Y for the treatment of unresectable HCC and metastatic colorectal cancer.[56–58] Initial studies evaluated CT findings after TARE. The treated areas tend to exhibit decreased attenuation on postcontrast images. The extent and heterogeneity of these areas of decreased attenuation logically vary according to the arterial level of microsphere infusion (whole liver, lobar, or selective), as well as with the size and vascularity of the target lesions. Larger hypervascular masses display preferential accumulation of the device, thus lessening the distribution of spheres to the surrounding parenchyma. These changes reach their peak 2 months after treatment and may spontaneously resolve after 6 months. The findings are nonspecific and can also be noted with external beam radiotherapy.[59,60] As with other forms of hepatic embolotherapy, lack of tumor enhancement is a potential indicator of favorable response. In a similar fashion, after radioembolotherapy, accurate functional imaging techniques that increase detection of treatment failures have the potential to allow early reintervention.[61] Metabolic imaging with FDG-PET is as an accurate way to evaluate response to radioembolization.[62] A consideration unique to ^{90}Y embolization is the acquisition of Bremsstrahlung scans, which are broad-spectrum secondary gamma-ray emissions produced as a result of the interaction of the high-energy beta emissions with tissue. Review of these scans combined with anatomic CT scans can depict extrahepatic deposition of microspheres or help elucidate the distribution of microspheres in the tumors (Fig. 39.5).

Large patient-cohort studies investigating the role of ^{90}Y TARE in HCC patients showed a median survival time of 16.9 to 17.2 months for patients at intermediate stages of the modified Barcelona Clinic Liver Cancer (BCLC) staging system. The median survival for patients classified as advanced stage by the BCLC staging without and with portal vein invasion was 10 to 12 months.[63–65] Objective response rates range from 35% to 50%. Because of the minimal embolic effect of ^{90}Y microspheres, radioembolization can be safely performed in patients with portal vein occlusion.[66] Studies comparing TARE with TACE have all been retrospective. These limited reports suggest that TARE offers less toxicity and at least equivalent time-to-progression compare with TACE.[67,68]

As mentioned previously, liver exposure to larger radiation doses can lead to RILD. This condition is characterized by the development of ascites, hepatomegaly, and elevated liver function tests weeks to months after therapy. The incidence of RILD after radioembolization is approximately 4%, and it is most commonly observed between 4 weeks and 4 months after injection.[69] Accurate interpretation of diagnostic studies is critical to differentiate RILD from disease progression. Changes in whole-liver morphology, signs of hepatic vascular congestion, and ascites suggest RILD as the underlying etiology.

KEY POINTS Radioembolotherapy

- This technique allows delivery of substantially higher radiation doses than external beam radiotherapy.
- Two radioembolotherapy devices are currently approved for use in the United States.
- Current data show a good safety profile and suggest equivalent time-to-progression compared with transarterial catheter embolization for hepatocellular carcinoma patients at intermediate stages of the Barcelona Clinic Liver Cancer staging system.

PORTAL VEIN EMBOLIZATION

Technical Background

Surgical resection remains the best curative option for patients with primary and metastatic disease confined to the liver.[70,71] However, extensive hepatic resection requires sufficient amounts of remaining liver tissue to avoid post-surgical hepatic failure. Thus, patients with limited liver remnant volumes may not be considered candidates for resection owing to the increased risk of posthepatectomy complications.[72,73] Portal vein embolization (PVE) has emerged as an important tool in the preoperative management of patients with small, anticipated future liver remnant (FLR) before major hepatectomy.[74,75] Embolization of the portal vein branches supplying the liver segments to be resected redirects blood flow to the nondiseased liver. This redistribution induces hypertrophy of the FLR, making it possible for these patients, not previously considered candidates, to safely undergo major hepatectomy. Extension of the preoperative embolization to segment IV to optimize hypertrophy is now performed in the majority of patients, and should be anticipated by the diagnostic imager.[76]

The range of reported mean absolute FLR increase for PVE in general was 46% to 70%, depending on the particle type used for embolization.[76] Whereas TACE leads to cell necrosis, PVE causes mostly apoptosis, so patients do not experience postembolization syndrome. Fibrin glue, Gelfoam, thrombin, particles, coils, and absolute ethanol all have been successfully used as embolic agents for PVE. In the United States, the most commonly used

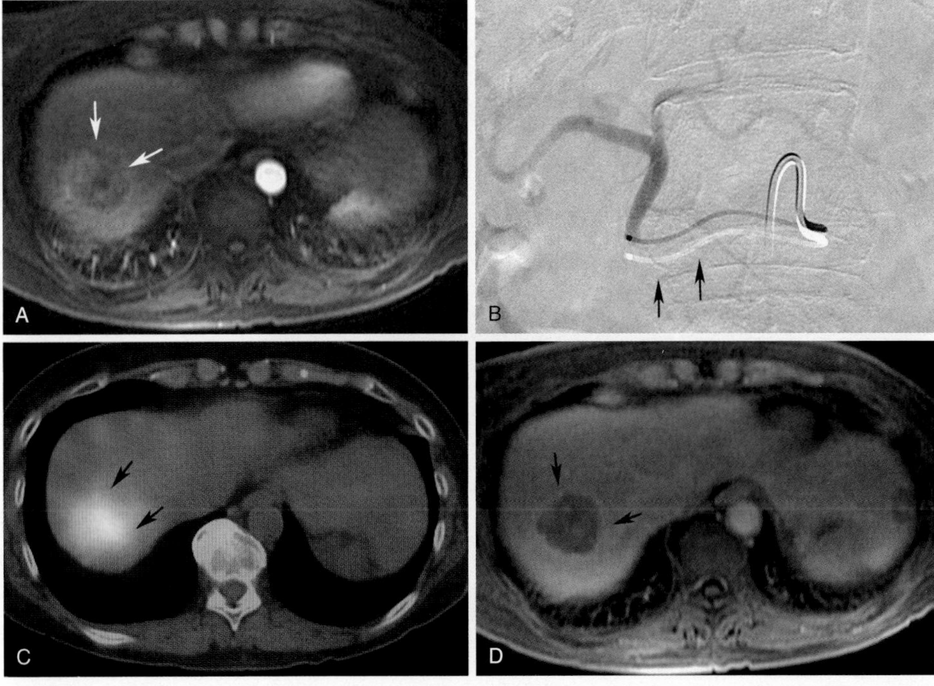

FIGURE 39.5. Transcatheter arterial radioembolization in a 71-year-old woman with diagnosis of metastatic neuroendocrine carcinoma. **A,** T1-weighted gadolinium-enhanced magnetic resonance imaging (MRI) study obtained before the radioembolization shows a mildly hypervascular right hepatic mass (*arrows*). **B,** Anteroposterior selective proper hepatic angiogram using a 3-Fr microcatheter (*arrows*) during delivery of yttrium-90 (^{90}Y) resin microspheres. **C,** Fused single-photon emission computed tomography/computed tomography *Bremsstrahlung* scan of the right liver immediately after delivery of ^{90}Y radioembolization shows homogeneous uptake in the right liver mass, suggesting adequate distribution of the microspheres (*arrows*). **D,** T1-weighted gadolinium-enhanced MRI study obtained 3 months after radioembolization shows uniform lack of enhancement throughout the right hepatic mass (*arrows*), consistent with treatment response.

agents include a combination of particles and embolization coils.[76] Recent studies have confirmed improvements in the postoperative course after PVE. Because of these improvements, an increased number of patients previously considered to have unresectable disease have become candidates for potentially curative hepatic resection. For this reason, PVE before major hepatectomy is now considered the standard of care in many comprehensive hepatobiliary centers worldwide.

Clinical Applications

PVE is indicated for patients with primary or metastatic liver disease who are otherwise hepatic resection candidates but are estimated to have small FLRs. These include patients with cirrhosis or advanced fibrosis with an FLR/total liver volume (TLV) of less than 40%,[77,78] patients with a history of extensive previous exposure to chemotherapy and an FLR/TLV of less than 30%,[79,80] and those with no underlying disease and an FLR/TLV of less than 20%.[75,81,82] It becomes obvious that, for optimal utilization of the technique, accurate determination of liver volumes is essential. Volumetric three-dimensional (3D) contrast-enhanced CT is essential for planning hepatic resection.[83]

3D-CT volumetric measurements are calculated by outlining the hepatic segmental contours and estimating surface measurements from each slice. Measurements should be standardized according to individual patient size, because larger patients require larger FLR than smaller patients.[84] The TLV is estimated using the following formula[84]:

$$\text{Total estimated liver volume (TELV)} = -794.41 + 1267.28 \times \text{body surface area}$$

Subsequently, standardized FLR is calculated by the ratio of FLR/TELV. Most imaging protocols require that the images be acquired immediately before PVE and approximately 1 month after the procedure to assess the degree of FLR hypertrophy. The degree of hypertrophy (DH) is also used as a predictor of postoperative course:

$$\text{DH} = \text{FLR/TELV (post-PVE)} - \text{FLR/TELV (pre-PVE)}$$

Patients whose DH is less than 5% have been shown to have a higher postoperative complication rate than patients whose DH is greater than 5%. DH, therefore, may be seen as a prognostic test to help determine whether or not the patient is ultimately resected[75] (Fig. 39.6). Particularly in those patients who do not show sufficient hypertrophy after PVE, the radiologist can help determine the need for additional embolization by identifying recanalized portal vein branches, which will show enhancement between the pre- and postcontrast CT sequences. Finally, the FLR should be carefully scrutinized for evidence of disease progression that would preclude surgical resection.

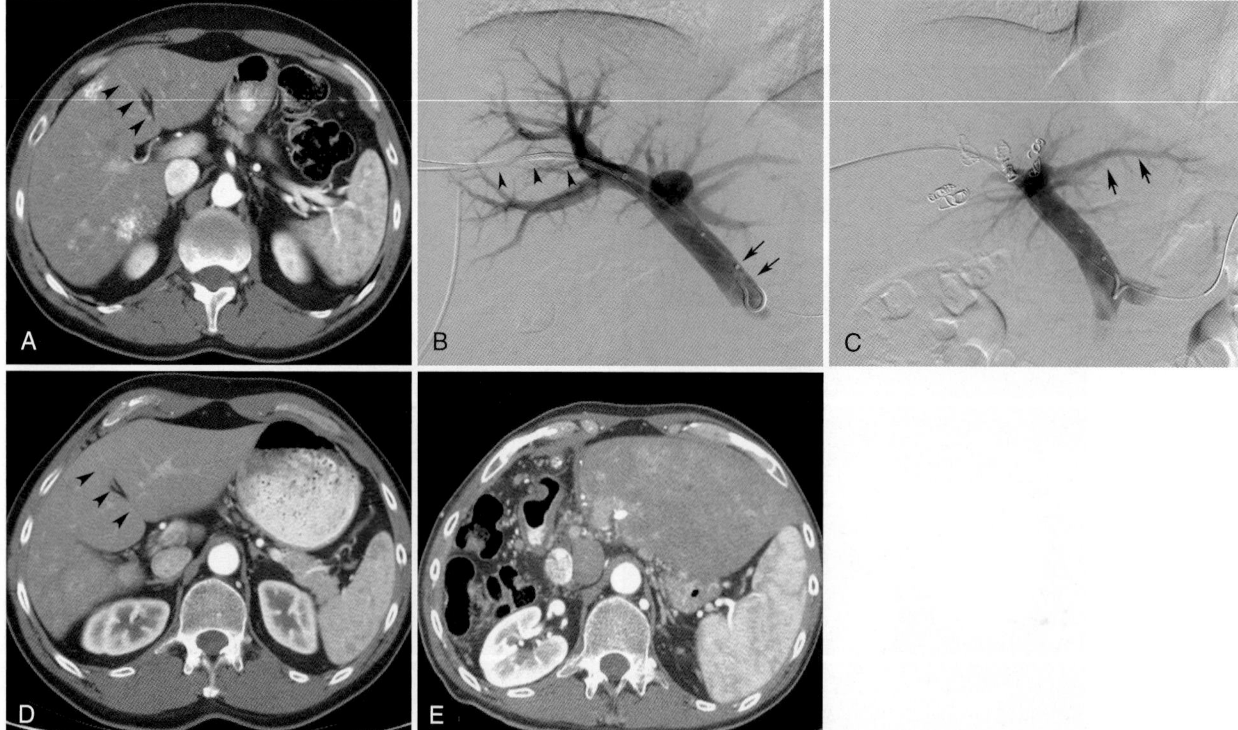

FIGURE 39.6. Transhepatic ipsilateral right portal vein embolization (PVE) extended to segment IV using tris-acryl particles and coils performed in a 47-year-old woman with colon cancer metastatic to the liver. **A,** Enhanced computed tomography (CT) scan obtained before PVE shows marginal future liver remnant (FLR) (FLR/total estimated liver volume [TELV] = 17%) (*arrowheads*). **B,** Anteroposterior flush portogram shows a 6-Fr vascular sheath in a right portal vein branch (*arrowheads*) and a 5-Fr flush catheter within the main portal vein (*arrows*). **C,** Final portogram shows occlusion of the portal vein branches to segments IV through VIII with continued patency of the veins supplying the left lateral lobe (*arrows*). **D,** Enhanced CT scan obtained 1 month after right PVE shows substantial FLR hypertrophy (FLR/TELV = 38%) (*arrowheads*). The degree of hypertrophy is 21%. **E,** Enhanced CT scan after right hepatectomy shows hypertrophy of the remnant liver.

In summary, interventional imaging and procedure are critical parts of the overall management of the oncologic patient.

KEY POINTS Portal Vein Embolization

- Portal vein embolization is indicated for patients with primary or metastatic liver disease who are otherwise hepatic resection candidates but are estimated to have small future liver remnants.
- Volumetric three-dimensional computed tomography is essential for optimal planning.
- The presence of patent vessels on follow-up in a patient with insufficient hypertrophy should prompt repeat embolization.

REFERENCES

1. Ahrar K, Matin S, Wood CG, et al. Percutaneous radiofrequency ablation of renal tumors: technique, complications, and outcomes. *J Vasc Interv Radiol*. 2005;16:679-688.
2. Ruarus AH, Vroomen LGPH, Pujik RS, et al. Irreversible electroporation in hepaticopancreaticobiliary tumors. *Can Assoc Radiol J*. 2018;69:38-50.
3. Cho YK, Kim JK, Kim WT, et al. Hepatic resection versus radiofrequency ablation for very early stage hepatocellular carcinoma: a Markov model analysis. *Hepatology*. 2010;51:1284-1290.
4. Erce C, Parks RW. Interstitial ablative techniques for hepatic tumours. *Br J Surg*. 2003;90:272-289.
5. Lee JM, Stitik FP, Carter D, et al. Local ablative procedures designed to destroy squamous-cell carcinoma. *Thorax*. 1975;30:152-157.
6. Murphy DP, Gill IS. Energy-based renal tumor ablation: a review. *Semin Urol Oncol*. 2001;19:133-140.
7. Gage AA, Baust J. Mechanisms of tissue injury in cryosurgery. *Cryobiology*. 1998;37:171-186.
8. Bageacu S, Kaczmarek D, Lacroix M, et al. Cryosurgery for resectable and unresectable hepatic metastases from colorectal cancer. *Eur J Surg Oncol*. 2007;33:590-596.
9. Seifert JK, France MP, Zhao J, et al. Large volume hepatic freezing: association with significant release of the cytokines interleukin-6 and tumor necrosis factor a in a rat model. *World J Surg*. 2002;26:1333-1341.
10. Sheen AJ, Poston GJ, Sherlock DJ. Cryotherapeutic ablation of liver tumours. *Br J Surg*. 2002;89:1396-1401.
11. Chu KF, Dupuy DE. Thermal ablation of tumours: biological mechanisms and advances in therapy. *Nat Rev Cancer*. 2014;14:199-208.
12. Chen MS, Li JQ, Zheng Y, et al. A prospective randomized trial comparing percutaneous local ablative therapy and partial hepatectomy for small hepatocellular carcinoma. *Ann Surg*. 2006;243:321-328.
13. Mulier S, Ruers T, Jamart J, et al. Radiofrequency ablation versus resection for resectable colorectal liver metastases: time for a randomized trial? An update. *Dig Surg*. 2008;25:445-460.
14. Goldberg SN, Gazelle GS, Compton CC, et al. Treatment of intrahepatic malignancy with radiofrequency ablation: radiologic-pathologic correlation. *Cancer*. 2000;88:2452-2463.
15. Goldberg SN, Grassi CJ, Cardella JF, et al. Image-guided tumor ablation: standardization of terminology and reporting criteria. *Radiology*. 2005;235:728-739.
16. Kim SK, Lim HK, Kim YH, et al. Hepatocellular carcinoma treated with radio-frequency ablation: spectrum of imaging findings. *Radiographics*. 2003;23:107-121.
17. Lim HK, Choi D, Lee WJ, et al. Hepatocellular carcinoma treated with percutaneous radio-frequency ablation: evaluation with follow-up multiphase helical CT. *Radiology*. 2001;221:447-454.
18. Goldberg SN, Solbiati L, Hahn PF, et al. Large-volume tissue ablation with radio frequency by using a clustered, internally cooled electrode technique: laboratory and clinical experience in liver metastases. *Radiology*. 1998;209:371-379.
19. Rhim H, Dodd 3rd GD. Radiofrequency thermal ablation of liver tumors. *J Clin Ultrasound*. 1999;27:221-229.
20. de Baere T, Risse O, Kuoch V, et al. Adverse events during radiofrequency treatment of 582 hepatic tumors. *AJR Am J Roentgenol*. 2003;181:695-700.
21. Livraghi T, Solbiati L, Meloni MF, et al. Treatment of focal liver tumors with percutaneous radio-frequency ablation: complications encountered in a multicenter study. *Radiology*. 2003;226:441-451.
22. Bandi G, Hedican SP, Nakada SY. Current practice patterns in the use of ablation technology for the management of small renal masses at academic centers in the United States. *Urology*. 2008;71:113-117.
23. Kunkle DA, Uzzo RG. Cryoablation or radiofrequency ablation of the small renal mass: a meta-analysis. *Cancer*. 2008;113:2671-2680.
24. Hegarty NJ, Gill IS, Desai MM, et al. Probe-ablative nephron-sparing surgery: cryoablation versus radiofrequency ablation. *Urology*. 2006;68(Suppl 1):7-13.
25. Atwell TD, Schmit GD, Boorjian SA, et al. Percutaneous ablation of renal masses measuring 3.0 cm and smaller: comparative local control and complications after radiofrequency ablation and cryoablation. *Am J Roentgenol*. 2013;200:461-466.
26. Jin GY, Lee JM, Lee YC, et al. Primary and secondary lung malignancies treated with percutaneous radiofrequency ablation: evaluation with follow-up helical CT. *AJR Am J Roentgenol*. 2004;183:1013-1020.
27. Higaki F, Okumura Y, Sato S, et al. Preliminary retrospective investigation of FDG-PET/CT timing in follow-up of ablated lung tumor. *Ann Nucl Med*. 2008;22:157-163.
28. Simon CJ, Dupuy DE, DiPetrillo TA, et al. Pulmonary radiofrequency ablation: long-term safety and efficacy in 153 patients. *Radiology*. 2007;243:268-275.
29. Howington JA, Blum MG, Chang AC, et al. Treatment of stage I and II non-small cell lung cancer: diagnosis and management of lung cancer, 3rd ed: American College of Chest Physicians evidence-based clinical practice guidelines. *Chest*. 2013;143:278-313.
30. Breedis C, Young G. The blood supply of neoplasms in the liver. *Am J Pathol*. 1954;30:969-977.
31. Ridge JA, Bading JR, Gelbard AS, et al. Perfusion of colorectal hepatic metastases. Relative distribution of flow from the hepatic artery and portal vein. *Cancer*. 1987;59:1547-1553.
32. Lewis AL, Dreher MR. Locoregional drug delivery using image-guided intra-arterial drug eluting bead therapy. *J Control Release*. 2012;161:338-350.
33. Yamada R, Nakatsuka H, Nakamura K, et al. Hepatic artery embolization in 32 patients with unresectable hepatoma. *Osaka City Med J*. 1980;26:81-96.
34. Maeda H, Seymour LW, Miyamoto Y. Conjugates of anticancer agents and polymers: advantages of macromolecular therapeutics in vivo. *Bioconjug Chem*. 1992;3:351-362.
35. Nakakuma K, Tashiro S, Hiraoka T, et al. Studies on anticancer treatment with an oily anticancer drug injected into the ligated feeding hepatic artery for liver cancer. *Cancer*. 1983;52:2193-2200.
36. Kan Z. Dynamic study of iodized oil in the liver and blood supply to hepatic tumors. An experimental investigation in several animal species. *Acta Radiol Suppl*. 1996;408:1-25.
37. Llovet JM, Bruix J. Systematic review of randomized trials for unresectable hepatocellular carcinoma: chemoembolization improves survival. *Hepatology*. 2003;37:429-442.
38. Llovet JM, Real MI, Montana X, et al. Arterial embolisation or chemoembolisation versus symptomatic treatment in patients with unresectable hepatocellular carcinoma: a randomised controlled trial. *Lancet*. 2002;359:1734-1739.
39. Lo CM, Ngan H, Tso WK, et al. Randomized controlled trial of transarterial lipiodol chemoembolization for unresectable hepatocellular carcinoma. *Hepatology*. 2002;35:1164-1171.
40. Lammer J, Malagari K, Vogl T, et al. Prospective randomized study of doxorubicin-eluting-bead embolization in the treatment of hepatocellular carcinoma: results of the PRECISION V study. *Cardiovasc Intervent Radiol*. 2010;33:41-52.
41. Poon RT, Tso WK, Pang RW, et al. A phase I/II trial of chemoembolization for hepatocellular carcinoma using a novel intra-arterial drug-eluting bead. *Clin Gastroenterol Hepatol*. 2007;5:1100-1108.
42. Brown KT, Do RK, Gonen M, et al. Randomized trial of hepatic artery embolization for hepatocellular carcinoma using doxorubicin-eluting microspheres compared with embolization with microspheres alone. *J Clin Oncol*. 2016;34:2046-2053.

43. Albert M, Kiefer MV, Sun W, et al. Chemoembolization of colorectal liver metastases with cisplatin, doxorubicin, mitomycin C, ethiodol, and polyvinyl alcohol. *Cancer*. 2011;117:343-352.
44. Akinwande O, Dendy M, Ludwig JM, et al. Hepatic intra-arterial injection of irinotecan drug eluting beads (DEBIRI) for patients with unresectable colorectal liver metastases: a systematic review. *Surg Oncol*. 2017;26:268-275.
45. Kobayashi K, Gupta S, Trent JC, et al. Hepatic artery chemoembolization for 110 gastrointestinal stromal tumors: response, survival, and prognostic factors. *Cancer*. 2006;107:2833-2841.
46. Jinno K, Moriwaki S, Tanada M, et al. Clinicopathological study on combination therapy consisting of arterial infusion of lipiodol-dissolved SMANCS and transcatheter arterial embolization for hepatocellular carcinoma. *Cancer Chemother Pharmacol*. 1992;31(Suppl):S7-S12.
47. Takayasu K, Arii S, Matsuo N, et al. Comparison of CT findings with resected specimens after chemoembolization with iodized oil for hepatocellular carcinoma. *AJR Am J Roentgenol*. 2000;175:699-704.
48. Choi BI, Kim HC, Han JK, et al. Therapeutic effect of transcatheter oily chemoembolization therapy for encapsulated nodular hepatocellular carcinoma: CT and pathologic findings. *Radiology*. 1992;182:709-713.
49. Kamel IR, Bluemke DA, Eng J, et al. The role of functional MR imaging in the assessment of tumor response after chemoembolization in patients with hepatocellular carcinoma. *J Vasc Interv Radiol*. 2006;17:505-512.
50. De Santis M, Alborino S, Tartoni PL, et al. Effects of lipiodol retention on MRI signal intensity from hepatocellular carcinoma and surrounding liver treated by chemoembolization. *Eur Radiol*. 1997;7:10-16.
51. Yu JS, Kim JH, Chung JJ, et al. Added value of diffusion-weighted imaging in the MRI assessment of perilesional tumor recurrence after chemoembolization of hepatocellular carcinomas. *J Magn Reson Imaging*. 2009;30:153-160.
52. Kamel IR, Liapi E, Reyes DK, et al. Unresectable hepatocellular carcinoma: serial early vascular and cellular changes after transarterial chemoembolization as detected with MR imaging. *Radiology*. 2009;250:466-473.
53. Dawson LA, Guha C. Hepatocellular carcinoma: radiation therapy. *Cancer J*. 2008;14:111-116.
54. Emami B, Lyman J, Brown A, et al. Tolerance of normal tissue to therapeutic irradiation. *Int J Radiat Oncol Biol Phys*. 1991;21:109-122.
55. Lawrence TS, Robertson JM, Anscher MS, et al. Hepatic toxicity resulting from cancer treatment. *Int J Radiat Oncol Biol Phys*. 1995;31:1237-1248.
56. Geschwind JF, Salem R, Carr BI, et al. Yttrium-90 microspheres for the treatment of hepatocellular carcinoma. *Gastroenterology*. 2004;127(5 Suppl 1):S194-S205.
57. Salem R, Lewandowski RJ, Atassi B, et al. Treatment of unresectable hepatocellular carcinoma with use of 90Y microspheres (TheraSphere): safety, tumor response, and survival. *J Vasc Interv Radiol*. 2005;16:1627-1639.
58. Stubbs RS, Cannan RJ, Mitchell AW. Selective internal radiation therapy (SIRT) with 90yttrium microspheres for extensive colorectal liver metastases. *J Gastrointest Surg*. 2001;5(3):294-302.
59. Marn CS, Andrews JC, Francis IR, et al. Hepatic parenchymal changes after intra-arterial Y-90 therapy: CT findings. *Radiology*. 1993;187:125-128.
60. Murthy R, Nunez R, Szklaruk J, et al. Yttrium-90 microsphere therapy for hepatic malignancy: devices, indications, technical considerations, and potential complications. *Radiographics*. 2005;25(Suppl 1):S41-S55.
61. Rhee TK, Naik NK, Deng J, et al. Tumor response after yttrium-90 radioembolization for hepatocellular carcinoma: comparison of diffusion-weighted functional MR imaging with anatomic MR imaging. *J Vasc Interv Radiol*. 2008;19:1180-1186.
62. Flamen P, Vanderlinden B, Delatte P, et al. Multimodality imaging can predict the metabolic response of unresectable colorectal liver metastases to radioembolization therapy with yttrium-90 labeled resin microspheres. *Phys Med Biol*. 2008;53:6591-6603.
63. Salem R, Lewandowski RJ, Mulcahy MF, et al. Radioembolization for hepatocellular carcinoma using Yttrium-90 microspheres: a comprehensive report of long-term outcomes. *Gastroenterology*. 2010;138:52-64.
64. Sangro B, Carpanese L, Cianni R, et al. Survival after yttrium-90 resin microsphere radioembolization of hepatocellular carcinoma across Barcelona Clinic Liver Cancer stages: a European evaluation. *Hepatology*. 2011;54:868-878.
65. Galle PR, Forner A, Llovet JM, et al. EASL clinical practice guidelines: management of hepatocellular carcinoma. *J Hepatol*. 2018;69:182-236.
66. Kulik LM, Carr BI, Mulcahy MF, et al. Safety and efficacy of 90Y radiotherapy for hepatocellular carcinoma with and without portal vein thrombosis. *Hepatology*. 2008;47:71-78.
67. Salem R, Gordon AC, Mouli S, et al. Y90 radioembolization significantly prolongs time to progression compared with chemoembolization in patients with hepatocellular carcinoma. *Gastroenterology*. 2016;151:1155-1163.
68. McDevitt JL, Alian A, Kapoor B, et al. Single-center comparison of overall survival and toxicities in patients with infiltrative hepatocellular carcinoma treated with Yttrium-90 radioembolization or drug-eluting embolic transarterial chemoembolization. *J Vasc Interv Radiol*. 2017;28:1371-1377.
69. Kennedy AS, McNeillie P, Dezarn WA, et al. Treatment parameters and outcome in 680 treatments of internal radiation with resin 90Y-microspheres for unresectable hepatic tumors. *Int J Radiat Oncol Biol Phys*. 2009;74:1494-1500.
70. Poon RT, Fan ST, Lo CM, et al. Improving survival results after resection of hepatocellular carcinoma: a prospective study of 377 patients over 10 years. *Ann Surg*. 2001;234:63-70.
71. Imamura H, Seyama Y, Kokudo N, et al. Single and multiple resections of multiple hepatic metastases of colorectal origin. *Surgery*. 2004;135:508-517.
72. Shirabe K, Shimada M, Gion T, et al. Postoperative liver failure after major hepatic resection for hepatocellular carcinoma in the modern era with special reference to remnant liver volume. *J Am Coll Surg*. 1999;188:304-309.
73. Shoup M, Gonen M, D'Angelica M, et al. Volumetric analysis predicts hepatic dysfunction in patients undergoing major liver resection. *J Gastrointest Surg*. 2003;7:325-330.
74. Madoff DC, Abdalla EK, Vauthey JN. Portal vein embolization in preparation for major hepatic resection: evolution of a new standard of care. *J Vasc Interv Radiol*. 2005;16:779-790.
75. Ribero D, Abdalla EK, Madoff DC, et al. Portal vein embolization before major hepatectomy and its effects on regeneration, resectability and outcome. *Br J Surg*. 2007;94:1386-1394.
76. Madoff DC, Abdalla EK, Gupta S, et al. Transhepatic ipsilateral right portal vein embolization extended to segment IV: improving hypertrophy and resection outcomes with spherical particles and coils. *J Vasc Interv Radiol*. 2005;16:215-225.
77. Farges O, Belghiti J, Kianmanesh R, et al. Portal vein embolization before right hepatectomy: prospective clinical trial. *Ann Surg*. 2003;237:208-217.
78. Kubota K, Makuuchi M, Kusaka K, et al. Measurement of liver volume and hepatic functional reserve as a guide to decision-making in resectional surgery for hepatic tumors. *Hepatology*. 1997;26:1176-1181.
79. Azoulay D, Castaing D, Krissat J, et al. Percutaneous portal vein embolization increases the feasibility and safety of major liver resection for hepatocellular carcinoma in injured liver. *Ann Surg*. 2000;232:665-672.
80. Adam R, Pascal G, Castaing D, et al. Tumor progression while on chemotherapy: a contraindication to liver resection for multiple colorectal metastases? *Ann Surg*. 2004;240:1052-1061. discussion 1061-1064.
81. Abdalla EK, Barnett CC, Doherty D, et al. Extended hepatectomy in patients with hepatobiliary malignancies with and without preoperative portal vein embolization. *Arch Surg*. 2002;137:675-680. discussion 680-681.
82. Vauthey JN, Pawlik TM, Abdalla EK, et al. Is extended hepatectomy for hepatobiliary malignancy justified? *Ann Surg*. 2004;239:722-730. discussion 730-732.
83. Vauthey JN, Chaoui A, Do KA, et al. Standardized measurement of the future liver remnant prior to extended liver resection: methodology and clinical associations. *Surgery*. 2000;127:512-519.
84. Vauthey JN, Abdalla EK, Doherty DA, et al. Body surface area and body weight predict total liver volume in Western adults. *Liver Transpl*. 2002;8:233-240.

CHAPTER 40

Complications in the Oncologic Patient: Chest

Edith M. Marom, M.D.; Amir Onn, M.D.; and Mary Frances McAleer, M.D., Ph.D.

INTRODUCTION

With advances in cancer therapy, iatrogenic diseases of the chest are increasingly encountered. They are predominated by those affecting the lungs, which are an important cause of patient morbidity and mortality. In the cancer patient, iatrogenic pulmonary disease could be as a result of chemotherapy, radiation therapy (RT), or stem cell transplantation (SCT). Recognizing these patterns of disease is important because the radiologist may be the first to notice these changes, which at times may be reversible if identified in a timely manner.

CHEMOTHERAPY-INDUCED NONINFECTIOUS LUNG DISEASE

The problem of drugs adversely affecting the lungs remains a major challenge to all primary care physicians. Symptoms are usually nonspecific, with patients presenting with dyspnea, nonproductive cough, and fever, which can begin weeks to years after the medication is first taken. Unfortunately, drug-induced respiratory disease remains a disease of exclusion, because the majority of drugs responsible for this effect cannot be identified by any specific test. Diagnosis requires a high index of suspicion, because infection, radiation pneumonitis, and recurrence of the underlying disease can manifest clinically and radiographically in a similar manner. There is underreporting of drug toxicity, and thus, the true incidence of drug-induced respiratory disease is unknown, although it is estimated to be less than 10%.[1,1a] To complicate matters, only a few patients are treated with single drugs. Thus, how much of an observed reaction is related to one agent or another versus synergy with other drugs, oxygen, or radiation often remains unknown. Prompt diagnosis of drug-induced lung toxicity is important, because early drug-induced lung injury will often regress with cessation of the therapy or with initiation of steroid therapy before pulmonary fibrosis is able to develop. For an updated list of generic drugs, types of reaction, and radiologic manifestations with references, the reader is referred to the routinely updated website Pneumotox (www.pneumotox.com).[2] In this reference and in Table 40.1, the reader will find some of the effects of drugs on other chest structures such as those causing pleural effusions, lymphadenopathy, or cardiomyopathy.

The lungs have a limited number of histopathologic responses to injury (see Table 40.1) that mimic many other pulmonary conditions.[1] The radiologic appearance of drug toxicity corresponds to the histopathologic finding. Owing to these nonspecific findings, diagnosis relies on correlation with clinical, laboratory, and radiologic information.[3] Even bronchoalveolar lavage (BAL) can only suggest an iatrogenic cause by helping to exclude infection and malignancy. Sometimes, cell composition in the lavage and elevation of a specific population (e.g., lymphocytes, neutrophils, or eosinophils) may suggest a more specific diagnosis.

As an aid for interpretation of the chest images, it is helpful to divide drug toxicity into acute and delayed presentation. Acute-onset, chemotherapy-induced lung injury is usually caused by noncardiogenic pulmonary edema/diffuse alveolar damage, hypersensitivity-type reaction, or pulmonary hemorrhage and occurs after the initial dose of chemotherapy. Radiographic findings usually include diffuse or scattered ground-glass opacities (GGOs) or consolidative opacities with or without septal thickening (Fig. 40.1).

Delayed-onset, chemotherapy-induced lung injury usually presents more than 2 months after the completion of treatment or during prolonged treatment and is often caused by chronic interstitial pneumonia, which can lead to fibrosis. The more common histologic patterns seen are usual interstitial pneumonia (UIP) or nonspecific interstitial pneumonia (NSIP).[3] The pattern most commonly encountered is that of NSIP, which appears as bilateral lower lobe–predominant heterogeneous or consolidative opacities on chest radiographs, and initially as scattered GGOs or consolidative opacities with lower lobe predominance on thin-section chest computed tomography (CT) (Fig. 40.2). Although intralobular septal thickening and traction bronchiectasis can be seen with NSIP, when present, these findings are much more likely to be from UIP.[4,5] Organizing pneumonia with fibromyxoid connective tissue plugs that fill distal airspaces, as well as terminal or respiratory bronchioles, is another nonacute form of drug toxicity. When associated with a known causative agent, this finding should be termed bronchiolitis obliterans organizing pneumonia (BOOP) caused by the name of the drug (e.g., BOOP caused by amiodarone).[3–5] Radiographic findings of drug-induced BOOP on chest radiographs are bilateral scattered heterogeneous or consolidative opacities in a peripheral distribution, and on chest CT there are unilateral or bilateral areas of consolidation, with either peripheral or the more typical peribronchovascular distribution and a lower

TABLE 40.1 Histologic Patterns Associated With Drug Reactions

FINDING	DRUG
Noncardiogenic pulmonary edema	Carbamazepine, gemcitabine, taxanes, cyclophosphamide, methotrexate, vinblastine
Alveolar hemorrhage	Bevacizumab, rituximab
Alveolar proteinosis–like reaction	Mitomycin C
Diffuse alveolar hemorrhage	Carbamazepine, methotrexate, gemcitabine
Diffuse alveolar damage	Gemcitabine, methotrexate, bleomycin, cyclophosphamide, gefitinib, erlotinib, immune checkpoint inhibitors
Organizing pneumonia	Bleomycin, cyclophosphamide, immune checkpoint inhibitors
Bronchiolitis obliterans syndrome	Busulfan
Usual interstitial pneumonia–like pattern	Bleomycin, gemcitabine, methotrexate, busulfan, cyclophosphamide
Diffuse cellular interstitial infiltrates with or without granulomas	Bleomycin, methotrexate
Nonspecific interstitial pneumonia	Bleomycin, taxanes, gemcitabine, methotrexate, imatinib, immune checkpoint inhibitors
Desquamative interstitial pneumonia	Busulfan
Acute or chronic eosinophilic pneumonia	Bleomycin, methotrexate
Pulmonary venoocclusive disease	Bleomycin, busulfan
Pulmonary nodules	Bleomycin, vinblastine
Pneumothorax/ pneumomediastinum	Bleomycin
Hilar/mediastinal adenopathy	Bleomycin, immune checkpoint inhibitors
Pleural effusion	Methotrexate, cyclophosphamide, imatinib, immune checkpoint inhibitors
Cavitations	Bevacizumab
Pulmonary thromboembolism	Bevacizumab, thalidomide
Cardiomyopathy	Doxorubicin, 5-fluorouracil, trastuzumab

(Modified from www.pneumotox.com; and Flieder DB, Travis WD. Pathologic characteristics of drug-induced lung disease. *Clin Chest Med.* 2004;25:37-45; and Broder H, Gottlieb RA, Lepor NE. Chemotherapy and cardiotoxicity. *Rev Cardiovasc Med.* 2008;9:75–83.)

lobe predominance.[6] Rarely, BOOP may have a nodular appearance that can be confused with metastatic disease.[7]

When clinical suspicion for drug toxicity is high, thin-section CT should be performed, especially in conjunction with a normal chest film, so that treatment can be initiated for reversal of the process. Often, however, these findings are detected incidentally on routine follow-up chest CT scans. Radiologists may thus be the first to suspect drug toxicity and must alert the clinician to this possibility before end-stage fibrosis develops.

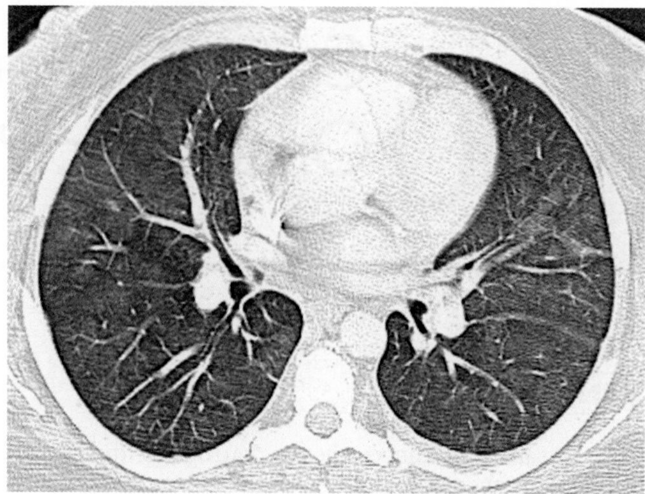

FIGURE 40.1. Acute drug toxicity. A 40-year-old woman with shortness of breath and fever during the month of new salvage chemotherapy with PTK787, a tyrosine kinase inhibitor, for acute myeloid leukemia. Chest computed tomography (CT) scan shows diffuse bilateral ground-glass opacities. Autopsy performed 9 days after the CT scan demonstrated acute interstitial pneumonitis with diffuse alveolar damage.

KEY POINTS Drug Toxicity

- Diagnosis is by exclusion.
- Early toxicity manifests as symmetrical airspace disease: consolidative or ground-glass opacities (GGOs).
- Delayed toxicity usually manifests as scattered peripheral consolidation or GGOs, with lower lobe predominance.
- Radiologist should alert clinician to drug toxicity probability before irreversible fibrosis formation.

CHEMOTHERAPY-INDUCED INFECTIOUS LUNG DISEASE

Drugs that are used to combat cancer target dividing cells, affect the bone marrow, and cause a decrease in neutrophils that results in infections. Other drugs that are often used to treat hematologic malignancies in conjunction with chemotherapeutic agents have immunosuppressive properties. Corticosteroids cause a broad suppression of the immune system.[8] Diagnosis of pneumonia depends on clinical symptomatology with radiographic findings. The type of pathogen producing the pneumonia, whether bacterial, viral, or fungal, depends mainly on the patient's immune status and the combination therapy they received. Given the inability of the severely immunocompromised patient (e.g., SCT recipients or prolonged neutropenia in patients with hematologic malignancies) to mount an adequate inflammatory response, the classic radiographic findings of each type of pneumonia may differ from those found in immunocompetent patients, and chest films may even appear normal. CT may disclose more subtle changes, such as minimal GGOs, bronchial thickening, or nodules, and in select cases may show the typical appearance for a specific group of pathogens.[9] Such findings may lead to the correct selection of antibiotic therapy and improved outcomes.[10,11]

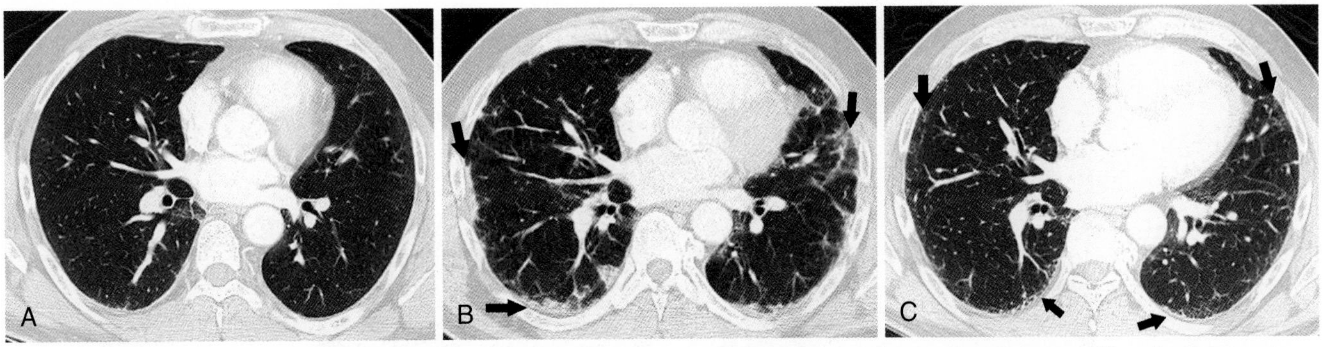

FIGURE 40.2. Bleomycin drug toxicity. A 49-year-old man with Hodgkin lymphoma developed increasing shortness of breath after completion of the first cycle of chemotherapy with doxorubicin, bleomycin, vinblastine, and dacarbazine (ABVD) that progressed after the second cycle. **A**, Baseline contrast-enhanced chest computed tomography (CT) scan before therapy. **B**, Chest CT scan obtained 2 weeks after the second course of ABVD chemotherapy shows interval development of mid to moderate lower lobe–predominant peripheral consolidative and ground-glass opacities (*arrows*). Bronchoscopy did not show any organisms. Bleomycin was discontinued, and the patient was treated with steroids with clinical resolution of shortness of breath. **C**, Chest CT scan 4 years after completion of chemotherapy shows that some of the acute changes that were seen in **B** resolved, although nonreversible peripheral bleomycin-induced pulmonary fibrosis remained (*arrows*).

Bacterial Pneumonia

The main source of pathogens is the patient's endogenous flora.[12] With the introduction of extended-spectrum beta-lactams, there has been a decrease in bloodstream infections because of gram-negative rod bacteremia and an increase in infections because of gram-positive cocci,[13] although nosocomial bacterial pneumonias are still predominated by gram-negative rods.[14] There is a low predictive yield to determination of the type of bacterial pneumonia from the chest radiographic or even chest CT appearance in the immunocompromised patient population.[15] In SCT recipients, bacterial pneumonia most commonly manifests as pulmonary nodules (81%), in a tree-in-bud distribution, lower lobe predominant, asymmetrically distributed consolidation (69%), and GGOs (35%), usually symmetrically distributed.[16] The majority of patients demonstrate a combination of these findings (73%), with another 15% of patients having pulmonary nodules only and 12% consolidation only on CT (Fig. 40.3).

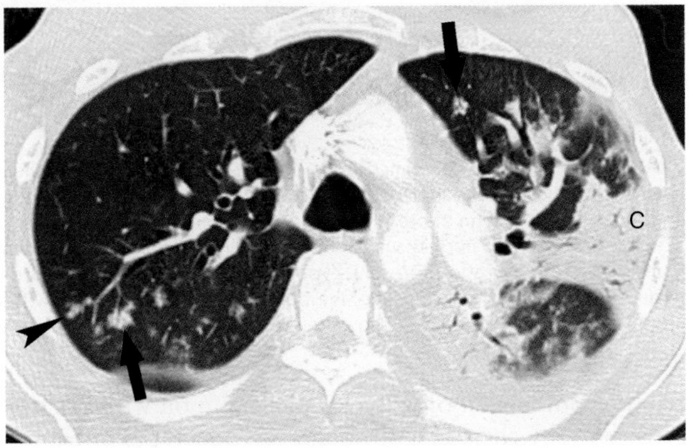

FIGURE 40.3. Gram-negative bacterial pneumonia. A 25-year-old man with T-cell large granular lymphocytic leukemia presents with neutrophenic fever. Contrast-enhanced chest computed tomography (CT) scan shows left upper lobe consolidation (C), peribronchovascular nodular opacities (*arrows*), and tree-in-bud nodules (*arrowhead*). Cultures from bronchoscopy that was performed on the day of the CT scan grew *Enterococcus* and *Serratia marcescens*.

Viral Pneumonia

DNA viruses such as herpes simplex, varicella, and cytomegalovirus (CMV) have long been recognized as causing severe respiratory infections in patients with hematologic malignancies.[17] These patients are also exposed to community seasonal respiratory viruses such as adenovirus or influenza A, which can be life-threatening in such immunocompromised patients.[18] Radiographically, one viral infection cannot be differentiated from another. They tend to be symmetrically distributed in the lung, usually with lower lobe predominance and a combination of GGOs or consolidative airspace disease (Fig. 40.4) in addition to small centrilobular nodules and consolidative opacities.[18–22] The mortality rate can be high, and early diagnosis is essential because early treatment improves survival. Of this group, airspace disease is the most common finding, seen in 90% of patients with CT-documented pneumonia.[18,21,22] The early changes of lower lobe–predominant peribronchial thickening and peribronchial GGOs or tree-in-bud opacities are more

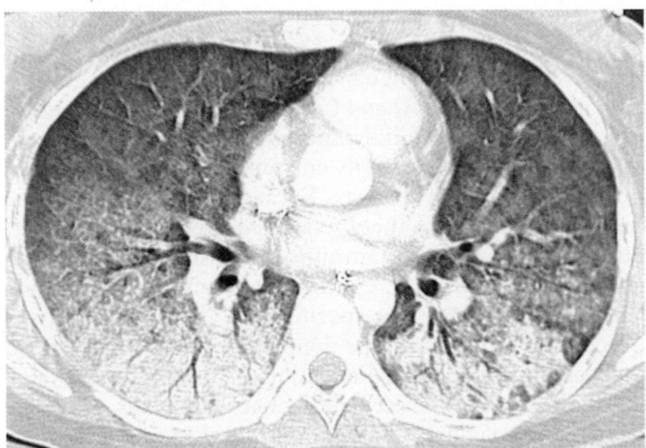

FIGURE 40.4. Viral pneumonia. A 19-year-old woman with acute lymphocytic leukemia, treated with hypercyclophosphamide, vincristine, doxorubicin, and dexamethasone for relapse, who presented with an abnormal chest radiograph, fever, shortness of breath, and hypoxemia. She had high cytomegalovirus antigenemia. Contrast-enhanced chest computed tomography scan shows diffuse airspace disease with lower lobe consolidation, whereas the rest of the lung shows diffuse ground-glass opacities.

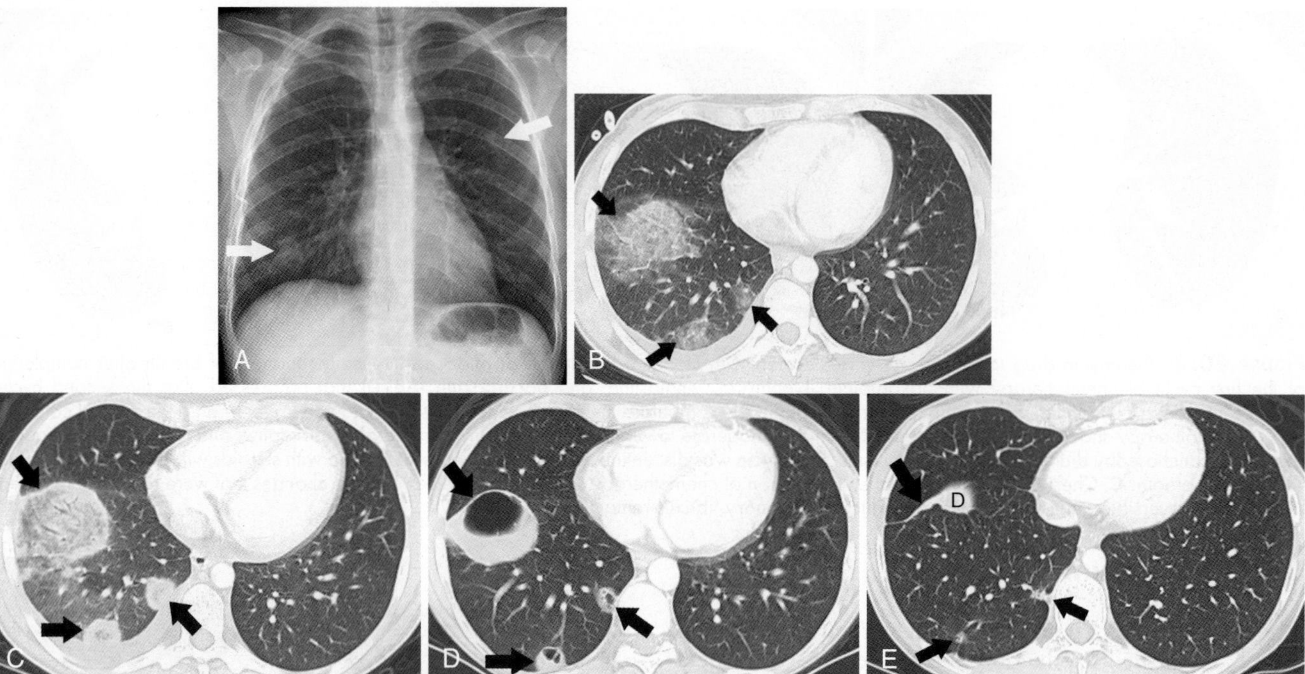

FIGURE 40.5. Fungal pneumonia. A 23-year-old woman with acute myeloid leukemia after stem cell transplantation presented with neutropenic fever. Chest radiograph at presentation shows a minimal heterogeneous opacity in the right lower lung (*right arrow*) and left upper lobe (A). Contrast-enhanced chest CT scan at presentation (B) shows ground-glass nodules and mass (*arrows* in B), which ten days later (C) progress to the "reversed halo sign": a ground-glass nodule surrounded by a ring of consolidation (*arrows* in C). Core biopsy from the mass showed 90-degree branching hyphae, confirmed with culture to represent *Zygomycetes.* Contrast-enhanced chest CT scan 1 month after C (D) shows interval cavitation of the pulmonary nodules (*arrows* in D). By this time, the patient was asymptomatic, with recovered counts and complete remission from leukemia. Contrast enhanced chest CT scan 3 years later (E) shows resolution of the nodules with persistent scars (*arrows* in E). D, partial averaging of the right hemidiaphragm.

readily appreciated on a lateral plain film or, with greater sensitivity, by chest CT, although early bacterial pneumonia may have a similar appearance.

Fungal Pneumonia

Opportunistic invasive fungal pneumonias are associated with high morbidity and mortality rates[23–25] and are typically found in patients with prolonged, severe immunocompromise, as can be seen with hematologic malignancies and SCT recipients but is rarely encountered in patients with solid malignancies. Although invasive pulmonary aspergillosis (IPA) and *Candida* are the most common, other angioinvasive molds, such as *Fusarium* and *Zygomycetes* species, are increasingly encountered in these severely immunocompromised hosts. Because early institution of high-dose antifungal therapy is associated with improved outcomes,[10,26] early recognition of invasive fungal disease is important. However, cultures of respiratory secretions are neither sensitive nor specific, and lavage and invasive procedures often cannot be done in these patients because of coagulation abnormalities and thrombocytopenia.[27,28] Thus, diagnosis of invasive pulmonary fungal disease relies heavily on imaging.[29] CT is often used in an attempt to identify fungal pneumonia in a timely fashion because some of these typical imaging findings cannot be detected by chest radiographs.

The "halo sign," a nodule surrounded by GGOs, is seen in 92% of patients with IPA at presentation.[10] The presence of large nodules (>1 cm) and visualization of the halo sign are most suggestive of fungal infection.[16] There have been attempts to differentiate pulmonary zygomycosis (PZ) from IPA, because this distinction has important therapeutic implications: specifically, voriconazole, the preferred drug in the treatment of IPA,[30] has no activity in zygomycosis.[2] The presence of the "reversed halo sign" (Fig. 40.5), a focal round area of ground-glass attenuation surrounded by a ring of consolidation, or the presence of multiple nodules (>10) is more commonly seen with PZ than with other invasive fungi.[31,32] Although these CT findings of the reversed halo sign and halo sign are not pathognomonic for fungal infections and can be seen, for example, with cryptogenic organizing pneumonia, infarction, or malignancy, when observed on imaging of a febrile, severely immunocompromised patient, these should be considered invasive fungal pneumonia until proved otherwise.

Pneumocystis pneumonia (PCP), once a major cause of morbidity and mortality in patients treated for hematologic malignancies, has been largely prevented by the use of antimicrobial prophylaxis. Chest radiographs at presentation can be normal and later nonspecific, with bilateral, perihilar reticular and poorly defined GGOs, which often progress to alveolar consolidation in 3 to 4 days.[33] Thin-section CT usually reveals scattered ground-glass attenuation that can be associated with interlobular septal thickening, findings that can resemble viral pneumonia such as CMV pneumonia. In an attempt to differentiate the CT appearance of CMV from PCP in patients without human immunodeficiency virus, apical distribution and a sharply demarcated mosaic pattern are found more frequently in PCP, whereas small nodules or unsharp demarcation of GGOs and lower lobe predominance are more likely to be seen in CMV pneumonia.[34]

Tuberculosis

Although patients immunosuppressed from chemotherapy are at risk for tuberculosis (TB), the incidence of TB in even the most severely immunosuppressed patients, such as SCT recipients, is proportional to the incidence of TB in the general population. The imaging appearance of TB in this population is identical to that in the general population.[35,36]

KEY POINTS Chemotherapy-Induced Pneumonia in the Severely Immunocompromised Host

- Bacterial pneumonia most commonly manifests as a combination of consolidation/ground-glass opacities (GGOs) with tree-in-bud lower lobe–predominant nodules.
- Viral pneumonia most commonly manifests as diffuse lower lobe–predominant consolidation/GGOs with or without centrilobular nodules.
- The presence of large nodules (>1 cm) and visualization of the halo sign are most suggestive of fungal infection.

STEM CELL COMPLICATIONS

Pulmonary complications develop in 30% to 60% of SCT recipients and are the immediate cause of death in approximately 61% of cases.[37–39] The donor source may be the patient (autologous), a sibling or unrelated person (allogeneic), an identical twin (syngeneic), or a genetically unrelated umbilical cord blood sample.[40] Although syngeneic grafts have lower treatment-related mortality and do not develop graft-versus-host disease (GVHD), they have a greater risk of malignant recurrence. Thus, the overall mortality is similar for syngeneic and allogeneic SCT. When evaluating the complications associated with SCT, chest imaging findings are generally nonspecific. Often, the patient will have a normal chest radiograph, and thus, the CT findings may prove to be of value. The correct interpretation of the CT scan depends on knowledge of the patient's immune recovery, because specific pulmonary complications tend to occur within well-defined time periods after transplantation.[41,42] Despite recovery to normal cell counts within a month, complete immunologic recovery occurs within 1 to 2 years in patients without GVHD. Complications after SCT are categorized into early (≤100 days from transplantation) and late (>100 days from transplantation) complications, according to time of presentation relative to the date of transplantation.

Early Complications

Early complications are subdivided into (1) the preengraftment period, with the onset of marrow suppression and development of neutropenia, and phagocytic recovery usually occurring within the first month after transplantation, and (2) the early phase, approximately 30 to 100 days after transplantation. During the early phase, cell counts are normal, although their function is not.

Preengraftment Period (Days 1–30)

This period immediately following transplantation, with its profound neutropenia, is predominated by infectious complications, most commonly bacterial and fungal, with associated imaging findings as described previously. The bacterial pathogens encountered include gram-negative enteric flora, gram-positive cocci, and gram-positive skin commensals, along with those related to indwelling catheters. When the period of neutropenia is prolonged, the patient is at high risk for invasive fungal infections, most commonly *Candida* and *Aspergillus*.[43]

Noninfectious complications during this period include pulmonary edema, periengraftment respiratory distress syndrome (PERDS), diffuse alveolar hemorrhage (DAH), and drug-induced injury (Fig. 40.6). It is difficult to differentiate radiographically between these conditions, because the main imaging finding related to these noninfectious complications is that of airspace disease, with bilateral symmetrical GGOs or consolidative opacities, with or without septal thickening.[44] Pulmonary edema occurs secondary to the large amounts of intravenous fluids administered with the conditioning regimen before SCT. PERDS is seen in approximately 5% of autologous SCT cases and refers to the pulmonary component of the engraftment syndrome.[45] Clinically, the syndrome is characterized by rash, fever, and diarrhea, thought to be caused by a complex interaction between the conditioning-related endothelial damage and the cytokine release associated with neutrophil and lymphocyte recovery. Corticosteroid treatment usually leads to rapid recovery.[45] DAH is associated with a mortality rate of 40% to 100%, but less than 20% of cases report hemoptysis. Thus, diagnosis of DAH relies on demonstration of more than 20% hemosiderin-laden macrophages in BAL fluid, in the absence of infection.[46] Early diagnosis and steroid therapy may improve outcome. Drug-induced injury occurs in 10% of SCT recipients, and its radiographic manifestations are as described previously.

Early Phase (Days 30–100)

Because of the impaired function of the SCT recipient's marrow cells, infections continue to be a threat during this phase. Bacterial infections are common, particularly in patients with indwelling catheters. Prophylactic antifungal medication has significantly reduced the occurrence of *Candida* infections, although a wider variety of invasive molds resistant to this prophylaxis is seen. Nevertheless, IPA continues to be the most common invasive fungus encountered during this period[43] (see Fig. 40.6). The early phase is the period in which CMV reactivation is common. With the availability of effective antiviral medication and initiation of therapy based on CMV viremia before disease manifests, CMV mortality has decreased. Consequently, CMV pneumonia is radiographically less often seen.[43] Similarly, PCP, previously encountered during the early phase, is now rarely seen owing to routine antimicrobial prophylaxis.[42]

Of the noninfectious complications during this period, idiopathic pneumonia syndrome (IPS) is the most common. Hence, IPS is the most common cause of diffuse radiographic abnormalities between 30 to 180 days after SCT, although its incidence has recently decreased to approximately 10%.[44,46] CT scan findings include airspace

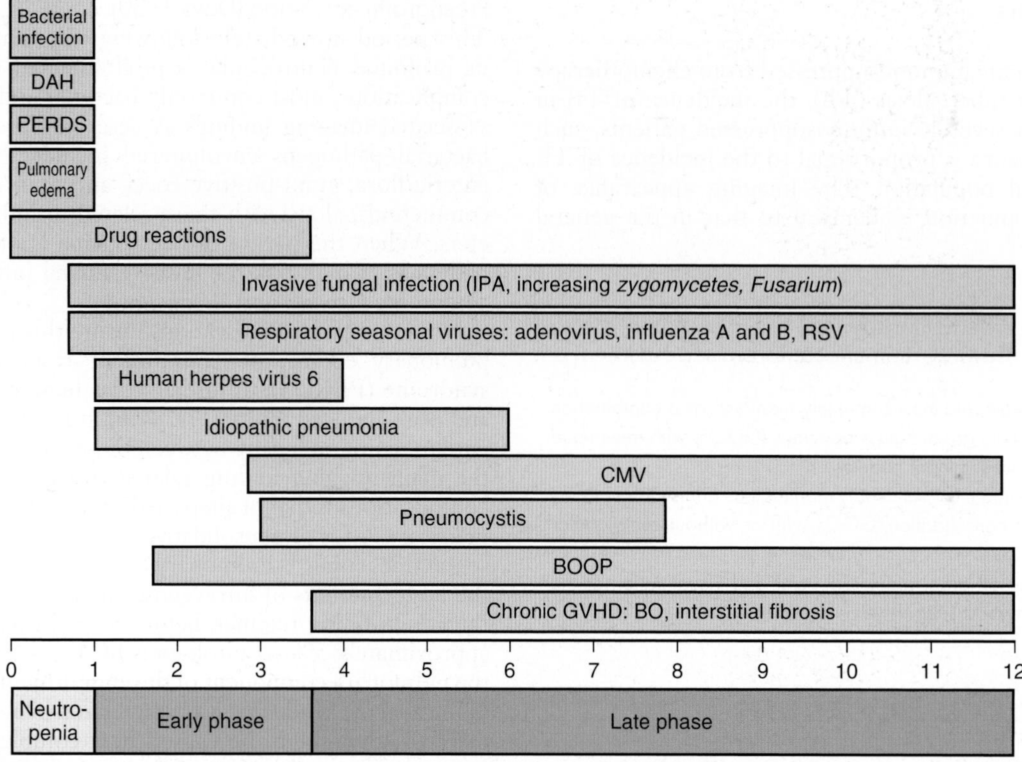

FIGURE 40.6. Timeline of infections after stem cell transplantation. *BO*, Bronchiolitis obliterans; *BOOP*, bronchiolitis obliterans organizing pneumonia; *CMV*, cytomegalovirus; *DAH*, diffuse alveolar hemorrhage; *GVHD*, graft-versus-host disease; *IPA*, invasive pulmonary aspergillosis; *PERDS*, periengraftment respiratory distress syndrome; *RSV*, respiratory syncytial virus. (Modified from Worthy SA, Flint JD, Muller NL. Pulmonary complications after bone marrow transplantation: high-resolution CT and pathologic findings. *Radiographics.* 1997;17:1359-1371; Hiemenz JW. Management of infections complicating allogeneic hematopoietic stem cell transplantation. *Semin Hematol.* 2009;46:289-312.)

disease with a lower lobe predominance, a pattern seen with noncardiogenic pulmonary edema.[44] IPS is a diagnosis of exclusion and is defined by the presence of widespread alveolar injury in the absence of lower respiratory tract infection. The pathogenesis of IPS is attributed to lung tissue injury from cytokine release. Mortality is approximately 70%, and treatment is supportive, because IPS does not respond to steroid therapy.[44,46]

Other complications during this period include a variety of manifestations of early GVHD and are, thus, usually seen in allogeneic SCT recipients. Early GVHD can present in the form of BOOP, characterized by the presence of granulation tissue within the alveolar ducts and alveoli, observed from 1 month to 2 years after transplantation.[44,46] Chest radiographs show nonspecific bilateral regions of consolidation, which may be nodular and even migratory. CT scans reveal scattered focal peripheral and/or peribronchovascular consolidation, with a lower lobe predominance.[47]

Late Complications

Late complications result from GVHD (see Fig. 40.6). Histologically, within the first 6 months, there is infiltration of the perivascular zones and alveolar septa by mononuclear cells and ongoing lymphocyte-mediated injury to the large and small airways. The interstitial process will cause exudation of fluid to the alveoli, which may form airspace granulation tissue. If not cleared, it will progress to the irreversible stage of fibrosis. A similar process occurs in the airways. The lymphocytic infiltration causes damage to the bronchus that, if allowed to continue, leads to intraluminal granulation tissue, as seen in BOOP. This process is still reversible but, if not treated, may progress to form concentric or luminal obliterative scars, which will disrupt normal airflow. This effect is known as bronchiolitis obliterans (BO) (Fig. 40.7).[48] Thus, from about 4 months after SCT, GVHD is to be excluded in a patient with respiratory complaints. Although pulmonary GVHD usually accompanies GVHD in extrathoracic sites, up to 30% of GVHD cases may occur in the lungs alone.[48] Early recognition of pulmonary GVHD, while the disease is still reversible, is important.

CT plays an important role in late SCT recipients who present with pulmonary complaints. This imaging modality not only helps to exclude pulmonary infection but may also show findings suggestive of GVHD. Early findings are nonspecific and include scattered GGOs or consolidative opacities, similar to the ones discussed in the context of drug-induced BOOP. Irreversible findings to look for include interstitial thickening/fibrosis or findings seen in BO, namely bronchiolar thickening, bronchiolectasis, and air trapping (Fig. 40.8). Thus, in the search for early pulmonary GVHD, expiratory CT scans are used to search for air trapping. Patients with chronic GVHD remain at risk for pulmonary infection, because their immune recovery may be prolonged for years.[46] Organisms include encapsulated bacteria, as well as invasive fungal molds such as *Aspergillus* species and *Zygomycete*,

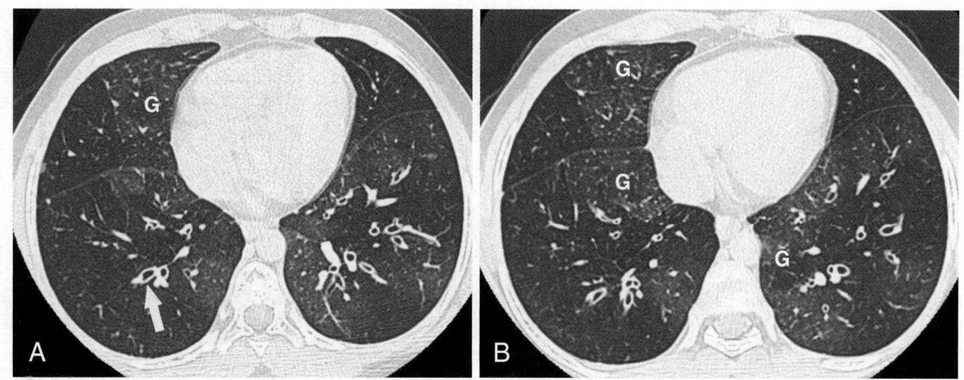

FIGURE 40.7. Bronchiolitis obliterans. A 10-year-old patient 3 years after stem cell transplantation for acute lymphoblastic leukemia and chronic graft-versus-host disease with bronchiolitis obliterans. **A**, Inspiratory contrast-enhanced chest computed tomography (CT) scan shows mosaic appearance of the lungs, with segmental scattered regions of ground-glass opacities (G) and lower density areas adjacent to them. Lower bronchi are dilated and thickened (*arrow*). **B**, Expiratory contrast-enhanced chest CT scan shows that the low-density regions of the lungs persist, despite the expiratory phase, consistent with air trapping in these regions. Bronchi to the ground-glass regions (G) remain patent, and, thus, at this expiratory phase, these ground-glass regions become slightly denser, accentuating the mosaic appearance.

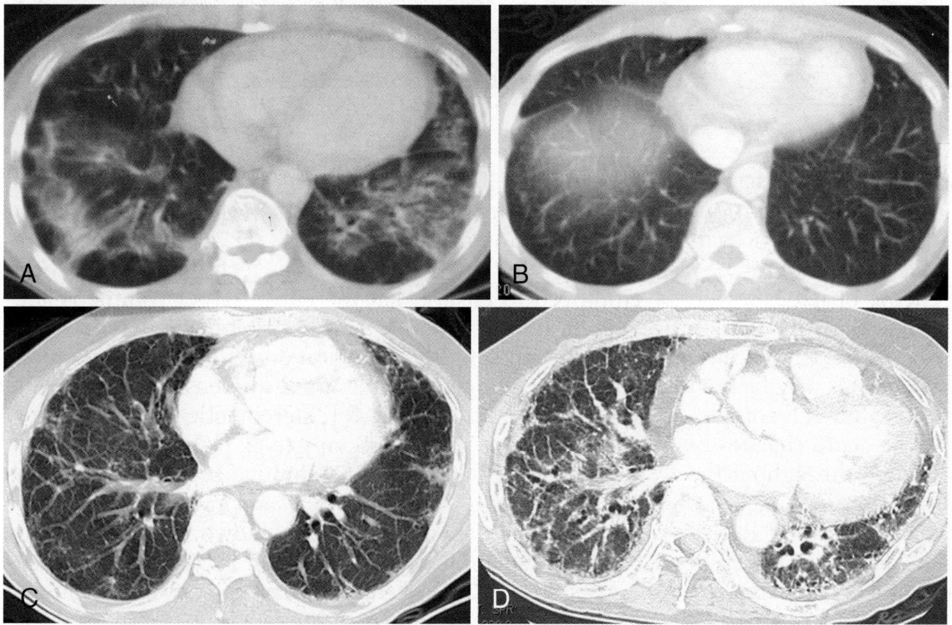

FIGURE 40.8. Graft-versus-host disease (GVHD). A 43-year-old patient with chronic severe GVHD affecting the lungs 10 years after stem cell transplantation (SCT). **A**, Chest computed tomography (CT) scan 2 years after SCT shows bilateral consolidation and ground-glass opacities centered around bronchi. Wedge biopsy 1 week after this chest CT scan showed inflammation consistent with GVHD. **B**, Chest CT scan after treatment with steroids 6 months after **A** shows resolution of inflammation. **C**, Chest CT scan 3 years after **B**, after multiple episodes of pulmonary exacerbations and infections, shows interval development of peripheral pulmonary fibrosis with traction bronchiectasis and intralobular septal thickening. **D**, Chest CT scan 1 year after **C** shows progression of pulmonary fibrosis.

especially in those patients with severe GVHD treated with high-dose corticosteroids and/or other immunosuppressive regimens. CMV reactivation is now more commonly delayed to this late period, but CMV pneumonia is rarely encountered, owing to treatment of viremia before the disease manifests clinically.[46]

KEY POINTS Stem Cell Transplantation Complications

- One to 30 days after stem cell transplantation (SCT), patients are severely neutropenic, and the most common complication is bacterial or fungal pneumonia.
- Thirty to one-hundred days after SCT, white blood cell function is impaired; thus, fungal pneumonia is still common, but early graft-versus-host disease (GVHD) in the form of bronchiolitis obliterans organizing pneumonia can be seen.
- Late complications after SCT are caused by GVHD, which can manifest as scattered symmetrical consolidation/ground-glass opacities, air trapping, interstitial thickening, and fibrosis.
- Because treatment of GVHD is immunosuppressive, patients are at risk for fungal and bacterial pneumonia.

RADIATION-INDUCED LUNG DISEASE

Radiation-induced lung disease (RILD) is common after RT but can mimic other inflammatory and infectious pulmonary conditions. To distinguish between these possibilities, one must be familiar with the expected timeline of pulmonary changes after RT and those associated with specific RT plans. When assessing for RILD, one refers to the last day of radiation administration to document changes. Within 4 to 12 weeks, transient radiation

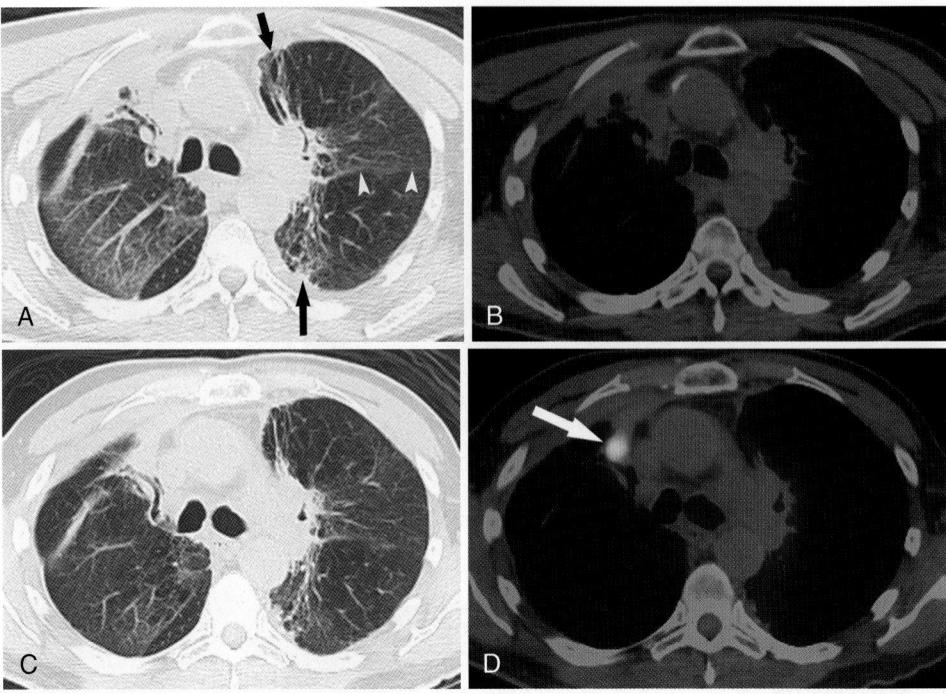

FIGURE 40.9. A 69-year-old man 3 years after radiation therapy of synchronous small cell and squamous cell lung cancer. **A**, Non–contrast-enhanced chest computed tomography (CT) scan shows radiation-induced fibrosis (*arrows*) with traction bronchiectasis crossing through the fissure (*arrowheads*) in the left paramediastinal region. **B**, Fused positron emission tomography (PET)/CT scan from the time of **A** shows no abnormal 2-[18F] fluoro-2-deoxy-D-glucose (FDG) activity and no evidence of recurrence. **C**, CT scan performed 6 months after **A** does not show a significant change in the appearance of the bilateral paramediastinal radiation fibrosis. **D**, Fused PET/CT at the level of **C** shows new focal FDG activity within the radiation fibrosis (*arrow*). Core biopsy confirmed recurrence of squamous cell cancer.

pneumonitis is expected histologically. Chest film changes are usually evident 6 to 8 weeks after standard-fractionated radiation doses of above 40 Gy, but similarly fractionated doses below 20 Gy rarely produce pneumonitis.[49–51] These changes manifest as heterogeneous opacities within the radiation portal, progressing to consolidation, which is usually most severe 3 to 4 months after RT.[52] Because of the greater sensitivity of CT scans, GGOs may be seen within the treatment portal by 3 weeks after RT completion and progress to consolidation. The acute changes of RILD may be homogeneously distributed throughout the radiation portal or scattered focally within it, sometimes in a nodular fashion, mimicking malignancy.[53,54] Rarely at this stage RILD can be seen outside of the radiation portal owing to a lymphocyte-mediated hypersensitivity reaction.[55,56] Chest radiographs may be normal or show heterogeneous peripheral opacities, but CT shows peripheral or peribronchial multifocal GGOs or consolidative opacities, which may be migratory, that have been biopsy-proven to represent BOOP.[56,57]

RILD may heal or, more commonly, progress to fibrosis within 6 to 12 months after RT. In most patients, the radiation fibrosis stabilizes 12 months after RT completion, although in some patients these changes may continue to evolve for up to 2 years before they stabilize.[49,58–62] Radiographically, these findings manifest as traction bronchiectasis, retracting consolidative opacities with volume loss. These changes are within the radiation field, with a clear boundary between the irradiated and the nonirradiated lung. With conventional two-dimensional RT, radiation is delivered in opposed parallel orientation (e.g., anteroposterior and posteroanterior opposed beams). Because of the limited beam orientations, relatively large volumes of surrounding lung are exposed, and RILD in this setting is identified by pulmonary abnormalities with a sharp border that crosses anatomic boundaries, such as the fissure (Fig. 40.9). This pattern of lung injury is unusual for other types of pulmonary injury, such as that resulting from infection or malignancy.

Since the 1990s, newer RT techniques have been employed to ensure that the entire target volume is adequately treated or even treated to higher radiation doses, while minimizing the radiation dose to normal structures. These techniques include three-dimensional conformal RT, intensity-modulated RT, stereotactic body radiotherapy, and heavy particle therapy (e.g., proton therapy).[63–66] Regardless of the radiation technique used, the local damage to the lung is histologically and radiographically the same within the radiation field. However, owing to the complex radiation portals produced by these newer techniques, the shape of RILD may be unusual, centered around the tumor, similar to the radiation portal produced by these more targeted radiation techniques, with an end result of either a scarlike or a masslike opacity that must be recognized by the radiologist to avoid misinterpretation of RILD for recurrence of malignancy or infection.[67]

Early identification of recurrence or persistence of malignancy within the radiation field is difficult and requires knowledge of the CT appearance of RILD in conjunction with the date of the last radiation dose. With the newer radiation techniques, it is essential for the radiologist to have the radiation plan if recurrence is to be identified early. Positron emission tomography (PET)/CT can also be helpful in this assessment. Although there have been no prospective large studies following patients for RILD with PET/CT scans, smaller studies and our experience show, that, while radiation pneumonitis is evolving, increased 2-[18F] fluoro-2-deoxy-D-glucose (FDG) is seen within the radiation field, thereby rendering recurrence difficult to appreciate, because FDG-avid tumor cannot be easily differentiated from inflammatory changes within the radiation treatment field. There is no exact date at which the inflammatory changes become less avid, although 3 to 6 months after radiation the inflammatory changes typically start to subside, and by 12 months they are not typically present.[49] When assessing PET scans for recurrence within the radiation field, one should look not only at the amount of FDG uptake, but also its pattern.[68] Recurrence is typically focal, whereas inflammatory RILD changes are mostly diffuse and conform to the radiation portal. Thus, early signs for recurrence include: (1) alteration in stable contours of radiation fibrosis, (2) failure of contracture of an area of radiation pneumonitis 4 months or more after radiation delivery, (3) filling of radiation-induced ectatic bronchi by soft tissue, and (4) focal FDG activity within the radiation field after the more diffuse activity has subsided.[69,70]

Traditionally, the heart has been viewed as a radiation-resistant organ. However, with improved survival rates of some malignancies, some patients may live to suffer long-term complications, including coronary artery disease, valvular disease, conduction abnormalities, pericardial effusion, and cardiomyopathy years after RT.[71] Long-term survivors of radiation may also suffer from secondary malignancies within the radiation port, including breast cancer, sarcoma, or skin cancers.[72]

Key Points Radiation-Induced Lung Disease

- Radiation-induced lung disease (RILD) can be detected radiographically 6 to 8 weeks after completion of radiation therapy (RT) above 40 Gy.
- RILD in the form of consolidation within the radiation port is most severe at 3 to 4 months after completion of RT.
- RILD progresses to fibrosis within 6 to 12 months after completion of RT and stabilizes within 2 years.
- RILD from newer radiation may mimic tumor or scar, and interpretation is enhanced by viewing the radiation plan.
- On positron emission tomography, recurrence within the radiation field shows focal 2-[^{18}F] fluoro-2-deoxy-D-glucose activity, whereas uptake of RILD is typically more diffuse within the radiation portal.

TREATMENT-ASSOCIATED MALIGNANCY

The incidence of a subsequent malignant neoplasm secondary to therapy of a first malignancy is not common, with an approximately 6% absolute risk at 45 years for all diagnoses, which translates into 1.88 absolute excess risk/1000 patient-years follow-up.[73,74] The greatest risk is in survivors of Hodgkin disease, with a 7.6% cumulative incidence at 20 years and a 5.13 absolute excess risk/1000 patient-years follow-up.[74,75] On multivariate analysis, the relative risk of any second malignancy is 2.3, with soft tissue sarcoma having the greatest relative risk (10.3), followed by breast cancer in female survivors (4.9), and then leukemia (4.0).[74] Approximately 80% of secondary malignancies are solid tumors, and approximately 50% of secondary solid tumors in female survivors are breast cancers.[73] Whereas the risk of secondary leukemia plateaus at 14 years after the primary tumor diagnosis, the risk of solid tumors continues to rise.[73,76]

There are both patient-related and treatment-related risk factors for development of secondary malignancies. Patient-related factors include age at diagnosis, genetic factors, and possibly gender, although this last factor is disputed in the literature.[74,75] The relative risk of second malignancy is inversely related to age at diagnosis, with patients younger than 20 years at first diagnosis having a 10.7 relative risk of developing a second tumor versus a relative risk of 2.4 in patients older than 50 years. The absolute risk of developing any second malignancy (per 10,000 person-years), conversely, is directly related to age at diagnosis, with patients younger than 20 years having an absolute risk of 71 versus 211 for patients older than 50 years.[75] However, both the relative risk and the absolute risk of developing breast cancer as a second malignancy are inversely related to age at diagnosis, with relative risk for survivors of first malignancy diagnosed at younger than 15 years being 112 compared with less than 1 if diagnosed at older than 40 years, and the absolute numbers being 82 versus 18 for the same patient groups.[75]

The most common treatment-related risk factors for development of secondary malignancy are RT and chemotherapy. The data for secondary malignancy from radiation have been extrapolated from survivors of radiation injury (e.g., atomic bomb and Chernobyl) and cohort studies. Most radiation-induced second malignancies occur in or near the radiation field, present after a long latency (from a few years to decades), and affect tissues with increased radiation sensitivity (e.g., breast and thyroid).[73] The median times to development of leukemia, non-Hodgkin lymphoma, and solid tumors are 5.3, 7.1, and 13.8 years, respectively, among patients who developed these second tumors.[75] Data for secondary malignancy from chemotherapy have been extrapolated mainly from cohort studies, comparing patient populations in pre- versus postchemotherapy eras. The type of secondary malignancy has also been found to vary depending upon the class of chemotherapeutic agent used, with alkylating agents among the more common offenders. The incidence of chemotherapy-induced secondary malignancy appears to plateau at approximately 5 years after initial diagnosis.[73]

Because the chest is often irradiated in the treatment of Hodgkin disease or breast cancer, and because subsequent solid malignant neoplasms secondary to therapy of a first malignancy are often incorporated in routine chest CT scans, particular attention should be paid to these organs—the thyroid gland, breast tissue, and chest wall—on the follow-up of patients, so that early detection may hopefully improve outcome.

Key Points Treatment-Associated Malignancy

- Malignancy develops after a latency of several years to decades.
- More common tumors encountered are thyroid cancer, breast cancer, sarcoma, and leukemia.
- Treatment of a first cancer in patients younger than 20 years increases the risk for development of treatment-related subsequent cancer.
- Both radiation therapy and chemotherapy can cause treatment-associated malignancy.

CONCLUSION

With the increased use of CT to follow up oncologic patients, the radiologist is often the first to encounter evidence of iatrogenic lung disease. Although iatrogenic lung disease has no specific radiographic pattern, when tied to the type of patient and the type and timing of a specific therapy the correct diagnosis can and should be made, particularly nowadays, when patient information is computerized and readily available. However, direct communication between clinicians and radiologists remains of utmost importance for improvement of interpretation, patient therapy, and outcome.

REFERENCES

1. Camus P. Rosenow 3rd EC. Iatrogenic lung disease. *Clin Chest Med.* 2004;25:XIII–XIX.
1.a Brahmer JR, Lacchetti C, Schneider BJ, et al. Management of immune-related adverse events in patients treated with immune checkpoint inhibitor therapy: American Society of Clinical Oncology clinical practice guideline. *J Clin Oncol.* 2018;36(17):1714–1768.
2. Philippe Camus. The Drug-Induced Respiratory Disease. version 690, September 5th, 2021, Dijon, France. Website. http://www.pneumotox.com
3. Flieder DB, Travis WD. Pathologic characteristics of drug-induced lung disease. *Clin Chest Med.* 2004;25:37–45.
4. Akira M, Inoue Y, Kitaichi M, et al. Usual interstitial pneumonia and nonspecific interstitial pneumonia with and without concurrent emphysema: thin-section CT findings. *Radiology.* 2009;251:271–279.
5. Silva CI, Muller NL, Hansell DM, et al. Nonspecific interstitial pneumonia and idiopathic pulmonary fibrosis: changes in pattern and distribution of disease over time. *Radiology.* 2008;247:251–259.
6. Lynch DA, Travis WD, Muller NL, et al. Idiopathic interstitial pneumonias: CT features. *Radiology.* 2005;236:10–21.
7. Akira M, Yamamoto S, Sakatani M. Bronchiolitis obliterans organizing pneumonia manifesting as multiple large nodules or masses. *AJR Am J Roentgenol.* 1998;170:291–295.
8. White DA. Drug-induced pulmonary infection. *Clin Chest Med.* 2004;25:179–187.
9. Ramila E, Sureda A, Martino R, et al. Bronchoscopy guided by high-resolution computed tomography for the diagnosis of pulmonary infections in patients with hematologic malignancies and normal plain chest X-ray. *Haematologica.* 2000;85:961–966.
10. Caillot D, Casasnovas O, Bernard A, et al. Improved management of invasive pulmonary aspergillosis in neutropenic patients using early thoracic computed tomographic scan and surgery. *J Clin Oncol.* 1997;15:139–147.
11. Caillot D, Latrabe V, Thiebaut A, et al. Computer tomography in pulmonary invasive aspergillosis in hematological patients with neutropenia: an useful tool for diagnosis and assessment of outcome in clinical trials. *Eur J Radiol.* 2010;74:e172–e175.
12. Murono K, Hirano Y, Koyano S, et al. Molecular comparison of bacterial isolates from blood with strains colonizing pharynx and intestine in immunocompromised patients with sepsis. *J Med Microbiol.* 2003;52:527–530.
13. Rolston KVI, Raad I, Whimbey E, et al. The changing spectrum of bacterial infections in febrile neutropenic patients. In: Klastersky JA, ed. *Febrile Neutropenia.* Berlin: Springer-Verlag; 1997:53–56.
14. Yadegarynia D, Tarrand J, Raad I, et al. Current spectrum of bacterial infections in patients with cancer. *Clin Infect Dis.* 2003;37:1144–1145.
15. Muller LM, Franquet T, Lee KS. *Imaging of Pulmonary Infections.* Philadelphia: Lippincott Williams & Wilkins; 2007.
16. Escuissato DL, Gasparetto EL, Marchiori E, et al. Pulmonary infections after bone marrow transplantation: high-resolution CT findings in 111 patients. *AJR Am J Roentgenol.* 2005;185:608–615.
17. Ljungman P, Griffiths P, Paya C. Definitions of cytomegalovirus infection and disease in transplant recipients. *Clin Infect Dis.* 2002; 34:1094–1097.
18. Franquet T, Rodriguez S, Martino R, et al. Thin-section CT findings in hematopoietic stem cell transplantation recipients with respiratory virus pneumonia. *AJR Am J Roentgenol.* 2006;187:1085–1090.
19. Gasparetto EL, Ono SE, Escuissato D, et al. Cytomegalovirus pneumonia after bone marrow transplantation: high resolution CT findings. *Br J Radiol.* 2004;77:724–727.
20. Kang EY, Patz Jr. EF, Muller NL. Cytomegalovirus pneumonia in transplant patients: CT findings. *J Comput Assist Tomogr.* 1996;20:295–299.
21. Franquet T, Lee KS, Muller NL. Thin-section CT findings in 32 immunocompromised patients with cytomegalovirus pneumonia who do not have AIDS. *AJR Am J Roentgenol.* 2003;181:1059–1063.
22. Horger MS, Pfannenberg C, Einsele H, et al. Cytomegalovirus pneumonia after stem cell transplantation: correlation of CT findings with clinical outcome in 30 patients. *AJR Am J Roentgenol.* 2006;187:W636–W643.
23. Dasbach EJ, Davies GM, Teutsch SM. Burden of aspergillosis-related hospitalizations in the United States. *Clin Infect Dis.* 2000;31:1524–1528.
24. Lionakis MS, Kontoyiannis DP. Fusarium infections in critically ill patients. *Semin Respir Crit Care Med.* 2004;25:159–169.
25. McAdams HP, Rosado de Christenson M, Strollo DC, et al. Pulmonary mucormycosis: radiologic findings in 32 cases. *AJR Am J Roentgenol.* 1997;168:1541–1548.
26. Greene RE, Schlamm HT, Oestmann JW, et al. Imaging findings in acute invasive pulmonary aspergillosis: clinical significance of the halo sign. *Clin Infect Dis.* 2007;44:373–379.
27. Kontoyiannis DP, Lionakis MS, Lewis RE, et al. Zygomycosis in a tertiary-care cancer center in the era of Aspergillus-active antifungal therapy: a case-control observational study of 27 recent cases. *J Infect Dis.* 2005;191:1350–1360.
28. Tarrand JJ, Lichterfeld M, Warraich I, et al. Diagnosis of invasive septate mold infections. A correlation of microbiological culture and histologic or cytologic examination. *Am J Clin Pathol.* 2003;119:854–858.
29. Ascioglu S, Rex JH, de Pauw B, et al. Defining opportunistic invasive fungal infections in immunocompromised patients with cancer and hematopoietic stem cell transplants: an international consensus. *Clin Infect Dis.* 2002;34:7–14.
30. Herbrecht R, Denning DW, Patterson TF, et al. Voriconazole versus amphotericin B for primary therapy of invasive aspergillosis. *N Engl J Med.* 2002;347:408–415.
31. Chamilos G, Marom EM, Lewis RE, et al. Predictors of pulmonary zygomycosis versus invasive pulmonary aspergillosis in patients with cancer. *Clin Infect Dis.* 2005;41:60–66.
32. Wahba H, Truong MT, Lei X, et al. Reversed halo sign in invasive pulmonary fungal infections. *Clin Infect Dis.* 2008;46:1733–1737.
33. Rossi SE, Erasmus JJ, Volpacchio M, et al. "Crazy-paving" pattern at thin-section CT of the lungs: radiologic-pathologic overview. *Radiographics.* 2003;23:1509–1519.
34. Vogel MN, Brodoefel H, Hierl T, et al. Differences and similarities of cytomegalovirus and pneumocystis pneumonia in HIV-negative immunocompromised patients—thin-section CT-morphology in the early phase of the disease. *Br J Radiol.* 2007;80:516–523.
35. Akan H, Arslan O, Akan OA. Tuberculosis in stem cell transplant patients. *J Hosp Infect.* 2006;62:421–426.
36. McAdams HP, Erasmus J, Winter JA. Radiologic manifestations of pulmonary tuberculosis. *Radiol Clin North Am.* 1995;33:655–678.
37. Afessa B, Peters SG. Chronic lung disease after hematopoietic stem cell transplantation. *Clin Chest Med.* 2005;26:571–586. vi.
38. Roychowdhury M, Pambuccian SE, Aslan DL, et al. Pulmonary complications after bone marrow transplantation: an autopsy study from a large transplantation center. *Arch Pathol Lab Med.* 2005; 129:366–371.
39. Sharma S, Nadrous HF, Peters SG, et al. Pulmonary complications in adult blood and marrow transplant recipients: autopsy findings. *Chest.* 2005;128:1385–1392.
40. Armitage JO. Bone marrow transplantation. *N Engl J Med.* 1994; 330:827–838.
41. Wah TM, Moss HA, Robertson RJ, et al. Pulmonary complications following bone marrow transplantation. *Br J Radiol.* 2003; 76:373–379.
42. Worthy SA, Flint JD, Muller NL. Pulmonary complications after bone marrow transplantation: high-resolution CT and pathologic findings. *Radiographics.* 1997;17:1359–1371.
43. Hiemenz JW. Management of infections complicating allogeneic hematopoietic stem cell transplantation. *Semin Hematol.* 2009;46:289–312.

44. Franquet T, Muller NL, Lee KS, et al. High-resolution CT and pathologic findings of noninfectious pulmonary complications after hematopoietic stem cell transplantation. *AJR Am J Roentgenol.* 2005;184:629–637.
45. Capizzi SA, Kumar S, Huneke NE, et al. Peri-engraftment respiratory distress syndrome during autologous hematopoietic stem cell transplantation. *Bone Marrow Transplant.* 2001;27:1299–1303.
46. Afessa B, Peters SG. Noninfectious pneumonitis after blood and marrow transplant. *Curr Opin Oncol.* 2008;20:227–233.
47. Yotsumoto S, Okada F, Yotsumoto S, et al. Bronchiolitis obliterans organizing pneumonia after bone marrow transplantation: association with human leukocyte antigens. *J Comput Assist Tomogr.* 2007;31:132–137.
48. Yousem SA. The histological spectrum of pulmonary graft-versus-host disease in bone marrow transplant recipients. *Hum Pathol.* 1995;26:668–675.
49. Choi YW, Munden RF, Erasmus JJ, et al. Effects of radiation therapy on the lung: radiologic appearances and differential diagnosis. *Radiographics.* 2004;24:985–997. discussion 998.
50. Libshitz HI, Southard ME. Complications of radiation therapy: the thorax. *Semin Roentgenol.* 1974;9:41–49.
51. Movsas B, Raffin TA, Epstein AH, et al. Pulmonary radiation injury. *Chest.* 1997;111:1061–1076.
52. Libshitz HI. Radiation changes in the lung. *Semin Roentgenol.* 1993;28:303–320.
53. Pagani JJ, Libshitz HI. CT manifestations of radiation-induced change in chest tissue. *J Comput Assist Tomogr.* 1982;6:243–248.
54. Libshitz HI, Shuman LS. Radiation-induced pulmonary change: CT findings. *J Comput Assist Tomogr.* 1984;8:15–19.
55. Roberts CM, Foulcher E, Zaunders JJ, et al. Radiation pneumonitis: a possible lymphocyte-mediated hypersensitivity reaction. *Ann Intern Med.* 1993;118:696–700.
56. Arbetter KR, Prakash UB, Tazelaar HD, et al. Radiation-induced pneumonitis in the "nonirradiated" lung. *Mayo Clin Proc.* 1999;74:27–36.
57. Crestani B, Kambouchner M, Soler P, et al. Migratory bronchiolitis obliterans organizing pneumonia after unilateral radiation therapy for breast carcinoma. *Eur Respir J.* 1995;8:318–321.
58. Chu FC, Phillips R, Nickson JJ, et al. Pneumonitis following radiation therapy of cancer of the breast by tangenital technic. *Radiology.* 1955;64:642–654.
59. Gross NJ. Pulmonary effects of radiation therapy. *Ann Intern Med.* 1977;86:81–92.
60. Roswit B, White DC. Severe radiation injuries of the lung. *AJR Am J Roentgenol.* 1977;129:127–136.
61. Rubin P, Casarett GW. Clinical radiation pathology as applied to curative radiotherapy. *Cancer.* 1968;22:767–778.
62. Smith JC. Radiation pneumonitis. *Am Rev Respir Dis.* 1963; 87:647–655.
63. Fraass BA, Kessler ML, McShan DL, et al. Optimization and clinical use of multisegment intensity-modulated radiation therapy for high-dose conformal therapy. *Semin Radiat Oncol.* 1999;9:60–77.
64. Galvin JM, De Neve W. Intensity modulating and other radiation therapy devices for dose painting. *J Clin Oncol.* 2007;25:924–930.
65. Timmerman RD, Forster KM, Chinsoo Cho L. Extracranial stereotactic radiation delivery. *Semin Radiat Oncol.* 2005;15:202–207.
66. Welsh JS. Basics of particle therapy: introduction to hadrons. *Am J Clin Oncol.* 2008;31:493–495.
67. Koenig TR, Munden RF, Erasmus JJ, et al. Radiation injury of the lung after three-dimensional conformal radiation therapy. *AJR Am J Roentgenol.* 2002;178:1383–1388.
68. Inoue T, Kim EE, Komaki R, et al. Detecting recurrent or residual lung cancer with FDG-PET. *J Nucl Med.* 1995;36:788–793.
69. Bourgouin P, Cousineau G, Lemire P, et al. Differentiation of radiation-induced fibrosis from recurrent pulmonary neoplasm by CT. *Can Assoc Radiol J.* 1987;38:23–26.
70. Libshitz HI, Sheppard DG. Filling in of radiation therapy-induced bronchiectatic change: a reliable sign of locally recurrent lung cancer. *Radiology.* 1999;210:25–27.
71. Stewart JR, Fajardo LF, Gillette SM, et al. Radiation injury to the heart. *Int J Radiat Oncol Biol Phys.* 1995;31:1205–1211.
72. Doi K, Mieno MN, Shimada Y, et al. Risk of second malignant neoplasms among childhood cancer survivors treated with radiotherapy: meta-analysis of nine epidemiological studies. *Paediatr Perinat Epidemiol.* 2009;23:370–379.
73. Moppett J, Oakhill A, Duncan AW. Second malignancies in children: the usual suspects? *Eur J Radiol.* 2001;38:235–248.
74. Neglia JP, Friedman DL, Yasui Y, et al. Second malignant neoplasms in five-year survivors of childhood cancer: childhood cancer survivor study. *J Natl Cancer Inst.* 2001;93:618–629.
75. Ng AK, Bernardo MV, Weller E, et al. Second malignancy after Hodgkin disease treated with radiation therapy with or without chemotherapy: long-term risks and risk factors. *Blood.* 2002; 100:1989–1996.
76. Bhatia S, Yasui Y, Robison LL, et al. High risk of subsequent neoplasms continues with extended follow-up of childhood Hodgkin's disease: report from the Late Effects Study Group. *J Clin Oncol.* 2003;21:4386–4394.

CHAPTER

41 Complications in the Oncologic Patient: Abdomen and Pelvis

Chitra Viswanathan, M.D.; Dhakshinamoorthy Ganeshan, M.D.; and Revathy B. Iyer, M.D.

INTRODUCTION

Treatment of cancer requires a multimodality approach, with most patients receiving chemotherapy, radiation, surgery, or a combination. It is important to understand the sequelae, complications, and imaging findings of each of the therapies to guide management of the oncologic patient. Preexisting conditions can also predispose a patient to such complications.

The efficacy of chemotherapy has allowed many patients with previously unresectable disease to proceed to surgical resection. However, chemotherapeutic agents used in treatment do have adverse effects. Chemotherapeutic side effects can occur at any time during the course of therapy. Late effects are increasingly being recognized. The field of immunotherapy has advanced cancer care. Along with the increasing use of immune-related agents, there is also increasing knowledge of immunotherapy-related adverse events (irAEs).

Radiation complications occur in an acute (<30 days) or chronic (>90 days) timeframe.[1] The effects of radiation depend on the duration and dose of radiation therapy. Each organ has a specific dose tolerance that, when exceeded, can lead to injury. The combination of radiation and chemotherapy may also increase the extent of injury.

Surgical changes lead to possible infection and inflammation, and eventually, fibrosis. Knowing the normal postoperative appearance can be helpful in excluding recurrent disease.

Cross-sectional imaging (computed tomography [CT], magnetic resonance imaging [MRI]) and now positron emission tomography (PET)/CT are valuable tools in the management of the oncologic patient.

HEPATOBILIARY, SPLEEN, AND PANCREAS

Liver

Chemotherapy Change

Hepatic steatosis is seen with administration of all chemotherapy agents, especially irinotecan and oxaliplatin.[2] It can be focal or diffuse; when diffuse, it is called chemotherapy-associated steatohepatitis. Knowing the different imaging appearances and characteristic sites can aid in differentiating between liver metastases and fatty infiltration. Clues that a focal lesion may represent fatty infiltration are localization to the falciform ligament, porta hepatis, or gallbladder fossa and a geometric, well-defined shape. Ultrasound findings include increase in echogenicity. On CT, there is decreased attenuation of the liver (Fig. 41.1). MRI with in- and out-of-phase imaging is very useful in confirming the diagnosis.[2]

Hepatitis is associated with immune checkpoint inhibitors, such as with anti–cytotoxic T-lymphocyte–associated protein-4 (CTLA-4) agents such as ipilimumab and the tyrosine kinase inhibitors.[3,4] Imaging findings include hypoattenuating lesions, periportal edema, and enhancing parenchyma on CT and 2-[^{18}F] fluoro-2-deoxy-D-glucose (FDG) uptake on PET/CT. The timing of the onset of hepatitis tends to differ depending on the agent used. Treatment includes steroids.[5]

Portal vein thrombosis has also been seen with patients undergoing preoperative chemotherapy.[6] Portal vein thrombosis is seen on CT as a filling defect within the portal vein. On ultrasound, there is echogenic thrombus within the portal vein. Branch portal vein thromboses can cause wedge-shaped areas of perfusion change, which need to be distinguished from development of metastatic disease (Fig. 41.2). Treatment is conservative and consists of anticoagulation.

The effect of chemotherapy on small vessels can lead to peliosis, sclerosing cholangitis, and sinusoidal obstruction syndrome. Sinusoidal obstruction syndrome has been described after stem cell transplantation and also after treatment for colorectal liver metastatic disease with oxaliplatin.[7] Clinically, the patients have hepatic failure and jaundice. CT findings include heterogeneous appearance of liver with narrowing of the right hepatic vein, periportal edema, and ascites (Fig. 41.3).[5] Ultrasound examination shows ascites; reversal of hepatic venous flow is a late sign.[8] This can be distinguished from hepatic graft-versus-host disease (GVHD) by its early presentation in the first 20 days after stem cell transplant.[7]

Pseudocirrhosis, or regenerative nodular hyperplasia, can occur after treatment with chemotherapy and is associated with drugs such as oxaliplatin, trastuzumab, paclitaxel, doxorubicin, and capecitabine. There is regenerating liver parenchyma without bridging fibrosis. This is in contrast to the form of pseudocirrhosis induced by an infiltrating tumor that causes fibrosis and occurs before the administration of chemotherapy. On CT, there is nodularity of the liver contour, caudate lobe enlargement, and a decrease in liver volume. Portal hypertension may occur.[9]

Changes that have been observed after intraarterial chemotherapy infusion are chemical hepatitis, gastrointestinal ulceration, sclerosing cholangitis, and biliary cirrhosis.[10]

Radiation Change

Radiation-induced liver disease occurs in approximately 5% to 10% of people who received whole-liver irradiation in doses exceeding 30 to 35 Gy.[11] Patients usually present 2 to 8 weeks (up to 4 months) after radiation exposure with hepatomegaly, ascites, and elevated liver enzymes.[12] Pathologically, there is venoocclusive disease with congestion of the central portion of the lobule, with sparing of the larger veins. The radiologic picture is a clear demarcation—also known as the straight border sign—between the area that has received radiation and that which has not been irradiated.[13] This can be differentiated from vascular changes, focal fat infiltration, and fibrosis by its nonanatomic distribution.[14] In the acute and subacute phases, the area that has been irradiated is seen on CT to be lower in attenuation than the adjacent liver, likely because of edema (Fig. 41.4). On MRI, the irradiated area has low signal intensity on T1 weighted imaging and high signal intensity on T2 weighted imaging because of edema. Chronic changes can occur, with fibrosis and volume loss. Usually, patients have resolution of findings in 3 to 5 months, but a small portion progress to liver failure.

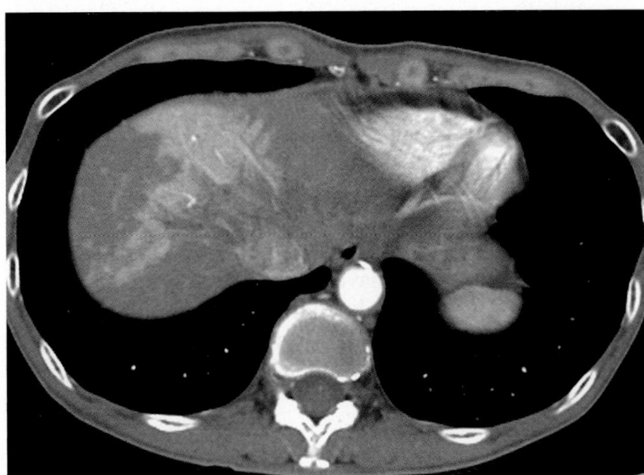

FIGURE 41.1. Axial contrast-enhanced computed tomography scan of the liver from a patient with lung cancer receiving chemotherapy with erlotinib shows perfusion abnormality and fatty infiltration. Changes were not seen before chemotherapy.

Surgical Change

Postoperative fluid collections after hepatic resection are abscess, postoperative seromas, and bile duct leak. At our institution, these are usually drained percutaneously. Over time, these collections and the perfusion change along the hepatic surgical margin will resolve. It is important to distinguish between postsurgical change and recurrence of tumor by reviewing the initial imaging study in the postoperative period. Over time, the remaining liver may regenerate.

Image-guided thermal radiofrequency or microwave ablation is used in the treatment of metastatic disease to

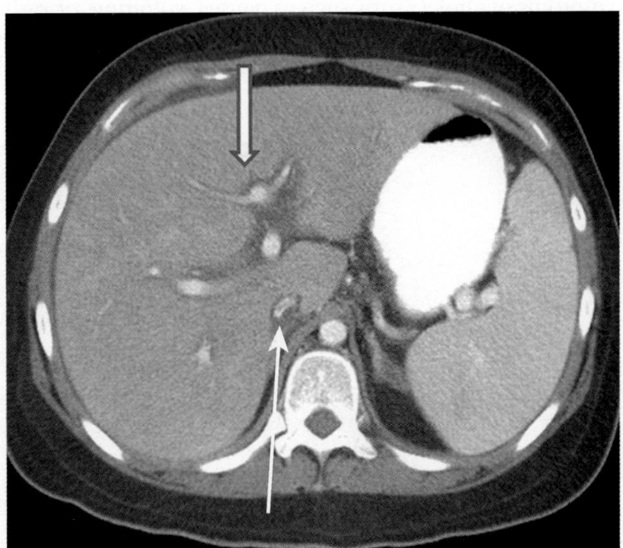

FIGURE 41.3. Axial contrast-enhanced computed tomography scan of the liver from a patient with colorectal carcinoma. There is periportal edema (thick arrow) and narrowing of the right hepatic vein (thin arrow).

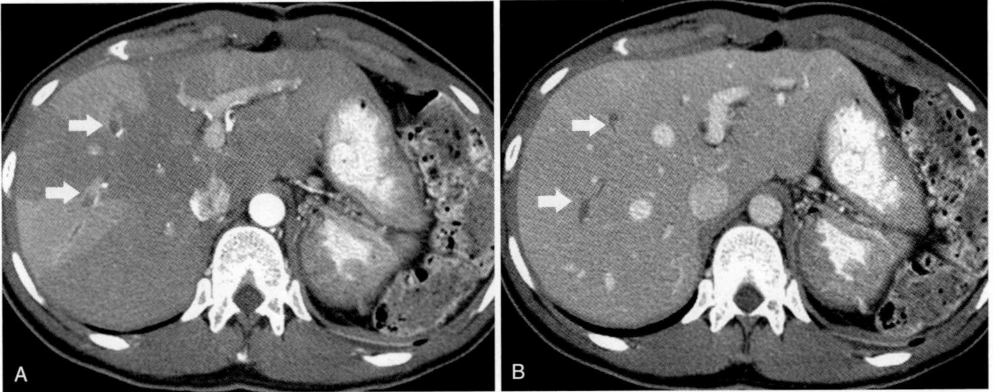

FIGURE 41.2. Axial contrast-enhanced computed tomography scans of the liver from a patient with colorectal carcinoma. **A,** Arterial phase scan shows wedge-shaped perfusion abnormalities and filling defects within the portal veins (arrows). **B,** In the portal venous phase the perfusion abnormalities are no longer visualized, but the portal vein filling defects are still seen (arrows).

the liver.[15] On CT and MRI, the ablation defect site is a low-density area in the place of the treated metastasis. There may be hypervascularity surrounding the surgical site initially, which usually resolves within 3 months. Both intrahepatic and extrahepatic complications can occur, depending on the location of the tumor intervention. Examples of complications include hemorrhage, vascular injury, biliary injury including bile leakage or biloma, gastrointestinal injury, cholecystitis, and, rarely, tumor seeding. It is important to distinguish these changes from recurrence, which is any change in the size of the cavity, mass effect, nodularity, and enhancement (Fig. 41.5).

Gallbladder

Chemotherapy Change

Cholecystitis is a complication of therapy resulting from the immunosuppression caused by conventional chemotherapy, immunotherapy, hepatic arterial infusion of chemotherapy, and hepatic arterial embolization. Patients may have classical symptoms of cholecystitis such as nausea, vomiting, or right upper quadrant pain. On imaging, the findings are much like the other causes of cholecystitis: pericholecystic fluid and thickening, gallbladder enlargement, and sonographic Murphy's sign.[16] One potential pitfall that may occur is pericholecystic fluid and thickening caused by therapy.

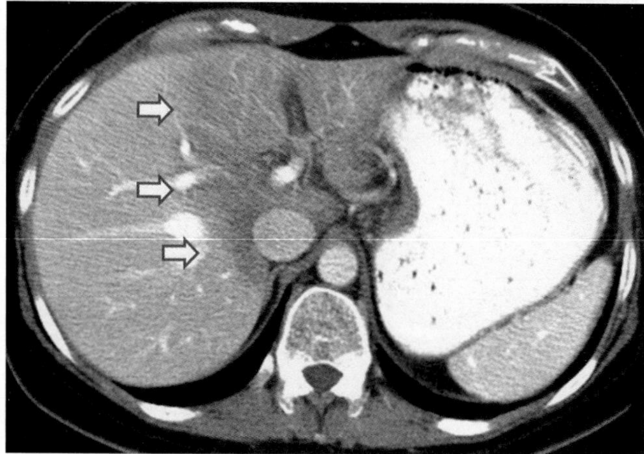

FIGURE 41.4. Axial contrast-enhanced computed tomography scan of the liver from a patient with gastric carcinoma. There is a well-demarcated line (*arrows*) between the liver in the radiation field and the liver outside of the radiation field. This line is indicative of radiotherapy.

Spleen

Chemotherapy Change

Certain chemotherapeutic agents, particularly oxaliplatin, can cause hepatic injury and portal hypertension, with resultant enlargement of the spleen and any adjacent splenules. This can be observed on routine screening CT with progressive enlargement of the spleen over the course of therapy. This finding has been seen to resolve within 2 years of cessation of therapy, which is suggestive of reversibility.[17]

Splenic rupture is a rare complication of stem cell transplant or treatment with granulocyte–colony stimulating factor (G-CSF), which is administered for therapy-induced neutropenia.[18] In splenic rupture, patients usually present with abdominal pain and left shoulder pain. On CT, there is irregularity of the spleen, splenomegaly, and high-density fluid surrounding the spleen and in the abdomen, consistent with hemoperitoneum. Treatment usually consists of intravenous hydration and resection of the spleen.[19]

Radiation Change

Radiation to the spleen is used for diseases such as lymphoma, hypersplenism, or splenomegaly. Radiation to adjacent organs can also impact the spleen. The spleen is very radiosensitive, and atrophy can result at small doses of approximately 4 to 8 Gy. Higher doses can result in fibrosis. Long-term effects that have been reported are functional asplenia and sepsis. Embolization of the spleen is now used more commonly. CT examination shows low-density areas with the spleen consistent with infarct. Eventually, the spleen will decrease in size.

Surgical Change

Splenectomy is performed for lymphoma, myelodysplastic disease, or other hematologic malignancy to obtain total local control. If the spleen is also adjacent to tumors of the pancreas, retroperitoneum, peritoneum, or kidney, it may be removed as well. Occasionally, in the postsurgical bed, small splenules will develop or remain behind.

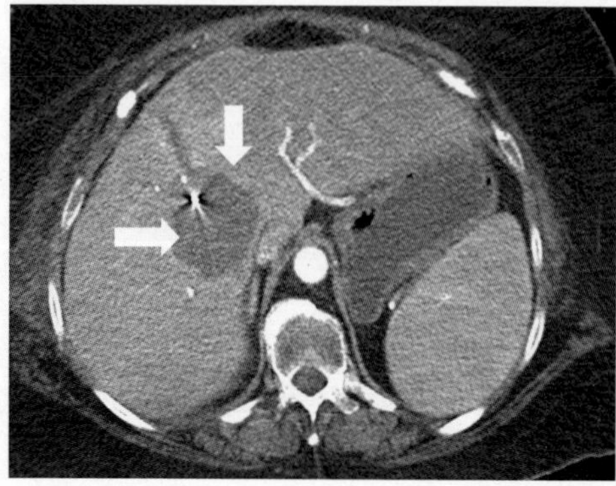

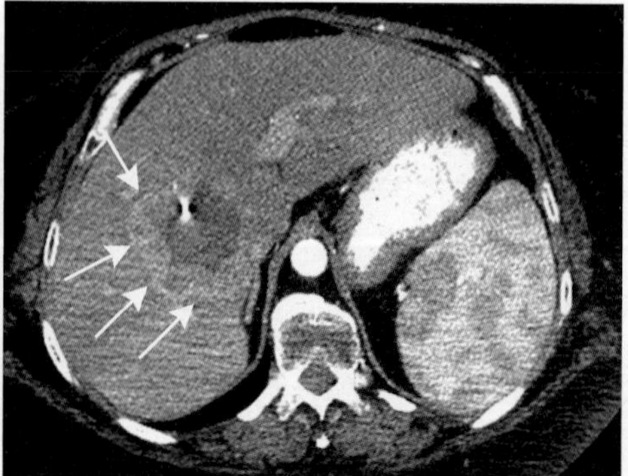

FIGURE 41.5. Axial contrast-enhanced computed tomography scans of the liver from a patient with colon carcinoma. **A,** A well-demarcated low-density region (*arrows*) indicates the site of radiofrequency ablation (RFA). **B,** Within 1 month, there is now nodularity and enhancement of the periphery of the cavity, consistent with recurrent tumor (*arrows*). Note the new scalloped shape of the RFA cavity, indicative of tumor involvement.

Pancreas

Chemotherapy Change

Chemotherapy-induced pancreatitis can occur during treatment. Many drugs can cause pancreatitis. Drug use history and timing of symptoms are critical in these patients. Pancreatitis can also occur as a complication in 2% to 7% of patients treated with hyperthermic intraperitoneal chemotherapy.[13] Pancreatitis and elevated amylase can occur after transarterial chemoembolization or yttrium-90 therapy.[20] Clinically, the patients present with abdominal pain and elevated amylase and lipase. The imaging appearance on CT, MRI, and ultrasound is similar to that of acute pancreatitis from other etiologies. Pancreatitis can be focal or diffuse. Both interstitial and necrotizing pancreatitis subtypes are seen on imaging.[21]

Pancreatic atrophy has been seen in patients receiving sunitinib, and is associated with a poor prognosis.

Radiation Change

Radiation injury to the pancreas can occur as a result of therapy directly or owing to irradiation for lymphoma or tumors of adjacent organs. Radiation treatment can also induce pancreatitis owing to damage of acinar cells. At the late stages, there may be fibrosis. Pancreatic atrophy as result of radiation may lead to endocrine insufficiency and diabetes.[22]

Surgical Change

Postoperative changes that are commonly seen at CT after pancreaticoduodenectomy are pneumobilia (particularly in the left lobe), normal jejunal loop, and postoperative fluid collections. CT is especially useful for the diagnosis of postoperative abscess, leaks, biloma, biliary obstruction, pancreatitis, and bowel obstruction.[23]

Key Points Liver, Spleen, and Pancreas

- Hepatic steatosis because of chemotherapy can be diffuse or focal. Knowledge of the typical location of fatty infiltration and magnetic resonance imaging or ultrasound can be helpful in confirming this diagnosis.
- Radiation change of the liver has a characteristic appearance and should not be mistaken for recurrent tumor.
- Enlargement of the spleen can be a result of chemotherapy-related sinusoidal obstruction syndrome, and patients who are receiving these agents should have follow-up of spleen size.
- Recurrent pancreatic tumor can be distinguished from radiation change with biopsy.

DIGESTIVE SYSTEM

Chemotherapy Change

Chemotherapeutic agents cause immunosuppression, which can lead to the bowel complications of *Clostridium difficile* infection, enterocolitis, and typhlitis. *C. difficile* infection and colitis can present with a spectrum of findings ranging from diarrhea to pseudomembranous colitis to fulminant colitis. Stool culture or endoscopy is used for diagnosis. CT scan findings include diffuse thickening of the bowel and mesenteric stranding. Treatment is antibiotic therapy.[24]

Typhlitis or neutropenic colitis can be seen in children and adults being treated for hematologic malignancies or undergoing immunosuppressive therapies. On CT, typhlitis is seen most commonly as bowel wall thickening greater than 3 mm and inflammation of the terminal ileum and cecum, but can sometimes be seen in the entire bowel. Pneumatosis and fluid/abscess can also be seen. Ultrasound may be a useful imaging tool. Imaging is also helpful in determining extent and excluding other etiologies of pain.[25] Treatment is supportive and consists of intravenous fluids, antibiotics, and, if necessary, G-CSF or surgery for bleeding.

Acute GVHD occurs within the first 100 days after transplant, and chronic GVHD occurs within 100 days after transplant. Acute GVHD clinically presents with cramping and diarrhea, which can be bloody. The diagnosis is usually made by endoscopy, but it can be seen on CT as bowel wall thickening (Fig. 41.6). Chronic GVHD affects the small bowel and colon less commonly than acute GVHD. Patients can have malabsorption, sclerosis of the intestine, and fibrosis.[24]

Immune checkpoint inhibitors are now more integrated into cancer care, such as bevacizumab for colorectal and ovarian cancers, ipilimumab for melanoma, and nivolumab for refractory lung and renal cell tumors. They affect the blood supply adjacent to the tumor and may have a system-wide thrombogenic effect. Perforation and fistulas, pneumatosis intestinalis, and enterocolitis are complications of

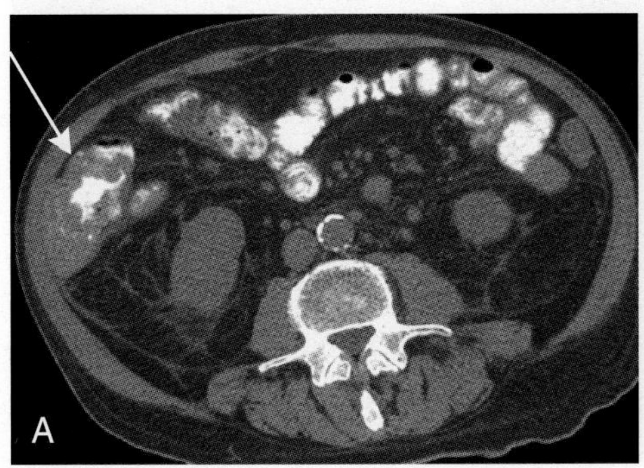

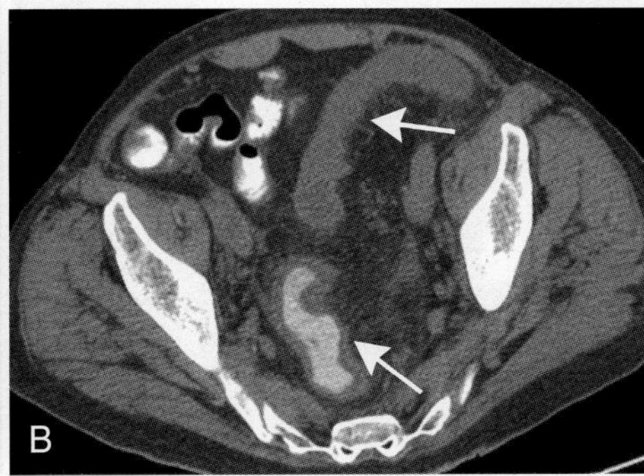

Figure 41.6. Axial contrast-enhanced computed tomography scans from a patient with leukemia 150 days after allogenic stem cell transplant. There is diffuse thickening of the cecum (*arrow*) and transverse colon **(A)** and rectosigmoid (*arrows* in **B**), which was biopsy-proven graft-versus-host disease.

treatment with the antivascular epithelial growth factor (VEGF) agent bevacizumab, anti–epidermal growth factor receptor agents, and the anti–CTLA-4 agent ipilimumab (Fig. 41.7).[16] The colitis seen with immunotherapy is associated with two patterns, with 75% of cases having a diffuse colitis pattern and approximately 25% of cases having a segmental colitis with diverticulosis pattern.[26] Imaging features include mesenteric vessel engorgement, colonic wall thickening, and mucosal hyperenhancement.[27]

Radiation Change

Esophagus

Radiation effects on the esophagus occur at doses greater than 45 Gy and can last weeks to months. The earliest sign is abnormal motility, which can be observed at barium examination. Mucosal edema and fistula may occur within the first month after therapy. Strictures can also be seen as smooth narrowing with tapered margins.[28] At CT, inflammatory change is seen as enhancement in a central ring or diffuse esophageal thickening. On PET/CT, esophageal radiation change can be FDG-avid and can sometimes be difficult to distinguish from residual tumor; endoscopy may be performed for diagnosis.[29]

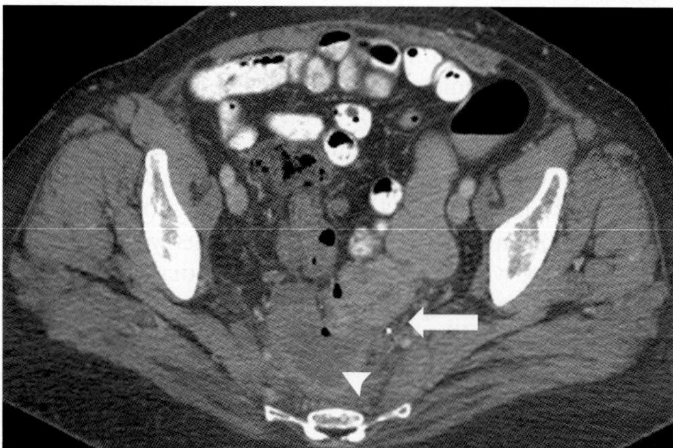

FIGURE 41.7. Axial contrast-enhanced computed tomography scan from a patient with ovarian cancer treated with a vascular endothelial growth factor–tartrate-resistant acid phosphatase agent shows a fistula between the rectum (*arrow*) and abscess cavity (*oval*).

Stomach and Duodenum

Radiation injury to the stomach and duodenum can occur as a result of therapy directly to these organs or owing to irradiation for tumors of the pancreas. Effects can happen after radiation of 50 Gy, and the fixed position of the duodenum and stomach contributes to the susceptibility to injury.[30] Diffuse inflammatory change, ulcers that do not heal, fixed narrowing, and deformity are all seen with radiation injury. CT may show wall thickening and perigastric or periduodenal fluid.

Small and Large Bowel

The small and large bowel receive radiation doses in cancer therapies for the retroperitoneum, abdomen, and pelvis. Administration of chemotherapy can increase the incidence of injury and the risk of severe complications. The most common sites of injury are the cecum, terminal ileum, rectum, and sigmoid colon.

The small bowel is the most radiosensitive, with minimal and maximal tolerance doses 45 and 65 Gy, respectively. In the treatment of gynecologic and urologic malignancies, the sigmoid and rectum can receive close to the entire dose of radiation, and rectal injuries are therefore more common than injury to small bowel.[31] Because radiation injury is a vascular insult, progressive ischemia can occur in the wall. There are acute and chronic entities to radiation-induced enteropathy. Acute changes occur in the short term after radiation exposure, with CT findings of enhancement and thickening of the bowel wall.[32] Chronic radiation injury may occur months to years after the exposure and can result in submucosal edema, ulceration, fibrosis, adhesions, and fistula formation. Small bowel studies can show diffuse thickening and straightening of the small bowel folds and separation of bowel loops in the acute setting, and tethering of bowel loops at the later stages.[33] On barium study, strictures, ulcerations, protrusions, and circumferential narrowing can be seen with radiation injury to the rectum (Fig. 41.8). There may be widening of the presacral space. CT is helpful in excluding recurrent disease, identifying fistulas, and evaluating for obstruction. CT findings in radiation injury are similar to those seen on fluoroscopy, with bowel wall thickening, fixation, and increased mesenteric density consistent with fibrosis or edema. Bowel perforation may occur but is rare.[32]

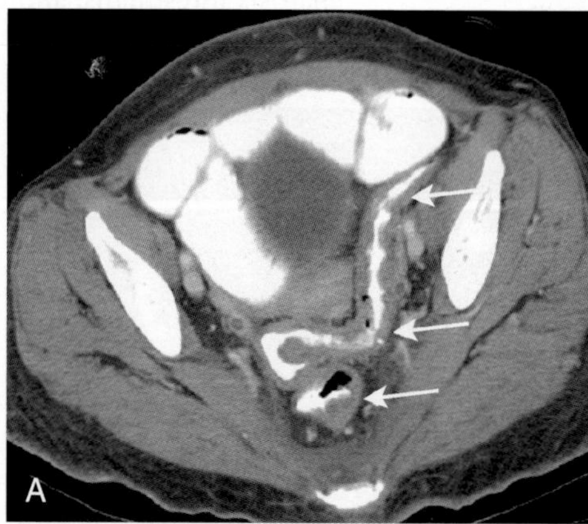

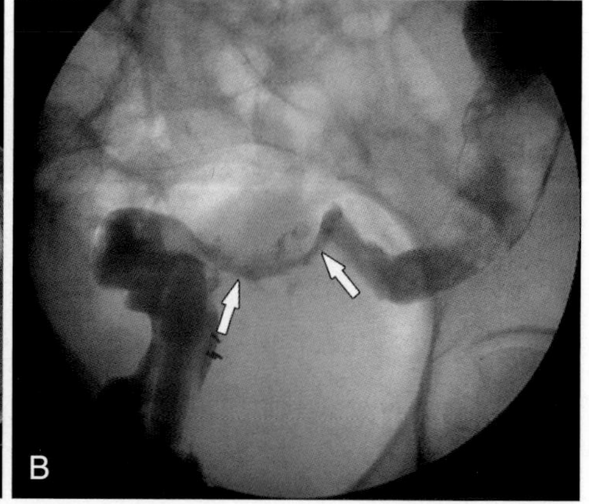

FIGURE 41.8. A, Axial contrast computed tomography scan from a patient with cervical cancer who has received radiotherapy shows diffuse thickening of the rectum and sigmoid (arrows) because of radiation enteritis. There is also presacral soft tissue thickening and dilatation of the small bowel. **B,** Image from barium enema in the same patient shows narrowing and stricture of the sigmoid and rectum (arrows) because of radiation enteritis.

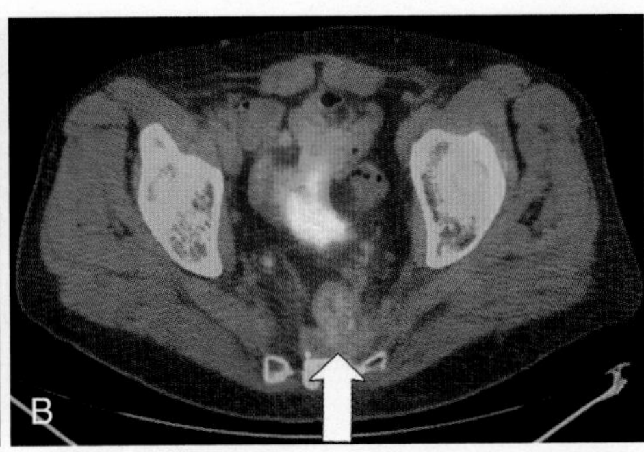

Figure 41.9. Axial contrast-enhanced computed tomography and fused positron emission tomography (PET)/ computed tomography (CT) scans from a patient with rectal cancer. **A,** Soft tissue thickening (*arrow*) adjacent to the surgical site had increased over time. **B,** There is no evidence of 2-[^{18}F] fluoro-2-deoxy-D-glucose avidity to this region on PET/CT (*arrow*), indicating posttreatment fibrosis.

Surgical Change

CT scan of the abdomen and pelvis is the optimal postoperative tool to evaluate for pneumoperitoneum, obstruction, abscess, or leak. Water-soluble contrast is used in cases of possible leak or obstruction. Postsurgical changes can sometimes cause bowel wall thickening and peritoneal stranding, which can confound the picture when searching for recurrent tumor. Alterations in anatomy as a result of surgery may lead to obstruction of bowel loops that are adjacent to recurrent tumor or adjacent to lymph nodes.

One problematic region is the pelvis after radiation and abdominal pelvic resection. MRI can be used to aid in diagnosis. In recent times, PET/CT has shown high specificity in evaluating for recurrent tumor (Fig. 41.9). However, it should not be performed within 4 months of radiotherapy or surgery.

Key Points Bowel

- Bowel wall perforation, colitis, fistulae, and pneumatosis can occur with specific chemotherapeutic agents. Knowledge of therapy can lead to accurate diagnosis and cessation of therapy.
- Radiosensitive bowel areas are most commonly the terminal ileum, cecum, rectum, and sigmoid colon.
- Radiation can cause increased soft tissue and spiculation of the bowel folds, widening the presacral space. This can be distinguished from tumor or abscess by computed tomography or positron emission tomography/computed tomography.

GENITOURINARY SYSTEM

Chemotherapy Change

Kidney

Renal injury can result from administration of chemotherapy and immunotherapy. The mechanism of injury is intrarenal or systemic microvascular thrombi, resulting in endothelial swelling and microvascular obstruction. Some drugs can cause renal tubular injury that leads to renal failure.[34] Acute interstitial nephritis, podocytopathy, and hyponatremia are side effects noted with the immune checkpoint inhibitors.[35]

Treatment for hypercalcemia as a result of cancer can also cause acute renal failure that can progress to end-stage renal disease.

Stem cell transplant is a confirmed cause of renal injury, occurring most frequently in patients who have received myelosuppressive agents for allogenic transplants. The incidence of acute renal failure requiring dialysis in this population ranges from 36% to 70%. Chronic renal disease as a result of stem cell transplant can occur in 15% to 20% of patients.[36]

Renal ultrasound is helpful in excluding other causes of obstruction or disease. In acute renal disease, increased echogenicity, loss of differentiation of the corticomedullary junction, or enlargement of the kidneys can be seen at ultrasound. In the chronic stages, renal atrophy may be present.

Bladder

Bladder function may be affected by chemotherapy owing to excretion of active metabolites in the bladder potentiating the effects of radiation. Cyclophosphamide is a major cause of toxicity, inducing leukocyte infiltration and submucosal hemorrhage. Irritation on voiding, bladder contracture, and hemorrhagic cystitis (HC) can occur. HC can be transient or persistent, minor or major. On imaging, there may be bladder wall thickening or echogenic material representing hematoma or clot. Treatment is supportive. Bladder fibrosis and contracture has also been reported after HC. Neurogenic bladder may occur.[37] Secondary malignancies of the bladder have been reported after cyclophosphamide administration.[38]

Reproductive System

Chemotherapy is associated with impairment of infertility.[39] The testicle is very sensitive to cytotoxic therapies. In women, amenorrhea and early menopause can occur. The ovaries may decrease in size owing to chemotherapy. There is also an increased risk of infections to the genitourinary system as a result of neutropenia and thrombocytopenia.

Immunotherapy agents also have side effects, and more effects are becoming known. Of the immunotherapy agents, ipilimumab has a known fertility risk. A rare but severe complication reported with the use of the anti–programmed cell death protein-1 agent pembrolizumab is epididymoorchitis.[40]

Radiation Change

Kidney

The kidneys are radiosensitive, and bilateral doses of 28 Gy have been shown to cause complications of renal failure.

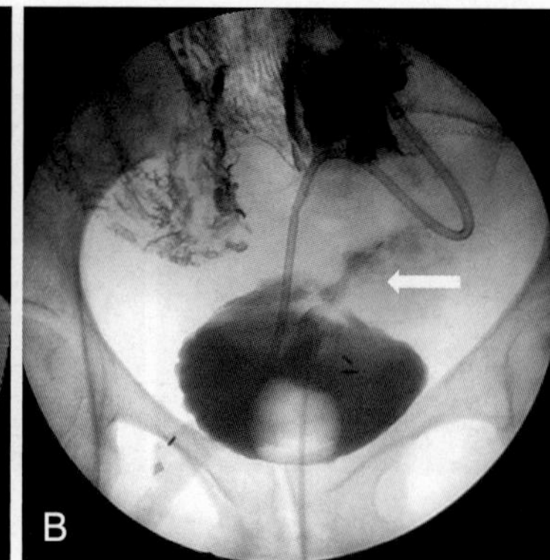

FIGURE 41.10. Axial contrast-enhanced computed tomography (CT) and cystography scans from a patient with cervical cancer who has received radiotherapy. **A,** CT scan shows diffuse thickening and irregularity of the bladder, with a lamellated appearance (*arrow*). Cervical radiation seed, radiation proctitis, and presacral soft tissue thickening are also present. **B,** Cystography scan shows that, on filling of the bladder with contrast, there is irregularity of the bladder wall along with extraluminal contrast, indicating a leak (*arrow*). This was caused by perforation of the bladder from radiotherapy.

Acute renal failure was seen at 6 to 12 months, and chronic disease presented at greater than 18 months. On intravenous pyelograms and CT, there are signs of diminished or absent renal function with delayed nephrograms.[41] In chronic disease, the kidney will be small and contracted, with a smooth border.

Bladder

Radiation effects on the bladder occur in an acute fashion in the first 3 to 6 months after therapy, and late reactions occur after 3 to 6 months when therapy is completed. Hypofractionated and accelerated techniques and doses higher than 70 Gy increase the risk of radiation injury. The risk of injury is also increased by concomitant administration of chemotherapy and other drugs.

The reported incidence of acute radiation change varies from 23% to 80%. Late effects are much more severe, and are seen in patients receiving radiation therapy for cervix and prostate cancer. Approximately 20% of patients suffer from late effects, with 10% developing the long-term effect of a small and contracted bladder. A small portion of patients require cystectomy. On CT and MRI, a small contracted bladder with wall thickening will be seen (Fig. 41.10). Cystogram may show a trabeculated bladder, and perforation may occur owing to friability of the bladder soft tissue. Radiation changes can be distinguished from recurrent tumor by using imaging, of which MRI is the superior modality. There may be high signal intensity in the bladder wall on T2-weighted imaging in patients with mild injury. Increased bladder wall thickening with a low-signal inner layer and a higher-signal peripheral layer (a lamellated appearance) may indicate more severe injury. Fistulas and sinus tracts may develop. The bladder wall can enhance with contrast for up to 2 years after irradiation.[42]

Ureter/Urethra

Strictures and fibrosis of the ureter are uncommon complications of radiation, and the incidence is low in external beam radiation. It does occur in 1% to 3% of patients who receive brachytherapy for gynecologic malignancies. Continued surveillance of renal function is advised, because the risk of ureteral narrowing increases from 1% at 5 years to 2.5% at 20 years after therapy. The typical site of strictures is at the ureterovesicular junction, but higher strictures can occur where the ureters cross the iliac vessels. The appearance on imaging is a smooth, long tapering of the ureter that may exceed 5 cm, but this cannot be distinguished from recurrence on imaging alone. Reflux may also occur as a result of bladder wall fibrosis.

Urethral strictures are also rare and occur in doses greater than 60 to 70 Gy. The risk of radiation injury in patients who have had transurethral resection of the prostate (TURP) is higher, 5% to 15% versus up to 5% in patients who have not had TURP. Urethral strictures are demonstrated on retrograde urethrograms. Some patients may require surgery for complex or recurrent strictures.[42]

Prostate and Seminal Vesicles

Posttherapeutic effects that can be seen in the prostate at imaging are decreased T2 signal intensity, shrinkage of the prostate, and normal zonal anatomy indistinctness. The seminal vesicles may also decrease in size, and also have decreased T2 signal intensity on imaging.

Testes

The testicles are extremely sensitive to radiation, and a limited dose should be used whenever possible. Doses as low as 2 to 3 Gy can result in azoospermia. Late recovery can sometimes occur. Sperm banking is encouraged for these patients. On imaging, there may be testicular atrophy.[41]

Uterus, Cervix, Vagina, and Vulva

The uterus and cervix may receive up to 200 Gy in therapy for gynecologic malignancy. The uterus can decrease in size. Ulceration of the endometrial cavity may result in an indistinct appearance and low signal intensity on T2 weighted imaging. Distention of the endometrial cavity can persist long after radiation has been completed.[43] Uterine necrosis is a rare complication.[44] Development of a high-grade endometrial cancer or sarcoma may occur many years after therapy.[32]

After radiotherapy, the cervix may atrophy and completely disappear with higher doses. Cervical os stenosis is a complication that may occur 3 to 6 months after therapy. Residual tumor may decrease in size and develop calcification. This needs to be distinguished from recurrence (Fig. 41.11).

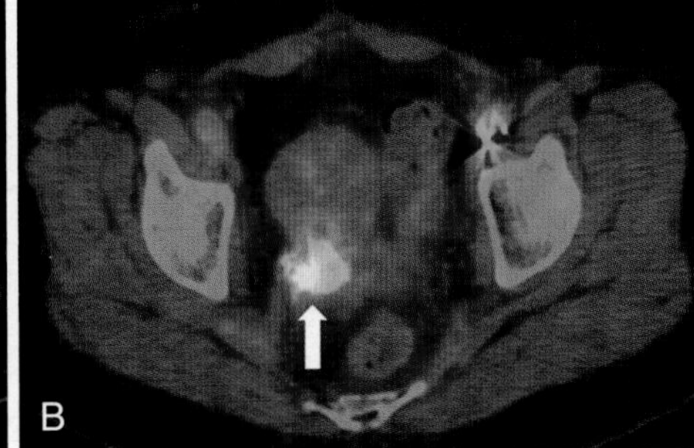

FIGURE 41.11. Axial computed tomography (CT) and fused positron emission tomography (PET)/CT scans from a patient with cervical cancer treated with radiation therapy. **A,** Axial CT noncontrast scan shows a nodular calcified mass in the right parametrium (*arrow*) after treatment. **B,** Fused PET/CT scan shows 2-[^{18}F] fluoro-2-deoxy-D-glucose uptake in this mass (*arrow*). Biopsy showed fibrosis consistent with treatment effect.

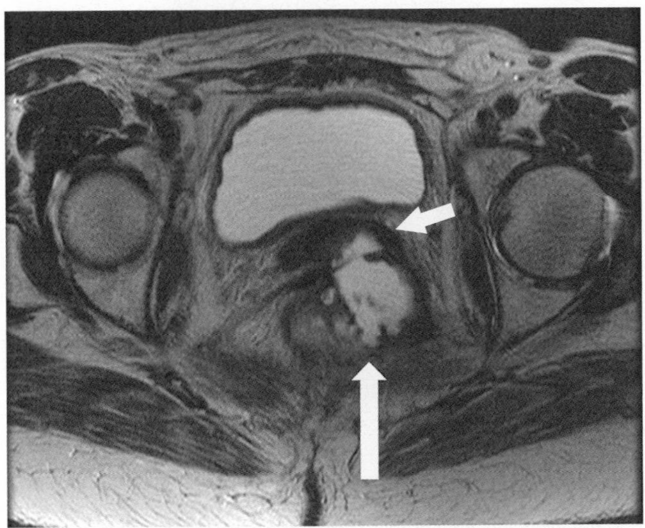

FIGURE 41.12. Axial T2-weighted magnetic resonance imaging study from a patient with anal cancer shows high–signal intensity fluid in the vagina (*short arrow*), a large rectovaginal fluid cavity, and communication with the rectum (*long arrow*), consistent with rectovaginal fistula.

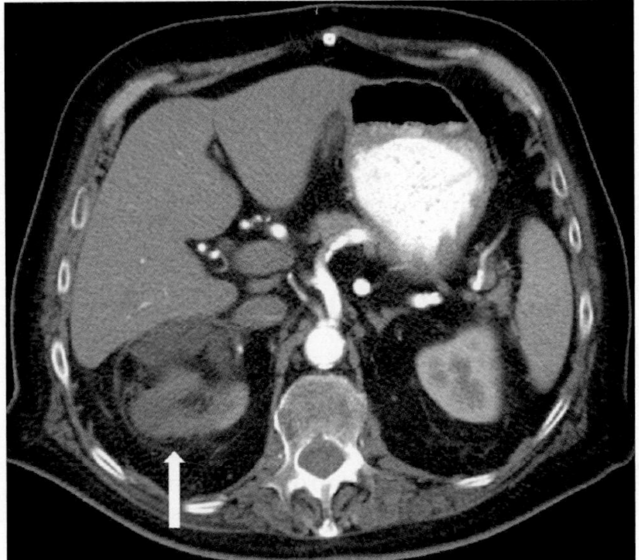

FIGURE 41.13. Axial contrast-enhanced computed tomography scan from a patient with renal cell carcinoma after radiofrequency ablation (RFA) shows low attenuation of the kidney (*arrow*), consistent with ischemia. There is soft tissue anterior to the kidney, which is a result of RFA changes.

The vagina can tolerate up to 140 Gy to the upper surface and 100 Gy to the lower surface. Vaginal atrophy, thinning, and fibrosis become more severe with higher doses of radiation therapy. A rectovaginal fistula can develop at doses of 80 Gy, and vesicovaginal fistulas usually occur at 150 Gy. Fistulas can be evaluated with fluoroscopy (Fig. 41.12) or, increasingly, with pelvic MRI, which usually better shows the fistulous connection.

Ovaries

Radiation of the ovaries can result in infertility and endocrine abnormalities. Small doses of 1.8 to 2 Gy per day or a total dose exceeding 24 Gy can lead to permanent ovarian ablation. For this reason, reimplantation of the ovary into the paracolic gutter is performed to reduce the risk of radiation injury.[45]

Surgical Change

Kidney/Proximal Ureter

Postoperative complications can arise after nephrectomy, partial nephrectomy, or radiofrequency ablation. The complications consist of hematoma, arteriovenous fistula, urinomas, ureteral injury, or pseudoaneurysm. CT is the best tool for evaluation of these complications and distinguishing postoperative change from recurrence of tumor (Fig. 41.13). Ultrasound and CT angiography are also useful for evaluation of the vasculature.[46]

Bladder/Distal Ureter

Surgical injury to the bladder or ureter may occur during partial cystectomy or surgery for prostate, rectal, or gynecologic tumors. In addition, the bladder or reconstructed bladder can take on an unusual appearance, which needs to be distinguished from recurrent tumor. CT can be very useful in this regard. Postsurgical complications include leak, hemorrhage, and urinomas. Postsurgical ureterovaginal fistulas can occur after hysterectomy.[46]

Prostate

Postsurgical fibrosis caused by radical prostatectomy can sometimes be extensive and a cause of urethral stricture. These changes can be difficult to distinguish from recurrence between the bladder and the membranous urethra. MRI with dynamic enhancement images in the postprostectomy bed may be useful because the recurrent tumor may enhance.

Ovaries/Testes

The ovaries may occasionally be transposed into the iliac fossa or higher in the pelvis for patients who require radiation or surgery. Large postoperative hydroceles can occur after testicular resection and simulate recurrent mass.

Key Points Genitourinary

- Fistulas resulting from radiation or chemotherapy are better evaluated with magnetic resonance imaging.
- Changes because of radiofrequency ablation in the kidney can be distinguished from recurrent tumor by use of computed tomography.
- Radiation change can be distinguished from recurrent tumor in the postprostatectomy bed by use of dynamic imaging.
- Ovarian transposition may mimic masses in the upper pelvis, and correlation with patient history is essential in avoiding misdiagnosis.

MUSCULOSKELETAL SYSTEM AND VESSELS

Bone

Chemotherapy Change

Chemotherapy and bone marrow or stem cell transplantation can cause regenerating hematopoietic marrow, with reconversion of yellow to red marrow. On MRI, there is decreased T1 signal and increased signal on T2-weighted imaging and short tau inversion recovery images, with mild enhancement after contrast administration. This may be difficult to distinguish from metastatic disease on T1 and T2 sequences, and chemical shift imaging or gradient echo imaging can help differentiate. On PET/CT, there is diffuse FDG uptake by the marrow, which most likely represents treatment response or marrow-stimulating agents (Fig. 41.14).[34] If there is persistent concern for recurrence, a bone marrow biopsy can be performed.

In children, chemotherapeutic agents such as methotrexate and ifosfamide can interfere with skeletal development. Methotrexate can cause a constellation of symptoms such as osteoporosis, scurvy-like findings, fractures, and periosteal reaction; changes are usually reversible. Side effects resulting from ifosfamide usually occur in patients who have had renal resection or impaired renal function as a result of Wilms' tumor. Findings in the long bones are identical to those seen in rickets.

Immune checkpoint inhibitors can cause arthritis as an irAE. Manifestations of immune-related arthritis include psoriatic arthritis, rheumatoid arthritis, monoarthritis, oligoarthritis, or polyarthritis.[47]

Radiation Change

Radiation changes in the bone marrow can be seen after 1 to 2 weeks of radiotherapy at doses as low as 16 Gy, with changes occurring at 6 months with doses as low as 8 Gy. The findings can be seen on MRI with increased T1 signal throughout the marrow or on PET/CT as a photopenic area corresponding to the radiation field. In children, this finding can be reversible, and the marrow may eventually return to normal signal intensity on imaging. In adults, this may be irreversible. The stages of radiation change in bone are gradual and are termed radiation atrophy. The first stage, demineralization, starts a year after therapy and may progress to an alteration in the trabecular pattern over 3 to 5 years. Continued progression at 5 years can lead to the development of lytic areas in the bone. Radiation atrophy can be distinguished from recurrent disease because it is limited to the radiation field, lacks periosteal reaction, and has delayed onset after irradiation. CT is helpful in further evaluation.

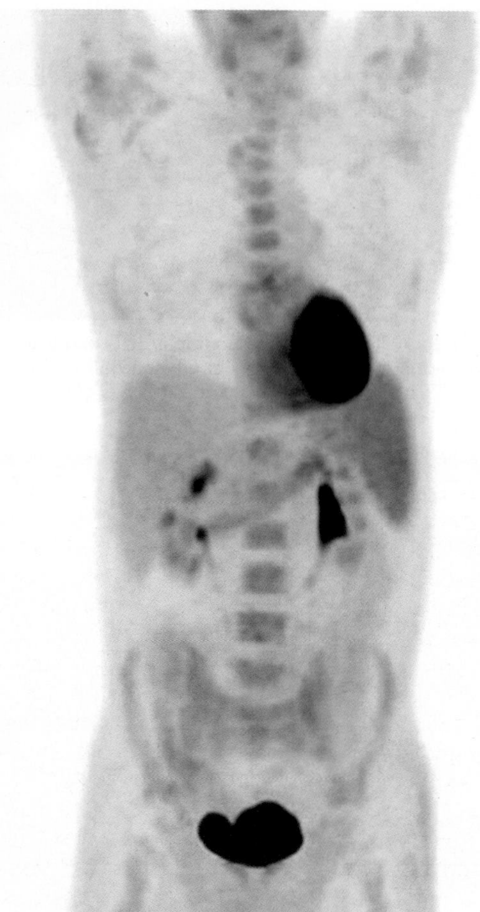

Figure 41.14. Coronal image from 2-[^{18}F] fluoro-2-deoxy-D-glucose–positron emission tomography/computed tomography from a patient with lymphoma receiving chemotherapy shows diffuse uptake throughout the spine and pelvic bones consistent with treatment effect. Patient had complete metabolic response to chemotherapy (uptake with the heart, kidneys, and bladder is physiologic).

In children, radiation can interrupt the growth plate, interfering with chondrogenesis. This effect is most profound in early childhood and puberty. The changes may not be evident until the child reaches puberty. Radiation to the abdomen for Wilms' tumors or neuroblastoma can lead to spinal changes, most commonly scoliosis. Kyphosis can develop. Children who have long-bone irradiation for tumors such as osteosarcoma can have radiation effects at the growth plate, with metaphyseal fraying, scoliosis, and epiphyseal widening. Limb length abnormalities may be seen. Orbital irradiation for retinoblastoma can result in abnormal orbital development. Slipped capital femoral epiphyses can occur in patients who receive irradiation to the proximal femurs for abdominal or pelvis malignancy and can present 1 to 8 years posttreatment.[48]

Osteonecrosis can occur in patients who receive radiation, corticosteroids, chemotherapy, or a combination of therapies. The primary malignancy itself can also be a sole cause. Unilateral or bilateral avascular necrosis (AVN) has been seen with doses of 30 to 40 Gy 1 to 13 years after radiation therapy. The imaging appearance of osteonecrosis caused by radiation or chemotherapy is similar to that of other etiologies.[49] Radiography is nonspecific in the early stages of AVN.

Radiation-induced fractures are caused by normal or physiologic stress on abnormal bone, and most fractures because of radiation are insufficiency fractures. Fractures heal slowly, and they have a high incidence of nonunion. Resorption of fracture fragments may occur. There can be abnormal callous formation. Insufficiency fractures of the sacrum are common in women who have received pelvic irradiation. Bone scan is the most sensitive test, with CT and MRI also useful for further evaluation. Insufficiency fractures of the pubis are less common than those of the sacrum. Other fractures that can occur are at the clavicle, rib, humerus, acromion, or any long bone. Imaging and timeframe may be helpful in excluding radiation-induced sarcomas.[49]

Vertebral body collapse can also occur as a result of radiation and chemotherapy, owing to the abnormal content of the bone before therapy and the loss of volume owing to therapy. MRI is helpful in distinguishing posttreatment collapse from metastatic collapse.

Muscle

Chemotherapy Change

Intraarterial chemotherapy has been reported to cause muscular edema or necrosis. This usually occurs when a catheter is placed peripherally, rather than centrally, within a supplying artery. The changes can be best seen at MRI as increased T2 signal within the muscle.

Immune checkpoint inhibitors such as ipilimumab are associated with muscular changes and myositis. Findings include diffuse increased intramuscular metabolic uptake on PET/CT and enhancing intramuscular foci on CT.[50]

Radiation Change

Radiation-induced changes can be seen as early as 6 weeks at doses of 60 to 65 Gy and usually resolve within 12 to 18 months. In some instances, changes can persist long after therapy has been completed, progressing to atrophy or fibrosis. MRI shows T2 signal increase in the muscles and skin of the radiation field.[51] Chronic changes of muscle atrophy such as fatty replacement or asymmetry can be present.

Nerves

Injury to the nerves has been reported with radiation to the shoulder, spine, and pelvis. Brachial plexus neuropathies with shoulder irradiation present similar to spinal cord symptoms because of radiation, within 1 to 4 years. Lumbar plexus neuropathies can present in patients who have received pelvic irradiation.[52] Imaging may be helpful in excluding recurrence as a cause.

Vessels

Chemotherapy Change

Conventional chemotherapeutic agents are associated with cardiotoxicity because of their vascular effects. The newer targeted therapy agents also have vascular complications. The VEGF inhibitors are associated with hypertension and arterial and venous thrombosis. Tyrosine kinase inhibitors have a high association with arterial thrombosis.[53]

Radiation Change

Radiation vasculopathy can develop at doses as low as 20 Gy, and the risk increases with dose and time. This has been seen in patients who undergo pelvic radiation for cervical or uterine cancer.[43] There can be enhancement of normal tissue owing to abnormal vessels for up to 18 months after radiation.

Fat

Ipilimumab has been associated with retroperitoneal fat opacities, thought to be because of lymphocytic infiltration. These may be diffuse or focal; when focal, they may mimic malignancy.[50]

Key Points Musculoskeletal, Nerves, and Vessels

- Fatty marrow changes are commonly seen after therapy.
- Avascular necrosis can result from therapy and from the primary tumor itself.
- Insufficiency fractures of the sacrum are common in women who have received pelvic irradiation; these have a characteristic appearance on bone scan.

SECONDARY TUMORS

Radiation-induced osteochondromas (cartilaginous exostosis) are benign tumors that have been reported to have an incidence of 6% to 12%. They may be small and can be located within any irradiated bone. They may cause symptoms of pain as they grow and can be resected if symptoms persist or size increases.[41]

Secondary malignancies can be induced by treatment, especially in children. There is a higher rate of leukemia, lymphoma, myelodysplastic disorders, and solid tumors. Radiation-induced tumor is a complication that can occur as early as 2 to 3 years after therapy and present as late as 50 years after therapy, with the average latency time of 10 to 15 years. Osteosarcomas are most common after bone irradiation, and malignant fibrous histiocytomas are more common after soft tissue irradiation. Soft tissue secondary tumors are more common.[54] The secondary sarcoma usually occurs within or adjacent to the radiation site. Imaging

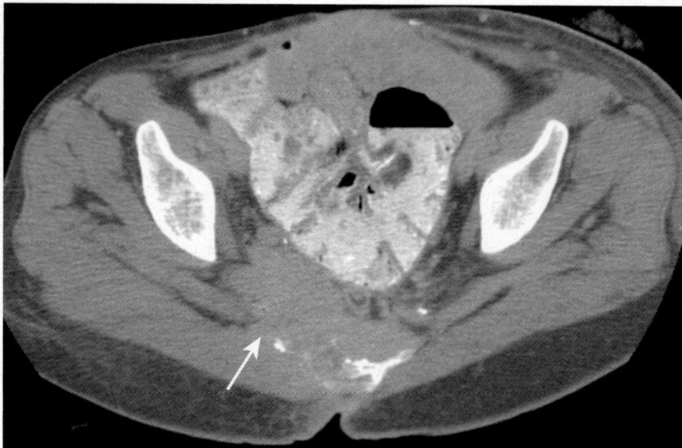

FIGURE 41.15. Axial contrast-enhanced computed tomography scan from a patient with history of radiation to the pelvis for endometrial carcinoma 30 years ago, now with radiation-induced sarcoma. There is a soft tissue mass causing bony destruction of the sacrum (*arrow*).

can be helpful in evaluating for new bone loss, destructive changes, soft tissue masses, or abnormal enhancement within the radiation field (Fig. 41.15). Distinguishing these changes from osteomyelitis may be difficult and require biopsy.

CONCLUSION AND IMPORTANT POINTS

Pseudoprogression, the enlargement of target lesion as a result of treatment response, is not specifically discussed in this chapter on complications of therapy, but it is an important sequela of treatment with immunotherapy. It has be seen with use of agents such as nivolumab, ipilimumab, and pembrolizumab, for example.[55]

Knowing the sequelae and understanding the imaging appearance of the differing oncologic therapies is crucial for radiologists to guide patient management.

KEY POINTS

- Splenomegaly and portal hypertension may result from chemotherapy.
- Bowel wall perforation and fistulas occurring during treatment should be conveyed to the clinician because they impact patient care.
- Radiation to the bowel can result in strictures, bowel wall thickening, dilatation, and fistulas.
- Magnetic resonance imaging may be helpful in evaluating for radiation injury and fistulas.
- Positron emission tomography/computed tomography can be used to distinguish posttreatment effect from recurrent tumor.
- Secondary malignancies that develop after chemotherapy or radiation include hematologic malignancies and solid tumors.

REFERENCES

1. Cox JD, Stetz J, Pajak TF. Toxicity criteria of the Radiation Therapy Oncology Group (RTOG) and the European organization for research and treatment of cancer (EORTC). *Int J Radiol Oncol Biol Phys*. 1995;31(5):1341-1346.
2. Kammen BF, Pacharn P, Thoeni RF, et al. Focal fatty infiltration of the liver: analysis of prevalence and CT findings in children and young adults. *AJR Am J Roentgenol*. 2001;177(5):1035-1039.
3. Howard SAH, Krajewski KM, Thornton E, et al. Decade of molecular targeted therapy: abdominal manifestations of drug toxicities—what radiologists should know. *AJR Am J Roentgenol*. 2012;199(1):58-64.
4. Birch JC, Khatri G, Watumull LM, et al. Unintended consequences of systemic and ablative oncologic therapy in the abdomen and pelvis. *RadioGraphics*. 2018;38(4):1158-1179.
5. Reynolds K, Thomas M, Dougan M. Diagnosis and management of hepatitis in patients on checkpoint blockade. *Oncologist*. 2018;23(9):991-997.
6. Donadon M, Vauthey JN, Loyer EM, et al. Portal thrombosis and steatosis after preoperative chemotherapy with FOLFIRI-bevacizumab for colorectal liver metastases. *World J Gastroenterol*. 2006;12(40):6556-6558.
7. Schouten van der Velden AP, Punt CJA, Van Krieken JHJ, et al. Hepatic veno-occlusive disease after neoadjuvant treatment of colorectal liver metastases with oxaliplatin: A lesson of the month. *Euro J Surg Oncol*. 2008;34(3):353-355.
8. Elsayes KM, Shaaban AM, Rothan SM, et al. A comprehensive approach to hepatic vascular disease. *Radiographics*. 2017;37(3):813-836.
9. Young ST, Paulson EK, Washington K, et al. CT of the liver in patients with metastatic breast carcinoma treated by chemotherapy: findings simulating cirrhosis. *AJR Am J Roentgenol*. 1994;163(6):1385-1388.
10. Ragnhammar P, Hafström L, Nygren P, et al. A systematic overview of chemotherapy effects in colorectal cancer. *Acta Oncol*. 2001;40(2-3):282-308.
11. Dawson LA, Normolle D, Balter JM, et al. Analysis of radiation-induced liver disease using the Lyman NTCP model. *Int J Radiat Oncol Biol Phys*. 2002;53(4):810-821.
12. Khozouz RF, Huq SZ, Perry MC. Radiation-induced liver disease. *J Clin Oncol*. 2008;26(29):4844-4845.
13. Itai Y, Murata S, Kurosaki Y. Straight border sign of the liver: spectrum of CT appearances and causes. *Radiographics*. 1995;15(5):1089-1102.
14. Takamatsu S, Kozaka K, Kobayashi S, et al. Pathology and images of radiation-induced hepatitis: a review article. *Jpn J Radiol*. 2018;36(4):241-256.
15. Wong SL, Mangu PB, Choti MA, et al. American Society of Clinical Oncology 2009 Clinical Evidence Review on Radiofrequency Ablation of Hepatic Metastases From Colorectal Cancer. *J Clin Oncol*. 2010 Jan 20;28(3):493-508.
16. Chang ST, Menias CO, Lubner MG, et al. Molecular and clinical approach to intra-abdominal adverse effects of targeted cancer therapies. *RadioGraphics*. 2017;37(5):1461-1482.
17. Overman MJ, Maru DM, Charnsangavej C, et al. Oxaliplatin-mediated increase in spleen size as a biomarker for the development of hepatic sinusoidal injury. *J Clin Oncol*. 2010;28(15):2549-2555.
18. Masood N, Shaikh AJ, Memon WA, et al. Splenic rupture, secondary to G-CSF use for chemotherapy induced neutropenia: a case report and review of literature. *Cases Journal*. 2008;1(1):418.
19. Benguerfi S, Thepault F, Lena H, et al. Spontaneous splenic rupture as a rare complication of G-CSF injection. *BMJ Case Reports*. 2018;2018 bcr2017222561.
20. Krishnamurthy P, Brown M, Agrawal S, et al. Acute pancreatitis as a complication of trans-arterial chemoembolization of hepatocellular cancer-case report and review of literature. *J Gastrointest Oncol*. 2017;8(1):E26-E30.
21. McGettigan MJ, Menias CO, Gao ZJ, et al. Imaging of drug-induced complications in the gastrointestinal system. *Radiographics*. 2016;36(1):71-87.
22. Gemici C, Yaprak G, Ozdemir S, et al. Volumetric decrease of pancreas after abdominal irradiation, it is time to consider pancreas as an organ at risk for radiotherapy planning. *Radiat Oncol*. 2018;13(1):238.
23. Gervais DA, Fernandez-del Castillo C, O'Neill MJ, et al. Complications after pancreatoduodenectomy: imaging and imaging-guided interventional procedures. *Radiographics*. 2001;21(3):673-690.
24. Davila M, Bresalier RS. Gastrointestinal complications of oncologic therapy. *Nat Clin Pract Gastroenterol Hepatol*. 2008;5(12):682-696.
25. Khoury NJ, Kanj V, Abboud M, et al. Abdominal complications of chemotherapy in pediatric malignancies: imaging findings. *Clin Imaging*. 2009;33(4):253-260.

26. Nishino M, Hatabu H, Hodi FS. Imaging of cancer immunotherapy: current approaches and future directions. *Radiology*. 2018;290(1):9-22.
27. Widmann G, Nguyen VA, Plaickner J, et al. Imaging features of toxicities by immune checkpoint inhibitors in cancer therapy. *Curr Radiol Rep*. 2016;5(11):59.
28. Libshitz HI, Southard ME. Complications of radiation therapy: the thorax. *Semin Roentgenol*. 1974;9(1):41-49.
29. Bruzzi JF, Munden RF, Truong MT, et al. PET/CT of esophageal cancer: its role in clinical management. *Radiographics*. 2007;27(6):1635-1652.
30. Singh AK, Tierney RM, Low DA, et al. A prospective study of differences in duodenum compared with remaining small bowel motion between radiation treatments: implications for radiation dose escalation in carcinoma of the pancreas. *Radiat Oncol*. 2006;1:33.
31. Iyer R, Jhingran A. Radiation injury: imaging findings in the chest, abdomen and pelvis after therapeutic radiation. *Cancer Imaging*. 2006;6:S131-139.
32. Maturen KE, Feng MU, Wasnik AP, et al. Imaging effects of radiation therapy in the abdomen and pelvis: evaluating "innocent bystander" tissues. *Radiographics*. 2013;33(2):599-619.
33. Coia LR, Myerson RJ, Tepper JE. Late effects of radiation therapy on the gastrointestinal tract. *Int J Radiat Oncol Biol Phys*. 1995;31(5):1213-1236.
34. Humphreys BD, Soiffer RJ, Magee CC. Renal failure associated with cancer and its treatment: an update. *J Am Soc Nephrol*. 2005;16(1):151-161.
35. Wanchoo R, Karam S, Uppal NN, et al. Adverse renal effects of immune checkpoint inhibitors: a narrative review. *Am J Nephrol*. 2017;45(2):160-169.
36. Schwartz CL. Long-term survivors of childhood cancer: the late effects of therapy. *Oncologist*. 1999;4(1):45-54.
37. Torrisi JM, Schwartz LH, Gollub MJ, et al. CT findings of chemotherapy-induced toxicity: what radiologists need to know about the clinical and radiologic manifestations of chemotherapy toxicity. *Radiology*. 2011;258(1):41-56.
38. Ritchey M, Ferrer F, Shearer P, et al. Late effects on the urinary bladder in patients treated for cancer in childhood: a report from the Children's Oncology Group. *Pediatr Blood Cancer*. 2009;52(4):439-446.
39. Dohle GR. Male infertility in cancer patients: review of the literature. *Int J Urol*. 2010;17(4):327-331.
40. Quach HT, Robbins CJ, Balko JM, et al. Severe Epididymo-orchitis and encephalitis complicating anti-PD-1 therapy. *Oncologist*. 2019;24(7):872-876.
41. Libshitz HI, DuBrow RA, Loyer EM, et al. Radiation change in normal organs: an overview of body imaging. *Eur Radiol*. 1996;6(6):786-795.
42. Marks LB, Carroll PR, Dugan TC, et al. The response of the urinary bladder, urethra, and ureter to radiation and chemotherapy. *Int J Radiat Oncol Biol Phys*. 1995;31(5):1257-1280.
43. Hricak H, Yu KK. Radiology in invasive cervical cancer. *AJR Am J Roentgenol*. 1996;167(5):1101-1108.
44. Marnitz S, Kohler C, Fuller J, et al. Uterus necrosis after radiochemotherapy in two patients with advanced cervical cancer. *Strahlenther Onkol*. 2006;182(1):45-51.
45. Husseinzadeh N, Van Aken ML, Aron B. Ovarian transposition in young patients with invasive cervical cancer receiving radiation therapy. *Int J Gynecol Cancer*. 1994;4(1):61-65.
46. Patel BN, Gayer G. Imaging of iatrogenic complications of the urinary tract: kidneys, ureters, and bladder. *Radiol Clin North Am*. 2014;52(5):1101-1116.
47. Pundole X, Abdel-Wahab N, Suarez-Almazor ME. Arthritis risk with immune checkpoint inhibitor therapy for cancer. *Curr Opin Rheumatol*. 2019;31(3):293-299.
48. Fletcher BD. Effects of pediatric cancer therapy on the musculoskeletal system. *Pediatr Radiol*. 1997;27(8):623-636.
49. Jones DN. Multifocal osteonecrosis following chemotherapy and short-term corticosteroid therapy in a patient with small-cell bronchogenic carcinoma. *J Nucl Med*. 1994;35(8):1347-1350.
50. Bronstein Y, Ng CS, Hwu P, et al. Radiologic manifestations of immune-related adverse events in patients with metastatic melanoma undergoing anti-CTLA-4 antibody therapy. *AJR Am J Roentgenol*. 2011;197(6):W992-W1000.
51. Ikushima H, Osaki K, Furutani S, et al. Pelvic bone complications following radiation therapy of gynecologic malignancies: clinical evaluation of radiation-induced pelvic insufficiency fractures. *Gynecol Oncol*. 2006;103(3):1100-1104.
52. Klimek M, Kosobucki R, Luczyńska E, et al. Radiotherapy-induced lumbosacral plexopathy in a patient with cervical cancer: a case report and literature review. *Contemp Oncol (Pozn)*. 2012;16(2):194-196.
53. Cameron AC, Touyz RM, Lang NN. Vascular complications of cancer chemotherapy. *Can J Cardiol*. 2016;32(7):852-862.
54. Dracham CB, Shankar A, Madan R. Radiation induced secondary malignancies: a review article. *Radiat Oncol J*. 2018;36(2):85-94.
55. Borcoman E, Nandikolla A, Long G, et al. Patterns of Response and Progression to Immunotherapy. *Am Soc Clin Oncol Educ Book*. 2018(38):169-178.

CHAPTER 42

Pulmonary Embolic Disease and Cardiac Masses and Tumors

Gregory Gladish

PULMONARY EMBOLISM

Pulmonary embolism (PE) and deep vein thrombosis (DVT) are common problems in patients with cancer owing to local and humoral effects of the tumor as well as to the effects of therapy. The diagnosis of venous thromboembolic disease is challenging because of nonspecific clinical signs, symptoms, and laboratory evaluations. Computed tomography (CT) angiography has taken a central role in the diagnosis of PE. CT provides the opportunity to identify PEs and to assess the severity of involvement and hemodynamic effects. Treatment of venous thromboembolism in cancer patients generally follows the standards used for nononcology patients. However, treatment can be complicated in patients with cancer because of drug interactions and continued stimulus for thrombus formation. PE remains a challenging problem in the management of patients with cancer.

EPIDEMIOLOGY AND RISK FACTORS

PE results from the migration of thrombi formed in the systemic venous system, usually from the pelvis or lower extremities, into the pulmonary arterial system.[1,2] These thrombi form as a result of abnormal veins, abnormal blood flow, or abnormalities of the coagulation system, all of which are frequently present in patients with cancer. Central venous catheters are a significant risk factor for thrombus formation, with up to 4% of patients with central venous catheters developing catheter-related thrombus.[3] The majority of upper-extremity DVTs are associated with catheters.[4] Abnormalities in the coagulation system that predispose to venous thrombus formation[1,2] include various coagulation factor abnormalities and cancer-associated hypercoagulability. Chemotherapeutic agents such as methotrexate, doxorubicin, thalidomide, and hematopoietic stem cell–stimulating agents can promote thrombus formation. Venous thromboembolism rates are highest in patients on chemotherapy, with an incidence as high as 28% in patients with malignant gliomas.[3] The frequency of presentation of venous thromboembolism is more closely related to the frequency of the tumor in the population, with most seen in patients with lung, colon, and prostate cancer.

Cancer patients are also at greater risk for poor outcomes after PE. For example, they are four to eight times more likely to die after a PE event.[5] The 1-year survival for patients with cancer and venous thromboembolism is approximately one-third that of patients with cancer without venous thromboembolism.

ANATOMY

DVTs occur most often in the pelvic and lower extremity veins.[1,2] The fragments that detach and embolize are typically tubular in shape and can vary from less than 1 mm in diameter to up to 2 cm in diameter. The larger-diameter thrombi may tend to be longer and may have branching components.

Once detached, emboli flow through the venous system until they encounter an impeding structure or reach a vessel that is too small to permit their passage, commonly a pulmonary arterial branch. Emboli may be captured *en route* to the pulmonary arterial system in trabeculations within the right atrium,[6–8] in a congenital Chiari network located at the base of the right atrium, or while passing through a patent foramen ovale. Thrombi that pass through the foramen ovale can embolize to systemic structures, including the brain.

Emboli that reach the lungs become lodged at arterial branch points or may reach an arteriole of lesser diameter than the embolus (Fig. 42.1). Larger and more elongated emboli will commonly be captured at branch points and may extend into multiple lobes and segments of the pulmonary arterial tree (Fig. 42.2). The largest PEs may become lodged across the main pulmonary artery bifurcation and are called saddle emboli (Fig. 42.3). Usually, there is a small bandlike component extending across the pulmonary artery bifurcation, with larger components of thrombus extending into the right and left pulmonary arteries and lobar or segmental branches.

If the embolus completely occludes a segment of the pulmonary arterial system, it can result in pulmonary infarction.[9] This is relatively uncommon because of the parallel blood supply from the bronchial arteries. Pulmonary ischemia or infarction results in hemorrhage and edema within the affected portion of lung. The involved area typically extends out in a wedge-shaped pattern from the occluded arteriole and reaches the pleural surface (Fig. 42.4). The hemorrhagic phase is followed by necrosis and coagulation of the underlying lung architecture. The infarct typically evolves over several days to weeks and may resolve completely or result in a small area of scarring.

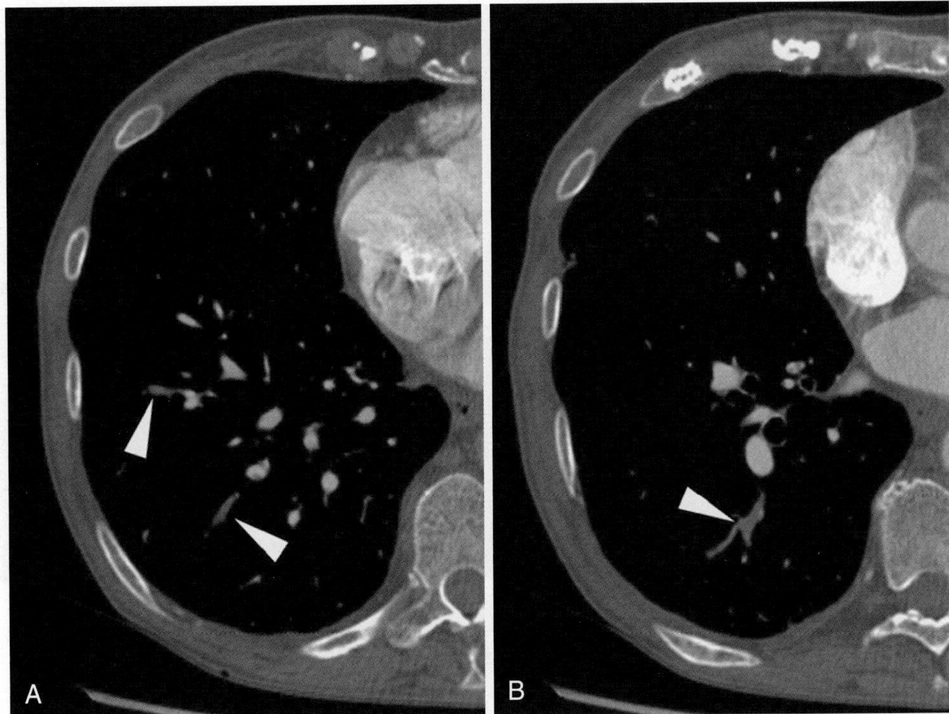

FIGURE 42.1. Distal pulmonary embolism. Small emboli (*arrowheads* in **A**, **B**) travel through the pulmonary arterial system until they become lodged in a vessel too small to permit further passage. These emboli typically completely fill the involved artery lumen.

KEY POINTS Anatomy

- Emboli are typically elongated "casts" of the vein of origin.
- Emboli tend to become lodged at branch points or become wedged in smaller-caliber arteries.
- Emboli can become entrapped in transit through the right heart chambers or pass through a patent foramen, causing systemic embolism.
- Wedge-shaped consolidation peripheral to an occluded vessel represents pulmonary ischemia or infarction and involutes over time.

CLINICAL PRESENTATION

DVT may be completely asymptomatic or may present with a variety of nonspecific symptoms, including asymmetrical extremity swelling or an erythematous tender mass along the venous structure.[10] PE may also be asymptomatic or cause nonspecific symptoms such as chest pain or dyspnea.[10,11] The acute onset of dyspnea is the most suggestive symptom and may be accompanied by a sense of impending doom. Emboli that cause right heart strain can produce systemic edema and abnormalities at cardiac auscultation.

Clinical history is helpful in suggesting PE.[1,10,11] Any recent period of prolonged immobilization, active cancer, or use of drugs associated with thrombosis should raise a suspicion of PE in patients with new dyspnea.

Patients with PE often have nonspecific laboratory abnormalities[1,2,10,11] such as elevated D-dimer levels, abnormal coagulation measurements such as prothrombin time, partial thromboplastin time, and the International Normalized Ratio, as well as elevated erythrocyte counts and hemoglobin levels and abnormalities of platelet number or function. These are typically abnormal related to the cause of thrombus formation, rather than a result of the thrombus or embolus itself. Arterial blood gas may show an increased difference between alveolar and arterial oxygen concentration, an increased A-a gradient, and pulse oximetry is often abnormal. These findings are nonspecific and indicate only an abnormality of pulmonary oxygenation, which may be the result of pneumonia, embolism, or tumor, among other possibilities.

PEs may be detected on routine imaging of cancer patients without suspicion of PE.[12–17] In patients without cancer, PEs are detected in up to 1% of outpatients and 3% of inpatients. Among patients with cancer, 3% to 4% of outpatients and over 6% of inpatients will have unsuspected PE at routine CT scanning. Unfortunately, up to 75% of these, including large central emboli, will not be seen at clinical interpretation,[13,14,16] particularly in patients with complex presentations of their underlying malignancy. The significance of subsegmental or smaller PE is unknown. Some studies have shown recurrence rates in patients with isolated subsegmental PE[13,18] similar to that of negative CT pulmonary angiography and much less than for patients treated for PE.[18] Other studies have shown that anticoagulation for unsuspected PE improves survival.[19] Further study is needed to determine the appropriate treatment of isolated subsegmental PEs in particular and unsuspected, asymptomatic PEs in general.

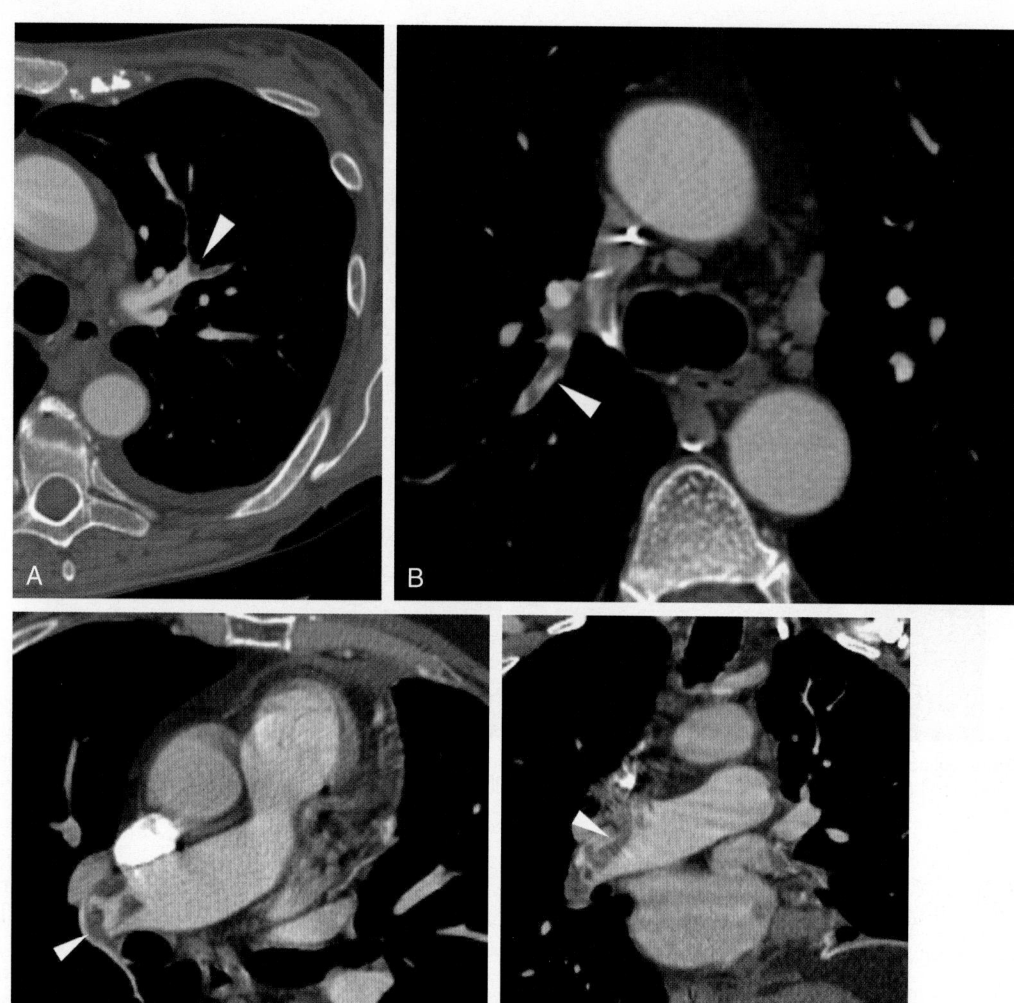

Figure 42.2. Proximal pulmonary embolism. Elongated emboli (*arrowheads* in **A–D**) often become lodged across more distal vessel branch points, such as at the lobar or segmental levels. These typically have a rounded eccentric appearance compared with the vessel cross-section. If they contact the vessel wall, they form acute angles with it.

SEVERITY ASSESSMENT

The size of PEs and the extent of involvement of the pulmonary arterial tree can impact the clinical symptoms and long-term outcome of these patients. More severe PEs are more likely to be associated with right heart strain and more likely to require aggressive intervention, including intensive care unit admission. Evaluation of pulmonary embolic disease, therefore, involves an assessment of the amount of thrombus and of any secondary effects.

Several scoring systems for the extent of pulmonary embolic disease have been proposed. These vary from simple assessment of the most proximal level of involvement[20] to detailed scoring of the number and severity of obstructed vessels,[21–23] and correlate with short-term outcomes and the use of intensive care unit admissions.[5,21,23–26] However, the risk of death from an acute episode of PE primarily depends on the hemodynamic state of the patient. Patients with cardiac shock have a high risk of death, normotensive patients with right heart dysfunction have an intermediate risk, and patients without heart dysfunction do not have a high risk.[27] Whereas cardiac shock is diagnosed clinically, right heart dysfunction may be evaluated with imaging.

Right heart dysfunction as a result of PE is represented in the development of pulmonary hypertension, right heart strain, and right heart failure. Assessment of these parameters at echocardiography or CT is predictive of survival to hospital discharge and the need for intensive care unit admission.[1,2,26,28–31] At CT, pulmonary artery diameter greater than 30 to 33 mm[32,33] or greater than the aortic diameter (Fig. 42.5) is suggestive of pulmonary hypertension. A right ventricle to left ventricle diameter ratio greater than 1.0:1 to 1.5:1 suggests right heart strain or right heart failure (Fig. 42.6).[34,35] Secondary signs of right heart strain and failure are less specific but include reflux of contrast material into the inferior vena cava (IVC) and hepatic veins and evidence of systemic edema, including hepatic congestion and subcutaneous edema.[36]

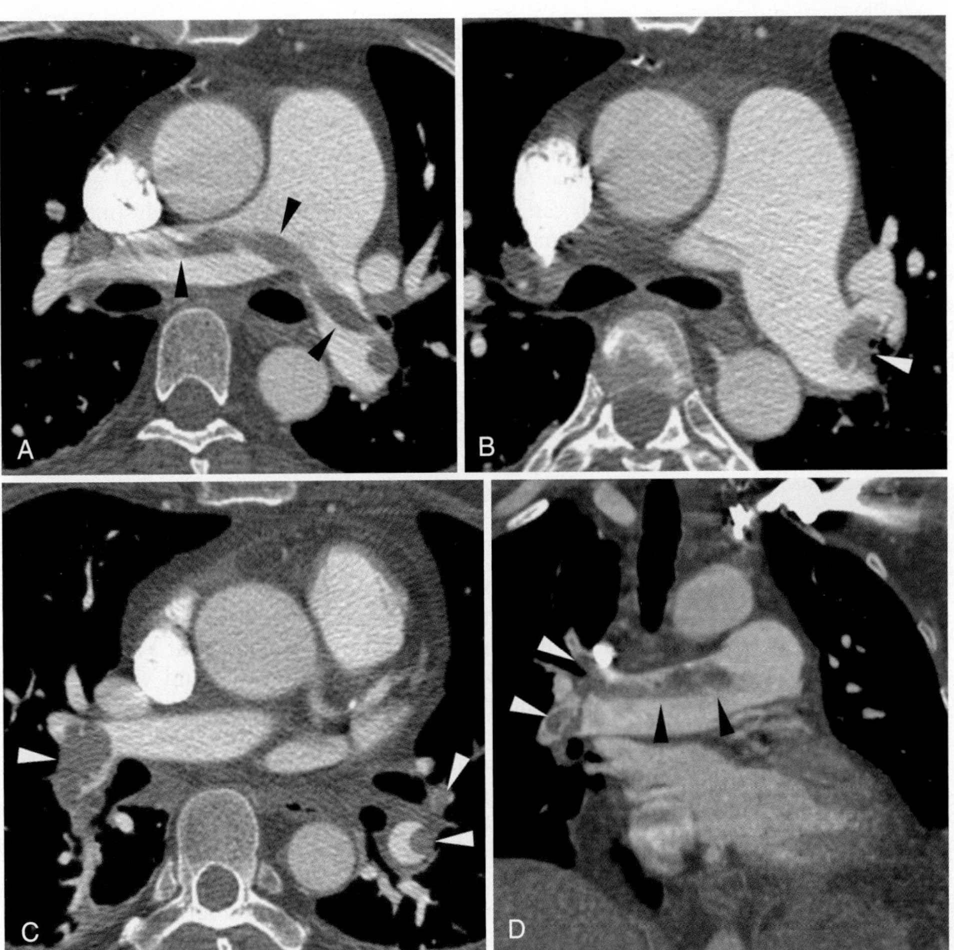

FIGURE 42.3. Saddle pulmonary embolism. Large emboli (*black arrow-heads* in **A**, **D**) can become lodged across the main pulmonary artery bifurcation. The clot may fill the majority of the vessel at this point, but among patients surviving to imaging, usually a bandlike component extends across the bifurcation, with larger components in the right and left pulmonary arteries (*white arrowheads* in **B–D**).

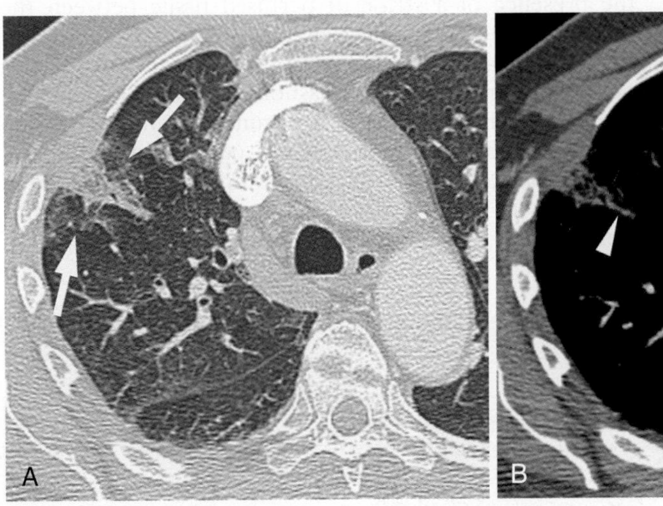

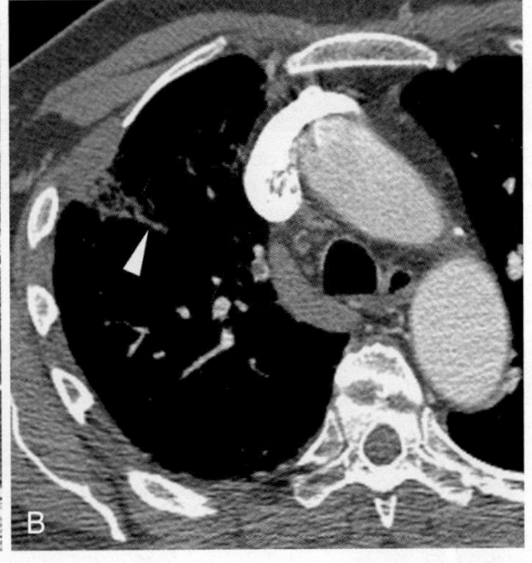

FIGURE 42.4. Pulmonary infarct. If arterial occlusion is complete, and collateral bronchial arterial flow is inadequate, ischemic injury or infarction occurs in the lung peripheral to the embolism. This causes focal consolidation (*arrows* in **A**) that is typically wedge-shaped, with the base along the pleural surface and the apex directed toward the affected artery (*arrowhead* in **B**).

These various methods of assessing the amount and severity of pulmonary arterial embolic disease and the effects of right heart strain are useful in identifying patients in need of more aggressive therapy and monitoring. They are not as helpful in predicting recurrent embolic disease. Therefore, identifying and ameliorating the inciting factors are important in the patient's long-term management.[1]

KEY POINTS Severity Assessment

- Scoring systems reflect the number of lung segments involved by emboli and predict the need for intensive management.
- Right heart strain, reflected in right ventricle or pulmonary artery dilatation, also predicts survival and need for more intensive management.
- Identifying inciting factors is critical in long-term management.

IMAGING

Traditionally, imaging for PE was previously done with chest x-ray and ventilation-perfusion (V/Q) scanning. Unfortunately, these methods are nonspecific and often do not provide a final diagnosis. Imaging now focuses on CT pulmonary angiography, which allows direct and noninvasive imaging of the pulmonary arterial tree. Imaging for DVT is predominantly done with ultrasonography. Venous-phase imaging in the lower extremity veins after CT pulmonary angiography has also been performed, but its radiation dose is high, especially relative to the nonionizing ultrasound examination.[37]

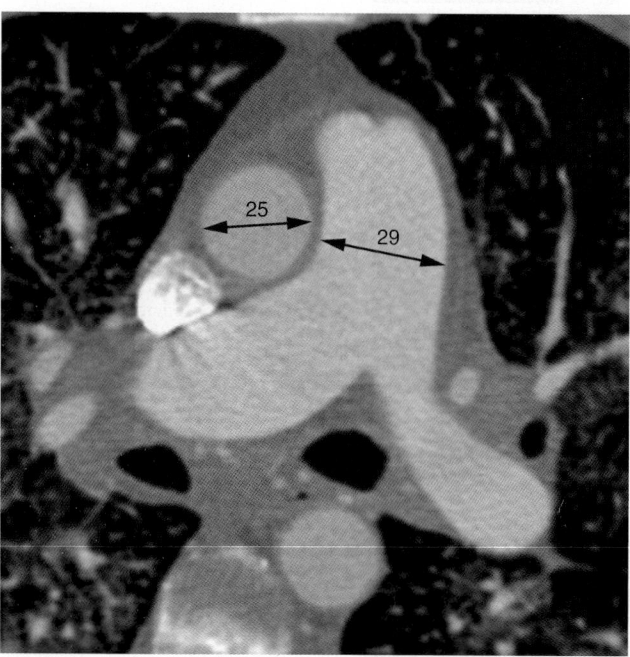

FIGURE 42.5. The diameters of the main pulmonary artery and aorta are measured at the level of the pulmonary bifurcation. A pulmonary artery diameter greater than 30–33 mm or greater than the diameter of the aorta indicates pulmonary arterial hypertension.

Chest Radiography

Chest radiography usually demonstrates some abnormality in patients with PE, but normal examinations are not uncommon.[11,38] The most common abnormal findings are focal pulmonary opacities and small pleural effusions, which can be seen with many etiologies of dyspnea.[1] The traditionally described radiographic signs, including the Hampton hump (a peripheral pleural-based wedge-shaped opacity), the Fleischner sign (widening of the pulmonary artery on the side of the embolism), and the Westermark sign (oligemia in the distribution distal to the PE), are nonspecific and at least as common in patients without emboli as in those with emboli.

Ventilation-Perfusion Scanning

V/Q scanning was long the standard for the initial detection of pulmonary embolic disease[39] and is highly sensitive but not very specific for the identification of emboli. Several large trials established the value of V/Q scanning in the identification of very high risk and very low risk patients, allowing their management without further imaging. Patients are categorized as high risk by the presence of two or more segments of V/Q mismatch, which is a perfusion defect larger than the ventilation defect or no ventilation defect. Patients have very low probability for emboli if they have normal perfusion or nonsegmental perfusion abnormalities related to the heart, hila, and diaphragm; perfusion defects smaller than the radiographic or ventilation lesion; multiple matched V/Q defects with a normal radiograph; one to three small segmental perfusion defects; the presence of a stripe of perfused tissue between the defect and the pleural surface; or a single matched defect with a matching chest radiograph abnormality in the mid or upper lung. However, at least one quarter of patients fall into the intermediate or indeterminate probability group and should have further imaging performed.[1] Although mostly supplanted by CT, it is an important alternative in patients with severe renal function compromise or significant contrast allergy history.

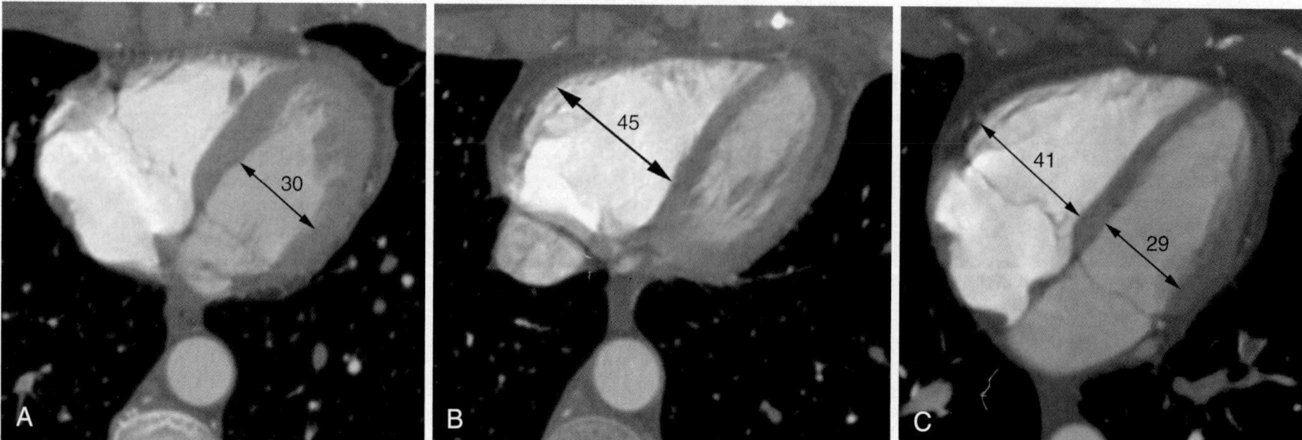

FIGURE 42.6. The transverse diameters of the left (LV; **A**) and right (RV; **B**) ventricles are measured at the widest point for each chamber. These are typically at different axial levels. A ratio of RV/LV diameters greater than 1.0:1 to 1.5:1 indicates right ventricular dilatation and dysfunction. **C**, The measurement can also be made on a single reformatted image in the long-axis view. In this view, the RV/LV ratio should be less than 1.0:1.

Computed Tomography

CT pulmonary angiography has emerged as the standard method of detection and identification of PE.[1,2,40,41] On modern scanners of 16 or more detector rows, scanning is easily accomplished in a short, single breathhold. A limited number of artifacts can simulate PEs, but CT pulmonary angiography probably is equivalent to invasive catheter pulmonary angiography for the detection of PEs down to at least the subsegmental level. CT has the advantage of providing alternate diagnoses in cases that are negative for PE.

Scanning technique should maximize contrast enhancement of the pulmonary arteries and provide sufficient resolution to visualize pulmonary arteries down to approximately 1 mm in diameter.[42,43] Short scan times are also important to allow adequate breathholding in dyspneic patients. Typically, scanning is performed at approximately 1-mm collimation, and the scan is acquired in as short a time as possible on the scanner. Radiation dose is a concern, and appropriate dose reduction strategies should be employed. These strategies include tube current modulation based on patient attenuation measurements and the use of anterior breast shields in premenopausal women.[44] The use of newer iterative statistical reconstruction techniques[45] and lower kilovolt techniques[46] can also reduce dose.

To obtain optimal vascular enhancement, a high–iodine concentration contrast material is administered at a relatively high rate.[41,47–49] Contrast material is typically 300 mg of iodine/mL or higher and administered at 4 mL/seconds or faster. This generally requires a 20-gauge or larger peripheral intravenous access and a relatively large upper extremity vein. Alternatively, the injection may be performed through a power-injectable central venous catheter. Scan timing after contrast injection is determined using bolus triggering with a detection region in the proximal main pulmonary artery and a 100 HU trigger threshold. Scanning begins 7 to 10 seconds after detection, to allow maximal enhancement and provide time for breathholding instructions. The amount of contrast media should allow an injection duration of the expected scan time plus the 7- to 10-second delay plus a margin of 3 to 4 seconds, up to a maximum of 150 mL of contrast media.

Scanning in a caudocranial direction is believed to reduce motion artifacts associated with suboptimal breathholding because the upper lungs are less affected by respiratory motion.[47,48] Although still used, its value is probably much less with 64–detector row or larger scanners because of the short scan duration.

A variety of artifacts may degrade the images of the pulmonary arteries.[47,48] The most significant is respiratory-related motion, which can usually be avoided with faster CT scanners. Both higher pitch and faster gantry rotation contribute to shorter breathhold requirements. Faster gantry rotations also improve the temporal resolution, which reduces the effect of any respiratory motion. Similarly, cardiac pulsations can cause motion artifacts in the adjacent parenchyma, seen most frequently in the left lower lobe. This can be minimized with faster gantry rotation times to minimize the amount of motion that occurs during a single image.

Another significant source of artifact is that of contrast interruption (Fig. 42.7) owing to inflowing of unopacified blood from the IVC during the examination.[50–52] The IVC inflow is accentuated during inspiration, whereas it is relatively stable during exhalation and during breathhold or Valsalva maneuver. This inflow during inspiration causes a short pulse of low-attenuation blood to be present in the pulmonary arteries a few seconds after the patient inhales. With faster scanners, this pulse of lower-attenuation blood can affect several centimeters of pulmonary arteries and simulate pulmonary arterial emboli. It may be recognized by its involvement of multiple vessels at the same level. This artifact appears to be increased by hyperventilation, so simple breathhold instructions may reduce its frequency and extent. When present, it may be necessary to repeat the examination. The repeat examination should be performed with a different breathhold timing to change the location

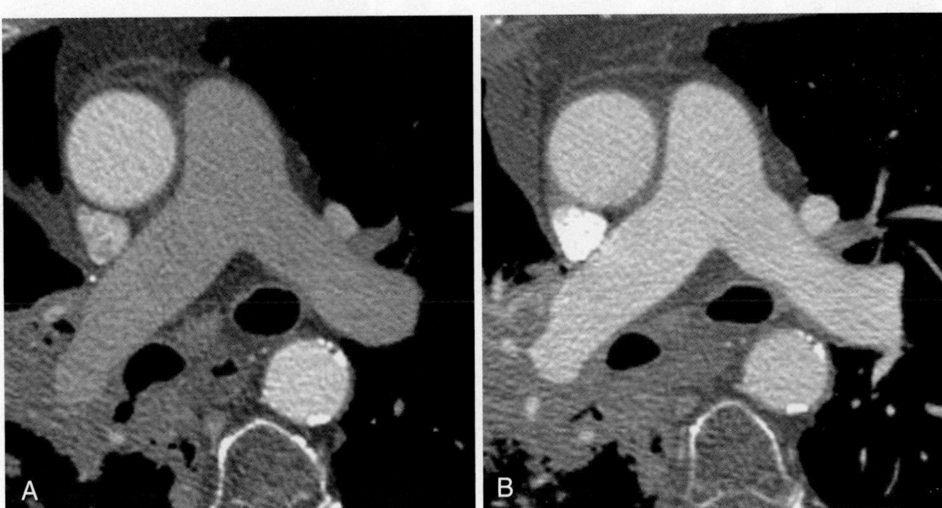

FIGURE 42.7. Contrast interruption artifact. Inflowing blood from the inferior vena cava is accentuated during inspiration and can significantly decrease pulmonary arterial enhancement. **A**, This may be seen as diffuse decreased attenuation in the pulmonary arteries compared with the aorta, or it may occur in a short segment of the pulmonary arterial tree, depending on the scan speed, duration, and breathhold timing. When a short segment is involved, the artifact typically involves all artery branches at that level. **B**, Repeating the examination with different breathhold timing or without breathholding can resolve the artifact.

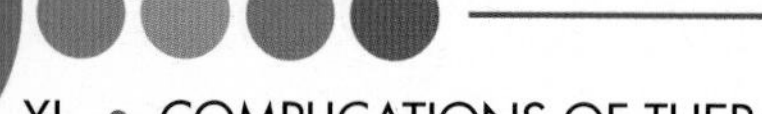

of the apparent filling defect or performed without breath-holding, particularly if a large portion of the central pulmonary system is affected on the initial scan.

PEs are identified as filling defects in the pulmonary arterial tree with sharp margins with the contrast column.[48,53,54] Acute PEs are typically located eccentrically and are rounded in contour or may fill a small vessel completely (see Figs. 42.1 to 42.3). Larger central emboli may have elongated or lobular components and often extend into multiple smaller branches. The CT equivalent of Hampton's hump may be demonstrated as a wedge-shaped peripheral focus of consolidation, with the base at the pleural surface and the apex directed to the occluded pulmonary artery (see Fig. 42.4).[9]

Over time, emboli may resolve or may become chronic and incorporate into the pulmonary artery wall. In that setting, the filling defect becomes crescentic in contour, and occluded segments may recanalize, showing small foci of contrast within the thrombus.[54] The filling defect may be reduced to a thin linear web within the vessel (Fig. 42.8). Some emboli retain their acute appearance, but persistence over greater than 6 weeks indicates a chronic embolism.

Assessment of obstruction severity and right heart strain should be performed in patients who have PE, using the criteria mentioned previously. CT also provides the opportunity to identify alternative diagnoses such as pneumonia or other lung disease, pericardial disease, or mediastinal disease that might contribute to dyspnea or chest pain. Such alternative diagnoses are found in the majority of patients without PE. With these advantages and its widespread availability, CT pulmonary angiogram has become the *de facto* standard for the evaluation for PE. It has very high sensitivity and specificity compared with V/Q scanning and has essentially the same sensitivity and specificity as conventional catheter pulmonary angiography, without the technical requirements and associated limited availability of that procedure. V/Q scanning still finds a role in patients for whom contrast administration is contraindicated.

Key Points The Radiology Report

- Presence of pulmonary embolism.
- Any alternative etiology for dyspnea.
- Description of extent of embolism, possibly including an obstruction score.
- Signs of right heart strain or pulmonary hypertension.

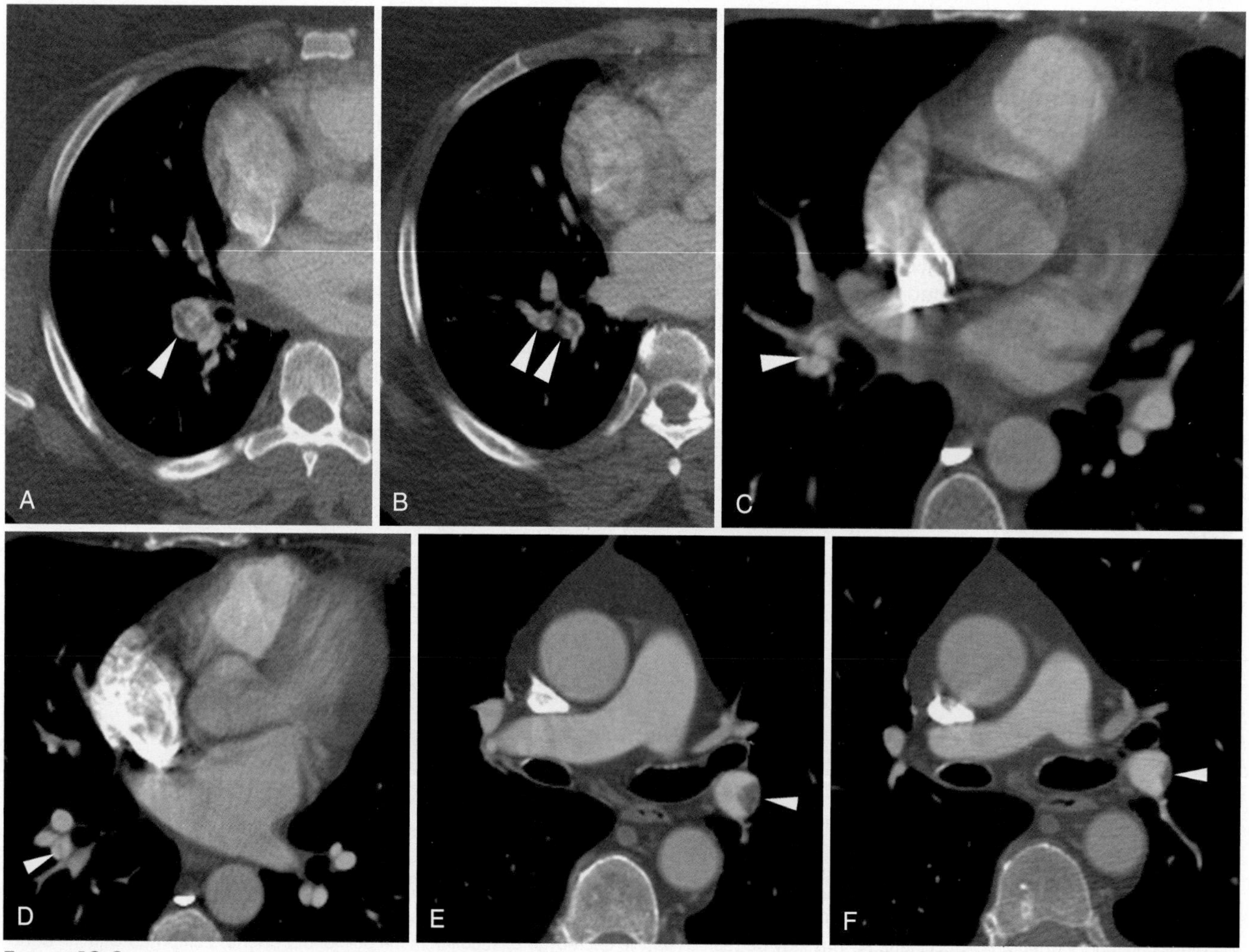

Figure 42.8. Chronic pulmonary embolism. As emboli *(arrowheads)* become chronic, they may recanalize (**A** and **B**) or form webs (**C** and **D**) within the artery lumen. **E**, An acute thrombus *(arrowhead)* in the left lower lobe. **F**, Several weeks later, the thrombus *(arrowhead)* is partly resolved but has developed a more eccentric appearance, with smooth margins and obtuse angles with the vessel wall.

TREATMENT

Treatment for PE and DVT depends on the hemodynamic status of the patient. This may range from therapy directed at removing the clot urgently, through intensive monitoring and supportive care, to long-term anticoagulation. Because there is a risk of fatality from any episode of PE, patients at a known high risk should undergo prophylactic treatment to prevent the development of thrombi and emboli. The appropriate therapeutic options depend on the overall clinical picture, including any planned or ongoing therapies, as well as the patient's immediate clinical status.

Patients with severe hemodynamic compromise require urgent therapy directed at removing the clot. This can include surgical embolectomy or systemic thrombolytic therapy. Catheter-directed thrombolytic therapy has received limited investigation but so far has not shown improvement in outcomes compared with systemic therapy.[2,55]

Surgical embolectomy for PE is primarily reserved for the most severely compromised patients.[56] European Society of Cardiology and British Thoracic Society guidelines suggest its use only for patients in cardiogenic shock or after failed thrombolytic therapy.[1,2] However, more recent reports suggest that the procedure may be more effective in patients with right ventricular compromise but without cardiogenic shock.[27] Other indications for surgery in patients who have cardiac compromise are those for whom thrombolytic therapy is contraindicated, such as after stroke or recent surgery or with other active bleeding, and those patients with paradoxical emboli or patent foramen ovale and emboli within the right heart chambers.

Thrombolytic therapy has predominantly been used in patients with evidence of cardiac dysfunction, particularly right heart dilatation or failure, and is probably not useful in patients without heart failure.[57] Minor bleeding complications are frequent, whereas major bleeding complications occur in 15% to 20% of patients, and intracranial hemorrhage or death occurs in fewer than 3% of patients.[56] The use of thrombolytic therapy alone does not appear to affect the rate of recurrent embolism and therefore may not change the long-term outcome in patients surviving to hospital discharge.[56]

Treatment of all acute PEs begins with early initiation of anticoagulation therapy. In patients with symptomatic embolism, survival is improved by early institution of anticoagulation therapy, usually in the emergency room.[58] A delay of 48 hours in achieving anticoagulation reduces overall survival. After initial rapid anticoagulation, transition to a long-term anticoagulation therapy can be achieved. Unfortunately, cancer patients have a higher risk of bleeding complications with long-term anticoagulation therapy, particularly with warfarin.[2,59] Recent trials have shown better long-term results with use of low molecular weight heparin (LMWH) injections rather than oral warfarin anticoagulation for the first 6 months after a PE event.[59,60] The CLOT (randomized comparison of low-molecular-weight heparin versus oral anticoagulant therapy for the prevention of recurrent venous thromboembolism in patients with cancer) trial found LMWH superior in its risk profile and equivalent in its prevention of recurrent PE.[61] There are no data on the need to continue anticoagulation after 6 months or comparing the use of specific agents after that time.

IVC filters have been used in the acute treatment of PE. Their effectiveness in the long-term setting is less certain, and there is no long-term mortality benefit for the addition of IVC filters to anticoagulation therapy. The use of IVC filters decreases the incidence of recurrent PE but is associated with increased risk of recurrent lower-extremity DVT. An additional complication in the setting of DVT is the development of postthrombotic syndrome, including pain, swelling, and skin changes in the affected limb. These symptoms can be difficult to distinguish from recurrent DVT. The use of graduated compression stockings is recommended and has been shown to reduce postthrombotic syndrome by up to 50%.[59]

The best treatment for catheter-related thrombosis is less clear. The incidence of symptomatic PE after catheter-related thrombosis is less than 10%.[4] There are no randomized, controlled trials to guide management using such catheters. It is not clear whether anticoagulation actually affects the resolution of catheter-associated thrombus. Catheter removal may have an effect on eventual thrombus resolution, but it need not be immediate removal. New catheters placed at different sites after a catheter-related thrombosis event frequently also develop catheter-related thrombus. As such, in the absence of catheter-related infections it is recommended that the catheter remain as long as it is needed and be removed once it is no longer necessary.[4,59]

Because of the significant mortality related to PE, prophylactic therapy is important. In postoperative patients, this includes compression devices and subcutaneous heparin in the immediate postoperative period.[27] The appropriate role and method of thromboembolic disease prevention in cancer patients is more complicated and not well established. Anticoagulation is probably appropriate in patients receiving chemotherapy combinations known to carry a high risk of venous thrombosis, but the needed duration of such therapy is unknown. The thrombosis risk must be weighed against complicating factors such as platelet dysfunction and drug-related coagulopathies in determining the appropriate treatment for a particular patient.

KEY POINTS Therapies

- Early anticoagulation is the mainstay of therapy for stable or unstable patients.
- Surgery is reserved for unstable patients, but it may be appropriate for stable patients with evidence of severe heart strain.
- Thrombolytic therapy is useful in unstable patients or those with heart strain, but it may not alter long-term outcomes.
- Inferior vena cava filters reduce the recurrence risk but increase the risk of lower extremity deep vein thrombosis and may not provide a long-term mortality benefit over anticoagulation alone.

CARDIAC MASSES AND TUMORS

Cardiac masses include metastatic tumor, benign and malignant primary tumor, thrombi and emboli, and endocardial vegetations. Although cardiac metastases are significantly more common than primary tumors, they usually occur late in the course of known cancer patients. Their imaging evaluation is usually focused on distinguishing metastasis from thrombus. Assessment of primary cardiac tumors focuses on identification of the likely tumor type based on location and imaging characteristics, as well as evaluating the need and potential for surgical resection.

EPIDEMIOLOGY AND RISK FACTORS

Primary cardiac tumors are rare, usually without any identifiable risk factors. The majority of primary cardiac tumors are benign myxomas and lipomas. Most primary cardiac malignancies are sarcomas, with angiosarcoma the most frequent histology. Approximately 10% of cardiac myxomas are familial, mostly as part of the Carney syndrome. Occasional cases of familial cardiac angiosarcoma have been noted. Sporadic myxomas are more common in women, whereas familial myxomas and primary sarcomas are more evenly distributed. Sporadic myxomas typically present in the sixth decade, familial myxomas in the third decade, and sarcomas in the fourth or fifth decade. Pulmonary artery sarcomas have an equal incidence in men and women, with a mean age at diagnosis of 50 years.[62]

Nontumor cardiac masses include thrombus and endocardial vegetations. Right atrial thrombi (Fig. 42.9) are usually related to central venous catheters, either initially arising on the catheter or at a site of endothelial injury near the catheter tip. Left atrial thrombi (Fig. 42.10) are usually attributed to atrial fibrillation and occur most often in the left atrial appendage because of stagnant blood pooling. They arise along the wall of the main left atrial chamber less often. Left ventricular thrombi (Fig. 42.11) usually develop at sites of ventricular infarct with aneurysm formation, most often at the ventricular apex. Thrombi in the right ventricle can occasionally be because of aneurysm but are most often entrapped emboli from systemic venous thrombus. Endocardial vegetations usually arise at the valve leaflet margins, but may occasionally be seen at any location in the heart.

Anatomic Distribution of Cardiac Tumors

Myxoma (Fig. 42.12) is the most common primary cardiac tumor.[63] Myxomas typically occur in the left atrium, or less often in the right atrium, and arise from the interatrial septum adjacent to the fossa ovalis. Larger tumors typically have a mobile component, which may protrude through the atrioventricular valve. These tumors are typically resected promptly because they can be fast-growing and because of the potential for mechanical valvular obstruction.

Lipomas (Fig. 42.13) are often identified incidentally at CT. Lipomas occur most often in epicardium along the atria or ventricles.[64] Lipomatous hypertrophy of the interatrial septum (Fig. 42.14) can be distinguished from lipoma by its wedge or dumbbell shape in the interatrial septum surrounding the fossa ovalis.

Although primary cardiac angiosarcomas (Fig. 42.15) are rare, they are the most common primary cardiac sarcoma, and the majority of primary right atrial masses are angiosarcomas.[65] Cardiac angiosarcomas present as diffuse wall thickening or focal masses involving the right atrium.[66] Most other histologic types of primary cardiac sarcomas (Fig. 42.16) tend to arise in the left atrium.[64] Primary cardiac lymphoma and rhabdomyosarcoma are more likely than other types to arise in the ventricles.[66]

Sarcomas of the pulmonary artery (Fig. 42.17) are most often leiomyosarcoma, but a variety of histologies occur at this location.[62] The tumor is usually confined to the lumen and wall of the pulmonary artery and can be difficult to distinguish from pulmonary artery emboli. However, at presentation they are often nearly completely filling the main or proximal pulmonary arteries in a pattern that is unusual for pulmonary embolism.[67]

KEY POINTS Common Primary Cardiac Mass or Tumor by Location

- Right atrium: Catheter-associated thrombus, angiosarcoma
- Left atrial appendage: Atrial fibrillation–related thrombus
- Left atrium: Myxoma, rarely sarcoma
- Right ventricle: Entrapped thromboemboli, sarcoma
- Left ventricle: Aneurysm-associated thrombus, sarcoma
- Cardiac valves: Endocardial vegetation

CLINICAL PRESENTATION

The clinical presentation of intracardiac thrombi depends on the cardiac chambers involved. Right heart thrombi are often asymptomatic and detected on thoracic imaging obtained for other purposes. They may result in pulmonary emboli with dyspnea. Left heart thrombi may also be detected incidentally but may present with stroke or other systemic embolism.

The presentation of cardiac tumor depends primarily on the location and size rather than histology. Tumor in the right atrium may cause tricuspid obstruction with resulting decreased cardiac output and systemic edema. An invasive right atrial angiosarcoma may extend to involve the tricuspid annulus, with resulting tricuspid insufficiency, or may involve the right coronary artery, resulting in ischemic chest pain.[66] Tumor of the left atrium may cause mitral obstruction with decreased cardiac output and pulmonary edema. Patients typically present with dyspnea or palpitations. Lipoma or lipomatous hypertrophy of the interatrial septum are most often asymptomatic but may be associated with arrhythmias.[64] Myocardial tumor involvement in the ventricles may be asymptomatic unless located at the valve or outflow tract. Even when smaller, myocardial tumors can affect the conduction system, with resulting arrhythmia. When large, overall ventricular function may be compromised, resulting in dyspnea and heart failure. Epicardial tumor may present with pericardial effusion, and rarely pericardial constriction. Tumors arising from the valves may interfere with valve function and cause symptoms of either insufficiency

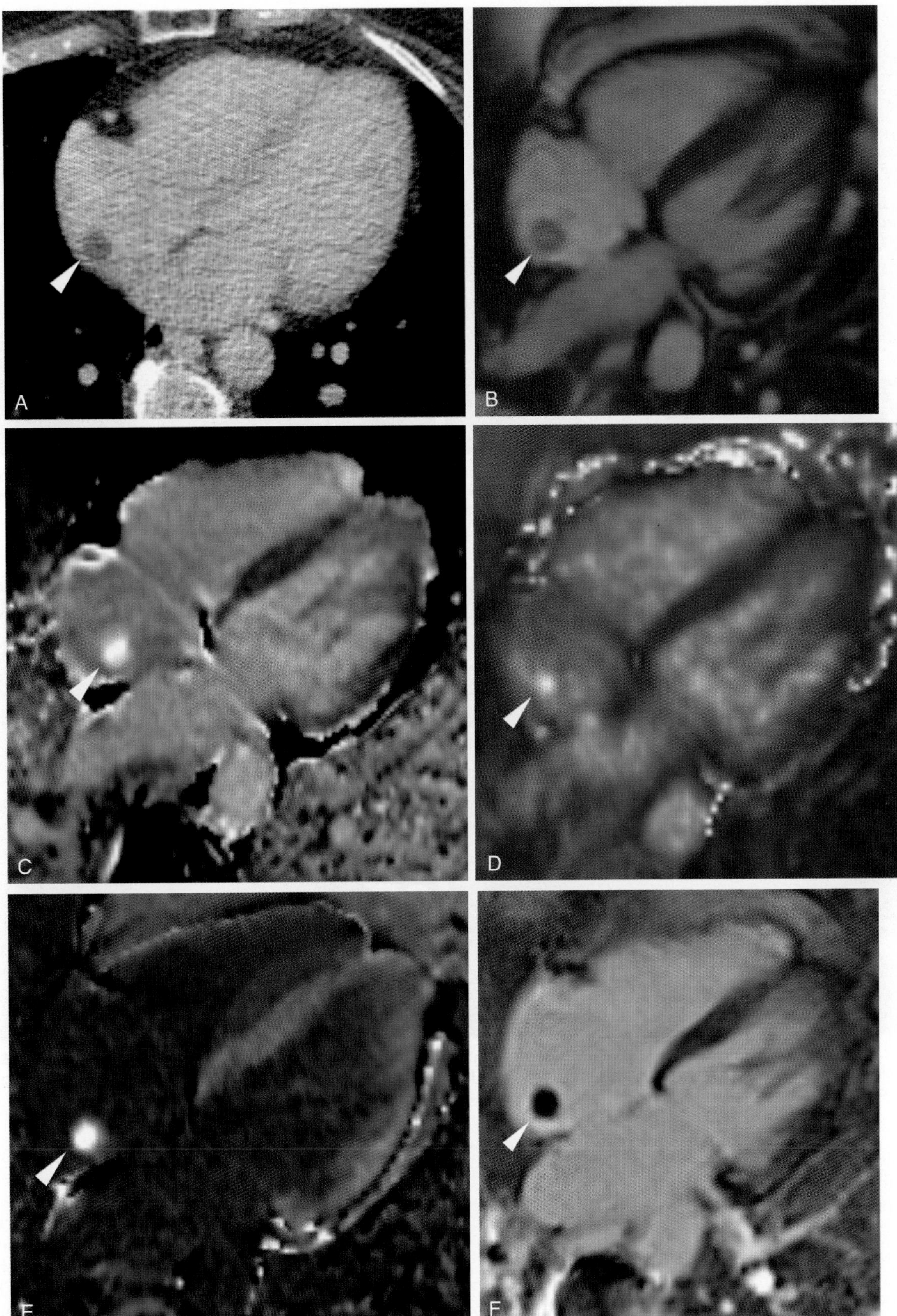

Figure 42.9. A 62-year-old woman with left rib chondrosarcoma and prior central venous catheter. **A**, At computed tomography, thrombus in the right atrium *(arrowhead)* is often most clearly seen on delayed images because early images during contrast injection often have significant mixing artifacts. These thrombi are usually related to central venous catheter placement and may be attached to the catheter or to the right atrial wall, often along the crista terminalis. White blood cine magnetic resonance imaging (**B**) shows the thrombus (*arrowheads* in **B–F**) along the right atrial wall with high signal on T1 map (**C**), T2 map (**D**), and postcontrast T1 map (**E**). Postcontrast imaging (**F**) demonstrates lack of enhancement.

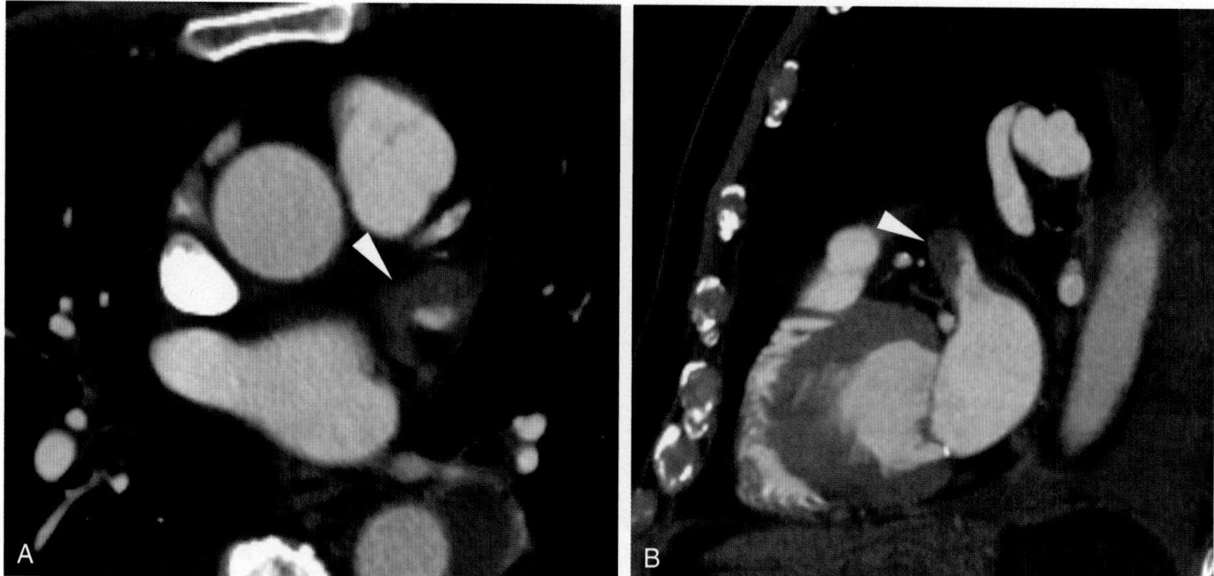

FIGURE 42.10. A 81-year-old man with lung cancer and left atrial appendage thrombus. Thrombi in the left atrial appendage (*arrowheads* in **A**, **B**) are related to poor function and slow flow in the appendage owing to atrial fibrillation. Flow artifacts can also be seen in this location as intermediate attenuation, often with a horizontal ill-defined margin. Flow artifacts resolve on delayed imaging, whereas thrombus will persist.

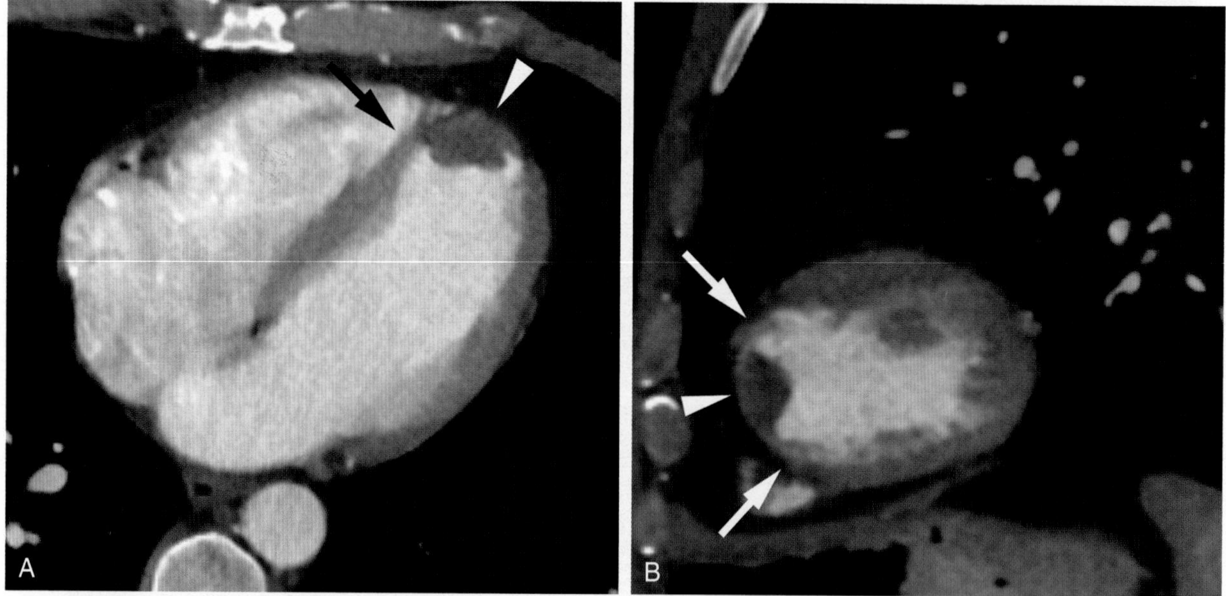

FIGURE 42.11. A 40-year-old man with testicular cancer and left ventricular thrombus. Thrombus in the left ventricle (*arrowheads* in **A**, **B**) is most often associated with infarct at the site of wall thinning (*arrows* in **A**, **B**) and motion abnormality. Thrombi with lobular or irregular margins have higher risk of systemic embolization.

or stenosis, depending on the size and exact location. Pulmonary artery sarcomas typically present with chest pain, dyspnea, or intractable congestive cardiac failure.[62]

KEY POINTS Clinical Presentation

- Pulmonary embolism from right heart thrombi.
- Systemic embolism from left heart thrombi.
- Tumor symptoms dependent on location and size:
  - Obstructive symptoms with heart failure and dyspnea.
  - Arrhythmia.

IMAGING EVALUATION

Both magnetic resonance imaging (MRI) and CT have been successfully used for imaging of cardiac tumors. Of the two modalities, MRI has a longer established history of successful evaluation of cardiac pathology.[68,69] The primary advantages of MRI have been the lack of ionizing radiation, the ability to gate the image acquisition to the cardiac cycle, high temporal resolution, and direct acquisition of arbitrary imaging planes. Additionally, assessment of perfusion and enhancement at MRI is effective in

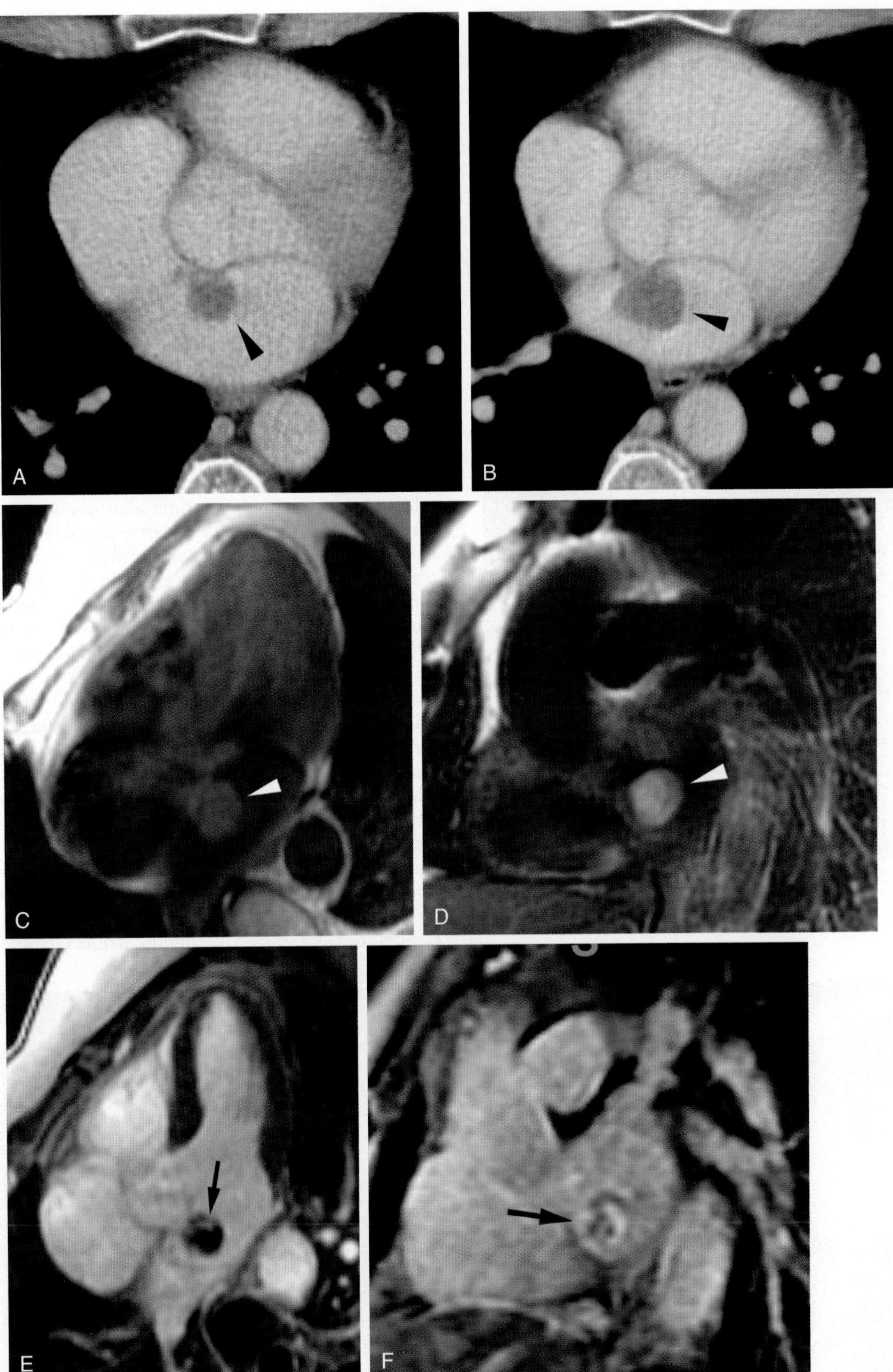

FIGURE 42.12. A 58-year-old woman with pancreatic neuroendocrine tumor and myxoma. Initial (**A**) and 2-month follow-up (**B**) computed tomography demonstrates a growing mass (*arrowheads* in **A–D**) attached to the interatrial septum between the aortic root and fossa ovalis, the most common location for myxoma. The mass has signal similar to muscle on double inversion recovery (**C**) and high signal on T2-weighted fat-saturated (**D**) images. Early postcontrast long TI (**E**) images show minimal enhancement (*arrows* on **E**, **F**), accentuated on delayed myocardial enhancement (**F**) images.

distinguishing tumor from nontumor masses. However, cardiac MRI can be more demanding than CT in terms of exam setup, patient cooperation, examination time, and technologist training.

Magnetic Resonance Imaging

Cardiac MRI uses a variety of acquisition sequences to evaluate the structure and function of the heart and provide tissue characterization. The most widely used techniques for cardiac tumor imaging include dark blood and white blood sequences, first-pass perfusion, and early and delayed postcontrast imaging. Dark blood imaging can be obtained with single-shot fast spin echo sequences that allow acquisition of multiple images at different slice positions during a single breathhold.[70] These sequences are typically used for anatomic survey and setup of imaging planes. White blood sequences are acquired as a series of images in each imaging plane to allow demonstration of the motion of solid structures and flowing blood. Steady-state free precession sequences have become the standard method of white blood cine imaging.[71] They are important for both anatomic and functional evaluation. First-pass perfusion and delayed myocardial enhancement imaging are used for tissue characterization, principally for distinguishing viable tumor from necrosis or thrombus. These require the use of gadolinium-based contrast media. Myocardial delayed enhancement imaging is best performed using a dose of 0.2 mg gadolinium/kg body weight and performed approximately 10 to 20 minutes after contrast administration. An inversion pulse is used to null the signal from normal myocardium, and the inversion time (TI) is selected using an inversion time scout sequence. The myocardial nulling increases the relative signal from tissues that have increased extracellular space, and therefore increased contrast media concentration compared with normal myocardium. This sequence can also be used immediately after contrast administration with a long inversion time (TI = 600 ms) to identify tissues with any enhancement and distinguish them from thrombus or necrosis.

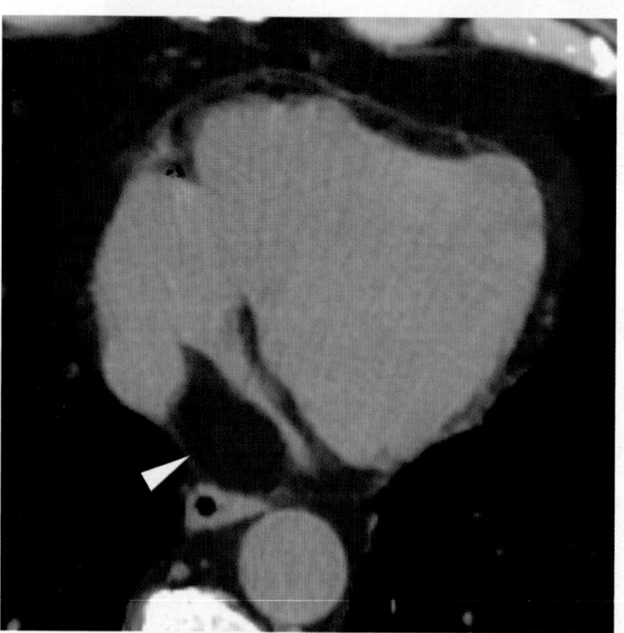

FIGURE 42.13. A 71-year-old man with prostate cancer and cardiac lipoma. Cardiac lipomas *(arrowhead)* are encapsulated fat attenuation masses that most frequently occur along the epicardium and atrioventricular grooves.

Most MRI sequences are performed with relatively thick slices, around 8 to 10 mm. As a result, it is necessary to select optimal imaging planes at the time of scanning. The commonly used imaging planes include 2-, 3-, and 4-chamber long axis views through the middle of the left ventricle and a stack of short axis images covering the ventricles or whole heart as necessary. Because many cardiac tumors and masses involve the right heart, vertical or inflow/outflow long axis images of the right ventricle are often useful. One or more of the long axis sequences may be acquired as a stack covering the whole chamber or heart

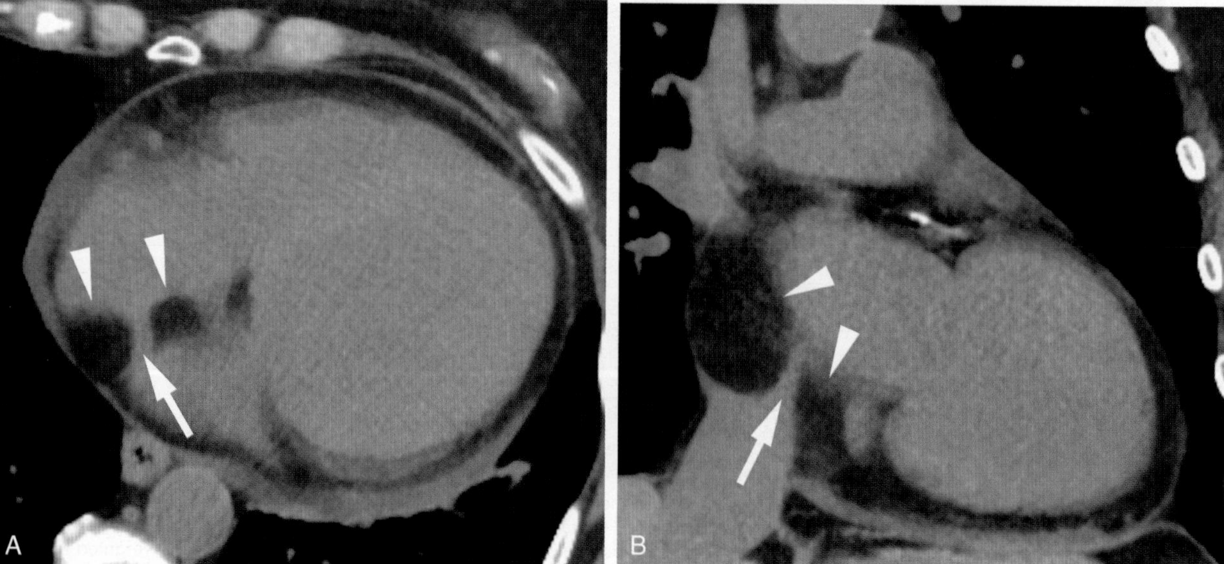

FIGURE 42.14. A 68-year-old woman with multiple myeloma. Lipomatous hypertrophy of the interatrial septum (*arrowheads* in **A**, **B**) is identified by its typical location and sparing of the fossa ovalis (*arrows* in **A**, **B**), creating a dumbbell appearance.

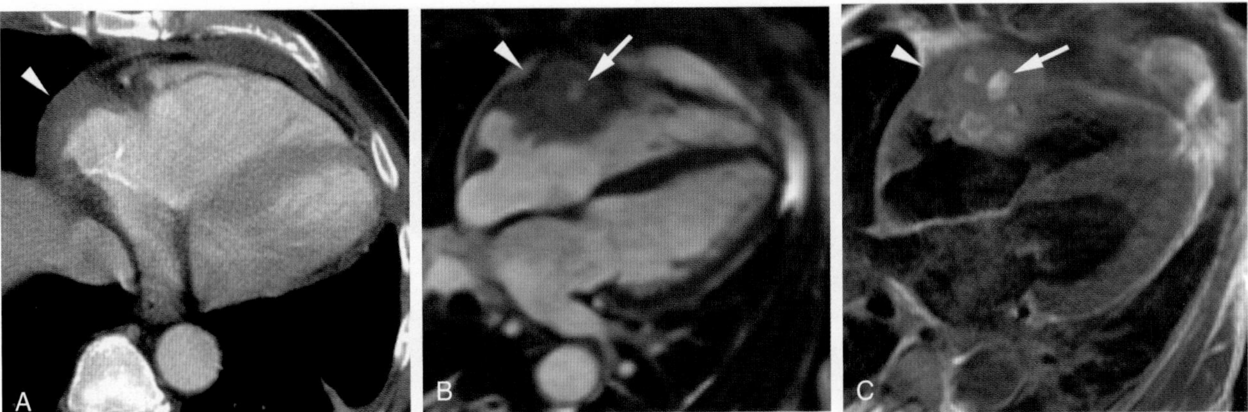

FIGURE 42.15. A 60-year-old man with cardiac angiosarcoma. Cardiac angiosarcoma is the most common primary cardiac malignancy and occurs most often along the free wall of the right atrium. The tumor (*arrowheads* in **A–C**) seen as wall thickening on computed tomography (**A**) had increased significantly at magnetic resonance imaging 4 months later. White blood cine (**B**) and double inversion recovery (**C**) reveal high signal vascular channels (*arrows* in **B**, **C**) within the tumor. Involvement of the right coronary artery and tricuspid valve are important features that would complicate surgical resection.

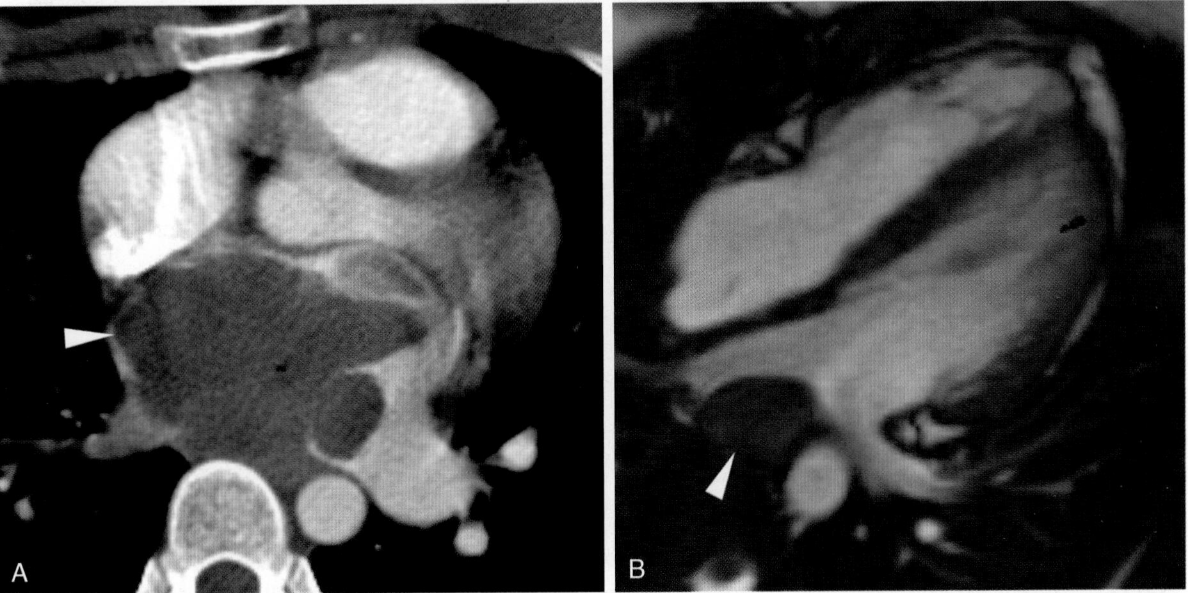

FIGURE 42.16. A 37-year-old female with spindle cell sarcoma of the left atrium. Large tumor (*arrowheads* in **A**, **B**) filling most of the left atrium on presentation (**A**) was suspected of being myxoma because of location, but the large size and multilobular configuration should prompt consideration of sarcoma. The mass was promptly resected because of concerns for obstruction or embolization, but was found to be sarcoma and had recurred at follow-up magnetic resonance imaging (**B**) 3 months later. Difficulty visualizing the entire wall of the left atrium at surgery makes curative resection difficult.

to provide complete anatomic evaluation. Because each slice is acquired during a breathhold, the optimal imaging planes and coverage should be identified before the exam, if possible, and reevaluated during the exam to minimize the total exam time.

Computed Tomography

Cardiac CT can be acquired with retrospective or prospective electrocardiogram gating. Because high or irregular heart rates can result in cardiac pulsation artifact even on gated CT, it is often effective to use short-acting beta-blockers to reduce the heart rate. In retrospective gating, images are acquired throughout the cardiac cycle, which allows generation of cine images allowing functional and motion assessment. The use of dose modulation provides optimal image quality at diastole, with lower dose and therefore noisier images through the remainder of the cardiac cycle to reduce total radiation dose. Prospective gating obtains images only at a selected cardiac phase, usually end diastole, in order to minimize total radiation dose.[72]

Intravenous contrast material is used to allow accurate delineation of the endocardial and epicardial contours, identification of intraluminal thrombus or mass, and visualization of the coronary arteries.[73] Contrast media is typically injected at 5 mL/second to optimize luminal enhancement and visualization of smaller structures, including coronary arteries. Optimal contrast timing may be achieved using bolus tracking. To reduce streak artifact from high-density contrast material in the IVC and right atrium, a saline bolus is used immediately following the contrast media, usually at a lower rate of 3 mL/second.

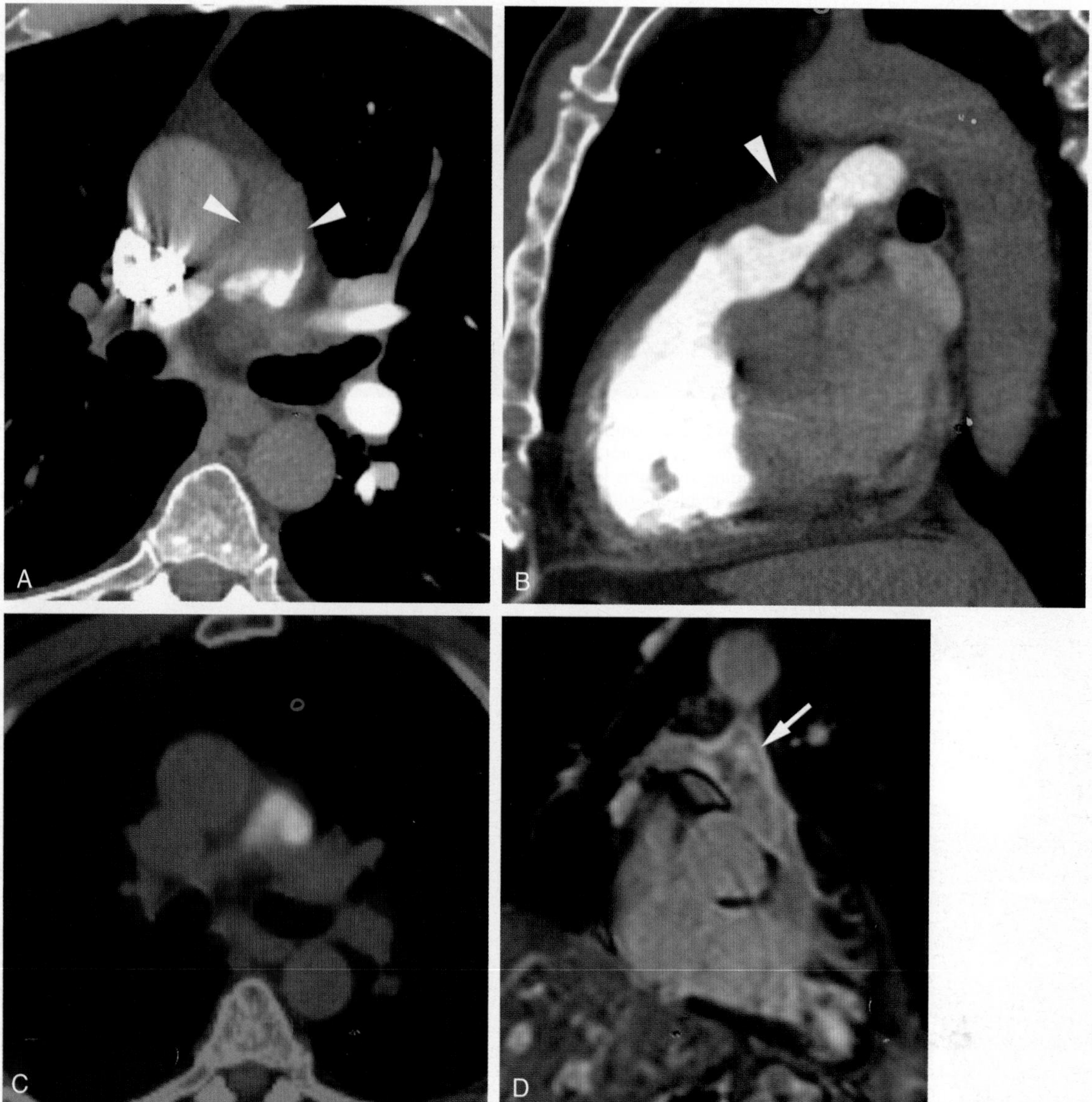

FIGURE 42.17. A 72-year-old man with a pulmonary artery sarcoma . The tumor (*arrowheads* in **A**, **B**) is attached to the mid wall of the main pulmonary artery separate from the bifurcation, unlike a saddle pulmonary embolus. Positron emission tomography (**C**) demonstrated (^{18}F)-fluorodeoxyglucose uptake, and magnetic resonance imaging demonstrates enhancement of the tumor (*arrow* in **D**), excluding thrombus.

Early scanning often has complex streak and flow artifacts in the right atrium lumen, so right atrial luminal tumors may be delineated better on delayed images obtained 60 to 90 seconds after the beginning of contrast injection.

Because the CT is obtained as a near isotropic volume, optimal imaging planes can be determined interactively with post processing software after the scan is completed. This simplifies and dramatically shortens the acquisition compared with MRI.

Cardiac Mass Assessment

Anatomic location and enhancement are important features in narrowing the differential for cardiac masses. Both MRI and CT are able to differentiate intracardiac thrombi and emboli from tumor based on characteristic locations and the lack of enhancement compared with both the intraluminal contrast material and the enhancing normal myocardium.[73,74] MRI is particularly helpful in the right atrium because mixing artifacts from inflowing blood limit assessment of right atrial structures at CT.

Although myxoma can be demonstrated at routine CT, cardiac gated MRI or CT may be needed for more complete evaluation.[63,64] These modalities can better delineate the attachment of the tumor and mobility of the tumor through the cardiac cycle to aid in surgical planning. Cardiac lipomas typically need no further evaluation after identification on conventional CT. If resection is considered because of local mass effect, then a cardiac gated MRI or CT may be useful.

Cross-sectional imaging is important in the evaluation of sarcoma patients to identify the local extent of involvement and to assess the potential for surgical resection. Cardiac gated MRI can demonstrate relationship of the tumor to myocardial, valvular, and coronary artery structures.[66,75] MRI has been the predominant imaging modality for the precise delineation of tumor extent because of its high temporal and spatial resolution, as well as its high tissue contrast. However, the increasing availability of cardiac gated CT and its ease of use make it valuable in the evaluation of response to therapy.

KEY POINTS The Radiology Report

- Tumor location and enhancement.
- Local tumor extent, including valve or coronary involvement.
- Valve obstruction/stenosis or insufficiency.

TREATMENT

Cardiac thrombi are treated with anticoagulation, similar to pulmonary or systemic thromboemboli. They may require prolonged or ongoing anticoagulation if the etiology of thrombus persists, as with left ventricular aneurysm or persistent atrial fibrillation. Thrombi with polypoid projections or mobile components are more likely to have subsequent embolic events than flat mural thrombi.[74] In patients with contraindications to prolonged anticoagulation, atrial appendage thrombi related to atrial fibrillation may be treated by ligation or occlusion of the appendage.[76]

Cardiac sarcomas frequently have metastases at presentation. Additionally, complete resection with negative margins is important for optimal outcomes in patients with tumor limited to the heart. Because complete resection is often difficult at presentation, aggressive chemotherapy is used prior to surgery to increase the opportunity for a negative margin resection. Surgery is typically offered only to patients with complete or nearly complete response to chemotherapy at all metastatic sites and substantial local tumor response.[77] Early resection may be contemplated when the tumor is causing symptoms, either obstructive mass effect or arrhythmia.[66]

KEY POINTS Therapy

- Anticoagulation for intracardiac thrombi may be prolonged or ongoing.
- Cardiac sarcomas are treated with chemotherapy to maximal response before considering curative surgery.
- Early surgery may be considered for symptomatic relief.

CONCLUSION

PE is a challenging complication in cancer patients. Cancer increases the risk of venous thromboembolism through local and humoral effects, and cancer treatments can contribute further. The presence of PE is most readily determined with CT pulmonary angiography, which provides information on the extent of embolic disease and heart strain. The development of PE is an indicator of poor prognosis in cancer patients, whether reflecting a later stage of disease or owing to the induced respiratory failure. Therefore, treatment and prevention of PE are important in the management of cancer patients.

Imaging of cardiac masses is important for the distinction of malignant tumors from benign tumors and thrombi in order to direct clinical therapy. Location and imaging characteristics are important in identifying thrombi and tumor types. Imaging is also important in monitoring response to therapy and determining appropriate timing for surgery. In patients where resection is considered, imaging can help determine the feasibility of surgery and plan the surgical approach.

REFERENCES

1. Guidelines on diagnosis and management of acute pulmonary embolism. Task Force on Pulmonary Embolism, European Society of Cardiology. Core Writing Group: A. Torbicki (Chairman), E. J. R. van Beek (Editor), B. Charbonnier etal., Internal reviewers: G. Kronik, J. Widimsky, *Eur Heart J*. 2000;21:1301–1336.
2. British Thoracic Society guidelines for the management of suspected acute pulmonary embolism. *Thorax*. 2003;58:470–483.
3. Lee AY, Levine MN. Venous thromboembolism and cancer: risks and outcomes. *Circulation*. 2003;107:I17–I21.
4. Jones MA, Lee DY, Segall JA, et al. Characterizing resolution of catheter-associated upper extremity deep venous thrombosis. *J Vasc Surg*. 2010;51:108–113.
5. Metafratzi ZM, Vassiliou MP, Maglaras GC, et al. Acute pulmonary embolism: correlation of CT pulmonary artery obstruction index with blood gas values. *AJR Am J Roentgenol*. 2006;186:213–219.
6. The European Cooperative Study on the clinical significance of right heart thrombi. European Working Group on Echocardiography. *Eur Heart J*. 1989;10:1046–1059.
7. Chartier L, Bera J, Delomez M, et al. Free-floating thrombi in the right heart: diagnosis, management, and prognostic indexes in 38 consecutive patients. *Circulation*. 1999;99:2779–2783.
8. Torbicki A, Galie N, Covezzoli A, et al. Right heart thrombi in pulmonary embolism: results from the International Cooperative Pulmonary Embolism Registry. *J Am Coll Cardiol*. 2003;41:2245–2251.
9. Sinner WN. Computed tomographic patterns of pulmonary thromboembolism and infarction. *J Comput Assist Tomogr*. 1978;2:395–399.
10. Bounameaux H, Perrier A, Righini M. Diagnosis of venous thromboembolism: an update. *Vasc Med*. 2010;15:399–406.
11. Stein PD, Terrin ML, Hales CA, et al. Clinical, laboratory, roentgenographic, and electrocardiographic findings in patients with acute pulmonary embolism and no pre-existing cardiac or pulmonary disease. *Chest*. 1991;100:598–603.
12. Storto ML, Di Credico A, Guido F, et al. Incidental detection of pulmonary emboli on routine MDCT of the chest. *AJR Am J Roentgenol*. 2005;184:264–267.
13. Engelke C, Rummeny EJ, Marten K. Pulmonary embolism at multidetector row CT of chest: one-year survival of treated and untreated patients. *Radiology*. 2006;239:563–575.
14. Gladish GW, Choe DH, Marom EM, et al. Incidental pulmonary emboli in oncology patients: prevalence, CT evaluation, and natural history. *Radiology*. 2006;240:246–255.
15. O'Connell CL, Boswell WD, Duddalwar V, et al. Unsuspected pulmonary emboli in cancer patients: clinical correlates and relevance. *J Clin Oncol*. 2006;24:4928–4932.
16. Ritchie G, McGurk S, McCreath C, et al. Prospective evaluation of unsuspected pulmonary embolism on contrast enhanced multidetector CT (MDCT) scanning. *Thorax*. 2007;62:536–540.
17. Hui GC, Legasto A, Wittram C. The prevalence of symptomatic and coincidental pulmonary embolism on computed tomography. *J Comput Assist Tomogr*. 2008;32:783–787.
18. Donato AA, Khoche S, Santora J, et al. Clinical outcomes in patients with isolated subsegmental pulmonary emboli diagnosed by multidetector CT pulmonary angiography. *Thromb Res*. 2010;126:e266–e270.

19. Sun JM, Kim TS, Lee J, et al. Unsuspected pulmonary emboli in lung cancer patients: the impact on survival and the significance of anticoagulation therapy. *Lung Cancer*. 2010;69:330–336.
20. Yusuf SW, Gladish G, Lenihan DJ, et al. Computerized tomographic finding of saddle pulmonary embolism is associated with high mortality in cancer patients. *Intern Med J*. 2010;40:293–299.
21. Mastora I, Remy-Jardin M, Masson P, et al. Severity of acute pulmonary embolism: evaluation of a new spiral CT angiographic score in correlation with echocardiographic data. *Eur Radiol*. 2003;13:29–35.
22. Miller GA, Sutton GC, Kerr IH, et al. Comparison of streptokinase and heparin in treatment of isolated acute massive pulmonary embolism. *Br Med J*. 1971;2:681–684.
23. Qanadli SD, El Hajjam M, Vieillard-Baron A, et al. New CT index to quantify arterial obstruction in pulmonary embolism: comparison with angiographic index and echocardiography. *AJR Am J Roentgenol*. 2001;176:1415–1420.
24. Engelke C, Rummeny EJ, Marten K. Acute pulmonary embolism on MDCT of the chest: prediction of cor pulmonale and short-term patient survival from morphologic embolus burden. *AJR Am J Roentgenol*. 2006;186:1265–1271.
25. Lu MT, Cai T, Ersoy H, et al. Interval increase in right-left ventricular diameter ratios at CT as a predictor of 30-day mortality after acute pulmonary embolism: initial experience. *Radiology*. 2008;246:281–287.
26. van der Meer RW, Pattynama PM, van Strijen MJ, et al. Right ventricular dysfunction and pulmonary obstruction index at helical CT: prediction of clinical outcome during 3-month follow-up in patients with acute pulmonary embolism. *Radiology*. 2005;235:798–803.
27. Carvalho EM, Macedo FI, Panos AL, et al. Pulmonary embolectomy: recommendation for early surgical intervention. *J Card Surg*. 2010;25:261–266.
28. Ocak I, Fuhrman C. CT angiography findings of the left atrium and right ventricle in patients with massive pulmonary embolism. *AJR Am J Roentgenol*. 2008;191:1072–1076.
29. Reid JH, Murchison JT. Acute right ventricular dilatation: a new helical CT sign of massive pulmonary embolism. *Clin Radiol*. 1998;53:694–698.
30. Schoepf UJ, Kucher N, Kipfmueller F, et al. Right ventricular enlargement on chest computed tomography: a predictor of early death in acute pulmonary embolism. *Circulation*. 2004;110:3276–3280.
31. Sukhija R, Aronow WS, Lee J, et al. Association of right ventricular dysfunction with in-hospital mortality in patients with acute pulmonary embolism and reduction in mortality in patients with right ventricular dysfunction by pulmonary embolectomy. *Am J Cardiol*. 2005;95:695–696.
32. Edwards PD, Bull RK, Coulden R. CT measurement of main pulmonary artery diameter. *Br J Radiol*. 1998;71:1018–1020.
33. Kuriyama K, Gamsu G, Stern RG, et al. CT-determined pulmonary artery diameters in predicting pulmonary hypertension. *Invest Radiol*. 1984;19:16–22.
34. Ghaye B, Ghuysen A, Bruyere PJ, et al. Can CT pulmonary angiography allow assessment of severity and prognosis in patients presenting with pulmonary embolism? What the radiologist needs to know. *Radiographics*. 2006;26:23–39; discussion 39–40.
35. Ng CS, Wells AU, Padley SPA. CT sign of chronic pulmonary arterial hypertension: the ratio of main pulmonary artery to aortic diameter. *J Thorac Imaging*. 1999;14:270–278.
36. Ghuysen A, Ghaye B, Willems V, et al. Computed tomographic pulmonary angiography and prognostic significance in patients with acute pulmonary embolism. *Thorax*. 2005;60:956–961.
37. Goodman LR, Stein PD, Matta F, et al. CT venography and compression sonography are diagnostically equivalent: data from PIOPED II. *AJR Am J Roentgenol*. 2007;189:1071–1076.
38. Worsley DF, Alavi A, Aronchick JM, et al. Chest radiographic findings in patients with acute pulmonary embolism: observations from the PIOPED Study. *Radiology*. 1993;189:133–136.
39. Sostman HD, Stein PD, Gottschalk A, et al. Acute pulmonary embolism: sensitivity and specificity of ventilation-perfusion scintigraphy in PIOPED II study. *Radiology*. 2008;246:941–946.
40. Remy-Jardin M, Pistolesi M, Goodman LR, et al. Management of suspected acute pulmonary embolism in the era of CT angiography: a statement from the Fleischner Society. *Radiology*. 2007;245:315–329.
41. Remy-Jardin M, Remy J. Spiral CT angiography of the pulmonary circulation. *Radiology*. 1999;212:615–636.
42. Patel S, Kazerooni EA, Cascade PN. Pulmonary embolism: optimization of small pulmonary artery visualization at multi-detector row CT. *Radiology*. 2003;227:455–460.
43. Schoepf UJ, Holzknecht N, Helmberger TK, et al. Subsegmental pulmonary emboli: improved detection with thin-collimation multi-detector row spiral CT. *Radiology*. 2002;222:483–490.
44. Kalra MK, Rizzo S, Maher MM, et al. Chest CT performed with z-axis modulation: scanning protocol and radiation dose. *Radiology*. 2005;237:303–308.
45. Prakash P, Kalra MK, Digumarthy SR, et al. Radiation dose reduction with chest computed tomography using adaptive statistical iterative reconstruction technique: initial experience. *J Comput Assist Tomogr*. 2010;34:40–45.
46. Heyer CM, Mohr PS, Lemburg SP, et al. Image quality and radiation exposure at pulmonary CT angiography with 100- or 120-kVp protocol: prospective randomized study. *Radiology*. 2007;245:577–583.
47. Hartmann IJ, Wittenberg R, Schaefer-Prokop C. Imaging of acute pulmonary embolism using multi-detector CT angiography: an update on imaging technique and interpretation. *Eur J Radiol*. 2010;74:40–49.
48. Wittram C. How I do it: CT pulmonary angiography. *AJR Am J Roentgenol*. 2007;188:1255–1261.
49. Yankelevitz DF, Shaham D, Shah A, et al. Optimization of contrast delivery for pulmonary CT angiography. *Clin Imaging*. 1998;22:398–403.
50. Gosselin MV, Rassner UA, Thieszen SL, et al. Contrast dynamics during CT pulmonary angiogram: analysis of an inspiration associated artifact. *J Thorac Imaging*. 2004;19:1–7.
51. Kuzo RS, Pooley RA, Crook JE, et al. Measurement of caval blood flow with MRI during respiratory maneuvers: implications for vascular contrast opacification on pulmonary CT angiographic studies. *AJR Am J Roentgenol*. 2007;188:839–842.
52. Wittram C, Yoo AJ. Transient interruption of contrast on CT pulmonary angiography: proof of mechanism. *J Thorac Imaging*. 2007;22:125–129.
53. Remy-Jardin M, Remy J, Artaud D, et al. Spiral CT of pulmonary embolism: diagnostic approach, interpretive pitfalls and current indications. *Eur Radiol*. 1998;8:1376–1390.
54. Wittram C, Maher MM, Yoo AJ, et al. CT angiography of pulmonary embolism: diagnostic criteria and causes of misdiagnosis. *Radiographics*. 2004;24:1219–1238.
55. Todoran TM, Sobieszczyk P. Catheter-based therapies for massive pulmonary embolism. *Prog Cardiovasc Dis*. 2010;52:429–437.
56. Samoukovic G, Malas T, deVarennes B. The role of pulmonary embolectomy in the treatment of acute pulmonary embolism: a literature review from 1968 to 2008. *Interact Cardiovasc Thorac Surg*. 2010;11:265–270.
57. Jenkins PO, Sultanzadeh J, Bhagwat M, et al. Should thrombolysis have a greater role in the management of pulmonary embolism? *Clin Med*. 2009;9:431–435.
58. Smith SB, Geske JB, Maguire JM, et al. Early anticoagulation is associated with reduced mortality for acute pulmonary embolism. *Chest*. 2010;137:1382–1390.
59. Coleman R, MacCallum P. Treatment and secondary prevention of venous thromboembolism in cancer. *Br J Cancer*. 2010;102:S17–S23.
60. Tran QN. Role of palliative low-molecular-weight heparin for treating venous thromboembolism in patients with advanced cancer. *Am J Hosp Palliat Care*. 2010;27:416–419.
61. Lee AY, Levine MN, Baker RI, et al. Low-molecular-weight heparin versus a coumarin for the prevention of recurrent venous thromboembolism in patients with cancer. *N Engl J Med*. 2003;349:146–153.
62. Sethi GK, Slaven JE, Kepes JJ, et al. Primary sarcoma of the pulmonary artery. *J Thorac Cardiovasc Surg*. 1972;63:587–593.
63. Grebenc ML, Rosado-de-Christenson ML, Green CE, et al. Cardiac myxoma: imaging features in 83 patients. *Radiographics*. 2002;22:673–689.
64. Grebenc ML, Rosado de Christenson ML, Burke AP, et al. Primary cardiac and pericardial neoplasms: radiologic-pathologic correlation. *Radiographics*. 2000;20:1073–1103; quiz 1110–1071, 1112.
65. Colucci WS, Schoen FJ, Braunwald E. Primary tumors of the heart. In: Braunwald E, ed. *Heart Disease: A Textbook of Cardiovascular Medicine*. 5th ed. Philadelphia: Saunders; 1997:1464–1477.
66. Araoz PA, Eklund HE, Welch TJ, et al. CT and MR imaging of primary cardiac malignancies. *Radiographics*. 1999;19:1421–1434.

67. Kauczor HU, Schwickert HC, Mayer E, et al. Pulmonary artery sarcoma mimicking Cardiovasc Intervent Radiol thromboembolic disease: computed tomography and magnetic resonance imaging findings. *Cardiovasc Intervent Radiol*. 1994;17:185–189.
68. Lanzer P, Botvinick EH, Schiller NB, et al. Cardiac imaging using gated magnetic resonance. *Radiology*. 1984;150:121–127.
69. Edelman RR. Contrast-enhanced MR imaging of the heart: overview of the literature. *Radiology*. 2004;232:653–668.
70. Vignaux OB, Augui J, Coste J, et al. Comparison of single-shot fast spin-echo and conventional spin-echo sequences for MR imaging of the heart: initial experience. *Radiology*. 2001;219:545–550.
71. Lee VS, Resnick D, Bundy JM, et al. Cardiac function: MR evaluation in one breath hold with real-time true fast imaging with steady-state precession. *Radiology*. 2002;222:835–842.
72. Desjardins B, Kazerooni EA. ECG-gated cardiac CT. *AJR Am J Roentgenol*. 2004;182:993–1010.
73. Boxt LM, Lipton MJ, Kwong RY, et al. Computed tomography for assessment of cardiac chambers, valves, myocardium and pericardium. *Cardiol Clin*. 2003;21:561–585.
74. Barkhausen J, Hunold P, Eggebrecht H, et al. Detection and characterization of intracardiac thrombi on MR imaging. *AJR Am J Roentgenol*. 2002;179:1539–1544.
75. Gilkeson RC, Chiles C. MR evaluation of cardiac and pericardial malignancy. *Magn Reson Imaging Clin N Am*. 2003;11:173–186.
76. Reddy VY, Sievert H, Halperin J, et al. Percutaneous left atrial appendage closure vs warfarin for atrial fibrillation: a randomized clinical trial. *JAMA*. 2014;312:1988–1998.
77. Ramlawi B, Leja MJ, Abu Saleh WK, et al. Surgical treatment of primary cardiac sarcomas: review of a single-institution experience. *Ann Thorac Surg*. 2016;101:698–702.

PART XII PROTOCOLS IN ONCOLOGIC IMAGING

CHAPTER 43 Protocols for Imaging Studies in the Oncologic Patient

Paul M. Silverman, M.D.

Well-thought-out protocols for imaging are critical to ensure that the resultant images have the best possible chance to answer the clinical question. In the case of oncologic patients, this usually hinges on whether disease is stable, has regressed, or has progressed and whether there are new sites of disease. Beyond these fundamental questions, our patients may have unexpected findings, as well as complications from therapy. The ability to answer such questions relies on high-quality images and, in the case of computed tomography (CT), the best quality titrated with the least radiation exposure, because patients generally go into a lifetime of surveillance. This is a significant challenge. In patients undergoing imaging for surgical intervention, especially for cure, these studies need to be directly targeted to the most likely sites of metastases (e.g., high-quality liver imaging for metastases in patients with orbital, choroidal melanoma) and have optimal image quality to detect metastatic disease.[1–5] Imaging with multidetector computed tomography (MDCT) can be performed in multiple phases, and developing protocols to detect hyper- as well as hypovascular metastases is critical in evaluating patients with tumors such as carcinoid, islet cell tumors of the pancreas, and a number of other primaries. Timing of the contrast bolus and subsequent imaging is critical in magnetic resonance imaging (MRI) as well as current MDCT scanning.[6–8]

The charts provide a selection of common protocols developed by authors of this textbook and used in their daily practice. The protocols were prepared January 2010. They are grouped together in one chapter rather than being individually recorded for the reader's convenience. They are simply provided for a reference within the context of this textbook, and scanning protocols should be developed and tailored to each individual physician's practice.

MULTIDETECTOR COMPUTED TOMOGRAPHY: COMPUTED TOMOGRAPHY IMAGING

Chest Protocols (MDCT 64 Slice)

Aorta (Gated Study)
Cardiac Tumor (Gated Study)
Chest with Contrast
Chest without Contrast
Coronary Artery Screening (Gated Study)
Esophageal Leak Protocol
Low-Dose Surveillance Chest with Contrast (Nodule or Lung Cancer)
Perfusion Chest without and with Contrast
Pulmonary Embolism Protocol
Superior Vena Cava Venogram
Chest with Contrast (Virtual Bronchoscopy)
Chest without Contrast (Virtual Bronchoscopy)

Abdomen/Pelvis Protocols (MDCT 64 Slice)

Abdomen with Contrast
Abdomen without Contrast
Abdomen without and with Contrast
Abdomen and Pelvis with Contrast
Abdomen and Pelvis without Contrast
Abdomen and Pelvis without and with Contrast
Adrenals: Abdomen with Contrast
Adrenals: Abdomen without and with Contrast
Adrenals: Abdomen and Pelvis with Contrast
Adrenals: Abdomen and Pelvis without and with Contrast
Adrenals: Chest and Abdomen with Contrast

Adrenals: Chest and Abdomen without and with Contrast
Adrenals: Chest, Abdomen, and Pelvis with Contrast
Adrenals: Chest, Abdomen, and Pelvis without and with Contrast
Angiogram/Venogram: Abdomen
Angiogram/Venogram: Abdomen and Pelvis
Appendiceal/Peritoneal: Abdomen and Pelvis without and with Contrast
Appendiceal/Peritoneal: Chest, Abdomen, and Pelvis without and with Contrast
Bowel Carcinoid: Abdomen and Pelvis without and with Contrast
Chest and Abdomen with Contrast
Chest and Abdomen without Contrast
Chest and Abdomen without and with Contrast
Chest, Abdomen, and Pelvis with Contrast
Chest, Abdomen, and Pelvis without Contrast
Chest, Abdomen, and Pelvis without and with Contrast
CT Colonography
CT Cystogram
Gastric: Abdomen and Pelvis without and with Contrast
Kidney Stone
Kidneys, Ureters, and Bladder for Barium
Liver: Abdomen without and with Contrast
Liver: Abdomen and Pelvis without and with Contrast
Liver: Chest and Abdomen without and with Contrast
Liver: Chest, Abdomen, and Pelvis without and with Contrast
Lymphoma with Contrast
Lymphoma without Contrast
Lymphoma without and with Contrast
Pancreas: Abdomen without and with Contrast
Pancreas: Abdomen and Pelvis without and with Contrast
Pancreas: Chest, Abdomen, and Pelvis without and with Contrast
Pancreatic Islet Cell: Abdomen without and with Contrast
Postcystectomy: Abdomen and Pelvis with Contrast
Postcystectomy: Chest, Abdomen, and Pelvis with Contrast
Postcystectomy: Chest, Abdomen, and Pelvis without and with Contrast
Renal: Abdomen with Contrast
Renal: Chest and Abdomen without and with Contrast
Renal: Chest, Abdomen, and Pelvis without and with Contrast
Renal + 3D: Abdomen without and with Contrast
Renal + 3D: Abdomen and Pelvis without and with Contrast
Renal + 3D: Chest and Abdomen without and with Contrast
Renal + 3D: Chest, Abdomen, and Pelvis without and with Contrast
CT Runoff
CT Runoff (Fast)
Enterography (Small Bowel): Abdomen and Pelvis with Contrast
Enterography (Small Bowel): Abdomen and Pelvis without and with Contrast
Enterography (Small Bowel): Chest, Abdomen, and Pelvis with Contrast
Enterography (Small Bowel): Chest, Abdomen, and Pelvis without and with Contrast
Urogram: Abdomen and Pelvis without and with Contrast
Urogram: Chest, Abdomen, and Pelvis without and with Contrast

Musculoskeletal (MSK) Protocols (MDCT 64 Slice)

MSK (Bridging Protocol) with Contrast
MSK (Bridging Protocol) without Contrast
MSK (Metal Protocol) with Contrast
MSK (Metal Protocol) without Contrast
MSK Operating Room Hi-Res Protocol (64 Slice)
Operating Room High-Res Protocol with Contrast
Operating Room High-Res Protocol without Contrast
Operating Room Standard Protocol (64 Slice)
Operating Room Standard Protocol with Contrast
Operating Room Standard Protocol without Contrast
MSK (Soft Tissue Protocol) with Contrast
MSK (Soft Tissue Protocol) without Contrast
MSK (Standard Protocol) with Contrast
MSK (Standard Protocol) without Contrast

MAGNETIC RESONANCE IMAGING PROTOCOLS

Chest Protocols (1.5 T)

Parathyroid
Heart/Cardiac
Superior Sulcus
Delayed Enhancement (Option)

Body Protocols (1.5 T)

Abdomen Single Phase with Liver Acquisition with Volume Acceleration (LAVA)
Abdomen for Large Patient
Pelvis
Abdomen Options
Triphasic Abdomen with LAVA
Triphasic Abdomen with LAVA and Eovist
Fast Dynamic Abdomen
Cholangiogram (magnetic resonance cholangiopancreatography [MRCP])
Kidneys with LAVA
Pancreas
Pancreas Options
Magnetic Resonance Angiography (MRA): Abdomen
Fluoro Triggering
Tandem Ovoid-Gyn Brachytherapy
Pelvis-Cervical Cancer with Gel
Rectum Staging
Pelvis with Dynamic
Routine Pelvis
Prostate with Torso Posteroanterior (PA)
Prostate with Torso PA
Prostate with Endorectal Coil
Testis
Pelvic Bone Tumor

Prostate with Endorectal Coil (Prostatectomy)
Lower Extremity Runoff
Abdomen Multiple Echo Recombined Gradient Echo (MERGE)
Active Surveillance Prostate
Options: Active Surveillance Prostate

Musculoskeletal Protocols (1.5 T)

Thigh
Thigh for Metal Artifact
Thigh (Optional Sequences)
Pelvis
Pelvis for Metal Artifact
Shoulder to Include Scapula
Shoulder to Include Scapula
Shoulder to Include Scapula for Metal Artifact
Shoulder to Include Scapula for Metal Artifact
T-Spine
L-Spine

REFERENCES

1. Einhorn LH, Burgess MA, Gottlieb JA. Metastatic patterns of choroidal melanoma. *Cancer*. 1974;34:1001–1004.
2. Zakka KA, Foos RY, Omphroy CA, et al. Malignant melanoma: analysis of an autopsy population. *Ophthalmology*. 1980;87:549–556.
3. Rajpal S, Moore R, Karakousis CP. Survival in metastatic ocular melanoma. *Cancer*. 1983;52:334–336.
4. Bedikian AY, Legha SS, Mavligit G, et al. Treatment of uveal melanoma metastatic to the liver. *Cancer*. 1995;76:1665–1670.
5. Collaborative Ocular Melanoma Study Group Assessment of metastatic disease status at death in 435 patients with large choroidal melanoma in the Collaborative Ocular Melanoma Study (COMS). COMS Report No. 15. *Arch Ophthalmol*. 2001;119:670–676.
6. Silverman PM. Liver metastases: optimizing detection with multislice CT (MSCT). *Cancer Imaging*. 2004;4(Spec. No. B):S108–S113.
7. Silverman PM, Roberts S, Tefft MC, et al. Helical CT of the liver: clinical application of an automated computer technique, SmartPrep, for obtaining images with optimal contrast enhancement. *AJR Am J Roentgenol*. 1995;165:73–78.
8. Silverman P. *Multislice (MSCT) Computed Tomography: A Practical Approach to Clinical Protocols*. Philadelphia: Lippincott Williams & Wilkins; 2002.

Visit ExpertConsult.com to view the protocols.

Index

Note: Page numbers followed by f refer to figures; page numbers followed by t refer to tables; page numbers followed by b refer to boxes.

C

D

H

M

N

O

Q

R

S

T

V

W

Y

Z